PATHOLOGY

Basic and Systemic

Neville Woolf
PhD, MMed(Path), FRCPath

Vice-Dean and Faculty Tutor
University College Medical School,
London, UK
and Former Bland-Sutton Professor of Histopathology

WB Saunders Company Ltd
London · Philadelphia · Toronto · Sydney · Tokyo

This book is printed on acid-free paper

W. B. Saunders   24–28 Oval Road
Company Ltd   London, NW1 7DX, UK

                  The Curtis Center
                  Independence Square West
                  Philadelphia, PA 19106–3399, USA

                  Harcourt Brace & Company
                  55 Horner Avenue
                  Toronto, Ontario, M8Z 4X6, Canada

                  Harcourt Brace & Company, Australia
                  30–52 Smidmore Street
                  Marrickville
                  NSW 2204, Australia

                  Harcourt Brace & Company, Japan
                  Ichibancho Central Building, 22-1 Ichibancho
                  Chiyoda-ku, Tokyo 102, Japan

A catalogue record for this book is available from the British Library

ISBN 0-7020-2291-8

Typeset by Phoenix Photosetting, Chatham, Kent
Printed and bound in Italy by Rotolito Lombarda, Milan

"I know death hath ten thousand several doors
For men to take their exits"
John Webster, "Duchess of Malfi"

Causes of Death Worldwide – 1990. The Global Burden of Disease Study

Number of deaths (thousands)	Causes	Rank
50467	All causes	
6260	Ischaemic heart disease	1
4381	Cerebrovascular disease	2
4299	Infections of lower respiratory tract	3
2946	Diarrhoeal diseases	4
2443	Perinatal disorders	5
2211	Chronic obstructive lung disease	6
1960	Tuberculosis (HIV positive individuals excluded)	7
1058	Measles	8
999	Road traffic accidents	9
945	Cancer of bronchus, lung and trachea	10
856	Malaria	11
786	Self inflicted injuries	12
779	Cirrhosis of the liver	13
752	Gastric cancer	14
589	Congenital anomalies	15
571	Diabetes mellitus	16
563	Violence	17
542	Tetanus	18
536	Nephritis and "nephrosis"	19
504	Drowning	20
502	War injuries	21
501	Liver cancer	22
495	Inflammatory heart diseases	23
472	Colo-rectal cancer	24
372	Protein-energy malnutrition	25
358	Oesophageal cancer	26
347	Whooping cough	27
340	Rheumatic heart disease	28
322	Breast cancer	29
312	HIV	30

The study of pathology is fundamental to the education of all health care professionals. Firstly it is the bridge leading from a study of the basic biological sciences to that of the practice of medicine. Secondly, within the context of clinical sciences, knowledge and understanding of the pathological basis of disease, with particular reference to causation, pathogenesis and possible natural histories are essential if the clinical manifestations of disease are to be interpreted and treated in a rational way.

However, as the tide of new factual knowledge rises ever higher, so does the medical curriculum tend to become more and more heavily overloaded. For this and other reasons, teachers in the medical sciences should be prepared both to review the objectives of their teaching programmes and to reassess the methods used for reaching these objectives.

It is a fact, albeit a regrettable one, that many students, perhaps the majority, are obsessively concerned with passing examinations which become for them the *raison d'etre* rather than a by-product of medical education. Even at this pragmatic level, it should be understood that the process of learning transcends the acquisition, partial retention and more or less accurate reproduction of a large body of factual knowledge. Real learning should be based on understanding and the ability to **use** knowledge in disparate contexts; it is one of the few of life's pleasures which does not lose its savour with passing time, provided only that we do not lose our sense of wonder as the mysteries of nature are made clear, however slow and tantalisingly incomplete this process seems.

This book attempts to make the study of pathology simple without, at the same time, losing too much of the challenging and thought provoking qualities of a subject currently in a most exciting phase of its evolution. In it I have attempted, in addition to providing a reasonably substantial body of factual knowledge, to develop some simple strategies for 'thinking about pathology', which I hope will help students gain access to their own 'knowledge banks'. Long experience has taught me that students at every level know far more than they think they do but often show deficiencies in accessing and organising this knowledge. This difficulty is experienced by many not only in the somewhat artificial situation of an examination but in 'real life' problem solving as well. Mastery of a subject lies in asking the right questions; if this is done the right answers usually present themselves.

In the pursuit of simplicity without superficiality many simple line diagrams have been included and it is hoped that these in themselves may prove to be a useful revision aid. They make use of a very limited number of visual patterns which students may be able to adapt for themselves for use in contexts not dealt with in this book.

Use of a small number of simple conceptual paradigms can be of considerable help in mastering a subject and in avoiding the necessity of attempting to commit long lists to memory.

● Use of the normal physiological background

Firstly it is often helpful to study a given disorder against the background provided by normal physiology. For example rather than trying to remember a list of the causes of jaundice or of osteomalacia or rickets, a consideration of the steps normally involved in the formation and transport of bile, or the synthesis, transport, metabolism and action of Vitamin D allows one to ask, in relation to each step, 'can something go wrong here?'

● Disturbances in dynamic biological equilibria can cause disease

Many pathological states can be represented, quite accurately, as expression of disturbances in a dynamic equilibrium. Increases in the size of cell populations such as occur in neoplasms may result either from an **increased drive to proliferate** or from a **decrease in the efficacy of those mechanisms which normally restrain excessive cell division**. This simple concept helps in understanding the role of oncogenes and tumour suppressor genes in the genesis of cancer.

However **the concept of an underlying disturbance of a normal dynamic equilibrium underlies many disease states**. Anaemia may represent either a failure in formation of red cells or increased destruction, and the very common disorder of bone remodelling, osteoporosis, may result either from excessive bone resorption, inadequate bone formation or a combination of these factors. Chronic peptic ulcer may occur either because of the upregulation of a potential injurious factor (e.g. gastric acid) or because of down regulation of the normal defence mechanisms of the mucosa. Wherever appropriate, the operation of this principle of disturbed equilibria is pointed out both in the text and in the figures.

● Generation, reception and transduction of signals at an appropriate level are intrinsic to normal cell behaviour

This is another 'mental framework' which can be very helpful in considering disease states. Cells do not function by accident and cell–cell communication is just as important as communication between people. We use words, facial expression and body language to communicate with others; cells use a variety of chemical species instead.

Serious functional disturbances may arise when a cell population is 'dumb' (cannot generate an appropriate signal) or 'deaf' (lacks the appropriate receptors to receive an important signal). Thus in von Willebrand's disease, a disorder characterised by abnormal bleeding due to decreased adherence of platelets to a damaged vessel wall, the failure in normal interaction between the platelets and the vessel wall is due to a failure by the vascular endothelial cells to secrete the protein (von Willebrand factor) which mediates platelet adhesion by binding to a receptor on the platelet. In a rather more uncommon disorder (the Bernard–Soulier syndrome), it is the receptor which is lacking and the functional disturbance in platelet/vessel wall interaction is just the same.

● The requirements of organs with a major secretory role

The maintenance of normality in many body systems depends on secretion of chemical signals at an appropriate level. The endocrine system represents an archetype of this principle in operation. In order to function normally, an endocrine gland requires:

- a normal drive in both qualitative and quantitative terms;
- an adequate number of functioning cells;
- adequate amounts of the required substrates;
- adequate amounts of the enzymes required for hormone synthesis.

If you know this, it becomes a simple matter to discuss the causes of hyper- or hypofunction or of hyperplasia or atrophy in a given endocrine gland. For example, in the context of the thyroid, the gland enlargement and hyperfunction seen in thyrotoxicosis are due to an increased and abnormal drive by thyroid stimulation immunoglobulins; in Hashimoto's thyroiditis, autoimmune mechanisms destroy much of the secretory tissue leading to hypofunction; in iodine deficiency, the lack of substrate leads to lack of hormone and thus to a negative feedback-mediated increase in drive leading to a goitre (thyroid enlargement); lastly in hereditary goitre, the absence of one or other enzyme concerned in hormone synthesis vitiates the normal functions of the other components of the synthetic pathway and leads to a deficiency of thyroid hormone and an increased, negative feedback-mediated drive on the thyroid.

● Things are more the same than they are different

The reaction patterns of cells are limited and thus the series of events occurring in response to a wide variety of unfavourable environmental and inherited factors are finite. The sets of processes which we learn about under the rubric of 'general pathology' are expressed in many tissues and under many different circumstances and are well worth knowing. Thus if you become familiar with the biological processes involved in, for example, wound healing, this knowledge can be applied usefully to help you understand and remember what is involved in such disparate situations as the formation of a connective tissue cap in atherosclerotic plaques, the scarring which occurs in some forms of interstitial lung disease, the formation of connective tissue stroma in certain neoplasms, the formation of new blood vessels in relation to malignancy neoplasms and in areas of hypoxia or ischaemia and in the organisation of thrombus. Systemic pathology is merely the processes of general pathology operating within defined anatomical territories.

● Learn pathology in a clinical context

It is sad but true that for some students pathology is a dull subject and its teachers even duller. The second proposition may be true; the first is certainly not. You should not attempt, in my view, to learn pathology as if it were a separate intellectual discipline. The symptoms your patients experience and the signs you elicit are but the expression of changes in molecules, cells and tissues. If you hear, for example, a rough systolic murmur at the right side of the sternum which radiates up towards the neck, you should be able to visualise the appearances of that patient's aortic valve and what effects the valve changes will have on left ventricular structure and function. You should be able to, and take pleasure in extrapolating from the clinical situation to the underlying changes in organs and tissues and similarly, you should be able to predict the clinical effects likely to occur as a consequence of functional and structural tissue changes.

For historical and vocational reasons you will be taught many different 'subjects' in the course of your medical training but it is vital that you should remember that the patient is ONE.

Neville Woolf

CONTENTS

ACKNOWLEDGEMENTS

Many colleagues have given me photographs of their material over the years. Their help, for which I am very grateful, is acknowledged below.

Professor M.J. Davies, St George's Hospital Medical School: Figures 18.9, 32.5, 32.18–32.20, 32.22, 32.28, 32.47, 32.49, 33.47.

Professor L.W. Duchen (deceased): Figures 45.1–45.13, 45.16–45.27, 45.29–45.32, 45.34, 45.35, 45.38–45.40, 45.42, 45.45–45.55, 45.58–45.67.

Dr G. Farrer-Brown: Figures 32.33, 32.36, 32.39, 32.40.

Dr D.F. Gleason: Figure 38.25.

Dr M. Griffiths, University College London: Figures 11.2b, 33.19, 33.29, 33.33, 33.34, 33.37, 33.38, 34.21, 40.8.

Professor P.G. Isaacson, University College London: Figures 42.5–42.7, 42.11.

Dr D. Lamb, University of Edinburgh: Figures 33.9, 33.11.

Dr A.J. Leathem, University College London: Figure 22.3.

Professor P. Luthert, Institute of Ophthalmology: Figures 46.1–46.6.

Dr M. Parkinson, University College London: Figure 36.16, 36.17, 36.26, 36.46, 37.8, 37.9, 38.14–38.18, 38.22–38.24.

Dr K. Patterson, University College London: Figures 41.3, 41.5, 41.10, 41.12–41.16, 41.22, 41.31–41.33.

Professor J.R. Pattison, University College London: Figure 17.14.

Professor P. Revell, Royal Free Hospital School of Medicine: Figures 32.51, 32.62, 32.73, 33.44, 34.11, 34.16, 34.19, 34.20, 34.35, 35.16, 35.22, 35.26, 35.27, 35.29, 35.31, 35.53, 36.4, 36.5, 36.44, 37.3, 39.8, 39.11, 39.13, 39.15–39.17, 39.22, 39.24, 39.38, 39.41–39.43, 39.48, 40.9, 40.35, 40.36, 40.40, 40.41, 42.8, 42.24–42.26, 42.29, 42.37, 43.5, 43.9, 43.10, 43.12, 43.16, 43.17, 43.22, 43.33, 43.39, 44.17, 44.22, 44.25–44.28, 44.31, 44.32, 44.34, 44.36, 44.38, 44.40–44.43, 45.43, 45.56.

Professor J. Rode: Figures 40.28, 43.20, 43.26–43.29, 43.31, 43.32, 43.36.

Dr K.V. Sanderson, formerly of St George's Hospital Medical School: Figure 43.19.

Dr A. Wotherspoon, Royal Marsden Hospital: Figures 42.12, 42.18–42.22.

The publishers are grateful for permission to reproduce the following tables:

Preliminary table Reproduced from Murray C.J.L. and Lopez A.D. (1997) *Lancet* **349**: 1269–1276, with permission.

Table 33.2 Reproduced with permission, from the *Annual Review of Immunology*, Volume 12, ©1994, by Annual Reviews Inc.

Table 35.7 Reproduced with permission from Triger D.R. and Wright R. (1992) In (Millward-Sadler *et al.*, eds) *Wright's Liver and Biliary Disease*, pp 229–244. W.B. Saunders, London.

Table 38.5 Reproduced with permission from Lytton B. (1989) Annual age-related incidence rates in North American Caucasians. In Fitzpatrick and Krane (eds) *The Prostate*, pp 85–90. Churchill Livingstone, Edinburgh.

Table 42.7 Reproduced with permission of Blackwell Science Ltd, from Pappermar, Kaiser Linge and Lennart K. (1979) Classification of Hodgkin's disease. *Histopathology* **3**: 295–308.

Table 42.8 Reproduced with permission from Bennett *et al.* (1985) Natural history and frequency of histological types in the UK. In Quaglino D. and Hayho F.J.G. (eds) *Cytobiology of Leukaemias and Lymphomas* vol 20, pp 15–32. Lippincott Raven.

Figures 36.14, 36.18, 36.21, 36.22, 36.25 and 36.27 are adapted from Turner D. (1978) *Recent Advances in Histopathology* **10**: 235.

To Lydia – Wife and Best Friend

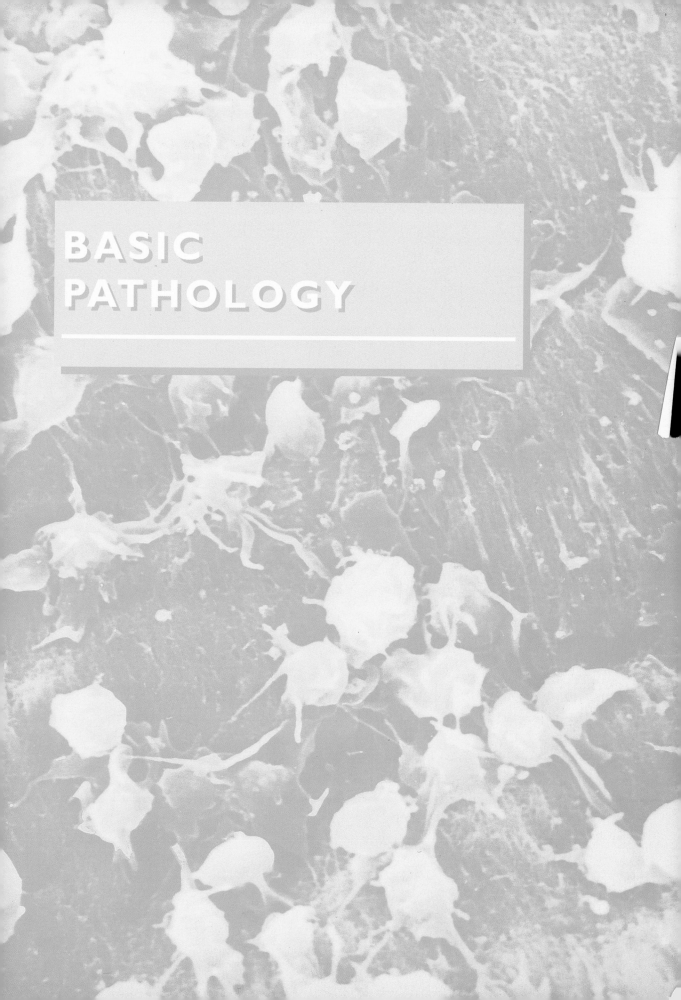

BASIC
PATHOLOGY

CHAPTER 1

The Nature of Pathology

Pathology is the bridge between the basic biological sciences and the practice of medicine. It is the study of the changes in structure and function that are produced either by injury, in its broadest sense, or by inborn errors.

It is important to realize that the reactions of cells and tissues are finite. This means that identical structural features may be found in both physiological and pathological situations and that morphology *per se* may be an unreliable guide to the cause of some particular change. For instance, the smooth muscle cells of the uterus increase enormously in size during pregnancy – a perfectly physiological state of affairs. However, if, for example, some obstruction to the normal outflow of urine were to occur, the smooth muscle cells of the bladder wall would also increase very greatly in size, providing a clear indication of some dysfunction in the lower urinary tract.

Even damage to and death of cells can be a physiological as well as a pathological phenomenon, and programmed cell death (**apoptosis**) is an important process in relation to events as disparate as morphogenesis in the embryo or surveillance against the development of cancer by removing cells with certain mutations in DNA (see pp 30–32). The same local tissue responses occurring as a result of 'pathological' cell injury may be seen under physiological circumstances. For example, the structural changes characteristic of acute inflammation are the inevitable consequences of a wide range of injuries, and yet these same histological changes may occur in association with perfectly physiological events such as the shedding of the endometrial lining of the uterus at the end of a menstrual cycle.

THE CONCEPT OF DISEASE

What is **disease**? Some have defined it as the condition in which the normal function of some part or organ of the body is disturbed. Others have maintained that disease does not exist except as a reaction to injury. These definitions are both valid and in no way mutually exclusive. Any individual disease can usefully be regarded, in terms of simple set theory, as the common set of a number of sets, most notably type of injury, type of reaction and the location of injury (*Fig. 1.1*). One can expand this simple concept to cover situations in which cells, tissues or organs are acted upon unfavourably either by injurious agents or by inborn errors acting alone or in conjunction with environmental circumstances. The sequence of events that follows

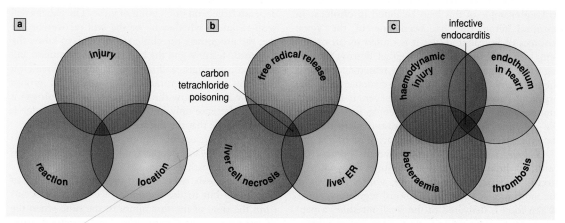

FIGURE 1.1 *Use of set theory to categorize disease. The chosen sets in this instance are shown in* **a** *and are the type of injury, its location and the type of local reaction. In example* **b**, *carbon tetrachloride initiates free radical release in the endoplasmic reticulum (ER) of the liver cells and this leads to lipid peroxidation and liver cell necrosis. In example* **c**, *a haemodynamic injury to the endothelium within the heart, such as might occur with a scarred mitral or aortic valve, will, in the presence of microorganisms in the blood, give rise to infected thrombi on the heart valve surface (infective endocarditis).*

may be dominated by the direct effects of the injurious agent on the cell (as in certain chemical injuries), or may be a combination of these direct effects, and the local and general cell and tissue reactions that may be elicited.

The functional disturbances produced by injury to cells are often mirrored by structural changes (**a lesion**), just as, in turn, structural damage may be followed by loss or alteration of some normal function. The sum of these effects finds its expression in the **symptoms** experienced by the patient and the signs observed by the physician (*Fig. 1.2*).

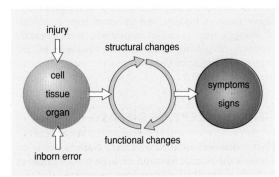

FIGURE 1.2 *Injury or inborn error may lead to functional and then structural disturbances within cells and tissues. These are expressed as the 'symptoms' experienced by the patient and the 'signs' observed by the physician.*

Severe Functional Disturbances Need Not be Accompanied by Significant Structural Changes

A direct relationship between disordered function and disordered structure is not always present and there may be very severe functional disturbances without any significant structural changes being present. A striking example of this is to be found in **cholera**. In historical terms this has been one of the worst scourges of humankind, yet it is caused by an organism, *Vibrio cholerae*, that cannot either destroy the lining cells of the gut wall or even penetrate between them. There is no microscopic evidence that the organism damages any tissue. However, if untreated, more than half of the infected people will die from the dehydration and electrolyte disturbances that are the consequence of the profuse watery diarrhoea that *V. cholerae* causes. This diarrhoea occurs because the epithelial lining cells of the intestine respond to a **toxin**, secreted by the organism, which behaves in the same way as a normal hormonal regulatory signal. When food is delivered to the small intestine, a peptide binds to a receptor site on the luminal membrane of the small intestinal epithelial cell and stimulates the adenylate cyclase system, with the result that about 2 litres of alkaline fluid are pumped into the small intestine (see pp 17–20).

Morphological Change Can Occur Without Significant Functional Disturbance

In other situations a considerable degree of morphological alteration may be present as, for instance, in some large benign neoplasms, but functional disturbance may be slight or absent.

GENERAL PATHOLOGY

General pathology is the study of the functional and structural changes that occur in cells and tissues as a result of direct damage by, or reactions to, a wide range of unfavourable circumstances. At any given time our knowledge of these is circumscribed by the techniques available to study these processes. Despite this reservation, it is probably true to say that the number of responses of the mammalian cell is finite. These responses represent, on the whole, either an increase or a reduction or loss in some of the components of a large, but not infinite, number of normal cell processes.

This general principle holds good only so long as **no change has taken place in the genome of the target cell or in the transcription of its genetic information**. If such changes have occurred, then a new range of phenotypic characteristics and new responses, not characteristic of this cell (at least in its adult or fully differentiated form), may be acquired. The words 'adult or fully differentiated' should be stressed because the acquisition of apparently new functions (such as the secretion of fetal antigens by the cells of some tumours) may be the expression of functions that were normal and appropriate at an earlier stage of the organism's embryological development.

Characteristics of a Disease

How one regards any individual disease process depends largely on one's point of view. The patient will wish to know whether he or she will recover or not (i.e. the prognosis); the clinician will wish to know the diagnostic features and the best mode of treatment; and the histopathologist will tend to classify the disease on the basis of its morphological features. All groups should want to know the basic cause (or **aetiology**) if possible, because only in the light of this knowledge is it conceivable that the disease can be avoided.

Another concept of importance is the pathogenesis of a disease. Many people tend to confuse the terms aetiology and pathogenesis.

Pathogenesis refers not to the actual first cause of the disease but to the sequence of events that occurs from the time of the first injury to the time when the disease expresses itself in functional and structural terms. Full understanding of pathogenesis is important because it may provide a number of novel therapeutic targets, which may lead to a beneficial alteration in the natural history of a given disease.

An example of the pathogenesis of a common and serious disease may be found in the natural history of coronary artery atherosclerosis, the complications of which are responsible for approximately 25% of adult male deaths in the UK.

In morphological terms it is a disorder characterized by the presence of focally distributed thickenings of the intima of large elastic and muscular arteries. These thickenings consist of a combination of proliferated connective tissue which forms a 'cap' to the lesion and a basal accumulation of lipid and tissue debris. As these plaque-like foci increase in thickness, they may produce a significant degree of narrowing of the vessel lumen. This may lead to regional underperfusion of the heart muscle, and the patient may experience chest pain provoked by exercise or cold and relieved by rest or vasodilator (**stable angina**). Not infrequently the plaque softens as its constituents undergo necrosis, and this may be followed by splitting of the connective tissue cap and exposure of the subendothelial elements of the plaque. This leads to adherence and aggregation of platelets, and within a very short time this mass of platelets and fibrin (a **thrombus**) may block the lumen of the artery.

The segment of ventricular wall supplied by this artery will thus be deprived totally of its arterial blood supply. In clinical terms this may be expressed as the onset of **severe central chest pain** or **serious ventricular arrhythmias**, which may prove fatal within a few minutes, as **low cardiac output** accompanied by peripheral vasoconstriction (**cardiogenic shock**), or as **chronic cardiac failure**.

In structural terms the morphological features of death of the underperfused muscle will develop over the next 24 hours or so. In most instances, if the patient lives, the dead muscle will be replaced by scar tissue. This, of course, lacks the contractile properties of muscle and may eventually stretch permanently, leading to the formation of a bulge or **aneurysm** on the wall of the left ventricle (see Chapter 32). If the patient died within a few minutes of the cutting off of the arterial blood supply, the structural changes that indicate cell injury or cell death do not occur.

Reducing the concentration of certain lipid classes in the plasma of patients with clinically overt coronary atherosclerosis by diet or drugs produces insignificant changes in the size of the lesions but has a highly significant lowering effect on the risk of both new clinical events and atherosclerosis-related death. **The lesion has not been removed but its natural history has been modified**.

THE STUDY OF DISEASE

HISTOPATHOLOGY: STUDIES OF DISEASED ORGANS AND TISSUES

Tissue pathology as a practical discipline has existed for little more than 250 years. Post mortem examinations,

chiefly for the gathering of anatomical knowledge, became almost fashionable in the later part of the renaissance as may be seen in some famous paintings such as Rembrandt's *The Anatomy Lesson of Dr Tulp*.

The primary motivation for all histopathological examinations is to delineate, as accurately as possible:

- structural tissue changes that correlate with the clinical expression of disease
- tissue changes that correlate with disturbance of normal physiological processes
- the sequence of events leading to the full-blown expression of an individual disease
- tissue changes occurring as a result of exposure to some known agent, living or non-living
- genetic or molecular abnormalities that may result in increased susceptibility to some disease or which result from some injurious agent

It is probably fair to say that the two greatest advances in attaining the objectives outlined above have been:

1) the introduction of the microscope and its application, in the second half of the nineteenth century to the study of normal and diseased tissues
2) the introduction of techniques derived essentially from **non-morphological disciplines** to the study of normal and diseased tissues. Such disciplines include:

- microbiology
- immunology
- biochemistry
- genetics
- physics
- molecular biology

Microscopy

The nineteenth century saw not only improvements in the primitive microscope described in the late seventeenth century by Antony van Leeuwenhoek but the development of knives of sufficiently high quality to section tissues very thinly and of dyes that stained particular tissue components in a reliable and reproducible fashion. It was this combination that led to the flowering of descriptive pathology, which occurred from about 1840 onwards.

Conceptually, a pivotal step forward was the recognition not only that the cell was the unit of living tissue, but that **gross pathological changes of all kinds were the expression of changes occurring within cells**. This, in brief, sums up the life work of the great German pathologist Rudolf Virchow (1821–1905), who is justly regarded as the father of modern histopathology.

The next advance was the extension of microscopic studies from samples derived from post-mortem examinations to samples of lesions occurring in patients who were still living (**surgical pathology**). At a stroke, this converted tissue pathologists from individuals who 'knew everything but always 24 hours too late to be of any use', to active colleagues of clinicians and important – indeed vital – participants in diagnosis and management. The application of techniques derived from the non-morphological disciplines referred to previously, has brought the art and science of surgical pathology to a considerable degree of sophistication.

Autopsy (Post-Mortem Examination)

The word autopsy means, literally, to see for oneself; such examinations have been, and in the writer's view still are, of great value, but there is no doubt that for many reasons the autopsy rate has declined steeply over the past three decades. Economic factors have played a part in this decline (especially in the USA), but much of it is due to changes in attitude in families of the deceased, in pathologists themselves and in clinicians, some of whom believe, quite incorrectly, that modern imaging methods have eliminated the need for post-mortem examination other than in medicolegal contexts.

In fact, the autopsy still has great value as:

- a means of **quality control** in relation to both diagnosis and treatment. Despite the increasing sophistication of the methods of clinical investigation during life, autopsy may reveal a considerable discrepancy between ante- and post-mortem diagnoses. Autopsy is also useful in evaluating the effects of new drugs, new operative techniques, new prostheses, such as heart valves or vascular grafts, and new diagnostic methods.
- a means of **education** for clinical students and clinicians in training
- a means of **discovering previously unrecognized disorders**. Two examples include the recognition of **familial hypertrophic cardiomyopathy** (see pp 370–372) as a result of forensic autopsies carried out by the late R.D. Teare in the late 1950s and, more recently, the recognition of **new variant Creutzfeld–Jakob disease**, which may be caused by eating beef products containing abnormal prion proteins (see pp 1142–1143).

Surgical Pathology

Surgical pathology is an indispensable component in the diagnosis and treatment of many disease states. Examination of biopsy material, including material suitable for cytopathology, provides:

- **essential diagnosis**: for example, is a lump in a woman's breast malignant or benign? Is a lymph node enlarged because of some reactive process or is it the expression of a malignant lymphoma? The decision reached in either of these cases has profound implications for correct treatment.
- **prognostic information**, especially in tumour pathology; the extent of disease and the degree of differentiation are useful indicators of the likely prognosis.
- **knowledge that throws new light on the pathogenetic processes that underlie certain disorders**. For example, specialized techniques may indicate the presence of immune complexes in many renal diseases (*Fig. 36.26*; see pp 652–653) and in inflammatory disorders affecting blood vessels (pp 396–410), or the inappropriate upregulation or downregulation of genes that regulate cell proliferation (pp 273–289).

For a high-quality diagnostic service to be maintained, it is essential that the pathologist should examine submitted tissues in their correct clinical context. Knowledge of the clinical data may affect both the selection by the pathologist of the most appropriate methods of examination and the interpretation of macroscopic and microscopic data. It is not only a discourtesy to submit tissues without adequate accompanying clinical information, but may not be in the best interests of the patient.

Intraoperative Consultation

While the 'turn-round' time from specimens reaching the laboratory to the report reaching the referring clinician has shortened significantly as a result of technical improvements, there are occasions when intraoperative consultation between clinician and surgical pathologist is appropriate. In such circumstances, the material may be examined by:

- making 'frozen sections' in which tissue blocks are rapidly frozen thus making the blocks hard enough for thin sections to be cut and then stained
- making 'touch' imprints of cut tissue on glass slides, taking smears of small portions of soft material or examining aspiration samples

In expert hands these methods, used singly or together, provide a high degree of diagnostic accuracy. Again, it is important to realize that such a transaction between clinician and pathologist is a consultative one and not an instruction from the former to the latter. There are occasions in which frozen sections are not only unlikely to provide the desired information but may also spoil the chances of obtaining an accurate diagnosis.

Cytopathology

This branch of diagnostic pathology is based on the correct premise that morphological changes in individual cells correlate with the pathological processes in the organs or tissues from which they come. Cells that may be examined microscopically in this way may:

- exfoliate naturally from epithelial surfaces and be found, for instance, in sputum or urine
- be dislodged from epithelial surfaces by gentle scraping or brushing as in the case of 'cervical smears'
- be obtained by fine-needle aspiration of organs such as the breast, lymph nodes, liver, lung or pancreas.

The ability to obtain material from deeply situated viscera in this relatively atraumatic way represents an enormous diagnostic advance.

Because of its relative simplicity, cytopathology has the power to transcend **diagnosis** in patients with clinical symptoms and to be useful also as a **screening procedure**. The widespread introduction of cytopathological examination of cervical smears from asymptomatic women, as pioneered by Papanicolaou, has been associated with a marked decline in the incidence of invasive cancer of the uterine cervix and in the number of deaths associated with this disease.

Electron Microscopy

Light microscopy has limitations: above a certain quite low magnification (about ×1200) the wavelength of light impairs resolution and the resulting image is blurred and, in effect, useless. The electron microscope overcomes this problem.

There are three principal types of electron microscope:

1) The **transmission electron microscope**, in which a beam of electrons is passed through an ultra-thin section of the material to be examined. The sections are 'stained' by being impregnated with heavy metals such as osmium, which bind differentially to various cell components.

2) The **scanning electron microscope**, in which surfaces are examined. This is accomplished by scanning a finely focused beam of electrons across the surfaces of tissues or other materials (such as computer 'chips'). This results in the generation of a secondary set of electrons which are 'collected' and form an image of the surface scanned in this way. This is often surprisingly informative and of great aesthetic charm.

3) The **analytical electron microscope**, in which the chemical composition of tissue components and of foreign material within tissue can be determined.

Transmission electron microscopy has provided an enormous amount of valuable information related to the microanatomy of cells and tissues. As a diagnostic tool it suffers from certain defects:

- The microscopes themselves and the microtomes used to cut the ultra-thin sections are expensive both to buy and maintain.
- Preparing the material and examining it is time consuming, labour intensive and, therefore, costly in the context of our current cost-conscious world.
- The size of the samples that can be examined is very small.

Despite this, there are selected areas in which the use of transmission electron microscopy, as an adjunct to light microscopy and immunohistology, is very useful. Such areas include renal biopsies in patients with glomerulonephritis, neoplasms in which the histogenesis may be uncertain, peripheral nerve and muscle biopsies, and tissues in cases of certain storage diseases in which characteristic inclusions may be seen.

Immunohistochemistry

The usefulness of immunohistochemistry is based on the highly specific binding reactions that occur between antibodies and their homospecific antigens. If a fluorescent molecule, a dye or an enzyme, which can then be demonstrated histochemically, is linked with antibody, the localization of the particular antigen within tissue sections can be demonstrated quite clearly (*Fig. 1.3*).

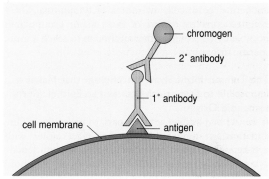

FIGURE 1.3 *Visualization of a specific antigen in a cell is possible using antibodies linked to a chromogen.*

The range of antigens that can be demonstrated in paraffin-embedded material is wide, and includes:
- hormones
- receptors
- cell adhesion molecules such as cadherins
- connective tissue matrix proteins
- plasma proteins
- oncofetal antigens (see pp 268–269)
- enzymes
- components of the cytoskeleton
- leucocyte antigens
- immunoglobulin components such as light and heavy chains of various types, secretory components and the J chain
- oncogenes and their products
- nuclear proliferation antigens
- a large number of infectious agents including bacteria, viruses, protozoa and fungi

Immunohistochemistry in Tumour Diagnosis

One of the most important applications of immunohistochemistry in diagnostic pathology lies in the field of tumour recognition. Situations in which immunohistochemistry may be of great help include the following commonly encountered situations.

The Biopsy Contains a Secondary Tumour Deposit but there is no Clinical Indication of the Primary Site in Which the Tumour has Arisen

Such a deposit might be, for example, an adenocarcinoma with no morphological features suggesting its site of origin. If the latter were, say, the prostate, it would be possible to demonstrate this by treating the section with an antibody reacting with prostate-specific antigen.

The Tumour is so Poorly Differentiated as to Make Its Lineage Quite Uncertain

Use of an appropriate range of antibodies would make it possible in most cases to determine, in the first instance, whether the tumour was of epithelial (carcinoma) or connective tissue origin (sarcoma), neuroendocrine, germ cell, melanoma or lymphoma. Once assigned correctly to one of these major groups, it is possible by employing other antibodies to reach a more specific diagnosis.

The Tumour Might Show Morphology that Makes it Impossible to Distinguish Between an Epithelial or a Lymphoid Origin

It should be possible, at a first pass, to make this differentiation by using antibodies that react either with cytokeratins (present in epithelial cells) or with leucocyte common antigen (LCA) (present in all lymphoid cells). If the cells bind the antibody to LCA, it is possible to go further and to determine whether they are B cells, T cells or of monocyte–macrophage origin (see pp 99–101).

Micrometastases Might be Present, for example in Bone Marrow of Lymph Nodes, but are not Recognized in Conventionally Stained Tissue Sections

The use of appropriate antibodies in the context of a given tumour may show such occult metastases. The presence of such deposits has definite implications for prognosis. For example, immunohistochemistry shows occult micrometastases in the bone marrow of 25–30% of patients with breast cancer in whom clinical and other pathological data suggest localized disease. More than 80% of such patients with bone marrow micrometastases go on to develop overt secondary deposits. Of those in whom micrometastases are not seen, only 33% develop overt secondary deposits.

The Degree of Expression of Certain Antigens may Provide Prognostic Information and also Predict the Response to Certain Forms of Treatment

In breast cancer the greater the degree of expression of the epidermal growth factor receptor on tumour cells, the more aggressive the behaviour of the tumour is likely to be. In tumours such as cancer of the breast or prostate, where the growth of tumour cells is, at least in part, regulated by hormonal stimuli, the degree of expression of receptors for these stimuli predicts the response to hormonal ablation. These features can be detected by immunohistochemical methods.

Histochemistry

Whenever some cell component or product is localized by a chemical reaction, a histochemical procedure has been applied. Indeed, the dye methods used universally by tissue pathologists are, strictly speaking, examples of the application of histochemistry. By convention, which is not always logical, both common staining methods and the immunohistological methods referred to previously are excluded from the rubric of 'pure' histochemistry.

Many chemical species can be localized in this way in tissue sections or in cytological preparations. These include:

- enzymes
- various lipid classes
- proteins and glycoproteins
- metals
- carbohydrates

It is impossible in this context to give more than one or two quite random examples of the use of histochemistry in tissue pathology.

Enzyme histochemistry (which can be carried out only in frozen sections) can be used, for example, in the intraoperative diagnosis of Hirschsprung's disease (see p 550), in which there is a segmental loss of ganglion cells and an increase in acetylcholinesterase-positive nerve fibres in the large gut submucosa. Staining intraoperative biopsy material for this enzyme is helpful in establishing a tissue diagnosis and in determining the extent of bowel involvement. Similarly non-viable heart muscle cells show loss of respiratory enzymes before morphologically recognizable features of cell death develop.

Molecular Techniques

In Situ *Hybridization*

Hybridization techniques of all kinds are based on the fact that nucleic acid bases in single strands of DNA or RNA anneal to each other in a **complementary** fashion. Thus adenine anneals only to thymine, and cytosine anneals only with guanine.

The use of a labelled nucleic acid probe allows the identification of complementary sequences in tissue. These complementary sequences may be part of the genome of the native cells, messenger RNA indicating the expression of certain genes or portions of the genome of pathogens such as viruses. With *in situ* hybridization, the targeted sequence can be identified microscopically in intact cells and tissues, and does not require prior extraction as is the case with the other commonly used methods based on hybridization – filter hybridization, such as Southern or Western blotting and the polymerase chain reaction (PCR). Although *in situ* hybridization does have the huge advantage that the sequence looked for may be seen in its microscopic context, it is much less sensitive than other hybridization methods. The labels associated with the probes may be either radioactive, such as ^{35}S, or non-radioactive, such as digoxigenin.

In situ hybridization has proved particularly useful in extending knowledge of the role of viruses in a variety of pathological processes. Examples of this application include:

- human papilloma virus in a variety of epithelial proliferative lesions involving the cervix uteri, vagina, vulva, penis and anus (see p 767)
- the detection of cytomegalovirus in a wide range of tissues, especially in patients suffering from the acquired immune deficiency syndrome (AIDS)
- Epstein–Barr virus, a herpesvirus, which has been implicated in the cause of the common and usually self-limiting disorder, infectious monocleosis, Burkitt lymphoma, nasopharyngeal carcinoma and other lymphoproliferative diseases
- the JC virus in the causation of progressive multifocal leucoencephalopathy. This formerly rare demyelinating disorder of the brain is associated with immune deficiency and has become increasingly common with the advent of AIDS.

Polymerase Chain Reaction

The introduction of the PCR has led to an enormous increase in our ability to identify small amounts of target DNA in tissues whether, in the final analysis, filter hybridization or *in situ* techniques are used. The target sequence must be known and must exist in double-stranded form for the PCR to be successful.

Each PCR cycle consists essentially of three phases:
1) denaturation of the double-stranded DNA at 94°C for 30–90 seconds so as to create two single strands.
2) the use of oligonucleotide primers, which are required to flank the target sequence. These primers must hybridize to the 3′ ends of both the sense and anti-sense strands of DNA. This annealing process takes from 30 to 120 seconds and is carried out at a temperature of 55°C.
3) the extension of the primers via the addition of free nucleotides. This is brought about by the action of the enzyme *taq* polymerase (a DNA polymerase derived from a microorganism, *Thermus aquaticus*, which lives in high temperature environments such as hot springs). Extension takes about 60–180 seconds to accomplish and is carried out at a temperature of 72°C. The extension of the flanking primers brings about the formation of additional target sequences which can act as templates for succeeding cycles. A reaction that runs for 30 cycles will, theoretically, amplify the target sequence a billionfold.

PCR can also be carried out on RNA but this requires that the RNA be converted to DNA by the use of a reverse transcriptase reaction. There are many modifications for PCR, such as nested PCR and *in situ* PCR to name but two, but these are beyond the scope of this text. Applications of PCR include:

- molecular genetic assays in haematological malignancies
- the detection of translocations (see pp 962–963) in both haematological malignancies and soft tissue tumours
- the detection of a wide range of microorganisms including bacteria, viruses, rickettsiae, protozoa and fungi. PCR has been used also to detect 'new' microorganisms such as *Tropheryma whipplei* (see p 524) and *Rochalimaea henselae*, the cause of bacillary angiomatosis.

SUMMARY

The introduction of all these techniques has brought closer the realization of the aims and objectives of tissue pathology as outlined on p 5. It is now possible not only to determine the lineage of cells involved in a pathological process, but to identify also the products which they are synthesizing and their state of activation. The methods of molecular biology, so fruitfully applied in the field of tissue pathology, can be used also to identify pathogenic microorganisms in tissues and to identify genomic alterations which may have profound effects in the genesis of many diseases.

CHAPTER 2

Cell Injury and its Manifestations

CELL ADAPTATION

Under most circumstances cells try to maintain a **steady state**. If their milieu is altered to some extent they will adapt to the change in circumstances without their function being significantly impaired (**cell adaptation**).

Obvious examples of this are to be found in situations where there is an alteration in the **functional demands** made on cells. An increase in demand usually leads to one or both of the following:

- an increase in **size** of individual cells (hypertrophy)
- an increase in **number** of cells (hyperplasia)

An example of such cellular adaptation is the marked increase in size of the cardiac muscle fibres that occurs when there is overload of cardiac muscle due to high pressure in the left ventricular outflow tract as, for example, in aortic valve stenosis or systemic hypertension. The increased size of individual cells leads to a significant increase in the thickness of the left ventricular wall. Conversely, when the demand for a function is reduced this may be mirrored by a marked **decrease** in cell size (atrophy). An example of this is the rapid muscle wasting that may follow immobilization of a limb in plaster following a fracture.

If the degree of change is so great that the cell cannot adjust to its changed milieu, then some **loss in its normal range of functions** is likely to occur. This may well be accompanied by characteristic structural alterations. These functional and structural changes are the correlates of **cell injury** and may be reversible. Irreversible injury is so severe as to lead to the loss of vital cellular functions and thus lead to the **death** of the cell (*Fig. 2.1*).

However, it is important to remember that **cell death is not always a pathological event**. It is also the means by which normal cell population numbers are maintained and plays a part in embryogenesis. This form of cell death which is a **programmed** phenomenon is known as **apoptosis** (see pp 30–32).

REQUIREMENTS FOR MAINTENANCE OF THE STEADY STATE

For a steady state to be maintained within a cell, it has to continue to perform a range of basic functions (*Fig. 2.2*).

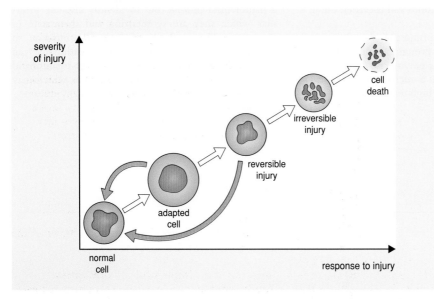

FIGURE 2.1 *The response to injury. Mild to moderate injury usually leads to adaptive changes on the part of the cell. If the severity of the injury is increased, first functional and then morphological evidence of injury appears. Very severe degrees of injury cause irreversible damage to vital cellular processes and death of the affected cell results.*

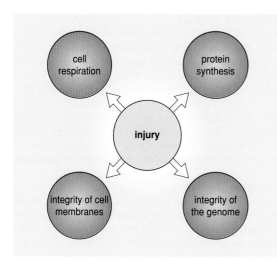

FIGURE 2.2 *The functional targets of injury. It is clear that these interrelate.*

These include:

- **Preservation of normal DNA templates.** Synthesis of nucleic acids, proteins, lipids and carbohydrates requires normality of the DNA templates, and subsumed within this must be the ability to excise and repair abnormal base linkages within the DNA molecule.
- **Normal enzyme content.** Normal amounts and types of enzymes are required for the assembly and reproduction of the cell's own organelles and membranes, and for the carrying out of a variety of other functions such as the degradation of a wide range of compounds.
- **Intact membranes and transmembrane proteins.** The transport of metabolites via energy-dependent transport systems requires intact membranes if osmotic and fluid homoeostasis are to be preserved.
- **Adequate supply of substrates and oxygen.** Aerobic energy production via oxidative phosphorylation and the production of high-energy phosphate bonds requires adequate oxygenation and normal amounts of suitable substrate. **Hypoxia** (a reduction of the amount of oxygen delivered to cells), often mediated via **ischaemia** (a reduction in the perfusion of a part relative to its needs), is one of the commonest and most important causes of both sublethal and lethal cell injury.

All these systems are intimately related to each other and their actions are interwoven. Because of this it is easier to identify the targets of cell injury in terms of anatomy than of function. Occasional exceptions exist where it is possible to identify the functional target precisely. This is seen in cyanide poisoning (in which cytochrome oxidase is inactivated leading to a block in aerobic respiration) and in relation to the action of certain bacterial toxins (see pp 17–21).

Despite these reservations, it is reasonable to consider the question of cell injury either in terms of the part of the cell microanatomy that is affected primarily, or in terms of the type of injury applied. Where possible, these two approaches should be combined.

SITES AND TYPES OF CELL INJURY

TYPES OF INJURY

There are many types of cell injury although the reaction patterns that result are limited. The outcome for any cell of an unfavourable environmental circumstance, for example hypoxia or anoxia, depends in part on the severity of the injurious factor and in part on the innate resistance of the cell. Thus **a given degree of injury will have different effects on different cell types**. Thus, for example, hypoxia of short duration is sufficient to cause irreversible injury to neurones but not to damage other cell types such as cartilage.

Common types of factors in the microenvironment that damage cells include:

- **Hypoxia**
- **Anoxia**
  These are most often caused by **ischaemia** in which perfusion by oxygenated blood is insufficient to meet the metabolic requirements of the affected organ or tissue.
- **Reoxygenation.** Reperfusion of acutely ischaemic tissue may have a considerable incremental effect on cell damage. This is believed to be due to the generation of oxygen free radicals (see pp 13–15)
- **Extremes of heat or cold**
- **Chemical agents** that produce cell damage in many different ways
- **Immunologically mediated mechanisms** operating through either the humoral or cellular arms of the immune system (see pp 125–131)
- **Infectious agents.** Bacteria may cause cell injury either by the release of toxic chemical species (see pp 17–21) or by eliciting cell-damaging immune responses, as in tuberculosis. Viruses may have a direct cytopathic effect (e.g. poliovirus) or may operate via immune-mediated mechanisms.
- **Irradiation**
- **Nutritional deficiencies**

SITES OF INJURY

The Nucleus

The nucleus, and hence the genetic constitution of the cell, may be altered in a number of ways.

Inherited and Congenital Abnormalities

The abnormality may be inherited and may involve a single gene only, as in sickle cell disease, in which case there will be no obvious morphological abnormality in the nucleus or its constituent chromosomes. However, distinct chromosomal abnormalities may be present. These may be expressed by:

1) **Alterations of the normal diploid number**, as in Down's syndrome or one of the other trisomy syndromes which, as a whole, lead to a large number of congenital abnormalities. These and other chromosomally determined disorders are discussed on pp 309–314.

2) **Alterations in the structure of individual chromosomes**

Abnormalities may occur in the form of chromosomal breakages. These produce syndromes such as **ataxia–telangiectasia** (complex intertwined bundles of abnormally and permanently dilated blood vessels) in the eyes and skin. This is associated with a severe immunological deficiency and extreme radiosensitivity of such a high degree that even diagnostic X-rays have been reported to be followed by leukaemia in affected patients.

There appears to be a very close link between such chromosomal breakage syndromes and an increased risk of developing leukaemia or other malignant conditions involving the lymphoid system. The greatest care should be exercised to prevent exposure of these, fortunately rare, patients to chemical or physical agents, such as irradiation, that are known to damage DNA. Other alterations may of course occur in the form of translocations of genomic material, or of deletions.

Toxic Nuclear Damage

Toxic nuclear damage occurs in the treatment of malignant disease with cytotoxic drugs. Such damage may arise in a number of different ways depending on the chemotherapeutic agent used. Some drugs, such as the alkylating agents (e.g. cyclophosphamide), combine directly with DNA, whereas others such as vincristine (the periwinkle alkaloid) damage the mitotic spindle. Others act as analogues of normal metabolites and block some of the enzyme-controlled steps in nucleic acid synthesis.

Nutritional Deficiencies and Nuclear Damage

Nutritional damage to the nucleus may be seen in the cells of patients with either folic acid or vitamin B_{12} deficiency, as seen in pernicious anaemia. The nuclei in these cells are larger than normal, but contain less DNA than is optimal for mitosis. These changes are present in many tissues but are most prominent among the red cell precursors in the bone marrow.

The Cell Membranes

Many functions are mediated via the cell membrane. These range from such vital matters as the maintenance of normal osmotic relationships between the intracellular and extracellular environments, to a variety of receptor and transduction functions.

Some inherited defects of membrane structure and function have been identified; two examples are given below.

Transport Defects

These include inability to transport the dibasic amino acids **lysine** and **ornithine** across the luminal membrane of the renal tubular epithelial cell, so that they appear in the urine in significant amounts. A similar inherited transport defect operates in **Hartnup's disease**, where there is a reduction in the ability to transport tryptophan from the gut across the small intestinal epithelium. Because tryptophan is an important source of nicotinic acid, a deficiency of the latter develops and leads to the appearance of the clinical signs of **pellagra**.

Receptor Defects

Several membrane receptor defects have been described. A paradigm of such defects is **familial type IIa hypercholesterolaemia** in which peripheral cells lack high-affinity receptors for low density lipoprotein (LDL), the molecule that transports most cholesterol in biological fluids. Failure to endocytose the LDL molecule at these receptor sites leads to a failure to control cell synthesis of cholesterol via its rate-limiting enzyme 3-hydroxy-3-methylglutaryl coenzyme A (HMG CoA) reductase as well as failure to catabolize circulating LDL.

The consequence is a grossly raised plasma concentration of LDL cholesterol, which is associated with abnormally early development of atherosclerosis and ischaemic heart disease (*Fig. 2.3*). The receptor protein is coded for by a gene on chromosome 19.

- **Heterozygosity** in respect of a mutation leads to a plasma cholesterol concentration of about twice the ideal and a risk of coronary heart disease striking in the fifth decade.
- **Homozygosity** leads to much higher plasma cholesterol concentrations and symptomatic coronary disease in the second decade. The relationship of the receptor defect to this disastrous scenario is made plain by the fact that transplantation of the liver can normalize the plasma cholesterol concentration in these homozygotes.

Complement-related Membrane Injury

If complement (see pp 111–114) becomes fixed to cell surface-bound antigen–antibody complex, its activation leads to the generation of a **membrane attack complex** mediated by components 8 and 9 of the complement sequence of proteins. This causes focal lysis of the cell membrane and escape of the cell contents into the extracellular environment.

An example of this is the red blood cell lysis following incompatible blood transfusions or other immune-mediated forms of haemolysis.

Electron micrographs of cell membranes following activation of complement bound to antigen–antibody complexes on the cell surface show rather uniform dark areas. These were at one time thought to be holes, but are now believed to be areas in which there is a local piling up of the lipid moieties of the cell membrane at sites where the C8 component of complement has

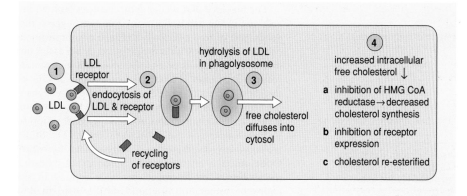

FIGURE 2.3 *Cell biology of familial type IIa hypercholesterolaemia. The diagram shows the course of events in normal cells that bind low density lipoprotein (LDL) at specific high-affinity receptor sites on the plasma membrane. This LDL is then endocytosed and broken down within phagolysosomes, with the consequent release of free cholesterol in the cytoplasm. The intracellular concentration of free cholesterol controls the level of activity of HMG CoA reductase. As intracellular free cholesterol rises, the enzyme is inhibited and cholesterol synthesis by the cell diminishes. Free cholesterol in the cytoplasm is esterified under the influence of acyl coenzyme A transferase. Patients with type IIa hypercholesterolaemia either lack receptors or have receptors which do not function adequately.*

become inserted into the membrane. Each 'hole' is a single complex containing one molecule each of complement components 5–8 and six molecules of C9. C8 opens and shuts a transmembrane channel; if this channel remains open then lysis occurs. The binding of C9 serves to jam this channel open.

FREE RADICALS AND CELL INJURY

It has become increasingly clear that the formation of free radicals is the common effector pathway for a number of different types of cell injury (*Fig. 2.4*) including:

- the injury associated with reperfusion following a period of ischaemia
- certain drug-induced haemolytic anaemias
- paraquat poisoning
- carbon tetrachloride (CCl_4) poisoning
- radiation injury (as in therapeutic irradiation)
- certain cellular correlates of ageing (e.g. accumulation of lipid products within cells – lipofuscins and ceroid)
- oxygen toxicity
- in atherogenesis where LDL within the arterial wall undergoes oxidative modification

What is a Free Radical?

A free radical is an atom or molecule that has a single unpaired electron in its outer orbit. Such chemical species are very active and not only react with molecules within the cell membrane, but often convert these to free radicals as well, thus forming a **positive amplification system** (*Fig. 2.5*).

Free radicals can arise in a number of ways. One of these is through the absorption of radiant energy. Thus

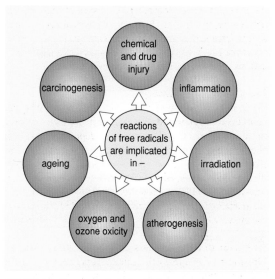

FIGURE 2.4 *Free radicals and cell injury.*

the cell damage that occurs in the course of therapeutic irradiation is, to a considerable extent, brought about by the generation of these radicals.

In a number of situations the reduction of molecular oxygen results in the gain of one rather than two electrons, with the formation of a highly reactive anion O_2^- known as **superoxide anion**. The generation of superoxide is an important part of the body's defences against bacterial infection, and bacterial killing by neutrophil leucocytes and macrophages cannot take place effectively without the formation of oxygen free radicals. This subject is dealt with in more detail in Chapter 5.

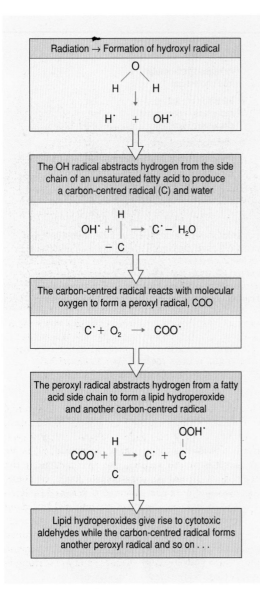

Radiation → Formation of hydroxyl radical

The OH radical abstracts hydrogen from the side chain of an unsaturated fatty acid to produce a carbon-centred radical (C) and water

The carbon-centred radical reacts with molecular oxygen to form a peroxyl radical, COO

The peroxyl radical abstracts hydrogen from a fatty acid side chain to form a lipid hydroperoxide and another carbon-centred radical

Lipid hydroperoxides give rise to cytotoxic aldehydes while the carbon-centred radical forms another peroxyl radical and so on . . .

FIGURE 2.5 Hydroxyl radicals damage cell membrane via a process of lipid peroxidation.

Another interesting model of free radical-mediated injury is carbon tetrachloride poisoning. CCl_4 is changed by mixed function oxidases into the free radical $CCl_3^{\bullet}$ in the smooth endoplasmic reticulum of liver cells. This leads to peroxidation of the phospholipids of liver cell membranes, first in the smooth endoplasmic reticulum, where the transformation of CCl_4 has taken place, and later in all the intracellular membranes. If the P450 enzyme system has been induced by previous administration of barbiturates, the amount of free radical formation will be increased and the degree of cell damage will be greater than would be expected for that dose of CCl_4.

The presence of scavenging mechanisms both within cells and in the extracellular environment suggests that generation of free radicals is a regular accompaniment of redox reactions within the cells and tissues and is not merely an occasional event associated with such abnormal circumstances as irradiation or poisoning. One of the most important scavengers is a group of enzymes, the **superoxide dismutases** (SODs), whose function is the catalytic dismutation of the superoxide anion to hydrogen peroxide and molecular oxygen. The SODs are so widely distributed as to suggest that the superoxide anion is an important byproduct of oxidative metabolism. The hydrogen peroxide formed in the course of dismutation reaction is further detoxified to water by catalases and peroxidase.

Effects of Free Radicals

The **peroxidation of unsaturated lipids in cell membranes** is an important effect of free radical action; other effects are protein (especially thiol-containing proteins) and DNA damage. The morphological correlate of such membrane lipid peroxidation is the formation of blebs on the plasma membrane of affected cells (*Fig. 2.6*). Functionally there is breakdown of the mechanisms normally controlling the entry of calcium to the affected cells and calcium accumulates in the form of deposits in mitochondria. Peroxidation is normally inhibited by hydrophobic scavengers such as **vitamin E and glutathione peroxidase**. Chain-breaking anti-oxidants like vitamin E are found in fresh vegetables and fruit, and it is interesting that diets high in these foodstuffs are associated with a reduced risk of atherosclerosis-related diseases and cancer.

Free radicals can also react with molecules in the ionic or water compartments of the cell. Molecules that have scavenging potential in ionic environments include such compounds as reduced glutathione, ascorbic acid and cysteine. In *ex vivo* circumstances the importance of these scavengers can be demonstrated by depleting their concentration within isolated cells. When this is done the functional and morphological changes that follow lipid peroxidation within membranes are reproduced precisely, even though no measures have been taken to increase the generation of free radicals.

The type of injury induced by the action of free radicals depends not only on the activity of the radicals generated, but also on the structural and biochemical environment. For instance, in the extracellular space, the **glycosoaminoglycans of connective tissue ground substance** may be degraded by free radicals; this might be important in relation to some of the destructive processes that occur in the joints (e.g. rheumatoid arthritis). So far as **plasma membranes** are concerned, uncontrolled activity of free radicals leads to blebbing of the membranes and a failure to maintain the normal fluid and ionic relationships between the intracellular and extracellular compartments.

a

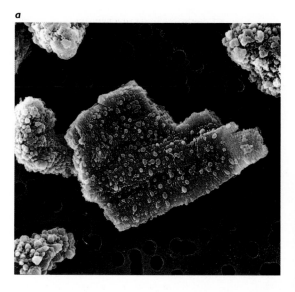

b

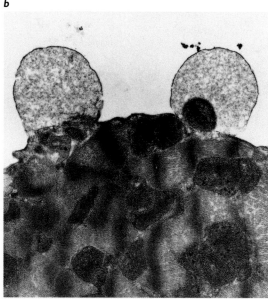

FIGURE 2.6 **a** *Scanning electron micrograph of isolated heart muscle cells from a rat. These cells have been treated with diamide, a compound that decreases the intracellular content of reduced glutathione and thus renders the cell more susceptible to free radical-induced damage. The cells are contracted and have numerous blebs on the plasma membrane. This morphological feature appears to be a common result of lipid peroxidation of cell membranes following free radical initiation. (Original magnification ×5300.)* **b** *Transmission electron micrograph of rat myocardium showing blebbing of plasma membrane caused by lipid peroxidation.*

LYSOSOMES AND CELL INJURY

Lysosomes are involved in disease in three main ways: storage diseases, lysosomal disruption and secretion of enzymes.

Storage Diseases

The first of these results from an inherited deficiency of one of the lysosomal enzymes that are responsible for the normal degradation and turnover of a wide range of molecules. The substrates that cannot be degraded accumulate in the lysosomes, mainly within phagocytic cells but also in liver parenchymal cells, neurones, fibroblasts and renal tubular epithelial cells. This group of disorders is known as the **storage diseases**.

Carbohydrates (e.g. glycogen), complex mucopolysaccharides and a wide variety of sphingolipids are some of the molecules that may accumulate in this way, and an equally wide range of clinical and pathological syndromes has been described. Cultured cells from affected patients usually show the same metabolic abnormalities. In some instances (e.g. Hurler's syndrome, one of the mucopolysaccharidoses) the inexorable advance of the disease has been halted by transplanting bone marrow from unaffected and histocompatible donors to the affected children.

Disruption of Lysosomes

The second way in which lysosomes are involved in cell and tissue injury is when there is release of intra-lysosomal enzymes into the cell cytoplasm. Lysosomal membrane rupture, mediated by a single mechanism, occurs in two apparently widely disparate diseases: gout and silicosis. In the first of these the neutrophil is the cell affected; in the second, the macrophage is the source of the released enzymes. In both of these, phagocytosis of crystalline material is followed by lysosomal fusion and the formation of abnormal hydrogen bonds between the particle surface and lysosomal membrane. The resulting perturbation of the lysosomal membrane leads to rupture, with spillage of the enzyme content into both the cell cytoplasm and the surrounding area (*Fig. 2.7*).

Secretion of Enzymes from Lysosomes

The third way in which lysosomes may be involved in a disease process is by secretion of lysosomal enzymes (usually from macrophages) into the immediate environment of these cells. The possibility that such events might be associated with the development of some forms of arthritis was mooted after the observation of Fell and colleagues that, if articular cartilage was incubated with an excess of Vitamin A, the glycosaminoglycan of the matrix was destroyed, although the cartilage cells themselves appeared to be viable. *In vivo*, injections of large doses of vitamin A or papain, both of which render lysosomal membranes unstable, into rabbits led to a loss of the rabbits' ability to prick up their ears; the histological correlate of this was once again a loss of the complex carbohydrate in the cartilage matrix. In

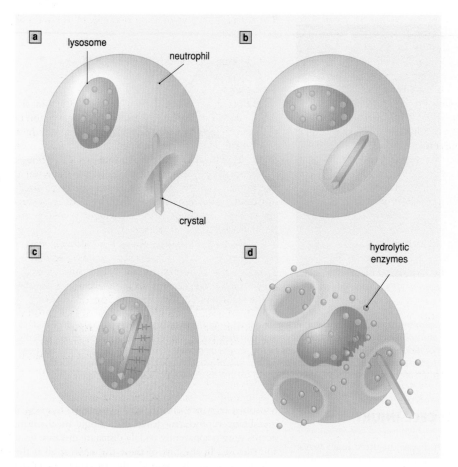

FIGURE 2.7 *Tissue injury resulting from intracytoplasmic release of lysosomal enzymes following the formation of abnormal hydrogen bonds between the lysosomal membrane and the surface of an ingested particle, as seen in gout and silicosis.* **a** *Phagocytosis of crystal.* **b** *The primary lysosome fuses with the phagosome.* **c** *Hydrogen bonds form between the crystal surface and the lysosome membrane.* **d** *As a result of this 'adhesion' between the crystal and part of the lysosomal membrane, the latter ruptures and spills its content of hydrolytic enzymes.*

humans, joint fluid from patients with rheumatoid arthritis contains lysosomal enzymes. These data have been interpreted as suggesting that the effector pathway for damage to the articular cartilage in the destructive arthritides is the inappropriate release of lysosomal enzymes. Clearly the instability of the lysosomal membranes in this situation is not due to either vitamin A intoxication or the presence of papain and, for the present, the pathogenesis of the lysosomal change remains obscure.

STRESS PROTEINS IN RELATION TO CELL INJURY

When cells of any type are exposed to environmental stresses, an increase occurs in the intracellular concentrations of a group of highly conserved proteins. The model of injury that has

been studied in most detail is heat: a temperature 5–10°C higher than is optimal for the cell type in culture. For this reason this group of proteins has been given the name of **heat shock proteins (hsps)**.

This is a misnomer because increases in the concentration of these proteins follow a range of stresses, including:

- fever
- ischaemia
- oxidant injury
- infection by certain microorganisms
- cancer
- a wide range of chemical species including transition metals (which cause the generation of free radicals), calcium ionophores, alcohol, metabolic poisons such as azide and various oxidants.

There is now considerable evidence that this response by cells is essentially a protective one. Not only do these proteins help the cell to withstand the stress that has caused the response but it equips them to resist stresses that are even greater in severity. In the context of cardiac ischaemia, this set of processes is called ischaemic preconditioning. Increases in the synthesis of certain stress proteins are found in many disease states.

The stress response, characterized by an increase in the production of specific proteins, is an example of **inducible gene expression**. With regard to the functions of stress proteins, it is believed that their common function is to act as **molecular chaperones** by:

- ensuring that other proteins produced by the cell are correctly folded
- taking part in the disassembly of certain oligomeric structures such as those involved in DNA replication.

Classification of Stress Proteins

The stress proteins are classified into four main groups, a division based on migratory behaviour during electrophoresis and on molecular weight (*Table 2.1*).

Table 2.1 Stress Proteins

Stress protein	Functions
hsp90	Regulates activity of other proteins by binding to them Prevents aggregation of refolding polypeptides (*in vitro*)
hsp70	Dissociates some oligomers Binds to extended polypeptides Has ATPase activity
hsp60 (also known as chaperonin)	Weak ATPase activity Binds to partly folded polypeptides and plays a part in their correct folding
hsp15–30	?

BACTERIAL TOXINS AND CELL INJURY

Many of the striking clinical features associated with certain bacterial infections are a result of the synthesis and release of highly active chemical species known as bacterial toxins. Included within this rubric are some of the most poisonous molecules ever identified. Two kilograms of the exotoxin of *Clostridium botulinum* would be sufficient to exterminate the entire world population.

Classification of Bacterial Toxins

Bacterial toxins are classified into two principal groups:

- **Exotoxins**
- **Endotoxin**

The defining criteria of these two groups are outlined in *Table 2.2*.

Actions of Bacterial Toxins

Exotoxins

Exotoxins differ functionally from endotoxin in the precise definition of their cellular targets. The action of an exotoxin might be likened to that of an arrow which always strikes the target at the same point. Endotoxin resembles, instead, a stone flung into a pool: although the stone makes contact with the surface of the water at one point, from this point ripples fan out in all directions and, in the same way, endotoxin produces a variety of functional perturbations brought about by the generation of many mediators.

Exotoxins exert their effects in the following ways:

- The toxin enters the cell via endocytosis. Within the cell it acts as enzyme. The commonest type of enzyme action is **irreversible adenosine 5′-diphosphate (ADP) ribosylation in which ADP ribose is transferred from nicotinamide adenine dinucleotide (NAD) to some intracellular protein,** the function of which is thus inhibited. The effects on cell function depend on which protein is ribosylated in this way (e.g. cholera toxin, diphtheria toxin).
- The toxin acts as **a lytic enzyme causing disruption of the cell plasma membrane** (e.g. α toxin of *Clostridium perfringens* causing 'gas gangrene').
- The toxin **inhibits neurotransmission** (e.g. acetylcholine at the motor end-plate is blocked by the toxin of *C. botulinum*).

Some Examples of Exotoxin Activity

Toxins that Function by Ribosylating Intracellular Proteins

Vibrio cholerae Toxin   *Vibrio cholerae* has been responsible for huge numbers of deaths during recorded history and still causes much disease.

This organism causes cholera, a disease characterized by the abrupt onset of **profuse, watery diarrhoea**. Patients may pass 11–30 litres of stool in a day. As a result they become dehydrated and suffer severe electrolyte disturbances.

This devastating pathophysiological effect is accomplished by the exotoxin produced by the vibrio; the organism itself fails to invade the tissues and remains within the gut lumen (*Fig. 2.8*).

Cholera toxin consists of two portions: a single A portion and a pentameric B portion. These operate by perverting a normal cell-signalling system:

- The **B portion** binds irreversibly to a GM1 ganglioside receptor on the luminal aspect of the small gut epithelial cell and activates the receptor. **This**

Table 2.2 Defining Criteria of Bacterial Exotoxins and Endotoxins

Characteristic	Exotoxin	Endotoxin
Secretion product of living microorganism	Yes	No
Part of structure of microorganism; often released from dead organisms	No	Yes
Basic chemical nature	Protein	Combination of lipid and a complex sugar (lipopolysaccharide)
Immunogenic	Yes	Weakly, if at all
Can be 'toxoided' (process by which toxic properties can be removed without impairing immunogenicity)	Yes	No
Heat labile or stable	Usually labile	Stable
Biochemical target	A precise intracellular process, membrane component or neurotransmitter	Several cell types and plasma protein cascade systems associated with inflammation

receptor is functionally coupled to adenylate cyclase via a stimulatory G protein, G_s.

- The adenylate cyclase system consists, functionally, of three parts:
  a) The GM1 receptor.
  b) The G_s protein, which is attached by farnesyl bonds to the plasma membrane. This G protein both binds guanosine 5′-triphosphate (GTP) and can act as a GTPase, thus constituting a molecular 'on–off' switch' for signal transduction.
  c) Adenylate cyclase which converts adenosine 5′-triphosphate (ATP) to adenosine 3′,5′-cyctic mono-phosphate (cAMP).

Normal Operation of the Adenylate Cyclase System

1) Binding of a ligand to the GM1 receptor produces a conformational change, which exposes a binding site for the G protein.
2) By diffusion within the membrane, the G protein associates with the ligand–receptor complex and is activated to displace guanosine 5′-diphosphate (GDP) and bind GTP.
3) Binding GTP causes the α portion of the G protein to dissociate from the ligand–receptor complex and exposes a binding site on the G protein for adenylate cyclase.
4) The G protein binds to and activates adenylate cyclase, and cAMP is produced.
5) The G protein now normally hydrolyses the GTP. This returns the G protein to its inactive conformation and it dissociates from adenylate cyclase. The production of cAMP therefore ceases.

- **The A portion of cholera toxin enters the small gut epithelial cell and irreversibly ribosylates the G protein. This inactivates its GTPase function and cAMP production thus continues in an uncontrolled manner.**

Such unregulated cAMP production has effects on both **villous** and **crypt** epithelial cells.

- At the villus, cAMP **inhibits entry** of water, sodium and chloride.
- In the crypt, cAMP **promotes the pumping out** into the gut lumen of water, sodium, chloride and bicarbonate.

The combination of these two effects is responsible for the water and electrolyte depletion seen in cholera and

FIGURE 2.8 (opposite) **a** *Activation of the adenylate cyclase system in small intestinal epithelium. (1) The inactive system showing a GM1 receptor, a G (stimulatory) protein complex which binds GDP and adenylate cyclase. (2) Binding of a ligand to the receptor exposes a binding site for the G protein. (3) Binding of the G protein to the receptor–ligand complex causes the exchange of GDP for GTP and leads to dissociation of the α subunit of the G protein, thus exposing a binding site for adenylate cyclase. (4) The α subunit of the G protein binds to adenylate cyclase, causing activation and the production of cAMP. (5) The α subunit of the G protein now acts as a GTPase and the GTP is exchanged for GDP, leading to dissociation of the α subunit from adenylate cyclase and cessation of cAMP production. This cycle of events is repeated as long as the ligand remains bound to the receptor. It ends (6) when the ligand dissociates from the receptor and the receptor returns to its inactive configuration.* **b** *The irreversible ADP ribosylation of the α subunit of the G protein leads to the latter being unable to function as a GTPase. As a result, activation of adenylate cyclase continues with continuing production of cAMP.* **c** *Cholera toxin causes sustained production of cAMP by small gut epithelium leading to blocking of water, sodium and chloride absorption by cells of villus and increased transport of water, sodium, chloride and bicarbonate into the gut lumen by crypt cells.*

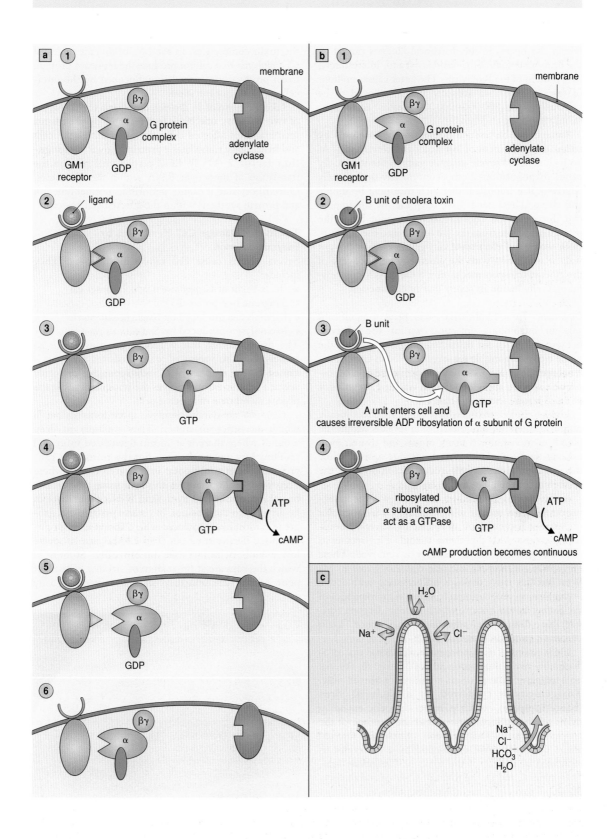

which also occurs in the diarrhoeal illnesses caused by the heat-labile toxin of *Escherichia coli* and, interestingly, by a protein of the Rotavirus. The latter causes millions of cases of diarrhoea annually and is believed to be responsible for 800 000–900 000 deaths each year, mainly in young children.

Patients can be rescued from this dire state only by adequate replacement of lost water and electrolytes. As both cholera and severe infantile gastro-enteritis usually occur in populations both economically and socially deprived, it is important that such treatment be simple and cheap. These needs have been met by the important discovery that cholera toxin does not block the passage of glucose from the gut lumen into the gut wall. Both water and electrolyte can gain access to the gut wall in association with the glucose. The discovery of the glucose transport mechanism is the basis for successful oral rehydration in severe diarrhoeal illnesses.

Diphtheria Toxin Diphtheria toxin plays a significant role in establishing infection within the pharynx because it is lethal for defending phagocytes and is the single factor responsible for severe disease in corynebacterial infections. It is extremely toxic for the cells of susceptible species: a single molecule reaching the interior of a cell is sufficient to kill that cell.

Unlike cholera toxin, which exerts its effect locally on gut epithelium, diphtheria toxin spreads within the bloodstream and affects many organs and tissues, most notably the heart, kidneys and nervous system, while the organisms themselves remain confined to the epithelium of the pharynx.

If the disease is established, treatment with neutralizing antibody (antitoxin) is mandatory. Of even greater importance is prevention of disease by actively immunizing infants with diphtheria toxoid. This retains its **immunogenicity** while **toxicity** is removed. These preventive measures have made diphtheria rare in the West but this rarity depends on persisting with active immunization programmes. In some of the republics of the former Soviet Union, which have undergone considerable disturbance, diphtheria has once again become a common disease.

Only strains of *Corynebacterium diphtheriae* that produce the toxin (toxigenic strains) cause diphtheria; non-toxigenic strains cause a mild sore throat only. **Toxigenicity is conferred by a bacterial virus (bacteriophage)**, which possesses the gene encoding the toxin, being incorporated into the genome of the corynebacterium. This situation, where an inserted phage codes for toxin production by a bacterium, is replicated in respect of the toxin of *Clostridium botulinum* types C and D, the toxin of *C. novyi* and the erythrogenic toxin of β-haemolytic streptococci.

The expression of the *tox* gene is normally regulated by a corynebacterial repressor protein which binds to the *tox* gene in the presence of ferrous iron. If the iron concentrations within the organism fall, production of

the toxin commences. In the case of mutant strains of *C. diphtheriae* that cannot produce the repressor protein, toxin production proceeds uninfluenced by the intracellular iron concentration.

Like the toxin of *V. cholerae*, diphtheria toxin consists of two portions: one binds to a receptor on the plasma membranes of affected cells; the other enters the cells and irreversibly ribosylates a protein known as **elongation factor 2** (EF-2). EF-2 plays a vital part on the translation of messenger RNA within the ribosomes. Once ribosylated it cannot perform its normal function and protein synthesis within the affected cell ceases.

Toxins that Damage Cell Membranes by Enzymatic Action

Several toxins cause cell injury in this way. They include:

- the α-toxin of *C. perfringens* which causes gas gangrene (see pp 20–21)
- haemolysins produced by *Staphylococcus aureus*
- haemolysins produced by *Streptococcus pyogenes*

The tissue damage that occurs in gas gangrene is an archetype of this variety of toxin-mediated injury. It is caused by the α-toxin of *C. perfringens*; this molecule acts as a lecithinase and cleaves the phospholipids in the plasma membrane of affected cells.

Clostridia are Gram-positive, spore-forming bacilli which are strict anaerobes. They multiply in deep wounds where there is abundant devitalized tissue and resulting low oxygen tension. For this reason, gas gangrene has been commonest in military practice where deep wounds, associated with much tissue destruction, become contaminated by the soil and clothing that can be driven into these tissues. In civilian practice, gas gangrene is most likely to occur where above-knee amputation has been carried out (*Fig. 2.9*) because of severe lower limb ischaemia (see pp 218–221). Stumps in which the flaps are at the margin of viability because of poor arterial perfusion may become contaminated by

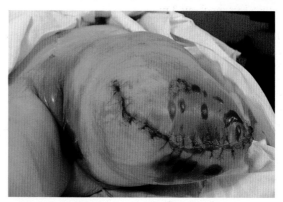

FIGURE 2.9 *Above-knee amputation for ischaemic lower limb. The patient developed gas gangrene as a result of contamination of devitalized tissues by* Clostridia. *Note the skin blebs.*

Clostridia derived from the patient's own large gut (auto-infection).

The presence of the toxin in material derived from wounds can be demonstrated by its lecithin-splitting properties. If cultures are set up using agar plates that incorporate egg yolk, toxin causes the appearance of an opaque zone of diglyceride in relation to the organisms (Nagler's reaction).

Toxins that Interfere with Neuro-transmission

Only two organisms produce toxins that act in this way: *C. botulinum* and *C. tetani*.

Botulinum Toxin The toxin of *C. botulinum* is one of the most toxic substances known: a dose of 1 μg is lethal to humans. The toxin is preformed in foods contaminated by the clostridium, which are then ingested by the victims. Unlike all the other forms of toxin-related injury discussed here, it is *not* necessary for an affected individual to be infected by the organism: a very small amount of the toxin suffices.

Botulinum toxin exists in eight antigenic forms (A, B, C1, C2, D, E, F and G), each of which is produced by a different strain of *Clostridia*. Botulism in humans is caused by toxins A, B, E and F; toxin type A accounts for about 60% of cases. Toxin A may occur in preserved fruits, vegetables and meat; B is usually found in meat and E in uncooked sea-food.

The toxin is carried in the bloodstream to peripheral neuromuscular junctions where it blocks the transmission of acetylcholine (ACh) by inhibiting its release from nerve terminals. The inevitable result is a flaccid paralysis of the affected muscles. Such paralysis may be widespread and is particularly lethal if muscles used in breathing are affected.

This action of the botulinum neurotoxin in blocking ACh transmission has led to use of the toxin as a therapeutic agent in certain dystonic disorders such as vocal cord spasm, eyelid spasm and spasmodic torticollis. Local injection of toxin at affected sites causes paralysis which lasts for about 3 months.

Tetanus Toxin *C. tetani* produces two toxins; the one responsible for the muscle spasms and contracture characteristic of tetanus is known as **tetanospasmin.**

The organisms most often enter the tissues as a result of deep penetrating wounds. In some parts of Africa neonatal tetanus occurs as a result of the practice of anointing the umbilical stumps of newborn infants with cow dung (a rich source of *Clostridia*). If the organisms can multiply within the tissues, the toxin released from them enters the motor nerves fibres by binding to ganglioside receptors. The toxin then travels in a cephalad direction up the axons until the anterior horn cells of the spinal cord are reached.

The toxin acts by blocking the transmission of **glycine** from inhibitory interneurones. This leads to a state of over-excitability of the motor neurones,

expressed in the form of spasms, rigidity and trismus (lockjaw).

The actions of **bacterial endotoxin** are discussed in the section on shock (see pp 368–389).

RADIATION AND CELL INJURY

All forms of radiation may be harmful to living cells. It is this fact that underlies the use of irradiation in the treatment of certain malignant neoplasms.

All of us are exposed to a certain amount of background radiation, the sources for this being:

- **cosmic radiation** derived from the sun and outer space. The higher the altitude the greater the degree of such exposure.
- **radioactive elements** present in the earth's crust, of which radium is the best-known example
- certain naturally occurring **radionuclides** present within the body

About 80% of the annual dose of ionizing radiation that we receive comes from these sources. The sources responsible for the remainder are:

- **radiation modalities** used in medical diagnosis and treatment
- **radioactive minerals** present in fertilizers and certain building materials
- **nuclear fall-out**
- **domestic products** such as television sets and smoke detectors

THE NATURE OF RADIATION

Basically, radiation is of two types: electromagnetic and particulate.

Electromagnetic Radiation

This represents energy that is propagated by wave motion. Forms of electromagnetic radiation that are relevant from the biological viewpoint include γ- and X-rays. γ-Rays are emitted spontaneously from radioactive materials; X-rays are produced artificially.

These forms have a short wavelength and are of high frequency. These attributes are associated with sufficient energy to ionize the materials through which they pass.

Particulate Radiation

This is brought about by the movement of sub-atomic particles. It occurs either because of the decay of radioactive substances or as a result of the acceleration of sub-atomic particles to very high speeds (e.g. in a cyclotron). When a substance has an unstable nucleus that decays with the consequent release of energy, it is said to be radioactive.

Radioactive Decay

This takes place in the form of:

- α**-particle emission.** When nuclei with high

atomic numbers decay, α particles are emitted and energy is released which is the expression of the kinetic energy of the particles.

- **β emission.** The most abundant radioactive isotopes are β emitters. β–Negative decay involves neutrons becoming transformed into protons. Energy release is related to the kinetic energy of neutrinos (uncharged particles with zero rest mass), β particles or γ-rays.
- **Electron capture.** The end–result of β decay is a nucleus lacking an electron. This gap becomes filled by electrons moving towards the nucleus from sites further away, this being accompanied by energy release. The movement of an electron from the inner shell to the nucleus, with resulting release of a neutrino, is known as electron capture.

γ Emission from radioactive sources is preceded by one of the processes mentioned above and is *never* the sole expression of radioactive decay.

Measurement of Decay and Ionizing Radiation

Decay is measured in the form of becquerels (Bq). It represents **one disintegration per second** and is *not* a measure of energy released. The unit of measure most used until recently is the curie (Ci). $1 \, Ci = 3.7 \times 10^{10} \, Bq$.

Ionizing radiation is measured in more than one way:

- as the unit of charge produced as rays ionize a given volume of air (roentgens). This is a unit of exposure, not a unit of absorption. It applies to X- and γ-rays.
- as the absorbed dose: 1 **rad** is the radiation dose resulting in the absorption of 100 ergs of energy per gram of absorbing substance. The SI system uses the **gray** (Gy) as the measure of dose absorbed. One gray is the dose of radiation in which there is absorption of 1 joule of energy per kilogram of absorbing substance. $1 \, Gy = 100 \, rad$.

In biological systems particulate radiation usually produces more damage than X- or γ-rays. For this reason additional units have been devised:

- The **rem** is the dose of any type of radiation that produces a biological effect equal to that of 1 **rad** of X- or γ-rays. 1 millirem = 1/1000 rem.
- In the SI system the **sievert** is the amount of any type of radiation producing a biological effect equal to that of 1 Gy of X- or γ-rays. 1 sievert = 100 rem.

THE BIOLOGICAL RESPONSE TO RADIATION

The biological response of cells and tissue to radiation depends on the interaction of:

- **Physical factors.** These include the total dose of radiation, the character of the radiation and the time over which administration occurs.
- **Chemical factors.** These may serve either to protect cells against radiation damage or to

potentiate that damage. The most active potentiating agent is molecular oxygen, which serves as a substrate for the generation of tissue-damaging oxygen free radicals (see pp 13–15). This is utilized in the treatment of certain malignant tumours in which attempts are made to increase oxygen tension within tumours by hyperbaric therapy before irradiation. Chemical species, such as sulphydryl groups, that act as free radical scavengers tend to protect cells against radiation damage.

- **Biological factors.** These are complex and not completely understood. An important consideration is the time during the cell cycle when exposure to radiation occurs (cells are most sensitive during the G2 phase (between DNA synthesis and mitosis) and during mitosis, and least sensitive during the S phase (when DNA is being synthesized)). Thus cells that are undergoing rapid division are likely to be more radiosensitive than those in which turnover is slow. Sublethal radiation injury can be repaired and the differing ability of cells to accomplish this is clearly related to their degree of radiosensitivity.

The relative sensitivity of normal organs and tissues to radiation is shown in *Table 2.3.*

Acute, Potentially Lethal, Damage Occurs after a Single Dose of Whole Body Irradiation of Sufficient Strength

A single dose of irradiation about 10 000 times the average daily background exposure (0.001 rad) is required before any functional or morphological changes occur. At this point (10 rad) specific functional and morphological abnormalities are noted in certain lymphocyte sub-populations.

- **100 rad.** This causes radiation sickness of mild degree associated with nausea and vomiting. The rate of division in haemopoietic cells decreases and there is a short-lived lymphopenia.
- **1000 rad.** This causes severe necrosis in the haemopoietic stem cell compartment with resulting pancytopenia. There is extensive loss of gut epithelium. This is severe radiation sickness, death occurring usually within 2 weeks.
- **10 000 rad.** This causes severe disturbances in central nervous system function. Death occurs within hours.
- **100 000 rad.** This dose kills most cells; death within minutes is likely.

Radiation Effects in Specific Tissues

Blood Vessels

Blood vessel damage is a common and important component of both acute and delayed damage associated with irradiation. In the acute phase there is dilatation and increased permeability of both arterioles and capillaries, this manifesting as erythema and oedema. At a slightly later stage endothelial cells undergo necrosis and

Table 2.3 Relative Radiosensitivity of Various Organs and Tissues

Very high	High	Intermediate	Low
Bone marrow	Kidney	Adult bone	Uterus
Testis	Liver	Adult cartilage	Vagina
Ovary	Lung	Mucosa of mouth	Pancreas
Breast (in childhood)	Heart	Oesophagus	Adrenal
Growing cartilage	Growing bone	Bladder	
Lens	Small bowel		
	Colon		
	Thyroid		
	Cornea		
	Pituitary		
	Spinal cord		
	Growing muscle		
	Salivary gland		
	Brain		
	Skin		
	Rectum		

there may be patchy necrosis of the smooth muscle cells of arterioles.

Months or years after exposure small blood vessels may still show damage in the form of sub-endothelial accumulation of ground substance and necrosis of the smooth muscle-rich media of arterioles. Depending on the part of the vascular bed affected, various secondary effects may occur:

- atrophic changes in the skin often associated with scarring of the sub-epidermal tissue
- interstitial scarring in the myocardium
- ulcer formation in the gut
- renal cortical atrophy associated with interstitial tissue scarring
- necrosis of white matter in the brain associated with increase in glial fibres; spinal cord damage

Skin

In the early stages (up to 4 weeks after exposure) there is likely to be erythema, loss of hair and dryness (due to death of hair follicle cells and sebaceous glands). Delayed injury is characterized by some degree of atrophy, dilatation of blood vessels, hyperkeratosis and a marked degree of homogenization of the dermal collagen.

Haemopoietic and Lymphoid Systems

These are very sensitive to radiation. Large doses of radiation, as stated above, cause severe lymphopenia, accompanied by a decrease in the size of spleen and lymph nodes. If the irradiation is not lethal, recovery takes place. In the long term, severe irradiation may cause leukaemia as demonstrated by the increased risk

seen in survivors of the nuclear attacks on Japanese cities in 1945 and nuclear accidents.

Heart

Radiation affects the heart of 2–9% of patients who receive treatment to the mediastinum for lymphoma and about 3% of those irradiated because of breast carcinoma. The most common expression of cardiac damage is pericarditis, which often goes on to scarring, thus producing constriction of the underlying myocardium. Interstitial fibrosis may also occur, and is attributed to vascular damage (see above).

Lung

A dose of 35–40 Gy administered in 3 to 40 fractions produces radiation pneumonitis in 10–15% of patients receiving irradiation to the chest area, usually about 8–15 weeks after exposure.

Initially damage affects the alveolar capillaries and the consequent increase in their permeability leads to oedema of the inter-alveolar septa. At a slightly later stage the epithelial cells lining the air spaces (alveolar pneumocytes types 1 and 2) are affected. Necrosis and desquamation of the type 1 cells occurs and type 2 cells tend to proliferate. The damaged air spaces often show an eosinophilic membrane plastered down on their walls (hyaline membrane). This is a non-specific sign of respiratory distress syndrome. Later (after 16 weeks) interstitial scarring develops, which causes restrictive lung disease.

All forms of radiation-induced lung damage carry an increased risk for the subsequent development of malignancy within the lung.

Gastro-intestinal Tract

The mouth shows evidence of radiation damage very early after therapeutic irradiation of the head and neck. Changes in the oral mucosa are similar to those described in the skin. Damage to the salivary glands leading to scarring and loss of secretory acini may gravely disadvantage patients, who may be left with permanent dryness of the mouth.

The principal change encountered in the rest of the gastro-intestinal tract following irradiation is denudation of the surface epithelium. This occurs because the radiation decreases the regenerative ability of the stem cell precursors of intestinal epithelial cells. The normal rate of loss of mature epithelial lining cells is not compensated for by the generation of new cells, and large areas of shallow ulceration result.

In the long term, strictures, chronic ulcers, fistulae and neoplasms may complicate irradiation of the gut. The small gut, colon and rectum are most commonly affected and it is believed that the most potent mechanism involved in long-term damage is radiation-mediated injury to small blood vessels in the gut wall.

Liver

Doses of 40 Gy or more are required before clinically obvious liver damage occurs. Such damage usually manifests about 3 months after exposure. The principal anatomical target is the venous drainage of the liver; terminal hepatic venules and the terminal portions of some sinusoids are chiefly affected. The endothelial cells of these vessels become swollen and in some cases necrotic, followed by fibrin deposition within the vessel lumina. Failing lysis of this fibrin, collagen strands grow into the vessels and obstruct their lumina. This situation (veno-occlusive disease) is not specific for radiation injury and also occurs in association with liver damage caused by certain chemical poisons. The end-result is congestion and, ultimately, necrosis, in the central part of the liver lobule (acinus zone 3).

Radiation-induced tumours in the liver have also been reported, particularly associated with use of thorium dioxide, an α particle-emitting imaging material. This collects in the fixed macrophages in the liver (Küpffer cells) and can cause many significant local changes including malignant neoplasms of the liver cells, bile ductules and blood vessels.

Endocrine System

Tumours have been reported following radiation in all endocrine glands. The thyroid is by far the most commonly affected gland, thyroid carcinomas having been reported in survivors of nuclear fall-out and in individuals who received therapeutic irradiation during childhood.

The Skeleton

The risk of radiation occurring in the skeleton depends largely on the age of the individual at the time of exposure. Growing cartilage and bone are radiosensitive; adult bone and cartilage are relatively resistant.

Many cases of malignant neoplasm of bone following radium exposure have been reported.

Testis and Ovary

The germinal epithelium in both sexes is very sensitive to irradiation. Acute radiation damage is expressed in the form of suppression of meiosis in both ovary and testis, followed by necrosis of germinal epithelium, the spermatogonia being most severely affected. Recovery tends to be slow.

Urinary Tract

The **urinary bladder** is very susceptible to radiation injury. Acute radiation damage is expressed in the form of suppression of the regenerative activity of epithelial stem cells, and this leads inevitably to ulceration. Scarring in the deeper portions of the bladder wall is an important and clinically most disadvantageous complication because the bladder's capacity may be greatly reduced. This leads to a crippling degree of increased frequency of micturition.

In the **kidney** radiation may cause vasodilatation, oedema of the interstitium and some degree of loss of the normal molecular sieving functions of the glomeruli, leading to proteinuria. Functional recovery from this phase is the rule, but after a long latent period progressive scarring of glomeruli and consequent loss of tubules may occur.

Breast

Irradiation of the breast is associated with an increased risk of breast cancer, the peak incidence occurring 15–20 years after exposure.

Nervous System

The mature nervous system is moderately resistant to acute radiation-mediated injury. Both the brain and spinal cord show necrosis associated with a degree of myelin loss. These changes are believed to be secondary to small blood vessel damage. In the spinal cord, severe post-irradiation damage may be expressed clinically in the form of paraplegia.

As in many other tissues, radiation increases the risk of subsequent malignancy.

Eye

The principal target for radiation damage to the eye is the lens. Opacities in the substance of the lens develop and may progress to full-blown cataracts.

SOME MORPHOLOGICAL EXPRESSIONS OF CELL INJURY

Injury of varying degrees of severity can often be correlated with morphological changes within the affected cells. The pathological literature of the nineteenth and early twentieth centuries abounds with graphic, but more or less meaningless, descriptive terms for cell injury such as **cloudy swelling** or **hyaline (glassy) degeneration**.

It is more logical to approach this subject by realizing that the commonest ways in which **sub-lethal** cell injury is manifested are by:

- alterations in **cell volume (acute cellular oedema)**
- accumulation of excess triglyceride (**fatty change**)

Changes in Cell Volume

The control of the volume of a cell within fairly narrow limits is one of the outstanding characteristics of mammalian cells. This control is exerted largely by sodium and potassium transport mechanisms, which are energy dependent and linked with membrane-bound enzymes.

If these control mechanisms break down, a large amount of isotonic fluid collects within the cell and the cell volume increases. The mitochondria also become swollen; it is for this reason that, on light microscopic examination, the cell cytoplasm appears granular. This increase in intracellular fluid content, or **acute cellular oedema** occurs particularly if the cells become **hypoxic**, but may also occur in the course of fever or cell injury by certain bacterial toxins and chemical poisons.

The normal cell has a higher potassium concentration and a lower sodium content than extracellular fluid. These differentials in respect of sodium and potassium are maintained by the ATP energy-dependent membrane transport system known as the **sodium pump**; part of this system is the ouabain-sensitive ATPase situated in the plasma membrane of the cell.

Hypoxia and the other forms of cell injury mentioned above cause a decrease in the production of ATP, and the ratio of ATP to ADP thus falls significantly. **This leads to a partial failure of the sodium pump.** Potassium ions diffuse out of the cell into the extracellular fluid, and the reverse applies to sodium ions, which enter the cell in large amounts. Because the hydration shell of sodium is greater than that of potassium, water enters the cells from the extracellular fluid as well. This will, of course, lead to an increase in cell volume.

The effects of hypoxia on the cell involve the following sequence of events (*Fig. 2.10*).

1) As the oxygen tension falls, mitochondrial phosphorylation decreases rapidly with a consequent fall in ATP.
2) This drop in ATP stimulates the activity of the enzyme **phosphofructokinase**.
3) This leads to an increase in the rate of anaerobic glycolysis.
4) This, in turn, causes an accumulation of lactate which, together with the increase in inorganic phosphate concentration, lowers the intracellular

pH. Morphologically this is believed to be reflected in the appearance of clumping of the nuclear chromatin.

5) At this point the decline in ATP will have produced its effect on the sodium pump, and the accumulation of sodium and water mentioned above takes place.

6) Protein production is also adversely affected at this stage, expressed in morphological terms by **detachment of polysomes** from the membranes

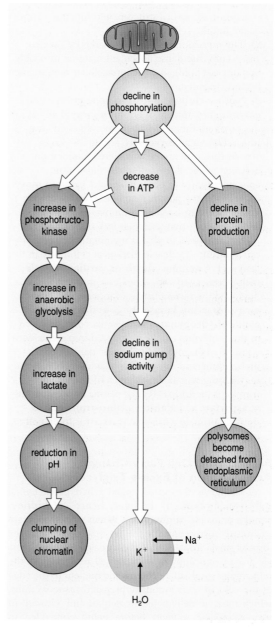

FIGURE 2.10 Effects of hypoxia on metabolic events within cells.

of the endoplasmic reticulum and scattering of both free and bound polysomes into monomeric ribosomes.

At this stage the process is still reversible: both the function and structure of the protein-secreting apparatus can be brought back to normal if the cell's oxygen supply is restored. By now the cytoskeleton also appears to be affected and the plasma membrane of the cells may show blebs or the appearance of microvilli.

7) If hypoxia continues beyond this point, the degree of cell damage may reach a point at which restoration of normal structure and function cannot occur and the cell will die.

8) The mitochondria become markedly swollen and accumulate dense flocculent material (probably calcium and lipid), and the intracellular membranes become fragmented.

9) Nuclear chromatin starts to undergo attack by enzymes (presumably of lysosomal origin) and as this proceeds the nucleus becomes digested away (this is known as **karyolysis**; see pp 29–30).

10) At this stage not only is there equilibration between extracellular and intracellular ionic concentrations, but other molecules begin to move freely across the plasma membrane so that dyes in the extracellular fraction can move into the cell, while the cell's own enzymes leak out (*Fig. 2.11*).

This alteration in plasma membrane permeability can constitute a valuable marker of cell injury in the patient. For example, **death of cardiac muscle cells** is associated with the release into extracellular fluid, and then into plasma, of intracellular enzymes such as **creatine kinase** and **β–hydroxybutyric acid dehydrogenase**. The plasma concentrations of these enzymes can be monitored in patients with a suspected diagnosis of ischaemic damage to the myocardium and can provide an additional method for assessing whether the degree of ischaemic damage is increasing. Raised plasma concentrations of **aspartate** and **alanine amino-transferases** similarly provide a valuable marker for **liver cell injury**.

Parenchymal Cell Fatty Change: Accumulation of Excess Triglyceride

Fatty change is the term applied when parenchymal cells, notably those of the **liver, heart** and **kidney**, contain stainable triglyceride. When the tissues are examined microscopically the fat may be seen in the form of small droplets or, if these coalesce, as large single drops that occupy most of the cell area and push the remaining cytoplasmic contents and nucleus to the edge of the cell. In conventionally prepared tissue sections, which must be dehydrated in alcohol and 'cleared' in various organic solvents before being embedded in paraffin wax, the fat droplets are dissolved away leaving intra-cytoplasmic spaces (*Fig. 2.12*). Therefore, the

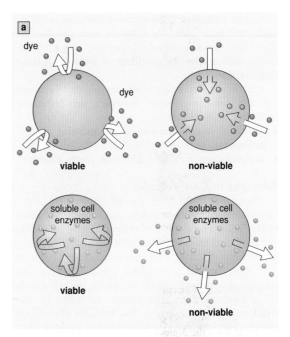

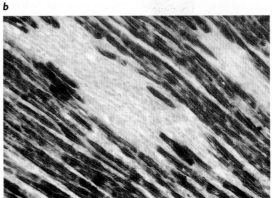

FIGURE 2.11 **a** *Lethal damage to cells is associated with change in permeability of the cell plasma membrane. The viable cell normally excludes dye molecules in the incubating medium. Lethal injury is associated with staining of the cells. Similarly, water-soluble intracellular enzymes do not leak out of a viable cell, but lethal cell damage is associated with escape of such enzymes into the intracellular fluid. The concentration of these enzymes can be monitored in samples of plasma.* **b** *Section of myocardium from rat treated with isoproterenol. Section treated to demonstrate succinate dehydrogenase (black). The presence of focal irreversible myocyte damage is shown by the pink areas, the enzyme having leaked out of the affected cells.*

presence of triglyceride cannot be confirmed by appropriate staining methods. The fat can, however, be demonstrated by cutting sections from blocks of tissue that have been frozen very rapidly. Staining these sections with dyes that dissolve preferentially in triglyceride, such as mixtures of Sudan III and IV or Oil-Red O, stains the fat-containing droplets a bright orange-red.

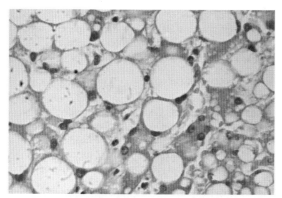

FIGURE 2.12 Section of liver embedded in paraffin and stained with haematoxylin and eosin. The liver shows severe, large-droplet form, fatty change demonstrated here by the presence of large intracellular vacuoles.

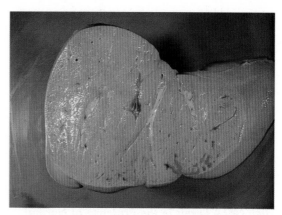

FIGURE 2.13 Liver showing severe fatty change. Note the characteristic pale yellow colour.

Macroscopic Features

Organs affected by severe fatty change are a pale yellowish-brown and may feel greasy (*Fig.2.13*).

In the **liver**, the degree of fat accumulation may be so great that blocks of tissue float in water or fixative solutions. The distribution of fat is usually diffuse in the organ as a whole, although not necessarily in individual liver acini.

In the **kidney**, fatty change shows up as a series of yellowish streaks in the cortex, as the accumulation of fat is non-uniform and tends to be confined to epithelial cells lining the convoluted tubules.

In the **heart**, severe fatty change is commonly seen as a pale and rather flabby myocardium. However, the fatty change sometimes seen in patients suffering from chronic anaemia produces a curious striped appearance, which is most obvious in the subendocardial layer of the interventricular septum in the papillary muscles. In a rare departure from the well-known tendency of morbid anatomists to characterize morphological alterations in terms of food, this appearance has been called '**tabby cat**' or '**thrush-breast**' striation.

Origin of the Excess Intracellular Triglyceride

The excess fat accumulating in affected cells is derived largely from the fat stored in adipose tissue and does not appear as a result of some 'unmasking' phenomenon of fat already present within the cell. A variety of experimental models can be used to demonstrate this. For example, if an animal is poisoned with phosphorus it develops acute liver damage associated with severe fatty change. Starving the animal before administration of the phosphorus, with resulting depletion of adipose tissue fat stores, prevents development of the fatty change, even though the liver cell damage occurs as before. Similarly cells grown in culture can accumulate triglyceride only if triglyceride is present in the culture medium.

The Causes of Triglyceride Accumulation within Liver Cells

The liver occupies a central place in fat metabolism, and the disorders (including various types of poisoning) that result in hepatic fatty change can be understood most easily in terms of disturbance of the various processes related to fat metabolism.

The liver cell normally receives fat in two forms and from two sources:

1) Non-esterified **free fatty acid** (FFA), derived from peripheral adipose tissue stores and released from adipocytes when lipolysis occurs.

2) The **chylomicron**, a large molecule synthesized within the small intestinal epithelium and which consists of triglyceride (90%), phospholipid and apoproteins B, C and E. If apoprotein B cannot be synthesized, then chylomicrons cannot be assembled and triglyceride derived from the diet accumulates within the intestinal epithelium (abetalipoproteinaemia). In the blood vessels draining the intestine, chylomicrons are acted on by a lipoprotein lipase, which removes some of the triglyceride. This is then either used to provide energy in muscle or stored in adipose tissue. The remaining portion of the chylomicron (the remnant particle) binds to a receptor on the liver cells (the ligand being apoprotein E) and is internalized by the liver cell.

Within the liver cell, hydrolysis of the chylomicron remnants takes place, liberating FFAs and glycerol. Acetate, from which additional FFAs can be synthesized, is also present within the liver cell. Irrespective of their origin, most of the FFAs are esterified to form triglyceride, some are incorporated into phospholipid, and others are incorporated into cholesterol esters. The triglyceride within the liver cell, which is kept in the form of a micelle by phospholipid, is then coupled to a lipid-acceptor protein or apoprotein and secreted from the liver in the form of very low density lipoprotein (VLDL).

It should therefore be clear that accumulation of excess triglyceride may reflect either one or both of the following:

- an increase in the amount of lipid being brought to the liver, particularly in the form of non-esterified fatty acids (NEFAs)
- an inability of the liver cell to carry out the functions outlined above in respect of the delivery to it of a normal amount of lipid

High NEFA Levels in the Presence of Normal Liver Cells

High plasma concentrations of NEFAs in the presence of normal liver cells are seen when there is a decrease in the energy normally supplied by carbohydrates. Increased fat catabolism is needed to make up for the energy shortfall, and this leads to lipolysis of the fat in adipose tissue stores and a rise in the plasma concentration of FFAs. This occurs in:

- **starvation**
- where there is a block in normal carbohydrate metabolism such as in **uncontrolled diabetes mellitus, galactosaemia** and some forms of **glycogen storage disease**

Normal Plasma NEFA Levels in the Presence of Injury or Abnormality of Liver Cells

Because of the large number of functions carried out by liver cells in respect of the FFAs delivered to the liver, the number of ways in which liver cell injury can be reflected by fatty change is correspondingly great. Liver cell injury affecting these particular functions (amongst others) includes:

1) **Anoxia due to severe congestive cardiac failure.** The cells first affected are those in the centrilobular zone. This gives the affected organ a mottled red and yellow appearance known as 'nutmeg liver'.

2) **Severe protein and calorie undernutrition.** In this condition (known as **kwashiorkor** when seen in children), the liver cell (because of a shortage of the necessary amino acid substrates) is not able to synthesize the lipid-acceptor proteins needed for the export of triglyceride in the form of VLDL. A marked degree of triglyceride accumulation may occur under these circumstances, so much so that the liver, when removed at post-mortem examination, may float in water or aqueous fixatives. Sequential liver biopsy studies have shown that hepatic fatty change of this type is completely reversible by a diet containing adequate amounts of protein.

3) **Chronic alcoholism.** This is one of the commonest causes of significant hepatic fatty change in over-privileged Western communities.

The metabolic effects on the liver cell of ingestion of excess amounts of alcohol are complex. It used to be believed that fatty change occurred as a consequence of malnutrition, especially with respect to protein intake, but this is now deemed unlikely. The substitution of large amounts of alcohol for part of the diet in healthy non-alcoholic volunteers produces fatty change in liver very rapidly; similar results have been obtained in baboons given large amounts of alcohol while being kept on an adequate diet. **Interference with oxidation of fatty acids is likely to be the most important cause of intracellular triglyceride accumulation in alcoholics, but there may also be an associated hyperlipidaemia (Frederickson type V) characterized by a rise in plasma triglyceride concentrations.**

4) **Other chemical and bacterial toxins.** Many chemicals are capable of inducing hepatic fatty change both in humans and experimental animals. These include CCl_4, puromycin, ethionine and phosphorus, to name only a few. The fact that CCl_4 can damage liver cells through the generation of free radicals has been mentioned earlier. There is some evidence that the metabolic events associated with this, which lead to the death of liver cells, are different from those that result in the accumulation of fat within the liver cell. CCl_4 reduces the secretion of protein by the liver cell, and the suggestion has therefore been made that the fat accumulates because of lack of secretion of adequate amounts of lipid-acceptor protein. However, work with other models such as **orotic acid** poisoning has shown that inhibition of protein secretion is not a prerequisite for intracellular fat accumulation and that the fault may be, at least in the early stages, a **failure of coupling** between triglyceride and lipid-acceptor protein.

The **decline in protein synthesis** that appears to be associated with some examples of both toxic and non-toxic hepatic fatty change may be brought about in a number of ways. For example, **puromycin**, an anti-biotic with a structure resembling the terminal portion of transfer RNA, is a powerful inhibitor of protein synthesis in the rat. Inhibition is accomplished by a decrease in the rate of **transcription** of ribosomal RNA, this being associated with a later effect on RNA maturation.

Ethionine, on the other hand, decreases protein secretion by acting as a drain on hepatic ATP. This is because ethionine, which is the ethyl analogue of the amino acid methionine, competes successfully with the latter for ATP and combines with the ATP to form S-adenosyl-ethionine plus inorganic orthophosphate. S-adenosyl-ethionine is inactive with respect to the transfer of methyl groups and simply acts as an adenosyl trap. Hepatic ATP is thus drained and there is a consequent reduction in messenger RNA synthesis, a break-up of polyribosomes and a decline in protein synthesis.

CHAPTER 3

Cell and Tissue Death

If changes in the environment are such that cells cannot achieve a new steady state, these cells die: the energy-dependent, organized interactions between DNA templates, membranes and enzyme systems break down and all cellular functions cease. Cell death occurs regularly under physiological as well as pathological conditions; for example, there is a high turnover of epithelial cells in the skin and small intestine. In many **diseases**, cell death is responsible for producing the symptoms and signs characteristic of that disease and the extent of such cell death may well determine the outcome.

The character of a given disease is often determined by the **type** of cell that dies. For example, in poliomyelitis the anterior horn cells of the spinal cord are the prime targets for destruction by the poliovirus. The patient thus develops a lower motor neurone type of paralysis in muscles whose motor nerve supply is related to the affected neurones. Many such examples could be given.

The **extent** of cell death has a significant effect on the natural history of certain pathological states. This is well shown in **myocardial infarction**. If the amount of cardiac muscle that undergoes irreversible damage is great (more than 35%), failure of the pumping function of the heart is likely to ensue and there may be a sudden and severe fall in cardiac output. It may not be possible to compensate for this by using inotropic drugs, and a balloon pump may need to be inserted into the patient's ascending aorta for output to be restored to near normal.

MORPHOLOGICAL CHANGES IN CELL DEATH

Cell death may be defined, in physiological terms, as the **irreversible breakdown of the energy-dependent functions of the cell**. For the histopathologist, cell death means the series of **morphological changes** that occur in relation to a cell or group of cells following lethal injury. The differences between functional cell death and cell death as morphologically defined are the expression of:

- elapsed **time** since the injury
- the unfettered action of **enzymatic degradation** and/or **protein denaturation**

Thus the cells of a piece of tissue removed at operation or biopsy and placed immediately in fixative are dead but show no morphological abnormalities indicative of cell death.

The morphological features seen in dead cells vary depending on which of the two processes – enzymatic digestion or protein denaturation – is dominant. Some degree of enzymatic degradation is nearly always present, and is manifested by various nuclear and cytoplasmic changes.

AUTOLYSIS

If enzymatic degradation is the dominant element, then dead cells are likely to be removed completely. This process may be accomplished by the activation of **enzymes that are normally present within the affected cell**. The process of **self-digestion** is known as **autolysis**.

Microscopic Features

Cytoplasmic Changes

The cytoplasm shows a decreased basophilia (indicating a loss of RNA and protein) and an increased affinity for acid dyes such as eosin. This increased eosinophilia is due to denaturation of some of the cytoplasmic proteins with exposure of basic groups that bind the eosin.

Loss of glycogen is noted when appropriate special stains such as the periodic acid–Schiff method are used; there may be some fragmentation and clumping of cytoplasmic contents.

Nuclear Changes

Irreversible damage to the nucleus shows itself in one of three patterns:

1) **Pyknosis.** The nucleus shrinks and becomes intensely basophilic. This stage is often followed by karyorrhexis.
2) **Karyorrhexis.** Here the nucleus undergoes fragmentation and the debris is either phagocytosed by other cells or just disappears.
3) **Karyolysis.** There is a gradual fading away of the basophilic nuclear material, presumably as a result of the activity of DNases.

The immediate result of these changes (as seen in a section stained with haematoxylin and eosin) is a highly eosinophilic cell that has lost its nucleus. Its survival in this form depends on whether further enzymatic digestion takes place (*Fig. 3.1*).

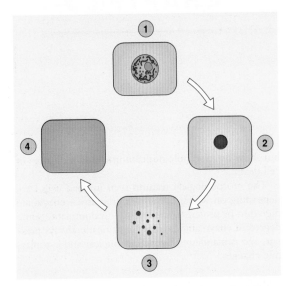

FIGURE 3.1 The progressive changes in nucleus and cytoplasm that accompany cell death. (1) Normal cells. Note relatively open chromatin network in the nucleus and slightly bluish tinge of cytoplasm which indicates ongoing protein synthesis. (2) The nucleus becomes contracted and stains intensely. This is known as pyknosis. The cytoplasm is pinker, showing that it binds eosin more avidly. (3) The nucleus breaks up, showing up as a more or less central area of dispersed chromatin (karyorrhexis). (4) All nuclear material has now disappeared (karyolysis) and the cytoplasm stains an intense red colour.

The enzymes are derived largely from lysosomes. The precise sequence of events leading to the activation and release of lysosomal enzymes is not known, but it is likely that a decrease in intracellular pH is an important factor. Release of lysosomal enzymes in cell death can be inferred from the following:

- Ultracentrifugal fractionation of dead cells shows that lysosomal enzymes are no longer particle-bound but present in the supernatant.
- There is evidence of enzymatic digestion of cell components in the form of loss of both DNA and RNA protein and glycogen.

HETEROLYSIS

If enzymatic digestion is accomplished by enzymes derived from cells other than dead or dying ones, the process is termed **heterolysis**. Here the enzymes are derived from the lysosomes of cells such as neutrophil polymorphonuclear leucocytes or mononuclear phago-cytes (macrophages). Heterolysis may occur as a result of **endocytosis**, in which phagocytes ingest portions of dead or dying cells and segregate them into phagocytic vacuoles (**phagosomes**). The lysosomes of the phago-cyte then fuse with the phagosomes to form secondary lysosomes in which enzymatic digestion of all or part of the ingested cell debris takes place. However, phagocy-tosis is not an absolute prerequisite for heterolysis,

which can take place as a result of the local release of lysosomal enzymes by phagocytes.

APOPTOSIS (PROGRAMMED CELL DEATH)

Normal **cell turnover** implies that all the fully differen-tiated cells populating a given tissue must die and be replaced in a controlled and 'programmed' manner. The term **apoptosis** (literally a 'dropping off', as in relation to petals and leaves) has been suggested for this controlled type of cell deletion which appears to play a role opposing that of mitosis in regulating the size of animal cell populations.

Apoptosis Differs from Necrosis

This form of cell death differs from necrosis in both negative and positive aspects. In contrast with necrosis there is *no*:

- breakdown in the mechanisms supplying cellular energy
- failure in the maintenance of normal cell volume
- rupture of plasma membranes
- acute inflammatory reaction elicited by the death

Microscopic Features

Morphological Changes in Apoptosis (Fig.3.2)

In structural terms apoptosis appears to take place in clearly defined stages:

- The affected cell separates from its neighbours.
- Characteristically the nuclear chromatin becomes condensed, and well-defined masses of chromatin form under the nuclear membrane.
- The cell then breaks up into a number of membrane-bound, ultrastructurally well-preserved, fragments (apoptotic bodies).
- These fragments are then either shed from epithelium-lined surfaces or are phagocytosed by other cells, where they undergo a series of changes resembling *in vitro* autolysis within phagosomes. This phagocytosis must involve a ligand–receptor interaction between the apoptotic bodies and the cells that engulf them; this is discussed (see pp 31–32) in the section on effector mechanisms.

In conventional histological sections, apoptosis is usually inconspicuous. This is because of the speedy nature of the changes and thus the short duration of the process as it affects a single cell (1–2 hours or less). Accurate assess-ment of the extent of apoptosis in tissue sections requires several thousand normal cells to be inspected as the pro-portion of recognizable apoptotic cells is less than 1%. Because the duration of time in which these cells can be recognized is so short, even a small proportion of apop-totic cells may be responsible for major reductions in the cell population of a given tissue.

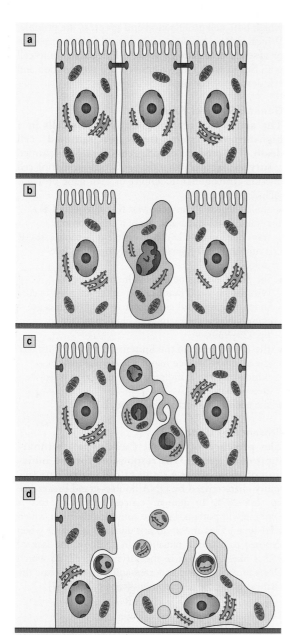

FIGURE 3.2 *Programmed cell death (apoptosis).* **a** *Normal.* **b** *The middle cell shrinks away from its neighbours. The nuclear chromatin is condensed along the nuclear membrane forming well-defined masses. The organelles, however, show no evidence of damage.* **c** *The affected cell now breaks up into several membrane-bound, ultrastructurally well-preserved, fragments (apoptotic bodies).* **d** *These are then engulfed either by neighbouring parenchymal cell or macrophages. Some apoptotic bodies are shed from epithelial surfaces in large numbers (e.g. in the small gut lining).*

The process is:
- energy dependent
- involves protein synthesis

Apoptosis is Involved in Both Physiological and Pathological Processes Affecting the Control of Cell Populations

Apoptosis appears to be involved not only in the turnover of cells in many healthy adult tissues but also in the focal elimination of certain cells during normal embryonic development. It occurs spontaneously in some untreated malignant neoplasms and also in some types of therapeutically induced regression of malignant tumours. It is implicated in both physiological involution and atrophy of various tissues and organs, some of which are listed below:

- **Organogenesis during embryonic life** (e.g. in the separation of digits during limb development).
- **Elimination of effete cells in cell populations with a high turnover**, such as the epithelial cells of the small gut.
- **Cell death following the removal of hormonal stimuli** (e.g. in the endometrial shedding phase of the menstrual cycle).
- **Clonal elimination of lymphocytes that might otherwise react with 'self' antigens**, and thus lead to autoimmune-mediated tissue damage.
- **Atrophy of hormone-dependent tissues** after removal of the stimulating hormone (e.g. the prostate after orchidectomy).
- **Atrophy of the secretory epithelial component** in exocrine glands after **prolonged duct obstruction** (e.g. the salivary and lacrimal glands and pancreas).
- **Spontaneous elimination of part of the cell population in certain tumours.**
- **Viral damage to cells.** This is seen in certain types of viral hepatitis.
- **Cytotoxic T lymphocyte-mediated cell death**, as in graft rejection.
- **Preventing genome instability** from developing in cells in which there has been a perturbation of the cell cycle.
- **Cell death associated with low doses of certain injurious stimuli** including therapeutic irradiation, cytotoxic drugs used to treat cancer, and heat.

Effector Mechanisms in Apoptosis

Some of the effector mechanisms may include the following and correlate with morphological and biochemical features:

- **Chromatin condensation is associated with chromatin cleavage**, first to fragments corresponding to the loop and rosette domains in which the chromatin is organized. Later these fragments are further broken down to mononucleosome and oligonucleosome size. This process is mirrored by the appearances seen when DNA from apoptotic cells is electrophoresed. Such DNA shows a characteristic 'laddered' pattern on electrophoresis, whereas that of necrotic cells is seen as an unstructured 'smear'. These features suggest that the **DNA is broken down by endonucleases**; indeed, some endonucleases have been identified in apoptotic cells. In addition, such cells contain a site-specific ribonuclease that cleaves RNA.

- Apoptotic bodies contain proteins that are insoluble in ionic detergents. **These proteins result from cross-linking brought about by a transglutaminase.**
- **Apoptosis may be blocked in several cell types by protease inhibitors.** Specific proteases are necessary for cell death to be brought about by cytotoxic T cells. The same is true in relation to the programmed cell death occurring in the hermaphrodite worm *Coenorhabditis elegans*, in which 131 of the 1090 cells undergo apoptosis. In *C. elegans* two gene products are necessary for apoptosis to occur, one of which (the product of *ced-3*) is a cysteine protease.
- **Engulfment of apoptotic bodies results from ligand–receptor interactions.** When macrophages engulf apoptotic neutrophils, two receptors on the macrophage surface become occupied. These are the vitronectin receptor (an integrin; see pp 43–44) and CD36 a thrombospondin receptor. These receptors bind thrombospondin which, in turn, acts as an intercellular bridge between the macrophage and the apoptotic body.

Genetic Regulation of Apoptosis

Because apoptosis involves protein synthesis, it is likely that the process is regulated, both positively and negatively, by the products of a number of genes. This hypothesis finds support from studies with *C. elegans* which contains:

- two genes that appear to **promote cell death** (*ced-3* and *ced-4*)
- one gene that **protects** the worm cells against apoptosis (*ced-9*).

The gene product of *ced-3* shows significant resemblances with the mammalian protein interleukin 1β-converting enzyme (ICE), while that of *ced-9* is similar to the product of the mammalian proto-oncogene *bcl-2* (see pp 273–282) with which it also shares functional similarities. Understanding of this subject is far from complete, but certain generalizations can be made.

Proto-oncogene Expression

Cells are rendered susceptible to apoptosis by expression of the proto-oncogene c-*myc*. Interestingly, c-*myc* encodes an essential part of the proliferative machinery of a cell and deregulation of this gene's expression is implicated in most neoplasms.

Myc-induced apoptosis occurs only in cells that have been deprived of growth-promoting factors or whose growth has been arrested with cytostatic drugs.

It has been suggested that c-*myc* induces a state in which both cell proliferation and apoptosis are possible. Which of these predominates depends on the presence or absence of additional factors. Indeed, in some cell populations with a high turnover, cell proliferation and cell death may coexist.

Genetic Survival Factors

The activity of certain genes protects cells in a high-turnover state from programmed cell death. The products of such genes should be regarded as **survival factors** rather than as factors promoting cell division (**mitogens**). Examples of such gene products include those of:

- the *bcl-2* gene. This gene was first discovered as a result of molecular analysis of a chromosome translocation (14 : 18) that is present in most cases of a human B cell follicle-centre lymphoma (see p 963).
- the proto-oncogene c-*abl*, which produces a tyrosine kinase. Translocation of the *abl* gene occurs in chronic myeloid leukaemia and in certain acute lymphoblastic leukaemias of childhood (see pp 929–930).
- the *LMP-1* gene of the Epstein–Barr virus. This has the ability to induce neoplastic transformation, which may result indirectly via induction of *bcl-2* (see p 963).
- the adenovirus early region gene E1b.

Presence of Gene p53

The presence of normal ('wild-type') tumour-suppressor gene *p53* is responsible for the initiation of apoptosis as a result of cell injury, especially injury characterized by DNA double-strand breaks (see pp 284–287). In human cancer treatment, this is extremely important, because tumour cells from which wild-type *p53* is absent do not undergo apoptosis when exposed to ionizing radiation. In addition, the lack of *p53* is likely to result in the survival of cells in which DNA mutations have occurred and thus to increase the chances of cancer development (see pp 284–287).

NECROSIS

Necrosis is the term commonly applied when cell death occurs in part of an organ or tissue and where continuity with neighbouring viable tissue is preserved. Various morphological forms exist. The differences between them, in some instances, mirror the dominance of one of the processes described above.

The morphological type may, as in the case of **caseation necrosis**, provide a clue to the cause of tissue injury.

COAGULATIVE NECROSIS

In coagulative necrosis, **denaturation of intracytoplasmic protein is the dominant process**. The dead tissue becomes firm and slightly swollen. The protein molecules within the cytoplasm become unfolded and this renders the tissue both more opaque than normal and more reactive with certain dyes such as eosin (*Fig. 3.3*). Microscopically, the cells show the signs of nuclear death described above, but the most noteworthy feature is the **retention of the general architectural pattern of the tissue**, despite the death of its constituent elements.

Coagulative necrosis occurs typically in ischaemic injury, such as may occur in the heart or kidney. However, for reasons that are not clear, ischaemic injury in the central nervous system leads to necrosis dominated by enzymatic digestion and liquefaction of the dead tissue.

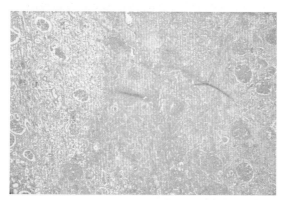

FIGURE 3.3 *This haematoxylin and eosin-stained section shows an infarct in the kidney. On the left, the renal tissue appears normal. On the right, the tissue appears acellular and stains homogeneously with the red eosin. Careful examination, however, shows the ghost outlines of glomeruli and some tubules.*

Caseation Necrosis

Caseation necrosis occurs characteristically in **tuberculosis**. It is a form of coagulative necrosis, in that no liquefaction has occurred. On microscopic examination the affected tissue appears completely **structureless** and exhibits a greater than usual affinity for dyes such as eosin. Caseation necrosis owes its somewhat unfortunate name (**caseous = cheese-like**) to its macroscopic appearance, large areas of caseous necrosis bearing some resemblance to white crumbly goat's cheese. On chemical analysis, large amounts of lipid are found to be present in these necrotic areas in addition to the coagulated protein.

LIQUEFACTION (OR COLLIQUATIVE) NECROSIS

In liquefaction necrosis the dominant factor is the effect of hydrolytic lysosomal enzymes. The end-result is a local accumulation of protein-rich, semi-fluid material. It is not particularly common as a primary event except, as mentioned above, in the brain. However, if necrotic tissue becomes secondarily infected by pus-forming organisms, liquefaction commonly takes place.

TRAUMATIC FAT NECROSIS

This is almost exclusively seen in the female breast, especially if the breast is heavy and pendulous. Essentially it results from the rupture of adipocytes with release of their contents. The released fat undergoes lipolysis and is converted to fatty acids and glycerol. Clinically the lesion appears as a hard lump in the breast, and may give the impression that a malignant neoplasm is present. On slicing the excised specimen a small central cystic area may be seen in which some oily droplets are present. At the periphery the adipose tissue is much firmer and also more opaque than usual.

Histological examination of the conventionally prepared material shows numerous granular macrophages containing phagocytosed lipid. Fatty acid crystals are also often present and these excite a foreign-body giant cell reaction (multinucleate cells formed as a result of the fusion of macrophages).

ENZYME-MEDIATED FAT NECROSIS

Another type of fat necrosis is seen in the peritoneal cavity as a consequence of **acute haemorrhagic pancreatitis**. In pancreatitis the enzymes secreted by the exocrine pancreas are released from the acini and ducts, and thus reach the interstitial tissues. The proteolytic and lipolytic enzymes damage cell membranes and convert the intracellular triglyceride into glycerol and fatty acids. These combine with calcium in the interstitial fluid to form **soaps**, which appear as small, intensely white and opaque patches on the adipose tissue of the pancreas, omentum and other areas of the peritoneum.

GANGRENE

Strictly speaking the term **gangrene** should be limited to necrosis of tissues associated with a superadded infection by putrefactive microorganisms. The responsible organisms include:

- *Clostridia* species (anaerobic, Gram-positive, spore-forming bacilli) derived from the gut or soil
- anaerobic streptococci
- members of the family Bacteroidaceae

Clinically, the term gangrene is often used to describe any black foul-smelling area that is in continuity with living tissues (*Fig. 3.4*). This state of affairs can be brought about primarily via the actions of bacterial toxins, or secondarily through a combination of ischaemia and superadded infection. True gangrene may occur, for example, in the gastrointestinal tract. This is most commonly due to the blood supply being cut off, which can lead to extensive necrosis. The presence of a resident population of potentially putrefactive organisms provides an ideal source for superadded infection.

Another example of true gangrene is so-called **gas gangrene**. This is a rapidly spreading form of tissue

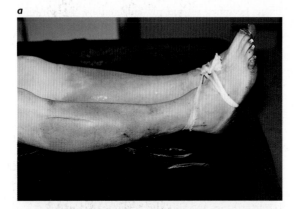

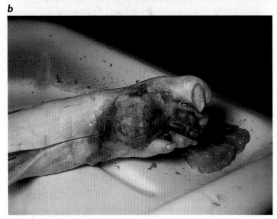

FIGURE 3.4 **a** *Lower limb ischaemia. The presence of ischaemia is shown by the well-demarcated bluish discolouration seen in both lower limbs.* **b** *Gangrene. Continuing severe ischaemia will lead ultimately to gangrene, evidenced in this photograph by black discolouration of the second toe and the dorsum of the foot.*

necrosis, often involving muscle, resulting from infection by saccharolytic and proteolytic *Clostridia*. These organisms make a wide range of toxins that are destructive to cell membranes and to the macromolecules of the interstitial ground substance. These toxins constitute the basis for the spreading that is so menacing a feature of gas gangrene. *Clostridia* infection of this type not infrequently complicates deep penetrating injuries sustained in battle. It may also occur as a rare complication of acute suppurative appendicitis, in strangulation of the gut, in the puerperium and in the stumps of mid-thigh amputations carried out for ischaemia of the lower limbs (see pp 218–221).

The presence of dead tissue as a result of injury, and the additional factor that the oxygen supply may be very poor, is a combination favouring the multiplication of these anaerobic organisms. The affected muscles and adjacent soft tissues are oedematous and often very painful. They may feel **crepitant** (crackly) on palpation because of the formation of gas bubbles (carbon dioxide) in the tissue as a result of fermentation of sugars by

bacterial toxins. The infection may remain localized or may become generalized (**septicaemia**). Evidence of such spread may be seen at post-mortem examination in the form of:

- bubbles in some of the solid viscera (most notably the liver) (*Fig. 3.5*)
- signs of haemolysis such as haemoglobin staining of the aortic intima

Gangrene brought about by ischaemia may occur, as already stated, in the gut and is also not uncommonly found in the lower limb. The background to this is usually severe atherosclerosis (see pp 327–347) of the large and medium-sized arteries of the limb. The stenosing lesions, which are composed partly of proliferated fibromuscular tissue and partly of lipid accumulations derived mainly from the plasma, then become complicated by superimposed thrombosis. Diabetic patients and cigarette smokers are particularly at risk. In younger patients ischaemic necrosis of the lower limbs may occur as a result of **thromboangiitis obliterans (Buerger's disease)**. In this condition an inflammatory process involves the whole vascular bundle (veins as well as arteries), leading to arterial occlusion.

If the limb is oedematous and a fairly thick layer of adipose tissue is present, the ischaemic necrosis may be associated with infection by putrefactive organisms. In this case the typical appearances of **wet gangrene**, with large blebs on the skin surface, occasionally accompanied by gas production, may be seen.

Where these do not occur, and where the arterial narrowing has progressed slowly over a long period, the appearances of so-called **dry gangrene** are seen. Starting at the most distal extremities the tissues become dessicated and black. The affected areas are very cold; there is no unpleasant smell and no bleb or gas formation. The black discolouration of the skin is due to staining by haemoglobin, which diffuses from the small vessels into the extravascular compartment. Not infrequently a line of demarcation forms at the junction between the living and dead tissues, and the latter may actually separate off (so-called **spontaneous amputation**).

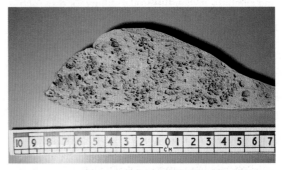

FIGURE 3.5 *Gas gangrene. The presence of many bubbles in this specimen of liver indicates clostridial septicaemia. The bubbles are due to the formation of carbon dioxide within the tissues.*

CHAPTER 4

Acute Inflammation I: Introduction

When living tissue is injured the surrounding areas undergo a series of changes resulting in **phagocytic cells and elements of circulating plasma entering the damaged area**. This process is **acute inflammation** and usually continues as long as the tissue injury persists.

Such reactions to injury are, in evolutionary terms, very ancient indeed and many of the processes now recognized as being involved in inflammation, such as chemotaxis and phagocytosis, are also present in simple unicellular and multicellular organisms. The acquisition of a complicated circulatory system has added very significantly to the complexities of the inflammatory response: it is the **changes** that occur in the **calibre** and **permeability** of arterioles, capillaries and venules (the **microcirculation**) that dictate the most prominent of the symptoms and signs of acute inflammation.

The acute inflammatory response is mediated via two pathways, one of which involves the microcirculation and the other, leucocytes. The process can be understood most readily if each of these pathways is viewed as a set of distinct operations (*Fig 4.1*). Thus the **changes** that occur in the microcirculation are:

- An **increase in the calibre** of arterioles, capillaries and venules. The inevitable result is an increase in the amount and speed of blood flow in the injured area, leading to **redness** and **heat**.
- An **increase in the permeability** of the affected blood vessels. This mediates the escape of larger amounts than normal of water and solutes and also of high molecular weight proteins such as fibrinogen, which normally do not form part of the extravascular interstitial fluid. This process, termed **exudation**, leads to **swelling** (inflammatory oedema).

The activities of phagocytic cells in inflammation are complex and involve several distinct steps, discussed in detail on pp 41–46, 57–59. They include:

- **Adhesion of neutrophils and monocytes to the endothelial cells** of microvessels in the affected area of tissue.
- **Migration of these leucocytes between endothelial cells** and through the basement membranes of microvessels to reach the extravascular fluid compartment.
- **Attachment to infecting microorganisms, or to dead or injured cells** and tissue elements.

- **Engulfment (phagocytosis) of the organisms, cell or tissue debris**, etc.
- **Killing of the phagocytosed organisms and digestion of cell or tissue debris.**
- **Effects on surrounding tissue of chemical mediators** secreted or otherwise released from phagocytes.

Is the Inflammatory Process Helpful or Harmful?

John Hunter, the famous London surgeon, stated in 1794 that 'inflammation in itself is not to be regarded as a disease but as a salutary operation consequent upon some violence or disease'. This is true, but not the whole truth. The overall biological significance of

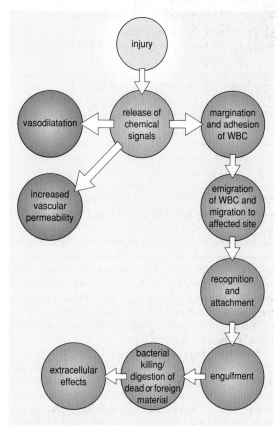

FIGURE 4.1 *Vascular and cellular pathways in acute inflammation. WBC, white blood cells.*

inflammation is, indeed, that of a defence mechanism, but it is equally true that some inflammatory reactions can have crippling or life-threatening consequences, for example the filling up of airspaces in the lung and the resulting blockage of gas exchange that occurs in various types of pneumonia.

CAUSES OF ACUTE INFLAMMATION

In general terms, any process that injures cells may cause an inflammatory reaction. Because acute inflammation associated with tissue invasion by pathogenic microorganisms such as bacteria or viruses is so common, there is a temptation to regard inflammation as being **synonymous** with infection. This is certainly not true. The acute inflammatory reaction has many other causes, which include the following:

- **Mechanical trauma,** such as cutting or crushing.
- **Chemical injuries,** such as those produced by acids, alkalis and phenols. An important cause of chemical injury of tissues in clinical medicine is the presence of physiological substances in inappropriate locations. For example, gastric juice is harmless in the stomach, its natural milieu, but produces a striking inflammatory response in the peritoneal cavity after perforation of a peptic ulcer.
- **Ultraviolet or X-irradiation.**
- Injury due to **extremes of cold or heat** (burns and frostbite).
- Injury due to a **reduction in the arterial blood supply** sufficient to cause death of the underperfused tissue (**ischaemic necrosis**).
- **Injury caused by living organisms such as bacteria, viruses, parasites, worms and fungi.**
- Injury produced by the **inappropriate or excessive operation of immune mechanisms**.

CLINICAL CHARACTERISTICS OF ACUTE INFLAMMATION

Anyone who has suffered from a common boil can give an excellent account of the clinical features of an inflammatory reaction. The affected area is **hot, red, swollen** and **painful** (*Fig. 4.2*). These are the so-called **cardinal signs** of inflammation and were described by the Roman physician Celsus in the first century of the Christian era as **calor, rubor, tumor** and **dolor** respectively.

The translation of these clinical observations into pathophysiological terms had to wait for the microscopic studies of Julius Cohnheim, who wrote a key paper on acute inflammation in 1867. Cohnheim studied the changes produced by mild injury in living tissues rather than in fixed or embedded material. Naturally he needed the most translucent possible preparations, so chose thin membranes such as the frog

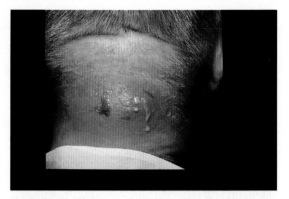

FIGURE 4.2 *Redness and swelling in acute inflammation exemplified by this patient with a carbuncle on the back of his neck.*

mesentery. Simply exposing the living mesentery on the stage of a microscope was sufficient to cause some irritation, and Cohnheim was able to see the rapid development of a series of changes in the small blood vessels. First the arterioles dilated and there was an obvious increase in and acceleration of blood flow in the whole vascular bed. Within a few minutes this accelerated blood flow slowed and large white blood cells began to line up along the walls of the venules, while the red cells flowed past. Then some of the white cells, which seemed to have become adherent to the venule wall, crawled through the blood vessel wall and thus reached the extravascular compartment. In some of the little blood vessels the blood flowed so much that columns of red cells appeared not to move at all; in these vessels the red cells were tightly packed together as if the plasma had been lost. Fifteen years later Cohnheim took up this last observation again, and suggested that the plasma had escaped from the affected vessels because of an **increase in the permeability of the vessel walls**. Cohnheim's powers of observation were so acute and his descriptions of the rapidly changing pattern of events were so beautiful that, despite the simplicity of the methods employed, they still stand as a model of scientific clarity and accuracy.

With the knowledge gained from these pioneering studies it is now possible to look at the cardinal signs of acute inflammation in the light of a series of events taking place in the microcirculation (*Fig. 4.3*).

REDNESS AND HEAT

The only logical explanation of these features is **persistent dilatation of small vessels and an increased blood flow in the affected area**. This involves increased filling of capillaries and venules, only part of the capillary network in any tissue being filled with circulating blood at any one time. As capillaries have no smooth muscle cells in their wall, they constitute a passive set of channels whose blood content depends largely on flow in feeding arterioles. **Thus the redness**

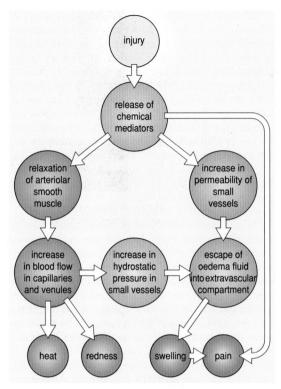

FIGURE 4.3 *Vascular events that underlie the cardinal signs of inflammation.*

and heat that are so striking a feature of acute inflammation must depend on an increase in the calibre of the arterioles feeding the injured area and this, in turn, must represent the result of **arteriolar smooth muscle relaxation**.

The tone of arterioles, acting as precapillary sphincters, is controlled in two ways:

1) Under normal circumstances the circular smooth muscle coat of the arteriole is under the control of the autonomic nervous system, in particular the sympathetic vasoconstrictor nerves. These nerves are largely responsible for controlling the blood pressure, cardiac output and distribution of blood flow among the different organs and tissues. Blushing in response to some embarrassing circumstance constitutes an easily observed example of this control system in operation.

2) However, the arteriolar smooth muscle cells also react to local chemical mediators, and the accumulation of such compounds at and around the site of injury is believed to play a dominant role in the arteriolar dilatation of acute inflammation. Support for this view comes from the fact that acute inflammation in tissue that has long been denervated shows no essential differences from the process in areas with normal innervation.

SWELLING

In simple terms the **presence of local tissue swelling must mean that something has been added to the bulk of the formed tissue elements or to the gel-like ground substance in that area**. Chemical analysis of such a swollen area shows that this increase in bulk is due to the local **accumulation of excess interstitial fluid**, which contains solutes and proteins derived from the plasma. This accumulation of fluid in the extravascular compartment is called **oedema** (*Fig. 4.4*).

In inflammatory oedema the fact that there has been a net transfer from the intravascular to the extravascular compartment can be shown by injecting a small amount of the dye 'Evans' blue' intravenously into a small animal. If, for example, a mild thermal injury is produced at some site, the skin at the site of injury shows blue staining. Because Evans' blue circulates in the plasma bound to albumin, this result indicates that albumin has passed from the small vessels into the extravascular compartment.

Exudation of Protein-rich Fluid in Inflammation

Inflammatory exudation is synonymous with the escape from small vessels of high molecular weight proteins. To understand this, we need to have some knowledge of normal routes of transport across endothelial barriers and the forces that determine the rates of such transport.

Endothelium of all types is permeable to a wide range of molecules. Most of the available data suggests the existence, in a functional sense, of a 'two-pore' system.

• The large-pore component appears to have a diameter of about 50 nm. Using the appropriate ultrastructural racers, the structural equivalent of the

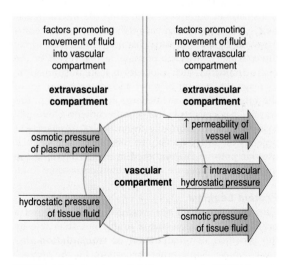

FIGURE 4.4 *Factors promoting the movement of fluid into and out of the microvascular compartment.*

large-pore system has been shown to be the plasmalemmal vesicles that are present in large numbers in endothelial cells and are concentrated along the luminal and abluminal membranes. Once these vesicles, which have a diameter of about 70 nm, have incorporated a large molecule by pinocytosis, they bud off from the luminal plasma membrane and travel across the endothelial cytoplasm towards the abluminal aspect of the cell. Here they fuse with the abluminal plasma membrane and discharge their contents.

- The structural equivalent of the 'small-pore' system is more equivocal, but the available evidence suggests that it may correspond to the junctions between adjacent endothelial cells, and has a diameter of 9 nm.

The mechanisms underlying the escape from the microcirculation of water and solutes on the one hand and plasma proteins on the other may well be different and merit separate consideration.

Ultrafiltration

Transport of water and solute across the endothelial cell barrier shows many of the features of ultrafiltration, in which the movement of fluid and electrolytes is controlled largely by physical forces. **There are two sets of such forces, which act in opposition to each other:**

1) Hydrostatic forces within the microcirculation tend to push fluid out into the extravascular tissue proteins and mucopolysaccharides.

2) The intravascular osmotic pressure exerted by the plasma proteins. The hydrostatic pressure of the extravascular tissues combines with plasma osmotic forces to push fluid back into the vessels.

Normally the resultant of these opposing sets of forces is a small net outflow of fluid from the microcirculation, which then drains from the extravascular compartment via the lymphatic channels. An increase in the intravascular hydrostatic pressure in the vessels of the microcirculation, such as occurs in acute inflammation, increases the amount of water and solute driven out of the vessels, although the oedema fluid produced in this way still has a relatively low protein content. Obviously **loss of protein** from the intravascular compartment potentiates this process, because the intravascular osmotic pressure falls and there is a corresponding rise in the osmotic pressure of the extravascular tissue fluid.

Protein Leakage

Chemical analysis of the exudate invariably shows a protein concentration that is simply not attainable by the processes of ultrafiltration or **transudation** discussed above. Some other mechanism for the appearance of relatively large amounts of plasma-derived protein must therefore exist.

That very large molecules escape from the microcirculation in the course of the formation of inflammatory oedema can be shown very elegantly in small animals by the technique of vascular labelling. This serves the additional purpose of identifying vessels in the injured area from which leakage has occurred. A few drops of indian ink are injected intravenously into a small animal such as a rat. Except in the liver and spleen where the endothelium is normally 'leaky', the tissues do not blacken and the vessels of the microcirculation are not outlined by the ink particles, which instead are taken up by phagocytic cells in the sinusoids of the liver and spleen. However, if a mild thermal injury is produced *after* the injection of the ink, some of the vessels in the injured area become outlined by the ink particles.

On microscopic examination, these particles can be seen to have crossed the endothelial cells and to be lying piled up against the basement membrane, which they do not cross. Careful examination shows that the vessels labelled in this way are small venules measuring up to about 80 or 100 μm in diameter; capillaries, larger venules and arterioles are not labelled when the injury has been mild. Identical appearances can be produced by an intradermal injection of small doses of histamine, 5−hydroxytryptamine or bradykinin. Therefore, it is not without interest that a sting from a nettle (which contains histamine) invariably produces local swelling.

It is not clear on light microscopy what cellular events underlie the passage of such large molecules as indian ink or ferritin across the normal endothelium. This question was answered by the electron microscopic studies of Guido Majno, who showed that, when small doses of histamine or other vasoactive substances were injected into the cremaster muscle of rats, the endothelial cells in venules contracted, creating gaps through which the particles of indian ink could pass. In due time the endothelial cells presumably relax and the gaps disappear, as carbon particles can be found lying deep to apparently intact interendothelial junctions. It is not too surprising that such contractile shortening of the endothelial cells should take place, as a combination of ultrastructural and immunocytochemical studies has shown that these versatile cells contain contractile filaments.

It should be emphasized that the change in microvascular permeability described above is what is seen when the injury is **mild**. In reality the alterations in vascular permeability following injury are more varied, both in nature and timing. The major factor affecting these changes appears to be the **degree of severity of the injury, which is reflected in the magnitude of the functional and structural change in the endothelial cells** (*Fig. 4.5*).

Patterns of Increased Vascular Permeability

Most of the data relating to this come from studies carried out in small animals, where the experimental conditions, in particular the type and severity of injury, are

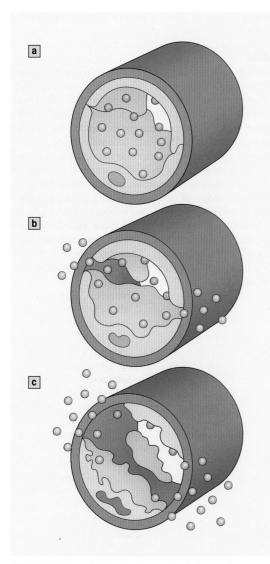

FIGURE 4.5 *Endothelial cell damage in relation to the escape of large molecules from the microvasculature.* **a** *Normal vessel.* **b** *If injury is mild, the endothelial cells contract and create gaps through which particles can pass.* **c** *In severe injury, the endothelial cells may be damaged or even killed, and the amount and duration of the escape of large molecules from the vascular compartment is greatly increased.*

clearly defined. It is likely that in human inflammatory disease the processes are much more complex. The patterns of increased vascular permeability following injury are characterized in terms of two variables:

- **The time between infliction of the injury and recordable changes in microvascular permeability.**
- **The duration of the change in vascular permeability.**

On this basis, then, three patterns can be observed: the immediate transient response, the delayed persistent response and the immediate persistent response.

Immediate Transient Response As its name implies, this response follows almost immediately on mild injury. The alteration in vascular permeability reaches a peak within 5 minutes or so and returns to normal within 15 minutes. Carbon labelling shows that the **escape of fluid is confined to small venules**. The development of leaky venules extends more widely than the immediate area of injury, suggesting that a chemical mediator is involved. Because the increase in vascular permeability can be blocked by predosing animals with antihistamine compounds, it is reasonable to suppose that this chemical mediator is histamine. **The short duration of the change strongly suggests that the increase in venule permeability is brought about by endothelial cell contraction** and that the endothelial cells are not seriously damaged.

Delayed Persistent Response This **response** takes longer to develop. In some instances the peak effect occurs about 4 hours after injury, while in others there may be an interval of up to 24 hours before the increased vascular permeability becomes maximal. Increased permeability of this type is not blocked by the prior administration of antihistamines. In cases where the peak effect is noted after 4 hours, labelling with carbon shows that **fluid and macromolecules escape from the capillaries**. When the reaction peaks later (e.g. 24 hours after injury), **both venules and capillaries are labelled**. Some of the affected capillaries contain small aggregates of platelets, and damaged and broken endothelial cells are also seen. While interendothelial cell gaps are found in affected venules, it is believed that these result from direct endothelial injury rather than from the operation of a chemical mediator such as histamine. A good example of the delayed type of response is to be found in **sunburn, which is mediated by ultraviolet radiation**. Exposure to sunlight on the first day of the holidays, while enjoyable, may be followed some hours after exposure has ceased by the onset of an uncomfortable inflammatory reaction.

Immediate Persistent Response The **immediate persistent response** is associated, in experimental situations, with the application of relatively powerful agents. The affected vessels begin to leak within a few minutes and permeability becomes maximal 15–60 minutes after injury. Labelling studies show that **small vessels of all types leak**, and electron microscopy reveals **severe damage to endothelial cells** and pericytes, with sloughing away of the former from their basement membranes. Until the endothelial cells have been replaced by ingrowth of new cells, derived from the uninjured part of the vessel lining, along the basement membrane, exudation will continue. It may therefore last for many days and be of impressive proportions. This type of response is seen in patients who have been badly burned or where severe mechanical trauma has been applied.

Blood Flow Patterns

Understanding how the fluid exudate forms in acute inflammation leads naturally to an understanding of why the flow of blood slows in some parts of the microcirculation in injured areas. This change in flow is associated with packing and sludging of red cells. Loss of water from the leaking venules and capillaries leads to an increase in the concentration of blood cells in these vessels. Although plasma proteins also escape from the vessels, loss of fluid may be so great as to increase the plasma protein concentration within these vessels; this will add further to the tendency for an increase in blood viscosity. Rouleaux formation by the red cells is enhanced, and the tendency of white cells to adhere to the endothelial surface of the postcapillary venules and to each other may also impair flow through the injured vessels.

PAIN

This is less well understood than the other cardinal clinical features of the acute inflammatory reaction and, indeed, may not always be present. Clearly the **local increase in tissue turgor** is one of the factors involved, and the denser the tissue affected, the greater the degree of pain. Palpating or squeezing an acutely inflamed area will either increase existing pain or produce pain where none existed; it seems reasonable to ascribe this also to an increase in local tissue pressure. However, some of the endogenous chemical compounds believed to be released in the course of genesis of the acute inflammatory reaction are capable of causing pain in their own right when injected subcutaneously or intradermally. Therefore, these may also contribute to the pain experienced in many inflammatory reactions.

CHAPTER **5**

Acute Inflammation II: Cellular Events and Chemical Mediators

In evolutionary terms, one of the first defences to develop against the presence of 'foreign' material, whether living or dead, was **phagocytosis** or **engulfment** by specialized cells. The migration of phagocytic cells to a site of injury remains one of the most fundamental components of the host's response. It is vital for a successful defence against invaders, especially when the injurious agent is a living microorganism. **The central role of the phagocytic cell is demonstrated by the increased susceptibility to infection shown by persons who have insufficient phagocytic cells or whose cells cannot seek out, engulf or destroy pathogenic microorganisms.**

Cell Population of the Inflammatory Exudate (*Fig.5.1*)

THE NEUTROPHIL

In the early stages of the inflammatory process most of the cells migrating to the injured area are **neutrophils**, although a small number of eosinophils and basophils may also be present. Neutrophils:

- are present in relatively large numbers in the blood
- can be replaced rapidly from precursors in the bone marrow
- move more quickly than other leucocytes.

The number of neutrophils present at sites of tissue damage depends on the severity of such damage and the nature of the injury. Physical injury rarely evokes a significant neutrophil response, whereas infection by certain organisms such as *Escherichia coli* or staphylococci elicits a striking response.

Neutrophils make up 40–75% of circulating white cells. They have a diameter of about 15 μm, characteristically segmented nuclei and granular cytoplasm. Two types of granule are present in the cytoplasm:

1) Larger granules that stain more densely with Romanowsky-type dyes and contain lysozyme (which accounts for about one-third of their content), lysosomal enzymes, peroxidase and certain cationic proteins, the last of which may be important signals for the recruitment of further neutrophils.

2) Smaller granules, which are also lysosomal in nature, also contain lysozyme (about two-thirds of their content), together with alkaline phosphatase and lactoferrin, an iron-binding protein, which inhibits the multiplication of bacteria.

The energy source of the neutrophil is glucose, which is normally stored as glycogen, and the cell can produce energy by glycolysis under anaerobic conditions, which is useful because oxygen tension may fall to a very low level in areas of tissue damage.

In general, the early peak of neutrophil migration to an inflammatory focus is followed some hours later by a further wave of cell migration, this time by mononuclear phagocytes (**macrophages**). This biphasic pattern of cell accumulation is found in most inflammatory reactions, but the precise timing may vary with the nature of the injury.

OPERATIONS BY THE NEUTROPHIL IN ACUTE INFLAMMATION

Adhesion of Neutrophils to Endothelium and their Subsequent Emigration

The mechanisms of emigration of neutrophils from the microcirculation are not completely understood. With the change in the dynamics of blood flow, the white cells, which are heavier than red cells, come to lie at the periphery of the column of flowing blood cells. Some **adhere** to the endothelium, a process known as '**margination**'. Adhesion of the leucocyte to the endothelium is clearly a pivotal step in emigration of the neutrophil from the microcirculation. The importance of adhesion is made plain by the existence of a rare inherited defect known as the **leucocyte adhesion deficiency syndrome**, in which adhesion of leucocytes to the microvascular endothelium cannot and does not occur. Patients suffering from this disorder have repeated episodes of life-threatening bacterial infection, because their neutrophils cannot emigrate from the vascular compartment.

Until recently the adhesion process was difficult to understand, because the **negative charges** associated with carboxyl groups of the sialic acid residues on the plasma membranes of the endothelial cells and the neutrophil might be expected to repel each other.

It is now known that there is a wide range of molecules that can cause cell–cell adherence as a result of a receptor–ligand interaction. Many of

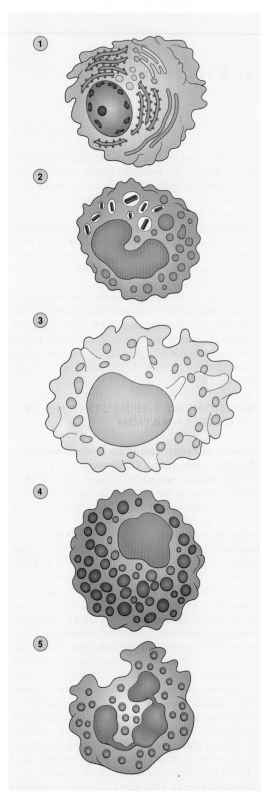

FIGURE 5.1   The cells involved in inflammation: (1) plasma cell; (2) eosinophil; (3) macrophage; (4) basophil; (5) neutrophil.

these have transmembrane domains and almost certainly mediate not only cell adhesion but transmembrane signalling as well. Some of these molecules are normally expressed on cell surfaces; others appear only after the cells that can produce them have been '**instructed**' to do so. Divalent cations, especially calcium and magnesium, appear also to play a part in adhesion; the pretreatment of experimental animals with chelating agents that remove these cations inhibits the margination and adhesion of white cells. It is also known that exposure of neutrophils to chemotactic factors decreases their negative surface charge and increases their adherence to endothelial cells. It has recently been suggested that exocytosis of lactoferrin from the specific granules of the neutrophil may also be a factor in neutrophil–endothelial adhesion, and there has been a case report in which neutrophils deficient in lactoferrin would not stick to endothelium when stimulated by chemotactic factors.

Adhesion Molecules on Endothelial Cells and Circulating Leucocytes

Adhesion molecules expressed on the **endothelial cell surface** are of two basic types (*Figs 5.2* and *5.3*):

1) **Selectins**, which derive their name from the resemblance of part of their structure to lectins. This is a series of proteins, widely distributed in nature, that bind with high affinity to sugars and that have a remarkable ability to distinguish between different sugars.

2) Members of the **immunoglobulin gene superfamily. This includes heavy and light chains of immunoglobulin, T-cell receptor α and β chains, major histocompatibility**

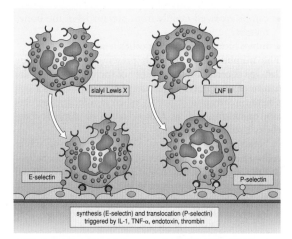

FIGURE 5.2   The 'rolling' phase of leucocyte adhesion to vascular endothelium, mediated by interaction between sugars on the leucocyte plasma membrane and selectins expressed on the surface membranes of endothelial cells.

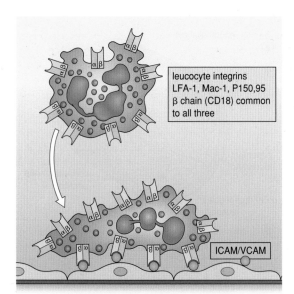

leucocyte integrins
LFA-1, Mac-1, P150,95
β chain (CD18) common
to all three

ICAM/VCAM

FIGURE 5.3 Flattening of leucocytes on the endothelium before emigration. Interaction occurs between β_2 integrins on the leucocyte surface and adhesion molecules of the immunoglobulin gene superfamily on the endothelium.

complex (MHC) class I and II peptides, β_2-microglobulin, CD4 and CD8 molecules on T lymphocytes, and certain adhesion molecules expressed on endothelium.

The Endothelial Selectins

The selectins are a family of glycoproteins that have certain structural features in common:

- an amino terminal lectin-like domain
- an epidermal growth factor-like domain
- many cysteine-rich tandem repeats similar to those seen in complement-regulating proteins
- a transmembrane region
- a short intracytoplasmic region

Selectins are *not* present on the surface of 'resting' endothelium but are expressed only after the endothelium has been stimulated by a number of chemical signals, including:

- bacterial endotoxin
- interleukin 1 (IL-1)
- phorbol esters
- thrombin
- tumour necrosis factor α (TNF-α)

Two endothelial selectins have so far been identified. These are:

1) **E-selectin, also known as endothelial leucocyte adhesion molecule 1 (ELAM-1).**

The ligand for E-selectin is believed to be a complex carbohydrate called **sialylLewisX**. This is present on the surface of the white cells (neutrophils and monocytes) that bind to E-selectin. The selectin itself starts to be expressed on the

endothelium within 30 minutes of stimulation, reaches its peak concentration somewhere between 2 and 4 hours after stimulation and is expressed for about 24 hours.

2) **P-selectin**, originally cursed with the name **platelet activation-dependent granule to external membrane protein (PADGEM).** This molecule is also present within the α granules of platelets. In the endothelium, P-selectin is synthesized constitutively and is stored in the curious rod-shaped cytoplasmic organelles known as Weibel–Palade bodies, from which it is transported to the luminal membrane when endothelial cells are stimulated.

The ligand for P-selectin has been identified as a sugar called **lacto-*n*-fucopentaose III (LNF-III)** which contains the sialylLewisX structure within its core. P-selectin binds neutrophils and monocytes and is maximally expressed on the endothelial surface membrane within 10–30 minutes.

Adhesion of neutrophils and monocytes to the endothelial selectins appears to be important in the early stages of the inflammatory reaction and is responsible for the phenomenon of the **leucocytes rolling along the surface of the endothelium** in the affected area.

Immunoglobulin Gene Superfamily of Adhesion Molecules

These receptors have been given this name because each contains several domains that resemble the structure of immunoglobulin. Three such molecules have so far been identified and cloned. They are known as:

a) **vascular cell adhesion molecule 1 (VCAM-1)**
b) **intercellular cell adhesion molecule 1 (ICAM-1) (CD 54)**
c) **intercellular cell adhesion molecule 2 (ICAM-2)**

All three are glycoproteins and it is the two ICAM molecules that are thought to be especially involved in the acute inflammatory reaction. Both are expressed constitutively by endothelial cells but, in the case of ICAM-1, the level of expression is very low, being increased in the course of acute inflammation by stimulants such as **IL-1** or **TNF-α**. Induction of high levels of ICAM-1 expression on endothelium takes 4–6 hours and reaches its maximum by 24 hours, at which point it reaches a plateau. Leucocytes bind to the ICAMs with high affinity; they then flatten and spread over the endothelial surface before migrating between adjacent endothelial cells.

The ligands on the surface of the neutrophils and monocytes which bind to the adhesion molecules of the immunoglobulin gene superfamily belong to a group known as the **integrins**.

Integrins are a family of cell surface proteins that mediate the adhesion of cells to:

- **extracellular matrices** such as fibronectin and vitronectin
- **fibrillar proteins** such as collagen and laminin, both of which are present in basement membranes
- **endothelial cells** in the inflammatory process

All integrins have two subunits, termed α and β. Eleven α subunits and six β subunits have been described, and these, in different combinations, form at least 16 integrins. Many cells express integrins, **some of the latter being clearly cell type-specific**. These include the **gpIIb/IIIa** molecule, which is expressed **only by megakaryocytes and platelets and which mediates platelet aggregation**. Three others, **LFA-1, Mac-1** and **p150,95** are expressed only on leucocytes and it is these that adhere to the endothelial ICAMs in the course of acute inflammation. They are known as the β$_2$-integrins; all three have the same β chain (CD18), although their α subunits are different.

Emigration

Once the neutrophils have come to lie in close contact with the plasma membranes of the endothelial cells, they put out pseudopodia. These enter the gap between two adjacent endothelial cells and force it open. The neutrophils then move into the basement membrane substance, through which they soon pass (*Figs 5.4* and *5.5*). This whole process takes from 2–9 minutes.

For reasons that are not clear, leucocytes from newborn infants and myeloblasts from leukaemic patients are not able to attenuate their cytoplasm sufficiently to squeeze through the interendothelial cell gaps. The chemoattractants responsible for this movement are believed to belong to a family of low molecular weight proteins known as the C-X-C chemokines (see pp 51, 54), of which IL-8 is probably the most important in this context.

Emigration Involves Movement

How Do Leucocytes Move Out of Microvessels and Through the Tissues Towards Sites of Injury or Infection? **The mechanisms responsible for leucocyte movement are also responsible for phagocytosis and for movement of the leucocyte's intracellular granules. They involve both the plasma membrane and the cytoplasm.**

Neutrophils move by crawling forward; this is accomplished by the protrusion of clear pseudopodia from the aspect of the neutrophil facing the direction of travel. The pseudopodia become transiently attached to their underlying substrate and, during this phase, the rest of the cell body is pulled forwards.

The movement of macrophages appears less polarized than that of the neutrophil, and macrophages extend a thin layer of plasma membrane and cytoplasm round the whole circumference of the cell. This phenomenon is known as '**ruffling**'. At the same time, macrophage cell surface that is not attached to the

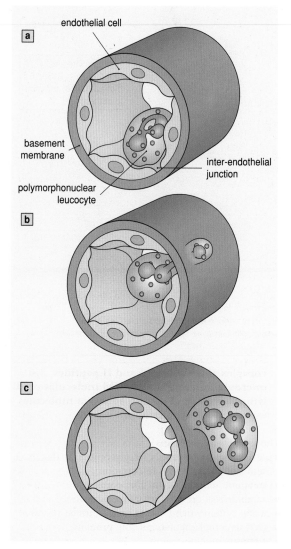

FIGURE 5.4 *Emigration of leucocytes from small blood vessels in acute inflammation.* **a** *Margination of white cells within the flowing blood occurs and granulocytes adhere to the endothelial cells.* **b** *The granulocyte inserts a cytoplasmic pseudopodium between adjacent endothelial cells.* **c** *The granulocyte has almost completely passed through the interendothelial gap and the underlying basement membrane, and will soon be seen free in the perivascular space.*

underlying substrate becomes covered with spiky projections, giving the plasma membrane a very 'restless' appearance.

Observations of moving leucocytes have suggested a dominant role for the **peripheral part of the cytoplasm**, which is obviously involved in the formation of pseudopodia. Heating activated leucocytes to 40°C leads to loss of pseudopodia. These cell fragments retain the capacity to move and even to respond to chemotactic signals, suggesting that the 'motor' that drives

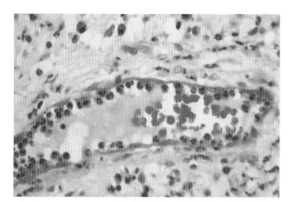

FIGURE 5.5 Small blood vessel in the serosa of an inflamed appendix showing pronounced margination of neutrophils.

movement in the leucocyte resides in this peripheral zone of the cytoplasm.

The fact that the **peripheral cytoplasmic zone** of an activated leucocyte always excludes cell organelles has led to the suggestion that it is in a **gelled** state. This suggestion is supported by studies in which aspiration of the plasma membrane of activated white cells with a micropipette shows that the peripheral zone of the cytoplasm exhibits **viscoelastic behaviour**. This means that initially there is resistance to the aspiration, but this phase is followed by one in which the peripheral cytoplasm flows freely into the pipette. This behaviour is characteristic of a gel.

The mechanical properties of this peripheral zone of cytoplasm are believed to be derived from its principal component: **actin filaments**. A compound, such as the fungal metabolite **cytochalasin**, which **inhibits the assembly of actin filaments from their monomeric subunits**, is a potent inhibitor of leucocyte movement, phagocytosis and granule movement.

Support for a **primary role for actin** in the mechanical responses of the white cells comes from a number of different sources:

- proteins that can gel actin *in vitro* are present in leucocytes (α-actinin and actin-binding protein)
- actin gel contracts in the presence of adenosine 5′-triphosphate (ATP)
- purified leucocyte myosin causes contraction of actin gels *in vitro*

The Architectural Arrangement of Actin Filaments in Activated Leucocytes Favours Movement

The actin filaments, which are arranged in a network, are attached to the inner side of the plasma membrane of the leucocyte on the **aspect that is attached to an underlying substrate**. Three-dimensional study of these organized actin networks has shown:

- features that are adapted for maximal extension of pseudopodia
- exclusion of cell organelles from this region

- a pore size that allows water, solutes and small molecules to penetrate through the meshwork

This arrangement of actin filaments is promoted by two proteins: **actin-binding protein** and α-**actinin**. Another compound that promotes actin filament assembly is the phosphoinositide, PIP$_2$.

Actin Filaments Assemble in Response to Chemotactic Signals

In the resting leucocyte, about half the actin content is in the form of filaments while the rest can be extracted easily from the cell by treatment with detergents. **When leucocytes are stimulated by chemotactic signals, the fraction of actin that resists solubilization by detergents rises.** What is of some interest is how the 50% of actin that is non-polymerized is kept in this state in the resting leucocyte, because this is certainly necessary if the leucocyte is not to become activated inappropriately. Two mechanisms have been suggested:

1) **A molecule sequesters monomeric actin molecules**. This molecule has been identified as **profilin**, a basic protein present in many cell types.
2) **A molecule binds to the growing ends of actin filaments** and prevents the addition of monomers to these ends. In addition some of the filaments that have already assembled are severed. The responsible molecule appears to be **gelsolin**, a protein that can be purified from leucocytes.

Myosin Powers the Contraction of the Leucocyte Cytoplasm.

There is abundant evidence that contraction of the peripheral zone of the cytoplasm in leucocytes is mediated by **myosin**. This includes the facts that:

- When extracted leucocyte gels contract, myosin concentrates in the contracted areas.
- The addition of myosin to actin gels causes the latter to contract.
- Anti-myosin antibodies inhibit the contraction of leucocyte cytoplasm extracts.

The mechanism responsible for the regulation of leucocyte myosin is thought to be similar to that which operates in smooth muscle and platelets. A calcium–calmodulin complex activates a myosin light-chain kinase which, in turn, phosphorylates the myosin light chain. One of the most fascinating differences, however, between the operation of contraction in muscle and in leucocytes is that in muscle the contractile apparatus is fixed so that only a 'switch on–switch off' mechanism is required. In non-muscle cells, especially leucocytes, the actin meshwork on which the myosin acts is built at different places within the cells and at different times in response to the demands of chemical signals.

Chemotaxis

Chemotaxis is the directional, purposive movement of phagocytic cells towards areas of tissue

injury or death or the sites of bacterial invasion. As its name implies, it is mediated by a series of chemical messengers. Chemotaxis must be distinguished from **chemokinesis**, a chemically induced increase in activity of phagocytic cells **which has no vectorial component**. Clearly a process of this sort must, as indicated above, have *two* aspects:

  1) **signals that attract the phagocyte** towards the appropriate area
  2) **the ability of the phagocyte to respond to the signal** by moving towards the point from which the signal has been generated (**reception** and **transduction**)

That phagocytic cells are capable of responding in a directed way to a variety of stimuli has been shown in a number of ways. In my view the most elegant of these is the system devised in Oxford by Henry Harris in which neutrophils are incorporated into clotted plasma between a coverslip and a slide. When such preparations are examined by dark-field microscopy, the cells show up as white spots against a black background, and movement in any direction can be recorded as white tracks by long exposure of a single photographic frame. Harris found that various bacteria were chemotactic under these experimental circumstances.

CHEMICAL MEDIATORS

Generation and Reception of Signals

Using *in vitro* systems, many substances are now known to be chemotactic for neutrophils, although, of course, their significance *in vivo* is less clear. These substances include **low molecular weight compounds** which are products of protein synthesis by invading microorganisms, and **endogenous compounds**.

Formylated Peptides

These low molecular weight compounds produced by microorganisms are the formylated peptides, which have methionine as the *N*-terminal residue. Formylated peptides have excited a considerable degree of interest. It is not certain whether such compounds as *f*-Met-Leu-Phe (formylated methionine-leucine-phenylalanine) have any role to play in inflammation as we know it, but is not without interest that, in prokaryotes, ribosomal synthesis of new proteins starts with formyl-methionine, which may later be cleaved. As eukaryotic protein synthesis does not proceed in this way (except, interestingly enough, in mitochondria), this provides a recognition system by which prokaryotic bacterial invaders could be distinguished from eukaryotic cells. Neutrophils certainly possess receptors for *f*-Met-Leu-Phe and the latter can also cause endothelial cells to express some adhesion molecules.

Endogenous Compounds

These may be classified as shown in *Table 5.1*. In this section we shall seek briefly to characterize these chemical mediators and to see how some of the systems interact with one another.

In theory no substance should be labelled a chemical mediator of acute inflammation unless, when given in a concentration likely to be found in human disease, it can reproduce the features of inflammation, and unless it can always be identified at sites of inflammatory reactions. However, it is not possible to operate with such a degree of certainty in many instances and some of the compounds discussed here retain for the present a putative rather than a proven role.

As outlined in *Table 5.1*, the main sources for **endogenous mediators** are the **plasma** and the **tissues**; these will be considered separately (*Fig.5.6*).

Table 5.1 Broad Groupings of Inflammatory Mediators

Source	Mediators
Activated plasma protein cascades	Complement system Kinin system Intrinsic blood clotting pathway Fibrinolytic system
Stored within cells and released on demand	Histamine 5-Hydroxytryptamine Lysosomal components
Newly synthesized in and released from cells on demand	Prostaglandins Leukotrienes Platelet-activating factor Cytokines such as IL-1 and TNF-α

MEDIATORS DERIVED FROM PLASMA

Endogenous mediators derived from plasma include those shown in *Table 5.2*. All these plasma systems are interconnected (see *Fig. 5.8*), the interconnections serving the purpose of **positive amplification loops** (see *Fig. 5.9*).

The Complement System

The complement system consists of about 20 different proteins which interlink functionally to play an important role in immune responses and inflammation. Activation of this system is discussed more fully in the section dealing with the immune system (see pp 111–114).

When activated, complement (*Fig.5.7*):
a) yields particles that coat, for example,

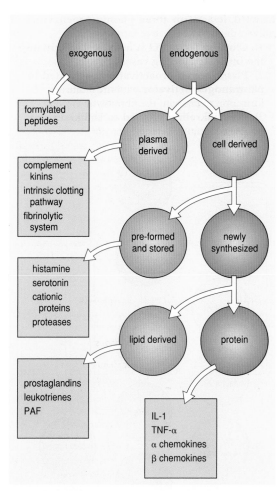

FIGURE 5.6 *A simple classification of the mediators of acute inflammation.*

Table 5.2 Plasma-derived Mediators in Acute Inflammation

System	Mediator in acute inflammation
Complement	C3a
	C5a
	C567 trimolecular complex
Kinin	Kallikrein
	Bradykinin and other short peptides
Clotting	Fibrinopeptides
Fibrinolytic	Plasmin

nate pathway can be activated by certain lipopolysaccharides derived from Gram–negative bacteria (endotoxins), by cobra venom and by polysaccharides derived from the cell walls of certain yeasts (zymosan). A number of aggregated immunoglobulins, notably immunoglobulin (Ig)A and IgE, will also act in this way, as will **plasmin**, a product of the fibrinolytic cascade, via both the classical and

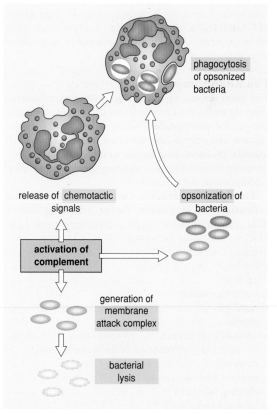

FIGURE 5.7 *Actions of complement in defence against infection.*

microorganisms and function as adhesion molecules for neutrophils and macrophages (**opsonins**)

b) leads to **lysis of bacterial cell membranes** via the membrane attack complex

c) yields biologically active fragments that influence the **vascular and cellular pathways of acute inflammation**

One of the most important chemotactic factors for neutrophils is the 5a component of the **complement cascade**, although a trimolecular complex of C567 also operates as an attractant for phagocytes, and some workers maintain that C3a also does.

The complement cascade can be activated in at least two ways. The first of these, known as the **classical** pathway, is through the **formation of antigen–antibody complexes to which C1q then binds.**

The second, known as the **alternate** pathway, operates via the **direct cleavage of C3 with consequent activation of the rest of the sequence. The alter-**

alternate pathways. In a later section we shall look at the interrelationship of these and other substances believed to operate as chemical mediators of the inflammatory reaction.

Mention has already been made of the role of some of the components of the complement cascade in relation to the chemotactic attraction of neutrophils and macrophages, and of the chief ways in which complement activation can be achieved. **However, the part played by the complement system extends beyond the bounds of chemotaxis to involve the vascular changes in the acute inflammatory reaction as well.** The increased vascular permeability produced by activation of the complement cascade has been attributed to the formation of what have been called '**anaphylatoxins**', which we now know are the cleavage products of C3 and C5 – **C3a** and **C5a**. If C3a and C5a are injected into human skin they cause local reddening and leakage from the microvasculature; C5a is 1000 times more active than C3a in this respect. Thus both C3a and C5a are deemed to be mediators of the vascular and cellular components of the inflammatory reaction, C5a being the more active, while the C567 complex exerts its effect solely in respect of chemotaxis. In addition C3 fragments can induce the release of neutrophils from bone marrow reserves, and C5a may induce the release of lysosomal enzymes. The effects of C5a on the microvessels are probably a result of its effect on mast cells, which are stimulated to produce large amounts of leukotriene B_4.

The Kinin System

The kinin system consists of a series of enzymatic steps that lead to the conversion of certain plasma precursors into active polypeptides. These share an **ability to induce change in the tone of vascular smooth muscle**. Some of these kinins, notably bradykinin, are powerful vasodilators and are also able to cause pain when injected intradermally.

The kinin-generating cascade starts with the activation of Hageman factor (clotting factor XII). Hageman factor can be cleaved by a number of different substances including:
- glass
- kaolin
- collagen
- basement membrane
- cartilage
- trypsin
- sodium urate crystals
- kallikrein (a later member of the kinin-forming cascade)
- plasmin (the fibrinolytic enzyme)
- clotting factor XI
- bacterial endotoxins

This wide range of activators signifies its central and important biological position. Once Hageman factor is

activated, **it acts on three plasma proenzymes** to convert them to their active form (*Fig. 5.8*):
1) **Clotting factor XI is activated to initiate the intrinsic clotting cascade**.
2) **Plasminogen proactivator is activated to plasminogen activator** with the ultimate formation of plasmin, the fibrinolytic enzyme.
3) **Prekallikrein is cleaved to kallikrein**, thus leading to kinin generation.

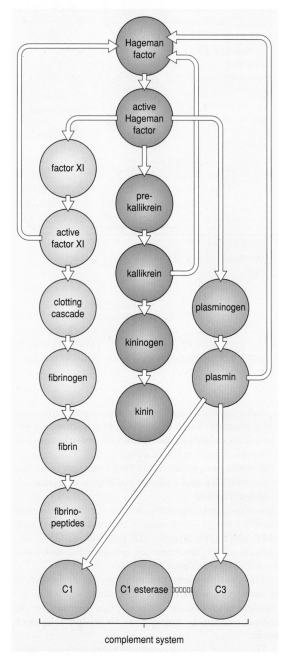

FIGURE 5.8 Interrelationships between the plasma cascade systems and acute inflammation.

Plasma **kallikrein** (which is itself chemotactic for neutrophils) cleaves a plasma substrate, kininogen, to release the active nonapeptide **bradykinin**. Bradykinin is a powerful hypotensive agent and produces both vascular dilatation and increases in vascular permeability in extremely small doses. Bradykinin is destroyed by two peptidases, and the other enzymes of the kinin-generating system can be interrupted at various points along the cascade. The precise role of the kinin system in inflammation has yet to be determined. Clearly it is not the only system involved, as patients with a deficiency of Hageman factor can still mount a normal inflammatory response. It may be that the kinin system is important because of its interrelationships with other inflammation-mediating plasma cascades.

The Clotting System

The activation of Hageman factor also activates clotting Factor XI. This active form of Factor XI feeds back to activate more Hageman factor, thus providing the third positive amplification loop. Of the three enzymes that act in this way – Factor XI, plasmin and kallikrein – the last is by far the most active on a molar basis. The fibrinopeptides released from fibrinogen by the action of thrombin may both induce vascular leakage and be chemotactic for neutrophils.

The Fibrinolytic System

Activated Hageman factor, as mentioned above, also triggers the fibrinolytic system, leading to the production of **plasmin**. Apart from its fibrinolytic powers, plasmin is well fitted to play an important part in the generation and maintenance of the inflammatory reaction. It feeds back to activate more Hageman factor and also digests the Hageman factor into particles that tend to activate prekallikrein rather than clotting Factor XI. Thus plasmin forms the second positive amplification loop in the kinin-generating system (kallikrein itself constituting the first) (*Fig. 5.9*). In some species, when fibrin is cleaved by plasmin, fibrin degradation products are formed which are chemotactic for neutrophils; these also have the ability to enhance vascular permeability. Plasmin also activates C1 to trigger the classical pathway of complement activation and can cleave C3 directly, thus also initiating the alternate pathway of complement activation.

MEDIATORS DERIVED FROM TISSUES

Preformed Compounds

Vasoactive Amines

The first of these to be linked with the acute inflammatory reaction was **histamine**. Histamine, which is formed by the decarboxylation of histidine, is found in the granules of mast cells and in the parietal cells of the stomach mucosa.

Mast cells are distributed throughout the body and

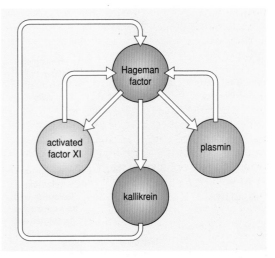

FIGURE 5.9 *Positive feedback mechanisms in relation to plasma-derived mediators of acute inflammation.*

can usually be found in relation to small vessels in the connective tissue. They are recognized by their metachromatic reaction with blue-violet dyes such as toluidine blue: their intracytoplasmic granules stain red. This reaction is due to the presence of sulphated mucopolysaccharides within these granules. In addition to histamine, the granules contain heparin, 5-hydroxytryptamine (in rats and mice) and a variety of other enzymes. The name 'mast' cell is rather curious; it is derived from the German name for these cells (*mästen*, meaning to stuff or fatten), presumably because of the large number of granules in the cytoplasm. They obviously have considerable pharmacological potential and play a significant part in the early phases of the acute inflammatory response and in type I hypersensitivity reactions (anaphylaxis) (see pp 126–128).

There is a wide range of non-cell-killing stimuli for the release of mediators from the mast cell granules (*Fig. 5.10*). These include:

- physical injury such as heat, mechanical trauma and irradiation
- chemical agents such as immunoglobulins, snake venoms, bee venom, dextrans, chymotrypsin and trypsin, certain surfactants and cationic proteins released from the lysosomes of neutrophils, C3a and C5a; and, in connection with type I hypersensitivity reactions, an antigenic challenge to IgE-coated cells.

The mechanism of release of granule contents depends on an increase in intracellular guanosine 3′,5′-cyclic monophosphate (cGMP) and a corresponding inhibition of adenosine 3′,5′-cyclic monophosphate (cAMP). Any treatment that increases the concentration of cAMP in the mast cell will inhibit release, not only of histamine but of certain other active substances that are not preformed within the cell but which are synthesized and released following on a rise in cGMP concentration.

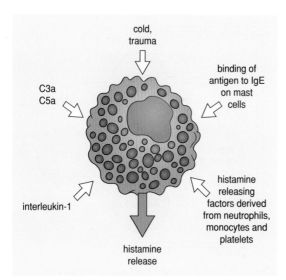

FIGURE 5.10 *Mechanisms leading to degranulation of mast cells and the release of histamine.*

Both histamine and, in small rodents, 5-hydroxytryptamine cause vascular dilatation and increased vascular permeability. However, as pointed out previously, when antihistaminic compounds are given, only the immediate phase of vascular permeability change is inhibited, suggesting that these amines are of significance only during this early period of inflammatory reaction.

Compounds Released from Lysosomes

The cell population of an acutely inflamed area can contribute a number of potential mediators derived from lysosomes. This applies not only to the neutrophils, but also to other cell types, notably platelets. Some of these candidates for the role of mediators are:

1) **Cationic proteins.** Some of these can attract mononuclear phagocytes when tested in *in vitro* systems, whereas others induce the release of histamine from mast cells and so have some effect on vascular permeability.

2) **Acid proteases.** The lysosomes of neutrophils contain many proteases, which are most active at approximately pH 3.0. In many areas of acute inflammation, the pH tends to fall because of the increased production of lactic acid consequent on the glycolysis occurring in the neutrophils. However, the pH does not usually fall so low as to provide the optimal condition for activity of these enzymes.

3) **Neutral proteases.** Although acid proteases play a limited role, the same is not true of the lysosomal enzymes active at neutral pH. It is believed that these are of considerable importance in causing tissue breakdown in a number of pathological situations. The range of targets that

may be attacked in this way is wide, because neutrophil lysosomes contain collagenases, elastases and enzymes that degrade cartilage and basement membranes. It may be that tissue damage caused by the exocytosis of lysosomal contents and the generation of oxygen free radicals occurs much more frequently and is of much greater significance than has hitherto been appreciated. Apart from the direct tissue damage that may be caused by release of lysosomal enzymes, some of these can also generate chemotactic fragments from C5 and produce kinins from plasma precursors. In addition, damaged or activated neutrophils release substances that attract other neutrophils by a mechanism independent of complement.

Acidic Lipids: the Products of Arachidonic Acid Peroxidation

In 1970 the discovery was made that certain 20-carbon-chain fatty acids were released in experimentally induced inflammatory states and in type I hypersensitivity reactions. These are known as prostaglandins (so named because they were first identified in seminal fluid). This was followed by a series of studies in which it was demonstrated that:

- peroxidation of arachidonic acid, a major constituent of the lipid in cell membranes, took place in many inflammatory conditions in a wide variety of species (including humans).
- injection of prostaglandins produced the vascular changes of the acute inflammatory response.

It is a matter of considerable interest that some potent anti-inflammatory drugs, most notably aspirin and indomethacin, selectively inhibit prostaglandin synthesis. Corticosteroids, the other major group of anti-inflammatory agents, do not inhibit prostaglandin synthesis. They stabilize membranes and in so doing may block the release of fatty acids from membrane phospholipids. Thus the supply of starting material for the synthesis of prostaglandins is cut off.

Arachidonic Acid can be Metabolized in Two Ways

First, the **stable prostaglandins**, such as prostaglandin (PG) E_2, the potent vasoconstrictor and platelet aggregator thromboxane A_2, and the dilator and antiaggregatory compound PGI_2 are all produced via two unstable endoperoxides. These are produced from arachidonic acid via an enzyme pathway known as the **cyclo-oxygenase pathway**. This cyclo-oxygenase system is blocked by aspirin and indomethacin. Both PGE_2 and PGI_2 have a strong vasodilator effect and also produce some increase in vascular permeability. Prostaglandins of the E series are hyperalgesic and also act synergistically with other pain-producing mediators of inflammation such as bradykinin.

Another pathway of arachidonic acid peroxidation exists which is known as the **lipo-oxygenase pathway**. This can occur in platelets, neutrophils and mast cells, and the initial step is the formation from arachidonic acid of an intermediate, 5-hydroperoxy-eicosotetraenoic acid (HPETE). From this intermediate, a family of compounds can be produced that are known as the **leukotrienes**. Much less is known about the inflammatory activity of these compounds than of the prostaglandins, but some are certainly chemotactic (most notably LT B_4) and others chemokinetic.

Leukotrienes C_4, D_4 and E_4 are now known to be identical to a compound discovered over 40 years ago known as **slow-reacting substance A**, which is remarkable for its ability to produce slow and sustained contraction of smooth muscle in contrast to the more rapid and short-lived effect of histamine.

This substance can be found in the lungs of sensitized guinea-pigs challenged with the appropriate antigen, and is believed to be the effector substance that causes contraction of bronchiolar smooth muscle, leading to narrowing and obstruction of small airways in type I hypersensitivity reactions. Interestingly, in view of the tendency for eosinophils to accumulate in the tissues of patients with type I hypersensitivity reactions, it is now known that eosinophils contain large amounts of **aryl sulphatase**, which can destroy slow-reacting substance A. Thus the eosinophil reaction in tissues, for so long regarded simply as a useful marker of allergic injury, can now be seen to be the expression of a protective function against excess leukotriene.

Platelet Activating Factor

The term platelet activating factor (PAF) is an example of terminology in science which tells the truth but not the whole truth. This compound, derived from membrane phospholipid, does activate platelets but has a wide range of other activities. In the context of inflammation it acts as a general upregulator of the processes so far described (*Fig. 5.11*).

PAF (1-O-alkyl-2-acetyl-sn-glycerol-3-phospho-choline) is generated after activation of phospholipase A_2 and is released at the same time as other membrane lipid-derived mediators.

Protein Mediators: the Cytokines

A wide variety of low molecular weight proteins is synthesized and released from cells active in inflammation and in determining immune responses. These are shown in *Table 5.3*; some that are active in the acute inflammatory process are discussed here.

IL-8 and Other Chemokines

Chemokines are low molecular weight proteins (8–11 kD) that are important in initiating and sustaining inflammatory reactions. Some preferentially attract neutrophils; others attract monocytes.

Chemokines are classified into two subfamilies: α and β.

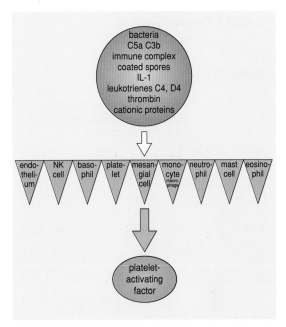

FIGURE 5.11 *Mechanisms leading to, and cell sources of, PAF release. NK, natural killer.*

The α Family This family is coded for by genes located on chromosome 4. These chemokines are characterized by an amino acid sequence in which the two terminal cysteines are separated by some other amino acid, thus giving the sequence **Cys–X–Cys**. Included in this group are IL-8, β-thromboglobulin *gro*-α, β and γ, and platelet factor 4.

α Chemokines are mostly produced by monocytes, although some are also produced by T lymphocytes, endothelial cells and platelets. **IL-8 mediates the rapid accumulation of neutrophils in inflamed tissues by inducing the formation of neutrophil-binding ligands on the endothelial cells of microvessels** in the injured area. The chemokine *gro* (MIP -2α or 2β) also acts as a neutrophil chemoattractant as well as promoting the release of lysosomal enzymes that contribute to the inflammatory response. **β-thromboglobulin** and **platelet factor 4**, which are released from activated platelets, stimulate the fibroblasts that take part in the organization of thrombi and haematomas.

β Chemokines The genes encoding β chemokines are located on chromosome 17. These mediators have a **cysteine–cysteine amino acid arrangement (Cys–Cys)**. They include:
- RANTES (Regulated on Activation, Normal T cell Expressed and Secreted). RANTES is a potent attractant for 'memory' T cells but not for naive T cells, and also attracts monocytes.
- Macrophage-activating factor (MAF)
- MIP-1α
- MIP-1β

Table 5.3 Peptide Cytokines

Cytokine	Source	Functions
Interleukins		
IL–1	Chiefly monocytes/macrophages but many other cells including epithelial and endothelial cells	A multifunctional protein; many of its activities are similar to those of TNF-α. Acts as an **endogenous pyrogen**. Induces magrophages to produce **additional IL-1 and IL-6**. Also induces glucocorticoid, prostaglandin and collagenase synthesis and release. Induces expression of adhesion molecules on vascular endothelium, thus stimulating leucocyte adhesion. Stimulates the production by macrophages of chemokines such as IL-8 which activate neutrophils
IL–2	T cells after stimulation by antigen or mitogen	Major growth factor for both helper and cytotoxic T cells and lymphokine-activated killer cells. Also involved in B-cell development
IL–4	Chiefly T$_H$2 cells	Pivotal in development of T$_H$2 subset; involved in B-cell help; causes switching of antibody production to IgE; growth factor for mast cells and stimulates production of VCAM
IL–5	T$_H$2 cells and activated mast cells	Stimulates growth and differentiation of eosinophils and thus promotes killing of helminths; promotes growth and differentiation of B cells and, together with other cytokines, induces synthesis of IgA and IgM in mature B cells
IL–6	Macrophages, fibroblasts, stromal cells in bone marrow, vascular endothelium and some T cells	Causes terminal differentiation of immunoglobulin-producing B cells; inhibits macrophage production of IL-1 and interferon-γ (IFN-γ); stimulates liver cells to produce acute-phase proteins such as fibrinogen, serum amyloid protein A, α$_2$-macroglobulin; promotes formation of osteoclasts
IL–7	Stromal cells in bone marrow and thymus	Stimulates proliferation of B-cell progenitors which show no rearrangement of heavy and light chain genes in germ cell line, and pre-B cells in which rearrangement of these genes has occurred but which have no surface immunoglobulin as yet. Stimulates mature T cells and enhances cytotoxicity
IL–9	T lymphocytes	Promotes proliferation of T cells
IL–10	T and B lymphocytes, macrophages, activated mast cells and epidermal cells	Downregulates production of cytokines including IL-1, IFN-γ and TNF-α by macrophages; inhibits nitric oxide (NO) production; stimulates B-cell proliferation, differentiation and activity
IL–11	Stromal cells	Promotes both lymphopoiesis and growth of haemopoietic cells
IL–12	Has two subunits: one produced by T, B, natural killer (NK) cells and macrophages; the other by activated macrophages and B cells	Strong stimulator of NK cells, growth factor for activated T cells and maturation factor for cytotoxic T cells; induces formation of IFN-γ and thus enhances formation of T$_H$1 cells

Table 5.3 Peptide Cytokines – *continued*

Cytokine	Source	Functions
Interleukins – continued		
IL–13	Activated helper and cytotoxic T cells	Suppresses proinflammatory cytokine, chemokine and growth factor production by macrophages and also downregulates the production of NO; enhances expression of MHC class II proteins and thus antigen presentation; causes human B cells to switch antibody production to IgE and IgG_4. Shares some features with IL-4
IL–14	T cells and malignant B cells	Induces proliferation of activated but not of resting B cells, and inhibits immunoglobulin production
IL–15	Epithelial cells	Stimulates T-cell proliferation by binding to IL-2 receptor
Interferons		
IFN–α and IFN–β	Leucocytes and fibroblasts	Antiviral; activates phagocytes
IFN–γ	T and NK cells	Antiviral; pivotal for development of T_H1 from T_H0 cells and inhibits development of T_H2 cells; it is the most powerful macrophage-activating factor (MAF) and is therefore important in cell/mediated immunity; increases expression of MHC class I and II proteins, thus enhancing antigen presentation; causes the expression of adhesion molecules on the surface of vascular endothelium (as does TNF-α); causes differentiation of cytotoxic T cells; antagonizes several IL-4 actions; promotes synthesis of IgG_{2a} by activated B cells
Cytotoxins		
TNF–α	Macrophages, mast cells and T cells. Macrophages stimulated to produce TNF by IFN-γ and migration inhibition factor (MIF). MIF production by T cells is stimulated by endotoxin	Derives its name because serum of animals given endotoxin produces haemorrhagic necrosis in tumours. At **high concentrations** (as may be induced by endotoxin), TNF acts systemically. It functions as a **pyrogen**, activates the **clotting** system, stimulates production of **acute–phase proteins** by the liver, inhibits myocardial contractility by stimulating production of NO, and over long periods causes cachexia. At **low concentrations** TNF-α upregulates the inflammatory response; it induces expression of the adhesion molecules ICAM-1, VCAM-1 and E-selectin, which promote adhesion and migration of leucocytes from the microvessels to the extravascular compartment. It enhances the killing of intracellular organisms such as *Leishmania*, and *Mycobacterium tuberculosis*. It activates several leucocyte types leading to the production by macrophages of various cytokines including IL-6, chemokines and TNF-α itself
TNF–β	Activated T cells	Shares many of the actions of TNF-α. Lyses tumour cells but not normal cells; activates neutrophils; increases adhesion of leucocytes to vascular endothelium and promotes their migration

Table 5.3 Peptide Cytokines – *continued*

Cytokine	Source	Functions
Colony stimulating factors		
Granulocyte–macrophage colony-stimulating factor (GM-CSF)	T cells, macrophages, mast cells, endothelium, fibroblasts	Stimulates growth of granulocyte and macrophage colonies; activates macrophages, neutrophils and eosinophils
G-CSF	Fibroblasts, endothelium	Stimulates proliferation of mature granulocytes
M-CSF	Fibroblasts, endothelium, epithelium	Stimulates growth of macrophage colonies
IL-3	T cells and mast cells	Stimulates growth and differentiation of haemopoietic precursors
Steel factor	Stromal cells in bone marrow	Causes mitotic division of haemopoietic stem cells (binds to the *c-kit* ligand)
Transforming growth factor β (TGF-β) This is a family of five closely related proteins. TGF-β is secreted in an inactive form and must be cleaved before it can bind to its receptor	Monocytes, T lymphocytes and platelets	Has an autocrine effect on monocyte–macrophages and regulates its own production by these cells. It also upregulates the production of IL-1, fibroblast growth factor (FGF), platelet-derived growth factor (PDGF) and TNF-α. It increases production of connective tissue matrix proteins and is a potent angiogenic factor. It has an immuno-suppressive effect by inhibiting the proliferation of T lymphocytes
Chemokines		
α Chemokines All have Cys–X–Cys amino acid sequence Includes IL-8 and *gro-α, β, γ*	Principally by monocytes, some also by T cells, endothelial cells and platelets	Induce rapid accumulation of neutrophils by mediating formation of neutrophil-binding ligands on endothelium
β Chemokines All have Cys–Cys amino acid sequence Includes RANTES and MAF	T lymphocytes and monocytes	Potent attractants for memory T cells and monocytes

These chemokines are produced by T lymphocytes and monocytes. MAF acts exclusively on monocytes, attracting them to sites of injury, activating them and regulating the expression of integrins on their surfaces.

IL-1 and TNF-α
IL-1 and TNF-α are peptides that have many activities in common.

IL-1 The principal sources of IL-1 are monocytes and macrophages but other cells such as endothelial cells and some epithelial cells may also produce this cytokine. IL-1 has a molecular weight of 17–18 kD

and is a potent regulator both of local events in the inflammatory process and of many systemic ones (*Fig. 5.12*). Its synthesis is stimulated by various microbial products, most notably bacterial endotoxin, and other cytokines.

1) **Locally,** it upregulates adhesion molecule expression on endothelial cells, leading to adhesion of both leucocytes and platelets and to stimulation of macrophage production of chemokines (such as IL-8) that activate neutrophils.
2) **Systemically**, IL-1 acts as an endogenous pyrogen (inducer of fever) and induces glucocorticoid synthesis and the release of

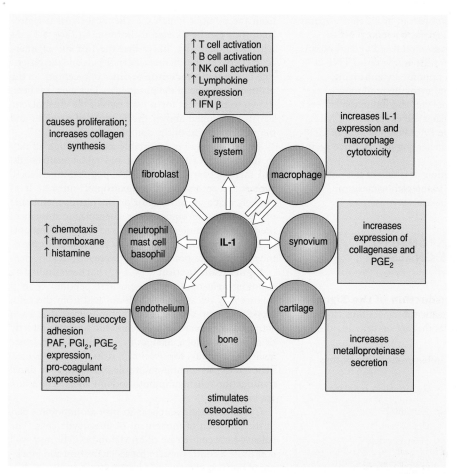

FIGURE 5.12 Targets and effects of interleukin 1. NK, natural killer; IFN, interferon; PG, prostaglandin.

prostaglandins, collagenase and acute-phase proteins.

It lacks the ability of TNF-α to produce necrosis of tumour cells and tissue injury, to increase the expression of MHC-coded proteins or to mediate the Schwartzmann reaction.

TNF-α TNF-α belongs to a family of ligands (currently with ten known members). Among many other functions mentioned below, all of these ligands bind to receptors on target cells that initiate signals for either cell proliferation or for apoptosis. TNF exists almost entirely as a secreted protein, but the others are transmembrane proteins that act chiefly through cell–cell contact.

TNF-α binds to two receptors, one a 55-kD and the other a 75-kD transmembrane protein (*Table 5.4*).

TNF-α is one of the cytokines produced in the greatest amounts by stimulated macrophages, especially if the stimulatory signal has been bacterial endotoxin.

Table 5.4 TNF-α and its Receptors

Receptor occupied	Effects
55 kD	Apoptosis
	Tumour cell lysis *in vitro*
75 kD	T-lymphocyte proliferation
	Skin necrosis
	Insulin resistance
Both	Bone resorption
	Haemorrhagic necrosis in tumours
	Endotoxic shock (see pp 387–389)
	Fever

1) It plays an important part in host defence against infections by Gram-negative bacteria, TNF-α production being greatly modulated by endotoxin. When endotoxin is present at low doses TNF-α mediates a protective response by enhancing macrophage killing and cytokine production, activation of B lymphocytes and induction of fever.
2) TNF both upregulates the expression of MHC class I proteins and the cytotoxic potential of CD8 T lymphocytes, thus increasing host defence against intracellular parasites.
3) At high concentrations it is one of the potent mediators concerned in the pathogenesis of endotoxin-related shock.

PHAGOCYTE RESPONSE TO CHEMOTACTIC SIGNALS

Reception and Transduction of the Signal

In the sense that chemotactic substances thus far identi-fied are soluble molecules that act on cells at a distance

Table 5.5 Effects of Inflammatory Mediators

Inflammatory event	Responsible mediator(s)
Dilatation of microvessels	Histamine
	Bradykinin
	Prostaglandins
Increase in microvessel permeability with production of oedema	Complement fractions C3a and C5a
	Histamine
	Bradykinin
	PAF
	Leukotrienes C_4, D_4, E_4
Chemotaxis	f-Met-Leu-Phe
	C5a, ?C3a
	Cationic proteins derived from neutrophils
	TNF-α, IL-8
Tissue damage	Lysosomal enzymes
	Oxygen free radicals generated by acute inflammatory cells
Pain	Bradykinin
	PGE_2
Fever	TNF-α
	IL-1
	Both act in this way by mediating production of prostaglandins

from the point at which the chemical signal is gener-ated, they can be likened to hormones (*Table 5.5*). As with hormones, it is likely that the first site of inter-action between the chemotactic molecule and the phago-cyte is a **specific receptor** or series of receptors on the plasma membrane of the phagocyte. This view has been shown to be correct for at least two of the chemotactic signals mentioned above: the formylated peptides and the 5a component of the complement system.

These peptides bind saturably and with high affinity to the surface of both human and rabbit neutrophils, and there appear to be definable populations of these peptide receptors on the neutrophil surface. It is unlikely that a single receptor on the plasma membrane of the phagocyte binds all the chemotactic substances mentioned, because exposing cells to excessive amounts of the chemotactic peptides does not appear to block their ability to respond to C5a; the reverse is also true.

Signal transduction (*Fig. 5.13*) has been studied by exposing neutrophils to chemotactic peptides. This is followed by release of arachidonic acid from the cells, suggesting that a membrane phospholipase has been activated. This increase in arachidonic acid may directly or indirectly induce changes in membrane ion perme-ability (especially for calcium). Ion fluxes are now believed to play an important role in chemotactic signal transduction, changes in both sodium and calcium flux are involved.

Cyclic nucleotides appear to play an important part in the initiation of movement of phagocytic cells. The balance between release of cAMP and cGMP may well constitute a control system for the activation and block-ing of both chemotaxis and certain other events (such as the release of active compounds from the granules of mast cells) in the acute inflammatory reaction.

cGMP enhances:
- chemotactic movement
- the release of pharmacologically active substances such as histamine and leukotrienes from mast cells
- the release of lysosomal enzymes and lymphokines from neutrophils and T lymphocytes respectively.

cAMP produces the *opposite* effect in each of these instances. The main effect of the cyclic nucleotides within the neutrophil is probably exerted on the cytoskeleton, the principal target being the microtubule system.

Microtubules are hollow fibres with a diameter of 24 nm; they appear to be inserted at the periphery of the cell in the region where the contractile microfila-ments are concentrated. The structural element of the microtubules is in equilibrium with the protein from which it is formed, which is known as **tubulin**. This is a dimeric protein which, when assembled into tubules, plays an important role not only in chemotaxis and cell secretion but also, in other cells, in mitosis.

A rise in the intracellular concentration of cGMP promotes assembly of the microtubules, and a rise in cAMP levels inhibits tubule assembly. Anything that

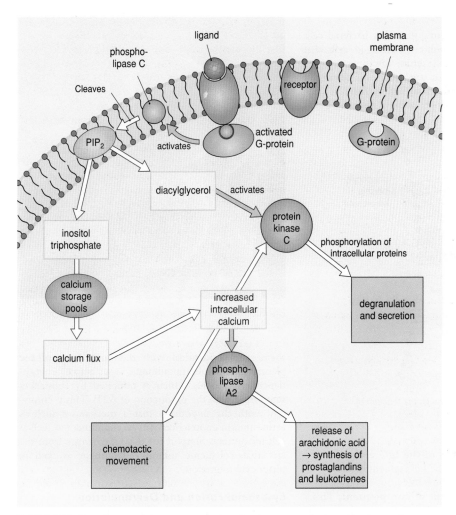

FIGURE 5.13 Transduction of chemotactic signals within leucocytes after ligand binding to the appropriate receptor on the leucocyte plasma membrane.

inhibits assembly of the microtubules will also inhibit the migration of neutrophils in response to chemotactic signals. This is the basis of an old treatment for acute gouty arthritis – colchicine. The acute local inflammation found in gout results from what might be regarded as a failure of normal neutrophil function. Sodium biurate crystals are deposited in the synovium as a result of an abnormality in uric acid metabolism. These 'foreign' bodies attract neutrophils, which engulf them in the normal way. However, abnormal hydrogen bonds form between the surface of the urate crystals and the phagolysosomal membrane, with resulting rupture of the membrane and spillage of the lysosomal enzymes into the extracellular space. It is this that causes the intense pain. Colchicine, through its interference with microtubule assembly, prevents phagocyte migration and interrupts this cycle of events. Vinca alkaloids, used in treating certain malignancies, act in the same way.

In contrast, drugs that *raise* the intracellular content of cGMP enhance the movement of phagocytes towards attractants. One such drug is levamisole, which can be shown to reverse chemotactic deactivation *in vitro*. More interestingly, levamisole has been shown to reverse the depression in movement of human neutrophils and monocytes induced by a number of viruses, including herpes simplex.

Phagocytosis

Once phagocytes have arrived at the site of tissue damage and/or bacterial invasion they must recognize which structures to attack and become attached to them. *In vivo*, phagocytes demonstrate remarkable selectivity as to what they will ingest, presumably by recognizing certain specific features on the cell surface. For example, mononuclear phagocytes (macrophages) ingest old or damaged red cells but disregard normal ones.

Opsonization

It has been known for a long time that bacterial cells coated with immunoglobulin or damaged cells that have interacted with fresh serum are phagocytosed more readily than those that have not. This coating of particles with proteins is called **opsonization** (preparation for eating, from the Greek *opsonein* meaning a 'relish') (*Fig. 5.14*).

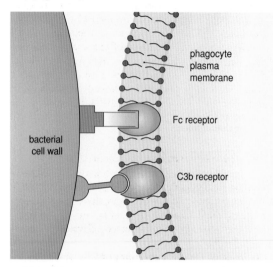

FIGURE 5.14 *Opsonization through the medium of immunoglobulin and C3b.*

The opsonins are either:
1) **Specific antibodies of the IgG class.** For opsonization to occur, the Fc fragment of the immunoglobulin must be intact.
2) The **C3b component of complement.** This is a non-specific activity of great biological value to the host, as invading microorganisms can be opsonized even on the first occasion that the host is infected with a particular organism.

The apparent restriction of opsonization to these two protein classes indicates that the plasma membrane of the phagocytic cell possesses specific receptor sites for the C3b subunit (one of the β_2 family of integrins) and for the Fc fragment of IgG.

Engulfment (*Fig. 5.15*)

Engulfment of the bacterium or foreign object takes place as a result of fusion of pseudopodia projecting from the phagocyte plasma membrane in the form of long finger-like projections. The pseudopodia fuse on the far side of the object to be phagocytosed, thus locking it within a membrane-bound vesicle or **phagosome**. The phagosome then buds off from the plasma membrane of the phagocyte and comes to lie within the cytoplasm of the neutrophil or macrophage. The membrane of this phagosome is obviously composed of part of the phagocyte plasma membrane which has become inverted; therefore the inner layer of the phagosome

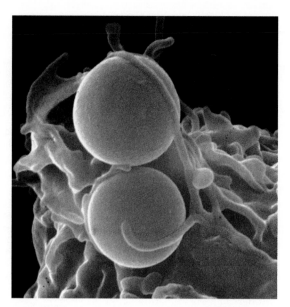

FIGURE 5.15 *Scanning electron micrograph of macrophage (ex vivo) engulfing small latex spheres.*

membrane is identical with the outer layer of the plasma membrane. Engulfment is an active, energy-dependent process which is inhibited by substances interfering with the production of ATP. This is consistent with the hypothesis that a mechanism such as actin–myosin contraction 'drives' engulfment as well as cell movement. Support for this view comes from the fact that colchicine inhibits engulfment as well as phagocyte migration.

Lysosomal Fusion and Degranulation

Once the phagosome has formed, lysosomal granules move towards it and apposition of their membranes, followed by membrane fusion, occurs. The lysosomal granules disappear as this happens (hence the expression 'degranulation of polymorphonuclear cells'). These events take place with great speed; fusion of lysosomes with phagosomes occurs more or less in concert with ingestion and ends when the process of ingestion is over. Compounds known to inhibit migration and phagocytosis also inhibit degranulation.

Metabolic Events Associated with Bacterial Killing

As well as triggering ingestion and fusion of phagosomes and lysosomes, recognition of an invading microorganism and attachment to it by the phagocyte is associated with a burst of oxidative activity (the **respiratory burst**). The results essentially in the step-wise **reduction of molecular oxygen to hydrogen peroxide**:
- This respiratory burst is associated with a 2–20-fold increase in oxygen consumption compared with a resting cell and a considerable increase in glucose metabolism via the hexose monophosphate shunt.

- The reduction of molecular oxygen is catalysed by a non-haem protein oxidase believed to be localized on the external surface of the phagocyte plasma membrane (which forms the **inner layer** of the phagosome membrane).
- The hydrogen donor for the reduction process is either reduced nicotinamide adenine dinucleotide (NADH) or reduced nicotinamide adenine dinucleotide phosphate (NADPH). The presence of one or other of these pyridine nucleotides is an essential link in the chain because, if regeneration from NAD to NADP cannot take place, hydrogen peroxide will not be formed. Hence adequate amounts of glucose-6-phosphate dehydrogenase (G6PD) are required within the cell if bacterial killing is to proceed in the normal way.
- In the reduction process the oxygen gains only one electron and is converted into an oxygen free radical, the **superoxide anion** (O_2^-). About 90% of the oxygen consumed in the respiratory burst is converted into superoxide anion.
- When two molecules of this anion react with each other, one is oxidized and the other reduced, forming **hydrogen peroxide** and oxygen in a dismutation reaction. This reaction is catalysed by the enzyme **superoxide dismutase**. Other highly reactive oxygen-derived metabolites have been identified or have been predicted to exist as a result of activation of phagocytic cells. These include an active hydroxyl radical (OH$^\bullet$), singlet oxygen and hypochlorous acid.

There is abundant evidence that phagocytes are unable to kill ingested organisms in the absence of the respiratory burst and without production of the superoxide anion. Both superoxide dismutase and catalase are capable of inhibiting phagocyte-mediated bacterial killing. However, superoxide appears to have little bactericidal effect on its own, and it is now widely believed that the most important bactericidal activity within the phagocyte stems from the production of hydrogen peroxide. Hydrogen peroxide by itself has significant bactericidal activity, but this is potentiated 50-fold when the hydrogen peroxide reacts with the myeloperoxidase (one of the phagocyte's lysosomal enzymes) and halide ions. The most likely product, in chemical terms, of the hydrogen peroxide–myeloperoxidase–halide complex is hypochlorous acid (HOCl).

The mechanism of bactericidal injury appears to involve halogenation or oxidation of the bacterial surface. It is also likely that decarboxylation of cell walls and/or cell membrane proteins occurs, with the local generation of toxic aldehydes. In addition to the activity of the hydrogen peroxide–myeloperoxidase–halide complex, there is a considerable body of evidence suggesting that hydroxyl radicals formed by the interaction between hydrogen peroxide and the superoxide anion are also important in bacterial killing; mannitol, a scavenger of hydroxy radicals, inhibits the bacterial activity of an acetaldehyde–xanthine oxidase system which can trap and reduce molecular oxygen, generating active oxygen free radicals.

Detoxification of Hydrogen Peroxide

As hydrogen peroxide can diffuse out of the phagosome, it is important that control mechanisms should exist to prevent lipid peroxidation of the cell's own membranes. The scavenger systems involved are catalase and, perhaps even more importantly, glutathione peroxidase. The activity of the latter implies a need for a constantly replenished supply of reduced glutathione. This, once again, emphasizes the importance of G6PD, as the reduced glutathione must be regenerated through coupling mechanisms linked to the hexose monophosphate shunt. Thus G6PD is involved in both the production and detoxification of bactericidal peroxides.

Other Mechanisms of Bacterial Killing

While the oxygen-dependent mechanisms described above are fundamental to the normal bactericidal activity of neutrophils and macrophages, there are other systems that are injurious to ingested microorganisms. These are related to various aspects of lysosomal function and include:

1) **Low pH within the phagolysosome.** The pH inside the vacuole is 3.5–4; this in itself may be bactericidal or bacteriostatic (preventing multiplication without killing organisms). In addition, the low pH promotes the production of hydrogen peroxide from superoxide.
2) **Lysozyme (muramidase).** This is a low molecular weight cationic enzyme which attacks the mucopeptide cell walls of some bacterial species.
3) **Lactoferrin.** This iron-binding protein inhibits the growth of a number of microorganisms.
4) **Cationic proteins** with antibacterial activity also enter the phagosome in the course of fusion and degranulation.
5) **Lysosomal hydrolases** entering the phagosome in the course of phagosome–lysosome fusion may have some antibacterial activity, but are probably more important in digesting the remains of organisms killed by other means.

DEFECTS OF NEUTROPHIL FUNCTION

Neutropenia

Even if the separate operations discussed in the above sections can be carried out normally, this is of no avail in protecting the host if there are insufficient cells to cope with the number of invading microorganisms. This occurs in various forms of bone marrow failure:

- drug or poison induced (e.g. chloramphenicol, benzene)

- infiltration of the marrow by large numbers of tumour cells
- bone marrow fibrosis
- other forms of marrow aplasia

Disorders of Migration and Chemotaxis

These may occur as a result of an intrinsic defect in the cell, from inhibition of locomotion or because of deficiencies in the generation of chemotactic signals.

Intrinsic Cell Defects

- **The 'lazy leucocyte' syndrome.** The precise point at which the defect occurs has not been identified.
- **Job's syndrome.** This typically affects fair-skinned, red-haired females and is characterized by recurrent 'cold' staphylococcal abscesses.
- **Diabetes mellitus.** Leucocytes from diabetic patients with poorly controlled diabetes show impairment of locomotion. This is at least partially reversed by adding insulin and glucose to the leucocytes.
- **Chediak–Higashi syndrome.** This rare congenital autosomal recessive disorder occurs in humans, cattle, mink and certain strains of mouse. In all species it is characterized by partial albinism, the presence of giant lysosomal granules in neutrophils, and increased susceptibility to bacterial infection. In humans death usually occurs in childhood and is often preceded by the development of a malignant process involving lymphoid cells. Two major defects have been documented in the neutrophils of patients suffering from this syndrome:
  1) Failure to show directed movement in response to chemotactic stimuli both *in vivo* and *in vitro*.
  2) A delay in intracellular bacterial killing which appears to result from a reduced rate of phagosome–lysosome fusion.

It has been proposed that this combination of defects results from a failure in the assembly of microtubules from tubulin; the addition of cGMP or agents that increase intracellular cGMP generation to the neutrophils might reverse the situation. The lysosomes in Chediak–Higashi leucocytes lack elastase and cathepsin G.

- **Leucocyte adhesion deficiency syndrome**: This is due to absence of the CD18 β subunit of the $β_2$ integrins expressed on the surface of leucocytes. This affects neutrophils only; monocytes, lymphocytes and eosinophils can make use of the $β_1$ integrin system, which involves binding of very late activation antigen 4 (VLA-4) on the leucocytes with VCAM on endothelium.

Inhibition of Locomotion

The serum of certain patients inhibits chemotaxis when added to neutrophils; certain drugs such as corticosteroids and phenylbutazone also do this.

Deficiencies in the Generation of Chemotactic Signals

The most important of these are deficiencies in the complement system.

Disorders of Phagocytosis

Opsonin Deficiencies

These include deficiencies of complement or of IgG. Some patients with sickle cell disease have opsonin deficiencies, apparently associated with failure of alternate pathway activation of the complement system.

Defects of Engulfment

These can be brought about certain drugs, such as morphine analogues, and under hyperosmolar conditions, such as may be seen in patients with diabetic acidosis.

Disorders of Lysosomal Fusion

This may occur after administration of certain drugs, such as corticosteroids, colchicine and certain antimalarials. Failure of lysosomal fusion in the neutrophils of patients with Chediak–Higashi syndrome is mentioned above.

Disorders of Bacterial Killing

The most important of these is **chronic granulomatous disease of childhood**. This is a rare disease of childhood, sometimes X-linked, characterized by recurrent bacterial infections involving skin, lung, bones and lymph nodes. Affected children show increased susceptibility to infection by a rather mixed bag of organisms including *Staphylococcus aureus*, *Aerobacter aerogenes* and certain fungi such as *Aspergillus* species. Draining lymph nodes are often enlarged and show proliferation of mononuclear phagocytes lining the sinuses or aggregations of mononuclear cells tightly packed together to form granulomatous foci.

The neutrophils in this condition respond normally to chemotactic signals and show no apparent difficulty in phagocytosis. However, once engulfment of the foreign organisms has occurred, the expected burst of respiratory activity does not take place and there is no superoxide or hydrogen peroxide production. Failure to produce reactive oxygen intermediates is due to a defect in the cytochrome b-245 oxidase system. This cytochrome has two subunits, large (92 kDa) and small (22 kDa).

The **X-linked** form of the disease is due to a mutation in the gene coding for the larger subunit. In most cases this results in failure to produce any gene product but in some cases a low level of gene product is present; these patients can be treated with interferon γ with some success.

About one-third of children with chronic granulomatous disease inherit the disease in an **autosomal recessive** pattern. The defect results either from a mutation in the gene encoding the smaller 22-kDa

KEY POINTS: Neutrophil Function as a Means of Host Defence

- As part of the host's system of defence against infection by pathogenic microorganisms, the role of the neutrophil is to **seek out, ingest and kill a wide range of these organisms**. These processes can be looked at most easily as a set of distinct operations, any of which can go wrong and thus render the neutrophil ineffective as a bacterial 'hunter–killer'.

- As with any instruction, that given to the neutrophil to emigrate from the local microvasculature and to proceed towards the invading microorganisms or the injured or dead tissue elements must involve the **giving** and **receiving** of an appropriate **signal**. **Transduction** of this signal must then take place, so that **migration** of the phagocytic cell **towards the point from which the signal emanated** can occur. This generation and reception of the signal and the vectorial movement by the neutrophil which follows is known as **chemotaxis**.

- Once the neutrophil has reached the invading microorganism or the dead or effete cells from which the chemotactic signal has been generated, a process of **attachment** between the neutrophil and the object to be phagocytosed occurs. This is facilitated by the latter being coated by either immunoglobulin or one of the components of complement C3b. **Phagocytic cells possess receptors for the Fc portion of immunoglobulin and for C3b.**

  In some instances, one of the acute-phase proteins, C-reactive protein binds to carbohydrates on certain bacteria and activates complement via the classical pathway, thus leading to coating of the organism by C3b. These coating molecules, which provide binding sites for the phagocytes, are called **opsonins** and the coating process is termed **opsonization**. The foreign material or organism is then engulfed by the plasma membrane of the phagocyte and comes to lie within a membrane-bounded vesicle called the **phagosome**. These two steps together constitute the process of **phagocytosis**.

- **Fusion then takes place between the membranes of the phagosome and a lysosome, resulting in the formation of a secondary lysosome or phagolysosome.** In this way the contents of the lysosome are released into the lumen of the phagosome. The morphological correlate of this operation is loss of granules in the cytoplasm of the neutrophil. If the occupant of the phagolysosome is a living organism, killing and digestion of that organism occurs. This is accomplished largely by **oxygen-dependent mechanisms**.

subunit or in the cytosolic components of the NADPH oxidase system.

Interestingly, neutrophils from patients with chronic granulomatous disease can kill certain pathogenic microorganisms such as streptococci and pneumococci. These organisms produce a certain amount of hydrogen peroxide themselves but do not produce catalase. Within the phagosome the concentration of hydrogen peroxide produced by the microorganism rises gradually until, in a sense, the organisms 'commit suicide'. However, bacteria that also produce catalase are safe from the effects of their own hydrogen peroxide.

The role of G6PD in the production and detoxification of hydrogen peroxide has been mentioned above. If the degree of deficiency of this enzyme is very severe, a clinical picture resembling that encountered in chronic granulomatous disease of childhood may be seen. Absence of myeloperoxidase brings about some reduction in the efficiency of intracellular, oxygen-dependent bactericidal mechanisms, but the functional defect is usually not very severe.

MONONUCLEAR PHAGOCYTES IN ACUTE INFLAMMATION

The cellular component of the inflammatory response includes another type of phagocytic cell apart from the neutrophil: the mononuclear phagocyte, which exists in two forms. An intermediate form, known as the **monocyte**, circulates in the blood, and when it migrates into tissues it either matures or differentiates into the tissue **macrophage**.

The monocyte has a half-life of about 22 hours, which is approximately three times as long as that of the neutrophil. Despite the fact that it can be regarded as an intermediate cell form, it possesses a range of functional activities shared with the mature tissue macrophage.

Monocytes and macrophages are derived from bone marrow. If the bone marrow is destroyed by exposing an animal to X-rays, injury fails to elicit any mononuclear cell response, whereas if the thymus is removed a normal response is produced. Within the tissue the transition from monocyte to macrophage brings with it a considerable structural and hence, by implication, functional increase in the phagocytic, lysosomal and secretory apparatus:

- the cell becomes larger
- the plasma membrane becomes more convoluted
- lysosomes increase in number
- both the Golgi apparatus and the endoplasmic reticulum become more prominent

There is a considerable degree of overlap in the phagocytic functions of the macrophage and the neutrophil, so it is not a surprise to find that the plasma membrane of the macrophage has surface receptors for the Fc fragment of immunoglobulin as well as for complement components.

Like the neutrophil, the macrophage depends on glycolysis for its energy needs in the course of phagocytosis and also exhibits a respiratory burst following bacterial engulfment. However, because it has a well-developed protein secretory apparatus, the macrophage can synthesize and replace depleted enzymes, and this allows it to act for a much longer time than the neutrophil.

Many pathogenic microorganisms are phagocytosed by the macrophage and a large number of these are destroyed within the phagosomes with a facility no less than that of the neutrophil. However, some organisms parasitize macrophages and multiply within the phagosomes. Such organisms include *Listeria, Brucella, Salmonella, Mycobacterium, Chlamydia, Rickettsia, Leishmania, Toxoplasma, Trypanosoma* and *Legionella*. This symbiotic relationship is destroyed by **activation of the macrophage**, which then becomes highly dangerous to its previous symbiotes.

Chemical Influences on Macrophage Function (see pp 52–54)

Macrophage chemotactic factors include those that have already been described in relation to the neutrophil, such as complement cleavage products, microbial products, *N*-formyl methionyl peptides and fibrin degradation products. In addition, however, there is an important group of chemical activators which trigger a wide range of macrophage functions apart from chemotaxis. These are called **lymphokines** and are secreted by activated T lymphocytes. The concept that sensitized T lymphocytes reacting with specific antigen can release products that activate macrophages, both *in vivo* and *in vitro*, is now well accepted. The lymphokines include a **macrophage chemotactic factor**, which can recruit macrophages into sites of infection, contact-type hypersensitivity or inflammation, a **migration inhibition factor**, which can immobilize macrophages in certain lesions, and factors that stimulate the secretion of hydrolytic enzymes by macrophages, rendering them capable of killing neoplastic cells and of limiting the ability of intracellular organisms to reproduce themselves. Other types of macrophage activation, for example via the action of complement cleavage products, lead to other forms of activity. This topic is discussed further in Chapter 14.

CHAPTER 6

Factors that Modify the Inflammatory Reaction

The processes described in Chapters 4 and 5 occur to a greater or lesser degree in all acute inflammatory responses to injury. However, it is obvious from personal experience that there are considerable differences between one inflammatory reaction and another and that these differences involve a number of variables; for example, a 'boil' on the neck differs very much from an area of 'sunburn'.

The outcome of an injury is the result of interaction between the injurious agent and the host, and variations in either of these may exert a considerable effect.

FACTORS RELATED TO THE INJURIOUS AGENT

These include:
- the amount or dose of the agent
- its strength (or, in the case of a pathogenic microorganism, its virulence)
- the duration of exposure in the case of physical or chemical agents
- the intrinsic nature of the agent

The amount of injury produced by any noxious agent, whether living or not, is a function of its inherent toxicity and the time for which it exerts its effect. Duration of exposure is of particular importance in injury produced by physical and certain chemical agents such as heat, cold, actinic rays, acids and alkalis. In injury produced by pathogenic microorganisms, the inherent power of the organisms to produce tissue damage is clearly of great importance, but here too the **dose** of the agent may determine the outcome of the infection.

MORPHOLOGICAL FEATURES

The intrinsic nature of the agent may produce a morphological reaction in the tissues that is quite distinctive. In some cases the type of structural change may be of considerable help to the histopathologist in making an aetiological diagnosis.

Suppurative Inflammation

For example, certain organisms, such as *Staphylococcus aureus*, tend to elicit an inflammatory response characterized by massive emigration of neutrophils to the site of infection. Many of these neutrophils die after phagocytosis of the invading microorganisms and release large amounts of lysosomal enzymes into the damaged area.

Because the organisms also produce substances (exotoxins) that damage tissues directly, the end result is a central area of liquefaction necrosis which contains tissue debris and many dead and dying neutrophils. This forms a rather thick, opaque, yellowish-green fluid, known as **pus**. Organisms that elicit this reaction are termed **pyogenic** (i.e. pus forming). The process by which such tissue necrosis associated with the formation of pus occurs is termed **suppuration** and the localized suppurative lesion is called an **abscess** (*Fig. 6.1*).

Membranous Inflammation

Corynebacterium diphtheriae and *Clostridium difficile* produce powerful exotoxins which kill surface epithelia. The fluid that exudes from the small subepithelial blood vessels is rich in fibrinogen. This is converted to fibrin and then becomes densely infiltrated by neutrophils. The end result is the presence, on the affected surface, of an opaque greyish-white membrane, consisting of a mixture of dead epithelial cells, fibrin and neutrophils. This type of reaction is described as **membranous** or **pseudomembranous**. In the case of the diphtheria organism, the target area is the pharynx and larynx; the clostridium causes pseudomembranous enterocolitis, particularly in patients whose bowel bacterial flora has been altered by previous antibiotic treatment.

Predominantly Macrophage Cellular Reactions

Salmonella typhi, the organism responsible for typhoid fever, does not elicit a neutrophil response, although *in vitro* it is chemotactic for the neutrophil. The lesions of typhoid, which may occur in the gut, lymph nodes, liver and less often at other sites, are therefore characterized by a cellular infiltrate in which the macrophage is the predominant cell.

Haemorrhagic Inflammation

Some organisms attack small blood vessels and thus produce lesions in which bleeding is a prominent feature. This is seen in certain rickettsial diseases such as typhus, in anthrax, and in some cases of pneumonia caused by the influenza virus.

Fibrinoid Necrosis

Inflammatory reactions resulting from the impaction or formation of antigen–antibody complexes in small blood vessels or from irradiation are characterized by a

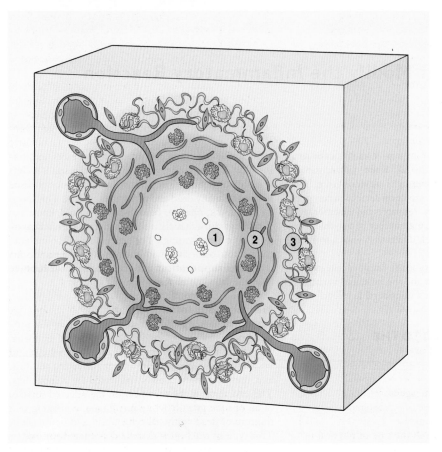

FIGURE 6.1 The architecture of an abscess showing the different zones: (1) liquefied dead tissue containing dead and dying neutrophils (pus); (2) fibrin and living neutrophils; (3) membrane composed of proliferating fibroblasts, macrophages, collagen fibres and new blood vessels.

tissue reaction in which both blood vessels and intercellular collagen show a curious form of necrosis. In sections conventionally stained with haematoxylin and eosin, the affected vessels or collagen fibres show a smudgy appearance and are deeply eosinophilic. Appropriate special stains show fibrin to be present in these areas, and this type of tissue damage is accordingly known as **fibrinoid necrosis** (see pp 129–130).

Extension of Inflammatory Processes

In cases in which the inflammatory reaction is due to infection by a pathogenic microorganism, the ability of the organism to spread through the tissues is an important modifying factor. Of prime importance in the natural history of the disease is whether the tissue reaction maintains a localized infection or whether spread to surrounding tissues or distant sites occurs. Factors that may influence this include:

- Release of **spreading factors** by infective agents. A wide variety of such agents exists, including exotoxins that can hydrolyse the mucopolysaccharide ground substance in the extracellular space, such as the hyaluronidase produced by both *Streptococcus pyogenes* and *Clostridium perfringens,* both of which characteristically cause spreading types of inflammation. Streptococci produce streptokinase, which lyses the polymerized fibrin laid down in the course of formation of the protein-rich inflammatory exudate; this too may inhibit attempts to localize the infection. The clostridia that produce **gas gangrene** (*C. perfringens, C. oedematiens* and *C. septicum)*, in addition to producing exotoxins such as hyaluronidase and collagenase which facilitate spreading of infection, also modify the local reaction by the release of powerful necrotizing toxins which break down muscle (see pp 20–21). The muscle carbohydrate is then fermented by appropriate enzymes also produced by these organisms, forming bubbles of gas which make the affected tissues feel crepitant (crackly).

- **Lymphatic blockage** may assist in localization of infection, presumably mediated by coagulation of lymph with the formation of fibrin, and appears to be inhibited if the invading pathogen (such as *S. pyogenes*) is able to elaborate lytic enzymes.

- The **susceptibility** of infecting microorganisms to the normal defensive process of **phagocytosis** is obviously an important variable in the shaping of events that follow infection. Some organisms have surface material (capsules) which makes phagocytosis difficult. This material may be carbohydrate in nature, such as the capsular polysaccharide of the *Pneumococcus*, or a protein. *S. aureus* has a protein (protein A) in its wall which combines with the Fc fragment of antibody attached to the organism and thus blocks attachment of this fragment to the Fc receptor on the phagocyte.

  S. pyogenes and *S. aureus* produce toxins that can kill the threatening phagocytes. These few examples serve to indicate the range of defensive options evolved by prokaryotes against phagocytosis and killing.

FACTORS RELATED TO THE HOST

Factors related to the **host** operate predominantly, but not exclusively, in relation to the injuries produced by microorganisms. Some of these factors may be inferred from material presented in earlier sections, especially in relation to chemotaxis, phagocytosis and bacterial killing (see Chapter 5).

The general physiological state of the host is clearly important; if the host is debilitated, undernourished or severely anaemic, infections that under normal circumstances might be regarded as fairly trivial may become life threatening. For example, measles, which occurs principally in childhood, is a disorder regarded as mildly unpleasant and inconvenient. In populations where malnutrition is rife, measles is a major cause of death in infants and children.

Just as defects in the phagocyte system render the host more susceptible to infection, so do defects in the B- and T-cell elements of the immune system. Such defects may occur as part of a congenital syndrome or may be acquired either through some disease process associated with immunosuppression (such as acquired immune deficiency syndrome or Hodgkin's disease). Immunodeficiency may also result from treatment in which immunosuppression is induced either deliberately (as in patients receiving allogeneic transplants) or as a side-effect (as in patients receiving cytotoxic therapy for malignant neoplastic processes, particularly those involving the lymphoreticular system).

CLASSIFICATION OF AN INFLAMMATORY REACTION

The classification of an inflammatory lesion can be regarded essentially as an exercise in simple **set theory**. The **sets** that can usefully be considered are:

- **duration** of the inflammatory reaction
- **type of exudate** associated with the particular type of injury. This may be:
  a) serous
  b) fibrinous
  c) haemorrhagic
  d) catarrhal
  e) purulent (suppurative)
  f) membranous or pseudomembranous
  g) a combination of the above
- The influence on lesion morphology and natural history of the **anatomical location** of the injury. This can be considered under the following simple headings:
  a) **solid tissue**
  b) **epithelium-lined surfaces**
  c) **serosal surfaces**

Examples of the use of a **common set** as an expression of a particular inflammatory reaction are shown in *Fig. 6.2*.

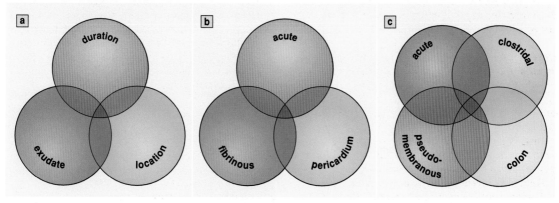

FIGURE 6.2 *Use of set theory to categorize inflammatory reactions.* **a** *chosen sets;* **b** *fibrinous pericarditis;* **c** *pseudomembranous colitis.*

DURATION OF INFLAMMATORY PROCESSES

If the duration of the inflammatory reaction is fairly short (e.g. days) it is termed **acute**. A reaction lasting for some weeks is termed **subacute**, and long-lasting inflammatory reactions (months or even years) are described as **chronic**.

TYPES OF EXUDATE (*Fig. 6.3*)

Serous Exudate

This is characterized by the outpouring of fluid with a rather low protein content, in particular of fibrinogen so that there is little formation of polymerized fibrin strands. This type of reaction is frequently seen in relation to surfaces lined by mesothelial cells, such as the joint spaces or pleural cavities. The fluid that accumulates in a common blister, such as that seen after mild repetitive trauma (e.g. chopping wood or rowing by those not used to the exercise), is a typical example of serous exudation. Similar serous effusions are seen not uncommonly as an expression of tuberculous pleurisy, particularly in young adults.

Fibrinous Exudate (*Figs. 6.4* and *6.5*)

This type of exudate is rather lower in volume than the serous type, and has a high protein content, with large amounts of fibrinogen that is converted to fibrin. It tends to occur particularly in relation to serosa-lined cavities such as pleura, pericardium and peritoneum. The mesothelial linings involved characteristically lose their moist, shiny-looking surface. This becomes dull, granular and opaque as the linings become covered by polymerized fibrin. Clinically, fibrinous serosal exudates are associated with pain elicited by movement of

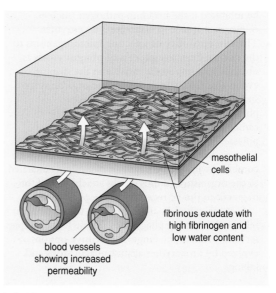

FIGURE 6.4 *Fibrinous exudates (high in protein, low in water) tend particularly to affect mesothelium-lined membranes.*

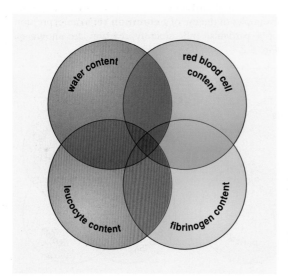

FIGURE 6.3 *The character of an inflammatory exudate is determined by the relative proportions of these components.*

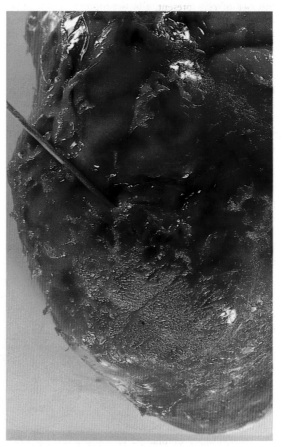

FIGURE 6.5 *Fibrinous pericarditis elicited by underlying myocardial necrosis due to ischaemia (infarct).*

the underlying viscera. Thus in patients with fibrinous pleurisy, inhalation causes a 'catch' in the breath due to pain. On clinical examination, auscultation reveals a creaking sound known as a 'friction rub'.

Two contiguous surfaces covered in fibrin tend to stick together, and, if the fibrin is not lysed later in the inflammatory process, bridges of scar tissue are formed, with permanent loss of function. One important example is postinflammatory stenosis of the aortic or mitral valves.

Haemorrhagic Exudate

This is usually an example of fibrinous exudation where damage to small blood vessels has been sufficiently severe to allow the escape of red cells from the lumen into the extravascular space. This may be seen in certain bacterial infections such as anthrax, in rickettsial infections such as typhus and rocky mountain spotted fever, and in some viral conditions such as influenzal pneumonia.

Purulent Exudate

As indicated above, certain pathogenic microorganisms elicit an inflammatory reaction in which the neutrophil is the dominant element. Largely because of the large number of cells present, the exudate is opaque. The organisms concerned often also liberate toxins that produce tissue necrosis, and the lysosomal enzymes liberated from the dying neutrophils cause liquefaction of the dead tissue, so that the centre of the lesion consists of the fluid material called pus. Not infrequently a combination of fibrinous and purulent exudation is seen, often in relation to serous surfaces such as the peritoneum. This is called a fibrinopurulent exudate.

Catarrhal Exudate

This variety of exudate is usually seen where mucous membranes are involved in inflammatory reactions. The exudate is initially serous in character, but this phase is followed by a profuse discharge of mucus from the glands of the mucosa which converts the exudate into sticky viscous material. An upper respiratory tract viral infection, such as a common 'cold', is a good example of such a reaction.

Membranous and pseudomembranous exudates are considered on pp 63, 535.

ANATOMICAL LOCATION AND THE INFLAMMATORY REACTION

The type of tissue in which injury and the consequent inflammatory reaction take place affects the course of events and hence the structural changes that occur.

Abscess Formation

If the injury takes place in the substance of what one might regard as a **solid block** of tissue such as the dermis, liver, kidney or brain, and the causal agent is a pyogenic organism, suppuration is likely to occur. The process takes two forms:

1) If the process is localized, the lesion with its necrotic pus-filled centre is termed an **abscess**.
2) If the inflammatory reaction is a spreading one, it is termed **cellulitis**.

An abscess has clearly defined zones that mirror the ongoing processes:

- The centre of the roughly spherical mass that constitutes the abscess is made up of partly or completely liquefied dead tissue admixed with the remains of dead and dying neutrophils.
- This is surrounded by a layer in which fibrin and living neutrophils are present.
- At the periphery of this is a membrane consisting largely of proliferating fibroblasts, new capillaries and young collagen fibres.
- This last layer represents the **repair process**, which is a possible line of development in the natural history of acute inflammation. This zone of fibroblastic proliferation serves as a barrier to further spread of the inflammatory process, but also prevents discharge of the abscess contents, without which healing cannot occur. It is often necessary, therefore, to lay the abscess open so that it may discharge adequately, or in some cases, such as the lung or brain, to remove the lesion completely with a rim of surrounding tissue.

Ulcers *(Fig. 6.6)*

In epithelium-lined tissue, such as the skin, gut, pharynx, larynx or trachea, a number of different reactions may occur. One, which was discussed above, is the pseudomembranous reaction, in which the surface epithelium becomes necrotic and, together with fibrin and inflammatory cells, forms part of a membrane which can be detached showing the raw, subepithelial tissue beneath. A more common type of inflammatory lesion in epithelial surfaces is the **ulcer**. An ulcer can be defined as a local defect in an epithelial surface, the defect being produced by the shedding of dead epithelial cells.

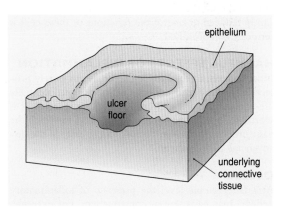

FIGURE 6.6 The basic architecture of ulceration: a local defect in an epithelial surface.

Inflammation on Serosal Surfaces

On serosal surfaces such as the pleura or peritoneum, the reaction is usually serous, fibrinous or fibrinopurulent. Because of the arrangement of the tissue in what are basically flat mesothelium-lined sheets, there is little or no tendency for the process to become localized other than by the 'glueing' together of contiguous affected membranes.

BIOLOGICAL EFFECTS OF THE INFLAMMATORY REACTION

ROLE OF THE EXUDATE

The outpouring of fluid exudate can be protective in a number of ways.

- **Dilution.** If the injurious agent is a chemical poison or if, in the course of infection, tissue-damaging exotoxins are released by the pathogen, the fluid exudate might **dilute** the toxin.
- **Bacterial killing by antibody and complement.** As exudation implies escape from the microcirculation of proteins as well as fluid and solute, antibodies and complement are likely to form part of the exudate and will contribute to the killing of microorganisms and/or the neutralization of their toxins.
- **Localization.** The transformation of fibrinogen to fibrin and the polymerization of the latter into tough strands may serve some **localizing function**, and the presence of fibrin assists the **phagocytosis** of non-opsonized organisms; this process is known as **surface phagocytosis**.

ROLE OF PHAGOCYTIC CELLS

At the risk of being repetitious, it must be said that the benefit accruing to the host through the action of phagocytic cells is obvious. The protective role of these cells as a primary means of defence against the consequences of infection is made clear by the greatly enhanced risk of serious infections in patients in whom either the number of circulating neutrophils is significantly reduced or one of the functions of these cells is seriously compromised.

HARMFUL EFFECTS OF INFLAMMATION

Inflammation, in the broadest sense, is not purely protective. It also forms the basis of a series of potentially life-threatening or functionally crippling diseases. It is worthwhile to examine some of the ways in which the basic processes considered above can operate to the disadvantage of the patient.

Oedema

At a fairly simple level the presence of inflammatory oedema may have serious consequences. For example, if the larynx is involved in a patient with a parainfluenza virus infection of the upper respiratory tract, laryngeal oedema may develop and obstruct normal airflow through the fairly narrow lumen of the larynx. The patient will experience great difficulty in breathing, the inspiratory and expiratory efforts will be accompanied by a loud noise (stridor) and the patient may become cyanotic through lack of oxygen. This event, which is comparable to being strangled, is a medical emergency. The patient may well require tracheostomy to restore normal airflow until the laryngeal oedema has subsided.

Cerebral oedema, which can occur as a consequence of inflammation as well as in certain other situations, may also have disastrous consequences. Swelling of the brain, within its rigid box, the cranium, means that any increase in pressure must be transmitted downwards and backwards through the only available potential avenue of escape, the foramen magnum. This displacement puts severe shearing stresses on the small perforating blood vessels at the base of the mid-brain and may cut off the blood supply to important areas. At post-mortem examination the presence of such displacement due to cerebral oedema may be expressed by the presence of deep grooves (formed by the pressure of the tentorium) on the mid-brain or of grooves produced in relation to the cerebellar tonsils if they have herniated through the foramen magnum.

Failure to Control Mediator Release

Very rarely, unpleasant consequences may arise from failure to control the generation of one or other of the chemical mediators of inflammation. One such example is a condition known as hereditary angioneurotic oedema, in which patients develop localized areas of oedema in a wide range of anatomical locations; the oedematous areas are often painful. This is believed to be due to the unrestrained activity of a kinin-like particle liberated in the course of activation of the C2 component of complement. Normally this is inactivated by an esterase, but in patients with this disease the inactivator substance is not synthesized.

Exudates can Cause Malfunction

In addition to the purely mechanical problems that may arise from inflammatory oedema, the presence of certain types of exudate in particular locations may produce profound and dangerous functional changes. In lobar pneumonia caused by *Streptococcus pneumoniae*, an exudate rich in fibrin is formed and this spreads through the pores of Kohn to involve large areas of lung tissue. The presence of the exudate causes some difficulty in oxygen diffusion and in gas exchange across the alveolar septa. Fortunately, in most cases blood oxygen levels are not significantly reduced, but if the process involves sufficient lung tissue a considerable disturbance in blood gases may occur. In underprivileged communities this condition is still an important cause of death, even though it has become much rarer in Western countries.

Phagocyte-mediated Tissue Damage

With respect to phagocytic cells, tissue damage may result either through some interruption of phagosome–lysosome fusion or, on a wider scale, through inappropriate triggering of some of their secretory or metabolic functions.

Examples of abnormalities in lysosomal fusion that might lead to tissue damage are found, in the case of the neutrophil, in acute gouty arthritis and, in the case of the macrophage, in silicosis. The former has already been discussed on p 15. In silicosis the silica particles are inhaled and deposited in the respiratory bronchioles. They are then phagocytosed in the normal way by macrophages and come to lie within phagosomes. Silicic acid forms on the surface of the silica particles and, when the primary lysosome fuses with the silica-containing phagosome, hydrogen bonds form between the silicic acid and the lysosomal membrane. This leads to rupture of the lysosomal membrane with spillage of its enzymes into the cytoplasm. The macrophage then dies and the lysosomal enzymes and the offending silica particle are released into the interstitial tissue. The lysosomal enzymes (which include collagenase and elastase) cause tissue damage, and the silica particle is once again available for phagocytosis, so the cycle starts again.

It is not unlikely that phagocytic cells may secrete lysosomal enzymes in response to a variety of stimuli. The potential ill effects of such secretion are avoided by the presence within both plasma and extracellular fluid of glycoproteins that inhibit the proteolytic effects of lysosomal enzymes. As in so many fields of pathobiology, the importance of such inhibitory mechanisms is discovered only when they fail. An example of this can be seen in the inherited condition known as **α₁-antitrypsin deficiency**. The ability to synthesize this protease inhibitor (in the liver) is governed by possession of a normal allelic pair of genes. Absence or mutation of both members of this pair renders the affected person homozygous for the deficiency; such people may develop destruction of the alveolar and bronchiolar walls in the lung leading to **panacinar emphysema** and may also have an enhanced risk for liver damage leading to **cirrhosis**. Absence or mutation of one member of the pair of genes (the heterozygous state) leads to an increased risk of lung damage if the subject is a smoker, although he or she will not as a rule develop signs of tissue damage if other potential noxious substances, such as smoke, are avoided.

Phagocytes Release Free Radicals

Another way in which tissue damage may be brought about by the action of phagocytic cells is by the release of oxygen-derived free radicals. Many experimental studies have shown that oxygen metabolites released from activated neutrophils and macrophages may be toxic to a wide variety of eukaryotic cells, including red cells, endothelial cells, fibroblasts, tumour cells, platelets and spermatozoa (see pp 13–15). Damage to endothelial cells, especially in the pulmonary capillary bed, can certainly be produced by oxygen-derived free radicals and this may be the most important pathogenetic mechanism underlying the respiratory distress syndrome seen in association with a number of clinical states.

Immune Complexes Cause Tissue Damage

Another area in which such a mechanism may be operative is the tissue damage that follows lodgement of antigen–antibody complexes in various locations. Such lodgement is often associated with the presence of phagocytic cells, and in experimental systems tissue damage may be avoided by the administration of superoxide dismutase, even though the normal inflammatory cell response takes place. Similarly in experimentally produced antigen–antibody complex-mediated injury in the lung, tissue damage can be reduced by administering catalase, whereas antiproteases have no such protective effect. Much work still remains to be done in humans to define the role of oxygen metabolites in tissue injury but it is almost certainly a major role-player in pathology (see also pp 13–15).

CHAPTER 7

The Natural History of Acute Inflammation I: Healing

A wide spectrum of biological events may follow tissue injury and the inflammatory reaction elicited by it. These include:

- a complete return to functional and structural normality (**resolution**)
- the replacement of lost tissue by scar tissue (**healing by repair**)
- persistence of the inflammatory process for weeks, months or years (**chronicity**)

Factors determining which of these will follow a given inflammatory reaction include:

- the nature of the injury
- the tissue target
- the host response

The spectrum of possible events is shown in *Fig. 7.1*. It involves the operation of one or more of the following processes which, in phylogenetic terms, are some of the oldest known. These are:

- **removal** via a number of different mechanisms of **foreign material** whether living or dead, exogenous or endogenous
- **clearance** from the tissues of the cellular and other elements of the inflammatory response
- **regeneration** of lost tissue components where this is possible
- **replacement** of lost tissue elements by **connective tissue** with an adequate blood supply

RESOLUTION

This term indicates that an inflamed area of an organ or tissue has returned to the **state existing before the injury that elicited the inflammatory reaction**. It implies that no significant loss of tissue has occurred: the injury was sufficiently severe that it caused inflammation, but not so severe that it produced tissue necrosis. Central to resolution is complete removal of inflammatory exudate. This process is accomplished largely via proteolysis, but phagocytosis of the exudate by macrophages also plays a part.

The natural history of lobar pneumonia provides a striking example of resolution. This is an acute inflammatory disorder affecting lung parenchyma and involving large areas of lung tissue in continuity. The sequence of events (*Fig. 7.2*) occurring in this disease is as follows:

- Invasion of the air spaces by *Streptococcus pneumoniae*

elicits a severe acute inflammatory reaction. This is characterized by the outpouring of an exudate, initially rich in fibrin and poor in cells, into the affected alveoli.

- This process spreads rapidly through the adjacent air spaces, involving extensive areas of lung tissue. Inflammatory cells migrate into the fibrin-rich exudate; while viable organisms are still present, most of these are neutrophils. The neutrophils engulf and kill most of the organisms, many neutrophils themselves dying in the course of this process.

  The affected lobes of the lungs of patients who die at this stage are red, fleshy and airless. Microscopic examination shows the dilatation of alveolar capillaries typical of acute inflammation, and air spaces filled with exudate. There is, however, *no* necrosis of the alveolar septa.

- Once the organisms have been cleared, the nature of the cellular infiltrate changes. Macrophages are recruited to the affected areas and become the dominant cellular element. The fibrin-rich element begins to undergo lysis, which is brought about largely by the action of plasmin. Plasmin is generated from plasminogen by plasminogen activator released from infiltrating macrophages.

- The macrophages phagocytose much of the cellular and bacterial debris. Secretion of lysosomal enzymes by reverse endocytosis accounts for the breakdown of the material that has not been phagocytosed. The lysed exudate drains from the lung tissue via the lymphatics; the protein content of this lymph is higher than that draining non-inflamed lung tissue. At the end of the sequence of events, all the exudate should have been removed and the air spaces return to normal both structurally and functionally. Failure to remove the exudate will trigger the process of organization, discussed below.

ORGANIZATION

If demolition of inflammatory exudate fails and the exudate persists, a set of processes known as **organization** is triggered. The exudate is infiltrated by numerous macrophages, followed by the migration of fibroblasts and new small blood vessels into the exudate. The whole process is more or less identical with the

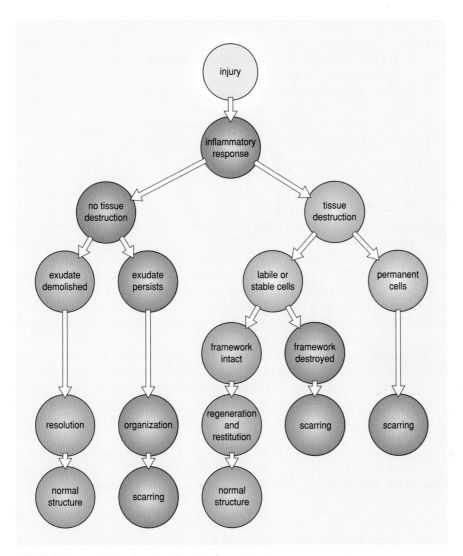

FIGURE 7.1 Possible natural history of acute inflammation.

repair of connective tissue that occurs in wound healing. Eventually the exudate is replaced by well-vascularized fibrous tissue and, finally, once the new blood vessels have died back, by dense collagen-rich scar tissue.

It is worth remembering that basic tissue processes such as this may occur in a number of different contexts. Thus organization is triggered not only by persisting inflammatory exudate, but also by unlysed blood clot or thrombus and by necrotic areas in tissue that cannot regenerate, such as the myocardium.

Some Clinical Consequences of Organization

Organization of persisting inflammatory exudate can lead to some highly disadvantageous clinical scenarios. Examples include:

- In the peritoneal cavity, persistence of exudate leads to the formation of fibrous tissue strands. These connect either adjacent loops of bowel or the serosal surface of segments of bowel and the abdominal wall. Such adhesions may lead to acute or subacute intestinal obstruction at some future time.
- Organization in other serosal cavities – the pleural cavity or pericardial sac may cause obliteration of these spaces. In **constrictive pericarditis**, which may follow tuberculosis, the heart becomes ensheathed in a thick unyielding layer of fibrous tissue. This interferes with both diastolic compliance (relaxation of the walls of the heart chambers during diastole) and systolic contraction, and leads to severe congestive failure which can be relieved only by surgical stripping of the fibrous tissue layer.

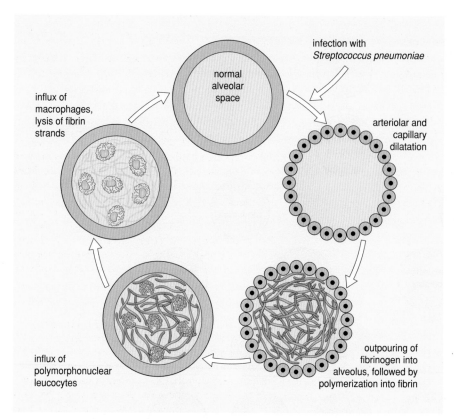

FIGURE 7.2 Natural history of lobar pneumonia terminating in resolution.

- In the lung affected by pneumonia, persistence of exudate leads to the affected air spaces becoming filled with connective tissue. This produces a solid meaty consistency instead of the normal spongy one characteristic of the lung; this is obviously associated with failure to ventilate the affected area and of normal gas exchange.

REGENERATION

Tissue that has been destroyed as a result of injury or inflammation must be replaced, if possible, by new living tissue. Ideally this is accomplished by a triggering of proliferation of the normal cellular constituents of the damaged organ or tissue, to replace the cells lost by injury.

If this tissue replacement takes place in an orderly fashion, not only are the lost tissue elements replicated but the normal architectural pattern is restored so that the tissue is 'as good as new'. This process is known as **regeneration** and operates most effectively in non-mammalian species such as the salamander, which can successfully replace amputated limbs.

Successful regeneration depends on two factors:

1) Lost cells must be of a type capable of being replaced by identical cells.
2) The normal architecture of connective tissue and blood vessels in the affected area must be either preserved or restored as it was before injury.

Influence of Lost Cell Type on Regeneration

In relation to regeneration, cells can be classified into three basic types:
1) **labile cells**
2) **stable cells**
3) **permanent cells**

Labile Cells

Labile cells are derived from the mitotic division of stem cells. The defining criteria of stem cells are that they:
- are not themselves terminally differentiated
- have no fixed limit on their capacity to divide during the lifetime of an animal
- give rise to daughter cells that can either remain stem cells or embark on a terminal differentiation pathway

Stem cell populations exist where a replacement mechanism is needed for differentiated cells that cannot themselves divide. These differentiated cells often have a rather short life and, hence, a high turnover rate. For example, a fully developed red blood cell cannot divide because it has no nucleus. The epidermis of the **skin** and the epithelium of the **small gut** are other striking examples of cell populations whose size is governed by stem cell activity.

Basically, labile cells fall into two groups:
1) **Covering epithelia.** These include:
   a) stratified squamous epithelium of the skin, mouth, pharynx, oesophagus, vagina and cervix
   b) transitional epithelium of the urinary tract
   c) gut epithelium
   d) lining epithelium of exocrine gland ducts
   e) endometrial gland epithelium and the lining of the fallopian tubes
2) **Blood and lymphoid cells**

In both these categories, cell loss is easily made good.

Stable Cells

Stable cells are normally quiescent and have a very low rate of turnover. When such cells are lost, replacement is carried out by means of mitotic division of **mature** cells; there appears to be **no stem cell compartment**.

Stable cells include liver cells, renal tubular epithelium, secretory epithelium of endocrine glands, bone cells and fibroblasts. Their loss is followed by a marked upregulation of cell division and the lost cells are rapidly replaced. For example, if 65% of a rat's liver is removed surgically, a burst of regenerative activity occurs and within two weeks the liver will have attained normal or near-normal size.

Such regeneration involves the upregulation of endocrine, paracrine or autocrine **mitogenic signals**, and possibly also of **receptor function, signal transduction** and **expression of DNA-binding proteins**. Many of these alterations in the level of function are regulated by increased expression of certain growth-promoting genes or proto-oncogenes, of which much more will be said in the section on the origins of cancer (see pp 273–289).

In liver and renal tubular epithelial regeneration, one of the most potent factors involved is a multifunctional cytokine, **hepatocyte growth factor (HGF) (scatter factor)**. HGF is encoded by a gene on chromosome 7 and has a structure resembling that of plasminogen and other blood proteases. It is produced by various cells including fibroblasts, epithelial and endothelial cells, Küpffer cells in the liver sinusoids and lipocytes (Ito cells) in the space of Disse, also in the liver.

Its production is increased by interleukin 1 (α and β) and by a humoral substance known as **injurin**, probably a glycosoaminoglycan, which shows increased plasma levels after partial removal of the liver. HGF exerts its effects by binding to a high-affinity receptor that is the gene product of a proto-oncogene c-*met*, expressed on a variety of cell types. Interestingly, liver cells show increased expression of c-*met* after liver injury, but this returns to normal soon afterwards. This suggests that normal tissue proliferation may be controlled by changes in the expression both of genes coding for mitogenic signals and of those that encode their receptors.

Permanent Cells

These cells, having been generated in sufficient numbers during fetal life, **never divide in postnatal life and cannot be replaced if they are lost**. Almost all nerve cells are permanent in this sense, as are heart muscle cells, the auditory 'hair' cells and the cells in the lens of the eye. Why these cells should behave in this way is not understood. Permanence in this context seems biologically unhelpful, although it may be that, in the case of the central nervous system, if neurones regenerated, establishment of the appropriate connections in the central nervous system might be difficult.

Preservation or Restoration of a Normal Stromal Framework is Essential for a Return to Normality

The replacement of lost cells by proliferation is only part of the process leading to a return to normal structure of an injured and inflamed tissue, albeit the most important. If the architectural arrangement of the connective tissue framework of an organ or tissue is destroyed, the arrangement of the regenerating cells will be disturbed; this can have serious consequences for the function of the affected tissue.

The natural history of some cases of liver necrosis is a good example of this type of event. The stable hepatocytes show a striking ability to proliferate by mitosis after injury sufficiently severe to lead to liver cell death. This is demonstrated by the regeneration following partial hepatectomy in the rat, mentioned above.

In certain cases of either acute massive necrosis or ongoing necrosis of relatively small numbers of cells, the connective tissue framework may either be destroyed or may collapse. In addition, the hepatic stellate cells (Ito cells) in the space of Disse may secrete connective tissue matrix proteins which form septa growing into the liver acini, producing marked architectural disturbance.

In these circumstances, the regenerating hepatocytes grow in the form of disorganized nodules, instead of being arranged in an orderly fashion in relation to sinusoids and bile canaliculi. Thus normal hepatic **mass** may be restored but not normal hepatic architecture.

This sequence of events leads, for example, to marked disturbance in blood flow patterns of the liver, in which blood is normally conducted from the terminal branches of the portal vein and hepatic artery to the terminal hepatic venules. This causes abnormally high pressure in the portal venous system (portal hypertension) and portal blood becomes shunted into the systemic circulation with profound and disadvantageous metabolic effects. This abnormal regeneration pattern and its functional consequences are important parts of the pathological and clinical picture seen in **cirrhosis** of the liver.

Both organization of exudate etc. and failure to restore the connective tissue framework to normal result in the formation of scar tissue. **Scarring is an essential component of wound healing**, which provides a useful model to study the events and controlling mechanisms that underlie scarring. This is discussed in Chapter 8.

The Natural History of Acute Inflammation II: Wound Healing

The biological objectives of wound healing are **twofold** (*Fig. 8.1*):

1) **To restore the integrity of epithelial surfaces, should this have been lost.** In this way, the underlying tissues are protected against:
   a) an abnormal environment leading to inappropriate drying or wetting of the exposed surface
   b) infection
   c) entry of non-living foreign material
2) **To restore the tensile strength of the subepithelial tissue.**

HEALING BY PRIMARY AND SECONDARY 'INTENTION'

Whatever the type of wound, the basic mechanisms involved in healing are the same, the differences described being largely of **degree** rather than of **kind**.

- **Primary intention** (*Fig. 8.2a*). By convention, the healing of cleanly incised, easily suturable wounds, where the edges are in close apposition, is termed healing by 'primary intention'.
- **Secondary intention** (*Fig. 8.2b*). Wounds in which there is extensive loss of epithelium, with a large subepithelial tissue defect that has to be filled in by scar tissue, and where the edges cannot be

brought together with sutures, are said to be healed by 'secondary intention'.

HEALING OF AN INCISED WOUND

Incision involves the division of:
- epidermis
- dermal connective tissue fibres and matrix
- subcutaneous tissue and, in some cases, deeper tissue layers
- blood vessels

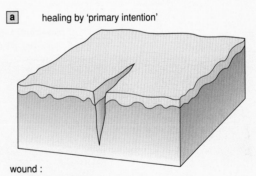

a healing by 'primary intention'

wound :
- is cleanly incised
- edges are in close apposition
- is easily suturable

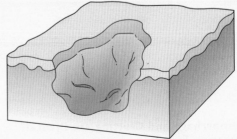

b healing by 'secondary intention'

wound is characterized by :
- extensive epithelial loss
- large subepithelial tissue defect which is filled by granulation tissue, this being followed by extensive scarring
- edges that cannot be brought together with sutures

FIGURE 8.2 *Healing by* ***a*** *'primary intention' and* ***b*** *'secondary intention'.*

epithelial regeneration / connective tissue repair

prevents:
- inappropriate wetting or drying of exposed subepithelial elements
- infection
- entry of non-living foreign material

restores:
- tensile strength of subepithelial connective tissue

FIGURE 8.1 *The basic components of wound healing and their biological purpose.*

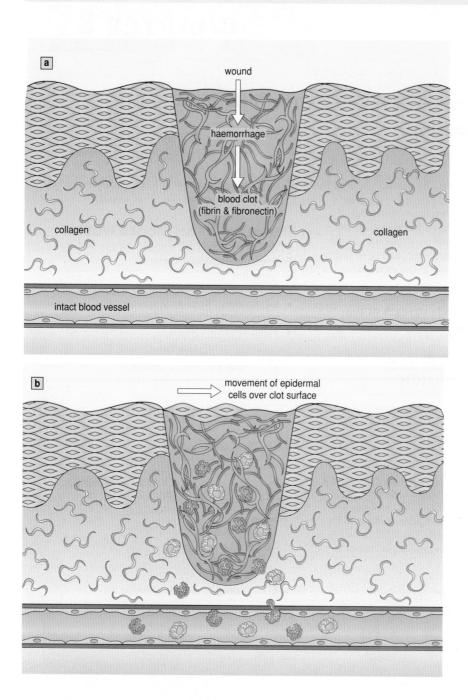

Haemorrhage and Clotting are Pivotal Triggering Events

Severing of blood vessels obviously leads to haemorrhage. This results in accumulation within the tissue defect of platelets and, pre-eminently among the plasma proteins, **fibrinogen** and **fibronectin**. Clotting mechanisms are activated; fibrinogen is converted to polymerized fibrin. This is stabilized by fibronectin binding to it by means of a glutaminase bridge.

The gel formed by fibrin and fibronectin acts in the early stages of healing as a 'glue', which helps to keep the severed edges of the tissue apposed.

Morphological Events in Healing *(Fig. 8.3)*

Morphological events can be considered under two headings:

  1) those that concern the **epidermis**
  2) those taking place within the **dermis**

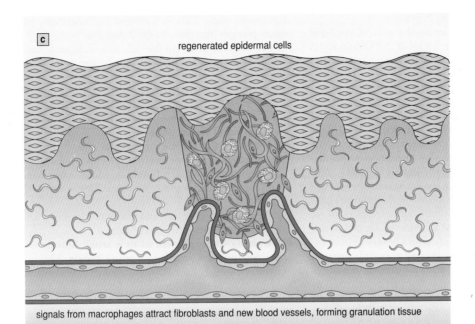

signals from macrophages attract fibroblasts and new blood vessels, forming granulation tissue

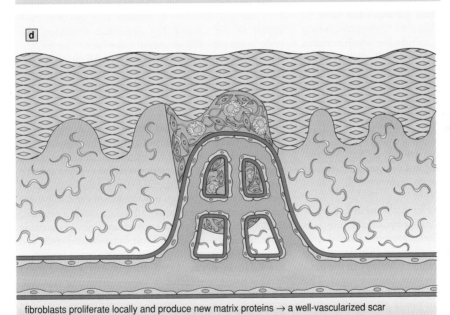

fibroblasts proliferate locally and produce new matrix proteins → a well-vascularized scar

FIGURE 8.3 **a–d** *The stages of wound healing.*

Epidermal Events

Within a few hours of wounding, a single layer of epidermal cells starts to **migrate** from the wound edges to form a delicate covering over the raw area exposed by the loss of epidermis.

This migratory process can be studied *in vitro* by observing the behaviour of epidermal cells when small cubes of excised skin are cultured at 37°C in appropriate nutrient media. Under these circumstances, the epidermal cells begin to spread over the five raw dermal faces and, eventually, the whole cube of dermal tissue is enclosed by epidermis like a small parcel. This spreading process is called **epiboly**. The idea that cell movement plays a significant part in this is supported by the fact that substances, such as cytochalasin B, that are known to interfere with cell migration inhibit epiboly.

Mechanisms Involved in Cell Migration

Epidermal cell migration across the area of epithelial loss depends on interaction between the keratinocytes at or near the wound edges and the extracellular matrix glycoprotein **fibronectin**.

The fibronectins are large two-chained glycoproteins which are present in plasma and tissues. They exert much of their effect by providing sites that act as ligands for receptors on a wide variety of cell types. This ligand–receptor binding mediates **cell matrix adhesion**. The binding sites often include the tripeptide **arginine–glycine–aspartate** (colloquially known as **RGD** sites). The receptors on cells, which serve as ligands for the RGD sequence, belong to what is known as the **integrin** family of receptors, which includes surface molecules on phagocytic cells that mediate adhesion to the endothelial cells in the microcirculation (see pp 43–44).

Differences between plasma and tissue fibronectins appear to be mediated by post-translational modifications, differences in splicing being particularly important. In relation to the epidermis in wounds, the type of splicing of fibronectin messenger RNA (mRNA) resembles that found in early embryogenesis.

Keratinocytes from **normal unwounded skin** do not possess receptors that bind to fibronectin, being tightly attached to basement membrane which contains laminin and collagen type IV. Those derived from wounds, however, express a fibronectin receptor. The activated keratinocytes preferentially adhere to the RGD sequences on the fibronectin and thus migrate across and, indeed, through the fibronectin-rich matrix.

Epithelial Cell Proliferation

Epidermal cell movement can provide an initial covering for very small wounds but, in most instances, epithelial re-covering cannot be accomplished without **proliferation** of epidermal cells.

The new cells are derived from the stem cell compartment of the epidermal cell population, which is made up of the basal cells just above the dermal–epidermal junction. From about 12 hours after wounding, there is a marked increase in mitotic activity in the basal cells, about three to five cells from the cut edges. The new epidermal cells grow under the surface fibrin–fibronectin clot and for a little distance down the gap between the cut edges to form a small 'spur' of epithelium which, afterwards, regresses. If the wound has been sutured, a similar downgrowth of new epidermis occurs in relation to the suture tracks. On occasion, these may form the basis of keratin-forming cysts within the dermis – so-called 'implantation dermoid cysts'.

Dermal Events

Cellular Infiltration

Within the first few hours after wounding a mild acute inflammatory reaction takes place with the usual influx of **neutrophils** into and around the wound (0–1 day after wounding). This is followed by migration of **macrophages** into this area (1–2 days after wounding) – a key event as these are the cells that orchestrate the complex interplay of chemical signals that now takes place.

Viewed in an operational sense the objectives of this phase of the healing process are:

- **To demolish and remove any inflammatory exudate and tissue debris**
- **To restore the tensile strength of the subepithelial connective tissue.** This involves:
  a) chemoattraction of fibroblasts, which synthesize and secrete collagen and other connective tissue proteins
  b) stimulation of these and resident fibroblasts to proliferate and secrete matrix proteins
- **To cause the ingrowth of new small blood vessels into the area undergoing repair.** This involves:
  a) budding of new endothelial cells from small intact blood vessels at the edges of the wound
  b) chemoattraction of these new endothelial cells into the fibrin–fibronectin gel within the wounded area

In a surgical incision, fibroblasts and myofibroblasts appear in the wound 2–4 days after wounding and endothelial cells follow about 1 day later. The infiltration of macrophages and fibroblast proliferation are followed, as stated above, by the ingrowth of new capillary buds derived from intact dermal vessels at the margins of the wound.

Formation of Granulation Tissue

Initially these buds consist of solid ingrowths of endothelial cells but they soon acquire a lumen. Local degradation of the basement membrane of the existing capillary is an essential starting step for the ingrowth of new vessels. At this stage newly formed capillaries have little basement membrane substance, and, compared with a normal capillary, are extremely leaky. This richly vascularized gel in which both inflammatory cells and collagen-producing fibroblasts are present is known as **granulation tissue** (*Fig. 8.4*).

This name, a misnomer, derives from the fact that, when the raw surface of a large wound is inspected, it shows a granular appearance somewhat like the surface of a strawberry.

Collagen Production

The ultimate development of tensile strength in a wound depends on:

- the production of adequate amounts of collagen
- the final orientation of the collagen

Collagen is the only protein that contains large amounts of the amino acids hydroxyproline and hydroxylysine. Within 24 hours of wounding, protein-bound hydroxyproline appears within the damaged area, and within 2–3 days some fibrillar material may be seen. However, this lacks the dimensions and the typical 64-

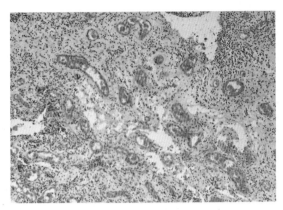

FIGURE 8.4 *Granulation tissue showing numerous new capillaries set in a background of mixed inflammatory cells.*

nm banding of polymerized collagen. Within a few weeks of the infliction of a surgical wound the **amount** of collagen in the wounded area is normal, although preoperative tensile strength is not regained for some months. This suggests that replacement and remodelling of the collagen formed early in wound healing is an important part of the whole process.

Each type of collagen (there are about 12, of which types I, II and III are the chief fibrillar collagens) consists of three peptide α chains wound round each other in a helical pattern. These chains are synthesized in the rough endoplasmic reticulum of the fibroblast following translation of the mRNA for each one. They then undergo post-translational hydroxylation of the proline and lysine moieties, and the hydroxylysine is then glycosylated.

Linkage of the three chains is accomplished by means of disulphide bonds. The three chains then become twisted into a helix and the molecule passes to the Golgi zone. Assisted by the microtubules, the soluble procollagen molecules are secreted into the extracellular environment. Solubility is conferred by the presence of an extra peptide. This is removed extracellularly by a peptidase and the cleaved molecules then assemble into fibres, which gain tensile strength by cross-linking. The typical periodicity of the collagen fibres is due to the staggered arrangement of the assembled molecules.

On some occasions, the control mechanisms that determine an appropriate amount of new collagen for healing a given wound are faulty, and excess collagen may be formed leading to the formation of a bulky scar which stands proud of the surrounding surface. This is known as a **keloid** (see pp 1104–1105).

HEALING OF WOUNDS WITH A LARGE TISSUE DEFECT

A large volume of tissue loss can occur in cases of severe trauma or extensive burns or, much less frequently, in relation to certain surgical procedures.

- **Qualitatively** there are few differences between the healing of such a wound and that of an incised wound.
- **Quantitatively** there are differences, as the formation of granulation tissue and ultimately of scar tissue is on a far larger scale than in incised wounds.

One feature of the healing process in large tissue defects not seen in relation to healing of incised wounds is **wound contraction**.

WOUND CONTRACTION

Two or three days after the formation of large open wounds, the area of raw tissue starts to decrease. This is the expression of a real movement of the wound margins and is quite independent of the rate at which covering by a new epithelial layer can take place.

Wound contraction occurs at a time when relatively little new collagen is being formed in the dermis and subcutaneous tissue. It seems, therefore, unlikely that shortening of collagen fibres at the wound margins is responsible for the contraction.

A currently favoured hypothesis is that the contraction is brought about by the action of cells appearing at the margins of the wound in the first few days. On electron microscopy, these show features suggesting both fibroblast and smooth muscle differentiation. This has led to the term **myofibroblast** being applied to them. Use of appropriate antibodies shows that these cells contain actin, but no smooth muscle-type myosin has been found within their cytoplasm.

In any circumstances, for a pulling force to be exerted there must be a connection between the object being pulled and whatever is applying the force. In wound contraction, the connection is thought to be provided by **fibronectin** molecules, which form bridges between collagen fibres on the one hand and receptors on the myofibroblasts on the other.

Strips of granulation tissue from healing wounds can be made to shorten *in vitro* by pharmacological agents that cause actin fibrils to contract. It has been postulated that a similar mechanism is responsible for the contracture of dermal connective tissue seen in such conditions as Dupuytren's contracture.

GROWTH FACTORS AND CYTOKINES IN WOUND HEALING

It is clear from what has been said above that the cellular events in wound healing must depend on a series of 'instructions' which:
- cause the cells concerned in repair, e.g. fibroblasts, epithelial cells and endothelial cells, to **migrate** into the wound.
- cause these cells and also the epithelial cells that must cover the raw surface to **proliferate**.

These instructions consist of a set of chemical signals

derived from a number of sources. Some, whose principal function is to exert a mitogenic effect on the cells to which they bind, are known as **growth factors**. The other, derived chiefly from inflammatory cells, are known as **cytokines, and these have many regulatory functions** (see pp 52–54).

GROWTH FACTORS

Growth factors are peptides that may reach their specific targets via one or more of three pathways (*Fig. 8.5*):

1) **The endocrine pathway**, where growth factors are synthesized at some considerable distance from their targets and are delivered to them via the bloodstream.

2) **The paracrine pathway**, where growth factors are synthesized and released by cells that are in the close neighbourhood of their targets.

3) **The autocrine pathway**, in which the same cells both synthesize and use the growth factor.

Growth factors can be divided into two groups depending on the phase in the life of a stem cell during which they operate: a **competence** growth factor is capable of moving a cell out of the G0 phase back into cycle, whereas a **progression** growth factor has a mitogenic effect only on cells that are not in the G0 phase.

Typical competence growth factors likely to be involved in the healing process are:

- **platelet-derived growth factor (PDGF)**
- **basic fibroblast growth factor (FGF)**

Progression growth factors are represented by such molecules as insulin-like growth factors 1 and 2 (the somatomedins) and epidermal growth factor (EGF).

Platelet-derived Growth Factor

The name platelet-derived growth factor is somewhat misleading in two senses. Firstly, although it is certainly stored in the α granules of platelets and released from them when the platelets are activated, PDGF is synthesized and secreted from other cells including:

- endothelial cells
- macrophages
- arterial smooth muscle cells
- cells from certain tumours

Secondly, **PDGF has a number of stimulatory functions apart from its, undoubted powerful, mitogenic effect.** In the context of healing, the most important of these is its ability to cause **chemotaxis** of mesenchymal cells into the wound (*Fig. 8.6*). PDGF also:

- increases intracellular synthesis of cholesterol and also the binding of low density lipoprotein (LDL) by increasing the number of LDL receptors expressed on the plasma membrane of the target cell
- increases prostaglandin secretion, initially by making more of the starting material (arachidonic acid) available and, later, by stimulating the synthesis of cyclo-oxygenase
- induces changes in cell shape accompanied by reorganization of actin filaments within the cells
- induces increased synthesis of RNA and protein
- is a potent vasoconstrictor

Thus PDGF can attract mesenchymal cells into the wound (with the exception of endothelial cells that do not possess the PDGF receptor) and

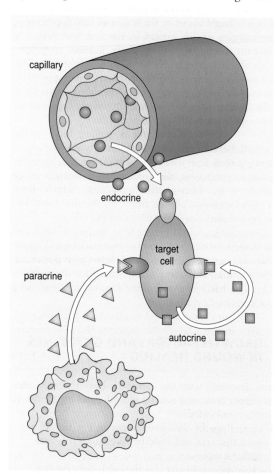

FIGURE 8.5 *Endocrine, paracrine and autocrine signalling pathways.*

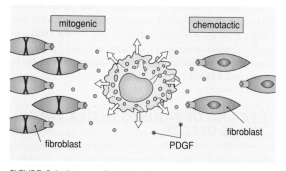

FIGURE 8.6 *Actions of platelet-derived growth factor (PDGF) in wound healing.*

acts as a mitogen for these cells and a stimulator of protein production.

PDGF and other growth factors bind to receptors which, after ligand–receptor interaction, act as tyrosine kinases. Transduction of the mitogenic signal from the cell membrane is followed, within a few minutes, by activation of the protooncogenes c-*fos* and c-*myc* (see pp 274–275) and also by the activation of genes coding for the production of the contractile protein actin and for the production of interferon β.

EGF and Transforming Growth Factor α

EGF is a 53-amino-acid polypeptide cleaved from a larger precursor protein. It was discovered in the salivary glands of baby mice. The factor was purified and is now known as EGF, although it **stimulates mitogenesis in connective tissue as well as in epithelial cells**. The salivary glands and lacrimal glands and Brunner's glands in the duodenum are all storage sites for EGF, which can be released in saliva, tears and duodenal 'juice'. Thus, 'licking one's wounds' in the literal rather than in the metaphorical sense may be of definite biological advantage, as may be the irrigation of the cornea by tears in corneal abrasion or ulceration. In rodents EGF may be found in the plasma, but in humans blood-borne EGF is concentrated within platelets, for the most part in α granules. As EGF protein is also found in the cytoplasm of megakaryocytes in the bone marrow, it seems almost certain that platelet EGF is derived from synthesis within megakaryocytes rather than by uptake from plasma.

In experimental wounds the application of EGF has been found to accelerate significantly the rate of epidermal regeneration. EGF also has a beneficial effect on the dermal component of healing in experimental wounds, causing an increase in proliferation of dermal connective tissue and in the tensile strength of incised wounds. In humans, also, topical application of EGF accelerates the healing of donor sites for skin grafts.

There is no evidence that EGF is produced by any of the cells taking part in the healing process, although, as already stated, platelets store EGF. However, another factor, known as **transforming growth factor α**, (TGF-α), shows a considerable degree of homology with EGF, and is produced in healing wounds by both epidermal cells and macrophages. **TGF-α binds to the same receptor on target cells as EGF, and has the same mitogenic effect. In this way TGF-α may be a direct mediator of wound healing** (*Fig. 8.7*).

Transforming Growth Factor β

TGF-β is a polypeptide produced by almost all cell lines in culture. In the presence of EGF it acts as a mitogen, but in some assays has also been found to inhibit growth. There is good evidence that macrophages in healing wounds express mRNA for TGF-β as well as for TGF-α. TGF-β has also been shown to be a powerful chemoattractant for monocytes, and its release

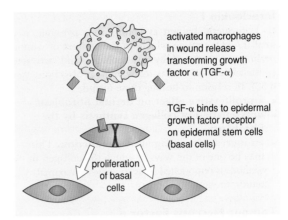

activated macrophages in wound release transforming growth factor α (TGF-α)

TGF-α binds to epidermal growth factor receptor on epidermal stem cells (basal cells)

proliferation of basal cells

FIGURE 8.7 *Epithelial regeneration in healing skin wounds.*

from the first wave of inflammatory cells migrating into the wound may act as a mechanism for recruiting additional monocyte–macrophages.

The pattern of expression of growth factors in healing wounds supports the idea that the macrophage plays a leading role in the healing process, as do observations that:

- Wound fluid stimulates cell division and promotes the ingrowth of new vessels.
- Ablation of macrophages in animals slows the process of wound healing.
- Macrophages in wounds also express other growth factors such as insulin-like growth factor 1.

CYTOKINES IN WOUND HEALING

Cytokine (see pp 52–54) is the term used for a group of protein cell regulators, which includes such members as:

- lymphokines
- monokines
- interleukins
- interferons

Growth factors could also, with some justification, be called cytokines: treating them as a separate class of regulator, as has been done here, is somewhat artificial, if convenient.

The four classes referred to above are low molecular weight proteins (usually less than 80 kDa). They tend to be produced rapidly and locally, and can act in an autocrine or paracrine fashion. They are produced by a wide range of cells and have many overlapping actions that are mediated by binding to high-affinity receptors on target cells. The response of an individual cell to a given cytokine is dependent on the cell type, other chemical signals being received at the same time and the local concentration of the cytokine.

Two cytokines that play a significant role in wound healing are:

- Interleukin 1 (IL-1)
- Tumour necrosis factor α (TNF-α) (*syn.* cachectin)

Interleukin I

IL-1, formerly known as endogenous pyrogen, is a small 17-kDa protein which, in the context of wound healing, is produced by macrophages and activated epithelial cells. IL-1 has many biological actions (see p 52). In relation to healing these include:

- **a proliferative effect on dermal fibroblasts**
- **upregulation of collagen synthesis by the fibroblasts**
- **an increase in collagenase production.** This may be one of the ways in which the collagen in wounds is remodelled so as to achieve maximal tensile strength

Tumour Necrosis Factor α

This is another monocyte–macrophage product which is released following tissue injury or infection. **It is the main factor responsible for macrophage-mediated tumour cell killing and is also responsible for the wasting (cachexia) seen in certain chronic bacterial and parasitic infections.** Its biological activity has a remarkable overlap with that of IL-1, although TNF-α does not appear to have the immunoregulatory functions of IL-1. Its receptors, however, are quite distinct from those of IL-1, and presumably the similarities in their actions indicate that they stimulate the same 'second-messenger' systems. The expression of TNF-α by monocytes and macrophages requires activation of these cells. This may be brought about in a number of ways:

- interaction with fibrin (which is always present in wounds)
- binding of TGF-β
- the action of interferon γ
- the action of endotoxin

TNF-α is a potent stimulus for the ingrowth of new blood vessels in healing wounds; it is not only chemotactic for endothelial cells but is also the agent responsible for the focal degradation of capillary basement membranes that precedes the migration of endothelial cells into a healing wound.

FACTORS THAT INTERFERE WITH WOUND HEALING

Failure to heal satisfactorily can be the result of either **systemic** or **local** factors.

SYSTEMIC FACTORS

Nutrition

Protein

The patient's state of nutrition is a potent factor in determining the success or failure of healing. There may be at least two explanations for this.

1) The undernourished patient shows evidence of depression of the immune system; wound infection and the inflammatory response that this elicits to this may delay healing.

2) A deficient protein intake may inhibit collagen formation and so inhibit the regaining of tensile strength. In this regard, sulphur-containing amino acids such as methionine seem to be particularly important; increasing the intake of this amino acid alone can partially offset the effects of a low protein intake on wound healing.

Vitamin C

Vitamin C holds the most prominent place, in historical terms, among the individual dietary factors affecting healing. It has been known since the seventeenth century that scurvy is associated with poor healing of wounds and fractures. It was not, however, until well into the twentieth century that vitamin C was discovered.

Once this was done, it was possible to examine the effects of vitamin C deficiency on experimental wounds. **Lack of vitamin C inhibits the secretion of collagen fibres by fibroblasts, due to a failure of hydroxylation of proline in the endoplasmic reticulum of the fibroblast.** In addition vitamin C concentrations in biological fluids appear to affect the production of galactosamine and hence the deposition of chondroitin sulphate in the extracellular matrix of granulation tissue.

Vitamin A

Vitamin A has important functions in relation to morphogenesis, epithelial proliferation and epithelial differentiation. In experimental wounds it will counteract the inhibitory effects of steroids on healing and, applied topically, it accelerates epithelial covering.

Zinc

A role for zinc in wound healing was discovered more or less by accident. In the course of a study on the effects of certain amino acids on wound healing, a phenylalanine analogue that had been expected to impair healing, instead accelerated it. Careful study of this analogue revealed that the sample used had been contaminated by zinc. Further studies showed that zinc does indeed accelerate the healing of experimental wounds. Zinc deficiency, such as is found in patients who have been on parenteral nutrition for long periods and in those with severe burns, is associated with poor healing and this is reversed by the administration of zinc, which is necessary for the function of many enzymes including nucleic acid polymerases.

Steroid Hormones

Many studies show that glucocorticoids have an inhibitory effect on the healing process and on the production of fibrous tissue. Indeed, advantage is taken of this by administering steroids in situations where inappropriate scarring is taking place, such as in interstitial fibrosis in the lung. It is still not clear whether steroids exert their effect indirectly by damping down the inflammatory process or whether they directly affect one or more of the mechanisms outlined in previous sections.

Age

Age is often stated to be a factor affecting the efficacy of wound healing. It is true that wounds tend to heal more rapidly in the young than in the elderly but it is difficult to be certain that it is age *per se* that is exerting an effect or whether delayed healing in the aged may be due to local vascular factors such as poor arterial perfusion.

Diabetes

The presence of diabetes, especially if control is poor, has an inhibitory effect on the healing process. In uncontrolled diabetes there is impairment of the neutrophil response to injury and infection. This reverts to normal (in the *ex vivo* situation) if insulin is added to the culture medium. In addition, diabetics may suffer from poor arterial perfusion and sensory neuropathy. The first of these impairs healing; the second makes repetitive injury more likely to occur. This is particularly noticeable on the soles of the feet where quite trivial injuries may develop into chronic non-healing ulcers.

LOCAL FACTORS

Foreign Bodies or Infection

The presence of infection or a foreign body increases the intensity and prolongs the duration of the inflammatory response to injury, and will inhibit a satisfactory conclusion to the healing process. It is worth remembering that fragments of dead tissue, such as bone, and other elements of the patient's own tissues that have become misplaced, such as hair or keratin, act as foreign bodies.

Excess Mobility

Even the least observant person will have noticed that a cut across a joint, such as an interphalangeal joint, takes longer to heal than one that is not subjected to frequent movement. Excess mobility in a wound inevitably increases the time taken for it to heal. This is of particular significance in relation to fracture healing (which is why the severed ends of the bone are immobilized), but applies in other tissues as well.

Perfusion and Venous Drainage

The degree of arterial perfusion and the efficacy of venous drainage play key roles in the healing of injured tissues. Where arterial perfusion is compromised by stenosis or occlusion of the supplying vessel, a quite trivial injury may give rise to a disproportionate degree of tissue damage, and healing may be delayed or even inhibited completely.

Adequate venous drainage is also important, and impairment of this may play a part in the genesis of chronic ulcers, which often occur on the anterior surface of the legs in elderly patients. This is the basis for the use of compression bandaging in the treatment of such ulcers.

Histological examination of the margins of these lesions suggests that drainage is compromised by the presence of cuffs of polymerized fibrin round the venules. This can, in part, be prevented by administration of the synthetic steroid stanozolol. Suboxygenation of normally perfused tissue, such as may occur in the presence of severe anaemia, will also lead to defective healing.

REPAIR IN SOME SPECIALIZED TISSUES

BONE (*Fig. 8.8*)

The processes involved in the early stages of fracture healing are basically the same as those described above. Thus, the tissue defect created by the fracture is, in the first instance, made good by well-vascularized connective tissue in a manner similar to that which occurs in the healing of large open wounds.

Once this stage has passed, important new features are imposed on the basic model of healing. These are necessary because bone, unlike soft tissues, requires mechanical and weight-bearing efficiency of a high order. These needs are met through the operation of two types of specialized cell:

1) The **osteoblast**, which lays down seams of uncalcified new bone (osteoid).

2) The **osteoclast**, a multinucleated cell, probably of macrophage lineage, which resorbs bone by releasing proteases into the local microenvironment and which, therefore, plays a key part in the remodelling of the new bone formed in the course of fracture healing.

Stages of Fracture Healing

Haemorrhage

When a bone is fractured, tearing of blood vessels takes place, **haemorrhage** results and the defect between the fractured ends of the bone becomes filled with blood clot and other plasma-derived proteins.

Inflammatory Reaction

As in any other tissue, the injury elicits an **acute inflammatory reaction**, although the degree of neutrophil infiltration is mild. The combined effect of haemorrhage and inflammatory oedema causes loosening of the periosteum from the underlying bone ends, resulting in a fusiform swelling at the fracture site.

Necrosis

Some degree of bone necrosis is almost inevitable and is due to cutting off the blood supply to some areas as a result of damage to blood vessels. It takes 24–48 hours for the first morphological evidence of bone necrosis to

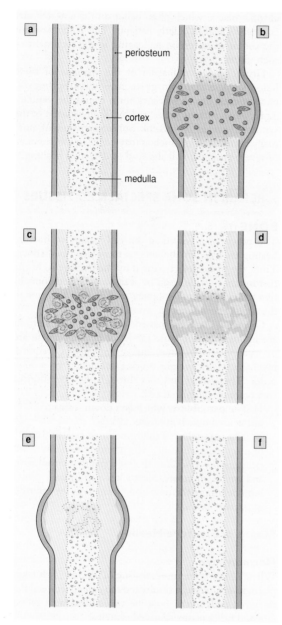

FIGURE 8.8 *Stages in the healing of fractures in long bones.*
a *Anatomy of long bone.* **b** *Fracture leads to bleeding from severed vessels. Blood clot accumulates in the gap and elevation of periosteum occurs, followed by a brisk inflammatory reaction.*
c *Granulation tissue is formed.* **d** *Osteoid and cartilage appear. This is known as the 'provisional callus'.* **e** *The callus is replaced by new bone. The ends are now firmly united.* **f** *The new lamellar bone is remodelled.*

supply. Some sites such as the **talus**, the **carpal scaphoid** and the **head of femur** are particularly likely to show significant ischaemic necrosis after fracture. Empty lacunae, the dead osteocytes having disappeared, are a reliable indication of bone necrosis.

Granulation Tissue

Macrophages now invade the fracture site and commence the process of demolition. This is followed by the formation of granulation tissue; about 4 days after fracturing the bone, the mass of blood clot is replaced by granulation tissue, which also extends upwards and downwards within the marrow cavity for a considerable distance from the fracture site. Within the granulation tissue small groups of cartilage cells are beginning to differentiate from connective tissue stem cells.

Formation of Provisional Callus

Provisional callus is the term used to describe a cuff of woven bone admixed with islands of cartilage. This serves to unite the severed portions of bone on their **external** aspect but not across the gap between the bone ends. The callus originates from two sources, and the relative proportions of these vary, depending on a number of factors.

The first and more important is the **periosteum**. The cells on its inner aspect proliferate and begin to lay down woven bone (i.e. bone in which the collagenous osteoid tissue is not deposited in a lamellar or 'onion skin' fashion but in a series of short bundles of parallel fibres, each bundle having a different orientation). Where the periosteum has been raised from the external surface of the bone (see above) the new woven bone fills the gap so that there are two cuffs of new bone around the periosteal aspect of the separated fragments. These cuffs then extend upwards and downwards until they meet, although there is, as yet, no direct union across the gap between the separated bone ends.

The degree of efficiency with which this **external callus** formation occurs depends on the adequacy of the blood supply around the fracture site. Some of the new blood vessels are derived from the periosteum itself, whereas others come from the muscle and other soft tissues that abut on the fractured bone. The amount of cartilage admixed with this periosteal new bone is small in human fractures that are healing well. However, it tends to be greater in cases where the local blood supply is poor or where the fractured bone ends have not been properly immobilized.

The second source of provisional callus is the medullary cavity where, following the formation of granulation tissue, fibroblasts and osteoblasts start to proliferate and lay down bone matrix. Some of this is deposited on trabecula of dead bone while the remainder forms new trabecula.

Healing Across the Fracture Gap

The provisional callus, as stated above, extends round the separated ends of the fractured bone but does not

become apparent, the marrow being the site of the first changes. Fat necrosis is seen and, if haemopoietic marrow is involved, the cells lose their nuclear staining. With respect to the bony tissue itself, the extent of necrosis depends on the anatomy of the local blood bridge the actual gap *between* the separated portions of bone. Well after the provisional callus has been formed, the clot that fills the gap between the fragments is invaded, first by granulation tissue capillaries and then by osteoblasts. Ossification within this gap may occur as a primary event, the osteoblasts being derived from the provisional callus. In some cases the bone ends are united by fibrous tissue and over a period of time this is replaced by woven bone. This takes far longer than direct ossification and is more likely to occur when the fracture has not been properly immobilized or in the presence of other factors likely to inhibit healing (e.g. infection or extensive and severe periosteal damage). Occasionally the fibrous tissue filling the gap is not replaced by bone (non-union) and weight-bearing by the affected limb is not possible. In cases of delayed or non-union, some improvement may be brought about by electrical stimulation, which appears to accelerate ossification at fracture sites.

Remodelling

Once union has occurred and the patient is bearing weight, the lumpy new cortical bone gradually becomes resorbed and smoothed out, and the excess medullary new bone is similarly removed with restoration of a normal medullary cavity. Woven bone, which is quite rapidly formed and much less efficient at weight bearing, is resorbed completely and is replaced by lamellar bone. This is a lengthy process: restoration to normal may take up to a year.

NERVOUS TISSUE

Central Nervous System

Most neurones cannot be replaced once they have been lost, although there is some evidence to suggest that a limited degree of regeneration can take place in the hypothalamic–neurohypophyseal system. In contrast with the peripheral nerves, where injury is not associated with any marked tendency towards scarring, necrosis within the central nervous system elicits the proliferation of glial cells and the formation of new glial fibres which, together with the ingrowth of capillaries, may constitute a physical barrier to the regeneration of new neuronal fibres.

Peripheral Nerves (see also pp 1171–1172)

When an axon is severed, the nerve cell shows chromatolysis (i.e. it swells and the Nissl granules, which represent zones of the endoplasmic reticulum studded with many ribosomes, disappear). The axon swells and becomes irregular, and its lipid-rich myelin sheath splits and later breaks up. The surrounding Schwann cells proliferate and accumulate some of the lipid released from the damaged myelin.

Soon new neurofibrils start to sprout from the proximal end of the severed axon and these invaginate the Schwann cells, which act as a guide or template for the new fibrils. The neurofibrils push their way down through the Schwann cells at a rate of about 1 mm per day. Eventually they may reach the appropriate end-organ and their myelin sheaths are reformed as a result of the secretory activity of the Schwann cells; in this way, a degree of functional recovery is attained. In some instances neurofibril sprouting takes place but the fibrils do not grow down existing endoneurial channels, and grow instead in a haphazard fashion. The end-result may thus be a tangle of new nerve fibres embedded in a mass of scar tissue, the whole being called a traumatic or 'stump' neuroma.

CHAPTER 9

The Natural History of Acute Inflammation III: Chronicity

If the inflammatory process lasts for months or years, it must, *ipso facto*, be termed **chronic**. Many important and common diseases are expressions of chronic inflammation. They are diverse in their origin and manifestations, but all share certain histological characters that are markers of a long-lasting process. Whatever the cause and characteristics of a chronic inflammatory reaction it represents a **failure to complete the natural history of acute inflammation** outlined in Chapters 7 and 8 (*Fig. 9.1*).

Chronicity may be defined in terms of:

- **Duration.** Any inflammatory process lasting for more than a few weeks is regarded as chronic.
- **Morphological appearance.** The main types of chronic inflammation have a characteristic microscopic appearance, which serves to indicate that they are chronic.
- **Biological processes involved.** These can be correlated with the microscopic appearances that are the expression of these processes.

CLASSIFICATION

Chronic inflammatory disorders are difficult to classify because they are so heterogeneous. This difficulty may be eased slightly by considering these chronic disorders as members of several major groups, as described below.

Following Significant Acute Inflammation
Conditions in which there has been a significant phase of acute inflammation (e.g. chronic peptic ulcer, chronic osteomyelitis). In such conditions formation of an inflammatory exudate and infiltrate continues, accompanied by attempts at healing.

Tissue Damage Caused by Non-Living Agents
Conditions where the tissue damage has been caused by the entry into the host tissues of **non-living** foreign material. Such irritants can persist within the tissue for a long time. If such foreign material is cytotoxic, the inflammatory response is dominated by the macrophage and by evidence of repair (e.g. pulmonary silicosis).

Granulomatous Inflammation
Conditions in which the acute inflammatory phase is short lived and mild, and the process is predestined by the nature of the injury to be chronic. The lesions in this group are also characterized by focal accumulation of macrophages and lymphocytes. Necrosis of a greater or lesser degree may be associated with macrophage aggregates and there may be extensive scarring. Cell-mediated immune reactions play a dominant role in the pathogenesis of this group of diseases, which includes such important conditions as tuberculosis and leprosy. This form of inflammation is known as **granulomatous inflammation** and is discussed in a later section.

Antibody-mediated Inflammation
Chronic inflammation dominated by the humoral effector arm of the immune system such as occurs in immune complex-mediated disorders (see pp 129–130).

Autoimmune Reactions
Chronic inflammatory disorders occurring as a result of autoimmune reactions and associated with autoantibodies in the plasma (e.g. rheumatoid disease, Hashimoto's thyroiditis).

Chronic Duct Obstruction
Chronic inflammatory disorders due to failure, as a result of duct blockage, to drain the normal secretions of exocrine glands as seen in chronic pancreatitis or chronic inflammation in salivary glands (sialoadenitis).

NON-SPECIFIC CHRONIC INFLAMMATION

Non-specific chronic inflammation occurs as a complication of an acute inflammatory process. It is the expression of failure of the sequence of events shown in *Fig. 9.1*, where the acute inflam-

Injury ⟶ Inflammation ⟶ Demolition ⟶ Resolution or Repair

FIGURE 9.1 *Natural history of acute inflammation terminating in resolution or healing.*

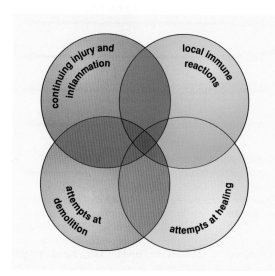

FIGURE 9.2 *Processes involved in non-specific chronic inflammation.*

matory reaction elicited by injury terminates in either resolution or repair (*Fig. 9.2*).

A number of objectives must be attained if complete healing of an acute inflammatory process is to occur.

Chronicity results from failure to reach one or more of these, which include:

- **Elimination of the injurious agent.** Persistence of injury is one of the most important factors in causing acute inflammatory reactions to become chronic.
- **Removal of the exudate** and any foreign material that is present. If suppuration has occurred, the pus must be drained adequately.
- **Adequate arterial perfusion and venous drainage** must be present. A classical clinical situation in which these factors are involved is chronic stasis ulceration of the lower limbs. In about 80% of patients with chronic leg ulcers there is evidence of vein disease and in about 33% there is also evidence of arterial disease. In about 40–50% of cases, venous ulceration is associated with evidence of previous deep vein thrombosis and in almost all cases there is incompetence of the communicating veins. **Thus there is a strong association between venous ulceration and failure of the calf pump due to vein abnormalities.** This is not uncommon, about 0.2% of the adult population being affected. In many cases, the ulcers are chronic so that, in terms of morbidity and health-care resources needed, this condition is important.

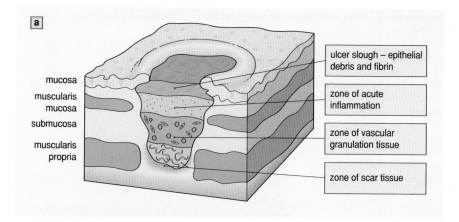

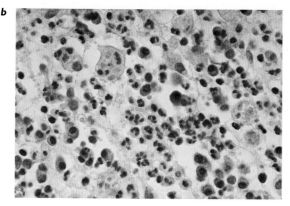

FIGURE 9.3 **a** *The architecture of chronic inflammation as exemplified by a chronic peptic ulcer.* **b** *Chronic inflammatory cell infiltrate showing a mixture of macrophages, neutrophils and plasma cells. Note the cellular debris within the cytoplasm of the two very large macrophages shown.*

- In appropriate anatomical locations, **drainage of exocrine gland secretions must be maintained** or re-established.

If all these conditions are not met, a type of pathological process is likely to develop in which there is a mixed morphological picture, well exemplified by chronic peptic ulcer.

Chronic Peptic Ulcer

This is a condition in which there is an imbalance between factors that promote acid and peptic digestion of the mucosa in the stomach and duodenum (**injury**) and those that protect the mucosa from such digestion (**defence**).

Table 9.1 describes the morphological appearances of such a chronic peptic ulcer from the mucosal surface outwards, and relates these to the biological processes operating in the lesion (*Fig. 9.3*). **Thus chronic peptic ulceration shows evidence of all the biological processes involved in an acute inflammatory response to injury, terminating in repair by scarring. In contrast, however, with what occurs in acute inflammation brought to a successful conclusion, these processes are not sequential but concurrent** (*Fig. 9.4*).

In the peptic ulcer model, chronicity is due to persistence of injury, which is associated in most cases with

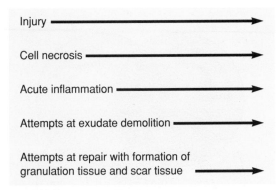

FIGURE 9.4 *Natural history of acute inflammation terminating in chronicity.*

infection by *Helicobacter pylori*. The zonal pattern described in relation to ulceration occurs in other chronic inflammatory lesions, such as chronic abscesses. In abscesses, the mechanism that can trigger chronicity is failure to drain pus.

THE MACROPHAGE IN CHRONIC INFLAMMATION

As in healing, the macrophage plays a dominant role in the natural history of chronic inflammation. Its impor-

Table 9.1 Morphological Features of Chronic Peptic Ulcer (from Mucosa Outwards) and Their Correlates in Terms of Process

Morphological features	Related biological processes
Loss of surface epithelium, underlying mucosal glands; stroma, musclaris mucosae and some of the muscularis propria. Epithelial and other debris is admixed with fibrin to form a greyish-white slough which can be seen on endoscopic examination.	Injury of sufficient severity to cause death of gastric or duodenal mucosa.
Immediately beneath this is a zone of acute inflammation infiltrated by neutrophils and some macrophages.	Typical acute inflammatory response to injury, which in this case is persistent.
Beneath this is a zone of vascular granulation tissue in which numerous large activated macrophages, lymphocytes and plasma cells are present. Many of the macrophages contain phagocytosed debris.	The macrophage infiltrate is a reflection of: • attempts at demolition of the exudate • the role of the macrophage as a secretory cell which orchestrates vascularization and repair The lymphocytes and plasma cells are evidence of tissue immune reactions elicited by local antigens.
A zone of scar tissue well vascularized in its more superficial part and consisting, more deeply, of dense fibrous tissue. Arteries in this 'ulcer bed' show intimal thickening due to hyperplasia of smooth muscle cells producing connective tissue matrix proteins. This is known as **endarteritis obliterans** and is seen in many chronic inflammatory lesions. Nerve bundles in this area are also unduly prominent.	This zone represents healing by repair. The process is clearly unsuccessful as necrosis and inflammation still continue. The changes in arteries and nerve bundles suggest the local release of growth factors.

tance in both these areas rests on the fact that it is a cell with power to:

- **phagocytose and scavenge living (microorganisms) and non-living foreign or effete material** (tissue debris, 'old' or abnormal red blood cells, immune complexes, modified lipoprotein)
- **kill many microorganisms**
- **synthesize and release tissue-damaging products**
- **synthesize and release mediators of acute inflammation and fever**
- **present antigens to both B and T lymphocytes and thus initiate immune responses**
- **become activated by signals released from lymphocytes following such antigen presentation**
- **release mediators that are chemoattractant for cells involved in repair and angiogenesis**
- **release growth factors**
- **regulate its own activities to a certain extent through the operation of autocrine loops**

Secretion of a wide range of products is an important part of the macrophage's functional repertoire (*Fig. 9.5*). Some of the secretion products of macrophages relevant to chronic inflammation and their main actions are shown in *Table 9.2*.

LOCAL IMMUNE RESPONSE

A common, indeed almost inevitable, feature of chronic inflammation is the presence of lymphocytes in the inflammatory infiltrate. Use of appropriate markers shows both B and T lymphocytes. These lymphocytes represent a local immune response to antigens released at the site of injury and inflammation; they reach such areas by emigrating from local microvascular channels. In some situations it has been demonstrated clearly that infiltrating lymphocytes react with antigen present in the lesions. This implies that there is a selective mechanism determining which lymphocytes remain within the chronic inflammatory lesion and which migrate back to the blood or lymph. In the case of the T cells, this mechanism involves the 'specific fit' of the T-cell receptors, and in B cells the configuration of surface immunoglobulin in relation to the local antigens (see pp 107–109, 110)

The Plasma Cell

The plasma cell is a reliable marker of chronicity in inflammatory reactions; it represents terminal functional differentiation of a B lymphocyte (see pp 95–96) that is now producing large amounts of immunoglobulin (*Fig. 9.6*).

The plasma cell measures 10–12 µm in diameter and has a single, slightly eccentrically placed, nucleus in which the chromatin appears to be fragmented and concentrated at the nuclear membrane, giving a clock-face or cartwheel appearance. There is a prominent perinuclear halo, known as the **hoff,** which is the site of the Golgi apparatus. In sections stained with haematoxylin and eosin, the cytoplasm is markedly basophilic, an expression of the abundant secretion of RNA. This can be confirmed by treating sections with pyronin, which stains the RNA red. On electron microscopic examination, the structure mirrors the predominant secretory function of the plasma cell, much rough endoplasmic

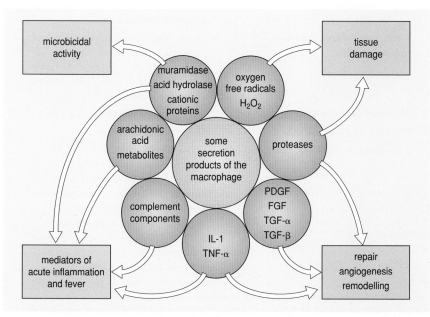

FIGURE 9.5 *Macrophage actions in chronic inflammation.*

Table 9.2 Macrophage Secretion Products in Chronic Inflammation

Product	Cell target	Main actions
Metabolites of arachidonic acid (prostaglandins and leukotrienes)	Smooth muscle, leucocytes	Upregulates acute inflammation; causes fever; implicated in pain
Lysosomal cationic proteins	Leucocytes	Chemoattractant
Oxygen free radicals and hydrogen peroxide, nitric oxide	Proteins and membrane lipids	Microbicidal; implicated in tissue damage
Metalloproteinases	Connective tissue matrix proteins	Connective tissue breakdown
IL-1	T and B lymphocytes, macrophages, osteoclasts, neutrophils, liver cells, endothelium	Induces proliferation of activated B and T cells; induces prostaglandin and cytokine release by macrophages; induces expression of adhesion molecules for leucocytes on endothelial surface; induces fever via prostaglandin release, causes osteoclast-mediated bone resorption; induces production of acute-phase proteins; upregulates production of IL-6, GM-CSF and IFN-β_1
IL-6	T and B cells, thymocytes, liver cells	Stimulates growth and differentiation of B and T cells and precursors of blood-forming cells; induces production of acute-phase proteins
IL-8	T cells, neutrophils	Chemoattractant
IL-10	T cells	Downregulates mononuclear responses in inflammation; inhibits IFN-γ production; increases T_H2 lymphocyte expression
GM-CSF	Neutrophil and monocyte precursors, macrophages, neutrophils and monocytes	Stimulates growth of neutrophil and monocyte precursors; activates mature neutrophils and monocytes
TNF-α and -β	T cells, macrophages, fibroblasts, endothelial cells	Activate phagocytic cells; play key roles in cachexia in cancer; induce expression of adhesion molecules; induce production of IL-1, IL-6, TNF-α, IFN-γ and GM-CSF; induce acute-phase proteins
PDGF and bFGF	Fibroblasts and smooth muscle cells	Chemoattractant and mitogen
TGF-α	Fibroblasts and epithelial cells	Mitogen; binds to EGF receptor
TGF-β	T lymphocytes, fibroblasts, endothelial cells	Inhibits T-cell proliferation; upregulates connective tissue matrix protein synthesis; promotes formation of new blood vessels; may either inhibit or stimulate connective tissue cell growth depending on local concentrations of other growth factors such as PDGF; has an autocrine effect on its own production by macrophages and on the production of other macrophage-derived polypeptides

bFGF, basic fibroblast growth factor; EGF, epidermal growth factor; GM-CSF, granulocyte–macrophage colony-stimulating factor; IFN, interferon; IL, interleukin; PDGF, platelet-derived growth factor; TGF, transforming growth factor; TNF, tumour necrosis factor.

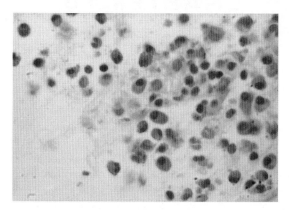

FIGURE 9.6 *Plasma cells representing a local immune response in chronic inflammation. Note the marked basophilia of the cytoplasm representing immunoglobulin synthesis.*

reticulum and a prominent Golgi apparatus being present.

The role of the plasma cell is to produce specific immunoglobulin (see pp 101–105); this can be confirmed by using appropriate fluorescein and peroxidase-linked antibodies, which bind to the immunoglobulin in the plasma cell cytoplasm.

SOME EXAMPLES OF NON-SPECIFIC CHRONIC INFLAMMATION

Some paradigms of chronic inflammation include:

- chronic osteitis (see pp 1069–1071)
- impaired drainage of normal secretions as in chronic pancreatitis or chronic sialoadenitis (see pp 636–638, 490–491)
- chronic pyelonephritis (see pp 676–678)
- chronic ulcerative colitis (see pp 545–548).

CHAPTER 10

The Immune System

It has been known for many centuries that a non-fatal attack of certain infectious diseases results in a diminution of the individual's susceptibility to that disease in the future. This degree of increased resistance against a specific infectious agent is known as **acquired specific immunity**. This phenomenon is the basis of many successful immunization programmes, some of which have led to the virtual eradication of some highly lethal infectious diseases such as poliomyelitis and smallpox.

While this has clearly been beneficial, the biological implications of acquired specific immunity are much more far reaching, as will be seen in later sections dealing with hypersensitivity and autoimmune disease.

The specific immune system present in most vertebrates is capable of:

- **Recognition** of what is foreign to the host, i.e. the ability to distinguish between **self** and **non-self**.
- Mounting a highly **specific response** to what is recognized as foreign.
- **Memory.** The existence of memory in the immune system can be inferred because a **subsequent encounter** with what has previously been recognized as foreign evokes a response that is both greater in degree and much quicker than that occurring on a **first encounter**.

What Does Immunity Mean?

Some conceptual difficulties arise when the word **immunity** is used to describe the whole range of activities in the immune system, since the commonly accepted meaning of the term is **a state in which there is absolute or relative freedom from some harmful condition.**

There is no doubt that the altered reactivity of a host following an encounter with some foreign species is, on the whole, extremely beneficial to the host in that it constitutes a powerful defence against the effects of pathogenic microorganisms (*Fig. 10.1*). However, the same mechanisms that operate to protect the host can be turned against it and cause serious damage to tissues. In this case, despite the dictum of Humpty Dumpty who declared that '**a word means precisely what I choose it to mean, neither more nor less**', the use of the word **immunity** seems less appropriate. Events mediated through the immune system that are harmful

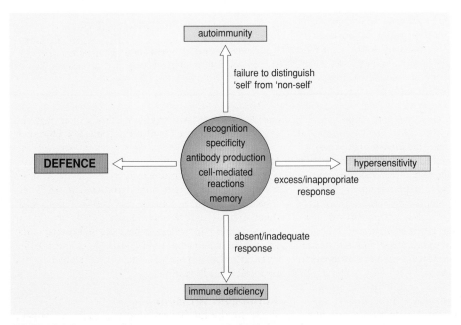

FIGURE 10.1 *Properties of the immune system: normal and abnormal.*

to the host clearly need to be identified in some other way; this problem is explored in subsequent chapters.

COMPONENTS OF THE IMMUNE REACTION

ANTIGENS

For an immune response to be generated, cellular elements making up the immune system must encounter a molecule that can be recognized as being of the '**non-self**' variety. Substances that are capable of inducing a specific response from these cellular elements are known as **antigens**. They are usually protein, polypeptide or polysaccharide in nature. The chemical sites on the cells of the immune system or on the specific globulins (antibodies) that are responsible for **recognition** of foreign chemical species are very small and will bind to only a few amino acids or sugar residues. This means that the part of an antigen eliciting specific recognition is correspondingly small. Most antigens in fact consist of many such areas, which are called determinants or **epitopes**. Each of these is capable of evoking a specific response.

What Confers Immunogenicity on a Molecule?

The ability of a chemical species to function as an antigen is related, in part, to its size. Most antigens have a molecular weight in excess of 10 000. About 2500 seems to be the limit below which foreign substances cannot elicit a response on the part of the immune system. However, it is possible for certain small molecules, which cannot act as antigens by themselves, to bind to a carrier, usually a protein. The complex formed by such binding can produce an immune response in which the antigenic determinant is the small 'passenger' molecule. These small molecules are known as **haptens**. The antibodies formed in response to the hapten–carrier complex can react specifically in solution with the free hapten (e.g. in sensitivity reactions to certain drugs) (*Fig. 10.2*).

Because of the 'foreignness' inherent in the concept of antigens, it is tempting to view them as chemical species derived entirely from the environment (**exogenous**). It is true that such exogenous antigens are involved in a wide spectrum of human diseases, including all infections and many hypersensitivity reactions such as asthma and hay fever. However, many antigens exist that are 'native' to the host; these **endogenous** antigens play an important part in many of the functions of the immune system in both health and disease. They may be classified as: **heterologous, autologous, homologous (iso-antigens)**.

Heterologous Antigens

These are antigens common to species that are unrelated phylogenetically. The existence of such antigens

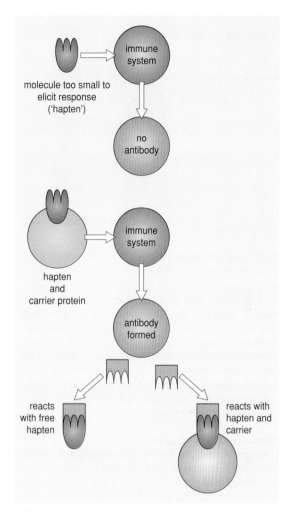

FIGURE 10.2 *Some molecules are too small to elicit a response from the immune system. Such molecules, known as haptens, can bind to a carrier protein, and together produce an immune response in which the antigenic determinant is the hapten.*

can lead to curious cross-reactions which may be important in the genesis of certain diseases. One such example is the cross-reactivity that exists between the M proteins of certain strains of β-haemolytic *Streptococcus pyogenes* and determinants present in heart muscle and many other human tissues (*Fig. 10.3*). As there is a known association between infections with these streptococcal strains and acute rheumatic fever, cross-reactivity between the bacterial and human antigens has been implicated in the pathogenesis of the disease. Absolute proof that this is the mechanism responsible is still lacking.

Autologous Antigens

These are the host's own normal constituents which, under most circumstances, are recognized as '**self**'.

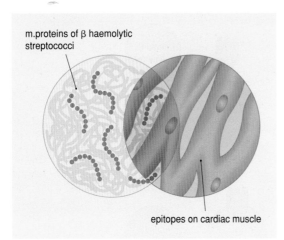

FIGURE 10.3 *Heterologous antigens. Common antigens in phylogenetically unrelated species.*

As a result of this they do not elicit an immune response from the host, a state known as **tolerance**. This state of tolerance can be broken down in a number of ways (see pp 134–136) and immune reactions can be mounted against one or more of the native tissue constituents. The disorders associated with this partial breakdown in the ability to distinguish between 'self' and 'non-self' are known as **autoimmune diseases**.

Homologous Antigens

These molecules, also known as **iso-antigens**, are the determinants that distinguish the tissue components of one **individual** from another. Their expression is genetically controlled, as can be seen from the mode of inheritance of one important group of such antigens: the ABO blood group system.

Consequences of an Encounter Between Host and Antigen

The introduction of an antigen into a host may give rise to one or more of three basic reactions (*Fig. 10.4*): antibody formation, clonal proliferation and specific tolerance.

Antibody Formation

This is the production of proteins of the globulin series which possess the ability to bind **specifically** to the antigenic determinant that has been introduced. Antibodies are produced by **plasma cells**, the fully differentiated form of **B cells**, one of the two major classes of lymphocytes.

The essential role of antibodies is in **defence** of the host against infections by extracellular, pathogenic microorganisms such as staphylococci and streptococci. In this type of response, known as the **humoral** type, bacterial toxins may be neutralized, complement-mediated cell lysis brought about, phagocytosis assisted

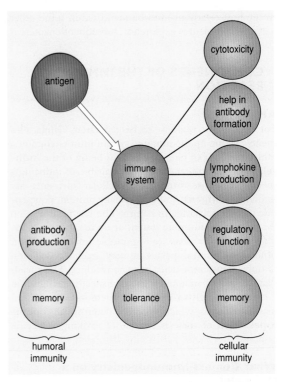

FIGURE 10.4 *Consequences of an encounter between antigen and host.*

through specific opsonization, and the entry of viruses to certain cells prevented.

Clonal Proliferation

This is the expansion of a clone of another class of lymphocytes, the **T cells**, which have a wider range of biological activities. These include the ability:

- directly to lyse foreign cells whose antigenic make-up has been modified by viral infection and certain tumour cells.
- to release a range of **non-antigen-specific** soluble products (known as **lymphokines**), some of which activate macrophages and others either 'help' or 'suppress' the function of one or both of the lymphocyte classes.

The antigen-induced proliferation of this class of lymphocyte and the range of activities carried out by them is known as **cell-mediated immunity**. In so far as defence against infection is concerned, this is most effective against **organisms that grow intracellularly such as viruses, certain bacteria (e.g. the organisms responsible for tuberculosis and leprosy) and fungi**.

Specific Tolerance

The induction of a state of **specific tolerance** to a given antigen can occur when the antigen is introduced to the host during fetal or very early neonatal life. A second exposure to such an antigen is not followed by antibody production or proliferation of sensitized lymphocytes.

CELLULAR BASIS OF IMMUNE REACTIONS

In the previous section it was stated that the response of elements of the immune system following exposure to foreign molecules, to which the host is not tolerant, has a **dual nature**, expressed by one or both of the following:

- the production of immunoglobulins that react specifically with the antigen (**antibodies**)
- the proliferation of lymphocytes that have a variety of other functions, some of which were listed above

The effector cell line in both reactions is the small lymphocyte. When an animal such as a rat is depleted of its small lymphocytes by repeated drainage of the thoracic duct, both sets of functions are lost.

Small Lymphocyte Classes: T and B Cells

How Were B and T Lymphocytes Discovered?

The existence of functions as different as the production of specific antibody globulins on the one hand and the wide range of activities characteristic of cell-mediated immunity on the other suggested that these might be carried by at least two distinct lines of small lymphocytes. The truth of this proposition began to emerge with the studies carried out by Miller in the mid-1960s on the role of the thymus, which up to that time had been regarded as a mysterious organ with no defined purpose. Miller found that if the thymus of mouse was removed in the neonatal period the following events occurred:

- There was a fall in the number of circulating lymphocytes.
- The ability to reject a tissue graft from a different strain of the same species (an allogeneic graft) was lost.
- There was a reduction in the antibody response to some antigens.
- After 3–4 months the animals died from a wasting disease, probably related to an inability to resist infection, as neonatally thymectomized animals kept under germ-free conditions did not succumb to this disorder.
- The mice became particularly susceptible to viral infection.
- The ability to mount an unimpaired antibody response to certain antigens was retained and plasma concentrations of immunoglobulins were not altered.

These data can be interpreted in the light of a series of elegant experiments in which immunological competence (e.g. the ability to reject allogeneic grafts) is first destroyed and then restored. For instance, if immunological competence is destroyed in an adult mouse by

irradiation of the bone marrow, it can be restored by transfer of bone marrow cells from an animal of the same species. If, in addition to irradiation of the bone marrow, the thymus is also removed, immunological competence cannot be restored by transfusion of bone marrow cells, although it can be by transfusion of adult spleen or lymph node cells.

Thus the role of the thymus appears to be in the **processing** of a population of small lymphocytes derived from the bone marrow. In the absence of the thymus these cells cannot develop their normal range of functions. Small lymphocytes processed in this way are known as **T lymphocytes** or thymus-derived cells (*Fig. 10.5*).

T Lymphocytes

T Cells Cannot Produce Antibody

While T cells clearly have a wide range of activities, they **cannot produce antibody themselves**. Another lymphocyte population is the precursor for the mature antibody-producing cell or **plasma cell**. The retention of the ability to produce antibody responses

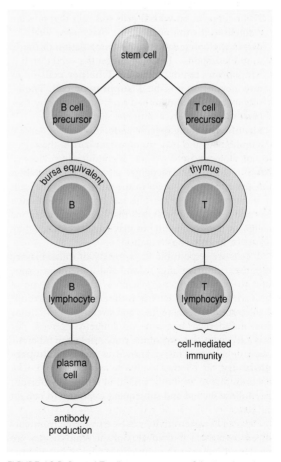

FIGURE 10.5 B- and T-cell compartments of the immune system.

to certain antigens following neonatal thymectomy suggests that the bone marrow stem cells destined to become plasma cells and produce immunoglobulin are processed in some place other than the thymus. The only species in which such an organ has been identified with certainty is the chicken, in which there is a localized mass of lymphoid tissue in relation to an outpouching of the cloaca. This is known as the bursa of Fabricius, and the small lymphocytes that are coded to transform into antibody-producing plasma cells on encountering the appropriate antigen are called **bursa-derived** or **B lymphocytes** (*Fig. 10.5*). It is still uncertain as to which tissues are the homologue in mammals of the bursa of Fabricius, but the processing of B-cell precursors is believed to take place in the haemopoietic system; some also occurs in **mucosa-associated lymphoid tissue** (**MALT**) (e.g. Peyer's patches in the intestine, pharyngeal tonsil, etc.).

T-cell Functions

In so far as defence against infection is concerned, T cells function in two ways:

1) On their own they act against pathogens that can survive and grow intracellularly.

2) In cooperation with B cells and cells that present antigens to the immune system, they play a vital part in the upregulation or downregulation of the immune response. In upregulation the subset of T lymphocytes responsible is the **T helper cell** and in downregulation it is the **T suppressor cell**. These subsets can be distinguished from each other by the possession of different antigens, and are thus identified by using specific antibodies.

T lymphocytes also play an important part in the rejection of allogeneic grafts. There is considerable evidence that T cells may also recognize certain tumour cells as non-self and destroy them in the same way as the cells of an incompatible graft. This variety of **surveillance** may also serve to suppress cells that have not undergone malignant transformation but may have been altered by viruses or spontaneous mutation.

T cells are responsible for a variety of inflammatory responses occurring after second and subsequent exposures to certain antigens or haptens. The archetype of this variety of T-cell activity is the set of skin reactions characterized by local redness and swelling 24–48 hours after intradermal injection of antigens derived, for example, from the organisms responsible for tuberculosis or leprosy. This is known as **delayed hypersensitivity**, in contrast with the virtually immediate reactions due to antibody which, in sensitized subjects, may follow second and subsequent exposure to certain antigens.

Delayed hypersensitivity can be transferred from sensitized to normal individuals only if lymphocytes are transferred, whereas the immediate type of hypersensitivity can be transferred via the medium of cell-free serum. Delayed hypersensitivity was originally defined in terms of the skin reactions described above, but the process – of which the skin lesion is only one expression – plays an important part in the production of many serious pathological lesions, such as those of tuberculosis.

Mode of Action of the T Cell

The functions outlined above are carried out either through:

- the medium of **cell-to-cell contact**, in the course of which virally infected cells, allogeneic graft cells or transformed cells are destroyed by the T cells
- through the **synthesis** and **secretion** of a number of active compounds known as **lymphokines**, which are concerned primarily with mediating interactions between cells:
  a) T cells with B cells
  b) T cells with macrophages

We have already seen in the section dealing with cytokines in inflammation that macrophages can also produce compounds that are capable of modulating the responses of the T cell. T cell-derived cytokines are shown in *Table 10.1*.

B Cells

B-cell Function

As stated earlier, the B cell operates through the production of antibody. Before the synthesis and secretion of such antibody takes place the small lymphocyte must undergo a series of morphological and functional transformations and mature into the **plasma cell** (see pp 89–91).

Lifespan and Circulation of Small Lymphocytes

The differing immunological roles of the T and B cells are also reflected in their other characteristics. The majority of circulating lymphocytes are T cells (70–80%) and this is likely to be an expression of their **long life** (a lifespan in humans of 5–10 years). It is presumably for this reason that thymectomy in adult life does not, as a rule, deprive the subject of immunological competence, as a long-lived population of memory T cells has already been established. B cells have a much shorter lifespan, although again it seems likely that there is a fairly long-lived subset of memory B cells.

The differing immunological functions of the two sets of lymphocytes are also mirrored in terms of their **relative mobility**. The primary role of the B cell is to produce large amounts of specific immunoglobulin. This is discharged into the lymph and thence into the bloodstream from the secondary lymphoid tissue (lymph nodes, MALT and spleen), where there are large concentrations of B cells.

Some aspects of T-cell function require cell-to-cell contact, and lymphokine-mediated T cell–B cell interaction requires relatively close proximity of the

Table 10.1 Peptide Cytokines Secreted by T Cells

Cytokine	Functions
Interleukins	
IL-2	Major growth factor for both helper and cytotoxic T cell and lymphokine-activated killer cells; also involved in B-cell development
IL-4	Pivotal in development of T_H2 subset; involved in B-cell help; causes switching of antibody production to IgE; growth factor for mast cells and stimulates the production of VCAM
1L-5	Stimulates growth and differentiation of eosinophils and thus promotes killing of helminths; promotes growth and differentiation of B cells and, together with other cytokines, induces synthesis of IgA and IgM in mature B cells
IL-6	Causes terminal differentiation of immunoglobulin-producing B cells; inhibits macrophage production of IL-1 and IFN-γ; stimulates liver cells to produce acute-phase proteins such as fibrinogen, serum amyloid protein A, α_2–macroglobulin; promotes formation of osteoclasts
IL-9	Promotes proliferation of T cells
1L-10	Downregulates production of cytokines including IL-1, IFN-γ and TNF-α by macrophages; inhibits NO production; stimulates B-cell proliferation, differentiation and activity
IL-12	Strong stimulator of NK cells, growth factor for activated T cells and maturation factor for cytotoxic T cells; induces formation of IFN-γ and thus enhances formation of T_H1 cells
IL-13	Suppresses proinflammatory cytokine, chemokine and growth factor production by macrophages and also downregulates the production of NO; enhances expression of MHC class II proteins and thus antigen presentation; causes human B cells to switch antibody production to IgE and IgG_4; shares some features with IL-4
IL-14	Induces proliferation of activated B cells but not of resting B cells and inhibits immunoglobulin production
Interferons	
IFN-γ	Antiviral; pivotal for development of T_H1 from T_H0 cells and inhibits development of T_H2 cells; it is the most powerful macrophage-activating factor (MAF) and is therefore important in cell-mediated immunity; increases expression of MHC class I and II proteins, thus enhancing antigen presentation; causes expression of adhesion molecules on the surface of vascular endothelium (as does TNF-α); causes differentiation of cytotoxic T cells; antagonizes several IL-4 actions; promotes synthesis of IgG_{2a} by activated B cells
Cytotoxins	
TNF-α	Derives its name from the fact that serum from animals given endotoxin produces haemorrhagic necrosis in tumours. At **high concentrations** (as may be induced by endotoxin) TNF-α acts systemically. It functions as a **pyrogen**, activates the **clotting system**, stimulates production of **acute-phase proteins** by the liver, inhibits myocardial contractility by stimulating production of NO, and, over long periods, causes cachexia. At **low concentrations** TNF-α upregulates the inflammatory response. It induces expression of the adhesion molecules ICAM-1, VCAM-1 and E-selectin, which promote adhesion and migration of leucocytes from the microvessels to the extravascular compartment. It enhances the killing of intracellular organisms such as *Leishmania* and *Mycobacterium tuberculosis*. It activates several leucocyte types, leading to the production by macrophages of various cytokines including IL-6, chemokines and TNF-α itself
TNF-β	Shares many of the actions of TNF-α. Lyses tumour cells but not normal cells; activates neutrophils; increases adhesion of leucocytes to vascular endothelium and promotes their migration

Table 10.1 Peptide Cytokines Secreted by T Cells – *continued*

Cytokine	Functions
Colony-stimulating factors	
GM-CSF	Stimulates growth of granulocyte and macrophage colonies; activates macrophages, neutrophils and eosinophils
IL-3	Stimulates growth and differentiation of haemopoietic precursors
Other	
TGF-β (a family of five closely related proteins, secreted in an inactive form that must be cleaved before binding to its receptor)	Has an autocrine effect on monocyte–macrophages and regulates its own production by these cells; upregulates the production of IL-1, FGF, PDGF and TNF-α; increases production of connective tissue matrix proteins and is a potent angiogenic factor; has an immunosuppressive effect by inhibiting the proliferation of T lymphocytes

FGF, fibroblast growth factor; GM-CSF, granulocyte–macrophage colony-stimulating factor; ICAM, intercellular adhesion molecule; IFN, interferon; Ig, immunoglobulin; IL, interleukin; MAF, macrophage-activating factor; MHC, major histocompatibility complex; NK, natural killer; NO, nitric oxide; PDGF, platelet-derived growth factor; TGF, transforming growth factor; TNF, tumour necrosis factor; VCAM, vascular cell adhesion molecule

interacting cells. **Thus the T cell must be mobile and able to travel constantly between the blood and the secondary lymphoid tissue where antigens are trapped by macrophages.** The bulk of this traffic occurs via the postcapillary venules in the lymph nodes. These venules can be recognized by their high, rather cuboidal, endothelium. T cells emigrate via the interendothelial cell gaps from the blood into the lymph node tissue where they can come into contact with antigens processed by macrophages and other antigen-presenting cells (APCs), and thus become stimulated to divide and differentiate.

NORMAL ANATOMY OF THE IMMUNE RESPONSE

Immune responses result from a series of cellular interactions that occur, for the most part, within the **peripheral lymphoid tissue**. The latter consists of a number of different elements:
- **lymph nodes**, which respond to antigens within the tissues reaching the nodes via lymphatics
- **spleen**, which responds to antigens within the blood
- **mucosa-associated lymphoid tissue (MALT)**, which responds to antigens at mucosal surfaces. This functional characteristic dictates the siting of 'native' MALT, normally found principally in the alimentary tract. In disease, MALT also occurs in salivary glands, lacrimal glands, the lactating breast and in the genitourinary system. **MALT is distributed in two forms:** component cells may

be distributed diffusely within the tissue compartment immediately beneath epithelia or they may be arranged in well-formed follicles (Peyer's patches).

LYMPHOCYTE 'TRAFFIC'
Expansion and activation of clones of lymphocytes sensitive to a particular antigen, and recruitment of these cells to required tissue locations, demands a series of pathways through which lymphocyte trafficking occurs. These pathways consist of:
1) An **extensive network of lymphatics**, some of which drain tissues and enter lymph nodes (afferent lymphatics) and others which drain nodes (efferent lymphatics). The lymph eventually enters the thoracic duct, from which it enters the bloodstream via the left subclavian vein.
2) **The blood.** Lymphocytes within the blood leave it again by migrating across vascular endothelium.

Migration
In lymph nodes, migration takes place across the so-called high endothelial venules (HEVs), postcapillary venules lined by endothelial cells that are taller than normal. Migration of lymphocytes is mediated by adhesion to this endothelium. This is due to a binding reaction between adhesion molecules on the surface of the lymphocytes and complementary molecules (so-called **addressins**) on the surface of the endothelium of the HEV. The lymphocyte surface ligand is one of the selectin family, **L-selectin**. The amino-terminal domains of this selectin recognize

oligosaccharides of the HEV addressin. The rest of the molecule consists of an epidermal growth factor-like sequence, several repeats of structures homologous with complement-binding proteins, a transmembrane domain and a short intracytoplasmic 'tail'.

In MALT, lymphocytes leave the blood by binding to an endothelial selectin which reacts with a lymphocyte surface ligand, CD44. This ensures that lymphocytes whose function is protection of mucosal surfaces by synthesizing dimeric IgA, will leave the bloodstream at functionally appropriate sites.

At sites where there is inflammation within tissues, lymphocytes leave the microvasculature via similar adhesion mechanisms involving inter-actions between surface sugars, integrins, selectins and adhesion molecules of the immunoglobulin gene superfamily such as ICAM-1 and VCAM.

FUNCTIONAL ANATOMY OF THE LYMPH NODE

A normal reacting lymph node consists of two sets of channels (lymphatics and blood vessels) and a number of functional cell compartments. It has a fibrous capsule from which septa penetrate into the substance of the node.

Anatomy of Lymph Flow

Just within the capsule is the marginal sinus surrounding the node parenchyma. Afferent lymphatics penetrate the capsule, entering the marginal sinus. From the marginal sinus, cortical sinuses are derived; these penetrate into the node breaking up into a series of fine arborizing channels. These small channels join to form larger sinuses (the medullary sinuses) and in turn the medullary sinuses join to form a single efferent lymphatic channel.

The sinuses, lined by phagocytic endothelial cells, also contain a resident population of macrophages. These two cell populations act as a filter for antigens in the afferent lymph.

Anatomy of Nodal Blood Flow

Blood enters the lymph node at the hilum via a single artery. This branches, forming successive generations of vessels of decreasing size until a fine network of capillaries has been formed. These drain into the high endothelial venules in which migration of lympho-cytes from the blood occurs. The high endothelial venules fuse to form larger veins, which ultimately unite in the region of the hilum to form a single draining vein.

The Cell Compartments of the Lymph Node (*Fig. 10.6*)

There are three types of lymphoid cells concerned with the regulation and mediation of immune responses:
1) **B lymphocytes**
2) **T lymphocytes**
3) **APCs (antigen-presenting cells)**

The two lymphocyte populations are both functionally and anatomically distinct. Each shows a spectrum of cells in different stages of differentiation and activation.

The B-cell Compartment

Most B cells are situated in the peripheral part of the node (**cortex**). The cells form rounded aggregates

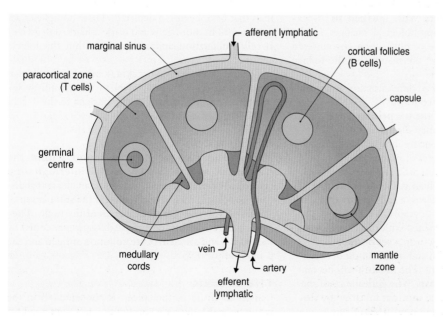

FIGURE 10.6 *Basic anatomy of a normal lymph node.*

known as **follicles**. In unstimulated nodes, these folli-cles are small and show no division into functional zones. When stimulated by antigens, they become enlarged and show a separation into two zones:

1) The **follicle centre**, which on low-power examination appears somewhat paler and more open than the second zone.

2) The **mantle zone**, which partially surrounds the follicle centre, usually on its capsular aspect; mantle zone lymphocytes show both IgM and IgD on their surfaces.

The principal cell components of the follicle cen-tre are centroblasts and centrocytes.

- **Centroblasts** are large, actively dividing, cells with rounded nuclei in which there are usually at least two nucleoli, touching the inner aspect of the nuclear membrane. The cytoplasm is small in amount and the cells tend to be clustered in the part of the follicle that is furthest from the node capsule.

- **Centrocytes** are smaller than centroblasts and tend to have rather irregularly shaped nuclei with a chromatin pattern rather coarser than that of the centroblast. Nucleoli are inconspicuous. In the course of B-cell proliferation elicited by antigenic stimulation, many B cells are eliminated by the process of programmed cell death (**apoptosis**). The cell fragments are engulfed by macrophages, present in large numbers within the follicle centres. These cells showing lymphocyte debris within their cytoplasm are known as **tingible body macrophages**.

B-cell Differentiation in the Follicle Centre

Differentiation of B cells within follicle centres is driven by encounters with antigen and is ex-pressed in a series of morphological changes in the small 'virgin' (in the sense of not having encountered antigen) B lymphocytes at the margins of the follicle centres.

Antigen-dependent B-cell differentiation and prolif-eration may take one of two forms:

1) If the immune response is a **primary** one, small B cells may be transformed directly into **immunoblasts**, differentiate into IgM-secreting plasmacytoid lymphocytes or plasma cells, and produce the IgM characteristic of the primary response. The immunoblast is a large cell with a somewhat vesicular nucleus, a large centrally placed nucleolus, and abundant cytoplasm which is basophilic in sections stained with the Giemsa stain.

2) In the **late primary** or in a **secondary** response, differentiation and proliferation occur within the follicle centre. The small B cells become converted to **centroblasts**. The appearance of the centroblast in the follicle centre is followed by that of the **centrocyte**. Two populations of centrocytes exist, one composed of small cells and the other of

larger cells. Ultimately these cells differentiate into immunoblasts from which plasma cells and B 'memory' cells are derived. **Lymphomas of follicle centre cell origin can express any of these differentiation patterns.**

The T-cell Compartment

The T-cell compartment is co-terminous with the cortical tissue lying *between* the follicles and is termed the **paracortex.** The high endothelial venules are sit-uated in this area. On examination of haematoxylin and eosin-stained sections, mature T cells appear as small lymphocytes morphologically indistinguishable from B cells. Cells that have encountered antigen and undergone transformation are, of course, much larger, both B and T variants being present in the para-cortex.

Antigen-presenting Cells (Accessory Cells)

There are two types of APC within lymph nodes: dendritic cells and interdigitating reticulum cells.

Dendritic Cells

Antigen-presenting cells in the follicle centres are called dendritic cells. These are small cells with elongated cytoplasmic processes forming a meshwork within the follicle centre. The follicular dendritic cells trap immune complexes, formed as the result of the reaction between quite small amounts of immunogen, homospecific circulating antibody and C3. The den-dritic cells express large numbers of receptors for IgG Fc and iC3b, and these enable the cells to trap the newly formed complexes effectively. The importance of complement in antigen localization in follicle cen-tres is shown by the failure of such localization in ani-mals that have been C3 depleted. These complexes act as powerful immunogens and cause a marked degree of B-cell proliferation and activation within the follicle centre.

Dendritic cells within the skin (Langerhans' cells) can process antigen and then travel in the lymph as so-called 'veiled' cells, which deliver antigen to the T cells in the paracortical areas of lymph nodes.

Reticulum Cells

The second type of APC is found within the paracortex and is known as the interdigitating reticulum cell. These cells have pale nuclei and abun-dant cytoplasm; their sole function is the stimulation of T cells within the paracortical areas of the node. They express large amounts of surface glycoprotein coded by the MHC, and also leucocyte common antigen and the β-integrin p150,95.

THE SPLEEN

Lymphoid tissue in the spleen is concentrated in the white pulp (Malpighian corpuscles) and is arranged for the most part around arterioles; this periarteriolar lymphoid sheath is divided into T- and B-cell zones. The T cells are arranged around the central arteriole, helper cells making up 70% and suppressor cells 30% of the T-cell population. The B cells are segregated from the T cells and consist of a germinal centre surrounded by a mantle zone.

The immune and non-immune functions of the spleen are discussed in the section on Splenic pathology (Chapter 42).

FUNCTIONAL ANATOMY OF MALT

MALT is characterized in terms of two functions:
- **transport of immunoglobulins to luminal surfaces**, as for example in the gut or respiratory tract
- **a specific pool of lymphocytes which appear to 'home' on to MALT**

In the gut, the site in which the functional anatomy of normal MALT has been studied most extensively, it is clear that there are three cell compartments:

1) **Peyer's patches in the small intestinal mucosa and their homologues in the large gut**
2) **lymphoreticular cells diffusely distributed in the lamina propria of the gut mucosa**
3) **intraepithelial lymphocytes**, which are chiefly suppressor T cells (expressing CD8)

Peyer's Patches

Each Peyer's patch shows a B-cell follicle centre partially surrounded by a mantle zone, thickest on the mucosal side of the follicle centre. Surrounding this mantle zone is another zone of small B lymphocytes known as the **marginal zone**, which is also thickest on the mucosal aspect of the patch. Marginal zone lymphocytes stretch up to involve the specialized epithelium (**dome epithelium**) over the patch, which can sample gut luminal constituents.

MALT Cell Population of the Lamina Propria

The mucosal lamina propria contains a mixed cell population in which macrophages, plasma cells and small lymphocytes are present. Mucosal plasma cells secrete equal amounts of both classes of IgA, two-thirds in dimeric form which can therefore bind to the secretory component, the complex being transported across the small gut epithelium into the gut lumen. Other immunoglobulin subclasses are also synthesized within plasma cells in the lamina propria but in considerably smaller amounts than IgA.

Intraepithelial T Lymphocytes

Under normal circumstances, lymphocytes are found between the epithelial cells lining the lumen of the small and large intestines. This lymphocyte population consists essentially of suppressor-type T cells, which differ in some respects from T cells found outside the gut. The function of this intraepithelial T-cell population remains to be clarified.

IDENTIFICATION OF T AND B LYMPHOCYTES

There are no morphological differences between lymphocytes of the T and B series. However, these cells possess a number of different surface markers and also respond to different sets of chemical species by polyclonal proliferation. These characteristics make it possible not only to distinguish between the two basic groups, but also to identify T-cell subsets such as **helper** and **suppressor** cells.

The outstanding feature of the B-cell surface is the presence of immunoglobulin, which can be identified by either immunofluorescence or immunoperoxidase techniques using antibodies prepared against these immunoglobulins. The T-cell population is identified by the immunohistological demonstration of a surface molecule known as CD3, which is responsible for transducing the signal that specific antigen has been recognized to the inside of the T cell (see p 108).

Other differences in cell markers, as defined by using monoclonal antibodies, define specialized T-cell subsets such as cytotoxic cells (CD8+) and helper cells (CD4+).

Normally each B lymphocyte is programmed to make immunoglobulin of only one specificity and it is this immunoglobulin on the B-lymphocyte surface that acts as a specific receptor for antigen.

In addition to the possession of surface components that can be recognized by treating lymphocytes with appropriate antibodies linked to a fluorescent dye, T and B lymphocytes respond to different sets of stimulating agents which cause them to proliferate and become larger and more primitive in appearance (this response is known as **blast transformation**).

ANTIBODIES (IMMUNOGLOBULINS)

Antibodies can be defined both in operational and chemical terms. In the **operational** sense they are molecules that bind specifically to the appropriate antigen and in so doing perform a range of tasks of great biological significance, even though these may not all be beneficial. Depending on the class of antibody involved, these operations include:
- **agglutination and lysis of bacteria (IgM)**
- **opsonization of such organisms**
- **initiation of the 'classical' complement pathway through the ability to bind the C1q component of complement avidly (IgM$_1$)**
- **blocking entry of the microorganisms from**

the respiratory tract, gut, eyes and urinary tract into tissues that lie deep to the epithelia (IgA)
- **killing of the infected cell via** antibody-dependent cell-mediated cytotoxicity in which antibody bound to antigen (e.g. viral antigen expressed on the surface of an infected cell) binds to Fc receptors of killer cells
- **neutralizing bacterial toxins and some of the bacterial products that otherwise enable the bacteria to avoid the effects of specific immunity**

From the **chemical** point of view it has been known since the studies of Tiselius and colleagues in the late 1930s that the antibody activity of the plasma resides in its **globulin** fraction, i.e. the group of plasma proteins that migrates most slowly on electrophoresis; antibodies are, in fact, also termed **immunoglobulins**.

STRUCTURE OF ANTIBODY

Immunoglobulin has a Y-shaped, four-chain structure. In the monomeric form, which is characteristic of three of the five major classes of immunoglobulin, the molecule consists of four polypeptide chains held together by disulphide bonds (*Fig. 10.7*). Two of these chains have a molecular weight of 22 000 and are known as **light chains**. The other two have molecular weights ranging from 55 000 to 72 500 depending on the immunoglobulin class and are called **heavy chains**. Each monomer has a pair of identical heavy chains and a pair of identical light chains.

The chemical and biological differences between the five classes of immunoglobulin are due to differences in their heavy chain structure and whether or not they exist as monomers (IgG, IgD, IgE), dimers (IgA) or pentamers (IgM). The heavy chain classes are shown in *Table 10.2*.

Two different classes of light chain exist and are known as kappa (κ) and lambda (λ). Pairs of one or other of these are found in all five classes of immunoglobulin.

Relationship Between Structure and Function in the Immunoglobulin Molecule

When a monomeric immunoglobulin molecule such as is illustrated in *Fig. 10.7* is treated with the proteolytic enzyme papain, it is cleaved just above the disulphide

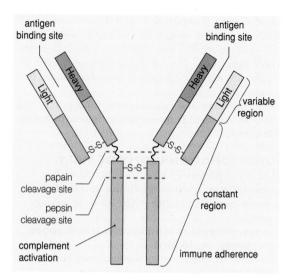

FIGURE 10.7 A monomeric immunoglobin molecule.

bridges between the heavy chains and thus splits into three fragments. The two fragments that contain the light chain are identical. Each possesses the ability to bind specifically to antigen and is known as the **Fab (fragment antigen binding)**. When the appropriate antigen is in solution, the union between these fragments and the antigen leads to the formation of a soluble complex, due to the fact that binding is **univalent**.

The third fragment has no power to bind to antigen, is easily crystallizable and is known as **Fc (fragment crystallizable)**. It is, however, the site of important biological functions such as **complement activation** and **immune adherence** to receptors on the surface of neutrophils and macrophages. Treatment of an immunoglobulin molecule with another proteolytic enzyme, pepsin, cleaves the molecule below the disulphide bond, as shown in *Fig. 10.7*, with the production of a divalent F(ab)$_2$ fragment and a dimer consisting of only part of the Fc portion (pFc).

Diversity of Antibody in Relation to its Structure

One of the most remarkable features of the antibody system is that each antibody has a combining site that matches with the epitope with which it binds specifically. Thus huge numbers of combining sites must exist. This diversity of antibodies is the expression of the great variability in the amino acid sequence which exists at the *N*-terminal or antigen-combining portion of both light and heavy chains; these portions of the chains are known as the **variable** regions.

Both light and heavy chains possess units of about 110 amino acids which are known as domains. These portions of the chain are usually folded, the folded loops being bridged by disulphide bonds. When amino acid sequencing is carried out on a monoclonal

Table 10.2 Immunoglobulin Classes

Immunoglobulin class	Heavy chain
IgA	alpha (α)
IgG	gamma (γ)
IgD	delta (δ)
IgE	epsilon (ε)
IgM	mu (μ)

immunoglobulin such as the proteins secreted by myeloma cells, the light chain is shown to have two domains: a variable one at the amino terminal end (V_L) and a constant one (C_L), each occupying about half the length of the chain. The heavy chain also has a variable domain at its amino terminal end (V_H). As this is about the same length as the variable domain found on light chains, only a quarter of the heavy chain is variable. The remaining three-quarters are divided into three constant domains ($C_H1,2,3$) (four in ε chains).

To form the combining site, the polypeptide domains in the light and heavy chains are folded into their unique shape by **weak non-covalent chemical forces that are determined by the amino acid sequences of each variable domain**. As the amino acid sequence determines the shape of the combining site, it is necessary only to vary this sequence to create a specific antibody, and thus it is easy to conceive how a vast number of antibody molecules can come into being.

The Genetic Basis of Combining Site Diversity

If a very large number of different combining sites can exist, does this mean that there is an equally vast array of genes to code for each of the possible amino acid sequences? Strict adherence to the one gene–one polypeptide view would mean just this, but in fact a quite different set of circumstances exists in relation to immunoglobulin chains. For each chain the variable and constant regions are coded for by a different gene. The complete gene coding for a heavy or light chain is not present in the germ cell line. Instead portions of each chain's gene are brought together during early development of the B cell, being physically translocated at this phase.

To encode the variable portion of a human κ light chain, two gene portions are required: a large V region and a small J region. The constant region is encoded by a single gene. There are about 70 V genes and five J genes. During B-cell development, translocation leads to one V gene joining with one J segment. After transcription, the VJ region transcript is spliced with the transcript of the constant region and this VJC messenger RNA is translated in the endoplasmic reticulum to form the κ light chain. Much the same occurs in relation to the arrangement of the genes coding for the variable regions of the λ light chains and the heavy chains. The heavy chains have, in addition to the V and J genes mentioned above, a D segment.

IMMUNOGLOBULIN CLASSES

Immunoglobulin G (IgG)

IgG is, in quantitative terms, the most important of the five main immunoglobulin classes, making up about 70–80% of plasma immunoglobulin. In structure it is monomeric and has the four-chain structure described above. It diffuses readily into the extravascular compartment and thus plays an important part in the neutralization of toxins and in opsonization of bacteria. However, to accomplish this it is necessary for more than one IgG molecule to bind to a small area on the bacterial cell wall so that multiple Fc fragments may be presented to the receptors on phagocytic cells. The coating of certain target cells with IgG can also attract cells of the lymphoid system that have Fc receptors but which are not specifically sensitized to any epitope on the target. These cells can kill the antibody-coated targets and are known as **K** or **killer cells**.

Two molecules of IgG bound closely together on an antigenic surface can activate complement by the allosteric rearrangement of part of the Fc fragment. This particular form of expression of biological activity varies within the IgG class; variations in the C_H2 region and four subclasses of IgG have so far been identified. IgG$_1$ and IgG$_3$ molecules readily activate complement when bound to antigen; IgG$_2$ antibodies are less efficient in this respect, and IgG$_4$ does not activate complement at all.

Of all the immunoglobulins, only IgG can cross the placental barrier and thus is the most important of the antibody classes in protecting newborn infants against infection.

Immunoglobulin A (IgA)

IgA appears selectively in the seromucous secretions of the gastrointestinal and respiratory tracts, and in tears, sweat, bile and breast milk.

Basically, it has the same four-chain structure as IgG, but the heavy chains have a higher molecular weight. IgA is dimerized by linkage to a small cysteine-rich protein known as the **J chain** within the plasma cell where it is synthesized. This dimer is then released into the lamina propria of the gut mucosa or the subepithelial tissues of the respiratory tract. It is then transported across the surface epithelium into the lumen. While in transit across the epithelium, the IgA becomes stabilized against proteolysis by attaching to a peptide known as the **secretory component**, which is secreted by epithelial cells.

The fact that dimerization takes place *within* the plasma cells ensures against the formation of dimers of **mixed specificity**, such as might occur if the process took place in the lamina propria. This avoids dilution of the antigen-combining efficiency of the molecule.

IgA is believed to act by inhibiting the adherence of coated microorganisms to mucosal surfaces and thus preventing them from entering the tissues. Both bacteria and viruses may be affected in this way; oral polio vaccines probably induce immunity by sensitizing the IgA-producing plasma cells in the mucosa of the gut. The role of the relatively large amounts of **monomeric IgA** in the plasma is still not clear.

Immunoglobulin M (IgM)

IgM is the largest of the immunoglobulins, with a molecular weight of 900 000. It consists of five basic four-chain units joined together to form a 20-chain molecule. This is held together by disulphide bonds between the five Fc fragments and a J chain, identical with that involved in the dimerization of IgA. The μ chain of IgM is the heaviest of all the immunoglobulin chains; about 10% of its weight is accounted for by carbohydrate. Because of its pentameric structure, IgM has ten potential antigen-combining sites, but in practice, perhaps because of some inherent rigidity in the pentamer, only five of these are usually involved in antigen binding at any one time. The possession of multiple binding sites gives IgM the ability to bind with great strength to antigenic surfaces on which there is a repetitive epitope pattern.

IgM antibodies are the first to be formed after immunization. Once IgG synthesis starts, the level of IgM falls. When antibodies are made that react with the antigen-combining sites on IgM (anti-idiotype antibodies), they are also found to react with the IgG antibodies appearing later against the same antigens. These results have been interpreted as suggesting that the differentiating clone of lymphocytes responding to an antigen first uses a pair of V_L and V_H gene segments in combination with a pair of C_L and C_μ gene segments to produce the IgM antibody. Later the same variable gene segments are used with C_L and C_H segments to produce IgG antibodies that have the same specificity as the IgM.

In so far as **complement activation** and consequent bacterial killing is concerned, IgM is the most effective of the immunoglobulins. Its very large size means that the molecule can cross capillary walls only with great difficulty and **it does not cross the placental barrier in significant amounts**. Thus, if IgM is detected in cord blood or in blood taken from an infant within the first few days of life, it is reasonable to assume that it represents an immune response on the part of the child itself and that intrauterine or neonatal infection has occurred. This inability to cross the placenta has direct relevance to the rarity of haemolytic disease of the newborn due to ABO group incompatibility.

Carbohydrate antigens such as A and B blood group substances elicit a prolonged response by IgM antibodies, and the usual switch-over to IgG production does not occur. Most people produce antibodies to blood groups that are not their own as a result of stimulation by plant carbohydrates that strongly resemble blood group substances. If IgM antibodies crossed the placenta, incompatibility between the ABO blood groups of mother and baby would inevitably lead to immune haemolysis of the infant's red cells.

Immunoglobulin D (IgD)

IgD is present in the plasma in only very small amounts. For a long time its function was uncertain, but it has been found that about half of all B lymphocytes have IgD on their surface, often in association with monomeric IgM. Both the coating immunoglobulin molecules appear to have the same idiotypic determinants (i.e. they have the same V_H and V_L regions on their respective light and heavy chains). It seems likely that they function as mutually assisting antigen receptors for the control of B-lymphocyte activation and suppression.

Immunoglobulin E (IgE)

IgE is present in only minute amounts in the plasma of most people. It has the ability to bind (via its Fc portion) to receptors on tissue mast cells, these cells having between 100 000 and 500 000 Fc receptors on their plasma membranes. When the appropriate antigen binds to the Fab portions of adjacent IgE molecules, a series of events is started which is not intrinsically different from that taking place when chemotactic signals bind to receptors on the neutrophil surface. In the case of the tissue mast cell, however, activation leads to a discharge of the cell granules, which include **histamine, leukotrienes** (products of arachidonic acid metabolism via the lipo-oxygenase pathway) and a factor chemotactic for eosinophils (*Fig. 10.8*). The release of these active compounds causes a local inflammatory reaction and, if the IgE antibody is bound to mast cells in the neighbourhood of bronchial smooth muscle, contraction of this smooth muscle. This reaction may be helpful in combating certain parasitic infestations.

Some people appear to have a genetically determined predisposition to produce large amounts of IgE-type antibody. This renders them more liable than others to a variety of unpleasant and even dangerous clinical expressions of large-scale release of mast cell granule contents, such as asthma, hay fever and urticaria. The antigens that trigger these reactions are called **allergens**, and those with a constitutional predis-

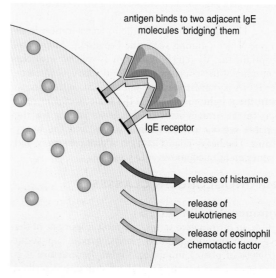

FIGURE 10.8 IgE-mediated degranulation of mast cells.

position to respond in this way are often spoken of as being **atopic**. This problem is explored in Chapter 11.

THE IMMUNE RESPONSE

The induction of a response to any antigen depends primarily on the **recognition** of a specific epitope by genetically programmed lymphocytes. This is followed by a monoclonal form of **cell proliferation**. Next **differentiation occurs**, which may lead to one or both of the following:

- antibody production
- initiation of one or more of the activities of the T-cell system

In addition there will be an increase in the number of cells programmed for recognition (or memory cells); this feature is responsible for the **increased speed** and **magnitude** of the reaction that takes place as a result of a subsequent exposure to the antigen concerned.

The functioning of such a system depends both on the nature of the antigenic **signal** and on the mechanisms that exist for the **reception** of such a signal.

THE SIGNAL

While both B and T cells may respond to the same antigen, the way in which this signal is presented is fundamental. B cells can recognize an antigen irrespective of the form in which it is presented. Thus these cells can bind free antigen in solution, antigens present on the membranes of cells, and antigens insolubilized in various ways.

In contrast, the vast majority of T cells can only bind antigen that is associated with the surface of a cell. Helper T cells and those that secrete lymphokines recognize foreign antigens that have been processed (with the exception of **superantigens**; see below) and then presented to them on the surface of macrophages and, perhaps, other accessory cells such as dendritic cells. In addition, however, a second signal is required. This is provided by a glycoprotein on the surface of the presenting cell that is coded for a gene sequence within the **MHC** (major histocompatibility complex).

The Major Histocompatibility Complex

The MHC is a set of genes encoding a number of cell surface glycoproteins of great importance in cell recognition. APCs such as the macrophage chiefly express MHC-coded surface glycoproteins known as class II histocompatibility antigens. The limitation of T-cell responses to antigens associated with specific classes of MHC-coded proteins is known as **haplotype restriction**.

T cells recognize antigen via receptors that have a wide range of variable regions mediating their ability to respond to an equally wide range of antigenic determinants. The T-cell repertoire develops during T-cell processing within the thymus.

- Cells that are selected for restriction to MHC class I molecule recognition almost all become cytotoxic T cells (CD8+).
- Those showing MHC class II restriction become T helper cells (CD4+).

Antigens expressed in association with MHC-coded proteins are processed within APCs and are then expressed on the surface membranes of the APC.

MHC Class I proteins consist of a heavy α chain and a β$_2$-microglobulin light chain (*Fig. 10.9*). **MHC class II-coded proteins** consist of α and β chains of more or less equal size. Both types of molecule show some similar features. Each has:

- two immunoglobulin-like domains
- a peptide-binding site formed by an eight-stranded β-pleated sheet and two α-helical regions.

Processed antigens are presented to the T cells within 'binding grooves' formed within the MHC-coded proteins. This groove is formed by the α helices and the β-pleated sheet portion in the outer domains of both classes of MHC-coded proteins.

A large number of possible alleles per locus exists in respect of the MHC genes and this has important implications in relation to finding compatible donor grafts for patients requiring transplants (see pp 140–142).

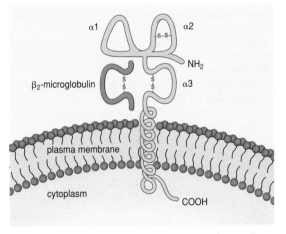

FIGURE 10.9 *Structure of MHC class I proteins, showing the* α *chain and* β$_2$*-microglobulin.*

Superantigens and the MHC

A small number of antigens can bind to MHC class II proteins without first being processed within APCs. These are known as superantigens. They have been implicated in a diverse group of disorders including rabies, acute T-cell responses to bacterial toxins such as those of *Staphylococcus aureus* which may cause the toxic shock syndrome or severe food poisoning, and acquired immune deficiency syndrome. It is also suggested that superantigens may be implicated in certain autoimmune diseases such as rheumatoid arthritis.

Superantigens appear to bind to MHC class II proteins outside the usual binding groove. The staphylococcal antigen that causes food poisoning (enterotoxin B) binds to the α_1 domain of the human MHC class II molecule and in so doing creates a novel binding site for the T-cell receptor. Whole T-cell subpopulations can be activated by superantigens, independent of antigen specificity. These T cells share a common Vβ chain configuration.

Antigen Processing

With the exception of the superantigens mentioned above, T cells recognize antigens that have been processed in some way within the APCs.

Processing Within Cells Expressing MHC Class II Proteins (Figs 10.10 and 10.11)

It is believed that exogenous soluble protein antigens are endocytosed by APCs. Within the endosome these proteins undergo unfolding and a limited degree of proteolysis as the early endosome undergoes progressive acidification. Antigen processing in these cells is blocked by treating them with chloroquine, which prevents acidification. This altered protein is later presented to the T cells in combination with the MHC class II proteins. A similar series of operations is involved in the case of microorganisms, whose antigens undergo proteolysis within phagolysosomes.

Meanwhile, the class II molecules are being assembled within the endoplasmic reticulum. α and β chains are complexed with a membrane-bound invariate chain with two functions:

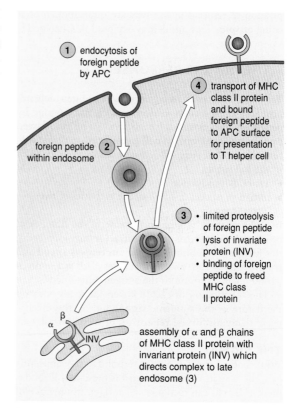

FIGURE 10.11 Processing and presentation by antigen-presenting cells (APCs) of antigens in association with MHC class II proteins.

1) It dictates the folding of the class II molecule.
2) It prevents premature binding of proteins to the class II molecule before the latter reaches the location of the intracellular processed antigen.

The vacuole containing the complex of class II and invariant chains now fuses with the endosome containing the partially proteolysed antigen. Cathepsins B and D, derived from the endosome, degrade the invariant chain. This frees the class II binding groove and allows the processed antigen to bind to the class II protein.

The antigen–class II protein complex is now transported to the cell surface.

Processing Within Cells Expressing MHC Class I Proteins (Fig. 10.12)

Virally coded proteins, presented on the surface of cells expressing class I MHC-coded proteins, can also pass through this process of proteolysis with the formation of peptides, some of which are recognized by T-cell receptors.

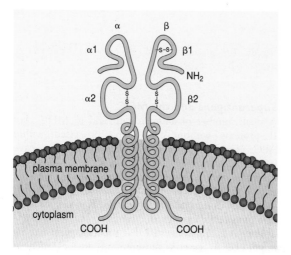

FIGURE 10.10 Structure of MHC class II proteins.

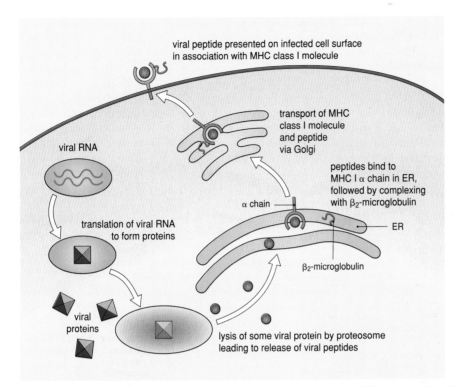

FIGURE 10.12 *Processing and presentation of viral antigens in association with MHC class I proteins. ER, endoplasmic reticulum.*

- Such proteins are degraded to peptides after being conjugated with ubiquitin by a complex of peptidases known as a proteosome. In the case of certain viral coat proteins, proteolytic degradation takes place within the lumen of the endoplasmic reticulum where there is a set of resident proteases.
- The peptides are then translocated into the endoplasmic reticulum of the infected cell by a transporter mechanism known as TAP1 and TAP2.
- In the endoplasmic reticulum the peptides cooperate with β_2–microglobulin and complex with newly formed class I heavy chains bound to membranes.
- The peptide MHC class I-coded protein complex is transported across the Golgi apparatus where it acquires some carbohydrate side-chains.
- The complex is then presented on the cell surface.

Other Molecules Concerned with Antigen Presentation

A third group of antigen-presenting molecules is said to exist in the form of certain class I-like β_2-microglobulin-associated proteins. Some of these are encoded by a gene located on chromosome 1 (unlike MHC genes which are situated on chromosome 6). One of these molecules, CD1b, presents lipids from the mycolic acid in the cell wall of *M. tuberculosis*. It has been suggested therefore that T cells may also recognize non-protein microbial antigens.

> **KEY POINTS: Antigen Presentation and the MHC**
> - Class I MHC molecules are present on virtually all nucleated cells in the body and signal to cytotoxic T cells.
> - Class II molecules are particularly associated with professional APCs, B cells and macrophages, and signal to T helper cells. Their expression may be induced in endothelial and some epithelial cells by IFN-γ.
> - The 'professional APCs' (B cells, macrophages, dendritic cells, Langerhans cells in the basal layer of the skin and, under certain circumstances, endothelial cells) present antigen more efficiently partly because of their ability to process endocytosed antigens and partly because they possess cell surface proteins that bind to counterstructures on the T-cell surfaces.

THE RESPONSE

Antigen Recognition by T Cells and T-cell Activation

The 'eyes' used by T cells to 'see' the antigens presented to them are receptors. The antigen-specific T-cell receptor is a membrane-bound molecule composed of two chains (most commonly an α and a β chain) linked by disulphide bonds (*Fig. 10.13*). Each chain is

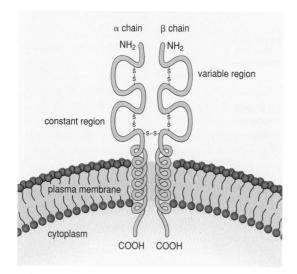

FIGURE 10.13 Structure of the T-lymphocyte receptor.

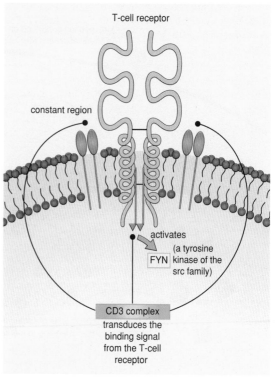

FIGURE 10.14 The T-cell receptor is associated with the CD3 complex, which mediates transduction of the binding signal received from the receptor.

folded into two immunoglobulin-like domains. One of these has a relatively constant structure; the other has a high degree of variability.

A less common type of receptor (TCR1) has γ and δ chains. In peripheral blood this receptor is found on only 0.5–15% of T cells. In the intestinal epithelium and skin it is more common. γδ T-cell receptors are particularly concerned with the recognition of mycobacterial antigens, especially the mycobacterial heat shock protein hsp65 which cross-reacts with a self-antigen.

The gene segments encoding the T-cell receptor β chains have V, D, J and constant segments just as in the heavy chain of immunoglobulin. These segments undergo rearrangement to form a continuous VDJ sequence, as happens in the course of development of B cells.

The CD3 Complex

Binding of antigen to an antigen-specific T-cell receptor is in itself insufficient for T-cell activation. In normally functioning T cells, the T-cell receptor is closely linked with a molecule known as CD3, which is made up of five peptide chains (γ, δ, ε, ζ and η). CD3 is responsible for transducing the signal received by the T-cell receptor to the interior of the T lymphocyte (*Fig. 10.14*). Two of the chains (γ and ζ) are associated with the Fc receptors I and III on natural killer (NK) cells and function as signal transducers in these cells as well.

Adhesion of T Cells to APCs Precedes Antigen Recognition

Antigen recognition by the T-cell receptor is preceded by a non-specific phase during which T cells adhere to APCs. Because APCs can present many different determinants on their surfaces and any T-cell receptor can

'see' only a few of these, the adhesion phase permits the T-cell receptor to 'sample' what is being presented. If the appropriate antigens are not present, adhesion between T cell and APC is broken.

Adhesion between T cells and APCs is mediated via a ligand–receptor bond. The adhesion molecules on the T cells are LFA-1 (an integrin; see pp 43–44) and CD2. CD2 binds to LFA-3 (another integrin) on the surface of the APC, and LFA-1 binds to ICAM-1 (see p 43).

T-cell Activation Requires Co-Stimulatory Signals

Another important bond between T cells and APCs is that between CD28, which is expressed on the surface of all T helper cells and most cytotoxic T cells, and B7, a molecule that can be induced on APCs and which is normally expressed at low densities on B lymphocytes. B7 is an important co-stimulatory signal for T-cell activation, the other being IL-1.

Before a resting T cell can be activated two signals are required.

- The first is the complex formed by the T-cell receptor, the antigen and the MHC-coded protein.
- The second is either B7 or IL-1. A T cell that is already activated will respond to a single signal.

Signal Transduction is Accomplished by Tyrosine Phosphorylation and Subsequent Activation of the Phosphatidylinositol Pathway

Activation of the T cell involves phosphorylation of CD3, which is carried out by two protein tyrosine kinases, both of which are related to the *src* proto-oncogene family (see pp 274–275, 277). This is followed, within 15 seconds, by the phosphorylation and activation of phospholipase Cγ which activates the phosphatidylinositol pathway with the release of inositol triphosphate from PIP-2 and diacyl glycerol. Thus there is much in common between the activation of T lymphocytes after antigen recognition and activation of neutrophils after binding of a chemotactic signal.

THE EFFECTS OF T-CELL ACTIVATION

T Helper Cells

T helper (CD4+) cells play a dominant role in cell-mediated immune response. They:

- **select the antigens and epitopes that are recognized**
- **determine which effector mechanisms will be used in the response to the chosen epitopes. These effector mechanisms include:**
  1) cytotoxic T lymphocytes (CD8+ or T_C cells)
  2) antibody and cells such as mast cells and eosinophils
  3) activation of macrophages and induction of delayed hypersensitivity such as occurs in granulomatous inflammation
- **assist the proliferation of appropriate cell types via the release of cytokines**
- **upregulate the functions of phagocytic cells such as macrophages and of other effector cells**

When 'virgin' T cells are stimulated they differentiate into T_H subsets. In the short term T_H0 cells arise which synthesize and release cytokines such as IL-2, IL-4, IL-5 and IL-10 and IFN-γ. In the longer term, as in chronic inflammation, two specialized subsets T_H1 and T_H2 differentiate:

- T_H1 cells promote macrophage activation and tend to respond well to the antigens presented by macrophages.
- T_H2 cells tend to promote the production of antibody and stimulate the activities of mast cells and eosinophils.

Both these subsets express some cytokines (IL-3, TNF-α and GM-CSF) in common. Expression of other cytokines is restricted to one or other T helper cell subset (*Table 10.3*).

The cytokines expressed by these subsets can oppose each other; the relative dominance of one or another in certain pathological situations, for example in tuberculosis, may have profound implications for the natural history of the disease.

Table 10.3 Cytokines Released by T_H1 and T_H2 Subsets

Cytokine	T_H1-produced	T_H2-produced
IL-2	+	0
IFN-γ	+	0
IL-4	0	+
IL-5	0	+
IL-6	0	+
IL-10	0	+

Amplification of T-cell Responses

The expansion of appropriate clones of T cells that follows antigen recognition depends on the synthesis and release of the cytokine IL-2, which acts as a growth factor. IL-2 produces its effect by binding to high-affinity receptors which are not present on the surfaces of resting T cells but are expressed within a few hours of T-cell activation following the T-cell receptor recognition of antigen. The importance of IL-2 production following antigen rejection is underlined by the effectiveness of the drug cyclosporin A, which is widely used in preventing rejection of allogeneic transplants. Cyclosporin blocks the transcription of the IL-2 gene, which normally follows T-cell activation (see *Fig. 13.8*).

T-cell-mediated Cytotoxicity

Cytotoxic (CD8+) T cells also synthesize and release cytokines. The output of cytokines in many instances resembles that of T_H1 cells; cells whose cytokine range is similar to that of T_H2 cells are thought to have regulatory rather than killing functions.

Killing of cells by lymphocytes takes place under three sets of circumstances; in each case a different population of lymphoid cells is involved:

1) MHC-restricted T lymphocytes (mainly CD8+) recognize specific antigens (for example, virally coded proteins) on the surface of cells. Binding takes place via the T-cell receptor as described previously.

2) Certain epitopes are recognized by receptors on NK cells. These cells are derived from large granular lymphocytes which constitute about 5% of blood lymphocytes in humans. They do not express CD3 but do express CD16 (an FcγIIIb receptor) and CD56, an adhesion molecule. Expression of class I MHC-coded proteins on the surface of a cell appears to protect it from NK cell-mediated lysis.

3) When a cell is coated with antibody that is recognized by lymphoid cells with the appropriate Fc receptors, binding occurs between the 'target' cell and the lymphocyte, and the former is lysed. This is known as **antibody-dependent cell-mediated cytotoxicity (ADCC)** and is carried

out by killer (K) cells. The term K cell is an operational one, i.e a lymphoid cell that kills by ADCC, and, in fact, covers several different cell types including both CD8+ and NK cells.

ADCC is not confined to lymphoid cells. Monocytes may also be cytotoxic to cells coated with antibody and eosinophil-mediated damage to antibody-covered schistosomes is also well recognized.

Mechanism of Lymphocyte-mediated Cytotoxicity

The basic mechanisms involved in lymphocyte cytotoxicity are believed to be similar in the three circumstances listed above. Most of our knowledge is derived from studies of NK cell activity.

- The cytotoxic cells adhere to appropriate ligands on target cells.
- The contents of vesicles in the cytotoxic cells are released into the space between the cytotoxic cell and its target. This process is calcium dependent.
- The vesicle contents so released contain **perforin**, a protein that structurally resembles complement component 9. The perforin becomes inserted into the membrane of target cells where it polymerizes to form a transmembrane channel rather similar to that of the complement membrane attack complex.

Complement membrane attack complex damages cells by causing lysis of their membranes. This is *not* the case with perforin, which instead induces **apoptosis** (programmed cell death) (see pp 30–32).

Other potentially cell damaging factors are present in cytotoxic lymphoid cells. These include:
a) a set of serine proteases known as **granzymes**; this contains a subset, the **fragmentins**, which are also thought to induce apoptosis
b) tumour necrosis factor β
c) adenosine 5′-triphosphate (ATP)

B-CELL ACTIVATION

Specific activation of B cells, with the resultant selection of a clone of antibody-producing cells, involves recognition of a homospecific antigen and, in the case of most antigens, assistance from the T-cell population.

Some antigens seem able to trigger B-cell responses in the absence of T cells and are called **thymus-independent antigens**. They are all polymers and include such molecules as pneumococcal polysaccharide, dextran, bacterial lipopolysaccharide, levan and others. The antibody response to these antigens is unusual in that it consists almost exclusively of IgM, very few memory cells are produced, and tolerance to these antigens is readily induced.

The actual recognition process is mediated by immunoglobulins on the surface of the appropriate B cell. The variable domains of these surface immunoglobulins fit precisely with the antigenic deter-

minant. Thus each lymphocyte is genetically programmed to bind one antigenic determinant. **It is this specificity of the variable regions of the surface immunoglobulins that determines which clone of B cells will proliferate and differentiate** (*Fig. 10.15*).

All B cells express IgM on their surface and about 70% express IgD. Only a relatively small fraction of the B-cell population expresses immunoglobulins of the other classes, and on these cells IgM is expressed as well. The nature of the immunoglobulin receptors on the B-cell surface has important implications for the future production of the antibody classes. B cells bearing IgM or IgM and IgD on their surface, when stimulated by the appropriate antigen, give rise to clones of cells that, when differentiated into plasma cells, produce IgM only. If immunoglobulin of one of the other classes is present in addition to surface IgM, then class switching occurs and IgG, IgA or IgE antibodies are produced, depending on which is present on the unstimulated B-cell surface.

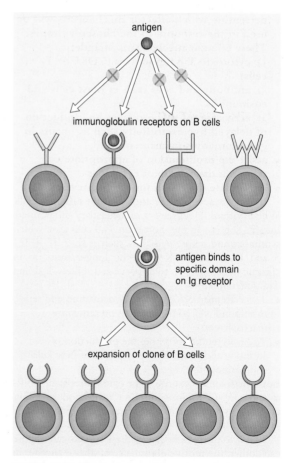

FIGURE 10.15 *Clonal selection in the immune response: result of the first exposure of B cells to antigen. Some of the clone will become memory cells and some effector cells.*

B- and T-cell Cooperation (*Fig. 10.16*)

As already stated, most antigens fail to trigger proliferation and maturation of B-cell clones without the active participation of T helper cells. Cooperation between the T helper cell and the B cell is a two-way process in which:

● Specific antigen is presented to the T_H cells by B cells, the processed antigen being presented in association with MHC class II coded proteins.

● The same B cells receive signals from the stimulated T_H cells which cause proliferation and differentiation into antibody-producing and -exporting cells.

Within the B cells antigen, which has bound to surface immunoglobulin, is internalized and processed and is then presented on the B-cell surface in association with MHC class II proteins.

Part of the T cell-mediated activation of B cells which then ensues is direct. Activating signals on the B-cell surface are 'triggered' by binding to appropriate ligands which are expressed on the T-cell surface after antigen has been presented. The most powerful of such activating signals is known as CD40.

In addition the T cell exerts powerful effects on B cells through its expression of cytokines including IL-2 and IL-4, which stimulate B-cell **proliferation**, and IL-4, IL-6, IL-10 and IFN-γ, which promote terminal **differentiation** into antibody-producing cells.

COMPLEMENT ACTIVATION

No account of the functional component of the immune response would be complete without some further consideration of the role of complement, which

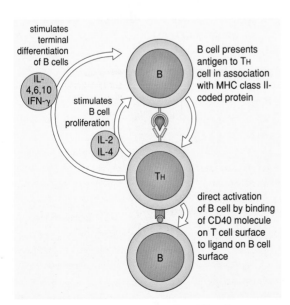

FIGURE 10.16 Cooperation between B and T_H cells.

has been alluded to in the section dealing with acute inflammation (see pp 46–48).

The complement system, which is involved in acute inflammation, phagocytosis and clotting, as well as in immune and hypersensitivity reactions, consists of sets of proteins. Some of these become activated sequentially to carry out the biological functions of complement, which include:

● killing of bacteria by membrane lysis

● promotion of phagocytosis by opsonization

● mediation of both vascular and cellular operations involved in acute inflammation

● processing of immune complexes which prevents precipitation of the complexes and promotes their removal from tissues and blood

● assistance in the binding of antigen to APCs and B cells

Other complement proteins group into superfamilies which share both genetic and functional characteristics. Such a grouping encompasses the **complement control proteins, six proteins that inhibit stable formation of the pivotal convertase complexes in both classical and alternate pathways of complement activation**. (*Fig. 10.17*). This superfamily consists of:

● factor H

● decay accelerating factor (CD55), which promotes breakdown of the C3 convertase formed in the course of classical pathway activation

● C4-binding protein

● membrane co-factor protein (CD46), which promotes the cleavage of C3b

● complement receptors 1 and 2

These proteins are coded for by a closely linked gene cluster on chromosome 1 and all share a common feature in the form of a 60-amino-acid domain known as a short consensus repeat, which may be repeated many times in an individual member of the group.

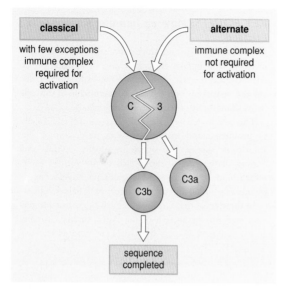

FIGURE 10.17 *C3 cleavage is the pivotal event in complement activation.*

In the course of complement activation, each activated component acquires the ability to activate several molecules of the next protein in line. Thus a marked amplification of the original step occurs, one activated molecule of C1 leading to a cascade in which thousands of molecules of the proteins 'further down the line' are activated.

The activation of the complement system takes place through the operation of one or both of two pathways, which ultimately converge after activation of C3. The first of these is known as the **classical** and the second as the **alternate** pathway of activation.

THE CLASSICAL PATHWAY

Each of the nine protein components in the classical pathway is designated by a number prefixed by C. C1 consists of a trimolecular complex consisting of the subunits C1q, r and s. For classical activation to occur (*Fig. 10.18*), bound IgG or IgM antibodies are essential, because **C1q** binds to the CH_2 of the Fc portion of these immunoglobulins. C1q has a collagen-like stem from which grow six peptide chains, each with a terminal subunit that binds to the Fc portion. For activation

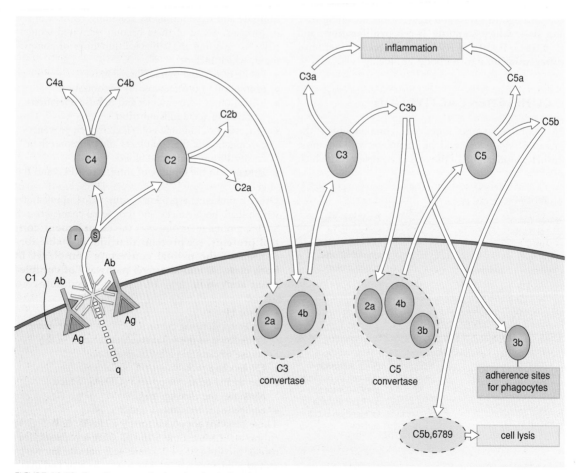

FIGURE 10.18 *Complement activation: the classical pathway.*

to occur, at least two of the subunits must bind to CH_2; this is much more easily accomplished with the pentameric IgM than with monomeric IgG.

Thus IgM antibodies to red cells have a much greater haemolytic potential: 'one hit' provides sufficient Fc binding sites to activate **C1q**. In the case of IgG a greater number of hits is required for antibody molecules to be bound close enough to each other to provide the dual binding sites required for **C1q** activation. C1q forms a calcium-dependent complex with the r and s components, and the whole, when activated, acquires esterase activity and binds first C4, which is cleaved into C4a and C4b, and then C2, which is cleaved into C2a and C2b. C1 activation is regulated by C1 inhibitor. The C4b2a complex is the convertase for the cleavage of C3, which leads to release of **C3a** (chemotactic for phagocytes and causes histamine release from mast cells) and **C3b**, which is bound to the surface membrane of the cell to which the antibody is attached. Formation of the C4b2a complex is inhibited by C4-binding protein.

C3b exhibits the phenomenon of **immune adherence** binding to a receptor on the plasma membrane of both neutrophils and macrophages. In this way it acts as an **opsonin**.

The final phase of complement activation is the formation of a membrane attack complex. This phase starts with the non-enzymatic binding of C5 to C3b. This entity is then cleaved by the convertase C4b2a3b. One of the cleavage products, C5a, is strongly chemotactic for phagocytic cells. The other, C5b, then forms a trimolecular complex with C6 and C7, which is also chemotactic for phagocytic cells. The final binding of one molecule of C8 with six of C9 leads to lysis of the cell membrane to which the antibody had originally bound.

The fundamental difference between classical and alternate pathways of complement activation is that the latter does not require the presence of immune complexes, but it should be remembered that there are circumstances in which classical pathway activation occurs in the absence of such complexes.

Such activating factors include certain polyanions, microorganisms (including *Mycoplasma* and retroviruses (not including human immunodeficiency virus).

THE ALTERNATE PATHWAY

The alternate pathway of complement activation (*Fig. 10.19*) can be triggered by:

- many strains of both Gram-positive and Gram-negative bacteria
- the polysaccharides of certain cell walls (e.g. bacterial endotoxins)
- some aggregated immunoglobulins such as IgA which cannot bind C1q, and by a positive feedback mechanism from C3b formed in the course of classical activation

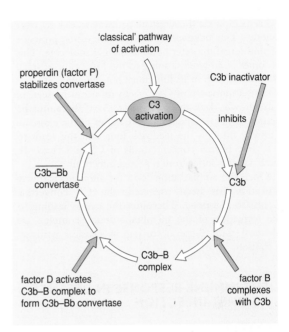

FIGURE 10.19 *Complement activation: the alternate pathway.*

- cells infected by certain viruses including Epstein–Barr virus, which causes infectious mononucleosis and is implicated in the causation of Burkitt's lymphoma and nasopharyngeal carcinoma
- trypanosomes and fungi
- miscellaneous factors including heterologous red cells, dextran sulphate and certain carbohydrates

In the classical pathway, C3 is activated by the formation of the convertase C4b2a. In the alternate pathway, the convertase is formed by the action of certain proteins on C3b and factor B, a molecule with a molecular weight of 100 000 which complexes with C3b produced by either the classical or alternate pathways. Factor B has some similarities to C2 and, like C2, is coded for by the MHC. The C3bB complex is activated by an enzyme known as factor D, which cleaves factor B giving Ba and Bb. **The resulting complex C3bBb is the active convertase for C3** and is stabilized by factor P (properdin).

If the convertase forms or is deposited on a foreign surface, amplification of the alternate pathway occurs. The stabilized convertase can now act on C3 to produce more C3b, which together with factors B and D leads to the production of more convertase and still more activation of C3. Thus there is a positive feedback loop with tremendous amplifying potential, kept under control in normal individuals by a C3b inactivator.

Under normal circumstances, a small amount of C3bBb convertase is generated in the plasma, but the inherent lability of this convertase together with the action of C3b inactivator prevents a 'runaway' amplification occurring with ultimate depletion of C3. Thus

C3 activation via the alternate pathway is 'ticking over quietly'. The 'tickover' occurs because of the presence of an internal thioester bond in the C3 molecule. This becomes hydrolysed, leading to the formation of small amounts of C3b or its functional homologue C3i.

The importance of C3b inactivation can be seen in patients who lack the inactivator. As C3b cannot be destroyed, there is continual activation of the alternate pathway through the feedback loop and this leads to very low plasma concentrations of C3 and factor B. Such patients suffer from repeated infections.

Once the amplification loop for alternate pathway activation has been triggered, the C5 convertase C3bBb3b is formed. Thereafter the events leading to the formation of the membrane attack complex are identical with those occurring in classical pathway activation.

THE IMMUNE RESPONSE IN DEFENCE AGAINST INFECTION

BACTERIA
In general terms bacteria are pathogenic because they:
- attach to host cell surface components
- proliferate within the host
- can, in some instances, avoid being phagocytosed
- may release toxins
- may invade tissues and cause tissue damage, in part mediated only by local toxin release.

These operational steps can all provide targets for host defence. Some are based on the specific immune responses described in previous sections and some on triggering of the same defence mechanisms **via pathways that do not require lymphocyte-mediated recognition of specific bacterial antigens**. These pathways include:
- **triggering of the alternate pathway of complement activation (see pp 113–114) by C-reactive protein, and mannan-binding protein (which has some structural resemblance to C1q).** The release of the active fragments C3a and C5a activates mast cells which, in turn, release histamine, leukotriene B_4, eosinophil chemotactic factor and IL-8. This results in:
  1) initiation of the vascular component of the inflammatory reaction
  2) chemotaxis of phagocytes
  3) activation of phagocytes
- **Activation of NK cells, monocytes–macrophages and neutrophils by components of the bacterial cell wall, such as lipopolysaccharide, peptidoglycan and lipoteichoic acid, and by factors released from bacteria such as f-Met-Leu-Phe.** The activated cells release a range of cytokines which both activate phagocytes and upregulate endothelial adhesive properties, thus promoting the defence

mechanisms embodied in the cellular phase of acute inflammation.

Role of Antibody in Defence Against Bacterial Infection
The ways in which antibody may act to counter infection have already been referred to (see pp 101–102). These mechanisms may be deployed against the pathogenic steps referred to on p 115, as shown in *Table 10.4* (see also *Fig. 10.20*). The mechanisms involved in bacterial killing by **phagocytes** have already been described in the section on inflammation (see pp 58–59).

Cell-mediated Immunity in Bacterial Infections
The ways in which T cells cooperate with B cells so that the latter produce antibody are discussed in an earlier section (see p 111). In defence against infection, host cell-mediated immunity is of great importance, particularly in relation to bacterial species that grow *inside* cells and appear able to resist intracellular killing. Important examples in the context of human disease include:
- *Mycobacterium tuberculosis*
- *Mycobacterium leprae*
- *Salmonella typhi*
- *Brucella abortus*
- *Listeria monocytogenes*

In relation to defence against facultative intracellular parasites such as the bacteria named above, cell-mediated immunity is expressed in the form of cooperation between appropriately stimulated T lymphocytes and macrophages. This is a process that is at once specific and non-specific:
- Its specificity resides in the fact that T cells become activated after recognizing their homospecific antigen (in association with an appropriate MHC-coded antigen); this is supported by a fact that immunity against an organism such as *M. tuberculosis* can be transferred from one animal to another only through lymphocyte transfer.
- The non-specific part of the process is mediated through the activation of macrophages by the cytokines (**lymphokines**) synthesized and released by activated T cells. Such soluble factors recruit macrophages to the site of infection, immobilize them at this site, increase their ability to kill intracellular organisms (possibly by enhancing the oxygen-dependent bactericidal function), and can even increase the number of C5a receptors on the surface of blood monocytes. Once macrophages have been activated as a result of the release of lymphokines by T cells responding to antigenic determinants on a specific organism, they acquire the ability to deal more effectively, not only with the organisms that elicited the T-cell response, but with other bacterial species as well.

Table 10.4 Antibodies May Block Bacterial Pathogenicity at Different Stages

Pathogenic step	Antibody
Attachment	Antibodies directed against bacterial attachment molecules, fimbriae and some bacterial capsules
Proliferation of microorganisms	Antibody coating may initiate complement-mediated lysis of cell membranes Antibodies may block receptors and transport mechanisms needed for uptake of relevant substrates
Mechanisms for avoidance of phagocytosis	Antibodies can combine with bacterial M proteins and capsules, thus opsonizing the organisms. The opsonins bind to Fc and C3 receptors on phagocytes Antibodies can neutralize immunorepellant chemical species liberated by the organisms
Synthesis and release of bacterial toxins	Antibody can neutralize the toxins. Neutralization is accomplished either by binding to the biologically active site on the toxin molecule or by stereochemical blocking of a binding site on the substrate for the toxin. Some of the most successful immunization programmes are based on the eliciting of neutralizing antibody (e.g. immunization against diphtheria in which a modified form of the toxin (toxoid) is used as the immunogen)
Invasion mediated by the synthesis and release of spreading factors by the organisms (e.g. hyaluronidases)	Invasion is countered by neutralizing antibodies

VIRUSES

As in the case of bacterial infections, some non-specific mechanisms exist to combat viral infection. These include:

- **Interferon production**. There are three types of interferon, α, β and γ. IFN-α is coded for by a family of genes (about 20 of them) on chromosome 9, chiefly in leucocytes. IFN-β is coded for by a single gene on chromosome 9, chiefly in fibroblasts, and IFN-γ is coded for by a single gene on chromosome 12, chiefly in activated T lymphocytes.

  Infection of a cell by a virus leads to the production of IFN-α and IFN-β, which activates mechanisms in adjacent cells that enable them to resist viral infection. The interferons are species-specific but not virus-specific. Interferons are discussed more fully in the sections dealing with viral infections (see pp 189–191).

- **Activation of NK cells**. Activated NK cells are important in the response to certain viral infections, most notably herpesvirus species with a special emphasis on cytomegalovirus. It is not clear which molecules the NK cells recognize on the surface of infected cells but their activity is certainly upregulated by increased local production of IFN-β. Interestingly, there is an *inverse* relationship between NK cell killing of infected cells and the expression of MHC class I-coded proteins on their surfaces.

Specific Immune Mechanisms in Viral Infection

Viral infections are followed by adaptive immune responses in the same way as bacterial infections. As in the latter, this response is characterized by:

- activation of T lymphocytes with expansion of clones of both helper and cytotoxic T cells
- activation and differentiation of B cells with antibody production

Role of Antibody in Viral Infections

Viruses are obligate intracellular parasites and, inside cells, are not exposed to antibody, but antibody can nevertheless play a significant role in combating viral infection, particularly when free virus is present in the bloodstream. This function is exercised in a number of different ways:

- **Antibody binds to free virus.** This may block **binding** of the virus to its target cell, inhibit **entry** of virus to that cell or stop the **uncoating** of the virus once it has gained entry to the target cells (see pp 183–184).
- **Antibody and complement may bind to free virus.** This may lead to lysis of the viral envelope.
- **Antibody may bind to cells infected by a virus.** This may lead to ADCC.
- **Antibody and complement may bind to a virally infected cell.** This may lead to lysis of the cell or to its opsonization and subsequent phagocytosis.

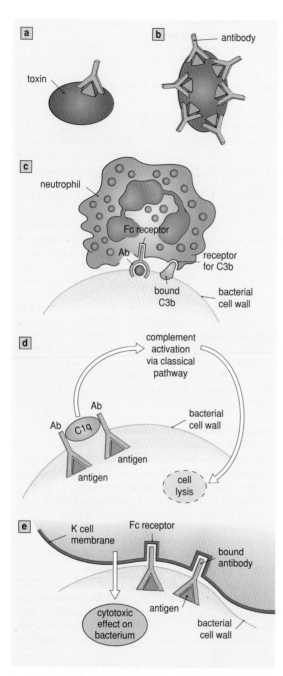

FIGURE 10.20 *Protective actions of antibody.* **a** *The neutralization of bacterial toxins: antibody binds with toxin near its biologically active site and blocks the toxin's reaction with its substrate.* **b** *Antibody can block the entry of viruses and bacteria into cells by coating them and preventing their adherence to mucosal surfaces.* **c** *Bound immunoglobin acts as an opsonin and enhances phagocytosis.* **d** *Complement-mediated lysis of a bacterial cell.* **e** *Antibody-dependent cell-mediated cytotoxicity (ADCC): the role of antibody in the binding of 'killer' lymphocytes (killer cells) to a bacterial cell.*

Cell-mediated Mechanisms

Once viral entry to target cells has been achieved, cell-mediated immunity plays a dominant role in the modulation of recovery from viral infections. Specifically sensitized T cells may counter the effects of invasion of cells by viruses in a number of ways:

1) **Direct destruction of infected cells by cytotoxic T cells** (*Fig. 10.21*). Recognition of these infected cells by T cells involves alteration of the normal cell surface by the expression of virally encoded antigens. In addition, as has already been mentioned, MHC class I surface antigens coded for by the HLA-A, -B or -C loci of the MHC are needed before recognition by the T cells can occur. The importance of the MHC-coded part of the signal can be shown *in vitro*, where T cells that are cytotoxic for cells of a certain strain infected by a virus will not kill cells of another strain infected by the same virus.

While this system is clearly beneficial in terms of viral elimination, there are circumstances when cytotoxic T-cell activity damages host cells and tissues. In a very real sense, certain viral diseases, in both morphological and pathophysiological terms, are the expression of T cell-mediated attack on virally infected cells (e.g. hepatitis B).

2) **Release of lymphokines from activated T cells.** This will attract macrophages to the site of infection. These macrophages are activated by the lymphokines and may kill the infected cells,

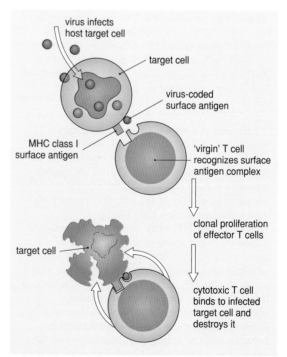

FIGURE 10.21 *Cytotoxic T cells in antiviral immunity.*

phagocytose free viral particles, or discourage the spread of virus from cell to cell.

3) T cells may release interferons which can block viral messenger RNA transcription and which render the cells adjacent to those infected unable to permit the replication of virus.

PROTOZOA AND HELMINTHS

Protozoa

Protozoal infections constitute a major cause of morbidity and death in many parts of the world, as shown in *Table 10.5* which gives the prevalence of four protozoal infections.

Both humoral and cell-mediated mechanisms may be involved in the immune reactions to protozoa. When the organisms are blood-borne, as in malaria and trypanosomiasis, antibody and complement appear to play a dominant role, whereas parasites that develop in tissues, such as *Leishmania*, usually elicit cell-mediated immunity.

In this group of infections it is quite common for elimination of the parasites by the immune system to be incomplete. Thus, although able to resist a second infection, the host may still be harbouring a small number of living parasites. This state is known as **premunition (concomitant immunity)**.

Antibody-mediated defence is of greatest importance in **African trypanosomiasis** and **malaria**. In the former the parasites are free in the blood; in the latter red blood cells are parasitized. Antibody coating of trypanosomes leads either to complement-mediated

cell lysis or to phagocytosis, the antibody functioning here as an opsonin. In malaria, antibody blocks invasion of the red cells or opsonizes them in the same way as trypanosomes.

In Chagas' disease, which causes chronic damage to heart muscle, and in the various forms of leishmaniasis, where the parasites reside within macrophages, T cells release cytokines such as IFN-γ which upregulate the killing power of the macrophages. Parasite killing is carried out by TNF-α, reactive oxygen species (free radicals) and nitric oxide.

Antigenic Variation in Evasion of the Immune Response

In the case of two important parasitic infections, **malaria** and **trypanosomiasis**, the effectiveness of antibody and complement in destroying the parasite may be overcome by the organisms varying their surface antigens into a form that cannot be bound by existing antibody. The trypanosome achieves this by expressing in a **constant sequence** alternative genes that code for surface glycoproteins. When sufficient antibody is present in the plasma to bring about complement-mediated lysis of organisms, the next gene in sequence is expressed and the surface antigens are altered. In due time, when new antibody has formed, the process is repeated; this can occur up to 20 times. Such a system clearly gives the trypanosome a great advantage in terms of survival.

Helminths

Helminth infestations are even more numerous than protozoal infections, schistosomiasis and hookworm infestations, affecting about 200 million individuals.

Two striking features of the immune reactions elicited by helminths are:
   1) the production of large amounts of IgE
   2) a sharp rise in the number of circulating eosinophils

Both these features suggest expression of the cytokines produced by T_H2 lymphocytes; indeed, antibodies to IL-4 reduce the IgE production in such infestations, and antibodies to IL-5 decrease the eosinophilia.

Degranulation of IgE-coated mast cells in the neighbourhood of the worm leads to the release of histamine (which can affect vascular permeability) and of a factor chemotactic for eosinophils. In *in vitro* culture systems, eosinophils can be shown to kill antibody-coated schistosomules, the cytotoxicity being associated with release of basic protein from the electron-dense core of the eosinophil granules.

Table 10.5 Protozoal Infections

Disease	Protozoon	No. infected
Malaria	*Plasmodium* (*vivax, malariae, ovale* and *falciparum*)	100 million
Tropical sore	*Leishmania tropica*	
Kala-azar	*Leishmania donovani*	10 million
Espundia	*Leishmania braziliensis*	
Chagas' disease	*Trypanosoma cruzi*	
Sleeping sickness	*Trypanosoma gambiense* and *rhodesiense*	

CHAPTER 11

Disorders Related to the Immune System

All the biological mechanisms that make up the immune response may go awry in one way or another. The disorders that arise from such defects can be understood most easily if they are classified in relation to the **individual functions** that fail and, in the case of **congenital immune deficiency**, in relation to the **ontogeny of the immune system**.

Defective or harmful immunological responses include the following:

- **Response to the introduction of an antigen may be inadequate.** As a consequence the host is unable to mount an effective defence against infection. Such a defective reaction may be **congenital** or **acquired** (sometimes deliberately induced) and is known as **immune deficiency**.
- **The immune system may react to an inappropriate extent on encountering an antigen.** Such a response may produce tissue damage by a variety of mechanisms. For this group of, on the whole, harmful reactions, the term **hypersensitivity** is used.
- **The immune system may lose the ability to distinguish between self and non-self** and as a result mount reactions against the antigens of the host. This process is known as **autoimmunity**.
- Many **neoplastic proliferations** of the elements of the immune system can occur. Both the B- and T-cell systems may give rise to such disorders.

IMMUNE DEFICIENCY

Immune deficiency can involve:

- **specific** afferent (antigen presentation and recognition) or efferent (T-cell activation and antibody production) pathways of the immune system described in Chapter 10
- **non-specific** effector mechanisms such as the complement system and bacterial killing by phagocytes

Recognition that definite and measurable defects in the functions of the immune system can cause a reduced ability to combat infection dates back to 1952, when it was observed that a child suffering from repeated infections had no immunoglobulin (Ig) in his plasma. Since then a wide variety of immune deficient states has been described.

Disorders of specific immunity may arise at any point in the differentiation of the B- and T-cell system. **The functional defect produced depends on the point in the differentiation process at which a block occurs:** the further back this point is the broader the range of functions that is affected (*Fig. 11.1*).

PRIMARY IMMUNE DEFICIENCY

Stem Cell Deficiency: Defects Arising before Lymphoid Cells are Processed by the Thymus or Bursa Equivalent

A deficiency in the number of stem cells produced leads to a deficiency or absence of the precursors of the B and T cells destined to undergo processing in the thymus or bursa equivalent. In its most severe form, known as **reticular dysgenesis**, there is complete failure of development of other bone marrow cells in addition to

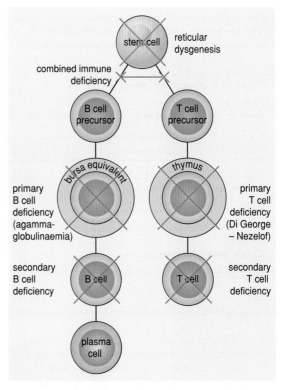

FIGURE 11.1 *The cellular components of the immune system and the sites of immune deficiency.*

the obvious gross defects in B and T cells. Such infants may die within the first week of life, usually due to overwhelming sepsis.

Severe Combined Immune Deficiency

A more common variety of primary immune deficiency arising in the 'pre-thymus, pre-bursa' phase is **severe combined immune deficiency (SCID)**. This may be inherited in either an X-linked or autosomal recessive pattern. In about half the sufferers the condition is due to lack of the enzyme **adenosine deaminase**. These patients may be helped by blood transfusions, as donor red cells contain this enzyme.

The thymus is usually very small or even absent. When it can be found at post-mortem examination, there is a gross lack of thymic lymphocytes and complete absence of Hassall's corpuscles. Lymphoid tissue in the gut and other peripheral sites is also markedly atrophic.

The combined defect, which affects both the B- and T-cell systems, is expressed by low immunoglobulin levels and a low blood lymphocyte count (fewer than 1.0×10^9 per litre). Affected children can neither produce antibodies nor mount an effective cell-mediated reaction against intracellular bacteria or viruses. Normal immune function can be established by grafting bone marrow from a sibling with an identical or near-identical major histocompatibility complex. Blood transfusion and treatment with thymic extracts may also improve the situation, but many of these children die within the first year or two of life, often as a result of pulmonary infections caused by agents that are normally not particularly virulent (opportunistic infections). A common example of such an infection is that caused by the protozoon *Pneumocystis carinii*. This organism proliferates within the alveolar spaces, filling them with material that has a foamy appearance on microscopy and is eosinophilic in sections stained with haematoxylin and eosin. The use of special staining methods based on the use of silver salts shows the presence of many protozoa. (*Fig. 11.2*).

Other forms of SCID are discussed in Chapter 42 (see pp 944–945).

Other Forms of Combined Immune Deficiency

Two other forms of combined immune deficiency exist which are difficult to explain in terms of the development and maturation of the immune system. These are **ataxia telangiectasia** and **Wiskott–Aldrich** syndrome.

Ataxia Telangiectasia

This fortunately rare syndrome, which is inherited as an autosomal recessive trait, consists of a triad of features:

1) Cerebellar degeneration and spinocerebellar atrophy, leading to the appearance of choreoathetoid movements early in life.

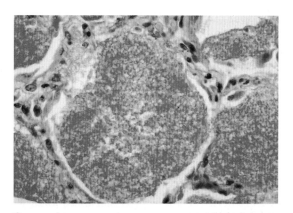

a

b

FIGURE 11.2 **a** This section of lung from a child with SCID shows the alveoli to be filled with foamy material which stains a magenta colour (the section has been stained by the periodic acid–Schiff method in which fuchsin binds to 1–2 glycol groups). The appearances are typical of Pneumocystis carinii pneumonia. **b** This section also shows the lung in P. carinii infection. It has been stained with silver salts (Grocott method) which show the Pneumocystis as black circles).

2) The appearance at a somewhat later stage (between the ages of 5 and 8 years) of leashes of dilated blood vessels, especially in the skin on the flexor surfaces of the forearms, and in the conjunctiva (telangiectases).

3) Diminished resistance to infection. Plasma levels of IgE and IgA are lower than normal and there is also depression of cell-mediated immunity. Affected patients tend to have repeated infections of the sinuses and respiratory tract, which may lead to the development of bronchiectasis.

Ataxia telangiectasia is, in addition, one of a small number of syndromes associated with **chromosomal breakages.** Like the others in this group (Bloom's syndrome and Fanconi's anaemia), there is an increased risk of the development of malignant neoplasms derived predominantly from lymphoid cells. This is the commonest cause of death in sufferers of ataxia telangiectasia.

Wiskott–Aldrich Syndrome

This is a strange combination of clinical features characterized by:

- low platelet count
- eczema
- recurrent infection

Patients have low levels of IgM and, in keeping with this, a poor response to polysaccharide antigens. IgA and IgE concentrations are raised and the IgG level is usually normal.

In addition, some depression of cell-mediated immunity is also present. T-cell numbers and effectiveness decline progressively and it takes a few years before the lymphocyte count is seriously diminished. Both T cells and platelets show absence of certain surface glycoproteins (CD43, which is a ligand for intercellular adhesion molecule ICAM-1) and it has been suggested that a defect of glycosylation, especially of sialidation of these cell surfaces, is present. As with ataxia telangiectasia, there is an increased risk of malignant neoplasms of the lymphoreticular system (5% of the patients die in this way).

The syndrome is inherited as an X-linked recessive trait, and signs and symptoms of the disease usually appear in the first few months of life (*Fig 11.3*).

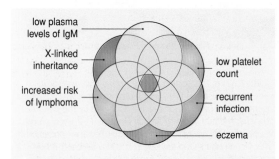

FIGURE 11.3 *The combination of clinical and laboratory findings that constitute the Wiskott–Aldrich syndrome.*

Primary Deficiencies of T-cell Function

Di George's and Nezelof's Syndromes

In both of these syndromes there is a selective T-cell deficiency due to failure of the thymus to develop normally as a result of defects in the development of the third and fourth pharyngeal pouches. Affected infants have grossly defective cell-mediated immunity and may succumb to viral infections such as measles. Bacterial infections elicit an antibody response but this is subnormal, presumably owing to lack of the normal cooperation between the T and B lymphocytes.

In addition to the thymic hypoplasia, infants with Di George's syndrome suffer from:

- cardiac defects
- cleft palate
- an abnormal facies

- hypocalcaemia due to absence of the parathyroids

Most cases show deletion of genomic material on chromosome 22 but the disorder is not an inherited one. Complete Di George's syndrome (i.e absence of the thymus) is rare and many of the sufferers have a very small but histologically normal thymus. In such cases the initially low number of T lymphocytes in the blood increases as the child grows and cell-mediated immunity may reach normality by the age of 5 years.

In Nezelof's syndrome, the same immune defects exist but only the thymus is affected. This disorder is inherited either in an autosomal or X-linked recessive fashion.

Infections with viruses and intracellular bacteria are particularly dangerous to these children, and even the bacille Calmette–Guérin (BCG) vaccine used against tuberculosis may have very serious results.

Primary Deficiencies of B-cell Function

Primary failure of normal B-cell function may result from:

- absence of B cells
- failure of B cells to differentiate into plasma cells
- inability of plasma cells to make one or other class of immunoglobulin

Any of these will be reflected in an absence or very low plasma concentrations of immunoglobulin. Children with this disorder show a tendency for repeated infections of pyogenic organisms (such as *Staphylococcus aureus*, *Streptococcus pyogenes* and *Streptococcus pneumoniae*, and also fall victim to opportunistic infections (e.g. *P. carinii*). Cell-mediated immunity is normal. Some cases are familial and sex-linked; others are sporadic.

Bruton's Congenital Agammaglobulinaemia

Several immune deficiency syndromes, including SCID and the Wiskott–Aldrich syndrome, are associated with abnormalities located on the X chromosome; Bruton's congenital agammaglobulinaemia is one of these.

The defect occurs at the pre-B-cell stage and thus B cells fail to mature and there is an absence of mature B cells in the circulating blood. The defect is associated in many cases with failure of rearrangement of the V_H genes. The affected gene on the X chromosome encodes a cytoplasmic tyrosine kinase which belongs to the *src* family of proto-oncogenes (see pp 274–275) and which is presumably concerned with signal transduction. How a failure in the function of this tyrosine kinase interferes with normal B-cell maturation is not yet known.

Affected males have very low plasma immunoglobulin concentrations. The morphological correlate of this situation is a lack of lymphoid follicles and germinal centres in nodes (*Fig 11.4*) and, not surprisingly, an absence of plasma cells in the tissues.

Repeated infections by pyogenic organisms occur in these children: *S. aureus*, *S. pyogenes*, *S. pneumoniae*, *Haemophilus influenzae* and *Neisseria meningitidis*. There

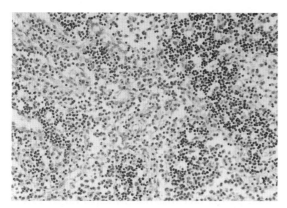

FIGURE 11.4 *The disorganized lymph node with a complete absence of germinal centres and poorly formed lymphoid follicles characteristic of infantile hypogammaglobulinaemia.*

is also an increased risk of infection by the protozoon *P. carinii* (see pp 119, 452) and by the intestinal parasite *Giardia lamblia*, which causes chronic diarrhoea. Purely cell-mediated responses to infection are normal.

IgA Deficiency

This is a common immune deficiency in Caucasians (1 in 700 population) but is very rare in other ethnic groups. IgA-bearing lymphocytes fail to mature into plasma cells. In most cases there are no symptoms but there is an associated defect in IgG_2 and IgG_4 production in about 20% of individuals with IgA deficiency. The combined defect is associated with an increased risk of recurrent pyogenic infections.

Common Variable Immunodeficiency

This term provides an umbrella for a number of different conditions affecting males and females equally and which are all characterized by hypogammaglobulinaemia and a tendency to develop recurrent infections. The defective immune response may be associated with several different sets of circumstances:

- failure of marrow pre-B cells to mature
- failure of circulating B cells to differentiate into plasma cells (possibly due to defective signalling from T cells)
- failure in about 30% of cases of T cells to respond to polyclonal activators
- presence, in a small proportion of cases, of T cells with marked suppressor activity for B cells

Transient Hypogammaglobulinaemia of Infancy

Newborn infants are protected against infections by maternal IgG that has crossed the placenta. By the age of 3 months, when much of this IgG has been catabolized, the infants start to synthesize their own. In some this immunoglobulin synthesis is delayed for long periods and the infants are thus at risk, especially for res-

piratory tract infections. The deficiency situation usually rights itself by the age of 4 years.

X-linked Hyper-IgM Syndrome

These patients are deficient in respect of IgA and IgG but synthesize large amounts of IgM. They are not only at increased risk of recurrent pyogenic infections but form IgM antibodies, which can be cytotoxic, to various blood cells including neutrophils and platelets.

The tissues of affected individuals show infiltration by large numbers of plasma cells containing IgM.

The functional defect is a failure to switch immunoglobulin class production from IgM to IgG and IgA. This appears to be due to failure of one of the ligand–receptor interactions necessary for class switching: the binding of a ligand on T_H cells to the CD40 protein on the surface of B cells. This results from a mutation in the gene encoding the CD40 ligand, which is located on the X chromosome.

Deficiencies Related to Non-specific Immune Functions

Phagocyte Defects

These can be expressed as:
- failure to respond to chemotactic signals
- failure of lysosomal fusion
- failure of bacterial killing

These defects are discussed in some detail in Chapter 5 in the sections on neutrophil function in acute inflammation (see pp 59–61), and further reference to them will not be made here.

Defects in Complement Function

As each component of the complement sequence appears to be coded for separately, it is theoretically possible for any one of them to be absent from the plasma. In some instances, instead of a component being absent, it is present at a reduced level, suggesting that the fault lies in a regulatory gene rather than in the one coding for that specific component.

Difficulties may also arise when certain inhibitors of complement activity are absent. As pointed out previously (see p 114), absence of C3b inhibitor results in continuous high-level activation of the alternate pathway, with depletion of C3 and thus an ultimate decline in the efficacy of the complement system. Absence of C1 inhibitor, inherited as an autosomal dominant trait, leads to unfettered production of C2 kinin activity, which causes painful swollen patches in the skin and oedema in the gut and respiratory tract. This is known as **hereditary angiooedema**. Sudden death from airway obstruction is a constant threat in these patients.

SECONDARY IMMUNE DEFICIENCY

Immune deficiency may occur in postnatal life as a result of the operation of a number of factors.

Age

In both infancy and old age there is a relative lack of effectiveness of the immune response. The transfer of maternal IgG across the placenta tends to compensate for this in infants.

Malnutrition

This may be associated with defective immunity in relation both to B- and T-cell function, and is, alas, very common. It has been suggested that this may explain the relatively high mortality rate associated with diseases such as measles in underprivileged communities.

Neoplastic Disorders of the Immune System

Neoplastic B-cell proliferation, such as occurs in the majority of lymphomas, myelomatosis and chronic lymphocytic leukaemia, is associated with a decline in antibody responses. However, in Hodgkin's disease the patients exhibit various manifestations of a deficiency of cell-mediated immunity and are more susceptible to infections caused by mycobacteria, viruses and fungi.

Iatrogenic Immune Deficiency

Suppression of immune reactions may be produced *deliberately* under two sets of circumstances:

1) Where an attempt is made to reduce the reaction to allografts. This is discussed in more detail in a later section (see pp 145–147).
2) In certain disease states, such as systemic lupus erythematosus, where tissue damage is being caused by failure to distinguish between self and non-self antigens (autoimmune disorders), 'damping down' the immune response by the use of appropriate drugs reduces the effects of the reaction and can improve the clinical state of the patient.

Iatrogenic immune suppression can also arise as a side-effect of treatments that are not aimed primarily at the components of the immune reaction. X-rays and cytotoxic drugs used in the treatment of malignant neoplasms may produce immune suppression, as may corticosteroids.

Infections

Good evidence exists that certain viral infections can cause immune suppression in both humans and other species. In some of these (e.g. measles), this effect has been ascribed to a direct cytotoxic effect on certain lymphocyte subsets. Malaria and the lepromatous form of leprosy are also associated with a decreased ability of the immune system to eliminate infecting microorganisms. In the latter, macrophages are seen to contain very large numbers of apparently healthy mycobacteria.

Acquired Immune Deficiency Syndrome

In recent years, increasing attention has been focused on a newly recognized form of acquired immune defi-

ciency, known as the **acquired immune deficiency syndrome (AIDS)**. **AIDS is the end-result of infection by a retrovirus known as human immunodeficiency virus (HIV)** of which two strains, HIV-1 and HIV-2 are recognized. Most cases are caused by HIV-1, but HIV-2 infections are common in west Africa.

HIV is an RNA virus closely related to the **lentiviruses**. Like other retroviruses, its single-stranded RNA genome is copied as double-stranded DNA via the viral **reverse transcriptase** system, and this DNA is then inserted into the genome of the host cell.

The consequences of HIV infection are predicated by the fact that the principal target cell is the T helper lymphocyte, as the CD4 molecules on the T cells bind with an envelope glycoprotein gp120 on the surface of the virus. Other target cells are macrophages, dendritic cells in lymphoid tissues, antigen-presenting Langerhans cells in the skin and neuroglia, all of which may express CD4 on their surfaces.

Infection of CD4+ cells leads ultimately to their destruction and a progressive fall in their numbers. This in turn exposes the affected individual to infection by a number of agents of low virulence, this situation being termed opportunistic infection. Agents commonly involved include *P. carinii* **(causing pneumonia),** *Mycobacterium tuberculosis, Mycobacterium avium intracellulare, Toxoplasma gondii, Cryptosporidium parvum* **(which causes chronic diarrhoea) and** *cytomegalovirus.*

Infection with HIV occurs via:

- **Sexual intercourse.** In some parts of Africa where large proportions of the population have been infected, the common route is via heterosexual intercourse. In the West, risk appears to be associated chiefly with homosexual anal intercourse in males where infected lymphocytes may be present in the semen of one partner and enter the tissues of the other partner via abrasions in the anal or rectal mucosa.
- **Intravenous drug abuse.**
- **Transfusion of infected blood or blood products** (e.g. commercial Factor VIII administered to haemophiliac patients). This risk is significantly diminished by testing donor blood for anti-HIV antibodies and by heat treatment of products such as factor VIII. It must be remembered, however, that seroconversion of an infected individual may take up to 3 months, during which time the blood will be infective despite the absence of antibodies.
- **Vertical transmission from infected mother to infant** via the placenta.

The HIV Virus

Like all retroviruses the single-stranded RNA genome of HIV contains *gag, pol* and *env* genes.

- The *gag* gene encodes a protein that becomes cleaved into four nucleocapsid constituents known as p24, p17, p9 and p7. p24 elicits the formation of antibodies in the infected host which assist the diagnosis of HIV infection.
- The *pol* gene encodes reverse transcriptase, an RNA-dependent DNA polymerase which uses RNA as its template for the formation of DNA.
- The *env* gene encodes a glycoprotein with a molecular weight of 160, which becomes cleaved into two closely linked envelope glycoproteins gp120 and gp41. Gp120 binds to CD4 and enters cells that express this molecule on their surface (*Figs 11.5* and *11.6*).

In addition, the HIV genome contains other genes that are important in the natural history of infection:

- The *tat* gene. This is a transactivator gene which upregulates transcription of the viral genome.
- The *vpu* gene, which is required for efficient virion budding.
- The *vif* gene, which controls infectivity of free, rather than cell-bound, virus.
- The *rev* gene, which acts post-transcriptionally and promotes the transport of viral messenger RNA to the cytoplasm of the infected cell.
- The *nef* gene, the function of which is uncertain.

Also important are long terminal repeats which, in addition to containing regions that bind products of *tat* and *nef*, contain core enhancer elements (NK-κB) which are activated when latently infected T cells or macrophages are stimulated.

Results of HIV Infection

Once gp120 has bound to CD4, fusion occurs between the lipid bilayers of the viral and cell membranes, and the virus enters the cell. The viral genome becomes uncoated and the viral reverse transcriptase makes a single-stranded DNA copy of the virus's RNA genome. Complementary strands of DNA are synthesized, which anneal and may then be inserted into the host cell's genome as a provirus.

This provirus may be transcribed with the production of new HIV RNA, and this may be translated in the endoplasmic reticulum of the host cells with the formation of new complete virions which bud from the host cell's plasma membrane and are released into

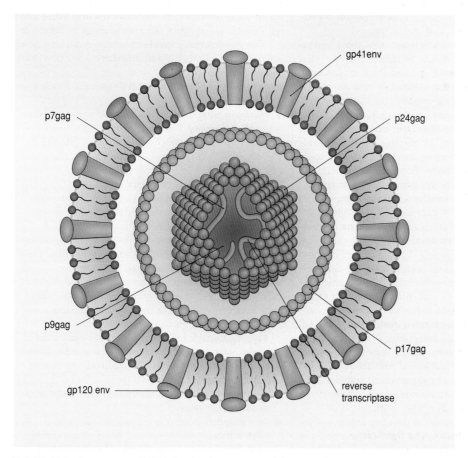

FIGURE 11.5 *The structure of HIV-1 showing the genome and the outer glycoprotein coat.*

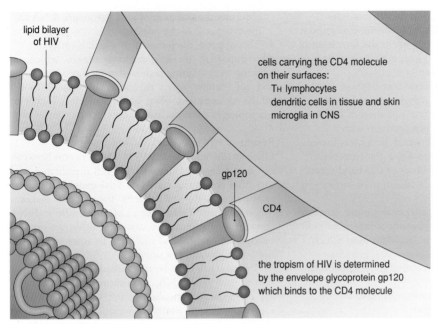

lipid bilayer
of HIV

cells carrying the CD4 molecule
on their surfaces:
TH lymphocytes
dendritic cells in tissue and skin
microglia in CNS

gp120

CD4

the tropism of HIV is determined
by the envelope glycoprotein gp120
which binds to the CD4 molecule

FIGURE 11.6 The tropism of HIV is determined by the envelope glycoprotein gpr120 which binds to the CD4 molecule.

the extracellular environment. This is termed a **productive** infection.

In some cases, the provirus is not transcribed and no new virus is made following integration of the viral genome copy. This state is described as **latency**. Latency is overcome if the infected T cells are stimulated either by other viruses or by increased concentrations of cytokines such as tumour necrosis factor α. **It is latency that is responsible for the, often long, symptom-free interval occurring in individuals infected by HIV.** During the latent period, some proviral transcription may be proceeding in the macrophage and follicular dendritic cell compartment.

HIV infection is followed by an immune response in which antibodies to p24 and the envelope glycoproteins are formed, and which is accompanied by production of gp120-specific cytotoxic (CD8+) T cells. This response combats the viraemia. Virus plus antibody and complement are trapped in lymph nodes by follicular dendritic cells, which present viral antigens within germinal centres (see p 100) and cause hyperplasia of the B-cell zones, which is later followed by atrophy.

Most of the antibodies formed during this phase fail to prevent infection of susceptible T cells. A major problem is the fact that the gp120 region of the viral genome is extremely variable and mutates readily and frequently. This has until now prevented active immunization against AIDS, as a vaccine prepared against one variant will have no effect against another.

In individuals who go on to develop serious consequences of HIV infection, **the pivotal event is a decrease in the number of circulating T$_H$ (CD4+) cells. This has effects that transcend T-cell func-tion; macrophages, B cells and natural killer cells all** show impairment of the normal range of functions.

The mechanism/s involved in the death of CD4+ cells is far from clear. Possibilities that have been canvassed include:

- increased susceptibility of HIV-infected T cells to apoptosis
- failure in antigen presentation, leading to a depleted pool of memory T cells
- direct cytopathic effect of the virus on infected T cells

Clinical Natural History of HIV Infections

Infection may be followed by:

- An acute early syndrome characterized by fever, myalgia and joint pain. This is the correlate of viraemia, and the nucleocapsid antigen p24 can be identified in the patient's plasma. This clinical phase occurs in 50–70% of infected individuals.
- An asymptomatic phase in which antiviral antibodies are present in the plasma. At this stage the affected individuals can transmit the disease to others despite their lack of symptoms. Hypergammaglobulinaemia is usually encountered at this stage and the B cells of affected individuals secrete immunoglobulin spontaneously in culture. The number of CD8+ cells specific for HIV antigens is increased in the blood. This phase may continue for years.
- In a proportion of infected individuals, mild constitutional symptoms may develop, associated with **persistent generalized enlargement of lymph nodes**.

- As the number of CD4+ cells in the circulating blood falls to below levels of 400 per mm^3, patients develop **AIDS related complex** (ARC). This consists of:
  a) fever lasting longer than 3 months
  b) weight loss
  c) diarrhoea
  d) anaemia
  e) night sweats

  At this stage, the patient may develop superficial fungal infections, such as candidiasis, which are particularly likely to affect the mouth and oesophagus.
- **Full-blown AIDS**.

At the stage of full-blown AIDS the CD4+ cell count is likely to be 200 per mm^3 or less. Clinical manifestations (*Fig. 11.7*) are predicated on the basis of:

1) **Immune deficiency**, which lays the patient open to a wide range of opportunistic infections (see *Table 11.1*).

2) **An increased risk of developing certain malignant neoplasms, most notably Kaposi's sarcoma** (see p 1031) and non-Hodgkin's lymphoma (including 'primary' lymphoma of the brain) and invasive squamous carcinoma of the uterine cervix.

3) **The direct effects of HIV infection within the nervous system** (see pp 1119–1121). These include:
- progressive encephalopathy associated with dementia
- a range of opportunistic central nervous system infections, including toxoplasmosis and cryptococcal meningitis (caused by the fungus *Cryptococcus neoformans*)
- peripheral neuropathies
- vacuolar changes in the spinal cord

HYPERSENSITIVITY

The introduction of a foreign antigen into an immunologically normal host induces a state of **altered reactivity**, expressed by antibody production and/or the proliferation of sensitized T cells. In such a **primed** host, a second encounter with the same antigen will produce a reaction that is greater both in degree and in speed of response. On some occasions this second reaction may be excessive in degree and cause tissue damage. Such injurious reactions are subsumed within the term **hypersensitivity**.

Hypersensitivity reactions are best classified on the basis of the **mechanisms** involved in their production.

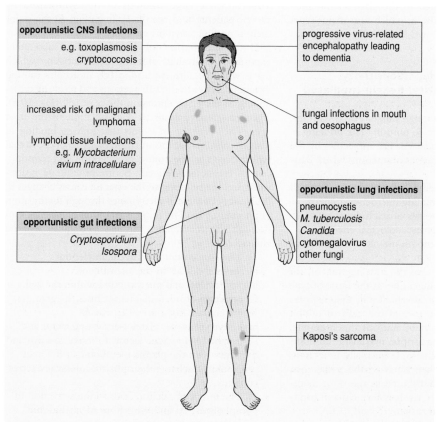

FIGURE 11.7 *Important clinical effects of AIDS.*

Table 11.1 Opportunistic Infections Commonly Occurring in Patients with AIDS

Group	Agent	Target
Bacteria	*Mycobacterium tuberculosis*	Lungs and other organs
	Mycobacterium avium intracellulare	Lymphoid and other tissues
	Nocardia	Lungs, meninges
	Salmonella	All tissues
Viruses	Cytomegalovirus	Lung, gut, eye, brain
	Herpes simplex	Local or disseminated
	Varicella zoster	Local or disseminated
	Papova viruses	Brain causing progressive multifocal encephalopathy
Fungi	*Candida*	Mouth, oesophagus, trachea and lung
	Cryptococcus	Brain and meninges
	Coccidioides	Disseminated
	Histoplasma	Disseminated
Protozoa and helminths	*Toxoplasma gondii*	Brain and lung
	Pneumocystis carinii	Lung and other tissues
	Cryptosporidium parvum	Gut
	Isospora belli	Gut

This approach is embodied in the classification proposed by Gell and Coombs, in which four major types of immunologically mediated tissue injury are recognized.

Type I (Immediate Hypersensitivity, Anaphylactic Sensitivity, Reagin-mediated Allergy)

In this type of reaction a foreign antigen reacts with IgE bound to mast cells via the Fc portion. The bridging of the Fab portions of two adjacent IgE molecules by the antigen sets off a complex series of reactions which basically results in:

- The release of preformed contents from the mast cell granules into the surrounding microenvironment.
- The synthesis of metabolites of arachidonic acid, which have powerful pharmacological effects, notably in relation to smooth muscle tone, which is greatly increased.

An excessive IgE response to the introduction of, for the most part, harmless antigens lies at the heart of type I hypersensitivity. In those affected by it, there is, presumably, a failure on the part of the cells to inhibit responses of B cells to certain antigens. Such people, who are spoken of as being **atopic**, make large amounts of IgE which is specific for some normally innocuous protein. This antibody then binds to the tissue mast cells, which are widely distributed in the skin, membranes of the nose, mouth, trachea, bronchi and bronchioles, gut and lymphoid tissues.

The surface of a mast cell is studded with between 100 000 and 500 000 receptors (FcεRI) to which the inappropriately large amounts of IgE synthesized by allergic patients bind, via the Fc fragment. At this point there is no functional disturbance.

Disturbance occurs only on a second or subsequent exposure to divalent homospecific antigen, which reacts with the adjacent bound IgE molecules causing 'bridging' between the Fab portions and resulting cross-linking of the Fc receptors on the mast cell (*Fig. 10.8*). This cross-linking leads to degranulation of the mast cells. The sequence of events that follows binding of antigen to IgE is not dissimilar, in many respects, to that which occurs in the course of reception and transduction of chemotactic signals. Serine proesterase is activated and the resulting serine esterase causes changes in the fluidity of the cell membranes through methylation of phospholipids. The result is an influx of calcium ions through the membrane; this has two quite separate effects.

1) The concentration of cyclic nucleotides increases and leads to the assembly of microfilaments and microtubules within the cell. Contraction of microfilaments causes the granules, which contain histamine, heparin, 5-hydroxytryptamine, platelet-activating factor and eosinophil chemotactic factor, to move towards and then fuse with the plasma membrane of the mast cell, and to discharge their pharmacologically active contents.

2) The influx of calcium leads to the activation of phospholipase A_2 and the release of arachidonic acid. With arachidonic acid as a starting point, a two-branched cascade occurs (*Fig. 11.8*).

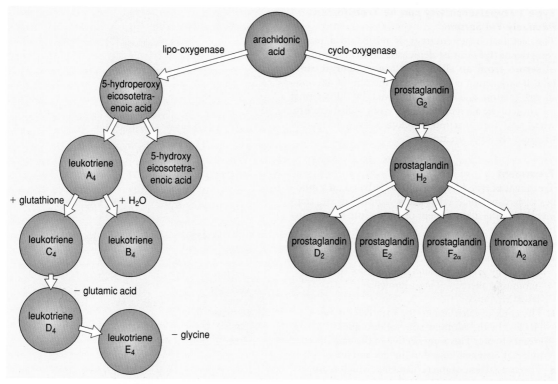

FIGURE 11.8 Arachidonic acid metabolism in the activated mast cell membrane.

- One pathway (the **cyclo-oxygenase** pathway) leads to the formation of prostaglandins via the endoperoxides prostaglandin (PG) G_2 and PGH_2.
- The second pathway, catalysed by the enzyme **lipo-oxygenase**, leads to the formation of powerful inflammatory mediators known as the **leukotrienes**, by converting arachidonic acid via 5-hydroperoxy-eicosotetraenoic acid (5-HPTE). A number of such leukotrienes is formed. These include B_4 (see pp 50–51), C_4, D_4 and E_4. The mixture of C_4, D_4 and E_4 constitutes what was formerly known as **slow-reacting substance A** (SRS-A), a powerful and long-acting agent for the contraction of smooth muscle.

The release of these powerful agents leads to a number of different clinical expressions mediated, at least in part, by the route of exposure to the offending antigen and thus the location of the affected mast cells. These include:

- Allergic rhinitis (hay fever).
- Extrinsic allergic asthma, dominated by bronchospasm. The small airways in asthma show evidence of inflammation in the form of infiltration by T cells, macrophages and, especially, eosinophils. Migration of eosinophils is determined largely by the local release from T cells of interleukin (IL) 3, IL-5 and granulocyte–macrophage colony-stimulating factor (GM-CSF). IL-5 is particularly powerful in this context, promoting eosinophil migration in a number of different ways. Eosinophils contain a protein known as **major basic protein** which upregulates bronchial responsiveness to allergens and is also toxic for bronchiolar and bronchial epithelium. The presence of large amounts of IL-5 in the affected airways suggests a T_H2 type of response to antigen, which seems to be associated with the atopic state.

- Atopic conjunctivitis, caused by spores, danders, pollens and faeces from the house dust mite *Dermatophagoides pteronyssinus*.
- Atopic dermatitis resulting from a variety of allergens (e.g. penicillin, heavy metals, local anaesthetics, etc.).
- Urticarial angio-oedema, characterized by intensely itchy skin papules and often related to insect bites or food allergies.
- Gastrointestinal disturbances such as pain, vomiting and diarrhoea, usually related to food allergies. Mucosal mast cells, which, presumably, are involved in this syndrome differ from the more widely distributed connectve tissue mast cells in that they:
  a) are induced to proliferate by IL-3
  b) release less histamine
  c) release relatively more leukotriene C_4 and less prostaglandin D_2.

Type I Hypersensitivity can be Transferred Passively Via Serum

The fact that hypersensitivity is related to a plasma component (IgE) can be demonstrated by the **transfer of serum from an allergic to a non-allergic subject**. If such serum is injected into the skin of the non-allergic person and this is followed by intradermal injection of the allergen at the same site, a characteristic wheal and flare reaction develops very quickly (the Prausnitz–Kustner reaction).

Treatment

Treatment of type I hypersensitivity is based on a number of factors which relate fairly logically to the steps involved in the development of the specific hypersensitivity:

- The specific allergen should be avoided if possible.
- The tendency to react to the allergen can be reduced by giving repeated injections of small amounts of allergen. This is known as desensitization.
- The entry of calcium into the mast cell can be blocked by the administration of disodium cromoglycate. This is ineffective in the case of mucosal mast cells found in the gut and lung.
- The contraction of microfilaments, which is an essential precursor of mast cell degranulation, can be inhibited by the use of corticosteroids.
- The effects of histamine can be blocked by administration of antihistamines.
- Smooth muscle contraction can be inhibited by isoprenaline or adrenaline.
- The adenosine 5′-cyclic monophosphate (cAMP) to guanosine 5′-cyclic monophosphate (cGMP) ratio can be increased by the use of theophylline or compounds that inhibit the enzyme phosphodiesterase and thus raise intracellular cAMP concentrations. As cAMP increases, the intracellular events described above are damped down.

Type II Hypersensitivity (Cytotoxic Hypersensitivity)

In this type of reaction, tissue damage arises primarily from the presence of circulating antibody directed against some tissue component and the binding of that antibody to its specific epitope. Once such binding has occurred, damage to and death of the affected cells can come about through the operation of a number of effector mechanisms (*Fig. 11.9*) (see also Chapter 10).

- Lysis of the cell membrane may occur as a result of activation of the complement system.
- The cell to which antibody has bound may be phagocytosed by macrophages via the adherence mechanisms mediated through C3b or the Fc portion of immunoglobulin.
- The antibody-coated cells may be killed by killer cells (antibody-dependent cytotoxicity).

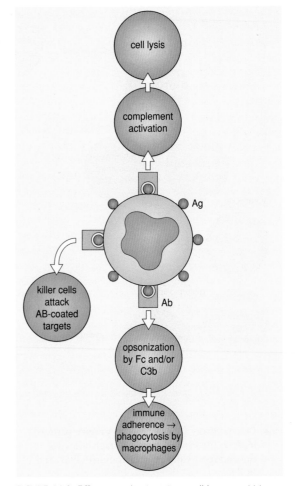

FIGURE 11.9 *Effector mechanisms in type II hypersensitivity.*

Cytotoxic hypersensitivity is of particular clinical importance in relation to the cells of the blood as in:

Immune haemolysis which is an archetypal type II reaction. It may occur under three different sets of circumstances: **incompatible blood transfusion, haemolytic disease of the newborn** (*Fig. 11.10*), **and autoimmune haemolytic disease**. These are described in Chapter 41.

Other examples of autoimmune type II hypersensitivity are considered in Chapter 12.

Drug-induced Type II Hypersensitivity

All varieties of hypersensitivity can be elicited by drugs, but here only those operating through type II mechanisms are considered. Even in this restricted frame of reference, diverse mechanisms may be involved.

In one form, the drug or part of it binds to a carrier (which may be a cell such as the red cell or platelet) and thus acts as a hapten. When binding

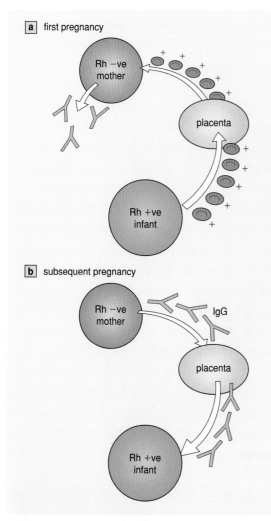

a first pregnancy

Rh –ve mother

placenta

Rh +ve infant

b subsequent pregnancy

Rh –ve mother

IgG

placenta

Rh +ve infant

*FIGURE 11.10 Haemolytic disease of the newborn. **a** Rhesus (Rh)-positive red cells from the fetus leak into the maternal circulation at parturition and cause the mother to produce antibodies directed at the Rh antigens. **b** In subsequent pregnancies, if the infant is Rh positive, the IgG antibodies against Rh antigens cross the placenta and cause haemolysis of the fetal red blood cells.*

takes place between the resulting antibody and the drug-related antigenic determinant, the carrier cell can be destroyed via one of the mechanisms already described. A classical example of such a reaction is the purpura that occurred in some people after taking the hypnotic drug Sedormid. The drug acted as a hapten bound to platelets, and the antibody formed in response bound to the drug and destroyed the innocent platelet by means of complement-mediated lysis. *In vitro*, the platelet lysis can be demonstrated only if the drug is added to a mixture of platelets and the patient's serum.

A totally different mechanism appears to operate in the case of a small number of drugs. Antibodies are formed, which, instead of binding with the drug, react with **self** antigenic determinants and thus, by implication, are elicited by them. An example of this is the very widely used antihypertensive agent α-methyldopa. In a number of patients taking this compound, the red cells become coated with an antibody which binds with **one of the antigens of the rhesus system (e)**. The reason postulated for these findings is that the interaction of the drug with the red cell membrane has revealed antigenic determinants that are normally masked.

Type III Hypersensitivity (Immune Complex-mediated Hypersensitivity)

The union of antibody and antigen in very finely dispersed or soluble form is known as an **immune complex**. Such complexes are capable of eliciting an inflammatory reaction, usually by the activation of complement and the consequent attraction of neutrophils and platelets (*Fig 11.11*). The tissue injury itself is largely due to:

- release of lysosomal enzymes from the neutrophils
- vasoactive amines released from aggregated platelets
- formation of platelet aggregates that can occlude vessels of the microcirculation

The role of the complement system in bringing about these events is thus a key one.

The effect of immune complexes can be reduced greatly if the actions of C3 and later components of the complement sequence are inhibited. The *size* of the complexes is of considerable importance in determining the type of reaction that occurs.

- **Large complexes** are usually phagocytosed, although phagocytosis may be preceded by an inflammatory reaction if the complex is localized within tissues.
- **Very small complexes** may circulate in the plasma and pass harmlessly through the glomerular filter into the urine.

The nature of the complex is, at least in part, governed by the relative proportions of antigen and antibody. If there is **antibody excess** or **mild antigen excess**, the complexes are rapidly precipitated and tend to be localized to the site of antigen introduction, thus giving local tissue reactions. If there is **moderate to gross antigen excess**, the complexes formed are soluble. They can thus circulate widely and become deposited in relation to the basement membranes of small blood vessels (e.g. the glomerular capillaries), in the joints and in the skin.

Immune complex localization in such sites can produce a spectrum of lesions, those affecting small blood vessels showing characteristic features as described on the following page. Tissue reactions in response to immune complexes are influenced by whether the complexes are formed **locally** or are **within the circulation**.

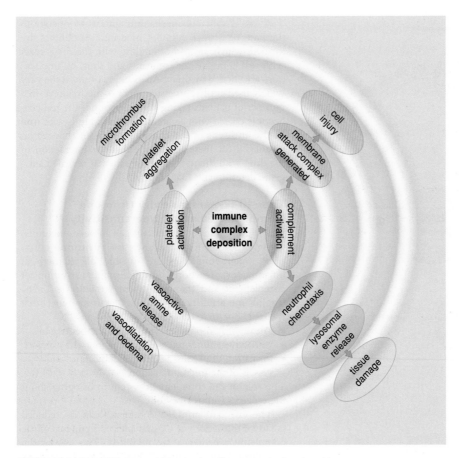

FIGURE 11.11 Type III hypersensitivity: results of immune complex deposition.

Microscopic Features of Small Blood Vessel Lesions Caused by Immune Complex Deposition

There may be extensive necrosis of smooth muscle cells associated with deposition of fibrin and immunoglobulin. This type of reaction is called **fibrinoid necrosis** (Fig. 11.12). When viewed microscopically in sections stained with haematoxylin and eosin, the necrotic portions of the blood vessel walls show a great affinity for the eosin and stain bright red with a curious 'smudged' appearance. These changes may involve the whole circumference of the vessel wall or only a segment of it. If sections containing such lesions are treated with the appropriate fluorescein-linked antisera, the presence of fibrin, immunoglobulin and, in most instances, C3 can be demonstrated.

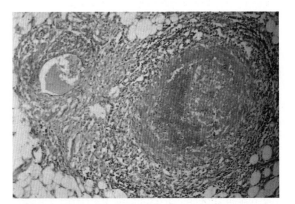

FIGURE 11.12 A blood vessel from a patient with immune complex-related arteritis. The vessel shows severe fibrinoid necrosis, associated with a florid perivascular inflammatory reaction.

Local Formation of Complexes

For local complex formation the essential precondition is a **high concentration of circulating antibody**, leading to rapid precipitation of antigen at or near its point of entry to the tissues. The archetype of this situation is the **Arthus reaction**, described by Maurice Arthus, who found that injection of antigen into the skin of hyperimmunized rabbits produced local reddening and oedema of the skin at the injection site within 3–8 hours. In some instances the inflammatory reaction was so intense that local necrosis occurred with the formation of a slough.

Microscopically such a lesion is characterized by an intense neutrophil response, and the antigen is often precipitated by antibody within small venules. The Arthus reaction can be blocked by depleting the animal of complement or by the use of specific antineutrophil sera.

Arthus-type reactions occur in human disease. Local formation of immune complex with a resulting inflammatory response is the pathogenetic mechanism operating in a number of human disorders, including rheumatoid disease and farmer's lung pp 441–442).

Immune Complexes Formed in the Circulation

Soluble complexes within the circulation are usually formed under conditions of **moderate to gross antigen excess**. This results in solubilization of the complexes which, if they are of appropriate size, can produce lesions in a wide variety of sites. Examples include serum sickness (*Fig. 11.13*) (see p 652) and various forms of glomerulonephritis (see pp 652–654).

Type IV Hypersensitivity (Cell-mediated Reactions)

Tissue injury resulting from the activity of sensitized T cells is common and includes some of the most widespread and serious disorders, such as tuberculosis and leprosy (see pp 157–168). Such injury occurs under three main sets of circumstances:

1) **Hypersensitivity reactions elicited by a number of microbial agents.** These include **bacteria** (tuberculosis and leprosy), **viruses** (smallpox, measles and herpes) and **fungi** (candidiasis, histoplasmosis). The **delayed** skin reactions induced by the injection of tuberculoprotein into the dermis of persons previously exposed to *Mycobacterium tuberculosis*, and hence having some degree of cell-mediated immunity, are highly characteristic. The interactions of sensitized T cells with macrophages, through the medium of lymphokine production have already been described (see pp 97, 109). The tissue reactions characteristic of some of the pathological expressions of cell-mediated reactions are considered in more detail in the section dealing with granulomatous inflammation (see pp 151, 155, 159–160).

2) **Rejection of tissue or organ grafts.**

3) **Contact dermatitis**, as seen after exposure to

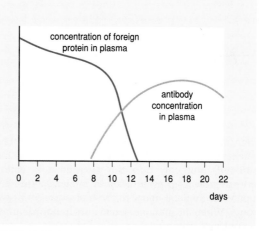

FIGURE 11.13 *Antigen and antibody concentrations in serum sickness. Pathogenic immune complexes are formed during the period of antigen excess.*

certain chemicals, plant products and metals (e.g. watchstrap dermatitis). Contact dermatitis is induced by complex antigens which are formed as the result of binding between the foreign substance and a carrier protein derived from the host's skin.

Stimulatory Reactions Caused by Antibody (Called Type V by Some Writers)

The concept that certain types of cell hyperfunction may be brought about as a result of immune reactions is a fairly new and obviously exciting one. The example most often cited is that of **thyrotoxicosis** (Graves' disease). This condition is characterized by:

- an enlarged thyroid gland
- increased plasma concentrations of the hormones produced by the thyroid
- the clinical features that arise from such an increase in hormone concentration (e.g. weight loss, tremor, anxiety, increased basal metabolic rate)

A significant proportion of patients show, in the plasma, an immunoglobulin that has a stimulatory effect on mammalian thyroid epithelium.

Antibodies that **block** thyroid function bind to the **glycoprotein** component of the receptor; those that **stimulate** thyroid activity bind to the **ganglioside** portion. Other models of antibody-mediated 'switching on' of cell functions have been described, but their relevance in clinical practice has yet to be established.

CHAPTER 12

Autoimmune Disease

Fundamental to the successful operation of an immune system is the ability to distinguish between **self** and **non-self**. Not only does this discriminatory ability serve to protect against invasion by foreign species, but it prevents immune injury to the host organism's own tissues. When the immune system loses its normal unresponsiveness (**tolerance**) to self components, this state is known as **autoimmunity**.

Tolerance to Self is Normally Induced in the Perinatal Period

Normally **tolerance** to self is induced during development of the fetus and in very early neonatal life. Exposure of the immune system to potential antigens during the perinatal period, when that system is developing rapidly, leads to a failure to respond to those antigens when the animal becomes mature in the immunological sense. For instance, the injection of cells from one strain of mouse into newborn of another strain suppresses the ability of the recipient strain, in adult life, to reject a skin graft from the donor strain.

It is possible that exposure of immature lymphoid cells to a specific antigen might lead to the **deletion** of that particular clone and thus account for the immunological unresponsiveness in later life. Such tolerance is just as highly specific as any other aspect of immunological reactivity. If, for example, the pituitary is removed from a tree frog larva while its immune system is developing and the excised tissue is kept alive by transplanting it into another tree frog larva, the animal from which the organ was removed will be found to regard its own pituitary as **foreign** after the neonatal period.

Induction of Tolerance in Adult Animals

Tolerance can be induced in adult animals as well as in neonates. This can be brought about under two sets of circumstances which, one might have imagined, would be mutually exclusive.

- The first of these, known as **low zone tolerance**, is induced when repeated **low** doses of certain antigens are used. Such tolerance is induced most easily by antigens that are **weakly** immunogenic, but can occur with strongly immunogenic antigens provided that antibody synthesis is inhibited during antigen dosage by an immunosuppressive drug such as cyclophosphamide.
- Tolerance can also be induced by the use of

repeated **high** doses of antigen (**high zone tolerance**). The **state** of the antigen is also of some importance in experimental induction of tolerance. Proteins that are soluble rather than in a macromolecular or aggregated form are more easily able to induce tolerance. The avoidance of antigen processing by macrophages before presentation to lymphocytes is also more likely to lead to tolerance of that antigen than to an immune response.

In low zone tolerance, only T cells are unresponsive; in high zone tolerance both B and T cells are involved. High zone tolerance is much more likely to maintain immunological unresponsiveness to **self** antigens than the **low zone** variety, because tolerant T cells could be bypassed by a change in one or more of the determinants in an antigen complex to which they had been made tolerant.

Another possible mode of maintaining tolerance to self antigens is via the operation of **suppressor T-cell activity**. Any reduction in the population of suppressor cells is associated with a tendency to form antibodies against self components. Neonatal thymectomy, which greatly reduces the population of suppressor T cells, exacerbates the autoimmune haemolytic anaemia that is characteristic of the New Zealand Black mouse. Similarly, the injection of thymocytes from young unaffected members of the same strain delays the appearance of the anaemia.

There are some self components to which tolerance does not normally develop but which do not elicit the formation of autoantibodies.

It is possible that there is a small number of self tissue components to which the immune system has never been exposed and to which, therefore, tolerance never develops. Such antigens are spoken of as being **secluded** and probably include lens protein and the antigens of sperm and the myocardium. Damage to tissues containing these antigens and their subsequent release elicits the formation of autoantibodies and this may be associated with immune-mediated injury to the parent tissue.

AUTOIMMUNITY

The concept that some diseases could be due to immune reactions mounted against self antigens stems from three very important sets of observations:

1) The first was the recognition that certain haemolytic anaemias were associated with the presence of antibodies that were cytotoxic to the patient's red cells.

2) This was followed by the discovery, in 1956, that the serum of patients suffering from a disorder of the thyroid known as Hashimoto's thyroiditis contained antibodies that bound to thyroglobulin and also to certain components of thyroid epithelium.

3) At about the same time, workers in the USA produced an experimental thyroiditis in rabbits by injecting extracts of thyroid tissue. Since then, autoimmunity has been invoked as the pathogenetic mechanism in a large number of diseases.

It is not always easy to establish absolute criteria that indicate that a specific disease has an autoimmune origin. Factors suggesting that this may be the case include:

- **Indirect** evidence of immunological disturbance, such as increased levels of immunoglobulins in the plasma.
- **Direct** evidence of autoimmune reactivity as shown by autoantibodies in the plasma and blast transformation *in vitro* of lymphocytes exposed to self antigen.
- Tissue changes characterized by infiltration by lymphocytes, mononuclear phagocytes and plasma cells, all of which mediate immune reactions.
- Clinical and serological associations with other autoimmune diseases in either the patient or their family.
- The occurrence of a similar disease in animals that can be shown to be mediated by immune mechanisms.

Do Autoantibodies Change Tissue Function and Structure?

Effector mechanisms for the production of tissue damage in autoimmune disorders are essentially the same as those that operate in hypersensitivity. Many autoimmune diseases are associated with the presence of either circulating autoantibody or soluble immune complexes, and these can be grouped roughly into two divisions: **organ specific** or **multisystem**.

Organ-specific diseases can be still further subdivided:

- Those in which there is a specific lesion in a target organ and the accompanying autoantibodies are directed against a specific component of that organ.
- Those where the lesions tend to be restricted to a single organ but the autoantibodies are not organ specific and, indeed, sometimes not species specific (e.g. primary biliary cirrhosis, where the *in vivo* target is intrahepatic bile duct epithelium but the antibody reacts *in vitro* with all mitochondria). The pattern of autoantibody production in such organ-specific diseases shows a considerable degree of overlap.

It should be clear from what has been stated about the effects of the antibodies that bind to the thyroid-stimulating hormone (TSH) receptor in the thyroid (see pp 240–241) and those that are implicated in autoimmune haemolytic anaemia that the features of certain disorders are due directly to the binding of autoantibody (*Table 12.1*).

Another striking example of such a situation is the disease **myasthenia gravis**, in which muscle contraction is impaired either by blocking of the acetylcholine receptors on the voluntary muscle or by actual destruction of the receptor, which can be shown to be stripped from the membrane of the muscle cells after they have been cross-linked by autoantibodies (*Fig 12.1*).

Some of the autoantibodies directed against acetylcholine receptors appear to be produced by the thymus. Thymocytes obtained at thymectomy from patients suffering from myasthenia gravis produce antibodies against acetylcholine receptors when cultured, and such antibodies have been shown to produce the muscle changes of myasthenia when injected into rats. The thymus contains a substance on some of its cells that resembles the acetylcholine receptor, and this substance is immunogenic in cell culture systems.

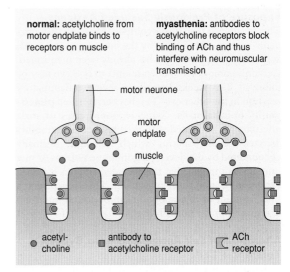

FIGURE 12.1 *At the motor endplate, acetylcholine normally binds to receptors on muscle cells. If antibodies to these receptors are present in sufficiently high titres, the binding is blocked and muscle stimulation to contract does not occur.*

The Presence of Autoantibody in the Blood need not Indicate Autoimmune Disease

It is worth remembering that autoantibodies in the plasma do not necessarily signify autoimmune disease. Such antibodies are found in a number of healthy people and may have no pathogenetic significance. In addition, autoantibodies may occur as a **result, rather than the cause, of tissue damage**. For instance, antibodies that react with human heart muscle are often found in the serum of patients who have undergone open heart surgery.

Many autoimmune diseases exist in which autoantibodies are present in the patient's plasma, but for which no pathogenic role has as yet been identified. If autoantibodies are not responsible for the tissue damage that occurs in some autoimmune diseases, it is necessary to invoke some other mechanism. It seems likely that the guilty party in these instances is either the T or the K cell. In Hashimoto's thyroiditis, where the antibodies reacting with thyroglobulin and thyroid microsomes can cross the placenta, there is no evidence of damage to the thyroid in children of sufferers from this disease, and in the experimental form of this disease caused by injected thyroid extracts of complete Freund's adjuvant, **the disease can be reproduced in non-immunized animals only by the transfer of lymphoid cells from affected animals, not by transfer of plasma**.

Possible Mechanisms for the Production of Autoimmunity

Loss of tolerance to self components leading to autoimmunity could, theoretically, occur in a number of ways.

Exposure of Previously Secluded Antigens

The possibility that tissue components exist that normally are not encountered by the immune system, such as sperm and lens proteins, has already been mentioned. Certainly some cases of open trauma to one eye may be followed 2–3 weeks later by a severe inflammatory reaction in the other eye. This has been termed **phacogenic ophthalmitis**. Similarly, some cases of male infertility are associated with the presence of antibodies directed against sperm, which are not normally encountered by the developing immune system. At one time it was thought that this secluded antigen situation existed in relation to thyroglobulin. This is incorrect; a small amount of thyroglobulin can be found in lymph draining from the normal thyroid.

Alteration of Self Antigens so as to Bypass Tolerant T Cells

Tolerance is due in many cases to the failure of T cells to respond to a certain antigenic determinant and thus to help appropriate B cells produce antibody. It is likely that this type of unresponsiveness can be overcome by some alteration in the **carrier** molecule, which might be accomplished by alteration of some of the determinants on the carrier or by addition of new ones.

In experimental autoimmune disease, extracts of **unaltered** tissue components do not, as a rule, elicit an autoimmune response. When such extracts are altered, either by treating them with certain chemicals or by incorporating them in Freund's adjuvant, autoantibodies are formed and the characteristic type of tissue damage occurs. However, there is no evidence that such alteration of self antigens plays a role in spontaneous

autoimmune disease, although low density lipoprotein molecules within the arterial intima which have undergone oxidative modification elicit the formation of autoantibodies. Such autoantibodies are found in many 'normal' individuals.

Modification of self antigens can occur in association with the use of certain drugs and probably as a result of some viral infections. One of the best known of the drug reactions (see pp 907–908) is the autoimmune haemolytic anaemia occurring in some patients treated with the antihypertensive agent α-methyldopa. In affected patients, autoantibodies are produced against the e antigen of the rhesus system, presumably as a result of some modification of the red cell surface by the drug or one of its metabolites.

The autoantigens may be directly modified and thus made immunogenic or, in some cases, there may be alterations in some molecule concerned in **associative recognition**. This is a phenomenon in which one membrane component provides help for the immune response to another. The appearance of a new helper determinant, either by drug-related modification of an existing molecule or by the insertion of a new antigen as a result of viral infection, may confer immunogenicity on a pre-existing cell component.

Cross-reactions in Bypassing Tolerance

There is no doubt that the immune system encounters certain exogenous antigens that share antigenic determinants with native tissue antigens. Normally tolerance for these determinants would be expected. In just the same way as T-cell tolerance can be overcome by a modification in the carrier molecule associated with an autoantigen, the presentation of one of these 'shared' determinants on a totally different carrier brings normal immunological unresponsiveness for that antigen to an end.

Rheumatic fever, a multisystem inflammatory disease which affects the heart most severely, follows an infection by certain strains of β-haemolytic streptococci. The antibodies produced as a result of such an infection also bind to antigenic components of heart muscle. Some patients with this disease develop a neurological syndrome characterized by abnormal, jerky, involuntary movements (**Sydenham's chorea**). Their serum contains antibodies that can be shown by immunofluorescence to bind to neurones, and this binding can be inhibited by prior absorption of the serum by streptococcal cell membranes. A similar mechanism is believed to operate in the encephalitis that sometimes followed the use of rabies vaccine containing heterologous brain tissue.

Idiotype Bypass

T helper cells with specificity for the idiotype on a certain B-cell receptor play a role in the stimulation of that B-cell clone. If, perhaps as a result of an infection, an antibody was formed with an idiotype that cross-reacted with the receptor of a potentially autoreactive T or B cell, then an autoimmune response might occur. Cross-reacting idiotypes have been found in certain autoimmune diseases such as rheumatoid arthritis and systemic lupus erythematosus (SLE).

Inappropriate Ia Expression

Most organ-specific antigens appear on the surface of the cells as class I but not as class II major histocompatibility complex (MHC)-coded molecules. As a result they cannot communicate with T helper cells and cannot act as immunogens. It has been suggested that if class II genes could become derepressed, MHC class II-coded proteins would be synthesized and appear on the surface of cells, thus rendering them able to present antigen to T helper cells. Thyroid epithelial cells in culture can be persuaded to express Ia molecules (HLA-DR) on their surfaces after stimulation by phytohaemagglutinin, and the epithelial cells from thyroid glands of patients suffering from Graves' disease bind anti-HLA-DR antibodies, suggesting that such inappropriate expression of MHC class II proteins can take place in 'real life' as well as in cell culture systems.

Impaired Regulation of T Cells

There can be little doubt that B cells from normal individuals have the potential to produce autoantibodies. It has been shown, for example, that normal lymphocytes in culture will produce immunoglobulin (Ig) M antibodies of the type seen in rheumatoid disease when stimulated with non-specific mitogens, and normal mice will also produce autoantibodies when injected with non-specific lymphocyte activators. In these situations the autoantibodies formed combine with antigens that are widely distributed. These include DNA, IgG phospholipids, red blood cells and lymphocytes themselves. It has been suggested that these antibodies form a group whose production is an inherent property of the immune system.

Regulation of these potentially autoreactive B cells is probably one of the functions of the T-cell population. The normal dormancy of autoreactive B cells could be regarded as being the result either of the **action** of T suppressor cells, **lack** of activity on the part of appropriate T helper–inducer cells, or both.

Certainly there is a reduction in the number of suppressor T cells in some autoimmune diseases, and in one such disease, **multiple sclerosis**, clinical exacerbations and remissions parallel changes in the suppressor T-cell population. We cannot be absolutely sure, however, that the decrease in the number of suppressor T cells is responsible for the activation of autoreactive B cells. Indeed, it is possible that the reduction in the T-cell subpopulation may be caused by the autoantibody; soluble immune complexes, for example, can impair both the function of suppressor cells and the expression of their markers.

An **excess** of T helper cells has been recorded in a strain of mouse prone to develop a disorder resembling human lupus erythematosus. Such excesses have not yet been described in human autoimmune disease. However, increased T helper cell **activity** has been noted in procainamide-induced lupus erythematosus. This may be due to an inhibition of adenosine 5'-cyclic monophosphate (cAMP) formation by the drug or its metabolites. A decline in intracellular cAMP concentration stimulates helper cells.

α-Methyldopa, on the other hand, which can cause autoimmune haemolysis, stimulates cAMP formation, an effect that inhibits suppressor cells. Thus autoimmunity could arise from either stimulatory or inhibitory effects on T-cell subpopulations.

Possible Role for Anti-idiotype Antibodies

Possible mechanisms for the activation of dormant, potentially autoreactive, B lymphocytes are discussed above. Such cells, as already stated, tend to produce autoantibodies that react with widely distributed antigens. In autoimmune states associated with the presence of highly specific autoantibodies, a normally regulated immune network seems essential. Examples include **myasthenia gravis**, in which there are antibodies directed against the insulin subunit of the acetylcholine receptor, antibodies against the insulin receptor in type I **diabetes mellitus**, and the thyroid-stimulating antibody found in primary **thyrotoxicosis**.

It has been suggested that the autoantibody binding to the acetylcholine receptor in myasthenia gravis may be an anti-idiotype antibody. An **idiotype** is a serologically identifiable configuration in the antigen-binding region of an antibody. An anti-idiotype reacts specifically with this site (*Fig. 12.2*). Binding between

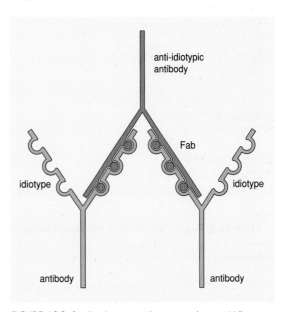

FIGURE 12.2 Binding between idiotypes and an anti-idiotype antibody.

idiotype and anti-idiotype can be inhibited by the antigen that originally elicited the formation of the first antibody, and, similarly, the anti-idiotype can inhibit binding between the antigen and the specific combining site on the first antibody.

In myasthenia gravis, acetylcholine plays the role of a ligand that binds both to its normal receptor and to its corresponding antibody. Thus both the receptor and the antibody must have similar ligand-binding structures. An anti-idiotype that combines with the ligand-binding structure in the variable region of the antibody can also bind to the corresponding structure in the receptor. Such an antibody has been described as 'a key that fits two similar but not identical locks'.

That this view is valid has been shown in experimental models in which eliciting anti-idiotype antibodies leads to a myasthenia-like syndrome.

SOME EXAMPLES OF AUTOIMMUNE DISEASE

The clinical and pathological features of autoimmune diseases encompass a wide spectrum:

- **organ-specific disease associated with organ-specific antibodies** (as seen in Hashimoto's thyroiditis)
- **disorders limited to one organ or tissue but where the antibodies are not organ specific** (such as primary biliary cirrhosis)
- **non-organ-specific or systemic diseases, where lesions may be found in many organs and a wide range of autoantibodies may be encountered** (e.g. SLE, rheumatoid arthritis)

The range of these disorders is illustrated in *Tables 12.1–12.3*. These disorders are considered in other chapters, and only one example is discussed briefly here.

SYSTEMIC LUPUS ERYTHEMATOSUS

SLE is a multisystem autoimmune disease in which the lesions appear to be produced by immune complexes and which is characterized by a generalized excessive autoantibody production. There is a strong predilection for the disease to occur in females (female:male ratio 9:1) and Negro females in the USA appear to be particularly at risk. An increased risk also seems to be conferred by the HLA antigens DR2, DR3 and BW15. Additional evidence of a genetic component comes

Table 12.1 Organ Specific Autoimmune Disorders with Autoantibodies Reacting Only with Antigens in the Affected Organ (*Fig 12.3*)

Disease	Antigen
Hashimoto's thyroiditis	Thyroglobulin
Primary myxoedema	Thyroid peroxidase
Thyrotoxicosis	TSH receptors on cell surface
Addison's disease	Hydroxylases in adrenal cortical cells
Pernicious anaemia	Intrinsic factor
Insulin-dependent diabetes mellitus	Islet cell cytoplasmic antigen; insulin
Goodpasture's syndrome	Basement membranes of glomeruli and lung
Myasthenia gravis	Acetylcholine receptors on muscle
Idiopathic thrombocytopenic purpura	Platelet antigens
Pemphigus vulgaris	Desmosomes between prickle cells
Pemphigoid	Epidermal–dermal basement membrane
Autoimmune haemolytic anaemia	Red cell membrane antigens
Phacogenic uveitis	Lens
Sympathetic ophthalmia	Uveal tract antigens

Table 12.2 Organ Specific Autoimmune Disorders without Organ-specific Autoantibodies (*Fig. 12.4*)

Disease	Antigen
Primary biliary cirrhosis	Mitochondria
Chronic active hepatitis	Smooth muscle, nuclear lamins
Ulcerative colitis	A lipopolysaccharide

Table 12.3 Multisystem Autoimmune Disorders (*Fig 12.5*)

Disease	Antigen
Sjögren's syndrome	Single-stranded RNA (Ro), duct epithelium, mitochondria
Rheumatoid arthritis	IgG
Scleroderma	DNA topoisomerase, centromeres
SLE	Double-stranded DNA, single-stranded DNA, histones, Sm (Smith) antigen (an extractable nuclear antigen), ribonucleoprotein, Ro (another small ribonucleoprotein), cardiolipin
Discoid lupus erythematosus	Nuclear antigens
Mixed connective tissue disease	DNA
Wegener's granulomatosis	Antigen in neutrophil cytoplasm (ANCA anti-neutrophilic cytoplasmic antigen)
Dermatomyositis	Extractable nuclear antigens

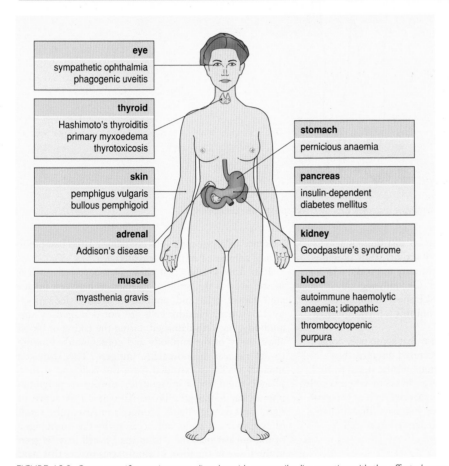

FIGURE 12.3 Organ-specific autoimmune disorder with autoantibodies reacting with the affected organ.

from family clustering of cases and from a high degree of concordance in monozygotic twins.

The tissues most frequently involved are the **skin**, where there is a highly characteristic erythematous rash in the 'butterfly area' of the face, the **joints** (with the production of a polyarthritis) and the **kidney**, where a life-threatening glomerulonephritis may occur (*Fig. 12.5*). Other tissues such as the pleura and pericardium are not infrequently involved and increasing attention has recently been paid to the effects of the disease on the central nervous system. In about half the cases, small warty excrescences may be seen on the heart valves (Libman–Sacks endocarditis).

Two views have been put forward to explain the hyperactivity of the B cells in SLE.

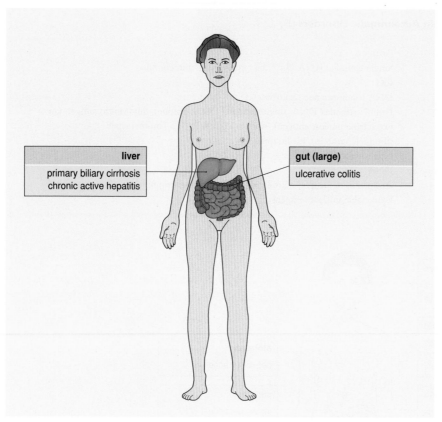

FIGURE 12.4 Organ-specific autoimmune disorders with no organ-specific autoantibodies.

1) The first of these postulates that there is a decline in suppressor T-cell activity, thus allowing B cells an unfettered opportunity to produce large amounts of autoantibodies. Certainly a good number of patients with SLE show evidence of decreased T-cell activity, but this is by no means a universal phenomenon.

2) The second suggestion is that some polyclonal activation of B cells has occurred directly, thus bypassing the need for a non-specific signal from T helper cells. Such activation can occur when B cells are exposed to lipopolysaccharides such as bacterial endotoxins, and it has been suggested that similar lipopolysaccharides can be derived from cell membranes.

Antibodies Found in SLE

These are discussed in the section dealing with glomerular lesions in multisystem disease (see pp 688–691).

The LE Cell Phenomenon

In 1948, long before the concept of autoimmunity had been recognized, Hargreaves found that when blood was taken from patients with SLE, heparinized and allowed to incubate for between 40 and 60 minutes at 37°C, smears made from the buffy layer showed the presence of phagocytic cells containing large basophilic masses composed of nuclear material.

It is now known that these phagocytosed nuclear masses arise as the result of interaction between nucleated blood cells and antibodies against deoxyribonucleoprotein. Healthy cells are not damaged by this antibody, but cells damaged during the taking of blood allow entry of the antibody and consequently binding to its nuclear homospecific antigen. The damaged nucleus swells, is extruded from the cells and is then phagocytosed by a phagocyte, usually a polymorphonuclear leucocyte. There is no good evidence of significant damage being produced *in vivo* as the result of cytotoxic antibody, but occasionally the homologue of the nuclear material within the LE cell may be seen in the tissue in the form of amorphous masses that stain a purplish blue with haematoxylin and which are found in relation to the necrotic lesions characteristic of SLE.

Animal Models of SLE

Our understanding of the processes involved in SLE has been improved by the finding of a number of animal models of the disease. Three of these exist in different strains of mouse (NZB/W, BXSB and MRL/1) and one in the dog.

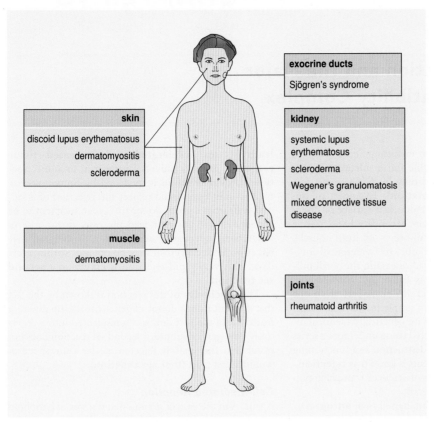

FIGURE 12.5 Non-organ-specific autoimmune disorders.

The hybrid strain produced by mating New Zealand Black (NZB) with New Zealand White (NZW) mice has for many years been the classical model for SLE. The NZW parent produces large amounts of antibody when immunized with DNA, but does not develop the disease, and the NZB parent is similarly free from SLE, although it tends to develop autoimmune haemolytic anaemia. Thus at least two genes must be involved in producing the greatly increased degree of susceptibility of the hybrid.

This hybrid shows a decline in suppressor T-cell activity fairly early in life. This is then followed by the appearance of antinuclear antibodies and the onset of autoimmune disease. The picture is complicated by the fact that both parent strains are infected with leukaemia virus and there is similar evidence of viral infection in canine lupus and in some human patients. In the NZB/W hybrid, the predilection for females noted in humans is also present and 50% of the female mice are dead by the age of 9 months. Males, on the other hand, usually live for 14–15 months before death on this scale occurs. Early castration and treatment with sex hormones can alter this state of affairs; an ovariectomized female given androgens will survive much longer than her untreated counterpart. In other murine SLE models, sex hormones do not appear to influence the situation. The MRL/1 mouse has a

recessive gene which, when homozygous, codes for a tremendous degree of lymphocyte proliferation, and in the BXSB mouse, the factor that accelerates the development of the lupus syndrome appears to be associated with the Y chromosome. Thus, even in the mouse, SLE appears to be a destination that can be reached by a variety of paths, some of which may involve infection.

Drug-induced SLE

A lupus-like syndrome, although usually without significant renal involvement, has been described following administration of a number of drugs, including the antihypertensive agent hydralazine, procainamide and isoniazid. Withdrawal of the drug is usually followed by significant regression of clinical and pathological features. Antibodies reacting with double-stranded DNA are not present, antibodies to nucleoprotein (which fix complement rather poorly) being most prominent. The risk of developing drug-induced SLE appears to be associated with the HLA antigen DR4; it has been suggested that the basic defect in these patients is an inability to acetylate hydralazine or amine groups, thus leading to an accumulation of metabolites that might alter the antigenic properties of certain cell constituents as a result of covalent binding.

CHAPTER 13

Transplantation and the Major Histocompatibility Complex

There are many situations in medical practice where it is clear that prolongation of life and an adequate quality of that life can be obtained only by replacement of a defective organ (**transplantation**). Examples of this include chronic renal failure due to a variety of disorders, intractable cardiac failure secondary to ischaemia or to one of the primary disorders of heart muscle, chronic respiratory failure due to widespread pulmonary fibrosis or widespread disease in the small pulmonary vessels, bone marrow failure and chronic liver failure. However, the transfer of a 'spare part' from one individual to another is not a simple matter and, unless the donor and the recipient are genetically identical or, at least, very similar, the grafted tissue undergoes a series of changes that result in its destruction as a functioning entity. This sequence of events is known as **rejection**.

Like every other branch of science, transplantation has its own jargon. Thus a graft:
- taken from the patient him/herself is an **autograft**.
- where both donor and recipient are genetically identical (syngeneic), as in the case of identical twins, is an **isograft**.
- where donor and recipient are of the same species but not identical in genetic make-up (allogeneic) is an **allograft**.
- where donor and recipient are *not* of the same species (xenogeneic) is a **xenograft**, e.g. monkey to human.

REJECTION

The events that take place in allograft rejection can be studied easily in a model system where skin from one strain of mouse is grafted on to a mouse of another strain. The grafted skin becomes normally vascularized in a few days, but shortly after this it becomes infiltrated by lymphocytes and macrophages, and the blood flow through the part begins to diminish. By 10 days or so after the transplant, the graft is necrotic and is sloughed off leaving a bare area of exposed dermis.

What is the Evidence that Rejection is Immunological in Nature?

First and Second Set Reactions
In granuloma formation, the **second contact with the responsible antigen (such as schistosome ova)** leads to an **accelerated and increased tissue response**; this is a universal pattern in immune reactions. If graft rejection is mediated by immunological mechanisms, one would expect the rejection of a second graft from a given donor to a given recipient to be accelerated and this is indeed the case. In the case of mouse skin, adequate vascularization of the graft may never occur and necrosis may be obvious within a few days. This very rapid rejection is known as a **second set reaction**.

The **specificity** of this reaction is shown by the fact that if a graft from a donor of genetic make-up different from that of the first donor is transplanted into a previously skin-grafted mouse, a second set reaction does not occur and the graft is rejected at the same speed as would a first graft (**first set reaction**).

Cell-mediated Reaction
Again, as in the case of granuloma, transfer of lymphoid cells from an animal that has had an allograft to an animal that has not, results in the second animal showing accelerated rejection of a graft from the original donor animal. In animals that have been thymectomized during the neonatal period, allografts survive for prolonged periods. The ability to reject such grafts at a 'normal' speed is restored by the injection of lymphocytes from a genetically identical normal animal.

Antibody Production
Humoral antibodies that react with donor cells can be found in the blood of the recipient after rejection.

All these data indicate that **rejection is immunologically mediated**. The success of isografts between animals with an identical genetic constitution suggests that the antigens responsible for rejection are determined genetically.

THE MAJOR HISTOCOMPATIBILITY COMPLEX (*Fig 13.1*)
The basis of rejection is the recognition by the recipient's immune system of a group of glycoprotein antigens on the surface of the donor cells known as **histocompatibility antigens**. In some ways, this is a misleading name because it obscures the fact that these antigens play a vital role in the regulation of immune responses in general.

The major histocompatibility complex (MHC) has been studied extensively in mouse and humans; in the

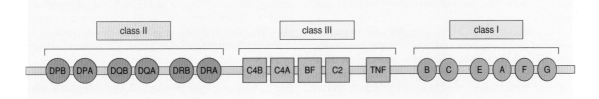

FIGURE 13.1 Principal genes of the MHC on chromosome 6.

latter it is made up of a group of genes on the short arm of chromosome 6. In the mouse there are at least 20 transplantation loci, but the most important of these is the H-2 locus. This provokes intense allograft rejections, which are difficult to suppress. The H-2 locus in fact consists of at least three loci, two of which code for the very 'strong' transplantation antigens H-2K and H-2D. The third locus codes for H-2L.

All lymphoid cells contain large amounts of the H-2K/D antigens; liver, lung and kidneys have moderate amounts; and brain and voluntary muscle have rather little.

Antigens of this group have been termed **class I molecules** (see p 105) and can be identified on lymphoid cells by the cytotoxicity of antibodies that react with them. The mouse histocompatibility complex, however, also codes for another group of antigens, called **class II molecules** or **Ia antigens**. These antigens were recognized by T helper cells and are thus the signals that stimulate a variety of T-cell functions. They cannot be identified by means of a panel of antibodies. However, when lymphocytes from animals that differ in respect of the genes determining Ia antigens are mixed together they undergo 'blast' transformation and mitosis.

The MHC in Humans and Transplantation

As stated above, the MHC in humans is located on the short arm of chromosome 6. The dominant group of antigens governing rejection reactions is spoken of as the HLA system. HLA stands for human leucocyte antigen, as the class I molecules have been delineated through the effect of their homospecific antibodies against human leucocytes, which, of course, constitute an abundant source of nucleated cells. The combination of genes coding for transplantation antigens which is inherited from each parent is known as the **haplotype**.

Class I Molecules

Class I molecules are coded for at three major loci: A, B and C. HLA-A and -B probably constitute the homologues of the 'strong' transplantation antigens H-2D and H-2K in the mouse, and readily induce the formation of complement-fixing cytotoxic antibodies, which can be used for tissue typing. These antibodies can be found in the plasma of patients who have had blood transfusions and in multiparous women who have

become immunized against fetal antigens defined by paternally derived genes.

The A and B gene products act as cell surface recognition markers for cytotoxic T cells. They usually present viral antigen on the surface of infected cells, thus enabling the cytotoxic T cells (CD8) to eliminate the virus by destroying infected cells. In kidney grafts, class I antigens are present on vascular endothelium, on tubular epithelium and on interstitial and mesangial cells.

HLA Typing

HLA typing in respect of these class I antigens is done by setting up an individual's lymphocytes against a panel of known antibodies in the presence of complement. Binding of antibody to its homospecific antigen on the surface of the lymphocyte leads to cell membrane damage; this is monitored by testing the cells' ability to exclude dyes such as trypan blue or eosin. A marked degree of polymorphism exists in respect of the major histocompatibility loci. There are 24 alleles for HLA-A, 42 for HLA-B and 11 for HLA-C.

Class II Molecules

Class II molecules were originally defined by the HLA-D locus. This is now known not to be a single locus and has been split into DR, DQ and DP, each of which codes for class II molecules. There are six DP alleles, 20 DR and nine DQ. Class II antigens are expressed on the surfaces of B lymphocytes, monocytes and macrophages, and other antigen-presenting cells.

The antigens coded for by the D genes are recognized by performing the **mixed lymphocyte reaction test**. In this test, lymphocytes, for example from a patient awaiting a renal transplant, are mixed with an equal number of lymphocytes drawn from a potential donor. The donor cells are pretreated either by irradiation or with mitomycin, which prevents them undergoing blast formation in response to the D antigens on the surface of the recipient's lymphocytes, should these be different from the donor's. Blast transformation of the potential recipient's cells is detected by measuring the uptake of tritiated thymidine, which is greatly increased if blast transformation occurs. Unfortunately this test takes 5 days to perform and thus is of no practical use if transplantation of a cadaver kidney is being contemplated. Newer serological methods are now available, however, for the detection of D and DR antigens.

The products of the MHC complex show a marked degree of polymorphism and it is virtually impossible, other than in the identical twin donor–recipient situation, to obtain a complete match of the MHC-encoded antigens. Nevertheless, the closer the match in respect of the histocompatibility antigens, the greater are the chances of long survival of the graft.

From the point of view of a surgeon wishing to undertake a transplantation procedure, **the most important factor in predicting the success or otherwise of the outcome is the degree of matching between the class II antigens, especially DR, of the potential donor and the recipient**. When the donor is a sibling of the recipient with good HLA matching, the chance of 10-year survival in the presence of appropriate immunosuppression is now about 90%. However, if the donor and recipient are not siblings, the same degree of HLA-A and -B matching gives a success rate over a 10-year period of only 60–70%. The explanation given for this discrepancy is that when brothers and sisters share a common heritage of HLA-A and -B antigens from one of their parents, they are likely to have inherited most or all of the genes that lie between these two loci. While individuals who are not related seem to be identical at their A and B loci, they may well have many genes in between that are not identical.

MECHANISMS INVOLVED IN ALLOGRAFT REJECTION

In humans, the system that has been studied most extensively is the renal allograft. Here, rejection can be seen to occur at different times after transplantation and the events at these different stages probably mirror different mechanisms (*Fig 13.2*).

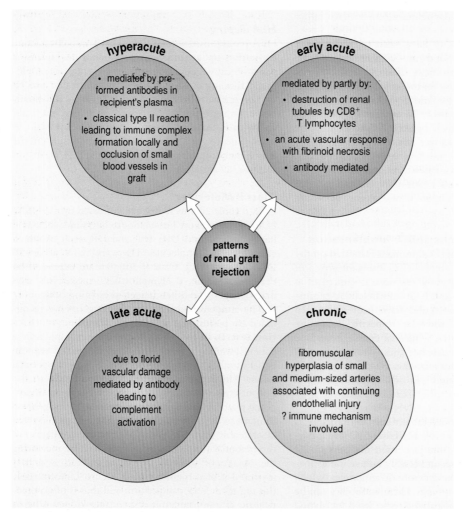

FIGURE 13.2 Patterns of renal graft rejection.

Thus rejection may be:

- **Hyperacute** – the graft may be rejected within minutes or hours.
- **Acute** – usually occurring within the first few weeks of the life of the graft.
- **Chronic** – usually manifesting some months or even years after transplantation. It may follow several episodes of acute rejection or may appear as an insidious decline in the function of the transplanted kidney with no history of acute rejection episodes.

Hyperacute Rejection

This takes place within minutes of the graft being inserted. It is characterized by the presence of small thrombi and of sludged red cells in the glomeruli. **It is a classical example of a type II immunological reaction.** Preformed antibodies, present either as a result of ABO incompatibility between donor and recipient or because the recipient has formed antibodies as a reaction to previous blood transfusions, bind to endothelial cells in the small vessels of the donor kidney and activate complement.

This in turn activates platelets and the clotting system, leading to occlusion of the vessels in the transplanted kidney and to ischaemic necrosis. The process is irreversible and the failed graft must be removed. Fortunately, hyperacute rejection is rare (0.5% of all rejections).

The events of hyperacute rejection are, in morphological terms, quite spectacular. The donor kidney, instead of being pink and firm as it is perfused by the recipient's blood, becomes blue, mottled and flabby. Angiography shows occlusion of the intrarenal small vessels, and over the next day or so complete cortical necrosis develops.

Light microscopic examination of biopsy specimens shows extensive occlusion of the small vessels by fibrin and platelets, this process extending into the glomeruli. Immunohistology shows immunoglobulin (Ig) G and C3 bound to the endothelial surfaces of the small blood vessels.

Early Acute Rejection

This takes place 7–10 days after transplantation. The affected donor kidney shows a dense infiltration by lymphocytes (*Fig. 13.3*) which, using appropriate markers, are shown to be cytotoxic T cells.

Acute rejection is common. A kidney showing acute rejection is not necessarily doomed to fail and many patients have one or more acute rejection episodes during the first few weeks after transplantation.

Acute rejection manifests in a number of ways:

- oliguria
- a rise in serum creatinine concentration (which may be the only evidence of rejection)
- fever
- some swelling and tenderness of the kidney
- the presence in the urine of protein, lymphocytes, tubular epithelial cells and interleukin (IL)-2

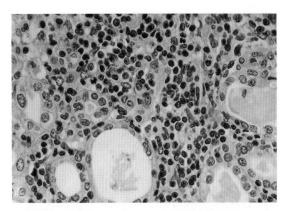

FIGURE 13.3 Acute early rejection. This renal allograft was rejected 10 days after transplantation. The renal tubules (RT) and the peritubular blood vessels are surrounded by immunologically competent cells, the majority of which are T cells. These are exerting a direct effect on the constituents of the graft.

Unlike hyperacute rejection which is entirely antibody mediated, the mechanisms involved in acute rejection are diverse. Renal biopsy can be a helpful guide to the pathogenesis and progress of the kidney following treatment for the rejection. Thus acute rejection can be the result of a cellular response mediated by T cells or a vascular response mediated by antibody.

Cellular Response Mediated Via Recipient T Cells

The principal targets for such a reaction are the tubules and interstitial tissues.

Light microscopic examination of renal biopsies shows severe oedema of the interstitial tissue, associated with a dense mononuclear cell infiltrate. Many grafts not undergoing rejection show some cells in the interstitium but the infiltrate seen in rejection episodes is much more extensive and severe. The T lymphocytes and macrophages which make up the infiltrate are often seen to be invading the walls of the tubules and evidence of tubular necrosis (see pp 681–683) is frequently present. Immunohistological examination shows the T cells to be activated and to be producing IL-2 as well as other activation and proliferation markers.

The reaction occurs because of a reaction by the recipient's T cells to antigens present on donor vascular endothelium and on dendritic cells present in the donor kidney interstitium. There is no evidence of binding of either IgG or C3. Recognition of donor antigens by recipient T helper cells is followed by the release of a number of lymphokines including IL-2. IL-2 is not synthesized by cytotoxic T cells and, therefore, a cytotoxic T-cell response in acute rejection depends on IL-2 synthesis by the helper-cells (*Fig. 13.4*). In this connection, it is not without interest that the most effective immunosuppressive drug in common use, cyclosporin A, inhibits the synthesis of

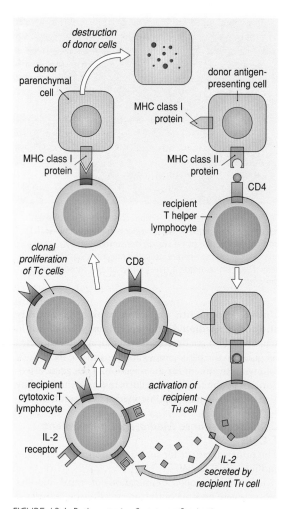

FIGURE 13.4 *Pathogenesis of acute graft rejection.*

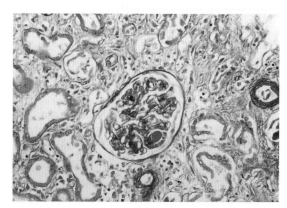

FIGURE 13.5 *Acute late rejection showing vascular damage (left) and red-staining fibrin masses within the glomerular capillary tuft.*

likely that T cells are also involved (CD8 cells are found in relation to the damaged endothelium). Once there is evidence of fibrinoid necrosis and/or thrombosis in the small blood vessels and glomerular capillaries, the outlook for long-term survival of the graft is bleak.

Acute Late Rejection

This occurs in patients who have been immunosuppressed with prednisolone and azathioprine. This regimen damps down the T-cell response but is not completely effective in stopping antibody production. The rejection takes place between 11 days and 6 weeks after operation and is characterized by florid vascular damage, which appears to be mediated by antibody and complement (*Fig. 13.5*). The immunoglobulins and complement can be identified within the vessel walls by immunofluorescent techniques.

Acute Transplant Glomerulopathy

About 4–10% of allogeneic kidney transplants develop a rather characteristic lesion in the glomeruli of the donor kidney. Clinically, the patient presents with evidence of an acute rejection episode, no different from any other.

The affected glomeruli show occlusion of the capillary lumina by swollen endothelial and mononuclear inflammatory cells (*Fig 13.6*). This glomerular lesion is often accompanied by evidence of either tubulointerstitial rejection or, in a minority of cases, by signs of vascular rejection. The pathogenesis is not known.

Chronic Rejection

Chronic rejection is responsible for about 8% of the kidneys rejected in the first year after transplantation and for the vast majority of those rejected at a later stage. Because chronic rejection is basically ischaemic in nature, most of the affected patients become hypertensive.

Chronic rejection can occur years after transplantation. The most prominent histological feature is fibro-

IL-2 and the expression of HLA class II antigens (*Fig. 13.8*).

Acute Vascular Response Mediated by Antibody

The clinical and laboratory findings are, for the most part, identical with those of acute cellular rejection but an additional feature, seen in some cases, is platelet sequestration within the transplanted kidney.

Cell infiltration in this type of rejection is concentrated on and between the vascular endothelial cells of the donor kidney. In severe cases, small blood vessels show fibrinoid necrosis extending into glomerular capillary tufts with resulting thrombosis.

IgG and IgM antibodies are often bound to the donor endothelium, as are C1q and C3 components of complement. **The presence of the former suggests classical pathway activation of the complement system.**

While it is clear that an antibody-mediated reaction with subsequent complement activation occurs, it is

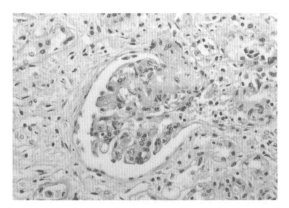

FIGURE 13.6 *Acute glomerulopathy. Capillary lumina in glomerulus largely obliterated by swollen endothelial cells.*

muscular hyperplasia of the intimal lining of small and medium-sized vessels in the kidney, with eventual occlusion leading to ischaemic necrosis of the glomeruli supplied by the affected vessels (*Fig. 13.7*). This too is thought to be mediated via the reaction of antibodies binding to HLA antigens on the endothelium of vessels in the donor kidney. Antibody and complement may also be seen to be deposited within the glomeruli.

Arterial Changes in Chronic Vascular Rejection

The arteries most commonly affected are the arcuate and interlobular arteries. The intima is grossly thickened, the whole circumference of the vessel wall being involved. Intimal thickening is due partly to the presence of cells and partly to connective tissue, which is rich in mucins. Lipid-laden macrophages are also present.

As the lesion ages, so the amount of collagen in the intima increases and the vessels become stiff and non-compliant. The pathogenesis of this arterial lesion is unclear. There is no direct evidence for the involvement of immune mechanisms but, equally, there is no doubt that the closer the match between donor and

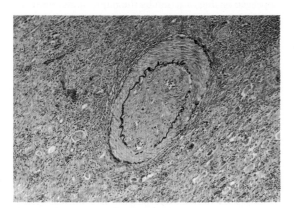

FIGURE 13.7 *The lumen of the medium-sized artery shown is occluded by an overgrowth of fibromuscular tissue (section stained by elastic/Van Gieson method).*

recipient in terms of histocompatibility antigens, the lower the risk of chronic vascular rejection.

Serial renal biopsies have shown that development of the intimal thickening of chronic vascular rejection is associated with the presence of mural thrombi on the endothelial surface of affected vessels. This tells us two things:

   1) The chronic vascular changes are likely to be due to continuing or recurrent endothelial injury leading to the formation of these thrombi in the affected vessels.

   2) The intimal thickening itself is likely to be mediated by growth factors released from the thrombi.

Glomerular Changes in Chronic Rejection

Glomerular damage as part of chronic transplant rejection occurs in about 4% of all grafted kidneys. Clinically, it is expressed in the form of a moderately heavy proteinuria (> 1 g per day) and the loss of protein may be so great as to lead to the nephrotic syndrome.

On light microscopy of renal biopsy material, the walls of the glomerular capillaries are seen to be thickened, due in part to widening of the subendothelial region with interposition of mesangial cell cytoplasm. This results in a double-contour basement membrane similar to that of mesangiocapillary glomerulonephritis. In addition there is some increase in the mesangial matrix and mesangial cell population.

AVOIDING REJECTION

The chances of rejection may be reduced essentially in two ways:

   1) **Good matching between donor and recipient.** The perfect match would be one in which the haplotypes of both donor and recipient are identical as, for example, in the case of monozygotic twins. This situation is rare.

   2) **Suppression of the immune responses of the recipient.**

Immunosuppression by Drugs

Azathioprine

This compound, which is broken down in the body to 6-mercaptopurine, is particularly helpful in inhibiting T cell-mediated rejection. It interferes with enzyme systems involved in nucleic acid synthesis and is thus most likely to affect cells that are actively replicating. In the first days after transplantation, the cells most likely to be undergoing clonal expansion are the T cells, and the drug thus inhibits lymphocyte proliferation. However, it is by no means specific for these cells and will affect other cell systems in which replication is a prominent feature.

Cyclosporin A

This is a fungal product which, unlike azathioprine, has no effects on the replicating cells of the bone marrow. It selectively penetrates antigen-sensitive T cells in the GO and G1 phase and inhibits an RNA polymerase, leading to blocking of the production of IL-2 by T_H cells, which is required for the clonal expansion of cytotoxic T cells (*Fig. 13.8*). It is now regarded as the first-line drug in the prevention of allograft rejection. At certain dose levels it is nephrotoxic and thus its blood concentration must be monitored carefully.

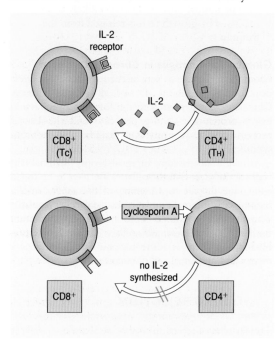

FIGURE 13.8 The action of cyclosporin A in preventing graft rejection.

Tacrolimus (FK506)

This is another fungal product which also suppresses lymphokine production by recipient T_H cells.

Rapamycin

This fungal macrolide differs from the previously mentioned compounds by interfering with the intracellular signalling pathways of the IL-2 receptor.

Biological Immunosuppression

Increasing attention is being paid to the potential for **selective immunosuppression by biological methods** that might lack the toxic effects of drugs. Such approaches include the use of:

- Monoclonal antibodies against T_H (anti-CD4) cells or activated T cells (anti-CD25, the IL-2 receptor).
- Monoclonal antibody conjugated with a toxin, such as ricin; the complex is targeted against CD5, a molecule expressed on activated T cells.

- A lymphokine complexed with toxin (e.g. diphtheria toxin); for example, IL-2 plus toxin would lock on to the IL-2 receptors on activated T cells and kill the cells.

Effects of Immunosuppressive Treatment

The survival of renal allografts depends, in the majority of cases, on adequate immunosuppression. Such immunosuppression is not without problems, which may be caused in a number of ways and have a number of effects.

Nephrotoxicity

There may be a direct nephrotoxic effect of the immunosuppressive agent. Cyclosporin A, for example, can cause acute nephrotoxicity at high dosages. In such cases there may be vacuole formation in the cells of the proximal tubules and hyalinization of arterioles.

Chronic nephrotoxicity can also occur as a result of cyclosporin treatment. This takes the form of interstitial fibrosis and tubular atrophy. The fibrosis shows a peculiar 'striped' pattern, being focal in distribution.

The use of antilymphocyte globulin to combat rejection occasionally leads to serum sickness associated with a diffuse endocapillary proliferative glomerulonephritis similar to that which can occur after streptococcal infections.

Infection

Immunosuppression must increase the risk of infection. Any variety of infectious agent may be involved. Viral inclusions may be seen, commonly as a result of cytomegalovirus infection.

Hypertension

Hypertension is quite common following renal transplant, being seen in about 50% of patients. It has been suggested that cyclosporin may contribute to this. The vasoconstriction associated with cyclosporin does not appear to be due to action by the renin–angiotensin system and is very responsive to restriction of the patient's sodium intake.

Hyperlipidaemia

Hyperlipidaemia is seen in about 60% of post-transplant patients. The hyperlipidaemia is of the combined type, both cholesterol and triglyceride being increased. As patients have both hyperlipidaemia and high blood pressure following transplantation, it is not surprising that they show an increased risk of cardiovascular events, such events being responsible for 30% of the deaths that occur in these patients.

Post-transplant Neoplasia

The concept that immunosurveillance may play a role in inhibiting the development of malignant neoplasms gains some support from the fact that post-transplant patients have an increased incidence of such tumours. In order of frequency, the tumours that complicate renal transplantation are:

1) squamous carcinoma of the skin
2) B-cell lymphomas, especially those associated with infection by the Epstein–Barr virus
3) Kaposi's sarcoma
4) cancer of the cervix uteri

BONE MARROW TRANSPLANTATION AND GRAFT VERSUS HOST REACTIONS

Thus far only the question of graft rejection by the recipient has been considered. Another aspect of the transplantation problem is what has been termed **graft versus host (GvH) reaction**. This is a major factor in bone marrow transplantation, which is used in patients with aplastic anaemia, immunological deficiencies and those whose bone marrow has been ablated by therapy, for example for acute leukaemia.

The basis of a GvH reaction is the fact that competent lymphoid cells are transferred from a donor to a recipient who is unable to reject them. If the donor cells survive long enough to recognize the recipient's cells as 'foreign', they will mount immunological reactions against the recipient's cells, hence the term 'graft versus host'.

- In mice there will be an inhibition of growth (so-called 'runting'), haemolytic anaemia and splenomegaly.
- In humans, GvH reaction is characterized by fever, weight loss, rashes, splenomegaly, anaemia and diarrhoea. Cyclosporin A reduces the frequency of GvH reaction and recently some success has been obtained by treating the bone marrow sample that is to be transplanted with monoclonal anti-T cell antibodies so that cells capable of responding to recipient antigens are removed.

HLA RELATIONSHIPS WITH DISEASE

Why do some people get certain diseases and others not? For many years geneticists have tried to answer this question. Apart from the various familial disorders for which the inheritance patterns have been worked out, some associations, although rather weak, have been noted, for example the relationship between ABO blood groups and gastric carcinoma. In 1963 an association was noted between susceptibility to spontaneous murine leukaemia and certain antigens of the H–2 system, and in 1967 an association was described between certain HLA antigens in humans and the risk of developing Hodgkin's disease. These early reports have led to considerable exploration of the relationships between human haplotypes and various diseases.

In considering this question it must be remembered that a number of genes not directly concerned with transplantation reactions are closely linked to the HLA complex on the short arm of chromosome 6. These include:

- the gene determining factor B (which is involved in the alternate pathway of complement activation)
- genes for controlling the production of the second and fourth components of complement (failure to produce these proteins increases the risk of immune complex-mediated disease)
- a gene controlling production of the enzyme 21-hydroxylase
- a gene encoding the heat shock protein hsp70
- genes encoding tumour necrosis factors α and β

The Distribution of HLA Genes is Non-uniform on a World-wide Basis

The prevalence of various HLA-determined antigens varies between populations. For instance, A30 is found in 28% of black-skinned people, in only 5% of Caucasians and not at all in Japanese people. Aw24 occurs in 58.5% of Japanese, in 18% of Caucasians and in only 6% of black-skinned people. HLA-B8 occurs in 16% of Caucasians, but in less than 0.5% of Japanese.

Linkage Disequilibrium

Sometimes the alleles of two or more loci, for instance A1 and B8 or A1, B8 and DR3, occur together more frequently than would be expected if their association was only random. This is known as **linkage disequilibrium**.

Several explanations have been offered for this phenomenon.

1) At some point in the course of evolution, a particular combination of alleles may have conferred some selective advantage. This, while not provable, gains a little support from the fact that the frequency of certain alleles and haplotypes differs between populations living under different environmental conditions. Thus the haplotypes that show linkage disequilibrium in European Caucasians are quite different from those occurring in West African Negros.

2) Some haplotypes have arisen relatively recently (in evolutionary terms) and there has been insufficient time for equilibration to occur by random recombination.

3) As a result of migration, some 'foreign' haplotype or gene has been introduced into a population, leading to linkage disequilibrium in the genetic pool of that population. Many generations of random breeding may be required before this effect vanishes.

Linkage and Association in Human Disease

The appropriate distinction between linkage and association should be made in considering genetic relationships in human disease. The term **linkage**, strictly speaking, applies to a situation where gene loci are close to each other on a particular chromosome. The presence of such linkage can be recognized only by carrying out family studies on more than one generation to see whether certain characteristics are transmitted together. Not many human diseases have been shown to be linked to the HLA system in this way.

Those that have been found include

- 21-Hydroxylase deficiency, which leads to congenital adrenal hyperplasia (see pp 240, 839).
- Deficiencies of the second and fourth components of complement.
- Some cases of haemochromatosis in which regulation of iron absorption is defective and large amounts of iron become deposited in parenchymal cells in various tissues, most notably, from the functional point of view, the liver and heart.

The term **association** refers to a relationship between two separate characteristics. This can be recognized by examining a sufficiently large number of cases of a certain disease and an equal number of controls. For example, HLA-B27 occurs more frequently in patients with ankylosing spondylitis (95%) than in a randomly selected control population (5%).

The most striking association with HLA-determined antigens is to be found in disorders in which immune mechanisms are implicated: the rheumatic diseases and a group of diseases characterized by chronic inflammation and abnormal immunological reactions.

Family Studies in Autoimmune Diseases Suggest a Genetic Influence

Two striking family studies reported in 1982 can be quoted as strong support for the operation of genetic factors in autoimmune disease. The two families between them contained 70 relatives and 23 spouses. In one family the patient originally identified had autoimmune haemolytic anaemia and hypothyroidism. Five relatives had hyperthyroidism and three others had ulcerative colitis. In the second family, the proband had autoimmune thrombocytopenia. Four of her relatives had rheumatoid arthritis, SLE, autoimmune thrombocytopenia and asthma. There was no evidence of autoimmune disease in the spouses. Other studies also show evidence of this type of familial clustering. Even more suggestive is evidence obtained from studying identical twins. The concordance of SLE in identical twins ranges from 50 to 60%. In type I diabetes, the concordance is also about 50% with respect to insulin requirement.

Ankylosing Spondylitis

The most convincing of all HLA associations with disease is that between HLA-B27 and ankylosing spondylitis. It might be better here to use the term 'the spondyloarthropathies', because, although ankylosing spondylitis is the archetype, a number of other arthritides involving the spine, sacroiliac and axial joints have this association. This group of disorders includes:

- ankylosing spondylitis
- Reiter's disease
- psoriatic arthritis
- post-*Shigella*, post-*Salmonella* and post-*Yersinia* arthritis
- spondylitis associated with inflammatory bowel disease

The B27 antigen is found in more than 90% of Caucasian patients with ankylosing spondylitis and in only 5% of Caucasian controls. Possession of the antigen confers a risk of developing the disease that is 80–90 times greater than that in the control population. Even so, individuals with the B27 gene stand a chance of only 5–20% of developing ankylosing spondylitis. Some 50% of first-degree relatives of spondylitics with B27 also have the antigen, and 30% of them develop either ankylosing spondylitis or some other spondyloarthropathy. The relative risks of developing one of these diseases in association with HLA-B27 are shown in *Table 13.1*.

Table 13.1 Relative Risk of HLA-B27 Associated Spondyloarthropathies

Disease	Relative risk
Ankylosing spondylitis	87.4
Reiter's disease	37.0
Post-*Salmonella* arthritis	29.7
Post-*Shigella* arthritis	20.7
Post-gonococcal arthritis	14.0

The prevalence of B27 in different populations correlates quite well with the risk of developing the disease. B27 is virtually absent in Japan and ankylosing spondylitis is very rare among the Japanese. Conversely, there is a tribe of native Canadians in British Columbia (the Haidas) in whom the prevalence of B27 is more than 50%. This tribe also has a very high prevalence of ankylosing spondylitis. The presence of B27 in the haplotype confers a lower increment of risk relative to the control population in respect of the other spondyloarthropathies than it does in relation to ankylosing spondylitis (*Table 13.1*).

One problem in relation to the association between B27 and ankylosing spondylitis is the different prevalence of the disease between the sexes. Males are affected five times as frequently as females, but the distribution of B27 is the same in both sexes.

Rheumatoid Arthritis

Classic rheumatoid arthritis (see pp 1075–1081) is associated with the class II antigens Dw4 and DR4. These are present in 25% of the control population and in 45% of those with the disease. The DR4 association is strongest for patients with severe erosive changes in the articular cartilage and underlying bone, and who have rheumatoid factors in the plasma. Patients with rheumatoid arthritis who are treated with gold or D-penicillamine, and who develop an immune complex nephritis as a result, have an association with HLA-B8 and -DR3.

A group of other diseases, in all of which immune mechanisms appear to be implicated, have associations with antigens of both the class I and class II variety.

Coeliac Disease

Coeliac disease (see pp 522–524) is characterized by malabsorption associated with subtotal or total atrophy of the villi in the duodenum and jejunum. Patients are sensitive to the gliadin fraction of gluten and, when this is withheld from the diet, both their symptoms and the appearance of the gut mucosa improve markedly. Such patients have a strong association with HLA-B8 (this being present in 60–81% of the patients and in only 16–22% of controls). DR3 is found in 79% of the patients, and D7 in 45%.

Myasthenia Gravis

Myasthenia gravis, which has already been discussed in relation to anti-idiotype antibodies, appears to exist in two forms with respect to its genetic associations. The early-onset type associated with thymic hyperplasia has an association with B8 and DR3. The adult-onset type, which is usually associated with a tumour of the thymus (thymoma), does not show any strong HLA association.

Juvenile Diabetes

So-called juvenile diabetes, which is usually early in onset and associated with a need for insulin, shows associations either for B8 and DR3 or for B15 and DR4. The presence of DR3 increases the relative risk to 3.3 and that of DR4 to 6.4. Being homozygous for either of these antigens increases the relative risk to 10 and 16 respectively, and if both DR3 and DR4 are present the relative risk rises to 33. The presence of an antigen coded for an allelic variant of the factor B gene (BF1) is eight times more common in patients with juvenile diabetes than in the general population. It is not known whether DR3 and DR4 *per se* confer increased susceptibility to diabetes mellitus or whether they may be linked with some, as yet unknown, susceptibility gene.

Genes Other Than Those Coding for HLA Antigens May Show Associations with Certain Autoimmune Diseases

Correlations have been found between genes that specify certain phenotypic markers of immunoglobulins and some autoimmune diseases. One of these phenotypes, called Gm, is a polymorphic marker on the Fc portion of immunoglobulin. Its variants are associated with thyrotoxicosis (Graves' disease), myasthenia gravis and type I diabetes mellitus. The use of these markers, and of certain others, in association with HLA typing may greatly strengthen our recognition of a genetic compo-

nent to certain diseases. For example, there is a recognized association between Graves' disease and HLA-B8/DR3. When Gm typing is added to the study of these patients, much stronger associations are found.

Possible Mechanisms Underlying the Association with HLA Type and Disease Susceptibility

Various explanations have been proposed to account for the associations between certain diseases and HLA type.

- The 'molecular mimicry' hypothesis, according to which histocompatibility antigens might show partial homology with some of the determinants of certain microorganisms and that this might lead to cross-reaction phenomena. For instance, cross-reactions have been shown between certain *Klebsiella pneumoniae* antigens (the bacterial nitrogenase) and B27, and between the urease produced by *Proteus mirabilis* and DR4.

- Certain HLA antigens might be susceptible to alterations as a result of events such as viral infection, exposure to toxins and neoplastic transformation, and this alteration might lead to a loss of tolerance of the HLA surface antigens.

- Genes, associated with the HLA complex and which determine the degree of immune reactivity, are involved in HLA-associated diseases and determine the immune over-reaction that is a feature of many of the disorders.

It may be that the undoubted complexities in this area could be simplified if the genes associated with increased susceptibility to certain diseases were divided into two classes:

1) Those related to the regulation of the immune response

2) Those related to the effector arm of the immune system

In this scheme the former would determine whether or not autoantibodies were formed, and the latter would determine the development of lesions. The two varieties of gene would be unlinked, to explain the **presence of autoantibodies but the absence of disease** (such as may be seen in the relatives of some patients with autoimmune diseases). Only when **both classes** of gene are inherited does the disease develop.

Regulation of Immune Responses

An example that is cited to support this view is the frequent association between the HLA antigens B8 and DR3 and autoimmune disease. Both of these have independently been associated with abnormalities of immune regulation in individuals without any evidence of autoimmune disorder.

Lymphocytes from normal individuals who have the HLA-B8 antigen respond less well to T-cell mitogens such as phytohaemagglutinin than do the cells of those without this HLA antigen. Not all HLA-B8 subjects show this defect, which suggests that HLA-B8, by itself, may be insufficient to produce it. HLA-B8 is the commonest phenotype in the 'healthy', autoantibody-producing relatives of patients with autoimmune diseases.

Normal individuals with HLA-DR3 have lymphocytes showing some impairment of suppressor cell function when tested *in vitro*, and the number of immunoglobulin-secreting B cells is increased relative to that in DR3-negative persons. *In vitro*, possession of the DR3 allele is associated with abnormalities of phagocytosis by macrophages, and defects in Fc receptor function have been reported in normal individuals with the HLA-B8/DR3 haplotype. DR4, the allele associated with classical rheumatoid arthritis, is said to correlate with the ability of lymphocytes from normal persons to mount an immunological response *in vitro* when exposed to collagen.

In connection with some autoimmune disorders (SLE, primary biliary cirrhosis and type I diabetes), clinically healthy first-degree relatives show impaired function of T suppressor cells, another indication of the influence of the genetic constitution of an individual on immune regulation.

The Effector Arm of the Immune Response in Autoimmune Disease

The elimination of immune complexes may well be mediated by the binding of C3b to its appropriate cell surface receptor, this being followed by binding and phagocytosis of the complex. The number of these receptors for C3b is genetically determined, and is reduced both in patients suffering from SLE and in their clinically healthy first-degree relatives. Thus one might possibly view systemic lupus as a disorder characterized by a genetically determined propensity to form autoantibodies in large amounts and a genetically determined inability to eliminate the immune complexes formed as a result of the presence of autoantibodies at appropriate concentrations.

It is also not without interest that some relatives of patients with autoimmune diseases show mild changes in their tissues of a type characteristic of the disease process; for example, a moderate degree of villous atrophy of the small intestinal mucosa is found in about 10% of the asymptomatic first-degree relatives of patients with dermatitis herpetiformis.

CHAPTER 14

Granulomatous Inflammation

Granulomatous inflammation is a special type of chronic inflammatory reaction characterized by the local accumulation of large numbers of macrophages, some of which may have undergone striking morphological and functional changes (*Fig. 14.1*). It occurs when either a living pathogen or some foreign material (e.g. beryllium) cannot be eliminated from the host by the processes of phagocytosis and killing or digestion.

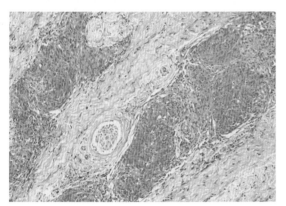

FIGURE 14.1 Well-formed granulomas in the skin of a patient with sarcoidosis. The lesions consist characteristically of aggregates of activated macrophages admixed with lymphocytes, which can hardly be seen at this magnification.

The cell biology of the macrophage dictates many of the features of this type of inflammation, which is expressed in the form of some of the most widespread, common and serious infective diseases. At any given moment, just three of these – tuberculosis, leprosy and schistosomiasis (bilharziasis) – affect more than 200 million people on a world-wide basis.

Viewed superficially there are marked differences between many of the granulomatous disorders in respect of their tissue and clinical manifestations. Some, such as tuberculosis, may cause extensive tissue destruction if local, whereas others show only focal or more diffuse infiltration by macrophages. The common factor is, however, the macrophage, with:

- its role in antigen presentation
- its reactions to the soluble products secreted by sensitized T lymphocytes

- its capacity to function as both a phagocyte and secretory cell

CELL BIOLOGY OF THE MACROPHAGE

Ultimately the macrophage is derived from the bone marrow. A precursor cell in the marrow, the **promonocyte**, is released into the circulation as a **monocyte**. After 12–32 hours, this cell migrates into the tissues, where it undergoes maturation to form the **macrophage**. The term macrophage was coined by Metchnikoff in the late nineteenth century. Its literal translation is '**big eater**', a term that could refer equally to its large size, its ability to engulf large particles, and its great reserve capacity for phagocytosis. As pointed out previously (see pp 61–62), the macrophage possesses certain inbuilt advantages over the neutrophil. It:

- has a longer natural lifespan
- can resynthesize the membranes and intracellular enzymes lost during phagocytosis (which the neutrophil cannot)
- can ingest particles that are far larger than those that can be coped with by the neutrophil
- can undergo mitotic division

PHAGOCYTOSIS AND ENDOCYTOSIS

The macrophage can ingest a wide variety of substances that exist within its cytoplasm in membrane-bound vesicles (the phagosomes). Large particles are engulfed in phagocytosis. This process is triggered by close contact between the plasma membrane of the macrophage and the object to be engulfed, and this is aided by the process of **opsonization**. Like the neutrophil, the macrophage has surface receptors for the common opsonins immunoglobulin (Ig)G and the 3b component of complement. Binding to these receptors starts a series of membrane and intracytoplasmic events leading to the formation of pseudopodia, which surround the target particle. Other receptors have been described for activators of the alternate complement pathway and for **lectins**, a family of proteins that bind with exquisite specificity to a variety of sugars expressed on the cell surface.

The expression of some of these receptors can be influenced profoundly by factors external to the macrophage. Monocytes have hardly any receptors for the chemotactic C5a component of complement.

However, if they are incubated in a medium containing lymphokines, expression of this receptor starts in a short time and eventually some 40 000 receptors can be found on the plasma membrane.

BACTERIAL KILLING

Just as with the neutrophil, ingestion of particles within phagosomes is associated with a respiratory burst and fusion of the phagosome with lysosomes. If the ingested particle is a microorganism it may be killed, the most important mechanism being the oxygen-dependent one described earlier (see pp 58–59). It seems likely that an additional microbicidal mechanism exists in the inducible pathway for nitric oxide (NO) synthesis.

NO is synthesized in a wide variety of cells from the amino acid L-arginine via operation of a NO synthase. In vascular endothelium, NO synthesis is constitutive (i.e. it proceeds constantly), and its synthesis and local release constitute an important mechanism for regulating vascular tone.

NO can, however, be synthesized in many other cell types, via an inducible rather than a constitutive pathway, and the macrophage is one of these. It is believed that triggering of this inducible pathway is not only important in the killing of certain pathogens but is one of the pathogenetic factors involved in septic shock.

However, for some organisms, the mere fact that engulfment by a macrophage has taken place is far from being a death warrant. *Mycobacteria* (including those responsible for tuberculosis and leprosy), *Brucella,* *Listeria, Salmonella, Toxoplasma, Leishmania, Chlamydia, Rickettsia* and *Legionella pneumoniae* are among those that maintain a symbiotic relationship with the macrophage unless the latter becomes activated, usually as a result of interaction with the soluble **lymphokines** released from activated T cells, most notably interferon γ.

FATE OF MACROPHAGES IN GRANULOMATOUS INFLAMMATION

Once a macrophage has migrated to a site of infection or tissue injury a number of possible fates await it (*Fig. 14.2*):

- The material phagocytosed may prove toxic to the macrophage and the cell may die, with release of its intralysosomal contents into the surrounding extracellular milieu.
- If the inflammatory stimulus disappears, macrophages that have gathered in response to its presence migrate from the site and the lesion resolves.
- Ingestion of non-toxic but undegradable material leads to conversion of the macrophage into a very long-lived form which persists in the tissue together with its intracytoplasmic load.
- Macrophages can undergo conversion into so-called **epithelioid cells** and fusion to form multinucleate giant cells or **macrophage polykaryons**.

Epithelioid Cell Transformation

In many granulomas (most notably in those occurring in tuberculosis and sarcoidosis) some of the aggregated

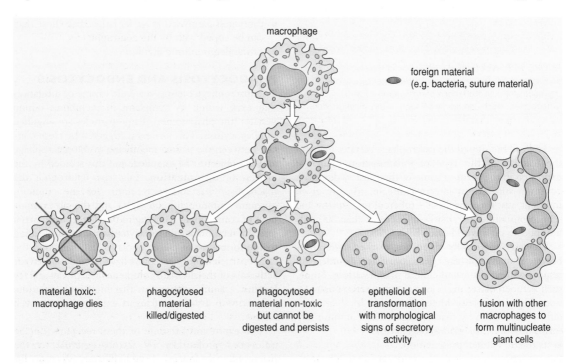

FIGURE 14.2 *The possible results of encounters between macrophages and foreign material (living or dead).*

macrophages, which account for most of the bulk of the lesion, can be seen to have undergone a series of morphological changes which have led to them being called **epithelioid cells**. This is a rather unfortunate term, coined by pathologists in the late nineteenth century who thought that there was some resemblance between these cells and squamous epithelium.

In essence the morphological changes involved include elongation of the cells, which appear to be in close contact, the cell boundaries being indistinct on light microscopy. When examined with the electron microscope, the plasma membranes of adjacent cells are seen to be closely applied to one another and often interdigitate. **The epithelioid cell has much more rough endoplasmic reticulum, much more plasma membrane and a much more developed Golgi apparatus than the untransformed macrophage, features that suggest the cell has become differentiated towards the secretory rather than the phagocytic end of the spectrum of macrophage activity.** Indeed:

- Epithelioid cells are only one-tenth as effective in phagocytosis as non–activated macrophages.
- There is less expression of surface receptors such as those for Fc and C5a.
- Phagocytosed material is seldom, if ever, seen in the cytoplasm and, by differentiating in this way, the epithelioid cells appear to have lost the normal ability of the macrophage to react with extracellular particles, although they retain the ability to express HLA-DR-coded antigens on their surface receptors and thus still have the potential to interact with T lymphocytes.

Histochemical studies have shown that the epithelioid cell contains the expected number of lysosomal enzymes, muramidase (lysozyme) and, rather surprisingly, angiotensin-converting enzyme. The role of this enzyme in granulomatous inflammation is not known, although it has been suggested, as a result of studies of schistosomiasis in the mouse, that it may inhibit further migration of macrophages and that its secretion may be controlled by T lymphocytes.

Activation of human macrophages by exposure to interferon γ leads to the expression of the enzyme 1α–hydroxylase. This causes the activation of circulating 25-hydroxycholecalciferol to the active form of vitamin D, 1,25(OH)$_2$ cholecalciferol. Macrophages have receptors for this metabolite, which activates them still further but tends also to shift responses in granulomatous inflammation from T$_H$1 towards T$_H$2 lymphocyte expression. Active vitamin D production may be so great in granulomatous disorders such as sarcoidosis and tuberculosis as to cause hypercalcaemia (*Fig. 14.3*).

Functions of the Activated Macrophage
The range of secretory products of the activated macrophage has been outlined on p 90. This, apart from its phagocytic powers, gives the cell a central role

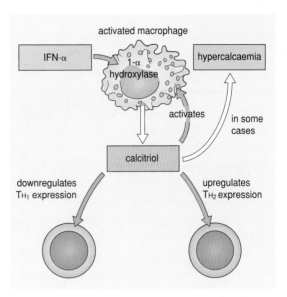

FIGURE 14.3 *Calcitriol and macrophage/lymphocyte interactions.*

in inflammation, healing and immunity (*Fig. 14.4*), its functions encompassing:

- production of fever
- expression of mediators of acute and chronic inflammation
- microbicidal activity
- a role in the preferential selection of T$_H$1 or T$_H$2 responses
- a role in lymphocyte activation via antigen processing and presentation and interleukin 1 production
- tissue breakdown through secretion of metalloproteinases, tumour necrosis factor α and oxygen free radicals
- a role in connective tissue matrix formation and remodelling

Multinucleated Giant Cell Formation (Macrophage Polykaryons)
The continued presence of any foreign material, whether living (as in the case of the organisms responsible for tuberculosis or leprosy) or non-living, tends to elicit a response in which the macrophage in one or other of its functional and morphological forms is the dominant element.

The simplest example of this is seen in the presence within the dermis of unabsorbed suture material. In this situation, as in many other types of granulomatous inflammation, some members of the local macrophage infiltrate fuse to form multinucleated giant cells. Classic morphological pathology teaches us (quite wrongly) that there are two distinct forms of the multinucleate giant cell: the **foreign body giant cell** and the **Langhans' giant cell**.

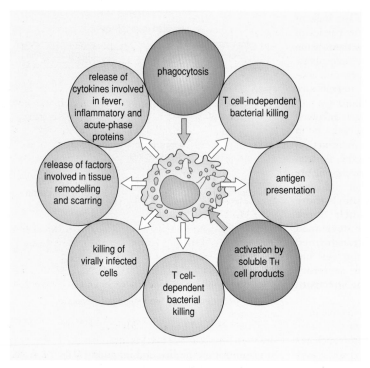

FIGURE 14.4 Roles of the macrophage.

The former has its many nuclei dispersed more or less evenly through the cytoplasm. It commonly appears in response to the presence of **exogenous** foreign material such as sutures or of misplaced **endogenous** material such as hair, cholesterol crystals or keratin, which have escaped from their normal confines and lie free in an inappropriate environment.

The so-called Langhans' giant cell has multiple nuclei, which tend to lie at the periphery of the cell in a horseshoe pattern, leaving a clear zone of cytoplasm in the centre. The archetypal situation in which this variant is found is in chronic infective granulomas such as tuberculosis. In fact the Langhans' cell merely represents a later stage in the development of the macrophage polykaryon; it has a greater content of lysosomal enzymes and a more highly developed Golgi apparatus than the foreign body giant cell. If microtubule function in the latter is interfered with by adding colchicine, transformation into the Langhans' variant is blocked.

How Do Multinucleated Giant Cells Form?

In certain experimentally induced chronic inflammatory lesions the fusion of macrophages to form multinucleate giant cells takes place only when the population of macrophages first elicited by the injurious agent is reinforced by the arrival of new macrophages. If a glass coverslip is placed in the subcutaneous tissues of a mouse, within a very short time

the glass becomes covered with macrophages. If the coverslip is removed at this time and placed within a diffusion chamber into which no further cell migration can occur and the whole apparatus is returned to the subcutaneous tissue, no fusion of macrophages takes place, despite the fact that mitotic division occurs. If holes are made in such a diffusion chamber so that cells can gain access to it, macrophage fusion can be seen to occur.

In addition to the recruitment of fresh macrophages, an additional factor that stimulates macrophage fusion and thus the formation of giant cells is the attempt by two or more cells to endocytose the same material. Once such fusion has occurred, the resulting cell can fuse with other macrophages and hence acquire the impressive number of nuclei commonly seen in some granulomas (see *Fig. 15.1*).

Role of the Multinucleated Giant Cell

Giant cells in chronic inflammatory lesions behave like other multinucleated cells in that their nuclei enter the mitotic cycle in a near-synchronous fashion. This is likely to lead to pooling of genetic material, and some of the resulting chromosomes are defective. Polyploidy is present in some nuclei and this appears to shorten the lifespan of the cell. It has been suggested that formation of the polykaryon, with the implication that its lifespan will inevitably be shorter than that of the unfused macrophage, is one of the ways in which the multiplication of macrophages in a chronic inflammatory focus can be controlled.

It is probably unwise to accept too uncritically the thesis that the multinucleated giant cell merely constitutes a stage of the macrophage's path to oblivion. One recent study compares the bone resorptive activity of mononuclear and multinucleated macrophages derived from the rat. The polykaryon variants bound and degraded significantly more bone than the mononuclear cells, suggesting that, at least in the frame of reference provided by osteoclast formation, existence in a multinucleate form confers some advantage.

CLASSIFICATION OF THE GRANULOMATOUS RESPONSE

In terms of the processes involved, the question of how to classify granulomatous reactions has been considered in two ways.

CELL KINETICS

The first type of classification is based on the cell kinetics of the lesion, granulomas being classified as of either **low** or **high turnover** type.

An aggregate of macrophages whose presence has been elicited by some persistent irritant will remain until the irritant is cleared (which may, of course, be never). The cell population is maintained, firstly, by continuing migration of macrophages to the site of the irritant. If this migration is balanced by death of macrophages, either within the lesion or by emigration to draining nodes, then the lesion will remain more or less **constant in size**.

Another mechanism for maintaining the cell population within the lesion is mitotic division of the aggregated macrophages. The number of successful mitoses is usually restricted to two or three, so that in the long term this mechanism cannot be very effective.

Lastly, the macrophages that have aggregated at the site of the irritant may become immobilized and remain *in situ* for prolonged periods, with few changes in the cell number due to either death or division.

In the so-called **low turnover** type of granuloma, the aggregated macrophages, as indicated above, remain for a long time within the lesion and there is little new migration of macrophages and little cell death or mitotic division. The irritant, which is typically non-toxic to the macrophage but poorly degradable by it (e.g. barium sulphate, carageenan), persists within the cells in relatively large amounts. Epithelioid cells are usually not present in such granulomas and the presence of lymphoid cells, which might suggest the involvement of immune mechanisms, is distinctly unusual.

In contrast, the macrophage population in the **high turnover** type of granuloma needs constant replenishment in order to compensate for the high death rate and the relatively short lifespan of the cells originally forming the lesion. The causative agents are usually highly toxic for the macrophages (e.g. mycobacteria, silica) and can be identified in only a small proportion of these cells. Such granulomas show evidence of functional heterogeneity within the macrophage population, and epithelioid cell transformation is a common phenomenon. Some of the most important disorders affecting humans are characterized by this high turnover type of granulomatous inflammation, amongst them tuberculosis and leprosy.

INVOLVEMENT OF IMMUNOLOGICAL MECHANISMS IN GRANULOMA FORMATION

As most granulomas of clinical significance are of the high turnover variety, additional methods of classification would be useful in understanding the pathogenesis. Recently some writers have attempted to classify granulomas on the basis of whether or not immune mechanisms are involved in their formation.

Granulomas without Evidence of Immunological Mechanisms

The major feature of such granulomas is the **lack of specific recognition of the irritant by the immune system and, therefore, the lack of an enhanced response on a second exposure to that irritant.** Thus no matter how great the frequency of exposure, the lesions always appear at the same time after the irritant has entered the host, and the size of the lesions is the same on each occasion. It is impossible to transfer reactivity from one animal to another with either serum or cells, and immunosuppressive measures do not affect the development of the lesion.

An experimental model of this type of reaction which has been studied extensively is the granuloma that follows the injection of small plastic beads into the tissue. *In vitro* the beads activate Hageman factor and generate kinin activity in normal human and mouse plasma. When such beads are injected into pigeons, which lack Hageman factor, no granulomas are formed. Agents such as talc and silica, which cause granulomas of this type, are believed to operate via similar mechanisms.

Granulomas in which Immunological Mechanisms are Involved

The fundamental difference between granulomas in which immune mechanisms play a part and those described above is that in the former case the first exposure to an irritant induces an altered state of reactivity. This expresses itself in the form of an accelerated and more severe reaction on second and subsequent exposures to the irritant. Formation of the granuloma can be inhibited by measures designed to suppress immunity and the altered reactivity can be transferred from animal to animal by either cells, serum or both.

Mechanisms Underlying the Induction of 'Immunologically Mediated' Granulomas

Much of the basic knowledge relating to immunologically mediated granulomas has been derived from studies of the tissue reactions to infestation by the helminth *Schistosoma* (bilharzia), which is a parasite affecting more than 100 000 000 people. The worms themselves induce no lasting tissue response, but many of the eggs they lay do not escape from the body of the host and it is these eggs that induce granuloma formation. When eggs of *Schistosoma mansoni* are injected into the tissues of a mouse, no inflammatory response is seen for 48 hours (a fact possibly related to the presence of anti-Hageman factor activity in the eggs).

Macrophages and eosinophils start to accumulate around the eggs about 60 hours after injection; this occurs at much the same time as delayed hypersensitivity can be demonstrated in the mouse foot pad following injection of soluble schistosomal egg antigens. Priming of the mouse host by prior intraperitoneal injection of *S. mansoni* leads to faster and more severe granuloma formation. A similar enhancement of the reaction can be seen on first exposure to *Schistosoma* in mice who have received injections of spleen or lymph node cells from an animal with schistosomal granulomas (**passive transfer**).

It is possible to culture living granulomas isolated from the livers of infected mice. These studies have demonstrated the secretion of two lymphokines from the cells of the granuloma: **macrophage migration inhibiting factor** and a factor that promotes the activity of eosinophils. In addition, lysosomal enzymes and a factor that stimulates fibroblast proliferation and the synthesis of collagen can be identified in the culture fluid. Very little antibody globulin can be isolated from these lesions. These data indicate the importance of cell-mediated immunity, at least in this model, and also show that such a granuloma carries within itself the means by which both necrosis and scarring can be brought about.

Scar Tissue Formation in Granulomas

The formation of scar tissue in and around granulomas is probably controlled largely by the secretion of cells that make up the lesion. The degree of such scarring is determined by the balance between factors that stimulate fibroblasts and hence collagen formation, and those that work in a contrary way and lead to collagen breakdown. Both these sets of factors are governed, at least in part, by the macrophage. The macrophage can secrete substances that stimulate fibroblast division (e.g. IL–1), and fibronectin and platelet-derived growth factor, which it secretes as well, are also chemotactic for fibroblasts. On the other hand, macrophages can secrete enzymes that break down collagen, and fluid in which macrophages have been cultured has been described as able to inhibit collagen synthesis.

This brief general account of the nature of immunologically modulated granulomatous reactions sets the stage for consideration of some of the serious human disorders in which the development of such lesions is a dominant feature.

CHAPTER 15

Some Specific Granulomatous Disorders

TUBERCULOSIS

Tuberculosis is a disease of great antiquity, diagnosable lesions having been found in Egyptian mummies dating back as far as 3400 BC. The fact that tuberculosis is an infective disease was confirmed in 1882 by the great bacteriologist Robert Koch. In doing so he put forward three postulates, fulfilment of which is still regarded in many instances as being essential in ascribing the origin of a disease to an infective cause. **Koch's postulates** are:

1) The suspected organisms must be present in the lesions in all cases of the disease.

2) It must be possible to isolate the suspected organisms in pure culture from the lesions.

3) It must be possible to reproduce the disease by injecting or otherwise introducing the organisms into a healthy animal.

Epidemiology

The mortality and morbidity due to tuberculosis have decreased so sharply in the affluent countries of the West that it is difficult now to conceive of its overwhelming importance as a cause of death and misery even as recently as 40 years ago. In the USA at the beginning of this century, tuberculosis was the premier cause of death, being responsible for the death of 200 per 100 000 population annually. By 1965 it had dropped to eighteenth place and killed only 4.1 per 100 000 each year.

However, in countries that are less privileged economically, the prevalence of tuberculosis remains much as it was half a century ago, and it has been estimated that, on a world-wide basis, three to five million people die each year from this disease.

Unfortunately tuberculosis is showing signs of resurgence in the West, largely because of the emergence of multidrug-resistant strains of the responsible organism. In addition, the appearance of **acquired immune deficiency syndrome** (AIDS) has greatly increased the toll exacted by tuberculosis in economically underprivileged populations. In some parts of Africa almost 40% of deaths in individuals suffering from AIDS are due to tuberculosis.

When a sharp decline occurs in mortality and morbidity from any disease there is a natural temptation to regard this as a triumph for the art of medicine. In the case of tuberculosis this is true to only a very limited extent; much of the credit for the great improvement must go to socioeconomic factors. These include:

- improved housing with less overcrowding
- improved nutrition
- improved sanitation
- effective chemotherapy for sufferers of the disease
- early detection by mass miniature radiography and hence early treatment
- pasteurization of milk and tuberculin testing of dairy cattle leading to the virtual elimination of primary intestinal tuberculosis

Risks

It is important to recognize that certain segments of the population have a higher than average risk of developing tuberculosis. These include:

- **diabetics**
- patients on **immunosuppressive** treatment
- individuals suffering from **AIDS**
- patients with **silicosis**
- in Britain, Asian immigrants, who are many times more likely to develop the disease than indigenous Britons

The Organism and its Identification

Tuberculosis is caused by *Mycobacterium tuberculosis*. This is a slender, slightly curved, rod-shaped organism which can be stained only with some difficulty and which has the remarkable property, once it has been stained, of resisting decolourization by acid and alcohol. This '**acid fastness**' is related to the presence of large amounts of complex lipid substances (neutral fats, phosphatides and various long-chain fatty acids) in the capsule of the bacillus.

The organism is stained by the **Ziehl–Neelsen** method (hot carbolfuchsin with methylene blue or malachite green). The organisms stain red with the carbolfuchsin and this red colour is *not* removed by treatment with acid and alcohol (*Fig. 15.1*). The bacilli may also be stained with auramine, a dye that exhibits yellow fluorescence when exposed to ultraviolet light; it is often easier to identify the mycobacteria in material treated in this way than by conventional light microscopic methods.

Mycobacteria are aerobic and grow slowly in culture. The media used are the egg-based Lowenstein–Jensen medium and the agar-based Middlebrook 7H10 and 7H11. A positive culture is regarded as the 'gold

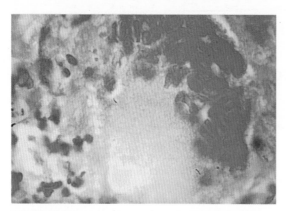

FIGURE 15.1 *A single red-stained mycobacterium within a multinucleate giant cell. The section has been stained by the Ziehl–Neelsen method using a methylene blue counterstain.*

standard' for the diagnosis of tuberculosis. More than 85% of the cases of tuberculosis in the USA confirmed by the US Centers for Disease Control and Prevention are culture positive. The major disadvantage of culture methods for the diagnosis of tuberculosis is that growth of the organisms is slow and colonies may not be visible for 4 weeks or more.

The sensitivity and specificity of direct examination of smeared material are much lower and are influenced by the amount of time and trouble put into doing the test and the population from which the samples were drawn. Sensitivity ranges from 22 to 80% (mean approximately 55%).

Recently molecular probes for mycobacterial DNA have been used in diagnosis. With chemical amplification of small amounts of DNA present in samples, the time taken to make a diagnosis can be reduced to a few hours and both sensitivity and specificity are increased in comparison with conventional staining techniques. A positive result with DNA probing in an individual with a positive smear test result gives a positive predictive value of close to 100% for culture. The combination of negative smear and negative probe results indicates that, in 94% of cases, mycobacteria will *not* be identified on culture of clinical samples.

How Does Infection Occur?

Mycobacteria are extremely resistant to drying and this means that infection can follow inhalation of dust in which infected dried sputum is present. At least five strains of the organisms exist:

1) human
2) bovine
3) murine
4) avian
5) reptilian

In humans the infection may be acquired in three ways:

1) inhalation
2) ingestion
3) inoculation

In communities where the dairy herds are free from mycobacterial infection, only the first of these is at all common or important.

Pathogenesis

The Lesions of Tuberculosis are the Result of the Interaction Between the Organisms and the Host's Immune System

Unlike organisms such as *Clostridium perfringens* or *Staphylococcus aureus*, which produce toxins that directly damage the tissues, the mycobacterium has not yet been shown to have any direct cytotoxic effect. Indeed, it survives and multiplies within macrophages in cell culture without any harm to the cultured cells.

The tissue damage that is so prominent a feature of tuberculosis is largely, if not entirely, mediated by the **specific altered reactivity of the immune system, which occurs as a result of introduction of the mycobacterium into the host**. This altered state of reactivity expresses itself in two ways:

- by enhanced resistance to infection and more effective **clearing** of the mycobacteria from the tissues of the host
- by the appearance of **hypersensitivity** through which tissue damage is caused, the likely mechanisms being locally released cytokines and direct action of cytotoxic T cells (*Fig. 15.2*).

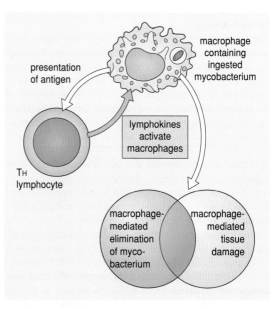

FIGURE 15.2 *The pathogenesis of tuberculosis. Mycobacterial antigens are presented to T_H lymphocytes by antigen-presenting cells which have ingested the organisms. The subsequent release of lymphokines activates the macrophages to eliminate the bacteria from the host tissues and to cause some degree of tissue damage. The relative severity of these two macrophage responses determines the outcome of the infection in each case.*

Virulence of Mycobacteria

While it is true that *M. tuberculosis* does not synthesize or secrete exotoxins, it is clear from many studies that **different strains exhibit differences in their ability to cause extensive disease**.

This increased 'virulence' is associated with the presence in the organisms of certain components that protect the organisms from intracellular killing:

- **'Cord' factor.** This is a surface glycolipid (trehalose-6-6'-dimycolate) which, when present, causes the bacteria to grow in 'cords' in media. Its presence is associated with the ability to induce granuloma formation and it inhibits neutrophil chemotaxis.
- **Sulphatides.** These are also surface glycolipids which, when present, inhibit fusion between phagosomes and lysosomes within macrophages that have ingested the organisms. This is likely to decrease antigen processing.
- **Lipoarabinomannan.** This is a lipopolysaccharide resembling endotoxin. It inhibits the upregulation of macrophage killing power by interferon γ, increases the output of tumour necrosis factor (TNF) α, associated with fever, weight loss and tissue destruction, and increases interleukin (IL) 10 secretion, which inhibits mycobacteria-induced T-cell proliferation.

TUBERCULOUS GRANULOMAS

The essential lesion of tuberculosis is the **tuberculous granuloma**. The development of tuberculous granuloma, or follicle as it is sometimes called, is the archetypal response of all tissues to the presence of *M. tuberculosis*. The extensive tissue destruction that may be found in this disease depends on the number of such granulomas, their growth and confluence, the degree of the characteristic **caseation necrosis** that occurs, and the attempts at repair which the long-continued presence of the lesions ultimately stimulates.

Evolution of a Tuberculous Granuloma

(*Fig. 15.3*)
Following the introduction of the bacilli into the tissues, there is a very mild, transient, acute inflammatory reaction in which neutrophils participate. The organisms are presumably engulfed by the local macrophage population and, in association with major histocompatibility complex (MHC) class II-coded membrane proteins, the mycobacterial antigens are presented to appropriate T helper (T$_H$) cells. Interaction between these two groups of cells leads to proliferation of specifically coded T cells and to the release of lymphokines from them. This is followed by infiltration by macrophages, which group together to form focal accumulations at the site of infection and then become immobilized at that site.

The whole process is subtly modulated by the immune system. One lymphokine is **chemotactic** for

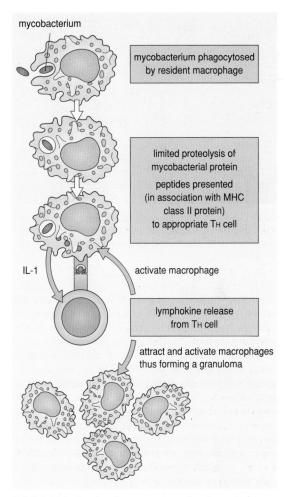

FIGURE 15.3 *Genesis of an immune-mediated granuloma.*

the macrophages, while another migration-inhibition factors (MIF) renders them relatively **immobile**. The fact that, in an **unprimed host**, bacillus-bearing macrophages travel from the site of infection in the tissue to the draining lymph nodes suggests that the full action of MIF takes some time to express itself *in vivo*. In addition, the stimulated T cells secrete **interferon γ**, which increases the expression of MHC class II-coded proteins on the macrophage membrane and thus can increase the ability of local macrophages to present antigen and upregulate the microbicidal properties of the macrophage.

Many of the macrophages then undergo **epithelioid cell** transformation. This, as described in Chapter 14, is associated with loss of the ability to phagocytose foreign particles. Some of the macrophages fuse, with the formation of multinucleate giant cells which mature and acquire the characteristic 'horseshoe' arrangement of nuclei found in the Langhans' giant cell (*Fig 15.4*). This mass of epithelioid cells becomes surrounded by a mantle of lymphocytes which can be shown, by use of

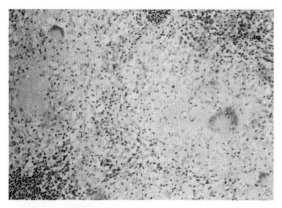

FIGURE 15.4 *Tuberculous granulomas occurring within a lymph node. Note the multinucleated Langhans giant cell in the lesion on the right-hand side of the picture, with its nuclei arranged at the periphery of the cell.*

appropriate antibodies, to be T cells. In granulomatous lesions lymphocytes in the centres of the lesions are likely to be T_H (CD4+) cells, whereas those at the periphery are more likely to be T_C (CD8+) cells.

Within 10–14 days, evidence of necrosis begins to appear in the centre of the lesion. The necrosis is coagulative in type and is characterized by the appearance of firm, allegedly cheesy, material (hence the name **caseation** necrosis). On histological examination, caseation necrosis shows virtually complete obliteration of normal cell and tissue outlines, all the tissue elements being merged into an amorphous mass of material (*Fig. 15.5*), which appears bright red in sections stained with haematoxylin and eosin.

What determines the central necrosis is not well understood. Presumably one of the important effector

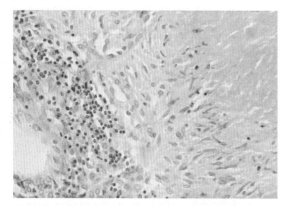

FIGURE 15.5 *A high-power view of part of a caseating tuberculous granuloma. On the right-hand side is an area of featureless, eosinophilic caseation necrosis. Immediately to the left is a zone occupied by macrophages that have undergone epithelioid cell transformation. Note the pale elongated nuclei. This zone is in turn bordered by a band of lymphocytes, which are likely to be CD8+ T cells.*

mechanisms is release of lysosomal enzymes from dying macrophages, which, of course, disappear from the centre of the lesion as the necrosis develops. It is believed that caseation necrosis is the morphological expression of a marked degree of delayed hypersensitivity, although evidence gained in experimental studies of mycobacterial infections in rats suggests that humoral factors also have a part in induction of the necrosis. In this situation it has been suggested that local formation of immune complexes in the centre of the lesions, where antigen is in excess, is a powerful influence in modulating the degree of necrosis. Such complexes are said to form if cell-mediated immunity declines, thus allowing the mycobacteria to proliferate. If complexes form under conditions of antibody excess, epithelioid cell transformation rather than necrosis tends to occur.

The type of T_H cell response probably plays an important part in determining whether extensive necrosis occurs or not. This is discussed in a later section (see p 162).

The sum of all these events constitutes the basic tissue response in tuberculosis.

Natural History of the Tissue Response

Experience has shown that different tissues and different individuals may react very differently to the presence of *M. tuberculosis*. Some lesions are small and heal readily; some may cause extensive local tissue destruction; and others may release organisms that can spread throughout the body. These differences are probably accounted for by interactions between:

- the virulence of the organisms
- the size of the dose of mycobacteria
- the degree of local and general resistance, which may be innate or acquired
- the type and degree of hypersensitivity which, as already stated, may correlate with the type of T_H cell response.

Some of these factors are discussed below.

Innate Immunity

This is difficult to disentangle from factors related to exposure to the organism and to unfavourable socio-economic circumstances. However, it appears that certain groups are inherently more susceptible to tuberculosis, notably North American Indians and the Negro races.

At an experimental level, where conditions are much easier to control, there is no doubt that strains of certain species of animals can be bred that differ markedly in their degree of resistance to infection by *M. tuberculosis*.

Age

In communities where there is a high prevalence of tuberculosis, the very young (aged under 5 years) and elderly appear to be more at risk for developing overt tuberculosis. In the UK, where the incidence of tuberculosis has been falling steadily, the increased risk in young children appears to have been eliminated. Those at greatest risk are socially and economically deprived middle-aged and elderly men, many of whom are poorly nourished and unsatisfactorily housed.

Immunosuppression

Immunosuppression associated either with certain disorders (such as AIDS) or with certain treatments (such as prolonged administration of high doses of corticosteroids) increases the risk of tuberculosis.

Effects of Previous Exposure to Mycobacteria

Previous exposure to mycobacteria is one of the most important factors in modulating the natural history of a tuberculous infection. A second infection produces tissue reactions that differ markedly from those seen after primary infection. This was first explored by Robert Koch in the course of studies of experimental tuberculosis in the guinea-pig. His observations have a significant bearing, not only on the natural history of the disease, but also on the evolution of the basic pathological unit – the tuberculous granuloma.

The Koch Phenomenon

If *M. tuberculosis* is injected subcutaneously into a guinea-pig that has not previously been exposed to the organism, no reaction is seen at the injection site for the first 10–14 days. Then a nodule develops and, if this is excised and examined histologically, tuberculous granulomas are seen. Meanwhile mycobacteria have been transported by macrophages to the regional draining nodes and in due time cause enlargement of these nodes and caseous necrosis within them. In time, infected macrophages escape from the nodes and the inoculated animals usually die from disseminated disease.

If the size of the initial dose was such that the animal survived at least 4 weeks and a second subcutaneous injection of *M. tuberculosis* is given at that time and at a different site, a nodule forms rapidly (within a few days), ulcerates and then heals. **No regional lymph node involvement occurs.**

These observations indicate that:

- The local tissue response to the second infection is much more rapid than that to the first.
- Local clearance of organisms by activated macrophages following a second infection is much more effective than after a first infection since the inflammatory process resolves quite rapidly.
- Macrophages containing viable organisms are immobilized at the site of the local infection: there is no evidence of spread to the draining lymph nodes in the second infection.
- Local hypersensitivity is increased after a second infection; rapid central necrosis leading to ulceration may occur.

These events have been interpreted as being due to the development of altered reactivity on the part of the host immune system. **This leads to an increased ability to clear the infecting organisms from the tissue and thus to an enhanced resistance to the infection (immunity), and to an increased tendency for tissue damage, probably also mediated by immune mechanisms, to occur (hypersensitivity).** It must be said, however, that in the light of the failure of certain large-scale trials of the efficacy of vaccination using attenuated strains of *M. tuberculosis*, some workers have challenged this view of the Koch phenomenon.

Favourable Aspects of the Altered Reactivity of the Immune System

The altered reactivity that occurs after infection with *M. tuberculosis* is largely, but not entirely, expressed in the form of cell-mediated reactions (delayed hypersensitivity). T_H cells with appropriate receptors encounter bacterial antigens expressed on the surface of macrophages or other antigen-presenting cells and proliferate. T_H cells release lymphokines (see pp 97, 162), which include factors chemotactic to the macrophage and factors that tend to immobilize them at the site of bacterial lodgement (MIF). **The macrophages become better able to kill intracellular organisms**, and the symbiotic relationship that can exist between mycobacteria and virgin macrophages is largely ended. **This aspect of the altered immune state is obviously favourable for the survival of the infected host**, although the enhanced resistance to the mycobacteria is not nearly as effective as that seen, for example, after smallpox or diphtheria.

Hypersensitivity to Components of the Mycobacterium

Most now agree that **the chief factor modulating the degree of tissue destruction in tuberculosis is hypersensitivity to some antigenic components of the bacillus**. In addition to its role in causing caseation necrosis, hypersensitivity is probably also associated with the very severe constitutional effects that accompany the lodgement of large numbers of the bacillus. It is most likely that these effects are mediated by release of large quantities of **TNF-α**. The liquefactive necrosis that tends to occur when there is active local proliferation of mycobacteria may be associated with the same phenomenon.

Such liquefied tissue debris usually contains very large numbers of mycobacteria and shows a marked tendency to rupture into adjacent tissue planes or into bronchi, lymphatics and blood vessels. Sometimes such debris tracks down through a tissue plane and may present as a soft mass at a point some distance away. Such a lesion is spoken of as a '**cold abscess**' because it consists of a localized mass of what looks like pus but lacks the heat and redness normally associated with abscess formation.

Relationship Between Immunity and Hypersensitivity

The relationship between enhanced resistance to infection by the mycobacterium and the tissue-damaging hypersensitivity reactions is one of the most difficult questions to answer satisfactorily.

Is the difference between these two expressions of altered reactivity (allergy) merely a quantitative one or is the 'protective face' of altered reactivity distinct from the 'tissue-damaging' hypersensitivity? At present there is no definite answer to this problem but there is evidence that the second of these possibilities is the correct one:

- The degree of **protection** produced by vaccination with an attenuated strain of the organism (bacille Calmette–Guérin (BCG) vaccination) is not related to the degree of **hypersensitivity** produced. For example, a guinea-pig immunized in this way and reacting to a skin dose of tuberculin (mycobacterial protein) at a titre of 1/10 000 is likely to survive an intramuscular challenge with live mycobacteria for about 99 days. An animal treated in the same way but reacting to tuberculin at a titre of only 1/10 is likely to survive a subsequent challenge for 250 days.
- It is possible to induce protection against a challenge with live bacilli by injecting a guinea-pig with bacilli extracted using methyl alcohol without hypersensitivity developing.
- Hypersensitivity can be induced without any protection against live bacilli being conferred at the same time. This can be accomplished by injecting mycobacterial protein together with some of the bacillary lipids.
- In both mice and humans, two types of response can be seen following exposure to mycobacteria. In humans who show the first of these responses, the injection of tuberculoprotein is followed by a fairly rapid reaction which peaks at 48 hours, resolves rapidly, itches but is not painful, and is often seen in recipients of BCG vaccine in the UK. The other pattern of response develops a little more slowly, peaks at 72–96 hours, lasts for 2–3 weeks, often shows evidence of necrosis and is often seen in those with a history of previous tuberculosis. The first pattern is believed to be associated with a higher degree of resistance to infection, the second with a greater degree of hypersensitivity. The basis for an individual developing one or other of these responses may well be previous exposure to mycobacteria other than the major pathogens *M. tuberculosis* and *M. leprae*. There are some 30 species of mycobacteria. The two major pathogens are usually encountered only following contact with patients who have open tuberculosis or leprosy. Many of the other species are common in the environment and may be encountered frequently. It has been suggested that when there has been a

'moderate' exposure to such more or less harmless mycobacteria via the oral route, that the first type of skin response is likely to develop. Where there has been 'excessive' exposure to these mycobacterial species, a high degree of hypersensitivity is found and BCG vaccination confers little protection.

> ### KEY POINTS: Caseation Necrosis
> The balance between cell-mediated immunity (as manifested by an enhanced ability to clear mycobacteria from host tissues) and the tissue damage related to hypersensitivity determines the natural history of tuberculous infections. The tissue damaging component is the major contributor to the clinical expressions of tuberculosis.

The Effect of TNF-α Differs Depending on Whether Infection Causes a Pure T_H1 Response or a Mixed T_H1 and T_H2 Response

In animal models of tuberculosis, necrosis of granulomatous lesions is accompanied by the release of large amounts of TNF-α. Similarly direct injection of TNF-α into tuberculous granulomas also causes necrosis.

At the same time, secretion by macrophages of TNF-α is a vital component in defence against *M. tuberculosis*, shown by the fact that mice in whom the gene encoding TNF-α has been 'knocked out' in the embryo show greatly increased suceptibility for tuberculosis.

Thus TNF-α has a double role and can be either helpful or harmful in the context of a tuberculous infection. The factor determining which of these operates in a given case appears to be the type and degree of priming of the host by mycobacteria, and, in particular, what type of T_H cell response occurs in the course of such timing. Two types of T_H cells exist: T_H1 and T_H2; their secretion patterns are shown in *Table 15.1*.

A **pure T_H1 response** is characterized by increased resistance to *M. tuberculosis*, whereas a mixed T_H1 and

Table 15.1 Secretion Patterns of T_H1 and T_H2 Lymphocytes

T_H1	T_H2
Interferon γ	IL-3
IL-2	Met-encephalin
TNF-α	IL-4
TNF-β	IL-5
Granulocyte–macrophage colony-stimulating factor	IL-6
IL-3	IL-10

T$_H$2 response, in which a much broader range of cytokines is expressed, is characterized by extensive necrosis occurring in tuberculous granulomas.

PATTERNS OF TUBERCULOSIS

First Infection-type Pulmonary Tuberculosis (Childhood Tuberculosis)

The lodgement of *M. tuberculosis* in a child's lung is usually followed by the development of a small lesion, often measuring not more than 1 cm along its longest axis. This lesion is almost always situated just beneath the pleura, either in the basal segment of the upper lobe of the lung or in the apical segment of the lower lobe. Classically this parenchymal lesion is known as the **Ghon focus**.

As might be expected in a primary infection, macrophages laden with organisms travel to the draining hilar lymph nodes and, just as in the guinea-pig experiments described by Koch, these nodes become enlarged and show caseation necrosis. It is a characteristic feature of childhood infection that, irrespective of the lodgement site of the organisms, there is a relatively inconspicuous local tissue response which tends to be overshadowed by involvement of the draining lymph nodes. The combination of this inconspicuous parenchymal lesion and the prominent lymphadenopathy is known as the **primary complex** or **Ghon complex** (*Fig. 15.6*).

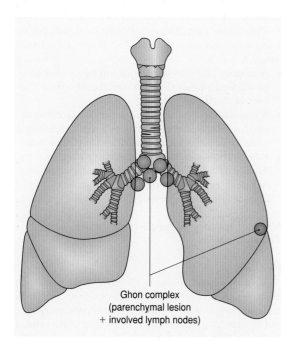

Ghon complex
(parenchymal lesion
+ involved lymph nodes)

FIGURE 15.6 Primary infection with Mycobacterium tuberculosis.

Natural History of the Primary Complex

Healing

Most lesions, in both the lung parenchyma and hilar nodes, will heal. This may be brought about by one of the following:

- Complete replacement of any areas of caseation necrosis by fibrous tissue.
- More often, by the local walling off of the necrotic area by scar tissue followed by deposition of calcium salts in the caseous material (**dystrophic calcification**). Organisms may survive in these calcified foci and, even years later, if immune regulatory mechanisms become less efficient may start to proliferate.

Exudative Responses

If high-grade hypersensitivity develops following infection, a severe exudative type of response occurs. This is characterized by the outpouring of a fibrin-rich exudate in which scanty epithelioid and giant cells may be found. This type of reaction may also manifest in the form of a large pleural effusion with a massive accumulation of serous fluid in which the cell population is scanty and the number of organisms that can be isolated is very small.

Spread

If the primary reaction is dominated by caseation and softening of the necrotic material, then spread to distant areas may occur. Such spread may take place via the bronchi or bloodstream (**haematogenous spread**). It occurs most often after softening of the caseous lymph node component of the primary complex. The organisms may reach the blood either by direct involvement of small blood vessels or via thoracic duct lymph.

Miliary Tuberculosis

If the number of organisms released into the circulation is large and the host resistance is low, the systemic spread of the mycobacteria is expressed by the development of very large numbers of small granulomatous lesions. These are more or less equal in size, and stud the **lungs** (*Fig 15.7*), **kidneys**, **spleen**, **brain**, **meninges**, **adrenals** and, to a lesser extent, the liver. The rather distressing habit of pathologists of an earlier day to describe lesions in terms of food led to these lesions being compared with millet seeds, hence the term **miliary tuberculosis**.

Classically we tend to associate miliary tuberculosis with childhood infection, but it is far from uncommon in the elderly receiving immunosuppressive therapy and in patients suffering from AIDS. These patients show both diminished resistance to the infection and diminished hypersensitivity, the latter being expressed in terms of negative skin reactions to intradermal injections of tuberculoprotein. Bone marrow or liver biopsy

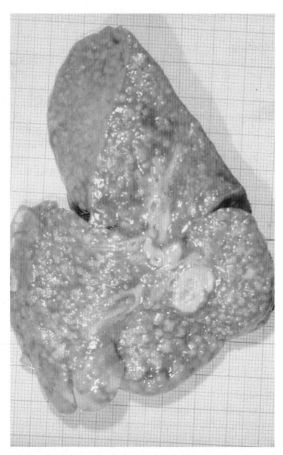

FIGURE 15.7 *Lung from a child showing widespread miliary lesions throughout and a larger lesion, which probably represents the primary focus.*

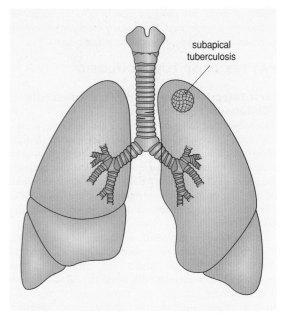

FIGURE 15.8 *The typical 'adult' or secondary type of infection in the lung is usually expressed in the form of a subapical lesion associated with much tissue destruction.*

may be useful diagnostic procedures in such cases, as the lesions are so widespread that the chances of obtaining a positive result on biopsy are quite high.

'Organ' Tuberculosis

If the dose of mycobacteria reaching the bloodstream is small, a different result may be seen, in both children and adults. Disseminated organisms may lodge and cause lesions in only one organ or tissue and the clinical picture will be determined by the site of such lesions. For example, a patient with tuberculous granulomas in the brain might present with the clinical features of a space-occupying lesion. Many tissues can be involved in this way, some of the most commonly affected being the kidneys, adrenals, fallopian tubes, bones, joints and tendon sheaths.

Adult-type Pulmonary Tuberculosis

In adult pulmonary tuberculosis the parenchymal lesions usually start in the subapical region of the upper lobe, where they are known as **Assmann foci** (*Fig. 15.8*). Apart from the fact, which may well be quite irrelevant, that the bacilli are obligate aerobes and that the ventilation in this part of the lung is said to be greater than in other segments, the reason for this localization is not known. The prominent lymph node involvement seen in primary infections is not present, although microscopic lesions may be seen.

The origin of adult-type infections is still poorly understood and controversial. The lesions might arise from:

- A primary infection which, for unknown reasons, has elicited a tissue response which differs from that seen in childhood.
- A second infection in someone previously exposed to *M. tuberculosis* and who has, as a result, developed some degree of both immunity and hypersensitivity.
- Reactivation of a previous infection owing to a decline in the efficiency of cell-mediated immunity as a result of malnutrition, overindulgence in alcohol, immunosuppression, etc.

Natural History of Adult-type Pulmonary Tuberculosis

Healing

As with childhood lesions in the lung, if the host has a high degree of immunity the lesions may heal with some scarring and calcification. Appropriate antimicrobial therapy reduces the amount of scar tissue formed and if there has been cavitation (see below) the end-result may be a smooth-walled cavity with very little peripheral fibrosis (*Fig. 15.9*).

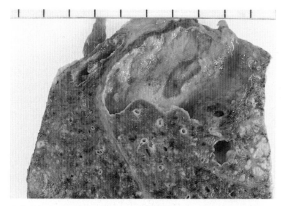

FIGURE 15.9 *A large cavitating subapical lesion in an adult. Intrapulmonary spread has occurred in this patient, as shown by the presence of numerous smaller lesions in the lung parenchyma.*

Softening and Cavitation

Softening of the caseous material may occur and, if this is associated with erosion into a bronchus, a **cavity** develops (*Fig. 15.10*). Apart from the destruction of lung tissue that this entails, cavitation is an extremely unfavourable development. Direct communication of the lesion with a major airway increases oxygen tension and thus favours multiplication of the bacilli, as they are obligate aerobes. The patient will cough up infected material and thus be a danger to those in contact with him or her, and a natural pathway will have been created for spread within the patient's own lung via the ramifications of the bronchial tree.

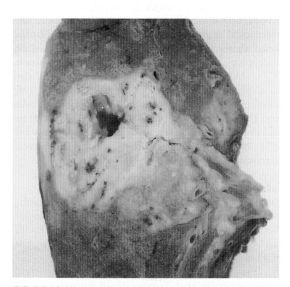

FIGURE 15.10 *A large upper lobe lesion in an adult. The focus shows abundant caseation necrosis and there is early cavitation within the centre of the lesion. The affected area is adjacent to a main bronchus, and a communication has probably been established between the large airway and the affected portion of lung parenchyma.*

Blood vessels in the cavity walls are frequently involved in the inflammatory process; sometimes they become blocked by small thrombi but not infrequently they become eroded; this is followed by bleeding, which may be massive.

Caseating lesions within the lung parenchyma are sometimes associated with involvement of the **pleura**. This may be expressed in the form of a **serous effusion** or a persistent **fibrinous exudate**, which may lead to obliteration of the pleural cavity by the processes of organization and repair. Occasionally the affected pleural cavity contains abundant, partly liquefied, caseous material; this situation is known as a **tuberculous empyema** (*Fig. 15.11*).

Spread (*Fig. 15.12*)

In addition to spread via the bloodstream, which can follow the same patterns as described for childhood infection, an important aspect of spread in adults involves natural anatomical pathways. If a bronchus is eroded, spread of infected material may occur by inhalation, with distal extension of the inflammatory process within the lung. This usually leads to a patchy tuberculous bronchopneumonia, but if the number of bacilli is very large and there is high-grade local tissue hypersensitivity, a massive degree of caseation can take place which may involve several segments of lung tissue or even a whole lobe.

Spread of infected caseous material can also occur in a proximal direction with involvement of the larynx. The patient may swallow some of the infected material and tuberculous involvement of the bowel may follow.

LEPROSY

Leprosy is a chronic infectious disease of humans caused by **Mycobacterium leprae** (one of the first bacterial pathogens to be recognized). It affects principally the skin, the nasal mucosa, the peripheral nerves and the testes, having a predilection for tissues that are relatively cool.

The organism has much the same morphological features as any other mycobacterium, but is more easily decolourized by acid than *M. tuberculosis*. Thus a modification of the Ziehl–Neelsen method is used which takes account of this (the Wade–Fite stain). Also, unlike *M. tuberculosis*, the leprosy bacillus is an obligate intracellular parasite and cannot be cultured in any known medium. However, it does survive and proliferate in the footpad of the mouse and in the nine-banded armadillo.

Leprosy is a rare disease in Western communities, but on a world-wide basis it is estimated that there are more than 11 million sufferers, 60% of these in Asia. In India alone there are 3.5 million lepers.

Transmission of leprosy is from person to person. The infectivity rate is low, only 5–10% of contacts actually developing the disease. The period between exposure to

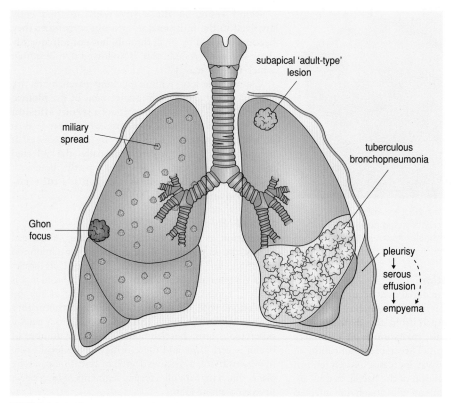

FIGURE 15.11   The spectrum of intrapulmonary and pleural manifestations of tuberculosis.

the organisms and the first appearance of tuberculoid lesions is about 3–6 years, although much longer incubation periods (10–20 years) have been reported in relation to the lepromatous form of the disease.

Local Tissue Responses in Leprosy Depend on the Degree of Cell-mediated Immunity

The tissue responses of the host to infection with *M. leprae* cover a wide spectrum. At the two extremes are the types of response that have been characterized as **lepromatous** and **tuberculoid** leprosy.

Lepromatous Leprosy

In the lepromatous form of leprosy there are widespread lesions in the skin and mucous membrane. The lesions consist of poorly organized infiltrates comprising very large numbers of macrophages, which look foamy, and smaller numbers of lymphocytes, plasma cells and mast cells (*Fig. 15.13*). When sections of such lesions are stained appropriately, acid- and alcohol-fast bacilli can be seen in enormous numbers within the macrophages, being arranged either in compact masses or in bundles, somewhat similar to cigarettes in a pack (*Fig. 15.14*). Ultrastructural studies show that the organisms are also contained within the Schwann cells ensheathing the cutaneous nerves. One gram of tissue from a lepromatous area may contain as many as 10^7 bacilli.

Tuberculoid Leprosy

In this form of the disease the lesions are far scantier and involvement of peripheral nerves is quite common. On histological examination, in contrast to the lepromatous form, there are tightly packed and well-organized macrophage granulomas with no evidence of caseation (*Fig. 15.15*). Lymphocytes are numerous; the macrophages have often undergone epithelioid cell transformation; and occasional multinucleate giant cells may be seen. Acid-fast bacilli are extremely difficult to find in these lesions; it may be impossible to see any on light microscopic examination, although electron microscopy may reveal some bacterial remnants.

Intermediate Forms

Between these two poles a large number of intermediate forms of tissue response exists. The more closely they resemble the lepromatous type, the more bacilli can be identified in sections, the reverse being true the more closely they resemble the tuberculoid type.

Lepromatous and Tuberculoid Leprosy Represent Two Extremes of the Cell-mediated Response

In tuberculoid leprosy, the type of lesion present and the fact that cutaneous hypersensitivity can be demonstrated by the use of antigen extracted from leprous

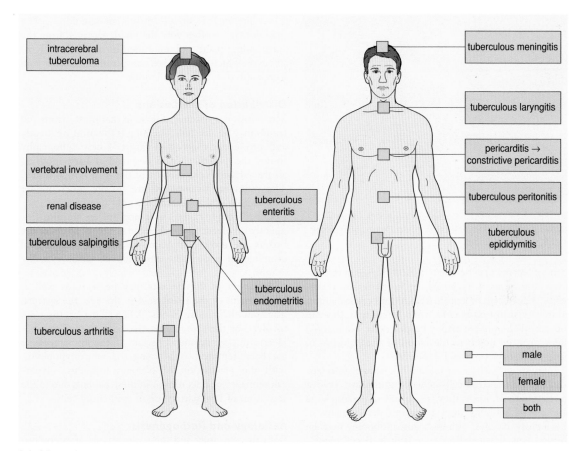

FIGURE 15.12 *The patterns of organ involvement seen in tuberculous infections that spread.*

tissue suggests that some cell-mediated immunity is present. This is not of a degree sufficient to eliminate the mycobacteria from the host. In lepromatous leprosy, the absence of well-formed epithelioid cell granulomas, the absence of skin hypersensitivity, and the absence of effective microbicidal function on the part of the infiltrating macrophages all suggest the opposite: poor or absent cell-mediated immunity.

This impression is strengthened by the observation that lymphocytes from patients with lepromatous leprosy fail to respond by undergoing blast transformation in the presence of *M. leprae in vitro*, whereas those from patients suffering from the tuberculoid form of the disease respond strongly. The relative failure of T cell-directed microbial elimination seen in the lepromatous

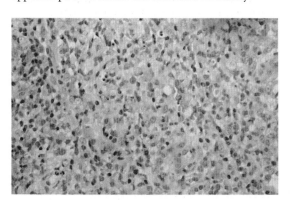

FIGURE 15.13 *Lepromatous leprosy. There are no well-formed granulomas; instead the lesion shows sheets of plump macrophages admixed with lymphocytes.*

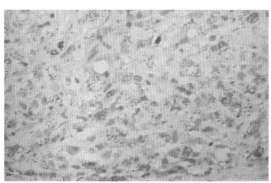

FIGURE 15.14 *Section from a lepromatous lesion stained by the Wade–Fite method to identify acid- and alcohol-fast bacilli. Note the large numbers of intracellular organisms. This is the expression of a poor degree of immunity and an inability to clear the host's tissues of organisms.*

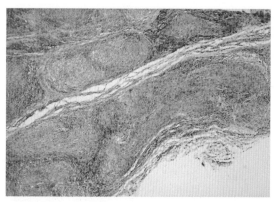

FIGURE 15.15 Section of a peripheral nerve showing well-formed granulomas in a case of tuberculoid leprosy. Organisms in such a lesion are scanty.

form of leprosy may be due to a local change in the relative proportion of T-cell subsets in the lesions themselves. The T cells in lepromatous lesions consist almost entirely of **suppressor cells** while, in contrast, those in tuberculoid lesions are mainly **helper cells**. No marked differences are noted in the blood of these groups of patients in respect of the T-cell subsets.

Interestingly, whereas patients with lepromatous leprosy exhibit impaired cell-mediated immunity, at least in relation to *M. leprae*, they are capable of making large amounts of antibody directed against determinants of the leprosy bacillus, although autoantibodies may be formed as well, suggesting some fault in B-cell regulation. In some patients, immune complexes are formed and these occasionally deposit in small subcutaneous blood vessels giving rise to slightly tender nodules (**erythema nodosum leprosum**). The killing of organisms in patients with lepromatous leprosy by appropriate antimicrobial agents can lead to an increase in cell-mediated immunity, and there may be a change in the character of the lesions with some progression occurring towards the tuberculoid type. This suggests that the local T-cell deficiency may be related in some way to the antigen load.

SARCOIDOSIS

Winston Churchill once wrote of Russia that it was a 'riddle, wrapped in a mystery, inside an enigma'. The same might be said of sarcoidosis.

Sarcoidosis is a disease of unknown aetiology which is fairly common in northern Europe, with the highest incidence in Sweden. It is characterized morphologically by well-formed epithelioid granulomas which show little or no central necrosis. These may be present in any organ or tissue. Multinucleated giant cells in the granulomas often show calcified bodies within the cytoplasm. These are sometimes star-shaped (hence the name **asteroid bodies**), or rounded and basophilic.

Their presence is not diagnostic of sarcoidosis. The granulomas are often very sharply demarcated from the surrounding tissue and are cuffed by a mantle of lymphocytes which is much less conspicuous than that seen in relation to tuberculous lesions.

Distribution of the Lesions

Sarcoidosis is a systemic disease in that most organs and tissues may be affected. The lung is the most frequently and prominently involved target. Chest radiography shows the presence of widespread miliary mottling associated with enlargement of the hilar lymph nodes. The pulmonary symptoms are usually much milder than radiological appearances would suggest.

Other lymph nodes, liver and spleen are also frequently involved. In the skeleton the small bones of the fingers are most conspicuously affected; radiological examination shows the presence of small cyst-like lesions.

A variety of skin lesions may be seen, as well as involvement of the uveal tract in the eye, the lacrimal gland and the salivary glands. When all the last three are involved at the same time, the triad is spoken of as Heerfordt's syndrome. On rare occasions sarcoidosis has been reported as affecting the neurohypophysis, with the production of diabetes insipidus. Hypercalcaemia is not uncommon in these patients due to the activation of 1α-hydroxylase in epithelioid cells.

Aetiology and Pathogenesis

Both the aetiology and the pathogenesis of sarcoidosis are poorly understood. One of the major difficulties is the fact that the basic pathological unit, the epithelioid granuloma, is non-specific and, as described previously, is a tissue reaction found after exposure to a large number of irritants, both living and non-living. While it is likely that the tissue response in sarcoidosis is an expression of cell-mediated immunity, we cannot be sure of this. In this connection it is not without interest that patients usually show diminished skin hypersensitivity as judged by their lack of response to tuberculoprotein.

Suggestions have been made that sarcoidosis may be the result of:

- A mycobacterial infection in a patient with altered cell-mediated immune reactions.
- A non-specific reaction to a wide variety of irritants. This would account for the histological features but would not explain the peculiar clustering of lesions that constitutes the clinical syndromes of sarcoidosis.
- Infection by an agent not as yet identified. Evidence that might be interpreted as supporting this view is derived from experiments in immunologically deficient mice. If such animals are injected with material from the lesions of a patient with sarcoidosis, they will develop large numbers of epithelioid cell granulomas. Material from these can

then be transferred to another immunologically deficient mouse, with the same results.

SYPHILIS

Syphilis is an important sexually transmitted disease. It is alleged that the disease was unknown in Europe until the last decade of the fifteenth century when Columbus's sailors were said to have introduced it on their return from the first voyage to the Americas. A large-scale outbreak was recorded after the siege and capture of Naples by Charles VIII of France in 1495–1496. The French called syphilis 'the Italian disease' and the Neapolitans dubbed it the 'French pox'. This episode tells us more about people than it does about syphilis.

The name syphilis is derived from a poem by Girolamo Fracastoro, who died in 1533, in which an amorous and presumptuous shepherd boy named Syphilus was visited by the disease as a punishment for having taken his pleasure with the goddess Aphrodite. The poem, now entitled 'Syphilis or a Poetical History of the French Pox', was translated into English in about 1680 by Nahum Tate, the poet laureate of the day, who is perhaps better known for having provided Shakespeare's King Lear with a happy ending in which Cordelia marries Edgar and lives 'happily ever after'.

The Organism

Syphilis is caused by a spirochaete, *Treponema pallidum*. This is a corkscrew-shaped bacillus which is resistant to ordinary staining methods and which, as yet, cannot be cultured in artificial media or in tissue culture systems. It can be maintained in the tissues of living animals; the rabbit testis is most frequently used for this purpose. The spirochaetes can be seen in fluid taken from ulcerated lesions in the early stages of the disease either by using dark-field microscopy or by impregnating the organisms with certain silver salts.

T. pallidum spreads widely throughout the body of infected subjects, aided by its invasive properties. These probably derive, in part, from the mucopolysaccharide capsule, which is antiphagocytic and may also downregulate the T-cell response. In addition, the treponema possesses enzymes that attack the constituents of the intercellular ground substance.

The organism is very sensitive to heat and drying; stories of syphilis having been acquired via the medium of 'cracked tea cups' and the like are thus inherently improbable. Other than in congenital syphilis, where the infection is transplacental, direct contact is required.

T. pallidum shows considerable ability to **adhere** to the surface of a number of cell types. Only the tapered end of the organism adheres to subjacent plasma membranes, suggesting the presence of a receptor in this part of the bacterial cell wall.

The Immune Response to Infection

Within 1–3 weeks of the first lesions of syphilis appearing, an immune response in the form of antibody production can be demonstrated. Two interesting groups of antibodies have been identified. The first of these forms the basis for widely used diagnostic tests: the VDRL (Venereal Disease Research Laboratory) and Wassermann reactions.

Wassermann Antibodies (Anticardiolipin)

The Wassermann antibody is an immunoglobulin M molecule which reacts with a constituent of the lipid membranes of many cell organelles, notably mitochondria. The antigen is diphosphatidylglycerol, often called **cardiolipin** because a common source is an alcoholic extract of beef heart. The presence of this antibody in serum is not an absolutely reliable indicator of syphilis as biological false-positive reactions may occur in association with a number of non-treponemal and nonvenereal diseases, including:

- malaria
- leprosy
- glandular fever
- trypanosomiasis
- some other treponemal disorders (e.g. yaws, pinta and bejel)
- mycoplasmal pneumonia
- some autoimmune haemolytic anaemias
- systemic lupus erythematosus
- following some Coxsackie B virus infections

Initially this wide range of disorders capable of eliciting the presence of the anticardiolipin antibody and the wide distribution within tissues of cardiolipin suggested that antibody formation was secondary to tissue damage and was not related to any specific antigen associated with *T. pallidum* itself. Cardiolipin has, however, now been shown to be present in *Treponema*, and it may be that this bacterium-associated cardiolipin acts as the antigen. Anticardiolipin antibodies do not react with intact organisms, and the case must still be regarded as not proven.

Antibodies Binding Specifically with Intact T. Pallidum

These antibodies can be detected in two ways:
1) by the **immobilization** of organisms in suspension
2) by the **fluorescent antibody** technique. In this group there are antibodies that react with all treponemas and others that react only with *T. pallidum*.

Natural History

As already stated, apart from the congenital form of the disease, syphilis is contracted as a result of direct sexual contact with an infected person. Minute abrasions of the skin and mucous membranes in areas making such contact facilitate entry of the organisms into the tissues.

After a 3–4-week incubation period, the primary lesions appear at the site of infection. Such a lesion is usually situated in the genital region, but in those who prefer the more recherché forms of sexual congress they may be found on the lips, tongue, fingers or anus. In at least half the patients, the disease will follow a course lasting many years if untreated. The natural history in these cases appears to fall into three clearly defined and separable stages, which have been termed primary, secondary and tertiary.

Primary Syphilis

The primary lesion usually occurs within 1 month of infection; occasionally the incubation period may be longer. The lesion, an indurated papule which is usually painless but often ulcerates, is known as a **chancre** (*Fig. 15.16*)

In microscopic terms the tissue response is that of a localized inflammatory reaction characterized by a dense cellular infiltrate in which plasma cells, lymphocytes (both T and B cells) and macrophages are prominent. The endothelial linings of small blood vessels in affected areas show a marked degree of swelling. This, if extreme, can lead to virtual obliteration of their

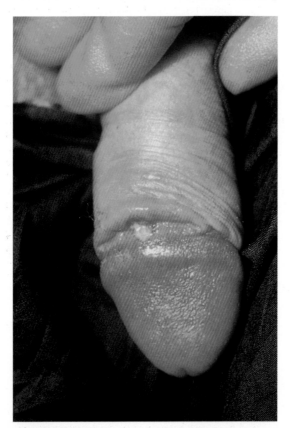

FIGURE 15.16 Primary syphilis: a chancre. This lesion is expressed as a small painless ulcer, in this case at the junction between the glans and the shaft of the penis.

lumina and patchy local ischaemia, which may contribute to ulceration of the chancre. The draining lymph nodes are usually enlarged.

Organisms are usually plentiful in the tissues at this stage and can be found in the fluid that oozes from ulcerated chancres. Local clearance of organisms appears to be effective, as the chancre heals spontaneously. In about half the patients the disease progresses no further, but in the others widespread dissemination of the treponema occurs and within a few weeks to a few months the next stage of the disease appears.

Secondary Syphilis

This stage commonly occurs within 2–3 months after exposure to infection. A generalized skin rash appears; the face, palms and soles are particularly likely to be involved. The rash usually consists of many reddish or copper-coloured papules, but other types of lesion have been described.

The mucous membranes of the mouth and pharynx show the presence of whitish patches, some of which break down to give the lesions known as 'snail track' ulcers. In the moist cutaneous and mucocutaneous areas of the anus, vulva and perineum, flat papules develop which are known as **condylomata lata**. These contain large numbers of organisms and are very infectious. Generalized slight enlargement of lymph nodes is common, those in the epitrochlear region and those related to the posterior border of the sternomastoid being involved most frequently. Immune complexes may be formed, which can give rise to lesions in a number of different places, the most noteworthy being the kidney where glomerulonephritis may occur. Fever, muscle pains and a general malaise occur quite commonly.

Both these symptoms and the various lesions disappear spontaneously after a few months and such patients no longer constitute a hazard to their sexual partners. A fairly high grade of immunity has now been established, but complete clearance of organisms usually does not take place. The treponemas appear to enter a latent phase, which may last for many years. Presumably this latent period is brought to an end when some diminution in cell-mediated immunity occurs, although it is not known how this comes about.

Tertiary Syphilis

Unlike the tissue responses seen in the primary and secondary stages of syphilis, the lesions that occur when the latent period comes to an end are very destructive and may lead to situations that can be crippling or even life threatening.

Two basic tissue responses are seen in the tertiary stage of syphilis:

1) A special type of coagulative necrosis known as **gummatous necrosis**.
2) Inflammatory damage to small blood vessels in a wide variety of sites. This may lead to necrosis of

the areas of tissue that they perfuse. Affected vessels show a severe degree of endothelial thickening with reduction of the lumina, and are cuffed by plasma cells and lymphocytes.

Gummatous Necrosis

A gumma may occur anywhere in the body. The clinical features that arise from their presence will depend on their anatomical situation. The gumma is an area of rubbery coagulative necrosis which bears some superficial resemblance to caseation necrosis. However, the centre of a gumma does not show the complete obliteration of cell and tissue outlines that is so characteristic a feature of caseation. The borders of the gumma show the presence of plump fibroblasts, macrophages and lymphocytes. Blood vessels at the periphery show narrowing of their lumen and this may contribute to the necrosis. Treponemas are very scanty and difficult to demonstrate in lesions. Healing of the gummas differs from the healing seen in tuberculosis. Fibrous bands criss-cross the necrotic area and coarse scarring results. Sites of predilection for such necrosis to occur include the liver, testis, subcutaneous tissue and bone (especially the tibia, ulna, clavicle, skull, nasal and palatal bones) (*Fig. 15.17*). The resulting lesions, especially in bone,

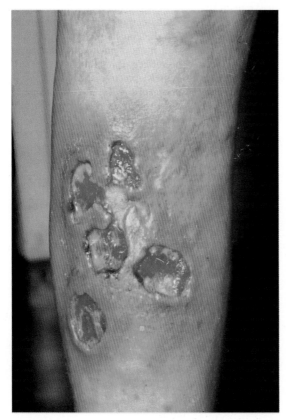

FIGURE 15.17 Gummatous ulcer on the anterior surface of the leg. These are large, deep, rather 'punched-out' lesions.

can lead to bizarre and striking clinical and pathological pictures.

The pathogenesis of gummatous necrosis is still unknown. It has been suggested that it is a hypersensitivity phenomenon.

Small Blood Vessel Disease

Small blood vessels in a variety of sites show periadventitial cuffing by lymphocytes and plasma cells. Endothelial cells swell and may proliferate and this can lead to obliteration of the lumina.

Such changes in the small blood vessels have a particularly baneful effect on the cardiovascular system. The ascending and thoracic parts of the aorta are the chief targets. The vasa vasorum in the adventitia and their extensions into the outer tunica media become cuffed by inflammatory cells. This is followed by destruction of both the elastic laminae and the smooth muscle cells in the media, and this inevitably leads to loss of the normal recoil of the aortic wall. The weakening of the aortic wall can lead to local dilatation of the vessel or **aneurysm** formation. The intimal surface of a vessel affected in this way often shows a curious wrinkled pattern, which has been likened to the appearance of tree bark. Any destructive process associated with scarring of the media of large elastic arteries shows this feature, which is therefore not diagnostic of tertiary syphilis.

Not infrequently the weakening process in the aortic media extends proximally to involve the aortic root, which becomes dilated as a result. This will give rise to incompetence of the aortic valve with consequent regurgitation of blood during diastole. Apart from the obvious dilatation of the aortic ring, the commissures between the valve cusps are widened and the cusps themselves show a characteristic cord-like thickening along their free edges which, presumably, is due to the alteration in haemodynamics. As with the wrinkling of the intimal surface mentioned above, these appearances of the aortic valve can occur in any condition that gives rise to dilatation of the aortic root (e.g. ankylosing spondylitis) and are not diagnostic of syphilis. Before the introduction of penicillin treatment for syphilis, aortic valve disease of this type was a common cause of both left ventricular failure and sudden death. Its frequency in Western countries has declined very steeply.

Syphilis and the Central Nervous System

The lesions of tertiary syphilis occurring in the central nervous system fall into two distinct groups:

1) Lesions that involve the meninges and their small blood vessels lead to a chronic meningitis, patchy gummatous necrosis and severe narrowing of arterial lumina as a result of swelling of endothelial cells. Lesions tend to occur early in the tertiary stage and have even been recorded in the secondary stage of the disease.

2) So-called **parenchymatous neurosyphilis**

occurs late in the tertiary stage and involves degeneration of the neuronal elements themselves.

Meningovascular Syphilis   Syphilis may involve either the leptomeninges or the pachymeninges; the former are affected more frequently. Leptomeningitis occurs most often at the base of the brain; the meninges become swollen and thickened, and occasionally small patches of gummatous necrosis may be seen. Cranial nerve involvement is not uncommon and the process may also obstruct the foramina of the fourth ventricle and thus cause hydrocephalus. Pachymeningitis may occur over the surface of the cerebral hemispheres and also in relation to parts of the spinal cord, where blood vessel involvement can cause patchy necrosis. These conditions are now seen very rarely.

Parenchymatous Neurosyphilis   Two quite distinct sets of lesions and clinical syndromes can be encountered. The first is termed **tabes dorsalis**, and is characterized by degeneration of certain sensory fibres in the posterior nerve roots and posterior columns of the spinal cord. This leads to atrophy, the posterior columns are seen to be shrunken and greyish in colour (instead of white) at post-mortem examination. The overlying leptomeninges are thickened and the posterior nerve roots are also atrophic.

On microscopic examination the posterior columns show fibre loss and demyelination. Similar changes may occur in more proximally situated parts of the nervous system (e.g. the optic discs and the third cranial nerve). The degeneration leads to severe loss of function, especially in relation to deep pressure sensation, vibration sense, position sense and coordination. Patients may develop a characteristic unsteady and 'stamping' gait, as they cannot feel the ground beneath their feet. Deep tendon reflexes disappear and there may be episodes of very severe shooting pains in the limbs, known as 'lightning pains'. The lack of sensation may lead ultimately to disorganization of large joints such as the knee (Charcot's joints).

The pathogenesis of tabes dorsalis is still unknown. It is not likely to be related to proliferation of the organisms at a time when cell-mediated immunity is deficient, as organisms are very scanty in the lesions.

The second type of parenchymatous lesion seen in neurosyphilis is known as **general paresis of the insane**. It was once one of the commonest causes of long-term admission to mental hospitals. General paresis of the insane is a chronic treponemal inflammatory disorder in which, in contrast, to tabes dorsalis, it is reasonably easy to identify the organisms. The brain becomes shrunken and the cerebral cortices are disorganized, the graphic term 'windswept cortex' being applied by some writers. The structural changes in the brain consist essentially of degeneration of nerve cells and their fibres, especially in the grey matter, with an associated proliferation of astrocytes and glial fibres. The small intracerebral blood vessels show the expected perivascular cuffing by lymphocytes and plasma cells, and swelling of the endothelial lining.

In the early stages the clinical picture is characterized by deterioration in personality and changes in mental function. This may express itself in the form of delusions, which may be at once bizarre and grandiose. If unchecked by treatment, the mental changes may proceed inexorably to complete dementia. Disturbances related to other functions may also be seen. These include tremors of the lips and tongue, general weakness, minor convulsive seizures and disturbances of finer movements.

Congenital Syphilis

The presence of treponemas in the blood of a pregnant woman exposes the fetus to the hazard of transplacental infection. This usually occurs in about the fifth month of pregnancy. Depending on the degree of maternal spirochaetaemia, the fetus may be aborted or the child may die at birth, the lesions of congenital syphilis may appear early in the neonatal period, or the infection may remain latent for quite long periods.

If the infection is sufficiently severe to cause lesions in the perinatal period, the clinical picture tends to be dominated by skin and mucous membrane lesions in which severe loss of surface epithelium may occur. These lesions are intensely infective and contain relatively vast numbers of organisms. Typical inflammatory changes are seen at the growing ends of bones and in relation to the periosteum. Severe deformities of bone may result, including the formation of periosteal new bone over the anterior surface of the tibia giving rise to a **sabre-like** appearance.

The **liver** may be diffusely affected by the syphilitic inflammatory reaction and this leads to an equally diffuse form of scarring where individual liver cells or small groups of such cells are surrounded by fine trabecula of fibrous tissue. Severe interstitial fibrosis may be seen in the **lung**, leading to a marked narrowing of air spaces and, in the most severe cases, to a relatively airless lung. The **cornea** is often the seat of an inflammatory reaction and the **teeth** can show a characteristic deformity, the incisors being 'screwdriver' or 'peg' shaped (Hutchinson's teeth).

If the congenital infection manifests after a prolonged latent period, the features are usually similar to those seen in the tertiary stage of an acquired infection, although the presence of inflammation of the cornea together with these features should suggest the possibility of transplacental infection.

CHAPTER 16

Amyloid and Amyloidosis

'Amyloid is a nineteenth century term in search of a twentieth century definition'
(George Glenner, NEJM)

Amyloidosis **is a disparate set of disorders** which show a single common feature: **extracellular deposition of proteins arranged in the form of β-pleated sheet fibrils.**

Credit, if that is the appropriate word, for the introduction of the term amyloid (*L. amylum* starch) goes to Rudolph Virchow in 1854, although recognition of the pathological features of amyloidosis occurred long before. By 1854 a number of terms had been used to describe what we now call amyloid, the commonest of which were 'waxy' or 'lardaceous' degeneration because organs in which large amounts of amyloid are deposited are:

- larger
- firmer
- paler

than normal.

Amyloid shows the same reaction with iodine as does starch; Virchow therefore coined the term amyloid (literally 'starch-like') for this reason. Only 5 years after the introduction of the term amyloid, Friedreich and Kekulé showed that amyloid was not a carbohydrate but was instead proteinaceous. Retention of the term amyloid is a tribute, therefore, to the conservatism of the medical profession where matters of nomenclature are concerned.

Identification of Amyloid in Tissue

As already stated, organs in which there is abundant amyloid deposition are **larger, paler and much firmer than normal**. They do indeed appear somewhat waxy and the cut edges of solid viscera are much sharper than normal (*Figs 16.1a* and *b*). It is sometimes possible to recognize the sites of amyloid deposition by staining portions of tissue with Lugol's iodine, the amyloid staining a rich brown colour.

Microscopic Features

Amyloid can be recognized by:

a) **Its eosinophilia and apparent lack of structure**, as seen in sections stained with haematoxylin and eosin (*Fig. 16.2*).

b) **Its ability to bind the dye Congo Red**, which stains amyloid orange-red (*Fig. 16.3*). **In polarized light, Congo Red-positive material has characteristic green–yellow birefringence, termed dichroism** (*Fig. 16.4*).

This is fairly sensitive method and, apart from electron microscopic examination of the tissue, is the most reliable everyday diagnostic method. Treatment of sections with potassium permanganate helps to differentiate between two forms of amyloid: **amyloid of immunoglobulin light chain origin and amyloid derived by cleavage of an acute-phase reactant, serum amyloid A (SAA).** In the case of the latter, Congo Red binding is abolished by permanganate treatment.

c) **Its ability to exhibit metachromasia** when sections are stained with **methyl violet**, the amyloid staining **red.** This is not a very satisfactory method because the dye does not bind permanently to the amyloid and tends to leach out into the mounting medium.

d) **Electron microscopy** shows amyloid not to be structureless but to consists of bundles of fibrils (*Fig. 16.5*) varying in width from 7 to 14 nm and measuring up to 1600 nm in length. High-resolution electron microscopy shows pentagonal subunits along the filaments. These consist of **amyloid P component**, a glycoprotein coded for on chromosome 1.

P component belongs to a family of pentameric glycoproteins known as the **pentraxins**, of which the acute-phase reactant C-reactive protein is a member. Amyloid P concentration in plasma increases under the same circumstances as other acute-phase proteins; its physiological role has not been determined, although *in vitro* it has some inhibitory effect on elastase.

It binds in a calcium-dependent fashion to a number of ligands including fibronectin and amyloid fibrils, but the significance of this is not yet known.

The close association of the P component with amyloid fibrils in systemic amyloidosis can be made use of, as serum amyloid P component linked with radioactive iodine, when injected intravenously, binds to the amyloid deposits. Thus it may be possible to use scintigraphy to diagnose amyloidosis, to locate the deposits and to monitor their extent.

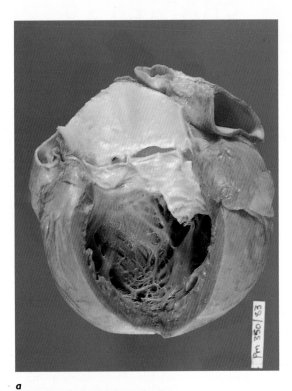

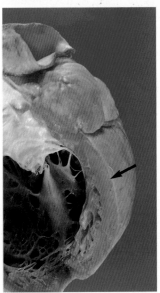

a

b

FIGURE 16.1 **a** *Cardiac amyloidosis. A grossly enlarged and dilated heart from a patient who died from amyloidosis of immune origin. Although the heart has not been fixed, note its pallor and how well its shape is maintained, this being particularly evident in respect of the left auricular appendage. This maintenance of shape is an indication of the increased stiffness of the walls of the heart chambers.* **b** *A closer view of the specimen in which, in addition to the features already described, it is possible to see how sharp the cut edge of the left ventricle is. This is another indicator of increased stiffness.*

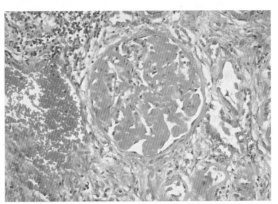

FIGURE 16.2 *Renal amyloidosis. The centre of the field of this microphotograph of a haematoxylin and eosin-stained section is occupied by a glomerulus. The structure of the glomerular capillary tuft is virtually obliterated by featureless, eosinophilic material, which represents amyloid deposited within the basement membranes of the capillaries.*

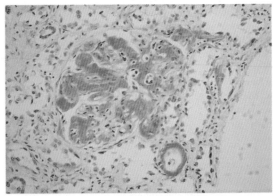

FIGURE 16.3 *Renal amyloidosis. This section has been stained with Congo Red. There is abundant orange staining within the single glomerulus shown and similar staining can be seen in an afferent arteriole close to the glomerulus.*

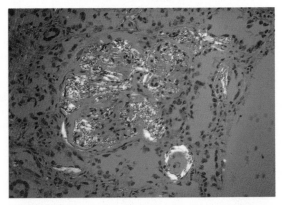

FIGURE 16.4 *Renal amyloidosis. This shows the same Congo Red-stained abnormal glomerulus and arteriole seen in Fig. 16.3, photographed in polarized light. Areas that previously appeared orange now show a green and gold birefringence, characteristic of amyloid.*

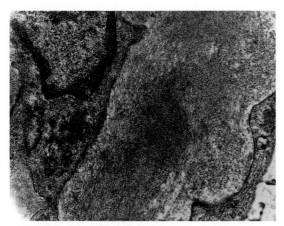

FIGURE 16.5 *Renal amyloidosis. Transmission electron micrograph of part of a glomerular capillary wall showing a fine meshwork of amyloid fibrils in the basement membrane running diagonally across the field between an epithelial cell on the left and an endothelial cell on the right.*

The β-pleated Fibril is the Unifying Feature of the Amyloidoses

It is well known that diseases associated with amyloidosis are widely disparate. Equally, modern methods of protein analysis show the existence of several widely differing amyloid proteins, each one characteristic of a certain group of disorders. The common and unifying factor in this complex situation is the fact that **all amyloid proteins have a β-pleated sheet structure** (*Fig. 16.6*).

Mammalian proteins, indeed vertebrate proteins in general, normally exhibit an α-helical structure, and β-pleating to this extent is not normally seen. **The β-pleated configuration causes:**

- the characteristic reactions with Congo Red
- the fibrillar ultrastructure
- the relative resistance of amyloid fibrils to dissolve in normal physiological solvents and to proteolytic digestion

CLASSIFICATION

Classification of the amyloidoses is most rationally based on identification of the protein precursor involved.

Older classifications of the amyloidoses were, quite understandably, based on clinical and pathological criteria but show certain inconsistencies:

1) **Primary amyloidosis** was defined by the presence of a tendency for nodular deposition of amyloid with a special predilection for mesenchymal tissues and, most importantly, an absence of any recognizable preceding or concurrent disease. The only distinction between this and the entity known as amyloidosis associated with myelomatosis was the presence in the latter of osteolytic lesions. In fact, both the distribution pattern of the amyloid and the protein involved are identical.

2) So-called **secondary amyloidosis** was characterized as such by the fact that it either followed or was associated with a wide range of **identifiable diseases**, many of which were chronic inflammatory disorders.

It seems more rational, therefore, to propose a scheme of classification based on simple set theory (*Fig. 16.7*).

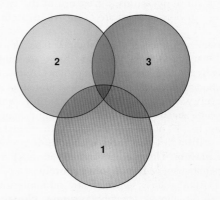

classification of amyloidosis

1. nature of the protein involved (e.g. immunoglobulin light chain)

2. anatomical distribution

3. inherited or acquired?

FIGURE 16.7 *A basis for classification of the amyloidoses. 1, The nature of the protein involved (e.g. immunoglobulin light chain); 2, anatomical distribution; 3, whether inherited or acquired.*

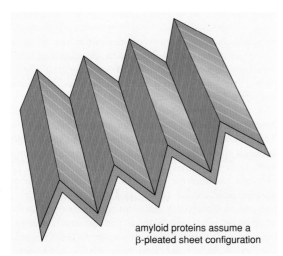

amyloid proteins assume a β-pleated sheet configuration

FIGURE 16.6 *Diagram of amyloid protein showing the characteristic β-pleated sheet fibril arrangement.*

Any individual case of amyloidosis can be regarded as representing the common set of three sets, which are:

- **the nature of the amyloid protein**
- **whether the amyloidosis is acquired or inherited**
- **the distribution pattern of the amyloid deposits**

SYSTEMIC AMYLOIDOSIS

Amyloidosis of Immune Origin (AL type)

In terms of the above criteria, this form of amyloidosis shows the following general characteristics:

- **The protein precursor is an immunoglobulin light chain and/or its homologous amino-terminal fragment.**
- **The disorder is acquired.**
- **The amyloid is systemically distributed.**

Amyloidosis of immune origin occurs in association (not surprisingly, in view of the nature of the amyloid protein) with **a monoclonal proliferation of B lymphocytes or plasma cells which, in some cases, is overtly neoplastic**. The most striking of these is **myelomatosis**, which accounts for about 20% of cases of this type of amyloidosis. Amyloidosis of immune origin is also found in association with Waldenström's macroglobulinaemia, heavy chain disease and even, in some patients, with agammaglobulinaemia.

The Amyloid Protein

Analysis of amyloid proteins in amyloidosis of immune origin shows them to consist of:

- **an intact immunoglobulin light chain**
- **the amino-terminal fragment of such a chain**
- **on some occasions, a mixture of the two**

These amyloid proteins are called **AL proteins**. The majority of the light chains found in amyloidosis of immune origin are of the **lambda** (λ) type, although in myelomatosis **kappa** (κ) light chains are more frequently found in the plasma of patients. Anti-idiotypic antibodies raised against the amyloid protein of a given patient with AL amyloidosis react only with that patient's amyloid light chain, indicating patient specificity. In 90% of patients with this form of amyloidosis, **the antibodies also react with soluble proteins in the plasma**. This plasma reactant is an intact circulating light chain or **Bence Jones protein**.

Thus the cellular source of amyloid fibrils of the AL variety is almost certainly a **single clone of B lymphocyte-derived cells** whose protein product circulates in the plasma in the form of Bence Jones protein. Deposition of these light chains as amyloid fibrils requires their **conversion from a normal α-helical to a β-pleated sheet configuration**. Thus amyloidogenesis, in this context, **must be a two-step process**. Step 1 is the secretion of excess amounts of a single type of light chain (monoclonal) and step 2 is conversion to the β-pleated form.

How Do Soluble Light Chains Undergo This Change?

Progressive proteolytic cleavage of certain λ light chains can yield Congo Red-binding fibrils. Electron microscopy shows these to be identical with amyloid fibrils.

Not all λ light chains behave in this way. Thus, inherent in the variable portion of some λ light chains is the capacity to assume a β-pleated sheet configuration when that part of the light chain is enzymatically cleaved.

The features that separate so-called 'amyloidogenic' light chains from those that cannot be induced to form amyloid fibrils is not known. No light chain protein unique for AL has been described but the variable region of λ IV appears to be associated with the development of amyloidosis, and amino acid substitutions in this region have been reported to lead to changes in hydrophobicity of the protein which might promote self-aggregation. What is quite certain is that the characteristic features of amyloid depend on its configuration: β-pleated fibrils such as the natural product of the silk moth and synthetically created β-pleated fibrils derived from poly-L-lysine show the same tinctorial and ultrastructural features as amyloid.

Clinical Features (*Fig. 16.8*)

Amyloidosis of immune origin is a disorder of middle life and old age, and affects males more often than females. Some 90% of patients show a plasma or urinary monoclonal immunoglobulin associated with a Bence Jones protein and, in some cases, only a Bence Jones protein is present. The bone marrow contains an excess number of plasma cells. While the clinical expressions are protean, certain symptom complexes strongly suggest amyloidosis.

Neuropathy

Both a peripheral and an autonomic neuropathy resembling that seen in diabetics may occur and manifestations of the latter, such as impotence, orthostatic hypotension, disturbances of gastrointestinal motility and dyshidrosis, may be prominent. A peripheral neuropathy with a characteristic 'glove and stocking' distribution may also be seen, and can be associated with intermittent attacks of pain.

Restrictive Cardiomyopathy

This is caused by extensive infiltration of the amyloid between the heart muscle fibres. It leads to a marked increase in the stiffness of the heart muscle and, thus, to a lessening of diastolic compliance. The clinical features of right-sided cardiac failure tend to dominate the picture and an incorrect diagnosis of constrictive pericarditis may be made when these patients are first seen. Patients with cardiac amyloidosis are extremely sensitive to digitalis, and fatal arrhythmias have been recorded following the administration of digitalis. Even in the absence of digitalis treatment, this variety of

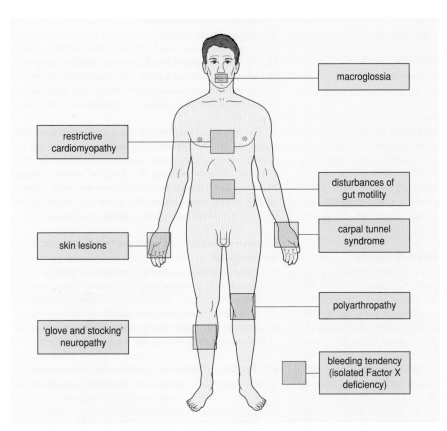

FIGURE 16.8 Spectrum of clinical features in amyloidosis of immune origin.

cardiac amyloidosis is strongly associated with an increased risk of arrhythmias, conduction disturbances and sudden death. Pulmonary deposition of amyloid has also been described in association with amyloidosis of the heart, and its presence strongly indicates an immune origin for the amyloidosis.

Skin Manifestations

There are two main changes in the skin. The first is known as 'pinch purpura' and is due to deposition of amyloid in the basement membranes of small blood vessels within the skin. Pinching of affected areas results in the formation of small haemorrhages. In addition, nodules of amyloid may be seen within the dermis, giving an appearance somewhat resembling small drops of white candle wax on the skin (*Fig. 16.9*). Areas of baldness and patchy thickening of the skin similar to what is seen in scleroderma may also occur.

Polyarthropathy

Large joints tend particularly to be sites of amyloid deposition and the distribution of the arthropathy is similar to that seen in rheumatoid disease.

Enlargement of the Tongue (Macroglossia)

This may be an early manifestation.

Isolated Deficiency in Clotting Factor X

Some patients develop a coagulation disorder characterized by Factor X deficiency. This Factor X deficiency appears to be due to very rapid clearance from the blood. For this to occur two criteria must be fulfilled: (1) the amyloid in the particular case must have binding sites for Factor X; and (2) there must be sufficient amyloid

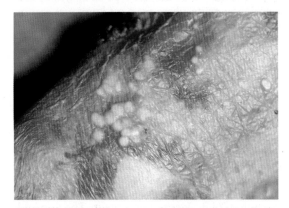

FIGURE 16.9 Skin lesions in a patient with amyloidosis of immune origin. Note the patchy intradermal haemorrhages and the well-defined, intensely white nodules that mark the amyloid deposits in the dermis.

exposed to the circulating blood for such binding to take place. The spleen is a likely candidate site for the exposure of amyloid to blood. Certainly, the removal of large, amyloid infiltrated, spleens in some patients affected with Factor X deficiency corrects the clotting defect.

Carpal Tunnel Syndrome

Carpal tunnel syndrome results from pressure on the median nerve and is expressed in the form of tingling in the median nerve distribution, followed ultimately by atrophy of the muscles in the hand that are supplied by this nerve. The carpal tunnel is affected not only in immune-mediated amyloidosis of the AL type but in one of the hereditary neuropathic amyloidoses and also in some patients who have been on long-term haemodialysis for chronic renal failure.

Haemodialysis-associated Amyloid

After 7 years on dialysis, 30% of patients develop carpal tunnel syndrome; this proportion increases to 50% after 10 years. The amyloid is derived from β_2-microglobulin. Amyloidosis of this type develops only in the presence of a persistently high plasma concentration of this protein, a situation that is particularly likely to develop if cuprophane membranes are used for the dialysis. β_2-Microglobulin shows some degree of homology for the constant region of both light and heavy chains of immunoglobulin and the protein is shed continuously from cell membranes into the plasma before being catabolized in the kidney. In very high concentrations, isolated and purified β_2-microglobulin can be precipitated as a material with a fibrillar ultrastructure and a capacity to bind Congo Red; it can therefore be regarded as a naturally 'amyloidogenic' protein.

Reactive Systemic Amyloidosis ('Secondary' Amyloidosis)

The basic characteristics of this form of amyloidosis are as follows. **The protein precursor of the amyloid (which is known as the AA type of amyloid) is a circulating acute-phase reactant known as serum amyloid A (SAA). This is a 12.5-kD protein produced chiefly by the liver, although messenger RNA for SAA has been detected in a number of tissues in the mouse.**

Under basal circumstances SAA is present in only very low concentrations. In the face of tissue injury and/or inflammation the concentration of SAA rises very sharply (sometimes more than 1000-fold), the signals that upregulate production being interleukin (IL) 1, tumour necrosis factor-α and probably IL-6. While the biological role of SAA as an acute-phase protein is still unknown, it is worth noting that SAA is an apolipoprotein in the HDL$_3$ fraction of high density lipoprotein. The amyloid protein itself (AA) appears to be a cleavage product of SAA, 28 amino acid residues at the carboxy-terminal having been removed from the SAA.

The disorder is acquired in most cases, and is associated with a wide range of chronic inflammatory diseases and some neoplastic ones. However, AA protein deposition in the same distribution pattern as for reactive systemic amyloidosis occurs in association with the autosomal recessive disorder, familial mediterranean fever (see p 180).

The distribution pattern is a systemic one: the kidneys, liver, spleen and adrenals are sites of predilection. The main cause of death in this variety of amyloidosis is chronic renal failure. Many other tissues may be involved and biopsy of the rectal mucosa or the gum can be a useful way of establishing a firm tissue diagnosis.

Disease Associations of Reactive Systemic Amyloidosis

- **Chronic inflammatory diseases in which infection is known to play a part.** The most common of these are tuberculosis, leprosy, syphilis, chronic osteomyelitis and bronchiectasis.
- **Chronic inflammatory diseases in which infection probably plays a part**, e.g. Reiter's syndrome, Whipple's disease.
- **Chronic inflammatory diseases of uncertain aetiology** such as rheumatoid arthritis and its variants, other connective tissue disorders, ulcerative colitis and Crohn's disease.
- **Long-standing paraplegia**, probably because of the high risk of recurrent urinary tract infections.
- **Neoplasms, especially renal adenocarcinoma.** Reactive systemic amyloidosis has also been reported with various other solid tumours and in association with Hodgkin's disease.

Chronic inflammatory diseases constitute the major causally related association of reactive systemic amyloidosis. With the advent of antibiotic treatment, the incidence of such disorders as chronic osteitis and bronchiectasis has declined and the introduction of successful chemotherapy for **tuberculosis** has led to a fall in the frequency of tuberculosis-associated amyloidosis. However, in parts of the world where tuberculosis still occurs on a large scale, it remains a far from negligible cause of amyloidosis.

Leprosy, because of the large number of sufferers world-wide, still ranks high as a cause of reactive systemic amyloidosis and is responsible for a significant proportion of the deaths caused by this disease.

In Western countries, the most common group of disorders associated with reactive amyloidosis is **rheumatoid disease**. In systemic-onset juvenile arthritis the frequency of amyloidosis is estimated to be 10% and morbidity and mortality in these patients is high because of the baneful effect on the kidneys: the patients first develop a nephrotic syndrome and ultimately chronic renal failure.

The association between **long-standing para-plegia** and a high risk of reactive systemic amyloidosis has been known for many years; in one series of paraplegics coming to autopsy, the prevalence of amyloidosis was found to be 40%.

Pathogenesis of Reactive Systemic Amyloidosis

The pathogensis of reactive systemic amyloidosis is still unclear. **Overproduction of SAA is clearly necessary for amyloidosis to develop but it does not appear to be a sufficient cause and other factors must play a part.** What these may be is still being debated. At the genetic level, more than one gene can code for SAA and it is possible that one form may be more 'amyloidogenic' than another. In some patients with juvenile arthritis-associated amyloidosis, a restriction fragment length polymorphism on the gene that codes for serum amyloid P component has been found to correlate with the risk of developing amyloidosis. It is possible that this component may exist in two structural forms, one of which may promote the deposition of AA by masking proteolytic sites on the SAA molecule.

It has also been suggested that an '**amyloid enhancing factor**' may exist. This is a blanket term for what is probably a group of chemical species that can be extracted both from the tissues of animals in which amyloidosis has been induced and from human tissues in which amyloid fibrils are present. It appears in the tissues of experimental models before there is microscopic evidence of amyloid deposition.

Some Specific Patterns of Organ Involvement in Amyloidosis

This form of amyloidosis involves:
- **The spleen** (see pp 985–986).
- **The liver.** The liver is enlarged in amyloidosis, sometimes hugely so, and is firm and pale. Amyloid is usually deposited in the space of Disse (between the liver cells and the sinusoidal endothelium). Because amyloid fibrils resist digestion, the cords of liver cells eventually become atrophic but, owing to the large functional reserve of the liver, the clinical effects of hepatic amyloidosis are not usually great.
- **The kidney.** In the kidney the amyloid is seen to be deposited in the walls of the glomerular capillaries, and in relation to the basement membranes of the arterioles and renal tubules. In most cases the kidney is enlarged, firm and pale on naked-eye examination (*Fig. 16.10*) but in a few cases secondary ischaemic changes dominate the picture and this may lead to irregular scarring and shrinkage of the kidney. Amyloidosis involving the glomeruli leads first to the appearance of the nephrotic syndrome (see p 651) and proceeds inexorably to chronic renal failure.

Hereditary Systemic Amyloidoses

These disorders are rare, affecting fewer than one person per 100 000 population per year in the USA.

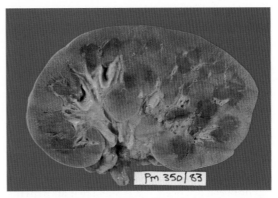

FIGURE 16.10 Renal amyloidosis. The kidney is enlarged and shows marked pallor of the cortex, contrasting with the much darker colour of the medulla.

Nevertheless they constitute experiments of nature in which there is much of interest to study, not only in relation to amyloidosis, but also in connection with genetically determined diseases of late onset.

The syndromes associated with hereditary amyloidosis can be divided into **three** main groups. These are:

1) A **neuropathic** group characterized by progressive systemic polyneuropathy. This occurs in three forms, the classification being predicated partly on the distribution of the neuropathy and partly in relation to the location of the affected families. Thus there is:

    a) A group in which the lower limbs are first and predominantly affected. This has been found in Portugal, Japan and Sweden.

    b) A group in which the nerves of the upper limb are particularly affected. This has been found in Germany and Switzerland.

    c) A group in which the neuropathy affects the face. This has been reported only in Finland.

2) A **cardiopathic** form, which has been found in one Danish family and in a kindred in the Appalachian region of the USA of German–Irish–English origin.

3) A **nephropathic** group in which two forms have been reported:

    a) familial mediterranean fever

    b) urticaria–deafness syndrome

With the exception of familial mediterranean fever, which is inherited in an autosomal recessive fashion, all these disorders are of the autosomal dominant variety.

Amyloid Proteins in Hereditary Systemic Amyloidosis

With one exception – the Finnish variety of familial amyloid polyneuropathy where the amyloid precursor protein has been described as being antigenically and structurally similar to **gelsolin**, an actin-depolymerizing protein – in both the neuropathic and cardiopathic forms the amyloid protein consists of an abnormal form of a plasma protein known until recently as **prealbumin**. This is a misnomer: the sole connection of prealbumin with albumin is that it migrates in front of albumin in electrophoretic strips.

Prealbumin has now been renamed **transthyretin**, a name that has the virtue of telling us something about its function:

- *trans*port of about 25% of plasma *thy*roxine
- transport of *retin*ol (vitamin A)

The transthyretin molecule has 127 amino acid residues and about 20 years after polyneuropathic amyloidosis had first been described, it was found that **all patients with the Portuguese form show a single amino acid substitution in the transthyretin molecule: methionine for valine at position 30.** About 20 mutations have now been discovered in the transthyretin molecule, indicating point mutations in the gene coding for this protein. Each of these is associated with a fairly distinctive clinical picture, although a certain degree of overlap is present.

The significance of mutations in the gene coding for transthyretin has been confirmed by a study in which mice were made transgenic by introduction of a mutant transthyretin gene cloned from a patient with the familial Portuguese type of polyneuropathy. Amyloid deposition started in these mice at 6 months of age and by 2 years was extensive.

The tertiary structure of transthyretin is unusual in that it is normally β-pleated. The molecule tends to form dimers and this is followed by fusion of a pair of dimers to form tetramers. **The presence of a mixture, within a single tetramer, of normal and mutated forms of the protein appears to promote the joining up of several hundred tetramers to form an amyloid fibril.**

Senile Cardiovascular Amyloidosis and Transthyretin

A transthyretin amyloid precursor has also been identified in the non-familial and quite common disorder of senile cardiac amyloidosis. Cardiac amyloidosis of this kind occurs frequently in old individuals, about 25% of subjects over 80 years being affected.

The patients present with signs and symptoms of congestive cardiac failure, often with a low-voltage electrocardiogram, recurrent syncope and a high risk of arrhythmias. Although this disorder is most commonly termed senile cardiac amyloidosis, there is increasing evidence that extracardiac sites are frequently involved and that the condition should be regarded as a variant of systemic amyloidosis.

Other forms of amyloid in the elderly that involve only the cardiovascular system are:

- Isolated atrial amyloidosis in which the amyloid protein precursor appears to be atrial natriuretic peptide.

- Aortic amyloidosis, which was found to be present in 100% of patients in a necropsy study of patients aged over 80 years. The amyloid is deposited mainly in the inner one-third of the tunica media. The nature of the protein precursor is still unknown but it does not react with antisera raised against transthyretin.

Nephropathic Forms of Familial Systemic Amyloidosis

Familial Mediterranean Fever

This is by far the commonest form of hereditary systemic amyloidosis, with one clinic alone in Israel caring for more than 1500 patients suffering from this disorder. Its biochemical basis is unknown, although a deficiency of an inhibitor for C5 has been suggested as the cause. The disease is transmitted as an **autosomal recessive** trait and is seen in Jews of Sephardic ancestry, Anatolian Turks, Armenians and Middle Eastern Arabs. The gene frequency is very high, reaching 1 in 22 among North African Jews and 1 in 14 among Armenians living in Los Angeles. Recently a gene believed to be responsible was mapped to the short arm of chromosome 16.

Familial mediterranean fever expresses itself in one or both of two forms:

1) Rather short-lived (24–48 hours), self-limiting febrile attacks associated with pain mimicking that of peritonitis, pleurisy or synovitis.

2) Amyloidosis which, in some of the groups mentioned above, may manifest itself very early in life. In the youngest fatal case reported, the patient died at the age of 5 years from renal failure, the amyloidosis having been obvious since the age of 2 years. Very few affected patients have survived beyond the age of 40 years, unless treated at an early stage or given a renal transplant.

The amyloid protein in familial mediterranean fever is of the AA type, and plasma concentrations of SAA are usually raised between attacks, although they also increase very steeply during febrile bouts. The amyloidosis obviously has a preclinical phase as it is only when glomerular function has been compromised significantly that proteinuria appears. **Early diagnosis is important because the development of amyloidosis can be inhibited in 90% of patients by administration of 1–2 mg colchicine daily.** Not only can amyloid deposition be inhibited *ab initio* but even in patients with established proteinuria the process can be halted in most, and even reversed in a small number.

Colchicine was tried because of its known stabilizing effects on inflammatory cells. Whether this is the reason for its effectiveness in familial mediterranean fever is unknown but it has undoubtedly brought great benefit to this group of patients.

Familial Nephropathic Amyloidosis with Febrile Urticaria and Nerve Deafness

In 1962 Muckle and Wells described an unusual syndrome in a single English family which was transmitted as an autosomal dominant condition and which, over four generations, affected nine of the 18 individuals at risk.

The syndrome showed itself during adolescence and its first expression was in the form of febrile attacks associated with an itchy or painful urticarial skin rash and with malaise, rigors and pains in the limbs. The second manifestation was progressive nerve deafness, followed in some patients by the onset of proteinuria leading to a nephrotic syndrome and eventually to death from chronic renal failure. Autopsy showed widespread amyloidosis, the kidneys being particularly affected. Interestingly, in view of the nerve deafness, no amyloid was found in the inner ear or cochlear nerve.

Extraction of the amyloid protein from the fixed tissues of a single patient and subsequent sequence analysis showed it to be homologous with AA protein in respect of 28 of its amino acid residues.

LOCALIZED AMYLOIDOSIS

Endocrine-related Amyloid

It has been known for a long time that certain endocrine glands, most notably the pituitary and the pancreatic islets, can be infiltrated by amyloid under certain circumstances. In the case of the pituitary, age seems to be the most important associated factor, whereas pancreatic islets frequently show the presence of amyloid deposition in patients with non-insulin-dependent diabetes mellitus.

Certain neoplasms of endocrine glands are associated with the presence of amyloid deposited solely within the stroma of the tumours and **not** appearing systemically. One of the tumours most consistently associated with stromal amyloid deposits is the **medullary carcinoma of the thyroid**, which is derived from the parafollicular or thyrocalcitonin-producing cells of the thyroid gland. **The amyloid precursor protein in this case is the 9–19 amino acid portion of the calcitonin molecule.**

The situation in relation to the amyloid appearing in the islets of patients with non-insulin-dependent diabetes and with insulin-producing islet cell tumours is equally intriguing. In acidic solutions, freezing and thawing of insulin can produce fibrils and it was initially thought that islet of Langerhans amyloid was related to the insulin molecule. More recent analysis has shown that, both in islet cells tumours and in diabetes, the amyloid shows homology with the vasodilator **calcitonin gene-related peptide**.

Intracerebral Amyloidosis

Central nervous system amyloidosis is by far the commonest localized form of the disease occurring in Alzheimer's disease, the commonest form of dementia. It is also found in the spongiform encephalopathies, in the dementia occurring in some boxers and in some hereditary haemorrhagic syndromes. Dementia-associated amyloidosis is discussed in Chapter 45 (see pp 1138–1140, 1141–1143).

Cystatin C

This was the first cerebral amyloid protein to be characterized biochemically. It is found as the principal protein in the amyloid fibrils deposited in the cerebral blood vessels in an autosomal dominant disorder known as **hereditary cerebral haemorrhage with amyloidosis of Icelandic type (HCHWA-I)**. This disorder has been found in 128 individuals in eight families in a certain area of Iceland and is characterized by the presence of amyloid in small arteries and arterioles in the cerebral cortex and leptomeninges. The patients usually die before they reach the age of 40 years from massive intracerebral haemorrhage. Cystatin C is an inhibitor of cysteine proteases and can normally be found in urine, where it is termed 'trace' protein. It is a 13-kD basic protein, related to kininogens, and is present in body fluids. It is produced in the brain, pancreas, thyroid and adrenals. The amyloid protein starts at position 11 of the normal cystatin C and there is substitution of glutamine for leucine at position 68. Whether this substitution represents a point mutation or is, instead, a normal genetic polymorphism is not known.

CHAPTER 17

General Pathology of Viral Infection

Viruses are obligate intracellular parasites, accounting for 60% of all infectious illnesses. The spectrum of disease caused by viruses ranges from trivial disorders to lethal or crippling situations. The range of tissue responses they evoke is similarly wide.

GENERAL CHARACTERISTICS OF A VIRUS

Size
As a group, viruses constitute the smallest infectious agents known. The largest ones are just visible with the light microscope, but the majority can be seen only on electron microscopy, their diameters ranging from 20 to 300 nm (1 nm = 10^{-3} µm).

Genome
Each true virus contains only a **single** nucleic acid as its genome, either DNA and RNA; the type of nucleic acid forms one of the bases for viral classification. The nucleic acid is covered by a symmetrically arranged protein shell, known as the **capsid**. The capsid consists of clusters of polypeptides that form ultrastructurally recognizable units called **capsomeres**. The arrangement of the capsid falls into two distinct structural patterns. It may confer either an **icosahedral** (20-sided) appearance to the virus or a **helical** one. All viruses in which the nucleic acid is **DNA** are icosahedral (apart from the **poxviruses**); **RNA** viruses may be either icosahedral or helical.

Infective Particle
The mature infective virus particle is called a **virion**. In the case of some viruses this may refer to the nucleic acid genome and the capsid only, but in others these are surrounded by a glycoprotein **envelope**. Most DNA viruses have no envelope (with the exception of the **herpesviruses**); most RNA viruses are enveloped (with the exception of **picornaviruses** and **reoviruses**).

INTERACTION BETWEEN VIRUS AND HOST SPECIES

The production of a viral illness involves several steps. The virus must have an appropriate route of access to the host and there must be a mechanism or mechanisms for the virus to reach its ultimate target, for example the anterior horn cells in poliomyelitis. Routes of access to the host include the skin and subcutaneous tissues, the conjunctiva, the respiratory tract, and the genital and gastrointestinal tracts. These and the possible outcome of viral entry are shown in *Figs 17.1* and *17.2*.

Viruses and the Target Cell
The effects of a disease-causing viral infection stem from:
1) **Changes produced directly by the virus in the host cell:**
   - the virus may **damage** or **kill** the infected cell
   - the virus may **persist within the cell without injuring it** (persistent infection)
   - the virus may **transform** the cell, rendering it capable of an indefinite number of passages in culture, and of forming tumours in susceptible animals (tumorigenicity) (see pp 301–304)
2) **Host tissue reactions to these changes**
3) **Responses of the immune system**, both to the presence of the virus and to the cellular changes it has produced

Transmission of Viral Infections
This may be:
- **Vertical**, i.e. the infection is transmitted from mother to child either *in utero* or perinatally
- **Horizontal**, i.e. from person to person via **respiratory** (aerosol borne), **gastrointestinal** (faecal–oral), **genitourinary** (sexual) or **percutaneous** routes

Entry into the host by any one of these routes must be followed by entry into susceptible host cells and viral replication within them. This is accomplished by an overlapping sequence of discrete steps.

I Virus Attaches to Cell Surface Membrane
Contact between viruses and target cells occurs more or less randomly. However, **attachment** of the virion to a cell surface will not take place **unless the surface membrane of the cell has a specific viral receptor site which is complementary to an attachment site on the viral surface.** The complementarity of ligands on the viral surface and receptors on the cells reflects configurational similarities and is almost certainly, in evolutionary terms, a matter of chance. It is of

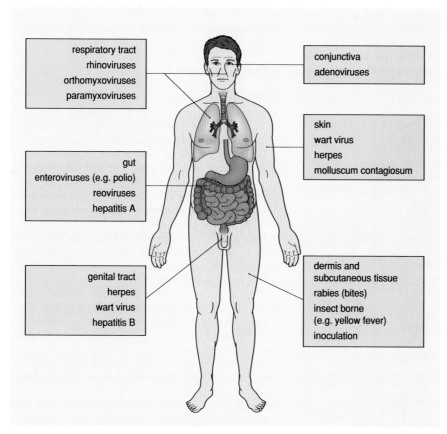

FIGURE 17.1 Portals of entry of some human viruses.

fundamental importance in determining cell tropism and viral pathogenicity.

This is well illustrated in the case of poliovirus. For poliovirus to attach to a target cell, the latter must possess a specific **lipoprotein receptor** on its plasma membrane. This is present in neurones and cells lining the intestinal tract in primates but is absent from those of rodents. The poliovirus virion will, therefore, attach to cells of primates but not to those of rodents, which cannot therefore be infected by poliovirus.

Similarly the influenza virus attaches to cells because of the presence of a specific glycoprotein receptor, **N-acetylneuraminic acid** (**NANA**) on the cell surface. The receptor on the target cell is a binding site for a **haemagglutinin** (so called because it causes red cells to clump) carried on the envelope of the influenza virus. This receptor can be destroyed by treating cells in culture with bacterial neuraminidase (sialidase); influenza virus will not attach to cells that have been treated in this way.

Epstein–Barr virus, a herpesvirus causing infectious mononucleosis and also implicated in the causation of two neoplastic diseases, Burkitt's lymphoma and nasopharyngeal carcinoma, binds to the receptor for the third component of complement (C3R) on B lympho-cytes; rabies virus recognizes acetylcholine receptors and human immunodeficiency virus (HIV) binds to the CD4 receptor on T helper lymphocytes.

Not all viral attachment is specific. Both orthomyxo-viruses and paramyxoviruses attach to sialic acid residues of host cell surface glycoproteins and glyco-lipids found on the membranes of most cells including those *not* susceptible to infection.

2 Virus Penetrates the Cell

Once attachment to the plasma membrane of the target cell has occurred, the virion becomes engulfed within the cell by a process akin to receptor-mediated endocy-tosis. This is a temperature- and energy-dependent step and can be inhibited by treating the target cells with various metabolic poisons. In the case of some enveloped viruses, the viral envelope fuses with the plasma membranes of the cell and the nucleoplasmid is released directly into the host cytoplasm.

3 Viral Nucleic Acid is Uncoated

The term 'uncoating' denotes physical separation of viral nucleic acid or, in some instances, the nucleocap-sid from outer structural proteins, this being accompa-nied by loss of infectivity. Sometimes uncoating commences during the attachment stage. More commonly, however, it occurs within the host cell cytoplasm and lysosomal enzymes are thought to play a part in the process. In the case of a few viruses of the **reovirus** family, uncoating may never be completed.

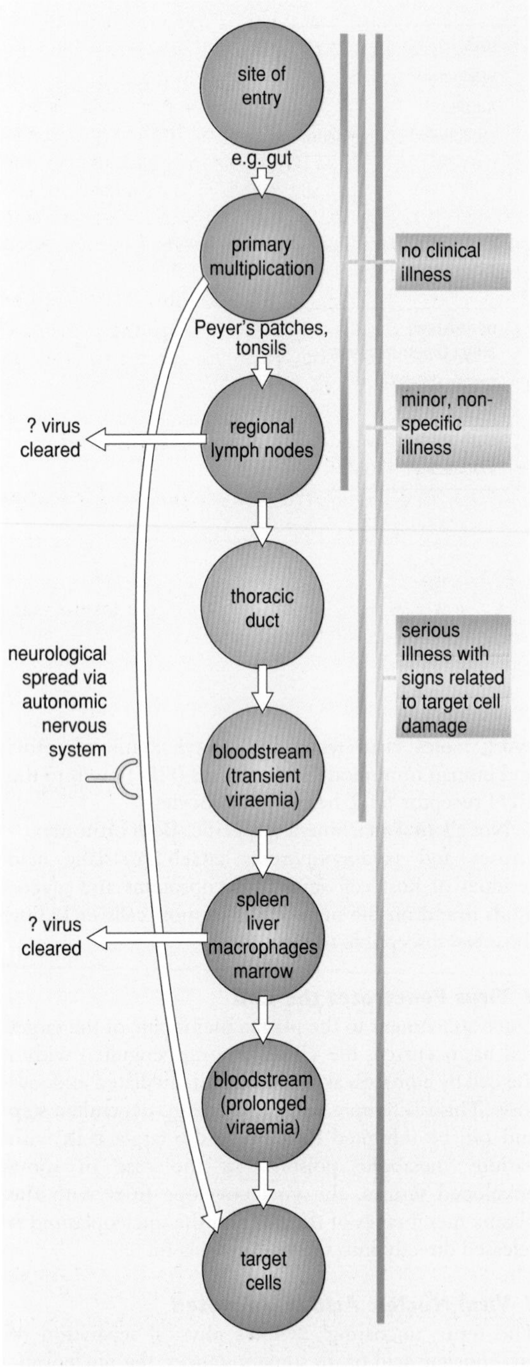

From this point, the events in viral replication differ according to whether the nucleic acid genome is DNA or RNA.

4 Viral Replication

DNA Virus Replication

The viral DNA is transcribed in two stages, giving rise to messenger RNA (mRNA) at two points in time, characterized as **early** and **late** (*Fig. 17.3*).

Early transcription from the viral DNA takes place in the nucleus of target cells. The mRNA produced reaches the cytoplasm and is then translated by the host ribosomes into **early proteins**. These are required for the synthesis of **new viral DNA**, which again takes place in the host cell nucleus.

Late mRNA is then transcribed. This leaves the nucleus and is translated in the cytoplasm into **late proteins**, which constitute the material from which the capsomeres are made.

These proteins then enter the nucleus and the virions are assembled there before leaving the host cell. This last move is accomplished by a bursting open of the cell, with release of the new virions into the surrounding extracellular environment.

All DNA viruses replicate in this way, with the exception of the poxviruses which do so entirely within the host cell cytoplasm. The polymerases concerned in the transcription of viral DNA are derived from the host cell in most instances. The poxviruses, however, have their own DNA-dependent RNA polymerase.

FIGURE 17.2 Pathogenesis of a viral disease such as poliomyelitis.

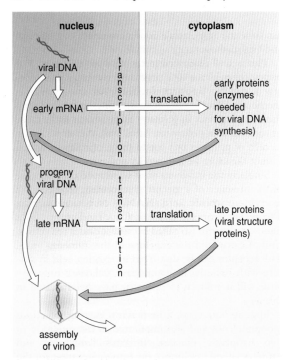

FIGURE 17.3 Replication of a DNA virus.

RNA Virus Replication

With two exceptions, all classes of RNA viruses **replicate within the cytoplasm of the host cell**. **Orthomyxoviruses** (responsible for influenza) and **retroviruses** replicate within the host cell nucleus. Because normal cells do not copy RNA, the RNA viruses need to have their own RNA-dependent polymerase for replication to take place. The details of RNA replication vary depending on the nature of the viral RNA, and both new viral RNA and mRNA are produced from the original viral genome.

After uncoating, the viral RNA may serve as its own mRNA. This is then translated, resulting in the formation of an RNA polymerase, which in turn is necessary for the formation of a replicative intermediate form of the viral RNA. This is double stranded, containing one strand from the parent RNA and one that is complementary to it.

At this time a series of **inhibitors** is formed; these effectively switch off the normal synthetic processes of the host cell.

From the double-stranded 'replicative' RNA, single-stranded viral RNA molecules are formed. These may then function in three ways:

1) They may serve as templates for further viral RNA synthesis.
2) They may serve as mRNA for capsid protein synthesis.
3) They may themselves become encapsidated forming mature virions.

Retroviral Replication

In one group of RNA viruses, the **retroviruses**, which cause acquired immune deficiency syndrome and are also known to produce neoplasms in many animal species, the pattern of replication is different. Genetic information derived from the virus is inserted into the **host genome** and this inserted segment must, of course, be DNA. The existence of this DNA means that **viral RNA must be copied into DNA**. For viral replications to occur, new mRNA must be transcribed from this newly formed DNA in order for new viral proteins to be synthesized.

The formation of the DNA replica from the viral RNA is accomplished by a unique enzyme system known as **RNA-dependent DNA polymerase (reverse transcriptase)**. This DNA replica, the proviral DNA, is then integrated into the host cell DNA. Transcription from the provirus is mediated by host cell RNA polymerases. The transcribed RNA then serves both as mRNA for the synthesis of viral antigens and as genomic RNA which is packaged into new virions.

The properties of an archetypal retrovirus, HIV-1, are described on pp 122–125.

During all the events that follow penetration of the virions into the host cells, virus particles

cannot be detected within the infected cells. This is known as the **eclipse phase**. Its length varies from virus to virus, ranging from minutes in the case of certain bacterial viruses (**bacteriophages**) to hours in the case of some viruses infecting more complex life forms.

Once the viruses have been assembled they are **released** from the infected cell. This may occur by:

- bursting or lysis of the host cell
- budding from the host cell membrane

In the latter case the host cell is not destroyed. Where release occurs by budding, the virus frequently becomes enveloped. The viral glycoproteins constituting the envelope are inserted into the plasma membrane of the host cell in the form of spikes. Beneath this there may be a matrix protein (M protein) which serves as an attachment point for the nucleocapsid. This altered segment of the host cell plasma membrane is wrapped round the nucleocapsid and the completed virion can then bud off from the cell in which replication has taken place (*Fig. 17.4*).

Morphological and Functional Effects of Viruses on Host Cells

The range of structural changes produced by viral infections is extensive (see *Fig. 17.5*).

No Change

Cells in which the viral infection is of the **latent** variety show no structural abnormalities.

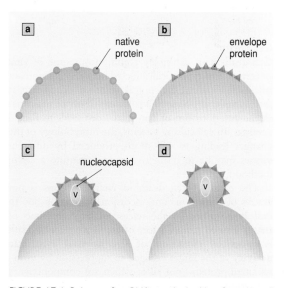

FIGURE 17.4 Release of an RNA virus by budding from the cell surface. **a** *Surface membrane of the host cell with 'native' proteins.* **b** *A segment of the host cell membrane expresses the virally coded envelope proteins.* **c** *The nucleocapsid adheres to the altered segment of the host cell surface membrane.* **d** *The altered segment of the cell surface membrane becomes wrapped round the nucleocapsid.*

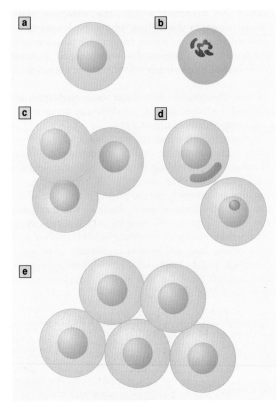

FIGURE 17.5 The effects of viruses on their target cells. **a** No change (latency); **b** cell death; **c** cell fusion; **d** formation of inclusion bodies; **e** cell proliferation.

Cell Death

Cell death is an extremely common outcome of viral infection. The type of cell affected may play a dominant role in determining the clinical pattern of the disease, as for example in poliomyelitis where death of neurones in the anterior horn of the spinal cord leads to flaccid paralysis. In cell culture systems, the morphology of the changes leading to cell death produced by different viruses may be so distinctive as to constitute a useful method for diagnosis.

The cause of cell death in viral infections is not always obvious. On some occasions it may be due to **cell lysis** caused by the release of large numbers of newly formed virions. More often, however, cell death is caused by **cessation of the normal synthetic activity** of the target cell due to suppression by virus-specified proteins, not all of which are components of the virion.

Cell death is not always caused directly by replicating virus. In some instances, the presence of a virus within a cell may lead to the expression of virally coded proteins on the cell surface. These are recognized as foreign by the immune system and immune-mediated lysis of the infected cells follows (see pp 115–116).

Alterations to Cell Surface Membranes

Some viruses, especially certain members of the paramyxovirus group, cause **fusion** to take place between infected and non-infected cells, with the formation of multinucleated giant cells. This is seen not uncommonly in the tissues of patients suffering from **measles**, the giant cells being found chiefly, but not exclusively, in lymphoid tissue (*Fig. 17.6*). The highly characteristic mulberry-like giant cells are known as **Warthin–Finkeldey cells** and may be useful in the diagnosis of measles in tissue sections from patients dying from measles pneumonia.

Formation of Inclusion Bodies

An inclusion body is a localized change detected on light microscopy in the staining properties of either the nucleus or cytoplasm of cells that have been infected by certain viruses. **They are rounded, sharply demarcated areas which usually show a marked affinity for acid dyes and are thus strongly eosinophilic in sections stained with haematoxylin and eosin.**

Intracytoplasmic inclusions are found in cells infected by poxviruses, paramyxoviruses and reoviruses. In one of the rhabdoviral infections (rabies), pathognomonic inclusions are present in neurones within the brain and spinal cord (**Negri bodies**).

Intranuclear inclusions may be present in cells infected by herpesviruses (*Fig. 17.7*) and adenoviruses.

Inclusion bodies can be helpful in the diagnosis of certain viral infections. For example, if difficulty were experienced in distinguishing between a severe case of chickenpox (varicella) and smallpox, examination of cells scraped from a lesion would reveal intranuclear inclusions in the former and intracytoplasmic ones in the latter. These criteria for diagnosis have been largely superseded by electron microscopy. Most inclusion bodies have been shown either by immunofluorescent or electron microscopic studies to be sites of viral synthesis within the cell. However, on some occasions, as

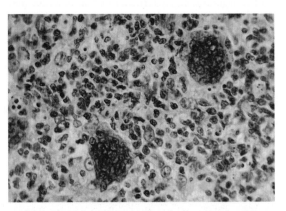

FIGURE 17.6 Multinucleate Warthin–Finkeldey giant cells in lymphoid tissue in a case of measles.

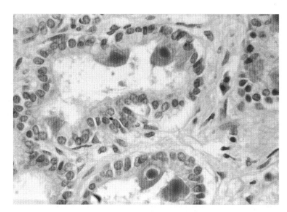

FIGURE 17.7 Intranuclear inclusions in pancreatic ductules in a case of cytomegalovirus infection.

in the case of herpesvirus infections, the inclusions do not consist of viral elements and may represent accumulations of byproducts of viral replication.

Cell Proliferation

Independent of any oncogenic effect, some viral infections can cause cells to proliferate. This is seen in a very common self-limiting disorder, **infectious mononucleosis**, in which the patients, usually young adults, present with malaise, sore throat and enlarged lymph nodes.

Infectious mononucleosis is caused by a herpesvirus, the **Epstein–Barr virus**, of which the target cell is the B lymphocyte. B lymphocytes proliferate and develop new antigens on their cell surface membranes. These virally coded antigens elicit a cytotoxic T-cell reaction which brings the virus-induced B-cell proliferation to an end.

Neoplastic Transformation

Viruses are directly implicated in the causation of many neoplastic disorders in non-human species and in some human tumours. This question is discussed in the section dealing with oncogenesis (pp 301–304).

NATURAL HISTORY OF VIRAL INFECTIONS

Viral infections may be divided into two main groups:
1) Infections that cause lesions **only at the portal of entry** (e.g. influenza and other viral infections of the respiratory tract).
2) Infections associated with **systemic spread**. In this case, viruses travel from the **portal of entry** to the **target organ**, producing the typical disease (e.g. poliomyelitis). In certain viral infections, both local and systemic lesions may occur.

Many of the effects of a viral infection (whether local or systemic) depend on the rate at which viral replication proceeds and whether the infected host cells are killed, either from lysis or from inhibition of their own synthetic processes by viral proteins.

Acute Productive Infections

Where a virus replicates actively within an infected cell and new viruses are released from such a cell, the infection is spoken of as being **productive**. This may lead to the patient experiencing an acute illness, often febrile, the clinical picture of which will be modified by the nature of the cells that are killed. Within a few weeks either the virus is eliminated or the infected person dies.

Not all acute infections, however, produce a clinically apparent disease. In many instances viral infections are subclinical and the only objective evidence that they have occurred is the presence of appropriate antibodies in the plasma.

Failure of Viral Elimination

Failure to eliminate virus from an infected host may lead to a number of different situations. Such infections can be:
- **Latent**, in which the virus is not normally detected. The infection persists in an occult, quiescent form with episodes of reactivation in the form of acute, self-limiting illnesses.
- **Chronic**, in which virus may be detected continuously in the host; symptoms may be mild or absent. This is seen typically in infants infected *in utero* by hepatitis B virus (HBV).
- **Persistent** and **slow** infections, in which the infection persists and causes a prolonged disease which is slow to develop and often inexorable in its progress.
- **Oncogenic**, in which part of the viral genome is incorporated into the host genome, resulting in malignant transformation.

Latent Infections

True latency implies the **persistence of virus in such small amounts that ordinary methods fail to**

detect its presence. However, the virus will usually appear if the infected tissue is cultured, and may be identified by means of labelled viral probes.

Latent infections tend to occur particularly with viruses of the **herpes** group. Amongst the commonest clinical expressions of this are the 'cold sores' or 'fever blisters' affecting many people at frequent intervals throughout their lives (*Fig. 17.8*). These are due to infections with the **herpes simplex virus**, which produces clusters of little vesicles, usually at the mucocutaneous junctions of the lips. The vesicles rupture, leading to painful ulcers that heal without scarring.

At various times, often in association with fever, sunburn, menstruation, etc, the vesicular lesions recur, always at the same site. Between these clinical episodes the virus can be recovered only with difficulty or often not at all.

The virus remains latent within the cells of the trigeminal ganglion between attacks and is released from the cells of the ganglion when they are cultured. The trigeminal ganglion is believed to harbour the herpesvirus in about 80% of adults.

Another virus of the herpes family, the **varicella zoster virus**, provides another common example of latency with occasional reactivation. The latter manifests as herpes zoster or shingles. This is characterized by a painful rash, usually limited to an area of skin or mucous membrane served by a single sensory ganglion. It occurs for the most part in individuals over 50 years of age and is **found only in those who have had chickenpox (varicella) in the past**.

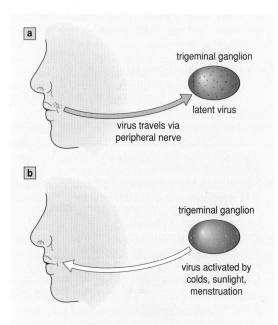

FIGURE 17.8 *Herpes simplex: an example of latency in viral infection.* **a** *Primary infection leading to latency.* **b** *Recurrent infection following activation of latent virus ('cold sore').*

Zoster and varicella are two distinct manifestations of infection by a single virus. Varicella represents the primary infection, and zoster the reactivation of the virus that has lain latent in sensory ganglia since the attack of the varicella, which may have occurred many years before.

Zoster is infectious to those who have not had varicella; infection in such an individual leads to an attack of chickenpox, not of shingles.

Zoster seems to increase in frequency in relation to X-irradiation and a similar increase is seen in patients suffering from Hodgkin's disease. This suggests that the expression of infection and the appearance of clinical manifestations are controlled by the state of immunity of the host. However X-irradiation of mice does not seem to have this effect.

Persistent Infections

These may be due to:
- well-characterized viral agents such as measles or hepatitis virus
- agents of unknown nature

In the first situation the virus is not eliminated from the host and goes on replicating inside infected cells, usually at a rate that does not cause any direct tissue damage. Often the infected individual will **carry** the virus in blood or other tissue fluids; such a patient may be a dangerous source of infection to others. Roughly one-third of patients who have an acute episode of hepatitis due to HBV will become carriers, and there are many more carriers with no history of a diagnosable episode of jaundice.

It is estimated that there may be as many as 300 000 000 carriers of HBV in the world. Obviously there is a considerable risk of the virus being passed on through the medium of blood transfusions, etc., and screening of donors for this and, indeed, other carrier states is clearly important. Other types of viral infection in which this asymptomatic carrier state can develop include **cytomegalovirus** and **Epstein–Barr virus** infection.

In some instances chronic asymptomatic infections may lead eventually to the appearance of serious, clinically apparent, disease. An example of this is **lymphocytic choriomeningitis** in the common household mouse. The virus (one of the **arenavirus** family) is transmitted vertically from generation to generation, the infection being acquired *in utero*. This infection appears to be associated with low zone tolerance in which T lymphocytes are tolerant but B lymphocytes are not. Low levels of antibody to viral antigens are produced which eventually cause the appearance of glomerulonephritis in old mice. The tolerance that develops is associated with the fact that the lymphocytic choriomeningitis infection occurs during the perinatal period. If mature, immunologically competent, mice are infected with this virus, they develop a severe inflammation in the brain (**encephalitis**).

A rather different type of chronic infection is seen in a small number of patients as a result of infection with **measles virus**. The disease, which follows the very long-continued localization of measles virus in the brain, is known as **subacute sclerosing panencephalitis**. The peak incidence of this, happily rare, condition is during adolescent life. Affected patients present with increasing reduction of intellectual function, motor abnormalities and fits. An inexorable downward path is followed by death within a year of the appearance of symptoms. The patients' brains show degenerative features with loss of myelin and a mild increase in the supporting glial fibres. There is also evidence of an encephalitis in the form of a perivascular lymphocytic infiltrate. Cerebrospinal fluid contains high titres of measles antibody and viral antigen, and nucleocapsid material can be identified in cells within the brain as well as within lymph nodes. It has been suggested that the disorder is an expression of an aberrant T-cell response to the presence of virus in the brain, but this is still a matter of debate.

Slow Progressive Infections
The term 'slow virus infection' was introduced to describe certain very slowly developing and chronic diseases in sheep, originally observed in Iceland, caused by members of the **lentivirus** group: **visna** and **maedi**.

In animals, slow virus infections occur in three disorders:

1) Maedi produces a slowly progressive pneumonia in Icelandic sheep.
2) Visna produces a progressive demyelinating disease, also of sheep.
   Both these diseases are caused by retroviruses and are transmissible with incubation periods of several years.
3) Aleutian mink disease is a slowly developing syndrome caused by chronic infection by a member of the **parvovirus** group. There is a humoral immune response but this does not succeed in eliminating the virus.
   Soluble immune complex formation is a prominent feature and most affected animals develop an immune complex-mediated glomerulonephritis. Other evidence of a disturbance in the regulation of the immune response is present in the form of hypergammaglobulinaemia and antibodies directed against red cell antigens.

Slow Infections may be Caused by Conventional Viruses
Subacute sclerosing panencephalitis, described above as a chronic infection, could just as well be regarded as a slow virus infection, because the onset of symptoms usually follows on a considerable period after the original measles infection.

Another slow viral infection in humans is **progressive multifocal leucoencephalopathy**, a rare disease of the brain leading to focal demyelination in many areas of the white matter. It is caused by infections with members of the **papovavirus** group and occurs only in patients who are immunosuppressed. Such immunosuppression may be seen in patients with neoplastic disease involving the lymphoid system, such as Hodgkin's disease, and also in those who are receiving cytotoxic chemotherapy in the course of treatment for malignant disease. The papovaviruses that have been isolated from the brains of affected individuals (the JC virus) are widespread, at least in Europe and the USA, and papovavirus infections in the general population are usually acquired fairly early in life.

Creutzfeldt–Jakob Disease and Other Transmissible Spongiform Encephalopathies
There is a group of slow, relentlessly progressive, disorders of the central nervous system occurring in both humans and animals, which, while being clearly **transmissible**, do not appear to be caused by agents with the characteristics of true viruses or indeed of any living agent. These disorders have been termed the **spongiform encephalopathies** because of the histological changes seen in the central nervous system. They are discussed in Chapter 45 (see pp 1141–1143).

Transforming Infections
Viruses can produce **malignant neoplasms** in a variety of animal species and play a part in the induction of some human neoplasms. They can also induce transformation of cells (chiefly of connective tissue origin) in culture. Viral transformation of this type is discussed in Chapter 28.

PROTECTIVE RESPONSES OF HOST CELLS AGAINST VIRAL INFECTIONS

Interferons
The term **viral interference** is used to describe the situation in which a viral infection in an animal appears, in some way, to protect against subsequent infections by another virus.

In 1957, Isaacs and Lindemann showed that cells infected with inactivated influenza virus released soluble compounds into the culture medium. These soluble compounds inhibited the replication of normal influenza virus within other cells. The blanket term 'interferon' (IFN) has been applied to these host-coded proteins, which inhibit viral replication and constitute an important line of defence against viral infections.

Many interferons exist which are classified broadly into three groups known as
1) IFN-α, which is released chiefly from leucocytes
2) IFN-β, released chiefly from fibroblasts
3) IFN-γ, released by activated T lymphocytes

Despite this tendency to identify certain interferons predominantly with certain cell types, it is likely that all cells can produce α and β interferons when suitably stimulated.

The most important inducers of IFN-α and IFN-β release are viral infections, although the production can be triggered by rickettsiae, protozoa, bacterial endotoxins and even certain synthetic polynucleotides (poly I (polyriboinosinic acid) : poly C (polyribocytidilic acid)).

Interferons produced by viral infection are species specific (i.e. chick interferon will not protect rat or monkey cells against infection), but are not virus specific. They appear between 12 and 48 hours after infection and shortly after their appearance viral replication starts to decline. They are extremely powerful; it has been estimated that fewer than 50 molecules of interferon per infected cell suffice to inhibit viral replication.

The stimulus to interferon production in virus-infected cells appears to be foreign double-stranded RNA formed in the course of viral replication. How this induces the formation of the interferons is not known (*Fig. 17.9*).

Action of Interferon

The protective effect of interferon is not limited to a single virus because, unlike antibody, it does not interact directly with the virus. The interferon secreted by an infected cell diffuses from that cell and binds to a membrane receptor on the surface of neighbouring non-infected cells. IFN-α and IFN-β bind to the same receptor, that for IFN-γ being quite distinct. IFN binding triggers tyrosine kinase activity, leading to the transcription of genes encoding enzymes that block viral replication.

There is no inhibition of viral attachment or penetration of the cell to which the interferon has bound. The protective effect is mediated by blocking the translation of viral mRNA in the host cell polyribosomes. There are two ways in which this can be done.

1) Cells to which interferon has bound contain increased amounts of an adenine trinucleotide, which activates a ribonuclease that can destroy certain mRNAs.

2) Bound interferon stimulates a protein kinase which phosphorylates and thus inactivates a protein initiation factor and thus inhibits synthesis of viral protein.

In both these situations double-stranded RNA is required, so that the inhibition of translation occurs only in cells infected by a virus (*Fig. 17.10*).

Other Effects of Interferon

In addition to the protection of cells against viral infection outlined above, the interferons have other actions. At high dose levels some interferons, especially IFN-α can inhibit cell proliferation and this has drawn attention to a possible role for them as **antitumour agents**. Unfortunately, high doses of interferons are associated with a number of unpleasant side-effects such as nausea, loss of hair, fever, and depression of platelet and leuco-

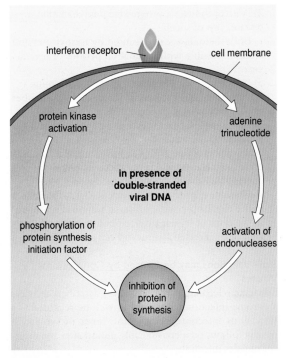

FIGURE 17.9 *Production of interferon in a cell infected by a virus.*

FIGURE 17.10 *Interferon binds to a non-infected cell and blocks translation of the viral messenger RNA.*

cyte production by the bone marrow. The interferons also have an effect on some immune functions, being associated with increased T-cell and natural killer cell activity and decreased antibody formation.

Protective Response of the Immune System

The ways in which the elements of the immune system respond to viral infections are discussed in Chapter 10.

A BRIEF CLASSIFICATION OF VIRUSES

Most known viruses can be separated into clearly defined groups on the basis of a number of criteria:
1) The type and form of the nucleic acid genome.
2) The size and morphology of the virus.
3) The natural method of transmission from host to host.
4) Susceptibility to a variety of chemical and physical agents.
5) Viral preference for certain hosts, tissues and cells.
6) The diseases they cause (see *Table 17.1*)

DNA-CONTAINING VIRUSES

Poxviruses

The poxviruses are divided into two subfamilies depending on whether they affect vertebrates or not. In humans the variola virus caused **smallpox** (now eradicated), and others cause **vaccinia** (cowpox), **alastrim** and a curious disorder characterized by waxy nodules on the skin and trunk known as **molluscum contagiosum**.

Many poxviruses infect non-human species exclusively, but some, such as the viruses causing **orf**, **cowpox** and **monkeypox**, may, rarely, cause disease both in animals and humans.

Some poxviruses, notably vaccinia, produce a growth factor that shows homology with both epidermal growth factor and transforming growth factor α; indeed the vaccinia growth factor has been shown to enhance wound healing. This growth factor production by poxviruses may be associated with the recognized ability of some of them to cause proliferative lesions in

KEY POINTS: Poxviruses
- The viruses of the pox group are the largest and most complicated known.
- They are brick-shaped or elliptical and contain double-stranded DNA.
- The nucleocapsid is enveloped by a double membrane.
- Poxviruses are unique in that they replicate solely within the cytoplasm of the host cell, where the site of the viral replication may appear as an inclusion body.

Table 17.1 Viruses and the Diseases They Cause

Disease	Virus
General diseases, in which blood spread of viruses occurs and many organs are affected	Vaccinia
	Measles
	Rubella
	Chickenpox
	Yellow fever
	Dengue
	Enteroviruses
Localized diseases	
Nervous system	Poliovirus
	Coxsackie
	Echoviruses
	Rabies
	Insect-borne encephalitides
	Herpes simplex
	Mumps
	Measles
	Vaccinia
	Papovaviruses (JC and BK)
Respiratory tract	Influenza
	Parainfluenza
	Respiratory syncytial virus
	Adenovirus
	Viruses causing the common cold
Skin and mucous membanes	HSV type 1 (mainly oral)
	HSV type 2 (mainly genital)
	Molluscum contagiosum
	HPV (warts)
	Herpes zoster
Eye	Adenovirus (conjunctivitis)
	Herpesvirus (keratoconjunctivitis)
	Enterovirus 70 (epidemic haemorrhagic conjunctivitis)
Liver	Hepatitis A
	Hepatitis type B
	Hepatitis type C
	Hepatitis type D
	Hepatitis type E
	Yellow fever
	In the newborn:
	Herpesvirus
	Enteroviruses
	Rubella virus

contd

Table 17.1 Viruses and the Diseases They Cause – *continued*

Disease	Virus
Localized diseases – *contd*	
Salivary glands	Mumps
	Cytomegalovirus
Sexually transmitted diseases	HSV
	Hepatitis B
	HPV
	Molluscum contagiosum
	HIV-1 and HIV-2
	Cytomegalovirus
Gastrointestinal tract	Rotavirus
	Norwalk virus
	Enteric adenoviruses

HSV, herpes simplex virus; HPV, human papillomavirus.

> ### KEY POINTS: Herpesviruses
> - Viruses of this group are large (the nucleocapsids measuring 90–110 nm and the enveloped forms 120–200 nm in diameter).
> - The viral genome consists of double-stranded DNA.
> - The capsid possesses icosahedral symmetry and is surrounded by a lipid-containing envelope.
> - There is little DNA homology among the different herpesvirus types and even different strains of the same type show considerable DNA differences. This has made possible the epidemiological tracing of different strains.
> - The virus forms intranuclear inclusion bodies (known as Cowdry type A bodies), which are rich in DNA and virtually fill the nucleus.

animals (e.g. Shope fibroma) and humans (molluscum contagiosum).

Herpesviruses

Herpesviruses may be classified on the basis of their biological activities. Thus we have:

- α **herpesviruses** which grow fast, are cytolytic and tend to establish latent infections in neurones.
- β **herpesviruses** which are slow growing and cause enlargement of the cells they infect (cytomegaly). They become latent in secretory epithelium and in renal tubular epithelium.
- γ **herpesviruses** infect lymphoid cells and cause them to proliferate (e.g. Epstein–Barr virus (herpesvirus 4)).

Herpesviruses are responsible for **cold sores** and **genital blistering** (herpes simplex virus) (*Fig. 17.11*), **chickenpox** (varicella) and **shingles** (zoster), **infectious mononucleosis** (Epstein–Barr virus) and cytomegalo-

virus-associated disorders, some of which occur in the context of intrauterine infections of the fetus with severe consequences. Herpesvirus type I can also produce a severe **encephalitis**, **keratoconjunctivitis** characterized by keratitis and/or corneal ulceration, and **Kaposi's varicelliform eruption** (a severe and extensive blistering disorder of the skin that tends to occur in those with chronic eczema). The Epstein–Barr virus (a γ herpesvirus) probably also plays a role in the induction of Burkitt's lymphoma (see pp 968–969) and nasopharyngeal carcinoma (see pp 303, 415). Evidence has also appeared recently that a novel type of herpesvirus (herpesvirus VIII) is implicated in Kaposi's sarcoma.

Adenoviruses

Adenoviruses can be divided into seven main groups on the basis, *inter alia*, of the animal species whose red cells they agglutinate. They can be further subdivided into 33 subtypes on the basis of antigenic differences in hexon and fibre proteins. Of the subtypes that cause infection in humans, many exhibit **latency** and may survive in lymphoid tissue such as the tonsil for many years.

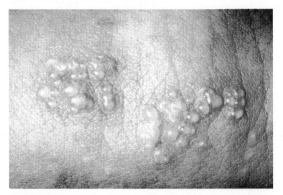

FIGURE 17.11 *Typical crops of blisters found in herpes simplex infections.*

> ### KEY POINTS: Adenoviruses
> - Like the herpesviruses, the adenoviruses are also medium sized (70–90 nm).
> - They contain double-stranded DNA and are icosahedral.
> - Most of the 252 capsomeres are hexons but 12 are pentons in which the cytotoxic potential of these viruses resides. From the pentons that form the corners of the virion, fine fibres project, each terminating in a knob-like structure. These terminal knobs are responsible for the agglutination of red blood cells and for adhesion to host cells.
> - The nucleocapsid is not enveloped and the virus resists treatment with ether.
> - Viral replication occurs within the host cell nucleus.

The disorders caused in humans by adenoviruses are summarized in *Table 17.2*.

Papovaviruses

This family derives its name from its three members:

- *PA*pillomavirus
- *PO*lyomavirus
- *VA*cuolating virus in monkeys

Gene products of these viruses may bind with proto-oncogenes and activate them. For example, the middle T antigen of simian virus 40 (SV40) complexes with the *c-src* gene product and activates its tyrosine kinase function. Similarly, gene products of both polyoma and papilloma viruses can bind with the gene products of tumour suppressor genes and inactivate them (see p 285).

Parvoviruses

Human parvovirus B19 is the cause of a number of diseases.

KEY POINTS: *Papovaviruses*

- These viruses are small (43–53 nm) and contain double-stranded DNA arranged in a circular pattern.
- In animals, papillomaviruses cause a variety of neoplasms; in humans they cause the common wart and almost certainly have a role in the pathogenesis of cervical neoplasia and other squamous neoplasms of the genital region.
- Polyomavirus infections (JC virus) are also associated with **progressive multifocal encephalopathy**, a rare degenerative condition of the cerebral white matter seen in immunosuppressed patients, usually with malignant lymphomas (see p 1119).

KEY POINTS: *Parvoviruses*

- As their name implies (*parvus* small), these are very small viruses with a diameter of about 20 nm.
- They contain single-stranded DNA and their replication takes place in the nucleus of the infected cell.
- Parvovirus infection in humans causes:
  a) temporary erythroid aplasia in patients with chronic haemolytic anaemia (e.g. sickle cell disease)
  b) a common rash illness of childhood (erythema infectiosum or 'fifth disease')
  c) one variety of gastroenteritis occurring particularly in cold weather ('winter vomiting disease')

Table 17.2 Adenoviral Diseases

System affected	Disease
Respiratory tract	**Acute febrile pharyngitis**: affects infants and children most commonly; usually caused by group C viruses. Patients complain of stuffy nose, cough, sore throat and fever.
	Pharyngoconjunctival fever: symptoms as above but conjunctivitis is also present. This disorder tends to occur in outbreaks in closed communities such as children's summer camps. Usually caused by group B viruses.
	Acute respiratory disease: characterized by fever, pharyngitis, cough and malaise. Tends to occur in young military recruits and is associated with overcrowding and fatigue. Caused by group B viruses.
	Pneumonia: this is a complication of acute respiratory disease. It may affect children as well as young adults and the mortality rate among the former is high (8–10%). Severe adenoviral pneumonia also occurs in immunocompromised individuals such as post-transplant patients.
Eye	**Mild self-limiting conjunctivitis** associated with respiratory and pharyngeal syndromes.
	Follicular conjunctivitis resembling that caused by *Chlamydia*; self-limiting.
	Epidemic keratoconjunctivitis: acute conjunctivitis associated with enlargement of the preauricular nodes. This is followed by corneal inflammation with the formation of subepithelial corneal opacities, which last for up to 2 years.
Gut	**Infantile gastroenteritis**: this can occur in the presence of infection by two adenovirus serotypes (40 and 41).
Other	**Acute haemorrhagic cystitis**: this occurs in boys and is particularly associated with infections by types 11 and 21.

Hepadnaviruses

There is only one virus in this group that causes disease in humans: the virus causing hepatitis B. There are many types, however, that cause hepatitis in animals such as woodchucks, squirrels and ducks. The virus and its effects are discussed in the section on liver diseases, as are the other hepatitis viruses (see pp 571–578).

RNA-CONTAINING VIRUSES

Picornaviruses

Enteroviruses include:

1) Three types of **poliovirus**.
2) Twenty-nine types of **coxsackievirus**.
3) Thirty-two types of **echovirus** (*e*nteric *c*ytopathic *h*uman *o*rphan virus). The term 'orphan' refers to the fact that for some time they were regarded as 'viruses in search of a disease'.

The enteroviruses cause a wide range of diseases in humans, including **poliomyelitis, aseptic meningitis, myocarditis (chiefly in the newborn), myositis, herpangina and upper respiratory tract infections**.

Infection occurs via both the **alimentary** and **respiratory** tracts, the former being much more important in the case of poliovirus infection. There is no natural animal host. This has interesting implications in respect of poliovirus, of which there are only three types. Vaccines have been prepared against all of these and it is quite possible that, following widespread immunization, the disease may be eliminated in a similar way to smallpox.

Most poliovirus infections are symptomless but the virus, which is cytocidal, may spread to involve the anterior horn cells with resulting paralysis. (The pathogenesis of full-blown poliovirus infections of this kind is shown in *Fig. 17.2*).

Rhinoviruses, of which there are 113 types, cause the common cold.

KEY POINTS: Picornaviruses

- Picornaviruses (*pico* small) are very small (2–30 nm), non-enveloped, icosahedral viruses.
- They contain single-stranded RNA and are resistant to treatment with ether.
- This family includes important human pathogens, including the viruses responsible for poliomyelitis and the common cold.
- The picornaviruses are divided into two genera: the **enteroviruses** and the **rhinoviruses**.

Orthomyxoviruses

The acute respiratory disease caused by the influenza virus in humans can be fatal and may occur in very large-scale local epidemics, usually every 2–4 years, or even on a world-wide basis (pandemics) every 10–20 years. A single influenza virus infection does *not* confer lifelong immunity to the disease. An important part of the reason for this curious epidemiological behaviour lies in the fact that the **viral genome is continually changing**.

Minor changes in the haemagglutinins of a particular strain may occur as a result of a series of point mutations; over a long period, this process is called **antigenic drift**. From time to time a much more fundamental change occurs in which multiple alterations in the antigenic make-up of the viral strain, probably as a result of recombination of genome segments, appear suddenly. This is known as **antigenic shift**. The appearances of new subtypes of influenza virus as a result of antigenic shift are likely to be associated with the occurrence of pandemic outbreaks. Of the three types of influenza virus – A, B and C – A is the most likely to undergo antigenic shift and is responsible for most epidemics of influenza. Type B and C viruses do not undergo antigenic shift, C being the most stable.

The pathogenesis of influenza is shown in *Fig. 17.12*. Sporadic cases are usually fairly mild and self-limiting. Sometimes, especially in the elderly, severe pneumonia supervenes. This is most commonly due to a secondary bacterial infection, although in rare instances it is a primary viral pneumonia, in which intrapulmonary haemorrhage is a conspicuous feature.

KEY POINTS: Orthomyxoviruses

- As defined currently, the orthomyxoviruses contain only viruses that cause human influenza.
- They are medium sized with a helically arranged capsid, contain single-stranded DNA and are enveloped. The lipid envelope is somewhat unusual in that it is studded with spike-like projections called peplomers. These are of two varieties, the first being a viral haemagglutinin which binds to the NANA on the surface membrane of most cells, and the second being a neuraminidase.
- In morphological terms they are pleomorphic, some viruses being spherical in shape whereas others are filamentous.
- The arrangement of the RNA is distinctly unusual. Instead of being a continuous thread, it exists in the form of eight segments, each of which represents a single gene. These eight gene segments code for 10 or 11 viral proteins, this being explained by the pattern of splicing of two of the mRNAs.

Paramyxoviruses

Viruses of this group cause:

- sore throats and croup (parainfluenza virus)
- measles
- mumps
- infections of the lower respiratory tract (respiratory syncytial virus)

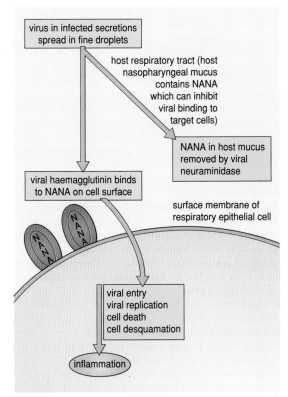

FIGURE 17.12 Pathogenesis of influenza. NANA, N-acetylneuraminic acid.

KEY POINTS: Paramyxoviruses

- These viruses were originally grouped with the orthomyxoviruses because of the morphological features that they share.
- They are roughly cuboid in shape.
- They are somewhat larger than orthomyxoviruses, but share with them a number of characteristics such as the presence of haemagglutinins and neuraminidase (which, in contrast to what is seen in the influenza virus, coexist on the same 'spike' on the envelope).

In animals, paramyxoviruses cause Newcastle disease in birds, distemper in dogs, and rinderpest in cattle.

One of the interesting characteristics of viruses of this family is that they promote cell fusion with the formation of multinucleate cells (see p 186). This feature has been used extensively in the production of hybrid cells, the virus employed for this purpose being Sendai virus (which causes parainfluenza in mice). The ability to promote cell fusion is conferred on the virus by its possession of a spike on the envelope glycoprotein. This glycoprotein is also necessary for penetration of the target cell, and strains that lack the F glycoprotein are not infective.

Rhabdoviruses

Rabies

Many warm-blooded animals such as dogs, foxes, bats, skunks and jackals are reservoirs for rabies virus. Victims of the disease are infected by the bite of a rabid animal, the virus being present in the saliva. The rabies virus appears to have a special affinity for nervous tissue and travels slowly up the peripheral nerves to reach the central nervous system where it causes the encephalitis characteristic of the disease.

In experimental rabies infections, where it is possible to examine specimens of peripheral nerves, viral particles have been seen in the axons on electron microscopy.

KEY POINTS: Rhabdoviruses

- Viruses of this group have a curious shape, being flattened at one end and rounded at the other.
- The genome consists of single-stranded RNA.
- The nucleocapsid is enclosed in an envelope which bears spikes of about 10 nm in length.
- This group includes the rabies virus, which causes one of the most serious of all viral infections.

Arenaviruses

Arenaviruses derived their name from the Latin word *harenaceus* meaning 'sandy'. This term was coined because of the electron–dense granules that can be seen within the virions on electron microscopy.

The natural hosts of arenaviruses appear to be rodents, which are often persistently infected. Humans are infected more or less by accident on exposure to rodent excretions. The resulting infections include some of the most lethal viral disorders known: Lassa fever and Argentinian and Bolivian haemorrhagic fevers. The natural host of the Lassa fever virus is a West African rodent, the multimammate rat, which is persistently but apparently harmlessly infected.

Another example of arenavirus infection in animals discussed earlier in this chapter is the virus that causes **lymphocytic choriomeningitis** in mice (see p 188).

Coronaviruses

Viruses of this family include several which, in many, cause the common cold. They are medium sized, rather pleomorphic, viruses which have widely spaced club-shaped peplomers in their lipoprotein envelope; it is the arrangement of these 'clubs' that gives this virus its distinctive appearance and its name.

Togaviruses

Togaviruses are spherical, closely enveloped, RNA viruses which contain single-stranded RNA. They multiply within the cytoplasm of their target cells and mature by budding from cytoplasmic membranes. All the togaviruses, with the exception of rubella, belong to a larger grouping known as the **arboviruses** (*arthropod-borne* viruses). Arthropods are not only the vectors for these viral infections, but are the primary natural **hosts** in which viral multiplication occurs before transmission to a secondary vertebrate host by insect bite. These vertebrates act as a **reservoir** for the viruses and are unaffected by the presence of the arboviruses. However, when humans, an unnatural host, are infected, serious and often lethal disorders arise, such as **yellow fever**, various encephalitides and some of the haemorrhagic fevers (*Fig. 17.13*).

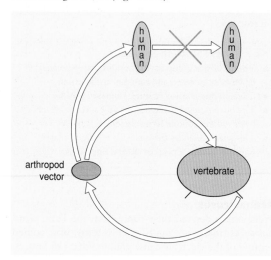

FIGURE 17.13 *Vector and vertebrate reservoirs for viral infections such as yellow fever.*

In human infections, the virus in the saliva of the insect, in the course of biting, is injected into capillaries. Viral multiplication occurs in the first instance in the vascular endothelium and in the fixed phagocytic cells of the reticuloendothelial system. There is a short-lived viraemia, which may be followed by a variety of clinical developments, depending on the precise nature of the virus and its localization. In the haemorrhagic fevers, bleeding occurs from many sites and death may result from hypovolaemic shock. In yellow fever, the liver and kidneys are affected, leading to jaundice and impaired renal function. There is massive necrosis in the mid-zones of the liver lobules and, as a consequence, a decrease in the synthesis of clotting factors formed in the liver.

Rubella

Rubella virus is a member of the togavirus family, but is not transmitted via an insect vector and is classified as being in the genus **Rubivirus**. Infection by the rubella virus has no serious consequences unless it occurs *in utero*, especially in the first 3 months of pregnancy. When this happens there is a high risk that the infant

will be born with a wide range of congenital defects, most notably in the heart, ears (nerve deafness) and eyes (cataract). Many other organs may be affected, and hepatitis and pneumonia in the neonatal period are quite common. The risks are so serious that rubella occurring in the first 3 months of a pregnancy constitutes good grounds for termination of that pregnancy. To prevent intrauterine infection with the rubella virus, girls may be immunized with an attenuated viral vaccine in their early teens. Alternatively, the vaccines may be given to all children in an attempt to eliminate the infection altogether.

Reoviruses

The acronym *reo* is derived from *r*espiratory, *e*nteric and *o*rphan. This is because the initial sites of isolation were the respiratory and gastrointestinal tracts, and because no diseases were known to be associated with this group of viruses (hence 'orphan'). Three genera are known, of which only two, **rotavirus** and **orbivirus**, cause disease in humans.

- **Orbivirus** is an arbovirus and causes Colorado tick fever.
- **Rotavirus** has a curious double-layered capsid, the outer layer appearing smooth on electron microscopy and the inner layer symmetrically 'roughened'. This gives the virion a wheel-like appearance, hence the name (L. *rota* wheel) (*Fig. 17.14*).

Rotaviruses are an important cause of gastroenteritis, mainly in young children (see pp 538–539), and of a similar syndrome in a variety of young animals. Diagnosis of gastroenteritis caused by these viruses can be made by examining stool samples either by electron microscopy, as the highly characteristic virions are present in large numbers in the faeces, or by immunological methods.

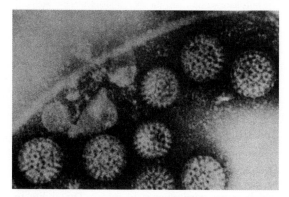

FIGURE 17.14 *Transmission electron micrograph of rotavirus in the stool of an infant with severe diarrhoea. The typical wheel-like appearance of this virus is due to the presence of a double-layered capsid, the outer layer being smooth and the inner layer being symmetrically roughened on electron microscopy. (Photograph by courtesy of Professor J. Pattison.)*

Retroviruses

Retroviruses occur in many vertebrate species and are implicated in many diseases. All have a diploid RNA genome which encodes **reverse transcriptase** (RNA-dependent DNA polymerase). The retroviral genome consists of at least three genes: *gag*, *pol* and *env*.

Gag encodes a precursor protein that is cleaved, yielding internal structural proteins; the reverse transcriptase is encoded by *pol* and the two disulphide-linked envelope proteins by *env*.

The retrovirus family is divided into three sub-families:

1) **Oncovirinae**, which includes tumour-producing viruses.
2) **Lentivirinae**, which includes HIV and the non-primate viruses causing Maedi and Visna.
3) **Spumavirinae** or foamy viruses.

Human Retroviruses

Four major classes of human retroviruses are recognized:

- human T-cell lymphotropic oncoviruses: HTLV-1 and HTLV-2
- human T-cell lymphotropic lentiviruses: HIV
- foamy viruses: these may be implicated in causing a granulomatous thyroiditis (de Quervain's thyroiditis) but this is not proven.
- endogenous retroviruses

Only HIV and HTLV are clearly linked with human disease (see pp 122–125).

Oncornaviruses

These are oncogenic RNA viruses belonging to family Retroviridae and responsible for the production of a wide variety of neoplasms of connective, lymphoid and haemopoietic tissue in a number of different animal species. They are also capable of inducing malignant transformation in cultured cells. This involves insertion of part of the viral genome into the genome of the target cell. As the viral genome consists only of RNA, clearly some mechanism must exist for transcribing DNA from the viral RNA; this is accomplished via the action of a virally coded enzyme system known as **reverse transcriptase**. The activity of these viruses is discussed in Chapter 28 (see pp 276–279).

CHAPTER 18

Disorders of Blood Flow: a Basis

Disorders of blood vessel are expressed in the form of:
- underperfusion of tissues (ischaemia)
- abnormal bleeding (see pp 911–912, 913–918, 921–924)

ISCHAEMIA

Ischaemia is the term used to define a state in which the arterial perfusion of an organ or tissue is insufficient to cater for the metabolic needs of that tissue. The circumstances that modulate the appearance of ischaemia in any vascular bed and the effects that it produces will be considered in Chapter 19.

Pathophysiology

ATHEROSCLEROSIS

Any pathological change causing either narrowing or blockage of an artery is likely to produce ischaemia in the tissue supplied by that vessel and distal to the point of narrowing or occlusion. In arteries, such narrowing is brought about by a widely prevalent disease of the wall of large elastic and muscular arteries known as **atherosclerosis**.

Eventual occlusion of the arterial lumen is caused by **platelets**, first adhering to an abnormal vascular surface and later aggregating one with another to form a plug that is capable of blocking the artery. Such a plug, which can form within a few seconds, is known as a **thrombus**. The process of thrombus formation is known as **thrombosis**.

In arteries, thrombosis is a frequent complication of atherosclerosis. Indeed, many workers hold the view that platelet deposition on the artery wall is intimately involved in the progression of atherosclerotic lesions.

In the West the complications of atherosclerosis kill more people than any other single disease, including all the forms of cancer. More than 150 000 patients die each year in Britain alone from the effects of coronary artery narrowing and occlusion, roughly one person for every 3 minutes of the day. Put another way, rather more than one-quarter of all deaths occurring in Britain are due to atherosclerosis.

Atherosclerosis is discussed fully in Chapter 32 (see pp 327–346).

THROMBOSIS

A thrombus is a solid mass or plug formed within the heart, arteries, veins or capillaries from the components of the streaming blood.

It is a matter of regret that thrombi and clots are often spoken of as being synonymous. It is important that the fundamental differences between the two processes should be appreciated (*Fig. 18.1*). In **clotting**

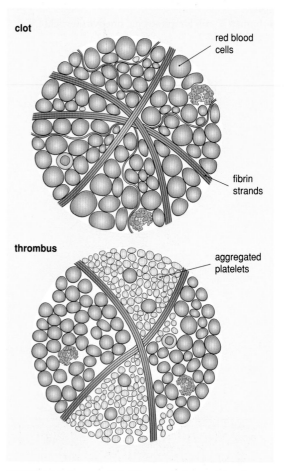

clot

red blood cells

fibrin strands

thrombus

aggregated platelets

FIGURE 18.1 *The essential differences between clot and thrombus. In the former the only process involved is conversion of soluble fibrinogen to insoluble polymerized fibrin. In the latter the various phases of platelet activation constitute an essential element.*

the activation of a protein cascade system within the blood leads to the generation of thrombin and thus to the conversion of the soluble plasma protein fibrinogen to the insoluble fibrin polymer (*Fig. 18.2*). **Thrombosis**, on the other hand, is characterized by a series of events involving the blood **platelets, which in essence involve the same mechanisms responsible for normal haemostasis**.

Platelets and Haemostasis

The contribution of platelets to haemostasis is mediated via a number of steps (*Fig. 18.3*):

- **adhesion of platelets to the underlying vessel wall**
- **release of pharmacologically active compounds**
- **aggregation (platelet to platelet) to form a plug**
- **provision of co-factors for clotting**

Adhesion

The platelet adheres to damaged endothelial cells or to exposed subendothelial components of the vessel wall. This is mediated through binding of vessel wall-derived ligands to glycoprotein receptors on the platelets.

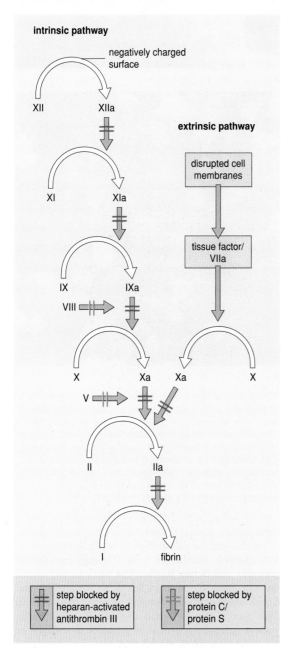

FIGURE 18.2 *The intrinsic and extrinsic clotting pathways showing the points at which the cascade is interrupted by either antithrombin III or the protein C–protein S system.*

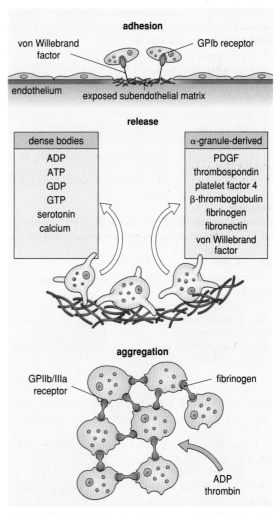

FIGURE 18.3 *The three phases of platelet activation: adhesion, release and aggregation. GP, glycoprotein; ADP, adenosine 5′-diphosphate; ATP, adenosine 5′-triphosphate; GDP, guanosine 5′-diphosphate; GTP, guanosine 5′-triphosphate; PDGF, platelet-derived growth factor.*

Collagen that is exposed when a vessel is damaged binds to a glycoprotein receptor (GP Ia), and von Willebrand's factor (**vWf**), a large multimeric glycoprotein synthesized by the endothelial cells, binds to GP Ib (*Fig. 18.4*).

Thus either deficient production of vWf (as is seen in von Willebrand's disease) or an absent Ib receptor (Bernard–Soulier syndrome) must lead to defective adhesion of platelets and will be reflected in an abnormally prolonged bleeding time.

Von Willebrand's disease is inherited for the most part as an autosomal dominant trait with variable penetrance. It is characterized by a prolonged bleeding time associated with defective platelet adhesion. vWf also carries Factor VIII in the plasma and prevents its premature degradation. Thus a patient with von Willebrand's disease shows depressed concentrations of Factor VIII in the plasma as well as defective platelet ahesion. The platelets themselves are normal, as are all their post-adhesion functions.

Laboratory Findings
- prolonged bleeding time
- low plasma concentration of vWf
- low plasma concentration of Factor VIII
- defective ristocetin-induced platelet aggregation. Ristocetin is an antibiotic, now withdrawn, because it causes thrombocytopenia, that causes aggregation of normal platelets *in vitro*.

Release
Adherent platelets undergo a marked shape change (*Fig. 18.5a* and *b*), releasing several preformed and newly

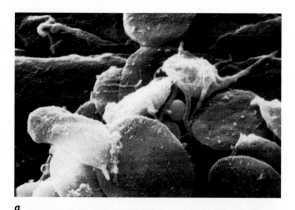
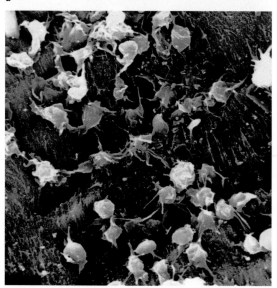

a

b

FIGURE 18.5 **a** *Scanning electron micrograph of platelets adhering to arterial endothelium. Some of the platelets quite clearly have retained a disciform appearance, whereas others have undergone a shape change and have contracted and put out pseudopod-like processes.* **b** *Scanning electron micrograph of platelets adhering to damaged endothelium in an ex vivo 'Baumgartner' chamber. The platelets seen here in a monolayer have all undergone shape change and have thus, by implication, released their granule contents.*

formed molecules which may affect both the haemostatic process and the metabolism of the underlying vessel wall. Platelets contain two types of storage granules: **α-granules** and **dense bodies**, the latter having a dark electron-dense centre and a less dense peripheral zone. A wide range of active chemical species is released from these (see *Table 18.1* and *Fig. 18.3*). The release reaction is usually triggered by exposure to collagen or thrombin (*Figs 18.6a* and *18.6b*).

In addition to the release of stored compounds, probably mediated via the activation of protein kinase C, **collagen and thrombin also initiate the release**

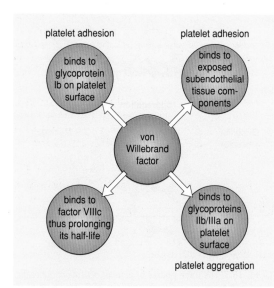

platelet adhesion — binds to glycoprotein Ib on platelet surface

platelet adhesion — binds to exposed subendothelial tissue components

von Willebrand factor

binds to factor VIIIc thus prolonging its half-life

binds to glycoproteins IIb/IIIa on platelet surface

platelet aggregation

FIGURE 18.4 *von Willebrand factor has roles in relation to platelet adhesion and aggregation, and in prolonging the half-life of Factor VIII$_c$.*

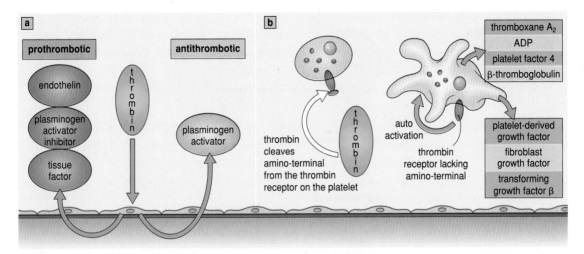

FIGURE 18.6 **a** *Some effects of thrombin on endothelium. Thrombin upregulates the synthesis and release by endothelium of certain prothrombotic molecules such as endothelin, plasminogen activator inhibitor 1 (PAI-1) and tissue factor. It also upregulates production by endothelial cells of the antithrombotic plasminogen activator.* **b** *Platelet activation by thrombin. Thrombin activates platelets by binding to a specific receptor on the platelet surface. It cleaves the amino-terminal from the receptor. The truncated receptor now acts as an auto-activator for the platelet, causing release of stored compounds from within the granules.*

Table 18.1 Compounds Released from Platelet Granules Following Activation

Granule type	Contents
α-Granule	PDGF, thrombospondin, platelet factor 4, β-thromboglobulin, fibrinogen, fibronectin, vWf, etc.
Dense body	ATP, ADP, GDP, GTP, serotonin, calcium

of arachidonate from the platelet membrane, the **first step in the synthesis of prostaglandins, including the powerfully antiaggregatory prostacyclin and the equally powerful proaggregatory thromboxane A$_2$** (*Fig. 18.7*).

Aggregation
This is the adhesion of platelets to other platelets, forming a mass of activated cells. It is accomplished by the formation of fibrinogen bridges between adjacent platelets. The fibrinogen molecule binds to heterodimeric receptors formed by a rearrangement of two platelet surface glycoproteins known as IIb and IIIa, which are members of the integrin family (see *Fig. 18.3*). This receptor also binds to vWf and may thus make a contribution to platelet adhesion as well. **The stimuli for aggregation are ADP and thromboxane A$_2$.** These also activate more platelets, with the release of more of these two compounds so that there is a positive feedback effect and rapid accumulation of platelets at sites of injury.

Provision of Co-Factors for Clotting
Platelets also interact with clotting cascade proteins such as Factors V, VIII, IX and X. Once platelets have been activated, phospholipids, normally present on the internal layer of platelet plasma membranes, are 'flipped' to the external aspect of the cell, playing an important part in the activation of prothrombin by Factor Xa, and in the activation of Factor X by the Factor IXa–VIIa complex.

Microanatomy of the Platelet
Of all the cells in the circulating blood, platelets are the most sensitive to a wide range of chemical and physical agents. For instance, minute amounts of catecholamines, which cause little or no response in neutrophils, monocytes, lymphocytes or red cells, can trigger irreversible changes in the platelet.

Understanding platelet physiology and pathology is made easier if we have some knowledge of the structure of the platelet; because it is so small, only ultrastructural studies are capable of providing this essential information.

The platelet circulates in the blood in the form of a flat disc. If such a disc is cut in the equatorial plane, **four major zones** can be seen on examination with the electron microscope (*Fig. 18.8*). These are:
1) The **peripheral** zone
2) The **sol-gel** zone
3) The **organelle** zone
4) The **membrane** zone

The Peripheral Zone
This consists of the surface membranes and structures closely associated with the surface.

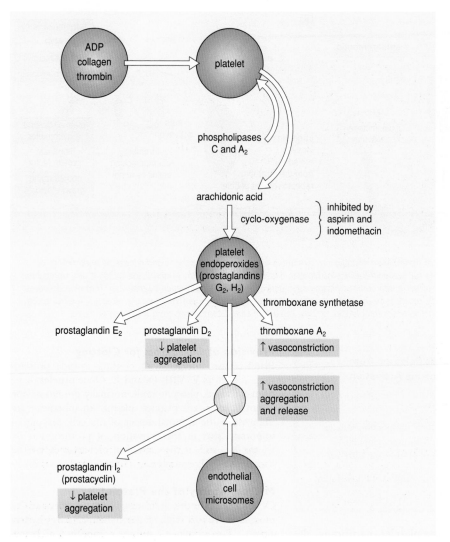

FIGURE 18.7 *Platelet activation causes arachidonic acid to be cleaved from membrane phospholipids and stimulates arachidonic acid metabolism with release of prostaglandins and thromboxanes.*

The Glycocalyx and its Receptors

There is an **exterior coat** or **glycocalyx** which is rich in glycoproteins. This houses the receptors for the signals that trigger platelet activation and the substrates for adhesion and aggregation reactions. Several different glycoprotein receptors have been identified, some of which clearly serve important roles in relation to platelet–platelet and platelet–vessel reactions (see above).

Platelets from patients with **thrombasthenia** lack glycoproteins IIb and IIIa and thus cannot bind fibrinogen and aggregate normally.

In **Bernard–Soulier syndrome**, platelets aggregate normally but fail to adhere to damaged blood vessels *in vivo*, or to bovine fibrinogen or the antibiotic ristocetin *in vitro*. This indicates that the glycoprotein Ib, which is absent from these platelets, is the receptor for vWf.

The Submembrane Filaments

Another component of the peripheral zone is the area that lies just deep to the unit membrane. It contains a system of filaments, which appear to be similar to microfilaments. They are believed to contribute to maintenance of the normal discoid shape of the unstimulated platelet and also interact with other elements of the platelet's contractile system.

The Surface-connected Canalicular System

An important element of the peripheral zone is the open canalicular system. This is a series of invaginations of the cell surface which ramify deeply within

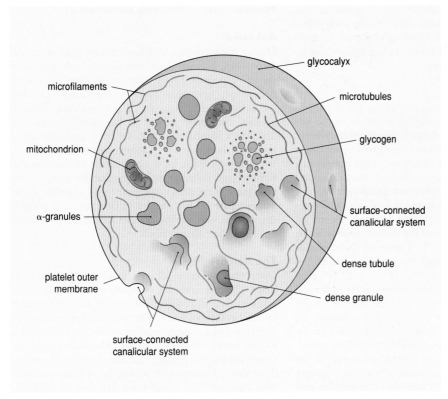

FIGURE 18.8 Microanatomy of a platelet.

the platelet and thus markedly increase its surface area in a manner analogous with the structure of a sponge. Its functions are closely interrelated with those of the membrane system, but structurally it shares the same features as other portions of the cell surface membrane.

The Sol-Gel Zone
Early studies with the phase contrast microscope suggested that the formed elements within platelets float in a fluid suspension. It is now known, as a result of ultrastructural studies, that fibres of various types are present in the cell matrix, and that changes in the state of polymerization and movement of these fibres are intimately related to maintenance of the discoid form and to internal contraction. At least three systems of fibres are present within the matrix:

1) The **submembrane fibres** mentioned above.
2) **Microtubules**, which are arranged as a circumferential band near the peripheral zone, suggesting that their role is to contribute to the support of the discoid shape of the unstimulated platelet. Agents such as colchicine, which interfere with the assembly of microtubules (see pp 56–57), dissolve platelet microtubules and cause loss of the discoid shape.
3) **Microfilaments** exist in a dynamic balance of sol-gel transformation and, like microfilaments in other cells, appear to consist of actin and myosin.

The Organelle Zone
Like many other cells, platelets contain mitochondria, lysosomes and peroxisomes. There are, in addition, two other types of intracytoplasmic organelle which are peculiar to the platelet.

The α-Granule
The contents of this organelle are listed above in *Table 18.1*. A rare defect (**the grey platelet syndrome**) is characterized by the absence of α-granules. These platelets lack all the proteins listed above. None of these is essential for platelet aggregation so long as the plasma concentration of fibrinogen is adequate. The only abnormalities noted are a somewhat prolonged bleeding time and easy bruising.

The Dense Body
This, as its name suggests, is much more electron-dense than the α-granule. Its contents are also listed in *Table 18.1*.

Dense bodies may be absent from platelets in a number of rare inherited syndromes, including the Hermansky–Pudlak syndrome (associated with albinism and accumulation of partly oxidized lipid in macrophages) and the Wiskott–Aldrich syndrome (see p 120). The lack of releasable ADP has its main effect on **aggregation**, but the bleeding problems in these patients are generally not severe as aggregation can be induced via other pathways.

The Membrane Zone

Two elements make up this part of the platelet structure. The first of these, referred to above, is the so-called **surface-connected open canalicular system**. This is a series of invaginations of the surface membrane which tunnel through the cytoplasm of the platelet in a serpentine manner. These channels remain open whether the platelet is inactive and discoid in shape, or activated, contracted and changed in shape. This suggests that the canaliculi serve not only as a means for increasing the surface area of the platelet susceptible to chemical signals, but also as a series of conduits for secretions produced by platelets in the course of the **release** phase of activation.

In addition to these channels, there is an additional membrane-related system of tubules known as the **dense tubular system**. These tubules consist of smooth endoplasmic reticulum derived from the parent megakaryocyte. In some areas within the cell the membranes of the dense tubular system and those of the open canalicular system are closely apposed in a manner similar to the relationship between sarcotubules and transverse tubules in muscle cells.

The role of these membrane systems can be appreciated most easily if the platelet is considered as being in some respects rather like a muscle cell, in that both types of cell contract on stimulation. The contraction of platelet actin and myosin, as in other situations, is modulated by calcium flux. In the platelet, calcium is sequestered in the dense tubular system when the cell has not been activated. Signals reach the platelet interior via the open canalicular system and the connections between this and the dense tubular system lead to the extrusion of calcium from the dense tubular system into the cytoplasm. This is followed by contraction of actomyosin and a change in the shape of the platelet. When the platelet is not activated by a chemical signal, the cytoplasmic calcium is maintained at low levels by the operation of a calcium pump which transports cytoplasmic calcium into the dense tubular system, and which appears to be essential for maintaining the platelet in its resting discoid form. If there is a rise in the intracellular concentration of adenosine $3',5'$-cyclic monophosphate (cAMP), the activity of the calcium pump is enhanced. Interestingly, chemical agents that appear to inhibit platelet activity, such as the antiaggregatory prostaglandins E_1 D_2 and I_2, act by stimulating platelet adenylate cyclase to produce a rise in intracellular cAMP levels. In addition to a role in modulating contractile functions, the dense tubular system also appears to be the site of prostaglandin synthesis within the platelet.

Mechanisms of Platelet Activation

Adhesion

During the formation of a haemostatic plug or arterial thrombosis, platelets react with exposed subendothelial tissue components. They then change from the normal disc shape, becoming more rounded, and put out pseudopodia. Alternatively, if polymerizing fibrin is present, they may adhere to the fibrin strands and undergo a similar shape change, this probably being brought about by local accumulation of thrombin, which is responsible for the conversion of fibrinogen to fibrin. How collagen influences platelet behaviour is not clear. There does not appear to be a specific collagen receptor on the platelet surface, and it is possible that several sites on the platelet membrane are cross-linked by the collagen fibril.

The Release Phase

Once platelets have adhered to collagen fibrils their shape changes and the contents of the intracellular granules are discharged. Some of the compounds released at this point are believed to be deeply involved in the next phase, **aggregation**, in which platelets stick to one another to form a clump. Many substances can cause platelets to aggregate (at least *in vitro*) and most of these also induce granules within the platelets to release their contents. The compounds likely to be operating in real life as opposed to the laboratory include **ADP**, which can be released from activated platelets, damaged red cells or injured cells of the vessel wall, or formed from ATP, which is also released from platelets. Another powerful aggregator of platelets is **thrombin**, which can exert its effect via a number of different pathways. In addition, an important group of both proaggregatory and antiaggregatory compounds can be released from activated platelets as a result of metabolic pathways that have **arachidonic acid**, derived from the platelet surface membrane, as their starting point.

Products of Arachidonic Acid Metabolism in the Platelet

In platelets that adhere to collagen or are acted on by thrombin or some other agent capable of inducing the release reaction, two phospholipases, C and A_2, act on membrane phospholipids. Phospholipase C cleaves phospholipids releasing diacylglycerol and phosphatidylinositol triphosphate, whereas phospholipase A_2 frees the arachidonate from phosphatidylinositol (aided by monoglyceride and diglyceride lipases) (*Fig. 18.7*).

The arachidonate is converted via the cyclooxygenase pathway to the prostaglandin endoperoxides, prostaglandin (PG) G_2 and PGH_2. These are then converted to thromboxane A_2 under the influence of thromboxane synthetase. Other products formed in platelets from prostaglandin endoperoxides include PGD_2 and PGE_2. PGD_2 is a powerful inhibitor of platelet aggregation because of its ability to stimulate adenylate cyclase. Thromboxane A_2 and its endoperoxide precursors are all platelet-aggregating agents and also cause contraction of vascular smooth muscle.

Just as certain prostaglandins are powerful agents for inducing aggregation of platelets, so the most potent inhibitors of aggregation are the prostaglandins that stimulate the adenylate cyclase system and thus produce an increase in the cAMP content of the platelet. One of these, PGI_2, is produced by stimulated endothelial cells. Its effects are directly opposite to those of thromboxane A_2 and it is the most powerful inhibitor of platelet aggregation known. PGI_2 formed locally, may affect the extent of platelet accumulation at that site, although it seems unlikely that it can act as a circulating hormone.

Platelet Factor 3 and Surface Glycoprotein Receptors

As stated earlier, when platelets undergo the release reaction, a phospholipoprotein called platelet factor 3 becomes available on their surface. This accelerates the generation of thrombin by taking part in two steps of the intrinsic clotting pathway: the interaction of Factors VIIIa and IXa to form Factor Xa from Factor X, and the interaction of factors Xa and Va to form thrombin from prothrombin.

FACTORS PROMOTING THROMBOSIS

Thrombosis may be likened to haemostasis occurring in the wrong place and at the wrong time. It is harmful rather than beneficial.

The very complexity of the interrelating processes involved in platelet adhesion, release and aggregation suggests that a number of different circumstances may influence platelet–vessel wall behaviour. In the 1860s, when thrombosis was recognized (but not the existence of the platelet), Rudolf Virchow suggested that the factors likely to promote thrombus formation fell naturally into **three** major groups:

1) changes in the intimal surface of the vessel
2) changes in the pattern of blood flow
3) changes in the constituents of the blood

These are known as **Virchow's triad**. Thrombosis may occur on the basis of one of these factors or a combination of them.

Changes in the Vessel Wall Surface

Changes in the surface of the vessel wall are recognized to be of major importance in the pathogenesis of arterial thrombi. The most important of these changes is undoubtedly unstable **atherosclerosis**, the lesions of which are described in Chapter 32 (see pp 327–346) (*Figs 18.9* and *18.10*).

However, injury (in the broadest sense), inflammation or neoplasms may also be associated with thrombosis-inducing damage to the vessel wall. Of all the components of the vessel wall, the one most likely to be implicated in thrombus formation is the **endothelial cell**. In any situation where there is actual loss of

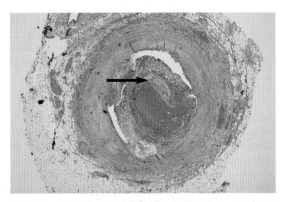

FIGURE 18.9 Occlusive coronary artery thrombus (stained red) which resulted from fissuring of the cap region (blue) of an atherosclerotic plaque.

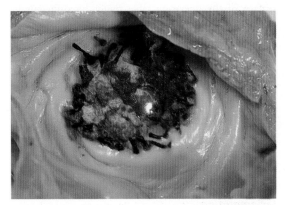

FIGURE 18.10 Thrombosis occurring in relation to a valvular prothesis (Starr–Edwards valve). Most of the metal ball of the 'ball in cage' valve is covered by thrombus. It is likely that both an abnormal surface and abnormal flow patterns have contributed to the thrombosis.

endothelial cells with exposure of the subendothelial collagen, platelet adhesion is the inevitable sequel. This certainly happens in complicated atherosclerotic plaques when either splitting ('deep injury') or fraying ('superficial injury') of the connective tissue plaque 'cap' occurs. Endothelial cell desquamation can also take place in the rare inherited metabolic disorder **homocystinuria**, and it has been claimed that endothelial cells can be identified in significant numbers in the blood after smoking.

One of the most persistent dogmas of vascular pathology is that platelets do not adhere to intact endothelium. However, in some experimental models such adhesion has been seen. This has followed infusions of the enzyme neuraminidase, which alters the proteoglycans in the luminal glycocalyx of the endothelial cell, and has also been noted in animals exposed to fresh cigarette smoke. A reduction in the amount of PGI_2 (prostacyclin) produced by aortic rings from rats exposed to fresh cigarette smoke has also been reported. These data, scanty as they are, suggest that certain factors may alter the structure and function of endothelium in such a way as to promote platelet–vessel wall interactions, without it being necessary for focal necrosis of endothelium to take place.

Trauma to the endothelium of a sufficient degree to cause thrombosis can occur under a number of circumstances. At a rather extreme level, thrombosis can occur after burning or freezing (e.g. capillary thrombosis in 'frostbite'). Mechanical trauma to endothelium occurs in association with the presence of indwelling cannulas. Another type of much less easily provable endothelial trauma has been suggested as one of the factors involved in the production of postoperative venous thrombi in the lower limb. During anaesthesia there is loss of normal muscle tone, and the dead weight of the limb and the hard surface of the operating table might be sufficient to cause trauma to the venous endothelium. There is no direct evidence for such trauma at the moment, although surgery certainly appears to be a potent thrombogenic stimulus as far as the veins are concerned.

Chemical injury to vessel walls certainly occurs, as seen in cases where thrombosis may follow infusion of certain compounds into veins. This fact is made use of in treating both varicose veins and haemorrhoids, where sclerosing chemicals are injected into the affected veins with the deliberate intention of causing thrombosis.

Inflammation

Thrombi occur frequently in situations where the vascular channels are involved in an inflammatory process. This may occur in the heart valves in patients with either rheumatic or infective endocarditis. Arteries involved in an immune complex-mediated inflammatory reaction, such as occurs in **polyarteritis nodosa** or **temporal arteritis**, are often thrombosed; both veins and capillaries passing through an inflamed area may also be affected in the same way.

Neoplastic Involvement

The invasion of small venules by malignant cells is often accompanied by thrombosis and there is evidence to suggest that fibrin formed in relation to the tumour cells in the course of this process may enhance their chances of survival and, hence, of multiplying.

Changes in the Pattern of Blood Flow

The important changes in blood flow pattern that are believed to increase the risk of thrombus formation are:
- changes in the **speed** of normal laminar flow
- **loss of the normal laminar pattern** of flow and its replacement by a **turbulent pattern**

Slowing of the speed of blood flow without loss of the normal laminar pattern appears to be of particular significance in relation to the formation of thrombi in

veins, while, in the **heart** and **arteries**, turbulence plays a more important haemodynamic role.

A reduction in the speed of blood flow may be either a general or a local phenomenon.
- The first of these may occur in patients with severe congestive cardiac failure, in whom the circulation time can be reduced significantly.
- Local slowing tends to occur particularly in the veins of the leg under a number of different circumstances, of which the most important are:
  a) prolonged dependence of the limb
  b) reduced muscle pumping activity
  c) proximal occlusion of the venous drainage

These circumstances are most likely to arise in a patient immobilized in bed, especially after surgery. With respect to the development of venous thrombosis, hospital is a very high-risk area. Dissection of the deep veins of the calf has shown the presence of thrombi in more than 30% of medical patients coming to necropsy and about 60% of surgical patients. The clinical diagnosis of such thrombi is difficult; only a small minority are correctly diagnosed during life by the presence of some swelling and tenderness in the affected calf and by pain in the calf being elicited on dorsiflexion of the foot (Homans' sign). Rational prevention related to minimizing changes in the pattern of blood flow, which is likely to be much more useful than treatment of an established thrombus, should include routine physiotherapy with exercises emphasizing calf and thigh muscle contraction, early postoperative ambulation, and avoidance of prolonged dependency of lower limbs.

Stasis of blood can also occur in the heart and large vessels such as the aorta if either the cardiac chambers or a segment of a major artery are abnormally dilated. This is found in aortic and other arterial **aneurysms**, in the dilated chambers of the heart in a disorder of heart muscle known as **congestive cardiomyopathy**, and in the dilated atria of patients with mitral valve disease, especially if there is associated atrial fibrillation. A situation rather similar to this occurs in patients in whom a large segment of the left ventricular wall has been rendered severely ischaemic following coronary artery occlusion (**myocardial infarction**). The dead heart muscle is replaced by scar tissue which is non-contractile, and this can lead to local disturbances of flow during ventricular systole and the formation of thrombi over the area of lost cardiac muscle.

Turbulent flow is of particular importance in relation to areas where arteries branch and to narrowed segments of arteries, chiefly due to atherosclerosis. The haemodynamics at points of branching are such that platelets tend to collect on the outer walls of branches. This has been demonstrated by introducing extracorporeal shunts, made of either glass or plastic, into the arterial system of animals, and then studying the sites at which platelets preferentially accumulate. In such a model system, the wall surface is uniform and thus the effect of flow can be studied in isolation.

Changes in the Constituents of the Blood

Platelets

It seems obvious that platelet function should be considered in relation to the three main components of their behaviour: adhesion, release and aggregation. In addition, their **concentration** within the blood should be determined, because a low platelet count is associated with abnormal bleeding and a high one with an increased tendency towards thrombosis.

In the laboratory it is common practice to measure the aggregatability of platelets to a given stimulus. ADP, collagen and thrombin are added to a suspension of platelets in a cuvette and the turbidimetric changes resulting from aggregation measured. Platelet adhesiveness can also be measured: the suspension of platelets (of known concentration) is passed at a constant rate across glass beads and the drop in platelet numbers occurring as a result of this passage is determined. The release reaction can be monitored by measuring changes in concentration of two products derived from the α-granules: platelet factor 4 (an antiheparin factor) and β-thromboglobulin. If sufficient care is taken in the sampling of the blood, a rise in the concentration of these compounds is *prima facie* evidence of thrombosis having taken place. However, the half-lives of both platelet factor 4 and β-thromboglobulin in plasma are very short and thus the timing of the sampling is critical.

A **hypercoagulable state** is one in which **the normal haemostatic equilibrium is tilted in such a way that thrombosis is favoured**.

In terms of the processes involved, an increased risk of thrombosis may therefore be due to:

- **Upregulation of platelet–vessel wall interactions.** The most important cause of this is atherosclerosis associated with either superficial or deep injury to the plaque cap. The presence of prosthetic heart valves or synthetic grafts also increases platelet reactions with the underlying vascular surface. Thrombosis may also be the consequence of endothelial damage in the rare inherited disorder of metabolism, homocystinaemia.
- **An increase** (which may be general or, more frequently, local) **in procoagulant factors**, most notably fibrinogen and Factor VII.
- **A decrease in natural anticoagulant factors** such as antithrombin III or the protein C–protein S–thrombomodulin system.
- **Increased viscosity of the blood**, as may occur in individuals with raised blood levels of fibrinogen or as a result of grossly increased plasma concentrations of immunoglobulins such as may be seen in plasma cell dyscrasias like multiple myeloma. Similar increases in viscosity are seen in patients with polycythaemia.

- **The presence of anticardiolipin antibodies** (lupus anticoagulants).
- **The presence of stasis** in the venous circulation, especially when associated with surgical trauma.
- **The release into the blood of procoagulant compounds released from malignant tumours**, especially adenocarcinomas.
- **An increase in the platelet count** (thrombocytosis).
- **An increase in platelet adhesiveness and aggregatability.**

INHERITED DISORDERS THAT INCREASE THE RISK OF THROMBOSIS

Deficiency of Antithrombin III

This disorder is inherited in an autosomal dominant fashion. The majority of the affected individuals are heterozygotes whose plasma, therefore, contains 50% of the normal concentration of functional antithrombin III. In patients with a deficiency of antithrombin III, there is an increase in the concentration of prothrombin fragments. This gives support to the view that the coagulation system is in a constant state of very low-grade activation, normally regulated and restrained by antithrombin III.

Antithrombin III deficiency causes recurrent episodes of mainly venous thrombosis. As is usual with venous thrombi, the leg veins are most frequently affected and complicating pulmonary emboli are common. In women the thrombi are often seen for the first time during pregnancy or in association with oral contraceptive use. In men there is often a history of antecedent injury or surgery. With increasing age, the frequency of the episodes of thrombosis increases.

Protein C Deficiency

Protein C deficiency is an autosomal dominant disorder. It is associated with a life-long increased risk of thrombosis. It occurs in two forms. In the first, the **amount** of the protein in the plasma is decreased; the functional deficit is proportional to the reduction of the protein concentration. In the second form, the amount of protein C in the plasma is normal but there is **a gross functional defect**. Levels below 65% of normal are usually associated with an increased incidence of thrombosis.

Clinically affected heterozygotes suffer from thrombosis in the deep leg veins and also have episodes of superficial thrombophlebitis.

Rarely the disorder may occur in a homozygous form. In this case the affected children have a devastating thromboembolic diathesis starting in infancy and involving the renal and mesenteric veins and dural sinuses. The clinical picture may be complicated by purpura fulminans in which there is widely distributed skin haemorrhage associated with the presence of fibrin plugs occluding small skin vessels.

Protein S Deficiency

This disorder presents with much the same clinical picture as protein C deficiency. It too is inherited as an autosomal dominant trait.

Deficiencies in both proteins C and S can occur in association with acquired diseases. Both these molecules are dependent on vitamin K for their activation and may thus be functionally impaired in patients with vitamin K deficiency from any cause.

Protein C Resistance

A syndrome characterized by recurrent familial venous thrombosis has been recognized, in which all the anticoagulant factors are present in normal concentration, but in which there is **abnormal resistance to the normal biological effect of activated protein C** (*Fig. 18.11*). This phenomenon has been found by one group of workers in about one-third of patients referred for evaluation of venous thromboembolism. The abnormality is inherited in an autosomal dominant fashion and confers a sevenfold increase in the risk of developing venous thrombosis.

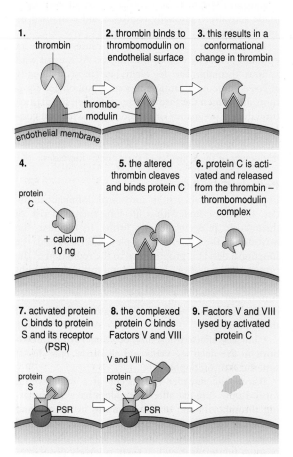

FIGURE 18.11 *Normal working of the protein C–protein S system shown in nine steps.*

The existence of this disorder implies that there must be a dysfunctional co-factor for activated protein C. This co-factor has been identified as Factor V, which now seems to have an anticoagulant as well as a procoagulant role.

Recently a mutation has been identified in the gene encoding Factor V which correlates with the presence of resistance to activated protein C. It is a single point mutation at nucleotide position 1691, at which there is a G→A substitution. In Holland where this mutation (Factor V Leiden) was identified, its frequency in the population appears to be about 2%, which is at least tenfold higher than that of all other genetic risk factors for thrombosis put together. The combination of this mutation with other risk factors for thrombosis may be very powerful; for example, women with mutated Factor V who take oral contraceptives have a 30-fold increased risk of thrombosis.

Inherited Disorders Affecting the Fibrinolytic Pathways

These are rare and include:

- dysfibrinogenaemia
- dysplasminogenaemia
- defective release of plasminogen activator from the vessel wall

Raised Plasma Fibrinogen and Factor VII$_c$ Concentrations

The Northwick Park Heart Study, a prospective study relating certain factors to coronary heart disease risk, has shown a strong positive association between plasma concentrations of fibrinogen and Factor VII$_c$ and the risk of a first episode of coronary heart disease.

Fibrinogen levels increase with:

- increasing age
- obesity
- use of oral contraceptives
- onset of the menopause
- diabetes
- cigarette smoking

With the exception of smoking, the same factors are associated with increased plasma levels of Factor VII$_c$. In addition, there is a positive association between a diet high in fat, leading to high plasma cholesterol concentrations, and raised plasma levels of Factor VII$_c$. Whether high plasma concentrations of fibrinogen are entirely 'acquired' or whether there is a genetic component is still not known.

ACQUIRED DISORDERS AND ENVIRONMENTAL FACTORS THAT INCREASE THE RISK OF THROMBOSIS

Oral Contraceptives

The introduction of oral contraceptives was followed by the recognition that both arterial and venous thrombosis might complicate their use. Users of 'the

Pill' in its original form had a three- to fivefold increased risk of developing a myocardial infarct or a stroke, and oral contraceptives appeared to act synergistically with other known risk factors such as cigarette smoking or diabetes mellitus.

This increased risk of thromboembolic disease correlates with the amount of oestrogen in the preparation. A reduction in oestrogen content has been associated with a decrease in, but not abolition of, the increased risk of thrombosis. Contraceptives raise the plasma concentrations of fibrinogen and vitamin K-dependent clotting factors by about 10–20% and there is also a decrease in plasma antithrombin III levels. Factor XII and prekallikrein levels increase, producing an increased contact factor-mediated fibrinolysis potential.

Malignancy

In addition to disseminated intravascular coagulation (see pp 915–917), patients with certain types of malignancy are at increased risk of thromboembolic disease.

Mucin-secreting adenocarcinomas, especially carcinoma of the pancreas, appear to be a risk factor for recurrent episodes of venous thrombosis. There is some evidence that venous thrombosis occurring for no very obvious cause may be followed by the clinical presentation of one of these tumours. Malignant cells may release tissue thromboplastin and there is also evidence that mucins released from certain adenocarcinomas, and proteases released from other tumours, can directly activate Factor X without involvement of the extrinsic clotting pathway.

The Nephrotic Syndrome

Venous thrombosis, particularly involving the renal vein, commonly complicates the nephrotic syndrome (average incidence 35%). Arterial thrombosis has also been recorded as an association but is much rarer.

The cause is not yet clear, although quantitative changes in some clotting and anti-clotting factors have been noted. One of the most striking of these is a decline in the plasma concentrations of antithrombin III, the levels of which fall proportionally with the decline in serum albumin concentration.

Correlations Between Risk Factors for Clinically Evident Thrombotic Events and Platelet Function

Prostaglandins

The results of epidemiological studies among the Eskimos of north-west Greenland suggest that alterations in the plasma concentrations of certain lipids may influence the balance between thromboxane A_2 and PGI_2. The incidence of ischaemic heart disease in this Eskimo community is very low. They have low levels of cholesterol and of low density lipoprotein in the blood and correspondingly high levels of high density lipoprotein. This plasma lipid pattern is not genetic in

origin but appears to be brought about by diet. In addition, platelet aggregatability is lower than in age- and sex-matched Danes and the bleeding time is prolonged. One of the outstanding features of the Eskimo diet is a high intake of eicosapentaenoic acid (EPA), which is present in fish; Eskimos have high plasma concentrations of this fatty acid and low concentrations of arachidonic acid. EPA is a starting point for the synthesis of PGI_3, which is antiaggregatory, but the thromboxane derived from EPA is said not to be proaggregatory. Diets rich in cod liver oil, which contains large amounts of EPA, have been shown to reduce the tendency to thrombosis in extracorporeal shunts inserted into rat aortas.

Platelet Aggregation and Plasma Lipid Patterns

Other evidence that the pattern and concentrations of plasma lipids may influence platelet behaviour is derived from patients with type IIa hyperlipidaemia. Their platelets are many times more sensitive to doses of aggregating agents such as collagen, ADP or thrombin than are those of normal subjects, although the lipid composition of the platelets themselves differs little, if at all. However, platelets from patients with hyperlipidaemia convert more arachidonic acid to thromboxane A_2 than do those from normal subjects.

Rabbits fed a diet high in saturated fat have an increased aggregatability of platelets in response to a standard dose of thrombin. This change takes place before any increase in the cholesterol concentration in the artery wall can be demonstrated. Similar data have been obtained from human studies.

Cigarette Smoking and Platelet Function

There is a strong positive correlation between heavy cigarette smoking and the risk of one of the major clinical manifestations of occlusive arterial disease. Cigarette smoking could operate as a risk factor in a number of ways; smoking experiments have yielded conflicting data on platelet aggregatability, but some studies suggest that smoking may have an effect on the adhesion of platelets to the underlying arterial wall.

EVOLUTION OF VENOUS THROMBI

The process of thrombus formation in a non-inflamed vein is usually termed **phlebothrombosis**. When thrombosis occurs in a vein that is inflamed, it is spoken of as **thrombophlebitis**. The latter is most commonly seen in superficial veins.

The site of initiation of the process is usually the valve pocket. If these areas are examined in sections of thrombosed veins, small clumps of platelets can be seen adhering to the luminal surface. It is a moot point whether this is preceded by damage to the endothelium in this area. Thus far, no positive evidence that such damage occurs has been presented, but the technical problems in carrying out such a study are daunting and it is, perhaps, too early to write off endothelial injury as being an important starting point for the process of venous thrombosis. Some workers have noticed the presence of leucocytes rather than platelets in these valve pockets and it is possible that these cells could bring about changes in the endothelium.

Once platelets have aggregated, clotting factors are activated locally and fibrin strands stabilize the platelet aggregate and help to anchor it to the underying vein wall. A second phase then begins in which a further batch of platelets is laid down over the initial aggregate. At this stage of thrombus development, platelets can be seen to have aggregated in the form of laminae which project from the surface of the initial aggregate and lie across the stream of blood. As a result of the forces exerted by the streaming blood, these platelet laminae are bent in the direction of flow and form a somewhat coralline structure (*Figs 18.12* and *18.13*). Between the platelet laminae are large numbers of red cells, some fibrin strands and a moderate number of leucocytes.

The laminar arrangement of the platelets, coupled with shortening of the fibrin strands between the laminae, gives rise to a curious 'rippled' appearance when the thrombi are viewed from above. The appearances are reminiscent of what one sees when a wind has blown across a beach and produced rippling of the sand. In both instances the 'ripples' lie concave to the direction of the force; in the case of the platelet laminae this force was the bloodstream. These elevated ridges on the surface of the thrombi are known as **lines of Zahn** in commemoration of the pathologist who first described them. They are clearly visible with the naked eye, but may be seen best with the aid of a hand lens. The more rapid the streaming of the blood in the segment of vessel where thrombosis has occurred, the more prominent are the lines of Zahn. They are seen most easily, therefore, in large arteries such as the aorta.

At this stage the process may come to an end. The

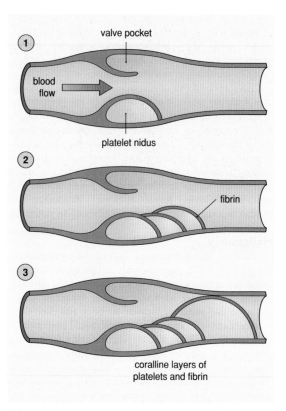

FIGURE 18.13 *Evolution of a venous thrombus.*

thrombus will then become covered by new endothelial cells and be incorporated into the structure of the underlying vessel wall. However, if the deposition of platelets and fibrin continues, a third phase ensues. As the coralline mass of platelets admixed with clotted blood continues to grow, the stream of blood through the affected segment slows still further and occlusion may ultimately occur. This phase is mediated predominantly by activation of the coagulation pathways rather than by platelet adhesion and aggregation, which appears to be the dominant element in the arterial system where blood flow is much faster (*Fig. 18.14*).

Once a segment of vein is occluded in this way, the flow of blood cephalad to the occlusion stops. Thus a stagnant column of blood exists between the point of occlusion and the point cephalad to it where the next venous tributary enters (*Fig. 18.15*). This stagnant column of blood coagulates and forms what is termed a 'consecutive clot' in continuity with the original thrombus. This is the first step in a process known as **propagation** of the thrombus. This process may occur in two basic patterns:

1) As mentioned above, consecutive clot forms between the original occlusion and the tributary immediately cephalad to it. At this point blood enters from the tributary and passes across the surface of the clot. Platelets then adhere to the

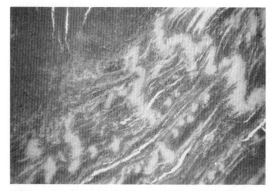

FIGURE 18.12 *Micrograph of a section through a venous thrombus stained with haematoxylin and eosin. The laminae of platelets appear as pale pink, rather wavy, bands; the red cells that constitute the greater part of the cell content are orange in colour.*

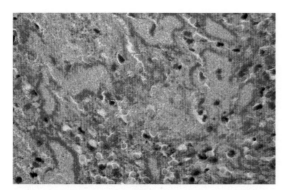

FIGURE 18.14 Section from an arterial thrombus stained by the Lendrum picro–Mallory method in which fibrin strands appear red, red blood cells yellow and platelets mauve. In contrast to venous thrombi, the bulk of the material here consists of platelets.

fibrin meshwork and aggregation follows with the formation of another small platelet thrombus. If this too grows enough to occlude the lumen, propagation may occur again and another segment of vein may fill with fresh clot. In effect, a long segment of venous drainage of the limb can become occluded in a series of 'jumps' or episodes of clotting, each of which is triggered by the adhesion of platelets. The mixed mass of platelet thrombi and consecutive clot is anchored to the underlying vein wall only at sites where there has been adhesion of platelets.

2) If the venous return from the limb as a whole is slowed down, propagation by the formation of consecutive clot may occur on a massive scale. Cephalad to the original occlusive platelet–fibrin thrombus, a long cord of clotted blood may form which fills the vein lumen and which is anchored only at its origin. With the eventual shortening of fibrin strands that takes place more or less inevitably after the formation of any clot, this mass of clotted blood comes to lie quite loosely within the lumen except at the point where the original thrombus is attached. If the thrombus becomes dislodged from its attachment point, then the whole mass is carried away in the systemic venous circulation until impaction takes place within the pulmonary arteries (pulmonary embolism).

Natural History of Thrombi

Lysis

Some thrombi may undergo lysis through the action of plasmin and 'like some insubstantial pageant faded, leave not a wrack behind' (*The Tempest*, William Shakespeare). From the pragmatic point of view this is clearly the most desirable outcome, especially in relation to **occlusive thrombi** within the arterial tree. It is not without interest that plasminogen activator, which

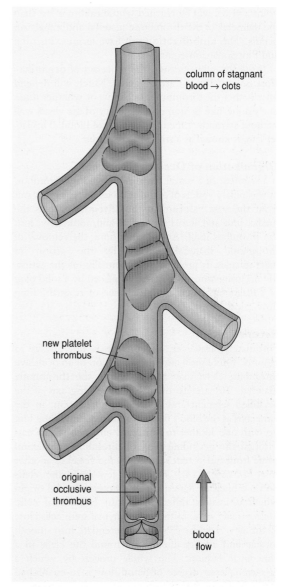

FIGURE 18.15 Propagation of a venous thrombus.

converts plasminogen to the active form plasmin, is present in greater concentrations within venous intima than within arterial intima. If spontaneous lysis is unlikely, the process can be initiated by treating patients with lytic agents such as streptokinase or genetically engineered plasminogen activator.

Embolization

Thrombi may become detached from the underlying vascular wall, be it vein, artery or heart. When this occurs, the detached portion of thrombus travels at high speed in the systemic venous circulation (if its origin is a vein) or within the systemic arterial circulation (if the site of origin was an artery or the heart). At some point a vessel will be reached whose calibre is less than the diameter of the thrombotic material and impaction occurs. This **embolization** can have serious structural and functional consequences.

If the thrombus persists, the processes of **organization** (see pp 70–71) are triggered. Much will depend on whether the thrombus is occlusive or whether it lies in a plaque-like fashion on the surface of the vessel wall without seriously impeding the flow of blood. This latter case is known as a **mural thrombus**.

Organization of Occlusive Thrombi

If a segment of a vessel remains plugged by thrombus, new capillary vessels of granulation tissue type grow out from the vasa vasorum in the adventitia, across the media, into and across the intima and, ultimately, into the thrombus itself. At the same time, the removal of thrombotic material, largely by the action of macrophages, is proceeding. Eventually, at the worst, the occlusive thrombus may be replaced by a solid plug of collagenous tissue and all chance of re-establishing flow is lost.

Recanalization

Fortunately, however, the picture is not always so gloomy. Quite soon after the formation of an occlusive thrombus, clefts may appear within the thrombotic material. These clefts often lie in the long axis of the occluded segment and hence, by implication, in the same axis as the blood flow. Not infrequently they link up with one another to form new channels which pass through the occluding plug of thrombus–granulation tissue from one patent segment of the vessel to another (*Figs 18.16–18.18*). Within a few days the clefts become lined by flattened cells of mesenchymal origin which ultimately differentiate into endothelial cells. Occasionally some of the mesenchymal stem cells close to the new vascular channels differentiate into smooth muscle and arrange themselves round the clefts in a concentric fashion. The whole process by which a greater or lesser degree of blood flow is re-established through the occluded segment of vessel is known as **recanalization**.

Organization of Mural Thrombi

In this situation the pattern of organization is different because the pathophysiological circumstances differ so much from those that obtain in an occluded segment of a vessel. Because flowing blood passes over the surface of the mural thrombus, the superficial portion of the thrombus is the seat of infiltration by oxygenated plasma, and granulation tissue-type capillaries derived from the vasa grow only very slowly, if at all, into the thrombus. The lack of this feature may be mediated, in part at least, by the normal intramural tension within the affected part of the vessel.

Many of the platelets disaggregate and are either washed away by the passing stream of blood or phago-

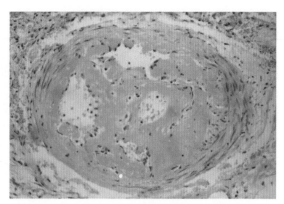

FIGURE 18.16 *Recanalization. The thrombus shown here is 8 days old. Note the clefts within the pink-staining substance of the thrombus. Some of these contain red blood cells and some are lined by flattened mesenchymal cells.*

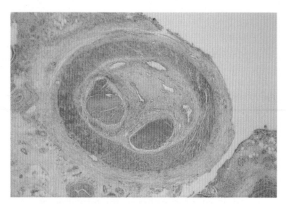

FIGURE 18.17 *Recanalization. This section is from the anterior tibial artery of an 18-year-old man with Buerger's disease (see p 405). The arterial lumen is occluded largely by cellular connective tissue but several recanalization channels can be seen. The two largest ones are occluded by recent thrombus and this occlusion precipitated ischaemic necrosis (gangrene) of the foot on the affected side.*

cytosed. In arteries this means that, within a short time, the major part of the remaining thrombus consists of a spongy mass of polymerized fibrin which tends to become packed down on to the surface of the underlying vessel wall. Within a few days the surface of the thrombus becomes partly covered by a layer of flattened cells. Originally it was thought that these were new endothelial cells but there is some evidence to suggest that the cells making up the early neointima are smooth muscle cells.

As in other situations where organization is taking place, the mass of fibrin and platelets becomes vascularized. An unusual feature, however, is the fact that the new vascular channels, which can be seen within a few days of the thrombus being formed, are derived from the main lumen of the vessel and grow down into the

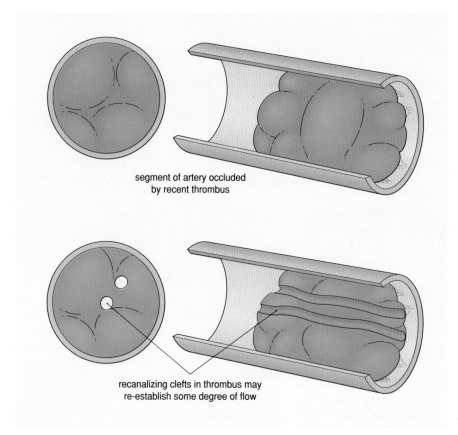

segment of artery occluded
by recent thrombus

recanalizing clefts in thrombus may
re-establish some degree of flow

FIGURE 18.18 Recanalization of an occlusive thrombus.

thrombus rather than upwards across the media from the vasa vasorum.

The picture is further complicated by the interaction of PDGF with smooth muscle cells in the underlying vessel wall. The major part of the proliferation of smooth muscle cells that ensues after the formation of a mural thrombus appears to take place on the luminal aspect of the thrombus, so that the thrombus eventually lies deep within the thick new intima (*Fig. 18.19*). The possibility that this process may play a part in the growth of atherosclerotic plaques is discussed in Chapter 32.

EMBOLISM

An embolus is an abnormal mass of material, either solid or gaseous, which is transported in the bloodstream from one part of the circulation to another and which finally impacts in the lumen of vessels too small a calibre to allow the embolus to pass.

Emboli may consist of:
- thrombus
- mixed thrombus and blood clot
- air
- nitrogen
- fat
- small pieces of bone marrow
- debris from the base of atherosclerotic plaques
- groups of tumour cells (embolization constitutes an important means of tumour spread)

Most major emboli are derived from thrombus.

Thrombus-derived Emboli
Roughly 99% of emboli are derived from thrombus or from thrombus mixed with blood clot such as is found in the veins of the lower limb.

Pulmonary Emboli
When the origin of the embolus is a venous thrombus, the end-result must be impaction in the pulmonary arterial tree. These emboli are discussed in Chapter 33 (see pp 474–476).

Systemic Emboli
Most thrombotic systemic emboli are derived from the left side of the heart. The thrombi may arise in the atrial appendages (this being particularly likely to occur in patients with atrial fibrillation). Intraventricular thrombi

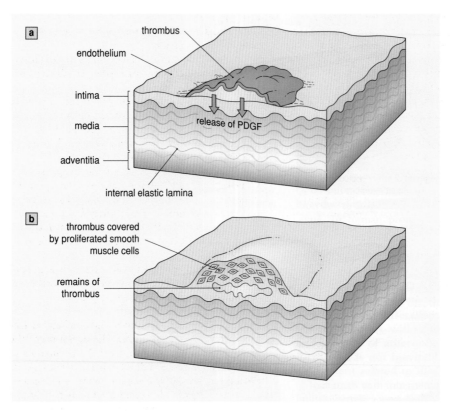

FIGURE 18.19 Organization of a mural thrombus. PDGF, platelet-derived growth factor.

may occur as a consequence of transmural myocardial infarction or in congestive cardiomyopathy, a muscle disorder in which the myocardium is flabby and the ventricles are dilated. There is a marked decrease in the systolic ejection fraction and thus a volume overload on the ventricular muscle. In life, the presence of these thrombi can be detected by echocardiography.

Thrombi affecting the heart valves, and of a size sufficient to give rise to significant emboli, are usually related to the presence of **infective endocarditis**, a disorder produced by the combination of haemodynamically induced endocardial injury and bacteraemia. The infected thrombi, or **vegetations** as they are often called, may be bulky and friable. Portions of the vegetations can break off readily and travel in the systemic arterial circulation until they impact. This may, of course, occur in a large number of places, but the brain, lower limbs, spleen and kidneys are favoured sites. When an infected thrombus impacts, it may set up a localized inflammatory reaction leading to partial destruction of the wall of the vessel in which impaction has taken place. This leads to dilatation of the affected arterial segment, and rupture followed by haemorrhage may occur. Such a lesion is termed a **mycotic aneurysm**, a misleading term as fungi have nothing to do with the pathogenesis (*mycos* mushroom).

Small **platelet thrombi** occur quite commonly in relation to atherosclerotic plaques at the point in the neck where the common carotid artery divides. Emboli derived from these platelet masses lodge in the cerebral circulation, often in small vessels, where they may give rise to permanent or transient neurological deficiencies.

Gaseous Emboli

Air may be introduced into the systemic circulation under a number of circumstances. These include:

- operations on the head and neck where a large vein is opened inadvertently
- mismanagement of blood transfusions where positive pressure is being used to speed up the flow of blood
- during haemodialysis for renal failure
- following insufflation of air into the fallopian tubes in the course of investigation of infertility
- interference with the placental site during criminal abortion

The air enters the right side of the heart where, in the right ventricle, it is whipped up into a frothy mass. This mass can block the flow of blood through the pulmonary arteries. The clinical picture that develops mimics closely that of massive pulmonary embolization by thrombus derived from the leg veins. In some cases the froth may gain access to the systemic arterial circulation and impact there. The most frequent site for this is the brain, but cases have also been reported of embolization of vessels supplying the spinal cord, with patients being investigated for infertility becoming quadriplegic following tubal insufflation. As little as 40 ml of air can have serious clinical results and 100 ml can be fatal, although there have been rare cases in which 200 ml have been tolerated. If air embolism is suspected as the cause of death, it is necessary to place the heart and pulmonary arteries under water when they are opened, in order to detect the escape of the air bubbles from the blocked vessels.

Nitrogen embolization occurs in decompression sickness, which is also known as 'caisson disease'. It affects persons whose occupation causes them to work at very high atmospheric pressures and who may then be returned too quickly to normal atmospheric pressure (deep sea divers, tunnellers, etc.).

At high pressures, inert gases, of which nitrogen is the most important, are dissolved in the plasma and in interstitial tissue, especially adipose tissue. If the person at risk returns too quickly to normal atmospheric pressure, the gas comes out of solution and small bubbles are formed within the interstitial tissues and blood, platelets often being associated with gas bubbles in the latter situation. These bubbles coalesce to form quite large masses and the clinical features are produced either by emboli in the circulating blood or by the presence of bubbles in the interstitial tissues, especially in tendons, joints and ligaments. When this happens the patient complains of excruciating pain (the syndrome being known as '**the bends**'). The central nervous system may be affected and the sudden onset of respiratory distress has also been described. Symptoms may be relieved by placing the patient in a compression chamber and forcing the gases back into solution. Once this has been done, slow and careful decompression should avoid a recurrence.

Occasionally the presence of nitrogen emboli in the systemic circulation is followed by ischaemic damage to the ends of long bones (aseptic necrosis), this being associated with secondary damage to the articular cartilages and joints.

Fat Emboli

Fat embolism is a common event occurring in 90% of patients who have sustained significant trauma. Significant clinical consequences are, happily, quite rare. It has been associated with:

- fractures of the long bones
- severe burns
- severe and extensive soft tissue trauma
- hyperlipidaemia
- ischaemic bone marrow necrosis in patients with sickle cell disease
- joint reconstruction
- cardiopulmonary bypass

- acute pancreatitis
- intramedullary nailing in the course of certain orthopaedic procedures

The fact that the syndrome can occur in the absence of trauma suggests a multifactorial pathogenesis, which is discussed below.

The two major theories of the pathogenesis of the fat embolism syndrome may be summed up as:

1) The **mechanical theory**, in which it is suggested that bone marrow-derived fat globules enter the venous system and lodge in the pulmonary vasculature as fat emboli. Droplets smaller than about 7–10 μm may pass through the pulmonary capillaries and eventually lodge in the systemic circulation. Indeed urinary fat droplets are so common after injury that their presence is of little or no value in the diagnosis of fat embolism syndrome.

2) A **biochemical theory**, in which it is suggested that circulating free fatty acids directly affect the cells lining the air spaces and thus produce abnormalities in gas exchange.

As is so often the case, mechanical and biochemical factors probably act synergistically. The operation of the biochemical pathway would explain the occurrence of fat embolism syndrome in the absence of trauma. A rise in the level of circulating catecholamines, which is seen in a number of pathophysiological situations including trauma and sepsis, promotes the release of free fatty acids from adipose tissue stores. In addition, increases in the acute-phase protein, C-reactive protein, causes chylomicrons to coalesce and form large fat globules.

Thus, in patients with fractures, especially multiple fractures, fat globules are thought to enter veins at the fracture site which have been torn at the time of injury. These globules are then carried in the systemic venous circulation to the lungs, where they may impact in small vessels and cause the sudden onset of respiratory distress some 24–72 hours after injury (*Fig. 18.20*). In such patients it may be possible to identify droplets of fat in the sputum or in bronchial lavage specimens by staining smears with fat-soluble dyes such as Oil Red O. In patients with fat embolism syndrome, 63% of the lavage cells have been found to contain fat droplets, whereas fewer than 2% of such cells taken from patients with other clinical syndromes show the presence of fat.

Clinical fat embolism syndrome always manifests with pulmonary dysfunction in the form of hypoxaemia and tachypnoea. This is the first manifestation of the syndrome. There is convincing evidence that following, for example, reaming and intramedullary nailing of the femoral bone marrow compartment for the repair of fractures, material that can be detected by means of echocardiography passes into the right side of the heart, and can cause the fat embolism syndrome.

Some patients present with predominant involvement of the central nervous system. They may become

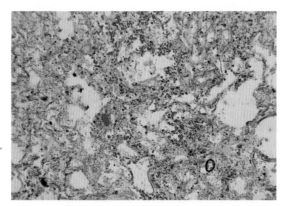

FIGURE 18.20 Fat embolism. A frozen section from the lung of an elderly man dying 24 hours after extensive soft tissue trauma. Note the numerous red-stained droplets blocking the alveolar septal capillaries.

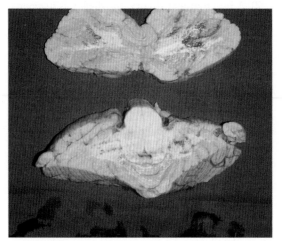

FIGURE 18.21 Sections through the cerebellum of a patient who, a few days after fracturing a long bone, lapsed into a coma and died. Note the numerous small haemorrhages, principally within the white matter.

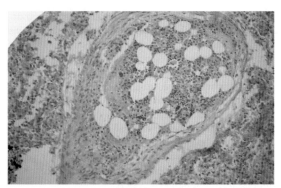

FIGURE 18.22 Bone marrow embolism. A small branch of the pulmonary artery is occluded by a cellular mass in which several punched-out spaces are visible. These represent the places where fat has been dissolved out in the course of processing the material. The cells consist of blood cell precursors. This pathological picture is most likely to be seen in middle-aged or elderly individuals in whom cardiopulmonary resuscitation has been unsuccessful, and in whom rib fracture has occurred in the course of attempted resuscitation.

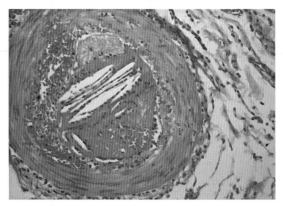

FIGURE 18.23 A small artery occluded by an atheromatous embolus. The clue to the nature of the embolus is provided by the cigar-shaped spaces within the embolus which represent where crystalline cholesterol has been dissolved out in the course of processing.

agitated at first and then lapse into coma; a high proportion of such patients die. At autopsy, if they have survived the onset of unconsciousness for a day or two, the brain shows oedema and **many tiny haemorrhages** (*Fig. 18.21*). These occur in both the grey and white matter but are more easily seen in the latter site. Frozen sections of brain stained with fat-soluble dyes show the presence of fat globules within the lumina of cerebral capillaries. There may be two explanations for the cases in which the nervous system is affected predominantly. The cerebral embolization may be due to the passage of emboli through a patent foramen ovale between the cardiac atria, an abnormality that is present in 20–34% of individuals, or the emboli may be derived from the small droplets that can pass through the pulmonary capillaries.

As mentioned above, fat emboli occur more frequently than does the **fat embolization syndrome**. When autopsies were carried out on Korean war battle casualties dying within 4 weeks of having been injured, evidence of fat embolization was found in 90% of cases. However, in only 1% could any part of the clinical picture in these patients be attributed to fat emboli.

Bone Marrow Emboli

Bone marrow emboli are not infrequently found on histological examination and post-mortem samples of lung tissue from patients who have had episodes of cardiac arrest due to ventricular fibrillation and in whom attempts at resuscitation included external cardiac massage (*Fig. 18.22*). In middle-aged and elderly people, in whom the costal cartilages have long since become ossified, repeated pressure on the rib cage usually results in the fracture of several ribs and it is from these sites that bone marrow is squeezed into the veins. The clinical effects, if any, of such emboli are unknown.

Emboli Derived from Atheromatous Debris

Atheromatous emboli obviously occur only in the systemic arterial tree. They are derived from plaques which ulcerate and in which there is a massive basally situated pool of lipid and tissue debris, as described in Chapter 32. The emboli are usually found incidentally on histological examination of tissue and can be recognized easily because they consist of a mixture of thrombotic material and lipid-rich debris in which highly characteristic, cigar- or torpedo-shaped, cholesterol crystals are present (*Fig. 18.23*).

CHAPTER 19

Ischaemia and Infarction

Ischaemia may be defined as the state existing when an organ or tissue has its arterial perfusion lowered relative to its metabolic needs (*Fig. 19.1*). This definition is often broadened to include the functional changes produced by such a diminution of perfusion. An **infarct** is a **morphological** entity: a large localized area of tissue necrosis brought about by **ischaemia**.

ISCHAEMIA

Ischaemia is most often caused by some local interference with the perfusion of the organ or tissue concerned. On some occasions, however, the ischaemic state may be generalized. This occurs only rarely and is associated with a fall in cardiac output. While acute reductions in cardiac output are by no means uncommon, they are not often expressed in the form of ischaemic changes in individual tissues.

Rarely, gangrene of the extremities may be seen following either extensive myocardial infarction or the sudden onset of a ventricular arrhythmia, both of which may be associated with a severe drop in cardiac output. Disorders of cardiac rhythm, including pathological changes in the conducting system, are not uncommon causes of cerebral ischaemia. An obvious and important example of this is **complete heart block**, in which sudden periods of unconsciousness (Stokes–Adams attacks) occur. If adequate perfusion of the brain is not restored within 3–4 minutes, irreparable damage to the neurones occurs.

Local Causes of Ischaemia

The most important of the pathological bases of acute ischaemia – thrombosis and embolism – were described in Chapter 18. In addition, arterial perfusion may be interfered with by spasm of the smooth muscle in the vessel wall or by pressure on the vessel from without. However, it is worth remembering that interruption of arterial blood flow is not the only way in which ischaemia may be produced: pathological changes affecting veins and capillaries can also lead to underperfusion of tissues.

Ischaemia due to Venous Occlusion

The pathogenesis of ischaemia due to venous occlusion is outlined in *Fig. 19.2*. It should be obvious from this that ischaemia on such a basis is likely to occur only in certain anatomical situations where it is not possible for the blood to bypass the obstruction via collateral drainage channels, and that, because of the local interruption to venous return, the affected tissues are likely to be **intensely congested** and possibly even **haemorrhagic**. The circumstances under which **venous infarction** is likely to occur include:

- Extensive mesenteric venous thrombosis, leading to infarction of the small intestine.
- So-called strangulation of hernias, where entrapment occurs leading to oedema and pressure on the draining veins.
- Cavernous sinus thrombosis, which may lead in turn to thrombosis of the retinal vein and, ultimately, to blindness.
- Thrombosis of the superior longitudinal sinus within the dura. This can occur in severely dehydrated children and leads to patchy haemorrhagic necrosis in the cerebral cortex.
- A very rare variant of thrombosis in the iliofemoral system, which may be followed by gangrenous changes in the lower limb.

Ischaemia due to Capillary Obstruction

This can occur as a consequence of physical damage to the capillaries, as in 'frostbite'. Capillaries may be occluded rarely by parasites, as in cerebral malaria, by abnormal red cells as in sickle cell disease or in certain autoimmune haemolytic anaemias, by fibrin where disseminated intravascular coagulation has occurred, by antigen–antibody complexes, by fat or gas emboli or by external pressure, such as is seen in 'bed sores'.

Arterial Obstruction

Obstruction of arterial inflow may be followed by a spectrum of functional and/or structural changes which range from no effect to extensive tissue necrosis. If neither functional nor structural changes can be observed, it can be inferred that the collateral arterial supply to the target area is good and that no significant reduction in perfusion has occurred.

Functional Evidence of Ischaemia

Functional disturbances are usually noted when the collateral supply is good enough to maintain adequate perfusion only as long as the metabolic demands of the tissue are at a basal level. If these demands are

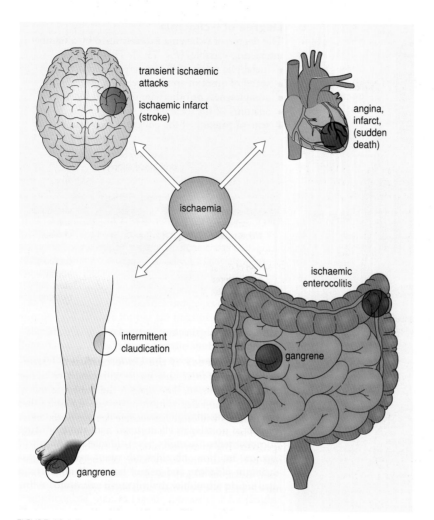

FIGURE 19.1 Principal anatomical targets for ischaemia.

increased, as for example in the heart or the muscle of the lower limb during exercise, then a state of ischaemia will be produced and the patient will experience either substernal pain (**angina pectoris**) or a cramp-like pain in the calf (**intermittent claudication**). Cessation of activity leads, in most instances, to disappearance of the pain.

The eventual changes in the function of an organ or tissue that has been rendered ischaemic may result either from **loss of cells** or from **abnormal or deficient behaviour on the part of surviving cells**. In ischaemic myocardium, for example, there is a marked tendency for electrical disturbances to occur and these frequently give rise to fatal arrhythmias such as ventricular fibrillation. Indeed, at least half the patients who die during their first clinically apparent episode of myocardial ischaemia, die in this way. Similarly the presence of ischaemic sensory nerve bundles may lead to qualitative abnormalities in the sensory patterns interpreted within the central nervous system, and it has

been suggested that this mechanism may underlie the phenomenon of persistent pain in patients with limb ischaemia.

Structural Changes Caused by Ischaemia

If the degree of ischaemia is greater than that described above, then structural damage to cells and tissues will occur. This may take the form of patchy loss of parenchymal cells, such as is seen in the myocardium of patients with a long history of angina pectoris, or massive necrosis. In either event, if the patient survives the ischaemic episode, the lost tissue is replaced, except in the case of the brain, by fibrous tissue in a manner identical with that occurring in repair (see Chapter 8).

The degree of postischaemic necrosis is proportional to the degree of ischaemia, which, in turn, depends on the balance between the needs of an individual tissue and the degree to which arterial perfusion is compromised. When the ischaemia is slow in onset and chronic in nature, a characteristic feature is the tendency for cell

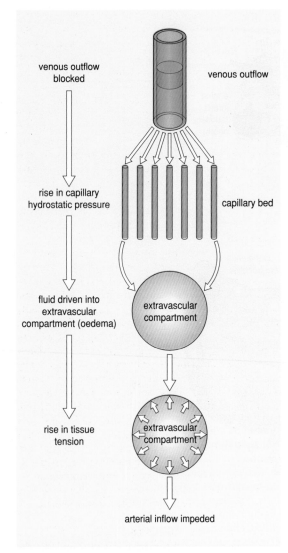

FIGURE 19.2 *Pathogenesis of ischaemia due to venous occlusion.*

death to affect either individual cells or small groups of cells.

Initially these may show the changes of intracellular oedema (see pp 25–26) or fatty change, but eventually they die and are replaced by small foci of fibrous tissue. When such chronic ischaemia occurs in the heart, it gives the muscle a curious flecked appearance because of the 'drop out' of small numbers of cells and their replacement by collagen fibres. In chronic lower limb ischaemia, the dermal papillae of the skin become flattened and both the epidermis and the dermis are thinned. Skin appendages such as hair follicles, sweat glands and sebaceous glands may also disappear. As a result of these changes, the skin appears shiny, hairless and dry.

Degree of Ischaemia

The degree of ischaemia is determined by a number of interacting variables (*Fig. 19.3*). These include:

- metabolic needs of the underperfused tissue
- speed of onset of arterial occlusion
- completeness or otherwise of arterial blocking
- anatomy of the local blood supply
- state of patency of the collateral blood supply

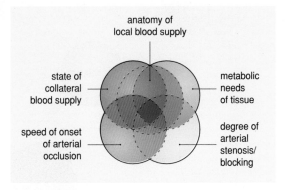

FIGURE 19.3 *Factors influencing the degree of ischaemia.*

Metabolic Needs of the Underperfused Tissue

Tissues vary in their capacity to withstand a reduction in arterial perfusion. The brain is the most sensitive in this respect, and deprivation of oxygen for more than 3–4 minutes will cause irreversible damage to the nerve cells. The myocardium is also very susceptible to damage following underperfusion. It is doubly unfortunate that both brain and heart have, on the whole, rather poor collateral blood supplies and that neither heart muscle cells nor neurones are able to regenerate.

Speed of Onset of Arterial Occlusion

If arterial occlusion takes place very rapidly as, for example, when an atherosclerotic coronary artery plaque ruptures, the effects are more severe than with slow narrowing of the same segment of artery, because there is little or no time for collateral vessels to open.

Completeness of Arterial Blocking

Other things being equal, complete occlusion of an arterial lumen causes more extensive damage to the affected area than severe stenosis. It must be equally obvious that the more proximally the occlusion is situated in a given arterial tree, the greater will be the area of tissue affected by ischaemia.

Anatomy of the Local Blood Supply

Some organs or tissues have no collateral blood supply; the arteries that perfuse such parts are known as 'end-arteries'. The retina is an example of such a tissue. It is supplied by a single vessel, the central retinal artery, which branches only once it has reached the retina. If occlusion of the central retinal artery occurs and is not rapidly relieved, irreparable ischaemic damage will be produced within the retina. The smaller arteries within the cerebral cortex also function as end-arteries. In contrast, some tissues, such as the lung, have a **double** arterial supply. Occlusion of one part of this blood supply need not lead to necrosis of the underperfused area because the supply from the other source may be sufficient to maintain tissue viability.

Patency of the Collateral Blood Supply

A good collateral supply, in the anatomical sense, can compensate for blockage in the main arterial tree only if the collateral vessels themselves are neither stenosed by atherosclerotic plaques nor in spasm.

INFARCTION

An **infarct** can be defined as a **fairly large area of tissue necrosis** (usually coagulative in type) **which results from ischaemia**. Blood may seep into the ischaemic area for some time, partly as a result of back flow from venules and escape of blood through the walls of vessels in the local microcirculation that have been damaged during the ischaemic process. Thus many infarcts contain a good deal of blood in the early stages of their natural history. In spongy tissue such as the lung, the escape of red blood cells and fibrin is a conspicuous feature and the ischaemic lung tissue becomes firmer than normal. At necropsy, infarcts of this type can be appreciated as wedge-shaped lumps on the pleural aspect of the lung. When the lung is cut into, the infarcted area tends to bulge and to stand proud of the surrounding normal lung. This outpouring or 'stuffing' of blood into the devitalized areas is merely an epiphenomenon and is not the core event in infarction. Failure of pathologists to appreciate this led to the introduction of the archaic and essentially unhelpful term 'infarct', which is derived from the Latin verb *infarcire* meaning 'to stuff'.

With the passage of time the dying cells often swell. This tends to squeeze blood out of the interstitial tissue in the infarcted area and the infarct becomes much paler. In the heart, for example, it takes 24–36 hours for this process to become complete. The pallor is a useful marker for the macroscopic diagnosis of infarction at necropsy. However, because this pallor takes a considerable time to develop, it may be difficult to make such a necropsy diagnosis in the early stages of the natural history of a myocardial infarct. The application of enzyme histochemical methods to this problem can be of great assistance in arriving at an accurate diagnosis on macroscopic examination of the heart (see p 350), but even these techniques fail to identify necrotic muscle tissue unless the patient has survived for 6–9 hours after the cutting off of the blood supply to an area of the myocardium.

The division of infarcts into '**pale**' and '**red**' varieties other than in the brain is pointless. Many infarcts start off as red and become pale as the blood is squeezed out of the infarcted area by swelling of the dying cells. Cerebral infarcts are usually pale *ab initio* (unless they are embolic in origin) and infarcts in the spongy lung tissue remain red and undergo repair while still at that stage.

The dead parenchymal cells in the infarcted area undergo autolysis and the diapedesed red cells lyse. At the same time a brisk inflammatory reaction occurs at the margins of the infarct, and first neutrophils and then macrophages infiltrate the necrotic tissue. Breakdown products of haemoglobin – haematoidin (bile pigment) and haemosiderin (aggregated molecules of ferritin) – may be seen in relation to the infarcted area and are ingested by macrophages. At this stage, usually about 1 week after cutting off of the arterial supply, an infarct in a solid organ is generally firm in consistency and a dull yellow in colour, with a red zone of hyperaemia at the margins.

The presence of large numbers of macrophages corresponds with what is seen in the **demolition** phase of an inflammatory reaction, and is of equal importance in the context of infarction. In some tissues, for example the **heart**, dead parenchymal cells are removed rapidly and there is an equally rapid replacement of these cells, first by granulation tissue and then by scar tissue. In other situations, such as the **kidney**, the infarcted area persists, sometimes for months, before being replaced by scar tissue (*Fig 19.4*). Histological examination of such an area shows the 'ghost outlines' of the architectural elements of the tissue, the tubules and glomeruli, although the constituent parenchymal cells are clearly dead. A slow but progressive ingrowth of connective tissue occurs even in these cases and, eventually, the infarct becomes converted to a fibrous scar in which calcium salts may be deposited (dystrophic calcification).

The sequence of events described above may be interrupted at any time by the death of the patient.

Infarction at Specific Sites

This is discussed under the appropriate anatomical locations.

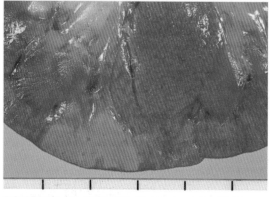

FIGURE 19.4 Renal infarct. The ischaemic zone appears as a wedge-shaped area of pallor which stands out strikingly against the red-brown background of the unaffected renal tissue.

CHAPTER 20

Abnormal Accumulations of Fluid and Disturbances of Blood Distribution

Among the most important requirements for good health is that there should be a normal quantitative relationship between intravascular and extravascular fluid. A disturbance in this relationship can produce life-threatening situations in certain anatomical situations, notably the lung and brain. Closely associated may be alterations in the distribution of blood in various tissue beds leading, for one reason or another, to local increases in the amount of blood present in a given organ or tissue.

OEDEMA

Oedema may be defined as an abnormal accumulation of fluid in the extracellular space. (This, therefore, excludes the increases in cytoplasmic sodium and water considered in the section on cell injury.) From a simple clinical point of view, the recognition of oedema depends on the identification of this excess fluid within the interstitial tissues.

Factors Controlling Distribution of Extra-Cellular Body Water

Total body water is approximately 49 litres. Of this, the intracellular component accounts for about 35 litres, and this varies very little. The intravascular compartment contains about 3 litres, and a further 11 litres are present in the extravascular compartment. **The maintenance of a relatively constant relationship between intravascular and extravascular water depends on a number of factors:**

1) Those that tend to cause fluid to **leave the vascular compartment**:
- **Increased intravascular hydrostatic pressure.** An increase in hydrostatic pressure within the vascular compartment may produce profound changes in fluid distribution. For instance, severe mitral stenosis will lead to a chronic rise in the pulmonary venous pressure and hence to a rise in pulmonary capillary pressure. If such a patient takes severe exercise, the resulting increase in pulmonary artery pressure may be sufficient on its own account to overcome all other relevant homoeostatic mechanisms and fluid will pass from the pulmonary alveolar capillaries first into the alveolar walls and then into the air spaces themselves.

- **Increased colloid osmotic pressure in the extravascular compartment.** If this is increased, more fluid tends to leave the microvasculature.
2) Factors that, under normal circumstances, tend to **keep fluid within the vascular compartment**:
- The **osmotic pressure of the plasma proteins**, of which albumin, with its relatively low molecular weight and high concentration relative to other plasma proteins, is the most important. A fall in the plasma concentration of albumin, due either to **reduced synthesis**, as in chronic liver disease, or to **excessive loss**, as in certain forms of kidney disease, may be associated with quite severe oedema.
- **Selective permeability function of endothelium.** Normally albumin does not leave the vascular compartment in significant amounts. Should the permeability barrier function of the capillary wall become impaired, there will be a decline in the plasma concentration of albumin and a corresponding increase in the protein content of the fluid in the interstitial tissues.
- **Tissue tension** in the interstitial tissue. This tends to limit the egress of fluid from the microvasculature. Normally this tension is low (less than 1 kPa).

All these physical factors can be summed up in the following mathematical expression:

$$J_v = k[(P_c - P_i) - \Pi_c - \Pi_i)]$$

where J_v is the local rate of fluid flux along the length of a capillary; k is the capillary hydraulic permeability; P_c is the capillary hydraulic pressure; P_i is the hydraulic pressure; and Π_i is the colloid osmotic pressure in the interstitial fluid.

Under normal circumstances there is a **nett loss** of fluid from the vascular compartment to the interstitial tissue but no oedema develops. This is because the excess fluid enters the lymphatic channels and drains away from the site where it might otherwise accumulate, eventually returning to the blood via the thoracic duct. Should the normal flow of lymph be obstructed, oedema fluid will collect.

Indeed, some of the most striking examples of local oedema occur in the context of lymphatic obstruction, this being known as lymphoedema. Examples of lymphoedema include the severe chronic swelling of the upper limb seen in some women following removal of the breast and axillary contents for carcinoma of the breast (radical mastectomy) and the spectacular oedema that may occur in the tropics in individuals infected with the helminth *Wuchereria bancrofti*.

Types of Oedema Fluid: Transudate and Exudate

Oedema may be either **local** or **systemic**. The characteristics of the oedema fluid depend on the mechanisms predominantly involved in its formation (see *Table 20.1*). If the collection of fluid in the interstitial tissues is associated with an increase in **vascular permeability** then the fluid will contain large amounts of macromolecular proteins including fibrinogen and is termed an **exudate**. If the mechanisms involved are predominantly **hydrostatic** then the protein content of the oedema fluid will be low; such fluid is spoken of as being a **transudate**.

In practical terms the three most important factors causing oedema are:
1) raised intracapillary pressure
2) low plasma oncotic pressure
3) retention of salt and water

The coexistence of any two of these is likely to be associated with oedema of considerable severity.

Table 20.1 Characteristics of Exudates and Transudates

Characteristics	Exudate	Transudate
Total protein	High	Low (1 g per 100 ml)
Protein pattern	As in plasma	Albumin only
Fibrinogen	++ (and clots)	Nil
Specific gravity	1.020	1.012
Cells	++	Few mesothelial cells

Systemic Oedema

Cardiac Oedema

Although the systemic oedema caused by congestive cardiac failure has been recognized for many centuries, the mechanisms involved are by no means simple or easy to understand. There is not only a redistribution but a general retention of fluid, this being shown by an increase in body-weight of the patient. The distribution of the excess fluid is determined largely by gravity. When the patient is ambulant, the legs are first involved and swelling of the ankles at the end of the day is often the first sign reported. When the patient is confined to bed, the oedema appears in the sacral or, less commonly, in the genital region. The oedematous areas pit readily on finger pressure.

It would be tempting to ascribe this oedema purely to failure of the pumping function of the ventricles leading to an increase in venous pressure and a consequent increase in capillary hydrostatic pressure with the formation of a transudate. However, this would be not only a gross oversimplification, but also wrong, although this mechanism does contribute to the development of cardiac oedema.

Doubt as to a significant role for back pressure in cardiac oedema arises from three observations:
1) There is often an increased **plasma volume** in heart failure, which may occur before there is any rise in central venous pressure.
2) Oedema frequently occurs **before the rise in central venous pressure**.
3) The **degree of oedema is not proportional to the height of the central venous pressure**.

The most important mechanism in causing the oedema of cardiac failure is **excess retention of sodium and water by the renal tubules**. Failure of the heart as a pump leads initially to a fall in mean capillary pressure. This will in turn lead to a reduction in renal perfusion, aggravated by vasoconstriction mediated by the sympathetic nervous system. This relative renal ischaemia causes an increase in the production of renin and thus of angiotensin I. The rise in angiotensin levels causes an increased release of aldosterone from the zona glomerulosa of the adrenal cortex and retention of sodium and water. At first, such retention has a good effect because it allows the mean filling pressure in the circulation to be increased. The increased filling of the heart stretches the heart muscle fibres and thus leads, in terms of Starling's law, to increased force of contraction. In due time, however, any advantage arising from sodium and water retention is lost.

Once cardiac filling pressure and hence stretching of muscle fibres exceeds a certain point, there is no further increase in cardiac output; indeed there is a decline in the work output of the cardiac muscle. Excess accumulation of fluid in the lung (pulmonary oedema) may ensue and this may interfere with gas exchange in the alveoli.

Renal Oedema

Oedema related to renal disorders occurs under two different sets of circumstances, associated with the nephritic and the nephrotic syndrome.

Oedema Associated with Acute Glomerulonephritis (the Nephritic Syndrome)

Oedema is often a presenting feature in this disease, although it is usually not severe. The face and eyelids are affected predominantly, although on some occasions the ankles and genitalia may be involved as well. There is no entirely satisfactory explanation for either the cause of the oedema or its distribution. However, it is likely that the control of sodium excretion in the urine is multifactorial and that states of sodium retention may exist in which there is no associated disturbance of plasma volume. Although in most examples of systemic oedema the kidney behaves as if it were responding to a low plasma volume stimulus, there are other vasoactive stimuli, including circulating catecholamines, aldosterone and intrarenal hormones such as prostaglandins or kinins, that may influence renal tubular handling of sodium. It has been suggested that the primary mechanism responsible for **nephritic oedema** is a fall in glomerular filtration rate, tubular reabsorption of sodium remaining more or less normal. The resulting increase in extracellular fluid volume would normally be followed by a brisk natriuresis but this response appears to be blunted in acute glomerulonephritis. The oedema fluid in acute glomerulonephritis has the characteristics of a transudate, indicating that no significant change has occurred in the permeability of the microcirculation.

Oedema Associated with the Nephrotic Syndrome

The nephrotic syndrome encompasses a group of features that most notably includes **heavy proteinuria** (in excess of the ability of the liver to synthesize albumin) leading to **hypoalbuminaemia** and a resulting **decrease in plasma oncotic pressure**. While this loss of plasma protein certainly plays a part in the genesis of the systemic oedema encountered in this syndrome, other mechanisms also operate, including excess retention of sodium by the renal tubules. This is partly due to increased aldosterone production by the adrenal cortex, but some workers believe that non-systemic intrarenal mechanisms related to sodium reabsorption are also of importance.

Nutritional Oedema

Oedema is a well-recognized feature of prolonged starvation. There is no correlation between the degree of oedema and the concentrations within the blood of albumin and other plasma proteins; indeed, oedema associated with starvation may be seen in the presence of normal concentrations of plasma protein. It has been suggested that the explanation for this variety of oedema lies in the loss of subcutaneous adipose tissue. This leads to a subcutaneous connective tissue of much looser texture than normal and an associated decline in the tissue tension within it. Bed rest is usually followed by a brisk diuresis and consequent lessening of the degree of oedema.

An important and, regrettably, common variant of nutritional oedema occurs in **kwashiorkor**, resulting from protein and calorie undernutrition in young children in economically deprived communities in Africa, Asia, and Central and South America. These children, who fail to grow normally, are anaemic and have grossly fatty livers. They often exhibit a curious combination of **oedema** (associated with hypoalbuminaemia), **mucocutaneous ulceration** (the skin of the inner thighs often looks as if it has been scalded), and **depigmentation of the hair**. Adequate nutrition in terms of the protein content of the diet can produce a complete return to normal.

Oedema due to Chronic Liver Disease

This is discussed in Chapter 35 (see pp 616–618).

Pulmonary Oedema

This subject is discussed in Chapter 33 (see pp 446–451).

Local Oedema

Local oedema may occur as a result of three types of pathological disturbance. Firstly, a **local increase** in the **hydrostatic pressure within the microcirculation** may be operating. This can occur in pregnancy, in patients with occlusive venous thrombosis, and in those with varicose veins where the valves are incompetent giving rise to increased pressure in the superficial plexus of draining veins. Secondly, **increased local vascular permeability** can result in local oedema, as in acute inflammation and type I hypersensitivity reactions such as urticaria and angioneurotic oedema.

Lymphoedema

The maintenance of the interstitial fluid volume within narrow limits requires normal lymphatic drainage, and any obstruction to the normal flow of lymph as a result of surgery or inflammation may cause quite severe local oedema. For example, some patients who undergo radical surgery for the removal of carcinoma of the breast and have the axillary tissue dissected and removed develop severe and intractable oedema of the arm on the side of the operation. The inflammatory disease classically associated with lymphatic obstruction is infestation by the nematode worm *Wuchereria bancrofti* (filariasis). In its adult form the worm inhabits the lymphatics in the groin. While it is alive the presence of the parasite produces little disability, but when it dies there is a brisk local inflammatory reaction which leads, eventually, to lymphatic obstruction. The resulting oedema of the lower limbs and the genitalia is severe and chronic – so severe that the condition is sometimes spoken of as **elephantiasis**. Sometimes lymphoedema may develop as a result of congenital malformations in the lymphatic drainage; an autosomal dominant variety of this is known as Milroy's disease.

HYPERAEMIA AND CONGESTION

These two terms, which are used more or less as synonyms, mean that there is a **greater amount of blood than normal** in a given organ or tissue. Clearly there can be only two mechanisms for this: an **increased inflow** or a **diminished outflow** of blood (*Fig. 20.1*)

Increased inflow of blood must be achieved by arteriolar dilatation and is known as **active hyperaemia**. It is seen in areas involved in acute inflammation, after exposure to excess heat, in flushing, and at the margins of areas of ischaemic necrosis.

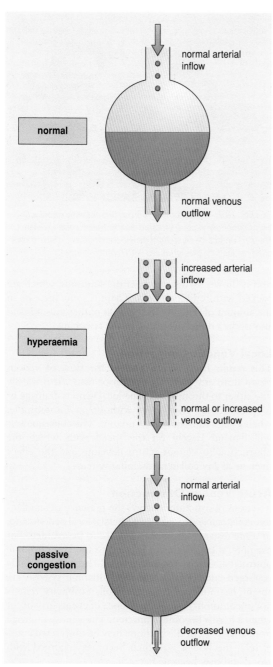

FIGURE 20.1 *Abnormal accumulations of blood in vascular beds arise either because of increased arterial inflow (hyperaemia) or diminished venous outflow (passive congestion).*

Diminished outflow is essentially an obstructive phenomenon. The obstruction may be functional rather than structural. An example of this is to be found in some patients with chronic bronchitis in whom the resultant hypoxia causes reflex constriction of the pulmonary arterioles. This leads to a rise in pulmonary artery pressure and hence, in due time, to a rise in central venous pressure and congestion of various organs. Because of the basically obstructive nature of the phenomenon, congestion of this type is generally spoken of as **passive**. As in the case of oedema, passive congestion can be generalized or local.

Generalized Venous Congestion

In its acute form, generalized venous congestion may be seen in many patients who die suddenly from a variety of causes; it represents the sudden accumulation of blood behind a failing ventricle with resulting engorgement of the affected organs or tissues. However, in clinical practice, generalized venous congestion is most often manifest in its chronic form, the basic cause being, once again, a failing ventricle. The mechanisms involved in the accumulation of blood are covered earlier in the discussion relating to cardiac oedema (see p 223). It results partly from the rise in pressure in the pulmonary and systemic veins, and partly (in so far as the pulmonary circulation is concerned) from the shift of blood from the systemic to the pulmonary circulation as a result of peripheral vasoconstriction.

Generalized venous congestion also occurs in a variety of pulmonary disorders associated with a rise in pulmonary artery pressure. This leads to a compensatory increase in the muscle mass of the right ventricle (hypertrophy due to pressure overload). In time the right ventricle may be unable to maintain a normal output in the face of the pulmonary hypertension and when this happens there is a rise in systemic venous pressure, and congestion in organs such as the liver and spleen. This form of cardiac failure is known as **cor pulmonale** and may be the result of disorders affecting the bronchioles and alveoli, thoracic movements or pulmonary vasculature.

Morphology and Pathophysiology of Cor Pulmonale

The characteristic change seen in cor pulmonale is **right ventricular hypertrophy** secondary to pulmonary hypertension. The pulmonary circulation is a low pressure system where an increase in cardiac output (as with exercise) produces no increase in pulmonary artery pressure until the flow has increased several times the normal. Once this level has been exceeded, there is a fairly steep, linear rise in pressure in proportion to the increase in flow. This ability of the pulmonary arterial bed to accept increased blood flow of a very considerable degree without a concomitant rise in pressure has important clinical implications. More than 50% of the pulmonary vascular bed must be destroyed or obstructed before pulmonary hypertension will be present at rest. Of course, any decrease in the pulmonary vascular bed will mean that smaller rises in cardiac output are required to raise the pulmonary artery pressure, and the more severe the reduction in capacity of the pulmonary circulation, the less the rise in cardiac output will need to be. Pulmonary hypertension, however, is quite common in the absence of destruction of part of the pulmonary vasculature. It arises as a result of pulmonary vasoconstriction, which occurs in the pulmonary arterioles as a response to hypoxia. This is frequently seen in diseases associated with chronic obstruction to air flow, such as chronic bronchitis.

Morphological Changes of Chronic Venous Congestion

Generally speaking, chronically congested organs are swollen, darker in colour, and firmer in consistency than normal.

The Lung

> #### *Microscopic Features*
> Marked engorgement of the alveolar capillaries is seen, each capillary being stuffed with blood. This distension of the capillaries gives the alveolar septa a beaded appearance. Quite often small intra-alveolar haemorrhages are seen due to rupture of the overdistended capillaries. This may be so marked a feature (especially in patients with severe pulmonary venous hypertension, as in mitral stenosis) that the patient coughs up blood-stained sputum (**haemoptysis**). The red blood cells break down and the iron-containing moiety of haemoglobin becomes converted to a yellow-brown crystalline pigment known as haemosiderin. This pigment is engulfed by alveolar macrophages, which then become known as **siderophages** or 'heart failure cells'. With the passage of time the congested alveolar septa become thicker than normal. In the early stages of chronic pulmonary venous congestion this is due largely to the presence of oedema fluid within the interstitial tissue of the septa. Later, fibrosis occurs within the septa and the lung tissue becomes much firmer than normal. The combination of a significant degree of iron pigmentation and interstitial fibrosis in longstanding pulmonary congestion is known as **brown induration** (*Fig. 20.2*).

The Liver

The structural changes seen in the chronically congested liver of a patient suffering from cardiac failure result from a combination of two processes. These are, firstly, a rise in pressure in the hepatic veins, central veins and sinusoids, and, secondly, poor perfusion of that part of the hepatic lobule which is furthest from its arterial supply. The morphological features are discussed in Chapter 35 (see pp 609–610).

The Spleen

The congested spleen is moderately enlarged (up to 250 g) and is of firmer consistency than normal. The cut surface is smooth and firm and the red pulp is a dark, purplish colour. On microscopic examination conges-

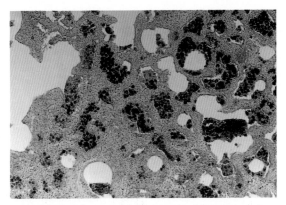

FIGURE 20.2 Section of lung from a patient with sustained high pulmonary venous pressure due to mitral valve disease. The section has been stained by the Perl method, which shows haemosiderin as blue granules within macrophages.

tion is shown by distension of the sinusoids, which are packed with red blood cells. There is some increase in the amount of reticulin in the walls of the sinusoids and also in the connective tissue in the trabecula.

Local Venous Congestion

This results from obstruction to the flow of venous blood from any part of an organ or tissue. It is usually due either to thrombosis in the local venous drainage or to pressure on veins from without as, for example, when a large tumour mass is present. The consequences will depend largely on the speed with which the obstruction to venous return develops and the effectiveness of any collateral draining systems.

Acute Venous Obstruction

If venous obstruction is acute, the presence of an effective collateral drainage system is vital if local oedema and, in some instances, haemorrhage are to be avoided. For example, if large veins in relation to the brain become obstructed, their tributaries will become severely engorged and, because collateral draining systems are absent, haemorrhage from the swollen tributary veins is not uncommon. A similar sequence of events may occur when a hernia becomes impacted. The venous drainage from a segment of the intestine may be obstructed completely; the bowel wall then becomes engorged with blood and may become necrotic.

When local venous obstruction is chronic, the collateral veins usually become markedly distended and may, under certain circumstances, rupture. This is seen in **portal hypertension**, which may occur as a result of disturbances in hepatic lobular architecture brought about by the processes involved in cirrhosis, as a result of pathological changes in the portal tracts, or as a result of obstruction to the portal vein itself. The rise in portal vein blood pressure leads to distension of the short gastric veins and of the anastomotic veins at the lower end of the oesophagus; this confers a risk of serious haemorrhage.

CHAPTER 21

Pigmentation and Heterotopic Calcification

PIGMENTATION

The pigments that may accumulate in excess amounts within the tissues or that may occur in abnormally small amounts can be separated into endogenous and exogenous groups.

Endogenous pigments are those produced within the body; there are three main types:
1) Melanin
2) Pigments derived from haemoglobin
3) Pigments associated with fats

MELANIN

Melanin constitutes the colouring matter of the hair, skin and eyes. It is also normally present in the leptomeninges, the nerve cells in the substantia nigra and the adrenal medulla. Limited pigmentation due to melanin may also occur in the juxtacutaneous mucous membranes of the vulva and mouth. Melanin-producing cells may also be found in small numbers in the ovary, gastrointestinal tract and urinary bladder.

Identification of Melanin in Tissues

As anyone who has moles and freckles will know, melanin usually produces a yellow-brown colour in the tissues where it is deposited. If present in very large amounts, the local area of tissue may appear black. On histological examination the melanin appears as brown intracellular granules. It possesses the ability to reduce solutions of ammoniacal silver with the consequent deposition of black granules of silver on the melanin granules. Substances that can do this are spoken of as 'argentaffin'. Where pigmentation is very heavy the melanin can be removed from the tissue sections by bleaching them with oxidizing agents such as hydrogen peroxide.

Site of Production

Melanin is produced by specialized cells, the **melanocytes**, which can be seen in the greatest numbers in the basal layer of the epidermis. They are of neural crest origin and migrate to their various permanent homes during embryonic life. The average number of skin melanocytes is 1500 per mm², the number varying from 2000 per mm² in the forehead and cheeks to 800 per mm² in the skin of the abdomen. The number of melanocytes in the skin is constant (relatively) regardless of race. The darker skin of black people, for example, is due to increased activity of the melanocytes, not to increased numbers.

Melanin is synthesized in small membrane-bound bodies known as melanosomes, which are to be found in the Golgi apparatus. The melanin granules are transferred from the melanocytes to the neighbouring epidermal cells. At the point of contact between the dendritic process of the melanocyte and the plasma membrane of the epidermal cell, there is considerable excitation of the latter and clumps of pigment are taken into the epidermal cell and come to lie in a perinuclear position.

Formation

The basic starting point for the synthesis of melanin is the amino acid tyrosine (*Fig. 21.1*).

The most important functional aspect of the melanocyte is its complement of tyrosinase. Absence of this enzyme results in complete inability to synthesize melanin. The resulting syndrome is **albinism** (absence of pigmentation in skin, hair and conjunctiva). All normal melanocytes contain tyrosinase but not all are actively engaged in producing melanin. For this reason it is sometimes necessary to employ special means for the identification of melanocytes. This may be done by incubating the tissue sections in a solution of either dopa or tyrosine. If tyrosinase is present within the cells, melanin will be produced.

Clearly the intensity of skin colouring depends not only on the number of melanin-producing cells present in any site but also on their activity. This appears to be related to certain hormones of the pituitary and, to a lesser extent, the gonads.

The pituitary secretes a hormone, **melanocyte-stimulating hormone (MSH)**, which shares part of its amino acid sequence with adrenocorticotrophic hormone. In Addison's disease, where there is destruction of adrenal tissue due to either autoimmune processes or tuberculosis, there is loss of normal feedback mechanisms because of the fall in adrenal activity. Additional MSH is secreted by the pituitary; skin and mucosal pigmentation is thus a common feature of the disease.

Abnormalities in Melanin Pigmentation

Generalized Hyperpigmentation

There are a number of diseases in which hyperpigmentation occurs.

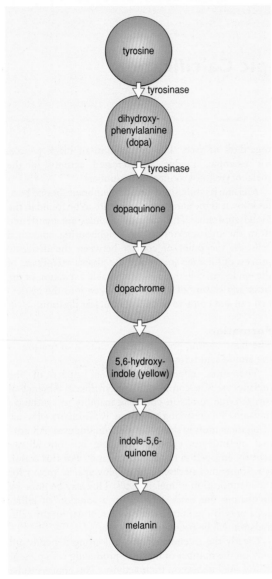

FIGURE 21.1 Synthesis of melanin.

- Addison's disease
- Acromegaly
- Large doses of oestrogens given for treatment of prostatic cancer. These sometimes cause generalized hyperpigmentation. In addition, the effects of oestrogen may be the reason for the hyperpigmentation that sometimes occurs in chronic liver disease, in which it is alleged there is inadequate hepatic breakdown of oestrogen. In pregnancy, the nipples and genitalia become darker and there is sometimes a blotchy hyperpigmentation in the butterfly area of the face. This is known as chloasma.
- Chronic arsenical poisoning

- Haemochromatosis in which excess storage of iron in parenchymal cells occurs
- In association with chlorpromazine administration. A curious violet-grey pigmentation occasionally develops after treatment with this drug; it may affect the eyes and parts of the skin exposed to sunlight.

Focal Hyperpigmentation

This may occur in a number of situations:
- **Freckles**, which are probably genetically determined.
- **Café au lait spots** are large hyperpigmented macules. Unlike common freckles, these show an increase in the number of melanocytes. They are found in two rare systemic conditions: firstly, neurofibromatosis, a condition characterized by the presence of multiple tumours derived from the fibrous element of the nerve sheath, and secondly, Albright's syndrome, which consists of a triad of polyostotic fibrous dysplasia, hyperpigmentation, and sexual and skeletal precocity.
- **Peutz–Jeghers syndrome** is a rare syndrome inherited as an autosomal dominant. It has two main characteristics: a curious focal hyperpigmentation involving the lips and the circumoral skin, and multiple polyps in the gastrointestinal tract, which may cause acute or subacute intestinal obstruction.
- **Lentiginosis** is the presence of multiple hyperpigmented spots characterized by an increase in the number of melanocytes. This has been reported to be associated with hypertrophic cardiomyopathy in a few cases.
- Focal hyperpigmentation can result from exposure to ionizing radiation, ultraviolet light, heat (*erythema ab igne*) and chronic irritation (as in itchy dermatoses).
- Tumours arising from melanocytes are most commonly seen in the skin but may occur at any of the sites in which melanocytes have been described. Most of these are benign – the 'moles' of various kinds – but a small proportion are malignant (mostly *ab initio*). These are termed 'malignant melanomas'. Other skin tumours may accumulate melanin and this may cause some concern as to their nature. This type of pigmentation is common in seborrhoeic warts and basal cell carcinoma.

Hypopigmentation

Albinism

This, as already mentioned, is due to a **deficiency of tyrosinase**. In classical cases the skin is very white, the hair pale, the irides transparent and the pupils pink. Such extreme cases are fortunately rare among humans. These patients tend to suffer from the skin tumours believed to be associated with exposure to sunlight, thus emphasizing the importance of melanin as a protective agent against the effects of ultraviolet light.

Focal hypopigmentation (**vitiligo**) is very common and is characterized by the presence of well-demarcated areas of depigmentation. Histological examination shows either paucity or absence of melanocytes.

PIGMENTS DERIVED FROM HAEMOGLOBIN

In this section we shall restrict our consideration to the iron-containing pigments.

Excess iron, which may be either localized or systemic, is initially stored in the form of **ferritin.** This is a micellar structure about 5.4 nm in diameter which consists of a ferric core surrounded by a shell of protein subunits. Ferritin cannot be seen under the light microscope and does not give positive reactions with the staining methods commonly employed for the recognition of iron. It may, however, be seen fairly easily with the electron microscope.

With further increases in intracellular iron accumulation, the ferritin molecules aggregate to produce a coarse crystalline yellow-brown pigment which is easily seen on light microscopy. This pigment is known as **haemosiderin**. These crystals are about 36% iron and can be identified with certainty by applying the Prussian blue method (also known as Perl's or Turnbull's reaction). This involves treating either tissues or tissue sections with a mixture of hydrochloric acid and potassium ferrocyanide. The iron in the tissues is present in a trivalent form and a blue precipitate of ferric ferrocyanide is produced. This method is both easy and sensitive.

Localized Deposition of Haemosiderin

Localized deposition of haemosiderin always implies that there has been haemorrhage at the site of the pigmentation. Haemosiderin pigmentation is therefore frequently seen in relation to bruises, organizing haematomas, fracture sites and haemorrhagic infarcts as well as certain tumour-like lesions such as sclerosing haemangioma in the dermis and pigmented villonodular synovitis in the large joints.

The cells of the renal tubules can convert haemoglobin to haemosiderin, and haemosiderinuria may sometimes follow haemoglobinuria.

One of the most frequent local depositions of haemosiderin seen at autopsy is in the lungs. This is usually associated with high pulmonary venous pressure as in 'tight' mitral stenosis or left ventricular failure. Sometimes severe pulmonary haemosiderosis will be caused by immune injury of the Gell and Coombes type 2 variety. This is accompanied by acute immune-mediated injury to the glomerular basement membranes and is known as Goodpasture's syndrome.

Generalized Haemosiderosis

If the body is overloaded with iron, haemosiderin is formed in excessive amounts and deposited in a wide range of tissues. The total quantity of iron normally present in the body is 4–5 g, and this level appears to be controlled by powerful homoeostatic mechanisms.

Normal Western-style diets contain 10–15 mg of iron per day; only about 10% of this is absorbed. There is a normal loss of about 1 mg per day through shedding of cells from the gastrointestinal tract, skin, etc. Females lose about 200–300 mg per year as a result of menstruation.

There are two basic morphological patterns for the deposition of the excess haemosiderin:

1) Parenchymatous deposition
2) Deposition in the cells of the reticuloendothelial system. This pattern is seen following parenteral iron administration or repeated blood transfusion.

The possible mechanisms that might account for the accumulation of excess iron in the body are:

- increased absorption of iron
- decreased excretion (although there is no evidence for this as yet)
- impaired utilization
- excess breakdown of haemoglobin with release of iron

Haemochromatosis is discussed in Chapter 35 (see pp 594–597).

PIGMENTS ASSOCIATED WITH FATS

This group of endogenous pigments is termed the **lipofuscins** (L. *fuscus* dark or sombre). These are often also spoken of as 'wear-and-tear' pigments because they appear to accumulate as a manifestation of ageing.

Lipofuscins are yellowish-brown granular pigments which appear within atrophic parenchymal cells, particularly in the liver and heart of old people. When present in large amounts they impart a brown colour to the affected organ or tissue. Such organs are spoken of as showing **brown atrophy**. These pigments are deemed to represent the breakdown products of membranes of 'worn out' organelles. With ageing of cells, autophagic vacuoles are formed in increasing number as active metabolic organelles become 'redundant'. With these autophagic vacuoles, the lipid portions of the membranes tend to resist lysosomal digestion. These lipid remnants undergo auto-oxidation to form a variety of lipoperoxides and aldehydes with a yellow colour. The pigment remains within lysosomes and appears to produce no ill effects on the tissues.

EXOGENOUS PIGMENTATION

Exogenous pigmentation can occur, but tends to be of social rather than pathological significance. The commonest example is to be found in tattoo marks. Occasionally the long-continued use of external medications containing metals, for example silver-containing ear drops, produces pigmentation.

HETEROTOPIC CALCIFICATION

Heterotopic calcification is the deposition of calcium salts in tissues other than osteoid and enamel. There are two main varieties: **dystrophic** and **metastatic calcification**.

DYSTROPHIC CALCIFICATION
In dystrophic calcification, serum calcium levels are normal and calcium salts are deposited in dead or degenerate tissues. This occurs in the following sets of circumstances:
- caseous necrosis (calcification is the hallmark of old caseation)
- fat necrosis
- thrombosis
- haematomas (e.g. subdural haematoma or myositis ossificans)
- atherosclerotic plaques
- chronic inflammatory granulation tissue (e.g. constrictive pericarditis)
- Mönckeberg's sclerosis of the medial coat of muscular arteries
- degenerate colloid goitres
- cysts of various kinds
- degenerate tumours (e.g. uterine leiomyomas)

METASTATIC CALCIFICATION
Here the fundamental defect is a **raised blood calcium level**. This may result from the removal of calcium from the bones as, for example, in hyperparathyroidism or from excess calcium derived from the gut. Occasionally, as in renal osteodystrophy, the precipitating factor appears to be high blood phosphate concentration.

This type of calcium deposition occurs at a variety of sites:
- **The kidney**. Deposition occurs round the tubules and damages them. Ultimately this may lead to renal failure. These patients often show an inability to acidify the urine. Stone formation in the renal pelvis and ureter is often associated with nephrocalcinosis.
- **The lung**. Calcium is deposited in the alveolar walls.
- **The stomach**. The calcium is deposited around the fundal glands. It has been suggested that because these glands secrete hydrochloric acid, the tissues are left relatively alkaline and this is said to favour calcium deposition.
- **Blood vessels**. The coronary arteries are most affected.
- **The cornea.**

Causes of Metastatic Calcification
There are five common causes of metastatic calcification:
1) **Primary hyperparathyroidism**. Here the parathyroid is overactive and does not respond to normal negative feedback control. It is most commonly associated with a benign neoplasm (adenoma) but also occurs when the glands are hyperplastic and, very rarely, in association with malignant tumours of the parathyroid. The excess secretion of parathyroid hormone upregulates osteoclastic resorption of bone and thus leads to hypercalcaemia.
2) **Excessive absorption of calcium from the bowel**, which may be due to hypervitaminosis D or vitamin D-sensitive states such as idiopathic hypercalcaemia of infancy or even through excessive milk drinking.
3) **Hypophosphatasia**.
4) **Destructive bone lesions**. Hypercalcaemia in this context is usually associated with osteolytic secondary deposits of malignant neoplasms. It is worth remembering that hypercalcaemia may be associated with malignancy in the absence of bone deposits. This is known as humoral hypercalcaemia of malignancy and, in many instances, is due to the synthesis and release from the tumour cells of a parathyroid hormone-related peptide.
5) **Renal tubular acidosis**.

IDENTIFICATION OF HETEROTOPIC CALCIFICATION
On histological examination calcium salts appear as granules which stain a deep blue colour with haematoxylin. They typically form encrustations on such structures as elastic fibres in the lung or arteries.

Calcium stained with alizarin red shows a magenta colour. More commonly the von Kossa method is used, in which silver impregnation forms the basis of the stain. What it shows is, in fact, phosphate and carbonate, but because these are almost always associated with calcium when in its particulate and insoluble form, it constitutes a fairly effective method for the demonstration of calcium.

CHAPTER 22

Neoplasia: Disorders of Cell Proliferation and Differentiation

In communities where undernutrition, malnutrition and infectious diseases are no longer a major problem, neoplastic disease comes second only to cardiovascular disease as a cause of death. In the UK neoplastic disease will kill over 100 000 people in the next 12 months. The commonest malignant neoplasms in men and women respectively are shown in *Figs 22.1* and *22.2*.

DEFINITIONS

The term **neoplasia** is derived from two Greek words: '**neos**' meaning 'new' and '**plassein**' meaning 'to mould'. This is usually translated as **new growth**,

although this phrase begs certain important questions as to the essential nature of neoplasia.

Neoplasia is, in fact, not easy to define; many pathologists regard the best available definition as that suggested by Willis:

> 'A neoplasm is an abnormal mass of tissue, the growth of which exceeds and is unco-ordinated with that of the normal tissues, and which persists in the same excessive manner after cessation of the stimulus which has evoked the change.'

If we attempt to analyse this definition in operational terms it becomes clear that there are at least three types of disturbance of cell behaviour inherent within it, each

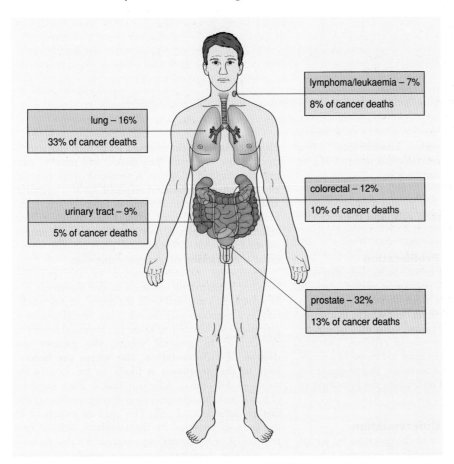

lymphoma/leukaemia – 7%

8% of cancer deaths

lung – 16%

33% of cancer deaths

colorectal – 12%

10% of cancer deaths

urinary tract – 9%

5% of cancer deaths

prostate – 32%

13% of cancer deaths

FIGURE 22.1 *Excluding skin tumours, five tumours account for 75% of cases of malignancy in males.*

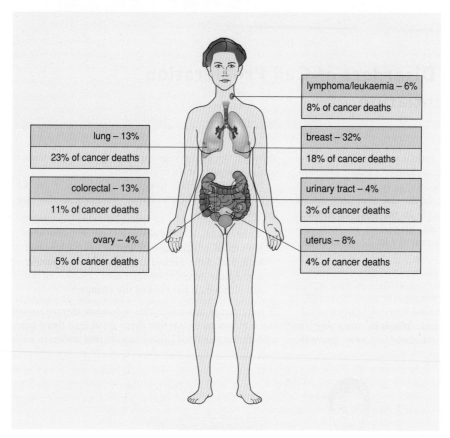

FIGURE 22.2 *Excluding skin tumours, seven tumours account for 80% of cases of malignancy in females.*

of which deserves separate consideration. This approach enables us to regard neoplasia in terms of a set of disorders showing a disturbance in:

- **cell proliferation**
- **cell differentation**
- **the relationship between cells and their surrounding stroma**

Disturbances in Cell Proliferation

Neoplasia involves defects in the mechanisms that normally maintain a given cell population within relatively narrow limits. This escape from normal control gives rise to a population of dividing cells which, in a sense, is **immortal** in that cell division occurs for a far greater number of times than in a normal cell line. The end result is a focus made up, in most instances, of a single type of cell in numbers that are totally inappropriate for the anatomical location. This leads to the formation of a mass or tumour.

Disturbances in Cell Differentiation

Differentiation is the sum of the processes by which the cells in a developing multicellular organism achieve their **specific set of functional and morphological**

characteristics. Cells sharing a set of such characteristics become organized into tissues, and these in turn may be arranged as organs. A fertilized ovum contains all the genetic information required for that organism and is, thus, totipotent in terms of future structure and function. A differentiated cell such as a muscle or liver cell obviously expresses only a small part of the genetic information; thus differentiation must involve a progressive **restriction** of genomic expression.

Impairment of differentiation of the cell line involved is extremely common in the formation of a neoplasm. At a practical level, the degree of differentiation in a neoplasm may, in many but not all instances, give useful information as to the likely natural history of the disease. **In general terms, the poorer the degree of differentiation, the worse the behaviour of the neoplasm is likely to be**. Loss of the ability to differentiate fully may lead to the acquisition of functional characteristics quite foreign to those of the mature differentiated cell. This may be expressed in the form of secretion by the neoplastic cells of fetal proteins or of hormones inappropriate for that particular cell type (**ectopic hormone production**) (see pp 265–267).

Disturbances in the Relationship Between Cells and their Surrounding Stroma

There is a disturbance in the relationship between cells that make up the neoplasm and the normal tissue that surrounds them. In many cases the cells of a neoplasm grow as a compact mass in an expansile fashion (**benign neoplasms**); in others the constituent cells **invade** the surrounding tissues and may spread to distant sites (**malignant neoplasms**).

CLASSIFICATION OF NEOPLASMS

In theory, neoplasms might be classified in a number of different ways. Some of the criteria that have been tried in the past include:

- aetiology
- embryogenesis
- organ of origin
- histogenesis or cytogenesis (tissue or cell of origin)
- biological behaviour

On a practical day-to-day level, the most useful of these are the cell type from which the neoplasm originated and biological behaviour. The latter is obviously of particular importance in determining the outcome of the disease in an individual. The pathologist who examines tissue removed in the course of biopsy or excision of a neoplasm will try to predict the biological behaviour on the basis of morphological appearances.

HISTOGENESIS AND CYTOGENESIS

As already stated, the cell and tissue types from which neoplasms arise, where it is possible to determine this, constitute the basis of the most commonly used classifications (*Table 22.1*).

At the simplest level these tissues of origin can be divided into two: **epithelium** and **connective tissues**. However, a much greater degree of subdivision is both possible and desirable. It is worth bearing in mind that, even at this basic level of grouping, certain difficulties may arise in correct attribution of a given neoplasm to one or other of these categories. For instance, neoplasms arising from mesothelial cells that line serosal cavities may show morphological characteristics suggestive of both epithelium and connective tissue. A more frequent problem in practice is that the cell population of a neoplasm may be so poorly differentiated as to make it very difficult or even impossible for the pathologist to identify the original cell type. In this situation, the use of immunological methods to identify either specific antigens or specific cell products may be helpful (*Fig. 22.3*).

BIOLOGICAL BEHAVIOUR

From the point of view of the patient, the most important characteristic of a neoplasm is its behaviour pattern. Essentially, all neoplasms, with only a few exceptions, are divided on this basis into two main groups: **benign** and **malignant**.

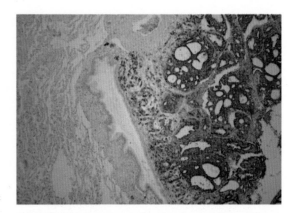

FIGURE 22.3 *Metastatic adenocarcinoma in the lung. The section has been treated with an antibody reacting with prostate-specific antigen. The binding of the antibody to the tumour cells (as shown by the brown staining) indicates a prostatic origin for the secondary tumour in the lung.*

Malignant neoplasms arising from **epithelium** are called **carcinomas** and those that have their origin from **connective tissue elements** are called **sarcomas**.

While this division into benign and malignant relates to the behaviour of a given neoplasm in operational terms, the behavioural characteristics, as stated above, are reflected to a considerable extent in the morphological appearances of the lesion.

Benign Neoplasms

Use of the word 'benign' does not imply that such neoplasms are clinically unimportant or that they may not constitute a serious hazard. In the context of neoplastic disease, the word **benign** means that the cells making up the neoplasm **show no tendency to invade the surrounding tissue** and, by the same token, **never spread to distant sites (metastasis).** The growth pattern of a benign neoplasm is an **expansile** one, often associated with the formation of a capsule derived from the surrounding connective tissue (*Figs 22.4* and *22.5*) and with some pressure atrophy of surrounding parenchyma. The growth rate is often low and few, if any, cells undergoing mitotic division are seen.

Malignant Neoplasms

The absolute criterion of malignancy is **invasiveness**. Instead of the expansile growth pattern characteristic of benign neoplasms, malignant cells separate from one another and grow out in an irregular pattern into the surrounding tissue (*Figs 22.4* and *22.6*). In many instances the malignant cells gain access to vascular channels – either lymphatics, blood vessels or both. Once such vascular invasion has occurred, groups of malignant cells can be carried in the blood or lymph until they impact at some distance from the primary growth. From the site of impaction the malignant cells emigrate into the extravascular compartment and may

Table 22.1 A Classification of Tumours

	Behaviour		
Tissue of origin	Benign	Intermediate	Malignant
Epithelium			
Covering and protective epithelium	Squamous, transitional and columnar cell papilloma		Squamous and transitional cell carcinoma; adenocarcinoma
Compact secreting epithelium	Adenoma: if cystic, cystadenoma; if papillary and cystic, papillary cystadenoma		Adenocarcinoma: if cystic, cystadenocarcinoma
Other epithelial neoplasms		Basal cell carcinomas; salivary and mucous gland neoplasms; carcinoid tumours (argentaffinoma)	
Connective tissue			
Fibrous	Fibroma		Fibrosarcoma
Nerve sheath	Neurilemmoma Neurofibroma		Neurofibrosarcoma
Adipose	Lipoma		Liposarcoma
Smooth muscle	Leiomyoma		Leiomyosarcoma
Striated muscle	Rhabdomyoma		Rhabdomyosarcoma
Synovium	Synovioma		Synoviosarcoma
Cartilage	Chondroma		Chondrosarcoma
Bone			
Osteoblast	Osteoma		Osteosarcoma
Unknown		◄———— Giant cell tumour ————►	
Mesothelium	Benign mesothelioma		Malignant mesothelioma
Blood vessels and lymphatics			Angiosarcoma
Meninges	Meningioma		Malignant meningioma
Specialized connective tissue			
Neuroglia and ependyma		◄——— Astrocytoma, oligodendroglioma ———► Ependymoma	
Chromaffin tissue	Carotid body tumour; phaeochromocytoma		Malignant variants
Lymphoid and haemopoietic tissue		Myeloproliferative disorders	Malignant lymphoma of varying degrees of differentiation, Hodgkin's disease; plasmacytoma; multiple myeloma syndrome; Waldenström's macroglobulinaemia; leukaemias
Melanocytes			Malignant melanoma
Fetal trophoblast	Hydatidiform mole		Choriocarcinoma

Table 22.1 A Classification of Tumours – *continued*

Tissue of origin	Behaviour		
	Benign	Intermediate	Malignant
Embryonic tissue			
Totipotential or pluripotential cell	Benign teratoma		Malignant teratoma
Kidney			Nephroblastoma
Liver			Hepatoblastoma
Unipotential cell			
Retina			Retinoblastoma
Hindbrain			Medulloblastoma
Sympathetic ganglia and adrenal medulla	Ganglioneuroma		Neuroblastoma
Unipotential embryonic cells in pelvic organs			Juvenile rhabdomyosarcoma (botryoid sarcoma)
Embryonic vestiges			
Notochord			Chordoma
Enamel organ		Ameloblastoma	
Parapituitary residues		Craniopharyngioma	

form new deposits of neoplastic tissue (**secondary deposits** or **metastases**). The mechanisms involved in tumour spread are discussed in Chapter 25.

From the morphological point of view, malignant cells and the structures they form tend to show evidence of **increased cell proliferation** and **incomplete differentiation**.

Increased Cell Proliferation

This is expressed in the form of an increased number of

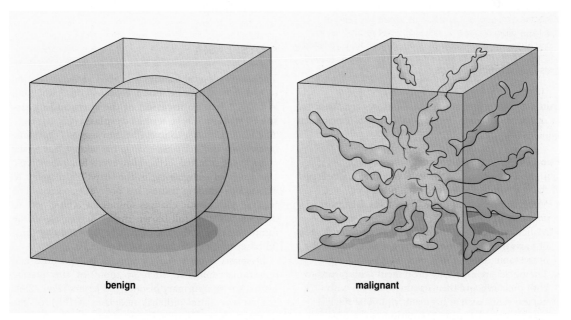

benign   malignant

FIGURE 22.4 Benign and malignant neoplasms are, in general, distinguished from each other by their growth patterns. Benign tumours have an expansile growth pattern whereas malignant ones are infiltrative.

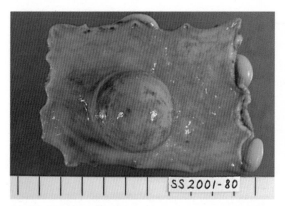

FIGURE 22.5 A lipoma (benign neoplasm arising from adipose tissue) of the caecum. The lesion shows the typical well-defined edge of a benign neoplasm. The mucosa is stretched over the mass and is thinned but not invaded.

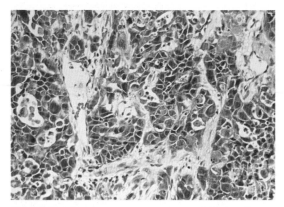

FIGURE 22.6 Invasive squamous carcinoma of the bronchus. While the tumour cells can still be recognized as being of squamous origin because of their shape and relationship with one another, they show features of malignancy both cytologically and in the form of breaching of the basement membrane and invasion of subepithelial tissue.

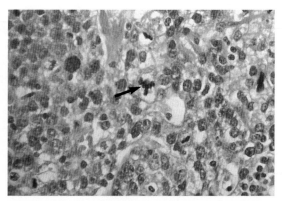

FIGURE 22.7 Poorly differentiated squamous carcinoma of the uterine cervix. The tumour cells are barely recognizable as being of squamous origin (compare with Fig. 22.6). Atypical mitoses are present, including a tripolar one (T) in the centre of the field.

mitoses. Not infrequently these mitoses are abnormal in appearance, with tripolar, quadripolar or annular spindles (*Fig. 22.7*).

Poor Differentiation

This shows itself both at the level of individual cells and in the relationship of cells to each other.

- Malignant cells tend to be larger than their normal counterparts.
- Malignant cells tend to show a much greater degree of **variation in size and shape** than normal cells of the same origin.
- The nuclei are especially prominent with regard to both their size and their staining reaction with nuclear stains such as haematoxylin. The nuclei occupy a much greater proportion of the total cell volume than is normal; this is termed an increase in the **nuclear:cytoplasmic ratio.** The DNA

content of the nuclei of malignant cells may be much greater than normal, and chromosomal analysis not infrequently shows loss of normal ploidy.

As stated above, loss of differentiation involves the patterns of cell arrangement as well as the morphology of individual cells. The normal orderly relationships between cells tend to disappear and structures, such as ductules or glands, formed by malignant cells may differ considerably from their normal non-neoplastic counterparts. In other instances the neoplasm may be so poorly differentiated that no recognizable structures are formed and the malignant cells grow in disorganized sheets or islands.

DYSPLASIA

The morphological features described above in relation to malignancy may be found, especially in epithelium, at a stage when **no invasion of the surrounding tissue is evident**. This is termed **dysplasia** (Gk. *dys* bad). The finding of dysplastic epithelium suggests that some irreversible and heritable change has taken place in the genome of affected cells. However, full phenotypic expression of malignancy, in the shape of an ability to invade surrounding tissues, has not yet occurred. The finding of dysplastic changes sounds a warning note to the clinician that full-blown malignancy may, in the future, develop at the site of the dysplasia and that careful observation of the patient is required.

Dysplasia is particularly common in squamous and transitional epithelia, such as those of the uterine cervix, the skin, urinary bladder and larynx (*Fig. 22.8*).

Dysplasia (intraepithelial neoplasia (CIN)) of the uterine cervix can usually be diagnosed by microscopic studies on cells exfoliated from the epithelial surface and collected on a spatula ('cervical smear

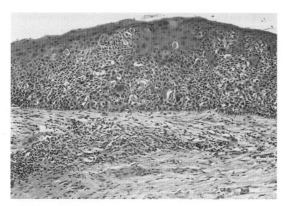

FIGURE 22.8 Intraepithelial neoplasia of severe degree (carcinoma in situ) of the larynx. Note loss of the normal orderly pattern of the stratified squamous epithelium, and variation in the size and staining of cells. The basement membrane remains intact.

cytology'). Such cytological diagnoses can be confirmed histologically by taking very small biopsies under direct vision (colposcopic biopsy). If the dysplastic process is severe and widespread within the cervix, the patient may be treated by a wide cone-shaped excision of cervical tissue in which, it is hoped, all the dysplastic epithelium is removed. Freedom from epithelial dysplasia in the lines of excision is checked by histological examination.

In some cases of epithelial dysplasia, the whole thickness of the epithelial covering shows dysplastic change; for these situations, the term **carcinoma** *in situ* (CIN-3) is often used. Dysplasia represents a continuum of change which, as already stated, may end in frank malignancy.

Some Lesions that may be Confused with True Neoplasms

Hamartoma

The term *hamartoma* is derived from the Greek word 'hamartanein' which means 'to make an error'. Hamartomas are tumour-like masses which may grow to a considerable size but which lack the autonomy and persistence of the excessive growth characteristic of a true neoplasm. In a hamartoma the elements that make up the lesion are fully differentiated and are normally found in the organ or tissue in which the hamartoma occurs. However, the way in which these elements are put together differs considerably from what is found in normal tissues.

These lesions may be found in a wide range of anatomical locations and may consist of a wide variety of differentiated tissue elements. The lung is not an uncommon site for the development of a hamartoma; in this situation, well-demarcated masses of cartilage measuring up to 2–3 cm in diameter may be found. On histological examination, such lesions show the presence of small slits within the cartilage which are lined by bronchial-type epithelium. Thus the lesion consists of some of the elements of the normal bronchial wall. In easily inspected tissues such as the skin, where hamartomatous lesions are common, it is clear that a hamartoma may be present at birth, but its growth phase may not occur until much later.

The commonest hamartoma is vascular in type. There is a wide range of these, from the flat 'port-wine stain' to large, raised, complex masses of abnormal vascular spaces.

Hamartomas may form part of some inherited syndromes. An interesting example is the Peutz–Jeghers syndrome (see also p 527) in which multiple hamartomas involving the glands and muscle of the intestinal wall may be present.

Heteroplasia

Heteroplasia is the differentiation of part of an organ or tissue in a way that is quite foreign to the part. It can be distinguished from metaplasia as there is no change from one fully differentiated form to another. Instead the anomalous differentiation takes place from the stem cell stage. For instance, gastric mucosa might be found within the wall of a Meckel's diverticulum in the distal part of the ileum or in the gallbladder wall. Similarly, anomalous masses of pancreatic tissue sometimes occur in the wall of the small intestine; it is of interest that these usually consist of ductal and acinar tissue only; islets of Langerhans are infrequent.

Occasionally heteroplasia may be expressed in the form of quite large and complicated masses in which several differentiated tissues may be seen. For example, a large mass on a patient's face has been described which contained ectopic liver, pancreatic tissue and gut epithelium. Such heterotopic masses have been termed **choristomas**.

STRUCTURAL FEATURES OF COMMON NEOPLASMS

BENIGN EPITHELIAL NEOPLASMS

Epithelial neoplasms show two basic growth patterns which are largely, although not entirely, dictated by their own anatomical relationships.

1) Neoplastic epithelial cells tend to grow in sheets covering a surface. Very often this mass of cells has a wavy irregular outline and is called a **papilloma** (*Figs 22.9* and *22.10*).
2) Cells grow as solid islands or masses, separated from each other by stromal connective tissue. This growth pattern is seen most often in neoplasms derived from ductal or glandular epithelium and is known as an **adenoma**.

Three main types of papilloma are described, consonant with the three main varieties of covering epithelium: **squamous, transitional** and **columnar**.

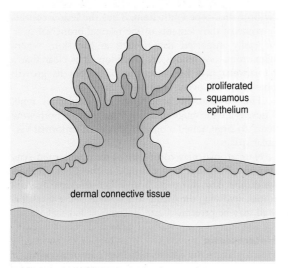

FIGURE 22.9 A papilloma of the skin.

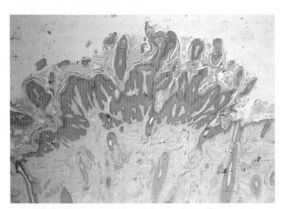

FIGURE 22.10 A papilloma of the skin showing many finger-like processes projecting from the skin surface.

Genesis of an Adenoma

Benign neoplasms arising from gland or duct epithelium are termed adenomas. The basic structure of adenomas is based on the tendency of the proliferating cells to form small groups, which usually surround a lumen. In many instances this lumen is reduced to an inconspicuous slit and it may be impossible to see any lumen at all on light microscopy. This latter appearance is particularly common in adenomas arising within endocrine glands.

The neoplastic acini have no draining duct systems. This absence of drainage, if combined with active secretion by the cells of the tumour, may lead to accumulation of the secretions, with distension of the lumina and eventual **cyst** formation. Such a neoplastic cyst derived from acinar or ductal epithelium is called a **cystadenoma**. If cyst formation is accompanied by continued proliferation of the lining cells, the increase in the area of the lining will result in the appearance of papillary infoldings which project into the lumen, a so-called **papillary cystadenoma.** Such neoplasms are frequently encountered in the ovary but may occur at many other sites.

The macroscopic appearances of a typical adenoma are those of a clearly demarcated and usually rounded mass, often with a thin fibrous tissue capsule and with some compressed normal tissue around it. If the acinar or ductal lumina are small, the adenoma appears solid when cut into, and is usually paler and more homogeneous in texture than surrounding tissue. If the gland or duct lumina are large and secretion has been a marked feature, this is usually easy to see when the lesion has been sectioned; either a single large cyst or many small ones may be present.

A common site for adenoma formation is the large bowel. Because of the peristaltic contractions, the localized islands of proliferated colonic glands may be pushed into the lumen. In the early stages of this process, the small mass of glands will appear as a small lump standing a little proud of the surrounding mucosal surface. With the passage of time, the adenoma may be pushed into the lumen, dragging with it a pedicle of subepithelial tissue containing blood vessels and conective tissue fibres. Such a lesion is called a **polyp** (*Fig. 22.11*).

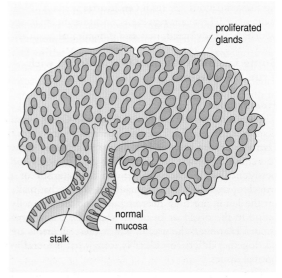

FIGURE 22.11 A colonic polyp.

CHAPTER 23

Non-neoplastic Disturbances in Cell Growth and Proliferation

Not all quantitative changes in a given cell population are neoplastic. Indeed, changes involving both **increases (hyperplasia)** and **decreases (involution)** in the cell population occur under both physiological and pathological circumstances. Hyperplasia is distinguished from the changes in cell growth and proliferation that occur in neoplasia by the fact that in neoplasia **normal mechanisms of control of cell proliferation do not operate**.

THE CELL CYCLE

Cells proliferate essentially by **undergoing mitosis**. However, the process of mitotic division occupies only a small part of the cell cycle. The length of the cell cycle will determine, to an extent, the characteristics of a tissue in terms of its cell kinetics.

- After mitosis (**M phase**), which usually takes 1−2 hours, the daughter cells enter a gap phase which is known as **G1**. The length of this phase differs from cell type to cell type, and varies greatly.
- The cell then enters a phase in which DNA is synthesized (**S phase**); during this, the content of DNA is doubled. This S phase lasts from 7 to 12 hours.
- After synthesis of DNA is complete, there is a second gap phase, known as **G2**, which lasts, as a rule, from 1 to 6 hours.

In human tissues, the M, G2 and S phases are relatively constant in length. **The differences in cell cycle time which characterize different tissues are a function of variations in the length of G1, which may last for days or even years.** In cell culture models, arrest of the cell cycle occurs only in the G1 phase (see p 285). This finding implies that once a cell has passed out of the G1 phase, the cell cycle proceeds to completion. In fact, the **point of no return** occurs late in the G1 phase and is known as the **restriction point**. This point in the cycle probably corresponds with the genetically programmed switching on of DNA polymerase synthesis.

In any given tissue, not all the cells are actually within the cell cycle; most fully differentiated cells **opt out**. When a cell leaves the cell cycle the commonest event is an advance down the pathway of differentiation which must end, in most cases, in obsolescence and cell death. For instance, a daughter cell arising in the course of mitotic division in the basal layer of the epidermis migrates upwards into the malpighian layer where it begins to synthesize keratin. Eventually it moves to the horny layer of the epidermis and dies, being shed from the skin surface as a flake of keratin. There is, however, an alternative. Cells can leave the cycle **temporarily** and, under certain circumstances, re-enter it much later. Such 'resting' cells are said to be in G0, although clearly it is not easy to distinguish between such cells and those in which there is a very long G1 phase.

That part of the cell population which remains within the cell cycle is known as the **growth fraction (stem cell compartment)**. The proliferative activity in any tissue is a function both of the length of the cycle and the size of the growth fraction.

HYPERTROPHY AND HYPERPLASIA

Excess growth with *no* escape from normal control mechanisms may be expressed in two ways (*Fig. 23.1*).

1) In **hypertrophy** the increase in the bulk of tissue or organ results from an increase in the **size of the individual cells** of which the tissue is composed. In pure hypertrophy there is **no increase** in the **number** of cells.

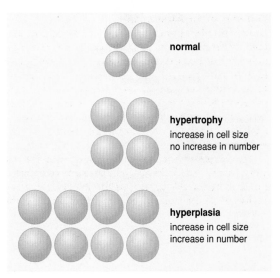

normal

hypertrophy
increase in cell size
no increase in number

hyperplasia
increase in cell size
increase in number

FIGURE 23.1 Hypertrophy and hyperplasia.

2) In **hyperplasia** there is an increase in the **number** of cells making up a given tissue. An increase in cell size is not infrequently seen as an associated feature.

Hypertrophy and hyperplasia can, in most instances, be recognized as being caused by some specific stimulus. Once the stimulus is removed, there is a reversion to normal. This stimulus is often a physiological one, such as an increased demand for a function that will lead to an increase in cell number, cell size or both. Both can be regarded as **adaptation phenomena**.

HYPERPLASIA

In many instances, hyperplasia constitutes a **demand-led** physiological event, the increase in cells being the response to an increased functional need. This is seen, for example, in such tissues as the breast and thyroid at the time of puberty or pregnancy. The negative feedback mechanisms that appear to control these phenomena will act in a wide range of circumstances, even when the circumstances themselves are pathological.

Operation of this negative feedback is seen quite commonly in the field of **endocrine hyperplasia**. Some examples are given below.

Congenital Adrenal Hyperplasia

The clinical pictures associated with congenital adrenal hyperplasia (*Fig. 23.2*) make themselves apparent in infancy and early childhood. They are characterized by:

- masculinization in the female
- precocious puberty in the male
- a salt-losing state may also be part of the syndrome

The basic defect is an enzyme deficiency in the cells of the adrenal cortex responsible for the synthesis of cortisol and aldosterone. These cells lack either a C21 or a C11 hydroxylase and as a result there is a block in the pathways leading to the synthesis of cortisol and aldosterone from cholesterol. The abnormally low concentration of these hormones in the plasma causes increased secretion of adrenocorticotrophic hormone by the pituitary; the adrenal cortex responds by increasing the number of functional cells. However, because the block in hormone synthesis persists, the dammed back precursors are diverted to another metabolic pathway in the cortex, and large amounts of androgenic steroids (which are responsible for the virilization) are formed.

Thyroid Hyperplasia

Thyroid hyperplasia (*Fig. 23.3*) may occur as a result of:

- the operation of normal negative feedback mechanisms controlling the levels of **thyroid-stimulating hormone (TSH)**

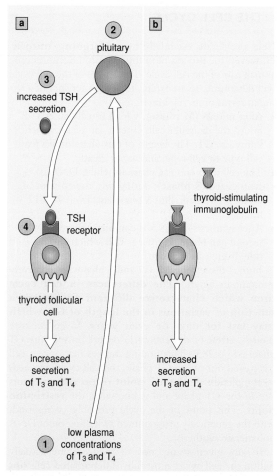

FIGURE 23.3 *Thyroid hyperplasia due* **a** *to increased drive controlled by negative feedback and* **b** *to abnormal drive (in the form of thyroid-stimulating immunoglobulin). TSH, thyroid-stimulating hormone; T₃, tri-iodothyronine; T₄, thyroxine.*

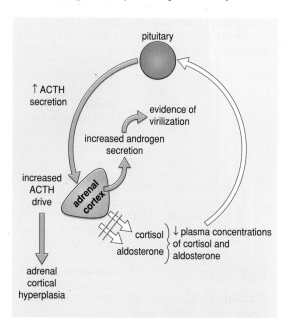

FIGURE 23.2 *Feedback mechanisms in congenital adrenal hyperplasia. ACTH, adrenocorticotrophic hormone.*

- the existence of **abnormal stimuli**

Many cases of hypothyroidism are associated with the structural changes of hyperplasia irrespective of the mechanism causing the hypofunction. Abnormally low secretion of thyroid hormones may arise from:

- a lack of secreting tissue (as in cretinism)
- a lack of substrate, as in iodine-deficiency goitre
- a lack of enzymes required for the various steps in hormone synthesis (dyshormogenetic goitre)

In all of these, the low circulating levels of thyroxine will lead to an increased output of TSH from the pituitary and hence to hyperplasia of the thyroid tissue.

Similar morphological changes may occur in **hyperthyroid** patients being treated with thiouracil or carbimazole. These compounds block the synthesis of thyroxine and the pituitary responds by secreting more TSH. The patient becomes clinically and biochemically euthyroid on this treatment, but the gland itself may become more hyperplastic.

Endocrine hyperplasia can occur not as the result of an increased normal drive controlled by negative feedback, but through the operation of abnormal drives. An example of this is primary hyperthyroidism (Graves' disease) in which the abnormal drive is a **thyroid-stimulating immunoglobulin** which binds to the TSH receptor on the surface of the thyroid acinar epithelium.

Pancreatic Islet Hyperplasia in Infants with Diabetic Mothers

Maternal diabetes is a potent risk for perinatal mortality unless appropriate measures are taken. These infants tend to be fat, flabby and rather cushingoid in appearance. On histological examination of the pancreas, there is a striking degree of islet cell hyperplasia.

Initially this was viewed as the result of the operation of normal feedback mechanisms: the high maternal blood glucose concentration was deemed to induce a greater than normal degree of insulin secretion by the fetal islets and, hence, hyperplasia. However, this is an oversimplification of a much more complex problem, since the islet cell hyperplasia seen in the infants of diabetic mothers is also seen in the stillborn infants of mothers who are destined to become diabetic, sometimes many years later, a state known as prediabetes.

Hyperplasia in the Target Organs of Hormones

Breast

An increase in the size of the breasts in the female is a normal feature of puberty, and also occurs during pregnancy and lactation. These changes are hormone induced and consist of an increase in both the epithelial elements and the rather specialized connective tissue elements that surround the breast ducts and demarcate the breast lobules from the interlobular connective tis-

sue. One of the most important factors in this change is oestrogen.

In clinical practice, breast hyperplasia of a rather different sort is common. This may manifest as a localized lump within the breast or as a generalized lumpiness in a fairly large area of the breast. It is not infrequently spoken of as **chronic mastitis**, a very poor term since the process is not inflammatory in nature. It is, instead, a mixture of hyperplastic and involuntary changes which are probably due to hormonal imbalance. The structural changes are basically an increase in the number of ducts within individual lobules (this is called **adenosis**) and in the number of cells lining individual ducts, with a consequent 'heaping up' of the epithelial cells (so-called '**epitheliosis**'). In any single case the histological appearances will depend on the relative proportions of these three changes and the secondary effects (such as cystic change) that result from them.

Prostate

Enlargement of the prostate is an extremely common event in males over the age of 60 years. Both the fibromuscular and ductal elements are involved. This is discussed more fully in Chapter 38 (see pp 743–745).

Non-specific Reactive Epithelial Hyperplasia

The lining epithelia of the skin, mouth, alimentary and respiratory tracts frequently become hyperplastic when any persistent irritant is applied to them. The irritant can be simple trauma, for example when a corn develops in response to the rubbing of ill-fitting shoes. Similarly, an incorrectly fitted denture can produce marked thickening of the squamous epithelium of the alveolar margin. Chronic inflammatory disease of the skin is often associated with thickening of the epidermis, and epidermal hyperplasia of a very marked degree can develop in response to the presence of certain intradermal lesions such as insect bites. At times this reactive epidermal hyperplasia may be so extreme as to raise suspicions that the process is neoplastic rather than reactive. It is humiliating to have to confess that the nature of the mitogenic stimulus in these situations is not understood.

HYPERTROPHY

Isolated hypertrophy occurs only in **muscle**. Clearly the stimulus that elicits this response is an increased workload. Work-related hypertrophy occurs in **smooth muscle** in a number of pathological circumstances, particularly where there is partial obstruction to the normal process of the contents of any hollow muscular organ. Some examples are given below.

The Urinary Bladder

Any obstruction of the outflow of urine as, for example, in postinflammatory urethral strictures or with enlargement of the prostate will lead to an increase in size of the muscle fibres and a considerable degree of thickening of the bladder wall. Because of the orientation of the muscle in the bladder, this leads to a woven or trabeculated pattern being seen when the mucosal lining of the bladder is inspected at cystoscopy.

The Gastrointestinal Tract

The gut, an archetype of a muscular tube, shows muscle hypertrophy proximal to chronic obstructions arising from any cause. In the **oesophagus** this is seen in association with:

- postinflammatory scarring
- carcinoma
- obstruction due to disorders of innervation (cardiac achalasia)

In the **stomach**, muscle hypertrophy may not only result from some obstructive lesion but may also **cause** obstruction. This is seen in **congenital hypertrophic pyloric stenosis** (*Fig. 23.4*). In this condition, affected infants, the vast majority of whom are male, present soon after birth with projectile vomiting shortly after feeding. On deep palpation of the abdomen, a small lump may be detected. At operation this is seen to be a thick ring of muscle around the pyloric opening. It is treated by dividing the muscle from the serosal aspect without damaging the mucosal lining. In this way the hypertrophied muscle ring is opened up and the obstruction is relieved.

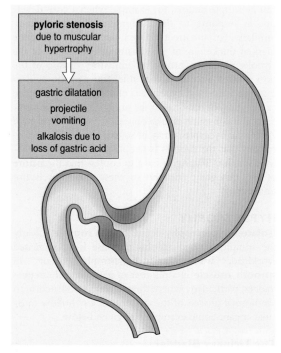

FIGURE 23.4 Pyloric stenosis. In infancy this is a congenital lesion, probably resulting from incoordination of the muscle of the pyloric sphincter.

The Heart

Cardiac hypertrophy is commonly encountered in clinical practice. It is due to an increased workload. It may be of two types, each of which is mirrored in the appearance of the heart. In **high pressure overload**, such as is seen in aortic valve stenosis, systemic hypertension or, much more rarely, coarctation of the aorta, there is a marked degree of left ventricular hypertrophy which is associated with a left ventricular cavity that is either normal in size or smaller than normal. In the case of **high volume overload**, the increased workload stems from an increase in end-diastolic volume (such as occurs in aortic or mitral incompetence); this is inevitably associated with a left ventricular cavity of large capacity.

ATROPHY

Just as there may be an increase in the bulk of a tissue or organ as a result of hyperplasia or hypertrophy, there may also be a decrease. If the diminution in bulk is acquired, it is spoken of as **atrophy** and this, as with hyperplasia and hypertrophy, may occur as a physiological phenomenon or in abnormal or pathological circumstances.

PHYSIOLOGICAL ATROPHY

This can occur at any time of life including the gestation period, but is associated particularly with early life. In the fetus, many structures are formed during embryonic development which undergo regression during the later stages of gestation. These include the notochord, the branchial clefts and the thyroglossal duct. Persistence of these structures to a greater or lesser degree may occur, and patients may present (in the case of the latter two) with masses in the neck, the true nature of which is revealed on histological examination after surgical removal.

In the neonatal period, the ductus arteriosus and umbilical vessels either disappear completely or remain merely as cords of fibrous tissue. Similarly, the fetal adrenal cortex undergoes a considerable degree of atrophy soon after birth.

Atrophy of the thymus occurs normally as adult life is entered, and in late middle and old age there is a significant decline in the amount of lymphoid tissue.

In the same way that increased functional demand can lead to hypertrophy and/or hyperplasia, a decrease in demand will lead to a degree of atrophy. This can be seen to a marked extent in voluntary muscle if a limb is immobilized as, for example, after a fracture. Muscle bulk decreases very rapidly, and when the period of immobilization is over a considerable amount of exercise may be required to restore it to normal. Similarly, starvation is associated with some degree of atrophy of the gut, the enterocyte lining being particularly affected.

Osteoporosis

A common and important example of atrophy is osteoporosis. This has been defined as a condition in which the mass of bone tissue per unit volume of 'anatomical' bone is reduced, with a decrease in the number and size of the trabeculae in cancellous bone. There is no defect in the mineralization of such osteoid matrix as is present, in contradistinction to **osteomalacia**, where the bone tissue mass is normal but the degree of mineralization is subnormal. This subject is discussed fully in Chapter 44 (see pp 1039–1047).

LOCALIZED ATROPHY

Localized atrophy may occur in the following circumstances:

- ischaemia
- pressure
- denervation

CHAPTER 24

Cell Proliferation and Differentiation in Relation to Neoplasia

In the examples of non-neoplastic expansion of cell populations considered in Chapter 23, all share one common feature: increased cell proliferation **ceases** following removal of the stimulus that has evoked it. In contrast, the proliferation of cells seen in neoplasia appears to be **autonomous**; it is not demand-led and a continuous application of an exogenous drive towards cell division is not present.

TRANSFORMED CELLS

Characteristics of Transformed Cells in Culture

Many of the data on the growth characteristics of neoplastic cells have been derived from cell culture systems. Although these are useful, care must be taken not to extrapolate too uncritically from these to the *in vivo* situation.

Transformed Cells Show Loss of Contact Inhibition

When normal cells are grown in a monolayer, their proliferation ceases once the culture has reached confluence. In other words, once each cell is in contact with a neighbour, cell division ceases. This is known as **contact inhibition**. In contrast, monolayer cultures of neoplastic cells of the same type (e.g. fibroblasts) do not show this characteristic. Instead of cell division coming to an end once the cells have reached confluence, it continues and the cells heap up in a multilayered fashion.

How does Contact between Normal Cells Cause Them to Stop Proliferating?

It has been suggested that cells of any given line:
- **recognize** each other
- **exchange information** that regulates cell division
- **adhere to one another** (homotypic adhesion)

Recognition of cells by their homologues certainly does occur: if two types of embryonic cells are mixed in culture, each type will segregate itself from the other. However, there are no hard data to indicate that failure of recognition is an important factor in the loss of contact inhibition that occurs with neoplastic cells.

Transformed Cells Differ from their Normal Homologues in Respect of their Surface Membranes

Neoplastic transformation appears to be associated in most instances with change in the surface membrane glycoproteins. One type of surface change can be detected by the use of a family of proteins known as **lectins**. These proteins, which are widely distributed throughout many phyla, are able to bind the different sugars on cell surfaces with exquisite specificity. One such lectin derived from **wheatgerm** can agglutinate neoplastic cells in suspension but cannot do this to their normal homologues. This change in lectin agglutinability is associated with binding to the sugar N-acetyl-glucosamine on cell surface membranes. As transformed cells do not appear to synthesize more N-acetyl-glucosamine than their normal counterparts, it seems reasonable to suggest that something has been lost from the surface of the transformed cells with resulting exposure of the lectin-binding sugars.

This view finds support from two studies. In the first, normal cells were treated with trypsin to remove some of the surface protein. They then became agglutinable by wheatgerm lectin. In the second, transformed cells in culture were treated with a monovalent wheatgerm lectin which bound to the N-acetyl-glucosamine residues, thus, in a sense, masking them. When cells treated in this way were cultured in a monolayer, contact inhibition was shown to be restored.

Possible Mechanisms for Autonomous Growth

The loss of contact inhibition shown by transformed cells in culture is an expression of disordered regulation of growth. It sheds no light, however, on the question of how transformed cells have escaped the normal mechanisms of growth control.

As in the case of regeneration, two basic possibilities exist:

1) There may be a **failure in some inhibiting mechanism that normally restrains excessive cell proliferation**

2) abnormal growth may represent a response to growth factors and may encompass:
- excessive amounts of growth factor
- overexpression of growth factor receptors
- abnormal regulation of signal transduction following growth factor–receptor interaction

'Autocrine' Growth Factors and Autonomous Neoplastic Cell Proliferation

In addition to their escape from the mechanisms normally controlling cell proliferation, transformed cells in culture also require **lower concentrations of growth factors for optimal growth and multiplication** than do their normal counterparts. It has been suggested that autonomous growth (and indeed some other phenotypic characteristics of malignant transformation) is due to the production of polypeptide growth factors which act on the same cells that produce them by binding to appropriate receptors on the surface membrane. This process, in which the secretory cells are activated by their own secretion products, has been called **autocrine secretion** (*Fig. 24.1*). It plays an important role in many tumours.

Many types of tumour, when cultured, release polypeptide growth factors into the culture medium; these same tumour cells often possess specific receptors for the released peptide. Each type of growth factor acts on a specific membrane receptor, which in turn, through phosphorylation of proteins downstream, transduces the signal generated by binding between the peptide and its receptor, into a mitogenic response.

Such a signalling system might be modulated in three ways:

1) By the level of expression of the growth factor.
2) By the level of expression of the membrane receptor.
3) By the level of expression of the postreceptor signalling pathway.

The peptides so far identified as functioning in this 'autocrine' fashion, include:

- transforming growth factor α (TGF-α)
- **platelet–derived growth factor** (PDGF)
- bombesin (gastrin-releasing peptide)

The autocrine action of a growth factor in malignant cells was first described in rodent cells transformed by either the Kirsten or the Molony mouse sarcoma viruses. The peptide identified is structurally related to epidermal growth factor (EGF) (see p 81) but distinct from it, and has been named TGF-α. It is released by a number of human neoplasms.

There is a very close relationship between the release of TGF-α and the transformed state. This can be demonstrated using a temperature-sensitive mutant of the mouse sarcoma virus as the transforming agent. If the target cells are not cultured at a temperature suitable for the mutant virus, transformation does not take place and there is *no* release of the TGF into the culture medium.

Molecules showing a considerable degree of homology with **PDGF** are released by a number of neoplasms. In humans these include:

- malignant connective tissue neoplasms of bone (**osteosarcoma**)
- malignant neoplasms of glial cells in the brain
- a cell line derived from human bladder cancer

In animal cell lines growth factors are released after transformation by a variety of RNA viruses. Many of these cell lines also possess receptors for PDGF, and such receptors may be targets for growth inhibition. For example, antibodies against PDGF block tritiated thymidine incorporation into cells transformed by the simian sarcoma virus. Transformed cells secreting only small amounts of PDGF form small tumours when inoculated into nude (athymic) mice. In contrast, tumours that secrete large amounts of the growth factor into culture medium produce large masses in the nude mouse model.

Similar data come from studies of another growth factor known as **bombesin**. This is a tetradecapeptide that is produced and released by most human small–cell carcinomas of the lung ('**oat cell carcinoma**'). Monoclonal antibodies that are specific for the *C*-terminal end of the bombesin molecule prevent bombesin from binding to its receptor and, in this way, inhibit the growth of small–cell lung cancer, in both culture and xenografts in nude mice.

An increase in the output of the effector peptide may not be necessary for increased autocrine activity. An increase in the number or binding affinity of the **receptors** will increase the autocrine effect of the peptide in the absence of any increase in its synthesis or secretion. Thus, human squamous carcinomas derived from the head and neck have been shown to have very large numbers of receptors for EGF on their surface membranes and, in some tumour cell lines, the affinity of these receptors is very high.

In some cases of human breast cancer, where transformation has involved activation of a cellular

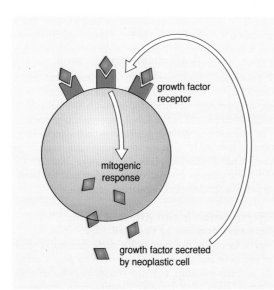

FIGURE 24.1 *'Autocrine' control of neoplastic cell proliferation. Transformed cells secrete growth factors that bind to receptors on the surface membrane of the same cell. Binding to these specific receptors generates a mitogenic signal.*

growth factor
receptor

mitogenic
response

growth factor secreted
by neoplastic cell

oncogene known as *her* or *neu*, the gene codes for a truncated version of the EGF receptor. This abnormal receptor cannot bind its ligand at the cell membrane, but appears to be able to generate a mitogenic signal independent of ligand binding.

Other growth factor receptors also appear to be able to act as tyrosine kinases (and thus as initiators of mitosis) in the absence of their appropriate ligands.

Autocrine Peptides can Inhibit Growth as well as Stimulate It

Growth factors may be multifunctional. Some, depending on circumstances, may downregulate or upregulate cell growth and may also have effects on the immune system. For example, TGF-β has an effect on T lymphocytes that is ten times more powerful, on a molar basis, than that of the widely used immunosuppressant cyclosporin A.

Transforming Growth Factor β

The TGF-β family includes at least three dimeric proteins secreted in an inactive form (TGF-β1–3). Either an acidic medium or cleavage by serine proteases is required for these peptides to become activated. These growth factors are related to a larger family of peptide signals, including factors responsible for morphogenesis in bone, müllerian inhibiting factor and inhibin. TGF-β is widely distributed throughout adult tissues and binds to receptors on many different cell types. TGF-β1 is the most potent of the three types.

- TGF-β **stimulates** the growth of fibroblasts in culture in the presence of PDGF.
- If EGF is present, the TGF-β inhibits the growth of these same fibroblasts.
- Similarly TGF-β can stimulate the growth of osteoblasts but this mitogenic effect is reversed by other peptide growth factors such as EGF, PDGF and tumour necrosis factor α.

Thus the context in which a peptide signal operates may significantly modify its effect.

TGF-β **inhibits** the growth of most epithelial cell lines (including malignant cells) in culture. In other contexts (e.g. wound healing, atherogenesis) TGF-β promotes the growth of fibrous tissue matrix.

DIFFERENTIATION

Neoplasia and Disordered Cell Differentiation

Cancer is a set of diseases that arise in the first instance from normal cells which, by one means or another, are **transformed**. But from which normal cells? Because one of the cardinal features of neoplasia is the ability of a given cell population to go on proliferating in a relatively autonomous manner, the cells from which the neoplasm arises must have the ability to respond to mitogenic signals (normal or abnormal) and divide. In most normal cell populations, cells that have this characteristic are found in the **stem cell compartment** and hence, by implication, are **undifferentiated** cells.

When a stem cell divides, one of its daughter cells may well retain the ability to divide. The other, by mechanisms that are not understood, becomes committed to differentiation and, ultimately, to death.

By definition, the process of differentiation requires that, for each type of differentiated cell, a **heritable** pattern of **read-out** of the genome must exist. As all cells in the body possess the same genetic information, differentiation similarly implies that, in each type of cell, genes are expressed that are not expressed in other cell types.

If the stable differences between cell types depend on the particular genes that are expressed in the form of protein synthesis, then, clearly, there are several levels at which this control can be exercised. These include:

- **transcriptional control** (when and how often a gene is transcribed)
- **RNA processing control** (determining how the primary messenger RNA (mRNA) transcript is spliced)
- **RNA transport control** (determining which mRNAs are exported to the cytoplasm for translation)
- **translational control** (determining which mRNAs are translated by ribosomes)
- **degradation control** (the selective destabilization of some mRNA molecules in the cytoplasm)
- **control of protein activity** (some proteins may be sequestrated or inactivated after synthesis)

In most instances, it is the first of these – transcriptional control – that is the most potent mechanism. Such expression is controlled by a series of gene regulatory proteins which recognize short, precisely defined, stretches of DNA, to which they bind. While, clearly, there must be enormous numbers of such regulatory proteins, a comparatively small number of structural motifs (e.g. zinc-finger motifs, leucine-zipper motifs and helix-loop motifs) is employed in the DNA recognition process.

In eukaryotes, gene regulatory proteins form large complexes which activate the promoter region of genes. One *Drosophila* gene, for example, has 20 000 nucleotide pairs in its controlling region and has binding sites for 20 different regulatory proteins.

Differentiation is also Affected by the Microenvironment of the Cell

Genetic factors in the form of heritable patterns of gene transcription and translation undoubtedly play a major role in differentiation, but the process may be affected in other ways. For instance, **interaction between mesenchymal and epithelial elements** is important in the development of many organ systems, including the pancreas, lung, kidney, salivary glands, breast, pituitary and liver.

Pancreatic epithelium alone, cultured from the developing rat pancreas, will not differentiate. If the same cells are seeded on to a filter, on the other side of which are mesenchymal cells in culture, then differentiation occurs. This suggests that a chemical differentiating signal is released from the mesenchymal cells. The effect of mesenchymal cell extracts is destroyed by trypsin and periodate oxidation, but not by ribonuclease or deoxyribonuclease. The signal is therefore presumably a glycoprotein. In cell culture systems, alteration of the medium may be sufficient to bring about profound changes in differentiation. Such a medium change may cause, for example, cartilage cells that synthesize type II collagen to revert to fibroblasts, which secrete type I collagen. The mechanism responsible for this switch is not known.

Cell–cell interactions also appear to play a role in differentiation. If mixed embryonic cells are cultured, cells of each type will segregate. It may well be that growth factors play a part in differentiation as well as in regulating the cell population size. For example, **EGF** causes granulosa cells from the ovary to differentiate into luteal cells.

METAPLASIA

Changes in Differentiation Patterns do not Necessarily Imply Neoplastic Transformation

A complete change in differentiation from one fully differentiated form to another occurs not infrequently in cells subjected to chronic irritation or to changes in the hormonal milieu. This is known as **metaplasia**. One of the commonest forms is a change from cuboidal or columnar epithelium into squamous epithelium. Such metaplastic change may occur under the following circumstances:

1) The pseudostratified ciliated columnar epithelium of the bronchi may change into squamous epithelium. This occurs in cigarette smokers, patients with chronic bronchitis, and in chronic abscess cavities in the lung, which can become lined by epithelium.
2) Squamous metaplasia is common in chronic cervicitis. The metaplastic epithelium may spread down into the cervical glands and fill the lumina. This process is called 'epidermidalization' by some, and may be mistaken for invasion by squamous carcinoma by the inexperienced.
3) The transitional epithelium of the renal pelvis and urinary bladder may undergo squamous metaplasia in the presence of chronic infection. This is seen very often in Egypt where schistosomal cystitis is common. The presence of stones seems to increase the likelihood of metaplasia.
4) The columnar cell lining of the gallbladder sometimes undergoes squamous metaplasia in the presence of gallstones and chronic inflammation.

5) Prostatic ducts, which are normally lined by columnar epithelium, undergo squamous metaplasia in patients treated with oestrogens for prostatic carcinoma.
6) A deficiency of vitamin A may be associated with squamous metaplasia of the nose, bronchi and urinary tract. In addition, keratin formation is accelerated and increased in amount in the skin and conjunctiva.

Is there any Identifiable Mechanism that Causes Metaplasia?

Recent experiments on cultured cell lines suggest that metaplasia can be caused by agents that interfere with DNA methylation; this supports the idea that such methylation plays a part in keeping the state of expression of genes stable. If, for example, cells are grown for a few cycles in the synthetic nucleotide analogue 5-aza-cytosine, the analogue becomes incorporated into the DNA in place of some of the cytosine residues. The 5-aza-cytosine is incapable of being methylated and also inhibits the action of the methylating enzyme. This breaks the chain of events in which the pattern of DNA methylation of a gene is passed from one cell generation to the next. When cultured cells resembling fibroblasts are treated in this way, they differentiate into a variety of cell types including skeletal muscle cells, to which they would never give rise under normal circumstances.

Cellular Differentiation in Malignant Neoplasms

Cancer cells are cells that are **not fully differentiated**. Because fully differentiated cells are unlikely to be able to 'regress' so far as differentiation is concerned, it is likely that the cancer cells are blocked at some stage in the maturation process. Unlike most normal cells that have progressed down the pathway toward full differentiation, these partly differentiated cells **still retain the capacity to divide**.

The degree of differentiation in neoplasms may be related to the precise point at which transformation occurs in the time-dependent sequence of events in which different genes are switched to the 'on' and 'off' positions after the stem cell has divided. This is particularly applicable to the liver, where there is marked heterogeneity in respect of differentiation in neoplasms induced by chemical carcinogens. Such neoplasms vary from very well differentiated lesions in which the constituent cells can be distinguished only with difficulty from those of normal liver, to highly malignant, very poorly differentiated, neoplasms in which the hepatic origin is difficult to determine.

The Microenvironment in which Malignant Cells Grow is Involved in the Maintenance of the Malignant State

Malignant teratomas are neoplasms arising from multipotent cells and can express a variety of differentiation

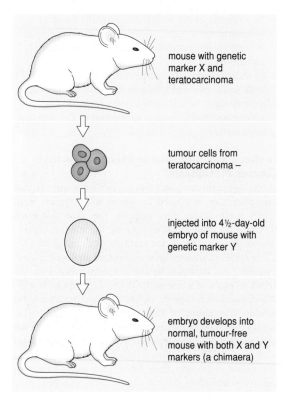

mouse with genetic marker X and teratocarcinoma

tumour cells from teratocarcinoma –

injected into 4½-day-old embryo of mouse with genetic marker Y

embryo develops into normal, tumour-free mouse with both X and Y markers (a chimaera)

FIGURE 24.2 Normal differentiation of malignant cells when transferred to a different microenvironment.

patterns. The commonest site of origin is in the gonads. Strains of mice exist in which malignant teratoma occurs in about 1% of the males. If cells from such a neoplasm are injected into the peritoneal cavity of unaffected mice of the parent strain, large cystic bodies develop. These are called embryoid bodies and contain both cancer cells and differentiated cells, suggesting that both the differentiated and cancer cells arise from a single precursor.

If teratoma cells from mice with certain genetic markers are injected into 4.5-day-old embryos of mice with a different set of genetic markers, the embryos develop into **completely normal mice** which express the genetic markers of both the embryo and teratoma cells (a **chimaera**) (*Fig. 24.2*). None of these chimaeras develops teratocarcinoma. This shows that the microenvironment of the embryo is able to convert the **neoplastic** teratoma cells into fully differentiated normal cells.

If, on the other hand, single teratocarcinoma cells are injected subcutaneously into adult mice, large neoplasms regularly develop at the injection site. Thus the differentiation signals provided by the embryo are lacking in the adult subcutaneous tissue.

KEY POINTS: Cancer

- Most cancers are monoclonal (derived from a single transformed cell).
- Most cancers are initiated by changes in the DNA of the target cell (genetic) rather than by changes in the expression of unaltered genes (epigenetic).
- The development of most cancers is a multistep process in which several mutations affect the target cell genome.
- The progression of cancer requires successive rounds of mutation and natural selection.
- Once cancer initiation has occurred, development of the tumour can be promoted by factors that do not affect the cellular DNA.
- Cancer incidence varies greatly from country to country and this may reflect different exposures to certain environmental factors.

CHAPTER 25

Relationship of Neoplastic Cells with their Environment: Tumour Spread

The ability of malignant tumours to invade and destroy surrounding tissues and to colonize distant sites has been recognized since the time of Hippocrates. Indeed, the term **cancer** was derived from the crab-like, macroscopic appearance of certain malignant neoplasms in which processes of tumour tissue can be seen to penetrate the surrounding stroma. While a number of morphological and behavioural characteristics are used to differentiate between **benign** and **malignant** neoplasms, **the only absolute criterion is the ability of a malignant neoplasm to invade surrounding tissue and to colonize distant sites (metastasis)**.

ROUTES OF SPREAD

Malignant neoplasms can spread by the following routes:
- **directly** through the tissues adjacent to the primary growth (*Fig. 25.1*)
- via the **lymphatics**
- via the **bloodstream** (*Fig. 25.2*)
- through body cavities (**transcoelomic**)

Invasiveness is the prerequisite for spread to distant sites; the processes involved are only now beginning to be understood.

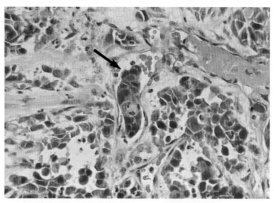

FIGURE 25.2 *Vascular invasion. The centre of the field is occupied by a small blood vessel, the wall of which consists of a single layer of endothelial cells. The presence of red blood cells within the lumen helps it to be recognized as blood vessel. A mass of tumour cells similar to those seen outside the vessel is also present within the lumen.*

DIRECT SPREAD

Direct spread involves the invasion of tissues adjacent to the original lesion; such spread occurs more or less in continuity with that lesion. It represents the coordination of a number of different processes, some of which favour invasion and metastasis and others that tend to inhibit these events. Most of our knowledge in this field is derived from the study of tumour cell lines in culture and their use in certain animal models. This means that caution should be exercised in extrapolating too far from these laboratory findings to the human situation, although some supportive evidence from human studies has accrued.

The processes believed to be involved in invasion and metastasis are summarized below.

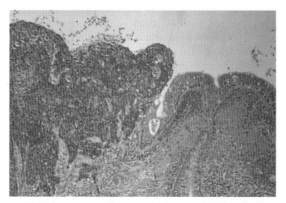

FIGURE 25.1 *Direct spread. Section from bronchus at the site of origin of a bronchial carcinoma. The surface epithelium in the right-hand side of the picture is normal. The left-hand half shows a darkly staining mass of tumour cells extending irregularly into the underlying bronchial wall.*

> **KEY POINTS: Processes Involved in Invasion**
> - aquisition of an **adequate blood supply** for the tumour
> - a **decrease in the adhesion of tumour cells one to another**
> - the **adhesion of tumour cells to basement membranes and extracellular matrices**
> - **proteolysis** of extracellular matrix
> - **active movement of tumour cells** through the extracellular matrix

Acquisition of New and Adequate Blood Supply for the Tumour: Angiogenesis

Ingrowth of new blood vessels (**angiogenesis**) is required for sufficient expansion of the primary mass of tumour cells. If new capillaries do not grow into the tumour, it will be unable to expand more than a few millimetres in any direction (*Fig. 25.3*)

The greater the new blood supply acquired by the tumour, the greater the risk of metastatic spread. For example, in excised breast cancers each increase of ten in the total number of microvessels identified in 200 microscopic fields was found to be associated with a 1.59-fold increase in the risk of metastases.

The new blood vessels that grow into the primary tumour are derived from adjacent venules and capillaries and not from arterioles, arteries or veins. The ingrowth of these new vessels is stimulated by chemical signals such as **basic fibroblast growth factor, transforming growth factor α and a polypeptide known as angiogenin, first isolated from cultured tumour cells and known to show considerable homology with tumour necrosis factor α. The process is inhibited by transforming growth factor β1.**

The resting endothelial cells in capillaries and venules adjacent to the tumour are stimulated to:

- **degrade their own basement membranes**
- **migrate into and through the extravascular stroma**
- **form capillary sprouts which become luminated**

It is interesting that the processes involved in the formation of these new blood vessels by endothelial cells (**proliferation, motility, proteolysis**) are functionally indistinguishable from those that occur in the invasion of extracellular matrices by malignant cells. The great difference, however, is that when the stimulus for new blood vessel growth is removed, the endothelial cells revert to their resting state. Proteolysis, which is a pivotal process in the migration of both tumour and endothelial cells, is also important in relation to the acquisition of a lumen by the new blood vessels. For a solid sprout of endothelial cells to become luminated, there must be a net balance in favour of proteolysis. Agents that inhibit proteolysis, such as some of the **tissue inhibitors of metalloproteases** (TIMPs) block angiogenesis.

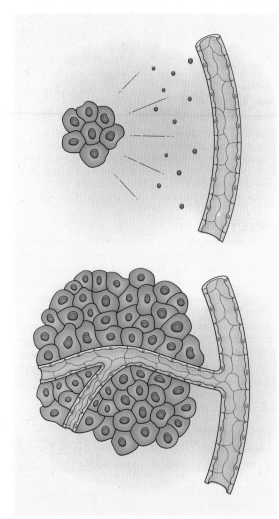

FIGURE 25.3 Angiogenesis is necessary for tumour progression. The colony of tumour cells at the top has secreted angiogenic factors (shown in green) which cause the ingrowth into the tumour cell mass of new blood vessels derived from neighbouring venules. The acquisition of this new blood supply permits a much greater degree of tumour cell proliferation.

Decrease in Adhesion of Tumour Cells to One Another (Loss of Homotypic Cell Adhesion)

Malignant cells infiltrating the tissue adjacent to the primary tumour mass are shed from the original primary. **This implies that cell-to-cell adhesiveness in malignant neoplasms is reduced in comparison with that of normal cells of the same type**. A number of mechanisms is involved in such adhesion:

- Normal epithelial cells develop well-established points for anchorage with each other (desmosomes), but these appear to be either totally lacking or partially deficient in malignant cells.
- It has been suggested that reduced adhesiveness of malignant cells may be due to an increase in the net negative surface charge of tumour cells. This could result from synthesis of abnormal amounts of a negatively charged sialomucopeptide or of normal amounts of a strongly negatively charged molecule of the same type.
- **Cadherins in relation to malignancy**. Cadherins are calcium-dependent cell–cell adhesion molecules. As long as they are functioning, inactivation of other cell adhesion systems seems to have little effect on the normal degree of adhesion between

cells. Cadherins are divided into a number of subclasses of which the most relevant to tumour invasiveness are the E-cadherins (epithelial cadherins). The degree of expression of these molecules has a marked effect on the ability of tumour cells to invade adjacent tissues (*Fig. 25.4*). Thus:

a) If DNA coding for E-cadherin is inserted into highly invasive cells, the cells revert to a non-invasive form.

b) Treatment of cells with antisense RNA specific for E-cadherin increases invasiveness.

c) Treatment of cells with antibody raised against E-cadherin increases invasiveness.

d) Carcinoma cell lines that show loss of E-cadherin expression are highly invasive.

e) There is an inverse relationship between E-cadherin expression and both loss of differentiation and invasiveness in some human tumours.

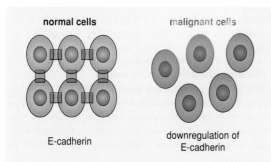

FIGURE 25.4 *Homotypic adhesion. Non-malignant epithelial cells adhere to one another partly through the agency of epithelial cadherins (red squares). In many tumours, E-cadherin expression is markedly downregulated, causing a reduction in the adhesiveness of cells one to another.*

Adhesion of Malignant Cells to Basement Membranes and Extracellular Matrices

For spread to occur, malignant cells must cross certain connective tissue barriers normally separating the epithelial and stromal tissue compartments from each other. One of the most important of these is the **basement membrane**. On one side of the basement membrane are attached the epithelial cells. On the opposite side is the interstitial stroma consisting of fibrillar and non-fibrillar connective tissue proteins and glycoproteins, and containing stromal cells of various types. In benign tissue remodelling, non-neoplastic proliferative disorders and intraepithelial neoplasia (carcinoma *in situ*), there is *no* breaching of the basement membrane. **The transition from *in situ* to invasive carcinoma is, however, marked by malignant cells crossing the basement membrane and thus reaching the stromal compartment.**

The basement membrane is a dense matrix of proteins and glycoproteins which does not have a pore size sufficiently large for tumour cells to penetrate. Thus breaches in the basement membrane must be accompanied by focal destruction of the matrix.

Tumour cell–basement membrane interaction involves three steps:

1) **attachment** of tumour cells to basement membrane components
2) **lysis** of the basement membrane matrix
3) **movement** of tumour cells through the breach created in the basement membrane

Attachment of Tumour Cells to Basement Membrane and Interstitial Stromal Matrices

Attachment of the tumour cells to basement membrane involves adhesion to matrix components such as **collagen, fibronectin and laminin** (*Fig. 25.5*). To bind to these matrix proteins, the tumour cells must express appropriate receptors. The **integrins** have a role of fundamental importance in the binding process. This family of dimeric adhesion molecules also plays an important role in inflammation and wound healing (see pp 43–44). Some of the integrins expressed by tumour cells and their binding matrices are shown in *Table 25.1*. The integrins bind to their respective adhesion molecules by recognizing the specific RGD (Arg–Gly–Asp) sequence.

Laminin is a cross-shaped glycoprotein molecule which is present in both the basement membrane and the interstitial stroma. In normal cells laminin receptors are found only on that aspect of the cell apposed to the basement membrane and are occupied by basement membrane laminin. Invasive cells, however, have laminin receptors diffusely distributed over the entire cell surface and these are often unoccupied. If such

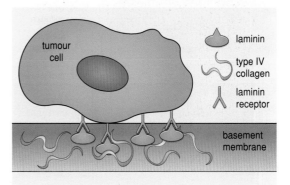

FIGURE 25.5 *Penetration through basement membranes by tumour cells is preceded by adhesion to basement membrane components. Tumour cells express receptors for the basement membrane protein laminin, and the ligand receptor interaction between laminin and its receptor on tumour cells is an important mechanism mediating binding.*

Table 25.1 Interaction between Matrix Proteins and Tumour Cell Integrins

Binding molecule on cell	Matrix protein or glycoprotein
VLA-2 ($\alpha_2\beta_2$)	Collagen and laminin
VLA-4 ($\alpha_4\beta_1$)	A variant of fibronectin
VLA-5 ($\alpha_5\beta_1$)	Fibronectin
VLA-6 ($\alpha_6\beta_1$)	Laminin
$\alpha_6\beta_4$	Laminin
$\alpha_v\beta_3$	Vitronectin

VLA, very late activation antigen.

tumour cells are treated with the receptor binding fragment of laminin, their capacity to invade is greatly reduced.

Proteolysis of Basement Membrane and Interstitial Stromal Matrices

Penetration by malignant cells of the basement membrane and interstitial stromal matrix requires dissolution of matrix proteins by degradative enzymes derived from the tumour cells (*Figs 25.6 and 25.7*)

This proteolysis is carried out in a highly organized manner with respect to both space and time; it is not simply an unbridled production of proteases by the tumour cells, because cell migration during invasiveness requires attachment and de-attachment to the matrix as the cell moves forward. The importance of

proteolysis can be demonstrated by the use of antibodies raised against the enzymes or of inhibitors of protease activity (TIMPs). **In both cases, invasion is blocked.** Conversely, there is positive correlation between the expression of several classes of proteinase by tumour cells and aggressive behaviour by the tumour.

The classes of proteolytic enzyme so far identified as being responsible for connective tissue lysis include:
- metal ion-dependent proteases (metalloproteinases)
- heparanases
- serine-dependent proteases
- thiol-dependent proteases

In connection with invasiveness, the metalloproteinases have been studied most extensively. There are three main groups of these, the division being based on substrate preference:
- interstitial collagenases
- gelatinases
- stromelysins

The gelatinases, which appear to be especially potent, degrade a wide variety of substrates. They are basically collagenases, which differ from other collagenases in that they have:
- **a unique region homologous to the gelatin-binding domain of fibronectin**
- **the ability to interact with TIMP-2**

There is a positive correlation between gelatinase (type IV) activity and invasiveness. Downregulation of this enzyme's activity (which can be accomplished with retinoic acid) has been shown to result in loss of invasiveness.

All the metalloproteinases are secreted in an inactive form and their activation is an important control step.

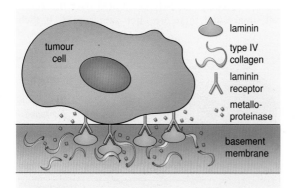

FIGURE 25.6

FIGURE 25.6 and 25.7 Binding to connective tissue matrix proteins is followed by proteolytic breakdown of these matrices and deattachment of tumour cells, which can then move through the breaches created by matrix protein breakdown.

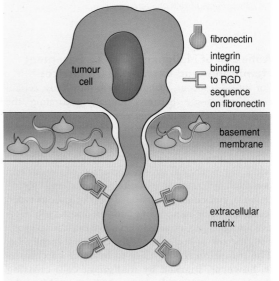

FIGURE 25.7

The *in vivo* mechanism whereby this activation occurs is still unknown.

Other Tumour-associated Proteolytic Enzymes

It has been known for 60 years that extracts from virally induced tumours in chickens can lyse plasma clots. Human sarcomas have been shown to have similar fibrinolytic properties. This fibrinolytic activity is now known to be due to the production by the tumour cells of **plasminogen activator**, a phenomenon that occurs in many cell lines following malignant transformation. There is some evidence to suggest that acquisition of the ability to produce plasminogen activator is associated with the ability to invade extracellular matrix. In this connection it must be remembered that some normal cells also produce plasminogen activator. Some of these cells (such as macrophages, neutrophils and trophoblastic cells) travel through the connective tissue matrix, whereas others (such as breast epithelium, Sertoli cells in the testis, thyroid and parathyroid epithelium, and β cells in the islets of Langerhans) are fixed.

Active Movement of Malignant Cells

Invasion and metastasis require active movement on the part of the tumour cells. Whether the movement involved in invasion is random (**kinesis**) or directed (**taxis**), or both of these, is not clear. Several factors have been identified as increasing one or other of these forms of movement (*Fig. 25.8*). These include:

- **Intact and fragmented molecules of the extracellular matrix** such as collagen or fibronectin
- **Tumour autocrine motility factor (AMF)**. This is a 64-kDa protein secreted by certain tumour cell lines. It binds to a glycoprotein receptor on the tumour cells, binding being followed by activation of a G protein-mediated signalling system. **Movement of the tumour cells appears to be associated with phosphorylation of the receptor**. The action of AMF can be simulated by treating tumour cells with monoclonal antibodies that bind to the AMF receptor.

  An interesting finding has been that the expression of the AMF receptor differs between melanoma cell lines of high and low metastatic potential. In cells with a high potential the AMF receptors are distributed over a localized area of the cell membrane; in cells with low metastatic potential, the receptors are distributed diffusely over the cell surface.

- **'Scatter factor'.** This protein, which is synthesized and secreted by fibroblasts, exerts a scattering effect on many epithelial cells in culture. This effect, which appears to be exerted in a paracrine fashion, occurs at picomolar concentrations. Scatter factor is a molecule resembling plasminogen in some respects and is identical to **hepatocyte growth factor**. It has a number of different functions, being able to induce motility in tumour cells, to induce

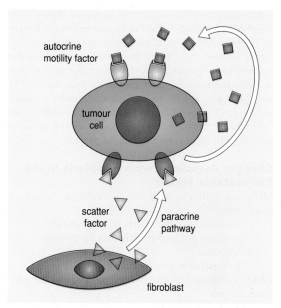

FIGURE 25.8 *Chemical signals stimulating active movement of tumour cells. Movement of tumour cells through connective tissues is mediated inter alia by an autocrine motility factor and a paracrine signal, in the form of 'scatter factor' derived from fibroblasts. The scatter factor binds to a receptor encoded by the proto-oncogene c-met.*

proliferation in epithelial cells and also to act as a morphogen in being able to induce tubule formation in some epithelial cell lines cultured in collagen gels. This multifunctional effect suggests that scatter factor binds either to separate receptors on different target cells or to a single receptor that is linked to multiple signalling pathways.

A ligand for scatter factor which has been identified is the gene product of a proto-oncogene called c-*met*. This product is a transmembrane heterodimer which has tyrosine kinase activity; it is widely expressed in normal epithelial tissue. It is interesting that the transfection of a mutated c-*met* oncogene into human osteosarcoma cells in culture leads to the cells becoming both tumorigenic and metastatic in athymic mice.

A Role for Mechanical Pressure in Direct Spread of Malignant Tumours

Invading cells tend to follow paths where the resistance is least and to spread along natural clefts or within tissue planes. This can be seen in cancer of the alimentary tract where, once the invading cells have reached the main muscle layers, the infiltrating columns of cells tend to avoid the muscle itself and pass instead through the connective tissue septa that separate the muscle fibres. On naked-eye examination, this gives the muscle a curiously segmented appearance, as if the muscle fibres were bricks and the intervening tumour-infiltrated septa, the mortar.

On the basis of these patterns of spread, it has been suggested that invasiveness can be accounted for largely by mechanical factors. If quick-setting dental plastic is injected into tissue samples, the plastic spreads along the zones of least resistance in a manner similar to that seen in some tumours. Such simple mechanical models do not, however, appear to explain the rapidly invasive behaviour of some malignant neoplasms. In addition, in cell culture systems, invasiveness can be shown to occur even though there is no mechanical pressure.

Changes Associated with Neoplasia in the Extracellular Matrix

Malignant cells can alter the extracellular matrix in three ways:
   1) Destruction of the matrix of tumour cells
   2) Increased production of matrix by the host ('desmoplasia')
   3) Synthesis of matrix by tumour cells
The first of these has already been discussed in the previous section.

Desmoplastic Response

The amount of stroma associated with malignant neoplasms determines, to a considerable extent, their consistency. The extreme hardness and 'gritty' feel of some tumours is due to the high proportion of fibrous tissue within them. The ancient Greek physicians recognized this phenomenon and coined the term **scirrhous** (rock-like) for such lesions. The biological purpose of desmoplasia is not clear. Its presence is certainly not necessary for invasion to occur; some invasive tumours have very little response, whereas others, notably breast, stomach and bile duct tumours, show a marked desmoplastic reaction.

Synthesis of Matrix

Some controversy exists regarding the origin of the fibrous tissue related to malignant tumours. Some workers, studying the stromal response to breast cancer cells, maintain that the new collagen is synthesized and secreted by the invading tumour cells. The results of other studies support a role for the host cells. Recently, myofibroblasts, which are not normally present in breast stroma, have been identified in the stroma of some breast cancers, and it has been suggested that malignant cells may, in some unknown way, either recruit or stimulate the formation of myofibroblasts, which then produce the excess connective tissue matrix found in tumours with a marked desmoplastic response.

Other Phenotypic Characteristics of Malignant Cells that may Contribute to Invasiveness

Loss Of Anchorage Dependence

With the exception of lymphocytes and haemopoietic cells, normal cells, when cultured, will grow only on a firm surface such as glass, plastic or solid agar. This type of growth is spoken of as being **anchorage dependent.** Many cell lines derived from malignant neoplasms or from cells that have undergone malignant transformation in culture can grow in suspension or in semi-solid soft agar. This growth feature in cell culture systems, more than any other, correlates with the ability of the cultured cells to produce malignant tumours when injected into animals of the appropriate species ('tumorigenicity').

Loss of Fibronectin from the Cell Surface

Fibronectin is a glycoprotein that has been identified as a component of the extracellular matrix of many cells in culture. It is also found in basement membranes and interstitial stroma in many animals and human tissues, and circulates in the blood (where it was originally called cold-insoluble globulin). Fibronectin can be found on the external surface of many cells, where it forms a fibrillary meshwork around and between them. It acts as an adhesive protein in cell-to-cell binding and in the binding of cells to their substratum. Malignant transformation is accompanied by a loss or marked reduction of cell surface fibronectin. The loss of this surface protein (and presumably the decreased adhesiveness that follows) may be an expression of one of the following:
- An increase in degradative enzymes on the surface of the malignant cells (see pp 252–253).
- A disturbance in the cytoskeleton, more particularly the microfilaments beneath the cell surface.

LYMPHATIC SPREAD

The invasion of lymphatic channels at an early stage of the infiltrative process is a characteristic property of carcinoma (malignant epithelial neoplasm). Malignant tumours derived from connective tissue cells (sarcomas) show a much greater tendency to invade the small blood vessels.

Invasion of the lymphatics may be made easier by the fact that basement membranes do not contain any type IV collagen or laminin. Because of this difference, it is possible, using appropriate antibodies, to determine whether the small vascular channels in tissue sections showing invasion by tumour are lymphatics or venules.

Little is known about the actual mechanics of lymphatic invasion. In certain experimental models, tumour cells have been seen to line up alongside the lymphatic channels and to enter the lymphatic by first pushing cytoplasmic processes between the endothelial cells and then travelling through the interendothelial gap in a reverse direction to that seen when leucocyte emigration occurs in inflammation. Such invasion is likely to make use of the mechanisms that have been discussed in relation to direct invasion of the tissues adjacent to a primary malignant neoplasm.

Once the malignant cells have gained access to the lymphatic vessel, they can grow along the lumen as a continuous cord which permeates the lymphatic drainage in that area and may extend quite widely. The presence of such intralymphatic tumour in a tissue section is, of course, an indicator of possible spread to regional lymph nodes. However, in some cases the presence of intralymphatic tumour in the absence of lymph node deposits may have an even more ominous prognostic significance, because it has been reported that patients with breast cancer in whom there is evidence of lymphatic permeation by tumour but no regional node deposits have an **increased risk** of developing distant metastases.

Lymphatic permeation is a particularly prominent feature of **carcinoma of the breast**. Lymphatic blockage occurs quite frequently in this situation. This results in diversion of lymph flow and may be accompanied by a similar diversion of groups of tumour cells, which may impact within the lymphatic drainage of the breast, producing satellite tumour nodules. Lymphatic blockage also causes lymphoedema of the tissues caudal to the block. In patients with carcinoma of the breast this produces an appearance of the skin which has been aptly termed **peau d'orange**. In the lung, extensive lymphatic permeation by tumour, often from a breast or gastric primary, produces the condition known as **lymphangitis carcinomatosa**. On chest radiography the lung shows a curious reticulated appearance. This is mirrored by the outlining of the subpleural lymphatic channels seen when the lung is removed at postmortem examination.

Malignant melanoma is another of the neoplasms that tend to permeate along the local lymphatic drainage. If the tumour cells are producing melanin, the cord of cells permeating the lymphatics may be seen as a black streak in the subcutaneous tissue.

Tumour cells enter the regional lymph nodes and gain access to the subcapsular peripheral sinus in the first instance. From here, the cells extend to involve the sinuses in the centre of the node. Within the node, tumour cells may be destroyed, remain dormant for long periods, or establish a growing focus with partial or total replacement of the node. For the last of these, acquisition of an adequate blood supply is important. Normal nodes have a dual blood supply, partly from hilar vessels and partly from transcapsular anastomoses. If the tumour nodules invade intranodal vessels, haemorrhage and necrosis may occur within the secondary deposit.

Tumour cells within lymph nodes may gain access to the bloodstream in a number of ways. These include:
- invasion of small intranodal blood vessels
- invasion of extranodal blood vessels by nodal deposits that have breached the lymph node capsule
- opening up of small lymphaticovenous communications
- via the thoracic duct

These connections between the lymphatic channels and the bloodstream work in both directions. If radioactively labelled tumour cells are injected into a periph-eral vein of a rat, tumour cells can be recovered from lymphatics within 1 hour. Thus, malignant cells within the bloodstream are not always trapped in the first capillary bed they encounter, but can escape into the lymphatic system.

BLOOD SPREAD

Apart from the connections between the lymphatic system and the blood vessels mentioned above, malignant cells may enter the bloodstream by invading either small new vessels within the substance of the tumour itself or the host blood vessels near the growing edge of the tumour. The newly formed vessels often have defective basement membranes and may lack normal perivascular connective tissue. Sarcomas often contain large, irregular, blood-filled channels, the linings of which consist partly or entirely of malignant tumour cells; these lining cells can, of course, be shed directly into the bloodstream. This may, in part, account for the predilection shown by sarcomas for spread via the bloodstream.

Permeation in continuity along invaded venous channels may be seen in certain malignant tumours. These include carcinomas arising from renal tubular epithelium (so-called **hypernephroma**) and carcinoma of the bronchus. In the case of renal adenocarcinoma, venous invasion may occur quite early and the tumour cells extend as a solid mass along the course of the renal vein. In rare instances, the inferior cava may be involved and cases have been recorded where tumour has grown up into the right atrium. When the left renal vein is involved in this way, the first clinical evidence of this occurrence may be the appearance of a left-sided scrotal mass consisting of dilated spermatic veins (**varicocele**). This is said to be due to the fact that the spermatic veins of the left side drain directly into the left renal vein. If the latter becomes blocked by tumour, hydrostatic pressure rises in the spermatic veins and they become distended.

METASTASIS

A growing colony of malignant cells that becomes established at a point distant from the original or primary lesion and with **no continuity between the primary lesion and the new deposit** is termed a **metastasis or secondary deposit**. The majority of metastases arise as a result of invasion of lymphatics or blood vessels, but in some instances they owe their existence to 'seeding out' of malignant cells across serosa-lined spaces such as the pleural and peritoneal cavities.

Metastasis is, fundamentally, an **embolic** process. It may be viewed as a series of events that occur sequentially (*Fig. 25.9*). Some of these have already been discussed. These events are:
- The **liberation** of cells from the primary tumour mass.
- The **invasion** of blood vessels or lymphatics.

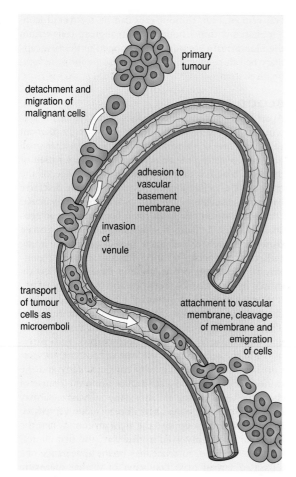

FIGURE 25.9 Outline of the operational steps involved in metastasis.

- **Transfer** of tumour cells as tumour emboli to distant sites.
- Their **adhesion to endothelium** in the vascular bed of some distant organ or tissue. The expression of appropriate adhesion molecules may be one of the important determinants for the localization patterns of metastasis seen in association with certain tumours.
- **Migration** from the vessels in which the emboli have impacted.
- **Survival** at the new site, which probably involves angiogenesis.
- **Multiplication** and **growth** to form secondary tumours.

Determination of the Extent of Spread (Staging) of Tumours Gives Useful Prognostic Information

As already stated, metastatic spread occurs as a result of invasion of lymphatic channels, the bloodstream and serosal cavities.

In patients with carcinoma, deposits of tumour in the regional nodes is a common occurrence. If the efferent lymphatic is invaded by the tumour cells, the stage is set for further extension to the next set of nodes, which may also become wholly or partly replaced by tumour. The extent of such nodal invasion is important in assessing the prognosis of patients with cancer and, despite the introduction of a number of new criteria in recent years, the presence or absence of lymph node metastasis remains one of the more reliable indicators of the natural history of an individual patient with cancer.

For instance, in one of the commonest malignant neoplasms encountered in clinical practice – carcinoma of the breast – absence of lymph node metastases after a careful search of the axillary contents is associated with a 5-year survival rate of 75–80%. The presence of lymph node deposits reduces this figure considerably, perhaps to approximately 50%.

A combination of assessment of direct spread and lymph node metastasis gives valuable prognostic information in carcinoma of the colon and rectum, and forms the basis of the Dukes' staging scheme for these tumours (see pp 558–559).

- If a colonic and rectal carcinoma penetrates the bowel wall no further than the main muscle coat (Dukes' stage A), the 5-year survival rate should be 80–90%.
- Penetration of the bowel wall by tumour through the muscle to reach the subserosa (Dukes' stage B) reduces the 5-year survival rate to approximately 50%.
- If the tumour is associated with lymph node deposits (Dukes' stage C) the 5-year survival rate is reduced to about 30%.

The occurrence of blood-borne metastases is the feature of malignant disease that is responsible for death in most fatal cases. It is obvious when considering an accessible tumour such as carcinoma of the breast, which can be apparently completely excised with relative ease, that it is the presence of **occult** metastases at the time of primary excision that will determine the outcome for the patient.

Much of our knowledge of this process comes from experimental systems such as transplantable breast cancers or malignant melanomas in mice. Once a transplantable tumour has grown to a few grams in weight, it starts to release several million malignant cells into the blood every day. Fortunately the presence of malignant cells in the blood (or lymph) does not mean that metastases will inevitably develop. An overwhelming majority of tumour cells released in the blood die very quickly.

In studies carried out using radioactively labelled malignant melanoma cells, it was found that only 1% of injected cells survived for 24 hours. After 2 weeks, only 0.1% had survived. However, at this stage deposits of secondary tumour could be seen in the lungs.

- While in the bloodstream the malignant cells may adhere to other tumour cells to form clumps, they may adhere to platelets or lymphocytes, and when they enter the capillary bed in which they may impact, they can adhere to the capillary endothelium. The greater the degree of clumping of tumour cells, the more likely is impaction and the greater the chances of a secondary deposit forming.

- After impaction in a small vessel, some tumour cells stimulate the production of fibrin; it has been suggested that this fibrin tends to protect the clump of malignant cells and enables them to proliferate. In animal models of the metastatic process, administration both of plasmin and anticoagulants have been shown to reduce the number of metastases consequent on intravenous injection of malignant cells.

- After impaction in small vessels, the malignant cells must emigrate from the vascular compartment into the perivascular tissues. It has been shown in experimental tumours that endothelial cells retract, leaving cell-free spaces through which the tumour cells can escape, using the same mechanisms to attach to basement membranes and penetrate them, as has been described in the section dealing with invasiveness.

- Within the extravascular tissues, a new and suitable microenvironment must be established if the colony of tumour cells is to grow and flourish. If the colony is to grow to a significant size, a new blood supply must become available both for nutrition of the tumour cells and for carrying away cellular waste products. The new blood vessels, as mentioned earlier, are derived from the host vasculature. The effect of this neovascularization can be shown in a number of animal models. For example, if tumours are implanted into the cornea of animals, initially tumour growth is slow. After about 1 week small capillaries begin to grow out from the iris into the cornea and, when these vessels reach the tumour, a marked spurt of tumour growth occurs. Implantation of normal tissues does not have this effect. Extracts from tumours applied to the chorioallantoic membrane of a fertilized chicken egg also show a considerable angiogenic effect.

Are Malignant Cells Homogeneous in Respect of their Tendency to Metastasize?

Only a small fraction of malignant cells released into the circulation from a primary tumour survive to establish secondary deposits. Does this mean that the successful cells have some special properties not shared by the other cells of the tumour?

This hypothesis has been tested in the mouse melanoma model. Malignant melanoma in humans frequently develops lymphatic and blood-borne metastases; non-human melanomas behave in much the same

way. Murine B16 melanoma, a tumour that arises spontaneously in a certain strain of black mice, can be transplanted from one animal of the strain to another and the cells can be grown in culture with relative ease. When B16 cells are implanted into the subcutaneous tissue of mice, the melanoma metastasizes at a low or moderate rate. To quantify the phenomenon of metastasis it is customary to inject a known number of tumour cells into the mouse tail vein and then to count the number of lung metastases. If the metastatic deposits are harvested and cultured, and these cultured cells then injected into mouse tail veins, the yield of metastases is greater. After, say, 10 cycles a cell line will have been established which has a much greater metastatic potential than cells from the original tumour line. **These data suggest that the original tumour cell population was not homogeneous in respect of the qualities needed to establish metastases** (*Fig. 25.10*).

This model may also throw some light on the common clinical observation that particular primary tumours metastasize preferentially to certain sites. For example, breast cancers commonly spread to lung, liver, bone and brain; lung tumours often spread to the brain and adrenals; and prostatic cancers frequently spread to bone. About 90 years ago, Ewing and Paget suggested that different patterns of metastasis were due to the fact that different tumour cells would thrive in certain '**biological soils**' but not in others. More recently the use of experimental models has suggested that properties of the malignant cells themselves also influence the pattern of their metastasis.

For instance, is the pattern of metastasis due solely to anatomical factors such as the vascular bed first encountered by tumour emboli?

If radioactively labelled B16 melanoma cells are injected into the tail veins of a batch of mice and also into the left ventricles of other mice, the initial distribution of the radioactivity suggests that the cells have indeed impacted in different sites in the two groups of mice. Within 24 hours, however, the distribution and number of surviving cells is the same, irrespective of the site of injection, and after 2 weeks the number of metastases in the lungs is the same in both cases. These results suggest that tumour cells destined to form secondary deposits in a particular organ can detach themselves from their initial impaction site and 'home' on to the favoured tissue. By cell selection procedures similar to those described previously, it has been possible to isolate a subpopulation of B16 cells that metastasizes only to one area of the brain, and another that preferentially colonizes the ovaries. Although the nature of this 'homing' mechanism is unknown, it appears to be related to the nature of the surface membrane of the malignant cell. A lung-metastasizing line of B16 cells was found to shed small membrane-bound vesicles into the culture fluid. These vesicles can be fused with a line that metastasizes poorly to the lung using polyethylene glycol. The cells enriched with vesicles now produce

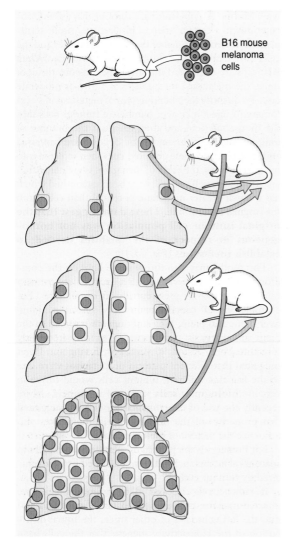

B16 mouse melanoma cells

*FIGURE 25.10 Heterogeneity of malignant cells in respect of their metastatic potential. **a** Cultured mouse melanoma cells injected into the tail vein of a susceptible mouse produce a small number of metastases in the lung. **b** If cells derived from these secondary deposits are injected into another set of mice, the yield of metastases is increased. **c** Repetition of this procedure leads to the identification of a subpopulation derived from the original tumour cells, with a very high metastatic potential.*

very large numbers of pulmonary metastases. Each of the melanoma cell lines that produce preferential metastases has been shown to have a specific pattern of cell surface proteins.

How far these observations relate to the behaviour of malignant tumours in humans is unknown, although there is increasing evidence that human tumours are heterogeneous with respect to features such as karyotype and DNA content, the presence of hormone receptors, antigenic determinants and cell surface con-

stituents, pigment synthesis (in the case of malignant melanoma), drug sensitivity, and growth in nude (immunosuppressed) mice.

Are there Genes that Determine Metastatic Phenotype?

The NM23 Gene

It is clear from studies such as those described above, that cell populations derived from a single tumour contain clones whose potential to form metastases varies. The screening of complementary DNA 'libraries' derived from tumours of 'high' and 'low' metastatic potential has shown that certain messenger RNAs (mRNAs) are present in different concentrations in these two classes of cell. The genes from which they have been transcribed have been investigated as possible regulators of metastasis.

Currently, the most interesting of these is **a *suppressor gene for metastasis* which has been called *NM23***. It was recognized in the first instance by the fact that in mouse melanoma cell lines mRNA for this gene was reduced in amount in cells of high as opposed to low metastatic potential. **In human breast cancer, poor survival is correlated with loss of expression of *NM23*, and increased expression is associated with a good prognosis.**

NM23 is coded for on the long arm of chromosome 17, a chromosome that is the site of a number of different genes involved in malignant disease, which include the important tumour suppressor gene *p53* which is located on the short arm. On the long arm are sited the loci for *NM23*, the retinoic acid receptor, TIMP-2, and the gene involved in hereditary breast and ovarian cancer.

The gene product of *NM23* is almost identical with that of the *awd* gene product in the fruit fly *Drosophila*. If *awd* expression is reduced, the development of several tissues is affected in postembryonic life when cells in the wing disc begin to divide and differentiate. It has been suggested that loss of NM23 may, in the same way, lead to a disordered state in which development may be abnormal or in which tumours may progress to become metastatic.

It is now known that the gene products of both *NM23* and *awd* are nucleoside diphosphate (NDP) kinases. NDP kinases play a part in two functions, either or both of which may be involved in malignancy:

1) The first of these is the assembly and disassembly of microtubules. Microtubule assembly requires that GDP be changed to GTP by transphosphorylation, which is catalysed by a microtubule-associated NDP kinase. Lack of this kinase could lead to an aneuploid state, as is frequently observed in metastatic cells.

2) The second is the fact that NDP kinases form complexes with a variety of G proteins which regulate many second-messenger pathways and may

thus be involved in the regulation of a number of pathways that could be related to development, oncogenesis and metastasis.

Mutation or Abnormal Expression of Oncogenes in Relation to Metastasis

In a variety of human malignancies, mutations or abnormal expression of the *ras* and *myc* oncogenes have been associated with aggressive behaviour. When mutated *ras* oncogene sequences were transfected into an immortal line of mouse-derived fibroblasts, the resulting cells produced metastases when injected into athymic mice. The induction of metastatic potential by activated *ras* genes appears not to be related to the ability of this gene to render mouse fibroblasts tumorigenic when injected into athymic mice.

Some Common Patterns of Metastasis in Human Tumours

The Liver

The liver is the site in which blood-borne metastases occur most frequently. Gastrointestinal and pancreatic tumours regularly metastasize there, which is not surprising in view of their venous drainage via the portal system. Other primary tumours that commonly metastasize to the liver are carcinomas of the lung, breast and genitourinary system, malignant melanoma and various sarcomas. Rare examples of transplacental metastases have been recorded in the liver.

The Lung

Tumours commonly producing metastatic deposits in the lung are carcinoma of the breast, carcinoma of the stomach, and sarcomas. Blood-borne metastases in this tissue may be single or multiple and tend to occur as well-demarcated rounded masses. Sometimes it may be difficult to distinguish between a single secondary deposit and a peripherally situated primary carcinoma of the lung. In a city-dweller, whose lung tissue is usually laden with carbon pigment, the absence of pigment from the centre of the tumour, which is characteristic of secondary deposits, may be helpful.

The Skeleton

After the liver and lungs, the skeleton is the most frequent site for metastatic deposits to occur (*Fig. 25.11*). The site of origin of the primary is commonly lung, breast, prostate, kidney or thyroid. Bony metastases may either elicit the production of new bone (**osteoblastic**) or destroy bone (**osteolytic**). In the former, the secondary deposits are very hard as a result of the abundant new bone formation and on radiography appear as radio-opaque shadows. Plasma alkaline phosphatase levels are high, reflecting active osteogenesis. Serum calcium and phosphate concentrations are usually normal. Such osteosclerotic secondaries are commonly seen in association with carcinoma of the

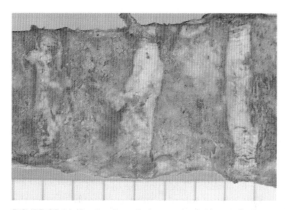

FIGURE 25.11 *Section through the vertebral column of a middle-aged woman dying from breast cancer. Note the presence of white tumour deposits in the vertebral bodies and sparing of the intervertebral discs.*

prostate. When this is the case, plasma concentrations of acid phosphatase (of tumour cell origin) are also much raised. Osteolysis shows itself on radiological examination by the presence of zones of radiolucency. Clinically, it draws attention to itself by pain or because of pathological fractures (fractures occurring after only slight trauma). If bone destruction has been extensive, hypercalcaemia may be present.

The mechanisms of tumour-mediated bone destruction are not well understood. Many tumours contain collagenase capable of degrading type I collagen. In organ culture systems where portions of breast cancer are incubated together with small pieces of mouse skull, osteolysis can be detected. This osteolysis can be inhibited by adding cyclo-oxygenase inhibitors such as aspirin to the culture medium. This suggests that the release of prostaglandins may play some part in mediating bone destruction.

The Brain

Secondary deposits occur quite frequently in the brain; the lung is one of the commonest primary sites. Often neurological and/or psychiatric disturbances produced by the metastasis are the first indication of the presence of cancer in these patients.

The Adrenal

Of all endocrine organs, the adrenal gland is the most frequently involved by metastatic tumour. The medulla is the most favoured site for metastases but nodules of secondary tumour may also be seen in the cortex. Common primary sites for adrenal secondaries include the lung and the breast.

TRANSCOELOMIC SPREAD

The term **transcoelomic spread** is applied to the sequence of events that follows invasion of the serosal lining of an organ by malignant cells. A local inflammatory response usually develops in relation to the infiltrating tumour cells and the malignant cells may become incorporated into the inflammatory exudate on the serosal surface.

These small groups of cells become detached from the main colony of tumour cells and can be swept away by the fluid portion of the exudate and float out into the serosal cavity. They settle on the walls of such a cavity, where some proliferate and set up small secondary deposits. These may elicit the formation of more exudation and the serosal cavity may, in time, come to contain a large volume of fluid.

This type of spread is most commonly seen in the peritoneal cavity of patients with gastric, colonic and ovarian carcinoma. The greater omentum may be so massively infiltrated that it becomes converted to a thick, firm, often rather gelatinous mass, which some, rather infelicitously, refer to as 'omental cake'. Deposits arising from gravitational seeding are especially common in the pouch of Douglas.

From time to time, gastric or colonic carcinoma may be associated with a highly individual pattern of transcoelomic spread in which the ovaries become involved preferentially. The ovaries become grossly enlarged and have smooth capsular surfaces and slightly mucoid cut surfaces. Much of the enlargement can be seen, on microscopic examination, to be due to a desmoplastic response in the ovarian stroma to the presence of the relatively scanty cancer cells. The classical jargon for these ovarian deposits is 'Krukenberg' tumours.

KEY POINTS: Tumour Spread

- The fundamental functional attribute of malignancy is invasiveness.
- Invasive cells show loss of homotypic adhesion, probably due to decreased expression of cadherins.
- Invasion is mediated by operation of a trio of linked processes:
  a) **adhesion** to connective tissue matrices
  b) **proteolysis** of matrix proteins
  c) **active movement** of tumour cells mediated by autocrine motility factor or 'scatter' factor
- The extent of spread, as determined by clinical and pathological examination (staging), has important prognostic implications.
- Patterns of metastasis are probably determined by both the biological characteristics of the 'soil' (tissues in which deposits occur) and the 'seed' (tumour cells).
- Tumour cells are heterogeneous in their ability to metastasize. This may correlate with the expression of certain genes (e.g. *NM23* and *ras*).

CHAPTER 26

Effects of Neoplasms on the Host

Both benign and malignant neoplasms can produce a wide variety of effects on the host. While the term 'malignant' rightly has ominous prognostic overtones, 'benign' lesions, while not invasive and having no metastatic potential, may, nevertheless have serious or even fatal consequences.

LOCAL EFFECTS

MECHANICAL PRESSURE OR OBSTRUCTION

In many cases the effects of neoplasms on the host depend on the interaction between the **site** of the tumour and its **size**. A large number of such instances exists; only a few examples are given in the following section.

In the gastrointestinal tract, the clinical presentation of a neoplasm is frequently related to the fact that the lesion may cause obstruction. This is usually, although not invariably, **chronic**. For example, in the case of a colonic or rectal tumour, the patient may complain of an alteration in the bowel habit. The obstruction may be due to the actual bulk of the neoplasm itself, but more often it is caused by the fibrous tissue response elicited by the presence of cancer cells (desmoplasia). In a few cases, a polypoid tumour mass may lead to intus-susception (see p 527).

Obviously the anatomical site of a neoplasm plays a major role in determining whether or not obstruction will occur. A small neoplasm in an unfavourable anatomical location can produce very serious obstruction. For instance, carcinoma in the common bile duct or head of the pancreas will produce a severe degree of cholestatic jaundice, associated with marked dilatation of the biliary passages above the obstruction and, not infrequently, with dilatation of the gallbladder as well (*Fig. 26.1*).

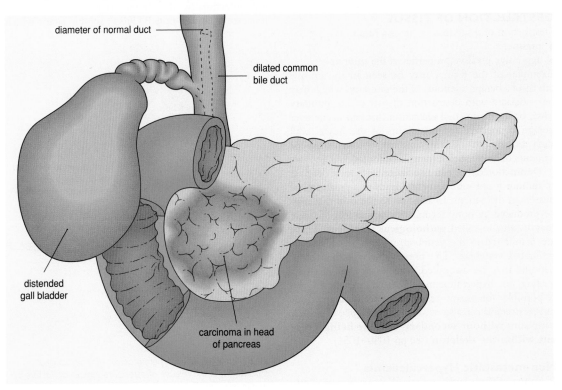

FIGURE 26.1 Carcinoma in the head of the pancreas compresses the common bile duct leading to dilatation of the bile drainage system and the gallbladder. The common presenting feature is cholestatic jaundice.

From the point of view of mechanical disturbances, one of the most serious locations for neoplasms to occur, apart from any question of their inherent malignancy, is within the cranium. One of the commonest intracranial tumours arises from the meninges (**meningioma**). The overwhelming majority of these are benign, but they can cause serious or fatal consequences as a result of the rise in intracranial pressure that they produce and the distortion of normal anatomical relationships that follows.

In some cases the type of obstructive phenomenon is determined by the **pattern of spread** of the neoplasm. This is seen very strikingly in carcinoma of the uterine cervix. Here the direct spread of tumour within the pelvis often involves the lower portions of the ureters, these being encased in a rigid sleeve of tumour and associated fibrous tissue. The obvious sequel is ureteric obstruction and in due time, if the obstruction cannot be relieved, chronic renal failure.

Another example of the role of anatomical location in determining the clinical picture may be seen, from time to time, in carcinoma of the lung occurring at the apices of the upper lobes. If such a neoplasm extends beyond the anatomical confines of the lung, it may involve either the brachial plexus or the sympathetic chain. In either instance there may be striking local neurological consequences, with unilateral Horner's syndrome in the case of sympathetic involvement.

DESTRUCTION OF TISSUE

Destruction of tissue may occur as a result of:
- pressure
- aggressive invasive properties of the tumour

Examples of the former may be seen in the erosive effects of a benign adenoma of the pituitary, which may be associated with destruction of part of the pituitary fossa, or in the mucosal ulceration that can occur over benign connective tissue tumours of the bowel wall such as smooth muscle tumours (leiomyomas) or tumours of nerve sheath (neurilemmomas).

Destruction of bone in association with local deposits of tumour is not infrequent and leads to a great deal of distress to the patient. In addition to the pain that may be produced by bony secondaries, actual loss of tissue may lead to so-called **pathological fractures**. These are manifested in the vertebral column as collapse of infiltrated vertebrae. The presence of multiple bony deposits may be associated with extensive osteolysis leading to hypercalcaemia. Skeletal metastases are responsible for many cases of hypercalcaemia, but hypercalcaemia can also occur in the presence of certain neoplasms **without secondary tumour being present within the skeleton** (see pp 1050–1051).

Non-metastatic Hypercalcaemia

If plasma calcium levels are raised, it seems reasonable to assume that the excess calcium has been released from bone and, in the absence of primary or secondary tumour actually within the bone, some other calcium-releasing mechanism must be invoked.

Some tumours (not of the parathyroid) have been found to secrete a parathyroid hormone-related peptide (PTHRP). This particular example of **ectopic hormone production**, which is considered in more detail later in this chapter, has been noted especially in tumours of the lung and kidney (*Fig. 26.2*). However, tumour-related hypercalcaemia can occur in the absence of both bony metastases and a raised PTHRP concentration.

Extracts of the tumours from these patients have an osteolytic effect *in vitro*. At least part of this effect is now thought to be due to prostaglandin (PG) production, either by the tumour cells or by cells associated with them. In a number of animal tumours, secretion of PGE_2 was noted and the hypercalcaemia could be prevented by the administration of a cyclo-oxygenase inhibitor such as indomethacin. PGE_2 can be shown to have a marked capacity for causing bone resorption in studies carried out *in vitro*. Several studies in humans have also indicated that increased secretion of PGE_2 is causally associated with hypercalcaemia.

Substances other than prostaglandins capable of inducing resorption of bone have also been found in association with certain tumours. Cultured cell lines of plasma cell tumour and from Burkitt's lymphoma (a B lymphocyte-derived tumour believed to be associated with infection by the Epstein–Barr virus) produce a non-prostaglandin, non-PTHRP, soluble factor which

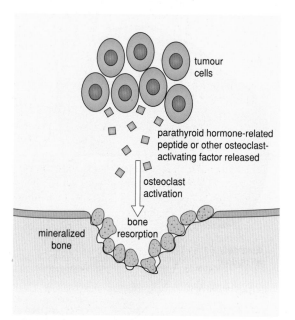

FIGURE 26.2 *Humoral hypercalcaemia of malignancy is associated with the release of osteoclast-stimulating factors by tumour cells. This is exemplified by the action of parathyroid-hormone-related peptide, the release of which causes severe hypercalcaemia due to bone resorption.*

can stimulate osteoclasts to resorb bone *in vitro*. This has been identified as the cytokine, tumour necrosis factor (TNF) β. In addition, some breast cancer cell lines have been shown to contain an osteolytic substance that does not appear to act by stimulating osteoclasts and which is not blocked by indomethacin.

HAEMORRHAGE

Most neoplasms involving surfaces lined by epithelium or lying subjacent to such surfaces will undergo a certain degree of ulceration, with resulting haemorrhage. In most instances the bleeding is slow and unspectacular, although none the less dangerous. The chronic blood loss may produce a severe microcytic anaemia of the type associated with iron deficiency. Occult bleeding of this type and degree is seen not infrequently in cancers of the right side of the colon or of the caecum. Indeed, the symptoms of vague ill-health associated with anaemia of this type may be the first and, for a long time, the only indication of the presence of a neoplasm. Occasionally, ulceration of a tumour may result in torrential haemorrhage, as for example in smooth muscle tumours of the stomach or intestine. Bleeding from these lesions may be so severe as to necessitate replacement of the total blood volume several times over.

INFECTION

Infection in relation to malignancy is common and may be the determining factor in the timing of a patient's death. Local infection tends to occur in any situation where the presence of a neoplasm causes obstruction to a drainage system with retention of secretions behind the obstruction. An example of this may occur in bronchial carcinoma, where narrowing or total blocking of the bronchus may cause damming back of the secretions derived from more distal parts of the bronchial tree. The retained secretions constitute an advantageous medium for the growth of organisms and this, coupled with the collapse of lung parenchyma distal to the obstruction, tends to lead to episodes of bronchopneumonia, which may be severe.

The role of malignant disease in promoting susceptibility to infection through immunosuppression has already been alluded to (see p 122) and will be considered further later in this chapter.

SYSTEMIC MANIFESTATIONS OF CANCER

FEVER

Episodes of fever are extremely common in patients with malignant disease, even in the absence of recognizable evidence of infection. Fever is particularly common in malignant disease involving the lymphoid system such as malignant lymphomas, the leukaemias and Hodgkin's disease, although it also occurs in cases of disseminated, solid, epithelial tumours. This effect is likely to be mediated by the release of cytokines such as interleukin 1 or TNF-α, either from the tumour cells or from infiltrating macrophages.

Occasionally fever may be the presenting feature of neoplasm. This is seen most notably in renal adenocarcinoma (hypernephroma), a tumour that is particularly prone to produce non-metastatic systemic disturbances.

CACHEXIA

Marked weight loss and wasting of tissue, especially muscle, is a well-recognized feature of the later stages of the natural history of many malignant neoplasms. This state is known as cachexia and understanding of its pathogenesis is still far from complete. Processes that have been canvassed as playing a role in the production of cachexia include:

1) **Anorexia.** Loss of appetite is a conspicuous feature in certain malignant disorders and appears not to be related to tumour bulk or location. Many reasons have been advanced to account for this, but none can be shown to operate in all instances of tumour-related anorexia.

2) **Malabsorption.** This may occur in association with neoplasms, such as medullary carcinoma of the thyroid, that secrete products that increase gastrointestinal motility. In most cases where malabsorption is present, the mechanism producing it is not known.

3) **The metabolic processes of the neoplasm.** In some experimental tumour models, the tumour gives the impression of 'growing at the expense of its host'; force-feeding of these animals results in tumour growth being stimulated in the absence of any weight gain in the host. However, when the dietary **constituents** are manipulated, a situation can be brought about in which tumour growth is minimal and host animal's weight is maintained. This is alleged to be because the metabolism of many tumour cells is dominated by anaerobic glycolysis, for which appropriate substrates are required. If such substrates are deficient in the diet, the rate of tumour progression slows down. There is little to suggest that these data, none of which is very recent, can be readily applied to the human situation.

4) **Is some cachexia-inducing product liberated from the neoplasm**? From time to time the suggestion has been made that some toxic product liberated from the neoplasm could be responsible for the nutritional changes seen. Decreased hepatic catalase activity can be shown to occur both in certain patients with malignant disease and in animals with experimentally induced tumours; this decline in catalase activity can be reproduced in animals injected with a polypeptide extractable from human gastric or rectal carcinoma. This extracted material also produces changes in

plasma iron concentrations, increases the levels of protoporphyrin in the liver, and may cause thymic involution.

Most of the changes associated with cachexia may be reproduced by injecting TNF-α into small laboratory animals. Indeed, one of the names given to TNF-α is **cachectin**. Patients with cancer do not as a rule show increases in the plasma concentration of TNF-α, but it is nevertheless possible that this peptide, perhaps working in concert with other cytokines, may play a significant role in cancer-related cachexia.

EFFECT OF NEOPLASMS ON THE IMMUNE SYSTEM

Patients with malignant disease, especially if this is related to the lymphoid system, appear to have their immune defences compromised. As a result, they are more prone to infection than expected. Depression of the defensive abilities of phagocytes is often present and patients, especially those with bone marrow involvement, quite commonly show a decline in the number of granulocytes.

Both humoral and cellular immune mechanisms may be depressed, a decline in the latter being associated with an increased liability to tuberculous, fungal and viral infections. It should not be forgotten that, in addition to the disease itself, treatment may cause a decline in the efficiency of the host's defences against infection, as both chemotherapy and irradiation have an immunosuppressive effect.

In addition to the immunosuppression associated with some cases of malignant disease, an association with autoimmunity has been recognized. Many patients can be shown to develop non-organ-specific autoantibodies directed against such 'self' components as smooth muscle, nuclei and nuclear fractions. Immune complex formation may also occur and some patients with malignant neoplasms present with an immune complex-mediated nephrotic syndrome (massive proteinuria, hypoalbuminaemia and oedema).

HAEMATOLOGICAL EFFECTS OF NEOPLASMS

Anaemia

Many patients with cancer show a diminished red cell mass at some stage of their illness. A number of possible mechanisms may be invoked to explain the presence of anaemia in any individual patient:

- **Iron deficiency anaemia** may result from occult blood loss associated with ulceration of a neoplasm involving an epithelial surface.
- A poor nutritional state may be associated with decreased folate intake, and, in the presence of malabsorption, such folate as is present may not be absorbed adequately, and **macrocytic anaemia** may result.

- Excess red blood cell destruction may occur as a result of an **autoimmune haemolytic anaemia**, with autoantibodies directed against components of the patient's own red cells. This tends to occur in association with neoplasms of the lymphoreticular system such as Hodgkin's disease and non-Hodgkin's malignant lymphomas. Why such an autoimmune reaction should occur is not understood.
- Lastly, anaemia may occur in association with malignant disease as a result of a **relatively decreased level of erythropoietin secretion**. Marrow cells from such patients appear to respond quite normally to erythropoietin in culture and the defect does not, therefore, appear to be a failure of response on the part of the red cell precursors.

Increased Red Cell Production

An increase in red cell mass is encountered not infrequently in association with certain neoplasms, most notably in:

- **renal adenocarcinoma**
- **cerebellar haemangioblastoma**
- **uterine fibroleiomyoma**
- **liver cell carcinoma**
- less frequently in ovarian carcinoma, adrenal tumours and carcinoma of the lung

The abnormal drive for red cell production seems to be due to the ectopic secretion of erythropoietic substances by the tumours.

Effects on Platelets and Clotting

In some patients with malignant disease there is a significant decrease in the number of circulating platelets and thrombocytopenic purpura may be seen. In some cases there is immune-mediated destruction of the platelets, but this is by no means always the case.

In contrast, an increase in clotting is quite often seen. This, of course, may itself contribute to the decrease in platelet count. Evidence of continued intravascular coagulation may be found in some patients by determining the level of fibrinopeptide A in the plasma. In one recent study, 60% of a group of patients with advanced cancer showed such evidence of intravascular coagulation. In these patients serial determinations of fibrin degradation products revealed an upward trend, which appeared to be related to progression of the neoplastic disorder. This intravascular clotting could be inhibited by giving oral anticoagulants such as warfarin.

In experimental tumour models, agents that promote clotting tend to promote tumour growth, whereas those that inhibit one or more aspects of the clotting process are associated with tumour regression.

Some malignant tumours are associated with a curious syndrome in which **recurrent migratory thrombophlebitis** occurs. Episodes of venous thrombosis involving both superficial and deep veins occur (see p 209). Carcinomas of the bronchus, pancreas, stomach and female genital tract are most frequently implicated and the thrombophlebitis may, in some instances, be the first indicator of occult malignancy.

ENDOCRINE EFFECTS OF NEOPLASMS

Hormonal effects associated with neoplasms fall into two main groups: appropriate and ectopic hormone production.

Appropriate Hormone Production

The neoplasms, whether benign or malignant, occur in endocrine glands and the hormones produced are **appropriate** in relation to the location of the tumour. For example, the fact that an adenoma of the β cells of the islets of Langerhans in the pancreas produces large amounts of insulin surprises no-one. Such tumours retain the normal biosynthetic pathways for the production of hormones and differ from normal cells only in their escape from normal 'feedback' controls. Examples of this type of endocrine disorder are given in *Table 26.1*.

Ectopic Hormone Production by Neoplasms

The second way in which hormonal effects may be experienced by patients with various forms of neoplasm is when hormones are secreted by the cells of tumours arising in **tissues not normally associated with hormone production**. This is termed **ectopic hormone production** and was first described in 1928 in a patient with a small-cell bronchial carcinoma who developed diabetes, hirsutism, high blood pressure and bilateral adrenal cortical hyperplasia (i.e. Cushing's syndrome). However, it was more than 30 years before it

was proved that the reason for such syndromes in patients with tumours arising outside the endocrine system was secretion of adrenocorticotrophic hormone (ACTH) by the tumours.

Although only a small proportion of patients with bronchial carcinoma of the small-cell variety show the clinical features associated with excess ACTH secretion, radioimmunoassay of extracts of such tumours show ACTH to be present in the majority. The disparity between the number of tumours that contain immunologically identifiable ACTH and those secreting 'active' ACTH arises because, in most cases, the hormone exists in the form of an inactive precursor or 'big' ACTH, which has less than 5% of the biological activity of ACTH secreted by the pituitary.

A wide variety of such '**paraendocrine**' syndromes has now been described. Some examples are given in *Table 26.2*.

Why are Ectopic Hormones Produced by 'Non-endocrine' Tumours?

One hypothesis suggests that the tumour cells involved in ectopic hormone secretion are derived from cells with potential endocrine functions that are normally present in many tissues and that would normally secrete amines such as serotonin and catecholamines.

Two groups of cells might fill this role:

1) **Neuroendocrine cells**, which are widely distributed in many tissues. The argentaffin cells in the gut, which can secrete serotonin and from which **carcinoid** tumours can arise, might be taken as an example.

2) A group of cells characterized as the **APUD**

Table 26.1 Effects of Appropriate Hormone Production by Neoplasms

Tumour	Hormone	Effect
Acidophil adenoma of the pituitary (see pp 829–831)	Growth hormone	Gigantism before puberty; acromegaly in adult life
Basophil adenoma of the pituitary	Adrenocorticotrophic hormone	Cushing's syndrome due to adrenal cortical hyperplasia and increased synthesis of cortisol
Chromophobe adenoma of the pituitary	Prolactin	Amenorrhoea Galactorrhoea Impotence
Adrenal cortical adenoma	Cortisol or aldosterone depending on cell type	Cushing's syndrome (cortisol) Conn's syndrome (aldosterone)
Parathyroid adenoma	Parathyroid hormone	Hypercalcaemia
Islet cell tumours of pancreas	Wide variety: commonest insulin and gastrin	Episodes of hypoglycaemia (insulin) Intractable peptic ulceration (Zollinger–Ellison syndrome in gastrin-secreting lesions)

Table 26.2 Ectopic Hormone Production by Tumours

Hormone	Principal tumours	Chief effects
Adrenocorticotrophic hormone	Bronchus Pancreas Thymoma Thyroid Ovary	Hypokalaemic alkalosis, weakness, thirst, polyuria
Antidiuretic hormone	Bronchus Duodenum Lymphoma Prostate Thymoma Ewing's tumour	Dilutional hyponatraemia
Thyroid-stimulating hormone	Lung Breast Choriocarcinoma	Hyperthyroidism
Melanocyte-stimulating hormone	Bronchus	Abnormal pigmentation
Parathyroid hormone	Bronchus (squamous) Kidney Liver Adrenal	Hypercalcaemia, vomiting, constipation, psychotic behaviour
Human chorionic gonadotrophin	Breast Bronchus Testis Stomach Pancreas Liver Ovary	Gynaecomastia; precocious puberty
Luteinizing hormone	Trophoblastic Malignant teratoma Bronchus	Gynaecomastia
Growth hormone	Lung Stomach Ovary Breast	Acromegaly; hypertrophic pulmonary osteoarthropathy
Glucagon	Kidney	Hyperglycaemia, etc.
Prolactin	Bronchus Breast	Galactorrhoea

series. The acronym APUD stands for *a*mine *p*recursor *u*ptake and *d*ecarboxylation, this name describing some of the outstanding characteristics of these cells. Associated with these is the ability to produce biologically active amines and peptide hormones. Such cells are present in small numbers in any individual location and could produce the 'ectopic' substance continuously. Clonal expansion of such a cell population, as would take place in

tumour formation, would obviously be associated with an increase in the total amount of hormone produced. This is sufficient in some instances to produce a recognizable biological effect.

It has been suggested that APUD cells are derived originally from the neural crest and migrate from there, principally to organs formed during development of the foregut. Support for this neural origin comes from the fact that:

- A number of the active substances secreted by so-called APUDomas are also secreted within the brain.
- Many APUD cells and the tumours arising from them express markers such as **neurone-specific enolase**.

This neural origin is no longer believed to apply to all cells and tumours in this group, some of which are thought to have an endodermal origin.

An example of an APUD cell is the parafollicular or C cell of the thyroid. This cell secretes the calcium-mobilizing hormone, **calcitonin**. The tumour arising from these C cells is known as a **medullary carcinoma**. It may occur as one of the genetically determined syndromes that can affect more than one endocrine organ simultaneously (see p 856) or as an isolated phenomenon. Most medullary carcinomas have amyloid in the stroma and the amyloid protein contains amino acids 9–19 of calcitonin (see p 181).

The '**oat cell carcinoma**' of the lung is an archetype of APUD tumours. It is one of the small-cell tumours that occur in the bronchi; the cells are arranged in a ribbon-like pattern in close relation to sinusoidal blood vessels. Electron microscopy shows the presence of dense-cored neurosecretory granules. These tumours are associated not only with a number of paraendocrine syndromes (see *Table 26.2*), but with some other systemic manifestations. The APUD concept has made a considerable contribution to our understanding of this area of pathology, but clearly cannot account for all cases of ectopic hormone secretion by neoplasms, such as the secretion of parathyroid hormone (PTH) by squamous carcinoma of the bronchus or by renal adenocarcinoma.

A complementary suggestion is that some cases of ectopic hormone production are due to the presence of excessive amounts of messenger RNA (mRNA) coding for the ectopic product in tumour cells. In some cells that are not known to make significant amounts of a polypeptide hormone, very small amounts of the inappropriate gene product may be found, suggesting that some transcription of the responsible gene may be occurring. Some workers have referred to this phenomenon as 'leakiness' of the gene. The difference between this situation and one in which large amounts of an inappropriate product are secreted by a neoplasm may be merely quantitative. Indeed, there is a considerable degree of homology between the mRNAs of normal cells and their neoplastic counterparts. The secretion of significant amounts of an 'ectopic' hormone may therefore simply represent an increase in gene expression via increased transcription.

NON-METASTATIC OSSEOUS AND SOFT TISSUE CHANGES

Clubbing

Clubbing of the fingers was first described more than 2000 years ago by Hippocrates. The angle between the nail and the cuticle becomes filled and the nail appears to 'float' on the nail bed. The curvature of the nail itself is altered, the nail being curved from front to back and having a rather 'beaked' appearance. In more severe instances, the periosteum over the terminal phalanges, wrists and ankles becomes thickened and new bone is formed from stem cells within the periosteum. In its most severe form, the complex of soft tissue and bony changes is termed **hypertrophic pulmonary osteoarthropathy (HPO)**.

Clubbing and HPO occur in association with a number of disease states. These include:
- the cyanotic forms of congenital heart disease
- chronic pulmonary sepsis
- infective endocarditis
- mesothelioma of the pleura
- carcinoma of the bronchus

The pathogenesis of this curious change is still far from clear. Some studies suggest that in affected patients the blood flow to the limbs is increased. Dividing the vagus nerve from the hilum of the affected lung relieves the condition in some instances, and is certainly associated with a reduction in blood flow to the affected part. Other studies suggest that there may be ectopic secretion of growth hormone in some cases of tumour-related HPO.

Interestingly enough, in view of the many systemic manifestations of small-cell carcinoma of the bronchus, HPO shows a strong negative correlation with this tumour. The commonest thoracic neoplasm to be associated with this syndrome is mesothelioma of the pleura. However, squamous carcinoma and adenocarcinoma of the bronchus have both been recorded as being the cause of HPO.

NON-METASTATIC CHANGES IN NERVE AND MUSCLE

Neuromyopathic changes associated with neoplastic disorders have been separated into three groups:

1) **Encephalomyeloneuropathy**, where degeneration of ganglion cells in the central nervous system is the dominant pathological feature.

2) **Myopathies** with or without features of myasthenia.

3) **Demyelinating** disorders.

In the first two there is no constant relation between progress of the neoplasm and that of the neurological condition. Indeed, neurological abnormalities may precede the diagnosis of tumour by up to 3 years or, at the other end of the spectrum, may appear after the tumour has been removed. The primary tumours most frequently implicated are carcinomas of the bronchus, breast, ovary, uterine cervix and colon.

The cause of these neurological conditions is unknown. They are not uncommon, an overall prevalence of neurological change of this type being recorded in 14% of patients with carcinoma of the bronchus (chiefly of the small-cell variety).

CUTANEOUS MANIFESTATIONS OF MALIGNANCY

Polymyositis and Dermatomyositis

This rather uncommon condition, encountered chiefly in the fifth and sixth decades of life, is associated with malignancy in 25–30% of cases. The muscular symptoms include pain and weakness, especially of proximal muscles such as those of the shoulder and hip girdles. Joint pain and stiffness are quite common. If the disorder is confined to muscle it is termed **polymyositis**, but the full clinical picture may include a striking rash as well. This ranges from a barely perceptible flush to a red or violaceous eruption, usually over the malar areas and the flush areas of the chest, back of neck and extensor surfaces of the arms and legs. Fine telangiectases (dilated small blood vessels) are almost always present on the cuticles.

If the disease appears when the patient is more than 40 years old, there is a 50% chance that it is associated with malignancy. The neoplasms associated with dermatomyositis are often those of the gastrointestinal tract, but carcinomas of the bladder, the bronchus and other endodermally derived tumours are not rare in this context. In cases associated with tumour, complete eradication of the tumour, where this is possible, cures the dermatomyositis.

Acanthosis Nigricans

In this condition, there is increased pigmentation of the skin, especially of the axilla, the back of the neck, and the periareolar region of the breast. In the early stages, despite the name **acanthosis**, there is little or no thickening of the skin, although itching is often present. Later the skin becomes thick, velvety and pigmented; the process may extend to involve quite large areas of skin. Acanthosis nigricans associated with malignancy appears most often in middle age when the age-related incidence of tumours is rising. About two-thirds of tumours associated with this skin lesion are carcinomas of the stomach.

Erythema Gyratum Repens

This is a rare but highly characteristic dermal accompaniment of malignancy. It appears as wavy irregular bands of red macropapules which coalesce to form a 'snake-skin' or 'wood-grain' pattern across the affected area of skin. This condition has been reported in patients with adenocarcinoma of the bronchus, small-cell carcinoma of the bronchus, and carcinomas of the breast, uterine cervix, tongue and gastrointestinal tract. In some cases, such as 'oat cell' carcinoma of the bronchus, the eruption usually occurs after obvious metastases have been diagnosed.

BIOLOGICAL MARKERS OF MALIGNANCY

The alterations in gene expression, whether qualitative, quantitative or both, that are part of the spectrum of malignant transformation may be associated with either the secretion of inappropriate substances or the expression of new antigens. Such biological markers can be helpful in diagnosis or in monitoring the progress of certain neoplasms.

These 'tumour markers' fall into three main groups:
1) hormones
2) isoenzymes
3) tumour-associated antigens

The first of these categories has already been described (see pp 265–267).

ISOENZYMES

Acid Phosphatase

An association between raised acid phosphatase concentrations in the plasma and carcinoma of the **prostate** has been known for many years. High plasma levels are particularly likely to be found in patients whose carcinomas have already metastasized, especially where secondary deposits are present in the skeleton.

Carcinoplacental Alkaline Phosphatase (PLAP)

This enzyme was discovered in the blood of a patient named Regan who had carcinoma of the bronchus, and it is termed by some workers the **Regan isoenzyme**. It is similar to the alkaline phosphatase found in the human placenta.

PLAP may appear in the blood of 3–15% of patients with malignant neoplasms. Primary tumours that can express PLAP include carcinomas of the bronchus, colon, pancreas and liver. Germ cell tumours may also express this enzyme.

The use of PLAP as a diagnostic test for the presence of malignant disease has proved disappointing. An increase in its concentration tends to occur late in the natural history of malignancy. False-positive results have been recorded in patients suffering from certain chronic inflammatory bowel diseases such as ulcerative colitis and also in those with cirrhosis of the liver. Low levels of the enzyme can be found in the plasma of some normal subjects. Nevertheless, as is the case with some other tumour markers, measurement of PLAP may give useful information about the natural history of certain tumours, most notably response to treatment and the appearance of recurrence or secondary deposits.

Tumour-associated Antigens

Alterations in the antigenic state of transformed cells is discussed further in Chapter 27. In some instances transformation and tumour growth may be associated with the appearance of antigens on tumour cells which are characteristic of the stage of fetal development and which are not present in fully differentiated adult cells. Such antigens are spoken of as **oncofetal antigens**.

α-Fetoprotein

α-Fetoprotein (AFP) is an $α_1$-globulin secreted in embryonic life, first by the **yolk sac** and later by the **fetal liver**. Secretion in the liver is established by the sixth week of embryonic life and reaches a peak of 3–4 mg/ml in the plasma by week 13 of intrauterine life. From this time on, the levels of AFP fall rapidly and in normal adults the amount that can be detected in the plasma by immunoassay is only about one-millionth of that present in fetal plasma.

In 1963 it was discovered that adult mice with transplantable liver cell tumours had high plasma concentrations of AFP. This observation was extended to humans with liver cell cancer 2 years later, and the presence of raised plasma concentrations of AFP has proven to be a fairly useful marker for this tumour. Subsequent studies have shown that AFP may appear in the plasma of up to 50% of patients with **malignant germ cell tumours**, there being a strong correlation between the presence of raised concentrations of AFP in the plasma and teratomas that contain elements histologically recognizable as showing **yolk sac** differentiation.

Carcinoembryonic Antigen (CEA)

This substance was discovered in 1965 to be present in fairly large amounts in malignant tumours of the large bowel. It is normally found in the gastrointestinal tract, liver and pancreas during the first 6 months of embryonic life. CEA is a water-soluble glycoprotein intimately associated with the glycocalyx on cell surface membranes. It can be localized to the luminal surface of the neoplastic cells that express it. Early studies suggested that the presence of raised plasma concentrations of CEA was specific for neoplasms derived from the endoderm. However, this is not correct.

Increased levels of CEA can be found in association with neoplasms of different histogenesis and may also occur in association with some non-neoplastic conditions. This last factor clearly limits the usefulness of CEA as a **diagnostic** marker. A further disadvantage is that CEA levels tend to be correlated with the extent of spread in certain neoplasms; before such spread has occurred, CEA concentrations may not be raised significantly. For example, in carcinoma of the colon or rectum, localized (Dukes' stage A) tumours are associated with increased CEA levels in only 40% of cases. In those cases of colorectal carcinoma where metastasis has occurred, 80–95% of patients have increased CEA levels.

The main application for the determination of CEA levels in the plasma is in the follow-up of patients with cancer after surgery and in monitoring the effects of therapy. After successful removal of a tumour associated with raised CEA concentrations in the plasma, the CEA concentration tends to fall to normal over a period of 2–4 weeks. If there is no tumour recurrence, these normal levels persist. A subsequent rise in the plasma concentration of CEA probably indicates either the presence of metastases or local recurrence of tumour. Such a rise of plasma CEA concentration may precede, by several months, clinical evidence of metastatic or recurrent disease.

Other useful tumour markers are discussed in relation to the appropriate tumours.

CHAPTER 27

Effect of the Host on Neoplasms

The effect of the host on the neoplasm must reside in the interaction between the host's immune system and the tumour; it is difficult to think of any other mechanism through which resistance to the progression of malignant disease might be mediated. This question might be examined in a number of ways:

1) Is there direct evidence that immune mechanisms modulate the behaviour of human neoplasms and cause them to regress?
2) Is there histological evidence that human neoplasms excite an immune response?
3) Is there any increase in the frequency of neoplastic disease in patients with immune deficiency states?

Tumour Regression

The first of these is extremely difficult to prove. It is true that in some instances malignant neoplasms regress, this having been noted most frequently in neuroblastoma and malignant melanoma. However, there is no direct evidence that such tumour regression is brought about by immune mechanisms, although in some cases of malignant melanoma that remain localized for a long time, there may be antibodies in the plasma that are cytopathic for the patient's tumour cells in culture.

Other clinicopathological oddities such as the prolonged survival of some patients with malignant disease, the frequency of clinically occult tumours found at necropsy, and the occasional regression of metastases after removal of the primary tumour have all been cited as possible expressions of an immune response. However, proof of the validity of this view is lacking.

Histological Features Suggesting an Immune Response to the Presence of Tumour

On histological examination, some tumours are seen to be infiltrated by lymphocytes, macrophages and plasma cells. This is especially common in carcinomas of the breast. In addition, a marked degree of hyperplasia of the macrophages lining the sinuses of lymph nodes draining a tumour may be seen, as well as epithelioid cell granulomas.

There is some evidence from prospective studies that these histological features may correlate positively with an improved prognosis, particularly in the case of breast cancer.

Immune Deficiency States and Malignancy in Humans

If it were true that immune reactions mounted by the host played a significant part in inhibiting the development and growth of malignant neoplasms, then one would expect **an increased frequency of malignant disease in patients with immune deficiency**. Up to a point, this is true: patients with inborn deficiency syndromes such as **ataxia telangiectasia**, the **Wiskott–Aldrich syndrome** and the **Chediak–Higashi syndrome** all show an increased frequency of malignant disease compared with their peers. However, most of these neoplasms primarily involve the lymphoid system.

In cases of iatrogenic immunosuppression, such as in patients who have received renal allografts, there is also an increase in the frequency of malignant disease; again, the vast majority of these are of the lymphoid system. There have been occasional reports, however, where recipients have received kidneys from patients dying with malignant disease. Although the donor kidneys were macroscopically free from tumour, tumours with histological characteristics of the donor's primary are said to have grown in some of these kidneys. In two cases the withdrawal of immunosuppressive drugs on which the patient had been maintained was reported to have led to regression of the tumour. These observations, scanty as they are, suggest that immunosuppression creates a favourable milieu for tumour progression.

Tumours can be Rejected by Animal Hosts

The possible role of cell-mediated immunity in controlling tumour growth can be studied most easily in relation to animal tumours induced by certain viruses. The most fully studied example is **polyomavirus**, a small DNA virus that infects many laboratory and wild mouse colonies.

- When large doses of the virus are injected into **adult** mice, no tumours result.
- Inoculation of the virus into **newborn** mice of the same susceptible strain produces large numbers of tumours.
- If, however, newborn mice are thymectomized and, when they have grown to adulthood, are inoculated with the polyomavirus, tumours occur in fairly large numbers.

Such experiments provide good evidence that **adult mice are protected against the oncogenic effect of the polyomavirus because they can mount an effective cell-mediated response**. The same sort of events are seen when mice of the C57BL strain, which are resistant to the oncogenic effect of the polyomavirus, are studied. Neonatal thymectomy or the use of repeated injection of antilymphocyte serum can make young mice of this strain develop polyoma-induced tumours.

While there is some evidence that cell-mediated rejection of some virally induced tumours can occur, the picture is by no means a simple one. If T cell-mediated immunity plays a major role in **immune surveillance** against tumour development, a high frequency of spontaneous tumour development would be expected in the '**nude mouse**', which is athymic. This is not so, although this mouse has been used with some success in studying transplantable tumours.

Tumour-associated Transplantation Antigens

A number of experiments in inbred strains of mouse indicate that **tumour rejection can occur as a result of the expression of certain antigenic determinants on the surface of the tumour cells which have nothing to do with the histocompatibility antigens** coded for by the major histocompatibility complex.

In general, tumours that have been induced by irradiation or chemicals have unique antigenic determinants on the cell surface which function as **transplantation antigens (TATA – tumour-associated transplantation antigen)** and can thus elicit rejection. Even two tumours produced by the same carcinogen in a single animal will have distinct transplantation antigens.

Tumours caused by viruses, however, show new antigens on the cell surface which cross-react with those on other tumours induced by the same virus. These virally induced TATAs appear not to be typical viral structural proteins.

Unfortunately, spontaneous tumours arising in both animals and humans show much less tendency to develop transplantation antigens on their cell surfaces, although some neoplasms appear to elicit a cell-mediated immune response which cannot be ascribed to allogeneic rejection mediated through the major histocompatibility complex. Tumours of this class include malignant melanoma, renal carcinoma and astrocytomas in the brain.

In melanoma, which has been studied in most detail, three classes of cell surface antigen have been identified.

1) Antigen distinctive for the particular patient's tumour.

2) Antigen specific for malignant melanoma cells, but which may be shared with cells of other malignant melanomas.

3) Antigens found on both tumour cells and some normal cells.

MECHANISMS BY WHICH THE IMMUNE SYSTEM CAN COMBAT TUMOUR GROWTH

A number of possible effector arms of the immune system may play a role in destroying tumour cells. These include:

- the macrophage system
- effector T cells
- antibodies that can promote antibody-dependent cell-mediated cytotoxicity
- natural killer (NK) cells

Macrophages

In culture systems, macrophages can be shown to destroy tumour cells. The precise mechanism is not clear, but does appear to involve cell-to-cell contact. The macrophages can be activated in two ways:

1) By contact with tumour antigen.

2) As a result of the release of activating factors from T cells that have been stimulated by contact with tumour antigens.

Such activation is associated with an increase in the number of Fc receptors on the surface of the macrophage and it is possible that coating of tumour cells by antibodies may help, through the binding of Fc to Fc receptors, to bring the macrophage into close contact with the tumour cell.

Effector T Cells

Cell killing by the T-cell arm is presumably carried out by cytotoxic T cells. The helper T cell may also play a part through its stimulatory effect on the cytotoxic subgroup.

The relative proportions of T helper and T suppressor cells may have some influence on the immune status of the host in respect of tumour cells. In certain transplantable tumours in animals, tumour growth is increased if there is a large population of T suppressor cells. It has been suggested that this comes about through an autoimmune reaction against the specific clone of cytotoxic T cells that bind to the tumour cells. This reaction is mediated by T suppressor cells, which recognize surface markers of a certain idiotype on the cytotoxic T cells and are themselves specifically cytotoxic for cells bearing that idiotype. In this way, the cytotoxic T cells are prevented from destroying the tumour cells.

Antibodies

Theoretically, as outlined earlier, humoral immune mechanisms could act in two possible ways in the destruction of tumour cells:

1) They could bind to tumour cells and initiate complement-mediated cell lysis. Such evidence as

we possess suggests that this is not a significant mechanism in tumour control.

2) They may adhere to the surface of tumour cells and thus attract potentially cytotoxic cells that have Fc receptors on their surface. These include macrophages, T lymphocytes and **NK cells**.

Natural Killer Cells

The NK cell constitutes a subset of the lymphocyte population that is believed by some workers to be derived from clones of immature pre-T lymphocytes. They are non-adherent, non-phagocytic and have Fc receptors on their surface. Their ability to kill tumour cells does not depend on the host being immunized against determinants on the tumour cells. It has been suggested that the NK cell can itself recognize several different types of determinant on cells that may exhibit cross-reactivity, and that this may explain its broad range of cytotoxic activity. The activity of NK cells is stimulated by interferon γ, which is released, in this context, by T cells and by NK cells themselves, the latter constituting a positive amplification loop.

Does Immune Surveillance Exist?

The original concept of immune surveillance was that malignant transformation of cells occurs frequently and that these cells are eliminated by immune mechanisms before clonal expansion can take place. In respect of 'spontaneously arising' neoplasms, this mechanism must clearly be deemed to fail in every case where a clinically or pathologically apparent neoplasm arises. However, in chemically or virally induced tumours in experimen-

tal animals, immune protection can be shown to be reasonably effective and it is possible that, in humans, immune mechanisms may be responsible for the fact that most people infected with the Epstein–Barr virus develop a self-limiting illness (infectious mononucleosis) and not a malignant lymphoma.

If immune protection is not effective in spontaneously arising neoplasms, how do the malignant cells that survive and form tumour masses evade the potential cytotoxicity inherent in immune effector mechanisms? It may be that many malignant cells are **poor immunogens** and natural selection processes would favour the survival of such cells in an antigenically heterogeneous tumour cell population. It is known, however, that it is possible for the host to develop an immune response to malignant cells but be unable to kill them. This '**blocking effect**' appears to be associated with the presence in the host plasma of tumour-specific antibodies. It has been suggested that in such instances the tumour cells constantly shed surface antigens which with the tumour antibody form circulating complexes that can bind to any killer cells with Fc receptors for the tumour antibody and thus prevent them from having a cytotoxic effect on the tumour cells themselves.

Another factor determining the effectiveness or otherwise of an antitumour immune response appears to be the actual **physical bulk of the tumour**. Small tumours are much more likely to yield to efforts to improve a host's immune response, and the removal of much of a host's tumour load, either by surgery or by other means, appears to be associated with an improvement in the effectiveness of the antitumour response.

CHAPTER 28

Oncogenesis and the Molecular Biology of Cancer

In operational terms cancer may be defined as a set of disorders in which there are three pivotal abnormalities in cell behaviour:

1) **A disturbance in the mechanisms that control cell proliferation.**
2) **A disturbance in cell differentiation.**
3) **A disturbance in the normal relationship between the proliferating cells and the surrounding connective tissue stroma.** This abnormality is expressed in the form of **invasiveness** and, ultimately, metastasis, and is, therefore a fundamental part of the malignant phenotype.

There are many epidemiological data that relate the risk of malignancy to a variety of environmental factors and there are clearly many different causes of cancer (see pp 290–304). Despite this, it is likely that the number of mechanisms operating at the cellular level is small and that these are mediated through abnormalities affecting **three classes of gene**:

- **oncogenes**
- **tumour suppressor genes**
- **mutator genes**

is discussed in a later section. Mutation or deletion of suppressor genes is clearly also a common feature of many neoplasms that are *not* inherited.

DOMINANTLY ACTING ONCOGENES

As already stated, neoplastic transformation arises from a disturbance in the dynamic equilibrium normally existing between growth-promoting and growth-inhibiting forces. In the same way as the speed of a motor car may be increased either because the driver presses on the accelerator or because the brakes have failed, so, in the cancer model, **the gene products of the dominantly acting oncogenes represent the accelerator and those of the tumour suppressor genes represent the brakes**. In this section some aspects of the dominantly acting oncogenes are considered.

The first point to appreciate is that proto-oncogenes form part of the **normal genome** and that they contribute to neoplastic transformation **only if they are qualitatively or quantitatively altered**. When they

Oncogenes, Suppressor Genes and Mutator Genes

The homeostatic control of growth and differentiation in cell populations, as in most other areas of biology, is the resultant of the interaction between growth-promoting and growth-restraining forces. These are the expression of transcription of **growth-promoting genes known as proto-oncogenes** and **growth-inhibiting genes, known as tumour suppressor genes** (*Fig. 28.1*). When there is a demand for expansion of cell populations in order to meet increased physiological needs, then upregulation of growth-promoting genes occurs.

More than 100 proto-oncogenes have been identified, although not all of these have been found to be mutated in human neoplasms. The number of tumour suppressor genes so far identified is much smaller. The existence of certain inherited neoplasms has provided much help in the identification of suppressor genes, and

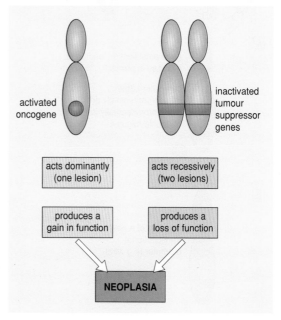

FIGURE 28.1 Some basic properties of oncogenes and tumour suppressor genes.

are not abnormally activated, the term cellular **proto-oncogene** is applied; when they are altered, the term **oncogene** is more appropriate. Such alteration (*Fig. 28.2*) may result in:

- **The encoding of abnormal gene products** as result of **point mutations** in the proto-oncogene. This is most likely to occur in relation to the *ras* proto-oncogenes which are mutated in 10–15% of human solid tumours.
- The overexpression of unaltered proto-oncogenes via a variety of mechanisms which include the presence of abnormally large numbers of copies of the gene (**amplification**) and **translocation** of a

proto-oncogene to a region where its transcription is significantly increased. The latter occurs in the Burkitt lymphoma where the c-*myc* proto-oncogene on the long arm of chromosome 8 is translocated to chromosome 14 and comes to lie adjacent to the gene encoding the heavy chain of immunoglobulin.

- **The formation of novel genes and the expression of chimeric gene products as a result of the fusion of proto-oncogenes with parts of other genes.** This occurs as a result of translocation of portions of chromosomes and is exemplified by the formation of the *bcr–abl* gene in chronic myeloid leukaemia in the course of translocation of *abl* from chromosome 9 to chromosome 22.

Proto-oncogenes are concerned with processes involved in cell division and proliferation (see *Table 28.1, Figs 28.3* and *28.4*). Thus different proto-oncogenes encode:

- **growth factors (*sis, int-2, IGF-1*)**
- **growth factor receptors with protein kinase (*erb-2, fms, met, trk, ret*)**
- **abnormally functioning growth factor receptors (*neu*)**
- **factors that act in the transduction of signals arising from ligand–receptor interactions:**

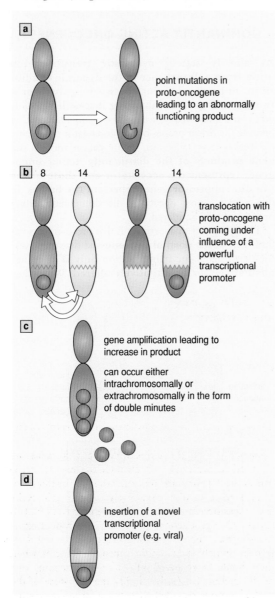

FIGURE 28.2 *Mechanisms of cellular proto-oncogene activation.*

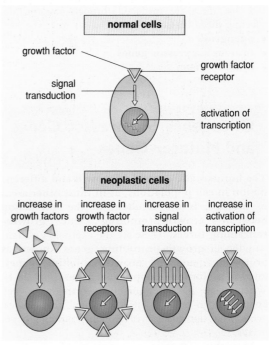

FIGURE 28.3 *Proliferation of normal cell populations results from a sequence of operations involving the binding of growth factors to receptors, transcription of the growth-promoting signal and activation of DNA transcription. The abnormal degree of proliferation in neoplastic cell populations results from the upregulation of one or more than one of these steps.*

Table 28.1 Functions of Some Oncogenes

Oncogene	Growth factor	Normal growth factor receptor	Abnormal growth factor receptor	Signal transducer	DNA-binding protein concerned with transcription
sis	+				
erbB1		+			
fms		+			
erbB2			+		
ras				+	
src				+	
myc					+
fos					+
jun					+

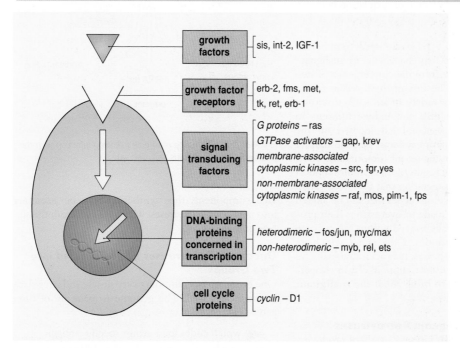

FIGURE 28.4 *The relation between the gene products of several proto-oncogenes and the operational steps involved in cell division.*

a) **G proteins (*ras*)**
b) **guanosine 5′-triphosphatase activators (GTPase) (*gap, krev*)**
c) **membrane-associated cytoplasmic kinases (*src, yes, fgr*)**
d) **non-membrane-associated cytoplasmic kinases (*raf, mos, pim-1, fps*)**
• **DNA-binding proteins concerned in transcription:**
a) **heterodimeric transcription factors (*fos–jun, myc–max*)**
b) **transcription factors (*myb, rel, ets*)**
• **cell cycle proteins**

Enzymes known as **cyclin-dependent kinases** are required to drive the cell through the events of the cell cycle. **Cyclins** are proteins whose concentrations change in a regular pattern during the cell cycle. Their function is to 'turn on' the kinases referred to above. Overproduction of cyclins, or production at inappropriate times, stimulates inappropriate cell division by switching on cyclin-dependent kinases when they should be switched off. The gene encoding one of the cyclins, D1 (active during the G1 phase of the cycle), is now regarded as being a proto-oncogene. The D1 gene is amplified in about 33% of oesophageal cancers, in 15% of breast cancers and is implicated also in the genesis of benign neoplasms of the parathyroid gland.

Through the Recognition of Oncogenes and Suppressor Genes we Begin to See the Molecular Basis for Cancer

The majority of malignant neoplasms have thus far been found to be **monoclonal**: that is the cells of which any neoplasm is composed are all descended from a single 'ancestor' cell. This ancestor cell was once a normal cell but at some point it must have undergone fundamental alterations conferring 'immortality' on the cell line and releasing it from the normal constraints on cell proliferation and growth. Just like normal cells, the progeny of malignant cells inherit the characteristics of their parents; **this suggests that the alterations mentioned above must have occurred in relation to the genome of the 'ancestor' cell**. This view is strengthened by the high degree of correlation between the mutagenic properties of a given compound and its potential carcinogenicity.

The realization that a relatively small number of molecular determinants may be active in malignant transformation has come from the convergence of two lines of investigation. The first of these relates to the mechanisms by which a variety of animal retroviruses can transform cultured cells and induce tumours in their host species. The second has focused on the effects, largely in cell culture systems, of gene transfer from the cells of human malignant tumours not obviously viral in origin. The results of these studies support the view stated above, suggesting that there is a group of functionally heterogeneous genes that can be altered by mutation, amplified, made to overexpress their protein products, or physically moved within the genome by chromosome translocations. These genes, which are known as **cellular oncogenes**, may act individually (in certain cell culture systems) or, more likely, in cooperation with one another to bring about the **malignant transformation of cells**.

Lessons from Oncogenic Retroviruses

There is a group of RNA viruses capable of producing tumours in their host species and of transforming certain cells in culture. These are known as **oncornaviruses** or **oncogenic retroviruses**.

The genome of these viruses is composed of **RNA** enclosed within a capsid which is, in turn, wrapped in a glycoprotein envelope. Once this virus infects a cell, the envelope and capsid are removed and the viral RNA is copied by the viral enzyme **reverse transcriptase** into a portion of DNA which is called a **provirus** (*Fig. 28.5*). The provirus is incorporated into the DNA of the infected cell and, by the normal processes of transcription, emerges as RNA molecules identical with the original viral RNA. This new RNA can act both as messenger RNA (mRNA) for viral proteins or as RNA for the genomes of new viruses. The

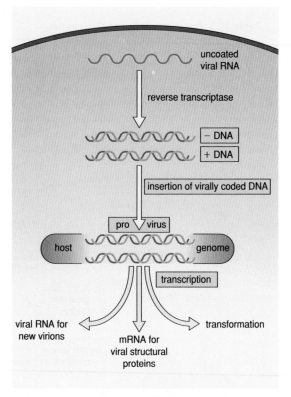

FIGURE 28.5 *The range of effects following infection with the oncogenic retrovirus, Rous sarcoma virus.*

viral components thus synthesized can be assembled into new complete viruses, which bud off from the surface of infected cells.

Oncogenic Retroviruses can be Divided into Two Groups

One group induces tumours very slowly and irregularly but replicates well. The genome is made up of three genes (*Fig. 28.6*):

gag, which codes for a group-specific antigen
pol, which codes for reverse transcriptase
env, which codes for envelope glycoproteins

Non-coding sequences at either end, known as **long terminal repeats** promote gene replication and expression.

These three genes contain all the information necessary for the manufacture of new viral particles within the infected cell. The group includes natural, 'wild' viruses, which typically produce malignancies of the lymphoma–leukaemia group in poultry, mice and cats.

The second group of oncogenic retroviruses can produce tumours in the appropriate host very quickly – in days or weeks. They are not common in the 'wild' state and most have been isolated from animal tumours. In contrast to the first group, inoculation is usually

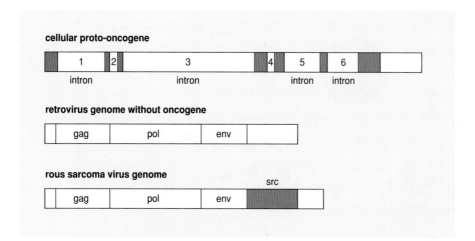

FIGURE 28.6 *Comparison between the arrangement of coding sequences (exons) in mammalian DNA and in the genome of oncogenic retroviruses. The differences support the view that retroviral oncogenes originated from cellular proto-oncogenes.*

required, because the viruses do not infect animals via natural pathways. Most of these viruses lack the full complement of genes necessary for **viral replication**. However, there is one noteworthy exception, the **Rous sarcoma virus**.

When the genome of the Rous sarcoma virus was dissected, it was found to have two distinct portions. The first contained the genes necessary for replication, *gag, pol* and *env*. The second contained a gene called *src*. The *src* gene has been found to be both *necessary* and *sufficient* for the virus:

- To cause sarcomas in appropriate hosts (poultry).
- To transform fibroblasts cultured in a monolayer (*Fig. 28.7*). On infection with the *src* gene, the normal orderly monolayer is lost and groups of cells pile up and form colonies many layers thick. This transforming gene codes for the production of a tyrosine kinase called pp60src.

The viral gene (**v-src**) is now recognized as belonging to a family of about 20 transforming genes known as **viral oncogenes (v-oncs)**, each of which is characteristic of a rapidly transforming oncornavirus. A number of v-oncs code for proteins that possess the ability to phosphorylate tyrosine in certain proteins. Another oncogene from the avian erythroblastosis virus (**erb b**) codes for a protein homologous with a portion of the cellular receptor for epidermal growth factor, and yet another, **sis** from the simian sarcoma virus, codes for a protein homologous with platelet-derived growth factor.

Homology Exists Between Viral Oncogenes and Cellular Proto-oncogenes in Other Species and Phyla

With cloned DNA copied from v-onc RNA by the use of reverse transcriptase, it is possible to scan the genome of any eukaryotic cell for the presence of matching sequences. This is known as DNA **hybridization** and

depends on the base-pairing relationship in double-stranded DNA. Adenine in one strand always pairs with thymine, and cytosine with guanine. Thus the sequence of bases in one strand must dictate the sequence in the other (*Fig. 28.8*). On this basis, it is possible to use a radioactively labelled sample of DNA as a tracer to see whether other samples of DNA contain matching sequences. **If the tracer used is the DNA copy of the whole or part of a v-onc RNA, one can investigate whether DNA from normal cells contains sequences that match with those in the v-onc.**

Southern Blotting

The identification of matching sequences in a DNA molecule, which may contain hundreds of thousands of base pairs, is made much easier by the application of a very sensitive hybridization method known as Southern blotting (*Fig. 28.9*).

- The cellular DNA is split into pieces by enzymes known as **restriction endonucleases**, which cleave DNA at specific sites defined by a base sequence that the enzyme can recognize.
- These portions of DNA can be separated by electrophoresing them in an agarose gel. After such treatment human DNA may give rise to more than 100 000 such fragments.
- The DNA fragments are then transferred from the gel to a sheet of nitrocellulose paper (hence the term 'blotting').
- A radioactively labelled sample of DNA (the probe), which is derived from the viral oncogene, may then be applied to the paper and thus small fragments of cellular DNA containing complementary base sequences can be identified.

Using this method, it has been shown that there are complementary sequences to **all retroviral v-oncs** in

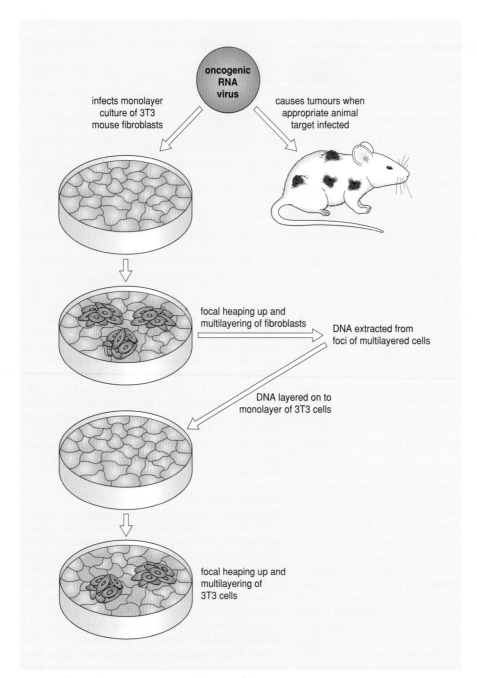

FIGURE 28.7 *The existence of actively transforming sequences in oncogenic retroviruses can be demonstrated either in the course of infection of the appropriate animal targets or by showing that infection of 3T3 murine fibroblasts in culture is followed by permanent and heritable changes in growth characteristics of the cells.*

restriction fragments prepared from DNA derived from widely disparate species (e.g. human, yeast, fruit fly). These normal genes, which are homologous with the v-oncs, are the **proto-oncogenes referred to in the previous section**.

The term 'proto-oncogene' implies correctly that **these constituents of the genome of normal cells have the potential for being converted into active genes capable of contributing to malignant transformation**.

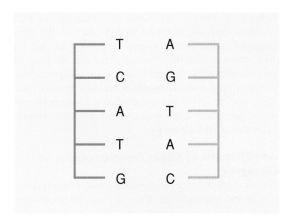

FIGURE 28.8 *Hybridization depends on the complementarity of base pairs (T anneals to A; C anneals to G). T, thymine; A, adenine; G, guanine; C, cytosine.*

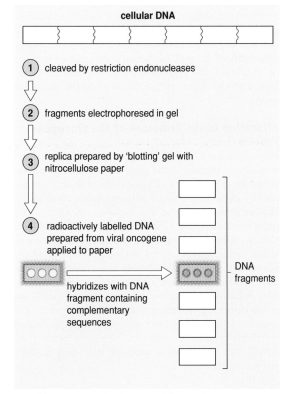

FIGURE 28.9 *Hybridization between single-stranded DNA copies of retroviral oncogenes and mammalian DNA shows homologies that serve the purpose of identifying cellular proto-oncogenes.*

Viral Oncogenes Originate from Cellular Proto-Oncogenes

In view of the homology between v-oncs and cellular proto-oncogenes, two mirror image possibilities exist to explain their relationship. Either the v-oncs are derived from cellular genes, or the reverse holds true. Several facts suggest that the first of these suggestions is correct:

1) The very high degree of conservation of the cellular proto-oncogenes during evolution (from yeasts to humans) supports the view that proto-oncogenes are not derived from viruses.

2) The structure of proto-oncogenes differs in some respects from their v-onc homologues. In v-oncs the nucleotide sequences coding for certain proteins usually occur in a solid block. In the proto-oncogene the information is split up, portions of the protein-coding sequences (exons) alternating with intervening sequences (introns). This is the characteristic structure of a vertebrate gene. Following transcription of the proto-oncogene, the mRNA corresponding to the introns is stripped away, leaving mRNA that is almost identical with the viral mRNA.

3) The fact that cellular proto-oncogenes code for growth factors, growth factor receptors or enzymes concerned with the modulation of these receptors suggests a physiological role for the proto-oncogenes in normal cells in relation to growth regulation, and hence a cellular rather than a viral origin.

The current view, therefore, is that v-oncs arise as a result of transcription from a cellular proto-oncogene, and that this cellular genetic material has been incorporated into the viral genome (see *Fig. 28.6*).

DNA from Chemically Transformed Cells and from Some 'Spontaneous' Human Tumours can also Transform Cells in Culture

When DNA is extracted from transformed cells and introduced into cultures of untransformed mouse fibroblasts (a technique known as **transfection**), foci of piled up transformed cells appear and these foci grow into tumours after inoculation into young mice. Thus certain varieties of chemically transformed cells carry oncogenic sequences in their DNA.

Even more interesting was the discovery that transfected DNA from biopsies of some human tumours produced exactly the same effect. Many types of human tumour cells have now been shown to develop transforming sequences in their DNA during progression from the normal to the malignant state. They include carcinomas of the bowel, lung, bladder, pancreas, skin and breast, fibrosarcomas and rhabdomyosarcomas, glioblastomas, neuroblastomas and various haemopoietic neoplasms. In all these experiments it should be borne in mind that the recipient cell (the 3T3 mouse fibroblast) differs significantly from the donor tumour cell, and it may well be that tumour-derived DNA samples that do not transform fibroblasts may possibly do so in other cell lines.

Some of the active oncogenes derived from human tumours have been isolated and cloned. In each case, as with the retroviruses, the transforming oncogene has been found to be closely related to a DNA sequence present in the normal cell genome (a proto-oncogene).

Successful transfection and transformation of cultured cells has been reported in respect of the oncogenes shown in *Table 28.2*.

How do Cellular Proto-oncogenes Become Activated?

Five separate mechanisms of cellular proto-oncogene (c-onc) activation have been discovered so far (see *Fig. 28.2*).

Over-expression of the C-onc Following the Acquisition of a Novel Transcriptional Promoter

Some proto-oncogenes can be activated by the addition of a strong transcriptional promoter. For instance, the avian leucosis virus (ALV) does not normally cause tumours but may occasionally do so after very long incubation periods. When the DNA of such rare tumours is analysed by Southern blotting, the ALV provirus sequence is found to hybridize to the same fragment as the v-onc, **v-myc**. This suggests that the ALV provirus must have been inserted into the host cell genome very near the proto-oncogene **c-myc** and that this proximity of the normally active ALV had activated the c-*myc*, the ALV having acted as a strong transcriptional promoter. This sequence of events is termed **insertional mutagenesis**.

Amplification of Either Proto-oncogene or Oncogene

A second mechanism of activation involves overexpression due to amplification of a proto-oncogene or oncogene. In human promyelocytic leukaemia the **myc** proto-oncogene has been found to be amplified between 30 and 50 times. Such amplifications have also been found in relation to a number of c-oncs in several different human tumour cell lines. Once there is an increased number of copies of the gene in a single genome, it is assumed that there is a significant increase in transcription and hence in the amount of gene product; this can be demonstrated using the Northern blotting method. In neuroblastoma, a malignant neoplasm of childhood, the aggressiveness of the tumour correlates with the degree of amplification of the oncogene n–*myc*.

Alteration in the Structure of the Oncogene Protein

Point mutations in the oncogene proteins have been recorded in relation to the products encoded by the **ras** genes. In the case of a cell line derived from a human bladder carcinoma, a single point mutation converts the **Ha-ras** proto-oncogene into a potent oncogene. This mutation causes the 12th amino acid in the 21-kDa protein coded for by **ras** to be changed from glycine to valine. Some studies carried out with oncogenes of the **Ki-ras** group have also shown that alteration of the gene product at position 12 leads to oncogenic activation. A human lung carcinoma oncogene of the Ha-*ras* group carries a mutation that alters the gene product at residue 61, and it has been suggested that the codons specifying residues 12 and 61 of the gene product are critical sites which, when mutated, will often produce oncogenic alleles.

'Enhancer Sequences' can Increase the Activity of Transcriptional Promoters

The level of transcription, and hence the amount of gene product, can be increased by the action of 'enhancer sequences', which increase the utilization of transcriptional promoters. The linked promoter may be a considerable distance from the enhancer sequence, which may be situated either upstream or downstream of the promoters. Such a mechanism is believed to operate in certain avian lymphomas, where retrovirus fragments are situated downstream from the **myc** proto-oncogene.

Table 28.2 Oncogenes that can Transform Cell Lines Following Transfection

Oncogene	Human tumour
Ki-*ras*	Carcinoma of thyroid, melanoma, acute myeloid leukaemia
Ha-*ras*	Carcinoma of colon, pancreas, lung
N-*ras*	Carcinoma of thyroid and genitourinary tract, melanoma
fos	Carcinoma of kidney, colon, lung, ovary
met	Osteosarcoma
mos	Carcinoma of breast
myc	Burkitt lymphoma, carcinoma of breast, colon, lung, ovary
sis	Glial tumours
ret	Carcinoma of thyroid
raf	Carcinoma of lung
int-1	Carcinoma of breast
trk	Carcinoma of thyroid
db1–mcf2	Carcinoma of breast, some B-cell lymphomas

Chromosome Translocation

Chromosome translocation can be associated with movement of a proto-oncogene to a different site in the genome. As a result of this change in position, the c-onc may become activated. This is believed to occur in Burkitt's lymphoma, in which translocations of material from chromosome 8 to chromosomes 2, 14 or 22 occur very commonly (the 8 : 14 translocation is the most frequent). The c-*myc* proto-oncogene has been located on chromosome 8 near the break point, and in chromosomes 2, 14 and 22 the genes that encode immunoglobulin chains are also present near the break point. When translocation occurs, the c-*myc* gene derived from chromosome 8 and the immunoglobulin genes that are being actively transcribed in B cells become juxtaposed. This appears in some cases to result in deregulation of the c-*myc* gene, possibly through the action of enhancer sequences contained within the immunoglobulin gene.

As stated earlier (see p 274), translocation may also be associated with the formation of novel genes as a result of the fusion of proto-oncogenes and genes on the chromosome to which the former are translocated. A classic example is the formation of a fused gene by the translocation of c-*abl* (which has tyrosine kinase activity) on chromosome 9 and a gene termed *bcr* (breakpoint cluster region) on chromosome 22. This occurs in chronic myeloid leukaemia and in some lymphoblastic leukaemias of childhood. The altered chromosome 22 is known as the **Philadelphia chromosome**.

Oncogenes and Multistep Carcinogenesis

Spontaneous and chemically induced tumours are believed to arise as a result of several steps, although the transformation of cultured fibroblasts on the 3T3 line by an oncogene such as Ha-*ras* appears to be a **single** event.

The explanation for this discrepancy lies in the nature of the 3T3 cells, which are removed from their progenitors by very many generations and which have been 'immortalized' as a line. If the oncogene is applied to a line not far removed from the ordinary rat fibroblast, the complete phenotypic picture of malignant transformation is not seen to develop, although one phenotypic change, **loss of anchorage dependence**, does occur. This implies that if the recipient cell line is normal, the *ras* oncogene requires cooperation from some other factor or factors before transformation can take place. Put another way, it could be said that one consequence of immortalizing a line of cells, as in the case of 3T3, is the activation of cell functions that can cooperate with the *ras* gene to create the complete transformation phenotype.

ras can Cooperate with Other Viral Oncogenes

The changes that occur when a cell line becomes established in culture and is thus 'immortalized' are poorly, if at all, understood. However, these changes can be mimicked by the action of certain DNA tumour viruses, notably polyomaviruses and adenoviruses, which contain true viral genes capable of inducing cells to grow continuously in culture. The polyomavirus genome codes for three proteins, which have been called the small, middle and large T antigens. The middle T antigen induces morphological changes in cultured cells and also loss of anchorage dependence. The large T antigen increases the lifespan of the cultured cells and also alters the dependence of these cells on certain serum factors.

When large T and the *ras* gene are transfected into a cell line that does not transform when the *ras* gene alone is used, a dramatic degree of transformation occurs and inoculation of transformed foci into nude mice produces rapidly growing tumours. Thus cooperation between a viral gene and a cellular one can convert normal cells into tumour cells.

Other Cellular Oncogenes can Cooperate with ras

The data referred to above shed no light on the possible mechanisms involved in the production of tumours where there is no obvious viral involvement. However, in some animal tumour lines, active **ras** oncogenes have been found to coexist with active **myc** genes. Transfection of both *ras* and *myc* into cell lines that are not transformed by either alone, again leads to a striking degree of transformation. It can be inferred that each of the genes must perform some distinct function that is needed for the genesis of tumours. Such experiments may provide some explanation, at the molecular level, for the multistep nature of carcinogenesis, in that each step may involve the activation of a distinct cellular gene.

The Action of Oncogenes

Obviously the next step in unravelling this puzzle is to find out how the gene products of active oncogenes induce and maintain the transformed phenotype. Proto-oncogenes encode proteins capable of acting in different parts of the cell (see pp 274–275) and are clearly implicated in all the steps involved in cell division. A striking example is provided by the actions of *ras* oncogenes, which are involved in many human tumours.

The ras Family

The retroviral homologues of human *ras* genes are the viral oncogenes of the Harvey (Ha-*ras*) and Kirsten (Ki-*ras*) rat sarcoma viruses. *ras* genes code for 21-kDa proteins which are attached to the inner suface of the plasma membrane by a lipid bond that is added after translation of the protein. They are homologues of G proteins and take part in signal transduction in the same way as do the G proteins. G proteins act as a sort of molecular 'on–off switch' by virtue of the fact that they can exist in two dynamically interconvertible states, bound to guanosine 5′-diphosphate (GDP) or guanosine 5′-triphosphate (GTP). **Only the GTP-bound form mediates a growth response.** The binding of a growth factor or other mitogen to its receptor leads to GTP being substituted for GDP and the ras protein becomes activated. The G protein's own inherent GTPase activity displaces the GTP and the ras protein becomes inactivated. Mutation of the *ras* gene leads to a loss of GTPase activity and thus the ras proteins are locked into a growth-stimulating mode.

TUMOUR SUPPRESSOR GENES

Genes whose products **normally inhibit** excessive cell proliferation are known as **tumour suppressor genes**. Mutation in or loss of these results in loss of their growth-inhibiting functions, so that unfettered cell proliferation is more likely to occur. **It is this loss of function that contributes to oncogenesis, a paradigm whose value has only recently been appreciated.**

The fact is that many tumours represent the phenotype associated with multiple genomic events which include, in a single neoplasm, inappropriate activation of proto-oncogenes and inactivation of tumour suppressor genes.

DETECTION OF TUMOUR SUPPRESSOR GENES

The effect of normally functioning tumour suppressor genes is essentially a negative or inhibiting one in respect of oncogenesis, so identification of these genes presents a different set of problems to those encountered in oncogene research.

The existence of tumour suppressor genes can be inferred in a number of ways:

• **Tumour formation is suppressed in hybrid cells resulting from fusion of malignant cells and their normal counterparts.**
• **Alteration or deletion of certain genes is associated with certain hereditary tumours.**
• **Loss of certain alleles identified by restriction fragment length polymorphisms can be detected in certain tumours (and pretumorous states such as familial adenomatous polyposis coli).**
• **Cloning of certain suppressor genes has been possible and their activities analysed in *ex vivo* systems.**
• **Transmission of wild-type suppressor genes into certain tumour cells in culture may restore a suppressed, non-tumorigenic phenotype.**

Hybrid Cells Express a Suppressed rather than a Transformed Phenotype

When cultured mouse tumour cells and their normal counterparts are fused by various methods, the resulting hybrid cells express the normal phenotype and lose their tumorigenicity. Over a period of time as these hybrid cells are repeatedly cultured, they may lose certain chromosomes or parts of chromosomes and, in this event, they revert to the transformed or malignant phenotype.

The reversion of the tumour cells to a normal phenotype after hybridization implies that the transformed state correlates with *loss* of certain genetic material which is restored by the contribution of normal cells to the hybrids. Such cell fusion studies may be useful in that they may indicate certain differences between normal and tumour cells in respect of surface or other markers, and it may also be possible to identify the chromosome that is carrying the putative suppressor gene in any given cultured tumour.

Certain Hereditary Tumours are Associated with Mutation or Loss of Alleles in Germline Cells

The paradigm for this hypothesis is **retinoblastoma**. This is a rare (1 in 20 000 infants and young children affected) malignant tumour which arises from the precursor cells (retinoblasts) of the photoreceptor cells in the eye, known as cones. Once the retinoblast differentiates fully, it stops dividing and appears no longer to be a target for oncogenic processes. This is reflected in the fact that retinoblastoma is not seen in older children or adults.

From the epidemiological point of view, it is clear that the tumour has two patterns of occurrence:
1) sporadic
2) familial

In the **familial** form the tumours:
• occur early (mean age 14 months)
• are bilateral
• may be associated with a family history of retinoblastoma
• are usually multiple (mean number of tumours 3)

In such a patient with retinoblastoma who has survived to adulthood and had children, about 50% of his or her offspring will also develop a retinoblastoma. Such data imply that the risk of the tumour is being transmitted from parent to offspring in an autosomal dominant fashion, possibly in the form of a mutated gene. In survivors there is an increased risk for developing second tumours later in life, most notably osteosarcoma.

This is in marked contrast to the sporadic form of the tumour which probably affects no more than 1 in 100 000 children. In **sporadic retinoblastoma** the mean age for tumours to occur is at 30 months, and the tumours are usually unilateral. Survivors show no increase in the risk for developing other tumours.

These epidemiological data were brilliantly interpreted by Alfred G. Knudson in 1971 on the basis of the assumption that a mutated gene in any individual may be acquired through two routes:

1) by inheritance from a parent
2) as a result of a somatic mutation

Knudson suggested that the differences in the risk of retinoblastoma arising from being born or not born into a 'retinoblastoma family' could be explained in the following way (*Fig. 28.10*):

- **All retinoblastoma tumour cells carry not one but two mutated alleles of the same gene.**
- **In familial retinoblastoma, one of the two required mutations is present from conception and must, therefore, be present in *all* cells of the body, including the retinoblasts.**
- **The second mutation could occur locally as a result of a somatic mutation in one of the already genetically abnormal retinoblasts.**
- **In sporadic retinoblastoma, *both* the mutations would have to be somatic mutations occurring locally in the retinal cells and the chances of this happening would be much less than is the case for a single somatic mutation. This would then explain the difference in risk.**

This **'two-hit'** hypothesis for the genesis of retinoblastoma embodies the important point that **both copies** of some gene of major importance must be lost or mutated if a tumour is to develop. Ten years after this

seminal paper, it was found that **retinoblastoma was associated with loss of part of the long arm of chromosome 13 (13q14). In patients with familial retinoblastoma this abnormality was found not only in tumour cells but in normal cells of all types throughout the affected child's body, whereas in sporadic cases the chromosomal abnormality was found *only* in tumour cells.**

The gene, which was presumably located somewhere in the deleted portion of chromosome 13, was given the name *RB* and the remaining parts of the Knudson hypothesis were confirmed. If inactivation of both copies of the *RB* gene is required for tumour formation, it follows that **normal *RB* must have a tumour suppressor function**. This view gains strength from the observation that abnormalities of the *RB* gene, due to either germline or somatic mutations, have been seen in association with both retinoblastoma and osteosarcoma (children with familial retinoblastoma have a much greater risk of developing osteosarcoma during adolescence and early adult life), breast, prostate, bladder and lung cancers.

Loss of function in both alleles of certain genes associated with tumour formation has now been seen in a variety of hereditary and non-hereditary tumours, some of which are discussed below.

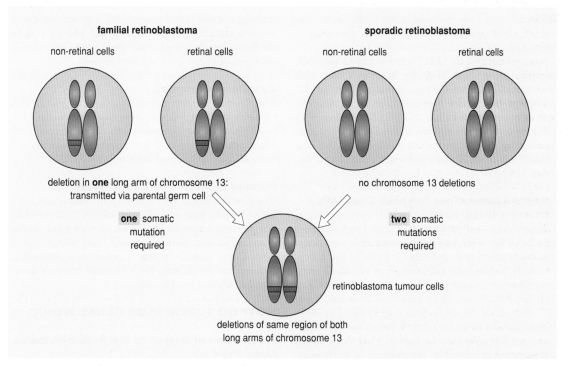

FIGURE 28.10 In familial retinoblastoma both retinoblasts and non-retinal cells show a mutation of one of the alleles encoding the RB protein at birth. Such an abnormality must be transmitted in the germ cell from one of the parents. In such circumstances only one further mutational event involving the second allele is required to produce the homozygous mutation required for tumour formation. In sporadic retinoblastoma, neither retinoblasts nor non-retinal cells show any abnormality of either allele of the RB gene at birth. Thus two mutational events, each involving one allele of the RB gene, are required before retinoblastoma occurs.

Wilms' Tumour

Wilms' tumour is a malignant tumour in which the constituents closely resemble elements of the embryonic kidney. Three genomic abnormalities appear to be associated with this lesion in a non-random fashion, these abnormalities being associated with certain 'marker' syndromes. Thus:

1) **In the WAGR syndrome (Wilms' tumour, aniridia, genitourinary tract anomalies, and mental retardation)**, there is a deleted region on chromosome 11 (11p13) in which a gene known as *WT-1* has been identified. *WT-1* codes for a nuclear protein that is believed to exert its suppressor function via regulating transcription.

2) **In 15–20% of sporadic Wilms' tumours and in Wilms' tumours associated with the Beckwith–Wiedemann syndrome,** there is a deletion in the region of 11p15.

3) **In some familial Wilms' tumours,** there is a deletion that does not map to either locus named above.

Neurofibromatosis Type I (NF-I)

All cases of NF-1 result from the inheritance of a mutant allele. The mutations often appear to arise paternally. Linkage studies suggest that the *NF-1* suppressor gene is located on the long arm of chromosome 17 (17q11.2). As with the mutant *RB* gene, mutated *NF-1* genes are found in all cells throughout the body, so that the restriction of tumour formation to a few sites is interesting.

The product of the *NF-1* gene is called **neurofibromin**, and it shows sequence homology both with mammalian and yeast GTPase-activating proteins. By binding to *ras*-encoded proteins (G proteins), neurofibromin increases the hydrolysis of GTP. Children with NF-1 are also at increased risk of developing neoplastic disorders of the bone marrow such as preleukaemic myelodysplastic syndromes and myeloproliferative disorders.

Familial Adenomatous Polyposis Coli (FAPC)

FAP is an inherited disorder in which multiple adenomatous colonic polyps develop in the second and third decades of life. The disorder is inherited in an autosomal dominant fashion and one or more of the polyps inevitably develops the full phenotype of colonic cancer in later life. Linkage studies have indicated that there is a APC locus, which appears to be deleted from the long arm of chromosome 5 (5q15–22). The APC protein appears to act as a link between surface membranes and the microtubular system. **This same locus seems to be involved in the genesis of both non-familial colonic adenomas and non-familial colorectal cancer.** Normal APC protein controls transcription by regulating β-catenin bonding to transcription factors TCF-1 and LEF-1. Loss of APC function causes loss of regulation by this pathway.

MECHANISMS OF ACTION OF TUMOUR SUPPRESSOR GENES

Some insights have been gained into this important area, partly by identifying the nature of the gene products of some tumour suppressor genes and partly through the interactions that occur between some tumour suppressor gene-coded proteins and proteins coded for by tumour viruses.

The products of tumour suppressor genes so far identified include:
- nuclear proteins
- cytoplasmic proteins
- membrane proteins

Nuclear Proteins

The gene products of some tumour suppressor genes, most notably *RB* and *p53* (see pp 284–287), are nuclear proteins as is the product of the putative Wilms' tumour locus (*WT-1*) on the short arm of chromosome 11 (11p13). Presumably these proteins act normally by:

- **regulating the expression of genes or the proteins they encode that are involved in cell proliferation or differentiation**
  or
- **controlling the biochemical mechanisms that regulate the initiation of DNA synthesis**

The protein coded for at 11p13, which is believed to be implicated in the genesis of some cases of Wilms' tumour, is a zinc finger protein; this suggests that it may act as a transcription factor. RB and p53 have been studied most extensively, and their mode of action is discussed in more detail in a later section.

Cytoplasmic Proteins

The product of the tumour suppressor gene *NF-1*, which is implicated in neurofibromatosis, is believed to be GTPase-activating protein which interacts with the p21 *ras* product and may thus regulate signal transduction pathways concerned with cell proliferation.

Proteins Expressed on Cell Surfaces

The gene known as *DCC* (deleted in colonic cancer) is located on the long arm of chromosome 18. Its product is a cell surface molecule which is a member of the immunoglobulin gene superfamily and which shows homology with neural adhesion molecules. Presumably, it influences the interaction between transformed cells and their neighbours.

HOW DO SUPPRESSOR GENES WORK?

Mechanism of Action of the Retinoblastoma Gene Product

The *RB* gene encodes a protein with a molecular weight of 105 kDa, which is known as p105–RB. The action of the RB gene product can best be understood against the background of the normal cell cycle (*Fig. 28.11*). **During G1 or G0, the RB pro-**

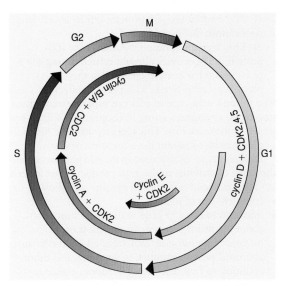

FIGURE 28.11   *The gene products of two important tumour suppressor genes, RB and p53, act as brakes on initiation of the S phase of the cell cycle and thus prolong the G1 phase. The cycle itself is driven by kinases which act only when bound to proteins known as cyclins and which are therefore known as cyclin-dependent kinases (cdk).*

tein forms a complex with the transcription factors E2F and DP1. **In the presence of this complex, transcription of S-phase genes cannot occur and the cell cycle cannot proceed**. The ability of the RB protein to maintain this complex with transcription factors depends on its degree of phosphorylation. Phosphorylation of the RB protein is mediated through the action of the cyclin–dependent kinases cdk-2 and 4, which are linked with cyclins D and E (*Fig. 28.12*).

Binding of some of the antigens of DNA viruses can inactivate the RB protein. In 1988 it was shown that p105–RB binds to the E1A transforming protein of adenovirus, to the large T antigen of SV40 virus and to the E7 protein produced by oncogenic strains of human papillomavirus (types 16 and 18) (*Fig. 28.13*). In the case of adenovirus, this binding is a prerequisite for transformation, and the site of binding on the E1A protein shows sequence conservation with sites on SV40, polyomavirus, BK virus and human papillomavirus transforming proteins. Interestingly, the E7 proteins of **non-oncogenic human papillomaviruses** bind to p105–RB with much lower affinity.

The *p53* Tumour Suppressor Gene

Mutations in this gene appear to be the commonest abnormality related to tumour suppressor genes in human neoplasms (*Table 28.3*). Thus far, the only tumour types in which a *p53* mutation has not been found are Wilms' tumour, testicular and pituitary neoplasms, and phaeochromocytomas.

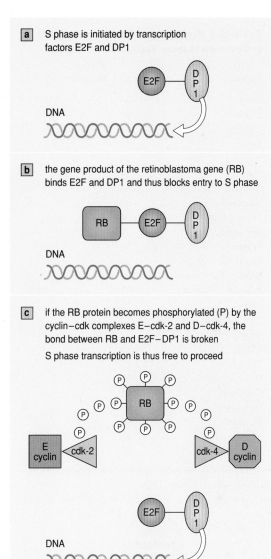

FIGURE 28.12   ***a*** *The S phase is initiated by the transcription factors E2F and DP1.* ***b*** *The gene product of the retinoblastoma gene (RB) binds E2F and DP1, and thus blocks entry to the S phase.* ***c*** *Phosphorylation of the RB protein breaks the link between RB protein and the transcription factors E2F and DP1. The latter can therefore initiate transcription of S-phase genes and G1 is terminated.*

Mechanism of Action of p53

The *p53* gene encodes a nuclear phosphoprotein with 375 amino acids. It is known to bind with transforming proteins of certain oncogenic viruses such as the large T antigen of SV40. Complexing the p53 protein with SV40 prolongs the protein's half-life from 6–20 minutes to several hours, and this stabilized form of p53 can be identified in cells by immunostaining. **The activity of p53 appears to be controlled by two factors:**

Table 28.3 Frequency of Abnormality of *p53* in Common Human Tumours

Tumour	*p53* Mutation (%)
Lung	56
Colon	50
Oesophagus	45
Ovary	44
Pancreas	44
Skin	44
Stomach	41
Head and neck	37
Urinary bladder	34
Sarcoma	31
Prostate	30
Liver cell	29
Brain	25
Adrenal	23
Breast	22
Endometrium	22
Mesothelioma	22
Kidney	19
Thyroid	13
Haematological neoplasms	12
Carcinoid	11
Melanoma	9
Parathyroid	8
Uterine cervix	7
Neuroblastoma	1

1) The level of the p53 protein, which is very low after mitosis but increases in G1.

2) The degree of phosphorylation. Like RB protein, p53 becomes phosphorylated during the S phase and it has been suggested that this phosphorylation blocks its suppressor effect.

The normal wild-type of p53 can suppress transformation by *ras* oncogenes acting in cooperation with c-*myc* in cell culture systems. This suggests that one function of p53 may be to inhibit the expression of c-*myc*.

Different types of alteration in the *p53* gene occur and the range of activities of the gene product is best looked at in this frame of reference. Tumours may show:

- complete loss of p53
- mutation of the *p53* gene with production of an abnormal protein. In carcinomas most of the mutations are missense mutations giving rise to an abnormal protein product; in sarcomas, it is more common to find deletions, insertions or gene rearrangements.

Most mutations in the *p53* gene are somatic mutations. However, in some families *p53* mutations may be found in the germ cell line. This occurs in a familial neoplastic syndrome known as the **Li–Fraumeni syndrome**, which is characterized by malignancy (often a sarcoma) appearing at a young age in probands with at least two first-degree relatives with malignant disease (breast, brain or adrenal cortical tumours).

The potency of the *p53* gene product is shown by animal studies. In transgenic mice carrying a mutant *p53* gene, 20% of animals develop tumours by 6–9 months of age. 'Knockout' mice with no *p53* genes develop malignant neoplasms within 3–6 months.

The Protein Coded for by *p53* Stimulates Production of Another Protein (*Fig. 28.14*)

The p53 protein acts as a transcription factor, 'switching on' the gene responsible for the encoding of another protein with a molecular weight of 21 kDa. This gene has at various times been called *cip-1* (cdk interacting protein 1) or *WAF1*.

The protein encoded by this gene in its turn inhibits the activity of enzymes that drive the cell cycle: the cyclin-dependent kinases (cdk) which phosphorylate the RB protein. In this way the complex formed by the RB protein and transcription factors E2F and DP1 remains in being.

p53 is Regulated by the Product of an Oncogene *mdm-2*

p53 protein is regulated by the protein product of another gene, *mdm-2* (murine double minute gene 2). *mdm-2* is a dominant oncogene; it enhances tumour production when overexpressed and its gene product binds to p53 protein and inactivates it so that the *cip-1* gene is not transcribed.

Thus some tumours could contain normal amounts of normal (wild-type) p53 protein so long as they over-

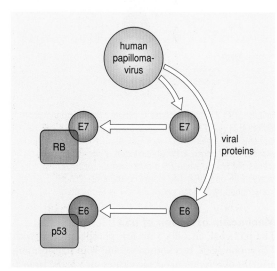

FIGURE 28.13 Both the RB and p53 proteins can be inactivated by protein products of oncogenic human papillomaviruses types 16 and 18. This inactivation of the gene products of two important suppressor genes may explain the oncogenic effect of these strains of human papillomavirus.

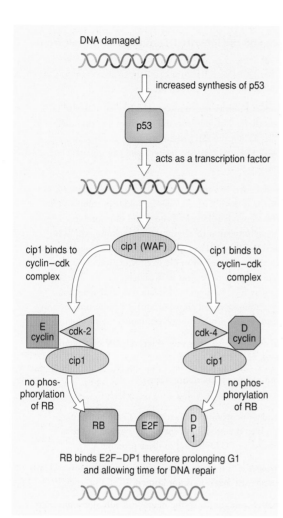

DNA damaged

increased synthesis of p53

p53

acts as a transcription factor

cip1 (WAF)

cip1 binds to cyclin–cdk complex

cip1 binds to cyclin–cdk complex

E cyclin   cdk-2   cdk-4   D cyclin

cip1   cip1

no phos-phorylation of RB

no phos-phorylation of RB

RB   E2F   D P 1

RB binds E2F–DP1 therefore prolonging G1 and allowing time for DNA repair

FIGURE 28.14 *p53 prolongs the G1 phase in cells with DNA damage by initiating transcription of a gene encoding the protein cip-1 (WAF-1). The latter protein prevents phosphorylation of RB protein by cyclin-cdk complexes (see Fig. 28.12c).*

KEY POINTS: Inactivation of p53

Inactivation of the p53 tumour suppressor gene protein can be due to:

- Mutation of the *p53* gene; this is the commonest situation in human malignancy.
- Degradation of p53 protein by virus-encoded products such as the E6 protein of human papillomavirus.
- Inactivation as a result of overproduction of *mdm-2* protein.
- Sequestering of p53 protein in cell cytoplasm so that it cannot act as a transcription factor.

express *mdm-2*. This occurs particularly in sarcomas in which 5–50-fold amplification of the *mdm-2* gene has been recorded.

Biological Role of p53

Experiments with 'knockout' mice, referred to above, have shown that p53 is not required for viability during either fetal or adult life. It seems likely that p53 plays little or no part in routine growth regulation but is **important in controlling uncontrolled growth such as occurs in malignancy**.

It has been suggested that a major function of p53 is to prevent chromosomal replication when DNA has been damaged, and some writers refer to p53 as 'the guardian of the genome' (*Fig. 28.15*).

Certainly, the level of p53 protein rises dramatically after irradiation:

- Arrest in the G1 phase in cells with damaged DNA would allow time for excision and repair, and thus would prevent the transmission of the altered DNA to daughter cells.
- In addition, the p53 protein can induce **apoptosis**, which again would eliminate cells harbouring genomic abnormalities.

The *p16* Gene

In 1992 it was shown that the short arm of chromosome 9 contains a susceptibility gene which is

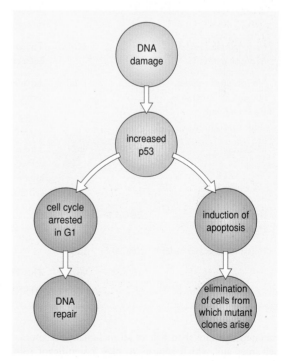

DNA damage

increased p53

cell cycle arrested in G1

induction of apoptosis

DNA repair

elimination of cells from which mutant clones arise

FIGURE 28.15 *In addition to its effect on the G1 phase, p53 protein induces apoptosis in cells with damaged DNA. Both these effects tend to decrease the chances of stem cell mutations being passed on.*

Table 28.4 Suppressor Genes, their Proposed Functions and the Inherited Tumours that Result from their Inactivation or Mutation

Inherited tumour	Gene	Site	Suggested function
Retinoblastoma Osteosarcoma	RB	13q14	RB gene product binds to two transcription factors, E2F and DP1, and inactivates them. This prevents the cell from entering the S phase from G1. When the RB protein becomes heavily phosphorylated, E2F and DP1 are released and can initiate transcription.
Osteosarcoma Breast cancer Glioma Li–Fraumeni syndrome	p53	17p13	p53 gene product acts as a transcription factor causing transcription of a gene known as cip-1. This encodes a 21-kDa protein which binds to cyclin-dependent kinases 2 and 4 and thus inhibits cyclin-dependent phosphorylation of certain targets including the RB protein. The RB–E2F–DP1 complex remains bound together and thus the cell cannot proceed from G1 to S. Mutation of p53 is one of the commonest genomic events in malignant disease. Certain viral antigens may bind with and inactivate p53, and aflatoxin, which can contaminate cereal crops, produces a point mutation in p53 which leads to the production of a mutant gene product.
Polyposis coli	APC	5q21	APC protein communicates between microtubules and certain cell surface proteins.
Nephroblastoma (Wilms' tumour)	WT-1	11p13	WT-1 protein acts as a transcription factor.
Neurofibromatosis type 1	NF-1	17q11.2	The gene product neurofibromin acts as a GTPase-activating protein. It binds to the product of the ras oncogenes and thus increases hydrolysis of GTP bound to these proteins.
Meningioma Acoustic neuroma	NF-2	22q11.1	The gene product is one of the proteins of the cytoskeleton and has been called merlin. Its function is not known.
No inherited tumour but somatic mutations associated with colorectal cancer	DCC	18q21	An adhesion molecule similar to the neural cell adhesion molecules found in the nervous system.
Melanoma	MTS-1	9p21	This is the first suppressor gene product shown to act directly on the cell cycle. It is a 16-kDa protein which binds to cyclin-dependent kinase 4 and prevents its activation by cyclin D1. This prevents the cell from progressing from G1 to S phase.
Breast (female) Breast and ovary	BRCA-1	17q	
Breast (female and male)	BRCA-2	13q	
?	MTS-2	9p21	This 15-kDa gene product also inhibits the activity of cyclin-dependent kinases.

mutated in more than half of all malignant melanoma cell lines and which appears to play a significant role in the genesis, in particular, of familial melanoma. Since that time, abnormalities at this locus have been reported in many other tumour types and, because the abnormalities include deletions, it has been sug-gested that another tumour suppressor gene is nor-mally present at this site. Early in 1994 the protein product of this gene was identified and called p16. p16 binds to one of the cyclin-dependent kinases (cdk-4) and thus inhibits its activation by cyclin D1. This is the first tumour suppressor gene product shown to act **directly** on the cell cycle. *p16* deletions have now been shown to be present in 50% of all cancers. Only in two types of tumour, colorectal cancer and neuroblastoma, have *p16* deletions not been found.

Tumour Suppressor Genes and Breast Cancer

About 5% of cases of breast cancer are familial. Two-thirds of these are believed to be associated with germline mutations in one of two genes known as *BRCA-1* and *BRCA-2*. The *BRCA-1* gene has now been isolated and localized to the long arm of chromosome 17. It is responsible for about one-third of cases of familial breast cancer and has been found in more than 80% of families in which breast and ovarian cancer occur together. The presence of a zinc finger domain close to the *N*-terminus suggests that the protein may be a transcription factor.

In high-risk families, female carriers of mutated *BRCA-1* genes have an 80–90% lifetime risk of developing breast cancer. It is not known how much risk is attached to such mutations in females from families with no documented history of high risk. A frameshift germline mutation (185delAG) is present in about 1% of Ashkenazi Jewish females, and they may be at high risk of developing breast cancer.

The second gene, *BRCA-2*, has not been isolated but has been mapped to the long arm of chromosome 13 close to the location of the *RB* gene. It is probably responsible for the same proportion of cases of familial breast cancer in females as *BRCA-1*, but differs from that gene by being involved in the genesis of familial breast cancer in males as well.

A list of the tumour suppressor genes currently known, their functions and the inherited tumours with which their deletion or inactivation are associated, is given in *Table 28.4*.

MUTATOR GENES

The gene products of normal mutator genes are involved in DNA repair. They were discovered during studies of hereditary non-polyposis colorectal cancer. The first mutator gene, *MSH-2*, was found to have strong homology with the *mut2* gene occurring in bacteria, and is located on the short arm of chromosome 2.

A second gene concerned with DNA repair is *MLH-1*, located on the short arm of chromosome 3.

CHAPTER 29

Oncogenesis

The many epidemiological data relating the risk of developing one or another malignant neoplasm to a variety of environmental factors indicate that there is no such thing as a single cause of malignancy. As discussed in Chapter 28, the number of final mechanisms involved in malignant transformation at the molecular level may, however, be rather small.

GENETIC FACTORS

The occasional clustering of certain types of malignancy in families and the presence of malignant neoplasms as part of some well-recognized inherited syndromes indicate that the genotype of an individual plays a part in determining susceptibility to malignant disease.

An increase in the liability of an individual to develop a malignant neoplasm may be inherited:

- as part of a clinical syndrome that may have diagnostic features of its own apart from the increased risk of malignancy. This may make it possible to recognize the individuals who are at risk and to take appropriate measures to reduce the chances of malignancy.
- as an increased likelihood of tumours developing as the only manifestation of a single gene abnormality.

The inherited syndromes associated with an increased risk of malignancy may be divided, essentially, into two groups:

1) Syndromes with a major, recognizable, chromosome abnormality.
2) Syndromes apparently determined by a single gene abnormality. These may be associated with an immunological defect, as in **ataxia telangiectasia** (see p 119), or there may be no identifiable defect in immunity.

CHROMOSOMALLY DETERMINED SYNDROMES

Three such syndromes associated with malignancy have been described:

1) **Down's syndrome** (mongolism) (see pp 309–310). An increased risk of developing acute leukaemia (myeloblastic : lymphoblastic risk 1 : 2) appears to be an integral part of the syndrome.
2) **Klinefelter's syndrome** (a type of male hypogonadism associated with the presence of an extra X chromosome) (see pp 312–314). Patients with Klinefelter's syndrome show an increased tendency to develop tumours of the male breast.
3) **Gonadal dysgenesis** in patients with a female phenotype and a male genotype (see p 754). Those with gonadal dysgenesis are more likely to develop tumours of the gonads.

However, this increased risk may be the secondary result of an interaction between an abnormal hormonal milieu and an unresponsive target organ rather than a primarily genetically determined type of carcinogenesis.

SINGLE GENE ABNORMALITIES

The syndromes associated with immune deficiencies have been considered already (see pp 119–120), so only some outstanding examples of such syndromes associated with an increased risk of malignancy and with *no* evidence of an immunological defect are mentioned here.

Xeroderma Pigmentosum

This rare condition, inherited in an autosomal recessive fashion, was first described by the famous dermatologist Kaposi in 1874. It is characterized by hypersensitivity to ultraviolet light and by a marked tendency to develop malignant skin tumours during childhood and adolescence. The skin of affected children appears normal at birth, but repeated exposure to sunlight results in a dry scaly skin with many areas of hyperpigmentation. These skin changes are followed within a few years by the appearance of a variety of skin tumours, some of which are malignant, such as squamous carcinoma. It is important for our understanding of this condition, to note that **unexposed** skin remains normal. Precise prevalence data are not available, but estimates of the frequency of xeroderma pigmentosum vary from 1 in 65 000–250 000 live births. The condition is most commonly encountered in North Africans. Protection from sunlight, either by suitable clothing or by barrier creams against ultraviolet light, can reduce the risk of tumour development; these are important measures to institute once the condition has been diagnosed.

Lack of the Enzymes Responsible for Excision Repair Leads to Perpetuation of Abnormal DNA Sequences

The nature of the intrinsic defect in individuals with xeroderma pigmentosum is of great interest. The main target for ultraviolet light within the cells of the epidermis is DNA. Absorption of photons by DNA results in the formation of a variety of new products, of which the most important are dimers formed by adjacent pyrimidine bases (usually thymine). Under laboratory conditions this phenomenon can be shown to occur in the DNA of cultured fibroblasts and bacteria. Normally the abnormal portion of the DNA which contains the thymine dimers is excised by an **endonuclease** and replaced by a new length of DNA some 100 nucleotides in length. In xeroderma pigmentosum, the endonuclease responsible for initiating this process of 'excision repair' is lacking and the change in DNA induced by the ultraviolet light is permanent.

Other syndromes in which DNA repair appears to be defective, and in which there is an increased risk of malignancy, are **ataxia telangiectasia** and **Fanconi's anaemia**, in which there is an increased risk of leukaemia, and **Bloom's syndrome**, which is also characterized by hypersensitivity to sunlight. In this last condition, unlike xeroderma pigmentosum, the increased risk of malignancy is not confined to the skin. The defect in repair, at the molecular level, has not been characterized in these three conditions.

The existence of these four rare syndromes indicates that **non-reparable alterations to the DNA of a target cell, however they may be caused, constitutes one of the initiating mechanisms of carcinogenesis.**

Familial Adenomatous Polyposis Coli and Related Disorders

This syndrome, which is due to the inheritance of an autosomal dominant gene, is rare and accounts for only a small proportion of the deaths due to colorectal cancer. Theoretically if one parent is affected, half the children may be expected to develop the disease. In practice, the penetrance rate is only about 80%, so that 40% of the children would show features of the disease.

Familial adenomatous polyposis is characterized by multiple polyps in the large gut which are not present at birth, and which appear between the ages of 10 and 20 years. The lesions are distributed fairly evenly through the large bowel, but the greatest concentration is to be found in the rectum, which is always involved. In their premalignant phase, the lesions show the features of adenomas on microscopic examination (see p 556).

Of patients with polyposis who present with symptoms attributable to the polyps, about 65% already have cancer of the large bowel. The average age at which cancer is diagnosed in these patients is 40 years (about 20 years younger than in the non-polyposis population). Death as a result of colorectal cancer also occurs at a much younger age in these patients than in the general population. The precise frequency with which patients suffering from polyposis coli develop colorectal cancer is not easy to assess, but some writers maintain that by the age of 60 years 100% of the victims of poly-

posis will have developed cancer of the large bowel. This gloomy prospect places a heavy burden of decision on the medical attendant of such a patient, because the only means of avoiding malignant transformation of one or more of the polyps is to undertake prophylactic resection of the whole of the large bowel, including the rectum.

Other inherited, multiple colonic polyp syndromes are **Gardner's syndrome** and **Turcot's syndrome**.

In Gardner's syndrome, which is also inherited in an autosomal dominant manner, there are multiple colonic polyps associated with tumours in skin, subcutaneous tissue and bone. The likelihood of a sufferer developing colorectal cancer is about 100%.

Turcot's syndrome consists of a combination of colonic polyps together with brain tumours. It is inherited in an autosomal recessive manner. There appears to be an increased risk of colorectal cancer, but the magnitude of this risk has not been established.

Familial adenomatous polyposis is associated with the inheritance of a malfunctioning *APC* gene, a tumour suppressor gene, on the long arm of chromosome 5 (see p 284 and p 556).

INCREASED RISK OF NEOPLASIA WITH NO 'PRECURSOR' SYNDROME

An increased risk of certain neoplasms developing may be inherited in the absence of any recognizable 'premalignant' or 'preneoplastic' syndrome such as polyposis or xeroderma pigmentosum. It is only rarely that these neoplasms occur in a pattern suggesting a major role for inheritance. They include retinoblastoma and phaeochromocytoma. Retinoblastoma and its molecular genetics are discussed on pp 282–283.

Phaeochromocytoma

This neoplasm arises wherever **chromaffin cells** are present, and is most common in the adrenal medulla. The tumour cells secrete noradrenaline and adrenaline, and patients may present with systemic hypertension. About 5–10% of these tumours are malignant. Most phaeochromocytomas occur sporadically, but it is thought that 10–20% are familial; these occur in association with one of a number of syndromes.

1) **An autosomally dominant tendency for phaeochromocytomas to occur.** These often occur in childhood and more than 50% are bilateral.

2) **Multiple endocrine neoplasia syndrome type IIa** (Sipple's syndrome), which consists of a **combination of phaeochromocytoma, medullary carcinoma of the thyroid and parathyroid adenoma or hyperplasia.** This syndrome is thought to be inherited as an autosomal dominant with a high degree of penetrance. The phaeochromocytomas occur between the ages of 30 and 40 years and there is an increased tendency for them to be malignant.

3) **Multiple endocrine neoplasia syndrome**

type IIb. In this variant there is **phaeochromo-cytoma, medullary carcinoma of the thyroid and neuromas affecting mucosal surfaces.** It is also transmitted in an autosomal dominant manner.
4) **An association between phaeochromo-cytoma and neurofibromatosis.**

CHEMICAL CARCINOGENESIS

Epidemiological studies dating back more than 200 years have established that many types of malignant neoplasm occurring in humans are causally related to environmental factors. Any such factor which can increase an individual's risk of developing a malignant neoplasm is spoken of as a **carcinogen**, although it might be more precise to refer to it as an **oncogen**. Such factors may be chemical, physical or viral. This section is concerned with the first of these.

The history of this field of oncological research starts with the observation, made in 1775 by Percivall Pott, a noted London surgeon, that there was a high preva-lence of cancer of the scrotal skin in chimney sweeps' boys. Anyone who has read *The Water Babies* by Charles Kingsley, a work of more than usually revolting sentimentality, will recall that the hapless children were sent up into the chimneys to sweep them and, conse-quently, were covered in soot.

Pott's writings were said to have inspired a ruling made by the Danish Chimney Sweepers' Guild in 1778 that its members should bathe daily. That this simple measure was effective is suggested by a study carried out by Butlin a century later, in which he showed that scro-tal cancer in chimney sweeps was comparatively rare outside England and attributed this to the habit of wearing protective clothing and bathing daily.

During the early industrial revolution, a similarly high prevalence of skin cancer was found in association with a number of occupations. Mule spinners in the Lancashire cotton mills, the fronts of whose garments were often soaked with lubricating oils, frequently developed cancer of the skin of the abdomen and scro-tum; workers engaged in the extraction of oil from shale appeared to be similarly at risk. All these observa-tions, relatively crude as they were, suggested that **coal tar** or one of its constituents might be responsible for the induction of such skin cancers and this led, ulti-mately, to the recognition of **polycyclic hydro-carbons** as a group of compounds with considerable carcinogenic potential.

Remote, Proximate and Ultimate Carcinogens: Carcinogenicity and Mutagenicity

Many of the substances that are called carcinogens on the basis of their ability to produce tumours in certain animal species are not themselves carcinogenic, but become so only after conversion in the body of the host to forms that are more active biologically (*Fig. 29.1*). In current terminology:

- The parent substance is called a **remote carcinogen** or precarcinogen.
- Its metabolites with greater carcinogenic potential are called **proximate carcinogens**.
- The final molecular species that interacts with the host DNA is termed the **ultimate carcinogen**.

This concept is of obvious importance when attempt-ing to identify the carcinogenic potential of new com-pounds before they are released for use, because the metabolites of such compounds must be tested for mutagenicity and/or carcinogenicity as well as the par-ent compounds (see below).

Normal cells transformed by carcinogens show permanent alteration of their phenotypes. This alteration is inherited from generation to genera-tion of the cell line and we can infer from this that **a permanent alteration to the genome of the trans-formed cell has occurred.** Such an alteration falls within the definition of a **mutation**. It is now known

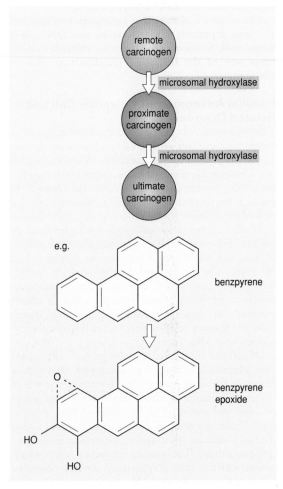

FIGURE 29.1 Activation of potentially carcinogenic compounds.

that most of the carcinogenic chemicals so far identified are also mutagens, although not all mutagens are carcinogenic. Nevertheless, the demonstration that a given compound is mutagenic sounds a warning that it may also be carcinogenic.

In testing for mutagenicity, the possibility that the test compound may be only a remote carcinogen must be taken into consideration.

Testing for Mutagens

Most tests for mutagenicity employ submammalian species. These include bacteria, bacterial viruses (bacteriophages), fungi and insects. All of these are useful because they have relatively small genomes and reproduce themselves quickly.

A commonly used test is the Ames test, in which the effects of the test compound on the histidine-requiring mutant of *Salmonella typhimurium* is assessed (*Fig. 29.2*).

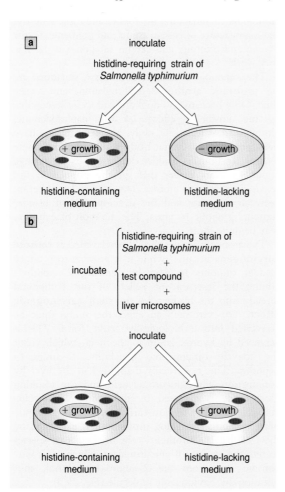

FIGURE 29.2 *Testing for mutagenicity using bacteria.*
a Normal results with a histidine-requiring strain of Salmonella typhimurium. *b The presence of colonies in medium lacking histidine indicates mutation of some bacteria to a state of histidine independence.*

Reversion of this strain, produced by a single base-pair substitution or insertion of a single base pair, can be detected quickly and easily. The possibility that metabolic conversion is needed before mutagenicity is expressed can be taken care of by preincubation of the test compound with liver microsomes.

Polycyclic Hydrocarbons in Relation to Carcinogenicity

Despite the recognized association between exposure to coal tar derivatives and skin cancer, it was not until 1915 that the experimental induction of coal tar-related neoplasms in animals was first carried out. By repeated applications of coal tar to the inside of rabbit ears, Yamagiwa and Ichikawa produced skin tumours in the areas of skin on which the tar had been painted. The next step was to be isolation of the substances in the tar that were responsible for the tumours. It was found that the compounds responsible were present in the higher boiling fractions obtained during the fractional distillation of coal tar. The fluorescence spectra of these fractions resembled that of the polycyclic hydrocarbon 1,2-benzanthracene.

This compound is only weakly carcinogenic in the skin-painting model but, using its characteristic fluorescence spectrum as a guide, Sir Ernest Kennaway and his colleagues were able in 1930 to isolate 50 mg of the powerful carcinogen 3,4-benzpyrene as the end-product of the fractional distillation of two tonnes of tar.

3,4-Benzpyrene is a major constituent of cigarette smoke and is also present in the exhaust fumes of petrol engines. Many other hydrocarbons have been tested since then. Not all are carcinogenic and, among those that are, there are distinct differences in their ability to induce tumours in experimental animals. Moderate or powerful carcinogenic compounds in this group include:
- 7,12-dimethylbenz(a)anthracene
- 3,4-benzpyrene
- 1,2,5,6-dibenzanthracene
- 3-methylcholanthrene

The Site of Application of Oncogenic Hydrocarbons and the Species Used Affect the Type of Neoplasm Produced

The classical model of experimental induction of tumours by polycyclic hydrocarbons is skin painting, which produces squamous tumours locally. However, the subcutaneous injection of 7,12-dimethylbenz(a)anthracene produces sarcomas in the rat and malignant tumours of the lymphoid system in newborn mice. Intraperitoneal injection in mice produces ovarian tumours; in rats, mammary tumours result.

Mechanisms of Action
Carcinogenic hydrocarbons act by binding to host macromolecules within both the cytoplasm

and the nucleus. They are activated by mixed-function oxidases to form epoxides which are more water soluble and more reactive than the parent compounds.

The carcinogenic potential of hydrocarbons seems to reside in certain double bonds to which oxygen is added (under the influence of mixed-function oxidases such as **aryl hydrocarbon hydroxylase**). The compounds formed are known as **epoxides** and it is these that appear to have the ability to bind to DNA as well as to macromolecules in the cytoplasm of target cells. This binding tendency is related to the fact that the epoxides are **electrophilic** (positively charged molecules that form covalent bonds with the negatively charged nucleophilic atoms in DNA, RNA and proteins). The greater the degree of DNA binding, the greater the carcinogenic potential of the hydrocarbon.

Cigarette Smoking and Lung Cancer

Almost certainly the most important of the polycyclic hydrocarbons in relation to neoplasms in humans is 3,4-benzpyrene, one of more than 3000 components in cigarette smoke.

There is now a vast literature supporting the existence of a direct causal association between cigarette smoking and lung cancer (chiefly of the squamous variety). If one were to regard the risk of a non-smoker developing carcinoma of the bronchus as an arbitrary level of **1**, the relative risk to an individual who smokes 20 or more cigarettes per day may be as great as **32**. Giving up smoking reduces the chance of carcinoma in that individual, and the longer the cigarette-free period, the greater the reduction in risk.

Clearly, not all smokers develop lung cancer (although about 10% do) and this raises the possibility that there may be some genetic contribution to the risk of an individual smoker developing cancer. This genetic component may be related to the inducibility of the enzyme **aryl hydrocarbon hydroxylase (AHH)** by the hydrocarbon substrate. It has been reported that differences exist in the inducibility of this enzyme; subjects in whom the enzyme is more readily induced may be at greater risk of developing a smoking-related tumour. Conflicting reports on the importance of AHH inducibility may be due to the fact that AHH measures the sum total of oxidation due to a number of P450 cytochromes and that the conversion of benzpyrene to a carcinogenic metabolite may be a function of only some of these enzymes. High-pressure liquid chromatography shows that benzpyrene is converted to more than 40 metabolites. One of these, a diol epoxide, is highly mutagenic and carcinogenic, and is found covalently bound to cellular DNA.

The ways in which individuals metabolize drugs may also be useful in delineating groups that may be more or less at risk of developing cancer after exposure to car-

cinogens. In a recent study, most patients with lung cancer were shown to be rapid metabolizers of debrisoquine, the pattern of distribution suggesting that this trait is inherited in an autosomal dominant manner.

Lung cancer is not the only neoplasm that appears to be causally associated with smoking: carcinomas of the oesophagus, pancreas, kidney and urinary bladder are others that also seem to be more common in smokers.

Aromatic Amines and Azo Dyes

2-Naphthylamine

As early as 1895, a high prevalence of carcinoma of the bladder was reported in men who had worked in an aniline dye factory in Germany. The causal nature of this association was soon confirmed and it is now known that several occupations carry an increased risk for the development of bladder cancer. These include aniline dye manufacture, the rubber and cable industry, the manufacture of certain paints and pigments, textile dyeing and printing, and certain categories of laboratory work.

The carcinogens identified in these situations are the **aromatic amines** 2-naphthylamine and benzidine. Only humans and dogs are said to be susceptible to the urothelial effects of the naphthylamine, although in at least one study, bladder tumours have been produced in the rat bladder after naphthylamine feeding. In humans bladder cancer occurs on average about 15 years earlier than in the population not exposed to aromatic amines. The average latent period between exposure and the development of bladder tumours is about 16 years. The duration of exposure may be quite short.

The aromatic amines should be classified as **remote carcinogens** because, while it is possible to produce bladder tumours in dogs by **feeding** 2-naphthylamine, the insertion of pellets of this compound directly into the bladder has **no such carcinogenic effect**. To exert such an effect the amine must be converted into a biologically active form. This is achieved by hydroxylation in the liver, which yields the actively carcinogenic metabolite, 2-amino-1-naphthol. This is normally detoxified in the liver by conjunction with glucuronic acid and the resulting glucuronide is excreted by the kidney. This glucuronide is said to be non-carcinogenic. The susceptibility of human and dog urothelium is explained by the fact that the urothelial cells in these two species secrete the enzyme β-glucuronidase, which splits glucuronic acid from the 2-amino-1-naphthol, thus releasing the carcinogenic molecule (*Fig. 29.3*).

2-Acetyl-Aminofluorene

This amine has excited considerable interest as an experimental model of carcinogenesis. It was developed as an insecticide in the 1940s, but before mar-

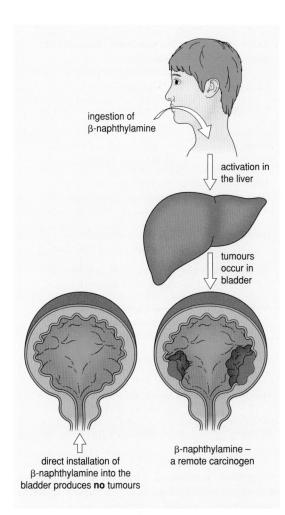

FIGURE 29.3 Ingestion of β-naphthylamine leads to cancer of the bladder. Instillation of the compound directly into the bladder does not. This indicates that the β-naphthylamine is activated in the course of metabolism and is thus a remote carcinogen.

keting was found to be carcinogenic. Unlike 2-naphthylamine or benzidine, which appear to produce tumours only in the bladder, 2-acetyl-aminofluorene produces neoplasms in a wide range of tissues including the liver, breast, lung and intestine. As with naphthylamine, this compound is also a remote carcinogen which undergoes hydroxylation in the liver to produce a proximate carcinogen of greater activity. The final step in the production of the ultimate carcinogen is probably esterification to form an *N*-sulphate ester, which is a highly reactive electrophilic compound.

Nitrosamines and Nitrosamides

The carcinogenic potential of this group of compounds has excited a great deal of interest since the discovery in 1956 that animals receiving dimethylnitrosamine in the

diet at a dose level of 50 parts per million developed liver cell tumours after 6–9 months of dosing.

Nitrosamines have the general formula

$$\begin{array}{c} R \\ \diagdown \\ \diagup \\ R^1 \end{array} N{-}N{=}O$$

in which one of the R groups is an alkyl radical and the other either an aryl or alkyl radical. In the case of the **nitrosamides**, one R is an alkyl radical and the other an amide or ester. The nitroso compounds, in animals at least, have proved to be potent and versatile carcinogens, producing tumours in a wide range of animal species and in many different tissues. An interesting feature of the individual compounds in this large group is their organotropy, many of them showing a marked degree of organ specificity.

In the case of nitrosamines, as with 2-naphthylamine, the parent compound is a remote carcinogen which requires metabolic activation. In the course of this activation, alkylating agents are formed and these bind to both the N7 and the O6 position on guanine, the latter probably being of more significance in so far as malignant transformation is concerned.

Nitrosamines can be formed in the gastrointestinal tract by the interaction of nitrous acid, derived from nitrites, with secondary amines. It has been suggested that the frequency of certain tumours, notably gastric carcinoma, may be related to the dietary intake of nitrites, which are present in large amounts in pickled, salted and smoked foods.

Nitrosamides do not require enzymatic activation to be rendered carcinogenic. Thus, instillation of methyl-nitrosourea into the rat bladder at an appropriate dosage results in the production of urothelial tumours in the majority of instances. An interesting aspect of nitrosamide activity is displayed by the compound ethyl-nitrosourea. When this compound, which has a half-life of only a few minutes, is given to a pregnant rat after the 11th day of gestation, the offspring develop malignant tumours of the brain at about the age of 9 months. Samples of brain taken from the litter at different ages and grown in culture show a stepwise development of the phenotypic evidence of malignant transformation.

Direct-acting Alkylating Agents

Alkylating agents can bind to DNA without any need for prior activation. This groups includes such compounds as mustard gas, β-propiolactone and several agents used in the treatment of malignant disease, such as cyclophosphamide, melphalan and busulphan. While the interaction of these molecules with DNA makes them useful as antitumour agents, this property constitutes a double-edged sword, because they also increase the risk of other neoplasms developing, most notably leukaemia and malignancies of the lymphoid series.

Some Naturally Occurring Chemical Carcinogens

The groups of chemical carcinogens considered thus far can hardly be looked on as natural environmental hazards, with the possible exception of nitrosamines derived in the gastrointestinal tract from dietary constituents. The marked influence that geographical factors have on the prevalence of certain neoplasms, such as carcinoma of the liver and oesophagus, suggests that these differences in tumour frequency may be affected by the existence of naturally occurring carcinogens in particular areas.

In relation to carcinoma of the liver (see pp 509–603), which is comparatively rare in Europe and North America but common in Asia and in certain parts of Africa, an interesting potential candidate for the role of naturally occurring carcinogen is a group of toxins produced by fungi, most notably *Aspergillus flavus*. The toxins derived from this mould, which may contaminate cereal and groundnut crops, are known as **aflatoxins**. Aflatoxins were discovered in 1960 when a large number of poultry, fed on groundnut meal imported from East Africa, died from extensive liver cell necrosis. When formal toxicological studies were carried out it was found that, at low dose levels, the toxin was capable of producing liver cell carcinoma.

The frequency of liver cell carcinoma is high in those parts of the world where there is a poor, largely agrarian, population heavily dependent on cereal crops for subsistence. Such crops may become contaminated by *A. flavus* and, indeed, epidemiological data indicate a positive correlation between aflatoxin consumption and the incidence of liver cell carcinoma. For example, in Thailand, where there was a ninefold difference in aflatoxin intake between two areas of the country, there was a sixfold difference in the frequency of liver cell carcinoma.

It appears that strong synergy exists between aflatoxin and chronic hepatitis B virus infection (see pp 600–601). Some of the proteins of hepatitis B virus mimic the action of tumour promoters. The resulting large population of dividing cells is more likely to acquire somatic mutations of one kind or another: **aflatoxin produces a point mutation at codon 249 of the *p53* gene leading to the production of an abnormal gene product** (see pp 285–287).

Occupational Carcinogens

The recognition that certain chemicals might be implicated in carcinogenesis stemmed directly from the observations of Pott and others (see p 292) that certain occupations carried a higher than normal risk for the development of certain neoplasms. A considerable number of occupational hazards of this kind is now known to exist (*Table 29.1*).

While it is impossible to give a detailed account of the 'occupational' neoplasms that have been recognized, a few general points of principle are worth considering.

Table 29.1 Some Occupational Hazards and their Associated Neoplasms

Chemical	Neoplasm
2–Naphthylamine	Urothelial malignancy (bladder, ureter, renal pelvis) (see p 714)
Arsenic	Cancers of skin and lung (see pp 458–464, 1020)
Asbestos (a fibrous silicate)	Mesothelioma, squamous carcinoma of lung (see pp 458–464, 470–472)
Ionizing radiation	Cancers of lung and bone, leukaemia (see pp 458–464)
Bischlormethylether	Small cell carcinoma of lung (see pp 461–462)
Nickel	Cancers of lung, paranasal sinuses, larynx (see pp 415, 418–419, 458–464)
Vinyl chloride monomer	Angiosarcoma of liver (see p 605)
Hardwood dusts	Adenocarcinoma of paranasal sinuses (see p 415)
Benzene	Leukaemia (see p 927)

In general, a neoplasm related to an occupational hazard does not differ from its non-occupational counterpart, either in clinical or structural terms. In some instances there may be associated histological features that may provide a clue as to the occupational aetiology, such as the finding of asbestos bodies in the resected lung of a patient with squamous carcinoma of the bronchus.

Sometimes the clue might reside in the unusual nature of the tumour or in the fact that it is of a type that is unusual at that particular anatomical site. An example of the first is **mesothelioma**, a neoplasm which, as its name implies, arises from the mesothelial cells of serosal linings. Mesotheliomas occur most commonly in the pleura, leading to a tremendous degree of thickening of the visceral pleura (see pp 470–472).

An example of the second type of situation, where a tumour unusual at a particular anatomical site is encountered, is **adenocarcinoma of the paranasal sinuses** in hardwood workers. Such a tumour otherwise only occurs rarely at this site.

No general rule appears to operate with respect to the age at which occupationally related neoplasms occur. It appears to be a function of two variables: the age at which exposure begins, and the latent period characteristic of the particular carcinogen. In a study of occupationally related cancer of the urinary bladder, the mean age at exposure was found to be 29 years and the mean latent period 16.6 years. Thus the tumours became obvious at a somewhat earlier age than is usual for bladder cancer.

CARCINOGENESIS AS A MULTISTEP PROCESS: TUMOUR INITIATION AND PROMOTION

In the late 1940s it was found that painting the skin with compounds such as croton oil, which are not themselves carcinogenic, greatly increased the yield of skin tumours in mice that had previously received a subcarcinogenic dose of the carcinogenic polycyclic hydrocarbon benzo(a)pyrene (*Fig. 29.4*). Croton oil *alone* produced no tumours and, if it was applied to the mouse skin *before* the hydrocarbon, *no* tumour-enhancing effect was noted.

The effect of the benzo(a)pyrene was described at that time as the **initiation of carcinogenesis**, and the enhancing effect of the croton oil was termed **promotion**. For many years this phenomenon was believed to be confined to the mouse skin model, but it is now thought that two-stage or multi-stage pathways in carcinogenesis exist in respect of a number of neoplasms, including liver, bladder, lung, breast, colon, oesophagus and pancreas.

If the term **promotion**, as originally defined in the mouse skin model, is to have an application in the wider field of carcinogenesis, it is important that common features should be demonstrated in both **operational** and **biochemical** terms between the mouse model and other chemically induced neoplasms.

Chemical carcinogenesis can be regarded, in operational terms, as a series of processes in which a normal cell and its progeny are converted into malignant cells (*Fig. 29.5*).

Initiation
The **initiation** phase involves a change in the genome of the target cell, this change being inherited by the progeny of that cell. The change in the genetic material, as indicated above, is usually associated with covalent binding of the active form of the carcinogen to DNA.

While **high doses** of initiating compounds can cause tumours to develop without the assistance of any other factors, **a low dose of the initiator will not be expressed in the form of phenotypically altered cells and may induce damage in the genome of only a small number of target cells**.

Characteristically, initiation:
- is a very rapid event
- is produced in a dose-related fashion after a single exposure to an initiating carcinogen
- occurs in only a small proportion of the target cell

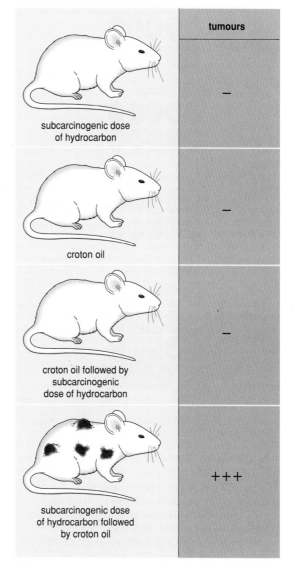

FIGURE 29.4 *Initiation and promotion of neoplasms in a mouse skin model.*

population. The number of cells affected is increased if rapid proliferation of the target cells is taking place.

Unless the DNA damage is quickly repaired, and provided the target cell is a 'stem' cell and not a fully differentiated one, the effect on the DNA is permanent and inheritable, even though there is no detectable change in the cell phenotype.

Promotion
The promotion phase in multistep carcinogenesis is brought about by agents that catalyse biochemical events in both normal and initiated cells, leading to an altered pattern of gene expression.

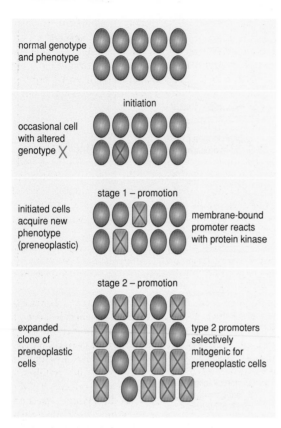

FIGURE 29.5 Initiation and promotion – a multistep process.

In the case of **initiated** cells, this results in the expression of cells with a new phenotype; these cells must be regarded as being **preneoplastic**.

- If exposure to the promoter is short-lived, the preneoplastic cells will not increase in number relative to their normal neighbours and the phenotypic changes that have occurred may not be identified easily because only a few cells are affected.
- If exposure to the promoting agent is continued or if the promoter is replaced by another agent capable of causing an increase in cell turnover and hence hyperplasia, there will be a concomitant increase in the number of the initiated and promoted (preneoplastic) cells and a histologically detectable tumour may develop. In the mouse skin model, such a tumour will be a benign papilloma.

It is believed that a further event is necessary for the benign focus of preneoplastic cells to be transformed into an invasive neoplasm. This event will also produce an inheritable change in the genome of affected cells and may involve either a further biochemical alteration of DNA, some transposition of genetic material, or activation of part of the genome to produce a portion of DNA capable of inducing malignant transformation (an oncogene) (see pp 273–276).

Promotion Itself is not a Single-stage Process

Promotion can be divided into two stages:

1) There is an early phase (stage 1 promotion), which can be brought about by diterpene esters such as 12−*o*-tetradecanoylphorbol-13 acetate (TPA).

2) A later, less specific, phase (stage 2 promotion) occurs, in which other compounds such as turpentine are active.

Specific inhibitors exist for each of these phases. In initiated skin, only a single exposure to promoters that have both stage 1 and stage 2 actions is required for tumours to develop. For the same result, multiple exposures to stage 2 promoters are necessary.

Promotion as a Biochemical Event

Different biochemical events underlie initiation, stage 1 promotion and stage 2 promotion (*Fig. 29.6*).

Initiating carcinogens react with cellular DNA, while the target for stage 1 promoters is the surface membrane of the cell. High-affinity receptors have been identified for TPA and other promoters on cell surface membranes in many tissues and in many species. The binding of a stage 1 promoter to such a receptor

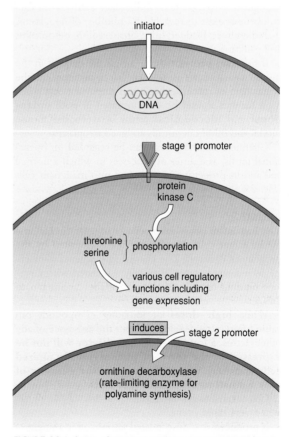

FIGURE 29.6 Some of the biochemical events in initiation and promotion.

sets off alterations in membrane phospholipid metabolism and in the structure and function of the membrane. The binding site for TPA appears to be the specific calcium- and lipid-binding protein kinase C.

When TPA binds to this enzyme and activates it, phosphorylation of serine and threonine residues in specific cell proteins occurs. **The state of phosphorylation of these proteins is the crucial factor mediating the activity of various hormone and growth factors.** Thus TPA is acting on the cell surface membrane in much the same way as insulin, epidermal growth factor or platelet-derived growth factor, all of which bind to another protein kinase (tyrosine kinase). The effects of TPA on these processes take place very rapidly, but are not by themselves sufficient to bring about tumour development. For this, stage 2 events are also necessary.

Stage 2 promotion is dependent on prolonged exposure to the promoting compound and on sustained cell proliferation, which enables the growth potential of the latent tumour cells to be expressed. Stage 2 promoters **induce enzymes**, the products of which increase the speed of cell division. The enzyme that appears to be particularly concerned is **ornithine decarboxylase (ODC)**, which is the rate-limiting enzyme for the synthesis of certain polyamines that have a role in the synthesis of DNA, RNA and protein. Further investigation has shown that most growth-promoting stimuli (e.g. growth-promoting hormones, epidermal growth factor, partial hepatectomy) induce ODC and also act as stage 2 promoters.

Not All Enhancers of Tumour Development are Promoters

Many factors other than stage 1 or 2 promoters can enhance the production of tumours. Some operate by increasing the efficiency with which the active metabolite of an initiating carcinogen is presented to the target cell, whereas others may modify the physiological response of the host to the presence of developing tumour cells. The latter include a wide range of factors, which may be nutritional or may affect immune surveillance mechanisms.

Initiation and Promotion Occur in Tumour Formation Apart from the Mouse Skin Model

In experimental bladder cancer, saccharin, cyclamates and some metabolites of tryptophan fulfil many of the criteria for labelling a compound as a promoter. Induction of ODC in cultured bladder urothelium has been shown after treatment of the cells with saccharin, and these data suggest that mechanisms similar to those identified in the mouse skin model may act in this different situation.

The importance of retaining the concept of initiation and promotion in relation to human neoplasms rests chiefly on the realization that a long period of promo-

tion may be part of the natural history of the development of many neoplasms. In some instances, the promotion process may be reversible and this may offer the chance to deploy novel treatment strategies such as the use of retinoids (which inhibit stage 2 promotion) to modify the natural history of neoplasms such as carcinoma of the bladder.

HORMONES AND NEOPLASIA

Recognition of the possibility that the hormonal milieu might play some part in the natural history of cancer dates back to 1895, when Beatson in Glasgow removed the ovaries from a woman with recurrent breast cancer and found that the tumour regressed. This observation suggested that at least some breast cancers were oestrogen dependent; this hypothesis has received considerable support from both human and animal studies.

A single dose of the carcinogen dimethyl-benz(a)anthracene, given either intravenously or via a stomach tube, produces carcinoma of the breast in rats. **If the animal has been ovariectomized before the carcinogen is given, no tumour is produced.** Ovariectomy has a similar inhibiting effect in relation to the tumours produced by the mouse mammary tumour virus. In addition, tumours occurring after administration of dimethyl-benz(a)anthracene regress following ovariectomy. In contrast, if prolactin levels in the rats are raised by giving them drugs of the phenothiazine group, there is an acceleration in the growth of breast tumours. Data of this type suggest that this model of breast carcinoma is hormonally dependent, but do not rule out the possibility that the hormones mentioned may also act as promoters.

Hormones in Human Breast Cancer

A link between ovarian function and human breast cancer is suggested by the increased risk encountered in those who had an early menarche, a delayed first pregnancy (or no pregnancies) and a prolonged period of menstrual activity.

While it is also true that ablation of ovarian function, whether by surgical, radiotherapeutic or pharmacological means, induces remission, at least temporarily, in a proportion of cases of breast cancer in humans, there is at best only conflicting evidence that patients (compared with controls) have high circulating levels of either oestrogen or prolactin.

A relationship has been noted between urinary levels of aetiocholanolone (C19 steroids) and the natural history of patients with breast cancer. When the levels of these steroids excreted in the urine are low, the prognosis is, in general, poor; these patients also show a poor response to removal of the ovaries.

Of equal interest has been the recognition of

oestrogen receptor sites on certain tumour cells. The oestrogen-binding protein is believed to form part of a two-step process in which oestradiol is bound in the cell and transported to the nucleus. **Absence of these receptors from the majority of cells in an individual breast cancer indicates that the response to endocrine therapy is likely to be poor.**

Carcinoma of the Endometrium

The suggestion that the development of endometrial carcinoma is influenced by oestrogenic steroids is supported by the following:

- Oestrogen-producing tumours of the ovary are frequently associated with endometrial hyperplasia and in some of these patients carcinoma of the endometrium supervenes.
- Carcinoma of the endometrium and of the breast occur in the same patient more frequently than would be expected if the association was a chance one.
- Administration of oestrogen-containing compounds (hormone replacement therapy) in postmenopausal women is associated with an increased risk of endometrial hyperplasia and carcinoma (see pp 758–761).
- There is an increased risk of endometrial carcinoma in obese females. It is said that 50% of patients with endometrial cancer weigh more than 82 kg (180 lb). This association is believed to be due to the fact that precursor steroids for oestrone, such as Δ-4-androstenedione, are converted in adipose tissue. This conversion rate is twice as high in postmenopausal women as in those still in active reproductive life, and obesity has a marked incremental effect.

  Conversion of Δ-4–androstenedione to oestrone is also increased in diabetic females; here too the risk of endometrial cancer is greater than in non-diabetic, age- and weight-matched peers.

It seems likely, therefore, that carcinoma of the endometrium can be regarded as one in which a certain degree of hormone dependency is present and in which oestrogenic steroids may also exert a promotional effect.

Other Neoplasms are Recognized in which Hormones Influence the Natural History of the Disease

Carcinoma of the prostate, like carcinoma of the breast and endometrium, is a neoplasm that has its peak incidence at a time when involution of the tissue could normally be expected. The prostate is clearly an hormone-dependent organ (see pp 743–744).

Another interesting example of the influence of hormones on tumour genesis is the rather curious **clear-cell adenocarcinoma of the vagina**, which occurred in the daughters of some women given diethylstilboestrol in the course of pregnancy (see pp 790–791).

PHYSICAL AGENTS IN ONCOGENESIS

ULTRAVIOLET IRRADIATION

The association between skin cancer and exposure to sunlight was reported more than 100 years ago. Epidemiological observations suggesting a role for ultraviolet light as the responsible agent were supported by the induction of skin tumours in rats exposed to ultraviolet irradiation in 1928. Because ultraviolet light is a low-energy form of emission and does not penetrate deeply, the skin absorbs most of the energy and hence is the primary target for this form of carcinogenesis.

Evidence of an aetiological role for sunlight in skin carcinoma is very strong. Most such neoplasms occur in exposed areas. They are relatively infrequent in dark-skinned races, in whom the ultraviolet radiation is filtered out by melanin, and are common in fair-skinned people. The prevalence of malignant tumours of the skin in the fair-skinned appears to be associated with the intensity of solar radiation and is increased in regions close to the Equator. The mechanism responsible for the induction of such neoplasms is likely to be associated with the production of abnormal thymine dimers in the DNA of the epidermal cells and perhaps the lack of efficient excision repair of the abnormal DNA, such as is seen in **xeroderma pigmentosum** (see pp 290–291).

The most common sunshine-related neoplasms are **basal cell carcinomas**, which may invade locally but almost never metastasize, **squamous carcinoma**, which may both invade the surrounding tissues and metastasize, and **malignant melanoma**, which is often highly malignant and is capable of spreading very widely.

IONIZING RADIATION

It has been recognized since the early part of the century that ionizing radiation constitutes a risk factor for the subsequent development of cancer (see pp 22–24). In humans this is seen under a number of different circumstances:

- There was an increased prevalence of both leukaemia and skin cancer in radiologists who, during the early days of diagnostic radiology, were inadequately protected.
- There is a greater than normal frequency of leukaemia and carcinoma of the thyroid, breast and lung among the survivors of the nuclear explosions over Hiroshima and Nagasaki.
- There is an increased risk of carcinoma of the thyroid in people who have had irradiation to the neck during childhood.
- There is an increased risk of osteosarcoma following

ingestion of bone-seeking radioactive substances (see p 1062)

- A thorium-containing contrast medium, **Thorotrast**, was used to outline the margins of abscess cavities in the 1940s. The prevalence of malignant tumours in patients investigated in this way is about twice as high as would normally be expected, with a sixfold increase in leukaemia and liver neoplasm.

The mechanisms by which ionizing radiation induces malignant transformation are not clear. Irradiation causes free radical generation (see pp 22–24) and these very active chemical species may react with elements of the target cell genome. Certainly irradiation can produce obvious changes in chromosome morphology and is mutagenic to cultured cells. In addition, in at least one model, a virus-induced leukaemia in the mouse, irradiation may activate viral oncogenes and bring about transformation in this way.

FOREIGN MATERIALS

Certain foreign substances are capable of inducing the formation of connective tissue neoplasms when implanted, usually subcutaneously, into the tissues of a variety of animals. The precise physical form in which these foreign materials exist appears to be of fundamental importance in relation to tumour induction. For example, sheets of certain plastics evoke a brisk fibrous tissue response when inserted subcutaneously, which eventually leads to the formation of low-grade fibrosarcomas. If the same plastic sheeting is ground up and then inserted into the connective tissue of the same species, no tumours result. Similarly, if holes are made in the sheeting before insertion, the likelihood of tumour formation decreases, this diminution of risk appearing to be associated with the size of the holes. This has been studied using millipore filters as the tumour-provoking agent. If the filter has a pore size greater than 0.22 μm, no tumours appear. The mechanisms involved in this curious form of oncogenesis are not known and there is, as yet, no evidence that the prosthetic materials widely used in surgical practice confer any increased risk of neoplasia.

VIRUSES AND NEOPLASIA

It has been known since 1908 that certain tumours in animals can be caused by viruses. It was recognized at that time that a variety of fowl leukaemia could be transmitted by cell-free extracts of tumour tissue. This discovery was followed by the pioneering studies of Peyton Rous, who found that cell-free extracts of chicken sarcomas produced identical tumours when injected subcutaneously into other chickens.

Viruses that are capable of inducing neoplasms are known as **oncogenic** viruses. Oncogenic viruses are found among both the **DNA** and the **RNA** viruses.

DNA ONCOGENIC VIRUSES

The best authenticated DNA oncogenic viruses come from three groups:

1) the **papova** group (see p 193)
2) the **herpes** group
3) the **hepatitis** group

The Papova Group

Papillomaviruses

The first virally induced mammalian neoplasm to be recognized was the so-called Shope papilloma, a curious warty lesion on the tails of Kentucky cotton-tailed rabbits. This neoplasm can be passaged in the same way as the Rous sarcoma but, in the case of the Shope papillomavirus, the host response makes a considerable difference to the natural history of an infection. If wild cotton-tailed rabbits are infected with the virus, tumours grow slowly, are usually benign, and free virus can be harvested from the horny layer of infected skin. If, on the other hand, domestic strains of the rabbit are infected, the tumours are rapidly growing, some of them become frankly malignant, and free virus cannot be harvested from the cells. Thus cell-free extracts from tumours in the domestic strain cannot be passaged.

In humans, papillomaviruses are the only ones that have been *proved* without doubt to cause neoplasms. The lesions associated with wart virus infections are the common skin wart, and anal and genital warts (**condylomata acuminata**).

Polyomaviruses

Polyomavirus, a large DNA virus, causes a wide variety of neoplasms in a variety of small animals (mice, rabbits, rats, hamsters) when they are infected in the neonatal period. Adult members of susceptible species are immune unless they have been neonatally thymectomized, an observation that suggests an effective degree of T-cell surveillance of cells transformed by the virus. A number of different tumours in various anatomical sites have been described as following infection with this virus, hence the name **poly**oma. There is no evidence of any involvement of polyomaviruses in the field of human neoplasia.

Simian Vacuolating Virus (SV40)

This virus was discovered in 1960 in the kidney cell cultures used to produce the first polio vaccine. In the course of immunization against poliomyelitis, some thousands of people had also been inoculated with the SV40 virus. Later it was shown that the virus could induce tumours in newborn hamsters and transform human cells in culture. However, no evidence has yet accrued that could lead to this virus being implicated in human neoplasia.

SV40 enters the affected cells through the action of its coat proteins; after uncoating, either the whole or part of the viral genome is inserted into the host DNA.

Transcription of the viral DNA takes place in two waves, the earlier messenger RNA being derived from codons responsible for transformation as well as for viral replication.

Herpesvirus in Neoplasia

Viruses of the herpes group are certainly responsible for the production of at least one important malignant neoplasm in poultry, and are probably involved in two or more neoplastic diseases in humans.

In chickens, a herpesvirus causes a variety of malignant lymphoma known as **Marek's disease**. Infection with this virus can be economically disastrous unless the birds have been immunized with an attenuated form of the virus, because, unlike most oncogenic animal viruses, the virus of Marek's disease spreads horizontally and is very contagious. Although the cell that undergoes malignant transformation is almost certainly a T lymphocyte, the virus invades epithelial cells in the skin in association with the feather sockets, and is shed from the skin.

ONCOGENIC RNA VIRUSES

The role of the oncogenic RNA viruses as a group is discussed in the section dealing with **oncogenes** (see pp 273–276). However, one RNA virus does merit consideration separately – the **mouse mammary tumour virus**. A viral aetiology for breast cancer in the mouse was first proposed following the observations of Bittner in 1936, who studied strains of mice known to have a high prevalence of carcinoma of the breast. Bittner found that the tendency to develop breast cancer could not be ascribed wholly to the genetic make-up of the hybrid strain he was studying and that the **female parent type** was the most important factor. Furthermore, if baby mice from a strain of high prevalence were delivered by caesarean section and suckled by a mother of a low prevalence strain, the young mice did not develop carcinoma of the breast to any appreciable extent when they grew to maturity. Conversely, when the progeny of a low prevalence strain were suckled by a mother of a high prevalence strain, the frequency of breast cancer in these young mice was uncharacteristically high (*Fig. 29.7*). These data suggested that the oncogenic agent was being **vertically** transmitted via the milk. Confirmation of this hypothesis came when viral particles were demonstrated on electron microscopy of the milk from high prevalence mothers.

In view of the commonness of breast cancer in human females, and the many recorded cases of breast cancer occurring in several members of one family, it is easy to understand why the possibility of a viral aetiology has been enthusiastically canvassed.

Some evidence that might link the data obtained from the mouse model to the human situation has come to light. Particles similar to those seen in the milk of strains of mice with a high cancer prevalence have

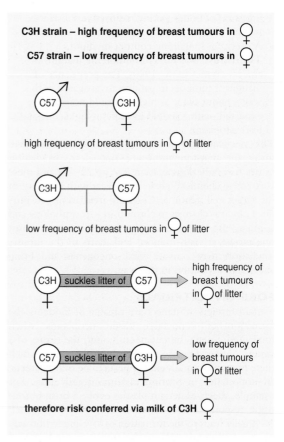

FIGURE 29.7 *Mouse mammary tumour virus.*

been identified both in human breast milk and in breast tissue. One report suggests that such particles can be found more frequently in groups of women in whom there is a higher than expected prevalence of breast cancer, such as the Parsee community in Bombay. Serum from some patients with breast cancer has been shown to contain antibodies that bind to the virus-like particles seen on electron microscopy of breast tissue. However, these data are far from being conclusive and the case for a viral factor in carcinogenesis of the human breast is not yet proven.

VIRUSES IN HUMAN NEOPLASIA

While viruses are thought to have a causal role in only a few types of human neoplasia, some of these are very common and thus up to 20% of human cancers, on a world-wide basis, may have a viral aetiology. Much of our appreciation of this fact is based on the striking geographical distribution of certain neoplasms and the concordance between this distribution and the prevalence of certain viral infections. Examples include

- hepatocellular carcinoma and hepatitis B infections
- human T-cell leukaemia virus (HTLV) type 1 infection and adult T-cell leukaemia

Epstein–Barr Virus and Neoplasia

Infections by the Epstein–Barr virus (EBV) have been implicated in a number of human neoplastic diseases, some of the most important of which are discussed below.

Burkitt's Lymphoma

This is described in Chapter 42 (see pp 968–969). It occurs with great frequency in certain parts of tropical Africa, the distribution being strikingly circumscribed to areas in which malaria is holoendemic and where climatic conditions favour the anopheline mosquito.

EBV infection is very common; about 90% of the world's population is believed to be infected. The virus binds to the CD21 receptor on B lymphocytes but can also infect epithelial cells.

If the EBV is as prevalent as epidemiological data suggest, it seems remarkable that Burkitt's lymphoma should, on the whole, be so circumscribed. The data suggest that the difference is to be found in the host response to EBV infection and, in view of the fact that malaria is known to be immunosuppressive, it seems probable that African Burkitt's lymphoma represents a malaria-related failure of immune surveillance. This view is strengthened by the observation that people who bear the **sickle cell trait**, and who are thus resistant to malaria, also have a reduced risk of developing Burkitt's lymphoma.

Translocation in Burkitt's Lymphoma

Burkitt lymphoma cells are characterized by a translocation, most commonly involving chromosomes 8 and 14. The breakpoint on the long arm of chromosome 8 is at the site of a proto-oncogene known as c-*myc*. In the course of the translocation the c-*myc* gene comes to lie adjacent to the gene encoding the heavy chain for immunoglobulin and is thus abnormally activated (see p 274).

Nasopharyngeal Carcinoma (See also p 415)

An association has also been found between EBV and a curious lymphoepithelial neoplasm found in the nasopharynx. Like Burkitt's lymphoma, this tumour shows a distinctive geographical distribution, being prevalent in China (especially southern China) and some other parts of south-east Asia. The clustering of cases of this tumour, not only within this area but within people originating from it, has been recognized for more than 300 years and, indeed, has led to the disease being termed Kwantung tumour by some, because it is so prevalent in Kwantung province.

On histological examination the neoplasm is seen to consist of two cell lines, one a poorly differentiated epithelial cell and the other a lymphoblastoid cell. EBV can be found in cell lines cultured from both these components and the patients show high titres of EBV antibodies.

Again the question arises as to why this widely prevalent virus should be related to a malignant neoplasm only in a circumscribed geographical area. There is no evidence of an **exogenous modifier** of the host response such as exists in the association between malaria and Burkitt's lymphoma, and the possibility remains that a genetic factor may be operating in the case of the nasopharyngeal carcinoma. Support for this view comes from the fact that emigration from the affected areas of Asia does not appear to lessen the risk and that clustering of human leucocyte antigen (HLA) A2 occurs in the people in high-risk areas.

EBV has also been implicated in:

- immunoblastic-type B-cell lymphomas in immunosuppressed individuals (e.g. in those with acquired immune deficiency syndrome)
- Hodgkin's disease (EBV sequences are found in Reed–Sternberg cells in many cases)
- certain rare T-cell lymphomas

EBV Effects on B Cells that may be Associated with its Malignant Potential

In human B lymphocytes in culture, infection by EBV results in immortalization of the cell line, an effect that appears to be due to six viral proteins, Epstein–Barr nuclear antigen (EBNA) 1, 2, 3A, 3C, LP, and the virally encoded lymphocyte membrane protein LMP-1. The LMP-1 protein is the only EBV-encoded protein that can transform cells in culture and it is presumably important in EBV-associated malignancy.

Carcinoma of the Uterine Cervix and Human Papillomavirus

Epidemiological studies indicate that there is an association between carcinoma of the uterine cervix and the individual level of sexual activity. Virginity, a currently unfashionable state, appears significantly to reduce the risk of cervical cancer and, conversely, an early start to sexual activity and widespread distribution of favours increase the risk of subsequent development of squamous carcinoma of the cervix.

Infection with most types of human papillomavirus, of which there are many, usually gives rise to benign and self-limiting epithelial proliferation (e.g viral warts on the hands and feet), but some strains, most notably 16 and 18, carry a considerable risk of malignancy especially in the genital region and most particularly of the uterine cervix (see p 767).

Over 90% of cases of frank cervical cancer and intraepithelial cervical neoplasia show signs of human papillomavirus infection. In young, sexually active women with normal cervical cytology, this frequency drops to about 25%.

The circular, double-stranded DNA, human papillomavirus genome encodes eight major open reading frames (ORFs). Three of these ORFs (E5, E6 and E7) encode proteins that, in cell culture systems, have transforming properties. E6 and E7 complex with and inactivate the p53 and retinoblastoma (RB) proteins respectively (see p 286). Thus intracellular expression of viral E6 and E7 proteins has the same effect as somatic mutations of the *p53* and *RB* tumour suppressor genes. E5 encodes a small protein localized chiefly in cell membranes; this appears to function by enhancing the activity of cell surface receptors for growth factors such as epidermal growth factor.

Hepatitis B Virus (HBV) (See also pp 573–577) This ubiquitous virus is responsible for one of the more serious varieties of infective hepatitis. The presence of a carrier state (which can be established by identifying the surface antigen of the virus in plasma) can be found in 10–20% of those who become infected with the virus. A significant positive correlation exists between the prevalence of the carrier state and the frequency with which liver cell cancer is seen. In addition, in parts of the world where prevalence of the tumour is high, the carrier rate is about 90% in those with liver cell cancer.

A virus resembling HBV has been found to cause hepatitis in woodchucks, and liver cell carcinoma is not infrequently seen in this species. DNA hybridization techniques have revealed woodchuck virus DNA incorporated within the liver cell genome, and similar observations in respect of the human virus have been made in relation to human cell lines derived from liver cell cancers. These data are strongly suggestive of an oncogenic role for human HBV.

The HBV genome consists of four ORFs: P (encoding reverse transcriptase), C (encoding the core antigen), S (three viral envelope proteins) and X (a transcriptional regulator).

The mechanism by which HBV contributes to malignant transformation is still unknown. Some have suggested that malignancy is due to the repeated cell death and regeneration characteristic of chronic infections. Evidence is beginning to accumulate that the virus may encode some transforming sequences, the current favourite being the X gene.

The X protein functions as a transcription regulator in an unusual and indirect way. It activates protein kinase C and *raf*-1-kinase, both of which play a key role in signal transduction. Thus X expression leads to a signalling cascade which nevertheless requires to be started off by a growth factor–receptor interaction. It has also been suggested that protein X might mimic the function of chemical tumour promoters such as phorbol esters (see pp 298–299), thus providing a large population of dividing cells in which somatic mutations are likely to become 'fixed'.

Human T-cell Leukaemia Virus

HTLV-1 infections are rare in most parts of the world. In the USA only 0.025% of the general population are carriers. In southern Japan, the Caribbean, parts of Africa and South America, the prevalence is much higher, reaching 30% in some areas of Japan.

The virus is linked with two diseases:
1) Adult T-cell leukaemia. There is a risk that 2% of infected individuals will develop this disorder during their lifetime.
2) A neurological disorder – tropical spastic paraparesis.

The chief cellular target is the T-helper cell (CD4), about 1–2% of peripheral cells being infected in a typical case. The possible mechanism of transformation by this virus is discussed in a later section dealing with lymphoma (see pp 928, 964).

CHAPTER 30

Genetic Disorders

All disease can be classified in the following way (*Fig. 30.1*). The disease may arise because of:
- a genetic abnormality acting alone
- an unfavourable environmental factor(s)
- a combination of the above

The term genetic disorders covers a set of diseases in which the manifestations are **either wholly or partly due to abnormalities within the genetic material**. The major classes of disease that fall under this rubric include:

- **Major chromosomal abnormalities**, some of which are associated with highly characteristic clinical syndromes such as Down's syndrome or Turner's syndrome. Such disorders may affect autosomal or sex chromosomes. Most of these genetic abnormalities occur as *de novo* events and are not inherited.

- **Single gene defects.** These are caused by a mutation in either a single allele or alleles of a pair. **Single** allele mutations that are expressed clinically are known as **dominant**; mutations that require **both** members of an allelic pair to be affected before the disorder is expressed are known as **recessive**. Either autosomal or sex chromosomes can be affected. The inheritance pattern gives valuable clues as to whether the disease is autosomal or recessive, and whether autosomal or sex chromosomes are involved.

- **Multifactorial disorders.** These are associated with certain congenital developmental disorders and with some common and important conditions,

including diabetes mellitus, atherosclerosis and its related clinical syndromes, and cancer. Many of these disorders involve an interaction between inherited and environmental factors. The relationship between these is complex and poorly understood.

- **Somatic genetic disorders.** These result from mutations arising in certain somatic cells, largely as a result of exposure to unfavourable environmental factors. Because they affect somatic rather than germ cells, these mutations are not inherited and thus cannot give rise to the disease in the succeeding generation. They are commonly associated with tumour formation and, as in the previous category, often involve interactions between the environment and inherited genetic susceptibility.

- **Mitochondrial genetic disorders.** These are rare and result from mutations in mitochondrial DNA, which is distinct from the chromosomal DNA within the cell nucleus. These disorders are transmitted only through the maternal line. The pattern of inheritance does not follow mendelian lines: all the offspring of an affected mother are affected.

CHROMOSOMAL DISORDERS

The Normal Karyotype

Normal human cells contain 46 chromosomes of which 44 are autosomal and two are sex chromosomes known as X and Y. The possession of a Y chromosome confers male sex. Thus females are XX and males XY in respect of their sex chromosomes. Each chromosome has a constricted area known as a centromere. The material above the centromere is known as the p (petit) or short arm and that below the centromere as the q (long) arm. The region at the end of each arm is known as the telomere. The position of the centromere (see *Fig. 30.2*) serves to divide chromosomes into three groups:

1) metacentric
2) submetacentric
3) acrocentric

The distribution of the chromosomes in these three groups is shown in *Table 30.1*.

When mitotic cell division occurs, each chromosome replicates, with each 'daughter' cell possessing the

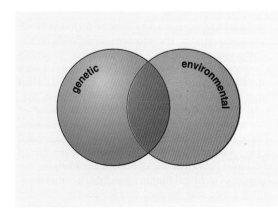

FIGURE 30.1 A classification of disease.

Table 30.1 Chromosome Types

Type based on position of centromere	Chromosome
Metacentric	1, 3, 16, 19, 20
Submetacentric	2, 4, 5, 6, 7, 8, 9, 10, 11, 12, 17, 18, 23, X
Acrocentric	13, 14, 15, 21, 22, Y

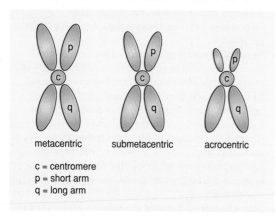

c = centromere
p = short arm
q = long arm

FIGURE 30.2 Three basic morphological types of chromosome.

normal diploid number (46 chromosomes). Division occurring in germ cells (meiosis or reduction division) leads to the formation of cells possessing half the normal complement of chromosomes (23 chromosomes or the haploid number). Ova and sperm thus contain one copy of each autosome and, in the case of sperm, either an X or a Y sex chromosome. All ova, of course, contain X chromosomes.

Analysis of Chromosomes (Karyotyping)

The number and morphology of chromosomes may be determined by studying samples of any tissue grown in cell or tissue culture. In many cases blood lymphocytes are used but data are also obtained from amniotic fluid cells, chorionic villus samples, bone marrow or fibroblasts derived from skin biopsy.

In the case of blood samples, T lymphocytes are induced to transform and proliferate by adding the mitogen phytohaemagglutinin to the culture. After 48–72 hours, mitosis is stopped in metaphase by colchicine, which interferes with the assembly of microtubular proteins forming the spindle. Swelling of the cells following the addition of a hypotonic solution serves to separate the chromosomes and a fixative is then added before spreading drops of the cell suspension on slides.

The smears are stained with the Giemsa stain, which produces a pattern of alternating dark and light bands. This allows the microscopic resolution of 300–500 bands which constitute the basis for categorizing the different regions of the chromosome. The stained bands are divided into seven groups from the centromere outwards and each band within a group is numbered also.

Thus the nomenclature used to describe a region on a chromosome uses:
- the **number** of the chromosome (e.g. 4)
- whether the region is on the **short (p) arm** or the **long (q) arm** (e.g. q).
- the **group** of the band (e.g. 3)
- the **number of the band within the group** (e.g. 4)

This region therefore would be called 4q34.

If the dividing cells are harvested during prometaphase instead of during metaphase, the resolution obtained by staining is greatly increased and up to 1500 bands can be identified.

Gene Mapping

Banding techniques are relatively crude. Ordinary Giemsa banding permits resolution of bands containing 4000–5000 kilobases (kb) of genomic DNA. Arresting cells in prometaphase improves this by a factor of two, but 2000 kb is still much larger than the size of most genes; for example, the cystic fibrosis gene is 250 kb.

More modern techniques have made it possible to map some genes to the correct regions of their chromosomes, and more than 2000 autosomal genes and more than 200 X-linked genes have been correctly assigned. Such gene mapping pays useful dividends, both in respect of prenatal diagnosis and in the cloning of genes recognized only as a result of their gross effects on phenotype.

The methods most commonly used in gene mapping are:
- *in situ* hybridization
- somatic cell hybridization

In Situ *Hybridization*

In situ hybridization is used to localize a cloned DNA sequence to a specific chromosome. It depends on the fact that a single strand, the cloned sequence (or probe) will anneal or bind to its complementary sequence on a denatured chromosome. The probe can be labelled either with a radioactive marker or a fluorescent dye. The labelled probe is then applied to a spread of prometaphase or, better still, interphase chromosomes.

The occurrence of hybridization can be demonstrated either by autoradiography or by examining the spread in ultraviolet light. The use of fluorescent labels has the advantages of technical simplicity and the fact that more than one probe may be used simultaneously, provided each is labelled with a different fluorescent marker. This technique is known as chromosome painting.

Somatic Cell Hybridization

The fusion of human cell lines with mouse cell lines results in the formation of hybrid cells that possess chromosomes from both human and mouse cells. When these hybrids are passaged they preferentially shed human chromosomes, in a random fashion. Eventually the hybrids become stable and will maintain their complement of human chromosomes for several passages. The establishment of several different hybrid cell lines provides a panel of cells that possess different complements of human chromosomes. Such hybrids may be used:

- to look for certain human proteins in cell homogenates. If the proteins are present, the cell line must contain the genes that code for them, and examination of the positive cell lines will narrow the possible gene localizations to a few chromosomes and, ultimately, indicate the chromosome on which the protein is coded.
- to hybridize DNA from the different cell lines to radiolabelled copies of probes that represent the gene, the location of which is being sought.

Genomic Imprinting and Chromosomes

Our ideas on the transmission of human genetic disorders are based largely on the theory that the parental origin of a mutant gene is irrelevant in so far as the expression of the abnormal phenotype is concerned. Thus in an autosomal dominant disease, affected fathers or affected mothers have a 50% chance of having an affected child. There are, however, some exceptions to this rule. Chromosomes, regions of chromosomes or even specific genes can be influenced in some way during germ cell lineage so that the expression of a phenotypic abnormality depends on the parental origin of the mutant gene or genes. This is known as genomic imprinting. Genomic imprinting may be expressed in the following ways:

- **The existence of chromosome sets.** In hydatidiform mole the chromosome number is normal but there are two haploid sets of chromosome derived from the father. In ovarian teratoma, the chromosome complement is also uniparental but this time both haploid sets are derived from the mother.
- **Uniparental chromosomes.** This term describes a situation in which both copies of an individual chromosome are derived from one parent. This is difficult to establish in humans but has been documented in two cases of cystic fibrosis and short stature in which both copies of chromosome 7 were maternally derived.
- **Deletion of the same regions of either paternally or maternally derived chromosomes produces different phenotypic effects.** The classical example of genomic imprinting in human genetic disease is embodied in two disorders that are cytogenetically identical but clinically distinct. These are:

1) The Angelman syndrome
2) The Prader–Willi syndrome

Angelman syndrome ('happy puppet' syndrome) is characterized by: severe motor and intellectual retardation, ataxia, a facies with a large mandible and protruding tongue, and hypotonia. Patients with the **Prader–Willi syndrome** show neonatal hypotonia, failure to thrive, obesity, short stature and mild to moderate mental retardation. In about 50% of the cases of each of these disorders there is a deletion of part of the long arm of chromosome 15 (15q11–13). The affected region appears to be the same in both disorders. In Angelman syndrome, the deletion affects the **maternally derived** chromosome; in Prader–Willi syndrome it is the **paternally derived** chromosome that is affected.

MAJOR CHROMOSOMAL ABNORMALITIES

Chromosome abnormalities, as well as causing some very well-recognized syndromes such as Down's syndrome or Turner's syndrome, are important causes of fetal loss. Spontaneous abortion occurs in about 15–20% of all pregnancies; 50% of these abortions are associated with chromosome abnormalities. It is estimated that, overall, about 6% of human conceptions show chromosomal abnormalities.

The frequency of chromosomal abnormality is 5.6 per 1000 births. The abnormalities are of the types shown in *Table 30.2*.

ABNORMALITIES IN CHROMOSOME STRUCTURE

Most structural abnormalities in chromsomes (*Fig. 30.3*) represent breakage of chromosomes, which may be followed by:

- loss of genetic material
- rearrangement of such material

Table 30.2 Chromosomal Abnormalities at Birth

Abnormality	Frequency per 1000 births
Abnormal number of sex chromosomes	2
Abnormal number of autosomes	1.7
Structural abnormalities (deletions, translocations, etc.)	1.9

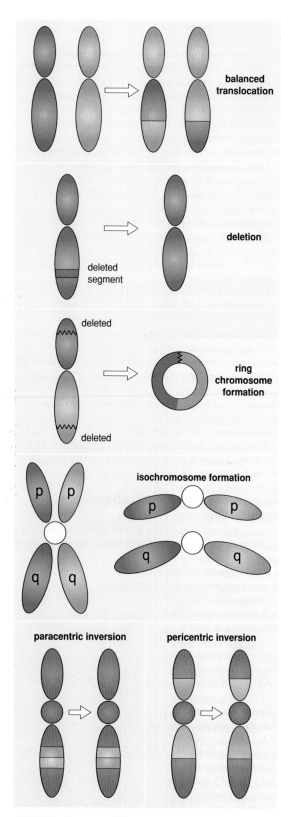

FIGURE 30.3 Structural abnormalities in chromosomes.

Deletions

This term covers the first possibility listed above in which a chromosomal break is followed by loss of the genetic material. Loss of chromosomal material cannot be seen on microscopy unless at least 4000 kb have been lost; thus visual identification of a deletion indicates the loss of a great deal of genetic material, which may have crippling effects on development or impair the chances of survival.

Deletion of the short arm of chromosome 5 produces a very characteristic syndrome of the newborn known as the **cri du chat** syndrome because of the typical mewing, kitten-like cry of affected infants. These children show:

- a round facies
- a small head (microcephaly)
- mental retardation

Ring Chromosome Formation

This results from breakages occurring at both extremes of a chromosome with fusion of the truncated ends. It should be regarded as a form of deletion. Usually there is significant loss of genetic material with serious consequences in respect of mental capacity and the chance of congenital malformation.

Translocations

In translocation, a segment broken from one chromosome is transferred to another. Different varieties include balanced and Robertsonian translocations.

Balanced Translocation

In this form segments break off from two separate chromosomes and are reciprocally transferred. As a result, no loss of genetic material occurs and the affected individual is phenotypically normal. These individuals are, however, at increased risk of producing abnormal offspring because the existence of translocated chromosomal material makes possible the formation of abnormal gametes during meiosis.

Robertsonian Translocation

This form occurs when there is a balanced translocation between two acrocentric chromosomes. The breaks usually affect a long arm in one of the chromosomes and the short arm in the other. The transfer of chromosomal material generally causes the formation of one very large chromosome and one very small one.

Isochromosome Formation

This is the end result of the loss of either a short or long arm of a chromosome and duplication of the lost material. The isochromosome consists either of two short arms or two long arms.

Inversion

This results from two breaks occurring within a single chromosome, this being followed by 180° rotation of the broken segment, which is then reincorporated into the parent chromosome. An inversion affecting only one arm of a chromosome is termed paracentric. If the breaks are on either side of the centromere, the inversion is called pericentric. Most inversions are without any phenotypic effect but may give rise to abnormal gametes.

ABNORMALITIES IN THE NUMBER OF AUTOSOMES

Such abnormalities fall into two groups:

1) **Aneuploidy**, in which the chromosome number is *not* an exact multiple of 23. Aneuploidy may be expressed in the form of one extra chromosome being present (**trisomy**) or of loss of one of a pair of chromosomes (**monosomy**). Aneuploidy may affect either autosomes or sex chromosomes. It is most commonly the result of non-disjunction of chromosomes during meiosis but can also occur as a result of delayed movement of one chromosome during anaphase so that it remains outside the nucleus (anaphase lag).

2) **Polyploidy**, in which there is an additional haploid set of chromosomes giving a total complement (69) which is a multiple of 23. This example of polyploidy (known as triploidy) is usually associated with early spontaneous abortion.

Syndromes Associated with Aneuploidy of Autosomes

Monosomy

Monosomy affecting an autosome is rare in live-born children because the amount of genetic information lost is generally too great to permit survival. Live-born children with monosomies are usually severely disabled and do not survive for long. An exception, however, is monosomy associated with chromosome 21, which is compatible with survival. It is not without interest that children with monosomy 21 develop severe respiratory difficulty when given oxygen during anaesthesia. This is believed to be related to the fact that the gene encoding superoxide dismutase (which catalyses the conversion of superoxide anion to hydrogen peroxide) is encoded on chromosome 21.

Trisomies

Down's Syndrome (Trisomy 21)

Down's syndrome is the commonest numerical chromosomal abnormality occurring in the newborn. It is also the commonest genetically determined cause of learning disability.

The overall frequency of Down's syndrome is 1 in 800 live births but this does not give a true picture of the risk which, to a considerable extent, is related to the **age** of the mother at conception. In women aged under 20 years at the time of pregnancy, the risk of Down's syndrome is 1 in 1550; in a mother who is aged 45 years or more, the risk is 1 in 28. The rate of increase in risk is very steep after the age of 35 years. Many Down's syndrome conceptions end in spontaneous abortion. In abortions occurring at 12 weeks the abortus of a mother over the age of 45 years shows a Down's syndrome karyotype in 1 in 13 cases.

Cytogenetics of Down's Syndrome Some 95% of infants with Down's syndrome show trisomy 21. This is due to non-disjunction of chromosome 21 at either the first or second meiotic division. Where the non-disjunction has taken place at the second meiotic division, the fetus carries two copies of one of the parental chromosomes 21 and one copy of the other parental chromosome 21. The cause of the non-disjunction or why it should be related to maternal age is unknown. In 95% of cases the non-disjunction affects the maternal chromosome 21.

About 4% of cases of Down's syndrome result from a Robertsonian translocation within either the maternal or paternal germ cell line (see p 308) of the long arm of chromosome 21 to either chromosome 22 or 14. Thus extra genetic material related to chromosome 21 is provided, as the fertilized ovum already contains two normal copies of chromosome 21. The translocation is present, in most cases, in the germ cell line of one of the parents and is inherited by the fetus. Because of the 'carriage' of the translocation in a parental germ cell line, there is a distinct risk that more than one child of these partners may be affected by Down's syndrome (see *Table 30.3*). In other instances the translocation occurs during formation of the gamete.

In the remaining 1% of cases of Down's syndrome, the cause is non-disjunction of chromosome 21 in the dividing cells of the zygote. Not all the cells are affected and the fetus contains some cells showing trisomy 21 and others that have the normal chromosome complement. This is known as **mosaicism.** Children with Down's syndrome in these circumstances tend to be less severely affected than when the non-disjunction occurs in the germ cell.

The clinical phenotype of Down's syndrome is summarized in *Table 30.4* (see also *Figs 30.4* and *30.5*)

Table 30.3 Risk of Recurrence of Down's Syndrome in a Parentage in which there is Translocation of the Long Arm of Chromosome 21

Translocation	Maternal carrier	Paternal carrier
14;21	15%	1%
21;22	10%	5%

Table 30.4 Clinical Features of Down's Syndrome

System affected	Clinical features
Face	The face tends to be flat with a low-bridged nose and oblique palpebral fissure and prominent epicanthic folds (hence the discarded term for Down's syndrome 'mongolism'). The mouth is often enlarged, possibly because of the enlarged protruding tongue. The tongue itself is coarsely furrowed and lacks the central groove.
Hands	There is a horizontal palmar crease, sometimes called a simian crease. The middle phalanx of the little finger is shorter than normal and, thus, the finger shows inward curving (clinodactyly).
Long bones	Long bones are shorter than normal and affected individuals are short. Abnormalities of the rib cage and pelvis may also be seen.
Cardiovascular	Approximately 40% of patients with Down's syndrome show congenital cardiac defects; these include endocardial cushion defects, atrial septal and ventricular septal defects.
Haematological	Patients with Down's syndrome show a marked increase in risk (10–20-fold) of developing acute leukaemia, which may be lymphoblastic or non-lymphoblastic.
Immune	There is an increased susceptibility to infections, especially those of the lung; the mechanism is unknown.
Central nervous system	Most individuals with Down's syndrome show a severe degree of mental retardation, the IQ being about 50. This is associated with a remarkable sweetness of disposition. Of those who survive into their forties, virtually all develop the neuropathological features of Alzheimer's disease (see pp 1138–1140). It is not without interest that the gene encoding the amyloid precursor protein found in the neuritic plaques of Alzheimer's disease is located on the long arm of chromosome 21, in the region believed to be of significance in bringing about the changes found in Down's syndrome.

Molecular Basis of Down's Syndrome   This is still not understood and probably will not be until all the genes on the long arm of chromosome 21 have been assigned correctly and the functions of their gene products worked out. The region that seems to be of functional importance in the expression of the facial, cardiac and neurological manifestations is 21q22.2 and 21q22.3. This is a large region capable of accommodating some hundreds of genes. Genes that have been assigned to this region include:

- GART, an enzyme implicated in purine metabolism
- ets-2, a proto-oncogene
- the gene coding for the cell surface receptor of interferons α and β
- the gene encoding the amyloid precursor protein implicated in Alzheimer's disease

Other Trisomies

Several other trisomies have been described. The two commonest of these, although much rarer than Down's syndrome, are trisomy 18 (Edwards' syndrome) and trisomy 13 (Patau's syndrome). Their fea-tures are summarized in *Table 30.5*. The combination of malformations in these syndromes is more severe than that in Down's syndrome, and affected infants seldom survive longer than 1 year. Many die within the first few weeks of life.

Syndromes Associated with Aneuploidy of Sex Chromosomes

Aneuploidy in respect of sex chromosomes is much commoner than that of autosomes. This group of disorders is best understood against a background of some general knowledge regarding the function and expression of sex chromosomes.

- The Y chromosome carries little genetic information other than the gene coding for testicular development (*sry* = sex-determining region on Y chromosome) and, thus, the determination of male sex.
- The X chromosome, in contrast, is large and carries abundant genetic information. Monosomy in respect of X (X0, Turner's syndrome) is certainly compatible with life but its mirror image (Y0) leads to a fetus that is not viable.

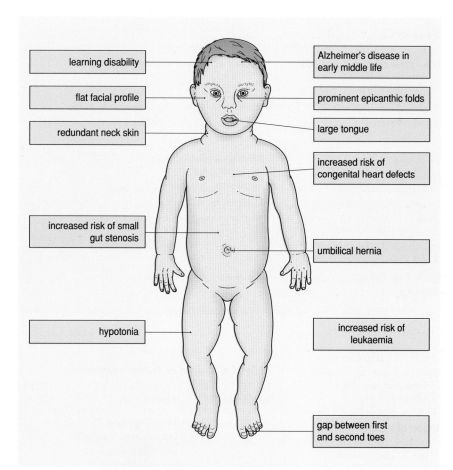

FIGURE 30.4 *Clinical features of Down's syndrome.*

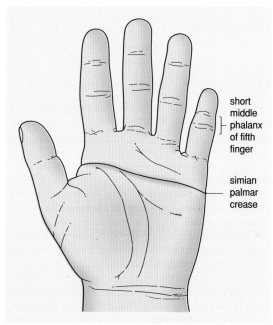

FIGURE 30.5 *The hand in Down's syndrome.*

- As the normal female possesses two X chromosomes, she would have a double dose of the genetic information carried on this large chromosome were it not for dosage compensation. This is brought about by inactivation of one X chromosome at about the 16th day of embryonic life, which occurs in every normal, eukaryotic, female, mammalian cell. This process is known as Lyonization (described by Mary Lyon in 1961). The inactivated X chromosome can be seen on examination of female cells in the form of the Barr body. This is a darkly staining small body closely apposed to the nuclear membrane. Because inactivation is random, all females are mosaics in that the X chromosomes in some cells are maternally derived, whereas those in other cells are paternally derived.
- The inactivation of one X chromosome is not total. Many genes distributed along the length of the chromosome are spared and continue to function. This is made clear in Turner's syndrome in which individuals with an X0 karyotype, and thus monosomy in respect of X, exhibit many

Table 30.5 Trisomies 18 and 13

	Edwards' syndrome (trisomy 18)	Patau's syndrome (trisomy 13)
Frequency	1 in 10 000 live births	1 in 10 000 live births
Chromosome	18: 90% due to non-disjunction; 10% due to mosaicism	13: 80% due to non-disjunction; 10% due to translocation in germ cell line; 10% associated with mosaicism
Clinical features	Mental retardation Prominent occiput Small lower jaw (micrognathia) Low set ears Short neck Overlapping fingers Congenital heart defects Kidney and intestinal defects 'Rocker-bottom feet' Hypertonicity	Small head (microcephaly) Mental retardation Small eye cavities (microphthalmia) Cleft palate and hare lip May have more than five fingers on each hand (polydactyly) Dextrocardia and, often, ventricular septal defects A variety of visceral defects

abnormalities. In the same way, the abnormalities that result from an individual having more than the normal complement of X chromosomes also indicate that inactivation is never complete.

- Inactivation of loci on one X chromosome is brought about by transcription of a gene on the X chromosome that is to be partially inactivated (this is known as acting in cis). The X-inactivation centre is localized to band 13 of the short arm of the X chromosome, and the gene that may be directly responsible for inactivation has been called the *XIST* (X-Inactive-Specific-Transcript) gene. Its exons show the presence of stop codons, suggesting that this gene does not itself produce protein. The messenger RNA transcribed from *XIST* spreads the inactivation signal to genes on the same chromosome that are capable of receiving it.

Turner's Syndrome

Turner's syndrome results from complete or partial monosomy of the X chromosome in a genotypic and phenotypic female. Several mechanisms exist through which this state of monosomy may be brought about (*Table 30.6*). The fact that distinct mechanisms exist is associated with differing phenotypic severity.

Frequency

Turner's syndrome is the commonest cause of primary amenorrhoea. The syndrome occurs in about 1 in 3000 live births. The X0 karyotype is probably much more frequent than this figure suggests, as the majority of conceptions with this karyotype end in miscarriage.

The clinical phenotype is summarized in *Table 30.7* (see also *Fig. 30.6*)

Table 30.6 Causes of Turner's Syndrome

Frequency (%)	Abnormality
53	Loss of an entire X chromosome, usually the paternally derived one. Karyotype 45X0
17	Complete deletion of the short arm (p) of the X chromosome resulting in the formation of an isochromosome of the long arm. Karyotype 46Xi(Xq)
10	Partial deletion of the short arm
20	Various abnormalities arising from mosaicism

Klinefelter's Syndrome

The defining criterion of this syndrome is the presence of more than one X chromosome in a phenotypic male. This arises most commonly on the basis of non-disjunction of the X chromosome in the mother, giving rise to the karyotype in the child of 47XXY. More rarely Klinefelter patients may have three or four X chromosomes.

Klinefelter's syndrome is both one of the commonest causes of male hypogonadism (see p 724) and one of the commonest chromosomal disorders affecting the sex chromosomes. It occurs in 1 in 600–850 live births.

Table 30.7 Clinical Features of Turner's Syndrome

Affected system	Abnormalities
General bodily appearance	Short stature, virtually never exceed 5 feet in height. Severely affected infants show peripheral lymphoedema, affecting principally the dorsum of the hands and feet. The neck is often webbed, due to distended lymphatic channels (cystic hygroma). These later resolve but the neck retains its webbed appearance. The chest is typically broad and the nipples widely spaced. The carrying angle of the forearm is usually increased (cubitus valgus). Pigmented naevi are common. The posterior hair line is low.
Cardiovascular system	There is an increased risk of: a) coarctation of the aorta b) bicuspid aortic valve and, consequently, aortic stenosis
Genitalia	Secondary sexual characteristics are poorly developed. The gonads develop as ovaries (because there is no Y chromosome), but do not reach normal size ('streak ovaries'). Both *in utero* and during the first 2 years of life, the decline in the number of primordial follicles that occurs in all females is much accelerated in girls with Turner's syndrome, so that there are no or very few oöcytes left by the age of 2 years. A writer in the *New England Journal of Medicine* has tellingly described this as the menopause occurring before the menarche.

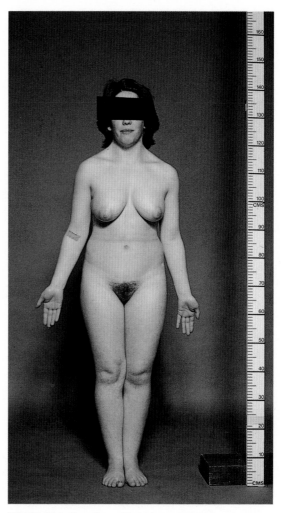

FIGURE 30.6 Turner's syndrome.

- patients have a eunuchoid appearance with a wide pelvis
- testes are atrophic and the penis small
- the distribution of body hair resembles that of the female rather than the male
- gynaecomastia may be present due because of high plasma oestradiol concentrations
- a minority of affected individuals shows some degree of learning disability

The diagnosis can be made easily by finding Barr bodies in the cells of a phenotypic male. Striking testicular changes occur which are described on p 724.

It is important to remember that the full-blown syndrome described above may not be present. Hypogonadism and infertility may be the only manifestations of Klinefelter's syndrome. Presumably because of the abnormal hormonal milieu, the risk of carcinoma of the male breast is increased in Klinefelter's syndrome.

In its fully expressed form, Klinefelter's syndrome causes a distinctive bodily appearance (*Fig. 30.7*):

- affected males are tall, most of this increased height being due to a disproportionate length of the lower limbs

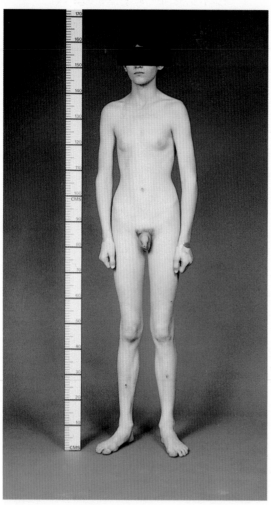

FIGURE 30.7 *Klinefelter's syndrome.*

XYY Syndrome

This syndrome occurs in about 1 in 1000 male live births. Most affected subjects appear normal but there is a tendency for them to be very tall and severely affected by acne. At one time it was suggested that the XYY syndrome was associated with aggressive behaviour and antisocial conduct. In fact only a small proportion of XYY individuals (1–2%) show such behaviour patterns.

'Superfemales': The Presence of more than Two X Chromosomes in a Phenotypic Female

This syndrome occurs in about 1 in 1200 female births. The commonest karyotype is 47XXX but cases occur in which there are increases in the X chromosome number beyond this point and, in these circumstances, there is a considerable risk of learning disability, which appears to increase in severity as the number of X chromosome increases. All individuals with a 49XXXXX karyotype are likely to suffer from learning disability.

Abnormalities of sexual development such as true and pseudohermaphroditism are discussed in a later section (see pp 724, 753–754).

CHAPTER 31

Single Gene Defects

As stated in Chapter 30, more than 4000 single gene defects have been recognized. These are caused by mutations that may affect either **autosomes** or **sex chromosomes** and which may be inherited in either a **dominant** or **recessive** pattern.

AUTOSOMAL DOMINANT DISORDERS

These are estimated to occur in 2–9 per 1000 live births. Pivotal to the concept of dominance is that a **single mutated allele is expressed despite the presence of a normal second allele**. This dictates the features of this group of disorders (*Fig. 31.1*).

KEY POINTS: *Autosomal Dominant Disorders*

- An affected individual normally has one affected parent. There are exceptions to this as mutations can occur *de novo* in the germ cell of one or other parent.
- Both heterozygotes for the mutation and homozygotes show the phenotypic abnormality. This is usually much more severe in the homozygous state (e.g. in familial hypercholesterolaemia; see pp 343–344).
- Both males and females are equally affected.
- The disorder shows itself in every generation.
- The marriage between an affected individual and a normal one confers a 1:2 risk of showing the phenotypic abnormality in each child of the marriage.

Penetrance and Expressivity

An individual inheriting a dominant mutant may be phenotypically normal. The gene is then spoken of as showing **incomplete penetrance**. For example if four-fifths of those inheriting the mutant gene are phenotypically abnormal, the gene shows 80% penetrance.

If *all* those in a sibship who inherit a mutant dominant gene show phenotypic abnormality, but there are differences in the severity of the abnormality, the gene is described as showing **variable expressivity**.

Some important autosomal dominant disorders are listed in *Table 31.1*. The values quoted in *Table 31.1* are approximations; differences in reported frequency exist. They apply to Europe only.

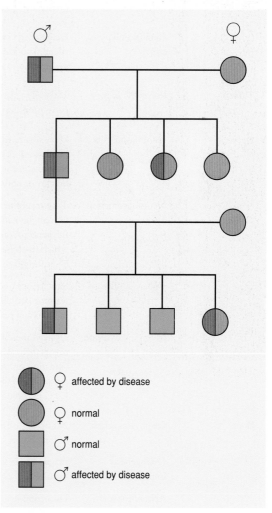

FIGURE 31.1 *Autosomal dominant inheritance pattern.*

AUTOSOMAL RECESSIVE DISORDERS

The defining criterion of an autosomal recessive disorder is that the disorder manifests only when both alleles at a given locus are mutated (*Fig. 31.2*).

The features of this group of disorders is shown in the summary box.

Table 31.1 Some Autosomal Dominant Disorders

System	Diseases	Features	Frequency per 1000 births	Text citation
Blood	Spherocytosis	Anaemia due to premature destruction of red cells	0.2	pp 893–894
Lipid metabolism	Familial hyperchole-sterolaemia	Low density lipoprotein receptor defect; premature atherosclerosis	2	pp 343–344
Large gut	Familial polyposis coli	Deletion in chromosome 5; multiple adenomatous polyps with inevitable progression to cancer	0.1	pp 284, 291, 556
Kidney	Polycystic kidney	Massively enlarged kidney with multiple cysts; progressive renal failure	1.0	pp 647–649
Nervous	Huntington's disease	Dementia in middle life associated with involuntary choreiform movements; abnormal trinucleotide repeat in gene on chromosome 4	0.2	pp 1140–1141
	Neurofibromatosis	Tumours of nerve sheaths; abnormal skin pigmentation; in type 1 deletion of the gene coding for neurofibromin, which interferes with guanosine 5′-triphosphate binding by *ras* proteins		pp 1167–1168
	Tuberous sclerosis	Skin lesions (sebaceous adenoma); learning disability; epilepsy; hamartomas in brain and heart	0.08	
	Myotonic dystrophy	Delayed muscle relaxation; cardio-myopathy; cataract; diabetes mellitus, etc. Mutation on chromosome 19 is expansion of the copies of a triplet CTG encoding a protein kinase	0.05	pp 1185–1186
Bone	Diaphyseal aclasis	Numerous cartilaginous exostoses at ends of long bones	0.5	
	Osteogenesis imperfecta	Fragile bones with increased risk of fractures	0.1	pp 1036–1037
	Achondroplasia	Dwarfism; deformity of bone; increased risk of fractures	0.04	p 1036
	Thanatophoric dwarfism	Severe skeletal deformities; early death	0.08	
Connective tissue	Marfan's syndrome	Mutation in gene encoding fibrillin on chromosome 15; long thin limbs; increased risk of aortic dissection	0.1	p 393
	Ehlers–Danlos syndromes	Variety of collagen defects giving hyperextensible joints and increased fragility of tissues	0.05	

Table 31.1 Some Autosomal Dominant Disorders – *continued*

System	Diseases	Features	Frequency per 1000 births	Text citation
Ear	Otosclerosis	Deafness occurring from time of adolescence onwards; changes in ossicles of middle ear	3.0	p 1207
	Dominant early childhood deafness	Deafness from infancy	0.1	
Eye	Dominant blindness	Blindness	0.1	
Teeth	Dentinogenesis imperfecta	Abnormal development of teeth	0.1	
Porphyrin metabolism	Acute intermittent porphyria	Acute abdominal pain and neurological disturbances; dark urine due to presence of porphobilinogen	0.01	

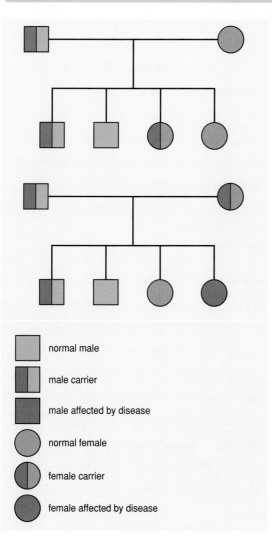

normal male

male carrier

male affected by disease

normal female

female carrier

female affected by disease

KEY POINTS: *Autosomal Recessive Disorders*
- Probands must be homozygous for the mutation.
- The affected individual must have phenotypically normal parents.
- Each parent must be heterozygous for the mutant gene (a carrier).
- Males and females are equally affected.
- One in four of an affected sibship will show the phenotypic abnormality.
- The disorder does not occur in every generation.
- Enzyme proteins are frequently affected.
- Penetrance is commonly complete.

Some common autosomal recessive disorders are listed in *Table 31.2*.

X-LINKED DISORDERS

Sex-linked disorders are all related to mutations within the X chromosome. With a few exceptions, the inheritance pattern in these disorders is recessive (*Fig. 31.3*).

Y chromosome genes are not homologous with those of the X chromosome and thus any deficiency in the male's X chromosome is not counterbalanced by production of normal amounts of normal gene product by the Y chromosome. Thus recessive mutations on the X chromosome are, for all practical purposes, expressed only in males.

If an affected male has children, all his daughters will be carriers of the mutant gene and all his sons will be both genotypically and phenotypically normal.

FIGURE 31.2 (left) Autosomal recessive inheritance pattern.

Table 31.2 Some Important Autosomal Recessive Disorders

Disorder	Features	Frequency per 1000 births	Text citation
Cystic fibrosis	Defect in chloride transportation due to mutation of gene on chromosome 7; viscid secretions, recurrent lung infections, failure to thrive	0.5–0.6	pp 641–642
Congenital deafness	Deafness from infancy	0.5	
Sickle cell disease	Point mutation on chromosome 6; valine substituted for glutamic acid in haemoglobin; haemolytic anaemia	0.1	pp 896–898
Adrenal hyperplasia	Enzyme deficiency leading to block in cortisol synthesis; precocious development of genitalia in males; virilism in females; may have addisonian crises	0.1	pp 240, 839
Phenylketonuria	Learning disability due to accumulation of intermediates of phenylalanine metabolism	0.2–0.5	
α_1-Antitrypsin deficiency	Chronic liver disease which may present in infancy; emphysema	0.1–0.5	pp 599–600
Recessive blindness	Blindness	0.1	
Cystinuria	Recurrent renal calculi	0.06	p 698
Tay–Sachs disease	Learning disability and blindness; occurs in Ashkenazi Jews; carrier state can be detected by screening	0.004	
Mucopolysaccharidoses	Accumulation of intermediates in macrophages leading to visceromegaly; mental retardation in some disorders	0.03	p 983
β-Thalassaemia	Anaemia; bone deformities; enlarged spleen	0.05	pp 901–903
Galactosaemia	Chronic liver disease starting in infancy and leading to cirrhosis and liver failure	0.02	pp 606–607
Homocystinuria	Learning disability; eye, bone and blood vessel abnormalities	0.01	
Metachromatic leucodystrophy	Defect in long-chain fatty acid metabolism; blindness; intellectual deterioration	0.02	p 1177
Friedreich's ataxia	Early onset of progressive unsteadiness and dysarthria; skeletal deformities, cardiomyopathy in some cases. Abnormal numbers of copies of triplet GAA in gene X25 on chromosome 9	0.02	p 1136
Spinal muscular atrophy	Progressive muscle weakness	0.04	p 1137
Wilson's disease	Involuntary athetoid movements and chronic liver disease associated with abnormal deposition of copper in basal ganglia and liver		pp 597–599
Some varieties of Ehlers–Danlos syndrome	Various collagen abnormalities; hyperextensible joints and fragility of connective tissues		
Neurogenic muscular atrophy	Progressive muscle weakness	0.01	

Some important X-linked disorders are listed in *Table 31.3*.

The Fragile X Syndrome

This is characterized by:

- severe learning disability occurring principally in males, although some 30–50% of female carriers show some degree of intellectual impairment
- a long face with prominent and everted ears
- large testes

This clinical picture is associated with a non-staining gap on the long arm of the X chromosome (Xq27.3). Special media are required for cell culture before this site shows up on microscopic examination.

Fragile X syndrome is the commonest cause of inherited learning disability, with a frequency of 1 in 1500 males and 1 in 2000 females.

The inheritance pattern originally suggested that this syndrome was inherited as an X-linked dominant syndrome in which penetrance is incomplete. This is an oversimplification: **phenotypically normal males can transmit the condition, not to their children but to their grandchildren**. This strange pattern has given rise to the concept of a **premutation** which needs processing through female meiosis before it can be expressed.

It is now believed that **mutation of a gene known as *FMR-1* is responsible for the fragile X syndrome. In affected individuals the striking abnormality in the *FMR-1* gene is an excess number of copies of the trinucleotide CGG** (which codes for arginine) in one of the 5′ exons of the gene. In normal individuals the median number of copies of this sequence is 30 (range 6–54).

Table 31.3 Some Important X-linked Disorders

Disorder	Features	Frequency per 1000 male births	Text citation
Fragile X syndrome	Learning disability; characteristic facies; large testes	0.9	pp 319–320
Muscular dystrophy (Duchenne and Becker type)	Progressive muscular weakness more severe in Duchenne type and leading to death in the third decade; complete or partial deletion of the gene encoding dystrophin	0.3	pp 1184–1185
Haemophilia A	Excessive post-traumatic bleeding due to lack of clotting factor VIII	0.1	pp 921–922
Haemophilia B	Abnormal bleeding due to deficiency of clotting factor IX	0.1	p 922
Ichthyosis	Thick skin with excessive keratin due to deficiency of a sulphatase	0.1	
Glucose-6-phosphate dehydrogenase deficiency	Haemolysis following ingestion of certain drugs		pp 895–896
X-linked agammaglobulinaemia	Increased susceptibility to infection		
Red–green colour blindness		8	
Diabetes insipidus			p 833
Lesch–Nyhan syndrome			p 1088
Childhood blindness	Blindness	0.02	

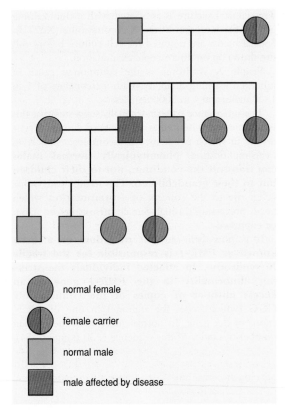

normal female

female carrier

normal male

male affected by disease

FIGURE 31.3 X-linked recessive inheritance pattern.

Phenotypically normal transmitting males and normal female carriers (those with the presumed premutation) have between 60 and 200 copies of the CGG sequence. This number remains stable in the course of male meiosis but **female meiosis leads to a very great expansion of the number of copies** and the development of full-blown fragile X syndrome in the sons and daughters of transmitting females. The presence of more than 140 repeats in the carrier indicates a very high risk of the syndrome developing. The fragile X syndrome itself is associated with increases of the copy number of CGG, ranging from 250 to 4000.

Other X-linked Disorders

Other inherited disorders characterized by excess copies of trinucleotide sequences include Huntington's disease (see pp 1140–1141) and myotonic dystrophy (see pp 1185–1186).

X-linked dominant disorders are very rare indeed. They include vitamin D-resistant rickets (see p 1045) in which abnormally large amounts of phosphate are lost in the urine and the bone is inadequately mineralized. The abnormal gene is expressed in both males and females (who receive it from affected heterozygous mothers). Fathers with this gene defect can transmit it only to their daughters.

MUTATIONS IN SINGLE GENE DEFECTS

Single gene defects may arise on the basis of the following.

GENE DELETIONS

An example of the effects of deletion of an entire gene is α-thalassaemia (see pp 899–901). Normal individuals have two α-globin genes. If one of these is deleted, there is reduced production of α-globin chains and an excess in haemoglobin of β-globin chains (HbH disease). If both α-globin genes are deleted, the fetus cannot make fetal haemoglobin and instead produces haemoglobin Barts, which has virtually no oxygen-carrying capacity. The condition hydrops fetalis is produced, leading to stillbirth or neonatal death. The deletion of a single α-globin gene results from unequal crossing over between homologous chromosomes 16 during meiosis.

PARTIAL GENE DELETION

If part of a gene is deleted some protein may still be encoded by the remnant even if this protein is grossly abnormal. This situation is exemplified by the X-linked muscular dystrophies of the Duchenne and Becker types. Both of these are caused by mutation in the dystrophin gene. This is the largest gene so far identified; it spans more than 2500 kilobases of genomic DNA and accounts for 1% of the whole X chronosome.

Duchenne-type disease is the more severe of the two. This has been ascribed to the fact that the partial deletion in Duchenne-type disease interrupts the reading frame as the deletion causes an **intracodon break**, thus creating a new reading frame to the 3' end of the messenger RNA (mRNA). Most deletions seen in the less severe Becker-type disease leave the reading frame intact by removing an entire codon or group of codons.

CODON DELETION

If a codon or a small set of codons is deleted, the reading frame will not be altered but the protein product of the affected gene will be deficient in one or more amino acids. This is known to occur in several haemoglobin variants, most of which involve the β-globin chain.

An important example of codon deletion is to be found in cystic fibrosis (see pp 641–642), in which the commonest mutation is the deletion of three nucleotides, CTT, from exon 10 of the gene encoding a chloride transporter (the cystic fibrosis transmembrane conductance regulator).

DUPLICATIONS AND INSERTIONS

While unequal crossing over during meiosis may lead to deletion of whole genes or parts of genes, it can also lead to duplications of genetic material. The effects of such duplications depends on whether disruption of the reading frame occurs or not. In the latter case there is little if any effect.

FUSION MUTATIONS

Unequal crossing over between non-homologous genes can result in the formation of fusion genes. The commonest example of this is in red–green colour blindness, which is quite common in males.

There are three pigment genes in humans:
- a blue pigment gene on chromosome 7
- red and green pigment genes situated contiguously at the tip of the X chromosome

Green colour blindness is about three times as common as red colour blindness. There are several mutational events leading to colour blindness. One is the formation of fusion genes consisting of parts of each of the red and green pigment genes. This results from unequal crossing over of these genes in the course of meiosis.

POINT MUTATIONS

Point mutation is defined as the **substitution of one base pair by another in double-stranded DNA**. If a purine is substituted for a purine, or a pyrimidine by a pyrimidine, the process is termed **transition**. If a purine is replaced by a pyrimidine, or vice versa, the process is termed **transversion**. Theoretically substitution of a base pair should lead to the encoding of a different amino acid. However, because of the degeneracy of the genetic code (see *Tables 31.4* and *31.5*) about one-third of all point mutations are not associated with an alteration in the encoded gene product.

Each amino acid is specified by the codon (triplet of nucleotides) in the mRNA molecule binding with three complementary nucleotides (anticodon) at the tip of a particular transfer RNA molecule.

RNA is composed of four nucleotides. Thus there must be 64 possible sequences, as shown in *Table 31.4*. Three of these sequences specify the termination of a polypeptide chain rather than coding for an amino acid. These three are known as stop codons. The remainder code for only 20 amino acids. Thus most amino acids are specified for by more than one codon (with the exceptions of methionine and tryptophan, which can be specified by only one codon each).

Point mutations may be divided into a number of different classes.

Missense Mutation

This is defined as a base substitution leading to the encoding of a different amino acid from that normally specified by the codon. Not all missense mutations have pathological consequences.

Table 31.4 The Genetic Code (mRNA Bases)

1st position (5′ end)	2nd position U	2nd position C	2nd position A	2nd position G	3rd position (3′ end)
U	Phe	Ser	Tyr	Cys	U
	Phe	Ser	Tyr	Cys STOP	C
	Leu	Ser	STOP	Trp	A
	Leu	Ser	STOP		G
C	Leu	Pro	His	Arg	U
	Leu	Pro	His	Arg	C
	Leu	Pro	Gln	Arg	A
	Leu	Pro	Gln	Arg	G
A	Ile	Thr	Asn	Ser	U
	Ile	Thr	Asn	Ser	C
	Ile	Thr	Lys	Arg	A
	Met*	Thr	Lys	Arg	G
G	Val	Ala	Asp	Gly	U
	Val	Ala	Asp	Gly	C
	Val	Ala	Glu	Gly	A
	Val	Ala	Glu	Gly	G

*AUG = a start codon for protein translation.

Table 31.5 Amino Acids, their Symbols, Abbreviations and Codons

Amino acid	Abbreviation	Symbol	Codons
Alanine	Ala	A	GCA, GCC, GCG, GCU
Cysteine	Cys	C	UGC, UGU
Aspartic acid	Asp	D	GAC, GAU
Glutamic acid	Glu	E	GAA, GAG
Phenylalanine	Phe	F	UUC, UUU
Glycine	Gly	G	GGA, GGC, GGG, GGU
Histidine	His	H	CAC, CAU
Isoleucine	Ile	I	AUA, AUC, AUU
Lysine	Lys	K	AAA, AAG
Leucine	Leu	L	UUA, UUG, CUA, CUC, CUG, CUU
Methionine	Met	M	AUG
Asparagine	Asn	N	AAC, AAU
Proline	Pro	P	CCA, CCC, CCG, CCU
Glutamine	Gln	Q	CAA, CAG
Arginine	Arg	R	AGA, AGG, CGA, CGC, CGG, CGU
Serine	Ser	S	AGC, AGU, UCA, UCC, UCG, UCU
Threonine	Thr	T	ACA, ACC, ACG, ACU
Valine	Val	V	GUA, GUC, GUG, GUU
Tryptophan	Trp	W	UGG
Tyrosine	Tyr	Y	UAC, UAU

Important examples of such mutations include:
- Sickle cell disease, in which GAG (encoding **glutamic acid**) in codon 6 of the β-globin gene is changed to CTG, which specifies the neutral and hydrophobic amino acid **valine** (see pp 896–899).
- α₁-antitrypsin deficiency, in which GAG (glutamic acid) in exon V of the gene is changed to AAG (lysine) at position 342 of the protein. The resulting protein is processed abnormally within liver cells and secreted only with difficulty by them. It is also not as effective as the more common M protein at combating neutrophil elastase.

Nonsense Mutations

A nonsense mutation is one that converts a codon specifying an amino acid to a **stop codon**. The nearer the 5′ end of the gene the mutation occurs, the greater will be the degree of truncation of the protein product.

A nonsense mutation in the second exon of the β-globin gene is one of the common causes of β-thalassaemia. A stop codon is produced in place of the mRNA specifying glutamic acid. This leads to a virtual absence of β-globin chains. Several nonsense mutations are also known to exist in the gene encoding Factor VIII in respect of haemophilia A. Patients whose haemophilia is caused by nonsense mutations are prone to develop antibodies to the human Factor VIII with which they are treated; presumably they produce no endogenous Factor VIII and thus recognize the Factor VIII given to them as 'foreign'.

Stop Codon Mutations

This is the exact opposite of a nonsense mutation in that it involves conversion of a stop codon into one encoding an amino acid. This is seen in one of the haemoglobinopathies, Haemoglobin Constant Spring, in which the normal stop codon found at position 142 on the α-globin gene (UAA) is altered to CAA, which encodes glutamine. The result is an unstable haemoglobin that is associated with the α-thalassaemia trait.

Frameshift Mutations

Frameshifts can occur as a result of point mutations as well as via partial gene deletions. Such frameshifts occur when either insertion or deletion of a single nucleotide disturbs the reading frame so that a new set of codons is specified near the 3′ end of the gene.

RNA Splice Mutations

Once transcription has occurred, the original product must have its introns removed for mRNA to be produced in a form suitable for translation. Most normal genes have a dinucleotide GT sequence at the 5′ end of the intron (this is called the **donor site**) and an AG dinucleotide at the 3′ end of the intron (the **acceptor site**). Mutations in the genomic DNA that alter either of these sites cause disturbances in normal splicing and the resulting mRNA is abnormal and non-functional. Several different splicing mutations have been described in the β-thalassaemias. If these mutations are homozygous, no β-globin chains are produced.

Consensus Sequence Mutations

Splicing defects can also occur as a result of mutations in consensus sequences. These are nucleotide sequences at the borders between introns and exons and, at the donor site, include the last three triplets in the preceding exon and the first six in the intron. At the acceptor site they consist of the last ten triplets of the intron and the first triplet of the exon. Several mutations in consensus sequences with consequent defects in splicing have been described in β-thalassaemia phenotypes.

Mutations leading to splicing defects can also occur in introns well away from consensus regions. These create new acceptor sites and thus alter splicing.

Transcriptional Mutations

Blocks of DNA upstream from the 5′ end of a gene play a significant part in regulating transcription of the gene. Several point mutations have been described in these promoter regions in relation to β-thalassaemia phenotypes.

MITOCHONDRIAL DISORDERS

The general characteristics of mitochondrial inherited disorders were described in the introduction to this section.

Examples of mitochondrial inherited disorders include:

KEY POINTS: Mitochondrial Genetics

- Each mitochondrion contains several copies of a circular chromosome made up of a rather small amount of DNA.
- Mitochondrial DNA encodes a number of protein components of the respiratory chain and oxidative phosphorylation system as well as some special types of RNA.
- The genome contains two RNA genes, 22 transfer RNA genes and 13 protein-coding sequences.
- The genetic code in mitochondria differs is some respects from that which in universal in all other organisms.
- Inheritance of mitochondrial genes in humans occurs entirely through the maternal line.
- Mitochondrial DNA has a high rate of mutations and the normal population shows considerable variation in respect of mitochondrial genes.

- Leber's hereditary optic atrophy. This is characterized by late-onset bilateral loss of central vision and by disturbances in heart rhythm.
- Myoclonus with ragged red fibres (see pp 1187–1188).
- Mitochondrial myopathy with encephalopathy, lactic acidosis and stroke (see pp 1187–1188).
- The Kearns–Sayre syndrome, in which there is paralysis of external ocular muscles (ophthalmoplegia), complete heart block, and pigmentary degeneration of the retina.

SYSTEMIC
PATHOLOGY

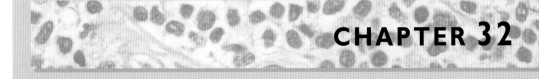

CHAPTER 32

The Cardiovascular System

Disorders of Blood Vessels

THE ARTERIES: ATHEROSCLEROSIS

In economically privileged populations such as those of Western Europe and North America, the process responsible for more deaths than any other is **athero-sclerosis**.

The term atherosclerosis is derived from two Greek words: *athere*, the literal meaning of which is gruel or porridge, and *sclerosis*, which means a hardening. On naked eye examination, most fully developed atherosclerotic lesions contain a region, situated deep within the arterial intima, that is soft, semi-fluid and yellow.

DEFINITIONS

In **morphological** terms, atherosclerosis can be defined as a disorder in which there are **focal lesions confined to large elastic and muscular arteries such as the aorta and the epicardial coronary, femoral and carotid arteries. Small arteries with a diameter of less than 300 μm are *not* affected.**

The lesions are focal areas of intimal thickening which consist of:

1) Collagen and matrix-rich connective tissue, forming a fibrous **'cap'** which lies immediately beneath the arterial endothelium.

2) Intraintimal accumulations of lipid derived largely from the plasma.

3) A basal zone or **'pool'** of necrosis that is rich in lipid. This varies in size from plaque to plaque. Within a plaque, the relative proportions of the connective tissue cap and the basal lipid-rich pool have important implications for the natural history of the lesion. Plaques in which the basal pool is of massive proportions and is separated from the artery lumen by a thin sheet of connective tissue are prone to undergo intimal injury followed, very often but not inevitably, by thrombosis.

This morphological definition emphasizes certain key features:

- The **focal distribution** of the lesions, which is governed by a set of complex haemodynamic factors.
- The predominantly **intimal** involvement of the artery wall.
- The **complexity** of individual atherosclerotic lesion and the **heterogeneity** existing within a plaque population.

Clinical effects depend on **four** mechanisms, which are outlined in *Table 32.1* and depicted in *Fig. 32.1*.

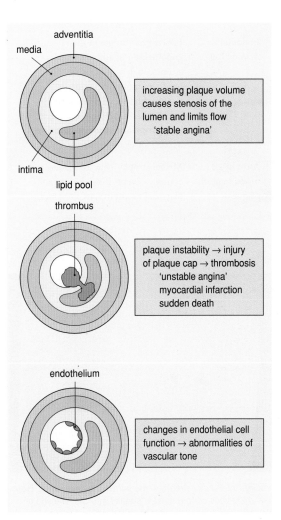

FIGURE 32.1 The effects of atherosclerosis.

Table 32.1 The Four Mechanisms Involved in the Development of Atherosclerosis

Mechanism	Event
Plaque volume	The primary processes involved in atherogenesis (lipid accumulation and connective tissue matrix production by smooth muscle cells) may cause plaque volume to become so great (> 75% of cross-sectional area of lumen) as to interfere with blood flow through the affected segment. This process is usually slow and leads to chronic symptoms such as **stable angina**.
Thrombosis	Injury to the plaque cap leads to thrombosis. Major episodes lead to **unstable angina, myocardial infarction** or **sudden death**.
Endothelial dysfunction	Functional changes in the endothelium of atherosclerotic arteries, such as inadequate production of nitric oxide or overproduction of endothelin 1, lead to abnormalities of tone so that **inappropriate vasoconstriction** occurs, for example on exercise.
Atrophy of media beneath plaque	Medial atrophy beneath plaques is a common event. If this is severe it may lead to **aneurysm** formation.

MORPHOLOGY OF ATHEROSCLEROSIS

FATTY STREAKS

The first macroscopically visible lesion is the **fatty streak**. This occurs early in life: some 40% of infants coming to necropsy between the ages of 1 month and 1 year show some degree of fatty streaking. Fatty streaking in the very young does *not* correlate with race, geographical location or, most importantly, with the prevalence of ischaemic heart disease.

Macroscopic Features

The fatty streak starts as a small yellowish dot about 1–2 mm in diameter, slightly raised above the surface of the surrounding intima. These dots occur in rows lying roughly parallel to the direction of blood flow and coalesce to form streaks along the long axes of the affected vessels.

In the young, fatty streaks tend to be concentrated in the arch and upper part of the ascending aorta in a 'fan-shaped' distribution, which narrows after 5–7 cm. From then, the streaks are concentrated along the posterior wall of the aorta (*Fig. 32.2*). Distal to the region where the main visceral branches arise, the pattern changes and the entire circumference of the aorta becomes involved in an apparently haphazard fashion.

Streak lesions are most conspicuous just above the mouths of the intercostal vessels whereas the curved and sharp-edged 'flow divider' region of these branch openings is spared. A similar distribution pattern occurs in hyperlipidaemic animals, as long as the cholesterol concentrations in the blood are in a 'steady state'. The determining factor for this localization of the fatty streaks appears to be the wall shear rate (the velocity gradient between the layers of blood in contact with and near to the artery wall). In regions where the wall shear rates are low, the intima is thickened and there appears to be a predilection for lipid deposition. The reverse holds for those areas (such as the flow-divider) where wall shear rates are high.

Microscopic Features

The lesions show mild, local intimal thickening associated with fat droplets, easily stainable with fat-soluble dyes in frozen sections. Most of this fat is intracellular, although some extracellular lipid may be sprinkled along the course of the internal elastic lamina that separates the intima from the muscular tunica media.

The cell population of the fatty streak is characterized by appropriate monoclonal antibody staining, which marks specifically either smooth muscle cells or macrophages, and by electron microscopy. **The major cellular component of the fatty streak is a**

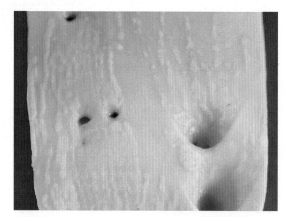

FIGURE 32.2 *Fatty streaks in the aorta of a young adult. Note how the lesions are arranged in parallel with the direction of blood flow and the concentration of lesions seen in the proximal part of the ostia of branches.*

monocyte-derived macrophage, which enters the arterial intima from the blood. The cytoplasm of the macrophages is distended by many droplets of lipid which are engulfed by these cells once they are within the intima and from which the term 'foam cell' is derived (*Figs. 32.3* and *32.4*). The other cell that is present is the arterial smooth muscle cell, which can be recognized on electron microscopy by the presence of a partial basal lamina and so-called 'dense bodies', which are the homologue of the Z bands seen in other muscle cells. The activities of these two cell types is fundamental to the genesis and progression of atherosclerosis and is discussed in a later section dealing with pathogenesis.

Progression of Fatty Streak to Fibrolipid Plaque: Does it Occur?

Most evidence supports the view that there is a progression from the fatty streak to the raised plaque but it is important to realize that this is *not* an inevitable progression and many fatty streaks either do not progress further or may undergo regression (see pp 336, 344). Progression from the fatty streak stage may be more likely to occur in individuals exposed to a set of unfavourable environmental factors.

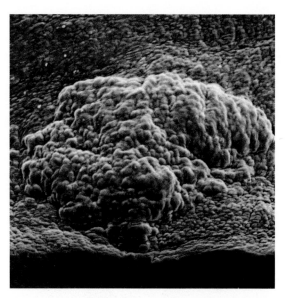

FIGURE 32.4 *Scanning electron micrograph of a fatty 'dot' in a human coronary artery. The lesion shows a subendothelial 'hump' (consisting of fat-filled macrophages) covered by intact endothelium.*

GELATINOUS LESIONS

Some have suggested that precursor of mature atherosclerotic plaques is the 'gelatinous lesion'.

Macroscopic and Microscopic Features

This is a small, translucent, blister-like, intimal elevation. Histological examination shows focal oedema only. Little if any stainable fat is present and is extracellular. There is an increased concentration within the affected areas of the intima of certain plasma proteins, most notably fibrinogen and albumin. Treatment of samples of such lesions with plasmin yields fibrin degradation products that are chemotactic for monocytes and can act as mitogenic signals for smooth muscle.

THE FIBROLIPID PLAQUE (RAISED LESION)

The fibrolipid plaque is the archetypal lesion of atherosclerosis, and its complications, most notably plaque fissuring, are the basis of the majority of cases of occlusive arterial disease.

Unlike the fatty streak, the extent of intimal involvement by fibrolipid plaques predicts the frequency and severity of clinical syndromes such as ischaemic heart disease, stroke and limb ischaemia in a given population. In addition, factors associated with an increased risk of these syndromes, such as hypertension, hyperlipidaemia, diabetes mellitus and cigarette smoking, are also associated with more extensive and severe involvement of the arterial tree by raised lesions.

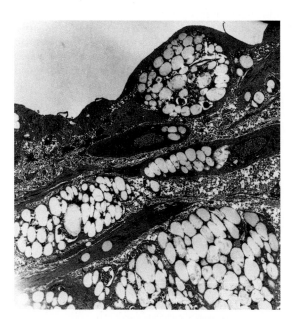

FIGURE 32.3 *Transmission electron micrograph through a fatty streak in a rabbit aorta. The endothelial surface is somewhat distorted by subendothelial aggregates of macrophages, the cytoplasm of which is distended by lipid droplets.*

MORPHOLOGICAL FEATURES

All raised lesions have the same two morphological elements:

- **a subendothelial connective tissue cap**
- **the 'atheromatous' basal pool** (*Fig. 32.5*)

Many morphological variants exist which either express differences in the relative proportions of the cap and the pool or relate to the presence of intimal injury and thrombosis. If the cap is thick, the plaque surface is a pearly white colour and is firm to the touch. If, on the other hand, the pool is large and the cap thin, the carotenoid pigment in the lipid gives the lesion a yellow colour and the plaque will be soft and easily deformable. **On this basis plaques may be classified as either 'fibrous' or 'lipid'.**

Lipid and Fibrous Plaques

The fibrous cap in an uninjured plaque consists of thick bands of collagen in which variable numbers of smooth muscle cells and macrophages can be identified. The use of monoclonal antibodies shows also the presence of variable numbers of T lymphocytes. Beneath this cap lies the atheromatous pool consisting of abundant lipid, mostly extracellular, and tissue debris. The margins of the pool usually show numerous lipid-filled macrophages. In some instances the lipid-rich pool is crisscrossed by strands of collagen forming a lattice between the underside of the plaque cap and the connective tissue beneath the pool. In others, no such lattice is present, the pool being a cavity filled with material which is semi-fluid at normal body temperatures. **This second type of pool is highly deformable by changes in haemodynamic circumstances and is strongly correlated with the risk of plaque fissuring and consequent thrombosis** (*Fig. 32.6*). Dystrophic calcification in the affected regions of the intima is common. This calcification is probably not of major patho-physiological significance, though occasional cracks may appear *in vivo* in relation to plates of calcium.

Eccentric and Concentric Plaques

A further important morphological feature is whether atherosclerosis involves the whole of the circumference of the affected arterial segment of artery (a **concentric** plaque) or only part of the circumference (an **eccentric** plaque) (see *Fig. 32.5a and b*). In concentric plaques, the media is splinted and alterations in muscle tone and hence in calibre are difficult to achieve. Eccentric plaque formation leaves part of the circumference of the arterial segment unaffected and, here, the media can

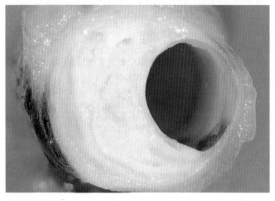

a

plaques are classified on the basis of:

- proportion of circumference of artery wall involved
  - all = concentric   • part = eccentric
- whether a large lipid pool is present or not
  - lipid-rich   • fibrous

concentric fibrous   concentric lipid

eccentric fibrous   eccentric lipid

b

FIGURE 32.5 **a** *Types of atherosclerotic plaque.* **b** *Eccentric coronary artery plaque showing sparing of part of the circumference of the artery wall.*

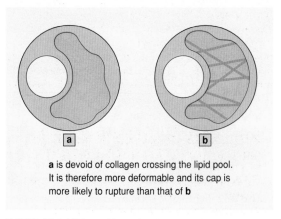

a is devoid of collagen crossing the lipid pool. It is therefore more deformable and its cap is more likely to rupture than that of **b**

FIGURE 32.6 High- and low-risk eccentric coronary artery plaques.

respond to vasomotor signals such as nitric oxide and various locally released neuropeptides.

About 12% of all the atherosclerotic plaques in the coronary arteries are both eccentric and lipid rich. Despite being in a minority, it is these lesions that are most commonly associated with acute thrombotic events.

In summary, the morphological and cytological features that correlate with a high risk of clinically significant thrombosis are:

- eccentric plaque
- large lipid-rich basal pool
- large population of macrophages
- small population of smooth muscle cells in the cap

MEDIAL CHANGES

The presence of raised intimal lesions is often associated with a marked degree of atrophy of the tunica media underlying the plaque and, when arterial samples are fixed at a pressure equal to the systolic blood pressure, plaques may bulge outwards into the atrophic media rather than inwards into the lumen. The internal elastic lamina beneath the plaque is often disrupted, with the broken ends of this thick sheet of elastic visible at the plaque margins. Medial atrophy makes it impossible to assess the **size** of an atherosclerotic plaque on angiography although it is, of course, possible to assess the **degree of stenosis** of the lumen.

ADVENTITIAL CHANGES IN RELATION TO ATHEROSCLEROSIS

In the underlying adventitia, new small vessels bud off from the vasa vasorum, and this vascularization may be sufficiently pronounced to be visible as a localized 'blush' on the adventitial surface beneath plaques. This plexus of new vessels fills readily on angiography, and may provide some small degree of collateral flow in segments where there is high-grade stenosis.

In addition, the adventitia may show a florid infiltrate of lymphocytes, plasma cells and monocytes–macrophages. This inflammatory reaction probably represents a local immune response to the presence of oxidized lipoprotein diffusing outwards from the basal pool. The free radical-mediated modification of the lipoprotein leads to the low density lipoprotein (LDL) molecule being perceived as 'foreign' by the immune system.

PROCESSES INVOLVED IN PLAQUE GENESIS AND NATURAL HISTORY

In terms of **process** (*Fig. 32.7*) rather than morphology, atherosclerosis results from:

1) **Excess infiltration and/or retention of cholesterol-rich, plasma-derived lipid within the arterial intima.**

2) **connective tissue (smooth muscle) cell proliferation associated with the synthesis and secretion of large amounts of collagen fibres and matrix proteins. This leads to the formation of the connective tissue cap.**

3) **necrosis of the cells, fibres and matrix at the plaque base, leading to the formation of the basal pool.**

INTIMAL LIPID ACCUMULATION AND FOAM CELL FORMATION

The artery wall normally contains a considerable amount of lipid, which increases with normal growth and ageing.

Atherosclerotic lesions of all types contain far more lipid than the normal arterial intima; for example, fatty streaks contain nearly nine times as much lipid as lesion-free aortic intima in children and adolescents, and four to five times as much as adult arterial intima. Between 65 and 80% of this intralesional lipid is cholesterol, the ratio of esterified : free cholesterol being high (about 3.5 : 1).

Lipid enters the arterial intima from the blood in the form of intact LDL, which has the

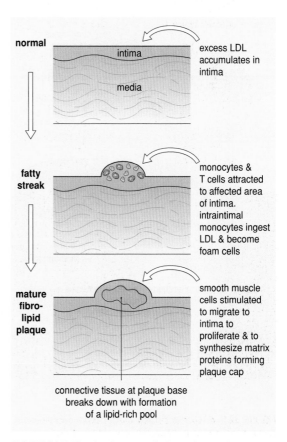

FIGURE 32.7 The development of atherosclerotic plaques.

highest cholesterol content of the lipoprotein classes. LDL within the arterial intima can be demonstrated immunohistochemically or by immunoelectrophoresis. As a result of haemodynamic factors, LDL accumulates preferentially in areas of the intima where lesions are most common. The concentration of intralesional LDL correlates positively with plasma concentrations of cholesterol and LDL in life.

The Fate of LDL within the Artery Wall

Most of the foam cells in atherosclerotic plaques are macrophages; their lipid content is derived from the LDL that enters the intima from the blood. More than 60% of LDL catabolism takes place via the LDL receptor pathway; the receptors are sites within coated pits in the plasma membranes of a number of cell types, most notably hepatocytes.

Evidence suggests that the formation of intimal foam cells does not make use of this pathway:

1) Foam cell formation occurs even in the absence of LDL receptors.

2) Macrophages fail to recognize native LDL.

3) Macrophages avidly bind and endocytose LDL that has been modified oxidatively.

If LDL is incubated in the presence of cultured macrophages, arterial endothelial cells or arterial smooth muscle cells, it undergoes important modifications:

1) LDL acquires the ability to bind to receptors on the macrophage known as scavenger receptors and, as a consequence, undergoes endocytosis. The

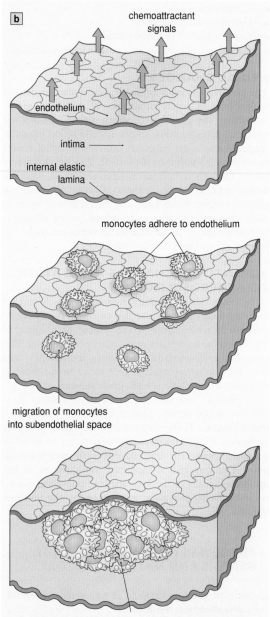

FIGURE 32.8 **a** LDL modification within the arterial intima and its functional effects. **b** Interaction between vessel wall and monocytes in fatty streak formation.

macrophages become distended by the large amounts of ingested LDL, becoming typical **foam cells**.

2) The LDL molecule becomes a chemoattractant for blood monocytes.

3) The LDL molecule causes monocytes entering the affected area of intima to lose much of their motility and thus to remain for long periods within the intima.

4) The LDL molecule becomes toxic for endothelial cells in culture.

These functional changes are due to peroxidation of polyunsaturated fatty acids as a result of free radical generation by endothelial cells and/or monocytes and macrophages. This is shown by the fact that **the effects of the incubation of LDL mentioned above are blocked if anti-oxidants are added to the *in vitro* system**.

Both the lipid and protein portions of the molecule undergo modification (*Fig. 32.8a* and *b*). In the lipid portion, lecithin is converted to lysolecithin, which is chemoattractant and cytotoxic. In the course of peroxidation of polyunsaturated fatty acids, a class of biologically active compounds – the **alkenals** – is generated. Alkenals interact with lysine residues of apoprotein B_{100}, the main carrier protein of LDL, and alters them in such as way **as to render the whole molecule recognizable by the scavenger receptor system of macrophages and by the host's immune system as no longer having the characteristics of 'self' antigen**.

Strong evidence supports the view that this sequence of events occurs during atherogenesis:

1) Treatment of hyperlipidaemic rabbits with the anti-oxidant probucol inhibits the development of fatty streaks, even though the compound has little effect on plasma cholesterol concentrations.

2) An inverse correlation exists between coronary heart disease risk and dietary intake of anti-oxidants.

CONNECTIVE TISSUE PROLIFERATION IN ATHEROGENESIS

Without a marked increase in intimal connective tissue, atherosclerotic plaques could not narrow the arterial lumen (*Figs 32.9* and *32.10*). The cell responsible for the striking growth of the intima both in atherogenesis and many other forms of arterial injury is the arterial **smooth muscle cell**.

The Intimal Smooth Muscle Cell can Exist in One or Other of Two Phenotypes

One of the most fascinating characteristics of arterial smooth muscle is its ability to exist in one or other of two phenotypes. **At one extreme is a smooth muscle cell whose function is almost entirely that of contraction and relaxation; at the other is a cell almost exclusively concerned with the proliferation, synthesis and secretion of a number of** **extracellular tissue components such as collagen, the microfibrillar portion of elastin and proteoglycans.** These are known as the **contractile** and **synthetic** phenotypes respectively (*Fig. 32.11*).

The expression of either of these phenotypes is controlled by a series of chemical signals (see *Table 32.2*). These may either 'drive' proliferation by means of the binding of mitogenic signals to appropriate receptors or, possibly, 'permit' cell proliferation via the removal of factors that normally inhibit cell proliferation. One model, for which compelling evidence exists, is that the proliferative activity of the synthetic phenotype is a response to receptor-mediated binding of growth factors, released in a paracrine fashion from neighbouring cells or originating in an autocrine manner from existing smooth muscle cells.

Growth Factors and Arterial Smooth Muscle Proliferation

Serum derived from whole clotted blood is mitogenic for arterial smooth muscle cells in culture; this effect is due to a factor released from platelets following their activation – **platelet–derived growth factor** (PDGF). This term is something of a misnomer because, whereas PDGF is certainly released from the α granules of activated platelets (*Fig. 32.12*), it can also be produced by:

- endothelial cells
- activated macrophages
- arterial smooth muscle cells themselves

In cell culture PDGF synthesis by smooth muscle cells is enhanced by both native and oxidized LDL. If this holds *in vivo*, it constitutes an additional nexus between lipid infiltration and the connective tissue response of the arterial wall.

PDGF is a cationic, dimeric protein (molecular weight 28 000–32 000). In platelets, it is stored in the α granules as a heterodimer containing both the A and B chains. The B chain of PDGF shows an 87% degree of homology with the gene product of the cellular proto-oncogene c-*sis*, expression of which is an important element in wound healing. In addition, several malignant tumour cell lines have been shown to secrete PDGF which, presumably, acts as an autocrine signal for their own proliferation.

The synthesis of PDGF by endothelium appears to be stimulated by coagulation factors such as thrombin and Factor Xa, following any event causing an increase in endothelial cell turnover, and by two cytokines: interleukin 1 and tumour necrosis factor α.

The growth factor binds to high-affinity receptors on arterial smooth muscle cells, fibroblasts and other mesenchymal cells, but not to endothelium. It is not only mitogenic for these cells **but also acts as a chemoattractant**. This property may account for the migration of medial smooth muscle cells into the intima, which occurs both in atherogenesis and in the intimal response to injury.

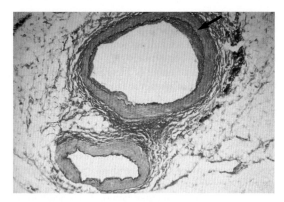

FIGURE 32.9 *Coronary arteries in infancy showing the thin intimal layer. The section is stained to show elastic tissue as black. The wavy internal elastic lamina (arrow) marks the boundary between intima and muscle-rich media.*

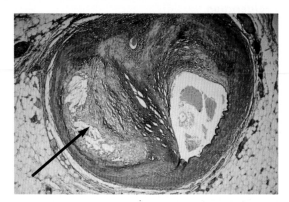

FIGURE 32.10 *Section through coronary artery in an elderly male. The lumen is greatly narrowed by a bulky plaque. The section has been stained to show collagen as blue and smooth muscle as red. Large amounts of new collagen have been formed in the lifetime of this lesion. Note the relatively small basal 'pool' (arrow).*

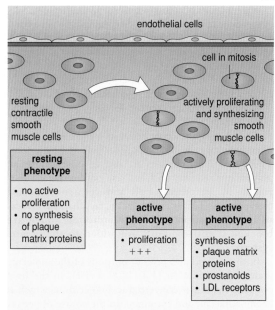

FIGURE 32.11 *Contrasting functional phenotypes of arterial smooth muscle cells.*

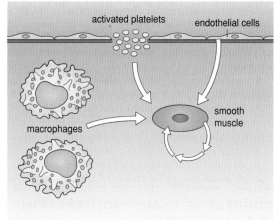

FIGURE 32.12 *Sources of platelet-derived growth factor in atherogenesis.*

Binding of PDGF to its receptor on cultured smooth muscle cells is followed by:

1) Transcription of the cellular proto-oncogenes c-*fos* and c-*myc*. The products of these genes, which in culture are activated within minutes of PDGF binding, are DNA-binding proteins, which play an important part in initiating cell proliferation.

2) Transcription of the gene coding for actin, a major muscle protein.

(These transcriptional events are probably mediated via the phosphorylation of several intra-cytoplasmic proteins, **a process that is, in turn, dependent on the PDGF receptor acting as a *tyrosine kinase* when bound with its ligand.**)

3) Activation of the phosphatidylinositol pathway, leading to changes in calcium distribution within the cells. This can regulate many metabolic pathways.

Growth-promoting Potential of the Macrophage

A potential growth-promoting role for the activated macrophage can be inferred from its observed behaviour in wound healing.

Allusion has already been made to the fact that the macrophage can secrete PDGF but this is not the only growth factor that these versatile cells can synthesize. Others identified include:

- **Fibroblast growth factor (FGF)**, a potent mitogen and stimulus for new capillary growth. It is certainly synthesized by activated macrophages but it is not clear whether the synthesized FGF is

Table 32.2 Regulation of Proliferation and Phenotype of Smooth Muscle Cell Growth Factors and Cytokines

Chemical species	Effect on smooth muscle cell proliferation	Effect on smooth muscle cell migration
Epidermal growth factor (EGF)	+	
Basic fibroblast growth factor	++	0
Heparin-binding EGF-like growth factor	++	+
Insulin growth factor 1	+	+
Interferon γ	+/−	
Interleukin 1	+	
Interleukin 6	+	
Platelet-derived growth factor	+	+
Thrombin	+	
Transforming growth factor α	+	
Transforming growth factor β	+/−	+
Tumour necrosis factor α	+	

secreted because the molecule lacks the signal peptide necessary for secretion to take place.

- **Transforming growth factor α (TGF-α)**, which binds to the receptor for epidermal growth factor (EGF); it has the same functional effects as EGF.
- **Transforming growth factor β (TGF-β)**, which is both a potent **inhibitor of cell proliferation** and **a powerful stimulus for the production of collagen**.

PLAQUE INJURY AND THROMBOSIS

In the vast majority of cases, the morphological correlate of potentially life-threatening events such as unstable angina or myocardial infarction is thrombosis arising in relation to plaques that have been termed 'unstable'. The antecedent to such thrombosis is plaque injury, which may be of two types: 'superficial' or 'deep' (*Fig. 32.13*).

SUPERFICIAL PLAQUE INJURY
Superficial injury can be defined as denudation of the surface endothelium and the most superficial strands of collagen of a fibrolipid plaque. It represents a progression of the process of focal endothelial denudation which is commonly seen on the surface of coronary artery plaques. When large areas of denudation develop, mural or even occlusive thrombi may form. This type of plaque injury is the antecedent of about 25% of the thrombi occurring in relation to damaged fibrolipid plaques. Plaques in which such superficial

injury occurs tend to be those in which the superficial collagen fibres of the plaque cap are separated by large numbers of foamy, lipid-filled macrophages.

DEEP INTIMAL INJURY (PLAQUE DISRUPTION)
The defining criterion of deep intimal injury is the development of a split or tear that extends from the

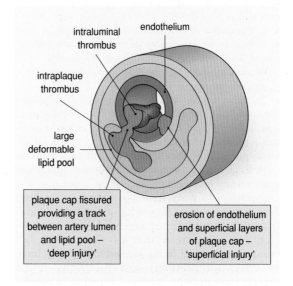

intraluminal thrombus

endothelium

intraplaque thrombus

large deformable lipid pool

plaque cap fissured providing a track between artery lumen and lipid pool – 'deep injury'

erosion of endothelium and superficial layers of plaque cap – 'superficial injury'

FIGURE 32.13 Deep and superficial plaque injury and thrombosis.

luminal surface of a plaque deep down through the connective tissue cap into the soft underlying atheromatous pool. Blood from the artery lumen enters the plaque and comes into contact with various thromboplastic components of the plaque, leading to activation of platelets and the clotting cascade. Thus the initial formation of thrombus takes place within the substance of the plaque itself and, in some instances, may never extend through the plaque fissure into the lumen of the artery. In other cases the thrombus grows up rapidly through the fissure into the lumen, where it may propagate in a cephalad or caudad fashion. Both mural and occlusive thrombosis may occur in this way. The intraplaque portion of such a thrombus is usually platelet rich while the intraluminal moiety is often relatively poor in platelets and rich in fibrin, a fact that may have considerable implications for the success of thrombolytic therapy.

The **unstable plaque** in which such fissuring is likely to occur is one in which there is a large lipid-rich pool (more than 40% of plaque volume), especially where this pool is lacking in collagen 'struts' passing from the undersurface of the plaque cap to the deep margins of the pool (see *Fig. 32.6*). Such a large, relatively unsupported, pool constitutes a highly deformable region within the plaque, and such deformation leads to a marked degree of stressing of the plaque connective tissue, particularly in the region where the cap connective tissue fuses with lesion-free parts of the arterial intima. In addition these lesions show a significant reduction in the ratio of smooth muscle cells to lipid-filled macrophages. This change in the proportions of these two cell types reflects an absolute increase in the volume of the plaque occupied by macrophages and a corresponding decrease in that occupied by smooth muscle cells. Plaque instability therefore appears to be a function of:

- The presence of a large amount of extracellular lipid
- A decrease in the number of smooth muscle cells, and thus a decrease in the amount of extracellular matrix protein, which might otherwise serve to stabilize the plaque
- An increase in the number of lipid-filled macrophages

An interesting question that arises from these data is whether these lipid-filled macrophages merely constitute a **marker** of unstable plaques or whether, which seems more likely, they actually mediate such instability. If this is the case, then the mechanisms employed by macrophages may include free radical generation and the secretion of metalloproteinases, such as has been demonstrated already in respect of stromelysin. This area of the natural history of atherosclerosis deserves much fuller investigation than it has received to date because **a reduction in plaque instability may have an effect on mortality and morbidity much greater than may be achieved by what is usually understood as plaque regression, i.e. a reduction of luminal stenosis seen on angiography.**

Epidemiological studies of the effects of substantial lowering of plasma lipid concentrations show a much greater reduction in the number of clinical events and in mortality rate than is indicated by angiographic improvements, providing support for the hypothesis proposed above.

Atherosclerosis II

EPIDEMIOLOGY: RISK FACTORS

There are major differences in the prevalence of atherosclerosis-related clinical syndromes between different countries and even between different groups within single countries. These differences correlate with the extent and severity with which major arterial beds are affected by fibrolipid plaques. These epidemiological data allow an examination of some factors that are believed to be implicated in *causing* or *aggravating* atherosclerosis and an assessment of the strength of the association between them and the degree of risk found in different populations.

This does not mean that the only determinant of occlusive arterial disease is the extent and severity of atherosclerosis. However, atherosclerosis is a *necessary* if not always *sufficient* precondition, and the extent of intimal involvement by raised lesions has a strong predictive value within whole populations for death from occlusive arterial disease. Support for this view comes from the finding that the decline in death rate from ischaemic heart disease in the USA has been accompanied by a significant reduction in the number and size of raised lesions seen in the coronary arteries at postmortem examination.

RISK FACTORS AND ATHEROSCLEROSIS

Risk factors have been described as **habits, traits or abnormalities associated with a sizeable increase in susceptibility to disease associated with severe or extensive atherosclerosis**. Not all factors having an association with such diseases conform to this: **age** and **sex**, which are important influences on atherogenesis, can hardly be regarded as habits, traits or abnormalities.

Age

Age has the strongest and most consistent association with atherogenesis. Lesions appear in the aorta in the first decade of life, in the coronary arteries in the second and in the cerebral vessels in the third. In the aorta, fatty streaks reach a peak at about the age of 30 years, occupying about 30% of the intimal surface. After this time involvement by fatty streaking either remains constant or declines, the decline being due in part to the replacement of fatty streaks by mature lesions. The latter, which appear as a rule in the third decade of life, increase progressively with age.

Sex

Clinical manifestations of atherosclerosis-related disease are much less frequent in middle-aged women than in men. After the female menopause and with advancing age, this difference between the sexes decreases, but never disappears. In the coronary artery tree in women, these data are mirrored by much less severe involvement by atherosclerosis. The reasons are not entirely clear. It is tempting to assume that female hormones are responsible and this suggestion gains support from studies indicating that hormone replacement therapy in postmenopausal women is associated with a decrease in the risk of ischaemic heart disease (IHD). However, in men who had had heart attacks, the use of oestrogen in a secondary prevention trial was not encouraging, new myocardial infarcts being more common in the group receiving hormone than in those having a placebo.

There do appear to be some differences between the sexes with respect to lipid metabolism. Mean concentrations of **high density lipoproteins** (correlated negatively with risk of IHD) are significantly higher in women than in men.

Race

There are striking geographical differences both in the prevalence of IHD and in the extent and severity of atherosclerosis. For instance, in the USA there is less extensive and severe atherosclerosis in black-skinned than in Caucasian populations, and in South Africa there is similarly less atherosclerosis in the indigenous black population than in either white Caucasians or Asian Indians. Are these differences racially mediated or due to differences in environment resulting from socioeconomic differences?

Within each racial group studied, there is a strong gradient for coronary atherosclerosis which correlates with plasma cholesterol concentrations. This suggests that race *per se* does not confer immunity from or increased susceptibility to atherosclerosis. This view is strengthened by data gained from studies of immigrants derived from 'low-risk' populations, for example the Japanese, who acquire the risk of the 'host' population. In these immigrants with increased risk (e.g. Japanese now resident in California) the distribution curve of plasma cholesterol concentration is shifted to the right, compared with those living in Japan.

Cigarette Smoking

There is a strong positive association between smoking more than 15 cigarettes per day and the risk of both ischaemic heart disease, stroke and peripheral arterial insufficiency. Doll has estimated that removing the 'cigarette smoking factor' could result in a 25% reduction in the rate of mortality from IHD in the UK.

In the long-running Framingham prospective study, **cigarette smoking acted most powerfully in respect of sudden death and acute myocardial infarction**, and the degree of risk correlated more closely with the number of cigarettes smoked daily than the duration of the habit. The increased risk decreases sharply after giving up smoking. These data have been interpreted as meaning that cigarette smoke-associated risk is mediated through an effect on platelet and clotting activity rather than by an increase in atherogenesis.

Many autopsy data show, however, that atherosclerosis, especially in the coronaries, is more extensive and severe in smokers than in non-smokers.

The cause of increased atherogenesis is not clear. Cigarette smoke causes morphological lesions in the major arteries of small animals which are consistent with **free radical**-mediated change, and, indeed, cigarette smoke contains a high concentration of free radicals (10^{14} per 25 ml 'puff'). Similar changes have been described in the umbilical artery endothelium of infants born to mothers who smoked.

Evidence also suggests a link between cigarette smoking and changes in platelet function and clotting parameters. Cigarette smoke causes microthrombi to form in small animal arteries and in humans, and is associated with shortened bleeding times and increased plasma concentrations of fibrinogen.

Prospective studies show that the concentration of fibrinogen is a reliable predictor of IHD risk. When smoking is discontinued, plasma fibrinogen concentrations decrease, reaching those of non-smokers after 5 years.

Diabetes Mellitus

Atherosclerosis-related disease is a major complication of diabetes mellitus. In Western countries, arterial disease accounts for more than 70% of deaths in diabetics. This increase in risk is especially marked in diabetic women who appear to lose the relative immunity from IHD normally present during reproductive life.

It is important to realize that diabetes operates as a powerful incremental risk factor for arterial disease only in those populations in whom a substantial 'background' level of atherosclerosis exists. Thus the presence of diabetes in 'low-risk' populations such as South African black-skinned does *not* significantly increase the risk of IHD and other atherosclerosis-related syndromes.

The coronary arteries of diabetics show increased involvement by both fatty streaks and fibrolipid plaques; in the aorta this is true only of fibrolipid plaques and the degree of difference is not statistically significant in all race or location groups.

The reason for the increase in risk of atherosclerosis-related clinical events in diabetics is not entirely clear.

- Common risk factors such as hypercholesterolaemia, high blood pressure and cigarette smoking are as common in diabetics as in non-diabetics, and are as strongly related to IHD in the diabetic as in the non-diabetic.

- However, for every risk factor and for every level of risk, data from the Multiple Risk Factor Intervention Trial show mortality from IHD in diabetics to be threefold higher than in non-diabetics. This suggests that additional risk factors are operating in diabetics.

Some **possible mechanisms** for the development of atherosclerosis-related disease in diabetics include:

1) Many diabetics show type IV hyperlipidaemia (see below). This may be associated with a decreased HDL concentration, which is in turn associated with an increased IHD risk.

2) Lysine residues of low density lipoprotein (LDL) may become glycosylated and this can lead to a decrease in receptor-mediated catabolism of LDL.

3) Glycosylation of fibrin makes it less susceptible to cleavage by plasmin.

4) Insulin resistance and high plasma insulin levels appear to promote atherogenesis. This may be an important contributor to the high risk of IHD found among Asian immigrants in Britain.

Systemic Hypertension

High blood pressure is an important risk factor for ischaemic heart disease in countries where atherosclerosis-related clinical disease is common. In countries where the risk of IHD is low, high blood pressure is associated with haemorrhagic stroke and renal failure but not with an increased risk of IHD.

There is no universal agreement as to what constitutes high blood pressure. In the British Regional Heart Study a twofold increase in risk was noted with systolic pressure greater than 148 mmHg, and a diastolic pressure greater than 93 mmHg increased this risk still further.

Post-mortem studies show that high blood pressure is associated with more extensive and severe involvement of the aorta and coronary arteries by fibrolipid plaques at all ages and in both sexes. The mechanism responsible for this increase in atherogenesis is not known but is likely to be a direct one because a rise in pressure in the pulmonary arterial system is also associated with an increase in fatty streaking.

HYPERLIPIDAEMIA AND ATHEROSCLEROSIS

HIGHER THAN IDEAL PLASMA CONCENTRATIONS OF CHOLESTEROL CONSTITUTE THE MOST IMPORTANT MODIFIABLE RISK FACTOR

There is a vast literature relating to the association between lipid metabolism and atherosclerosis. This subject is complex but can be summarized as follows:

1) Atherosclerotic lesions contain far more lipid, especially LDL, than does normal intima.

2) Increasing plasma LDL concentrations of various animals by dietary or other means leads to the formation of atherosclerotic lesions. Such lesions also occur in animals with inherited hyperlipidaemias.

3) Certain inherited hyperlipidaemias in humans cause greatly enhanced atherogenesis and a marked increase in coronary heart disease risk.

4) High mean LDL concentrations in a population are associated with a high risk of coronary heart disease. The converse applies when mean LDL levels are low.

5) An individual's plasma lipid profile is the result of interaction between genetic and environmental factors, the most important of which is diet.

PLASMA LIPIDS, LIPID TRANSPORT AND ATHEROSCLEROSIS

The chief plasma lipids are:
- triglycerides
- phospholipids
- cholesterol and its esters
- free fatty acids

Triglycerides are fatty acid esters of glycerol. Dietary triglycerides are absorbed mainly in the small gut. In its wall they are assembled into **chylomicrons** in which form they enter the circulation. Triglycerides are also derived from endogenous fatty acids being synthesized for the most part in the liver but also in the small intestine. The liver-derived triglycerides enter the blood in the form of **very low density lipoprotein** (VLDL). Dietary triglycerides are cleared from the plasma in about 12 hours and thus measurement in the fasting state gives a reliable indication of endogenous triglyceride in the plasma. Normal values in men are 0.5–2.0 mmol/l and up to 1.5 mmol/l in premenopausal women.

The chief **phospholipids** in plasma are:
- lecithin (phosphatidylcholine)
- sphingomyelin

While synthesis of these phospholipids occurs in most tissues, plasma phospholipids are derived mainly from the liver. Phospholipids play a key role as part of the lipid-transporting molecules (lipoproteins) in which they maintain non-polar lipids such as cholesterol esters and triglyceride in a soluble state. Plasma phospholipid concentrations range from 2.3 to 3.0 mmol/l, and are somewhat higher in females than in males.

Cholesterol is a sterol which, in humans, is found both in its free form and esterified with various long-chain fatty acids. Free cholesterol is the predominant form in most tissues, with the exception of the adrenal cortex, the plasma and atherosclerotic plaques. In these three situations cholesterol ester predominates. Under most circumstances, the bulk of newly synthesized cholesterol derives from the liver and the distal part of the small intestine.

Cholesterol is synthesized from acetate, an important early step being the **conversion of acylcoenzyme A**

(CoA) to mevalonate. The rate limiting enzyme for this reaction is *3-hydroxyl, 3-methyl glutaryl CoA reductase (HMG CoA reductase)*, which is subject to feedback suppression by cholesterol. The discovery of a group of compounds, the **statins**, that inhibit this enzyme has made possible for the first time major reductions in plasma cholesterol levels in hyperlipidaemic individuals. Plasma total cholesterol concentration normally ranges from 4.0 to 6.5 mmol/l.

Plasma Lipoproteins

With the exception of free fatty acids, lipids are transported in the plasma in the form of **lipoproteins**. These are macromolecules which contain specific carrier proteins or **apoproteins**. These interact with phospholipid and free cholesterol to form a polar, and hence soluble, outer shell within which is a non-polar core consisting of cholesterol esters and triglycerides. Apoproteins also regulate the reactions of plasma lipids with enzymes and bind to specific receptors on cell surfaces. Thus they determine the sites of uptake and the catabolic rates of such important lipid classes as cholesterol.

Plasma taken after a meal contains six different classes of lipoprotein which can be separated by high-speed centrifugation. The lipoproteins and their constituents are shown in *Tables 32.3* and *32.4*, listed in descending order of size. **Most plasma cholesterol is carried as LDL.**

High Density Lipoproteins

HDL consists of two subclasses (HDL$_2$ and HDL$_3$). More than 90% of the protein in HDL is apoprotein A (ApoA) and about 3–5% is ApoC.

HDL is synthesized in both the liver and small intestine and is secreted in a nascent form as bilayered discs. The nascent molecule contains ApoE and free, rather than esterified, cholesterol. In the plasma most of the ApoE is replaced by ApoA and the cholesterol becomes esterified as a result of the action of the enzyme **lecithin cholesterol acyl transferase** (LCAT). These changes are followed by the molecule becoming spherical.

It is believed that HDL normally plays a major role in **mobilizing tissue cholesterol**, a suggestion that is supported by the fact that, in the absence of HDL, cholesterol esters accumulate in the reticuloendothelial system (*Tangier disease*).

There is a strong *inverse* relationship between plasma HDL concentrations and the risk of IHD. **This is believed to be due to the participation of HDL in reverse transport of cholesterol from tissues (including the artery wall). The free cholesterol so removed is re-esterified and then transferred to LDL and intermediate density lipoprotein (IDL) via the action of a cholesterol ester transport protein.**

Factors that *decrease* plasma HDL concentration include:
- certain antihypertensive agents
- chronic renal failure
- obesity
- non-insulin-dependent diabetes mellitus

Factors *increasing* the plasma concentration of HDL include:
- moderate alcohol consumption
- genetic factors
- female sex
- fibric acid compounds
- physical exercise

Table 32.3 Protein and Lipid Proportions of Lipoprotein

Lipoprotein class	Protein (%)	Lipid (%)
Chylomicrons	1–2	98–99
VLDL	10	90
IDL	18	82
LDL	25	75
HDL$_2$	40	60
HDL$_3$	55	45

Table 32.4 Lipid Components of Lipoproteins

Lipoprotein class	Triglyceride (%)	Cholesterol (%)	Phospholipid (%)
Chylomicron	88	3	9
VLDL	56	17	19
IDL	32	41	27
LDL	7	59	28
HDL$_2$	6	43	42
HDL$_3$	7	38	41

Lipoprotein(a)

Lipoprotein(a) (Lp(a)) is a quantitative genetic marker, the concentration of which varies between individuals. Current interest in this molecule stems from epidemiological studies showing a significant correlation between high plasma Lp(a) concentrations and IHD risk. In patients who have had a coronary artery bypass graft, high concentrations of Lp(a) confer a high risk of graft stenosis.

Lp(a) consists of two proteins combined with a lipid component which resembles that of LDL. These proteins are:

1) Apoprotein B_{100}, the major apoprotein of LDL.
2) A protein called apoprotein(a) (Apo(a)), which has structural similarity with plasminogen.

Plasminogen contains a globular protease domain which, when activated, cleaves fibrin. This is followed by five domains called **kringles** (which are pretzel-like loops), the name being derived from the ancient Norse *kringla* – a ring. Such kringle domains are found in clotting proteins, fibrinolytic proteins, the complement system and fibronectin. Apo(a) is a giant mutant form of plasminogen and has 37 copies of kringle 4.

The mechanisms(s) responsible for the increased risk of IHD are not known; it is possible that increased atherogenesis results from Lp(a) blocking the activation of plasminogen to plasmin. This leads to failure of proteolytic activation of transforming growth factor β (TGF-β), an autocrine inhibitor of vascular smooth muscle cell proliferation. Support for this view comes from studies of transgenic mice that express the human apolipoprotein(a) gene. The arteries from these mice show inhibition of TGF-β and this correlates with excessive proliferation of arterial smooth muscle.

THE HYPERLIPIDAEMIAS

Increases in the plasma concentration of one or more of the lipoprotein classes is termed hyperlipoproteinaemia or hyperlipidaemia. Such a hyperlipidaemia may be predominantly or entirely genetically determined. Some of these are expressed in the form of clearly defined familial syndromes and are known as the **primary hyperlipidaemias**. Some occur in association with other disorders such as hypothyroidism or diabetes or certain drugs such as β-blockers and these are known as **secondary hyperlipidaemias**. It is estimated that more than 60% of the variability in plasma lipid concentration is genetically determined. In most of such cases, the genetic component is polygenic. Interaction between such abnormalities and environmental factors, most notably diet, is likely to be the commonest cause of hyperlipidaemia in the general population.

CLASSIFICATION: LIPOPROTEIN PHENOTYPES

Five **phenotypic** hyperlipidaemic patterns have been described, and form the basis of the commonly used World Health Organization (WHO) classification. This system has faults. Firstly, an approach based entirely on phenotype does not distinguish between primary and secondary hyperlipidaemias. Secondly, it throws no light on the mechanisms involved and, thirdly, it disregards the important **inverse correlation that exists between plasma concentration of HDL and the risk of occlusive arterial disease**. Despite these reservations, the WHO classification is worth knowing because it is used so widely (see *Table 32.5*) but **understanding of the mechanisms underlying the primary hyperlipidaemias is most easily gained in relation to normal lipid transport**. Once the basic physiology is appreciated, the application of 'Murphy's law' to each step indicates the metabolic failures expressed in the various hyperlipidaemias (*Table 32.6*).

NORMAL PATHWAYS OF LIPID TRANSPORT

There are two basic pathways of lipid transport:

1) An **exogenous** pathway that involves the transport of lipid from the gut to the liver (*Fig. 32.14*). In the course of this journey, fatty

Table 32.5 WHO Classification of Hyperlipoproteinaemias

Type	Plasma cholesterol	LDL cholesterol	Plasma triglyceride	Lipoprotein abnormality
I	Raised	Low or normal	Raised	Excess chylomicrons
IIa	Raised or normal	Raised	Normal	Excess LDL
IIb	Raised	Raised	Raised	Excess LDL and VLDL
III	Raised	Low or normal	Raised	Excess remnants (chylomicrons) and IDL
IV	Raised or normal	Normal	Raised	Excess VLDL
V	Raised	Normal	Raised	Excess chylomicrons and VLDL

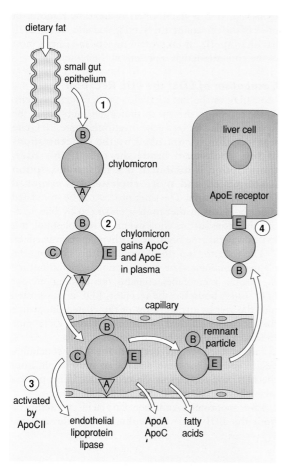

FIGURE 32.14 The exogenous pathway of lipoprotein metabolism.

acids are deposited in the adipose tissue stores and are also used as fuel by muscles.

2) An **endogenous** pathway in which lipoproteins synthesized and assembled within the liver undergo modifications and may interact with one another in the plasma.

THE EXOGENOUS PATHWAY AND ITS DISORDERS

The main lipid component of the diet is triglyceride, the amount of cholesterol ingested being comparatively small. ***This dietary fat is absorbed across the luminal aspect of the small intestinal epithelial cell and, within this cell, the lipid is assembled into the first of the lipoproteins –* the chylomicron.** This huge molecule, ranging in size from 100–1000 nm, consists predominantly of triglyceride. While the apoproteins (ApoB$_{48}$; ApoC and ApoA) constitute a comparatively small part of the molecule, they are functionally vital. This applies particularly to ApoB$_{48}$, without which no chylomicrons are formed and dietary lipid cannot be transported from the intestine via the lymphatics into the blood. When the chylomicron enters the plasma from the thoracic duct it gains some ApoE and more ApoC from HDL.

Once within the plasma the chylomicron is acted upon by a* lipoprotein lipase *derived from endothelium. This lipase splits fatty acids from the triglyceride and these fatty acids either fuel muscle activity or are deposited in the adipose tissue stores. What is left of the chylomicron is called a **remnant particle**. Failure of lipase activity leads to hyperchylomicronaemia and thus a grossly raised plasma triglyceride concentration. **This is the type I phenotype arising either from lack of lipoprotein lipase or from absence from the plasma of ApoC-II, which activates endothelial lipoprotein lipase.**

> ### KEY POINTS: The Characteristics of Type I Hyperlipoproteinaemia *are as follows:*
> - Rare, affecting less than one person per million population
> - Occurs in childhood
> - Main clinical features
>   Attacks of acute abdominal pain resembling acute pancreatitis
>   Eruptive xanthomata
>   Hepatosplenomegaly
> - Turbid plasma

Table 32.6 Causes of Hyperlipidaemia Phenotypes

Type	Primary	Secondary
I	Lipoprotein lipase deficiency; ApoC-II lack	Systemic lupus (rare)
IIa	Familial hypercholesterolaemia	Hypothyroidism; nephrotic syndrome
IIb	Familial combined hyperlipidaemia	Nephrotic syndrome; diabetes; anorexia nervosa
III	Familial type III hyperlipidaemia	Hypothyroidism; diabetes; obesity
IV	Familial combined hyperlipidaemia; familial hypertriglyceridaemia	Diabetes; chronic renal disease
V	Familial hypertriglyceridaemia; ApoC-II deficiency	Alcohol, β-blockers, diuretics, oral contraceptives

The next step is the clearing of chylomicron remnants from the plasma by binding to receptors on liver cells and subsequent internalization. This step also occurs in the handling of endogenous lipid, VLDL remnants being cleared from the plasma in exactly the same way. **Failure to do this is termed type III hyperlipoproteinaemia.**

The ligand is the ApoE protein which exists in three different isoforms, E_2, E_3 and E_4. E_3 and E_4 bind avidly to receptors on the liver cell but, *in vitro*, remnant particles containing ApoE$_2$ bind hardly at all. *In vivo*, most patients who are unable to clear remnant particles or VLDL from the plasma have inherited an E_2/E_2 genotype. Mice in which the ApoE gene has been knocked out in the embryo develop severe atherosclerosis.

It seems likely that some other factor is needed apart from the ApoE genotype before this form of hyperlipidaemia occurs, because the frequency of E_2 in the general population is about 1 in 100, whereas type III hyperlipidaemia occurs in only about 1 in 5000 of the population. The additional metabolic defects may arise from the presence of diabetes, obesity, hypothyroidism or other familial hyperlipidaemias.

> **KEY POINTS: Clinical features of Type III Hyperlipidaemia *include*:**
> - corneal arcus
> - xanthelasmata
> - yellow striae on palms
> - xanthomata, especially on knees and elbows
> - a broad band of lipid on electrophoresis in the β lipoprotein region
> - increased risk of vascular disease; 50% of patients have clinically apparent arterial disease
> - presence in many patients of hyperuricaemia and glucose intolerance
> - occasional occurrence of acute pancreatitis

THE ENDOGENOUS PATHWAY AND ITS DISORDERS

VLDL is assembled in the liver and then enters the bloodstream, where it undergoes considerable modification with the formation of IDL (*Fig. 32.15*) **and LDL.**

The liver is the chief site for synthesis of endogenous lipid. Within the hepatocyte both triglyceride and cholesterol are synthesized and exported into the blood in the form of **VLDL**. In structure and composition, VLDLs are similar to chylomicrons but are smaller and contain relatively less triglyceride and more cholesterol, phospholipid and protein. The protein component consists of ApoB$_{100}$, ApoC and ApoE, the first of these being essential for transport of the lipid from the liver. VLDL is acted on by a posthepatic lipase, and triglyceride is stripped away from it with the formation of **IDL**. The ApoC is transferred to HDL. Some of the IDL is removed from the circulation in exactly the same way as chylomicron remnant particles. The

remaining IDL is transformed to **LDL** by removal of most of the remaining triglyceride and also ApoE; LDL has only ApoB$_{100}$ in its protein moiety and carries most of the cholesterol that is present in the blood.

Catabolism of LDL: the LDL Receptor

Most LDL catabolism takes place via a receptor system. These receptors, present in the largest numbers in the liver, are coded for by a gene on chromosome 19. **Gene transcription is controlled by the concentrations of free cholesterol inside the cell. If this rises, transcription is inhibited; if it falls, transcription is stimulated and more cholesterol is removed from the plasma.** The latter process can be stimulated if bile acid loss in the stools is enhanced by bile acid-binding resins such as cholestyramine or Colestipol; it is in this way that the resins exert a hypolipidaemic effect.

The receptor is a single protein chain spanning the plasma membrane. The outer portion, which is outside the plasma membrane, contains the binding site for LDL. Once bound to the receptor, LDL is transported into the cell by invagination of the coated pit, which then becomes 'pinched off' from the plasma membrane to form a membrane-bound vesicle.

Fusion then occurs between the LDL-containing vesicle and the lysosome, and the receptor is split from the LDL and recycles to the cell surface. This process takes about 10 minutes.

First apoproteins and then fatty acids are removed from the LDL molecule within the vesicle and free

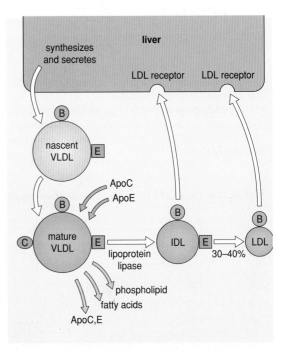

FIGURE 32.15 The endogenous pathway of lipoprotein metabolism.

cholesterol diffuses into the cytosol. The resulting increase in cytosolic cholesterol leads to:

- **Inhibition of the rate-limiting enzyme for cholesterol synthesis, HMG CoA reductase, and thus a 'switching off' of cholesterol synthesis.**
- **Inhibition of transcription of the gene coding for the LDL receptor.**

The intracellular free cholesterol is re-esterified following activation of acyl cholesterol acyl transferase (ACAT) and is stored in the cell. If large amounts of free cholesterol are delivered to the cell as a result of diets high in saturated fat, the expression of LDL receptors is inhibited thus leading to raised plasma concentrations of LDL cholesterol.

Type IV Hyperlipidaemia (Familial Triglyceridaemia)

This is characterized by **moderate hypertriglyceridaemia due to increased concentrations of VLDL**. The nature of the genetic abnormality is unknown but affected individuals have VLDL particles that are *larger* than normal and have a greater ratio of triglyceride : ApoB than normal. Free fatty acid flux into VLDL during synthesis in the liver is increased in these patients, and is aggravated if they have a high carbohydrate intake. There is a decrease in the amount of VLDL converted to LDL, and this maintains the LDL cholesterol concentration within normal limits.

> **KEY POINTS: Features of Type IV Hyperlipidaemia *include*:**
> - normal posthepatic lipolytic activity
> - hypertriglyceridaemia aggravated by dietary carbohydrate, corticosteroids and oestrogens
> - glucose intolerance and hyperuricaemia are common
> - conflicting views regarding an increased risk of atherosclerosis-related arterial disease

Type V Hyperlipidaemia

This is uncommon and has features of both types I and IV, as evidenced by the increased levels of both VLDL and chylomicrons. There is an increase in VLDL ApoB synthesis, as is also seen in type IV hyperlipidaemia, but the decrease in fractional catabolic rate of VLDL is more severe than in type IV.

> **KEY POINTS: Features of Type V Hyperlipidaemia *include*:**
> - unlike type 1, seldom presents in childhood
> - lipoprotein lipase activity normal
> - tendency for acute pancreatitis to develop. This is *the* major complication of this form of hyperlipidaemia, and every effort should be made to keep the triglyceride concentrations in the plasma down

> - hypertriglyceridaemia is aggravated by obesity and alcohol consumption
> - no increased risk of atherosclerosis-related arterial disease
> - eruptive xanthomata, glucose intolerance and hyperuricaemia

The foregoing types of hyperlipidaemia principally show hypertriglyceridaemia, although total plasma cholesterol, not LDL cholesterol, is raised in the type IV phenotype. Two of the most important primary hyperlipidaemias related to atherosclerosis show the presence of raised plasma LDL cholesterol, or of raised LDL cholesterol and triglyceride. These are:

- **type IIa hyperlipoproteinaemia (familial hypercholesterolaemia)**
- **type IIb hyperlipoproteinaemia (familial combined hyperlipidaemia)**

Type IIa Hyperlipidaemia (Familial Hypercholesterolaemia)

Familial hypercholesterolaemia (*Fig. 32.16*) is due to one of a number of mutations in the gene coding for the LDL receptor. Heterozygosity in respect of this mutation is quite common; 1 in 500 of the UK population is affected. Homozygosity is, fortunately, much rarer, only about 1 per million of the population being affected.

The mutations may result in a number of functional defects:

1) **Failure of receptor synthesis**
   - no receptors present (in homozygous form)
   - 50% of the normal number of receptors present (in heterozygotes)

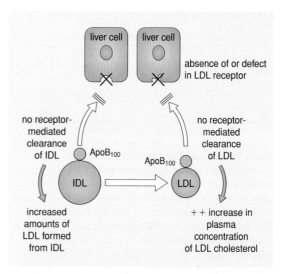

FIGURE 32.16 The basis of familial hypercholesterolaemia.

2) **Failure to transport receptors from endoplasmic reticulum via Golgi apparatus to cell surface**

3) **Failure of receptor to bind LDL**

4) **Failure of receptors to cluster in coated pits.** This prevents internalization after LDL binding. It is the rarest of the mutations and affects that part of the receptor molecule which lies within the cytoplasm.

Diet and drug treatment in patients homozygous for familial hypercholesterolaemia is without effect. The gross hyperlipidaemia can be controlled by plasma apheresis, the LDL being removed on a special column, or by liver transplantation, which supplies the patient with receptors on the donor liver.

Heterozygous familial hypercholesterolaemia is less severe, but quantitatively presents a much more important problem (0.2% of the population). **It frequently goes undiagnosed until the affected individual presents with premature IHD in early middle life. The IHD appears, on average, about 20 years earlier than in unaffected individuals.**

As with the homozygous form, skin and tendon xanthomata and corneal arcus occur but these tend to appear later in life than in homozygotes. Between the ages of 1 and 16 years the LDL cholesterol is about twice as high as in normal age-matched controls.

There is a mirror image of familial hypercholesterolaemia in which the LDL receptors are normal in number and function but where the ApoB is abnormal and cannot bind to the receptors. This rare defect is associated with a moderate degree of hypercholesterolaemia.

KEY POINTS: Features of Homozygous Familial Hyperlipiproteinaemia include:

- gross hypercholesterolaemia (18–20 mmol/l)
- virtually complete absence of receptor-mediated catabolism of LDL
- precocious development of atherosclerosis. Involvement of the aortic root is usually present by the time of puberty. Clinical manifestations of myocardial ischaemia may be present before the age of 10 years in patients lacking receptors, and about 25% of these die before the age of 25 years in the absence of appropriate treatment

---

Type IIb Hyperlipidaemia (Familial Combined Hyperlipidaemia)

Some 30% of survivors of myocardial infarction show an increase in the plasma concentration of both cholesterol and triglycerides. About half the relatives of these individuals are also hyperlipidaemic. They may show:

- **hypercholesterolaemia** (about 33%) (type IIa phenotype)
- **hypertriglyceridaemia** (about 33%) (type IV or V phenotype)

- **an increase in both lipid classes** (about 33%) (type IIb phenotype)

It is still not clear whether there is a single gene defect or whether inheritance is polygenic. Type IIb hyperlipidaemia is relatively common, being found in 0.5% of the general population, and is associated with at least 15% of cases of IHD. The nature of the genetic defect is unknown but **increased synthesis of ApoB$_{100}$ is certainly a feature**. There are no distinctive clinical features. Diagnosis depends on demonstrating the presence of multiple phenotypes within the affected family. The hyperlipidaemia is not often controllable by a low-fat diet alone but the excessive synthesis of ApoB$_{100}$ can be reduced by nicotinic acid.

CAN THE FORMATION OF ATHEROSCLEROTIC LESIONS BE PREVENTED AND, IF PRESENT, CAN THEY UNDERGO REGRESSION?

The significant differences existing among different populations with respect to the prevalence and severity of atherosclerosis show that plaque formation is not inevitable and is to a considerable extent related to lifestyle.

In animals with inherited hyperlipidaemias the use of lipid-lowering agents and/or antioxidants can inhibit lesion formation. Slow-channel calcium blockers also have this effect. In humans, a double-blind angiographic study demonstrated that individuals treated with the calcium antagonist, nifedipine, developed fewer new lesions in the coronary arteries over a 3-year period than those given a placebo.

The occurrence of lesion **regression** is much more difficult to demonstrate; it must be remembered that a decrease in risk of IHD should not necessarily be equated with shrinkage of atherosclerotic lesions. A decrease in risk following lipid lowering may well be due to a **qualitative change** in plaques involving a decrease in the bulk of soft, deformable lipid-rich pools. This might bring in its train a lessened risk of intimal injury and, thus, a lessened risk of acute thrombotic events.

THROMBOSIS AND ATHEROSCLEROTIC LESIONS

TYPES OF THROMBUS

Thrombi that occur in relation to plaques vary considerably in size as well as in the functional effect on the natural history of atherosclerotic plaques. They may be ultramicroscopic, microscopically identifiable and angiographically identifiable.

Ultramicroscopic Thrombi

Ultramicroscopic thrombi are visible only on electron microscopy (*Fig. 32.17*).

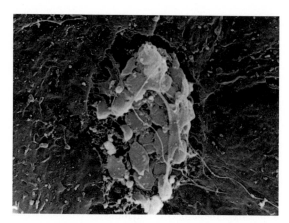

FIGURE 32.17 *Scanning electron micrograph of human coronary artery showing a focal erosion in the endothelial surface. The raw area is covered by adherent platelets which have undergone shape change and discharged their granule contents. Some aggregation has also occurred and an occasional strand of fibrin is present.*

Explanted hearts removed from recipients of cardiac allografts are an ideal source for the study of endothelium both over plaques and over lesion-free areas because they can be perfused at physiological pressures and fixed within a few minutes of removal. Coronary arteries from such hearts show the surface changes seen in animal models except that microthrombi are seen regularly rather than occasionally in relation to defects in the endothelium over human atherosclerotic plaques. These tiny thrombi do not, of course, encroach on the vessel lumen but probably stimulate further connective tissue growth within the plaque cap.

Microscopically Identifiable Thrombi

Many of the lesions regarded as being atherosclerotic consist, at least in part, of altered thrombi (*Fig. 32.18*). Evaluation of the possible contribution of mural throm-

bosis to the growth of human atherosclerotic plaques must be based on accurate identification of thrombus or its residua within the plaques; this may be done reliably by immunohistochemistry.

In this way both fibrin and platelets have been demonstrated in atherosclerotic lesions. Such incorporated remains of mural thrombi can be found in more than 40% of aortic plaques, the proportion rising in the arteries of patients who have died from acute IHD. Whether this represents an increased prothrombotic tendency in the period before death or a decreased ability to clear thrombi by means of lysis remains a matter of speculation.

Angiographically Identifiable Thrombi in the Coronary Arteries and Their Pathogenesis (*Figs. 32.19* and *32.20*)

The characteristics of the 'high-risk' plaque have been described in an earlier section of this chapter (see

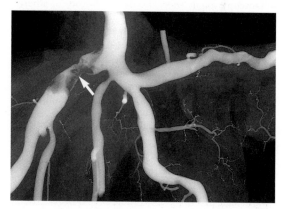

FIGURE 32.19 *Post-mortem coronary angiogram showing an irregular filling defect (arrow) representing acute thrombus formation.*

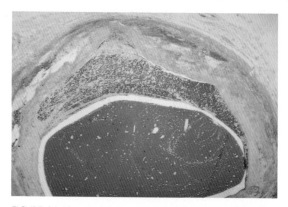

FIGURE 32.18 *Transverse section across a coronary artery. The section has been stained to show fibrin as red. A moderately large intramural thrombus is present. This is separated from the lumen by a thin layer of blue-staining connective tissue.*

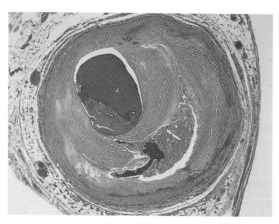

FIGURE 32.20 *Coronary plaque selected after angiography and showing intra-luminal and intraplaque thrombus. Both the lumen and the basal pool contain the barium used in post-mortem angiography (seen here as brownish material). This finding indicates a connection between the lumen and the pool.*

pp 330, 335–336). Cap disruption leading to fissuring extending from the artery lumen down to the lipid pool (**deep intimal injury**) is found in association with about 75% of acute major coronary artery thrombi.

Accumulation of lipid-filled foamy macrophages between thinned and separated collagen fibres within the upper layers of the plaque cap is the histological correlate of superficial plaque injury, which is found in the remaining 25% of cases of acute coronary thrombosis. It may be speculated as to whether this morphological appearance signifies breakdown of collagen by proteolysis or a reduction in collagen synthesis by smooth muscle cells, which appear to be sparse under these circumstances.

Significance of Thrombi in the Genesis of IHD and the Progression of Atherosclerosis

From the above it can be appreciated that ultramicroscopic thrombi and thrombi visible on optical microscopy might affect the natural history of atherosclerotic plaques purely as a result of their **growth-promoting functions**. The third type of thrombus, as already stated, is a major factor in the genesis of acute ischaemic syndromes but, in non-fatal cases, will also exert a growth-promoting effect and leave the surviving patient with more severe luminal narrowing in the affected segment than existed before the episode of plaque injury and acute thrombosis.

Ischaemic Heart Disease

In clinical terms ischaemic heart disease (IHD) expresses itself in a number of different forms. These include:

- **stable angina**
- **unstable angina**
- **variant or Prinzmetal's angina**
- **syndromes associated with acute myocardial necrosis**
- **sudden death**
- **chronic pump failure**

These are not distinct entities but form part of a spectrum of pathophysiological events of which the common pathological basis is atherosclerosis of the coronary arteries. In the more acute syndromes, atherosclerosis is usually complicated by thrombosis secondary to plaque injury.

Epidemiology

IHD is by far the commonest cause of death in the West. In Britain alone it accounts for some 140 000 deaths annually (roughly 27% of all deaths) and is a major drain on the resources allocated for health care.

Risk Factors

Although certain **inherited** characteristics, such as genetically determined hyperlipidaemia and diabetes mellitus, undeniably play a part in the genesis of IHD, it is fair to say that many of the most significant risk factors are linked to 'lifestyle'.

The most important risk factors have been discussed in the section dealing with atherosclerosis (see pp 336–340).

Data from the US 'Pooling Project' (1978) show the effects in males on the incidence of myocardial infarction and sudden death of being placed in the top quintile as opposed to the bottom in respect of the three most strongly predictive risk factors:

- plasma cholesterol concentrations
- diastolic blood pressure
- cigarette smoking

These are shown in *Table 32.7*. **Being in the top quintile for all three risk factors increased the risk by a factor of 8.6.** The use of multiple logistic functions (taking multiple risk factors into account simultaneously) greatly increases the accuracy with which the relative risk of a clinical event can be predicted. It is currently not possible to predict *absolute* risk for any individual on the basis of the risk factors so far identified. This may be because of risk factors yet to be recognized, or because of the difficulty in assessing the product of dose and time in relation to known factors. **However, it is possible to identify individuals who have a relatively low or high risk in terms of variables that can be modified, and those in the second group can be given advice and a regimen that offer the possibility of risk reduction.**

Secular trends in IHD mortality, particularly in the USA since the late 1960s, show that a nihilistic attitude to risk reduction is unjustified. The death rate in the USA from IHD has fallen steadily and markedly. This decline involves all sectors of the adult population. For those between the ages of 35 and 74 years, IHD mortality rates have fallen by more than 30%, resulting in more than 800 000 lives saved between 1968 and 1984. In the 1960s the USA ranked second in the world (just behind Finland) for IHD mortality. By the late 1980s, it ranked eighth out of the 27 economically developed countries studied.

Table 32.7 Effects of Being in the Top Quintile in Respect of Three Risk Factors	
Risk factor	Risk increment
Cholesterol	$3.7 \times$
Diastolic blood pressure	$3.3 \times$
Smoking	$5.2 \times$

This decline in mortality rate has been accompanied by an increase in the numbers being treated for hypertension, by a fall in mean cholesterol levels of about 4.2% and by a decrease in the number of cigarette smokers.

GENERAL PHYSIOLOGICAL FACTORS INFLUENCING THE EXPRESSION OF ISCHAEMIA

ENERGY REQUIREMENTS

The requirements of heart muscle for energy generation are high. Contraction requires large amounts of high-energy phosphates. There are considerable energy demands also for the maintenance of membrane integrity and of the high concentration gradients in respect of sodium, potassium and calcium ions that exist between the intracellular and extracellular milieu.

Cardiac muscle is poorly supplied with endogenous fuel stores, is well vascularized and is highly aerobic in its metabolism. This is why interruptions to the blood supply of the myocardium, even for comparatively short periods, produce catastrophic results. The lack of endogenous fuel stores is especially important. The mammalian heart, even at rest, removes some 80% of the oxygen available in coronary blood. Thus increased workloads necessitate a rapid increase in myocardial blood flow. The heart will use any fuel with which it is presented and is normally provided with a mixture of fuels. The relative proportions of these in the blood varies with the physiological state of the animal; for example, in the postprandial state the fatty acid concentrations will be low while in starvation the levels rise. It is often stated that the heart has a predilection for fatty fuels. This is not a property specific to heart muscle. Any tissue capable of oxidizing glucose and fatty acids will, when presented with a mixture of these, oxidize the fatty acids preferentially. This is simply inherent in the operation of the glucose–fatty acid cycle.

PATTERNS OF MYOCARDIAL BLOOD FLOW

Perfusion of the myocardium occurs during diastole due to the compression of intramyocardial vessels by contracting heart muscle during systole. **This diastolic flow is driven by the difference between the pressure in the aortic root above the closed aortic valve (as transduced along the epicardial arteries) and that obtaining in the left ventricular cavity.** While flow is directly proportional to the pressure-dependent drive and the time for which this is allowed to operate, it is inversely related to the resistance in the myocardial vascular bed. Increases of intramyocardial flow, such as occur during exercise, are mediated by relaxation of small arteries and arterioles within the myocardium; changes in the calibre of the much larger epicardial arteries, in the **disease-free state**, do not contribute much to resistance.

In functional terms, **the epicardial arteries are regional**: each major branch supplies an identifiable segment of the myocardium. In the dead human heart it is possible to demonstrate anastomotic flow by injection of media of low viscosity. However, in humans and in large animals such as the pig or dog, sudden blockage of a major coronary artery branch leads to necrosis of the segment of muscle supplied by that branch, indicating that coronary arteries are functional end-arteries.

GENERAL PATHOLOGY OF ISCHAEMIC MYOCARDIAL INJURY

It is not easy in human IHD to obtain data relating to the time-related functional, biochemical and ultrastructural changes that follow major coronary branch obstruction. Thus, most of our knowledge in this field is derived from studying the sequence of events following ligation of a major coronary artery branch in relatively large animals such as the pig or dog.

Within a few minutes a portion of the relevant area of the left ventricle wall ceases to contract, and in surviving animals a significant area of coagulative necrosis (myocardial infarct) develops over the next 12 hours. The size of any such infarct is influenced by the coronary artery anatomy in the individual animal and on the degree of collateral flow.

While ischaemic muscle ceases to contract within a few minutes of coronary artery ligation, the development of necrosis may be inhibited if flow can be re-established within 20–40 minutes; longer periods of ischaemia lead to irreversible damage.

BIOCHEMICAL CHANGES

Within seconds, oxygen tension falls in the ischaemic muscle; mitochondrial respiration declines and then ceases. Fatty fuels can be used only in the presence of oxygen and thus anaerobic glycolysis of glycogen becomes the only source of energy. This leads inevitably to a rise in the concentration of lactate which, in the ischaemic state, cannot be removed readily. The heart's glycogen stores are limited and anaerobic glycolysis is an inefficient means for the production of adenosine 5′-triphosphate (ATP). Intracellular ATP concentrations thus fall steadily, reaching almost zero after 40–60 minutes, and the creatine phosphate content falls to zero after about 15 minutes of ischaemia. This, coupled with the inhibition of myosin ATPase by hydrogen ions, leads to cessation of contraction.

The key to cell survival in ischaemia is **preservation of membrane integrity**. This may be lost as a result of the action of a number of potentially cytotoxic mechanisms, including lipid peroxidation of unsaturated membrane lipids. The damaging free radicals could be generated in a number of ways. Superoxide anion is generated in large amounts when electron carriers are highly reduced, such as is the case in ischaemia. Release of large amounts of endogenous catecholamine, known to occur under these circumstances, may also be associated with free radical generation, and other mechanisms such as oxidation of hypoxanthine and xanthine by xanthine oxidase may also produce superoxide and hydrogen peroxide. In relation to lipid peroxidation in ischaemic myocardium, a time of great potential danger is the **reperfusion phase**, whether this is established spontaneously or therapeutically induced by thrombolytic agents. During reperfusion, oxygen is readmitted to hypoxic tissues which contain high concentrations of reduced nicotinamide adenine dinucleotide (NADH) and hypoxanthine, and this combination of circumstances is likely to be associated with much free radical generation and consequent lipid peroxidation of cell membranes. In experimental ischaemia, additional myocardial damage certainly occurs during the reperfusion phase.

STRUCTURAL CHANGES OCCURRING IN ISCHAEMIC MYOCARDIUM

Between 15 and 40 minutes after perfusion has ceased, characteristic ultrastructural changes appear, with mitochondrial and membrane damage. Reperfusion causes the damage to become more severe; there is swelling of the muscle cells, the accumulation in mitochondria of hydrated calcium phosphate, and extensive sarcomere disturbance with smaller than normal distances between the Z bands. These 'contraction bands' are thought to be the result of the myocyte losing its ability to relax as a result of an abnormally high concentration of calcium within the cell.

Microscopic Features

Damage cannot be seen on light microscopy until at least 4–8 hours after coronary artery occlusion.

- The first easily recognizable feature is the presence of neutrophils in the interstitium. This may start as early as 4 hours after occlusion and may last for some days.
- Macrophages begin to infiltrate the ischaemic zone after about 4 days. Individual muscle cells undergo coagulative necrosis and stain much more deeply with eosin; this is followed by nuclear pyknosis and the loss of normal cross-striations.
- Within 4–5 days the dead cells disappear and cell debris is phagocytosed by macrophages. Repair of ischaemic tissue and its replacement by fibrous tissue depends on the ingrowth of capillaries from the viable myocardium at the periphery of the ischaemic tissue (Fig. 32.21).
- Collagen fibres begin to appear on about the ninth day and repair is usually complete within 6 weeks.

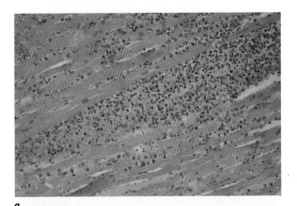

a

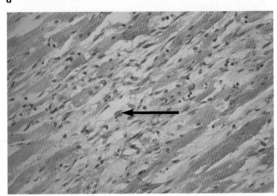

b

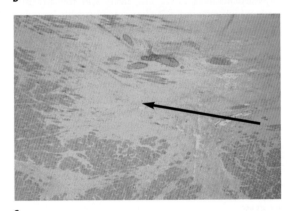

c

FIGURE 32.21 *Infarcted myocardium.* **a** *Necrotic myocytes have elicited a brisk acute inflammatory reaction.* **b** *At a slightly later stage the necrotic muscle cells are repaced by granulation tissue (arrow).* **c** *The repair process terminates in the formation of relatively acellular scar tissue (arrow).*

SPECTRUM OF ISCHAEMIC HEART DISEASE IN HUMANS

STABLE ANGINA

Stable angina occurs when increased myocardial demands for oxygen cannot be met. This may be caused by exercise, cold, eating, emotion, or a combination of some or all of these. Angina may also occur when myocardial oxygen demand remains constant but perfusion is decreased as, for example, in coronary artery spasm. **The term 'stable angina' is applied to the situation where it can be predicted that chest pain will occur once myocardial work, and hence oxygen demand, exceed a certain known level.**

Coronary Artery Pathology in Stable Angina

Coronary artery angiography shows **segments in which there is significant stenosis of one or more of the epicardial coronary arteries. The term 'significant' in this context means a reduction in diameter of the lumen of more than 50% compared with adjacent segments of 'normal' coronary artery. This degree of luminal reduction equates with a reduction in cross-sectional area of 75%.** The resistance of flow that an atherosclerotic plaque of such dimensions causes may be offset to a certain extent by a fall in resistance within intramyocardial vessels. However, there is a limit to this dilatation and eventually the plaque-mediated stenosis becomes flow limiting, usually when there is an increase in myocardial oxygen demand. Post-mortem angiography of such patients often shows the presence of multiple segments of stenosis.

Stenosis Morphology: Concentric and Eccentric Lesions

A post-mortem study of stenosed segments from patients with stable angina has shown that concentric lesions (see p 330) account for 76% of stenoses, the remaining 24% being eccentric. Over 60% of the concentric lesions are fibrous plaques with small lipid-rich pools at their base. In the case of eccentric lesions, half have large lipid-rich pools and half are fibrous. In addition to the stenosed segments described above, many patients with stable angina have segments in which the lumen is plugged by connective tissue containing multiple small vascular channels. These have been interpreted as being segments in which occlusive thrombosis occurred at some time in the past, the presence of the small channels representing recanalization of the thrombi.

UNSTABLE ANGINA

The feature that differentiates stable and unstable angina is the *unpredictability* **of chest pain in the latter.** Pain may occur at rest, and differs from time to time in frequency, intensity and character. **Over the first 3 months following the onset of unstable angina, 4% of patients will die suddenly, 15% will suffer myocardial infarction and many of the remainder will undergo spontaneous remission.** Treatment of unstable angina with aspirin reduces the frequency of sudden death and myocardial infarction, suggesting the involvement of thrombosis. The existence of patients whose unstable angina persists for years raises the possibility that there is more than one underlying pathophysiological mechanism.

Stenosis Morphology

Coronary artery angiography both during life and in post-mortem hearts shows two distinct morphological variants:

- In type I the luminal outline of the stenosis is smooth and resembles what is seen in the vessels of patients with stable angina.
- Type II shows a ragged luminal outline and/or overhanging edges, and the presence of contrast medium may be noted within the plaque substance.

Histological examination has shown that the type II lesion is a plaque in which acute changes are taking place. Most often they show splitting or fissuring of the plaque's connective tissue cap, and this is frequently associated with the presence of thrombus, both within the 'pool' at the plaque base and within the lumen, although the latter is not occluded at this stage. The myocardium of patients with unstable angina who have died and in whom such type II lesions are present, not infrequently shows the presence of platelet microemboli in intramyocardial vessels downstream of the unstable plaque.

Unstable angina associated with eccentric type I lesions is almost certainly due to localized spasm, and in a few cases may occur on the basis of spasm of lesion-free coronary arteries (variant angina). There are several possible causes for altered vasomotor responses at the sites of eccentric stenosing plaques. These include:

1) a decline in the production by the arterial endothelium of the powerful, endogenous vasodilator nitric oxide (NO) originally called **endothelium-derived relaxing factor (EDRF).**
2) a reduced response to NO, perhaps associated with intimal thickening which might block the access of the NO to medial smooth muscle cells
3) increased smooth muscle sensitivity to vasoconstrictors
4) adventitial inflammation, which may affect nerves in the adventitia
5) neutralization of NO within the intima by plasma constituents such as haemoglobin

Thus patients with angina may have any possible combination of fixed luminal stenosis due to the presence of plaques, dynamic stenosis, which will vary with medial muscle activity, and intraluminal thrombosis associated with plaque injury. In summary:

- Stable angina is associated with fixed stenosis.
- Patients with angina in which the degree of ischaemia is disproportionate to the myocardial oxygen demand usually have an element of dynamic stenosis superimposed on a fixed stenosis.

- Unstable angina is associated with major thrombus formation, spasm or a combination of these factors.

ACUTE MYOCARDIAL NECROSIS (MYOCARDIAL INFARCTION)

The diagnosis of **acute myocardial necrosis** depends on the recognition of a set of morphological features, and **no case of death from IHD should be classified as acute myocardial necrosis (infarction) in the absence of such morphological recognition**. The importance of this, apparently banal, point is emphasized because failure to appreciate it has led to a long, pointless and sterile controversy over the pathogenesis of myocardial infarction: many cases have been labelled as such without there being any evidence of myocardial necrosis.

In animal models myocardial necrosis cannot be recognized on light microscopic examination until 6–8 hours after the cessation of perfusion, and it is unlikely that human heart muscle will behave differently. Thus, in any post-mortem series of rapidly occurring deaths from IHD there will always be a number of cases in which a correct attribution cannot be made. In addition there are different macroscopic patterns of acute myocardial necrosis in which the underlying pathogenetic mechanisms are also different, and these must be recognized.

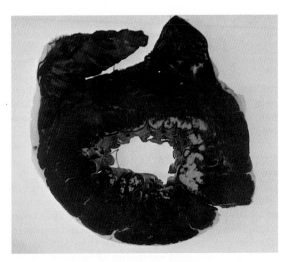

FIGURE 32.22 A transverse section through a heart treated with nitro-blue tetrazolium. Viable muscle is a dark purplish-blue colour. Non-viable myocardium shows no staining. In this case the ischaemic damage is confined to the subendocardial portion of the left ventricular wall.

Macroscopic Delineation of Acute Myocardial Necrosis

This is accomplished by a simple histochemical technique in which differentiation between viable and non-viable myocardium depends on the presence or absence of intracellular respiratory enzymes, e.g. succinic dehydrogenase. Transverse slices of unfixed post-mortem heart are immersed in a solution of nitro-blue tetrazolium together with some sodium succinate (to provide excess substrate) and incubated at 37°C for 7–8 minutes. In viable heart muscle the intracellular dehydrogenases mediate the donation of hydrogen to the yellow, soluble, nitro-blue tetrazolium. This leads to the precipitation of the dye as a purplish-blue insoluble 'formazan'. The necrotic areas, lacking intracellular enzymes, appear colourless against the purplish-blue background (*Fig. 32.22*).

Patterns of Acute Necrosis

Two major patterns of myocardial infarction exist (*Fig. 32.23*) which are known as transmural and subendocardial.

Regional Transmural Infarction (*Fig. 32.24*)

Regional infarcts are relatively large areas of coagulative necrosis confined to the territory of one major coronary artery branch. Thus, for example, occlusion of the anterior descending branch of the left coronary artery (taking account of some variation in coronary artery

anatomy) will lead to necrosis of the anterior wall of the left ventricle and the anterior two-thirds of the interventricular septum. Similarly, infarction of the posterior wall of the left ventricle and the posterior one-third of the septum is likely to be associated with occlusion of the right coronary artery.

Regional infarcts may be further subdivided on the basis of the amount (in terms of thickness) of ventricular wall that has undergone necrosis. Those that involve most of the thickness from endocardium to epicardium are called **transmural**, although they usually show a very thin layer of non-necrotic myocardium just beneath the endocardium, this area being perfused directly from the ventricular cavity. Those that involve less than 50% of the thickness of the ventricular wall, and in which the inner half of this wall is affected, are spoken of as **subendocardial**.

Subendocardial extension is often found at the margins of transmural infarcts.

Coronary Artery Pathology in Regional Transmural Infarction

Within the first hour of the onset of pain and electrocardiographic changes, the artery subtending the area that will later undergo necrosis is totally occluded in the vast majority of instances. In the hours that follow, some of the occluding thrombi undergo lysis and within 12 hours flow becomes restored in about 30% of cases. At this point the previously occluded segment often shows the characteristics of a type II lesion. Thus, a post-mortem examination carried out on a patient who survived for more than 24 hours after the onset of symptoms **may not accurately reflect the causal arterial pathology**. Despite this reservation, more

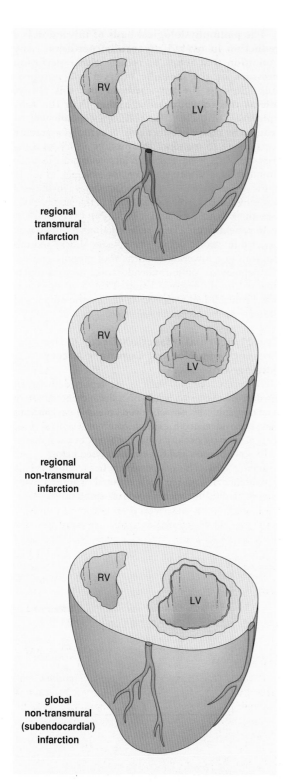

FIGURE 32.23 *Patterns of acute ischaemic necrosis.*

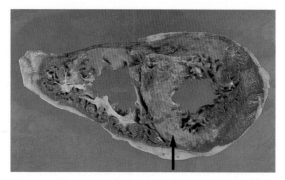

FIGURE 32.24 *Section through a heart treated with nitro-blue tetrazolium. The specimen shows regional myocardial infarction involving the anterior wall of the ventricle and much of the interventricular septum. These findings suggest occlusion of the anterior descending branch of the left coronary artery.*

than 90% of cases of full-thickness regional infarction do show the presence of thrombotic occlusion of the sub-tending artery at post-mortem examination, and it may well be that failure of thrombolysis and the resulting failure of any myocardial salvage may increase the risk of dying and thus skew the post-mortem sample in the direction of those cases in which the thrombus persisted.

Plaque Fissuring and Thrombus Propagation Most occlusive thrombi are associated with plaque fissuring. If the atherosclerotic plaque has a massive basal pool of lipid and tissue debris, and a relatively thin connective tissue cap, the risks of fissuring are enhanced (see pp 335–336). In some cases the fissures are narrow, whereas in others most of the plaque cap appears to have been lost. In either instance, the defect in the connective tissue cap is associated with a platelet-rich thrombus that has both intraplaque and intraluminal components. Downstream of the fissure and the platelet-rich plug, the thrombus consists predominantly of fibrin and incorporated red blood cells, suggesting that propagation has occurred. In a small number of cases thrombosis develops in the absence of plaque fissures, such thrombi forming in areas of high-grade stenosis. In a very small fraction, regional transmural infarction has been documented as being due to spasm, usually in relation to a stenosed segment, but occasionally in the absence of stenosing atherosclerosis.

Regional Subendocardial Infarction

Aspects of the pathogenesis of this lesion remain unclear, particularly in view of persisting uncertainties regarding the electrocardiographic criteria on which this diagnosis is based during life.

There is a lower frequency of occlusive coronary artery thrombi at post-mortem examination in these patients and angiographic studies suggest a greater degree of collateral flow than in hearts with regional transmural infarcts. Despite this, these patients run an increased risk of recurrent episodes of severe myocardial ischaemia.

Non-Regional Infarction

In non-regional infarcts the whole circumference of the left ventricular wall is involved (see *Figs 32.22* and *32.25*) and these lesions are usually subendocardial, although in some instances the necrosis may be more extensive and may approach the endocardium in a curious 'saw-tooth' pattern. Satellite foci of necrosis may be seen in association with this diffuse subendocardial lesion and in such cases the right ventricle may also be involved.

Non-regional infarction (diffuse subendocardial necrosis) occurs most frequently in patients with widespread coronary artery stenosis **but may be seen in the absence of coronary atherosclerosis**. Occlusive thrombosis is found in no more than 15% of patients with this pattern of necrosis who come to post-mortem examination.

The pathophysiological basis of this lesion is a reduction in overall myocardial perfusion. Any condition that tends to reduce either perfusion pressure or the diastolic interval will compromise flow to the myocardium and this always affects the subendocardial rather than the subepicardial muscle. The perfusion pressure will be reduced by means of either a fall in aortic root pressure (or a failure to transduce this pressure in severe coronary stenosis), or an increase in intraventricular diastolic pressure. Such situations occur, for example, in severe aortic valve disease or cardiogenic shock, in the end stages of dilated cardiomyopathy or in the presence of a very thick ventricular wall (*Fig. 32.26*).

In patients with a large transmural infarct there may be a fall in cardiac output (cardiogenic shock) and this can lead to a lowering in aortic root pressure and the development of diffuse subendocardial necrosis superimposed on the regional lesion. Thus, a vicious circle may be established with ever-falling cardiac output and ever-increasing myocardial necrosis.

Can Myocardial Infarction Occur in the Presence of a Normal Coronary Artery Angiogram?

Occasionally, regional infarcts are reported (between 1% and 3% of the total) in which the subtending artery is angiographically *normal*. Several possible explanations have been advanced for this uncommon event:

1) Coronary occlusion has occurred, but was due to embolization and the embolus lysed before angiography. This is a possibility but requires the existence of a source (such as mitral or aortic valve endocarditis) for such a coronary embolus.

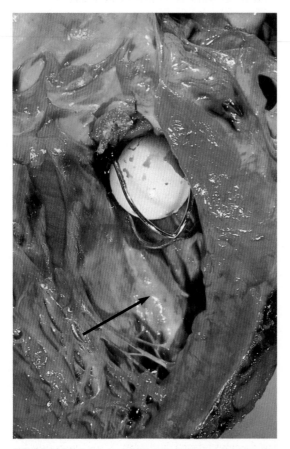

FIGURE 32.25 *Subendocardial ischaemic necrosis involving the interventricular septum. This shows as a large area of pallor (arrow). The patient, whose left ventricular function was severely compromised by mitral valve incompetence, developed ischaemic necrosis after valve replacement. The heart proved difficult to 'restart' after coming off cardiopulmonary bypass.*

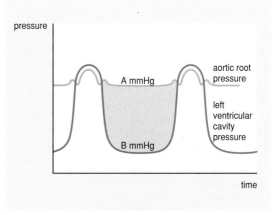

FIGURE 32.26 *Factors controlling perfusion of the subendocardial zone of the left ventricular wall. Perfusion 'drive' = A mmHg − B mmHg. Total diastolic perfusion = (A − B) × length of diastole, and is represented by the shaded area. Any decrease in (A − B) or in the length of diastole may lead to subendocardial necrosis.*

2) There may have been an acute plaque event followed by thrombus formation and thrombus lysis before angiography.

3) There may have been a coronary artery dissection that has now resolved.

4) The infarct may have been due to pure arterial spasm. Such an event may be triggered by cocaine abuse, although this is not the only trigger.

5) The affected area of coronary artery may have been 'bridged' by myocardial muscle.

Microscopic Evolution of Myocardial Infarcts

It is difficult to age myocardial infarcts on histological examination because areas may be found in a single infarct that clearly are at different stages of evolution, in terms of necrosis and repair.

Most muscle cells in a regional transmural infarct undergo coagulation necrosis, which is shown by a marked degree of eosinophilia. Within 36–48 hours, loss of cross-striations is seen; individual myofibrils begin to break down and appear as granular debris within the sarcolemma. These early changes are accompanied by an influx of acute inflammatory cells. These cells, chiefly neutrophils, may play a role in limiting the salvageability of the ischaemic myocardium, probably via the release of oxygen free radicals which can cause fatal injury to cell membranes, a situation that is particularly likely if reperfusion takes place. The extent of experimental myocardial ischaemic damage can be limited by pretreatment with non-steroidal anti-inflammatory drugs or by rendering the animals neutropaenic before inducing ischaemia.

In some cases, so-called 'contraction band' necrosis is evident. These localized deeply eosinophilic areas within individual cells represent telescoping of sarcomeres and tend to be seen most often where some degree of reperfusion has taken place. The speed with which **demolition of the necrotic tissue and its replacement by fibrous tissue** take place depends, to a considerable extent, on whether the ischaemia has rendered only the heart muscle cells necrotic or whether the under-perfusion has been so severe as to involve the connective tissue stroma and the intra-myocardial blood vessels.

Where the latter have also undergone necrosis the processes of demolition and repair are retarded; dead muscle fibres may persist in the centre of the infarct for weeks or months, and replacement of the whole area may be very slow indeed. In contrast, repair is much more rapid in those lesions where the stroma has not been rendered necrotic. Small, focal areas of necrosis are common especially near the margins of large infarcts and similar lesions may be seen, independent of the presence or absence of ischaemia in patients with **very high catecholamine levels, low plasma potassium concentrations and severe cardiac hypertrophy**. Some cells show a curious enlarged and vacuolated appearance with

disappearance of myofibrils which has been termed 'myocytolysis'. Their nuclei stain normally and the cells still retain their intracellular enzymes. These cells are thought to be teetering on the edge of survival but have lost their ability to maintain their normal volume, possibly through inhibition of the sodium-potassium ATPase pump.

Right Ventricular Infarction

Most cases of myocardial infarction affect the left ventricle alone; isolated right ventricular infarction is exceedingly rare and usually occurs in patients who have marked right ventricular hypertrophy. However, in patients with large posterior infarcts resulting from proximal occlusion of the right coronary artery, some extension of myocardial damage to involve the right ventricle is not uncommon.

Complications of Acute Transmural Infarction (*Fig. 32.27*)

Myocardial Rupture

This catastrophic development may occur in three forms: external cardiac rupture, rupture through the interventricular septum and rupture of the papillary muscle.

External Cardiac Rupture

This is the third most common cause of death in patients with transmural infarcts, and is responsible for 10–20% of fatal cases. It tends to occur relatively more commonly in older women.

The diagnosis of cardiac tamponade at post mortem is not always easy because haemorrhage into the pericardial sac may be agonal being associated with vigorous external cardiac massage in patients. However, the presence of a tense bulging pericardium due to the accumulation of 300–500 ml of blood can be regarded as unequivocal evidence of true tamponade.

Early rupture (within 48 hours) is associated with a slit-like tear in the myocardium at the junction of the viable and non-viable muscle. More commonly, rupture occurs between 5 and 10 days after the onset of symptoms and, in these cases, the rupture takes place through the infarct itself, blood tracking through the wall between the necrotic muscle bundles.

Rupture Through the Interventricular Septum

Septal rupture complicates antero- and postero-septal infarcts and may create a defect between 1 and 3 cm^2 in area. Such a defect imposes a sudden additional haemodynamic burden on a heart already functionally compromised by a large transmural infarct, and it is therefore not surprising that this complication carries a

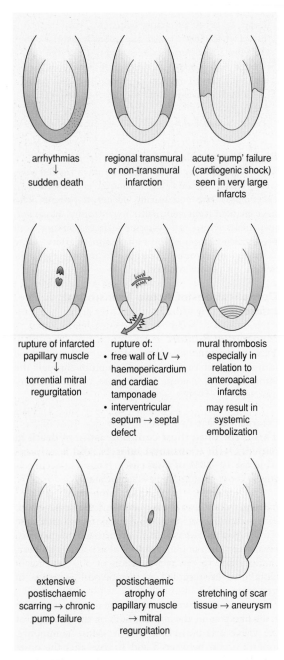

arrhythmias
↓
sudden death

regional transmural
or non-transmural
infarction

acute 'pump' failure
(cardiogenic shock)
seen in very large
infarcts

rupture of infarcted
papillary muscle
↓
torrential mitral
regurgitation

rupture of:
• free wall of LV →
  haemopericardium
  and cardiac
  tamponade
• interventricular
  septum → septal
  defect

mural thrombosis
especially in
relation to
anteroapical
infarcts

may result in
systemic
embolization

extensive
postischaemic
scarring → chronic
pump failure

postischaemic
atrophy of
papillary muscle
→ mitral
regurgitation

stretching of scar
tissue → aneurysm

FIGURE 32.27 Possible consequences of acute myocardial
ischaemia. LV, left ventricle.

high mortality rate. Initially, the septal defect has a
ragged outline but, in patients who survive long
enough to undergo surgical repair of the defect, the
edges become smoothed out as the infarct heals. The
fibrous tissue that has, by this time, formed round the
defect provides an anchorage for the insertion of
sutures.

Rupture of Papillary Muscle

Ischaemic damage to the papillary muscles is extremely
common, and is present in up to half of patients with
posterior infarction and in a sizeable proportion of
those with anterior infarction. In a small minority of
patients (less than 1% of fatal cases) part or all of the
papillary muscle becomes torn off and is swept up
towards the mitral orifice. **This leads to sudden
and torrential mitral valve regurgitation.** Postischaemic atrophy, as opposed to rupture, of the
papillary muscles is quite common and may also lead to
severe grades of mitral incompetence.

Intraventricular Thrombosis

Myocardial infarction often leads to non-moving (aki-
netic) segments of the ventricular wall. The resulting
stasis promotes the formation of intraventricular
thrombi. The larger the infarct, the greater is the risk of
such thrombi occurring; they are seen only in association with transmural infarction. Large anteroapical
infarcts have a 50% chance of being complicated by
mural thrombosis. The main adverse consequence is, of
course **systemic embolization**.

Extension and Expansion in Myocardial Infarcts

The term **extension** refers to the situation when an
infarct increases in size because of further episodes of
myocardial ischaemia. In a clinical context it can be
recognized by more widespread electrocardiographic
changes or decreasing left ventricular function in a
patient with an acute infarct.

Infarct **expansion**, on the other hand, refers to a
'stretching' of the infarcted area so that it increases.
There is *no* new ischaemic necrosis and thus thinning of
the left ventricular wall is the usual consequence.
Expansion may be due to sliding of necrotic cardiac
muscle cells in relation to each other or to actual tearing apart of the infarcted muscle bundles. The latter
mechanism tends to be associated with the formation of
a tear in the overlying endocardium.

Ventricular Aneurysm Formation

A true aneurysm of the left ventricle is a convex dilatation, the wall of which consists predominantly of collagen. Such lesions are the result of full-thickness
infarction and the stretching that occurs in the fibrous
tissue replacing necrotic muscle. The term includes
lesions with a wide base and which bulge diffusely from
the ventricular wall, as well as saccular lesions that have
a comparatively narrow neck. Patients may present
with recurrent or persistent re-entry arrhythmias, cardiac failure or systemic embolization as a consequence
of mural thrombosis.

The fibrous tissue wall occasionally undergoes
extensive dystrophic calcification. This is particularly
likely when there is a thin layer of thrombotic material
covering the luminal surfaces.

SUDDEN DEATH DUE TO MYOCARDIAL ISCHAEMIA

Sudden death means death occurring within 6 hours of the onset of symptoms in a previously symptom-free individual. **IHD accounts for 60% of such fatalities.** Even if the time period is reduced to 15 minutes, the proportion of cases due to IHD does not change. Some 40% of all deaths attributable to IHD fall into this category, a clinical problem of enormous magnitude considering the frequency of IHD. Half the patients dying suddenly from IHD are said to have been unaware that they had any cardiovascular disease. Such data re-emphasize the importance of **prevention** as opposed to treatment of established, clinically overt disease, if significant reductions in mortality are to be obtained.

PATHOPHYSIOLOGY OF SUDDEN DEATH

Sudden death due to IHD is almost entirely due to the occurrence of fatal ventricular arrhythmias – ventricular fibrillation usually preceded by increasingly frequent ventricular ectopic beats. Of patients who collapse and are successfully resuscitated, only about 16% develop a Q wave on electrocardiography and about 45% show raised plasma concentrations of intracellular cardiac enzymes. **Thus sudden ischaemic cardiac death is *not* merely a stage in the evolution of acute myocardial infarction.**

Pathological Changes in the Coronary Arteries in Sudden Death Due to IHD

For many years the pathogenesis of sudden death in IHD has been a matter for controversy. Post-mortem coronary angiography followed by detailed histological studies of the stenosed or occluded segments have shown the presence of type II lesions with plaque fissuring and consequent thrombosis in more than 90% of cases examined. The frequency of **occlusive thrombi** is low (about 30%) but the remaining 60% show mural thrombi of the type described in unstable angina. Intramyocardial platelet emboli (*Fig. 32.28*) and tiny foci of muscle necrosis have been found in up to 40% of cases. **Such data show that there is a common pathological basis for a significant proportion of cases of unstable angina and for sudden cardiac death due to myocardial underperfusion – plaque fissuring – and emphasize the importance of gaining a better understanding of this key event in the natural history of atherosclerotic plaques.** In patients in whom no new acute arterial lesion is found at necropsy, there is usually evidence of a healed myocardial infarct, often in a heart with left ventricular hypertrophy.

In the 'thrombotic' group, the arrhythmias arise

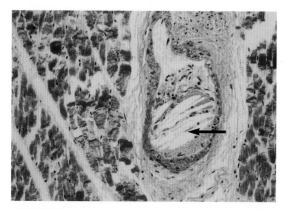

FIGURE 32.28 *Atheromatous embolism in an intramyocardial vessel. Note the cholesterol crystals (arrow) admixed with mauve-staining platelets.*

because of acute ischaemia of the myocardium. In patients with a scarred and/or hypertrophied myocardium, the arrhythmias arise on the basis of a re-entry tachycardia. The prognosis of patients in the second group is said to be worse than that of those in the 'thrombotic' group.

Disorders of the Heart Valves

ACUTE RHEUMATIC FEVER

Many processes cause dysfunction of the heart valves. The consequences of *acute rheumatic fever* in the form of **chronic valve disease**, dominated cardiological practice until the mid-1960s. In Western countries, acute rheumatic fever is now rare but a significant amount of cardiac surgical practice still consists of dealing with the chronic consequences of previous rheumatic episodes. In economically deprived communities rheumatic heart disease still contributes significantly to the burden of chronic ill-health.

DEFINITION

Rheumatic fever is a non-suppurative inflammatory disorder resulting from an immune-mediated reaction to cell wall components of β-haemolytic streptococci. In the acute phase many tissues may be affected but the heart valves are the principal target for chronic effects.

CHILDREN ARE THE CHIEF VICTIMS OF ACUTE RHEUMATIC FEVER

Acute rheumatic fever occurs mainly in childhood, most commonly affecting those between the ages of 5 and 8 years, although first attacks may occur up to the age of 20 years. Its pathogenetic relationship with chronic valvular disease is well established; the incidence of *new* cases of chronic rheumatic valve disease has declined in parallel with a very steep decline in the incidence of acute rheumatic fever in the countries of the West. **In the UK it is estimated that in the mid-1920s between 2.6 and 15% of all children had suffered an attack of rheumatic fever, while by 1975 only 400 hospital admissions per annum for acute rheumatic fever were recorded.**

This decline is a reflection of a number of factors. These include:

- improved socioeconomic circumstances
- the introduction of antibiotics for the treatment of streptococcal pharyngitis
- a decrease in the frequency of such streptococcal infections

Despite the decline of acute rheumatic fever in certain countries, the disease is still common in the Third World. Even in the USA there has been a recrudescence, apparently related to the consequences of economic deprivation including crowded living conditions which promote spread of infection and inadequate or no antibiotic treatment for streptococcal infections.

Clinical Features

Classically, the patients develop **a self-limiting sore throat caused by a β-haemolytic streptococcus (Lancefield group A)**. This is followed within 10 days to 6 weeks by the appearance of a syndrome characterized by features classified as being either *major* or *minor*. These are listed in *Table 32.8*.

A clinical diagnosis depends on the presence of *two major* or *one major and two minor* features. The acute disease is self-limiting in most cases, although a few patients die during the acute phase from cardiac failure, which is an expression of extensive and severe myocardial involvement. The risk of recurrence associated with subsequent episodes of streptococcal pharyngitis is high. While in an acute attack, joint involvement (in the form of a 'flitting' polyarthritis, i.e. one that involves one joint after another) is most conspicuous from the patient's point of view; it is the cardiac involvement that can lead to lifelong disability. The aphorism coined by Sir Thomas Lewis, that 'rheumatism licks the joints, but bites the heart', is an apt one. In some instances the onset may be subtle and insidious, lacking fever, arthritis and tachycardia. Such a mild clinical syndrome does not *per se* carry a reduced risk for the development of chronic valve disease.

Pathogenesis

When the prevalence of rheumatic fever was at its peak, only about 3% of patients with streptococcal sore throat were at risk of developing acute rheumatic fever; thus the immune reaction to streptococcal antigens is idiosyncratic. The response is elicited by antigenic cell wall components of the streptococcus and is a **systemic** one; there is no question of direct infection of the heart by the streptococci. The antigen(s) believed to be implicated are closely related to the fibrillary M protein of the **β-haemolytic streptococcus**. This protein confers the ability to resist phagocytosis; antibodies raised against it cross-react with antigens on the sarcolemma of the heart muscle cell. In addition, the serum of patients with acute rheumatic fever also contains antibodies against the polysaccharide antigen characteristic of group A streptococci, and these antibodies also react with glycoproteins in the connective tissue of the heart.

The Cellular Targets for this Immune Response are Multiple

Targets for the immune response in acute rheumatic fever include:

- heart muscle (sarcolemma and subsarcolemmal cytoplasm)
- heart valve connective tissue
- thymic cells
- human glomerular basement membrane
- neuronal cytoplasm of the subthalamic and caudate nuclei in the brain
- skin
- lymphocytes

These all share antigens with the cell wall of the streptococcus; for example, absorption of serum from a patient with rheumatic fever by streptococcal cell wall removes antibodies binding to neuronal cytoplasm. The appearance of antibodies directed against these 'self' antigens indicates that normal T-cell tolerance has been overcome, presumably because of the presentation of the antigens to the immune system on a different carrier. **While there is no doubt that acute rheumatic fever is associated with the presence of cross-reacting antibodies in the serum of patients, it is much less clear that these antibodies are responsible for the tissue damage.** The

Table 32.8 Clinical Features of Acute Rheumatism

Major	Minor
Pancarditis	Fever
'Flitting' polyarthritis	Prolonged P–R interval on ECG
Chorea	Raised erythrocyte sedimentation rate
Subcutaneous nodules	
Erythema	

injection of certain streptococcal antigens into mice is followed by the appearance of myocardial lesions and antistreptococcal antibodies. Passive transfer of *serum* from these mice to non-immune mice is *not* followed by the development of cardiac lesions, although such lesions occur if *lymphoid cells* are transferred from sensitized to non-immune mice. This suggests that tissue damage is mediated by T cells and that the presence of antibodies may be an epiphenomenon.

Pathological Features

Rheumatic fever produces a *pancarditis*, i.e. the pericardium, myocardium and endocardium may all be affected.

Pericardium

Rheumatic pericarditis is characterized by a fibrin-rich exudate, deposited on visceral and parietal pericardia, with strands of fibrin connecting the two layers. In fatal cases, parting the two layers of pericardium at post mortem shows the surface exudate to have a somewhat reticulated appearance sometimes called a '*bread and butter heart*'. In most cases the pericarditis resolves completely and is not followed by scarring and consequent constriction of the heart.

Myocardial Pathology

In about 1% of cases, death occurs during the acute phase; this is due to severe, diffuse, myocardial involvement giving rise to conduction disturbances and heart failure. At post-mortem examination, the heart has a globular shape owing to dilatation of the chambers and the myocardium feels flabby.

The intramyocardial lesions seen during this acute phase fall into two groups:

1) A **non-specific myocarditis** with oedema between the muscle fibres, focal collections of inflammatory cells in the interstitial connective tissue and, rarely, an arteritis involving small intramyocardial vessels.

2) A **specific granulomatous myocarditis**, in which variable numbers of small, highly characteristic lesions are found in the connective tissue between the muscle fibres. These are known as **Aschoff nodules** (*Fig. 32.29*).

Aschoff nodules may occur in the walls of all four chambers but are most common in the interventricular septum, the posterior wall of the left ventricle, the posterior papillary muscle, the pulmonary conus and the left atrium. The appearance of these lesions varies with the stage of their development.

The earliest stage is focal swelling of collagen fibres which show some alteration of the normal staining pattern. Often the lesions occur near small blood vessels or even within the walls of such vessels. Some studies have shown the presence of immunoglobulins bound to altered collagen but this is not always so. The next stage is the accumulation of cells round the altered collagen. These cells are of three main morphological types:

1) **Aschoff giant cells** which are multinucleated and have a basophilic cytoplasm.

2) So-called **Anitschkow myocytes. This is a misnomer since both these cells and the Aschoff giant cells are derived from macrophages rather than muscle.** The nuclei of these cells have a highly characteristic appearance with a bar of darkly staining chromatin running down the centre of the nucleus parallel to its long axis. From the sides of this bar small processes protrude giving the appearance of a caterpillar or a date-stone. When cut transversely this central darkly stained zone within a relatively pale nucleus has been termed an 'owl's eye' nucleus. Both this and the Aschoff giant cell react with antibodies raised against macrophage components.

3) **Lymphocytes**, 90% of which are T helper cells and the remainder either suppressor or cytotoxic T cells.

With the passage of months or even years, the Aschoff nodules become converted to small scars. Because of the chronicity of these lesions, **the presence of Aschoff nodules tells us only that there has been an episode of acute rheumatic fever but it has no implications that the process is active at the time of biopsy.**

In the case of the mitral valve, contraction due to the presence of scar tissue and fusion frequently affects not only the cusps but the **chordae tendineae** as well (*Fig. 32.30*), this resulting in a marked loss of the ability of the valve cusps to move up into position during ventricular systole. This makes a considerable

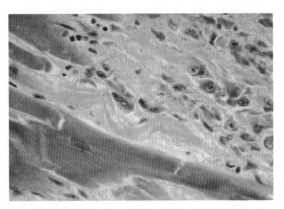

FIGURE 32.29 *Aschoff nodule in acute rheumatic carditis; intermyocyte connective tissue shows aggregates of macrophage-derived cells, some of which show very prominent nucleoli ('owl-eye' nuclei).*

Endocardial Pathology

In patients who have died during the acute phase of the illness, the endocardial changes are the least impressive. The affected valves are somewhat thickened as a result of oedema and there is usually a row of small (1–2 mm in diameter), flat, tan-coloured vegetations along the line where the cusps touch each other during closure of the valves. **These vegetations are platelet-rich microthrombi** occurring from contact-related trauma to the endocardial surface of the valves. Unlike the larger thrombotic vegetations of infective endocarditis, the tiny vegetations of acute rheumatic fever do not easily become detached and are, thus, not associated with embolic complications. Any valve may be affected; the mitral valve alone is the site of rheumatic endocarditis in about 50% of cases and the aortic valve is the next most frequently affected, this occurring either with coincident mitral valve lesions or alone.

Within a few days new blood vessels appear within the cusp at its base and extend deeply into the cusp substance. This vascularization is associated with an increase in fibroblast activity and the laying down of new collagen which is predominantly type III. This process is analogous to that occurring in wound healing. In many instances the degree of fibrosis is slight and self-limiting, and valve function is hardly if at all affected. In other instances the scarring continues relentlessly over years. This can lead to:

a) **contraction of cusp tissue leading to a decrease in cusp area** and thus to **incompetence** of the valve.

b) **thickening and stiffening of the cusp leading to a decrease in normal mobility and thus to incompetence**. This is particularly likely to occur in relation to the mitral valve.

c) **fusion of the commissures (the points at which adjacent cusps are inserted into the valve ring) by bridges of scar tissue. This leads to a decrease in the area of the valve orifices (stenosis)** and affects the mitral and/or the aortic valves most commonly.

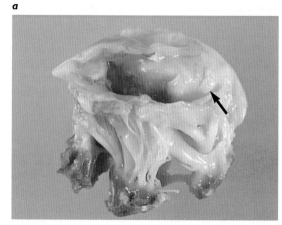

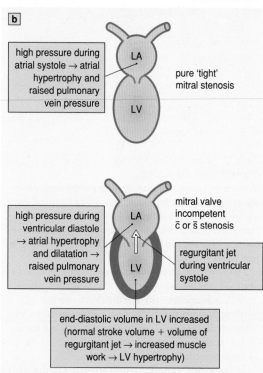

FIGURE 32.30 **a** *Post-rheumatic mitral valve disease. This surgically removed specimen shows fusion of the commissures (arrow) and marked thickening and shortening of the chordae tendineae.* **b** *Mitral stenosis and mitral incompetence. LV, left ventricle.*

contribution to the development of mitral valve incompetence.

Why the scarring of valves continues in some patients who have had acute rheumatic fever and not in others is still not well understood. In some instances it may be due to repeated immunological injury associated with recurrences of streptococcal infection, which may be subclinical. In others, the abnormal blood flow patterns across somewhat distorted valves may be associated with the occurrence of small mural thrombi, and the growth factors released from the platelets and other components of the thrombi may account for the increasing fibrosis.

CHRONIC RHEUMATIC VALVE DISEASE

Whichever valve is considered, the processes involved in chronic rheumatic disease are essentially the same:

- **commissural fusion**
- **cusp scarring**
- **dystrophic calcification**

These are the features of any postinflammatory valve disorder and are not *specific* for rheumatic heart disease.

MITRAL STENOSIS

Despite the equal sex incidence of acute rheumatic fever, mitral stenosis is more common in females (the reported female : male ratios vary from 1.5–4 : 1).

Fusion of commissures with reduction of the area of the mitral valve orifice is a major contributor to the stenosis but increased cusp stiffness and chordal fusion also play a part. In young patients in whom cusp retraction and dystrophic calcification have not yet developed, pure commissural fusion accounts for the stenosis, the valve cusps retaining most of their normal mobility. Auscultation in such cases shows the presence of a pronounced 'opening snap' associated with an abrupt halting of movement of the cusps. The commissural fusion may be treated effectively by splitting the commissures, so restoring virtually normal valve function. In a few children, congenital commissure fusion has been reported as being the cause of mitral stenosis. Stenosis is sometimes seen in the absence of commissural fusion where cusp stiffness and calcification are very marked, and obliteration of the interchordal spaces by scar tissue may also contribute significantly to stenosis.

Effects of Mitral Stenosis on the Left Atrium

The size of the left atrium in mitral stenosis varies from case to case. In some, the left atrium is normal in size while in others it is grossly dilated; these larger atria are almost invariably the site of intracavity thrombus formation. The reason for this variability in left atrial volume is not clear.

Left-sided intra-atrial thrombosis is clinically significant principally because of the risk of systemic embolization. This is potentiated by the presence of **atrial fibrillation**, which is frequently seen in association with left atrial dilatation and thrombus formation. The most frequent site for thrombi is within the atrial appendage from which part of the thrombus often protrudes into the main atrial cavity. Occasionally a sheet of thrombus forms over the whole of the left atrial wall and this thrombus may calcify, thus rendering the outline of the left atrial wall easily visible on radiography. The rarest form of atrial thrombus is a roughly spherical mass usually attached to the interatrial septum and this may on occasion block the mitral orifice in a ball-valve fashion.

Systemic Embolization in Mitral Stenosis

This occurs in up to 30% of cases and may be a presenting feature of mitral valve disease. The clinical syndromes resulting from embolization reflect, of course, the site of impaction of the emboli.

Atrial thrombi are by far the most common site of origin of emboli, but occasionally masses of calcified debris mixed with thrombus may break off from the abnormal valves themselves.

Pathophysiological Effects of Mitral Stenosis

Significant mitral valve stenosis leads inevitably to pulmonary *venous* hypertension with a concomitant rise in pulmonary wedge capillary pressure. This leads to pulmonary *arterial* hypertension which, in turn, both causes an increased workload on the right ventricle and is associated with increased lipid deposition in the intima of the pulmonary arteries.

The **morphological correlates** of these events are:

- Rather solid **brown lungs caused by** the presence of many haemosiderin-laden macrophages in the alveoli. The iron deposition is due to recurrent bleeding from congested alveolar capillaries.
- Numerous **fatty streaks** and, on occasion, some fibrolipid **atherosclerotic plaques** in the pulmonary arterial bed.
- **Right ventricular hypertrophy** due to the high pressure overload on this chamber.

Mitral Incompetence in Rheumatic Heart Disease

Pure mitral incompetence is seldom a manifestation of chronic rheumatic disease but occurs quite frequently in association with stenosis. Chief contributors to the incompetent state are cusp retraction due to scarring and thickening and fusion of the chordae tendineae.

In contrast with pure stenosis, where the left ventricle appears normal, the presence of incompetence is associated with **dilatation and hypertrophy of the left ventricle due to volume overload**. The degree of left atrial enlargement tends to be greater in the presence of mitral incompetence than in association with pure stenosis. Pulmonary venous and arterial hypertension occur in the same way as in pure stenosis but the survival times tend to be shorter and the morphological changes in the lung and right ventricle are, as a result, less striking than in pure stenosis.

Aortic Valve Changes in Chronic Rheumatic Heart Disease

Pure aortic stenosis is rare in rheumatic heart disease because the commissural fusion that causes it does not only narrow the valve orifice but renders it incapable of being closed. Thus the typical aortic valve abnormality in chronic rheumatic heart disease is **combined stenosis and incompetence**. If cusp scarring is present in the absence of commissural fusion then pure aortic incompetence may occur.

NON-RHEUMATIC VALVE DISEASE

AORTIC VALVE

Normal Anatomy and Function

The normal aortic valve has three half-moon–shaped cusps of equal size, giving the valve orifice a triradiate shape. In diastole each cusp overlaps its neighbours and thus the line of closure is not at the free edge of the cusps. The area between the line of closure and the free edge is known as the lunula and this often becomes fenestrated in later life, although this has no functional significance because of the overlapping of the cusps in diastole. **Overlapping of the cusps is essential for effective valve closure; this means that the cusp area must be greater than the area of the aortic root, (a ratio of 1.6 : 1 in the normal valve). If this ratio is decreased, the resulting mismatch between aortic root area and cusp area leads to regurgitation of blood from the aortic root into the left ventricle during ventricular diastole (i.e. aortic incompetence develops)** (*Fig. 32.31*).

In ventricular systole, the three cusps, being freely mobile, fold back into the aortic sinuses and there should be no pressure gradient between the left ventricular cavity and the aortic root when the valve is open.

Congenitally Abnormal Aortic Valve

Some 1–2% of the population has a congenitally bicuspid aortic valve. This functions quite normally during early life but even then can be diagnosed by the presence of a late systolic 'click' on auscultation, and by echocardiography. The two cusps may be equal or unequal in size and the appearance may be complicated by the presence of a bar of connective tissue which extends between the aortic surface of one cusp (usually the larger one) and the aortic wall. This is known as a **median raphe** and its presence should not be interpreted as evidence of the existence of a third cusp.

The passage of time affects all aortic valves. Fibrous thickening occurs along the line of closure, and small nodules (known as corpora Arantii) marking the central point of each cusp are almost always found in deceased patients aged 50 years or more. They have no functional significance. Calcification commonly affects the valve and is an important cause of stenosis in subjects aged more than 70 years). The calcium deposition begins in the sinus area and later extends to involve the cusps themselves. **The presence of abnormal closure patterns, as found in congenitally bicuspid valves, leads to the valve being significantly calcified much earlier in life than is the case with normal tricuspid aortic valves.**

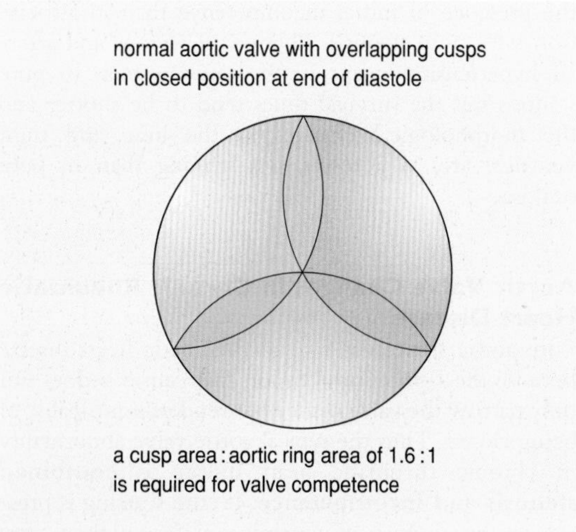

Aortic Stenosis

Four main types of aortic stenosis are listed in *Table 32.9* (see also *Fig. 32.32*). With respect to acquired causes, more than one may be found in a single individual.

Table 32.9 Main Types of Aortic Stenosis

1. True congenital aortic stenosis

2. Post-inflammatory aortic stenosis resulting from commissural fusion

3. Stenosis resulting from calcification of a congenitally bicuspid aortic valve

4. Stenosis resulting in old age from dystrophic calcification of a tricuspid aortic valve

---

True Congenital Aortic Stenosis

True congenital aortic stenosis results from failure of separation of the aortic valve cusps. Most commonly the valve ring is occupied by a dome-shaped sheet of fibrous tissue in which there is a small central orifice. It is the precise homologue of congenital pulmonary stenosis. More rarely, there may be what is called unicommissural stenosis in which there is an eccentrically situated orifice with an elliptical or 'teardrop' shape. Early surgery is needed in both these situations but some patients with the unicommissural variant may survive to adult life; in patients aged 15–35 years, this is the commonest type of aortic stenosis seen in the UK.

normal aortic valve with overlapping cusps in closed position at end of diastole

a cusp area : aortic ring area of 1.6 : 1 is required for valve competence

FIGURE 32.31 Normal aortic valve.

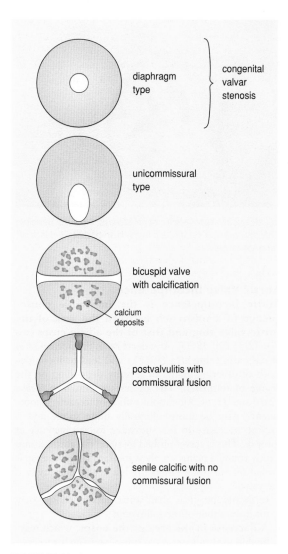

FIGURE 32.32 *Aortic stenosis.*

Congenital aortic stenosis accounts for **about 5% of the cases of congenital heart disease** seen in the UK. Stenosis affecting the left outflow tract may also occur as a result of subvalvar or supravalvar anomalies.

Post-inflammatory Aortic Stenosis

This is due to commissural fusion following rheumatic fever. In the UK it occurs mainly in immigrants from areas, such as Asia and the Middle East, where rheumatic heart disease is prevalent.

Calcified Congenitally Bicuspid Aortic Valve

This is the commonest single cause of isolated aortic stenosis in middle life. Only a small proportion of those with a congenitally bicuspid valve develop sufficient dystrophic calcification to cause stenosis; it is not known why some should be affected and others escape.

A typical patient will develop a short ejection systolic murmur in the aortic region between the ages of 20 and 40 years; the mean age for diagnosis of stenosis is about 50 years, although it may make itself apparent as early as 35 years and as late as 75 years.

Macroscopic Features

To make an accurate macroscopic diagnosis the *intact* valve should be inspected because, however marked the secondary changes, the **linear, slit-like valve orifice**, which *must* be present if there are only two cusps, will still be readily apparent (*Fig. 32.33*). A mild degree of aortic incompetence is often present in addition to the stenosis.

As in all types of aortic stenosis, there is a marked degree of concentric hypertrophy of the left ventricular wall with a normal or small, centrally situated, ventricular cavity. **This type of left ventricular hypertrophy is characteristic of a** *high pressure overload* **situation and is seen not only in aortic stenosis but also in patients with systemic hypertension and/or with coarctation of the aorta** (*Fig. 32.34*).

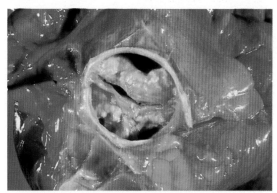

FIGURE 32.33 *Aortic stenosis superimposed on bicuspid aortic valve. Note the slit-like valve orifice, which is characteristic of the bicuspid state.*

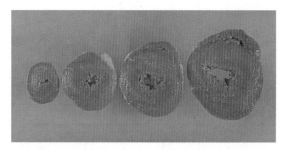

FIGURE 32.34 *Aortic stenosis imposed a high-pressure overload on the left ventricle leading to 'concentric' left ventricular hypertrophy in which the ventricular chamber is centrally placed and either normal or, more often, decreased in size.*

Patients with aortic stenosis run a considerable risk of dying suddenly, presumably related to the onset of serious ventricular arrhythmias. There is a considerable pressure gradient between the left ventricular cavity and the aortic root when the valve is open (*Fig. 32.35*) and myocardial perfusion is decreased. Thus subendocardial blood flow in the left ventricular wall may be seriously compromised. In addition 30–50% of patients requiring aortic valve surgery for stenosis have significant degrees of coronary artery narrowing.

Stenosis Due to 'Senile' Calcification of a Tricuspid Aortic Valve

This form is due to the presence of rigid crescent-shaped masses of calcium, deposited initially in the aortic sinuses, which fix the cusps in a semi-closed position. There is *no* evidence of commissural fusion (*Fig. 32.36*).

Most patients are older than 75 years but the condition can be seen in those aged 60–70 years. Some of these younger patients have a coexisting cause of accelerated dystrophic calcification such as Paget's disease of bone.

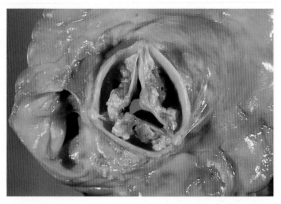

FIGURE 32.36 *Senile calcific aortic stenosis. Note the triradiate valve orifice, heavy calcification in the cusp pockets and lack of commissural fusion.*

Aortic Valve Incompetence

Aortic incompetence is the inevitable consequence of a mismatch between the area of the aortic valve ring and that of the aortic cusps (see *Figs 32.35* and *32.37*). Any decrease in the normal ratio of cusp area : ring area (1.6 : 1) will lead to incompetence of differing grades of severity depending on the degree of mismatch. The causes are shown in *Tables 32.10* and *32.11*. Alterations sufficient to cause incompetence may be morphologically quite subtle and it may be necessary to test the valve for competence at autopsy. This is accomplished by tying the aortic stump tightly round a mains supply water tap. When the tap is turned on, no water enters the left ventricular cavity if the valve is competent.

It should be clear that aortic incompetence may result from either of the following:

- A **decrease in the area of the cusps**, which may be due to shrinkage as a result of scarring, or to perforation
- An **increase in the area of the valve ring**

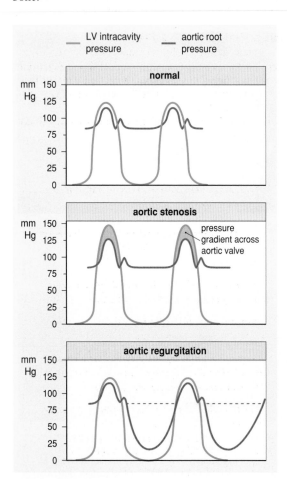

FIGURE 32.35 *Functional changes in aortic valve disease.*

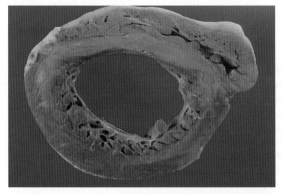

FIGURE 32.37 *The left ventricle in aortic incompetence. This imposes a high volume overload on the ventricle; hypertrophy is associated with a dilated left ventricular chamber.*

Table 32.10 Causes of Cusp Abnormality	
Perforation of cusps	Infective endocarditis
Retraction of cusps	Rheumatic disease
	Rheumatoid disease
	Ankylosing spondylitis

Table 32.11 Causes of Aortic Root Abnormality	
Inflammatory	Syphilis
	Rheumatoid disease
	Ankylosing spondylitis
	Non-specific urethritis
	Non-specific aortitis
Non-inflammatory	May have aortic dissection
	Marfan or non-Marfan familial
	No aortic dissection
	Idiopathic root dilatation

Cusp Abnormalities

Perforation of the cusps usually results from destruction of part of the cusp substance in the course of infective endocarditis (see pp 366–369). A decrease in the cusp area due to scarring may be the expression of chronic rheumatic valve disease. In ankylosing spondylitis a combination of cusp scarring and distortion of the aortic root may occur and a rather similar situation obtains in rheumatoid disease affecting the aorta.

Aortic Root Abnormalities

Dilatation of the aortic root is an important mechanism for aortic incompetence. The normal upper limit of the circumference of the aortic root is 10.5 cm and an increase may cause incompetence. If the circumference reaches 12 cm or greater then significant regurgitation *must* occur.

Aortic root dilatation today is most commonly encountered as a result of connective tissue dysfunction in the aortic root. This condition is called **idiopathic aortic root dilatation,** a name that emphasizes our ignorance of its aetiology. It is characterized by loss of both elastic lamina and smooth muscle cells, and evidence of inflammation is entirely lacking. In some cases accumulations of connective tissue mucins are present. Similar histological changes are seen in the aorta of patients suffering from Marfan's syndrome (associated with a mutation in the gene coding for the protein fibrillin), and in some cases of osteogenesis imperfecta.

Aortic root dilatation also occurs in association with certain inflammatory disorders. At one time tertiary syphilis was the commonest of these, but now inflammatory aortic root disease is more frequently seen in association with HLA-B27-associated disorders such as ankylosing spondylitis, Reiter's disease and, less frequently, rheumatoid arthritis.

In this group, there is destruction of the elastic fibres and muscle cells of the tunica media, associated with the presence of an inflammatory cell infiltrate of lymphocyte and plasma cells, concentrated around the vasa vasorum.

In inflammatory aortic root disease, dilatation of the root is associated with intimal changes; this appears irregular and 'cobble-stoned', because of scarring within the damaged media. The outermost layer (adventitia) is thickened as a result of also being involved in the inflammatory process.

Aortic root dilatation, especially that associated with inflammation, is associated with secondary changes in the aortic cusps. In syphilitic aortic valve disease, a prominent feature is widening of the commissures with resulting separation of the cusps. The regurgitant flow across the surface of the cusps tends to produce a linear, rolled, fibrous thickening at the cusp edges.

Mitral Valve Incompetence

The causes of mitral valve incompetence are most easily understood against the background of **the functional elements that together make up normal mitral valve closure**. These are listed in *Table 32.12* (see also *Fig. 32.38*, p 364).

A defect in any one of these may lead to mitral incompetence.

Table 32.12 Requirements for Normal Mitral Valve Function
1. **Active muscular narrowing of the valve ring,** the area of which is reduced by 50% during ventricular systole.
2. **Normal mobility of the mitral valve leaflets** so that they move upwards and abut one on the other.
3. **Normal area of the leaflets,** which, if too large, will prolapse into the left atrium.
4. **Normal support by the chordae tendineae** so that the leaflets do not prolapse into the left atrium as pressure increases within the left ventricle.
5. **Normal contraction of the papillary muscles** which hold the chordae and cusps in the correct position as the left ventricle changes shape during systole. It is also important that the direction of papillary muscle 'pull' remains correct.

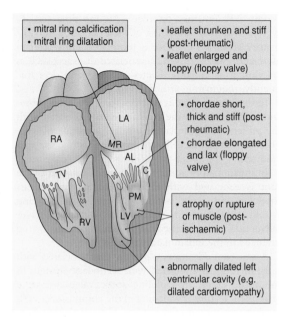

- mitral ring calcification
- mitral ring dilatation

- leaflet shrunken and stiff (post-rheumatic)
- leaflet enlarged and floppy (floppy valve)

- chordae short, thick and stiff (post-rheumatic)
- chordae elongated and lax (floppy valve)

- atrophy or rupture of muscle (post-ischaemic)

- abnormally dilated left ventricular cavity (e.g. dilated cardiomyopathy)

FIGURE 32.38 *Causes of mitral incompetence. AL, anterior leaflet; C, chordae; LA, left auricle; LV, left ventricle; MR, mitral ring; PM, papillary muscles; RA, right auricle; RV, right ventricle; TV, tricuspid valve.*

Mitral Ring Disease

Dystrophic calcification in the angle between the insertion of the valve leaflet and the ventricular myocardium is increasingly common after the age of 70 years (*Fig. 32.39*). Incremental risk factors are **female sex, the presence of diabetes mellitus and Paget's disease of bone**. The calcium is laid down in a J- or C-shaped mass which pushes up the leaflets and may exert a splinting effect on the mitral valve ring during systole. Some degree of incompetence may occur and, in rare cases, the calcium may encroach on to the ventricular septum and interrupt the conduction system, producing atrioventricular block (**Rytand's syndrome**).

Abnormalities of Mitral Leaflet Mobility

Leaflet mobility may be either restricted or abnormally great:

- *Restriction of movement is due to postinflammatory scarring* and is most commonly seen in chronic rheumatic disease where the loss of mobility is mediated by scarring and retraction of the valve cusps and shortening and fusion of the chordae tendineae.
- *Excessive cusp mobility*, resulting in prolapse into the left atrium during ventricular systole, may occur either as a result of lesions related to the cusps and chordae themselves or as a result of dysfunction of the papillary muscles.

The commonest intrinsic pathological lesion in the cusps and chordae resulting in prolapse is what has been called '**floppy mitral valve**'. About 5% of the population can be shown by echocardiography to have some degree of mitral valve prolapse, usually as a result of some degree of floppy change.

Macroscopic and Microscopic Features of Floppy Mitral Valve

The valve cusps are increased in area, dome-shaped and somewhat mucoid in appearance, this last feature being due to accumulation of mucopolysaccharide within the valve matrix (*Figs 32.40 and 32.41*). The chordae, which have a similar myxoid appearance, are elongated and sometimes have a 'waisted' appearance; these waisted areas are sites of potential chordal rupture.

On histological examination the central dense fibrous tissue core of the leaflet shows fragmentation and loss of collagen fibres. It is not known whether this represents an increased degree of collagen breakdown or a partial failure in collagen synthesis. The aetiology is unknown, although the association of floppy mitral valve with both Marfan's syndrome and osteogenesis imperfecta suggests an inherent connective tissue defect.

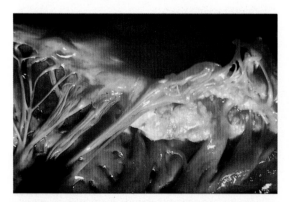

FIGURE 32.39 *Mitral ring calcification. Note the white shelf-like projection protruding from beneath the posterior mitral valve leaflet.*

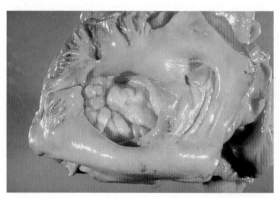

FIGURE 32.40 *Floppy mitral valve, seen from the left atrium. When pressure is exerted on the left ventricle the floppy mitral valve bellies up into the left atrium in a parachute-like fashion.*

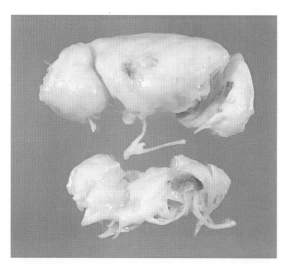

FIGURE 32.41 *Surgically removed floppy mitral valve showing the increase in leaflet area and thin stretched chordae.*

In the majority of patients with a floppy mitral valve, no significant degree of mitral regurgitation develops, the chief clinical expression being a 'click' heard on auscultation during mid-systole. This is thought to be due to the tensing of the chordae as they halt the upward movement of the valve cusps.

The increased cusp mobility may lead to injury to the endocardial surface during valve closure, and areas of endocardial erosion may occur. The exposure of subendocardial fibres and matrix leads to the occurrence of small thrombi. These may be bland, in which case the chief complication is breaking off of small emboli that can be associated with transient cerebral ischaemic episodes, or infected, leading to infective endocarditis.

The most serious complication is chordal rupture (*Fig. 32.42*) leading to the sudden onset of an often catastrophic and torrential mitral regurgitation.

Ischaemic Damage to Papillary Muscles

Postischaemic papillary muscle dysfunction is now one of the commonest causes of mitral incompetence. It may be acute rupture of the whole papillary muscle at its base occurring within a few days of the development of acute myocardial ischaemia. The free portion of the papillary muscle and its chorda prolapse immediately into the left atrium and a torrential regurgitant jet develops. This is fortunately a rare complication, and is found in only 1% of patients with myocardial infarction coming to post-mortem examination. The posteromedial papillary muscle is much more likely to rupture than the anterolateral. The development over longer periods of time of less serious degrees of mitral regurgitation associated with postischaemic scarring of the papillary muscles is common.

Abnormal Ventricular Function and Shape

Where the left ventricle is abnormally dilated, the papillary muscle base may be swung laterally so altering the line of pull on the cusps and producing incompetence. If the ventricular dilatation is associated with dilatation of the mitral valve ring, the incompetence is aggravated.

Acquired Pulmonary Valve Disease

The pulmonary valve may be involved in the chronic rheumatic process. This is rare, and isolated pulmonary stenosis from this cause is extremely uncommon.

The pulmonary valve may also be affected as part of the carcinoid syndrome as a result of the presence of metastasizing argentaffinomas. In the full-blown carcinoid syndrome, usually associated with hepatic metastases, the heart is involved in about 50% of the cases. The pathogenesis of this curious cardiac lesion remains unclear.

Macroscopic Features

The chief pathological change is fibrosis which affects the ventricular aspect of the pulmonary valve cusps to produce either diffuse or plaque-like thickening of the affected cusps. The most common functional consequence is stenosis of the pulmonary valve, although a degree of regurgitation may occur in some cases. The lesions are not necessarily confined to the valve cusps and may extend on to the mural endocardium of the right ventricle.

Microscopic Features

Histologically, the thickened cusps show the presence of a layer of rather acellular fibrous tissue that can be distinguished easily from the underlying valve connective tissue.

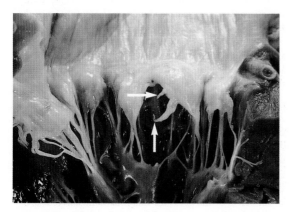

FIGURE 32.42 *Floppy mitral valve in a 74-year-old man. Two of the chordae have ruptured (arrows) and this precipitated the patient into severe pulmonary oedema.*

INFECTIVE ENDOCARDITIS

DEFINITION

Infective endocarditis is an inflammatory disorder affecting the endocardial surface of the heart as a result of infection with one or other of a wide range of pathogenic microorganisms.

It is expressed, morphologically, in the form of masses of thrombus containing the responsible microorganisms. These infected thrombi are known as **vegetations** (*Figs 32.43* and *32.44*).

The clinical and pathological patterns of infective endocarditis have undergone considerable change in the past 30 years. In the past the clinical picture was determined by the predominance of infections by two bacteria. These were *Staphylococcus aureus* **and** *Streptococcus viridans*, **the former being associated with acute endocarditis and the latter with a subacute clinical syndrome. It is now recognized that many pathogenic microorganisms cause infective endocarditis and, with this recognition, has come the realization that there is a similarly**

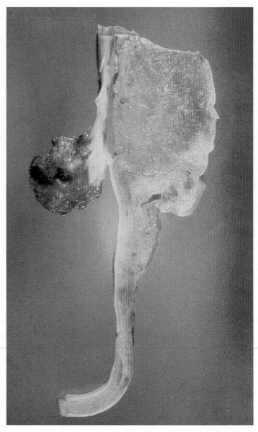

FIGURE 32.44 *Section through left atrial wall and intraventricular septum, showing a vegetation on the posterior cusp of the mitral valve.*

wide clinical spectrum, determined largely by the responsible organism.

Acute Endocarditis

This is a disorder of acute onset that can develop *without any pre-existing haemodynamic abnormalities in the heart*. Its course, in the pre-antibiotic era, was short with an inevitable fatal outcome within days. The heart valve lesions were destructive and often resulted in severe valve incompetence. Any emboli derived from the vegetations of acute infective endocarditis tended to cause pyaemic abscesses.

Sub-acute Endocarditis

This was a disorder with a slow insidious onset, usually associated with some pre-existing haemodynamic abnormality in the heart such as post-rheumatic valve disease, a congenital abnormality such as a ventricular septal defect or the presence of a prosthetic valve. It progressed slowly to produce further valve damage and was associated with a very high death rate in the pre-antibiotic era.

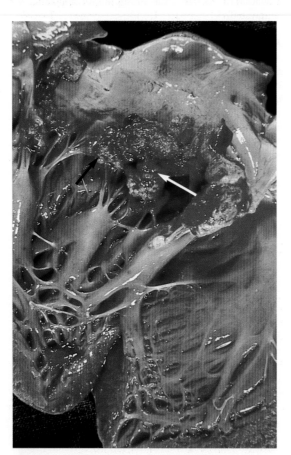

FIGURE 32.43 *Bulky vegetations on the mitral valve (arrow) in a case of staphylococcal endocarditis.*

The epidemiological picture of the disease as seen today shows:

- an increase in the mean age of patients
- a decreasing number of patients known to have pre-existing, acquired, valve disease
- an increase in the number of staphylococcal infections, some of which occur in the context of intravenous drug abuse

Pathogenesis

Two factors appear to interact in the causation of infective endocarditis: **small thrombotic masses** and **bacteraemia**.

Small Thrombotic Masses

Small thrombotic masses on endocardial surfaces may result from haemodynamic injury of the endocardial surface, something that is associated with high pressure jets of blood striking the endocardium, or turbulent flow in relation to endocardial surfaces.

Such injury occurs **in association with both acquired and congenital valve disease, particularly when the principal functional defect is incompetence**. Thus infective endocarditis is a definite risk in patients with:

- mitral valve prolapse from any cause
- congenital bicuspid aortic valve, where only a relatively mild degree of incompetence may be associated with infective endocarditis
- postinflammatory valve disease, especially when characterized by incompetence
- All prosthetic valves, however useful in restoring competence or relieving stenosis, are associated with abnormal haemodynamics and are thus at risk for developing surface thrombi

Haemodynamic injury can also occur at sites other than valves if high-pressure turbulent flow is present. This occurs in **congenital cardiac defects**, most notably small **ventricular septal defects** and the **tetralogy of Fallot** within the heart, and **patent ductus arteriosus** and **coarctation of the aorta** outside it. The importance of high-pressure flow in determining the occurrence of endocardial thrombi is emphasized by comparing the low risk of infective endocarditis in patients with the common **secundum type of atrial septal defect** where there is low-pressure flow between the atria, and the higher risk seen in small ventricular septal defects where there is high-pressure flow between the ventricles.

Generally the greater the degree of virulence of the responsible organism, the more likely endocarditis is to develop in the absence of a serious haemodynamic disturbance. Indeed, organisms such as *S. aureus* can cause infective endocarditis on valves that are macroscopically normal, or, at worst, show only mild age-related thickening (*Fig. 32.45*). It is a moot point as to whether, with advancing age, such an entity as an absolutely normal valve exists, as small erosions associated with

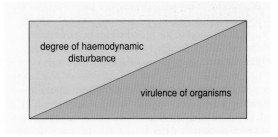

FIGURE 32.45 *Interaction between bacteraemia and haemodynamic disturbance in causation of infective endocarditis.*

platelet microthrombi can be detected on valves that are normal on naked-eye examination when appropriate methods of examination are used.

Bacteraemia

A full list of the organisms capable of causing infective endocarditis would comprise virtually all known pathogens. Various strains of the α haemolytic *S. viridans* still account for 40–50% of cases and streptococci of **Lancefield group D** for a further 10–20%. Staphylococci are responsible for another 15–25% of cases. Some of these are due to the virulent *S. aureus*, but much less virulent variants such as the coagulase-negative *S. epidermidis* can also cause endocarditis, especially in patients with prosthetic heart valves. Drug addicts have a higher incidence of endocarditis due to Gram-negative bacteria (which account for 6–8% of all cases of infective endocarditis) than individuals who are not so addicted. **In drug addicts there is a marked tendency for the right side of the heart to be affected, the tricuspid valve being the most frequent target.** Isolated pulmonary valve involvement does sometimes occur, as does involvement of both tricuspid and pulmonary valve from time to time. The diagnosis of right-sided endocarditis is not easy and is missed in a high proportion of patients because there may be no murmurs associated with tricuspid valve endocarditis. Infections by *S. aureus* are responsible for about half the cases.

Fungal endocarditis is usually due to infections with *Candida albicans* and is particularly liable to occur in:

- intravenous drug abusers
- patients with prosthetic heart valves
- immunosuppressed patients

How do the Bacteria Gain Access to the Bloodstream?

Transient bacteraemia is common and is associated frequently with minor invasive procedures such as:

- **dental work**, which is still a known antecedent of about one-third of cases of *S. viridans* endocarditis occurring in patients with pre-existing haemodynamic abnormalities, despite the recognition that antibiotic cover of such procedures can inhibit the development of bacteraemia.

- other forms of **invasive procedure** such as cystoscopy, prostatectomy and intestinal manipulations can all lead to invasion of the bloodstream by enterococci.
- the existence of staphylococcal infections of skin, lung or wounds may precede staphylococcal bacteraemia.

In patients with liver cirrhosis, in whom clearance of microorganisms from portal blood is ineffective, the risk of infective endocarditis is significantly increased.

The outcome of the bacteraemia, i.e. whether the organisms successfully colonize a heart valve or not, depends to a considerable extent on the adhesive properties of the organisms. Molecules on the bacterial surface may act as ligands for matrix proteins such as fibronectin, while in some cases the organisms possess surface molecules that bind to receptor sites on platelets.

Cardiac Lesions in Infective Endocarditis

Macroscopic Features

The characteristic lesion is the **vegetation**, a crumbling mass of thrombus adherent to the endocardium. Vegetations are often large and easily distinguished from the small, grey-brown, sessile lesions seen along lines of contact in acute rheumatic fever. In the atrioventricular valves vegetations generally appear on the atrial aspect, whereas semilunar valves are more usually affected on the ventricular aspects.

The vegetations may be single, sessile or polypoid, or multiple irregular masses of thrombus covering much of the surface area of the affected valve. In advanced cases of mitral valve endocarditis, the vegetations may extend upwards to involve the posterior wall of the left atrium, while in some cases of aortic endocarditis they may spread down to involve the interventricular septum or even the anterior leaflet of the mitral valve. In addition, the vegetations may burrow deeply into the tissues adjacent producing paravalvar abscesses, which may make valve replacement during this stage difficult and hazardous. Particularly in cases where the causal organism is highly virulent, destruction of the substance of the valve may occur, probably as a result of the proteolytic enzymes released by neutrophils. Such destruction may take the form of **cusp perforation** or, in the case of the mitral valve, of **chordal rupture**. Healing of the endocarditic process leads to scarring; rarely, aneurysm-like sacs may be seen in the aortic cusps or in the anterior leaflet of the mitral valve.

Microscopic Features

Vegetations can be seen to be composed of several distinct zones. The irregular material on the luminal surface is eosinophilic and finely granular, and consists predominantly of platelets and fibrin; it is from here that small emboli arise. Beneath this is a zone in which masses of organisms are seen. Acute inflammatory cells are scanty in this part of the infected thrombus. The part of the vegetation adjacent to the valve often shows some inflammatory cell infiltrate and the underlying valve is clearly inflamed and contains many newly formed blood vessels and proliferated fibroblasts as well as a brisk, acute, inflammatory cell infiltrate. Often there appears to be a layer of thrombus between the proliferating organisms and the acute inflammatory cells, giving an impression that the organisms occupy a relatively protected position.

Coronary artery embolization may result from the breaking off of small portions of vegetation, especially in patients with aortic valve endocarditis. These small emboli may lead to multiple small area of myocardial necrosis, particularly in the papillary muscles. In the majority of fatal cases an inflammatory infiltrate is seen in the interstitial tissues of the myocardium.

Natural History

Three distinct sets of processes are responsible for the clinical features and complications of infective endocarditis: **embolism**, **cardiac failure** due to a combination of the haemodynamic disadvantages of valve cusp damage leading to regurgitation and of myocardial damage, and **immune-mediated lesions**.

Embolic Complications

The friable nature of the vegetations, their constant exposure to high-pressure flow and the movement of the valves all combine to make systemic embolism common. Emboli containing pyogenic organisms may lead to the formation of metastatic abscesses. In most instances, however, the lesions produced by embolic impaction are bland. About 20% of patients experience cerebral embolization, a major contributor to death in patients with infective endocarditis. Renal emboli are more common (about 50% of patients) but produce much less severe clinical consequences. Major coronary emboli are not common except in patients with 'ball-in-cage' aortic valve prostheses. Sometimes, the organisms present in an embolus elicit an inflammatory reaction and slowly erode the wall of the blood vessel in which they have impacted. Such a lesion is called a **mycotic aneurysm**. These are especially likely to be formed in the intracranial vessels and, should they rupture, subarachnoid or intracerebral haemorrhages occur. It is likely, in addition to infected emboli, that the presence of immune complexes contributes to the arterial wall damage.

Cardiac Failure

This ranks alongside a major embolic event as a major cause of death in infective endocarditis. The chief factor is a **rapidly developing volume overload of the left ventricle**. This results from either the onset of valve regurgitation or the exacerbation of pre-existing valve incompetence. Valve incompetence in this context is due to perforation of a cusp or ulceration of the edge of the cusp, or, in the case of the mitral valve, to chordal rupture.

Even normal left ventricles do not adapt well to a rapid increase in volume load, and in patients with infective endocarditis myocardial function may already be compromised as a result of small intramyocardial emboli or immune complex-mediated small vessel damage. Low-grade vasculitic foci are often associated with small intramyocardial lesions characterized by small foci of necrosis of heart muscle; this is associated with a surrounding inflammatory reaction (Bracht–Waechter bodies).

Other Cardiac Complications

Other cardiac complications include:

- myocardial abscesses
- papillary muscle rupture causing torrential mitral regurgitation
- abscess within the valve rings, which is especially likely to occur in relation to the aortic valve. If associated with an aortic valve prosthesis, paravalvar leakage (*Fig. 32.46*) is likely to occur
- mycotic aneurysm affecting the sinus of Valsalva
- pericarditis, a rare complication occurring in about 8% of patients and probably due to immune complex localization
- progressive obstruction of ball-in-cage type of prosthesis by thrombus formation

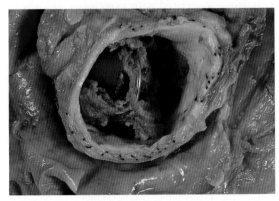

FIGURE 32.46 Infective endocarditis complicating an aortic valve prosthesis.

Immune Complex-mediated Complications

The prolonged bacteraemia, so typical of infective endocarditis, is associated frequently with circulating immune complexes. Almost any organ or tissue may be affected but the commonest targets are:

- **skin**, where purpuric haemorrhage due to vasculitis is quite common
- **joints**, where the localization of complexes causes arthralgia

- **kidneys**, where localization of immune complexes within the glomeruli is the cause of glomerulonephritis. The most common type seen is a focal mesangial-proliferative glomerulonephritis that occurs following lodgement of the immune complexes within the mesangial matrix with subsequent proliferation of mesangial cells. This form of glomerulonephritis has a wide range of clinical correlates that include:
  1) proteinuria
  2) a 'nephritic' syndrome
  3) a full-blown 'nephrotic' syndrome

In some instances the mesangial reaction extends into one of the capillary lobules giving the appearance termed focal, segmental proliferative glomerulonephritis.

Involvement of the kidney in patients with infective endocarditis is a serious event and renal failure secondary to such involvement accounts for about 25% of deaths from infective endocarditis. At post-mortem examination kidneys affected in this way show the presence of small subcapsular haemorrhagic lesions giving the appearance known as 'flea-bitten' kidney.

NON-BACTERIAL THROMBOTIC ENDOCARDITIS

Non-bacterial thrombotic endocarditis (NBTE) is defined as the presence of small, non-infected, thrombotic vegetations usually situated along the lines of closure of the affected valves. Strictly speaking both the endocarditis of acute rheumatic fever and the endocarditis associated with systemic lupus erythematosus fall, by definition, into this category, but these entities are usually considered separately and not under the rubric of NBTE.

NBTE may be found quite often at post-mortem examination, the frequencies quoted ranging from 0.3% to 9.3%. The vegetations themselves are usually somewhat larger than the small (1–2 mm in diameter) thrombi seen in acute rheumatic fever. Microscopic examination shows vegetations to consist of an admixture of platelets and fibrin, and the underlying valve usually shows no significant abnormalities, although it is probable that they are related to small defects in the endocardial lining. There is some controversy as to whether the aortic or mitral valve is most commonly affected.

Malignant disease, especially mucin-secreting adenocarcinoma, is a fairly common association and about half of the patients have a hypercoagulable state.

In most cases NBTE produces no clinical disturbance of any note, but embolic complications may occur and these are particularly likely to affect the cerebral circulation.

Disorders of Heart Muscle: The Cardiomyopathies

The term **cardiomyopathy** encompasses a set of disorders that are expressed in the form of **functional and/or structural abnormalities of the heart muscle**. Curiously, the defining criteria of cardiomyopathies are **negative** ones. Thus the diagnosis requires that the heart muscle disorder *not* be due to:
- the effect of volume or pressure overload from any cause including:
  1) valve disease
  2) congenital shunts
  3) high pressure in the systemic or pulmonary circulation
- ischaemic heart disease

Especially in the developing countries, cardiomyopathies account for a considerable proportion of patients suffering from heart disease but they are not uncommon in the developed world.

CLASSIFICATION

Aetiology and pathogenesis are poorly understood and this has made rational classification *within* the group difficult. Indeed, the World Health Organization appears to have added ignorance to the defining criteria, maintaining that once the cause of a cardiomyopathy is known the disease ceases to be a cardiomyopathy and should be termed instead a 'specific muscle disorder'. This is essentially unhelpful and most cardiologists prefer to continue using the term cardiomyopathy for syndromes of myocardial dysfunction occurring in the frame of reference outlined above. If a cause or an association can be identified, this should be used as a qualifying, descriptive, term such as in 'alcoholic dilated cardiomyopathy'.

At a simple level the cardiomyopathies can be classified as in *Table 32.13* in both morphological and functional terms. Some patients may show functional disturbances that cross the defining boundaries outlined in the table. Thus a patient with a dilated cardiomyopathy may have a disturbance of diastolic compliance with resulting difficulty in left ventricular filling. In addition, confusion arises when the cardiomyopathy manifests principally with disturbances in rhythm and conduction rather than with impaired systolic contraction or diastolic compliance.

HYPERTROPHIC CARDIOMYOPATHY

The defining criteria of hypertrophic cardiomyopathy are:
- **presence of left ventricular hypertrophy**
- **absence of dilatation of the left ventricular cavity**

The increase in ventricular wall thickness may be symmetric or, more commonly, asymmetric. Asymmetric thickening is expressed most frequently as disproportionate thickening of the interventricular septum (*Figs 32.47* and *32.48*).

The main functional problem in this disorder is **impairment of diastolic relaxation of the left ventricle, this being coupled with either normal or increased contractility of the ventricle, and an increased systolic ejection fraction** in some patients.

The common clinical presenting features are:
- **sudden death**
- **syncope associated with exercise**
- **anginal-type chest pain**
- **dyspnoea**

Outflow obstruction may appear to be present, although this is probably simply the reflection of the high pressures generated across the outflow tract in the late part of systole when most of the blood has already been ejected. Some of these patients present with congestive cardiac failure, which can also arise *de novo* in the absence of apparent 'outflow obstruction'.

Table 32.13 The Cardiomyopathies

Type	Functional abnormality	Morphological abnormality
Hypertrophic form	Decreased diastolic compliance and enhanced, abnormal, early systolic contraction	Thick, often asymmetric, left ventricular muscle with a small left ventricular cavity
Dilated form	Loss of systolic contractile force leading to increased end-systolic volume and, eventually, an increased end-diastolic volume	Dilated, thin-walled left ventricle with a large cavity
Restrictive form	Impairment of diastolic relaxation; may be partial obliteration of left ventricular cavity	Various patterns

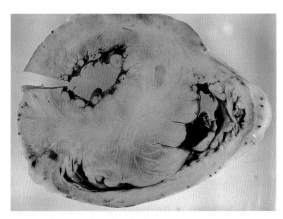

FIGURE 32.47 Hypertrophic cardiomyopathy. A transverse section showing gross hypertrophy of the interventricular septum and a relatively small left ventricular cavity size.

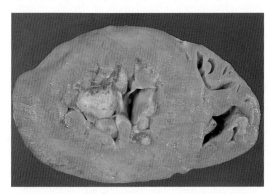

*FIGURE 32.48 Hypertrophic cardiomyopathy. This specimen shows the **symmetrical** variant of this condition.*

GENOMIC ABNORMALITIES IN HYPERTROPHIC CARDIOMYOPATHY

Hypertrophic cardiomyopathy tends to be concentrated in certain families; the inheritance pattern is that of an **autosomally transmitted disorder** with incomplete penetrance (15–35%). Inheritance is clearly not sex linked, although males appear to be affected twice as commonly as females.

In about 50% of cases, the disorder appears to be a reflection of **abnormalities in the heavy chain of β cardiac myosin**. More than 30 different point mutations in the gene that codes for this molecule have been described. Those producing the greatest changes in the nett molecular charge are associated with the most severe degrees of functional disturbance, and thus with the greatest risk of symptomatic disease. Linkage studies have identified four other genes, all on different chromosomes, that produce an identical phenotype. It seems likely that all these genes encode proteins related to myofibrillary structure and, indeed, it is suggested that an appropriate name for this set of diseases would be **myofibrillary dysgenesis**. Other families have been described in which there is an abnormality in a myosin-

binding protein. The result of the molecular abnormality is the formation of abnormal contractile filaments in the heart muscle cells with disturbance of their normal spatial arrangement. The heavy chain of β-myosin is transcribed in circulating lymphocytes and this provides a method for screening relatives of probands. The CMH-1 (heavy chain myosin) abnormality is fascinating in that, within a single family with the same gene mutation, there is a wide range of phenotypic expression extending from a minor asymptomatic echocardiographic abnormality to the fully expressed disease leading to sudden death.

Clinical Features

The commonest presenting feature is sudden death of one of the family members. Echocardiographic screening of relatives often reveals more cases. The risk of dying suddenly appears to be greatest during adolescence and subsequently decreases, although it never disappears.

Echocardiography is a most useful diagnostic tool, showing thickening of both the left ventricular wall and the small ventricular cavity.

Macroscopic Features

The heart usually shows a very significant degree of hypertrophy and is heavy for its volume, reflecting the combination of a thick ventricular wall and a normal or small left ventricular cavity.

The commonest variant shows asymmetric hypertrophy, the septum being the area disproportionately affected. In these cases, the ratio of the septum : free wall of the ventricle may be above 2 : 1 and the cut surface of the affected septum shows a characteristic **whorled** appearance similar to a uterine smooth muscle tumour (leiomyoma). The upper part of a hypertrophied septum may bulge out below the aortic valve leading to forceful contact being made during systole between this part of the septum and the anterior leaflet of the mitral valve. This may lead to thickening of the normally transparent endocardium over the septal bulge which appears as an opaque white patch.

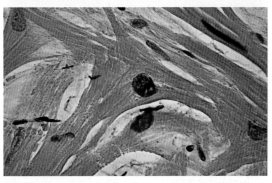

FIGURE 32.49 Disarray of cardiac myocytes in hypertrophic cardiomyopathy. The muscle cells are arranged in a typical whorled fashion.

Microscopic Features

The characteristic feature is **disarray of the heart muscle fibres** (*Fig. 32.49*). This occurs:

- within individual cells, which may show a marked degree of disorganization of the myofibrils
- at the cell–cell organizational level where there are bizarre shape changes of individual cells and abnormally sited cell connections. This leads to a highly characteristic whorled arrangement of heart muscle cells around a central focus of collagen.

There has been much controversy as to the specificity of muscle fibre disarray. Small foci of such disarray may be present in normal hearts while a few cases, clinically consistent with hypertrophic cardiomyopathy, may show no disarray. Cardiac pathologists resolve these problems partly by extensive sampling and partly by using a scoring system that allows quantitative assessment of myocardial abnormalities. As a rough approximation, abnormal myofibres are likely to account for 30% or more of the volume of myocardium examined in hypertrophic cardiomyopathy. As the hypertrophy increases, patchy scarring occurs, which may be of two types. The first is associated with focal myocyte loss; the second is interstitial and independent of myocyte loss.

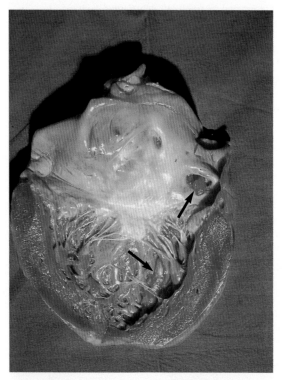

FIGURE 32.50 Dilated cardiomyopathy showing the typical globular appearance of the heart with marked dilatation of both atria and ventricles. Note the presence (arrows) of thrombi in the left ventricle and left auricular appendage.

DILATED CARDIOMYOPATHY

In dilated cardiomyopathy (formerly termed congestive cardiomyopathy) the principal functional abnormality is a **reduced ability of the ventricular muscle to contract during systole**. The failure is usually biventricular, although the left ventricle is *always* involved. The left ventricular ejection fraction falls (< 0.4) and thus **both end-systolic and end-diastolic volumes are increased markedly, leading to gross ventricular dilatation**. The clinical presentation is progressive congestive cardiac failure and the downhill course is relatively rapid. Sudden death, presumably due to the onset of ventricular arrhythmias, is also a feature. The ventricular cavity dilatation is associated with haemodynamic abnormalities, and mural thrombi within the cavities are quite common, as are resulting embolic phenomena. Disturbances of rhythm or conduction occur; left bundle branch block is particularly common.

Macroscopic Features

The characteristic feature is enlargement of the heart, in terms of both weight and volume. A mean weight of 630 g in men and 550 g in women has been recorded. Because of the volume increase resulting from gross dilatation of the chambers, ventricular **wall thickness** may be normal (*Fig. 32.50*).

In addition to marked chamber dilatation, an outstanding feature is general **flabbiness** of the myocardium: once the heart has been removed from the deceased, it virtually collapses and flattens as it is placed on a dissecting table. The myocardium may appear pale and some endocardial opacity due to thickening is common especially in the left ventricle. Mural thrombi may be present in any of the chambers.

Microscopic Features

Cardiac myocytes are hypertrophied, although their diameter may be normal or less than normal as a result of stretching. Nuclei are large and darkly stained and often show rather characteristic square ends. Large perinuclear vacuoles containing glycogen or lipid are often present. Some cells show separation or actual loss of myofibrils, and occasionally cells with such myofibrillar loss are invaded by macrophages.

Interstitial fibrosis is usually present and, in addition, there may be large areas of scarring where it is reasonable to suppose that heart muscle cells have been replaced by scar tissue.

Focal collections of lymphocytes and macrophages may be seen, and on occasion the histological features suggest an active inflammatory process. Such a picture may be difficult to distinguish from acute myocarditis, a term that is not easy to define or use appropriately. It should certainly be borne in mind that the presence of an inflammatory process need not be equated with infection. Myocardial necrosis associated with an inflammatory infiltrate may well be the result of a viral infection but can also occur in association with catecholamine-mediated damage, or as a result of treatment with anthracycline compounds such as Doxorubicin.

Aetiology

It is probably sensible to regard dilated cardiomyopathy as a set of disorders with many causes rather than as a single disease with a single cause; the functional and structural changes in the heart muscle may represent a common response to a wide range of insults. While the cause remains a mystery in many cases, many well-recognized disease entities and many drugs and chemicals have been associated with dilated cardiomyopathy. For instance, cobalt was recognized as a cause of dilated cardiomyopathy in 1967 when there was an 'epidemic' of the disorder in Quebec among men who consumed large amounts of beer to which cobalt sulphate had been added as a foam-stabilizing agent.

Associations with dilated cardiomyopathy include the examples shown in *Table 32.14*. In most cases, however, the cause of the cardiomyopathy is unknown. There have been repeated suggestions that at least some of these cases represent the end stages of an episode of acute viral myocarditis.

RESTRICTIVE CARDIOMYOPATHY

This is the least common of the three major types of cardiomyopathy in developed countries. Its main pathophysiological defect is a **decrease in the ability of the ventricular muscle to relax during diastole**, a feature it shares with hypertrophic cardiomyopathy. As a result diastolic filling is impeded and ventricular systolic filling pressure increases. Unlike hypertrophic cardiomyopathy, systolic function is essentially normal, and there is often no significant degree of ventricular hypertrophy. In some cases there is a reduction in the *size* of the ventricular chamber. This may be due to the presence of either mural thrombi or a gross degree of thickening of the endocardial layer, as is seen in the condition known as **endomyocardial fibrosis**. When this occurs, the term **restrictive–obliterative cardiomyopathy** is applied.

The morphological correlate of the restriction in diastolic compliance is a stiff ventricular wall. Such an increase in stiffness may arise because of:

- generalized scarring
- infiltration in the myocardium (e.g. amyloid)
- scarring of the superficial layers of the myocardium and thickening of the endocardium which has a 'splinting' effect on the ventricular wall

The single characteristic pathophysiological dysfunction may be the expression of a large number of quite disparate disease entities, ranging from such interstitial infiltrates as amyloidosis or adipose infiltration of the septum to rare disorders such as pseudoxanthoma elasticum. In many cases the cause of the cardiomyopathy is not determined. In this section, only those that can be diagnosed on morphological grounds are discussed.

ENDOMYOCARDIAL FIBROSIS

On a worldwide basis this is the most common form of restrictive–obliterative cardiomyopathy. It is found principally in tropical countries but may also occur in temperate zones, associated with eosinophilia. In the tropics, the disease affects chiefly young adults. Some show eosinophilia in the course of the disease but this is so common because of the many parasitic infestations in these patients that its pathogenetic significance remains unproven. The patients present with congestive cardiac failure. If the left ventricle is predominantly involved,

Table 32.14 Disorders Associated with Dilated Cardiomyopathy

Infective disorders	Bacterial, viral, protozoal
Familial neurological, neuromuscular or muscle disorders	Friedreich's ataxia, abetalipoproteinaemia, Duchenne muscular dystrophy, mitochondrial myopathy
Inborn metabolic errors	Wilson's disease, haemochromatosis, carnitine deficiency
Nutritional and metabolic disorders	Thiamine deficiency, protein malnutrition, diabetes mellitus, selenium deficiency
Autoimmune diseases	Dermatomyositis, progressive systemic sclerosis, systemic lupus erythematosus
Cardiotoxic drugs and chemicals	Alcohol, cobalt, cocaine, anthracyclines, lead, lithium, mercury

clinical findings of mitral incompetence and pulmonary hypertension may be present. If the right ventricle is the principal target, a large pulsatile liver, ascites and bilateral proptosis may be seen.

Macroscopic Features

The chief finding in the heart is a gross degree of **endomyocardial scarring** in the form of a thick, white, opaque layer of fibrous tissue confined more or less to the inflow tracts. This fibrous tissue often tethers and immobilizes the posterior leaflet of the mitral valve, causing mitral regurgitation. In the right ventricle, the apex of the chamber is often obliterated by the excessive endocardial fibrous tissue.

Microscopic Features

The thickened endocardium is seen to consist of acellular, hyaline, fibrous tissue with focal myxoid areas. The luminal surface shows the presence of organizing fibrin. In the early stages of the disease, focal necrosis of endocardial collagen has been described and there is a brisk infiltration of eosinophils in the granulation tissue which initially replaces the lost collagen. In the variant of this disorder that has been described in developed countries, the pathological findings are essentially similar but the heart valves are more often involved and eosinophilia is more consistently observed. This eosinophilia may be associated with such disparate entities as:

- eosinophilic leukaemia
- myeloblastic leukaemia following treatment with daunorubicin
- polycythaemia rubra vera
- parasitic infestations

A pathogenetic role for the eosinophil is supported by the finding in these patients of functional abnormalities of these cells which, it is suggested, release some tissue damaging factor(s).

AMYLOIDOSIS

Cardiac amyloidosis may cause a number of functional abnormalities, one of which is restrictive cardiomyopathy. This variant is seen most commonly in patients suffering from amyloidosis of immune origin in which the amyloid protein is either an intact light chain of immunoglobulin (most often the λ variety) or the amino-terminal end of such a light chain. There is extreme thickening of the ventricular wall and thus both diastolic filling and systolic ejection are compromised, in contrast to what occurs in endomyocardial fibrosis. Serious ventricular arrhythmias are also common.

Extensive deposition of amyloid in the heart may also be part of the inherited amyloidosis syndromes. The vast majority of these are inherited in an autosomal dominant pattern and the different syndromes are, for the most part, expressions of different point mutations

in the gene that codes for the thyroxine and vitamin A-transporting protein, **transthyretin**. The cardiomyopathy, if present, is usually only part of a multisystem disorder, with the exception of the amyloidosis encountered in a Danish kindred in which the heart is the principal target.

Macroscopic Features

The heart is usually considerably enlarged and very stiff. The myocardium has a pale, brownish, colour and the increased stiffness is evident also in the form of a very 'sharp' cut edge.

Microscopic Features

Extensive deposits of amyloid, staining positively with Congo red, are present in the interstitial tissues.

RESTRICTIVE CARDIOMYOPATHY ASSOCIATED WITH EXCESS IRON STORAGE

Excess iron storage may be seen in patients suffering from hereditary haemochromatosis and also in those with siderosis due to multiple blood transfusions or thalassaemia, sickle cell anaemia and other haemolytic states. Patients may present with a restrictive cardiomyopathy, but the dilated form is more common.

Macroscopic Features

The heart is dilated and the ventricular walls are thickened. The most striking feature is the rusty reddish-brown colour of the myocardium. Confirmation that this is due to iron deposition may be obtained by immersing a sample of myocardium in a mixture of potassium ferrocyanide and dilute hydrochloric acid. The presence of iron is shown by the rapid development of a bluish-green colour ('Prussian blue' or Perls' reaction).

ENDOCARDIAL FIBROELASTOSIS

The term endocardial fibroelastosis (EFE) is applied to a situation in which there is marked plaque-like thickening of the ventricular endocardium which may be several millimetres thick. **A characteristic feature is the presence of large numbers of elastic fibres lying tangentially to the surface within the thickened endocardium.** The disorder may be classified as primary or secondary.

Primary EFE is disease of infancy, the symptoms usually developing usually between 2 and 12 months of age. The clinical features are those of congestive cardiac failure and about 40% of cases have an apical systolic murmur, as heard in mitral regurgitation. The same process in the right ventricle may cause tricuspid regurgitation.

Macroscopic Features

In most cases, the left ventricle is dilated, although sometimes this chamber is normal or smaller than normal in size. The most striking feature is the presence of a thick white endocardium which obliterates the papillary muscles and may extend up to involve the mitral and aortic valves.

In the secondary form of EFE the thickening of the mural endocardium occurs in association with other types of cardiac malformation, usually those that produce obstruction in the left ventricular outflow tract such as aortic stenosis, coarctation of the aorta, hypoplastic left heart syndrome and anomalous origin of the coronary arteries.

Many different causes have been canvassed as being responsible for the highly characteristic morphological picture of EFE. The ultimate *mechanism* is likely to be a reaction to sustained high pressure within the ventricular cavity and/or decreased wall resistance leading to stretching of the wall.

OTHER ASSOCIATIONS

Restrictive cardiomyopathy may also occur in association with a variety of other disorders, including:
- sarcoidosis
- inborn errors of metabolism, especially those associated with storage of metabolites in the heart muscle cells
- Fabry's disease
- mucopolysaccharidosis type 1
- glycogen storage disease of a number of different types
- Gaucher's disease

MYOCARDITIS

DEFINITION

Myocarditis is a set of heart muscle disorders in which myocardial cell damage is associated with the presence of a significant interstitial inflammatory cell infiltrate. The occasional small focal groups of lymphocytes that are often found on histological examination of hearts at post mortem should *not* be regarded as constituting myocarditis.

CLASSIFICATION

Classification of myocarditis is difficult and rather unsatisfactory. At the morphological level one system broadly divides myocarditis into **two** groups: **acute non-specific myocarditis and granulomatous myocarditis**. The latter includes:

- tuberculous ⎫
- fungal ⎬ myocarditis
- rheumatic ⎪
- syphilitic ⎭
- sarcoidosis
- giant cell myocarditis of uncertain origin ('idiopathic')

Myocarditis has also been classified on the basis of the **pathogenetic mechanisms** involved, a difficult task because these are not known in many cases. In this system the myocarditis is classified as being:

1) post-infectious
2) drug related
3) immune-mediated of uncertain aetiology
4) miscellaneous, the cases being grouped on the basis of the histological appearance

POST-INFECTIOUS MYOCARDITIS

Infection is a major cause of myocarditis. In developed countries viral infections predominate. In South America infections due to the protozoon *Trypanosoma cruzi* are common and cause much chronic myocardial dysfunction.

A spectrum of clinical events may occur as a result of myocarditis, including:

1) An asymptomatic state that may progress no further or which, in some cases, may possibly lead to a dilated cardiomyopathy.
2) The rapid onset of severe, often fatal, cardiac failure, which is often dominated by diastolic dysfunction.
3) The onset of serious arrhythmias such as ventricular tachycardia, ventricular fibrillation and Stokes–Adams syncopal attacks. This may be associated with sudden death.
4) Chest pain in the presence of normal coronary arteries and normal left ventricular function.

THE PERICARDIUM

The pericardial sac that surrounds the heart is composed of two layers of connective tissue (visceral and parietal pericardia) each covered by a single layer of mesothelial cells. As with other serosa-lined cavities, pathological expressions of disease are limited to:

- **Accumulations of fluid within the sac**, giving rise to acute or chronic cardiac tamponade
- **Acute inflammation** characterized by fibrinous, serofibrinous, purulent or haemorrhagic exudates
- **Chronic inflammation**, often dominated by the repair phase giving rise to a thick layer of fibrous tissue which limits cardiac filling (constrictive pericarditis)

ACCUMULATIONS OF FLUID (EFFUSION)

Chronic Effusion

If the accumulation of fluid is slow, the pericardial sac can dilate to accommodate more than 1 litre of fluid before signs of tamponade appear, i.e.:

- congestive cardiac failure
- pulsus paradoxus
- heart sounds muffled on auscultation
- cardiac outline seen on radiography is greatly enlarged

Such effusions occur in:

- cardiac failure and other disorders giving rise to oedema
- involvement of the pericardium by tumour
- myxoedema

Acute Tamponade

This occurs most commonly in association with the rapid accumulation of pure blood within the pericardial sac (haemopericardium). This is the result of either:

a) rupture of the myocardium
b) rupture of the intrapericardial portion of the aorta

Myocardial rupture occurs in patients with full-thickness myocardial infarcts or, more rarely, as a result of trauma. Haemopericardium due to aortic rupture is seen in patients with type A dissections in which the blood within the aortic media tracks back towards the heart, finally bursting into the pericardial sac.

When fluid accumulates very rapidly, the parietal pericardium cannot stretch sufficiently quickly to accommodate it; thus pressure within the sac rises very rapidly causing acute tamponade. Cardiac output and blood pressure decline steeply and death is usually rapid. In these circumstances, 200–400 ml of blood are usually sufficient to cause death.

ACUTE INFLAMMATION (PERICARDITIS)

Infectious Pericarditis

This may be caused by viruses or bacteria.

Viruses

Coxsackie B, echoviruses, influenza, mumps and Epstein–Barr virus are those commonly implicated. Viral pericarditis is usually expressed in the form of an effusion which, in most cases, resolves within 1–2 weeks.

In young adults, acute pericarditis clinically similar to viral pericarditis may occur after an upper respiratory tract infection. This, too, is self-limiting. The 2–3-week interval between the infection and onset of pericarditis suggests the possibility of a hypersensitivity reaction.

Bacteria

Pyogenic organisms such as *Staphylococcus aureus*, streptococci and *Haemophilus influenzae* are most commonly involved. Pericardial involvement tends to occur as a complication of septicaemia, pyaemia, pneumonia, lung abscess, empyema or tumours of the oesophagus or bronchus that have ulcerated.

Tuberculous pericarditis is by no means rare in areas where the prevalence of tuberculosis is high. The pericardium may become involved either by direct spread from a caseous mediastinal node or by blood spread. In its early stages the pericarditis may be fibrinous but this often progresses to the formation of a haemorrhagic exudate. Chronicity is more or less inevitable and the associated abundant scar tissue formation leads to constrictive pericarditis with a consequent decline in ventricular filling.

Non-infectious Pericarditis

Acute non-infectious pericarditis occurs in a wide variety of disparate clinical and pathological situations including:

- **Acute rheumatic fever**, which is almost always accompanied by some degree of fibrinous pericarditis.
- **Myocardial infarction**: the pericarditis may manifest in two ways. It may develop very rapidly, presumably as an inflammatory response to necrotic heart muscle, or may appear only after 2–3 weeks in which case the mechanism is likely to be a hypersensitivity reaction (Dressler's syndrome). A similar sequence of events may occur after **cardiac surgery**, with pericarditis appearing only after an interval of some weeks.
- **Connective tissue disorders** such as **systemic lupus erythematosus** and **rheumatoid disease**. The pericardial involvement presents most commonly as an effusion but some cases become chronic, with eventual scarring and constrictive pericarditis.
- **Uraemia**
- Following **renal transplantation**. Fibrinous pericarditis is not rare in patients who have had a renal transplant. Most are due to uraemia, some to uraemia plus a viral infection (most commonly cytomegalovirus), some to cytomegalovirus infection alone and some to bacterial infection.
- **Postirradiation**
- Following **cardiac trauma**

Clinical Features

Fibrin on the pericardial surfaces shows itself in the form of acute onset of pain and fever. On auscultation a pericardial friction rub is heard. If fluid accumulates in significant amounts, thus separating the inflamed visceral and parietal pericardia, both the pain and the rub tend to disappear.

Macroscopic Features

The appearances seen in pericarditis (excluding the constrictive variety) depend on the relative proportion of fibrin and fluid in the exudate/transudate:

- If there is little fluid and abundant fibrin, the normally smooth and shiny surface of the pericardium is lost. It is usually easy to see the meshwork of deposited fibrin. Often there are fibrin 'bridges' between the visceral and parietal pericardia, and when these two layers are pulled apart the surface fibrin shows a reticulated appearance ('bread and butter' heart) (*Fig. 32.51*).
- Exudates in which fluid is the major component are most often serous in nature; haemorrhagic effusion suggests malignant involvement of the pericardium, tuberculosis or renal failure.

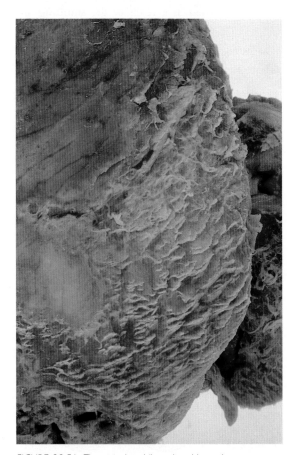

FIGURE 32.51 *The reticulated 'bread and butter' appearance of fibrinous pericarditis. The inflammatory reaction in this case is associated with myocardial infarction.*

CHRONIC PERICARDITIS

Constrictive Pericarditis

This results from a progressive scarring process that obliterates the pericardial cavity, encasing the heart in a thick layer of fibrous tissue which restricts atrial and ventricular filling. Tuberculosis is a common cause in populations in which the disease has a high prevalence. Where this is not the case, the cause of the pericarditis is often unknown.

Patients present with clinical features of congestive cardiac failure. Because right atrial filling is affected early, jugular venous pressure is raised and ascites and hepatomegaly are often conspicuous.

The cardiac shadow is normal or small on chest radiography, and the fibrous tissue obliterating the pericardial sac often shows dystrophic calcification. Surgical removal of a substantial amount of pericardium is the only effective means of treatment.

PERICARDIAL NEOPLASMS

The pericardium is involved in about 8.5% of cases of disseminated malignancy. The most common expression of pericardial tumour is a haemorrhagic effusion which may lead to cardiac tamponade; indeed malignant pericarditis is the second most common cause of tamponade. Neoplasms most commonly involving the pericardium are carcinomas of the lung and breast, malignant melanoma and lymphoma.

Primary pericardial neoplasms are very rare. The commonest are benign mesothelial tumours and cysts. Malignant mesotheliomas primarily involving the pericardium have been recorded but are extremely rare.

Congenital Cardiac Defects

DEFINITION

Congenital heart disease can be defined as all disorders in which a structural and/or functional defect in the heart or great vessels is present at birth.

One of these malformations, **congenitally bicuspid aortic valve** is common, affecting 1–2% of the population. It is expressed clinically in middle age in the form of aortic stenosis which occurs as a complication of the abnormal flow patterns created by the abnormal valve (see pp 360–362).

Without treatment, 60% of infants who have a congenital cardiac defect identified at birth would die in infancy, 25% in the neonatal period, and only about 15% would survive into their teens or adult life. Advances in treatment have changed this bleak outlook considerably, and thus early and accurate diagnosis is a matter of great importance.

CLASSIFICATION

The classification and nomenclature of congenital cardiac defects is not easy. They may be classified on the basis of:

- **the major functional disturbance**
- **the major embryological step that is disturbed**
- **the major morphological abnormalities**

In the section that follows, the first of these defects is emphasized. No pretence is made to a description of all known congenital anomalies of the heart; only the commoner defects and one or two examples of rarer types are included.

Difficulties in classification have given rise to some inconsistencies in the incidence figures reported in different series but there is reasonable agreement on the ranking of the commonest disorders. *Table 32.15* gives the frequency in **live-born children**, eight defects accounting for 75% of such cases of congenital heart disease.

Table 32.15 Distribution of Congenital Heart Defects in Live Births

Defect	Frequency (%)
Ventricular septal defects	32.5
Patent ductus arteriosus	11.9
Pulmonary stenosis	7
Coarctation of the aorta	6.3
Tetralogy of Fallot	5.9
Atrial septal defect	5.9
Aortic stenosis	5.1
Complete transposition of the great vessels	5
Hypoplastic left heart	2.8
Absent right atrioventricular connection, pulmonary atresia with intact septum, Ebstein's anomaly	2.5
Atrioventricular septal defect	2.4
Double-inlet atrioventricular connection	1.7
Persistent truncus arteriosus	1.1
Total anomalous pulmonary venous return	0.8

MAJOR FUNCTIONAL DISTURBANCES IN CONGENITAL HEART DISEASE

Some 80% of cases of congenital heart disease are associated with abnormal communications between the two sides of the cardiovascular system, or shunts, which may in turn be divided into two subclasses:

1) **Those in which there is flow of blood from left to right.**
2) **Those in which the flow of blood is from right to left. As unoxygenated blood is present in the systemic circulation from the outset, affected children are likely to show early development of cyanosis.**

LEFT TO RIGHT SHUNTS *(Fig. 32.52)*

The presence of such a shunt results in a volume overload of the right atrium, right ventricle and pulmonary vascular bed. Initially this is *not* associated with any increase in **pressure load** on the right side of the heart and patients **show no evidence of cyanosis**. The volume of the shunt can be calculated by measuring the cardiac output and the degree of increased oxygen saturation in the right atrial blood resulting from the left to right flow.

With the passage of time, continued high flow causes intimal hyperplasia in the small blood vessels of the lung and **irreversible pulmonary hypertension results**. This may be so severe as to cause *reversal* of the direction of flow through the shunt and the patient becomes centrally **cyanosed** as a result of the **shunting of**

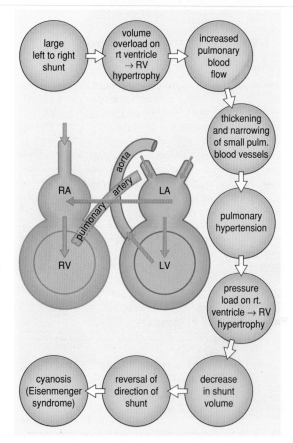

FIGURE 32.52 *Pathophysiology of left to right shunts (e.g. atrial septal defect).*

unoxygenated blood into the left side of the heart (*Eisenmenger's syndrome*).

The major causes of such left to right shunts are **ventricular septal defect** (VSD), **patent ductus arteriosus** (PDA) and **atrial septal defect** (ASD).

Ventricular Septal Defect

VSD is, with the exception of bicuspid aortic valve, the commonest congenital cardiac defect (1 in 500 live births). In about one-third of cases the defect is an isolated one; in the remainder it is associated with other abnormalities such as tetralogy of Fallot. The location of the septal defect varies from case to case. The majority are perimembranous (i.e. situated fairly high up in the septum in relation to its membranous portion). Other locations are within the main muscular part of the septum or very high in relation to the outflow tracts.

The pathophysiological effects of VSD depend greatly on the size of the defect. Small defects (i.e. those less than 0.5 cm in diameter) produce a low-volume shunt during systole. There is a high pressure gradient between the left and right ventricles and the flow produces a loud and sometimes prolonged systolic murmur. As always, where there is an abnormal high pressure jet, an increased risk for developing infective endocarditis exists. In most cases, the affected patients are asymptomatic and, as the heart grows, the defect tends to decrease in size and may even close spontaneously.

A large VSD has much more serious implications. A large volume of blood is shunted from the left ventricle and there is thus a significant degree of **volume overload** of the right side of the heart. The increased flow through the pulmonary circulation leads to a rise in pulmonary artery pressure and thus to hypertrophy of the right ventricle, expressed clinically in the form of a **right ventricular heave**. The effects of continued high flow on the small pulmonary blood vessels lead to intimal hyperplasia and a sustained rise in pulmonary pressure, which may be sufficient to cause cessation of shunting from left to right or even a reversal of the left to right flow pattern leading to **central cyanosis**. If the defect is very large, the affected child is seriously ill early in life and heart failure develops within a few weeks.

Patent Ductus Arteriosus

The Normal Ductus

The ductus arteriosus is a normal channel, rising from a point immediately distal to the origin of the left subclavian artery, that operates in fetal life to connect the aorta and pulmonary artery. This allows blood from the right ventricle to bypass the unexpanded and inactive fetal lungs. After birth, the lungs expand and pulmonary artery pressure falls. Flow through the ductus ceases within the first day or two of life, and is due initially to

spasm of the muscular layer of the ductus, which may remain probe-patent for some weeks. The functional muscle changes are, in part, due to decreased plasma levels of prostaglandin E_2 and may be potentiated by the administration of inhibitors of the cyclooxygenase system such as indomethacin.

Failure of Ductus Closure

The cause of **failure of ductus closure**, which is the basis of PDA, is unknown.

In the vast majority of cases (85–90%) PDA occurs as an isolated defect, but it may also be seen in association with stenosis of the semilunar valves of the outflow tracts, with coarctation of the aorta or with VSD.

The effects of PDA depend to a considerable extent on the diameter of the patent ductus.

- Where the defect is small, only a relatively small amount of blood is shunted from the aorta to the pulmonary artery. The resulting rise in pressure within the latter will be small. Because of the pressure gradient between the aorta and the pulmonary artery **throughout the cardiac cycle**, shunting of blood continues through the cycle and is associated with the presence of a continuous murmur, which has been called a 'machinery' murmur.
- A large-diameter PDA leads to a considerable rise in pressure within the pulmonary circulation and, as already described, shunt reversal may occur. As in the case of VSD, there is an increased risk of infective endocarditis.

If the ductus defect is an isolated one, early closure should be carried out. In a small proportion of cases, the affected child will depend on the patency of the ductus for maintenance of any pulmonary circulation since the pulmonary valve may have failed to develop (**pulmonary valve atresia**). In such instances, of course, closure of the ductus should not be carried out.

Atrial Septal Defect

Atrial septal defect accounts for about 30% of congenital heart defects encountered in adult life. The different types of atrial septal defect can be understood most easily in relation to the embryological development of the interatrial and atrioventricular septa.

The Normal Septum

Division of the common atrial canal starts with the formation of a septum, known as the **septum primum**, in which there is an opening called the **ostium secundum** which lies forward of and above the site of the foramen ovale. To the right of the septum primum, another septum, the **septum secundum**, grows downwards towards the endocardial cushions at the base of the atria. This, too, normally has an opening known as the **foramen ovale**, which lies adjacent to part of the septum primum. This part of the septum primum serves as a flap valve which in postnatal life becomes fused to the edges of the foramen ovale thus sealing the foramen. In about one-quarter of normal adults it is possible to insert a probe through the edges of the foramen ovale, but this incompleteness of the seal has no significance.

Defects

Atrial septal defects can be divided into three anatomical types:
1) ostium secundum defects
2) sinus venosus defects (rare)
3) ostium primum defects

Ostium Secundum Defect

This is the commonest type of atrial septal defect accounting for about 70% of all cases. It is three times as common in females as in males. In 20–30% of cases, associated prolapse of the mitral valve is found. Other lesions occurring in association with secundum-type ASD are pulmonary and mitral valve stenosis.

The defect is mid-septal in position, at the site where the flap valve normally contributed by the septum primum seals off the foramen ovale.

Small ASDs are tolerated well but if the defect is greater than 2 cm in diameter a substantial degree of left to right shunting will occur, resulting in a considerable degree of volume overload of the right side of the heart and a long-term risk of shunt reversal due to pulmonary hypertension. This rarely occurs before the third decade of life. Rheumatic fever may produce a combination of ASD and acquired mitral stenosis, known as the **Lutembacher syndrome**. In these cases the advent of pulmonary hypertension is hastened because of the high pulmonary capillary wedge pressure imposed by the mitral valve disease.

In contrast to VSD, flow through the atrial septal defect is rather *slow* and there is no pressure gradient between the two atria. Thus the increased risk for infective endocarditis that is present in patients with VSD is not seen in those with atrial septal defects.

Ostium Primum Defects

So-called ostium primum defects (5% of cases of ASD) are really due to atrioventricular septal abnormalities and are not truly defects of the interatrial septum at all. The connection between the two atria is often complicated by the presence of a cleft in the anterior leaflet of the mitral valve, which may produce mitral incompetence of varying degrees of severity. On examination of the atrioventricular connections once the valve leaflets have been stripped away, it is often difficult to tell whether there has been a common atrioventricular valve orifice or whether there is, in fact, a bridging tongue of tissue separating left and right atrioventricular connections.

The haemodynamic abnormalities seen here are similar to those of ostium secundum defects, with the addition of mitral incompetence. However, because of the mitral incompetence, the outlook for these patients is worse than that in those with an ostium secundum defect.

RIGHT TO LEFT SHUNTS (ASSOCIATED WITH CENTRAL CYANOSIS)

> Lesions that produce central cyanosis may be subdivided on the basis of whether they are associated with diminished pulmonary blood flow or not

Lesions Associated with Diminished Pulmonary Blood Flow

Tetralogy of Fallot (Fig. 32.53)

The most frequent and important of these is **tetralogy of Fallot.** As the name implies there are *four* morphological abnormalities:
1) Pulmonary valve stenosis and/or stenosis of the pulmonary infundibulum **causing obstruction to right ventricular outflow**.
2) A large, high, ventricular septal defect just beneath the aortic valve.
3) So-called overriding of the aorta across the ventricular septal defect.
4) Hypertrophy of the right ventricle.

The functionally important components are obstruction to the right outflow tract and the ventricular septal defect, which determine the size of the right to left shunt. Clinical severity is determined, in particular, by the degree of pulmonary valve or infundibular narrowing. The more severe the narrowing, the more right ventricular blood enters the aorta and the greater is the

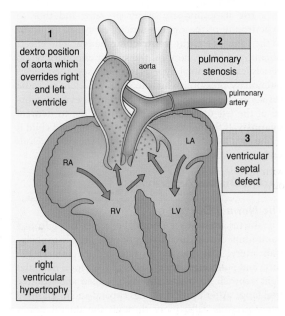

FIGURE 32.53 Tetralogy of Fallot.

degree of central cyanosis. In some cases, the degree of right outflow tract obstruction at birth is mild but, as the child grows, infundibular narrowing increases and, gradually, shunting of blood from the right to the left side develops.

Clinical Features

Most babies with tetralogy of Fallot are pink at birth and gradually become cyanosed as they grow. At about the age of 4–6 months hypoxic episodes may begin in which there is deep cyanosis, breathlessness and, not infrequently, loss of consciousness due to cerebral anoxia. These attacks are a result of spasm of the infundibulum, which prevents blood from the right ventricle reaching the lungs. With relaxation of infundibular muscle, recovery gradually occurs but some infants may die during these episodes or sustain brain damage. In between such attacks, the child may be completely acyanotic.

Not all affected children have hypoxic attacks. Instead they may fail to thrive and become increasingly cyanotic and limited in activity. A highly characteristic feature is that the children tend to *squat* after exercise, sitting with their knees up to the chest until they become less cyanosed and breathless. Squatting is believed to counteract the effects of exercise in two ways:

1) By reducing arterial blood flow to the legs; this helps to maintain the systemic vascular resistance. As a result, more blood enters the pulmonary circulation.

2) By slowing venous return from the legs; thus less desaturated blood enters the circulation and the 'oxygen debt' incurred during exercise can be paid off over a longer period.

Other clinical features include:

- a **right parasternal 'heave'** due to the presence of right ventricular hypertrophy
- **polycythaemia**, which parallels the degree of severity of desaturation by oxygen in the arterial blood
- **clubbing of fingers and toes**

Complications

Cerebral thrombosis is a real risk in severely cyanosed infants and may lead to cerebral infarction with hemiplegia. Because children with Fallot's tetralogy have a high haematocrit level anyway, it is important to ensure that they are well hydrated, or the viscosity of the blood will be further increased.

Cerebral abscess, interestingly, is usually not associated with the presence of infective endocarditis in these children. It has been suggested that, instead, it is due to some localized ischaemic cerebral damage resulting from thrombosis in small cerebral vessels and that these areas become infected if bacteraemia develops.

Infective endocarditis is a relatively frequent complication, occurring in about 14% of cases.

Pulmonary Atresia with Ventricular Septal Defect

This condition is only about one-fifth as common as tetralogy of Fallot. There is a high and anteriorly situated VSD but, instead of pulmonary stenosis, **there is complete obstruction to the flow of blood from the right ventricle into the pulmonary artery because either the pulmonary valve or the pulmonary valve together with the infundibulum is atretic.** Blood can reach the pulmonary circulation either via a patent ductus arteriosus or via aortopulmonary collateral vessels arising from the aorta. In the former case, closure of the ductus inevitably leads to complete cessation of perfusion of the lungs and death.

Clinical Features

The onset of cyanosis is earlier than in the tetralogy of Fallot, usually occurring in the neonatal period. The hypoxic attacks and squatting so characteristic of Fallot's tetralogy are not seen. Because no blood is flowing through the pulmonary valve there is no systolic murmur in the pulmonary area but, if perfusion of the lung is taking place via a ductus, there will be a continuous ductus murmur in the pulmonary area.

Ebstein's Anomaly

This a rare defect, occurring in less than 1% of congenital cardiac defects. **It is defined as the state existing when the posterior and septal leaflets of the tricuspid valve are not attached to the valve ring but to the endocardium of the right ventricle.** The leaflets themselves are often thickened and are inserted into chordae tendineae which are attached directly to the muscular wall of the right ventricle rather than to papillary muscles as normal. Thus the heart above the valve consists in part of atrium and in part of the upper part of the right ventricle. The valve is usually cone-shaped and is narrowed and incompetent. The part of the right ventricle below the valve is small and functionally rather ineffective in the first few days of life when the pulmonary vascular resistance is normally high, because of the presence of an incompetent tricuspid valve.

Lesions that cause Cyanosis but which are associated with increased pulmonary blood flow

Transposition of the Great Vessels (Aorta and Pulmonary Artery)

This is the second commonest congenital anomaly of the heart causing cyanosis. It is defined as the state in which **the aorta arises from the right ventricle and the pulmonary artery from the left ventricle**. The aorta, therefore, lies anterior to the pulmonary artery instead of posterior. In pathophysiological terms **there are two separate circulations**. While the ductus remains open, mixing of the blood can occur, but once ductal closure takes place, severe cyanosis becomes apparent. The children usually become severely acidotic. The conventional treatment is, in the first instance, to produce a defect in the atrial septum with a balloon **so as to get mixing of oxygenated and desaturated blood**. This can be followed by surgery at a later date to divert the systemic and pulmonary *venous* blood to the opposite sides. In some centres a direct arterial switch is performed as the first and only line of treatment. This variety of transposition is known as '**uncorrected transposition**' (*Fig. 32.54*).

Another type of transposition is so-called '*corrected transposition*' (*Fig. 32.55*). In this variety there is a mismatch between the atria and the ventricles, the right ventricle arising from the left atrium and the left ventricle from the right atrium. The aorta arises from the right ventricle and the pulmonary artery from the left ventricle. No communications are required for a normal circulation to be maintained and, in due time, the right ventricle responds to the peripheral resistance of the systemic circulation by becoming hypertrophied.

About 20% of children with transposition also have a large VSD and this considerably alters the functional situation. Cyanosis is minimal but progressive cardiac failure, which is refractory to medical treatment, soon develops.

Lesions in which there is *Common Mixing* of Blood within the Heart or Great vessels

Where such mixing occurs there is desaturation of arterial blood but the main problem arises from a high pulmonary blood flow and volume overload on the heart, which lead to heart failure. Cyanosis is usually minimal.

Persistent Truncus Arteriosus

This is a rare defect arising from a failure of the primitive truncus arteriosus (the common ventricular outflow tract) to divide into aorta and pulmonary artery. It is always accompanied by a VSD. Three types are described according to the way in which the pulmonary arteries arise. There is a single semilunar valve (the truncal valve) which may have four, three, two or even a single cusp.

In the early stages there is only minimal cyanosis despite the mixing that takes place in the truncus. The

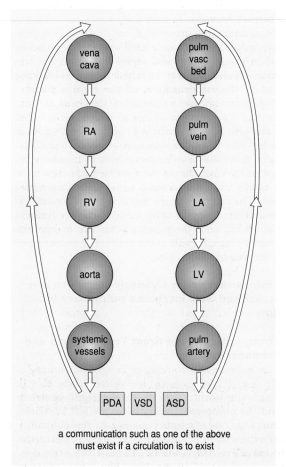

FIGURE 32.54 'Uncorrected' transposition of great vessels.

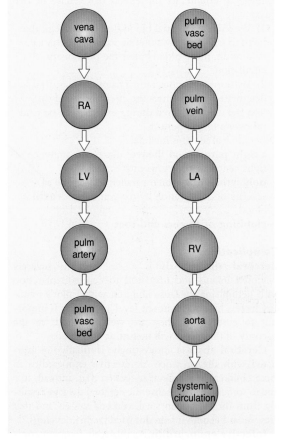

FIGURE 32.55 'Corrected' transposition of great vessels.

pathophysiological picture suggests the presence of a large left to right shunt with **high pulmonary blood flow**. The overloading of the pulmonary circulation leads to breathlessness and heart failure. As pulmonary vascular resistance falls (quite normally) in the first 2 weeks of life, so the pulmonary blood flow increases steeply to three or more times normal, and it is this which is so lethal. Without surgical treatment, the babies rarely live longer than 6 months.

Lesions that produce outflow obstruction not associated with cyanosis

Such lesions affecting the **left side of the heart** include **coarctation of the aorta** and **aortic stenosis (see pp 360–361)**.

Coarctation of the Aorta

Coarctation is defined as a stricture in the aorta in the region where the ductus arteriosus is inserted into it (*Fig. 32.56*). It is fairly common (6% of congenital cardiac anomalies) and occurs three times as commonly in males as in females. In females there is an association between Turner's syndrome and coarctation. About half the cases of coarctation have associated cardiovascular defects including bicuspid aortic valve, congenital aortic stenosis, ADS, VSD, mitral valve abnormalities and 'berry' aneurysms of the circle of Willis. The coarctation may be found just distal to the insertion of the ductus, which is the commoner site, or just proximal, the narrowing at this site usually being more severe.

Preductal Coarctation

If the narrowing is very severe, clinical problems appear in the first 10 days of life, once the ductus has closed. At this point there is a marked reduction in perfusion of tissues in parts of the body that derive their blood supply from branches of the aorta arising distal to the ductus insertion site. The clinical picture is dramatic: the babies are breathless, pale and collapsed with severe left-sided cardiac failure. Oliguria or anuria may supervene as a result of the grossly impaired renal perfusion and the infants are acidotic and hypoglycaemic. The situation may be retrieved temporarily by giving intravenous prostaglandins to open up the ductus and thus restore blood flow to the lower part of the body. Once the child's condition has improved, surgery must be undertaken and the narrowed segment of aorta resected.

Postductal Coarctation

This may be asymptomatic until adolescence or adult life. The most common presenting symptoms are headache, intermittent claudication and leg fatigue. Typically there is hypertension in the upper half of the body. Simultaneous palpation of the brachial and femoral pulses characteristically shows the latter to be smaller and delayed. There is usually a well-developed system of collateral vessels between pre- and post-coarctation levels and these may be so prominent as to be appreciated on clinical examination. The presence of collaterals may be inferred from notching of the ribs seen on chest radiography; this is due to dilated intercostal arteries. Patients who survive, without operation, into adult life may suffer from a number of different complications, including:

- congestive cardiac failure
- aortic rupture
- infective endocarditis
- intracranial haemorrhage

The mean lifespan of patients with coarctation that has not been repaired surgically is about 50% of normal.

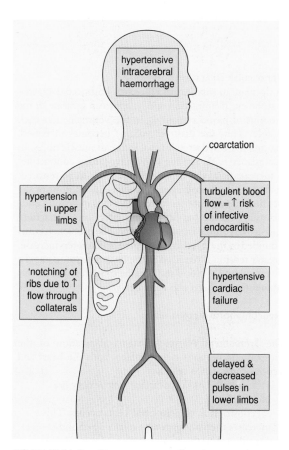

FIGURE 32.56 *Possible consequences of aortic coarctation.*

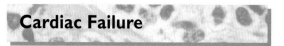

Cardiac Failure

Cardiac failure is **failure** by the heart, despite normal venous pressure, **to maintain an output adequate to meet the body's needs**. The basic mechanisms are shown in *Table 32.16* and their pathological correlates are discussed in the following sections.

Table 32.16 Basic Mechanisms of Cardiac Failure

Mechanism	Clinical picture	Examples
Heart muscle dysfunction	Left-sided failure Biventricular failure Left-sided failure	Loss of muscle as in ischaemic heart disease Dysfunction of muscle as in cardiomyopathy High systemic blood pressure
Outflow obstruction	Left-sided failure Right-sided failure	Aortic valve stenosis Pulmonary stenosis Pulmonary hypertension Pulmonary embolism
Obligatory high output		Severe anaemia Thyrotoxicosis Beriberi Left to right shunts Paget's disease of bone
Volume overload	Left-sided failure	Aortic valve regurgitation Mitral valve regurgitation
Inability of ventricles to fill adequately	Right-sided failure	Constrictive pericarditis Large pericardial effusions causing tamponade Restrictive cardiomyopathy
Disturbances of rhythm	Biventricular failure	

Heart failure may be acute or chronic, the former being the case when the onset of dysfunction is sudden. Thus, acute failure occurs in the context of:

- sudden onset of a serious arrhythmia such as ventricular fibrillation
- rapid and extensive loss of heart muscle as in some cases of myocardial infarction (cardiogenic shock)
- massive pulmonary embolization
- sudden onset of some mechanical dysfunction such as the acute mitral incompetence occurring with papillary muscle rupture or perforation of a mitral valve leaflet in infective endocarditis

Pathophysiology

Compensatory Mechanisms

As the cardiac output falls, a number of compensatory mechanisms involving the heart itself and the peripheral vascular system comes into operation (*Fig. 32.57*). As heart failure progresses, however, these mechanisms are overcome and become part of the pathophysiological problem. They include:

- ventricular dilatation
- ventricular hypertrophy
- neurohumoral activation involving the sympathetic nervous system, the renin–angiotensin system and atrial natriuretic peptides (ANPs)

Ventricular Dilatation

A decrease in myocardial efficiency leads to a decreased systolic ejection fraction and hence to an increase in the amount of blood remaining in the ventricle after each systole. Thus the diastolic volume becomes increased, causing increased stretching of the heart muscle fibres. In accordance with Starling's law, myocardial contractility is increased and the stroke volume tends to be restored. As heart failure progresses, however, the contour of the Starling curve becomes flattened so that increasing end-diastolic pressure has little or no effect on contractility and stroke volume falls significantly. The problem is compounded by the fact that, as ventricular diameters increase, greater tension is required in the myocardium to expel a given volume of blood and thus the oxygen requirements of the myocardium also increase.

Neurohumoral Activation

The Sympathetic Nervous System   Activation of the sympathetic nervous system affects both the heart and venous capacitance vessels:

1) heart rate and myocardial contractility are increased

2) constriction of peripheral veins occurs. This increases the venous return to the heart and contributes to the augmentation of ventricular function by the Starling mechanism.

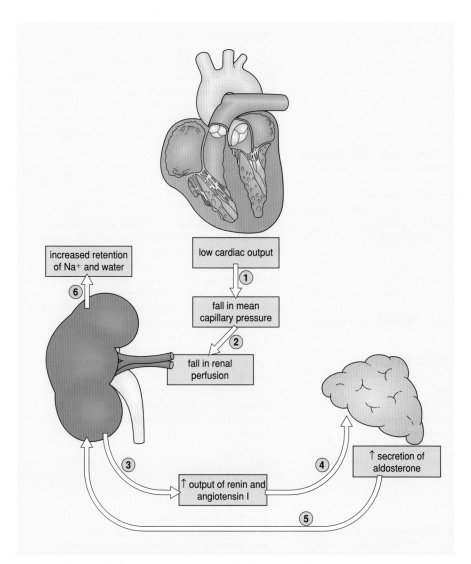

FIGURE 32.57 Mechanisms involved in causing the oedema of cardiac failure.

Unfortunately, sympathetic overactivity also causes arteriolar constriction, thus increasing the workload on the ventricles (afterload).

Renin–Angiotensin System **The combination of a reduced cardiac output and arteriolar constriction leads to decreased renal perfusion**. This activates the renin–angiotensin system with a resulting increase in retention of salt and water. In the early stages of heart failure, this increase in plasma volume increases venous return and helps to maintain stroke volume by the Starling mechanism. With progressive failure the increased venous pressure leads to both pulmonary and systemic oedema.

Atrial Natriuretic Peptides Sodium retention due to underperfusion of the kidneys is partly compensated for by increased output of ANPs. These are short-chain peptides that cause vasodilatation and increase sodium loss in the urine. Their concentration rises in cardiac failure, in an attempt to decrease both preload and after-load.

The clinical picture of heart failure is likely to be dominated by inadequacy of either the right or left ventricle.

RIGHT-SIDED CARDIAC FAILURE

The commonest cause of right-sided cardiac failure is left-sided failure. The syndrome also occurs in association with:

- chronic lung disease (cor pulmonale)
- pulmonary hypertension

- tricuspid or pulmonary valve disease
- left to right shunts (such as in ventricular septal defect)
- mitral valve disease with secondary pulmonary hypertension
- rare instances of isolated right-sided cardiomyopathy

Clinical Features
The clinical picture results from high pressure and distension in systemic veins and thus may include:
- a clinically detectable rise in jugular venous pressure
- an enlarged and tender liver due to chronic venous congestion. The resulting morphological appearance (known as nutmeg liver) is described on pp 609–610
- dependent subcutaneous pitting oedema owing to the increased hydrostatic pressure in the microcirculation which is aggravated by the effect of gravity
- the development of pleural transudates and/or ascites

LEFT-SIDED CARDIAC FAILURE

The commonest causes are:
- ischaemic heart disease
- inadequately treated systemic hypertension
- aortic stenosis and incompetence
- mitral incompetence. Pure mitral stenosis produces signs of left ventricular failure but does not cause the left ventricle itself to fail
- cardiomyopathies

Clinical Features
The clinical picture is dominated by pulmonary vascular congestion due to a failing left ventricle. Pressure in the left atrium increases and this is transduced to the pulmonary veins and capillaries. The rise in hydrostatic pressure in the pulmonary microvessels leads to formation of intra-alveolar oedema of varying grades of severity. Patients experience fatigue, exertional dyspnoea, orthopnoea and paroxysmal nocturnal dyspnoea.

Pulmonary oedema is detected clinically by the fine crackles heard at the lung bases on auscultation. On radiological examination, the lung shows a diffuse hazy appearance owing to the presence of intra-alveolar fluid, and there may be linear shadows (Kerley B lines) as a result of interstitial oedema.

Macroscopic Features
The morphological correlate of pulmonary oedema in the post-mortem room is a heavy congested lung. Fluid drips in large amounts from the cut surface.

Microscopic Features
The alveoli contain pink-staining material (oedema fluid); the alveolar capillaries are distended, looking rather like beads on a string. If the pressure in the alveolar capillaries is very high, microhaemorrhages may occur, leading to the accumulation of iron in alveolar macrophages (so-called heart failure cells).

Shock

Shock is defined as a clinical syndrome characterized by systemic underperfusion of tissues due to prolonged and severe hypotension.

If the circulation is regarded as a closed system in which a volume of fluid (the blood), controlled within fairly narrow limits, is propelled by a pump (the heart), it is clear that the major pathogenetic mechanisms capable of causing shock must be:
- a significant decrease in the **volume of fluid** within the system: **hypovolaemic shock**
- failure of the myocardial pump: **cardiogenic shock**
- a significant increase in the capacity of the system brought about by an abnormal degree of vasodilatation: **redistributive shock**, occurring most frequently in the context of bacterial sepsis

HYPOVOLAEMIC SHOCK

Hypovolaemia is caused by:
1) severe haemorrhage
2) loss of large amounts of body fluid such as is seen in severe diarrhoea or vomiting or where there is extensive loss of skin as in extensive burns.

The initial clinical picture is the expression of mechanisms that have evolved to compensate for the drop in cardiac output caused by the fall in blood or plasma volume. **The heart rate is increased and there is extensive peripheral vasoconstriction** brought about by the operation of vasoconstrictors such as catecholamines, vasopressin and the angiotensin system.

CARDIOGENIC SHOCK

This occurs when the myocardial pump fails to provide an output sufficient to maintain normal tissue perfusion. It is commonest in the context of acute myocardial infarction. Where the loss of ventricular muscle exceeds 35%, the compensatory mechanisms described previously prove inadequate and cardiac output falls significantly. Because of the low output, subendocardial necrosis occurs in the myocardium and this obviously further worsens myocardial pump function.

REDISTRIBUTIVE (SEPTIC) SHOCK

Septic shock may occur as a result of systemic infection with a variety of pathogenic microorganisms including Gram-negative and Gram-positive bacteria and, occasionally, viruses (dengue fever) and fungi (systemic candidiasis).

The patients show severe hypotension and, **unlike cardiogenic or hypovolaemic shock, their skin is warm**. This is due to **systemic vasodilatation,** the major factor in the pathogenesis of this syndrome and which is difficult or impossible to reverse with commonly used vasopressor agents.

Many of the lesions seen in fatal cases of septic shock are clearly ischaemic (e.g. renal changes causing acute renal failure (see pp 680–683) and ischaemic colitis) but others are associated with certain features specific for septic shock:

- **consumptive coagulopathy (disseminated intravascular coagulation** (see pp 915–916). This may show itself in a number of ways, including purpura as seen in meningococcal septicaemia
- **adult respiratory failure syndrome (ARDS)** (see pp 448–450)
- **reduction of the ventricular systolic ejection fraction and consequent ventricular dilatation.** This has been attributed to the release of a chemical species that depresses myocardial function

Prior to the fully developed septic shock syndrome, which carries a risk of dying of 80–90%, there is a phase that must be recognized clinically. This has been called the 'sepsis syndrome' and is characterized by fever, tachycardia and some evidence of inadequate tissue perfusion, which may be expressed as oliguria, alterations in mental status or hypoxaemia. At this stage, the mortality rate is much lower (10–20%).

Pathogenesis

Role of Endotoxin

Many of the features of septic shock can be understood on the basis of the action of bacterial endotoxin (lipopolysaccharide), which is a common component of the cell structure of many Gram-negative bacteria. Endotoxin consists of a lipid (lipid A) which is the 'toxic' portion of the molecule linked with a complex polysaccharide. It is heat stable and poorly immunogenic.

Most proteinacious bacterial exotoxins produce their effects by interacting either with some biochemical process within the target cells (e.g. cholera toxin), with some component of cell membranes (α-toxin of *Clostridium perfringens*) or with a neurotransmitter (tetanus or botulinus toxins). Endotoxin acts in a totally different fashion. While, under certain circumstances, it is directly cytotoxic, most notably on endothelium, it produces most of its effect by interacting with several different cell types and plasma protein cascade systems. This causes the release of many other chemical signals. Some are vasoactive causing vasodilatation and thus hypotension; others contribute to the pathogenesis of disseminated intravascular coagulation.

In terms of analogy, one might say that bacterial exotoxins are like arrows which hit a precise point on a biochemical target; endotoxin action might be likened to throwing a stone into a pond: from the point of impact, ripples spread outwards in many directions (see *Fig. 32.58*).

Endotoxin Interactions and Cytokine Production

Compounds released from interactions between endotoxin, certain cells and plasma protein cascade systems result in the release of:

- cytokines such as tumour necrosis factor (TNF) 1α, interleukin (IL)1, IL-6 and interferon (IFN) γ
- nitric oxide (NO)
- products of arachidonic acid metabolism such as prostaglandins, leukotrienes and platelet-activating factor

These are summarized in *Table 32.17* and in *Fig. 32.58*. Of these cytokines, one of the most important is TNF-α, which is responsible for many of the features of shock induced by both endotoxins and exotoxins. When injected in a purified form into small animals, TNF-α reproduces most of the features of septic shock. IL-1 and IFN-γ act in synergy with TNF-α.

Nitric Oxide in Septic Shock   NO is a major, if not the major, determinant of normal vascular tone. It is constitutively (normally) produced by vascular endothelium, its production being upregulated by such compounds as acetylcholine and bradykinin, which cause vasodilatation in normal arteries.

NO is derived from the amino acid L-arginine; its production is catalysed by the enzyme NO synthase, the constitutive form of which is present in endothelial cells.

NO can, however, be produced in cells not normally releasing NO, via an **inducible** form of the synthase. This form of NO production occurs in sepsis, major sources being macrophages, endothelial cells and vascular smooth muscle cells. **Induction can be brought about by endotoxin, certain exotoxins and cytokines.**

The inappropriately large amount of NO thus released causes marked vasodilatation, the vessels now being refractory to vasopressor agents. This refractory state can be overcome by the administration of inhibitors of NO synthase.

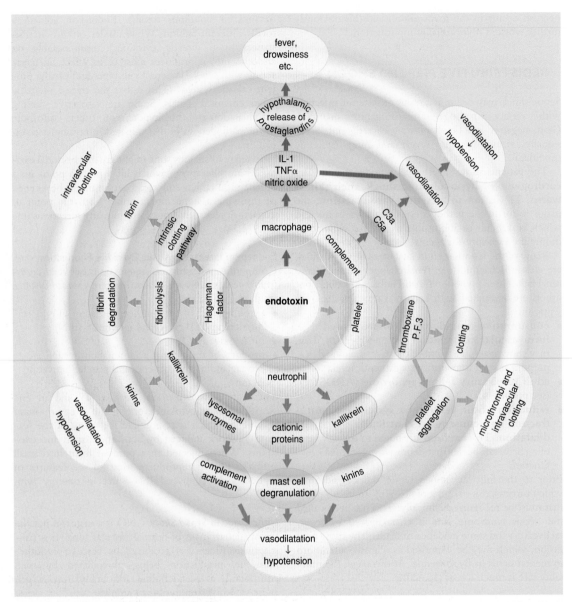

FIGURE 32.58 Endotoxins: interactions with cells and protein cascades.

Other Bacterial Toxins

The redistributive shock syndrome can occur also as a result of infections with certain Gram-positive organisms. The responsible molecules may be exotoxins such as staphylococcal enterotoxin, *exfoliatin*, which cleaves the junctions between epidermal cells causing Lyell–Ritter's disease (scalded skin syndrome) or toxic shock syndrome toxin 1, a product of some strains of *Staphylococcus aureus*.

These exotoxins function as **superantigens**, i.e. they can bind to and activate certain T cells without needing to be presented with a major histocompatibility complex class II protein. These T cells then release large quantities of cytokines such as TNF-1α and IFN-γ.

In addition, it is believed that some cell wall components of Gram-positive organisms, such as peptidoglycans and lipoteichoic acid, may exert a direct toxic effect.

Morphological Features of Shock

The pathological picture of shock is characterized by the results of poor perfusion due to ischaemia and by evidence of disseminated intravascular coagulation (microthrombi and haemorrhage). Virtually any tissue can be affected, although some are clearly more

Table 32.17 Septic Shock

Target for toxin interaction	Products released	Pathophysiological effects	Clinical effects
Macrophages	IL-1 TNF-α IFN-γ IL-6 NO released via inducible NO synthase	Phagocytes activated Prostaglandin release in hypothalamus All inflammatory reactions upregulated NO causes abnormal systemic vasodilatation	Fever Drowsiness Increased capillary permeability, especially in lung
Complement	C3a C5a	Vasodilatation Increased capillary permeability Phagocyte activation	Hypotension Capillary leakage
Platelets	Platelet-activating factor Thromboxane A_2 Platelet factor 3	Upregulation of inflammatory processes Aggregation of platelets Procoagulant effect	Vasodilatation causing hypotension Intravascular coagulation
Neutrophils	Cationic proteins Kallikrein Lysosomal enzymes	Mast cell degranulation Kinin production Complement activation	Hypotension Capillary leakage
Hageman factor	Kinin system activated Intrinsic clotting pathway activated Fibrinolytic pathway activated	Release of kallikrein and kinins Consumption of fibrinogen	Intravascular clotting Haemorrhage as a result of fibrinogen consumption Hypotension

Table 32.18 Pathological Features of Shock

Organ	Frequency (% of fatal cases)	Lesion
Lungs	50	ARDs (see pp 448–451, 680–683)
Heart	36	Affected more commonly in cardiogenic and hypovolaemic than in septic shock. Subendocardial necrosis seen, usually not regional (see p 352)
Kidneys	21.6	Acute tubular necrosis (see pp 680–683, 915–916). Occasionally renal cortical necrosis
Liver	56 in cardiogenic, 46 in hypovolaemic and 32 in septic shock	Hypoxic damage chiefly in zone 3. Septic shock tends to produce cholestasis associated with bile duct proliferation and cholangitis
Pancreas	6.4	Ranges from focal necrosis to extensive haemorrhagic pancreatitis
Gut	26 in septic shock, less in others	Petechial haemorrhages, erosions and acute ulcers in stomach and duodenum. Ischaemic enterocolitis of differing grades of severity
Brain	7	Ischaemic lesions in cerebral cortex
Pituitary	1–8	Haemorrhage and necrosis which may be sufficiently severe to cause Sheehan's syndrome (see p 824)
Adrenals	14	Haemorrhage with or without necrosis; haemorrhage may be focal or extensive as in Waterhouse–Friderichsen syndrome

vulnerable than others. The organs commonly affected are (in descending order of frequency) lungs, heart, kidneys, liver, pancreas, gut, brain, pituitary and adrenals. The pathological features are summarized in *Table 32.18*.

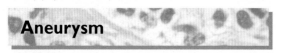

Aneurysm

Definition: 'True' and 'False' Aneurysms

Aneurysm is defined as an abnormal, permanent, segmental dilatation occurring in an artery, a vein or in the heart. The wall of a *true aneurysm* consists, at least in part, of the affected vascular segment. *'False'* aneurysm arises in relation to a ruptured vessel and its wall is formed from the connective tissue that surrounds the haematoma.

Aneurysms may be classified on the basis of:

- **location**
- **shape**
- **cause**

LOCATION

Aneurysms may occur in:

- arteries
- veins
- the heart – the wall of the left ventricle is the site invariably involved in aneurysm formation

In each case, it is pertinent to identify the affected vessel and, in the case of the aorta, it is equally relevant to state which part of the vessel is involved.

SHAPE

These lesions show two basic conformations:

1) **Saccular** (*Fig. 32.59*) – defined as a bag-like or spherical dilatation projecting from one aspect of the affected vessel. Saccular aneurysm is the structural correlate of a **process that weakens only part of the circumference of a vessel wall**. The aneurysm lumen is connected with lumen of the affected vessel by an opening that may be quite narrow in relation to the diameter of the main vessel lumen. Because of this, blood flow through the aneurysm is usually turbulent and thrombosis is common. Indeed, much of the aneurysm lumen may be filled with thrombus.

2) **Fusiform** (*Fig. 32.60*), which describes an elliptical dilatation of the vessel that is due to a **process causing weakening of the entire circumference of the affected segment of blood vessel**. Thrombus formation is also common in this type, and the lumen may be lined by a sheath of poorly organized thrombus.

CAUSE

The reaction patterns of blood vessel walls are limited and most causes of vascular disease can, on occasion, be associated with aneurysm formation. **Aneurysms are the expression of atrophy or necrosis of the**

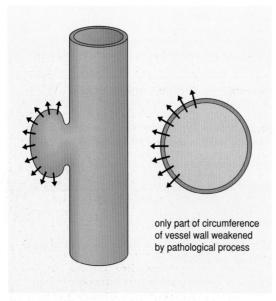

only part of circumference of vessel wall weakened by pathological process

FIGURE 32.59 Saccular aneurysm.

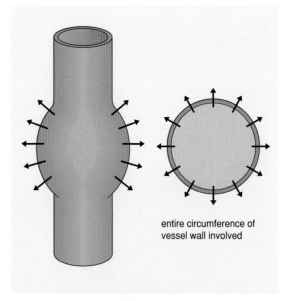

entire circumference of vessel wall involved

FIGURE 32.60 Fusiform aneurysm.

medial smooth muscle cells and destruction of elastic laminae in large vessels such as the aorta.

Aneurysm formation reflects **the interaction between the strength of an injury (which might be infection, inflammation mediated by immune mechanisms or physical forces such as hypertension) and the resistance of the vessel wall.**

AORTIC ANEURYSM

The aorta is the commonest site of aneurysm. Any part of the aorta may be affected. With the decline in the prevalence of tertiary syphilis, **atherosclerosis has become by far the most common association.** Thus the **abdominal aorta** is most often affected, largely because atherosclerosis is generally more severe in this part of the aorta.

This is a common lesion: 1–4% of the population aged over 50 years is affected. Aneurysms of the abdominal aorta occur 4–6 times more often in males than in females and it is clear that the prevalence in middle-aged and elderly males is greater than 4%.

Aortic aneurysm is not only common but is dangerous, having been likened to 'a U-boat in the belly – silent, deep and lethal'. **It is dangerous because of the risk of rupture, such rupture being the 13th most common cause of death in the USA.**

RISK FACTORS (*Table 32.19*)

Genetic Factors
Certain families show an increased risk of abdominal aortic aneurysm. Some 18% of patients with abdominal aortic aneurysm have a first-degree relative similarly

affected, whereas only 2.4% of the general population show this. **The diagnosis of aneurysm in a first-degree relative confers a 12-fold increased risk of an individual developing an aneurysm.**

A weak association has been reported between the risk of aortic aneurysm and the **haptoglobin 2–1 phenotype**; the polymorphism of this protein results from the existence of variant α chains. Aneurysm sufferers express the α^1 allele more often than healthy subjects. **Haptoglobins containing an α^1 chain accelerate the degradation of aortic elastin by elastases *in vitro* by two- to four-fold.** Homozygosity in respect of the α^2 allele appears to be protective.

In addition to the haptoglobin allele that is present on chromosome 16, another rare polymorphism on chromosome 16, which affects the gene that encodes **cholesterol ester transfer protein** (a molecule responsible for the transfer of cholesterol ester from high density lipoprotein to intermediate or low density lipoprotein), increases aneurysm risk.

Monogenic disorders of connective tissue in which aneurysm may occur are discussed separately.

The loss of elastic laminae in aneurysm suggests that elastolysis is involved in the pathogenesis. The elastin content of aneurysms is reduced markedly compared with that of the normal abdominal aorta. Tissue samples from atherosclerotic aneurysms show more proteolytic activity than do samples from aortas with atherosclerosis but no aneurysm. The clustering of aneurysms in certain families may be the expression of a genetically determined increase in the local production of proteolytic enzymes. It is not without interest that the gene for gelatinase (type IV collagenase A) also maps to chromosome 16 and is close to the genes described in the preceding section.

Pathological Features

Macroscopic Features
Abdominal aortic aneurysm is most frequent a few centimetres distal to the origin of the renal arteries. The normal infrarenal aortic diameter in men of 65–74 years is 2.01 ± 0.51 cm, and aneurysm diameter is commonly about 5–10 cm. Aneurysm size differs from case to case and the commonest morphological variant is a fusiform aneurysm. In the majority of patients the aneurysm is confined to that portion of aorta between the renal arteries and the bifurcation, but extension to involve one or both iliac arteries is not rare.

Thrombosis is extremely common. **The thrombus is unusual in that much of it fails to organize** and to be replaced by connective tissue. Thus it **appears as a laminated, gelatinous yellow-brown mass with a granular surface.** This granular surface layer represents the most recent deposition of platelets and fibrin which are easily recognizable on microscopic examination.

Factor	Comment
Table 32.19 Risk Factors for Aortic Aneurysm	
Age	Strong association with increasing age; frequency *doubles* between 50 and 80 years of age
Sex	Marked male predominance
Race	Caucasians are more often affected than Black-skinned
High blood pressure	Strong positive correlation (? because of incremental effect on atherogenesis)
Cigarette smoking	Strong positive correlation
Genetic factors	See main text

Microscopic Features

The most significant features within the aneurysm wall of an atherosclerotic aortic aneurysm are essentially *negative* ones:

- **atrophy of smooth muscle**
- **loss of elastic laminae**

The degree of loss of these aortic wall components correlates with aneurysm size and the degree of vessel wall dilatation. Some remnants of elastin and muscle may persist but, in the most severe cases, the wall consists essentially of fibrous tissue.

The adventitia is compressed and often shows lymphocytic infiltration. This is believed to represent a response to the presence of **oxidized lipid (*ceroid*), which acts as a foreign antigen and elicits the inflammatory response**. This response to ceroid may play a significant role in the pathogenesis of the variant form of abdominal aortic aneurysm known as 'inflammatory aneurysm'.

Pathogenesis

Atherosclerosis and proteolysis set the stage for **an interaction between systolic blood pressure and the weakened aortic segment which will lead to localized dilatation**. Once this begins the distending effect of the systolic blood pressure becomes more and more pronounced as a result of the physical effects of increasing the radius of the affected segment of the aorta. La Place's law states **that wall tension increases as the fourth power of the radius.** Thus, the wall tension in an aneurysm with a diameter of 6 cm is 12 times as great as that in the wall of a normal aorta with a diameter of 2 cm.

Complications

Rupture

The most important of the complications of aortic aneurysm is rupture. This is related to increasing wall tension and the aneurysm size.

Ultrasonographic studies show a median rate of expansion of aneurysm diameter of about 0.21 cm per year, although in some cases the rate of expansion is twice as great as this.

The risk of aneurysm rupture, in relation to size, is shown in *Table 32.20*. All aneurysms that rupture have a diameter of 5 cm or more at the time of rupture, but uncertainties about the natural history are translated into uncertainties as to the best treatment.

All vascular surgeons would offer elective repair to patients whose aneurysms are 6 cm or more in diameter (mortality rate about 5%, although some centres report only 1.5%). In contrast, emergency repair carries a mortality rate of more than 40%, with complications including such potentially disastrous entities as acute renal failure, acute lower limb ischaemia and colonic ischaemia.

The principal consequence of rupture is **haemor-**

Table 32.20 Risk of Aneurysm Rupture in Relation to Size

Diameter of aneurysm at first ultrasonographic examination	Risk of rupture over next 5 years (%)
Less than 5 cm	0
More than 5 cm	25

rhage. This may produce a number of clinical pictures, which it is not appropriate to discuss here.

Other Complications

Rarer complications include bacterial infection and embolization.

Bacterial Infection   The route for infection of an aortic aneurysm wall is via clefts in the thrombus and underlying plaque; the responsible organisms are blood-borne. Various *Salmonella* species and *Staphylococcus aureus* are most commonly involved. The vessel wall and the overlying thrombus show infiltration by acute inflammatory cells, and patients complain of low back pain associated with fever and a tender, pulsating, abdominal mass.

Embolization   Emboli impacting in peripheral vessels may complicate aortic aneurysm. These emboli may be derived principally from the mural thrombus associated with the aneurysm or may consist of a mixture of thrombus and the cholesterol-rich extracellular debris from a disintegrating atherosclerotic plaque. The pathological and clinical consequences depend on the size of the emboli and the site of impaction, but bluish-red discolouration of the toes and/or ankles associated with pain are not uncommonly seen.

'INFLAMMATORY ANEURYSM'

The term 'inflammatory aneurysm' describes an **aortic aneurysm characterized by a marked degree of fibrous thickening of the periaortic tissues,** and a florid inflammatory cell infiltrate in this scar tissue. The infiltrate consists of T and B lymphocytes and immunoglobulin-secreting plasma cells. There is a marked resemblance to what is seen in **chronic periaortitis and so-called idiopathic retroperitoneal fibrosis.** It may be that these are all facets of an essentially single disorder in which there appears to be an immune response in the periaortic tissues followed by marked fibrosis. The trigger in all these cases is still unknown, but the reaction seen in inflammatory aneurysm may be an exaggerated response to the presence of oxidized lipid.

The fibrous tissue surrounding the aneurysm can involve adjacent structures and compress some of these, with serious consequences. For example, the ureters may become narrowed leading to hydronephrosis and, eventually, to renal failure. It is interesting that the proliferation of fibrous tissue appears to affect the areas that lie in front of and laterally to the aorta, soft tissues on the posterior aspect being comparatively unaffected.

Rupture is less common in inflammatory aneurysm. When it does occur, not surprisingly, the posterior wall of the aorta is the most common site.

Patients often present with abdominal pain and weight loss and are found, on investigation, to have abdominal tenderness and a raised erythrocyte sedimentation rate. Modern imaging techniques such as magnetic resonance imaging can be helpful in the diagnosis and show the periaortic ring of fibrous tissue quite clearly.

ANEURYSMS OF THE THORACIC AORTA

While now much less common than those of the infrarenal portion of the abdominal aorta, aneurysms in this part of the aorta are not without significance.

ANEURYSMS OF THE SINUS OF VALSALVA

Aneurysms at this site may arise on the basis of either inherited or acquired disorders. One of the commonest inborn causes is defective insertion of the aortic base into the aortic ring leading to periaortic fibrosis and resulting in traction on the aortic wall. Monogenic inherited defects of connective tissue protein synthesis such as Marfan's syndrome and Ehlers–Danlos syndrome may also be associated with aortic sinus aneurysm.

The commonest **acquired** aneurysm affecting the aortic sinuses is associated with infective endocarditis, the lesions being known as mycotic aneurysms. These aneurysms are most commonly found in association with endocarditis affecting the aortic valve and, if they rupture, they do so into the right side of the heart, thus establishing a high-flow fistula between left and right sides. Mycotic aneurysms can affect any vessel in which infected emboli become impacted. The most common site, however, is in the vessels of the circle of Willis at the base of the brain.

ANEURYSMS OF THE AORTIC ROOT

Medial changes characterized by elastic lamina fragmentation, atrophy of muscle and the accumulation of connective tissue mucin within the aortic media are seen typically in aortic root aneurysm. This set of histological features is known as Erdheim's cystic medial necrosis. Some of these cases are undoubtedly due to Marfan's syndrome, whereas others may be a *forme fruste* of this condition, in which none of the other stigmata of Marfan's syndrome is present. If the genomic changes of Marfan's syndrome are not present in these patients, the lesions are termed **idiopathic**.

In aortic root aneurysm, the proximal portion of the ascending aorta is usually dilated in a fusiform fashion and this is often associated with dilatation of the aortic valve ring as well and, hence, aortic incompetence.

Marfan's Syndrome (*Fig. 32.61*)

Marfan's syndrome is usually inherited in an autosomal dominant fashion, although some cases occur as a result of new mutations. Its main features are:

- extreme tallness
- a longer arm span than normal
- a high arched palate
- long, rather spidery, fingers (**arachnodactyly**)
- tendency for dislocation of the lens to occur
- increased risk of aortic or mitral incompetence
- increased risk of aortic dissection (dissecting aneurysm)

The biochemical basis of Marfan's syndrome is failure to synthesize sufficient quantities of the protein fibrillin, which is normally present in many tissues. The gene (*FBN1*) has been mapped to chromosome 15, and the protein itself appears to associate with elastin in the tissues. Cloning of the gene reveals, in many cases, a point mutation with cytosine substituted for guanine.

Many other mutations have been identified in the fibrillin gene, which makes screening for Marfan's syndrome difficult.

Another monogenic connective tissue disorder associated with aortic aneurysm or aortic rupture is

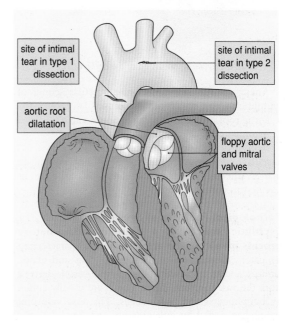

site of intimal tear in type 1 dissection

site of intimal tear in type 2 dissection

aortic root dilatation

floppy aortic and mitral valves

FIGURE 32.61 Cardiac complications of Marfan's syndrome.

Ehlers–Danlos syndrome type IV. In this condition, mutations have been described in the gene that encodes collagen type III (*COL3A1*) which maps to chromosome 2.

ANEURYSMS OF THE ASCENDING AND DESCENDING THORACIC AORTA

Until the antibiotic era, thoracic aortic aneurysms were common, most occurring as a result of syphilitic aortitis which was recorded as being present in 1% of autopsied adults (*Fig. 32.62*). Penicillin treatment for syphilis decreased the prevalence of tertiary syphilis, the phase of the disease in which vascular complications occur.

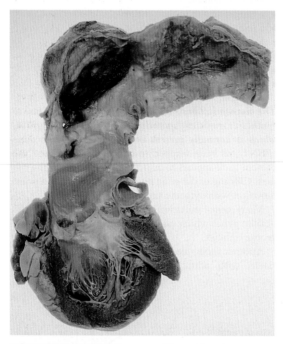

FIGURE 32.62 *Syphilitic aneurysm of the aortic arch.*

Aneurysm was the commonest vascular sequel of syphilitic aortitis, which can also cause:

- aortic root dilatation leading to aortic valve incompetence
- stenosis of the coronary artery ostia

Saccular aneurysms are much commoner in syphilis than in atherosclerotic aortic disease, 68% of the lesions having this configuration.

Pathological Features of Syphilitic Aortitis

Syphilitic aortitis is a chronic inflammatory process involving the arterial media, characterized by patchy destruction of the muscle cells and elastic laminae and by ingrowth of new blood vessels derived from the vasa vasorum. These vessels are usually cuffed by lymphocytes and plasma cells. The vasa vasorum, themselves cuffed by inflammatory cells, may be narrowed by intimal thickening. Small gummatous lesions

may be seen in the affected media, as may multinucleated giant cells. Muscle and elastin loss leads to scarring and this causes a characteristic wrinkled appearance in the aortic intima, described as a 'tree-bark' appearance.

About one-third of patients with this condition died as a result of aneurysm rupture. Syphilitic aneurysm, in the absence of associated aortic valve disease, is compatible with long life and some patients showed striking bone erosion caused by the aneurysms.

With the virtual disappearance of tertiary syphilis in Western countries, syphilis has become increasingly rare as a cause of aneurysm, being replaced by atherosclerosis.

Rarer causes of aneurysm in this part of the aorta include **tuberculosis, rheumatoid disease, giant cell arteritis and Takayasu (pulseless) disease.**

AORTIC DISSECTION (DISSECTING ANEURYSM)

Aortic dissection, given the inappropriate name 'dissecting aneurysm' by Laennec in 1819, is defined as **longitudinal splitting of the aortic wall, usually at the junction between the inner two-thirds and outer one-third of the media, the plane of cleavage being filled with blood.**

This results in 90–95% of cases, from **a tear in the intima and media which extends down to communicate with the potential plane of cleavage** (*Fig. 32.63*).

Blood flows down through this tear and cleaves the media. The rare instances of dissection in the absence of intimal tearing have been ascribed to rupture of vasa vasorum supplying the outer part of the media, but this is far from established.

The mortality rate in untreated patients is high: more than 75% in the first 2 weeks after presentation and more than 90% in the first 3 months.

The tearing should be viewed as the result of an interaction between **haemodynamic factors** that may produce the intimal–medial tear and the **resis-**

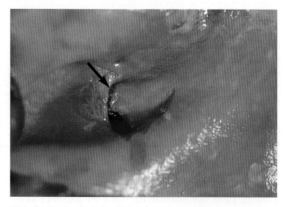

FIGURE 32.63 *An intimal tear (arrow) in aortic dissection.*

tance of the aortic wall to either normal or excessive haemodynamic stress.

Intimal tearing is most likely to be due to shearing stresses which could cause the intima and inner part of the media to become wrinkled up rather like a sleeve in relation to the arm. Once tearing has occurred, the two most powerful forces tending to propagate dissection are:

- **blood pressure**
- **steepness of the pulse wave**

Some 80% of patients presenting with aortic dissection are hypertensive and, in those coming to autopsy, 90% show the presence of left ventricular hypertrophy consistent with hypertension. The frequency of dissection appears to be greatest in patients with accelerated hypertension, although this is now rare as a result of better therapeutic control.

Decreased resistance of aortic connective tissues has been postulated as a risk factor for dissection, as described under the generic title 'Erdheim's cystic medial necrosis'. These changes have been recognized as occurring, both in well-recognized connective tissue disorders such as Marfan's syndrome and also as a normal concomitant of ageing. However, this does not rule out a quantitative difference between victims of aortic dissection and age-matched controls, although this would not be easy to establish.

Risk factors for aortic dissection are shown in *Table 32.21.*

The commonest site for intimal tearing is the ascending aorta. The site of tearing forms the basis for a classification of aortic dissection:

- **Type A:** the tear occurs in the ascending aorta. About 75% of cases are of this type.
- **Type B:** the tear is in the descending thoracic aorta. The dissection may either stop above the diaphragm or extend below this level.

The distinction is important because any dissection involving the ascending aorta is likely to be more serious and to require surgical intervention. Type A dissections tend to occur in younger patients, and are more often associated with anterior chest pain, neurological deficits (stroke, ischaemic peripheral neuropathy, and paraparesis or paraplegia), the development of aortic valve regurgitation, dissociation of arm pulses and blood pressure, cardiac failure and rupture into the pericardial cavity producing cardiac tamponade. Rupture may occur into the pericardial cavity (*Fig. 32.64*), but rupture into the left pleural cavity is not uncommon and, in some more fortunate patients, the haematoma may rupture back into the main aortic lumen resulting in spontaneous repair.

Table 32.21 Risk Factors for Aortic Dissection

Factor	Comment
Sex	Dissection occurs two to three times more commonly in males than in females.
Age	Peak incidence is between 50 and 70 years.
Race	In the USA there is an increased incidence in black-skinned compared with Caucasians.
Presence of systemic hypertension	See main text.
Pregnancy	Some 49% of dissections occurring in patients under 40 years are in pregnant women. Most of the affected individuals are primiparous and dissection tends to occur in the last trimester.
Monogenic connective tissue disorders	Marfan's syndrome is a major risk factor: 44% of patients with the syndrome have aortic dissection. There is a weaker association with Ehlers–Danlos syndrome.
Congenital disorders of aortic valve (bicuspid aortic valve) or aorta (coarctation)	Between 9 and 13% of patients with aortic dissection have a bicuspid aortic valve, compared with 1–2% in the general population. Coarctation is similarly associated with aortic dissection, partly because of the hypertension associated with this anomaly and partly because there is an association between coarctation and bicuspid aortic valve.
Miscellaneous	There is an association between Turner's and Noonan's syndromes and dissection.
Iatrogenic	Dissection has occasionally been reported in association with bypass cannulation, intra-aortic balloon counter-pulsation, etc.

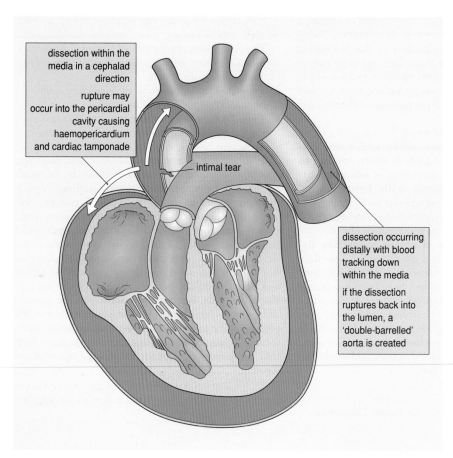

dissection within the media in a cephalad direction

rupture may occur into the pericardial cavity causing haemopericardium and cardiac tamponade

intimal tear

dissection occurring distally with blood tracking down within the media

if the dissection ruptures back into the lumen, a 'double-barrelled' aorta is created

FIGURE 32.64 Aortic dissection.

ANEURYSMS OF MEDIUM-SIZED ARTERIES

POPLITEAL ANEURYSMS

The second most common site for aneurysm formation is the popliteal artery. These aneurysms are usually associated with **atherosclerosis**. Popliteal aneurysms are often bilateral and it has been suggested that they are related to mild recurrent trauma.

SPLENIC ARTERY ANEURYSM

The usual male predominance is reversed in splenic artery aneurysm in which there is a 3 : 1 preponderance of females over males. In only 50% of cases are the aneurysms associated with atherosclerosis. Rupture is not common (about 8% of cases) and tends to be associated with pregnancy.

SO-CALLED 'BERRY' ANEURYSMS OF THE CIRCLE OF WILLIS

These are discussed in the section dealing with vascular disorders of the central nervous system (see pp 1150–

1153) as are the microaneurysms of Charcot and Bouchard, which play an important role in the pathogenesis of intracerebral haemorrhage.

Inflammatory Diseases Affecting Blood Vessels: The Vasculitides

VASCULITIS

Vasculitis is an umbrella term for inflammatory disorders of vessels accompanied by evidence of structural damage to the vessel wall. It is used irrespective of the size of the vessels involved and of the aetiology and pathogenesis of the inflammatory process. **In a number of instances the inflammation is associated with a florid degree of acute necrosis of the vascular wall; these variants are known as necrotizing vasculitides.**

CLASSIFICATION

The rubric of vasculitis covers a group of disorders in which the individual entities show significant differences related to (*Fig. 32.65*):

- **size of the vessels predominantly involved**
- **pathogenetic mechanisms involved**
- **aetiology (unknown in most instances)**
- **associated clinical features**

It is difficult, therefore, to classify the individual members of this heterogeneous group in a logical way.

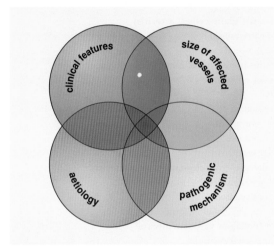

FIGURE 32.65 *Vasculitides are classified on the basis of the sets shown in the diagram.*

In the 1950s it was suggested that the generic term **necrotizing angiitis** should be used to cover the following clinical entities:

- hypersensitivity angiitis
- allergic granulomatous angiitis
- rheumatic arteritis
- periarteritis (polyarteritis) nodosa
- temporal arteritis

This classification omitted a number of disorders not as yet described, but it has proved to be a useful foundation for the more recent ones now used widely (see *Table 32.22*).

Pathogenesis

In such a heterogeneous group it is unlikely that a single set of pathogenetic mechanisms is operating. Nevertheless **evidence suggests that immune-mediated injury plays a significant role in many vasculitides**.

This derives from the observations that:

1) **The lesions that occur in animal models of immune complex-mediated disease closely resemble those seen in some types of human vasculitis.**

2) **Patients with various vasculitis syndromes show evidence of immunological disturbances in the form of:**

- circulating immune complexes
- autoantibodies in the plasma
- changes in the concentration and function of one or more of the components of the complement system
- changes in T cell and/or macrophage function

3) **Improvement is shown by some patients with vasculitis treated by immunosuppressive drugs.**

Immune-mediated mechanisms causing vasculitis may be of different types, including (*Fig. 32.66*)**:**

1) The formation of **pathogenic immune complexes** and their localization in one or other vascular bed (Gell and Coombes type III reactions).

2) **Immediate hypersensitivity reactions** mediated by immunoglobulin (Ig)E.

3) **Direct tissue damage mediated by antibody (Gell and Coombes type II reactions).**

4) **Tissue damage mediated by activation of white cells** as a result of binding of antibodies to white cell antigens.

5) **Tissue damage occurring as a result of cellular immune mechanisms, often accompanied by granuloma formation.**

Some vasculitis syndromes may result from the operation of more than one of these suggested pathways as, for example, systemic lupus erythematosus (SLE).

Vasculitis Related to Deposition of Pathogenic Immune Complexes

Vascular damage related to immune complex deposition has been studied in several model systems, some

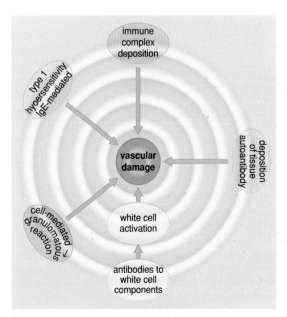

FIGURE 32.66 *Immune mechanisms involved in vasculitis.*

Table 32.22 Classification of Vasculitis

	Size of vessels	Disorders
Infective		*Agents:*
		Spirochaetes (syphilis, Lyme disease)
		Mycobacteria
		Pyogenic bacteria or fungi
		Rickettsia
		Viruses
Non-infective	Large, medium and small	Takayasu's arteritis
		Granulomatous ('giant-celled' arteritis)
		● cranial and extracranial
		● disseminated visceral
		● granulomatous arteritis of the central nervous system
	Medium and small	Thromboangiitis obliterans
		Polyarteritis
		● polyarteritis nodosa
		● microscopic polyarteritis
		● infantile polyarteritis
		● Kawasaki's disease
		'Pathergic–allergic' granulomatosis and arteritis
		● Wegener's granulomatosis
		● Churg–Strauss syndrome
		● necrotizing sarcoid granulomatosis
		Vasculitis of 'collagen vascular disease'
		● systemic lupus erythematosus
		● rheumatic fever
		● rheumatoid disease
		● dermatomyositis or polymyositis
		● systemic sclerosis
		● Sjögren's syndrome
		● Behçet's syndrome
		● relapsing polychondritis
	Small	Serum sickness
		Schönlein–Henoch purpura
		Drug-induced angiitis
		Vasculitis associated with malignancy
		Retroperitoneal fibrosis
		Mixed cryoglobulinaemia
		Hypocomplementaemia
		Inflammatory bowel disease
		Primary biliary cirrhosis
		Goodpasture's syndrome
		Transplant vasculitis

closely resembling human disease. Four of these models are described below.

Acute Serum Sickness Rabbits given a single intravenous injection of a foreign plasma protein develop, after about 14 days, a necrotizing arteritis and glomerulonephritis similar to that seen in humans with polyarteritis nodosa. The peak time for lesion development coincides with the formation of immune complexes when antigen is present in slight excess. Appropriate imnmunohistochemical studies show the antigen, rabbit immunoglobulin and complement within the vascular lesions. **Activation of complement, the release of vasoactive mediators such as histamine and neutrophils are essential components in lesion development. This is shown by the fact that depletion of complement or neutrophils and pretreatment with antihistamines inhibit forma-**

tion of the vascular lesions. A similar sequence of events occurs in human serum sickness, as, for example, in patients receiving injections of horse immunoglobulin. The clinical effects seen in such patients are clearly related to the development of immune complexes, and the increasing levels of circulating complexes are associated with a decline in the concentration of C3 and C4 and a corresponding increase in the plasma concentrations of C3a and C5a–Des–Arg showing complement activation.

Chronic Serum Sickness   Here, the foreign protein is injected in small doses every day for months. In this model the host response is variable. In some instances the animals appear tolerant of the foreign antigen; in others complexes are formed but are rapidly cleared; and in the rest a glomerulonephritis develops that is not accompanied by arteritis.

Intermittent Injection of Foreign Protein   If injections of foreign protein are given **intermittently**, a severe arteritis develops but no glomerulonephritis occurs.

Arthus Phenomenon   The last model of immune complex-mediated vasculitis is the **Arthus phenomenon**. Here, vasculitis occurs at the site of local injection of antigen in an animal presensitized to the same antigen. Preformed antibody complexes with the locally injected antigen in small blood vessels and complement and neutrophil activation result.

In terms of the development of vasculitis, the consequences of immune complex formation and localization are variable. This variability may relate to:
- **physical properties of the complex such as size and composition**
- **ability of the immune complex to activate complement** and the consequences flowing from this
- **release of local vasoactive factors** that can increase vascular permeability and thus allow the immune complexes to leave the circulation and gain access to the interior of the vessel wall

All of these may determine whether a complex persists or not.

Physical Properties of the Complex   The size and composition of immune complexes is determined largely by antigen and antibody concentrations and valencies. **Complexes formed at zones of slight antigen or slight antibody excess appear to be most damaging to tissue.** This may be due in part to a failure of clearance mechanisms and thus a longer 'life' for these complexes, and in part to the fact that they seem to be of a size associated with most effective complement activation.

Whether a complex damages tissue is also affected by the class, subclass and affinity of the antibodies concerned. IgM and IgG_1, IgG_2 and IgG_3 all activate complement effectively via the classical pathway. IgG_4, IgA and aggregates of IgE, in contrast, operate via the alternate pathway.

Complement Activation   Binding of complement components to immune complex may result in two very different biological consequences. These are:
1) **Elimination or clearance of the complex**
2) **'Switching on' the inflammatory response by the generation of chemical signals activating neutrophils, platelets and monocyte–macrophages**

Clearance of immune complexes (*Fig. 32.67*) is enhanced by deposition of many C3b molecules within the substance of the complex. Binding of C3b can lead to reduction in the binding of antigen to antibody and also in the Fc–Fc interactions that help to hold the elements of the complex together. In some circumstances C3b binding can promote solubilization of complex and its diffusion away from the site of formation.

More importantly, the bound C3b acts as an opsonin, facilitating binding of the complex to cells responsible for its clearance. Clearance takes place in two steps.

1) **Complexes coated with C3b bind to specific receptors present on the surfaces of many cell types including red cells, neutrophils, macrophages, B lymphocytes, dendritic reticular cells in the germinal centres of lymph nodes and the epithelial cells in the glomerulus.** The red cell is probably most important in quantitative terms. It acts efficiently to transport immune complex within the blood to the fixed tissue macrophages in the liver and spleen.
2) **In the liver and spleen the sinusoidal macrophages bind immune complex via their C3b and Fc receptors.** In this way, the complexes are separated from the red cells, which now return, minus their load of complex, to the circulation.

Thus failure of clearance can occur as a result of:
- **qualitative or quantitative defects in one or more of the components of complement involved in clearance** (some inherited deficiencies of complement)
- **failure of antibody to initiate complement activation**
- **lack of C3b receptors or blockade of these receptors if they are present** (e.g. in association with dermatitis herpetiformis (see p 997)
- **failure in the function of tissue macrophages**

Release of Vasoactive Mediators and Initiation of Acute Inflammation and Vascular Damage   Immune complex-mediated vessel wall damage is greatly enhanced by the local release of vasoactive mediators. **The**

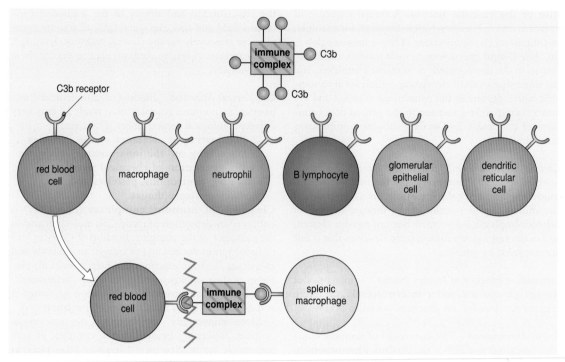

FIGURE 32.67 Involvement of complement in the clearance of immune complexes.

mediators not only increase vessel wall permeability, thus allowing the complexes to gain access to subendothelial tissues, but also attract cells such as neutrophils and platelets whose products have tissue-damaging potential.

Actual damage to the vessel wall may be due also, in part, to completion of the sequence of complement activation with production of the membrane attack complex, but is probably more likely to be mediated by the generation of free radicals and the release of lysosomal enzymes by neutrophils.

Immediate-type Hypersensitivity Reactions Mediated by IgE

In some cases of vasculitis, it has been suggested that immediate-type hypersensitivity reactions, associated with the participation of IgE in immune complex formation, may have a role. Serum IgE levels are increased described in several vasculitides including polyarteritis nodosa and the Churg–Strauss syndrome (see pp 405–406, 408).

Vascular Damage Directly Mediated by Antibodies

Direct tissue damage caused by cytotoxic antibodies certainly plays a part in the genesis of certain disorders (e.g. the **Goodpasture syndrome** and **immune-mediated haemolysis**). Evidence for this in vasculitis is much less strong.

In some patients with SLE, complement-fixing antibodies that bind to endothelial cell antigens are described. These can induce morphological changes in cultured endothelial cells. In the acute phase of Kawasaki's disease (see pp 408–409) IgM antibodies have been identified that lyse cultured endothelial cells pre-treated with interferon γ.

Anti-neutrophilic Cytoplasmic Autoantibodies and Vasculitis

Many cases of **systemic vasculitis**, as well as patients with **crescentic glomerulonephritis**, show no evidence either of immune complex deposition in lesions or of binding of antibodies to vessel wall autoantigens.

Recently **anti-neutrophilic cytoplasmic autoantibodies)** (ANCAs) (*Fig. 32.68*) have been identified in the sera of patients with:

- **Wegener's granulomatosis**
- **microscopic polyarteritis nodosa**
- **crescentic glomerulonephritis**
- **so-called 'leucocytoclastic' angiitis, seen most commonly in the skin**
- **Churg–Strauss syndrome**

Two types of ANCA have been characterized. Their names are derived from the immunofluorescence patterns seen after alcohol-fixed leucocytes are treated with sera from affected individuals.

c-ANCA   This antibody stains the entire **cytoplasm** of alcohol-fixed white cells. It reacts with a 29-kDa protein derived from primary lysosomes of neutrophils and monocytes.

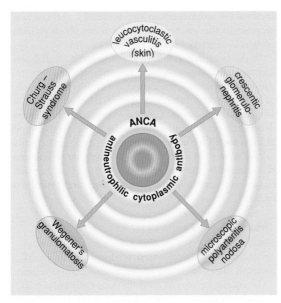

FIGURE 32.68 Antineutrophilic cytoplasmic antibodies are present in the plasma in these forms of vasculitis.

c-ANCA appears to be associated particularly with Wegener's granulomatosis, although it may also be present in some cases of polyarteritis nodosa. In the latter case the leucocyte antigen with which the antibodies react, appears to be different from that in Wegener's granulomatosis.

c-ANCA is a sensitive marker for Wegener's granulomatosis, but its specificity is low: about 50% of patients with c-ANCA in the serum do not have the condition. The hypothesis that it constitutes a pathogenetic mechanism rather than being simply a marker receives support from the facts that:

- relapses in patients with Wegener's granulomatosis are preceded by increases in the titre of c-ANCA
- treatment that produces changes in the serum concentration of c-ANCA can prevent relapses

p-ANCA   p-ANCA is an antineutrophil autoantibody that stains the **perinuclear region** of alcohol-fixed neutrophils. The specific antigen that usually binds this antibody is **myeloperoxidase**. p-ANCA tends to be associated with polyarteritis nodosa, the Churg–Strauss syndrome and crescentic glomerulonephritis.

How may Antineutrophil Antibodies Produce Vasculitis?
Two possible mechanisms are suggested:

1) **The antibodies may activate neutrophils:** sera containing ANCA and the immunoglobulin fractions of such sera cause degranulation of neutrophils with release of lysosomal enzymes. In addition, neutrophils treated with ANCA produce highly reactive oxygen free radicals, most notably superoxide. Priming of the white cells by tumour

necrosis factor α seems to be an important ancillary mechanism in this process.

2) Release of lysosomal enzymes from white cells **may lead to T cell-mediated immune reactions to these enzymes**.

Role of Infectious Agents in Vasculitis

In theory, any infectious agent could produce vasculitis via the mechanisms outlined above. In practice, only a minority of infections are followed by vasculitis. These include:

- **Herpesvirus** infections, which may directly affect endothelial cells which then express receptors for C3b and Fc on their surfaces
- **Mycoplasma** infections, which in both humans and other species are reported as being associated with vasculitis at sites distant from the primary infection
- **Rickettsial** infections, such as Rocky Mountain spotted fever, typically cause vasculitis chiefly involving the arterioles. This effect is a direct one as the rickettsiae multiply within the endothelial cells, which first become swollen and then necrotic. This necrosis is associated with small thrombi. The vasculitis is most obvious within the skin but occurs in many other organs and tissues. The clinical picture is correlated with the sites of blood vessel lesions
- **The human retrovirus, human T-lymphotropic virus I (HTLV-I),** infects human endothelial cells *in vitro*; this has been adduced to explain the lymphoma-associated vasculitis of the skin occurring in HTLV-I-related T-cell leukaemia. Vasculitis has also been recorded in a number of patients with human immunodeficiency virus (HIV) infections, especially where the brain is affected.

Vasculitis in Patients with Malignant Disease

Associations exist between various vasculitis syndromes and malignant disease. These include:

- hypersensitivity vasculitis occurring in association with a wide variety of malignant neoplasms
- a rather characteristic association between polyarteritis nodosa and hairy cell leukaemia
- granulomatous vasculitis in association with Hodgkin's disease

In most of these conditions vessel wall damage has been attributed to pathogenic immune complexes. However, in some, the vasculitis is associated with direct invasion of the affected blood vessels by tumour cells. This occurs exclusively in T-cell malignancies such as:

1) **HTLV-I–associated T-cell leukaemia**
2) **Mycosis fungoides**
3) **Lymphomatoid granulomatosis. In this disorder various tissues are the sites of infiltration by a mixed lymphocyte and plasma cell population. This cell infiltrate is**

often centred around blood vessels, which show a florid vasculitis. In a majority of cases the disease evolves into a frank T-cell lymphoma.

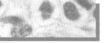

Major Vasculitides

VASCULITIS INVOLVING LARGE AND MEDIUM-SIZED BLOOD VESSELS

TAKAYASU'S ARTERITIS (PULSELESS DISEASE)

This is a chronic inflammatory disease that can involve both the systemic and pulmonary circulations. It most commonly affects the aorta and its major branches, including the coronary arteries.

Its clinical manifestations derive largely from a striking degree of fibromuscular intimal proliferation and from mural thrombosis. Both are the consequence of artery wall inflammation and are governed by what part of the vascular bed is particularly affected. For example, if the abdominal aorta is affected, either an atypical coarctation of the aorta or actual obstruction of the lumen may develop. The process may extend to involve the renal arteries and these patients may present with severe hypertension.

Epidemiology and Aetiology

Takayasu's arteritis has been reported in many parts of the world, most commonly in the Far East. It characteristically affects young women aged between 15 and 45 years. Its aetiology is still unknown and, although there have been reports raising the possibility of an immune-mediated mechanism, there is no specific set of immunological abnormalities. It is interesting, however, that Takayasu's arteritis has been reported in association with a number of disorders believed to have an immunological component, such as rheumatoid disease, ankylosing spondylitis, Reiter's syndrome, chronic inflammatory bowel disease, retroperitoneal fibrosis, Riedel's thyroiditis and scleroderma. There appears to be an association between the risk of this disorder and human leucocyte antigen (HLA) B5. Tuberculosis is another reported association.

Clinical Features

Clinical presentation depends on the location of the lesions, their severity and speed of progression, and the state of the local collateral circulation.

In the early stages, when the vascular inflammation is still active, there may be generalized symptoms such as fever, malaise, dizziness and arthralgia. At this time the erythrocyte sedimentation rate is raised and there is an increase in the concentrations of acute-phase proteins such as C-reactive protein and α_2-globulin.

In the later stages, where fibromuscular intimal proliferation and superimposed thrombosis dominate the pathological picture patients may complain of episodes of pallor of the fingers or entire hand, and later of weakness of the hands. Clinical examination may show, depending on which of the arterial trunks to the upper limbs is involved, either absent pulses or a weaker pulse in one wrist than in the other. A somewhat characteristic retinopathy may occur in which preretinal haemorrhage and arteriovenous anastomosis are prominent features.

Microscopic Features

In the active stages of the disease, there is a granulomatous panarteritis with patchy areas of destruction of medial smooth muscle cells and of the medial elastic lamellae. The cellular infiltrate is made up mainly of lymphocytes and plasma cells, although multinucleated giant cells may also be present in variable numbers.

The active inflammatory phase is succeeded by scarring of the affected layers of the artery walls. This is associated with adventitial and periadventitial fibrosis and a striking degree of fibromuscular intimal thickening. Ultimately the affected vascular segment is converted into a rigid tube with associated stenosis. This may have either a tapered or an undulating configuration, depending on the pattern of intimal hyperplasia.

In most cases arterial stenosis is the characteristic feature, but aneurysms may develop. Where the aortic root is severely affected, aortic valve incompetence may develop as a result of aortic root dilatation. This occurs in about 10–20% of patients.

Anatomical Classification

Takayasu's disease is classified according to the areas of the vascular tree predominantly affected, as shown in *Table 32.23* and *Fig. 32.69*.

GIANT CELL ARTERITIS: CRANIAL AND EXTRACRANIAL

Giant cell arteritis is the commonest of the vasculitides. It is a granulomatous inflammatory process that can affect any elastic and muscular artery in the body. It is most classically seen in the superficial temporal artery and other cranial arteries, where the chief clinical risk is of blindness. Because it responds well to steroids in most instances, prompt diagnosis and treatment are important. It is a disease of the elderly, the mean age of patients being 70 years, and is commonly associated with the clinical syndrome of **polymyalgia rheumatica**. This is characterized by:

Table 32.23 Topographical Classification of Takayasu's Disease

Type	Vessels affected
Type IA	Aortic arch and brachiocephalic vessels
Type IB	Aortic root and proximal part of the arch. This variant tends to be associated with aneurysm formation
Type II	Thoracic and abdominal portions of the descending aorta
Type III	This is a combination of types I and II
Type IV	Pulmonary arteries. This type usually occurs in association with involvement of systemic arteries

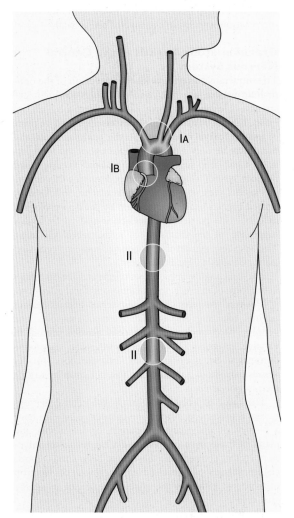

FIGURE 32.69 Distribution of lesions in Takayasu's disease.

- pain and stiffness in the shoulder and pelvic girdles without any evidence of muscle weakness or atrophy
- raised sedimentation rate
- non-specific general symptoms
- a prompt response to moderate doses of steroids.

The aetiology of giant cell arteritis is unknown. Affected subjects show increased prevalence of HLA-DR4. It is not unlikely that the condition is mediated by immune mechanisms but convincing evidence for this is still lacking.

Cranial Giant Cell Arteritis

Clinical Features

The clinical presentation of patients with giant cell arteritis affecting the **cranial arteries** is characterized by:

- headache
- tenderness over the scalp
- claudication symptoms referred to the jaw
- transient visual disturbances including blurring or actual loss of vision
- musculoskeletal symptoms
- non-specific features such as fever, malaise, weight loss and anaemia

Occasionally a swollen, pulseless and tender superficial temporal artery is palpable.

Tissue Diagnosis

Confirmation of a clinical diagnosis of temporal arteritis depends on the gold standard of a tissue diagnosis. However, the chances of obtaining a 'positive' biopsy depend on:

1) **The stage of the inflammatory process at which the biopsy is taken.** Once in the healing stage, the vessel wall may show no more than fibromuscular intimal thickening and some fragmentation of the elastic laminae, appearances that are non-specific.

2) **Sampling.** The inflammation is often focal and segmental with 'skip' lesions being present. The affected segments may measure no more than 300–400 μm in length. Failure to sample the affected area will inevitably lead to a false-negative diagnosis. Biopsies from the superficial temporal artery should measure at least 2–3 cm in length.

3) **Whether treatment with steroids had been started before the biopsy was taken.** In a recent study 82% of biopsies yielded a positive result if the procedure was carried out before starting treatment. If steroid treatment had been given for less than 1 week before biopsy, the positive yield fell to 60%; if the steroids had been given for longer than 1 week, only 20% of biopsies showed active inflammation.

Microscopic Features

The histological appearances can be classified under three headings.

1) **'Classic' acute granulomatous arteritis** shows an inflammatory process that is often focal and usually confined to the media. There is a mixed inflammatory cell infiltrate dominated by lymphocytes, plasma cells and macrophages. The giant cells, if present (they are by no means consistently so), are typically found in the region of the junction between the intima and media, and cluster around breaks in the elastic laminae. They are not a prerequisite for histological diagnosis and, in any event, may be found in a number of other arteritides. They may represent a non-specific reaction to damaged elastic tissue.

2) **In atypical (non-granulomatous) arteritis**, the cellular infiltrate is much the same as in the granulomatous variety but no giant cells are seen.

3) **Healed giant cell arteritis.** There is prominent intimal thickening (*Fig. 32.70*) and little or no medial inflammation, although medial scarring may be present. Collagenous replacement of the media extends between the breaks in the elastic laminae. There is a marked degree of fibromuscular intimal thickening, presumably triggered by the release of growth factors and cytokines released from the macrophages which accumulate in the media during the phase of active inflammation. These probably include the growth factor, PDGF coded for by the c-sis proto-oncogene, and cytokines such as TNF-α and IL-1 which exert their growth promoting effect by 'switching on' the expression of the c-sis gene.

Extracranial Giant Cell Arteritis

Despite the predilection of giant cell arteritis for the cranial vessels, it is important to remember that any large artery including the aorta may be involved. However, only 10–15% of patients present with

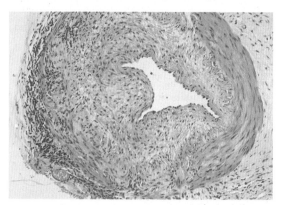

FIGURE 32.70 *Temporal arteritis. There is marked fibrocellular thickening of the intima and a brisk inflammatory reaction within the deeper part of the media and the adventitia.*

clinical disturbances related to the aorta and its major branches.

In these circumstances, **intermittent claudication** is the commonest presenting complaint and evidence of stenoses in the form of arterial bruits or pulse and/or blood pressure abnormalities is common. Complications arising from extracranial giant cell arteritis include:

- coronary involvement leading to myocardial ischaemia
- aortic valve incompetence
- aortic dissection
- aortic aneurysm accompanied, on occasion, by rupture

Only a small number of cases of disseminated visceral giant cell arteritis have been reported. These patients were somewhat younger than the average for giant cell arteritis and in no instance were the cranial vessels involved. It is not possible to judge whether this syndrome is truly related to the usual form of giant cell arteritis or whether, as seems likely, there is merely an apparent overlap because of the restricted range of tissue reaction patterns in the injured artery wall.

Granulomatous Angiitis of the Central Nervous System

The intracranial arteries, with the exception of the ophthalmic vessels, are not usually a target for giant cell arteritis. However, a form of granulomatous arteritis exists, in which **intracranial vessels** appear to be more or less **exclusively** involved. As the granulomatous element may be only a minor component of the total picture, it has been suggested that 'isolated angiitis of the nervous system' might be a better name for this entity.

Patients present with severe headache, followed by altered mental function and then by focal neurological deficits. This particular sequence is said to be highly suggestive of the diagnosis of intracerebral vasculitis. The systemic symptoms so conspicuous in 'ordinary' giant cell arteritis are absent here.

Cerebral angiography shows segmental abnormalities in the form of stenoses, irregularities and focal dilatations.

'Positive' biopsies show a segmental granulomatous angiitis affecting intracranial arteries, arterioles and venules. Multinucleated giant cells may be present in variable numbers. While the histological picture is dominated by granulomatous inflammation, smaller vessels may show a necrotizing vasculitis similar to that seen in polyarteritis nodosa.

The cause of isolated angiitis in the central nervous system is unknown. About one-quarter of patients have a history of malignant lymphoma or leukaemia and many of these have or have had a herpes zoster infection. In this connection, there have been some reports claiming that viral particles have been seen on electron microscopy, either in the affected vessels or in nearby glial cells.

The prognosis is very poor but in a few patients clinical remission has been induced by cyclophosphamide.

BUERGER'S DISEASE (THROMBOANGIITIS OBLITERANS)

In 1908 Leo Buerger, a urologist practising in New York, described a syndrome of vascular insufficiency that progressed to gangrene in the lower limbs of young adult males. **The features of Buerger's disease are both positive and negative:**

1) **Ischaemia, most commonly, but not exclusively, involving the lower limbs** and often progressing to gangrene
2) **Predominant prevalence in males aged between 20 and 45 years**
3) **Strong positive correlation with cigarette smoking**. It is not without interest that there has been a sharp increase in Buerger's disease in females, along with other smoking-associated disorders
4) **Absence of other stigmata of atherosclerosis and, with the exception of cigarette smoking, of recognized risk factors for atherosclerosis**
5) **Association with migratory thrombophlebitis**
6) **Involvement of medium-sized arteries and veins** in the affected part of the vascular bed

Epidemiology and Aetiology

The disorder occurs in all ethnic groups but is somewhat commoner in Orientals and Ashkenazi Jews. Patients show a greater prevalence of the HLA antigens A9 and B5 than control populations, and it is possible that an individual with a specific haplotype might react differently to one of the constituents of cigarette smoke. There is no doubt that cigarette smoke has a strong contributory role in the pathogenesis of Buerger's disease. In most instances the disease will worsen as long as the patient continues to smoke. Stopping smoking is followed by improvement of the clinical features, and resumption is followed by exacerbation within a few weeks or months. It has been shown that most patients with Buerger's disease have evidence of cellular sensitivity to human collagen (types I and III), sometimes with anticollagen antibodies in the plasma, although admittedly at low titres.

Of course, these findings do not necessarily mean that autoimmune reactions against collagen play a part in the pathogenesis of Buerger's disease, although their absence in patients with lower limb ischaemia believed to be due to atherosclerosis does reinforce the concept of a distinct identity for Buerger's disease.

Macroscopic Features

In most cases the samples of blood vessel examined by the pathologist come from amputation specimens and the inflammatory process is largely burnt out. At this stage the affected segments of blood vessel look like fibrous cords and scar tissue may form a sheath around the whole vascular bundle.

Microscopic Features

In the early stages of the disease, the affected vessels contain very cellular thrombi in which microabscesses may be seen. The vessel walls of both arteries and veins show transmural inflammation. The inflammatory process, unlike, for example, that found in giant cell arteritis, does not appear to be associated with breakage of the internal elastic lamina.

Recanalization of the occlusive thrombi often occurs and the residual thrombus undergoes organization, being converted into a somewhat cellular mass of connective tissue that markedly narrows the vascular lumen. Not infrequently, recanalized channels become occluded by subsequent episodes of thrombosis.

VASCULITIS CHIEFLY INVOLVING MEDIUM-SIZED AND SMALL VESSELS

POLYARTERITIS NODOSA

Polyarteritis nodosa is a disease of early middle life, the peak incidence being 40–50 years. Males are affected twice as often as females.

It is a life-threatening disorder. If left untreated the 5-year survival rate is less than 15%, and of fatal cases half die within 3 months of diagnosis. Treatment with steroids or immunosuppressive drugs has made a great difference to the outlook: 80% can now be expected to survive 5 years or more from the time of diagnosis.

Pathogenesis

Evidence so far available suggests that there is no single pathogenetic mechanism involved in polyarteritis nodosa. In some cases the lesions clearly show evidence of immune complex deposition and circulating complexes. The antigen most frequently identified, in both lesions and circulating complexes, is the surface antigen of hepatitis B. Indeed, hepatitis B has been associated with a number of vasculitis syndromes, ranging from vasculitis confined to the skin and associated with urticarial reactions to systemic necrotizing vasculitis. Other antigens involved in polyarteritis nodosa include tumour antigens (as in hairy cell leukaemia) and certain drugs.

Patients with polyarteritis nodosa, especially the microscopic variety, in which there is no evidence of either immune complex or antibody deposition, show **ANCA** in the serum.

Clinical Features

The clinical picture depends largely on the particular vascular beds involved (see *Table 32.24*), but presentation may be non-specific with **fever, headache, myalgia, weight loss,** etc.

Involvement of dermal vessels is reflected in the appearance of purpuric eruptions. Cardiac manifestations, as a result of involvement of the coronary arteries,

Table 32.24 Organ Involvement in Polyarteritis Nodosa

Organ	Frequency of involvement (%)
Heart	50–90
Kidney	70–80
Gastrointestinal tract	30–60
Joints and muscles	30–60
Nervous system	20–50
Skin	10–30
Lungs	< 10

are common. Where medium-sized arteries have been the chief target, **aneurysms** occur as a result of the segmental artery wall damage and these may be identified by angiography, being present in up to 50% of cases of classical polyarteritis nodosa.

Diagnosis
The gold standard for diagnosing polyarteritis nodosa is a positive biopsy. Any tissue that is accessible may be biopsied. Skin biopsy is obviously the easiest and least traumatic for both patient and physician, but an arteritis in this site does not necessarily indicate systemic vasculitis and is less valuable diagnostically than positive results from some other sites. Skeletal muscle is a common site for biopsy in patients with suspected polyarteritis nodosa, but yields rather disappointing results with a false-negative rate of 65%.

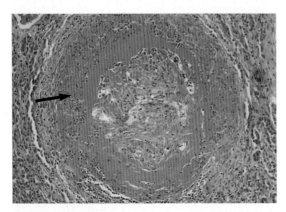

FIGURE 32.71 *Fibrinoid necrosis and arterial occlusion in polyarteritis nodosa.*

Microscopic Polyarteritis
This is an entity in which systemic vasculitis involving small vessels is associated with a **segmental necrotizing form of glomerulonephritis**. The term **microscopic polyarteritis** is applied to distinguish this entity from the classical form in which medium-sized vessels are characteristically involved.

Microscopic Features
The vascular changes depend on the stage in the evolution of the arteritic process at the time of biopsy.

In the early phases the picture is dominated by focal necrosis of the artery wall. In the case of the so-called microscopic form of polyarteritis nodosa, the necrosis affects arterioles and may extend to involve the entire wall thickness. The necrosis is characterized by brightly eosinophilic, rather fuzzy, material resembling fibrin (**fibrinoid necrosis**) (*Fig. 32.71*).

On immunohistological examination, anti-fibrin antibodies bind to this material, although in some cases immune complexes and bound complement can also be identified within the necrotic vessel wall. The damage is associated with a brisk inflammatory cell infiltration in which neutrophils are prominent. If the arteritis is segmental, then bulging of the affected part of the circumference is seen – the first stage of aneurysm formation. Thrombosis, either mural or occlusive, is an almost inevitable accompaniment of this stage of the vasculitis.

As **healing** commences, the inflamed necrotic vessel wall becomes infiltrated by fibroblasts and the infiltrate shows a relative increase in macrophages and lymphocytes and a decrease in the number of neutrophils. The fibroblasts and the connective tissue matrix proteins they produce may be seen **around** the affected vessel as well as within its wall, giving the nodular appearance which led to the use of the term 'nodosa' in this disorder. The progression of the healing process is marked, not only by scarring of the media of the affected vessel but also by fibro-muscular intimal proliferation, presumably due to the release of growth factors by the macrophages in the cellular infiltrate.

WEGENER'S GRANULOMATOSIS
Wegener's granulomatosis is a serious systemic disorder characterized by three main features (*Fig. 32.72*):
1) Necrotizing granulomatous lesions involving both the upper and lower respiratory tracts.
2) A systemic necrotizing vasculitis, which may involve many organs and tissues.
3) Glomerulonephritis, ranging from a focal necrotizing glomerular lesion associated with haematuria to a rapidly progressive, crescentic, proliferative glomerulonephritis giving rise to renal failure.

The disease can occur at any time from adolescence to old age but peak incidence is in early middle life (40.6 years). It is slightly more common in males than in

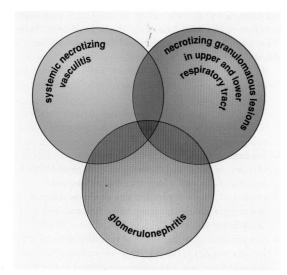

FIGURE 32.72 Principal features of Wegener's granulomatosis.

Table 32.25 Pattern of Organ Involvement in Wegener's Granulomatosis

Organ or tissue	Frequency of involvement (%)
Lung	94
Paranasal sinuses	91
Kidney	85
Joints	67
Nose or nasopharynx	64
Ear	61
Eye	58
Skin	45
Nervous system	22
Heart	12

females and there is a positive association with HLA-ĐR2, not seen in association with either polyarteritis nodosa or the Churg–Strauss syndrome.

Untreated, the disease carried a very poor prognosis: 82% of patients died within 1 year of diagnosis and 92% within 2 years. This bleak outlook has been transformed by the introduction of immunosuppressive treatment (a combination of cyclophosphamide and prednisone). There is also evidence that some patients, in whom cyclophosphamide treatment is no longer appropriate, may respond to antibacterial treatment with trimethoprim and sulphamethoxazole.

Clinical Features

The most common modes of clinical presentation relate to the respiratory tract. About two-thirds of patients complain of symptoms related to the upper respiratory tract such as sinusitis, nasal obstruction, nasal ulceration, severe otitis media and deafness. The remaining one-third have complaints related to the lower respiratory tract such as productive cough, haemoptysis and dyspnoea.

The kidneys are involved in more than 80% of cases, the clinical manifestations ranging from asymptomatic haematuria to rapidly progressive renal failure. Other systemic clinical features correlate with the pattern of organ involvement shown in *Table 32.25*.

Diagnosis

Although ANCAs are found in most patients with Wegener's granulomatosis, the **specificity** of this finding remains low. Patients with c-ANCA in their serum at a titre of more than 1/40 usually have a clinical and pathological picture consistent with Wegener's granulomatosis. Histological examination still provides the most secure base for diagnosis. The option most frequently yielding positive results is open lung biopsy.

Macroscopic Features

The pulmonary lesions of Wegener's granulomatosis are usually multiple and well circumscribed, varying in size from a few millimetres to several centimetres in diameter. The lesion centres consist of soft and friable grey, or sometimes haemorrhagic, material; the periphery is firmer.

Microscopic Features

Histological examination shows areas of coagulative necrosis surrounded by granulation tissue. In the necrotic zone, 'ghost' outlines of vessels may be seen in some areas, whereas in others the tissue architecture is completely effaced. Multinucleate giant cells may be present but well-formed granulomas are not seen as a rule.

The necrotizing vasculitis involves both arteries and veins, and is most clearly identified away from the necrotic areas by using elastic stains to demonstrate the vessel outlines. The vasculitic lesions may be very sparse or even absent in a given lung biopsy. Thrombosis in the affected segments of vessel is a common accompanying feature, and may lead to areas of infarction. Granulomas may be seen within the affected portions of the vessel wall or at its periphery, but are by no means an inevitable accompaniment of the vasculitic lesions.

Extrapulmonary Lesions

In the upper respiratory tract and skin the same combination of necrosis, granulomatous inflammation and vasculitis as described above may be seen. In other sites, necrotizing vasculitis dominates the histological picture and the lesions strongly resemble those seen in polyarteritis nodosa. In the kidneys, a focal and segmental necrotizing glomerulonephritis is seen and this may progress to a fulminating crescentic form with the rapid appearance of renal failure.

CHURG–STRAUSS SYNDROME (ALLERGIC ANGIITIS AND GRANULOMATOSIS)

This clinical and pathological entity is characterized by:
- **asthma and eosinophilia**
- **pulmonary and systemic necrotizing vasculitis**
- **extravascular granulomas**

It is found almost exclusively in patients with asthma or a history of atopy. Asthma usually precedes the onset of the vasculitis by some years. Eosinophilia is invariably present at some stage of the disease, the number of eosinophils frequently being greater than 5×10^9 per litre. During the vasculitic phases, the IgE concentrations may also be increased.

Patients often present with fever and weight loss; this is accompanied in about 70% of cases by pulmonary infiltration. The frequency of diagnosis depends on how strictly the three criteria above are applied. There is overlap between the Churg–Strauss syndrome and some of the other vasculitides.

Microscopic Features

Regardless of the organ affected, the typical lesions are:

1) Eosinophilic vasculitis involving small arteries, veins and, sometimes, capillaries. The vasculitic lesions are often focal and show patchy necrosis of the vessel walls associated with transmural and perivascular eosinophil infiltration.

2) Extravascular eosinophilic granuloma with a necrotic centre. Macrophages take part in the formation of these granulomas, which are much less well formed and cohesive than the epithelioid cell granulomas of, for example, sarcoidosis or tuberculosis. The centres become necrotic and surrounded by macrophages arranged in a palisaded fashion.

Visceral lesions outside the respiratory tract are found most often in the **gastrointestinal tract** and **spleen**, and less frequently in the **prostate** or **heart**. About half the patients also have skin and subcutaneous granulomas, but this last feature occurs in a number of other vasculitic and non-vasculitic conditions.

KAWASAKI'S DISEASE (MUCOCUTANEOUS LYMPH NODE SYNDROME)

This is an acute febrile disease occurring usually in children below the age of 5 years. It was first reported from Japan in 1967 but cases have also appeared in the USA.

It is associated with systemic vasculitis involving medium-sized arteries, most notably the **coronary arteries**, which may become the seat of aneurysms. This complication occurs in 5–10% of patients seen 2 months or more after the onset of symptoms.

The aetiology is still unknown, although there has been a suggestion that a mite-borne rickettsial infection may be responsible.

The acute phase of the disorder is characterized by:
- The onset of fever, generally lasting for 5 days or more.
- Bilateral congestion of the conjunctiva.
- Dryness, redness and fissuring of the lips and diffuse redness of the oral cavity mucosa and tongue. Frequently there is prominence of the papillae of the tongue giving the appearance known as 'strawberry tongue'.
- Acute swelling of the cervical lymph nodes, which is often painful. This is seen in about two-thirds of the Japanese cases and usually disappears as the fever declines.
- A polymorphous rash over the trunk and extremities.
- Reddening of the skin of the palms and soles which then becomes desquamative and spreads up to the wrists and ankles. This may be associated with oedema, which gives the affected area an indurated consistency.

Pathophysiology

The most important pathophysiological features are those affecting the cardiovascular system. In the acute stage both coronary arteritis and pancarditis may occur, and two-dimensional echocardiography shows coronary artery dilatation or aneurysm formation in 40% of cases about 10–12 days after onset of the disorder. Presumably there must be healing and reversal of this process, as within 30 days the prevalence of abnormal echocardiographic changes drops to 20% and within 60 days to 10%.

The natural history of the aneurysms appears to depend, at least in part, on the dimensions:
- If the diameter is less than 4 mm, regression is more or less the rule.
- If the diameter is greater than 8 mm, there is little possibility of regression and, at a later stage, stenosis or occlusion of the affected coronary artery segment can occur. Fortunately this last complication affects only 3–5% of all cases in which angiography has confirmed coronary dilatation.

These aneurysms, especially if they become complicated by thrombosis or are associated with marked intimal thickening, constitute a risk of ischaemic heart disease.

Other systemic disturbances include:
- diarrhoea (about 35% of cases)
- severe abdominal pain owing to gallbladder involvement
- rise in serum transaminase levels

- rise in acute-phase proteins
- leucocytosis with a shift to the left
- albuminuria, which may be associated with aseptic pyuria
- arthralgia or arthritis (25% of cases)
- aseptic meningitis (about 20–50% of cases)

Microscopic Features

There is acute vasculitis characterized by fibrinoid necrosis of the affected segments and an acute inflammatory cellular reaction. Within 2–4 weeks of the onset of symptoms, coronary aneurysms may have already developed and may be associated with segmental coronary artery stenosis and thrombosis.

VASCULITIS CHIEFLY INVOLVING SMALL BLOOD VESSELS

HYPERSENSITIVITY VASCULITIS

This term was used originally to characterize a group of vasculitides involving small blood vessels, both systemic and pulmonary, and to distinguish this group from polyarteritis nodosa. **Serum sickness**, now rare, and **drug-induced vasculitis** (not at all rare) are archetypal examples. The skin is most commonly affected (*Fig. 32.73*), but a wide range of organs may be involved.

The vascular damage within the skin is characterized by **fibrinoid necrosis** (*Fig. 32.74*) and a brisk **inflammatory reaction** in which the predominant cell is the neutrophil. One of the most characteristic microscopic features is karyorrhexis (nuclear fragmentation) of many of the white cells in the vasculitic lesions. It is this feature that led to the introduction of the term **'leucocytoclastic'** vasculitis.

When the cell infiltrate is predominantly neutrophilic, patients often show hypocomplementaemia. In some instances the cell infiltrate is predominantly lymphocytic and, in these, hypocomplementaemia is not a feature.

Many cases show immune complexes within the lesions. The number of antigens canvassed as playing a part in the formation of these complexes is formidable and includes **microorganisms, drugs and tumour antigens**.

Some types of hypersensitivity vasculitis present such characteristic clinical features as to make individual consideration worthwhile. These include Schönlein–Henoch purpura, essential mixed cryoglobulinaemia and hypocomplementaemic urticarial vasculitis.

Schönlein–Henoch purpura

This is a form of hypersensitivity vasculitis occurring predominantly in children and young adults; its cause

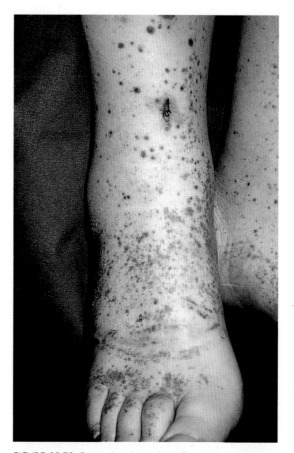

FIGURE 32.73 *Drug-related vasculitis affecting the lower leg and foot.*

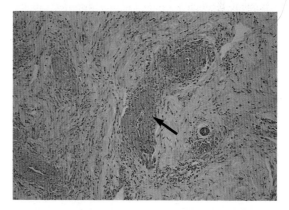

FIGURE 32.74 *Fibrinoid necrosis (arrow) and inflammation in small subcutaneous vessels in drug-related vasculitis.*

is unknown. The classical clinical presentation, which is seen in about 80% of patients, consists of three features.

1) Purpura characteristically involving the buttocks and extensor surfaces of the arms and legs
2) Arthritis

3) Abdominal pain, sometimes associated with intestinal bleeding. This is presumably a manifestation of mucosal or submucosal vasculitis.

The kidney is involved in about one-third of patients, this manifesting in the form of proteinuria, nephrotic syndrome or gross/microscopic haematuria. The glomerulonephritis, which is usually focal and mesangial proliferative in type, is often self-limiting, although episodes of haematuria may occur on and off for years. A few patients may go on to develop a rapidly progressive crescentic glomerulonephritis.

The histological correlate of the purpura is necrotizing vasculitis involving the small vessels of the dermis and associated with subepidermal haemorrhage. Immunohistological studies show IgA to be the predominant, often the only, antibody present both in glomerular and skin lesions. This has led to the suggestion of a relationship between Schönlein–Henoch purpura and the rather common IgA nephropathy (Berger's disease). The presence of C3 supports the hypothesis that the vasculitis is immune complex mediated.

Essential Mixed Cryoglobulinaemia

Cryoglobulinaemia may be found as part of a syndrome in which there is:
- widespread small vessel vasculitis often associated with severe glomerulonephritis
- purpura
- arthralgia

The affected vessels show deposits containing complement, IgG and IgM cryoglobulins. The latter is a rheumatoid factor showing anti-IgG activity. The clinical and pathological features resemble those of Schönlein–Henoch purpura but the disorder can be distinguished by the presence of cryoglobulinaemia, rheumatoid factor and hypocomplementaemia.

Hypocomplementaemic Urticarial Vasculitis

This is a syndrome characterized by:
- marked hypocomplementaemia
- recurrent skin lesions sometimes resembling urticaria, sometimes erythema multiforme
- arthralgia
- myositis
- abdominal pain
- an infrequent glomerulonephritis

Histological examination of the skin lesions shows a leukocytoclastic vasculitis similar to that seen in Schönlein–Henoch purpura. IgG complexes may be seen in the vessel walls in some cases.

Many other varieties of acute small vessel vasculitis overlap clinically and pathologically with the entities described above. The most notable of these are the vasculitides associated with the collagen–vascular diseases such as rheumatoid disease and SLE.

Disorders of Veins

NORMAL ANATOMY AND PHYSIOLOGY

Although veins are composed of the same cellular elements as arteries, architectural differences exist. The three layers of the arterial wall are also present in veins but are less well defined. Where the internal elastic lamina in arteries is clearly recognizable, its venous counterpart is not, and smooth muscle is less abundant in the venous tunica media than in arteries.

There is considerable variation in the amount of muscle in vein walls, which appears to be influenced by:
- calibre of the veins
- intraluminal pressure

When an individual assumes an erect posture the superficial veins in the lower limb become filled to capacity and their cross-section is circular. Thus, even a small incremental volume of blood (e.g. due to deep vein thrombosis or incompetent communicating veins) raises superficial limb vein pressure significantly.

In a very real sense, the veins are capacitance vessels in that at any given moment they contain about two-thirds of the circulating blood. However, this is not their only role. Because veins are richly innervated by the autonomic nervous system, rapid changes in the volume of blood in different parts of the circulatory system are controlled by reflex changes in venous tone. In this way cardiac output can be maintained in the event, for example, of blood loss.

Venous blood flow in the lower limb is produced by interaction between:
- the pressure drive produced by contraction of the calf muscles during walking or when the foot is dorsiflexed
- changes in intra-abdominal and intra-thoracic pressure

THE 'CALF PUMP'

The action of the calf muscles in venous flow has been compared with the actions of the left ventricle of the heart, with the deep intramuscular veins representing the left ventricular cavity and the superficial veins representing the left atrium. Under normal circumstances, as the calf muscles and muscles in the deep posterior compartment of the leg contract, blood is forced into the venous outflow tract, just as in the heart, blood is forced from the left ventricular cavity into the aorta.

The direction of venous blood flow is controlled by bicuspid venous valves. There are no valves in the inferior vena cava or common iliac veins. Valves are present in the external iliac veins in between 25 and 33% of individuals, with the number of valves increasing distally.

In diastole, blood flows from the superficial veins into the deep ones via the valved communicating veins.

As the superficial veins empty, so their intraluminal pressure falls. This pressure decrease is essential for the maintenance of healthy skin and subcutaneous tissue. **Thus the calf pump carries out two very important functions:**

- It is responsible for venous return from the lower limbs during exercise.
- It reduces superficial vein pressure and thus minimizes the effects of hydrostatic pressure on the veins of the skin.

DISORDERS OF VEIN PRESSURE

Most types of vein pathology arise on the basis of an absence of venous hypotension during exercise. This situation may arise because of:

1) **Abnormalities of the calf pump itself**, which include:
a) calf muscle weakness
b) a decrease in the capacity of the deep veins due, for example, to extensive deep vein thrombosis
c) valve incompetence within the deep calf veins
d) an abnormal degree of dilatation of the deep veins leading to secondary valve incompetence.
2) **Outflow tract obstruction**, which leads to dilatation of both the deep calf veins and communicating veins.
3) **Incompetence of the outflow tract in the absence of obstruction.** This is rare.
4) **Incompetence of the communicating veins** (analogous to mitral valve incompetence). If the valves of the communicating veins fail, then blood from the deep veins is expelled not only into the venous outflow tract but also backwards into the superficial veins.
5) **Incompetence of the superficial veins without associated incompetence of the communicating veins.** This is mainly a cosmetic problem. Incompetent superficial veins (varicose veins) contain only 5–10% of the blood passing through the lower limb, and seldom contribute to pump failure and skin damage unless present for many years.

DISORDERS OF VENOUS DRAINAGE

Common abnormalities of the limb venous drainage encountered in clinical practice are:
- varicose veins
- leg ulceration associated with venous hypertension
- deep vein thrombosis and its complications

VARICOSE VEINS

The World Health Organization defines varicose veins as *'saccular dilatations of veins, these being often tortuous'*. The channels involved are either:

- saphenous veins and their tributaries
- superficial veins

Epidemiology

How Frequent are Varicose Veins and why do They Occur?

In Europe and North America varicose veins affect about 2% of the population. If this figure is correct, in the UK alone there are more than one million individuals with varicose veins. There is a positive association with:

- **increasing age**, the peak incidence being between 50 and 60 years of age.
- **female sex**: varicose veins are found about four times as commonly in women as in men. This is believed to be due to the increased venous pressure in the lower limbs occurring during pregnancy.
- **obesity**
- **type of occupation**: a correlation, albeit not a very strong one, exists between occupations requiring long periods of standing and the risk of developing varicose veins.
- **heredity**: there is an increased frequency of varicose veins in the relatives of sufferers from this condition, although some controversy exists as to strength of the association.

Secondary Varicose Veins

Varicose veins associated with some other clearly defined factor are termed secondary varicose veins. Causes include:

1) **damage as a result of previous thrombosis**
2) **pelvic tumours**
3) **congenital abnormalities**
a) congenital absence of valves
b) *Klippel–Trenaunay* **syndrome**, a condition characterized by cavernous haemangiomatous malformations of the skin, varicose veins, and hypertrophy of the bone and soft tissue of a limb.

Pathophysiology

The most frequently affected part of the venous drainage is the long saphenous system. The main trunk is, however, rarely involved: the varicosities affect principally the tributaries of the long saphenous vein.

The affected veins are dilated, elongated and tortuous. On microscopic examination the most striking feature is scar tissue, which appears to invade the media and break the smooth muscle component of this layer into a number of separate bundles. An increase in fibrous tissue is also seen in the intima. These changes are patchy in distribution, and heterogeneity is a hallmark of varicose vein pathology.

Complications
These include:
- **Haemorrhage**
- **Superficial thrombophlebitis.** This presents as a tender, warm, red thickening along the course of a varicose vein. The patient may be pyrexial and feel unwell but serious post-thrombotic complications such as embolization do not usually occur.
- **Brown pigmentation of the skin of the lower legs.** This is the result of extrusion of red cells from venules into the surrounding connective tissue and consequent accumulation of haemosiderin in the dermis and subcutis. It is seen more commonly in patients with venous hypertension due either to previous deep vein thrombosis or to calf pump failure of some other type, and is a characteristic accompaniment of venous ulceration (see below).
- **Lipodermatosclerosis.** This term describes the progressive fibrosis of the dermis and subcutaneous tissue occurring as a result of prolonged venous hypertension. In its acute phase the patient complains of pain and a sensation of heat in the affected area. The skin appears hot, red and tense, and this appearance may easily be mistaken for cellulitis or superficial thrombophlebitis. In the fullness of time the skin becomes stiff and shiny, and on palpation fails to move on the underlying subcutis. The subcutaneous adipose tissue itself also feels hard and stiff and is, presumably, fibrosed.

VENOUS ULCERATION
A venous ulcer is defined as an ulcer of the lower limb caused by some abnormality in the veins and their blood flow patterns. It is not uncommon: about 0.2% of the adult population is affected. In many cases the ulcers are chronic so that, in terms of morbidity and healthcare resources, this condition is important.

In about 80% of patients with chronic leg ulcers there is evidence of vein disease and in about 33% there is also evidence of arterial disease. In about 40–50% of cases venous ulceration is associated with evidence of previous deep vein thrombosis and in almost all cases there is incompetence of the communicating veins. **Thus there is a strong association between venous ulceration and failure of the calf pump due to vein abnormalities.**

Capillary changes are seen in association with venous hypertension in the lower limbs.

Venous hypertension associated with calf pump failure may have a profound effect on dermal capillaries, which become dilated and tortuous. This is associated with a marked increase in the amount of fibrinogen leaving the vascular compartment in the affected areas of dermis and subcutaneous tissue. Some degree of cleavage of this fibrinogen must take place as both histological and immunohistological methods show increased amounts of fibrinogen/fibrin in the pericapillary areas. Similarly, there appears to be a decrease in the fibrinolytic activity of these sites in patients with chronic venous hypertension and ulceration. It has been suggested that pericapillary accumulation of fibrin produces a 'diffusion block' and that this leads to anoxic changes in the overlying skin, but proof of this is lacking.

DEEP VEIN THROMBOSIS
The aetiological and pathogenetic factors contributing to venous thrombosis have been discussed in detail on pp 206–208.

There are, however, clinical syndromes related to venous thrombosis, that are not discussed elsewhere and to which some allusion should be made. These are phlegmasia alba dolens and phlegmasia caerulea dolens.

Phlegmasia Alba Dolens ('White Leg')
This condition is almost always associated with iliofemoral venous thrombosis and a marked degree of lower limb oedema, the latter feature being responsible for the pallor of the limb. Patients complain of pain and swelling of the affected leg. It is strongly associated with pregnancy, the thrombosis being likely to occur either late in pregnancy or soon after delivery. The marked degree of oedema is believed to be due to lymphatic obstruction.

Phlegmasia Caerulea Dolens
This term describes a syndrome resulting from extensive thrombosis involving both the external and common iliac veins. Quite often, the internal iliac vein is affected as well. The affected leg is swollen, painful and cyanosed. This last feature is attributed to the marked degree of venous congestion that is present. The skin may show numerous small haemorrhages, and patches of gangrene may develop if the outflow tract obstruction is not relieved.

CHAPTER 33

The Respiratory System

The Nose, Paranasal Sinuses and Nasopharynx

This anatomical area is very commonly affected by inflammatory disorders, most of which are viral in origin, and much less commonly by neoplasms.

NORMAL STRUCTURE AND FUNCTION

The nasopharynx is lined by squamous epithelium. It has a large and varied normal microbial flora and may be temporarily colonized by many potentially pathogenic species.

The paranasal sinuses, eustachian tubes, middle ear and infraepiglottic portion of the airway are lined by respiratory epithelium composed of ciliated columnar cells and goblet cells. The subepithelial tissue contains mucous and serous glands. These regions are normally devoid of a microbial flora.

Defence Mechanisms

Several mechanisms have evolved to protect the upper airways against infections. These include:

- **Mechanical defences** such as sneezing, coughing and the gag reflex. In addition, the combination of viscous mucous secretions and ciliary action tend to trap foreign particles and propel them upwards (the so-called mucociliary escalator).
- **Local immunological defences** including abundant lymphoid tissue and the secretion of immunoglobulin (Ig) A at the mucosal surfaces.
- **Abundant blood vessels** which provide conduits for the rapid delivery of phagocytic cells.

Any circumstances that inhibit these defence mechanisms promote infection. Such circumstances include:

- type I hypersensitivity leading to allergic rhinitis
- irritation by chemicals
- trauma
- viral infections

All of these produce mucosal oedema, which tends to occlude the relatively narrow channels draining the middle ear and sinuses. In addition, viral infections cause a depression of ciliary function which may be of several weeks' duration. Such problems may be intensified by rapid changes in atmospheric pressure such as occur in the course of air travel.

INFLAMMATORY DISORDERS

These may be either infective or non-infective in origin, the majority of the latter being the result of type I (IgE-mediated) hypersensitivity.

Acute Nasopharyngitis (Common Cold)

Acute nasopharyngitis, although basically a trivial disorder, has economic significance because of its extreme commonness and, thus, the large number of working days lost. More than 200 strains of virus can produce the familiar clinical picture. These include:

- rhinoviruses (at least 110 strains)
- adenoviruses (31 strains)
- parainfluenza viruses (four strains)
- enteroviruses (60 strains)
- coronaviruses (three strains)

Interestingly, in view of their wide use, aspirin and acetaminophen suppress the formation of neutralizing antibodies to these viruses and increase viral shedding from the nasopharynx. While common colds are self-limiting, they may predispose to bacterial infections such as paranasal sinusitis.

Allergic Rhinitis

Allergic rhinitis (hay fever) arises on a basis of IgE-mediated hypersensitivity. The allergens most commonly involved are plant pollens but animal danders and house-dust mites may also cause hay fever and asthma (see pp 126–128, 432–436). Following exposure the affected nasal mucosa is reddened and markedly oedematous, the oedema causing nasal obstruction.

Microscopic examination shows, in addition to hyperaemia and oedema, an inflammatory cell infiltrate in which eosinophils are prominent.

Nasal Polyps

After repeated episodes of allergic rhinitis, polypoid lesions may develop within the nasal passages and, sometimes, within the paranasal sinuses. These striking lesions may measure up to 4 cm along their longest axis. They are not neoplastic but represent islands of oedematous mucosa. These contain hyperplastic mucous glands and a mixed inflammatory infiltrate in which plasma cells are prominent. Such polyps cause obstruction within the nasal passages and in so doing may impair drainage from the sinuses. This predisposes to recurrent attacks of sinusitis.

Sinusitis

Acute sinusitis is characterized by nasal congestion, a purulent nasal discharge, unpleasant breath, facial pain (typically increased on stooping forward) and, often, fever and other systemic manifestations of infection. Some predisposing causes have already been cited. Other contributing factors include deviation of the nasal septum, trauma, foreign bodies or neoplasms, and certain systemic disorders, most notably cystic fibrosis and Kartagener's syndrome (see p 424). Immuno-suppression from any cause increases the risk of sinusitis, which is often severe and refractory in patients with acquired immune deficiency syndrome.

The frontal and maxillary sinuses are most often involved in adults; in children, the ethmoidal sinuses seem to be particularly at risk.

The range of organisms implicated in acute sinusitis has not yet been delineated completely. This is because of the difficulty in obtaining relevant samples for culture. Certainly the results obtained from nasal culture correlate poorly with those obtained from sinus fluid. Direct puncture of the sinuses to obtain samples shows that the pathogens most commonly involved are *Haemophilus influenzae*, *Streptococcus pneumoniae* and *Moraxella catarrhalis*. Anaerobic organisms are obtained from culture in just over 25% of cases.

Most cases of sinusitis yield to treatment with antibiotics and decongestants but in a few cases extension to involve the orbit, the bony margins of the sinus or even the cranium occurs. In the last, thrombophlebitis of one of the intracranial sinuses may supervene.

NECROTIZING AND CHRONIC PROCESSES WITHIN THE NASOPHARYNX

Rhinoscleroma

This is a chronic inflammatory process affecting the nose, pharynx and larynx. It is caused by infection with *Klebsiella rhinoscleromatis*. The organisms multiply within macrophages and the characteristic diagnostic feature on microscopic examination is foamy macrophages in which the organisms can be identified by appropriate special stains.

Mucormycosis

This is the most common and important fungal infection of the sinuses. It is most likely to occur in patients with poorly controlled diabetes mellitus or in immunosuppressed individuals. The non-septate branching hyphae of the *Mucor* species invade blood vessels and

cause thrombosis. This results in necrosis of the affected tissues. The infection may spread to involve the orbit and brain.

Wegener's Granulomatosis

This is discussed in the section on vasculitis (see pp 406–408).

NEOPLASMS

Papilloma

Papillomas of the nose and sinuses occur most commonly in males, presenting as nasal stuffiness or nasal obstruction, or with bleeding from the nose. They are associated with infection by human papillomavirus (types 6 and 11).

Some examples, especially those occurring on the lateral wall of the nose, show a pattern in which the proliferating epithelium invaginates the fibrovascular core instead of growing outwards. This is called an **'inverted papilloma'** and must not be mistaken for carcinoma.

These tumours tend to recur and may invade the orbit or the skull.

About 3% show focal frank malignancy at the time of first excision; a further 3% may present with carcinoma months or years after the first excision with or without recurrences in the interim. In both cases, the prognosis is poor.

Juvenile Angiofibroma

This lesion occurs chiefly in males aged 10–20 years. This age and sex distribution has been interpreted as indicating androgen dependence; indeed, receptors for both testosterone and dihydrotestosterone have been detected in these tumours.

The tumours arise from erectile-like fibrovascular stroma in the posterior lateral wall of the roof of the nose.

Macroscopic Features

Lesions present as polypoid masses which characteristically bleed profusely when biopsy samples are taken.

Microscopic Features

The lesions consist of a mixture of blood vessels and fibrous stroma varying from dense collagen to a loose oedematous tissue in which stellate fibroblasts and numerous mast cells are present.

Natural History

Occasionally these lesions regress after puberty. In most cases, however, surgical removal or irradiation is required. Recurrence is a well-recognized phenomenon, most of the recurrences developing within the first 12 months after initial treatment. Sarcomatous transformation following treatment by radiation has been reported in a few cases.

Carcinoma of the Paranasal Sinuses

Carcinoma of the sinuses (usually squamous) is a rare tumour that tends to occur most frequently in the maxillary sinus. An increased risk has been found in nickel refiners.

The tumours remain clinically silent for quite prolonged periods and, at the time of diagnosis, many have invaded the bony margins of the affected sinus.

Adenocarcinoma of the Paranasal Sinuses

These occur chiefly in the ethmoidal sinus and in relation to the middle turbinate. There appears to be an increased risk in woodworkers.

Carcinoma of the Nasopharynx

Epidemiology

Carcinoma of the nasopharynx is one of the commonest malignant neoplasms and a leading cause of death in South Chinese adult males; it is also not uncommon in the countries of North Africa where children tend to be particularly affected. There is a bimodal age distribution with peaks occurring at 15–25 and 60–69 years.

Aetiology

Factors deemed to play a leading part in causation are genetic characteristics, environment and infection by the Epstein–Barr virus (EBV). Patients usually show IgG antibodies reacting with early EBV antigen, and IgA antibodies which are directed against the capsid antigen of the virus.

Natural History

Unfortunately the lesions tend to grow in a clinically silent fashion and are often irresectable at the time of diagnosis. Nasopharyngeal carcinoma shows a marked tendency to involve regional lymph nodes, and enlargement of cervical nodes may be the presenting clinical feature. Undifferentiated nasopharyngeal carcinoma is radiosensitive and the cure rate is about 50%. Younger patients tend to fare better than older ones; the prognosis is also improved if the lymph node involvement is on the same side as the tumour and is confined to the upper part of the neck.

Carcinoma of Minor Salivary Glands

Tumours arising from minor salivary glands occur in both the nose and the paranasal sinuses, especially the maxillary sinuses. In the sinuses most of these tumours are malignant, the commonest variant being adenoid cystic carcinoma. In the nose benign lesions are fairly common, pleomorphic salivary adenoma being the commonest.

Olfactory Neuroblastoma (Aesthesioneuroblastoma)

This is a variant of neuroblastoma arising either from neuroepithelial elements in the olfactory membrane or from neuroectodermal elements of the olfactory placode.

These tumours occur at any age, the peak incidence being at about 50 years.

Microscopic Features

It is important to distinguish between nasopharyngeal carcinomas that show evidence of keratinization (squamous carcinoma) and those that do not. The former lack an association with EBV and tend to occur in an older age group than the latter.

Non-keratinizing NPC may be further subdivided into two groups:
- undifferentiated
- non-keratinizing but obviously squamous tumours

Undifferentiated carcinomas tend to be associated with a prominent inflammatory cell infiltrate which has led to their being called (inaccurately) lymphoepitheliomas. The neoplastic epithelial cells show two growth patterns:
1) Well-defined aggregates
2) A diffuse pattern intermingled with the inflammatory cells. Before the introduction of immunocytochemistry into diagnostic pathology, this type was often confused with large cell lymphoma.

Electron microscopy and immunocytochemistry show the tumour cells to be unequivocally epithelial, probably arising from the basal layers of the pseudostratified and stratified epithelium.

Macroscopic Features

The tumours appear generally as reddish-grey, very vascular, polypoid masses in the roof of the nasal fossa. Rare cases have been reported in the nasopharynx and sinuses.

Microscopic Features

The commonest appearance is of a highly cellular tumour consisting of uniform small cells with round nuclei and scanty cytoplasm. Rosettes may be present.

Immunocytochemistry shows catecholamines and a variety of peptide markers including neuron-specific enolase and chromogranin to be present.

Electron microscopy shows neurofilaments and dense-core neurosecretory granules in the cytoplasm of the tumour cells.

The tumour cells commonly show an 11–22 translocation similar to that seen in Ewing's sarcoma (see pp 1065–1066), suggesting a common origin with other primitive neuroectodermal tumours.

Natural History

Local invasion tends to occur into the sinuses, orbit, palate, nasopharynx and base of skull. Distant metastases occur in about 20% of cases, involving chiefly the cervical nodes and the lungs. The 5-year survival rate is 50–60%.

Disorders of the Larynx

NORMAL STRUCTURE

The larynx is divided into three parts (*Fig. 33.1*):

1) **A superior or supraglottic region.** This includes the epiglottis, the aryepiglottic folds, the arytenoid cartilages and interarytenoid fold, the false vocal cords or vestibular folds, and the laryngeal sinuses.

2) **A glottic region.** This includes the true vocal cords and anterior commissure.

3) **An infraglottic region.** This portion lies below the true vocal cords.

The functional anatomy of the larynx dictates that pathological processes occurring at this site are expressed in the form of either:

- **abnormalities of phonation**, the commonest of which is **hoarseness**
- **obstruction to normal air flow** of differing grades of severity

DISORDERS OF DEVELOPMENT

Malformations and deformities of the larynx may be congenital or acquired. The commonest of the former is **laryngeal web**, which is usually a rather delicate membrane made up of epithelium and a few strands of connective tissue, stretching between the anterior portions of the vocal cords.

Laryngeal stenosis may also occur as a congenital abnormality, and is usually due to the presence of cysts or webs.

Acquired laryngeal stenosis may follow trauma or exposure of the laryngeal tissues to caustic substances, or may be the result of a wide range of inflammatory processes including tuberculosis.

Laryngocele is an abnormal enlargement of the laryngeal ventricle. It is a congenital abnormality but may be aggravated by any circumstances, such as persistent coughing, that cause intralaryngeal pressure to rise.

INFLAMMATORY DISORDERS

Laryngeal inflammation may be infective or non-infective in origin, the former being caused by bacterial, viral or fungal infections. As in inflammatory processes in general, the disorders may be acute or chronic, acute laryngitides being most commonly associated with obstruction to airflow whereas chronic inflammation is more likely to be expressed in the form of hoarseness.

Acute Infective Laryngitis

The most common and clinically important disorders that fall under this rubric are:

- **acute epiglottitis**
- **acute laryngotracheobronchitis**

In both of these disorders, **children are predominantly affected**. Since their airways are narrow, obstruction, due chiefly to oedema, is likely to be serious and may be life threatening if appropriate treatment is not promptly instituted.

Acute Epiglottitis

Despite its name, the inflammation in this condition affects not only the epiglottis, but also the posterior part of the tongue and pharynx, and the supraglottic portion of the larynx.

The illness starts with sore throat and difficulty in swallowing. Within a few hours, the affected child may be very seriously ill with evidence both of airway obstruction manifest by stridor, and a severe grade of toxaemia or septicaemia. Examination of the upper airway shows a reddened and inflamed pharynx but the most striking and characteristic sign is the presence of a gross degree of swelling and hyperaemia of the epiglottis, which has been likened to a bright red cherry.

In many cases, acute epiglottitis is due to infection with *Haemophilus influenzae* type B, which is also the commonest cause of bacterial meningitis in children under 5 years of age. This strain possesses a polyribose-ribitol-phosphate (PRP) capsular antigen. *H. influenzae* is a common commensal in the pharynx, **non-**

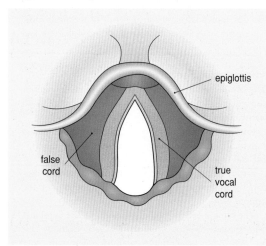

FIGURE 33.1 *The normal larynx as seen through a laryngeal mirror.*

epiglottis

false cord

true vocal cord

capsulated strains being isolated from the throats of about 50% of healthy children. Very few healthy individuals, however, are found to carry the capsulated type B strain. It is likely that significant infections occur chiefly in very young children, as by the age of 3–5 years, many children have circulating antibodies against the PRP capsular antigen. This antibody promotes both complement-dependent bacteriolysis and phagocytosis. The organism does not produce any exotoxin and the mechanisms involved in disease causation are not understood.

The microscopic changes are non-specific and are essentially those of any florid acute inflammation. Some superficial ulceration of the epiglottis associated with the presence of a fibrinopurulent exudate may be noted.

Acute Laryngotracheobronchitis

This disorder is a fortunately uncommon complication of infections of the upper respiratory tract, especially those caused by parainfluenza and influenza viruses. Children under the age of 3 years are most commonly and most severely affected. The chief pathological event is the occurrence of inflammatory oedema involving chiefly the subglottic region. The clinical correlates are:

- hoarseness
- cough, which has a 'barking' character
- stridor (due to airway obstruction)

Diphtheritic Laryngitis

Diphtheria is now extremely rare in the UK; this has resulted from the virtually universal immunization of infants by administration of diphtheria toxoid.

The disease is caused only by toxin-producing strains of *Corynebacterium diphtheriae*; the toxin enters cells and causes irreversible adenosine 5′-diphosphate ribosylation of **elongation factor 2**, a translocase that plays a vital role in protein synthesis (see p 20). It most commonly involves the fauces and tonsils, but the process may spread distally to involve the larynx. The local inflammatory process is characterized by the formation of a greyish-white pseudomembrane which consists of polymerized fibrin admixed with necrotic epithelium and acute inflammatory cells. This membrane can cause airway obstruction, which untreated may be fatal.

Chronic Infective Disorders of the Larynx

Tuberculous Laryngitis

Tuberculous laryngitis was a not uncommon complication of active open pulmonary tuberculosis. With the advent of effective drug treatment for tuberculosis, open pulmonary tuberculosis has become a comparative rarity in developed countries. As a consequence, the incidence of tuberculous laryngitis has declined steeply.

Affected patients present with hoarseness or loss of voice. Examination of the larynx shows nodular ulcerated lesions on the vocal cords, the appearance of which may be confused with laryngeal cancer. Microscopic examination of biopsy material shows typical granulomas in which caseation may or may not be present. The demonstration of *Mycobacterium tuberculosis* in such lesions is necessary for a firm diagnosis to be established.

Fungal Laryngitis

Fungal infections of the larynx are expressed clinically by chronic hoarseness and, microscopically, by granulomatous lesions from which mycobacteria *cannot* be isolated.

Fungal laryngitis is more common in the USA than in Europe; the two most common causes are *Histoplasma capsulatum* and *Blastomyces*.

The granulomatous lesions induced by fungal infections of the larynx may be associated with marked hyperplasia of the overlying squamous epithelium, which may be so gross as to lead to a mistaken diagnosis of cancer (pseudoepitheliomatous hyperplasia).

Acute Non-infective Inflammatory Disorders

Angioneurotic Oedema

In this condition, acute attacks of laryngeal oedema occur. These involve principally the upper parts of the larynx and are important because they can cause obstruction to the airway.

Angioneurotic oedema may occur in two forms:

1) **Hereditary** (inherited in an autosomal dominant fashion). It is associated with a mutation to the gene coding for the **C1 esterase inhibitor** which modulates the intravascular activation of complement via the classical pathway. The mutation leads either to a deficiency in the inhibitor or to an inhibitor that does not function normally.

The attacks may be triggered by mild trauma to the skin and soft tissues but occur more commonly in the absence of an obvious trigger. They may be preceded by an erythematous rash.

The laryngeal oedema may be so severe as to lead to complete airway obstruction and death. In milder cases, the airway oedema is accompanied by colicky abdominal pain. Because C1 activation cannot be controlled in these individuals, it is not surprising that the concentrations of C1, C2 and C4 in the plasma are low: they are consumed in the course of this inappropriate activation.

2) **Non-hereditary**, usually being associated with urticaria in an atopic individual.

Chronic Non-infective Inflammatory Reactions in the Larynx

Granulomatous reactions can occur in the larynx in a number of circumstances, including:

- as a consequence of trauma caused by laryngeal intubation
- as a result of Teflon injections into a paralysed vocal

cord. Such injections are used as a means of augmentation in the cords of patients with recurrent laryngeal nerve damage.

Pyogenic Granuloma

This florid nodular overgrowth of granulation tissue-type capillaries is not uncommon in the larynx. The lesion resembles quite closely a capillary haemangioma. It usually follows trauma to the larynx, this rubric including biopsy or intubation.

Vocal Cord Polyps

These rather common lesions result from mechanical damage to the connective tissue of the vocal cords. Such damage is most often the consequence of persistent misuse of the voice, hence the wide range of occupation-associated synonyms used for this lesion, such as 'singer's nodule', 'politician's nodule' and 'preacher's nodule', to name but a few.

Faulty voice production can lead to the cords being firmly pressed together at a time when rapid vibration is occurring. If repeated many times, this can cause congestion, oedema and focal haemorrhage in the cords.

The commonest site for such polyps is at the junction of the anterior and middle thirds of the cords on their medial aspect.

Patients with vocal cord polyps present complaining of hoarseness. Although vocal cord polyps are benign, they should always be examined microscopically to rule out the presence of carcinoma.

Microscopic Features

The pathological appearances depend on the relative proportions of a number of different processes that can contribute to the genesis of the polyp. These are:
- fibrosis
- ingrowth of new blood vessels
- focal haemorrhage resulting in the deposition of haemosiderin in the connective tissue of the cord
- the appearance in the extravascular tissue of **fibrinoid**, the staining characteristics of which resemble those of fibrin
- hyaline change in the collagen component of the stroma, leading to a featureless, eosinophilic appearance which may be confused with amyloid

---

LARYNGEAL NEOPLASMS

EPITHELIAL NEOPLASMS

These may be, as in any other anatomical location where epithelium occurs, either **benign** or **malignant**.

Benign Epithelial Neoplasms

The commonest benign epithelial neoplasms in the larynx are papillomas. These lesions occur in two main forms: juvenile and adult papillomas.

Juvenile Papillomas

These occur in young children. They are usually multiple and tend to recur after surgical removal. By the time of puberty the lesions tend to regress, although occasional examples may undergo malignant transformation. Almost half these lesions can be shown to contain human papillomavirus antigens (types 6 and 11). A proportion of such infections occurs in infants born to mothers with papillomavirus-related genital condylomata.

The papillomas are small, pink (as they are not keratinized) and finely lobulated lesions. Microscopic examination shows delicate frond-like processes covered by well-differentiated non-keratinizing squamous epithelium.

Adult Papilloma

In contrast with the juvenile variety, this is almost always a single lesion, keratinization is regularly seen and the epithelium covering the papillary processes may show evidence of dysplasia. Malignant transformation is reported in 2–3% of lesions.

Malignant Epithelial Neoplasms

Intraepithelial Neoplasia (Carcinoma in situ)

Evidence of intraepithelial cancer of the larynx is seen most often at the margins of frankly invasive squamous carcinoma. It may be the only lesion present in some patients, who present complaining of hoarseness and whose vocal cords show slight reddening. The criteria for diagnosis are the same as in any other squamous epithelium, i.e. the presence of atypia involving the epithelial covering of the cord. As in the case of the uterine cervix, the greater the proportion of the thickness of the epithelium that shows atypia, the more severe is the grade of intraepithelial neoplasia.

It is not easy to make a prognosis for the individual case and treatment is by excision of the affected area or by stripping away the epithelial covering of the true cord.

Invasive Squamous Carcinoma of the Larynx

More than 90% of malignant tumours of the larynx are squamous carcinomas (*Fig. 33.2*). They occur most frequently in individuals above the age of 50 years and account for 2.2% of all cancers in males and only 0.4% of those occurring in females; men are affected about 24 times as frequently as women.

Tobacco smoking appears to be the main risk factor, smoke from both pipe tobacco and cigarettes being implicated. In post-mortem studies, evidence of intraepithelial neoplasia or invasive carcinoma occurs ten times as frequently in males with a history of heavy smoking as in non-smokers. Experimental studies carried out in hamsters support a carcinogenic role for tobacco smoke and show a linear dose–response effect.

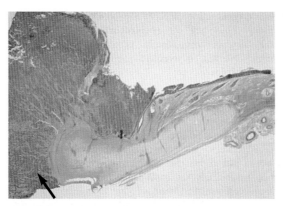

FIGURE 33.2 *Squamous carcinoma of the larynx. This low-power view shows the tumour to have invaded right through the laryngeal cartilage (arrow).*

The effect of smoking appears to be enhanced by heavy consumption of alcohol.

Classification

Classification of laryngeal squamous cancer is based on location, the different sites of origin having a significant effect on patterns of spread (see *Table 33.1*).

The Normal Lung

NORMAL ANATOMY OF THE LUNGS

The lungs are a pair of asymmetrical organs roughly conical in shape. Their combined weight is normally

Table 33.1 Classification of Laryngeal Carcinoma

Location	Frequency (%)	Behaviour
Glottic	60–65	**These lesions arise from the true vocal cords, the anterior portions being affected most frequently**. Because of the comparatively small number of lymphatics and the cartilaginous wall that surrounds the glottis, **the tumours tend to remain localized for long periods and lymph node metastases occur relatively late.** This eliminates the need for prophylactic node dissection in early cases where the tumours are small and the cord is not fixed and immobile. **High cure rates are obtained by either irradiation or surgical removal of the vocal cord lesions. The overall 5-year survival rate is 80%.**
Supraglottic	30–35	**These tumours involve:** • **the false cord** • **the laryngeal ventricle** • **the epiglottis (about one-third of cases)** There is a marked tendency to spread into the pre-epiglottic space but the laryngeal cartilage is seldom invaded. The glottis itself is seldom involved. This means that surgical removal is often possible without permanent loss of voice. **The main cause of treatment failure is spread to cervical lymph nodes, which occurs in about 40% of cases. The overall 5-year survival rate is 65%.**
Transglottic	< 5	**The defining criterion of these tumours is crossing of the laryngeal ventricle.** They show the greatest tendency to spread to cervical nodes and this spread may be clinically occult. Appropriate treatment is total laryngectomy together with prophylactic lymph node dissection. **The overall 5-year survival rate is 50%.**
Subglottic	< 5	**These tumours may:** • **be entirely subglottic (which is very rare)** • **arise from the true cord but extend for 1 cm or more into the subglottic region** The tumour frequently spreads to involve the thyroid gland, the cricoid cartilage and the trachea. Lymph node deposits within the neck occur in about 15–20% of cases but paratracheal nodal metastases are found in about 50%. **The overall 5-year survival rate is 40%.**

about 850 g in men and 750 g in women. Because they are attached only at the hilum, they are able to move fairly freely within the thoracic cavity. This freedom of movement may be partly or completely lost if inflammatory pleural exudates are not demolished in the recovery phase. Failure of demolition triggers the process of repair and, thus, the formation of bridges of scar tissue (or adhesions) between the visceral and parietal layers of the pleura.

The lungs are divided into their major subdivisions, the **lobes**, by clefts which are lined by the visceral pleura. The right lung has three lobes; the left two, although the inferior portion of the left upper lobe (the lingula) is the homologue of the right middle lobe and, not infrequently, is partly divided from its parent lobe by a fissure.

Each lobe is subdivided into further subunits. The first of these is termed the **bronchopulmonary segment**. This is a unit of tissue supplied by a first-generation bronchus distal to the main lobar bronchi and is roughly wedge shaped with its base at the pleural surface. The bronchopulmonary segments are important anatomical entities in relation to thoracic surgery because they can be resected with little haemorrhage and little leakage of air from adjacent raw surfaces.

Bronchopulmonary segments are further subdivided into **lobules**, which can be seen easily with the naked eye on the pleural aspects of the lung as roughly polygonal areas about 1 cm across, outlined by fine connective tissue septa. On section, these septa can be seen to extend for a little distance into the substance of the lung.

The **conducting airway system** starts with the **trachea**, which branches at the level of T4–5 into two main bronchi. The branching is asymmetrical: the left bronchus comes off at a much greater angle than the right (hence the increased risk of aspirated foreign material going down the right main bronchus) and is much longer and narrower than the right. Once the lobar bronchi enter the lung tissue, they divide repeatedly in two, each 'daughter' bronchus having a cross-sectional area of about three-quarters as great as that of its parent. The number of generations from main bronchus to acini varies, between 8 and 25, depending on the region of lung.

Classification of Conducting Airways

All conducting airways share certain features:
- they are lined by ciliated epithelium
- their walls contain smooth muscle

Nevertheless, certain size-related differences exist. The walls of all airways with a diameter of 1 mm or less are reinforced by cartilage, and these are called **bronchi**. Airways without cartilage in their walls are **bronchioles**. In humans and other primates, the last order of bronchioles is transitional in type in that, as well as

being conducting airways, alveoli open directly from them. These are the **respiratory bronchioles** and the airways immediately proximal to these, and which are not so alveolated, are known as **terminal bronchioles.**

Bronchi

Bronchi are lined by pseudostratified, ciliated, columnar epithelium (*Fig. 33.3*). In addition to the ciliated cells, there are small cells with rounded nuclei just above the basal lamina which are known, not surprisingly, as basal cells and which form the stem cell compartment of the bronchial lining. A third type of cell specialized for secretion is also present and is responsible for the production of the mucous 'blanket'. On light microscopy the bronchial epithelium appears to rest on a distinct eosinophilic layer often called the **basement membrane**, but which consists of a normal slender basal lamina together with a layer of closely packed collagen fibres. Beneath this lies a lamina propria, which contains loose connective tissue in which elastic fibres are prominent. The bronchial smooth muscle lies deep to the lamina propria and is arranged in bundles wrapped spirally around the bronchus. Loose connective tissue and the bronchial glands occupy the deep portion of the bronchial wall between the muscle and the cartilage.

In addition to the surface secretory cells the bronchial wall contains **mucous glands**, which are, quantitatively, the most important normal source of bronchial mucus. They are compound tubular glands draining into collecting ducts that discharge into the bronchial lumen with a frequency of about one duct per mm^2. Each gland contains three cell types: **mucous**, **serous** and **myoepithelial** cells, the last of which probably 'milk' the secretions towards the lumen.

The bronchial walls also contain neuroendocrine cells that secrete peptide hormones such as **bombesin**

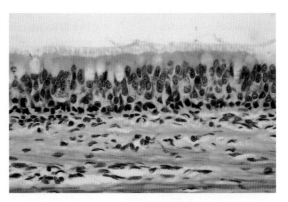

FIGURE 33.3 *Normal bronchial wall showing ciliated pseudostratified respiratory-type epithelium.*

and **calcitonin**. This is not without interest in view of the presence of bombesin in some cases of small cell carcinoma of the lung.

Bronchioles

As well as having no cartilage, bronchioles differ from bronchi in their simpler epithelial lining. This consists of two cell types: a **ciliated columnar cell** and a non-ciliated secretory cell – the **Clara cell**, which secretes a proteinaceous fluid in which two antigenically distinct proteins can be identified.

The Acinus

The basic structural unit for gas exchange is the **acinus**. This consists of the conducting airways and parenchyma distal to a single terminal bronchiole. An acinus is made up firstly of **respiratory bronchioles**, air spaces composed in part of muscular bronchiolar wall and in part of alveoli. There may be two or three generations of respiratory bronchioles within a single acinus and the degree of alveolation increases with each successive generation (*Fig. 33.4*). The most distal respiratory bronchioles lead into the **alveolar ducts**, conducting passages that are lined entirely by alveoli, and these, of which there may be two to six generations, in turn lead into the **alveolar sacs**, grape-like collections of spaces that end blindly. The final generation of alveolar ducts may give rise to as many as six alveolar sacs. The complexity of a single acinus is, therefore, considerable. Three to five acini may be present in a single lobule and there are about 300 million alveoli with mean diameters of 250 μm in the human lung.

Structure of the Alveolar Septum

Air within the alveolus is separated from the pulmonary capillary blood by the alveolar septum, and changes in the septal structure may affect gas exchange profoundly (*Fig. 33.5*). Starting from the alveolar lumen, the following structures may be seen:

- alveolar epithelium
- alveolar basement membrane
- interstitial space
- capillary basement membrane
- capillary endothelium

The non-cellular elements of this blood–air barrier are much thicker on one side of the alveolar space than on the other. On the thin side, the alveolar and capillary basement membranes are fused and there is no interstitial space. On the thick side, the two basal laminae remain quite distinct and are separated by an interstitial compartment of which the chief cellular constituent is a **mesenchymal cell resembling a fibroblast**, capable of secreting collagen and elastin.

Alveolar Lining Cells

There are two types of alveolar lining cells which are called type I (**membranous**) and type II (**granular**) pneumocytes. The type I cell accounts for about 40% of

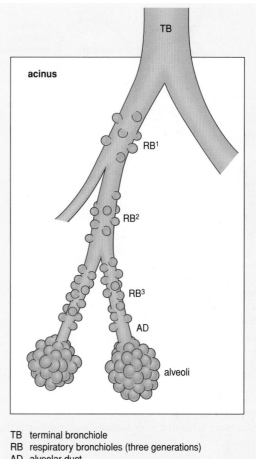

TB   terminal bronchiole
RB   respiratory bronchioles (three generations)
AD   alveolar duct

FIGURE 33.4 Anatomy of a normal lung acinus.

the cell population of the alveolus but covers more than 90% of the area of the alveolar basement membrane. This disparity between the number of cells and the area covered is because the cytoplasm is spread out very thinly over the basement membrane: the diameter of the cell is about 50 μm and the cytoplasmic thickness as little as 0.1 μm.

The type II cell is cuboidal with many stubby microvilli on its alveolar surface. In some animals it tends to be recessed into small hollows in the basement membrane but in the human lung it protrudes into the alveolar space. Type II cells cover only about 3% of the alveolar surface but they are very numerous and it has been estimated that, if all the type II cells in a pair of human lungs could be collected together, they would form a mass comparable in size to a human spleen. The cell has a prominent Golgi apparatus and contains characteristic secretory granules consisting of closely packed, whorled layers of membrane-like material with a marked affinity for osmium. This is the alveolar **surfactant**.

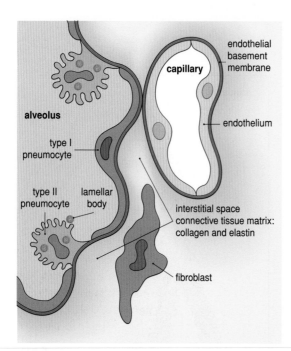

FIGURE 33.5 Structure of the alveolar wall and its relation to alveolar capillaries.

Surfactant

Pulmonary surfactant is an acellular material lining the alveolar surface. It consists largely of surface-active lipids and a carrier (or apo) protein which is lung specific. It is called surfactant because of its ability to lower the surface tension that would otherwise be generated by the presence of a fluid–gas interface in the alveolus. In the absence of surfactant (such as occurs in infantile respiratory distress syndrome), the alveoli cannot remain expanded and the lungs collapse.

NORMAL FUNCTION

The lung exists to allow the exchange of gases between the air and blood, oxygen being added to and carbon dioxide removed from pulmonary arterial blood. Thus partial pressures of these gases are maintained within a normal range in the systemic arterial blood (10.5–13.5 kPa for oxygen and 4.8–6.0 kPa for carbon dioxide) as is a normal acid–base balance.

Gas exchange takes place within specialized functional units known as **acini, which comprise the lung tissue distal to conducting airways known as terminal bronchioles**.

The major processes involved in gas exchange are **ventilation, perfusion** and **diffusion**; many important lung diseases interfere with one or more of the above.

VENTILATION

This is the movement of gases in and out of the lungs. Ventilation must be adequate in volume and appropriate in distribution in relation to perfusion of blood through the capillaries of the distal air spaces.

Ventilation depends on the rhythmic inflation and deflation of the lungs which is governed by:

- **natural elasticity of lung tissue**
- **lowering of surface tension by a phospholipid-rich compound (surfactant) secreted at the surface of the alveolar spaces**
- **contraction of the intercostal muscles and diaphragm, which decreases the intrathoracic and intra-alveolar pressure.** This decrease allows air in the mouth or nose at atmospheric pressure to flow into the distal air-spaces at subatmospheric pressures.
- **elastic recoil of lung tissue and relaxation of the diaphragm and muscles of the chest wall during normal expiration. These increase intrathoracic and intra-alveolar pressure,** and gas flow is thus reversed. Under conditions of forced expiration, however, the activity of the intercostal and abdominal muscles plays an important additional role.
- **depth, rate and rhythm of respiration,** controlled by the respiratory centre in the medulla oblongata, which responds to changes in the carbon dioxide concentration in cerebrospinal fluid, and by the carotid body in the neck, which senses the partial pressure of oxygen in blood.

Thus disturbances in ventilation can result from:

- **disorders of the conducting airways**
- **disorders of lung compliance**
- **disorders of the muscles of the chest wall and diaphragm**
- **disturbances in the respiratory drive**

PERFUSION

About 5 litres of blood per minute pass through the pulmonary circulation. In any vascular bed, blood flow equals the ratio of **driving pressure : resistance**. Mean pulmonary artery pressure is only about 15 mmHg and thus resistance in the pulmonary vasculature must be low (about one-tenth of that in the systemic arterial circulation).

This vascular resistance is regulated by the partial pressures of oxygen and carbon dioxide in the blood. **Hypoxia from whatever cause increases pulmonary vascular resistance.** A reduction in local carbon dioxide concentrations, such as occurs if a pulmonary artery is blocked, leads to a **decline in local ventilation**. This suggests a local homoeostatic mechanism which tends to match ventilation with perfusion.

Pulmonary blood flow may undergo significant alterations. **Increased flow occurs in:**

- exercise
- anaemia

- hyperthyroidism
- fever
- left to right shunts

Decreased flow occurs in:
- right to left shunts
- cardiac failure

Rather more significantly, **pulmonary vascular resistance is increased** in:
- **disorders with chronic airflow obstruction** such as chronic bronchitis and emphysema
- **where there is a significant reduction in the number and calibre of vessels** such as occurs after resection of large parts of a lung
- **inflammatory disorders affecting pulmonary vessels**
- **sustained pulmonary venous hypertension** such as occurs in mitral valve disease
- the rare condition of **'primary pulmonary hypertension'**

Ventilation–Perfusion Mismatch

Many disorders can affect the pulmonary circulation, but the **functional abnormality with the greatest effect on gas exchange is an imbalance or 'mismatch' between pulmonary capillary flow and ventilation of the distal air spaces**.

Ventilation and perfusion are not evenly matched, even in the normal lung. Both increase from the apex of the lung to its base, but the **ventilatory increase is much less than that of blood flow**.

Thus the ventilation : perfusion **ratio** tends to fall from apex to base. The lung apices are well ventilated in relation to blood flow, whereas the reverse applies at the lung bases. Nevertheless normal partial pressures of oxygen and carbon dioxide are maintained. However, in a number of common and important lung diseases, notably disorders of airflow obstruction, severe disturbances occur in ventilation–perfusion relationships, which can lead to hypoxaemia.

DIFFUSION OF GASES

Within the alveoli, almost all the movement of gas molecules is determined by **diffusion**. The transfer of gases from the alveolus into the pulmonary capillary (and vice versa) requires the molecules to pass through the lining epithelium of the alveolus, basement membranes, interstitial space and endothelial lining of the alveolar capillaries. Once the capillary lumen is reached, a second stage of diffusion involves transfer through the plasma and across the red cell membrane and, lastly, the combination of oxygen with haemoglobin. Gas transfer rates are influenced by:
- the available **surface area**
- the distance between the alveolar space and the capillary lumen, which in practice means the **thickness of the alveolar wall**
- the **molecular weight and solubility of the gases concerned**. Carbon dioxide has the same molecular weight as oxygen but is much more soluble and thus diffuses much more rapidly.

> **KEY POINTS: Reasons for Poor Diffusion**
>
> Low diffusion values occur in association with:
> - reduced lung volume
> - emphysema in which there is a decrease in the area available for gas exchange
> - interstitial (fibrosing) lung disease
> - disorders such as chronic air flow obstruction with abnormal distribution of ventilation/perfusion ratios

DEFENCE MECHANISMS IN THE RESPIRATORY TRACT

Some 10 000–20 000 litres of air enter the respiratory tract every day. This air may contain noxious gases, potentially injurious particles and infectious microorganisms ranging from fungi to viruses. It varies also in temperature and degree of humidification. After the skin, **the lung is the organ most exposed to the environment**. Faced with this potentially very hostile environment, it is not surprising how often, but how seldom, the lung is adversely affected by airborne noxae. The lung must be protected as far as is possible; the range of defence mechanisms available starts with the nose.

The Nose

During normal quiet breathing the nose contributes about 50% of the total resistance to air flow, most of which occurs in the anterior 2–3 cm. Mouth breathing reduces the resistance by about 30%. The very complex cross-sectional outline of the nose not only gives it a very large surface area in relation to its volume, but promotes **turbulent flow**, favouring the deposition of airborne particles. Particles deposited on the nasal mucosa are removed by ciliary action together with nasal mucus. The particle-laden mucus is moved in an anterior–posterior direction and collects on the soft palate, from which it is removed by a sucking action and often swallowed.

The nasal mucosa also operates a countercurrent heating and humidification system to make the air reaching the alveoli as near to body temperature as possible, and also ensuring that it is adequately humidified.

The Lower Respiratory Tract

The most important mechanism for the removal both of foreign materials and airway secretions is the so-called **mucociliary escalator**. This protects the conducting airways by trapping particles on a superficial mucous layer. The beating of the epithelial cilia in large conducting airways propels this mucous 'blanket' up the airways to and through the glottis where it is swallowed. The 'blanket' is two-layered, the upper layer consisting of mucus, and the deeper of watery periciliary fluid. Like the arms of a swimmer, as the cilia beat they are fully extended, their tips touching the deep surface of the mucus. In their recovery phase they bend, and this allows them to remain within the non-viscid fluid just above the epithelium.

The volume of secretions within the airway represents the net difference between the amounts secreted and reabsorbed. It may be as little as 10 ml per day. Secretion is increased in several diseases, notably **chronic bronchitis and asthma**, and is stimulated partly by reflex mechanisms and partly by the action of inflammatory mediators such as histamine and the leukotrienes.

Tracheal mucus velocity is **decreased**:
● in smokers
● in patients with chronic bronchitis and asthma
● during anaesthesia

The Immotile Cilia Syndrome (Primary Ciliary Dyskinaesia, Kartagener's Syndrome)

The importance of normal ciliary function is illustrated by a vivid experiment of nature: the immotile cilia syndrome. In 1933 Kartagener described an association between **bronchiectasis, sinusitis and dextrocardia**. Patients with this syndrome have defective mucociliary transport in the large airways, their cilia being either completely immotile or dyskinetic. Electron microscopy shows a variety of structural abnormalities, the most common being an abnormality of the arms (consisting of the protein **dynein**) that link the subunits of microtubules in the cilia.

Other Methods of Mechanical Clearance: Coughs and Sneezes

'Coughs and sneezes spread diseases.' They also serve a protective function in expelling foreign particles or excessive tracheal or bronchial secretions from major airways. The cough reflex becomes less sensitive in the elderly and is lost during unconsciousness from any cause including anaesthesia. This increases the risk of aspiration of stomach contents and, thus, of inhalation pneumonia.

Alveolar Clearance: Role of Alveolar Macrophages

Particles deposited in the most distal air spaces, the **alveoli,** cannot be removed by ciliary activity because **cilia are not found beyond the terminal bronchiole**. Acinar clearance is mediated by the **macrophage**.

Macrophages make up over 90% of the cells seen in bronchial lavage specimens and cover about 5% of the alveolar surface. The many secretory functions of the macrophage, which transcend its phagocytic role,

make it one of the most important actors in the drama of lung pathology. In a very real sense, the macrophage is a double-edged sword. It can certainly defend the lung tissues against both living and non-living foreign material, but it may also injure them via release of lysosomal enzymes or secretion of scar-promoting factors.

In defence, alveolar macrophages function by attaching to foreign particles and ingesting them. If they are living, they may be killed within phagolysosomes or processed so that their antigens may be presented to T helper cells in association with major histocompatibility complex class II-coded proteins. Non-living foreign material, depending on its nature, may undergo differing degrees of digestion or, in the case of metals, none at all. Most of these macrophages move proximally towards the terminal bronchioles where they can be incorporated into the mucous layer, which is transported centripetally by ciliary action.

Chronic Airflow Obstruction

Chronic obstructive airway disease (COAD, chronic obstructive pulmonary disease) is a set of disorders of either the conducting airways or acini, characterized by the **diminished ability to expire air**.

It is neither an aetiological nor a pathological diagnosis as airflow obstruction may occur as a result of a number of distinct pathological entities. Thus a patient presenting with COAD requires the same rigorous diagnostic investigation as, for example, a patient with jaundice or anaemia.

The expiration of air from the lung is determined by the same two major factors as flow in any other system:
● **the force that is applied**
● **the resistance to flow**
In the lung the **force** applied to the system is determined by elastic recoil of the lung tissue; the **resistance** to airflow depends largely on the **calibre** of the conduits through which the air flows. **Therefore, any pathological condition that tends to decrease either the elastic recoil or the airway calibre, or both, is likely to cause airflow obstruction.**

Airflow obstruction is demonstrated by measuring the forced expiratory volume in 1 second (FEV_1). The FEV_1 expressed as a percentage of the forced vital capacity (FVC) is a good indicator of obstruction. Normally FEV_1/FVC is 75%. With increasing obstruction to airflow, FEV_1 falls more than FVC, whereas in restrictive lung disease FEV_1 and FVC are reduced to the same extent and the FEV_1/FVC ratio remains unaffected.

KEY POINTS: Causes of Airflow Obstruction
The chief pathological causes of chronic airflow obstruction are:
- chronic bronchitis
- emphysema
- chronic asthma
- bronchiectasis
- cystic fibrosis

Although the most obvious morphological changes in all of these, other than in emphysema, occur in central airways, **obstruction to airflow is related to changes in the peripheral airways** and structural abnormalities are regularly found in these small air passages.

CHRONIC BRONCHITIS AND EMPHYSEMA

These two disorders account for the majority of patients in the UK who present with chronic airflow obstruction. The two conditions are quite frequently found in the same patients, emphysema occurring about twice as commonly in chronic bronchitics as in non-bronchitics. Chronic bronchitis and emphysema may exist as distinct entities in which chronic airflow obstruction may or may not occur, or they may occur together in one patient, in which case chronic airflow obstruction is almost certain.

How are Chronic Bronchitis and Emphysema Defined?
Chronic bronchitis is defined in clinical terms as the presence of chronic cough productive of mucus or mucopurulent sputum for at least 3 months over a period of at least 2 consecutive years.

Emphysema is defined in morphological terms as permanent overdistension of the air passages distal to the terminal bronchioles, associated with destruction of the walls of airspaces within the acini.

The nexus between these two conditions is an aetiological one: atmospheric pollution, of which the most significant element is cigarette smoking.

Epidemiology

International Differences
Death rates for chronic bronchitis and emphysema show considerable geographical variation. Part of this may be due to differences in diagnostic practice but much is genuine and related to differing degrees of atmospheric pollution. These diseases are common in

all industrialized societies, COAD being the fifth commonest cause of death in the USA. England and Wales rank sixth in the order of frequency published in the *World Health Statistics Annual* for 1986, with a death rate in individuals aged 55–64 years of 56 per 100 000 in males and 24 per 100 000 in females.

Age and Sex
In every country in which mortality rates from chronic bronchitis and emphysema have been recorded, there is a substantial excess in deaths from this cause among males. Similar trends have been found for other smoking-related diseases such as bronchial cancer. In the past 20–30 years, the differences in respect of cigarette smoking between males and females have decreased. One can expect, therefore, that the current difference between the prevalence rates of COAD in the two sexes will narrow, as it has already done with respect to lung cancer.

Aetiology
Several factors have been implicated in causing chronic bronchitis and emphysema. These include:
- cigarette smoking
- atmospheric pollution
- infection

Rarely, emphysema may be found as a result of a **genetic defect, α_1-antitrypsin deficiency**. Although only a small minority of cases of emphysema are due to this, it represents an experiment of nature that helps us to understand the pathogenesis of the more common varieties of this disorder.

Protease–Antiprotease Balance in the Lung
Destruction of the walls of airspaces, which occurs in emphysema, requires the breakdown of proteins such as collagen, types I and III, elastin, proteoglycans and fibronectin. This occurs as a result of enzymic activity. The sources within the lung for such enzymes, most notably **elastases** and **collagenase** are **neutrophils** and **macrophages**, both of which, when activated, release their intralysosomal enzymes. **Under normal circumstances this potentially tissue-damaging activity is counterbalanced by the action of protease inhibitors such as α_1-antitrypsin. Thus the integrity of the connective tissue framework of the lung parenchyma is maintained by a dynamic balance between the local concentrations of proteases and antiproteases.**

α_1-**Antitrypsin** is a glycoprotein synthesized in the liver cell. The molecule is shaped like a shepherd's crook, with a reactive methionine group exposed in the crook handle. The antiprotease activity resides in the methionine, which binds to proteases. However -SH- (thiol) groups in methionine are readily oxidized by oxygen free radicals. In this way excess free radical, such as occurs in cigarette smoking or exposure to other toxic gases, inhibits the antiprotease activity.

Genetically Determined α_1-Antitrypsin Deficiency α_1-Antitrypsin molecules vary because of the many different alleles encoding the protein. The most common and thus 'normal' genotype is PiMM (Pi = protease inhibitor), and the most serious genotypic abnormality is PiZZ. This is the expression of homozygous inheritance of an abnormal gene resulting in plasma concentrations of α_1-antitrypsin about 10% of normal. This decrease in plasma levels is due to failure of liver cells to export the abnormal molecule; the **abnormal α_1-antitrypsin thus accumulates within the liver cells**. The structural correlate of this transport failure is the presence within liver cells of rounded, eosinophilic, intracytoplasmic bodies which, because of their glycoprotein content, stain positively (a magenta colour) with the periodic acid–Schiff method.

About 3% of people in Britain are estimated to be carriers of the abnormal Z gene and about 1 in 5000 children are born with the PiZZ genotype, although fortunately not all of these develop lung or liver disease.

However, a significant number of people with the homozygous abnormal genotype will develop severe emphysema that is predominantly **basal in distribution** and that may manifest clinically under the age of 40 years. This is in marked contrast to what is seen in commoner varieties of emphysema, which chiefly affect older people and which initially affect the **upper** part of the lung. Only a very small proportion of patients with emphysema owe their disease to this inherited deficiency of normal protease inhibitors, but recognition of the mechanisms involved has had important implications for our understanding of the much more common disease related to cigarette smoking and atmospheric pollution. It is not clear whether cigarette-smoking heterozygotes (e.g. individuals with a PiMZ genotype) are more at risk of emphysema than smokers with a normal genotype. It seems likely that risk does not increase until α_1-antitrypsin levels are below 40% of normal.

Cigarette Smoking

As well as having other baneful effects on the respiratory tract (see the section on neoplasia, pp 458–468) cigarette smoking shows a strong positive correlation with mortality from chronic bronchitis and emphysema. A survey of cigarette-related disease in male British doctors, showed **a 38-fold difference in mortality between those who were non-smokers and those who had smoked more than 25 cigarettes per day**.

Other large-scale studies in the USA and Canada have given similar results. It is worth remembering that non-smokers may be adversely affected by cigarette smoke in their immediate environment (so-called 'passive smoking').

How May Cigarette Smoke Act in the Pathogenesis of Chronic Bronchitis and Emphysema?   One of the most significant characteristics of cigarette smoke is its large content of **free radicals** and **nitric oxide**. A single puff of cigarette smoke contains 10^{14} such radicals, which are likely to damage the lung tissue in the following ways:

- by increasing release of proteolytic enzymes from neutrophils and macrophages
- by interacting directly with cell constituents causing, for example, peroxidation of membrane lipids or cleavage of proteins
- by interfering with antiproteolytic defences in the lung

Atmospheric Pollution

Many epidemiological clues suggest that atmospheric pollution is a factor in the causation of COAD:

- Increasing prevalence of and mortality from chronic bronchitis and emphysema with increasing urbanization.
- Higher prevalence of emphysema seen at post-mortem examination on subjects living in areas with high levels of atmospheric pollution.
- Worsening in the clinical state of patients with chronic bronchitis at times of increased atmospheric pollution.

The factors in the urban environment that are responsible for this malign effect on airflow are not known precisely although, again, free radicals found, for example in motor vehicle exhaust fumes, are likely to play a significant role. Industrial smoke appears to have a considerable effect and the two great 'smogs' in London in 1952 and 1962 were both associated with a rise in bronchitis-associated mortality. It is interesting that the increase in mortality rate was less in 1962 than 10 years previously, and this has been attributed to a decrease in smoke by 1962. The atmospheric sulphur dioxide content was much the same at both times. The introduction of Clean Air Acts has led to a very marked decrease in atmospheric pollution in Britain.

Infection

Lung infections in early childhood may be significant in relation to the later development of chronic cough and airflow obstruction. Many studies have demonstrated a **strongly positive correlation between impaired respiratory function in adult life and a history of childhood respiratory infections**. In this connection, infections with **respiratory syncytial virus** appear to be particularly significant.

Pathological Changes in Chronic Bronchitis

The pathological changes in major airways in chronic bronchitis can be inferred logically from the clinical picture, characterized as it is by **chronic cough that is productive of mucoid sputum**.

The presence of abundant viscid sputum indicates quite clearly that the essential structural change *must* be an associated **hyperplasia of the mucus-secreting apparatus**. This is expressed by:

- an **increase in the volume of the mucous glands** in the trachea and bronchi
- an **increase in the goblet cell population** of the airways

The enlargement of tracheobronchial mucous glands found in chronic bronchitis was studied quantitatively by Lynne Reid, who calculated the **ratio of the thickness of the bronchial glands to the thickness of the bronchial wall** in bronchitics and non-bronchitics. **The bronchial wall was defined as the distance between the basement membrane of the bronchial epithelium and the aspect of the bronchial cartilage facing the bronchial lumen** (*Fig. 33.6*).

This ratio is referred to as the **Reid index**. The thickness of the glands is equivalent to the cube root of their volume, and thus, as the latter increases so does the Reid index.

In her study Reid reported that the ratios of gland : wall were **0.14–0.36 (mean 0.26) in non-bronchitics and 0.41–0.79 (mean 0.59) in chronic bronchitics**.

The Reid index has a considerable power in discriminating between bronchitics and non-bronchitics. **With an index of 0.36 or greater, only 6% of individuals are bronchitic. When, however, the index is 0.55 or more, 70% of the sample are bronchitic.** The glands themselves consist partly of mucus-secreting and partly of serous fluid-secreting cells. **The sputum of patients with chronic bronchitis differs from that of non-bronchitics in that it contains relatively more sulphated mucins than sialomucins, and hence is more viscid.**

'Goblet Cell Metaplasia' in Peripheral Airways

Although the mucous gland hyperplasia in large airways may be striking, it is not responsible for the overproduction of mucus causing obstruction in **peripheral airways**. Such obstruction is due to an **increased goblet cell population** within the **bronchioles**, normally accounting for up to about 1% of the surface cell population in these small airways. In chronic bronchitis there is an increase in the number of goblet cells and this is commonly referred to as **goblet cell metaplasia**. The presence of excess intraluminal mucus within the bronchioles may make a significant contribution to obstruction and it has also been suggested that this mucus may displace surfactant normally lining the bronchioles, thus altering the mechanical properties of the affected airways.

Other Changes in Small Airways in Chronic Bronchitis

There is increasing evidence that small peripheral airways are affected in the early stages of chronic bronchitis before symptoms have become obvious, and there are good correlations between structural changes in these air

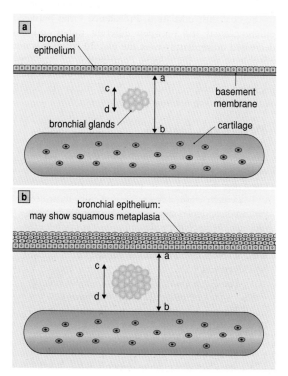

FIGURE 33.6 *The Reid index (gland : wall ratio) in **a** a normal bronchus and **b** a chronic bronchitic.*

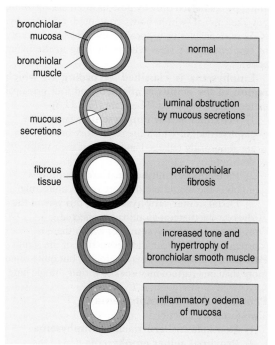

FIGURE 33.7 *Factors contributing to airway narrowing in chronic bronchitis.*

passages and disturbances in small airway function (*Fig. 33.7*). The changes commonly seen include **inflammation**, affecting both the lumen and the wall, **smooth muscle hypertrophy** and **peribronchiolar fibrosis**.

Microscopic Features

From the morphological data, it may be inferred that airflow obstruction may be due to:

- Intraluminal mucus accumulation
- Oedema of the bronchiolar wall
- An increase in smooth muscle tone and reactivity
- Peribronchiolar fibrosis leading to loss of tethering of small airways to the surrounding interlobular septa and thus to a greater degree of bronchiolar narrowing during **expiration**. Normally during expiration, narrowing of the small peripheral conducting airways takes place. The degree to which this occurs is controlled by the tethering of these airways to interlobular septa in the lung. The effect of peribronchiolar fibrosis on airway narrowing during expiration is due to loss of this controlling mechanism.

EMPHYSEMA

The definition of emphysema emphasizes the importance of the **lung acinus as the target in this disorder.** Formerly a clinical diagnosis of emphysema could be confirmed only by post-mortem examination, but the use of whole-body computed tomography, (CT) now enables us to localize and assess the severity of emphysematous areas within the lung in the living patient.

Emphysema is classified according to which region of the acinus is affected, and four principal patterns are recognized. These are (*Fig. 33.8*):

1) **Proximal acinar emphysema** (centriacinar emphysema), in which the respiratory bronchioles are abnormally enlarged and some of their walls destroyed.
2) **Panacinar emphysema.** Here, the process involves the whole acinus more or less uniformly.
3) **Distal acinar emphysema.** In this variant the alveolar ducts are predominantly affected.
4) **Irregular emphysema**, in which there is irregular enlargement and destruction of the acinus.

Pure forms of these types may be found, but quite often more than one pattern may coexist within a single lung.

Proximal Acinar Emphysema

Two forms are described:
1) Non-industrial **centriacinar emphysema**
2) **Proximal acinar emphysema** due to the inhalation of dust (simple coalminers' pneumoconiosis).

Non-industrial Centriacinar Emphysema

In this common variant the primary lesion is **dilatation and destruction of the respiratory bronchioles**, airways of the second and third order being most severely affected (*Fig. 33.9*). This distinguishes it from simple coalminers' pneumoconiosis in which the emphasis is on dilatation of the respiratory bronchioles.

Macroscopic Features

Classically the abnormal airspaces lie near the centre of the secondary lobules and for this reason centriacinar emphysema is sometimes called **centrilobular emphysema**. The lung surrounding the dilated airspaces is often normal and this normal tissue separates the emphysematous spaces from one another. The upper lobes are usually more extensively and severely affected than the lower lobes. Inflammation is commonly present in the airways supplying the emphysematous spaces and, in 60% of cases, these are narrowed. The walls of the emphysematous spaces nearly always show some chronic inflammation and fibrosis.

Centriacinar emphysema is the commonest form associated with chronic airflow obstruction. It is more common in men, probably because of the greater frequency of smoking.

Proximal Acinar Emphysema due to Dust

This lesion occurs in coalworkers and has been ascribed to the coal dust inhalation. Prevalence varies between different areas and between different mines and has decreased quite sharply over the past 30 years. It is not possible to assess the relative contribution of dust-suppressing measures in the mines because of the recorded decline in smoking (from 20.7% of miners in South Wales in 1960 to 6.2% in 1987).

Macroscopic Features

Appearances in proximal acinar emphysema are similar to those seen in centriacinar emphysema with the addition of carbon pigmentation in the form of numerous foci situated near the centre of the secondary lobules.

The emphysematous spaces are formed by dilated respiratory bronchioles and these are surrounded by accumulations of dust lying within the alveoli arising from the respiratory bronchioles. The distinction between this form of emphysema and the centriacinar variety is based on four criteria:

1) The distribution within the lung is more uniform than is the case with centriacinar emphysema.
2) The airways supplying the emphysematous spaces show neither inflammation nor scarring.
3) There is always a large amount of dust adjacent to the emphysematous spaces.
4) The affected respiratory bronchioles are dilated, not destroyed.

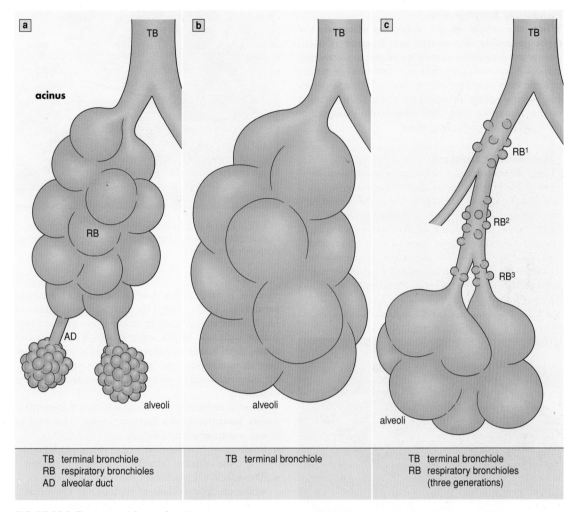

TB terminal bronchiole	TB terminal bronchiole	TB terminal bronchiole
RB respiratory bronchioles		RB respiratory bronchioles
AD alveolar duct		(three generations)

FIGURE 33.8 The principal forms of emphysema.

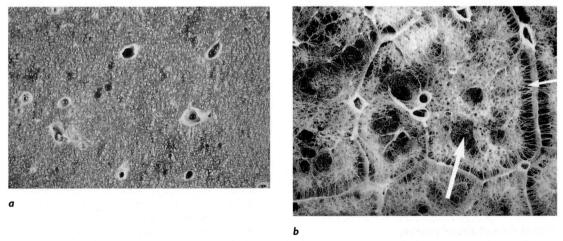

*FIGURE 33.9 **a** The cut surface of a normal lung. **b** Cut surface of lung showing a combination of centriacinar emphysema (large arrow) and paraseptal emphysema (small arrow).*

Panacinar Emphysema

When the whole of the acinus is affected, the term panacinar destructive emphysema is used. The word destructive should be added to distinguish this condition from the acinar overdistension occurring in some cases of asthma and in so-called 'compensatory emphysema' where there is permanent overdistension of the remaining lung after obstructive collapse, or removal, of part of the lung tissue.

Macroscopic Features

Lungs severely affected by panacinar emphysema are enlarged and fail to collapse when the pleural cavities are opened (Fig. 33.10). The appearances of the cut surface are best seen if the lung has been inflated with formaldehyde vapour before cutting. When this has been done, the cut surfaces show a gross degree of enlargement of the airspaces (Fig. 33.11). The distribution pattern may be variable, but the lower lobes tend to be more severely affected than the upper, in contradistinction to centriacinar emphysema.

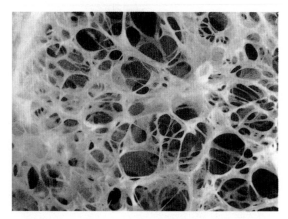

FIGURE 33.11 A portion of lung, inflated with formaldehyde vapour, showing severe distension of airspaces characteristic of panacinar emphysema.

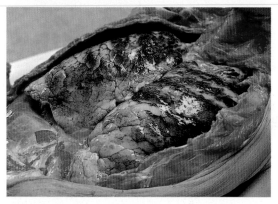

FIGURE 33.10 The anterior part of the chest wall of this severely emphysematous individual was removed at post-mortem examination. Note how bulky the lungs are and that they have failed to collapse when the pleural cavities were opened.

Microscopic Features

The most striking feature of panacinar emphysema is total disorganization of the architectural pattern of the acini. Normal alveoli are replaced by large, thin-walled, irregularly shaped spaces. Respiratory bronchioles cannot be identified in the affected areas and all distinction between them and the smaller, more distal airspaces is lost. The emphysema associated with α_1-antitrypsin deficiency is of this type.

Distal Acinar Emphysema

Distal acinar emphysema affects the peripheral part of the acinus and, because these areas often lie along septa, it is often referred to as **paraseptal emphysema** (Fig. 33.9b). This is the least common variety of emphysema and may occur either alone or in combination with one of the other types. When it occurs alone, distal acinar emphysema is usually most prominent along the posterior margins of the upper lobes in the subpleural region and is often associated with areas of scarring.

Its most characteristic clinical association is **spontaneous pneumothorax** in young males. This may be due to a combination of factors.

- Predominant localization within the upper lobes where the negative intrapleural pressure is greatest.
- The subpleural position of many of the lesions which predisposes them to rupture into the pleura tissue. As a result blebs form, which then subsequently rupture into the pleural space.

There is a classical association between the occurrence of spontaneous pneumothorax and habitus, tall thin individuals being most at risk. This emphasizes the importance of negative intrapleural pressure in the pathogenesis, because this pressure is highest in tall subjects and at large lung volumes. Carcinoma of the lung has been reported sporadically in association with bullous emphysema. The frequency of this association has been estimated as being between 2 and 6%.

Irregular Emphysema

Irregular emphysema is at once the most common and the least significant form of emphysema (Fig. 33.12). It is almost always associated with areas of scarring and, because scars are very common in the lung, this type of emphysema is frequently found at autopsy if a careful examination is made. Most lesions are not associated with any disturbance in lung function but occasionally, if there is widespread scarring, the irregular emphysema may be extensive and severe, and thus lead to airflow obstruction.

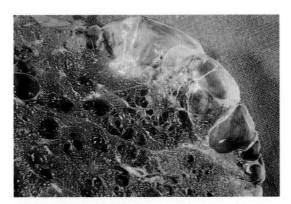

FIGURE 33.12 Irregular emphysema associated with subpleural bulla formation.

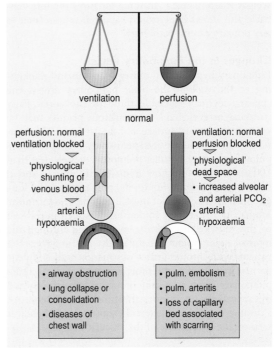

FIGURE 33.13 Causes of ventilation–perfusion mismatch.

CLINICOPATHOLOGICAL CORRELATES OF CHRONIC OBSTRUCTIVE AIRWAY DISEASE

KEY POINTS: Emphysema and Lung Function

Emphysema may affect lung function in a number of ways:

- **Loss of the elastic recoil of the lung tissue decreases the force of expiration.**
- **During expiration, the small airways narrow to a greater degree than normal.**
- **Loss of the walls in the acinar airspaces reduces the surface area available for gas exchange and thus decreases the diffusing capacity of the lung tissue.**

Where obstruction to airflow is severe, bronchiolar lesions may lead to a significant degree of underventilation of parts of the lung; this in its turn will lead to hypoxaemia as a result of a mismatch between ventilation and perfusion (*Fig. 33.13*).

Effects of Hypoxaemia on the Pulmonary Circulation

The presence of hypoxaemia from whatever cause produces constriction of the pulmonary arterioles and thus a **rise in pulmonary artery pressure**. If this persists, the increased afterload on the right ventricle causes hypertrophy and, ultimately, right-sided cardiac failure will supervene. This is the state known as **cor pulmonale**.

Cor pulmonale typically occurs in a patient with prolonged, severe and irreversible airflow obstruction but it may also be seen in bronchiectasis and **restrictive** lung disease.

KEY POINTS: Pulmonary Artery Pressure

Pulmonary artery pressure is determined by three factors:
1) **left atrial pressure**
2) **resistance to flow offered by the pulmonary vessels**
3) **flow of blood through the pulmonary circulation**

A sustained increase in any of these factors will be followed by a sustained rise in pulmonary artery pressure.

The right ventricular wall is **hypertrophied**, approaching or even equalling left ventricular thickness.

Measurement of the thickness of the ventricular wall at post mortem may give a misleading impression of the presence or absence of hypertrophy. Wall thickness is the expression of the wall **mass** divided by its **area**. Thus, if an hypertrophied right ventricle is dilated, wall **thickness** may be quite normal. A more reliable way in which to determine the presence of right ventricular hypertrophy is to remove the atria at post-mortem examination and then to dissect the right ventricle free from the interventricular septum and left ventricle. Right ventricular hypertrophy is deemed to be present if the weight of the isolated right ventricle is greater than 80 g and/or the ratio of the combined weight of the left ventricle and septum to the right ventricular weight is less than 2.1. In some instances the **left** ventricle also shows hypertrophy, apparently unrelated to any primary cardiac pathology.

Changes in the Pulmonary Vessels

Pulmonary hypertension causes dilatation and thickening of the wall of the main pulmonary artery; the appearances may resemble those of the aorta. Fatty streaking or even frank atheromatous plaques may be seen on the intimal surface and similar intimal changes may be present in the intrapulmonary branches of the pulmonary artery. Smaller pulmonary vessels (less than 100 μm in diameter) show an increase in muscle, and in slightly larger arteries (up to 800 μm) an abnormal longitudinal arrangement of muscle may be present in the intima. At a later stage some fibrosis is seen in relation to this muscle; this scarring may extend through the internal elastic lamina into the media. About 50% of the patients with chronic airflow obstruction and right ventricular hypertrophy also show structural changes in the pulmonary veins, consisting of medial hypertrophy and the appearance, in at least part of the circumference, of a distinct internal and external elastic lamina, such as is seen on the arterial side of the vascular bed.

The 'Blue Bloater' and the 'Pink Puffer'

The hypoxaemia that occurs in patients with chronic airflow obstruction (more commonly those with chronic bronchitis) may, in some patients, be associated with retention of carbon dioxide (hypercapnia). This usually occurs when the FEV_1 is less than 1 litre and probably results from a combination of ventilation–perfusion mismatching and alveolar hypoventilation.

Normally hypoxia acts as a stimulus to the respiratory centres to increase the respiratory **drive** but in some patients with severe chronic airway obstruction the ventilatory response to hypoxia is depressed. **These patients are more likely to develop pulmonary hypertension, secondary polycythaemia and cor pulmonale, and to become cyanosed.** As a result of the poor ventilatory response, carbon dioxide retention is particularly marked in these patients, for whom the term **'blue bloater'** was coined. These patients tend to have repeated episodes of respiratory insufficiency. They depend on the hypoxic drive to breathing to maintain adequate levels of ventilation and, **if treated with high concentrations of oxygen, the carbon dioxide retention may worsen and respiratory acidosis may develop**.

In other patients in whom cough and sputum production are less severe, and in whom emphysema often predominates, the respiratory drive is well maintained and the patients maintain normal oxygen tension until late in the course of the illness. However, dyspnoea occurs relatively early and may be severe. These are the so-called **'pink puffers'**.

It has been suggested that these two clinical states are the correlates of predominant chronic bronchitis in the case of the 'blue bloater' and of predominant emphysema in respect of the 'pink puffer'; this is almost certainly a gross oversimplification. Severe emphysema may be present in either of these two groups although, it is fair to say, detailed histological comparisons of the bronchiolar pathology in 'pink puffers' and 'blue bloaters' have not yet been made.

Other Associations of Airflow Obstruction

Loss of Weight

As emphysema increases in severity so body-weight decreases. A little more than one-quarter of patients with chronic airflow obstruction show this feature, which is marked by loss of muscle as well as of fat. The underlying mechanism is unknown, but it has been suggested that the patients have difficulty in eating and breathing at the same time.

Diaphragmatic Changes

Diaphragm area and mass are reduced in patients with emphysema. In some patients this is relatively more severe than the overall loss in weight and muscle bulk described above.

Peptic Ulceration

Chronic airflow obstruction is associated with an increased prevalence of chronic peptic ulceration, prevalence rates between 15% and 43% have been recorded. The ulcers occur both in the stomach and the duodenum, the distribution between these sites being no different from that found in the general ulcer population. It has been suggested that high carbon dioxide concentrations in the blood increase the secretion of gastric acid and this may well account for the particularly strong association between cor pulmonale, hypercapnia and peptic ulcer. An alternative explanation is the high prevalence of cigarette smoking in patients with chronic airflow obstruction.

Central Nervous System Effects of Hypercapnia

These vary from patient to patient, with a poor correlation between the partial pressure of carbon dioxide and cerebral effects. In some, increases in the partial pressure of carbon dioxide lead to dilatation of intracerebral blood vessels, an increase in cerebral blood flow and increased cerebrospinal fluid pressure. Cerebral oedema and papilloedema may be present, and patients may become drowsy or comatose and exhibit a 'flapping tremor' of the hands.

ASTHMA

The term **asthma** is defined in clinical terms as a syndrome characterized by **episodes of widespread narrowing of airways, associated with wheezing. It** is the common endpoint of interactions between certain genetic characteristics and a wide range of exogenous factors on the one hand, and the reactivity and muscle tone of the airways on the other.

The common thread that runs through all types of asthma is **hyper-reactivity of the airways**, and the pathological picture arises on the basis of three main sets of events:

1) **muscle spasm**
2) **inflammation of the airways with mucosal oedema**
3) **increased secretion of mucus**

Prevalence

Asthma is increasing in prevalence, especially in the second decade of life. In westernized societies the prevalence appears to range from 2 to 6%, and about half of these patients present before the age of 10 years. In certain, rather inbred, communities the prevalence is much higher and thus genetic factors can obviously be of considerable importance in asthma. What is of interest is the fact that certain communities (e.g. in Papua, New Guinea) previously had a very low prevalence of asthma which, with the advent of the somewhat mixed blessings of Western 'civilization', has increased sharply.

Pathology

Histopathologists have a biased view of the pathology of asthma because, for the most part, their experience is derived from fatal cases. This is mitigated to some extent by studies carried out on lungs from patients with asthma who have died from other causes.

Macroscopic Features

In patients who have died from acute severe asthma (**'status asthmaticus'**), the lungs are voluminous and do not collapse when the chest is opened; this finding indicates entrapment of air within the lung as a result of airway obstruction. The cut surface of the lungs characteristically shows sticky mucous plugs obstructing the small and medium-sized airways.

Microscopic Features

Many, although not all, of the histological features of asthma are mirrored in the sputum. Structural changes involve **both the lumen and the wall of the airways**.

Luminal Changes

The airway lumina are blocked by a mixture of non-sulphated epithelial mucins and a protein-containing serous component, which has exuded from the small subepithelial vessels in the airways (*Fig. 33.14*). The exudate is cellular and contains eosinophils, normal and degenerate respiratory columnar epithelial cells, arranged either in strips or singly, and some squamous cells, which presumably represent metaplastic change. This stripping off of

cells from the airway wall is *not* a post-mortem artefact, as the same cells are seen in the sputum of living asthmatic patients.

Mucous Membrane Changes

The bronchial mucosa of patients dying in **status asthmaticus** often shows extensive damage. Marked oedema is present between the epithelial cells, and many of the latter become detached from the airway wall leaving a layer of basal or reserve cells behind. It is from these reserve cells that regeneration of the epithelial lining occurs, the new epithelium consisting largely of **non-ciliated** columnar cells. Eosinophils may be present between the epithelial cells but mast cells are not easy to see because they are likely to have degranulated and discharged their pharmacologically active stored contents into the local microenvironment. They are, however, prominent in bronchial lavage specimens. A very typical feature is thickening of the subepithelial **basement membrane**. The reason for this is not understood but, in nasal polyps occurring in atopic individuals, similar basement membrane thickening is seen.

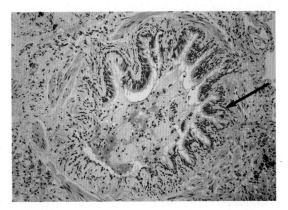

FIGURE 33.14 *Bronchiole from a patient dying in status asthmaticus. Note the virtual occlusion of the lumen by a mucous plug and the prominence of the basement membrane (arrow). The epithelial lining is convoluted, indicating the high degree of spasm.*

Microscopic Features

The inflammatory theme is continued in the **submucosa**, where there is **oedema and a marked degree of capillary dilatation**. An inflammatory cell infiltrate, consisting chiefly of eosinophils and lymphocytes, is also present.

The remaining part of the bronchial wall shows hypertrophy of the mucous glands and a considerable degree of **thickening of the muscle layer, which is due to hyperplasia as well as hypertrophy.**

The Sputum in Asthma

Sputum from asthmatics shows certain characteristic features and constitutes an area in which eponyms rage unchecked. The microscopically identifiable features described in such sputum are the three 'Cs'.

Charcot–Leyden Crystals

These are colourless hexagonal crystals consisting mainly of a lysophospholipase, which degrades lysophospholipids and is also involved in prostaglandin metabolism. They are derived from the granules of **eosinophils** and are found not only in asthma, but wherever there is an excess of eosinophils, whether in blood, tissue or secretions.

Curschmann Spirals

These are curiously twisted casts of airways which may be so large (longer than 1 cm) as to be visible with the naked eye. Microscopically they appear to consist of glycoprotein cores around which many fibrils are bound.

Creola Bodies

These consist of clumps of cells or isolated metaplastic cells.

Classification

The classification of asthma into its different types is closely intertwined with the pathogenetic mechanisms involved and raises some difficult questions.

Conventionally asthma is divided into two main groups:

1) **Intrinsic, which is associated with atopy and thus increased production of reaginic immunoglobulin (Ig) E antibody binding to mast cell membranes via its Fc portion.**
2) **Extrinsic, in which patients are usually not atopic and in whom the asthma may be provoked by a number of widely disparate triggers.**

The background to most cases is a system of airways that is hyper-reactive. Airway reactivity can be assessed quite simply by exercising, by asking the individual being tested to breathe cold air, or by challenging them with methacholine or histamine. In most, but not all, patients with asthma, such a procedure results in an **increase in airway resistance** as shown by a fall in FEV_1. This increase in resistance is short lived (about 30 minutes) and provides a useful model to study the mechanisms of the immediate component of asthmatic airway narrowing.

Patients who respond to exercise by developing bronchospasm have raised baseline levels of histamine in the plasma. These histamine concentrations are further increased on exercise, a response also reported in some control subjects. The use, before exercise, of antihistamines with a selective action on the H_1 receptor inhibits bronchospasm, suggesting that the release of histamine is a significant mechanism in the response of at least some hyper-reactive airways. Nevertheless, mediator release is not the only factor involved in bronchospasm and there may well be quantitative or qualitative differences in airway receptors in these asthmatics. Patients who have exercise-induced asthma also show a reduced sympathetic response to exercise and thus do not have the sharp increase in adenosine 3′,5′-cyclic monophosphate (cAMP) levels that normally occurs.

Exposure of patients with intrinsic asthma to their specific allergens causes both an immediate and a delayed reaction (*Fig. 33.15*). Inhalation of allergens in atopic patients with intrinsic asthma causes a dual response. The immediate phase can be blocked in the same way as exercise-provoked bronchospasm. The delayed phase usually starts during the period of recovery from the acute response and may continue for 24–48 hours. It is blocked, in most cases, by corticosteroids and cromoglycate. This pattern of response suggests that the prolonged phase is due to mucosal inflammation and oedema rather than to spasm, and bronchial lavage specimens taken at this time show the presence of large numbers of eosinophils and eosinophil cationic protein. The whole sequence of events suggests that antigenic challenge results in the release of both long- and short-acting chemical mediators (*Figs 33.16* and *33.17*).

Mediators that are likely to be involved and their actions in this context are shown in *Table 33.2*.

Triggering Factors in Asthma

More than 90% of children with asthma are atopic, producing excessive amounts of IgE, which becomes bound to mast cells by its Fc portion. When the homo-

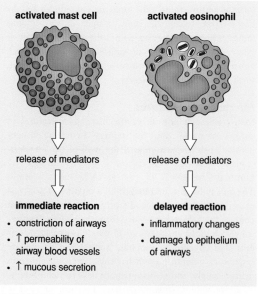

FIGURE 33.15 Immediate and delayed reactions in asthma.

Table 33.2 Chemical Mediators in Patients with Asthma

Action	Mediator
Constriction of airways	Histamine
	Prostaglandin D_2
	Leukotrienes C_4, D_4 and E_4
	Platelet-activating factor
	Thromboxane
	Bradykinin
	Eosinophil granule proteins
Damage to epithelium of airways	Eosinophil granule proteins
Vasodilatation, increased vascular permeability and oedema of airway wall	Histamine
	Prostaglandin D_2
	Leukotrienes C_4, D_4 and E_4
	Leukotriene B_4
Increased mucus secretion	Histamine
	Prostaglandin D_2
	Leukotrienes C_4, D_4 and E_4
	Eosinophil granule proteins
Activation of vascular endothelium in airways	Histamine
	Tumour necrosis factor
	Interleukin 1
	Interleukin 4
Recruitment and activation of leucocytes	Leukotrienes C_4, D_4 and E_4
	Leukotriene B_4
	Platelet-activating factor
	Interleukin 3
	Interleukin 5
	Granulocyte–macrophage colony-stimulating factor
	RANTES (regulated on activation, normal T-cell expressed and secreted)
Stimulation of nerves	Histamine
	Prostaglandin D_2
	Leukotrienes C_4, D_4 and E_4
	Bradykinin

specific allergen is encountered, it binds to the Fab portions of two adjacent molecules of cell-bound IgE, leading to the release of preformed compounds from mast cell granules and to the formation of a range of pharmacologically active compounds from phospholipids of the cell membrane. Allergens commonly triggering asthma attacks in atopic subjects are found in **house dust, pollens and animal danders**. The major allergen in house dust is derived from mites, *Dermatophagoides pteronyssinus* being the most frequent culprit in Europe. This mite lives mainly on skin scales and prefers the warm, rather humid, environment provided by a bed. The allergen itself is a glycoprotein excreted in the faeces of the mite.

Pollens and fungal spores are also implicated in the aetiology of asthma in atopic subjects, the former being associated with a seasonal pattern and with rhinitis, often combined with itchy conjunctivitis. Sensitivity to animal proteins, as detected by skin testing, is found in about 25% of asthmatics. The allergens in this case are animal proteins derived from hair particles, dander and urine. Contact with the offending animal species is likely to provoke rhinitis and conjunctivitis as well as wheezing.

Some attacks of asthma in atopics are provoked by certain foods and drinks, of which milk, eggs, fish, cereals, nuts and chocolate are the most frequent offenders. Sensitization is believed to occur as a result of

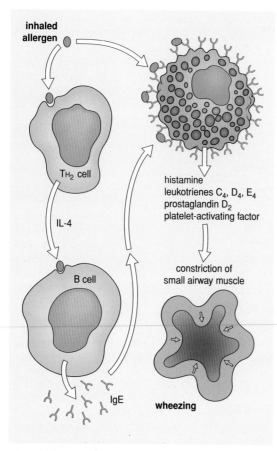

FIGURE 33.16 *Interactions between IgE and mast cells in the immediate phase of asthma.*

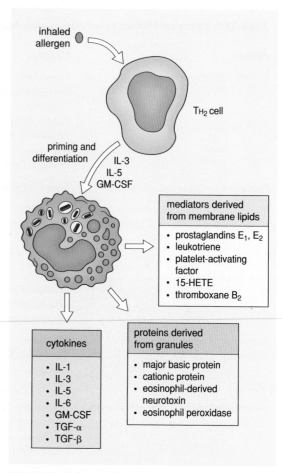

FIGURE 33.17 *Eosinophil products that may be acting in asthma.*

pinocytosis of antigenic proteins via the intestinal epithelium, and a subsequent encounter with the allergen may give rise to gastrointestinal disturbances as well as asthma.

Asthma may also be triggered by exercise, inhalation of cold air, emotion and certain drugs.

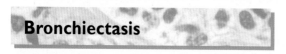

Bronchiectasis

Definition

Bronchiectasis is defined as a **permanent, abnormal dilatation of the bronchi** (i.e. airways that possess cartilage in their walls). The word **permanent** is an integral part of the definition since reversible dilatation of the bronchi may occur in the course of various bacterial and viral infections.

Prevalence

Before the introduction of modern imaging methods, the frequency of bronchiectasis in a population was not easy to determine because the diagnosis could be established only by bronchography or examination of surgically resected or post-mortem lung tissue. Studies carried out in Britain in the early 1950s suggested a prevalence of about 1.5 per 1000 population. No large-scale data have been collected since, but it is generally agreed that the prevalence of bronchiectasis in Western societies has decreased markedly. This has been attributed to:

- effective vaccination programmes which have markedly reduced the incidence of measles and whooping cough
- more effective treatment of respiratory infections in childhood
- a decline in the frequency of fibrocaseous tuberculosis

In Third World countries, however, where these have not happened, bronchiectasis remains a serious problem in children and young adults.

Aetiology and Pathogenesis

In some instances bronchiectasis may be the single or predominant pathological change in the lung; in others it may be a part of a more complicated picture, as in bronchiectasis associated with **obstruction of a major bronchus by carcinoma** or as a consequence of **cystic fibrosis**. Whatever the aetiological background, **dilatation results from the interaction of two basic mechanisms** (*Fig. 33.18*).

1) **increased dragging forces on the bronchial wall**

2) **postinflammatory weakening of the bronchial wall**

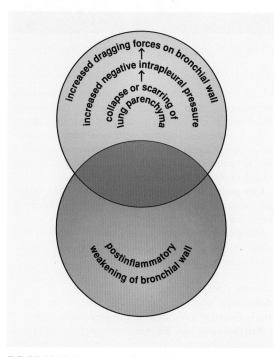

FIGURE 33.18 Pathogenetic factors in bronchiectasis.

Increased Dragging Forces on the Bronchial Wall
Negative intrapleural pressure is a powerful factor in maintaining the lung in an expanded state. If parenchyma in relation to a bronchus becomes airless, either through collapse or as a result of postinflammatory scarring, the effect of negative intrapleural pressure on that bronchus becomes greater and it tends to dilate.

This state of affairs can come about in a number of ways.

1) Infection involving the distal airways, either 'non-specific' bronchopneumonia or viral bronchiolitis (these days **adenovirus** is particularly important in this connection), may lead to obliteration of the affected airway and varying degrees of collapse. In addition, there will be chronic airflow obstruction caused by the airway obliteration. Secretions will accumulate in the dilated bronchi because the local airflow obstruction will make coughing relatively ineffective and the

distorted shape of the affected bronchi may contribute to impaired clearance of mucus.
2) Chronic lung infections may lead to loss of parenchyma and thus to an increase in the effect on the bronchi of negative intrapleural pressure.
3) Obstruction of a major bronchus by a neoplasm, foreign body or enlarged lymph node will cause collapse of the segment of lung parenchyma normally ventilated by flow through that bronchus. Obstruction alone is said to be unlikely to cause bronchiectasis unless infection of that part of the bronchial tree is also present.

Postinflammatory Weakening of the Bronchial Wall
Inflammation due to infection can produce a profound degree of damage to the bronchial wall associated not only with loss of bronchial epithelium but, in its most severe form, with damage to or loss of the bronchial cartilage.

Infection is more likely to occur if there are defects in mucociliary clearance. This may arise because of failure of ciliary function as seen in the various ciliary dyskinesia syndromes to which reference was made in an earlier section of this chapter (Kartagener's syndrome, immotile cilia syndrome with no dextrocardia, and Young's syndrome – infertility due to azoospermia associated with bronchiectasis in about 20% of the cases). The risk of bronchiectasis is considerably increased in conditions where local defence mechanisms are impaired, such as in **cystic fibrosis** (see pp 641–642), where obstruction due to the increased viscosity of bronchial secretions and infection tend to go hand in hand, and in whooping cough and measles.

Structural Changes Seen in Bronchiectasis

Distribution
The airways most often affected are those of the third and fourth order, because more proximal bronchi possess a cartilage layer of sufficient thickness to resist the dilating forces described. The distribution of dilated bronchi reflects, to a considerable extent, the aetiological processes involved in any individual case. Thus, bronchiectasis arising on the basis of **infection** tends to involve the basal segments of the lung; patients with **cystic fibrosis** have more generalized disease, whereas in **allergic bronchopulmonary aspergillosis** the bronchi in the hilar region appear to be the favoured target.

Macroscopic Features
Much has been made of the different shapes that dilated bronchi may assume in this disease, although these variations have no bearing on the aetiological processes involved or the resulting functional disturbances. Such terms as **cylindrical**, where the affected airways are

uniformly widened, **fusiform** where they taper, and **saccular**, in which there are local cystic dilatations easily seen with the naked eye, possess nothing more than descriptive value (*Fig. 33.19*). Macroscopically, the most striking feature is the fact that the dilated airways can be followed out to the pleural surface.

Microscopic Features

Where the process is active, the affected bronchi usually contain pus and any surviving mucosal lining shows the vascular and cellular features of acute and chronic inflammation, with cellular markers of chronicity such as lymphocytes and plasma cells being prominent. Lymphoid follicles may be seen in appreciable numbers and in these cases the term **follicular bronchiectasis** is used. In many instances there is extensive loss of the lining epithelium, the dilated bronchi being lined by either fibrous or granulation tissue. In others, the surviving epithelium shows either heaping up of columnar cells, giving a pseudostratified appearance, or squamous metaplasia.

Other Changes in the Lung

Bronchial arteries characteristically show hypertrophy of the muscular portion of their walls, and anastomoses not infrequently develop between these altered arteries and similarly sized pulmonary artery branches. This may be associated with loss of part of the alveolar capillary bed as a result of necrotizing inflammation and scarring. The combination of these vascular changes may make some contribution to the pulmonary hypertension and **cor pulmonale** that can complicate severe bronchiectasis, especially in patients with cystic fibrosis. If the necrotizing process within the airway walls destroys them totally, the lung parenchyma becomes secondarily involved and an abscess cavity into which several dilated airways open may form. Because the dilated airways often end blindly, the lung distal to them may show absorption collapse unless inflation can be maintained by collateral ventilation.

Complications

Local Complications

Infective exacerbations are marked by increased volume and purulence of sputum. Occasional progression to pneumonia may occur, and suppuration and abscess formation occur rarely. Empyema (a collection of pus in the pleural cavity) has been described but this is even less common these days than abscess formation, presumably because of the use of antibiotics. Old bronchiectatic cavities may be the site of invasion by **fungal** species, most notably *Aspergillus fumigatus*, which grow saprophytically within the cavity and seldom invade the surrounding lung tissue. Ultimately a ball-like colony of the fungus, or **aspergilloma**, may be formed. Such colonies appear as rubbery, grey or

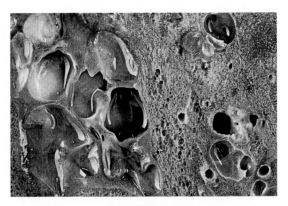

FIGURE 33.19 *Lung showing saccular bronchiectasis.*

reddish-brown masses which may undergo heterotopic calcification, thus gaining a gritty consistency. Histologically the colony consists of a dense mass of fungal hyphae held together with apparently structureless eosinophilic material. Haemoptysis is a common clinical manifestation. Disseminated aspergillosis may occur but, fortunately, is rare.

Cor pulmonale may complicate severe and extensive bronchiectasis and has been reported to occur in about one-third of fatal cases.

Massive haemoptysis, may occur, with bleeding from bronchial artery anastomoses where systemic blood pressure operates.

Systemic Complications

Metastatic abscess, especially in the brain, was a greatly feared complication in the preantibiotic era.

Amyloidosis, of the reactive systemic variety, is characterized by the deposition of AA amyloid protein, the β-pleated form of SAA, one of the acute-phase proteins. Its most baneful effect is on the kidney where it may produce proteinuria heavy enough to lead to the **nephrotic syndrome** and, in the end, to chronic renal failure (*Fig. 33.20*).

Restrictive Ventilatory Impairment

Restriction of ventilation may occur even when the chest wall is moving normally and there is no obstruction to airflow. This is due to an abnormal degree of **stiffness** or loss of compliance of the lung, which has many causes.

In this group of conditions, patients complain of chronic cough and shortness of breath, this eventually progressing to respiratory failure. **The decrease in forced expiratory volume in 1 second (FEV$_1$) is**

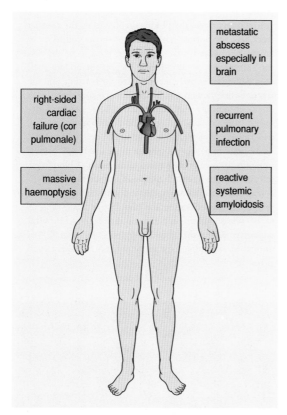

FIGURE 33.20 *Complications of bronchiectasis.*

proportional to the decrease in forced vital capacity (FVC) and thus, unlike chronic airflow obstruction, the ratio FEV_1/FVC remains within normal limits. Lung volume and oxygen-diffusing capacity are also decreased.

The principal pathological processes causing pulmonary restriction are **scarring (fibrosis), cellular infiltration of the lung tissue** and **interstitial oedema**. The most important is **pulmonary fibrosis**, which may be either **local** or **widespread**.

Local scarring, common in the apical or subapical region of the upper lobe, is associated with **tuberculosis, a reaction to rupture of apical emphysematous bullae, and connective tissue disorders such as ankylosing spondylitis**. In many instances, no explanation can be found. Local areas of scarring are also seen in relation to old infarcts and to some of the industrial lung diseases (pneumoconioses).

Diseases causing widespread scarring of the lung can be classified, in **anatomical terms**, depending on whether the basal regions are predominantly affected or whether they are spared (see *Table 33.3*).

Scarring may be:

- **intra-alveolar**, in which fibroblasts migrate from the interstitium through defects in the alveolar epithelial basement membrane

Table 33.3 Diseases Causing Lung Scarring

Bases involved	Bases spared
The organizing phase of diffuse alveolar damage	Sarcoidosis
Cryptogenic fibrosing alveolitis (usual interstitial pneumonia)	Extrinsic allergic alveolitis
Chronic oedema	Silicosis
Asbestosis	Chronic berylliosis
Acute idiopathic interstitial fibrosis (Hamman–Rich syndrome)	Histiocytosis X (eosinophilic granuloma)

- **interstitial**, in which all the fibrosis occurs in the interstitial spaces, the alveoli being more or less unaffected
- **obliterative** in which the lumina of several adjacent airspaces are effaced as a consequence of severe alveolar damage (e.g. paraquat poisoning)

Where scarring is advanced and extensive, these patterns can no longer be identified and the normal architecture of the lung is lost. Affected areas show the presence of many cystic spaces to which the descriptive term **'honeycomb lung'** has been applied. This is the morphological **'end-stage'** of several different diseases.

The interstitial lung diseases in which these features are displayed are a heterogeneous group of conditions that have in common, derangement of the walls of the distal airspaces and loss of functional alveolar–capillary units.

More than 100 causes are known but in more than 60% of cases the aetiological agent cannot be identified.

INTERSTITIAL LUNG DISEASES

Cryptogenic Fibrosing Alveolitis (Idiopathic Pulmonary Fibrosis)

This is a chronic inflammatory disorder, characterized by an alveolitis in its earlier stages and ending in severe interstitial fibrosis. It is the most frequent cause of 'honeycomb lung'. The aetiology is still unknown.

Its prevalence is thought to be 3–5 per 100 000 population and it presents chiefly in the fifth and sixth decades of life, but other age groups are not immune. Occasionally, a familial clustering is noted, the susceptibility to this disorder being inherited in an autosomal dominant fashion. Patients usually present with cough or dyspnoea, or both, and the disease runs an aggressive course with a high fatality rate within 3–6 years from the onset of symptoms.

Clinical Features

Physical examination usually reveals crackles on auscultation of the lung bases and clubbing of the fingers and/or toes is common. The chest radiograph typically shows a fine, diffuse mottling which is maximal at the lung bases. Lung function tests show **reduced lung volume** and a **reduction in diffusing capacity**, which is a reflection, at least in part, of actual loss of part of the alveolar capillary bed. Radioactive gallium scans (a marker of inflammation) show uptake in the lung parenchyma in about 70% of patients, the tracer being taken up chiefly by activated intra-alveolar macrophages.

Pathological Features

The structural changes seen in the lung depend very much on the stage of the disease when a biopsy is taken. Two basic histological patterns have been described:

- **usual interstitial pneumonitis (UIP)**
- **desquamative interstitial pneumonitis (DIP)**

Once thought to be distinct disorders, these conditions are now viewed as variants of a single disease with the **'usual'** type showing more evidence of damage to **alveolar walls** and the **'desquamative'** variety showing much more marked **intra-alveolar accumulation of activated inflammatory cells**. The latter is likely to have a good response to steroids and tends not to progress to end-stage fibrosis with honeycombing (the 5-year survival rate of DIP is 95%, that of UIP 55%).

Interstitial fibrosis carries a considerable increase (tenfold) in the risk of lung cancer; squamous carcinoma and adenocarcinoma are the most frequent types.

Microscopic Features

The disease starts with patchy inflammation within the alveoli. Bronchoalveolar lavage shows a three- to fourfold increase in the number of cells, with a marked increase in the proportion of neutrophils. These normally constitute only about 1% of the intra-alveolar cell population; in this condition neutrophils account for up to 20%. In contrast the proportion of macrophages, normally contributing 90% of the cells, falls to about 70%.

The inflammation leads to a progressive derangement of the alveolar wall and its lining. There is loss of the type 1 alveolar epithelial cells, these being replaced by proliferating type 2 cells and, in some areas, by cells resembling those of bronchiolar epithelium, which some think are atypical type 2 pneumocytes.

The interstitial matrix becomes expanded, partly due to the presence of masses of collagen fibres and partly because of a marked increase in the interstitial cell population of fibroblasts, myofibroblasts and true smooth muscle cells.

In its early stages the fibrosis involves only the alveolar septa, and the normal relationship of the alveoli to more proximal airways is maintained (*Fig. 33.21*). As the disease progresses, a considerable degree of architectural remodelling takes place secondary to the scarring, and the airspaces that remain are of irregular size and shape with thick, chronically inflamed walls. These distorted airspaces contain a mixture of cellular debris, mucin, macrophages and crystalline cholesterol derived from the membranes of destroyed cells. In the scarred areas there is some fibromuscular thickening of the walls of blood vessels and smooth muscle hyperplasia may be marked.

Vascular changes are associated with the presence of pulmonary hypertension and this, in its turn, appears to be related to the severity of the decrease in **vital capacity**. Where the latter is reduced to less than 50% of normal, raised pulmonary artery pressure is present even at rest.

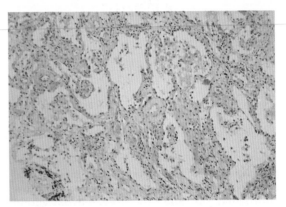

FIGURE 33.21 Section of lung showing moderate degree of interstitial fibrosis with some disorganization of lung architecture.

Pathogenesis

This disorder results from the interaction of two processes: **damage and repair** (*Fig. 33.22*).

Both the initial injury (to alveolar lining cells) and the repair leading to scarring are orchestrated by the secretory functions of **activated macrophages** (*Fig. 33.23*).

Activation of alveolar macrophages may be due to immune complexes, but this is as yet unproven. Once activated, macrophages release two neutrophil chemoattractants. These are an arachidonic acid metabolite (probably leukotriene B_4) and a high molecular weight peptide. The neutrophils cause local damage by generating oxygen free radicals and by the release of proteolytic enzymes such as elastase. Macrophages can, of course, behave in an identical fashion, thus contributing directly to local tissue damage.

Repair, too, can be ascribed to secretion products of the activated macrophage. These include:

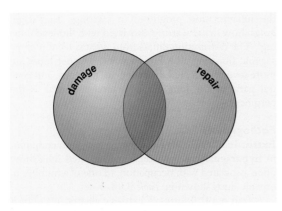

FIGURE 33.22 *Principal processes involved in cryptogenic fibrosing alveolitis.*

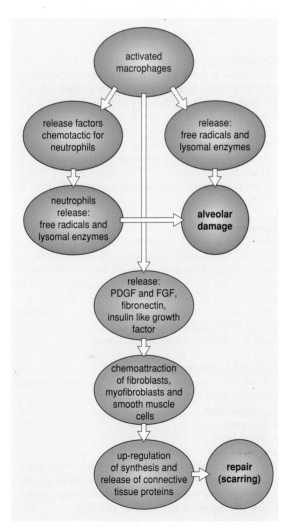

FIGURE 33.23 *Roles of the activated macrophage in the pathogenesis of cryptogenic fibrosing alveolitis.*

- **Fibronectin**, a multimeric glycoprotein which, among its other actions, signals fibroblasts to enter the cell cycle.
- **Platelet-derived growth factor (PDGF) and fibroblast growth factor.** Alveolar macrophages obtained from patients with idiopathic pulmonary fibrosis by bronchial lavage secrete four times more PDGF than those from normal non-smokers. Alveolar macrophages from patients in the prefibrotic stage of familial idiopathic pulmonary fibrosis also secrete more PDGF, fibronectin and more neutrophil chemoattractants than do macrophages from control subjects.
- **An alveolar macrophage-derived growth factor**, which induces fibronectin-primed fibroblasts to release an insulin-like growth factor (somatomedin).

Cryptogenic Organizing Pneumonia (Bronchiolitis Obliterans Organizing Pneumonia)

Restrictive lung disease is bedevilled by uncouth-sounding acronyms, such as BIP, LIP, GIP and BOOP:

- **BIP – bronchiolitis obliterans in combination with interstitial pneumonitis. The functional changes show both obstructive and restrictive features.**
- **LIP – interstitial pneumonitis associated with heavy lymphoid infiltrates. This condition is best considered in relation to malignant lymphomas of the lung.**
- **GIP – an interstitial pneumonia in which giant cells are prominent. Many examples of this occur in association with inhalation of fumes of hard metal alloys.**
- **BOOP (bronchiolitis obliterans organizing pneumonia) shows the same pathological picture as seen in postinfective pneumonias i.e. failure of resolution of the intra-alveolar exudate with consequent organization. However, the clinical picture is quite different: the insidious onset of dyspnoea, persistent cough and malaise with widespread opacities visible on the chest radiograph. The functional changes are predominantly those of a restrictive disorder but some patients also show obstructive features.**

Biopsy shows **intra-alveolar buds of fibrous tissue** with chronic inflammatory cells lying in the centres of the buds. Alveoli are principally involved but lesions also occur in respiratory bronchioles.

Extrinsic Allergic Alveolitis (Hypersensitivity Pneumonitis)

This is a chronic granulomatous disease of the lungs due to inhalation of organic dusts which act as foreign antigens and elicit a local hypersensitivity response.

Clinical Features

Induction of hypersensitivity probably takes a considerable time and there is a spectrum of clinical manifestations. At one extreme, there may be the sudden onset, within a few hours of exposure to the offending allergen, of fever and rigor, followed by cough, shortness of breath and, in some cases, the production of blood-stained sputum. Chest radiography at this time shows patchy lung infiltrates, which are usually transient. Recovery from mild attacks usually takes 2–3 weeks but recurrent attacks tend to be both more severe and prolonged; complete recovery from these may never occur. At the other extreme patients who are exposed to lower allergen concentrations may present simply with a history of increasing breathlessness over a long period.

Diagnosis depends on:

1) **a history of exposure to an allergen known to cause extrinsic allergic alveolitis**
2) **typical symptoms and, in particular, the characteristic time lapse between exposure to the allergen and the onset of symptoms**
3) **a restrictive ventilatory defect and impaired diffusion capacity**
4) **the presence in the patient's serum of specific precipitating antibodies to the suspected allergen**

Microscopic Features

The appearances depend on the **stage** of the disease at the time of examination; few reports exist as to microscopic appearances during the acute stages of a first attack.

Biopsy, usually performed after recurrent episodes of respiratory disability over a period of months or years, probably represents the disease in its **subacute** stage before chronic interstitial fibrosis has developed. Five microscopic features are said to be characteristic:

1) **The presence of epithelioid granulomata, usually with no evidence of caseation necrosis.** They are generally smaller than those seen in sarcoidosis. In contrast to what is seen in sarcoidosis, the hilar lymph nodes are not affected.
2) **An interstitial pneumonitis, the alveolar septa being infiltrated by macrophages, lymphocytes and plasma cells.**
3) Bronchiolar obstruction resulting from ulceration of the lining surface followed by ingrowth of granulation tissue into the airway lumina.
4) **Foamy macrophages within the alveolar lumen.**
5) In some cases, **foreign material** within the cytoplasm of macrophages and multinucleate giant cells.

Natural History

The granulomas usually resolve in about 6 months in the absence of further allergen exposure. In many cases, the inflammation progresses to scarring. 'End-stage' lungs show dense scarring associated with 'honeycombing'. The distribution differs from what is seen in cryptogenic fibrosing alveolitis in that the upper lobes are more severely affected than the basal portions, and central parts of the lung are as severely affected as the periphery.

Pathogenesis

Extrinsic allergic alveolitis is the common endpoint, in **hypersensitive** individuals, of repeated inhalation, often associated with occupation, of one of a number of organic dusts shown in *Table 33.4*.

A feature of all forms of extrinsic allergic alveolitis is the finding in patients' serum of **precipitating antibodies against the allergens that elicit that patient's symptoms. Many more individuals show the presence of these antibodies than actually develop the disease.** It seems likely that both humoral and cellular effector arms of the immune system are involved.

Sarcoidosis

Sarcoidosis is a multisystem granulomatous disease of uncertain cause. It is characterized by **enhanced** cellular hypersensitivity at sites of involvement (see Chapter 15).

Lesions can be found virtually at any site (*Fig. 33.24*), but the lung is the organ most frequently affected, 90% of patients with sarcoidosis showing pulmonary involvement. Of these, 20–25% show irreversible loss of lung function, and in 5–10% the disease is fatal.

Epidemiology

Sarcoidosis is found throughout the world and is most common in Sweden (prevalence 64 per 100 000) and amongst the black population of New York (80 per 100 000). In the USA generally, sarcoidosis is found 10–17 times as frequently in black populations as in white ones. There are no positive correlations between environment and risk, but it is not without interest that there is a decreased prevalence in smokers.

Clinical Features

The clinical onset of sarcoidosis of the lungs is usually insidious, with symptoms such as:

- **weight loss**
- **fatigue**
- **weakness**
- **fever**
- **erythema nodosum (a non-specific vasculitis with or without granuloma formation in the dermis and subcutaneous tissue. Often seen on the anterior surfaces of the legs**
- **dry cough**
- **dyspnoea**
- **exercise intolerance**

Table 33.4 Causes of Extrinsic Allergic Alveolitis

Antigen	Disease	Source
Thermophilic bacteria		
Micropolyspora faeni	Farmers' lung	Mouldy hay
Thermoactinomyces vulgaris	Grain handlers' lung	Mouldy grain
M. faeni, T. vulgaris	Mushroom workers' lung	Mushroom compost
T. sacchari	Bagassosis	Mouldy sugar cane (bagasse)
T. vulgaris, T. thalpophilus	Air conditioner lung	Contaminated water
Other bacteria		
Bacillus subtilis	Detergent packers' lung	Biological washing powders
True fungi		
Cryptostroma corticale	Maple bark strippers' lung	Mouldy maple bark
Aspergillus clavatus	Malt workers' lung	Mouldy malt
Aureobasidium pullulans	Sequoiosis	Mouldy redwood dust
Penicillium casei	Cheese washers' lung	Cheese mould
P. frequentans	Suberosis	Mouldy cork dust
Trichosporon cutaneum	Summer-type pneumonitis	House dust, bird droppings
Animal proteins		
Bird serum and excreta	Birdfanciers' lung	Pigeons, budgerigars
Poultry feathers and serum	Chicken/turkey handlers' lung	Chickens, turkeys
Rat urine and serum	Rodent handlers' lung	Rats
Porcine or bovine protein	Pituitary snuff takers' lung	Pituitary snuff

However, the disease may be symptomless and the diagnosis first considered after abnormalities found on routine chest radiography.

Classification

Chest radiography shows several different patterns and these are used to classify the disease into a number of different types.

- **Type 0 – no obvious thoracic involvement.** Occurs in 5–15% of patients.
- **Type 1 – bilateral hilar adenopathy often associated with paratracheal adenopathy.** About 50% of all patients with pulmonary sarcoidosis present with this radiological picture. These radiographic changes resolve in about 50–75% of patients so affected.
- **Type 2 – hilar lymphadenopathy plus pulmonary parenchymal involvement.** A number of different patterns of lung infiltration may be seen, including:
  1) fine reticular shadowing
  2) small nodular infiltrates
  3) confluent shadowing giving a 'ground glass' appearance
  4) large pulmonary nodules, some of which may show cavitation (very rare)

Approximately 25–50% of patients with pulmonary sarcoidosis present with type 2 disease.
- **Type 3 disease shows parenchymal infiltrates in the lung without any hilar adenopathy.** This pattern is seen more commonly in cases where the disease is more advanced and is often associated with pulmonary fibrosis. Initial presentation with this form occurs in only 10–25% of patients; resolution of the inflammatory process is infrequent (10–25%). The remodelling of airspaces associated with interstitial fibrosis may lead to the formation of cystic spaces, which may subsequently become colonized by *Aspergillus fumigatus*, leading to the formation of mycetomas.

Functional Abnormalities

Lung function changes occurring in sarcoidosis are similar to those seen in patients with pulmonary fibrosis due to other causes:
- Decrease in lung volume
- Decrease in diffusing capacity
- In addition, many patients show some evidence of airflow obstruction in the form of decreased flow at the end of expiration. This is believed to be related to the presence of granulomas in the walls of airways.

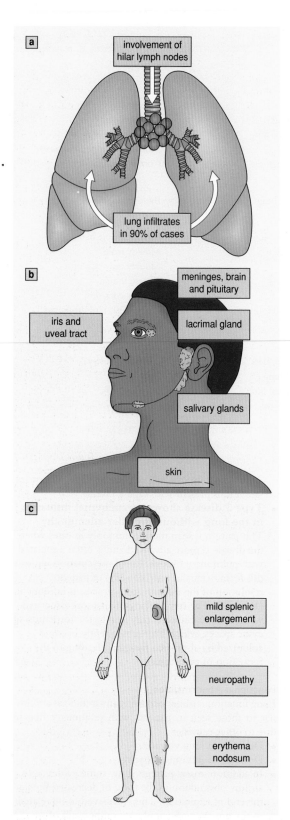

FIGURE 33.24 *Lesion sites in sarcoidosis.*

Microscopic Features
The diagnostic marker is the epithelioid cell granuloma.

The most striking abnormality in the majority of patients with sarcoidosis is the presence of sharply circumscribed, non-caseating granulomas. These may be present in the walls of the alveoli, bronchioles or blood vessels and their identification in samples obtained by transbronchial biopsy or, much more rarely, open lung biopsy is the so-called 'gold standard' for diagnosis. A marked degree of interstitial fibrosis is found in about 25% of patients but, in contrast to what is seen in cryptogenic fibrosing alveolitis, the fibrosis rarely extends into the airspaces themselves, and severe cystic change resulting from destruction of lung tissue and consequent remodelling is also rare.

Alveolar Cell Population in Sarcoidosis Suggests T Helper Cell Activation Much suggests that alveolitis is an essential element in the pathology of sarcoidosis. There is a three- to fivefold increase in the total cell population, most of these cells being lymphocytes and macrophages. There is a striking increase in the proportion of T helper cells. In the normal lung the T helper : suppressor ratio is 1.8 : 1. In active sarcoidosis this becomes 10 : 1. Some of this increase in the local T-cell population appears to be due to proliferation rather than to migration. T cells derived from bronchoalveolar lavage in sarcoidosis replicate spontaneously *in vitro* and also spontaneously release interleukin 2, which induces T-cell proliferation.

Changes in Blood Lymphocyte Population The blood shows a lymphocyte pattern completely opposite to that in the lung. These patients usually have **lymphopenia**, and the T helper : suppressor cell ratio is 0.8 : 1. Similarly the spontaneous release of mediators relevant both to granuloma formation and to polyclonal antibody formation characteristic of alveolar T cells in sarcoidosis does not occur from the blood derived T cells. The shift in the T helper : suppressor ratio in favour of suppressor cells may explain why many patients with sarcoidosis show negative results (anergy) when tests for cutaneous cellular hypersensitivity such as the tuberculin test are performed.

Activation of Alveolar Macrophages in Sarcoidosis In addition to increased numbers, intra-alveolar macrophages show behavioural changes suggestive of activation. For instance, when alveolar macrophages from patients with sarcoidosis are exposed to an antigen such as tetanus toxoid, and are then incubated with autologous T helper cells, the resulting degree of T-cell proliferation is much greater than normal, and it has also been suggested that these macrophages release more interleukin 1 than alveolar macrophages derived either from normal individuals or from patients with cryptogenic fibrosing alveolitis.

Quantitative Changes in the Blood Chemistry of Some Patients with Sarcoidosis are the Expression of Macrophage Activation About one in five patients with sarcoidosis show **hypercalcaemia** and about 55% show **an increase in the serum concentration of angiotensin-converting enzyme (ACE).** The hypercalcaemia is believed to be due to overexpression by activated macrophages of 1α-hydroxylase, this increasing calcitriol (1,25-dihydroxycholecalciferol) production. This leads to increased calcium absorption from the small gut and thus to hypercalcaemia and hypercalciuria. Corticosteroid therapy rapidly reduces the concentrations of both calcium and vitamin D_3, and this can be useful in distinguishing the hypercalcaemia of sarcoidosis from other types of hypercalcaemia.

The increased secretion of ACE by macrophages is by no means specific for sarcoidosis, and, because the level is raised in only about half the patients with sarcoidosis, it is not diagnostically useful. In patients in whom ACE concentration is raised at the time of diagnosis, ACE can be used to monitor the activity of the disease and the effect of treatment with corticosteroids. This can be especially useful in giving a forewarning of relapse in patients whose dose of steroids has been reduced.

Aetiology and Pathogenesis
The data presented above provide no clue as to the aetiology of this enigmatic disease. It is possible that there is, indeed, no single aetiology, and that sarcoidosis is the consequence of a 'built-in' **quantitative** abnormality of the immune system in which normal modulation of the consequences of antigen recognition does not occur. The increased concordance of sarcoidosis in monozygotic rather than dizygotic twins lends some support to this view.

Pulmonary Histiocytosis X (Eosinophilic Granuloma of the Lung)
This is one of a **set of diseases, the common element being proliferation of a mononuclear cell showing the immunohistochemical and ultrastructural characteristics of a Langerhans cell.** This mesodermal cell is normally found in the epidermis and thymus. It carries surface receptors for Fc and C3 and, like thymocytes, also binds the antibody T6 (CD1a). It has a single cleaved nucleus and very few lysosomes. Its most characteristic feature is ultrastructural: the Birbeck granule or X body which is a pentilaminar cytoplasmic inclusion with a constant width (40–45 nm) and 10-nm longitudinal periodicity in the central lamina. The skin Langerhans cell is believed to process antigens and transport them to the paracortical region of draining lymph nodes.

Other members of this disease set are Letterer–Siwe and Hand–Schüller–Christian disease, the former being the acute generalized, and the latter the chronic generalized, form of histiocytosis X.

Pulmonary histiocytosis is rare, occurring chiefly in young adults (20–40 years) and is somewhat more common in males than in females. The majority of the patients are cigarette smokers. Patients usually present with non-productive cough, exertional dyspnoea or, rarely, chest pain, and fever. Weight loss, wheezing and haemoptysis are occasionally seen. Spontaneous pneumothorax occurs in about 10%.

Chest radiography shows small irregular nodular shadows in the upper and mid-zones. The costophrenic angles are usually spared and this helps to distinguish the condition from idiopathic interstitial fibrosis.

Tests of lung function show a mixture of obstruction and restriction associated with a decreased diffusing capacity and exercise-associated hypoxaemia.

Microscopic Features
Biopsy material shows a cellular infiltrate both within the walls and lumina of alveoli and in the interstitial tissues around centriacinar bronchioles and small vessels in the interlobular septa. Early lesions consist of nodular collections of Langerhans cells mixed with eosinophils (hence the term 'eosinophilic granuloma'), although blood eosinophilia is not seen. With progression, some of the Langerhans cells become replaced with pigment-laden macrophages and eventually scarring occurs.

Bronchial lavage specimens contain Langerhans cells which can be identified by electron microscopy and these cells, when cultured, spontaneously secrete fibronectin and alveolar macrophage-derived growth factor, this being, perhaps, the common mechanism for pulmonary fibrosis.

Natural History
The natural history is variable and difficult to understand because the essential nature of the disease and its aetiology are still unknown. Some cases pursue a rapid downhill course with early death as the outcome, while others appear to resolve spontaneously. With others there is a gradual downhill course which may be interrupted by remissions but the disease may arrest at any point leaving patients with differing degrees of functional impairment depending on the extent and severity of the scarring. About one-third improve, one-third show no change and one-third deteriorate.

Pulmonary Lymphangioleiomyomatosis
This is a rare disorder found exclusively in females during reproductive life. It is characterized by an abnormal proliferation, which may be focal or diffuse, of rather immature smooth muscle cells. The proliferation involves all parts of the lung and the cells are believed to be derived from the walls of pulmonary lymphatics (hence the name of the condition). Similar changes may

be found in extrapulmonary situations in some patients. The sex and age distribution are so striking (as is the fact that the onset of menopause brings a halt to the progression of the disease in some patients) as to suggest that it may have a hormonal basis. Some studies have shown the presence of progesterone and oestrogen receptors on the proliferated smooth muscle, and treatment with oestrogen antagonists such as tamoxifen is now a well-established practice, although the response is variable.

Clinical Course

The normal course is a progressive decline in respiratory function punctuated by episodes of spontaneous pneumothorax, the accumulation of lipid-rich pleural effusions (chylous) and pulmonary haemorrhage due to the involvement of small veins by the process.

PULMONARY OEDEMA (INCLUDING ADULT RESPIRATORY DISTRESS SYNDROME)

As in any other tissue, quantitative relationships between intravascular and extravascular fluid in the lung are governed by the interaction of two principal factors (*Fig. 33.25*):

1) **intracapillary hydrostatic pressure**
2) **capillary permeability**

If either or both of these are increased, oedema will result, first within the interstitial tissue and then within the alveolar spaces. **The lung is deemed to be oedematous when there is more than 4–5 ml of fluid per gram of dry blood-free tissue. This will occur only when the volume of extravascular fluid overwhelms the capacity of pulmonary lymphatic drainage, which is the first line of defence against oedema.**

Increased interstitial fluid derived from small blood vessels is easy to understand; the responsible mechanisms are identical to those involved in oedema at other sites. How the excess interstitial fluid gains access to the alveolar space is less certain; it has been suggested that in high capillary pressure oedema it is due to leakage through the tight junctions between epithelial cells because of increased interstitial pressure.

There are major differences in the natural history of pulmonary oedema occurring principally as a result of **high pressure within the small blood vessels** or as a result of **increased permeability of the walls of the lung capillaries**. High-pressure oedema can be relieved as a rule if the cause of the increased pressure is removed. Oedema resulting from injuries that cause increased capillary permeability is much more difficult to relieve, tends to last longer, and is associated with a significant risk of interstitial lung fibrosis.

High-pressure Pulmonary Oedema

This is the most common type encountered in clinical practice. Many conditions cause increased pressure in the microcirculation of the lung (*Fig. 33.26*); of these, cardiac disease is the most important and common.

Cardiac causes of increased pulmonary capillary pressure include:

- **left ventricular failure** from any cause but, particularly, as a consequence of coronary artery disease and systemic hypertension
- ventricular and supraventricular **tachycardias**
- **high pressure in the pulmonary veins** as is seen in patients with mitral valve disease, left atrial myxomas and the very rare congenital condition of cor triatriatum
- constrictive pericarditis and pericardial effusion

Other disorders in which high pulmonary capillary pressure is either the sole oedema-producing mechanism or is a major contributor are:

- severe anaemia
- intravenous fluid overload
- veno-occlusive disease of the lung
- cerebral injury (including subarachnoid and intracerebral bleeding)
- renal failure
- effects of high altitude

In the last three, increased capillary permeability is also believed to play a part.

Cardiogenic Pulmonary Oedema

The salient features of this form of pulmonary oedema are shortness of breath, orthopnoea, cough and paroxysmal nocturnal dyspnoea.

Acute episodes may occur during which frothy, sometimes pink, sputum may be produced. The patients are usually understandably anxious and fright-

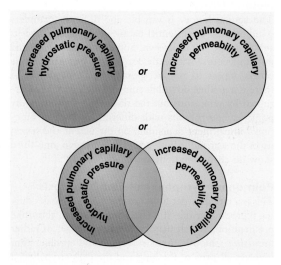

FIGURE 33.25 *Basic pathogenetic factors in the production of pulmonary oedema.*

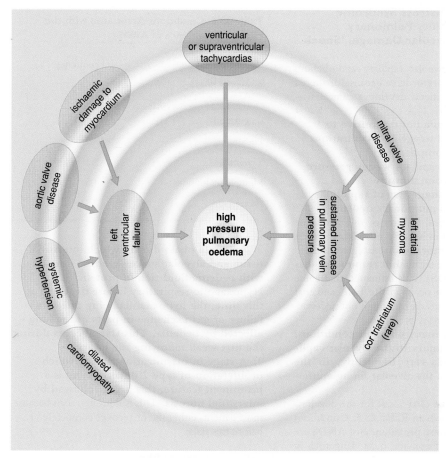

FIGURE 33.26 *Causes of high-pressure pulmonary oedema.*

ened. At auscultation there are bilateral basal crackling sounds, particularly on inspiration.

The functional effects of interstitial and intra-alveolar oedema are a **reduction in lung compliance** and in the **effective lung volume**. Hypoxaemia is almost always present and patients often show hypocapnia, although hypercapnia can occur in some elderly patients as the oedema worsens. Poor left ventricular output leads to poor oxygenation of peripheral tissues, resulting in metabolic acidosis.

Radiological abnormalities precede the appearance of symptoms; the earliest features are the appearance of blurring of the outlines of the larger pulmonary vessels and the presence of Kerley B lines (collections of fluid in the interlobular septa) which manifest as short horizontal linear shadows at the lung bases.

Macroscopic Features

At post-mortem examination, the lungs are reddened, heavy and **wet**; abundant watery, often bloodstained, fluid exudes from the cut surface.

Microscopic Features

The presence of oedema fluid is shown by pink-staining, sometimes rather granular, material within the alveolar spaces.

Prominence of the congested capillaries along the alveolar septa, rather like beads on a string, reflects the high pulmonary capillary wedge pressure.

Chronicity of high wedge capillary pressure leads to repeated small haemorrhages within the alveoli. The iron component of the haemoglobin within alveoli is phagocytosed by macrophages in the form of haemosiderin particles. These appear as browny-yellow granules within these macrophages, which have been called 'heart failure cells'. In cases of really long-standing pulmonary vein hypertension, such as used to occur in cases of mitral stenosis before valve replacement became a practicable procedure, the accumulation of haemosiderin could be so great that the lung appeared brown on naked-eye examination. In addition, such chronic oedema was associated with an increase in the stiffness of the lung due to interstitial fibrosis and smooth muscle cell proliferation.

Adult Respiratory Distress Syndrome (Increased Permeability Pulmonary Oedema, Diffuse Alveolar Damage, 'Shock Lung')

Extensive damage to alveolar capillary endothelium results in severe pulmonary oedema because of altered capillary permeability. Patients develop a clinical syndrome characterized by –

- **refractory hypoxaemia not responsive to increases in inspired oxygen concentrations**
- **reduction in lung compliance**
- **normal pulmonary capillary wedge pressure**
- **normal plasma oncotic pressure**
- **a chest radiograph suggestive of rapidly developing bilateral pulmonary oedema**

Clinical and morphological features of this syndrome are similar to those seen in infantile respiratory distress syndrome (**hyaline membrane disease**), and this led to the introduction of the term **adult respiratory distress syndrome (ARDS)**. It is estimated that some 150 000 cases per annum occur in the USA and that 60% of the affected patients die, although not necessarily all as a result of respiratory problems.

ARDS results from many different conditions, all of which produce injury to the alveolar capillary endothelium and, very frequently, to the type 1 pneumocytes of the alveolar lining epithelium as well.

Clinical conditions that carry a risk for the development of ARDS are shown in *Table 33.5*. Conditions associated with the **highest prevalence** of ARDS are seen in *Table 33.6*. Of these, the most dangerous in terms of high mortality rates are:

aspiration of gastric contents	93.8%
bacteraemia	77.8%
pneumonia	60%

About 60–65% of all patients who currently develop ARDS will die.

The evolution of ARDS occurs in three phases (*Fig. 33.27*). **These are:**
1) **A preclinical phase during which microvascular injury is taking place.**

Table 33.6 Conditions Associated with the Highest Prevalence of ARDS

Condition	Frequency (%)
Aspiration of gastric contents	35.6
Disseminated intravascular coagulation	22.2
Pneumonia	11.9
Trauma	5.3
Multiple transfusions	4.6
Bacteraemia	3.8

2) **An acute phase during which interstitial tissue and alveolar spaces become flooded with oedema fluid rich in protein. Hypoxaemic respiratory failure develops at this time, the hypoxaemia being due to a failure of gas exchange in parts of the lung affected by oedema. This stage occurs during the first week following the injury.**
3) **A stage of organization during which proliferation of type 2 pneumocytes is a prominent feature, this being followed by interstitial fibrosis.** This is not often seen because most patients either die or recover competely before this stage.

Preclinical or Injury Phase

Possible Mechanisms of Injury
Activated neutrophils probably play a key role in this phase. In some forms of ARDS neutrophils clump within small blood vessels and adhere to the endothelium. Experimental, increased permeability-type pulmonary oedema in animals can be inhibited by first inducing neutropenia. Similarly neutrophil-activating agents such as phorbol myristate acetate cause acute lung injury.

Table 33.5 Conditions that may Lead to the Development of ARDS

Primary lung damage	Secondary lung damage
Aspiration of gastric contents	Traumatic shock
Oxygen toxicity	Bacteraemia or septicaemia
Inhalation of other toxic gases (e.g. smoke, chlorine)	Extensive burns
Bacterial or viral pneumonia (particularly if requiring ventilation)	Multiple blood transfusions
Adverse drug reactions, notably bleomycin toxicity, other cytotoxics, salicylates	Fat embolism
Radiation damage to the lung	Acute pancreatitis
Certain poisons (e.g. paraquat)	Disseminated intravascular coagulation

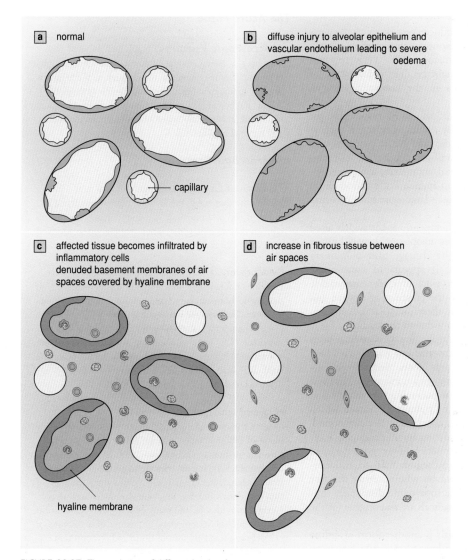

FIGURE 33.27 The evolution of diffuse alveolar damage.

Activated neutrophils can injure cells in many different ways. These include the release of:

- **proteolytic lysosomal enzymes** such as collagenase and elastase
- **cell-damaging oxygen free radicals**
- **compounds derived from arachidonic acid metabolism (leukotrienes and prostaglandins) following the activation of phospholipase A$_2$**
- **platelet-activating factor (PAF)**, another powerful lipid-derived autacoid, which upregulates inflammation and causes platelet activation

There is also evidence that **platelets** become sequestered in the lung as ARDS develops and as many as half the patients become thrombocytopenic.

Amongst compounds released from the activated platelet is PDGF. The release of PDGF may be significant in relation to the interstitial scarring that takes place in the later stages of ARDS.

There is obviously a complicated interaction between cells, cytokines and toxins in this preclinical phase of ARDS. At the risk of oversimplifying the problem, it might be helpful to regard these events as having an **afferent** and an **efferent** or **effector** component.

1) The **efferent** component is represented by the generation and release of compounds that are **intrinsically cytotoxic**, such as free radicals or lysosomal proteases, or which **upregulate** reactions associated with release of cytotoxic or vasoactive compounds.

2) The **afferent** limb of the process might be represented by the pathogenetic mechanisms that lead to the release of efferent limb cytotoxins.

Free Radicals and ARDS

Some causes of ARDS produce their effect by the generation of free radicals without the participation of neutrophils or other inflammatory cells. Thus **oxygen toxicity**, for instance, might be due to formation of **cytotoxic free radicals** in the course of oxygen metabolism.

Free radicals are thought also to be responsible for the lung damage caused by oxides of nitrogen such as nitric oxide and nitrogen dioxide. Nitric oxide, as well as having profound vasodilator properties, can also cause cell damage. Bacterial endotoxin, a well-recognized cause of ARDS, can induce both endothelium and macrophages to produce large quantities of nitric oxide.

Bleomycin, a chemotherapeutic agent widely used in treating certain malignant neoplasms, is well known to produce diffuse alveolar damage and pulmonary fibrosis in some patients. It appears to concentrate within the lungs and, *in vitro*, produces superoxide anions when incubated in the presence of oxygen and free iron. It seems likely, therefore, that bleomycin-related pulmonary damage is due to free radicals.

Many cases of fatal diffuse alveolar damage have been caused by ingesting the powerful and widely used herbicide **paraquat**. With large doses, death from pulmonary haemorrhage occurs within a few days. In most cases of accidental paraquat poisoning the victims survive long enough to develop pulmonary fibrosis which appears within 10–14 days of ingesting the compound. Paraquat is a powerful oxidizing agent, producing oxygen free radicals in the presence of oxygen. Paraquat causes more damage to epithelium than to endothelium. This can be lessened by administering the free radical-scavenging enzyme superoxide dismutase, supporting the idea that free radicals are responsible for the cell injury.

Radiation pneumonitis is another form of diffuse alveolar damage leading to lung fibrosis which may be due to the generation of free radicals within cell and tissue water. Its toxic effects, like those of other free radical-generating systems, are potentiated by a high oxygen concentration.

Activation Mechanisms for Neutrophils and Platelets in Situations in which a Risk of ARDS Exists

What factors cause activation of neutrophils and platelets in the clinical scenarios in which ARDS occurs? In some situations a single activation pathway may operate, such as, perhaps, **complement activation**, the release of C5a being brought about by the presence of leucocyte antibodies in **multiple blood transfusions**.

In others, for example **Gram-negative septicaemia**, multiple potential pathways exist through which neutrophil and platelet activation could be brought about. This is described in the section dealing with cardiovascular disease (see pp 387–390).

The Acute Phase

Macroscopic Features

The lung is heavy, reddened and airless. Unlike high-pressure pulmonary oedema, the cut surface of the lung is dry due to coagulation of the protein-rich oedema fluid. Again, unlike cardiogenic pulmonary oedema, blocks of tissue sink immediately when placed in fixative or saline, and are thus non-aerated.

Microscopic Features

Evidence of Capillary Leakage

During the first week, the alveolar septa are widened as a result of the accumulation of oedema fluid; the alveoli contain eosinophilic protein-rich material often admixed with abundant red cells.

Evidence of Cell Damage

Electron microscopic examination shows evidence of damage to both capillary endothelium and type 1 pneumocytes. The cells are swollen and show blebbing of the plasma membranes, suggesting free radical-mediated peroxidation. On light microscopy, cell debris is present within alveolar spaces and, in severe cases, both the epithelial and endothelial basement membranes are denuded of their cell covering.

Hyaline Membrane Formation

One of the most characteristic features during this early phase of diffuse alveolar damage is the presence of **hyaline membranes**. These appear 1–2 days after onset of oedema. Hyaline membranes are eosinophilic, apparently structureless, layers of material plastered along the walls of the respiratory bronchioles, alveolar ducts and alveoli. Electron microscopy shows them to be neither uniform nor completely structureless, consisting of a mixture of cell debris, a small amount of fibrin and glycoprotein.

Evidence of Microthrombus Formation

Capillary thrombi can be seen during the acute phase of diffuse alveolar damage and are probably a result of capillary endothelial damage.

The Repair Phase

The repair phase starts normally 2–3 days after the onset of acute changes. It consists essentially of two components: replacement of alveolar lining epithelium and interstitial fibrosis.

Replacement of Alveolar Lining Epithelium

Basement membranes denuded as a result of the death of the type 1 pneumocytes now become partly or fully covered by proliferating type 2 cells, which have a cuboidal appearance. The alveolar lining thus appears much more prominent than in normal lung.

Interstitial Fibrosis

In the acute phase the alveolar septa are widened, partly by oedema fluid and partly by a mixed cellular infiltrate in which macrophages are present. The release of cytokines and growth factors from these cells is, presumably, the mechanism for the interstitial fibrosis that follows. Some fibroblasts also migrate from the interstitium into the alveolar spaces via defects in the epithelial basement membrane and these lay down new connective tissue within the airspaces. In due time a new basement membrane is formed over these masses of connective tissue which become incorporated into the interstitial tissue.

Other Types of Pulmonary Oedema

In general, the concept of pulmonary oedema being due to an increase in either pulmonary capillary pressure or pulmonary capillary permeability serves us well, but certain types of pulmonary oedema do not fit into either of these categories and their pathogenesis is not clear.

Neurogenic Pulmonary Oedema

Pulmonary oedema occasionally follows trauma to the head, subarachnoid or intracerebral haemorrhage, and intracranial surgery. The common aetiological factor appears to be raised intracranial pressure.

To a certain extent the oedema may be mediated through a rise in pulmonary capillary pressure. Rises in intracranial pressure are associated with a major sympathetic discharge and a consequent rise in the level of circulating catecholamines. This can cause a rise in pulmonary capillary pressure by increasing the venous return and inducing severe peripheral vasoconstriction with a resulting pressure load on the left ventricle.

However, the oedema fluid may contain high concentrations of protein, as is seen in cases where the mechanism is an increase in capillary permeability, and neurogenic oedema may also occur in some patients in the absence of high pulmonary capillary pressure. Why an increase in the permeability of these vessels should occur in patients with increased intracranial pressure is a mystery.

High-Altitude Oedema

One of the risks in ascending to high altitudes (3000 m or more) is acute mountain sickness. The syndrome, which affects only some people at these altitudes, consists of lethargy, anorexia, nausea, dizziness and vomiting. In most individuals these symptoms resolve in a few days but a small number develop acute pulmonary oedema, which can make its appearance from as little as 3 hours to as much as 96 hours after the ascent. In some, cerebral oedema also develops and they may lapse into coma. The aetiology of high-altitude oedema is not known, although many theories have been canvassed. Hypoxia appears to play some part but by itself does not cause oedema. There is some evidence, from the high protein content of the oedema fluid and the presence of red cells within it, that a disturbance of capillary permeability is also involved.

Pulmonary Oedema in Uraemia

Chronic renal failure is not uncommonly associated with pulmonary oedema and this is almost certainly multifactorial in origin. Clearly a number of mechanisms could be involved:

- Retention of sodium and water can lead to circulatory overload.
- The high blood pressure often associated with chronic renal disease may lead to left ventricular failure.
- An element of increased capillary pressure is involved because the oedema fluid has a high protein content. The reason for this is not known.

The central portions of the lung are most involved, giving a rather characteristic 'butterfly' shadowing on chest radiography.

Pulmonary Oedema Associated with Re-expansion of Lung Tissue

In a small number of patients, rapid draining of a pneumothorax may be followed by the development of pulmonary oedema on the same side as the pneumothorax. A similar syndrome may follow rapid drainage of a pleural effusion. The cause is unknown but it has been suggested that a loss of surfactant occurs in the collapsed portions of lung. On re-expansion, leakage of fluid from the interstitium takes place across those portions of the alveolar wall that are devoid of surfactant.

Pneumonia

Definition

Pneumonia is defined as **acute inflammation of the lung parenchyma caused by living microorganisms**. It is characterized by filling of the alveoli by inflammatory exudate, so-called **'consolidation'**.

Pneumonia can and must be distinguished from immune-mediated intra-alveolar inflammation and from pneumonitis – parenchymal inflammation caused by physical agents such as radiation.

Clinical Significance

Pneumonia is the commonest **infective** cause of death in Western countries, accounting for roughly 56 deaths per 100 000 population annually in England and Wales. In Western communities pneumonia shows a marked predilection for the elderly, causing 30 times as many deaths in patients aged 75–84 years as in those of 55–64 years.

Pneumonia may be acquired in the community, the incidence being highest in infants and the elderly, or in **hospital (nosocomial infection)**. Pneumonia is the commonest hospital-acquired infection, the elderly once again being the most frequent targets. It is said to cause death in 0.5–5% of hospital admissions.

While this is far from unimpressive, it pales into insignificance when compared with the effect of pneumonia among **economically deprived children**. Worldwide, no fewer than **five million children die each year from pneumonia**; 96% of these deaths occur in Third World countries, highlighting once again the powerful nexus between economics and disease.

Classification

Pneumonia can be classified in a number of ways, each of which can make a contribution to rational treatment. Criteria that should be considered are described below and shown in *Fig. 33.28*.

The Causal Organism

Many microorganisms cause pneumonia. These include:

- bacteria
- *Mycoplasma*
- viruses
- ? protozoa

Precise identification of the responsible organisms may be difficult and, in some cases, impossible. Because prompt treatment with antimicrobial agents is essential, the clinical frame of reference of the pneumonia may give valuable clues as to the organism.

For instance, if the pneumonia occurs in a **previously healthy** individual, it is likely to be due to **Streptococcus pneumoniae**. If, on the other hand, it

supervenes on a **pre-existing viral infection** of the respiratory tract, *Staphylococcus aureus* or *S. pneumoniae* are likely suspects. A patient with chronic bronchitis is a candidate for pneumonia caused by either *S. pneumoniae* or *Haemophilus influenzae*, and patients with **acquired immune deficiency syndrome (AIDS)** are at risk of developing opportunistic lung infections such as *Pneumocystis carinii* pneumonia (*Fig. 33.29*).

Anatomical Distribution of the Inflammatory Process

The common anatomical terms used in describing pneumonia are **lobar pneumonia** and **bronchopneumonia** (*Fig. 33.30*).

In lobar pneumonia the inflammatory process involves one or more entire lobes and the

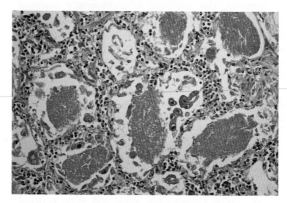

FIGURE 33.29 *Section of lung from a patient with AIDS. The alveoli are filled with* Pneumocystis carinii *(stained a magenta colour with the periodic acid–Schiff stain used here).*

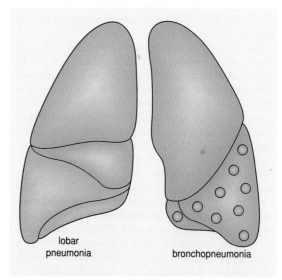

lobar pneumonia   bronchopneumonia

FIGURE 33.30 *Basic anatomical differences between lobar pneumonia and bronchopneumonia. In lobar pneumonia the lung parenchyma is involved in continuity so that a whole lobe or more than one lobe may show consolidation. In bronchopneumonia the lesions are focally distributed.*

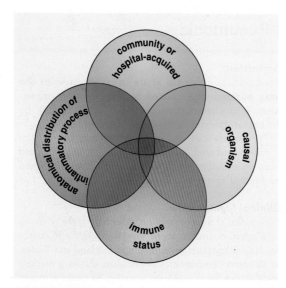

FIGURE 33.28 *Factors that interact to determine the type and severity of pneumonia.*

involvement is confluent rather than focal. Lobar pneumonia results from the spread of infected oedema fluid through the alveoli, this being halted only by the barrier of the pleura. In **bronchopneumonia** the involvement is **focal. The inflammatory process arises as a result of inhalation of organisms into small airways and the parenchymal inflammation is centred on these airways and involves the centriacinar alveoli.** It has been suggested that this pattern is due to rapid mobilization of neutrophils in the areas of lung tissue where the infecting organisms lodge and is thus associated with localization of the infection. Because the same organisms (e.g. *S. pneumoniae*) can cause either lobar pneumonia or bronchopneumonia, it has been suggested that the occurrence of one rather than the other depends on the relative balance between neutrophil-mediated localization and the rapid formation of infected oedema fluid.

Bronchopneumonia is commonest in infants, young children with debilitating disorders and the elderly; it is usually a **secondary** event, being preceded by some other condition tending to decrease the effectiveness of local and general defences against infection.

Other acute respiratory tract infections, notably viral ones such as influenza, and conditions predisposing to recurrent pulmonary infections, such as chronic bronchitis and cystic fibrosis, are important risk factors for bronchopneumonia. It may also result from aspiration of food or vomitus, obstruction of a bronchus by a foreign body or neoplasm, or inhalation of irritant gases. Surgery, particularly when carried out on the upper abdomen, is not an uncommon precursor of bronchopneumonia. The pathogenesis here is very complex, involving such elements as impairment of the ciliary activity due to anaesthesia, possible inhalation of infected material during unconsciousness, temporary depression of the cough reflex and restriction of aeration of the lower lobes of the lungs as a result of pain associated with movement of the abdominal wall.

Community Acquired Versus Nosocomial Infection

Nosocomial infection is a special problem following operation and in intensive care units. Patients are at risk for one or more of the following reasons:

- they are likely to be immunocompromised to some extent
- because of intubation of the respiratory tract
- because of alterations in bacterial flora as a result of treatment with antimicrobial agents

These hospital-acquired infections are more often due to Gram-negative aerobic bacilli or *S. aureus* than those acquired in the community.

Is the Patient Immunocompromised?

Patients whose immunological competence is impaired, either because of their disease or because of the use of cytotoxic or immunosuppressive agents, are at high risk of developing pneumonia. Some of these pneumonias are due to infection by organisms that 'normally' cause pneumonia, but many are a result of **opportunistic infection** by organisms that are normally non-pathogenic commensals.

To a considerable extent, the type of pulmonary infection likely to occur in an immunocompromised patient is dictated by the type of immune deficiency (*Fig. 33.31*).

Commonly encountered defects in defence against infection are:

1) **A quantitative or qualitative defect in respect of neutrophils.** Thus, too few neutrophils (neutropenia from whatever cause) or one of the many possible functional defects in these cells markedly increases the risk of infection. In the lung this may be manifested by infection with normal

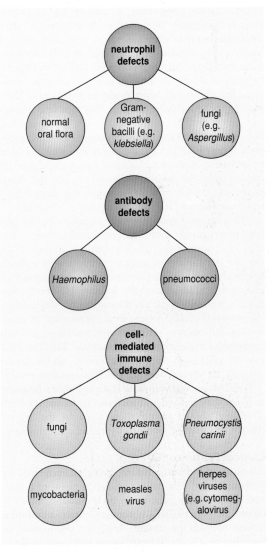

FIGURE 33.31 *The type of immune deficiency determines, to a large extent, the type of organism responsible for pneumonia.*

oral flora, with Gram-negative bacilli such as *Klebsiella* or fungi such as *Aspergillus* species.

2) **A defect in antibody formation.** Here pneumonococcal and *Haemophilus* infections are especially likely to occur.

3) **Defects in respect of cell-mediated immunity** are associated with a very wide range of pneumonia-causing organisms. These include fungi, *Toxoplasma gondii*, *Pneumocystis carinii* (seen particularly in patients with AIDS), mycobacteria, measles and herpes viruses such as cytomegalovirus and zoster.

SPECIFIC MICROBIOLOGICAL TYPES OF PNEUMONIA

Pneumococcal Pneumonia

Pneumococcal pneumonia is caused by a Gram-positive lanceolate diplococcus: *S. pneumoniae* (**the pneumococcus**). This is the most common cause of bacterial pneumonia. It is aerobic and facultatively anaerobic, growing on blood agar and producing α-haemolysis. There are some 82 different antigenic varieties, the distinction being made on the basis of their capsular, polysaccharide antigen. This capsule is important in conferring pathogenicity on the organism, because it protects the pneumococcus against phagocytosis. Types I, II and III are most commonly isolated from patients with pneumococcal pneumonia; type III appears to be the most virulent and to carry the worst prognosis. The neutrophil response in the affected lung tissue correlates with the infecting dose of organisms.

The frequency with which the organism can be isolated from patients' sputum depends on whether antibiotics have been given before isolation is attempted. In this case the chances of isolation are decreased and this has given rise to the impression that the prevalence of pneumococcal pneumonia has declined. However, even if it is impossible to culture the organism, pneumococcal antigen is usually present in the serum and in other biological fluids for 7–10 days after infection, and can be detected by immunoelectrophoresis. This can be a valuable adjunct to diagnosis because it can be carried out quite rapidly and does not yield false-positive results.

Pneumococcal pneumonia is slightly more frequent in males than females and increases in frequency with increasing age. It occurs most often in the winter months and may be preceded by a brief coryzal illness.

Clinical Features

Classically the onset is abrupt, being characterized by chills and fever. The patient often complains of unilateral, sharp, stabbing chest pain on inspiration, which is due to the presence of a fibrinous pleurisy, a common feature of lobar pneumonia but very uncommon in bronchopneumonia. Respiration is rapid and shallow, producing a reduction in the tidal volume, and much of the ventilation involves the bronchial dead-space.

Cough may be prominent and is often associated with blood-stained so-called 'rusty' sputum. This full-blown syndrome is rarely seen nowadays, probably because of early treatment with antibiotics.

Evolution of the Structural Changes in Lobar Pneumonia

Before the introduction of antibiotics, the evolution of the pathology followed a classical pathway (*Fig. 33.32*).

Congestion

This phase usually lasts less than 24 hours. The lung tissue is intensely red owing to a marked increase in blood flow through alveolar wall capillaries. In the rare cases coming to post mortem at this stage, the cut surface of the lung is wet, exuding blood-stained frothy fluid.

Microscopic Features

There is marked dilatation of alveolar capillaries and pale, eosinophilic oedema fluid in the alveolar spaces. These contain a few red blood cells and neutrophils, and Gram staining often shows fairly abundant pneumococci. Little, if any, fibrin can be seen within the alveoli at this stage.

Red Hepatization

This term derives from the **firm, 'meaty' and airless appearance of the lung at this stage**. The cut surface of the lung is dry and blocks of tissue taken from these areas sink immediately in fluid because of the lack of aeration. The pleural surface usually shows a fine, fibrinous exudate, which accounts both for chest pain and the 'friction rub' often heard on auscultation. The lung is still red, indicating that alveolar capillary dilatation is still present.

Microscopic Features

Examination of histological preparations readily explains the macroscopic features. Within the alveoli, coagulation of the original, fibrinogen-rich exudate has occurred and, as a result, the alveoli are filled with interlacing strands of polymerized fibrin. Often these strands can be seen to extend from one alveolus to another via the inter-alveolar pores of Kohn. Within the fibrin, neutrophils are much more numerous and may contain pneumococci.

Grey Hepatization

As the illness progresses the lung gradually becomes greyish-red (*Fig. 33.33*). The cause of this colour change is twofold:

1) A sharp decline occurs in the degree of hyperaemia, to the extent that there is a virtual shutdown of bloodflow through the inflamed segments of lung.

2) There is a continued migration of large numbers of inflammatory cells into the intra-alveolar exudate (*Fig. 33.34*).

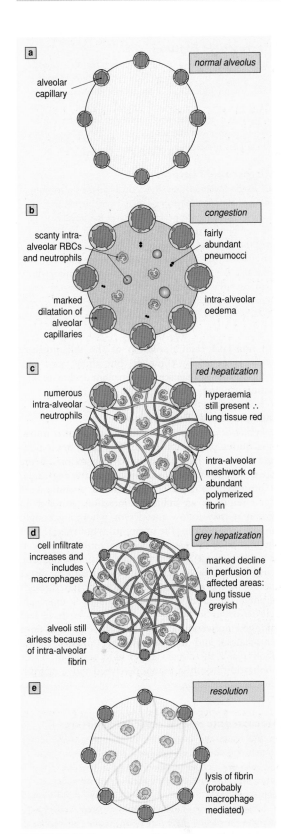

FIGURE 33.32 *The evolution of lobar pneumonia.*

(a) **normal alveolus**
alveolar capillary

(b) **congestion**
scanty intra-alveolar RBCs and neutrophils
fairly abundant pneumocci
marked dilatation of alveolar capillaries
intra-alveolar oedema

(c) **red hepatization**
numerous intra-alveolar neutrophils
hyperaemia still present ∴ lung tissue red
intra-alveolar meshwork of abundant polymerized fibrin

(d) **grey hepatization**
cell infiltrate increases and includes macrophages
marked decline in perfusion of affected areas: lung tissue greyish
alveoli still airless because of intra-alveolar fibrin

(e) **resolution**
lysis of fibrin (probably macrophage mediated)

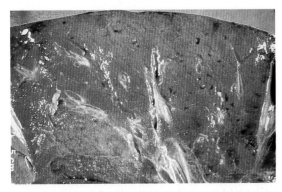

FIGURE 33.33 *Lung showing lobar pneumonia in the stage of early grey hepatization. Note how meaty and airless the normally spongy lung parenchyma appears.*

FIGURE 33.34 *Section of lung in lobar pneumonia (grey hepatization stage). Every alveolus is stuffed with neutrophils.*

Resolution

Lysis of the polymerized fibrin now occurs. Before the introduction of antibiotics, this usually occurred 8–9 days after the start of the illness and was associated with a sudden fall of the fever ('the crisis'), sweating, slowing and increase in depth of breathing, and general improvement in the patient's condition.

The importance of fibrinolysis in restoring functional normality to the affected lung tissue cannot be overemphasized, as exudate persistence triggers the processes of organization and scarring. It is likely that the lytic process is mediated via the release of **plasminogen activator** from activated macrophages within the exudate. Once the fibrin has been lysed, it is removed, partly via sputum but chiefly via lymphatic drainage.

Complications of Lobar Pneumonia

Localized

- **Breakdown of parenchymal tissue with abscess formation.** This is most likely to happen if the pneumonia has been caused by a type III pneumococcus.

- **Local spread of infection to the pleural space** leading to **empyema formation**.
- **Failure of resolution leading to scarring** of the affected areas of lung and thus permanent loss of ventilation (so-called 'carnification').

Generalized
In many cases of pneumococcal pneumonia there is bacteraemia during the acute phase. Acute endocarditis may develop, followed by a cerebral abscess if infected material breaks off from the inflamed heart valves and impacts within the cerebral circulation. More rarely pneumococcal **meningitis, peritonitis or arthritis** may be encountered.

Legionella Pneumonia
Legionella pneumonia was first recognized in 1976 in the course of an outbreak of pneumonia amongst delegates to a convention of the American Legion held in Philadelphia, Pennsylvania. Some 123 people were affected and 34 died. Since then, several other outbreaks and many sporadic cases have been reported. *Legionella* pneumonia is often lobar in distribution and many cases in the past may have been misdiagnosed as lobar pneumonia, from which an organism could not be isolated.

The cause is a minute coccobacillus staining poorly with Gram's stain: *Legionella pneumophila*. *Legionella* can be stained non-immunologically by a silver impregnation method (Dieterle stain), but this is not completely reliable. Fortunately some of its antigens resist inactivation by the methods used in tissue preparation and thus organisms can be readily demonstrated by using appropriate monoclonal antibodies.

Apart from *L. pneumophila*, there are at least 22 other species of *Legionella*; nine of these are also pathogenic for humans. *L. pneumophila* has at least 11 different serotypes, of which group 1 is the most important human pathogen. The organism can be cultured but its growth requirements are exacting. Complex media are needed and there are also precise requirements with respect to temperature and humidity. In human infections, the organism can be recovered from bronchial washings, pleural fluid, lung biopsy specimens or blood.

Mode of Infection
Legionella organisms are ubiquitous in warm moist environments, and outbreaks of infection, often in debilitated or immunosuppressed humans, commonly follow inhalation of bacteria from aerosols generated from contaminated air-conditioning systems (the water used to cool heat exchangers), shower-heads and similar sources. It is less easy to determine the source of infection in sporadic cases; patient to patient transmission does not appear to occur.

Macroscopic Features
The gross appearances of the lung resemble, to a considerable extent, those seen in lobar pneumonia. There is confluent pneumonia associated with fibrinous pleurisy and often with a blood-stained pleural effusion. Empyema is rare but small abscesses are seen in the affected portions of the lung in up to 25% of fatal cases seen at post-mortem examination.

Microscopic Features
Histological examination shows an alveolar exudate consisting of abundant fibrin strands and variable numbers of neutrophils and macrophages. Many of the inflammatory cells can be seen to have undergone necrosis, and necrosis of the epithelial cells lining the alveoli is also a prominent feature. At low magnifications it may be difficult to recognize the alveolar walls, but the use of appropriate connective tissue stains shows that, for the most part, the architectural pattern remains intact.

In non-fatal cases resolution of the inflammatory process is generally complete but there are some patients in whom a degree of permanent decline in lung function is noted; this is presumably due to fibrosis.

Staphylococcal Pneumonia
Staphylococcus pyogenes aureus is a rare cause of community-acquired pneumonia (1–2.5% of cases) but is a frequent cause of hospital-acquired pneumonia, being more or less equal with *Escherichia coli* in this regard.

Community-acquired staphylococcal pneumonia is often a sequel of an influenzal infection, although in children it may follow measles or whooping cough. The main reservoir for the organisms is humans (15% of the community carry staphylococci asymptomatically in the nose or throat). The organisms can infect the lung by inhalation or may reach the bloodstream by direct invasion of the skin or mucous membranes through abrasions. Infection via the bloodstream is especially likely to occur in patients in hospital who have had prolonged intravenous cannulation, those on long-term haemodialysis and intravenous drug abusers. Septic emboli reach the lungs, either as a result of direct embolization from the lesions described above or from tricuspid endocarditis.

Macroscopic and Microscopic Features
In fatal cases the lung is heavy and congested. The bronchi are acutely inflamed and there are many centrilobular foci of suppuration. In cases that are more advanced at the time of death, these suppurating foci may have coalesced to form abscesses which may exceed 1 cm in diameter. If some of these abscesses are subpleural, rupture into the pleural space may occur, causing empyema.

Long-term complications in surviving patients include scarring, bronchiectasis or large air-filled cysts known as pneumatoceles.

Klebsiella Pneumonia

Klebsiella pneumonia is caused by two members of the *Klebsiella* species: *K. pneumoniae* and *K. oxytoca*. *K. pneumonia* is a common inhabitant of the oral cavity, particularly in individuals with a poor standard of oral hygiene, and those most at risk for developing *Klebsiella* pneumonia include such individuals, the elderly and diabetics. The widespread use of antibiotics has increased the number of instances in which *Klebsiella* becomes dominant in the oral bacterial flora and this is believed to be associated with an increased frequency of pneumonia caused by *Klebsiella* species.

Macroscopic Features

Klebsiella is unusual among Gram-negative bacilli in that it tends to cause a confluent pneumonia with a predominantly lobar distribution. The pneumonia is usually unilateral and right sided, and the posterior segments of the upper lobes and the apical segments of the lower lobes are the preferred sites, consistent with the view that aspiration in the supine position of oropharyngeal contents, such as may occur in alcoholics, is an important pathogenetic mechanism. *Klebsiella* has a mucoid capsule and this gives the consolidated areas a characteristically slimy feel. Identification of the mucinous component of the capsule by appropriate special stains may be helpful in establishing the aetiology in lung tissue samples. Suppuration with lung abscess formation is likely to occur and, in some cases, necrosis of lung tissue may be extensive.

LUNG ABSCESS

An abscess is a local area of suppuration, walled off from surrounding tissue by a limiting membrane composed of granulation and fibrous tissue.

Pus-filled cavities in the lungs may be either abscesses or bronchiectatic cavities secondarily infected by pyogenic organisms. The distinction between these two can be made fairly readily if the essential differences in the pathogenesis are borne in mind.

In **abscess** formation the destruction of an area of lung parenchyma means that **several airways are likely to communicate with the abscess cavity**. In **bronchiectasis** each cavity is formed by **abnormal dilatation of a single airway** and thus it is not possible for multiple airways to communicate with a single cavity.

Abscess formation is either **primary** or **secondary**.

Primary abscess formation is not preceded by any other inflammatory process within the lung. Such abscesses are usually thought to be the result of aspiration of infected oropharyngeal contents; poor oral hygiene with sepsis, and any circumstance increasing the chance of aspiration, act synergistically.

The bacteria responsible mirror the mixed anaerobic flora of the oral cavity such as *fusiform* bacteria, *Bacteroides* and aerobes such as *Streptococcus milleri*.

Conditions that increase the risk of aspiration include any condition leading to loss of consciousness (e.g. alcoholic stupor); and dysphagia or primary oesophageal dysfunction, which are likely to be associated with regurgitation.

Primary abscesses are most commonly found on the right side, probably because the right main bronchus leads more directly off the trachea than does the left, and the most dependent parts of the lung are sites of predilection.

Secondary abscesses develop as a complication of a number of different conditions. Local predisposing factors include bronchial carcinoma, the presence of a foreign body in an airway, and bronchiectasis. One of the most important disorders to present as a lung abscess is bronchial carcinoma. Diagnosis in these cases may be far from easy because the tumour may not be visible on bronchoscopy, and it may be difficult to make a radiological distinction between the abscess and the tumour. Abscesses may also develop in the course of certain pneumonias most notably staphylococcal and *Klebsiella* pneumonias. Pneumococcal pneumonia used to be an occasional cause but, with effective antipneumococcal treatment, this is no longer so.

Natural History

Spontaneous rupture of the abscess into a bronchus is quite a common event in relation to lung abscess. This can be either helpful or harmful. Drainage of pus is likely to bring about a considerable improvement in the general condition of the patient. There is, however, a risk that infected material may be aspirated into other parts of the bronchial tree, thus spreading the infection within the lung.

Following drainage the empty cavity may become lined by epithelium, and communications between the cavity and airways may be sealed off leaving a cyst resembling a simple congenital cyst of the lung. Occasionally the airway communicating with a postinflammatory cavity may open only during inspiration and thus act as a one-way valve. As a result the cavity gradually increases in size and its fibrous wall becomes progressively stretched until a thin-walled, air-filled sac rather like an emphysematous bulla is formed. This is termed a **pneumatocele**.

Neoplasms of the Lung

PRIMARY MALIGNANT NEOPLASMS

Epidemiology

Carcinoma of the lung, which 30–40 years ago was a comparatively rare neoplasm, now poses a threat to life greater than any other tumour, causing some 35 000 deaths annually in the UK. In males in the UK it is the commonest significant malignant neoplasm, accounting for 30% of all cancer deaths. In females the incidence has also been rising steadily, and deaths from carcinoma of the lung have now overtaken those from breast cancer. The male : female ratio, previously about 7 : 1 has now fallen to 2 : 1. In the USA the annual death rate from carcinoma of the lung increased sevenfold between 1950 and 1988; thus during this time it is estimated that lung cancer killed 2.4 million people. The increase in men has now levelled off and some fall in male lung cancer mortality rates may be expected, but lung cancer incidence is still rising in women in parallel with cigarette smoking. This enormous increase in incidence over a comparatively short time strongly suggests that environmental factors are important in causation.

Cigarette Smoke as an Aetiological Factor in Lung Cancer

Strong epidemiological evidence exists to link cigarette smoking with lung cancer.

Case–Control Studies

These compare the frequency of a putative risk factor in a group of patients with a given disease with its frequency in a matched group of individuals without the disease. In a 1950 study (Doll and Hill) of males with lung cancer only 0.5% were non-smokers and 56% smoked more than 15 cigarettes daily. Estimated mortality in the smoking group appeared to relate strongly and positively to the **duration** of the smoking habit and to the **number of cigarettes smoked**.

Prospective Studies

Here, the fate of two cohorts is studied: one with and the other without the putative risk factor. Doll and Hill published in 1956 and 1964 the results of a classic prospective study based on the smoking histories of 41 000 British physicians. They showed that:

1) There was a marked and steady increase in death rate from lung cancer as the amount of smoking increased.
2) Mortality was significantly greater in cigarette smokers than in pipe smokers.
3) There was no significant difference between urban and rural dwellers.

4) In men who gave up smoking, death from lung cancer fell significantly and this fall continued as the time from cessation of smoking increased, although it took 10–15 years before the risk equalled that of non-smokers.

Other epidemiological evidence suggests that risk increases the earlier in life one starts to smoke. Some evidence also exists that 'passive smokers' (non-smokers exposed to cigarette smoke) have a higher risk of developing lung cancer than non-smokers not so exposed.

Evidence for a direct effect of cigarette smoke on bronchial epithelium comes from comparing biopsy and autopsy material from smokers and non-smokers. Material from cigarette smokers shows a much higher prevalence of squamous metaplasia than does that from non-smokers, and this metaplastic epithelium shows grades of dysplasia of varying degrees of severity suggesting that there is progression in some cases from metaplasia through dysplasia to frank carcinoma.

How Does Cigarette Smoke Influence the Risk of Lung Cancer?

Clearly cigarette smoke contains chemical carcinogens. Because smoke is so complex a mixture, the search for the responsible carcinogen(s) is likely to be difficult. However, some identified constituents are known to be carcinogens in appropriate animal models. These candidate carcinogens are derived from both the **main phases of cigarette smoke**: the tar (particulate) phase and the gas phase.

The **tar phase** contains a number of carcinogens. In the **neutral** phase there are the **polycyclic hydrocarbons**, 3,4-benzpyrene, dibenzanthracene and benzofluoranthenes. The polycyclic hydrocarbons were among the first chemical carcinogens to be discovered and can cause skin tumours when painted on to the skin of mice. When activated by mixed function oxidases, they become converted to highly reactive epoxides which bind to DNA. Some support for their relevance in human disease comes from epidemiological data which suggest that a switch, on the part of some of the smoking population, to the use of filters and low-tar cigarettes may be responsible for a lessening of risk in the past few years.

The **basic** fraction contains nitrosamines and nicotine, and the **acidic** phase is said to contain a number of **tumour-promoting** compounds.

The **residual** fraction of the tar phase contains cadmium, nickel and polonium-210, all of which are believed to have carcinogenic potential.

The **gas phase** of cigarette smoke contains large numbers of free radicals (about 10^{14} per 25-ml puff), nitric oxide, hydrazine, nickel carbonyl, vinyl chloride and nitrosodiethylamine, all of which have carcinogenic potential.

Carcinogenesis in the Lung may also be Related to Other Environmental and Occupational Hazards

Cigarette smoking is almost certainly the chief carcinogenic atmospheric pollutant, but some data relating to differences in incidence that occur on either a geographical or an occupational basis must be explained. For instance, the lung cancer risk, in some studies, is higher in urban than in rural areas and is greatest in big industrial cities. In the USA states that have the highest incidence of lung cancer are those in which chemical, petrochemical, shipbuilding and paper industries are established.

Some Specific Environmental Hazards Other than Cigarette Smoke

Asbestos There is a strong correlation between exposure to asbestos and the risk of lung cancer. As with the other asbestos-related neoplasm (mesothelioma), amphibole varieties of asbestos (see pp 468–469) are most dangerous. Synergy seems to exist between asbestos exposure and cigarette smoking, the lung cancer risk for smoking asbestos workers being some 14 times as great as that in non-smoking ones. Most asbestos-related cancers occur in the lower lobes, where the concentration of asbestos fibres is greatest.

Other Industrial Chemicals Apart from polycyclic hydrocarbons (encountered by workers in the petrochemical industry), other organic chemicals associated with an increased risk of lung cancer include mustard gas, vinyl chloride and chloromethyl ether. The risk is related to the total dose, and the majority of tumours are of the small cell variety. Increased risk also occurs in the metal refining and smelting industries, and **nickel, chromium and cadmium** have all been proposed as possible carcinogens.

Arsenic, a hazard to vineyard workers engaged in spraying grapes with arsenical insecticides, is also associated with an increased risk of lung cancer.

Ionizing Radiation Miners exposed to radon and other short-lived decay factors from radioactive elements have a risk of lung cancer 30 times as great as that in the general population, smoking being a powerful co-factor.

The course of events in these miners has been studied by repeated cytological examination of their sputum. The first change is the appearance of squamous cells, followed by the detection of cells that are frankly atypical. Such atypia precedes frank carcinoma by 4–5 years.

A Possible Role For Diet Recent data suggest that deficiencies in dietary intake of vitamin E and β-carotene may increase the risk of lung cancer. Formal trials of antioxidants have not, however, yielded positive results thus far.

Molecular Changes in Lung Cancer

ras Oncogenes

Oncogenes of the *ras* family have been found to be activated in a number of human neoplasms including lung cancer. There are three well characterized members of the *ras* family. These are:
1) H-*ras*
2) K-*ras*
3) N-*ras*

All three code for closely related **G proteins**. The G protein is inserted into the cell membrane and acts as a powerful molecular switch mechanism in transducing growth signals. The *ras* proteins acquire transforming potential when an amino acid at position 12, 13 or 61 is replaced as a result of a point mutation in the encoding *ras* gene. About one-third of **adenocarcinomas** of the lung are associated with a point mutation in codon 12 of the K-*ras* oncogene and this mutation indicates a poorer prognosis (12 of 19 Ki-*ras*-positive patients died compared with 16 of 50 Ki-*ras*-negative ones). Cultured, immortalized, human bronchial cells that harbour viral K-*ras* form poorly differentiated adenocarcinomas when injected into immunodeprived 'nude' mice. For some reason the K-*ras* point mutations seem to be associated particularly with **adenocarcinomas** rather than with other morphological forms of cancer.

Chromosomal Deletions in Lung Cancer

One morphological variant of lung cancer, small cell lung cancer, shows two types of genetic abnormalities. One of these is amplification of the c-*myc* oncogene. The other is a deletion of part of the short arm of chromosome 3, which appears to occur in all small cell carcinomas. Whether the deleted material represents a tumour suppressor gene is not known, but it is certainly a possibility.

Classification of Lung Cancer

The purpose of any histological classification of tumours is twofold:
- to delineate subtypes with either a better or worse prognosis
- to recognize, preferably as a result of biopsy rather than resection, those types for which a given treatment (e.g. resection versus chemotherapy) is most appropriate

The most commonly used classification is that published by the World Health Organization (WHO) (*Table 33.7*). It is based on light microscopic appearances and thus can be applied by all practising pathologists without the need for sophisticated methods.

The most important practical distinction to be made when examining biopsy material is that between small cell carcinoma and non-small cell carcinoma, because the primary treatment modalities and prognosis are very different. Small cell carcinoma appears to spread outside

Table 33.7 World Health Organization Histological Classification of Malignant Epithelial Tumours of the Lung

Frequency (%)	Type
25–40	**Squamous carcinoma** Variant: spindle-celled squamous carcinoma
15–25	**Small cell carcinoma** a) oat cell carcinoma b) intermediate cell type c) combined oat cell carcinoma
30–50	**Adenocarcinoma** a) acinar adenocarcinoma b) papillary adenocarcinoma c) bronchioloalveolar adenocarcinoma d) solid carcinoma with mucus formation
10–20	**Large cell carcinoma** Variants: a) giant cell carcinoma b) clear cell carcinoma
	Adenosquamous carcinoma
	Carcinoid tumour
	Bronchial gland carcinomas a) adenoid cystic carcinoma b) mucoepidermoid carcinoma
	Others

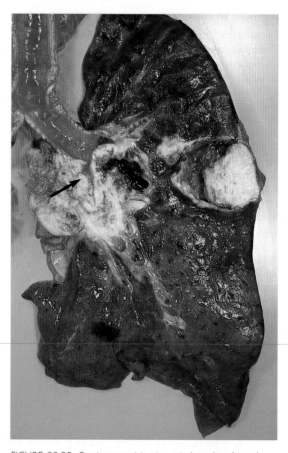

FIGURE 33.35 *Carcinoma arising in main bronchus (arrow) and extending deeply into the lung parenchyma.*

the confines of the lung at an early stage of its natural history, and is thus less likely to be amenable to resection.

Pathology

General Considerations

Most lung cancers, other than adenocarcinomas, arise centrally in the larger airways and in many resection specimens the site of origin can be identified on naked-eye examination (*Fig. 33.35*). The right lung is more frequently affected than the left and the upper than the lower lobes (except in the case of asbestos-related cancers where lower lobe tumours are commoner). Ulceration of the affected bronchus is often present; this causes the small haemoptyses that often call attention to the presence of cancer.

Growth into the airway frequently causes obstruction, leading to absorption collapse of the segment of lung distal to the obstruction. Obstruction also leads to impaired drainage of secretions from airways distal to the tumour; retention of such secretions increases the risk of infection and of bronchiectasis. Bronchial obstruction may also lead to 'endogenous lipid pneumonia', where lung parenchyma distal to the obstruction becomes consolidated as a result of the accumulation of large numbers of intra-alveolar lipid-filled macrophages. In large tumours, especially squamous carcinomas, central necrosis with cavitation may be a prominent feature and on radiography lesions may be mistaken for an abscess. Direct extension may involve the pleura and/or pericardium, and involvement of regional lymph nodes is seen in more than 50% of cases.

Squamous Carcinoma

Macroscopic Features

Squamous carcinoma is generally seen in relation to main or lobar bronchi, although peripheral examples are not rare. The cut surface of the tumour is greyish white and often rather friable. The appearance of its endobronchial component depends on the growth pattern, which may be predominantly exophytic (i.e. the tumour grows out into the bronchial lumen in a cauliflower-like fashion) or one where the tumour has partly destroyed the bronchial wall and spread extensively into the lung parenchyma.

Microscopic Features

Squamous carcinoma consists of irregular islands and strands of large malignant cells, often lying within a fairly dense fibrous stroma (*Fig. 33.36*). Giant nuclei with convoluted nuclear membranes and prominent nucleoli may be apparent, and atypical mitoses are common.

At least one of two histological features must be demonstrated before classifying an individual lung cancer as squamous. These are:

1) the presence of **keratin**
2) the presence of **intercellular bridges** or '**prickles**'

Keratinization may occur on an extensive scale with the formation of large laminated masses of keratin or may be comparatively slight with small central foci of keratin surrounded by concentric layers of tumour cells. Well-differentiated squamous tumours usually show abundant keratinization and the converse is true for poorly differentiated ones.

Intercellular bridging, regularly spaced cytoplasmic threads crossing the spaces between adjacent tumour cells, is one of the 'gold standards' for squamous differentiation. The bridges are cytoplasmic extensions of the tumour cells which are linked by **desmosomes** (button-like points of intercellular contact that hold adjacent plasma membranes together).

Where doubt exists as to squamous differentiation, some help may be obtained by the use of immunohistochemistry, **cytokeratins** 4, 10 and 13 in tumour cells being strongly suggestive of squamous differentiation, as is also **involucrin**, a soluble cytoplasmic precursor of the protein envelope of keratinized cells. These antigens can be identified by appropriate monoclonal antibodies.

If neither keratinization nor intercellular bridges can be found, the tumour is usually classified as a **large cell carcinoma**, although some of these may show evidence of squamous differentiation when examined by electron microscopy.

Small Cell Carcinoma

Small cell carcinoma usually runs a more aggressive course than other types of lung cancer, **early dissemination being a characteristic feature**. In most instances, the tumour has already metastasized by the time of diagnosis and is irresectable, although an initial response to radiotherapy and chemotherapy is not infrequent. **Of all lung cancers it is the one most frequently associated with paraneoplastic syndromes.**

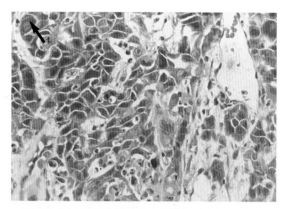

FIGURE 33.36 Squamous carcinoma showing intercellular bridges. An occasional tumour giant cell (arrow) is seen.

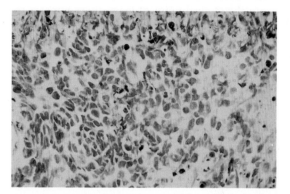

FIGURE 33.37 Small cell carcinoma. The small darkly staining cells are packed together, in this instance, into irregular nests and strands.

Microscopic Features

The cells, which are usually small (three to five times the size of a lymphocyte) or medium sized, are packed together in nests and strands (*Fig. 33.37*) and often show a ribbon-like arrangement. In bronchial biopsies the small cells may be seen to spread beneath intact lining epithelium. Stromal vessels may show deposition of purple material, which is tumour cell DNA. This finding, however, is not specific for small cell carcinoma and can occur in association with other highly cellular neoplasms. Clumps of the small dark tumour cells often show parallel orientation of their nuclei, giving an appearance similar to that seen with the crush artefact produced by less than optimal handling of small biopsies. This so-called 'streaming' of the tumour cells is very characteristic of the 'oat cell' variant of small cell carcinoma.

Small cell carcinomas often show evidence of neuroendocrine differentiation on ultrastructural and immunohistochemical examination.

On electron microscopy the hallmark of this is the presence of small cytoplasmic granules with a dense core, seen within 15–25% of the cells. The granules are circular and have a central electron-dense core surrounded by a clear halo. They average about 100 nm in diameter.

Immunohistochemical examination shows the enzyme neurone-specific enolase and the neural protein PGP 9.5 in many small cell carcinomas but this finding is not specific for small cell tumours. The presence of bombesin (gastrin-releasing peptide) has also been noted in many small cell carcinomas, as has synaptophysin (normally present in presynaptic vesicles). Low molecular weight cytokeratins can usually be identified but the higher molecular weight ones seen in squamous carcinoma are not present.

Intermediate Cell Carcinomas
From the clinical point of view, there appears to be no difference between the behaviour of the intermediate and oat cell variants of small cell carcinoma.

Microscopic Features
This variant has a cell population which in appearance and size lies between the 'oat cell' type and large cell carcinoma. Preservation tends to be better than in oat cell cancer and the 'streaming phenomenon' is not seen. The nuclei are larger and, because chromatin staining is not so intense, nucleoli are fairly easily seen. Neurosecretory dense-core granules are more easily found than in oat cell tumours.

Combined Oat Cell Carcinoma
This term is applied to cases in which oat cells are found in combination with squamous cell carcinoma (the most common combination) or with adenocarcinoma. This variant is more often seen in resected material or at post mortem than on biopsy.

Adenocarcinoma
Adenocarcinoma is the most frequent histological type occurring in women. In non-smokers with lung cancer, most of the tumours are adenocarcinomas, although smoking is a risk factor for this variant as well.

Macroscopic Features
Most adenocarcinomas occur peripherally, although some do arise centrally. Central scarring with or without the presence of dust pigment is quite common. It is virtually impossible to tell whether this scar tissue is elicited by the tumour or whether it preceded the tumour. Most pathologists now believe that true 'scar cancers' are rare and that the scarring seen in association with peripheral adenocarcinomas is, in most instances, a secondary phenomenon.

Microscopic Features
The criteria that must be satisfied before a lung cancer is classified as being an adenocarcinoma are:
- **the demonstration of mucin production**
- **the formation of tubular or papillary structures**

The presence of intracellular mucin can be demonstrated by the use of easy and commonly used staining methods (e.g. periodic acid–Schiff) It exists in the form of very small droplets or as somewhat larger vacuoles. Extracellular mucin accumulates within glandular lumina formed by the tumour cells.

The chief diagnostic difficulty is proving that a peripheral adenocarcinoma is **primary**, because the periphery of the lung is a common site for metastases to occur. The difficulty is compounded because adenocarcinomas arising in certain sites, most notably **the body and tail of pancreas, ovary and kidney**, may be clinically silent for a long time. On the basis of light microscopy alone it may be impossible to differentiate between one of these secondary deposits and a primary lung tumour, as both may show evidence of mucin production or assume a papillary pattern. In resection specimens, the problem may be somewhat easier: the presence of multiple tumours points towards a diagnosis of metastasis, whereas involvement of hilar nodes is more common in primary tumours. The presence of significant scarring in relation to a single peripheral tumour also supports the diagnosis of a lung primary.

Bronchioloalveolar Carcinoma
Although this tumour comes under the rubric of adenocarcinoma, it shows so many peculiarities that it merits separate consideration. It is not sex related, shows no predilection for any particular occupation or social class, and appears to be unrelated to cigarette smoking.

In the original WHO classification it was described as **'a highly differentiated adenocarcinoma originating in the peripheral part of the lung beyond a grossly recognizable bronchus and tending to grow upon the walls of pre-existing alveoli'**.

The outstanding histological feature is the presence of **'alveolar colonization' (i.e. growth of tall mucin-secreting cells, or cells with distinctive 'peg-like' luminal aspects, along the alveolar septa with no stromal reaction)**.

Mixed differentiation patterns may be seen, giving rise to the suspicion that there may be more than one cell of origin. What does appear to be important is the growth pattern of bronchoalveolar carcinomas along the alveolar septa, which allows viable tumour cells to spread through the lung via the airways (aerogenous spread) and thus give rise to satellite tumours at some distance from the site of origin.

Large Cell Carcinoma

Large cell carcinoma is rather unsatisfactorily defined on the basis of negative criteria as **'a non-small cell carcinoma in which neither squamous nor adenocarcinoma differentiation can be seen on light microscopy'**. Thus the diagnosis is made by excluding other better-characterized variants. The light microscope cannot be regarded as being in any way a final court of appeal, and use of electron microscopy and/or immunohistochemistry will remove a number of cases from the group of large cell tumours.

Microscopic Features

The tumours are usually composed of large cells which may assume various shapes. They have abundant cytoplasm and large irregular nuclei. Mitoses are common and multinucleate tumour giant cells are often seen. Where they predominate, the term **giant cell carcinoma** has been applied, although whether this is really a separate entity is still debatable.

Staging of Lung Cancer

The extent of spread of the tumour as shown by staging gives valuable information not only regarding the prognosis for an individual patient but also as to the most appropriate treatment.

Surgery is the best option for maximal survival. **Approximately two-thirds of lung cancers are inoperable at the time of diagnosis. Clearly, one wants to save such a patient from unnecessary surgery.** Part of the assessment for treatment involves factors such as the age of the patient, his/her general state of health and whether lung function is good or poor. All this having been said, however, **the ultimate decision must depend on whether or not the tumour can be shown to have spread to a point at which surgery should no longer be a favoured option**.

Staging a lung cancer has **two components**: intrathoracic and extrathoracic staging.

Intrathoracic Staging

This involves:

- **Assessment of the history and clinical findings.** For example, a patient with hoarseness, dysphagia or superior vena caval obstruction must have a significant degree of spread to the mediastinum.
- **Assessment by the use of imaging techniques.** The detection of mediastinal node enlargement on radiography indicates an inoperable lesion. Computed tomography (CT) has great advantages over conventional radiography for detecting nodal involvement and mediastinal invasion; CT has a sensitivity of 80–94% compared with the results obtained by mediastinoscopy and lymph node sampling, and the predictive value of a negative CT scan is of the order of 90–95%.

- If a pleural effusion is present, it should be examined **cytologically** after aspiration.
- **Mediastinoscopy.** CT has reduced the number of cases in which mediastinoscopy with lymph node sampling is appropriate. It remains, nevertheless, a useful step in preoperative staging.

Extrathoracic Staging

The chief modalities for extrathoracic staging in patients with lung cancer are clinical examination and biochemical screening.

Clinical Examination

This may show evidence of obvious extrathoracic spread in the form of organ enlargement (e.g. hepatomegaly) or signs (e.g. localizing neurological abnormalities) suggesting organ-specific abnormalities which can be followed up by imaging. If lymph nodes are palpable, this can be investigated by fine-needle aspiration and subsequent cytological investigation.

Biochemical Screening

This may produce evidence suggestive of spread. A **decrease in serum albumin concentration** is often a pointer to tumour dissemination and a **low serum sodium level points to a diagnosis of small cell carcinoma**, which is notorious for disseminating early. **Hypercalcaemia** may be due to the secretion of a parathyroid hormone-related peptide (PTHrP) by squamous cell carcinoma but may also be an indicator of bony metastases.

Pathological Staging

The most accurate evidence within the thorax is derived from careful examination of resected specimens. The system adopted for recording the stage of a given tumour is a modification of the **tumour–node–metastasis (TNM) system**. The results of follow-up suggest that gross involvement of any node in the mediastinum carries a poor prognosis in terms of survival. The precise limitations to carrying out resection in the face of some degree of mediastinal involvement are not yet certain.

OTHER PRIMARY EPITHELIAL TUMOURS OF THE LUNG

Carcinoid Tumours

Part of the cell population of the lower respiratory tract is made up of elements of the **diffuse neuroendocrine system**; these cells are present in the basal layer of the surface epithelium and in bronchial glands. Their numbers increase between bronchi and smaller airways, but they are seldom found in terminal bronchioles or acini. Electron microscopy shows numerous dense-core secretory granules, containing both peptide and steroid hormones. These include 5-hydroxytryptamine, bombesin (gastrin-releasing peptide), calcitonin and adrenocorticotrophic hormone (ACTH).

Carcinoids show neuroendocrine differentiation and account for about 1–2% of all primary lung neoplasms. Unlike bronchial carcinoma there is no predilection for either sex and the peak incidence occurs at a younger age than bronchial carcinoma. Neither smoking nor environmental pollution appears to act as a risk factor.

Sites of Predilection and Naked-eye Appearances

Carcinoids may occur either centrally or peripherally. In the former position, where the vast majority arise, they tend to draw attention to themselves by obstructing airways. The small proportion that are found peripherally may be asymptomatic.

Macroscopic Features

Typically, part of the tumour lies within the bronchial wall extending into the lung parenchyma, and part protrudes out into the bronchial lumen giving an appearance that has been likened to a dumb-bell or cottage loaf. The growing edge within the lung is often well defined and smooth, and is pseudoecapsulated by compressed lung tissue. The cut surface is either yellowish or a pale tan colour, an appearance seen in other endocrine neoplasms.

Microscopic Features

Most **'typical carcinoids'** are composed of a strikingly uniform cell population. The cells have dark, rather evenly stained, nuclei and inconspicuous small nucleoli. Cell outlines are very well defined and the cytoplasm is either clear or slightly granular.

A number of different architectural patterns may be seen. Most commonly the tumour cells are arranged in intertwining ribbons, cords or small islands, separated by narrow fibrous tissue septa containing thin-walled blood vessels. The degree of vascularization tends to be increased in peripherally situated carcinoids and, because the cells in these are often spindle shaped, peripheral carcinoid of this type can be mistaken for a primary malignant vascular neoplasm. In occasional cases islands of bone or cartilage may be seen in the stroma. Unlike carcinoids of mid-gut origin, the cells of bronchial carcinoids seldom display the **argentaffin reaction** (precipitation of silver salts in the absence of a reducing agent) but are frequently **argyrophilic** (silver salt precipitation in the presence of a reducing agent).

Confirmation of the diagnosis of one of these neuroendocrine tumours is most reliably and easily made by immunohistochemistry, where antibodies against the matrix protein, chromogranin, the enzyme, neurone-specific enolase and the neural protein PGP 9.5 bind to tumour cells. Peptide hormone or amine production by the tumour cells can be demonstrated quite frequently but clinical evidence of this is distinctly rare.

Natural History of 'Typical' Carcinoid

While all carcinoids should be regarded as potentially malignant, **only a very small proportion (6%) of typical carcinoids spread to local draining lymph nodes, and distant metastases are less common still**.

'Atypical' Carcinoids

The recognition of an atypical variant of lung carcinoid is important because these tumours behave in an aggressive manner, more than 70% of them eventually metastasizing. Atypical carcinoids, which account for about 11% of all lung carcinoids, show:

- nuclear pleomorphism with a coarser chromatin pattern and more prominent nucleoli than are seen in the 'typical' carcinoid
- a high mitotic rate
- areas of necrosis, which may be extensive

A number of other primary epithelial tumours may occur in the lung, arising chiefly from the bronchial glands. These are, however, rare and, like connective tissue, nerve sheath and vascular tumours, are best dealt with in specialist texts on lung pathology. An exception can, however, be made for the **bronchial adenochondroma**, which accounts for about 10% of all 'coin' lesions on chest radiography.

Adenochondroma (Chondroid Hamartoma)

For a considerable time, this lesion has been regarded as a **hamartoma** (a tumour-like malformation consisting of a disorganized proliferation of epithelial and connective tissue elements normally present in the lung).

Adenochondromas are, however, rare in childhood and continue to grow in adult life and thus

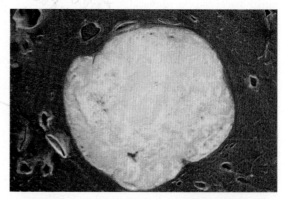

FIGURE 33.38 A well-defined mass consisting predominantly of cartilage. This is a typical adenochondroma (hamartoma) of the lung.

some writers now prefer to regard them as benign connective tissue neoplasms, the epithelial clefts that they contain being due to entrapment of epithelial structures within an expanding mass of neoplastic cartilage. Most are small to moderate in size (1–3 cm in diameter) (*Fig. 33.38*), but much larger examples sometimes occur. Other connective tissue elements such as bone, adipose tissue, fibrous tissue (sometimes dense, sometimes loose and myxoid) may be found. All are very well differentiated and are benign.

CLINICAL FEATURES OF LUNG CANCER

These result from the interaction of:
- **local spread** of the tumour
- **distant spread** of the tumour
- **paraneoplastic syndromes** (i.e. systemic effects not mediated by tumour spread)

Effects of Local Spread

Intrapulmonary Spread
Intrapulmonary growth may produce a number of effects (*Fig. 33.39*):
- **Cough** due to **irritation of bronchial receptors**
- **Haemoptysis** caused by **erosion of small blood vessels**
- **Airway obstruction** may cause **wheezing or, if the trachea is involved, stridor** and may also lead to **recurrent episodes of pneumonia** or to

bronchiectasis. Collapse of lung tissue distal to a bronchial obstruction may also be seen.
- Some patients complain of a dull aching type of **chest pain**. In cases of centrally situated tumours the mechanism responsible for this is not clear. In patients with peripheral carcinomas, chest pain is usually due to **involvement of the pleura**.

Direct Spread from the Lung to Neighbouring Tissues
Involvement of the pleura is likely to cause a **pleural effusion**.

Invasion of nerves cause effects related to the area supplied by the affected nerve. Involvement of the **recurrent laryngeal nerve** is associated with **hoarseness**, whereas that of the **phrenic nerve** causes **paralysis of the diaphragm**.

In carcinomas growing in the apical portion of the upper lobe (**Pancoast's tumour**), extension of the tumour may involve the **brachial plexus**, giving rise to **pain and weakness in the shoulder and arm** on the affected side, and the **sympathetic ganglia** may be similarly affected causing a **unilateral Horner's syndrome**. (Unilateral constriction of the pupil with slight ptosis and enophthalmos; some loss of sweating on the same side of the face is usually seen as well). This combination of effects, often associated with destruction of a rib, is known as **Pancoast's syndrome**.

Spread to the mediastinum with either involvement or **compression of the superior vena cava** gives rise to the **vena caval syndrome** (facial congestion, oedema of the face, neck and upper limbs, and distension of the veins in the neck and over the chest).

Chest pain or cardiac tamponade can follow

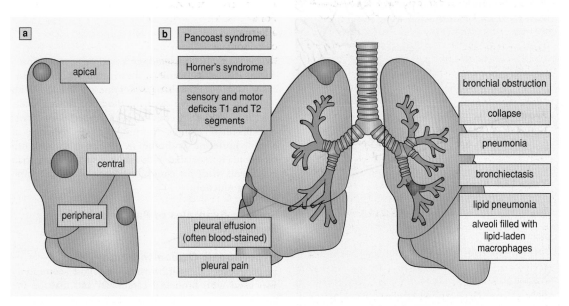

FIGURE 33.39 **a** *Principal sites within the lung at which carcinomas may arise.* **b** *Intrathoracic manifestations of bronchial carcinoma.*

invasion of the chest wall or pericardium respectively.

Effects of Distant Spread

The clinical effects of metastatic spread are, obviously, a function of the sites of the secondary deposits. The frequency with which local spread occurs is much the same for all histological varieties of lung carcinoma, but this is not the case with distant spread. Here it is the **small cell carcinoma that metastasizes to distant sites most frequently**, followed by adenocarcinoma and then by large cell carcinoma (see *Table 33.8*).

The commonest sites outside the thorax at which metastases, of all histological types, are found are shown in *Table 33.9*.

PARANEOPLASTIC SYNDROMES

Lung cancer may be associated with many systemic abnormalities unrelated to tumour spread (see *Table 33.10*). As these can sometimes be alleviated by tumour resection, it seems likely that they are mediated by tumour-derived chemical signals. In the endocrine and neuroendocrine syndromes that occur in patients with lung cancer, the chemical messengers are clearly the **peptide and steroid hormones** secreted, however inappropriately, by the tumour cells. In non-endocrine syndromes, the nature of the chemical messengers is still unknown.

Many hormones are produced by lung cancers (see *Table 33.11*), but in most cases their concentration is insufficient to produce the appropriate clinical syndrome. Small cell carcinoma is the histological type

Table 33.8 Residual Extrathoracic Disease at Post Mortem 1 Month After Lung Resection

Tumour type	Frequency of extrathoracic disease (%)
Small cell carcinoma	68.4
Adenocarcinoma	43.3
Squamous carcinoma	32.6

Table 33.9 Sites of Metastases

Site	Frequency (%)
Brain	44.7
Extrathoracic nodes	44.6
Liver	44.1
Adrenal gland	33.7
Bone	29.5
Kidney	23.6

Table 33.10 Paraneoplastic Syndromes in Lung Cancer

System	Condition
Non-endocrine	
General	Weight loss
	Fever
	Loss of appetite
Dermatological	Acanthosis nigricans
	Dermatomyositis
	Tylosis (marked hyperkeratosis of palms and soles)
Vascular	Thrombophlebitis migrans
	Non-infective thrombotic endocarditis
	Disseminated intravascular coagulation
Skeletal	Clubbing
	Hypertrophic osteoarthropathy
Nervous system	Cerebellar syndrome
	Peripheral neuropathies
	Myasthenia gravis-like syndrome
	Myositis
	Encephalopathy
Endocrine and neuroendocrine	
	Cushing's syndrome
	Inappropriate secretion of antidiuretic hormone
	Hypercalcaemia
	Gynaecomastia

most frequently associated with ectopic hormone production but other histological variants may also be associated with paraneoplastic endocrine syndromes. With increasingly sensitive assay methods becoming available, it is clear that a considerable number of lung cancers produce 'ectopic' hormones. The presence of ectopic hormone syndromes in patients with small cell carcinoma is associated with a shorter survival time than in patients with no clinical evidence of ectopic hormone production.

Specific Examples of Paraneoplastic Syndromes

Hypertrophic Osteoarthropathy

Hypertrophic osteoarthropathy is most commonly associated with bronchial carcinoma and may be the presenting complaint. About 12% of patients with bronchial carcinoma are so affected. Patients complain of wrist and ankle pain and swelling. On examination,

Table 33.11 Endocrine and Neuroendocrine Products of Lung Cancer

ACTH
Calcitonin
Parathyroid-related peptide
Antidiuretic hormone
Melanocyte-stimulating hormone
Growth hormone
Chorionic gonadotrophin
Insulin
Gastrin
Renin
Glucagon
Oestradiol
Erythropoietin
Histaminase
DOPA-decarboxylase
Carcinoembryonic antigen
α-Fetoprotein
Bombesin
Neurone-specific enolase

KEY POINTS: Neuromuscular Abnormalities Associated with Lung Cancer

The neuromuscular abnormalities described in association with lung cancer include:

- **Peripheral neuropathy**, which may be motor, sensory or mixed. Muscle weakness and wasting may be noted with loss of tendon reflexes and a 'glove and stocking' type of loss of sensation.
- **Autonomic neuropathy**, which may cause gastrointestinal and bladder disturbances and/or postural hypotension.
- **Cerebellar ataxia** characterized by nystagmus, dysarthria and impaired coordination.
- **Eaton–Lambert syndrome**, a **myasthenic** syndrome which differs from myasthenia gravis in that muscle function improves with repeated effort. This improvement with repetitive effort is mirrored by the changes seen on electromyography where there is an increase in the amplitude of, initially very small, action potentials.
- **Polymyositis–dermatomyositis**, which is a syndrome characterized by proximal weakness and by pain and tenderness in affected muscles. A purplish facial rash may be present and a variety of systemic symptoms may occur, including arthralgia, dysphagia and Raynaud's phenomenon.
- **Acute transverse myelopathy**, a very rare complication. It gives rise to a flaccid paraparesis with a sensory level and loss of control of sphincters. It can be difficult to distinguish this from secondary deposits in the spinal cord or from the effects of radiotherapy.

gross clubbing is usually present and there is thickening of the distal ends of the radius and ulna and of the tibia and fibula. This is due to a marked degree of periosteal new bone formation. The joints themselves may be hot and tender. Some degree of controversy exists as to the histological type of lung cancer most frequently associated with hypertrophic osteoarthropathy. All agree that small cell carcinoma is only rarely associated with the condition.

Blood flow in the calf and forearm is increased and, where clubbing of the fingers is also present, this hyperaemia extends to the distal phalanges and nail beds. The increased vascularity of the periosteum and subcutaneous tissue leads to localized oedema, which can involve adjacent tendons and ligaments.

The mechanisms responsible for hypertrophic osteoarthropathy remain a mystery. Some clinical evidence suggests that a vagal mechanism, as resection associated with vagal section or even suprahilar vagal section alone can result in symptomatic relief. Some response is also obtained when non-steroidal anti-inflammatory agents are used, suggesting that local prostaglandin release may play a part in producing the clinical features.

Non-metastatic Neuromuscular Syndromes

A wide variety of neuromuscular abnormalities has been described in association with lung cancer. **They are most commonly associated with small cell carcinoma** but can also be produced by other histological types. The mechanisms responsible are quite unknown.

Cushing's Syndrome

Cushing's syndrome was the first paraneoplastic endocrine syndrome to be described and is one of the commonest, accounting for about 2% of patients with lung cancer. Abnormalities in the metabolism of cortisol may be found in over 40% of patients with small cell carcinoma. The clinically affected patients do not usually present with a full-blown picture of Cushing's syndrome (see pp 840–842), and instead show anorexia, muscle weakness and mental slowing. **Urinary loss of potassium is the outstanding feature**, leading to **hypokalaemic alkalosis**. The syndrome occurs most commonly in patients with small cell carcinoma or, occasionally, with carcinoid tumours. The hormone responsible for the biochemical changes is usually 'big' ACTH, the precursor of the active ACTH molecule.

Occasionally, ACTH secretion is accompanied by secretion of melanocyte-stimulating hormone, which leads to a progressive increase in melanin pigmentation of the skin.

Inappropriate Secretion of Antidiuretic Hormone

Inappropriate secretion of antidiuretic hormone, usually by a small cell carcinoma, causes significant dilutional hyponatraemia (plasma sodium concentration of less than 120 mmol/l). Plasma osmolality is low (less than 260 mosmol per kg water) and urinary osmolality is high, being at least twice that of the plasma.

There may be no symptoms or the patient may complain of weakness, nausea, vomiting, anorexia and headache. Severe hyponatraemia causes confusion and forgetfulness and, at very low plasma concentrations of sodium (less than 115 mmol/l), fits and coma may occur.

Hypercalcaemia Not Associated with Bony Secondaries

Malignant disease is the commonest cause of hypercalcaemia in the hospital population. Although this is often due to destruction of bone by osteolytic metastases, severe degrees of hypercalcaemia may occur as a paraneoplastic syndrome. **In the case of carcinoma of the lung, squamous carcinoma is the variant most frequently associated with this syndrome.**

Ectopic production of true parathyroid hormone is very rare and most of these paraneoplastic hypercalcaemias are due to the secretion of PTHrP (see pp 262, 1051). Antibodies to the N-terminal end of PTHrP can reduce the hypercalcaemia and prevent bone changes in animal models of paraneoplastic hypercalcaemia.

Inappropriate Secretion of Chorionic Gonadotrophin

About 5% of patients with lung cancer develop gynaecomastia owing to the ectopic secretion of chorionic gonadotrophin. Any histological type of lung cancer can produce this hormone but the syndrome is said to occur most often in association with variants of large cell carcinoma.

The Pneumoconioses

Pneumoconiosis is legally defined as **permanent alteration of lung structure due to the inhalation of mineral dusts and the tissue reactions which follow this. It includes asbestos-related disease, coal miners' pneumoconiosis and silicosis.**

Mechanisms of Injury in the Dust Diseases

The lung reacts in different ways to the presence of retained dust particles. These reactions range from a trivial local aggregation of dust-filled macrophages at one extreme to diffuse or massive local fibrosis, with or without cavitation, at the other. The character and severity of these reactions depend on the interaction between three sets of factors (*Fig. 33.40*):

- **the intrinsic properties of the dust**
- **the amount of dust retained and the duration of exposure**

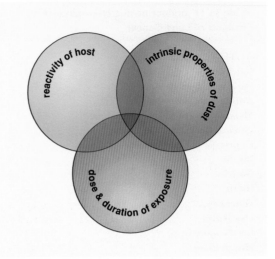

FIGURE 33.40 Interacting factors in dust diseases of the lung.

- **modifications, which may be the result of individual idiosyncrasy and immunological reactivity of the person exposed.**

Each of these factors poses complex problems, not as yet completely solved. However, it is clear that **in the encounter between the lungs and dusts of various types, the phagocytic cells within the lung are of crucial importance. Not only do they engulf the lung particles, but their reactions to the dust determine the reaction pattern of the tissues and thus the natural history of the disease.**

Sedimented dust particles on the lining of the peripheral airways and airspaces are engulfed by resident macrophages. If the particles are very numerous, alveolar clearance mechanisms are overloaded and dust-laden macrophages accumulate. Type 1 pneumocytes proliferate at this stage and grow over the macrophages, which are thus separated from the airspace lumen. Large aggregates of macrophages may bulge into the airspace, and even obliterate the latter. Meanwhile, a delicate supporting framework of fine reticulin fibres develops between the macrophages. If the dust is fibrogenic, these fine fibres are replaced by coarser collagen bands and a palpable nodule can develop.

ASBESTOS-RELATED DISEASE

Asbestos is a set of fibrous silicates, known for about 2000 years for their fire-resisting properties.

Physically, two forms of asbestos exist; the fibres may be either curly (**serpentine**) or straight (**amphibole**). Serpentine fibres tend to shear into short fragments while the straight, stiff amphiboles remain intact. The only important serpentine form is **chrysotile** (white asbestos – the name being derived from the Greek word for golden) The chief members of the amphibole group are:

- **crocidolite** (blue asbestos), the name of which is derived from a Greek word meaning **flaky**
- **amosite** (brown asbestos), from, *A*sbestos *M*ining *O*rganization of *S*outh Africa
- **anthophyllite**, from the Latin '**clove**'
- **tremolite**, from the town of Tremola in Switzerland

Asbestos, largely because of its heat-resistant properties, is used in the manufacture of a wide range of products. These include articles made from asbestos cement (corrugated roof tile), vinyl floor tiles, brake linings, wicks for oil heaters and many others.

Asbestos has also been used extensively for lagging boilers and pipes in ships and steam locomotives. Industrial exposure occurs under many circumstances, ranging from the mining process to stripping of asbestos lagging, and demolition of buildings in which asbestos has been used in the construction. The domestic use of asbestos products does not seem to constitute a hazard but **mesothelioma**, a malignant neoplasm arising from serosal lining cells, has been reported in the female relatives of some workers exposed to asbestos. It is believed that these women became exposed by washing asbestos-impregnated overalls belonging to their partners.

Pathological Expressions of Asbestos Exposure

Major intrathoracic lesions resulting from asbestos exposure are:

- **asbestosis – a form of interstitial fibrosis affecting mainly the posterior segments of the lower lobes**
- **benign pleural disease: pleural plaques, diffuse pleural thickening**
- **mesothelioma**
- **carcinoma of the lung**

While a not insubstantial number of cases of asbestos-related disease is seen in the UK at the moment (**500 deaths annually from mesothelioma and 150 from asbestosis**), the Asbestos Industry Regulations that came into force in 1970 have significantly reduced the dangers of exposure to asbestos.

How do Asbestos Fibres Reach their Intrapulmonary Targets?

Despite their considerable length (sometimes up to 200 μm), asbestos fibres appear to have little difficulty in reaching the ultimate destination within the chest: the parietal pleura. The 'falling speed' of a fibre and, hence, its tendency to sediment within the respiratory tract depend on the **square of its diameter** and are influenced hardly at all by fibre **length**. The curly serpentine fibres of chrysotile have a much greater cross-sectional area than amphibole fibres and thus penetrate for a much shorter distance down the airway than the latter. Because all types of asbestos have tissue-damag-

ing potential, this may account for the fact that chrysotile does not often cause lung disease. Fibre length does, however, have some effect on the final destination of the fibres: those with a length of 50–100 μm can reach the alveoli, whereas longer fibres tend to be deposited in the respiratory bronchioles and alveolar ducts.

The Fate of Inhaled Asbestos Fibres

Most inhaled asbestos fibres are ingested by macrophages and cleared from the lung either via the mucociliary escalator mechanism or via lymphatic drainage, chrysotile clearance being greater than that of amphiboles.

Asbestos Bodies

The asbestos body is the microscopic hallmark of asbestos exposure (*Fig. 33.41*). These structures, which may be found in the lung as little as 2 months after exposure, are about 80 μm long and are usually golden-yellow or brown in colour. The asbestos body consists of an amphibole fibre, either wholly or partly coated with layers of yellow-brown, iron-containing protein. This iron–protein coat is usually segmented, giving the effect of a bamboo cane, with swellings at one or both ends. The use of Perl's stain to demonstrate iron makes it much easier to see the asbestos bodies, especially if they are scanty. Uncoated asbestos fibres far outnumber asbestos bodies but they are difficult to see on light microscopy. In asbestosis there may be up to 100 000 000 amphibole fibres per gram of dried lung tissue.

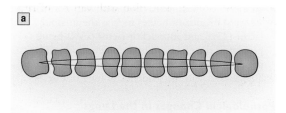

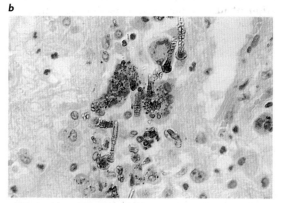

FIGURE 33.41 **a** *Diagram of an asbestos body.* **b** *Banded golden-yellow asbestos bodies within lung tissue.*

Asbestosis

The characteristic fibrosis affects chiefly the lower lobes. It is often associated with fibrous thickening of the pleura over the affected portions of lung, something not seen in the fibrosis of cryptogenic fibrosing alveolitis (see pp 439–441). It can take up to 20 years from the time of exposure for asbestosis to develop, but if exposure has been continuous over a substantial period, fibrosis may appear in as few as 5 years.

Asbestosis shows the same pathophysiological consequences as other diseases in which interstitial scarring occurs: **a reduction in pulmonary compliance and evidence of disordered gas exchange due largely to ventilation–perfusion mismatch**.

Pathogenesis

As with other forms of lung fibrosis, **activation of pulmonary macrophages, with release of cytokines, oxygen free radicals and growth factors, may provide a common pathway for the cell damage and subsequent scarring**. It is known that inhalation of asbestos fibres is followed by the activation of a complement-dependent chemoattractant for macrophages.

Bronchoalveolar lavage samples from patients with asbestosis show an increase in the number of intra-alveolar macrophages and lymphocytes in about 40% of cases. The intra-alveolar lymphocyte population shows a decline in the T helper : suppressor cell ratio and, in the blood, natural killer cells may show decreased function. Other abnormalities related to the immune system, reported in patients with asbestosis, include:

- an increase in the serum concentrations of immunoglobulins
- an increased likelihood, compared with normal subjects, of autoantibodies such as rheumatoid factor (23%) and antinuclear factor (25%) being present in the plasma. These autoantibodies are present in only about 3% of individuals exposed to asbestos but with no evidence of lung disease.

Pathological Changes in the Lungs

The earliest changes occur in respiratory bronchioles where there is maximal fibre impaction. Alveoli opening directly from these bronchioles show fine septal scarring associated with an increase in both septal and intra-alveolar macrophages and in type 2 pneumocytes. Some of the latter contain small intracytoplasmic, eosinophilic inclusions resembling Mallory's hyaline bodies (tangled bundles of intermediate filaments) seen within the hepatocytes in a variety of liver diseases. The significance of this is not known.

Subpleural areas are severely affected and eventually advanced disturbance of lung architecture with **'honeycombing'** is seen. Asbestos bodies may be seen both within alveoli and adjacent to areas of scarring. The pleural fibrosis that often accompanies intrapulmonary scarring due to asbestos shows no diagnostic features. Asbestosis is graded as shown in *Table 33.12*.

Table 33.12 Grading of Asbestosis

Criterion	Grade
Amount of lung substance involved	
	A – none
	B – less than 25%
	C – 25–50%
	D – more than 50%
Severity of fibrosis and distortion of lung architecture	
	From 0 (none) to 4 (severe)

Benign Pleural Disease

Asbestos exposure can lead to various forms of pleural disease, the commonest being the formation of well-defined localized **pleural plaques**. These are markers of asbestos exposure, not the forerunners of asbestos-related pleural tumours or of asbestosis, although they may be associated with the latter in a small number of cases. They can occur after exposure to any form of asbestos, the correlation with anthophyllite being strongest. There is also an epidemiological correlation with populations living in areas where the **soil** is contaminated with asbestos, such as Finland, Bulgaria and Greece, and with proximity to asbestos mines and processing plants.

The plaques appear as shiny, white, well-demarcated, thickened areas, chiefly on the parietal pleura, and look rather like the sugar icing on a Chelsea bun. Histologically they consist of dense collagen fibres, sometimes arranged in a 'basket-weave' pattern. The plaques often show some focal dystrophic calcification and small collections of lymphocytes and plasma cells.

Diffuse pleural thickening may also occur in some patients who have a history of asbestos exposure. It is much less clearly dose related than either asbestosis or malignant mesothelioma. The thick layer of scar tissue, involving the visceral pleura, may cause increasing difficulty with expansion of the lung, giving rise to shortness of breath on exertion. In instances of unilateral involvement, there may be some doubt, clinically, as to whether a malignant mesothelioma is present. In these cases pleural biopsy should resolve the difficulty.

Malignant Mesothelioma

Malignant mesothelioma is a neoplasm arising from the stem cell compartment of mesothelium. Thus the most common sites are the pleura and peritoneum, although sometimes the pericardium or tunica vaginalis of the testis may be involved.

Epidemiology

The very existence of mesothelioma was a controversial issue until the latter part of the 1950s when, not only did mesothelioma become established as a distinct entity, but its association with asbestos exposure was finally acknowledged. This followed a report of crocidolite exposure in 32 of 33 cases of malignant pleural mesothelioma. It is now accepted that the vast majority of mesotheliomas are caused by asbestos exposure, although a small number of cases apparently lacking this history are seen.

In Britain, the incidence of mesothelioma is still rising and will probably reach its peak about the year 2000. This reflects the long latent period between exposure and diagnosis of tumour (20–40 years).

Males are affected far more often than females – a reflection of their greater chance of occupational exposure. The tumour can occur at any age, but in view of its generally long latent period the majority of the patients present between the ages of 50 and 70 years.

Fibre Type and Size in Relation to the Pathogenesis of Mesothelioma

It is difficult to assess the potential tumour-inducing qualities of different forms of asbestos because many of those exposed have encountered a mixture of dusts. However, it is clear that **amphiboles are more dangerous in this connection than serpentines** and that, of the amphiboles, **crocidolite** has most tumour-inducing potential.

Fibre diameter and length, even within the same species of asbestos, both appear to be significant variables. Fibres with a **diameter less than 0.5 µm** and a **length of more than 8 µm** are cleared less readily than fibres of larger diameter, and are thought to have more oncogenic potential. The fibres are believed to work through the lung tissue and eventually to penetrate the visceral pleura and its lymphatics.

Mesothelioma has also been found to be linked causally with exposure to a form of fibrous silicate known as a zeolite, of which erionite is perhaps the best-known example. Erionite, consisting of very fine fibres, has been thought to be the culprit in a localized 'epidemic' of mesothelioma occurring in Anatolian Turkey where the erionite was used as a building material. In two villages 50% of all the deaths were recorded as being due to malignant mesothelioma, an annual incidence more than 900 times as great as normally expected.

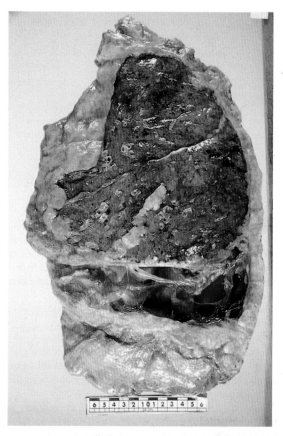

FIGURE 33.42 Malignant mesothelioma. The lung is surrounded by a thick sheath of yellowish-white tumour tissue which extends into the interlobar fissure.

Macroscopic Features

Mesothelioma can arise from either the visceral or the parietal pleura; the right side is more frequently involved than the left. The tumour grows over the pleural surface of the lung including the fissures, resulting in a striking appearance with the dark, somewhat compressed, lung tissue being surrounded by a thick layer of white tumour tissue, which may separate widely the upper and lower lobes (*Fig. 33.42*).

Microscopic Features

Mesothelial cells differentiate along several pathways. This is reflected in considerable diversity both within a single tumour and between different tumours. Tumours are usually classified as falling into one of four groups:

1) tubulopapillary ('epithelial')
2) sarcomatous, composed of spindle-shaped, collagen-producing cells
3) undifferentiated polygonal celled
4) mixed forms

The epithelial type shows some resemblance to adenocarcinoma of the underlying lung and its differentiation from this tumour may be difficult. If there is appropriately fixed material, transmission electron microscopy shows characteristic long, slender microvilli on the surface of the mesothelial cells, but these may be absent in poorly differentiated examples.

In practice, **the distinction between the epithelial type of mesothelioma and adenocarcinoma is usually made on the basis of certain features which are absent from the former.** The presence of neutral mucin in the tumour cells strongly supports a diagnosis of adenocarcinoma, as does the presence of two tumour markers, carcinoembryonic antigen and β_1 pregnancy-specific glycoprotein (SP1). Searching for asbestos bodies is unhelpful, as they are not usually found within mesotheliomas, although they are often present in the underlying lung tissue. In cases where there is difficulty in distinguishing reactive mesothelial cells from malignant ones, the presence of the epithelial antigens human milk fat globule 1 and 2 supports a diagnosis of malignancy, while positive staining for α_1-antichymotrypsin occurs in reactive cells but not in malignant ones.

Tumour Spread

Direct extension of mesothelioma to involve the pericardium and pleura over the diaphragm is common, as is the presence of a pleural effusion in more than 70% of epithelial and mixed forms of mesothelioma. Distant metastases occur in a number of sites, the commonest being:

- lymph nodes
- kidney
- liver
- central nervous system

Such metastases are twice as common in association with the sarcomatous variety of mesothelioma as in the epithelial or mixed forms.

Pathophysiology

As the tumour increases in bulk, it gradually ensheathes the lung in a jacket of tumour and fibrous tissue, causing a restrictive ventilatory defect and leading to increasing shortness of breath.

Pleural effusions, when present, are commonly blood-stained and have the high protein concentration characteristic of an exudate. The prognosis is uniformly bleak.

COAL MINERS' PNEUMOCONIOSIS

In the days when 'coal was king' 3000 miners were diagnosed each year as having occupationally related pulmonary disease. Studies after the Second World War into the epidemiology and pathogenesis of coal-related lung disease have fed through in the form of a variety of preventive measures. So successful have these been that the incidence of coal miners' pneumoconiosis has now fallen in the UK to fewer than 400 cases annually. Most of these are older members of the miners' cohort, the disease now being rare in miners who are less than 50 years old.

Coal miners' pneumoconiosis results from interaction between:

1) The **length and intensity of exposure** and, hence, the total bulk of dust inhaled.
2) The **nature of the coal dust**. The composition

of coal varies with its 'age' and geographical location. Thus it may be difficult to compare the degree of risk and the pathogenetic mechanisms operating in one coalfield with those found in another. Two types of coal exist: high rank (which contains more carbon and less mineral) and low rank (which contains less carbon and more mineral).

High-rank coal is more toxic to macrophages in culture systems than low-rank coals and, in the UK at least, this type appears to carry a greater risk of lung disease. In mines where the coal is of high rank, the development of pneumoconiosis appears to be related directly to the amount of coal dust inhaled during a working life. In low-rank collieries, the mineral content of the coal appears to be a more important factor.

Coal miners' pneumoconiosis is divided into two major pathological types:

- **simple**
- **complicated**

Simple Pneumoconiosis

Simple pneumoconiosis does not usually cause symptoms.

Macroscopic Features

The basic lesion is a small black macule, 2–5 mm in diameter, most numerous in the upper zones. These can be seen easily on both the pleural surfaces, where they cluster along the lymphatics, and the cut surface.

Microscopic Features

The lesions are usually star-shaped and consist of aggregates of dust-laden macrophages. The target area for their development is the centre of the lung acinus.

Mild centriacinar emphysema may be seen. Some authorities regard this as a distinctive form of focal emphysema causally related to the accumulation of coal dust, whereas some others do not accept that these lesions are essentially different from those of centriacinar emphysema found in the general population.

If the dust is fibrogenic, the macules may progress to become nodules which, unlike the former, are palpable. The nodule differs from the macule in that it has a much greater content of collagen. As this collagen increases, so the macule gradually loses its star-shaped appearance and becomes rounded.

Microscopic examination of nodules in polarized light usually shows the presence of small amounts of birefringent crystalline material, which may be mica or kaolinite. Nodular lesions are more likely to develop as a result of inhalation of low-rank coals with a higher mineral content.

Complicated Pneumoconiosis

Complicated pneumoconiosis also known as **progressive massive fibrosis**, defined as the presence of black collagen-rich nodules exceeding 1 cm in diameter.

Macroscopic Features

The lesions may be single or multiple and occur most commonly in the upper lobes and towards the posterior aspect of the lungs. When situated near the lung periphery, progressive massive fibrosis is often associated with pleural scarring and puckering. The nodules vary somewhat in shape; a striking feature is their well-demarcated margins, which makes them look almost as if they had been 'dropped' into the surrounding lung tissue.

The cut surface of the lesions is commonly homogeneously black and uniformly hard and rubbery. Some of the lesions, however, undergo central necrosis, which can lead to cavitation, and contain semifluid areas that may scintillate because of the presence of crystalline cholesterol.

Microscopic Features

Lesions consist of rather haphazardly arranged mixtures of dust and fibrous tissue. The connective tissue component has been shown to be rich in fibronectin. At the periphery of the lesions, dust-filled macrophages and a small number of chronic inflammatory cells may be seen. Small blood vessels in the adjacent tissue may show infiltration of their walls by lymphocytes and the lumina may be narrowed or even obliterated.

There appear to be two pathways for development of the lesions of progressive massive fibrosis:

1) fusion of several individual small nodules
2) enlargement of a single nodule

The first of these patterns seems to be associated with exposure to coal with a relatively high mineral content, the second with exposure to coal with a lower mineral content.

Caplan's Syndrome

Caplan described a syndrome characterized by nodular lesions in the lungs of coal miners with rheumatoid disease. These lesions appeared in miners in whom the total dust burden was thought to be relatively low and did not correlate with the degree of severity of the rheumatoid disease. It is now recognized that this syndrome is not confined to coal miners and may occur in patients with rheumatoid disease who have been exposed to silica–containing dusts.

Macroscopic Features

The lesions are often situated subpleurally. They are usually multiple, fairly large (up to 5 cm in diameter), round in shape and laminated in appearance.

Microscopic Features

The most characteristic feature is the presence of dust within the nodules, the dust being arranged in the form of circumferential bands. Apart from this feature they look very much like large rheumatoid nodules with a typical peripheral palisade of fibroblasts and macrophages, and a central zone of necrosis in which the dust is located.

SILICOSIS

This is a severe disabling chronic disease resulting from the occupational inhalation of silica or silicon dioxide. Silica should not be confused with the silicates, in which the anion is a combination of silicon and oxygen and the cation aluminium or magnesium.

Exposure to silica may occur in:

- mining in circumstances where drilling into siliceous rocks takes place
- quarrying
- manufacture of bricks, tiles and pottery
- foundry work
- sandblasting

Mechanism of Injury in Silicosis

It is believed that a major pathogenetic factor is a toxic effect on the lysosomal membranes of macrophages that have ingested the silica in a crystalline form. Crystalline silica is fibrogenic and cytotoxic to macrophages, whereas amorphous silica is harmless. Of the crystalline forms, tridymite is the most harmful and quartz the least.

Following engulfment of the silica dust within phagosomes, fusion of the phagosome and the primary lysosome takes place to form a secondary lysosome. In the case of silica ingestion, abnormal hydrogen bonds form between the surfaces of the silica particles and the lysosomal membranes, presumably because of the strong hydroxyl groups on the particle surfaces, which can act as hydrogen donors. This is followed by lysosomal rupture and the release of the lysosomal enzymes into the cytosol of macrophages. The macrophages, when studied in cell culture, round up, become immobile and soon disintegrate, liberating not only the cytoplasmic contents but also the offending silica particles, which can be ingested by other macrophages with a similar cytotoxic effect.

Microscopic Features

The evolution of silicotic nodules starts with focal laying down of collagen following the macrophage–silica interactions described above. As the nodules mature, the fibroblast population decreases and the nodules become hyaline and relatively acellular.

Macroscopic Features

On macroscopic examination the pleura is seen to be scarred and thickened, and the visceral and parietal layers often show adhesions.

The lung itself feels nodular and when cut, shows the presence of many small nodules (2–6 mm in diameter), which have a whorled pattern and which tend to be dark grey in colour. The lesions occur most frequently in the upper and posterior zones of the lungs. Liquefaction of the centres of these nodules seldom occurs in the absence of tuberculosis complicating the silicosis. Fusion of the nodules may occur, with the formation of much larger lesions.

Relationship Between Silicosis and Tuberculosis

Silicosis is a recognized predisposing factor for the development of tuberculosis. Inhalation of quartz by guinea-pigs is followed by reactivation of healing tuberculous lesions and is also followed by the occurrence of tuberculous lesions when guinea-pigs are exposed to normally non-pathogenic strains of *Mycobacterium tuberculosis*. Other mycobacteria such as *M. kansasii* and *M. avium intracellulare* also appear to be important pathogens complicating silicosis.

'Rheumatoid' Silicotic Nodules

In the presence of rheumatoid disease or in patients who have circulating rheumatoid factor in the absence of overt signs of rheumatoid disease, silicotic lesions show some deviation from the usual form. The lesions are larger than usual and frequently have central areas of necrosis.

Clinical Features

Silicosis is characterized by exertional dyspnoea, which starts insidiously and gradually increases in severity. This is accompanied by an irritating cough and, in the later stages, weight loss proceeding to emaciation may be present. Chronic bronchitis or tuberculosis may complicate the picture.

The chest radiograph is characteristic, with discrete opacities being present in the early stages. The small lesions may coalesce to form larger, more irregularly shaped, opacities measuring 1 cm or more in diameter and, eventually, shadows comparable with those seen in progressive massive fibrosis of coal miners may appear. The development of such lesions is associated with marked clinical deterioration.

Disorders of the Pulmonary Circulation

PULMONARY EMBOLISM

Pulmonary embolism is the commonest disorder affecting the pulmonary vascular system, accounting for 50 000 deaths annually in the USA. There are differing accounts of the frequency with which evidence of embolization is found within the pulmonary circulation at post-mortem examination but it is not less than 10% in unselected material.

Source of the Emboli

Most pulmonary emboli are derived from venous thrombi in the lower limbs. More than 80% of such occur in calf veins but it is the relatively small proportion involving larger thigh veins that account for most major clinical episodes of pulmonary embolization. Pelvic veins may be the site of origin in some patients who develop pulmonary embolization following gynaecological surgery, and some cases result from right atrial thrombi.

The risk factors for pulmonary embolism are obviously much the same as those for venous thrombosis (see pp 206–208). These include:
- **stasis** of venous blood
- **a hypercoagulable state**

Natural History

The clinical presentations of pulmonary emboli are essentially four in number:
1) massive pulmonary embolism resulting in sudden death or severe strain on the right ventricle
2) silent embolism with little or no clinical effect
3) medium-sized embolism giving rise to pulmonary infarction
4) recurrent embolism leading to a chronic rise in pulmonary artery pressure and, eventually, to congestive cardiac failure (**cor pulmonale**)

These effects of pulmonary embolism are the result of the interaction between three factors (*Fig. 33.43*).

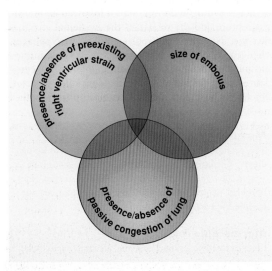

FIGURE 33.43 Factors determining the outcome in pulmonary embolization.

These are:

1) The **size of the embolus**, which naturally correlates with the size of the pulmonary artery that becomes occluded.

2) The **state of the pulmonary circulation**, with particular reference to the presence or absence of passive congestion associated with left ventricular failure or mitral valve disease.

3) The presence or absence of **right ventricular hypertrophy**.

Massive Pulmonary Embolism

Massive pulmonary emboli can occlude either the main left or right pulmonary arteries or the main pulmonary artery as it exits from the right ventricle. Obviously a large mass of thrombotic material is needed for this to occur. Because the diameter of the main pulmonary artery is greater than that of the femoral or iliac veins, occlusion is accomplished by coiling up of the embolus into a loose knot. At post mortem such an embolus can often be uncoiled and seen to be a cast of a considerable length of the venous drainage of the lower limb, the sites of valves often being clearly visible.

The patient may die suddenly, not infrequently while straining at stool, or may present with:

- right-sided heart failure associated with severe shortness of breath and a rapid pulse
- cardiovascular collapse with hypotension, syncope or coma

Such acute, severe syndromes are the expression of emboli that have obstructed more than 50% of the pulmonary circulation.

The pathogenetic mechanisms responsible for such life-threatening situations are still not understood. It is obviously tempting to ascribe the clinical effects of massive pulmonary embolization purely to obstruction that would be expected to throw a considerable strain on the right ventricle on the one hand, while the amount of blood that manages to pass the obstructing embolus would be insufficient to fill the left side of the heart and thus maintain a normal systolic arterial blood pressure. This may well be an oversimplification, as the inflation of a balloon catheter within one of the main pulmonary arteries, in a conscious individual, produces no symptoms, although there may be a slight (5 mm) increase in pulmonary artery pressure.

Additional factors operating in the massive pulmonary embolism syndromes may include:

a) release of vasoactive humoral factors such as thromboxane A_2 and leukotrienes from platelets accumulating at the site of impaction

b) presence of compromised cardiac function as a result of pre-existing cardiopulmonary disease

In patients with no pre-existing cardiopulmonary disease, reduction of the pulmonary vascular bed by 25% or more increases the right ventricular afterload. To compensate for this, the pressure in both the pulmonary artery and the right ventricle rises, a normal right ventricle being able to generate a pressure of approximately 40 mmHg. As right ventricular afterload increases acutely, the chamber dilates, tricuspid incompetence occurs and the right side of the heart becomes hypokinetic. This acute failure of the right ventricle leads to cardiogenic shock. In patients whose cardiac function is already somewhat compromised, smaller pulmonary emboli obstructing only one or two lung segments can exert the same haemodynamic effect as much larger ones.

So far as the blood gases are concerned, there is characteristically a reduced arterial partial pressure of oxygen, caused by a combination of ventilation–perfusion mismatching and shunting of blood through parts of the lung that are underventilated. Arterial partial pressure of carbon dioxide is usually normal or reduced.

Diagnosis of acute pulmonary embolism may present severe problems, which may be eased by the use of radioactive nuclide imaging. **A normal perfusion lung scan is sufficient to rule out a diagnosis of pulmonary embolism**, although, of course, defects in perfusion can be produced by many conditions other than pulmonary embolism. **Pulmonary embolism is, however, the only condition that produces a defect in perfusion without any accompanying defect in ventilation.** If, therefore, a ventilation scan is performed using a radioactive gas such as krypton or xenon, and this is normal in the face of defective perfusion, a confident diagnosis of pulmonary embolism may be made. The 'gold standard' for diagnosis remains pulmonary angiography.

Embolism Leading to Pulmonary Infarction

Pulmonary infarction occurs in some, but by no means all, instances where medium-sized emboli obstruct peripheral arteries in the lung. It is not altogether clear why only some of these emboli lead to the formation of infarcts, although in animal models medium-sized emboli do *not* cause infarction **in the absence of congestion of the pulmonary venous circulation**. Extrapolating from this model, one would expect to see a higher risk of pulmonary infarction in patients with left ventricular failure or with high pulmonary vein pressure secondary to mitral valve disease; in fact, this is the case. However, from time to time pulmonary infarction (confirmed histologically) occurs following embolization in patients who appear otherwise healthy with regard to the heart and lung.

Pulmonary infarcts occur more commonly in the lower than in the upper lobes of the lungs. This may be because pulmonary venous pressure is higher in the lower lobes when the individual is in the upright position.

Macroscopic Features

The infarcted area is usually wedge shaped, the base of the wedge being just under the pleural surface of the lung, and the occluded vessel at the apex of the wedge (*Fig.*

33.44). The lesion often has a dull bluish-red colour; one of its most striking features is the sharp demarcation from the surrounding lung tissue. Infarcted tissue is generally much firmer in consistency than normal lung and is swollen, usually standing proud of the surrounding tissue. At post mortem, infarction can be identified easily by running the fingertips over the pleural surface. The overlying pleura shows the presence of a fibrinous exudate, and a small pleural effusion is often present.

Microscopic Features

Histologically, one of two alternative appearances may be seen. The first is true necrosis, termed 'complete infarction' while the second and commoner finding is where the airspaces are filled with blood but the alveolar walls appear viable ('incomplete infarction'). Complete infarction is much rarer than the incomplete variety, probably because of the dual blood supply of the lung parenchyma, which receives blood not only via the pulmonary arteries but also from the bronchial arteries arising from the aorta. Complete infarcts become converted to inconspicuous fibrous scars, whereas incomplete infarcts may resolve completely, the affected area of lung becoming, ultimately, normally aerated once again.

The Fate Of Pulmonary Emboli

In occlusive emboli, the earliest reaction in the underlying vessel wall is dilatation of the adventitial vasa vasorum, followed by an inflammatory reaction with infiltration of neutrophils into the embolus at points of attachment to the vessel wall. In experimental models, the occluding emboli begin to retract within the first few hours. Not only does this allow blood to percolate past the embolus but it facilitates contact with blood-borne fibrinolytic agents. The ordinary processes of organization follow and whatever remains of the thrombus becomes converted to neointima, consisting of fibromuscular tissue. In the case of occlusive thrombi, **the combination of lysis, retraction and organization often leads to the formation of fibrous bands**, criss-crossing the lumen.

Non-occlusive or mural emboli usually organize into eccentric fibromuscular intimal thickenings.

Cor Pulmonale Occurring as a Result of Recurrent Pulmonary Embolization

Recurrent pulmonary embolization is often cited as a cause of pulmonary hypertension leading to right ventricular hypertrophy and congestive cardiac failure (**cor pulmonale**), although it is, in fact, very rare. It is suggested that this is the expression of showers of emboli which, individually, are too small to cause either acute strain on the right ventricle or pulmonary infarction. Ultimately the stimulatory effect on intimal connective tissue that all thrombi exert may produce a sufficient degree of obstruction to blood flow through the small

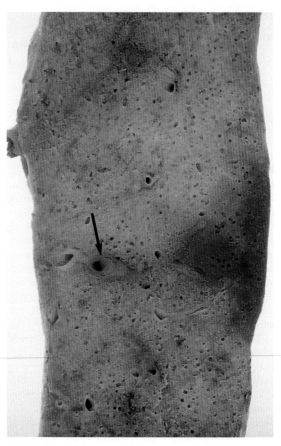

FIGURE 33.44 Pulmonary infarction secondary to embolization. Note the red, roughly wedge shaped, subpleural area of infarction. An embolus (arrow) can be seen in the feeding vessel.

vessels of the lung to lead to chronic pulmonary hypertension and congestive heart failure.

PULMONARY HYPERTENSION

Pulmonary hypertension is defined as a systolic/diastolic pressure in the pulmonary artery consistently exceeding 30/15 mmHg. There are many causes of pulmonary hypertension and, where possible, it is helpful to classify them in relation to the chief pathogenetic mechanisms involved (*Fig. 33.45*):

- **hyperkinetic** (increased pulmonary blood flow)★
    congenital heart disease characterized by major left to right shunts
- **pulmonary venous causes**
    left-sided heart disease
        left ventricular failure
        mitral valve disease
    pulmonary veno-occlusive disease
- **embolic**
    thromboembolic

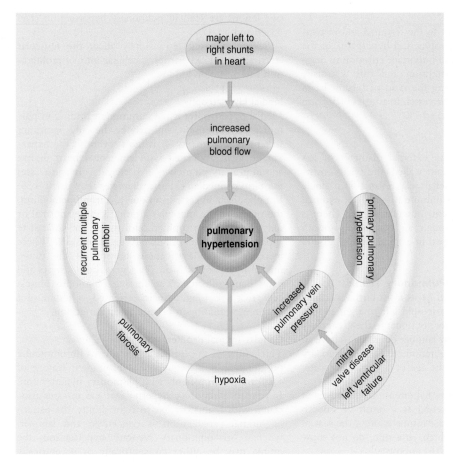

FIGURE 33.45 Causes of pulmonary hypertension.

parasitic (schistosomes)
tumour emboli
- **severe and extensive pulmonary fibrosis**
- **hypoxia**
- **'primary' pulmonary hypertension★**
- **pulmonary hypertension associated with cirrhosis of the liver★**

Entities marked with an asterisk are associated with a highly characteristic lesion known as **plexogenic pulmonary arteriopathy**.

Vascular Lesions of Pulmonary Hypertension

Vascular lesions seen in pulmonary hypertension are most easily understood against the background of the normal histology of the pulmonary vascular bed.

Normal Histology

The Pulmonary Trunk

Significant differences exist between the structure of the aorta and the main pulmonary trunk, these relating to the wide divergence in pressure between the two vascular beds. The intima of the pulmonary trunk is much thinner than that of the aorta; the architecture of the media is much more irregular; and elastic laminae are fewer in number and more widely spaced and irregularly shaped than in the aorta. During fetal and early postnatal life these differences are much less marked and by 9 months of age it is normally easy to distinguish histologically between the pulmonary trunk and the aorta. In certain forms of congenital heart disease, most notably post-tricuspid shunts, pulmonary hypertension persists after birth and the pulmonary trunk never loses its structural resemblance to the aorta.

Conducting Arteries

These are the arteries extending from the pulmonary trunk down to vessels having an external diameter of 1 mm and accompanying the airways. Their most striking feature is the large amount of medial elastic tissue, in contrast to the relatively scanty elastic seen in the pulmonary trunk. In vessels near the hilum of the lung there may be as many as 20 parallel elastic laminae but this number decreases as successive branches get smaller, there being only three or four laminae in the 1-mm diameter vessels.

Muscular Arteries

These arteries lie adjacent to the terminal and respiratory bronchioles. Hypertrophy and hyperplasia of the media in these vessels is an important criterion in diagnosing pulmonary hypertension and this is usually accomplished by measuring the ratio of the media to the external diameter of the vessel. In arteries of 300 μm or less, this should not exceed 7%.

Pulmonary Arterioles

These are vessels with an external diameter of less than 100 μm. They are thin walled, the wall consisting of a layer of endothelial cells resting on a single elastic lamina which is continuous with the external elastic lamina of the parent muscular artery. There is no media as such, although an occasional smooth muscle cell may be wrapped in a spiral fashion around the vessel.

Lesions Affecting the Pulmonary Trunk

If pulmonary hypertension exists from birth, as it may do in patients with post-tricuspid left to right shunts, the media of the trunk does not undergo the usual postnatal change and the elastic laminae continue to have an embryonic aortic configuration. If the pulmonary hypertension arises after the age of 1 year, this 'aortic configuration' is not seen.

In later-onset pulmonary hypertension, the media of the trunk becomes thickened as a result of smooth muscle hypertrophy and the intima is often the seat of atherosclerotic lesions, which, as a rule, do not show erosion and superimposed thrombosis.

The main forms of post-tricuspid shunts which can cause pulmonary hypertension from birth are:

- ventricular septal defects
- single ventricle
- a wide patent ductus arteriosus
- aortopulmonary septal defect
- persistent truncus arteriosus

Pretricuspid shunts in the form of high atrial septal defects or anomalous pulmonary venous drainage also cause pulmonary hypertension, but in these cases there is a long period of high pulmonary blood flow before pulmonary hypertension develops.

Lesions of the Conducting Arteries

The principal changes seen in these vessels in pulmonary hypertension are much more atherosclerosis than in age-matched controls, hypertrophy of the medial smooth muscle and an accumulation within the media of acid sulphated mucopolysaccharides, giving an appearance rather similar to what is seen in the aorta in patients with aortic dissection.

Lesions of the Muscular Arteries

The main determinant of vascular resistance in the pulmonary circulation is the state of tone of the muscular arteries, and it is here that the most striking and exten-

sive lesions are seen in pulmonary hypertension (*Figs 33.46* and *33.47*).

Several different lesions may affect the muscular arteries: medial hypertrophy, cellular intimal proliferation and dilatation lesions.

Medial Hypertrophy

Medial hypertrophy is the commonest finding in pulmonary hypertension, and may be the only significant structural abnormality. It is most severe in the hyperkinetic form associated with congenital heart disease and in primary pulmonary hypertension. In some cases the ratio of media : external diameter may reach 0.25. In pulmonary hypertension due to thromboembolism, the media of the muscular arteries is either normal or only mildly hypertrophied, and much the same state applies in hypoxic pulmonary hypertension. Where increased pulmonary venous pressure is the cause, medial hypertrophy is usually severe, both arteries and veins being affected. The finding of smooth muscle cells that are longitudinally oriented is also a not uncommon finding in pulmonary hypertension.

Cellular Intimal Proliferation

Thickening of the intima as a result of fibromuscular proliferation is a frequent and prominent feature of small arteries in patients with pulmonary hypertension. In primary pulmonary hypertension and in cases associated with high-flow left to right shunts, the pattern of intimal proliferation is concentric and laminar, whereas in pulmonary venous hypertension the intima may be either concentrically or eccentrically thickened but shows absence of a laminar pattern. In the remaining varieties, the intimal thickening is usually eccentrically situated giving a plaque-like appearance. The appearance of significant amounts of collagen within the thickened intima is regarded as evidence of increased severity of the pulmonary hypertension.

Dilatation Lesions

Dilatation lesions are found characteristically in hyperkinetic pulmonary hypertension, in patients with primary pulmonary hypertension and in cases where pulmonary hypertension is associated with chronic liver disease.

All of them occur proximal to an occlusive lesion in a muscular pulmonary artery. Three variants have been described, although all three may result from the same pathogenetic mechanism: a 'blow-out' of a segment of a weakened artery wall.

Plexiform Lesions These are aneurysmal dilatations typically affecting the smallest muscular arteries and arterioles. The wall of the sac is made up of a single thin elastic lamina with, in some instances, a few smooth muscle cells. The sac itself is filled with cellular connective tissue in which a number of endothelium-lined

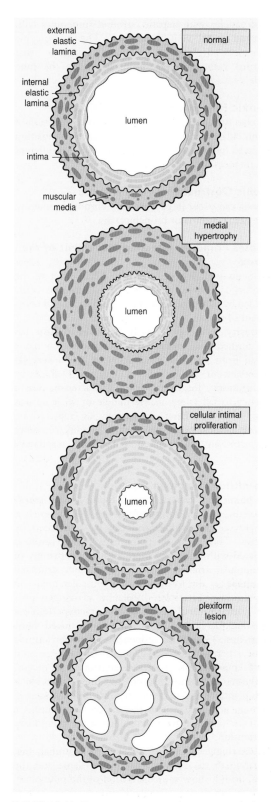

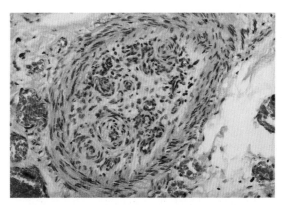

FIGURE 33.47 A muscular artery showing features of a plexiform lesion. The arterial lumen is filled with cellular connective tissue in which numerous small lumina can be seen.

channels can be seen. This picture is probably the expression of organization of a thrombus.

Simple Dilatation Lesions These are aneurysmal sacs similar to the lesions described above but without any of the cellular proliferation within the sac characteristic of the plexiform lesion.

Angiomatoid Lesions These consist of multiple, dilated, thin-walled vessels that link a severely hypertrophied muscular pulmonary artery with its capillary bed.

Fibrinoid Necrosis or Necrotizing Angiitis This is a rare lesion in pulmonary hypertension, occurring only when pulmonary artery pressure is both very high and has risen rapidly. As in other examples of fibrinoid necrosis affecting small arteries, there is evidence of smooth muscle cell necrosis, an accumulation of fibrin (which can be identified immunohistologically) and, often, an acute inflammatory reaction.

Lesions of the Pulmonary Arterioles

Normal pulmonary arterioles have no media but in pulmonary hypertension a muscular media may be formed. If the hypertension is sufficiently severe, changes similar to those described in relation to the muscular arteries may be seen. Grading of pulmonary vascular lesions is summarized in *Table 33.13*.

Is Hyperkinetic Pulmonary Hypertension Reversible by Correcting the Congenital Cardiovascular Defect?

In the case of congenital cardiac defects leading to pulmonary hypertension, it is essential to know whether the pulmonary hypertension is reversible before undertaking corrective surgery. The consensus view is that **grades 1–3 are reversible** but that **the presence of plexiform lesions or fibrinoid necrosis constitutes a contraindication to surgery**.

FIGURE 33.46 Changes seen in muscular arteries in the lung in pulmonary hypertension.

Table 33.13 Grading of Pulmonary Vascular Lesions

Grade	Pathological features
1	Medial hypertrophy
2	Grade 1 + cellular intimal proliferation
3	Grade 2 + intimal fibrosis
4	Grade 3 + plexiform lesions
5	Grade 4 + dilatation (angiomatoid lesions)
6	Grade 5 + necrotizing arteritis

SPECIFIC TYPES OF PULMONARY HYPERTENSION

Primary Pulmonary Hypertension

Primary pulmonary hypertension is a diagnosis that should be made only when all other recognized causes have been excluded, if necessary, by histological examination of open lung biopsy. A not inconsiderable number of patients with this clinical diagnosis have been found to be suffering from pulmonary hypertension due to recurrent pulmonary embolization.

It is a rare condition that can occur at any age but is more frequently found in children and young adults. Females are affected more commonly than males (1.7:1). About 30% of the patients have antinuclear factor in their serum and about 10% show Raynaud's phenomenon.

Microscopic Features

Microscopic features are the same as those seen in severe hyperkinetic pulmonary hypertension and, as in this condition, plexogenic changes and fibrinoid necrosis are often present. Marked medial hypertrophy and a high grade of intimal proliferation are seen, the latter being characterized by a concentric distribution and a laminar pattern. The cause of this disorder is not known but it is believed that the rise in pressure is due to vasoconstriction and that primary pulmonary hypertension is an analogue of essential systemic hypertension.

In pathophysiological terms, the patients show severe pulmonary hypertension and a reduced cardiac output. Exercise causes pulmonary artery pressure to rise steeply and the effect of this is to impair still further the function of the right ventricle; some patients experience syncope under these circumstances. Eventually, right-sided heart failure supervenes with oedema and ascites, but some patients die suddenly before this stage is reached. The only effective treatment is heart–lung transplantation.

Pulmonary hypertension with identical histological appearances has also been recorded in a small number of patients with hepatic cirrhosis, sometimes with associated portal vein thrombosis. The microscopic appearances (plexiform lesions) suggest that abnormal vasoconstriction is occurring in the lung vessels.

Hypoxic Pulmonary Vascular Disease

Hypoxia, from whatever cause, leads to constriction of the muscular arteries in the lung. Reduced ventilation leading to hypoxia occurs under a number of different circumstances.

Chronic Obstructive Airway Disease

Hypoxia can occur in patients with chronic bronchitis, emphysema, asthma or bronchiectasis.

Diseases Primarily Affecting Movement of the Thorax

In patients with **kyphoscoliosis**, if the onset of the deformity is very early in life, the situation is compounded by failure of development of the normal complement of alveoli.

Obesity associated with hypoventilation has been termed the 'Pickwickian' syndrome – a name derived from Dickens' description of Joe, a very fat boy-servant of Mr Wardle of Dingley Dell. Apart from gluttony, Joe's outstanding characteristic was a tendency to fall asleep in the middle of what he was doing; this has been interpreted as representing daytime apnoea, possibly related to obesity or, more likely, to an unexplained failure of respiratory drive.

High-altitude Hypoxia

Mild pulmonary hypertension is found among members of the native-born population in the Andes. It is more severe in children and can be aggravated by exercise. This form of pulmonary hypertension is associated with only very mild medial hypertrophy of the muscular arteries; the most prominent structural abnormality is the formation of a muscular media in the pulmonary arterioles. Inhalation of oxygen produces partial reversal of the pulmonary hypertension, suggesting that it is due to a hypoxia-induced vasoconstriction. Change of residence to a lower altitude produces permanent reversal, implying that regression of the muscularization of the arterioles can occur. With increasing age, some of these individuals develop intimal proliferation in small blood vessels in the lung, and this intimal fibrosis probably means a loss of the potential for reversibility of the pulmonary hypertension.

Interestingly, species of non-human mammals that are native to the Andes, such as the llama and the alpaca, do not show muscularization of the pulmonary arterioles and thus do not develop pulmonary hypertension, despite the fact that their entire lives are spent in a state of mild hypoxia.

Subacute Mountain Sickness in Children

Fifteen cases have been reported of the fairly rapid onset of fatal pulmonary hypertension in children of Han origin, born and normally resident at low altitudes, who had been moved to Lhasa, Tibet, which has an altitude of 3600 m. The illness usually starts with cough and progresses to congestive cardiac failure. At necropsy there is striking right ventricular hypertrophy, the weight of the right ventricle being four times that of age-matched controls. The pulmonary trunk is dilated and both muscular pulmonary arteries and pulmonary arterioles show medial hypertrophy. Children born in the Tibetan highlands are affected by this disorder only very rarely.

This disorder appears to be the human analogue of a disorder seen in cattle which is known as 'brisket' disease. Brisket disease affects cattle, especially calves, moved from a low to a high altitude and manifests as pulmonary hypertension associated with congestive cardiac failure, the oedema associated with this particularly affecting the chest region or 'brisket'. It has been suggested that both the infants and cattle are prone to develop subacute mountain sickness because of the persistence of fetal type muscular pulmonary arteries during the first few months of life.

Pulmonary Venous Hypertension

Pulmonary venous hypertension secondary to heart disease can occur in any patient in whom the left atrial pressure is raised. However, severe pulmonary vascular changes appear to be confined to cases of mitral stenosis.

Mitral stenosis differs from other causes of pulmonary hypertension in two essentials:

1) The vascular lesions often show **regional variations** within the lung.
2) **All categories of vessels are involved.** Thus histological changes are found not only in arteries but also in capillaries, veins and lymphatics. The high postcapillary pressure may also lead to other characteristic changes within the lung parenchyma, such as aggregates of iron-containing macrophages (haemosiderosis), patchy interstitial fibrosis and even such oddities as focal intra-alveolar ossification.

The **pulmonary trunk** is dilated and, together with the elastic conducting arteries, shows a degree of atherosclerosis more severe than in age-matched controls.

The **muscular arteries** show medial hypertrophy; the mean ratio of medial thickness to external diameter is about twice the normal value. Intimal fibrosis is also seen; it is of the eccentric variety and is often associated with the presence of thrombi.

Pulmonary **arterioles** develop a well-formed media and, in some instances, also show intimal thickening.

The pulmonary **capillaries** are grossly dilated and engorged with red cells, particularly in the lower zones.

The pulmonary **veins** show medial hypertrophy, and elastic laminae arrange themselves around the smooth muscle cells in a manner reminiscent of what is seen in arteries. This appearance is termed 'arterialization'.

Lymphatics, especially those in oedematous interlobar septa near the lung bases, are grossly dilated. These altered septa account for the Kerley B lines seen on chest radiography in patients with mitral stenosis.

Pulmonary Veno-occlusive Disease

This is a rare disease of unknown aetiology occurring principally in children and young adults. In adulthood, men are affected roughly twice as often as women, but this sex difference is not seen among affected children.

The basic pathological change is obliteration of the lumina of pulmonary veins by scar tissue, accompanied by a severe degree of medial hypertrophy; consequently it may be difficult to identify the affected vessels as veins. This can be accomplished by noting the **location** of the affected vessels. Intrapulmonary veins are sited along the interlobular septa, whereas arteries are found in the central part of the lung acini in relation to the airways.

Obstruction to the venous outflow results in severe interstitial oedema, which may be followed by fibrosis. Incorrect diagnosis of interstitial fibrosing lung disease can be made if care is not taken to examine the veins. Pulmonary haemosiderosis, not surprisingly in view of the very high postcapillary pressures that are achieved, is a prominent feature of veno-occlusive disease. It takes the form of intra-alveolar collections of iron-laden macrophages (a familiar feature of other types of vascular disease associated with high pulmonary vein pressure), and of encrustations of capillary basement membranes and elastic laminae in veins, seen as blue-staining deposits of iron and calcium.

Disorders of the Pleura

The number of disorders **primarily** affecting the pleura is small, consisting essentially of:

- infections occurring in the absence of underlying lung disease
- neoplasms, of which the only important example is malignant mesothelioma (see pp 470–472)

Pleural disease is much more commonly a **secondary** manifestation, either of local inflammatory or neoplastic disease within the lung or of a systemic disorder such as systemic lupus erythematosus.

PLEURAL EFFUSION

Most pleural disorders are expressed in the form of excess fluid (greater than 15 ml) within the pleural cavity (pleural effusion). Such effusions may amount to more than 1 litre. Effusion in this, as in other serosal cavities, is brought about by the same basic mechanisms that mediate oedema formation in other situations:

- **increased intravascular hydrostatic pressure** such as occurs in congestive cardiac failure
- **increased vascular permeability** associated either with inflammation or with the abnormally leaky vessels found when serosal linings are involved by tumour
- **decreased plasma oncotic pressure** occurring in hypoproteinaemic states as, for example, in the nephrotic syndrome
- **decreased lymphatic drainage** due to obstruction of or trauma to the thoracic duct, or tumour-related obstruction to lymphatics at the hilum of one of the lungs

With the exception of increased microvessel permeability, the effusions in all cases are transudates (i.e. the protein concentration is low). Where thoracic duct obstruction is the cause of the effusion, the excess pleural fluid is opaque and yellowish-white because of the presence of lipid. The lipid may separate out when aspirated pleural fluid has been allowed to stand for some time.

Characteristics of Pleural Effusions

In the pleura, as in other serosal cavities, the type of fluid depends on:

- the relative amounts of water and protein
- the type and concentration of cells present in the fluid

Thus effusions may be:

- **serous** (in which large amounts of fluid are present)
- **fibrinous** (in which large amounts of polymerized fibrin are deposited on the serosal surfaces)
- **serofibrinous**
- **purulent** (indicating bacterial or fungal infection)
- **haemorrhagic** (due to pleural involvement by tumour or, more rarely, an abnormal bleeding tendency or rickettsial infection). Haemorrhagic exudates must be distinguished from haemothorax, in which blood collects in the pleural cavity.

Haemothorax may result from leakage from an aneurysm of the thoracic aorta, aortic dissection or trauma to the chest.

Serous Effusions (Hydrothorax)

These are, for the most part, non-inflammatory in origin. Pleural inflammation may be associated with the outpouring of abundant fluid in which small fibrin clots may be seen; this is not uncommon in tuberculosis in young adults. Non-inflammatory serous exudates are seen most frequently in patients with congestive cardiac failure. In such cases the effusion is usually, but not invariably, bilateral.

Inflammatory Effusions

These are most commonly associated with lesions in the underlying lung tissue (inflammatory or non-inflammatory). **Infective lung lesions** associated with a pleural reaction include those of tuberculosis, pneumonia, lung abscess and infected bronchiectasis (see pp 436–438).

Bacterial seeding of the pleura leads to the formation of a purulent exudate in which the fluid is opaque because of large numbers of inflammatory cells. Infection may reach the pleura from:

- extension from the underlying lung
- the external environment as a result of penetrating injuries
- a subphrenic abscess
- the bloodstream in bacteraemic states
- oesophageal rupture resulting in mediastinitis
- thoracic surgery

If frank pus is present in the pleural cavity, this is described as **empyema**.

Non-infective processes causing effusion include pulmonary infarction, rheumatoid disease, systemic lupus erythematosus and uraemia.

Other important conditions, **pneumothorax** and **malignant mesothelioma**, are described on p 430 and pp 470–472 respectively.

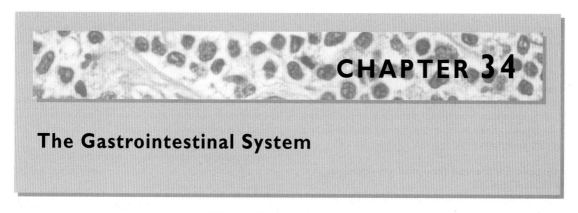

CHAPTER 34

The Gastrointestinal System

The Oral Cavity

NORMAL ANATOMY

The oral cavity is lined by stratified squamous epithelium similar to that of the skin. Within this single anatomical location, the epithelium varies in respect of the presence and/or pattern of keratinization. In addition, there are variations in the presence or absence of rete ridges: these are absent from the floor of the mouth and well marked in the palate and gum.

In view of the structural similarities, it is not surprising that many oral disorders are homologues of those found in skin and other squamous epithelium-covered surfaces (see pp 988–1033).

CONGENITAL AND INHERITED DISORDERS

MAJOR DEVELOPMENTAL ANOMALIES

Hare-lip and Cleft Palate

Facial clefts, of which more than 200 types are described, are common, occurring in about 1 per 800 live births. The basic mechanism is failure, at about the seventh week of gestation, of the facial processes to fuse, the gap between them normally being bridged by ectomesenchyme. Recent studies indicate that abnormalities in growth factors may be linked with malformations, for example, mutation of the transforming growth factor-α gene has been described in some cases of facial clefting.

The most common defect is clefting of the upper lip (**hare-lip**). This results from failure of fusion of the lower part of the median nasal process with the maxillary process. In more than 80% of cases, this clefting is unilateral and in two-thirds of these the cleft is left sided. There is some predilection for males: the male : female ratio is 3 : 2. This may be due to the fact that some cases of hare-lip are inherited in an X-linked recessive pattern.

The degree of clefting of the upper lip varies ranging from a small notch to one side of the philtrum to a large cleft extending into the nostril on the affected side.

Hare-lip may be an isolated defect, but in 50% of cases it is associated with a cleft palate. The lat-

ter also varies in severity. In some it is expressed merely as a bifid uvula, whereas in others there is complete clefting. Cleft palate, as an isolated defect, is less common than hare-lip, occurring in about 1 per 2500 live births. Unlike hare-lip, isolated cleft palate is more common in females.

Cleft palate is also found in about 40% of cases of a curious set of congenital anomalies, the **Pierre Robin syndrome**. This comprises:
- **an abnormally small mandible**
- **backward displacement of the chin**
- **a small tongue that is displaced posteriorly and downwards into the hypopharynx. This results in obstruction to the upper airway**

Cleft palate is seen also as part of the gamut of abnormalities associated with certain major chromosomal abnormalities, such as trisomies 13 and 18.

Hemifacial Hypertrophy

In this condition, both hard and soft tissues on one side of the face grow more rapidly than those on the other side. The teeth on the affected side and also half the tongue may be affected, the latter showing the presence of hypertrophied papillae.

FOCAL ABNORMALITIES

Fordyce's Granules

These are small yellowish-white granules situated either on the lateral part of the vermilion of the upper lip or in the buccal mucosa. They represent ectopic development of sebaceous glands. They are common, occurring in more than 50% of normal adults, and have no clinical significance.

Congenital Lip Pits

These are small fistulae connecting the surface squamous epithelium with underlying mucous glands. They are usually bilateral and occur on the lower lip. The pits may be associated with hare-lip, cleft palate and agenesis of the second premolars, or may be an isolated phenomenon. In the first of these, the abnormalities appear to be inherited in an autosomal dominant fashion.

Endogenous Pigmentation

Melanin pigmentation of the lips, oral mucosa and circumoral skin occurs in several conditions. These include **neurofibromatosis, fibrous dysplasia of** bone, **Addison's disease, haemochromatosis** and the **Peutz–Jeghers syndrome**. In the latter syndrome there is distinctive freckling of the vermilion of the lips, a useful sign of the possible presence of small intestinal hamartomatous polyps.

Multiple Endocrine Neoplasia Syndrome (MEN) Type IIb

For a description if this syndrome, see pp 856–872.

Congenital Epulis

This is a mass, present at birth, occurring in the gum. It consists of aggregates of large granular cells covered by well-differentiated squamous epithelium. In haematoxylin and eosin-stained material, these cells cannot be distinguished from those of granular tumour (see below). Electron microscopy suggests an origin from either fibroblasts or the perivascular pericyte. Unlike the cells of granular tumour, binding of the antibody to S-100 protein does not occur. The lesion occurs almost exclusively in females and is benign.

White Sponge Naevus

This is an autosomal, dominantly inherited disorder. The lesions appear as shaggy white patches on the oral mucosa; the buccal areas are most frequently involved. The thickened squamous epithelium of which the lesion is composed is extremely oedematous and tends to desquamate, the underlying surface being macroscopically normal. Microscopic examination shows the patches to be composed of well-differentiated but hyperplastic squamous epithelium in which there is marked intracellular and intercellular oedema.

INFLAMMATORY LESIONS OF THE MOUTH, LIPS AND TONGUE

Inflammatory lesions of the oral mucosa may be **infective** or **non-infective** in nature.

BACTERIAL INFECTIONS

Acute Ulcerative Gingivitis

This is a painful condition characterized by ulceration of the gum between the teeth and usually caused by a *mixture of* **spirochaetes** and **fusiform bacteria**. These organisms flourish in an anaerobic environment and thus tissue breakdown promotes their growth. Malnutrition enhances the risk of developing this disorder.

Actinomycosis

Actinomyces species form part of the normal mouth flora; their presence alone is not sufficient to cause disease. It is suggested that invasion of the oral tissues by these organisms occurs as result of abrasions, but the latter are very common whereas actinomycosis is comparatively rare.

The lesions present as firm mucosal swellings from which pus containing typical 'sulphur granules' exudes. These granules consist of colonies of Gram-positive filaments surrounded by eosinophilic club-shaped bodies, which may be immune complexes.

Microscopic examination shows the lesions to be abscesses with zones of central necrosis surrounded by granulation and fibrous tissue.

Tuberculosis

Oral tuberculosis is uncommon in the West. It is usually due to spread from a pulmonary lesion. The tongue is most frequently involved, showing irregular ulcers.

Syphilis

Syphilis affecting the oral cavity is now rare. This site can, however, be involved in all three stages of the disease:

- Chancres may occur on the lips or tongue.
- In the secondary stage, the mucosa may be involved by 'snail-track' ulcers.
- The gummatous lesions characteristic of tertiary syphilis may affect the tongue or palate.

VIRAL INFECTIONS

Herpes Simplex Virus (HSV)

In the oral cavity HSV type 1 is usually responsible for inflammatory lesions. These may occur in two forms.

Acute Herpetic Gingivostomatitis (Vincent's Angina)

This is most frequent in small children aged 1–3 years. The oral mucosa shows blisters and ulcers, associated with fever and enlargement of draining lymph nodes. Lesions usually heal within 2–3 weeks.

Herpes Labialis (Cold Sores)

This is the commonest **recurrent** disease produced by HSV-1. Localized clusters of vesicles occur usually at the junction between the skin and the lip vermilion. Vesicles rupture and painful ulcers form, which heal without scarring. Such lesions may recur repeatedly in the same location.

Recurrence is due to latency of the virus within trigeminal ganglion neurones. The virus becomes latent in these neurones because of the presence of a repressor for the viral IE (intermediate–early) gene.

Herpes Zoster

Varicella zoster virus most commonly affects the skin, but may involve the oral mucosa. The lesions are usually unilateral and initially take the form of painful vesicles on a reddened mucosa.

Coxsackie Virus Type A

Coxsackie viruses (named after the town of Coxsackie in the USA) are enteroviruses divided into two large groups, A and B. Certain strains of A virus (2, 4, 5, 6, 8, 10) cause **herpangina**, a disorder characterized by the abrupt onset of fever, sore throat, anorexia, dysphagia, and vomiting or abdominal pain. The oropharynx is reddened and shows discrete vesicles on the anterior pillars of the fauces, palate, uvula and tongue. The disorder is self-limiting.

Human Papillomavirus (HPV)

The most obvious evidence of HPV infection is the presence of warts. Some lesions show the typical microscopic features of an HPV infection such as koilocytosis, but in others such features are lacking. The possible role of HPV in relation to the causation of oral cancer is discussed later in this chapter.

Human Immunodeficiency Virus (HIV) and the Mouth

The oral manifestations of HIV are due chiefly to a decline in cell-mediated immunity, consisting principally of **infections and neoplasms**.

Oral infections in HIV-positive individuals may be bacterial, viral or fungal in origin. Of the fungal infections **candidiasis** is commonest, affecting between 50 and 70% of HIV-infected individuals. Lesions due to HSV and HPV are also seen, as is a curious condition known as **'hairy leucoplakia'**.

Hairy leucoplakia occurs almost exclusively in patients infected with HIV, although many, perhaps the majority, have no clinical features of acquired immune deficiency syndrome (AIDS) at the time of presentation. Most patients have had homosexual relationships or have been intravenous drug abusers. Patients present with white patches, usually sited on the lateral borders of the tongue, which have a corrugated or 'hairy' surface.

Microscopic examination shows the epithelial thickening and the hyperkeratosis characteristic of all types of leucoplakia. **The diagnostic hallmark is the presence within epithelial cells of herpes-type intranuclear inclusions, and cytoplasmic expansion or 'ballooning' is present in the deeper part of the epithelium.** Immunohistochemical studies show that the inclusions react with antibodies against HPV, but this is believed to be the result of a cross-reaction and that the aetiological agent is the Epstein–Barr virus. Associated infection with *Candida albicans* is very common, both yeasts and hyphae being seen in the surface keratin.

Bacterial infections leading most commonly to periodontal disease of differing grades of severity are also frequent.

The most common neoplasm to be associated with HIV infection is Kaposi's sarcoma (see pp 1031–1032). In patients with AIDS who have Kaposi's sarcoma, lesions are present in the oral cavity in about 50%, the palate being the site affected most frequently.

FUNGAL INFECTIONS

The most important fungus affecting the oral cavity is *C. albicans*.

Oral Candidiasis (Thrush)

This is most common in neonates and very young infants, although it may also occur in immunosuppressed adults. About 5–10% of neonates are affected, infection being acquired during delivery. Discrete white patches involving any part of the oral mucosa, including the tongue, are seen. In more severe cases, there may be extensive pseudomembrane formation; the white membrane consists of keratinous debris, containing many yeasts, overlying a denuded base.

Other Variants of Oral Candidiasis

Acute Atrophic Candidiasis Associated with a Painful Tongue

Painful reddened lesions develop on the tongue, associated with atrophy of the filiform papillae. They may occur as a consequence of prolonged broad-spectrum antibiotic treatment (e.g. in acne vulgaris) and also in individuals using steroid-containing inhalers for the treatment of asthma, or topical steroids in the mouth. Successful treatment requires removal of any such predisposing factor.

Candida Cheilitis (Inflammation of the Lips)

This may affect the angles of the mouth (*perlèche*) or the lip vermilion. It is most likely in association with excessive licking of the lips, or with the use of topical steroids.

Candida Leucoplakia

In this condition there are discrete areas of epithelial hyperplasia associated with *Candida* in the superficial layers. Lesions may occur anywhere in the oral or lingual mucosa. Patients complain either of pain or of a burning sensation in the affected areas. Some degree of cellular atypia may be seen in the hyperplastic areas and carcinoma has been reported as a late complication in some instances.

NON-INFECTIVE INFLAMMATORY LESIONS

Aphthous Ulcers

The commonest inflammatory lesions affecting the oral mucosa (up to 40% of the general population) are **aphthous ulcers**. They are most frequent in the first two decades.

Their cause is unknown, although some occur in association with chronic inflammatory bowel disease and Behçet's syndrome. Trauma, endocrine disturbances (including menstruation and pregnancy), stress and allergy have all been canvassed as predisposing factors, but remain unproven.

The onset is often abrupt and is marked symptomatically by localized discomfort or a burning sensation in the affected mucosa. On inspection, the mucosa shows areas of intense reddening associated with dilatation of the subepithelial blood vessels, which are easily seen with the naked eye. This is followed by epithelial breakdown and the formation of well-demarcated ulcers. At this stage the lesions, which measure 2–3 mm in diameter, are intensely painful. The disorder is self-limiting and the ulcers heal without scarring, usually within 1 week. Recurrence is a common phenomenon. Healing is accelerated by the local application of steroids and, indeed, if steroids are applied in the early stages, ulcer formation can be inhibited.

LEUCOPLAKIA

The term **leucoplakia**, derived from Greek, literally means 'white patch'. **The pathological basis for this appearance, in most instances, is epithelial proliferation and alterations in epithelial maturation leading to:**
- **an increase in the thickness of the epithelium**
- **increased amounts of surface keratin**

The term is a descriptive one, having no implications for the natural history of an individual lesion. Lesions may reflect benign, reactive hyperplasia or may show differing degrees of dysplasia, which may be so severe as to merit the label of carcinoma *in situ*.

Erythroplakia

This term is applied to **red velvety patches affecting the oral mucosa**. Increased redness in any situation is the correlate of increased local blood flow due to the vascular dilatation characteristic of acute inflammation. Erythroplakia is no exception to this general principle: microscopic examination shows a florid inflammatory reaction beneath the affected areas of squamous epithelium.

Aetiology

In most patients with leucoplakia, no specific cause can be identified. Some cases are associated with the use of tobacco in a variety of forms, including chewing tobacco. Other factors suggested include trauma, for example from poorly fitting dentures, and chronic exposure of the oral mucosa to dietary irritants.

Microscopic Features

There is a wide spectrum of appearances in patients with leucoplakia, depending on the presence and severity of:
- **disturbed maturation shown by the presence of abnormal keratinization**
- **an increase in cell proliferation leading to thickening of the oral squamous epithelium**
- **epithelial dysplasia**

In some cases there is hyperkeratosis associated with the presence of hyperplastic but orderly squamous epithelium, whereas in others there may be architectural and cytological disturbances suggestive of intraepithelial neoplasia. The latter include the presence of:
- enlarged nuclei that stain more darkly than normal
- an increased nuclear : cytoplasmic ratio
- mitoses above the level of the basal cells
- abnormal mitoses

Natural History

Severe dysplasia is relatively more common in erythroplakia, which carries a much greater risk of malignant transformation (about 50%) than leucoplakia. There is still controversy regarding the degree of risk of subsequent carcinoma in patients with leucoplakia, figures quoted ranging from as low as 1% to as high as 30%. These discrepancies are almost certainly due to failures of classification of the lesions. A risk of cancer developing in areas of leucoplakia of the order of 5–6% is probably realistic.

MALIGNANT TUMOURS

Epidemiology

Cancer of the oral cavity (including the tongue) accounts for about 4% of cancer deaths in males and about 2% in females.

There are marked geographical differences, oral cancer being most frequent in the Indian subcontinent. In the West, the mean annual incidence is about 4 per 100 000 for both sexes combined. Males are affected more often than females, a difference that is especially marked for carcinoma of the lip, which is ten times more common in males than in females. Carcinoma of the oral cavity is, in the main, a disease affecting middle-aged and elderly individuals, the incidence rising quite steeply after the age of 70 years.

Some 95% of malignant neoplasms affecting the oral cavity are, not surprisingly, squamous cell carcinomas.

Aetiology

Principal environmental factors implicated in the genesis of oral cancer are **tobacco** and **alcohol**.

Smoking increases the risk of oral cancer by two- to fourfold and, if this is combined with drinking, the relative risk becomes 6–15-fold. The use of tobacco appears to be more important, and the association is particularly clear in those who indulge in 'snuff dipping' (holding a pad of tobacco between cheek and gum or between lip and gum). Tobacco is also used, in Asia, as part of a mixture known as **pan**, which contains areca nut and, sometimes, lime. This is chewed and may well contribute to the increased frequency of oral cancer in South-East Asia.

Other Possible Aetiologial Factors
- **HPV infection.** Evidence of infection with type 16 HPV has been found in nearly 50% of oral cancers in some studies.
- **Exposure to sunlight.** On the basis of epidemiological studies, sunlight appears to play an important part in the genesis of cancer of the lip.

Cytogenetic Changes seen in Oral Cancer
Loss of multiple chromosome regions is seen in cell lines derived from squamous cell cancers of the head and neck. In descending order of frequency these include loss of:
- 18q (100%)
- 10p (80%)
- 8p (70%)
- 3p (60%)

Short arms of acrocentric chromosomes (13, 14, 15, 21, 22) are deleted in 70% of the cell lines examined and additional copies of 7p are found in 90% of the lines.

At the molecular level, amplification and overexpression has been noted in respect of the **epidermal growth factor receptor**, the **apoptosis-inhibiting gene**, ***bcl-2***, and some others. The high frequency of these aberrations suggests that these genomic alterations play a part in causing oral squamous cell tumours.

Pathological Features
The tongue, especially its ventrolateral surface, and the floor of the mouth are the sites most frequently affected, accounting for over 50% of cases. The least commonly affected regions are the dorsum of the tongue and the hard palate. Areas where the risk of carcinoma is greatest, have in common a lining of thin non-keratinized squamous epithelium with poorly developed or absent rete ridges and a narrow lamina propria. Where snuff-dipping or pan chewing are the aetiological factors, the tumours are sited either between cheek and gum or between lip and gum.

Macroscopic Features
These depend on the stage of presentation. Early in the natural history, lesions appear either as opaque white plaques or as irregular rather warty areas. In either case, there may be associated leucoplakic or erythroplakic lesions. At a later stage, the lesions tend to ulcerate, **the ulcers having a firm rolled edge and an indurated bed which can be readily palpated** (*Fig. 34.1*).

Microscopic Features
Most oral cancers are well differentiated, keratinizing, squamous carcinomas; many keratin 'pearls' are present. The infiltrating margins are marked by the presence of islands and strands of neoplastic epithelium which may spread both broadly and deeply within the subepithelial connective tissues.

In the tongue, carcinomas infiltrate deeply between the muscle bundles; in the floor of the mouth, the tumours are characterized by subepithelial spread on a broad front, and clinical judgement as to whether excision is complete may be difficult. Some oral carcinomas are poorly differentiated and these tend to have a worse prognosis. Such poor differentiation is particularly likely to be a feature of cancer at the tongue base.

Tumour Markers
Assessment of the degree of differentiation may be aided by the use of appropriate immunohistochemical reagents. For example, the presence of **involucrin**, a cytoplasmic envelope protein and a marker of terminal differentiation, is a common finding in well-differentiated tumours. **Similarly cytokeratin expression differs in well and poorly differentiated tumours.** Well-differentiated tumours commonly express cytokeratins 1 and 10 (or 4 and 13 if they are non-keratinizing), whereas cytokeratins 8 and 18 are characteristically found in poorly differentiated tumours.

Spread
The tendency for tumours to spread either deeply or widely within the subepithelial tissue has been alluded to above. Such local invasion, especially if the mandible is involved, presents a considerable obstacle to complete surgical excision.

Lymph node metastases are often present at the time of presentation, especially in relation to cancer of the tongue and floor of mouth. Node involvement follows, in general, the pattern of lymphatic drainage from the site of the primary lesion. The nodes most commonly

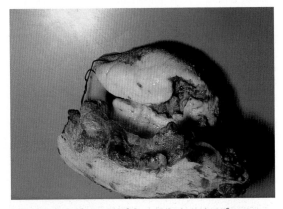

FIGURE 34.1 *Carcinoma of the tongue: a portion of tongue removed at surgery together with part of the mandible. Note the large irregular ulcer which represents the tumour at a rather late stage.*

involved are usually to be found in the submandibular group. Distant spread may involve:

- mediastinal nodes
- lungs
- liver
- the skeleton

Verrucous Carcinoma

This is a variant of squamous carcinoma, sufficiently distinctive as to be regarded as a separate entity. It occurs in a number of anatomical locations including the oral cavity, anal region, penis, vulva, vagina, cervix uteri and skin, especially the skin of the sole of the foot.

In the oral cavity the tumour occurs chiefly in elderly men, the commonest sites being buccal mucosa and gum of the lower jaw. The lesions commonly present as bulky, soft, cauliflower-like growths which often become infected and have an unpleasant smell.

Microscopic Features

On histological examination, verrucous carcinoma appears well-differentiated throughout. This feature helps to distinguish it from the more common squamous carcinoma. Another helpful feature is the very large size of constituent tumour cells.

The rete pegs of the markedly thickened epithelial lining grow down into the underlying tissues in a characteristically **bulbous pattern**, and true stromal invasion appears only at a relatively late stage in the natural history. Although the tumour has a papillary appearance, reminiscent of warty lesions, the connective tissue cores present in the papillae of a true condyloma are not seen here.

Reaching a correct diagnosis may be difficult, especially if only biopsy material is available. This is because of the extremely well-differentiated nature of the tumour. It is important, therefore, that the surgical pathologist should be aware of the naked-eye appearances of the lesion from which the biopsy has been derived. The tumour, despite its relatively benign cytological appearances, may penetrate deeply into the soft tissues of the cheek, may invade underlying bone and may gain access to perineural spaces.

Natural History

The main factors in determining the outcome in patients with oral cancer are:

- the **location** of the lesion (see *Table 34.1*)
- the **stage** (hence the importance of early diagnosis and careful follow-up of patients with leucoplakia or erythroplakia)
- the **histological grading**: poorly differentiated tumours carry a worse prognosis than well-differentiated examples

Table 34.1 Overall 5-year Survival Rates

Site	Survival rate (%)
Lower lip	90
Anterior part of tongue	60
Posterior part of tongue Floor of mouth Tonsil Gum Hard palate	40
Soft palate	20–30

Other Oral Tumours

Granular Cell Tumour

This lesion can occur in almost any site. However, the **tongue**, soft tissue of the chest wall and upper limbs seem to be sites of predilection. Granular cell tumour has also been encountered in the central nervous system, especially within the neurohypophysis.

This **benign tumour** was formerly called **granular cell myoblastoma** because of a fancied resemblance between its constituent cells and muscle cells. Granular cell tumours are now thought to be of Schwann cell origin.

Microscopic Features

The microscopic appearances are highly characteristic, the lesions consisting of sheets of large pink-staining cells with coarsely granular cytoplasm and small, centrally placed, nuclei. Material present within the cells stains a bright magenta colour with periodic acid–Schiff (PAS) stain. It is currently believed that the PAS-positive granular material represents glycolipid.

Despite the benign behaviour of virtually all these lesions, examination of the margins may show the presence of tumour cells in perineural spaces. About 20% of cases are associated with a marked degree of hyperplasia of the overlying squamous epithelium, which is termed pseudoepitheliomatous hyperplasia. Care should be taken not to confuse this appearance with squamous cell carcinoma.

The Salivary Glands

NORMAL FUNCTION AND ANATOMY

The functions of the salivary glands are mediated by their secretions which:

- **lubricate**, thus enabling chewing and swallowing to take place with ease. This is due to the high water and glycoprotein content of saliva

- **digest** complex carbohydrate through the medium of the amylase that is present in saliva
- **protect** against infection through the medium of secreted immunoglobulin A and also certain non-specific antibacterial compounds such as muramidase and lactoferrin
- **protect** the teeth against the low pH produced by acid-producing bacteria involved in tooth decay, as the secretions are alkaline

The glands themselves are classified as being either **major** or **minor**. Minor glands, of which there are many, are situated in the submucosa of the mouth, pharynx and upper part of the respiratory tract.

The **major** glands consist of three paired glands, named in accordance with their location:

1) The **parotid** glands located below and in front of the external ear. The gland is divided into superficial and deep portions by the facial nerve. Each gland drains via a main duct (Stensen's duct) which follows a rather tortuous path, crossing the masseter and buccinator muscles before entering the mouth.

2) The **submandibular** glands lying in the groove between the lower jaw and tongue. These drain via Wharton's duct, running for a distance of 5 cm between the mylohyoid, hyoglossus and genioglossus muscle and opening into the mouth through small caruncles lying on either side of the frenulum of the tongue.

3) The **sublingual** glands in the sublingual fossae of the mandible. The main sublingual gland drains via Bartholin's duct into a series of small openings on either side of the groove below the tongue. In some cases this gland's main excretory duct joins the main submandibular duct.

Microanatomy

Each of the major glands has a basically similar structure.

Microscopic Features

There is a **secretory apparatus** composed of groups (acini) of wedge-shaped cells, each acinus having a central lumen. In the parotid gland all the cells secrete a thin watery fluid rich in amylase. These **serous cells** have basally situated nuclei and rather granular basophilic cytoplasm. The granules (zymogen granules) contain amylase and stain magenta with the periodic acid–Schiff (PAS) stain.

The submandibular and sublingual glands contain **mucin-secreting acini** lined by cells with clear cytoplasm. In the submandibular gland, the acini are mixed, both serous and mucin-secreting cells being present. The sublingual gland consists of mucin-secreting acini only.

The glands have a lobular structure with many acini present in each lobule.

The acinar lumina drain into **intercalated ducts** lined by flattened or cuboidal epithelium. The intercalated ducts blend almost imperceptibly with another series of ducts known as **striated ducts**, also lined by cuboidal epithelium. They are given this name because there are striations on the basal aspect of the epithelial cells caused by invaginations of the membrane and the presence of mitochondria. The striation represents a specialized area of the epithelial cell surface which is concerned with water and electrolyte transport. Both these types of duct run within the lobules.

Striated ducts drain into **interlobular ducts**, which run in the connective tissue septa between the lobules. These are lined by columnar pseudostratified epithelium in which a few goblet cells are seen. More distally, these ducts become larger and eventually drain into the **principal excretory duct**, the lining of which becomes squamous near its orifice.

Between the epithelium and its basement membrane lie the **myoepithelial cells**. These are flat cells with long cytoplasmic processes. On the basal side of these cells are intracytoplasmic filaments consisting of actin, myosin and tropomyosin arranged in a pattern similar to that of smooth muscle. These cells, also found in relation to the ducts, are contractile. They increase the speed of the flow of saliva by contracting and increasing the pressure in the duct system.

The myoepithelial cell is a key cell in primary neoplasms involving the salivary glands. It exhibits both epithelial and mesenchymal characteristics, both of which may be expressed in salivary neoplasms, especially in pleomorphic salivary adenoma.

DISORDERS OF SECRETION

Secretions of saliva may be increased above the norm (**sialorrhoea** or **ptyalism**) or, more commonly, may be diminished or even absent (**xerostomia**).

Xerostomia

The importance of normal salivation becomes very clear when it is no longer present. Loss of the lubricating and protecting functions of normal amounts of saliva leads to:

- oral and pharyngeal infection
- ulceration of the oral mucosa
- severe and accelerated dental caries

Xerostomia may have either a **structural** or a **functional** basis. In the latter the dry mouth may be temporary as a result of fear (which increases sympathetic discharge), or of dehydration and hypovolaemia. The majority of cases of **functional xerostomia** are due to drug treatment. The compounds most commonly associated with a decrease in the amount of saliva are:

- antihistamines
- tricyclic antidepressants
- phenothiazines
- certain hypotensive agents
- some antiemetic agents

Withdrawal of the drug is followed by a return to normal salivation.

The structural bases of xerostomia involve loss of secreting tissue:

- following therapeutic irradiation of the head and neck. The damage to the secretory apparatus is permanent and the gland becomes fibrotic
- in Sjögren's syndrome, characterized by autoimmune inflammation resulting in loss of secretory cells

Mumps and sarcoidosis involving the salivary glands cause a reduction but not a cessation in the flow of saliva and, in the case of mumps, a complete return to normal function is the rule.

Sialorrhoea

Pathologically increased flow of saliva is most commonly associated with inflammation of the mouth or gum mucosa, such as aphthous or herpetic stomatitis. It is, of course, also a common accompaniment of teething in infants. More rarely it may be seen in association with mercury poisoning, pemphigus, epilepsy, Parkinson's disease or myasthenia gravis.

INFLAMMATORY DISORDERS

Inflammation of the salivary glands (sialadenitis) may be **acute** or **chronic**. The distinction is worth making because not only are the clinical presentations and natural history different but there is a much wider range of causative agents involved in chronic sialadenitis.

Acute Sialadenitis

Acute inflammation is usually the result of a bacterial or viral infection. In the former, the infection is usually an ascending one, the organisms involved usually being resident in the oral cavity. Such ascending infection is most commonly seen when saliva flow through the affected duct system is decreased.

In the past, acute sialadenitis was not uncommon in patients who had become dehydrated and debilitated after major surgery, but good practice should have made this a thing of the past. Nowadays, acute sialadenitis (the parotid is the gland most frequently involved) is seen mainly in association with chronic xerostomia.

The **usual clinical presentation** is of painful enlargement of one or both parotids. Examination of the duct orifices may show the presence of pus discharging into the mouth.

Salivary Calculi

In a few instances, acute sialadenitis may be due to impaction of a salivary calculus in a main excretory duct. Salivary calculi consist principally of calcium phosphate, with calcium carbonate being the second most abundant component. The submandibular ducts are affected two or three times more commonly than those of the parotid gland, and the calculi found in the former location are larger, as a rule, than those in the latter, because Wharton's duct is much more distensible than Stensen's duct.

Submandibular calculi are found in most instances within the main excretory duct but about 15% involve the intraglandular portion of the duct system. Frequently the stones can be palpated in the floor of the mouth and, in some cases, part of the stone protrudes from the orifice of Wharton's duct. Submandibular stones can grow to a quite considerable size before any symptoms occur. If the main duct is completely obstructed then, as tension increases within the duct system proximal to the obstruction, pain and swelling can occur, this being especially likely to be associated with meals.

Parotid calculi are more difficult to diagnose on radiography than those within the submandibular duct because they are much less radio-opaque. They are now believed to be the commonest cause of unilateral parotid swelling.

The presence of a calculus sufficiently large to obstruct a duct is associated with a decrease in secretion by the units draining into that duct. Thus, the recurrent swelling associated with meals, so characteristic of submandibular duct calculi, is absent here. Instead recurrent attacks of painful swelling of the parotid associated with inflammation are likely to occur.

Chronic Sialadenitis

Chronic Obstructive Sialadenitis

This occurs quite commonly in the submandibular gland, producing a highly characteristic microscopic picture.

Microscopic Features

- **Dilatation of the duct system.** The dilated ducts often contain eosinophilic glycoprotein. In some instances squamous metaplasia of the duct lining may be noted.
- **Expansion of the interlobular connective tissue** as a result of the growth of new connective tissue. Some fibrosis within lobules may also be seen.
- In secretory units draining into the affected part of the duct system, there is a **marked degree of acinar atrophy**, which may end in their disappearance. It is likely that this is mediated by programmed cell death or apoptosis.
- A mild to moderate **chronic inflammatory cell infiltrate**.

Chronic Recurrent Parotitis

This disorder of unknown aetiology affects principally children between the ages of 5 and 15 years, girls being more often affected than boys. It presents as recurrent episodes, lasting 7–10 days, of swelling and tenderness of the parotids; the episodes are associated with fever and malaise. There may be intervals of weeks or months between the attacks.

Histological examination of affected glands shows acinar atrophy and fibrosis associated with a marked degree of dilatation of the smallest ductules. These ductular changes, known as **sialectasis**, are associated with a highly characteristic appearance when radio-opaque material is injected into the parotid duct, the dilated ductules showing up as contrast medium-filled globules.

Sjögren's Syndrome

This is an autoimmune disorder characterized by an increase in B-cell activity and the appearance in the plasma of several antibodies, some organ-specific (e.g. antithyroid) and others non-organ-specific. Among the tissues affected are salivary and lacrimal glands, this exocrine gland involvement leading to dry eyes (**keratoconjunctivitis sicca**) and dry mouth (**xerostomia**); many other clinical features may be noted.

Sjögren's syndrome may present as an isolated syndrome (**primary**) or in a **secondary** form, associated with other autoimmune diseases. Of these, rheumatoid arthritis is by far the commonest. Other disorders associated with Sjögren's syndrome include **primary biliary cirrhosis, scleroderma, polymyositis** and **systemic lupus erythematosus**. Some differences between the two forms are shown in *Table 34.2*.

Epidemiology

The peak incidence is the fourth and fifth decades, women being much more commonly affected than men (F : M ratio 9 : 1). What triggers the autoimmune process is not known. Because viruses can alter cell surfaces with consequent loss of normal tolerance to these cells, much attention has been paid to the possibility of an infective trigger. Candidates include the Epstein–Barr virus and cytomegalovirus, but to date no hard evidence has emerged.

Epidemiological studies show antibodies to the p24 capsid glycoprotein of human immunodeficiency virus in a much larger proportion of patients with Sjögren's syndrome (30%) than in the general population (1–4%) and transgenic mice bearing the *tax* gene of human T-lymphotropic virus develop a disorder closely resembling human Sjögren's syndrome. In some humans with Sjögren's syndrome, the *tax* gene has been found to be present in epithelial cells of affected minor salivary glands. All these data lend some support to the view that a viral infection triggers this disorder, but proof is still lacking.

Microscopic Features
- **Focal chronic inflammatory cell infiltrates** adjacent to or replacing the acinar tissue. Such infiltrates are defined as **aggregates of at least 50 lymphocytes, plasma cells and macrophages**. These are found in both major and minor salivary glands and are the diagnostic benchmark in biopsies of minor salivary glands in the lip.
- **'Lymphoepithelial' lesions.** These consist of a chronic inflammatory cell infiltrate involving islands of epithelial and myoepithelial cells.

Lymphoepithelial lesions can and do occur without associated manifestations of Sjögren's syndrome, and may represent a separate clinical and pathological condition. Isolated lymphoepithe-

Table 34.2 Primary and Secondary Forms of Sjögren's Syndrome

Primary	Secondary
Associated with HLA-DR3	Associated with HLA-DR4
Eyes and mouth more severely involved	
More severe: swelling of salivary glands, systemic manifestations such as Raynaud's phenomenon, lymph node enlargement, lung and renal involvement	
Antibody pattern:	Antibody pattern:
Anti–SS-A (Ro): 75%	Anti–SS-A: 10%
Anti–SS-B (La): 40%	Anti–SS-B: 5%
Rheumatoid factors: 95%	Rheumatoid factors: 100%
Antisalivary gland: 25%	Antisalivary gland: 70%
Rheumatoid arthritis precipitin: 5%	Rheumatoid arthritis precipitin: 85%

HLA, human leucocyte antigen; SS, single stranded DNA.

lial lesions are seen most commonly in women in the fifth and sixth decades. About 20% of these cases progress to B-cell lymphoma derived from **mucosa-associated lymphoid tissue**.

TUMOURS OF THE SALIVARY GLANDS

Epidemiology
Any of the salivary glands may be the site of origin of primary tumours but most occur within the parotid gland. As a rough approximation, there are 100 parotid tumours for ten in the minor glands, ten in the submandibular glands and one in the sublingual glands. At least 80% of salivary gland tumours are benign and, of these, **pleomorphic salivary adenoma** accounts for the greatest number. A greater proportion of minor salivary gland tumours is malignant compared with those occurring in major glands.

Salivary tumours are rare, accounting for only 1–2% of all tumours. The only aetiological feature so far recognized is irradiation. Adults who as children received therapeutic irradiation of the tonsils and adenoids show an increased risk of salivary gland tumours, of which approximately one-quarter are malignant. An increase in the incidence of salivary gland tumours is also reported amongst survivors of the nuclear attacks on Hiroshima and Nagasaki.

Classification
Classification of salivary gland tumours is shown in *Table 34.3*.

Table 34.3 Classification of Salivary Gland Tumours

Tumour	Type
Adenoma	Pleomorphic adenoma
	Myoepithelioma
	Adenolymphoma
	Basal cell adenoma
	Oncocytoma (oxyphilic)
Carcinoma	Adenoid cystic
	Mucoepidermoid carcinoma
	Acinic cell carcinoma
Non-epithelial tumours	Haemangioma
Lymphoma	
Secondary tumours	

ADENOMAS

Pleomorphic Salivary Adenoma
This is the commonest major salivary gland tumour. Its former name was **mixed salivary tumour** because of the presence in the stroma of areas mimicking cartilage differentiation. It is now recognized as being entirely epithelial.

Although it may occur at any age, the peak incidence is in the fourth and fifth decades and there is a slight female preponderance.

Most arise in the superficial parotid above the facial nerve but about 10% occur in the deep part of the gland below the facial nerves, and these lesions may present late because they cause localized swelling only at a late stage.

Macroscopic Features
The lesions are rounded masses with a well-defined edge and a connective tissue capsule enabling the tumours to be shelled out from their bed. This is a dangerous practice, which cannot be too strongly deplored, because the lesions often show small projections jutting out from the periphery of the main mass. **If the tumour is enucleated, these projections are left behind and serve as foci from which multiple recurrent tumour nodules develop. The correct treatment, therefore, is a superficial parotidectomy** with a rim of normal gland surrounding the tumour mass.

In most instances, the tumour is firm in consistency and the cut surface may show the presence of small foci that resemble cartilage.

Microscopic Features
In general terms there is considerable variation in the microscopic structure, not only between individual tumours but within single lesions; multiple samples are necessary if a complete picture is to be obtained.

The **epithelial component**, believed to originate from intercalated ducts, may show:
- well-formed ducts lined by cuboidal epithelium, beneath which is a layer of flattened, more darkly staining myoepithelial cells
- compact masses of myoepithelial cells which may become widely separated from each other, extending out into the stroma and becoming elongated and spindle shaped. The morphological alteration in these may be so marked as to make it difficult to appreciate their epithelial origin.

In some instances they may show a superficial resemblance to smooth muscle cells whereas, in others they undergo hydropic degeneration and resemble chondrocytes. Squamous metaplasia may occur, with the myoepithelial cells merging with islands of typical squamous epithelium.

The stroma shows accumulation of basophilic material with the staining reaction of connective tissue mucins. This stromal appearance heightens the resemblance to cartilage. The myxoid stroma may be very bulky, only a few strands of myoepithelial cells breaking the monotony.

Natural History

This tumour is benign but has a tendency to recur, in the form of multiple tumour nodules, after inadequate removal. A small proportion (1–5%) will develop histological evidence of malignant transformation if left untreated for long periods (e.g. 15–20 years).

Adenolymphoma (Warthin's Tumour)

The term adenolymphoma should not be confused with any form of lymphoma. It is a monomorphic adenoma with a heavy lymphocytic infiltrate in the stroma.

Adenolymphoma accounts for about 8% of all tumours of the parotid, its commonest site. It is three to four times commoner in men than in women, and the peak incidence is in the sixth and seventh decades.

Macroscopic Features

These tumours form soft, well-defined, brown masses usually located superficially within the gland.

The cut surface is polycystic with papillary ingrowths of epithelium projecting into the cyst cavities and clefts.

Microscopic Features

The **clefts and cysts** seen on naked-eye examination are lined by a double layer of pink-staining epithelium. The inner layer consists of tall columnar cells with typically granular cytoplasm, whereas the outer one shows the presence of small cells that are either cuboidal or pyramidal in shape. In both layers, electron microscopy shows the presence of large numbers of mitochondria, accounting for the granular cytoplasm, and which is the common feature for **oncocytes** in all epithelial tissues. It is believed that these cells originate from the striated ducts described in an earlier section.

In rather more than 50% of cases, this epithelial lining is interrupted focally by the presence of goblet cells secreting epithelial mucins.

The **stroma** contains a florid lymphocytic infiltrate in which some normal lymphoid follicles with germinal centres are present.

Natural History

Adenolymphomas tend to grow slowly and are virtually always benign. A small number of reports of malignancy developing in these lesions exists. In these cases, malignant transformation has occurred exclusively in the epithelial component.

In about 10% of cases, tumours are bilateral, and multiple adenolymphomas have been reported in single glands.

For reasons that are not well understood, adenolymphoma may become infected and abscesses can occur within the tumour.

Oxyphilic Adenoma (Oncocytoma)

This is rare, accounting for no more than 1% of all parotid tumours; it is even less common in the other glands.

These lesions are well-defined, round or oval masses and have a pinkish cut surface. **Their defining criterion is the presence, on microscopic examination, of large epithelial cells in which the cytoplasm is eosinophilic and granular due to many mitochondria (oncocytes).** The architectural pattern is somewhat variable. In some instances the cells are arranged in solid clumps; in others there is obvious tubule formation.

CARCINOMA

Adenoid Cystic Carcinoma

About 15% of submandibular gland tumours are adenoid cystic carcinomas, in contrast with the parotid in which only 2% of all tumours are of this type. Some 15–20% of tumours in minor salivary glands are adenoid cystic carcinomas, the majority occurring in the palate. The tumour also occurs in the mucous glands of the upper respiratory tract.

Adenoid cystic carcinoma is slow growing but highly malignant. The growth pattern is most commonly, at least in part, infiltrative and this makes complete removal difficult and recurrence likely.

Macroscopic Features

Adenoid cystic carcinoma grows slowly and, at least in its early stages, appears circumscribed giving a false impression of benignancy. The cut surface of the tumour is uniform, with no areas of haemorrhage or cystic change.

Microscopic Features

While the biological behaviour of adenoid cystic tumours is in complete contrast to that of pleomorphic adenoma, the tumour cell population consists basically of the same cell types found in the latter – epithelial cells believed to be of intercalated duct origin, and myoepithelial cells. Myoepithelial cells make up the larger fraction of the tumour cell population and are arranged in a highly characteristic pattern.

The myoepithelial cells form compact masses within which mucoid material may accumulate to form rounded cystic spaces. It is this gland-like appearance that accounts for the inclusion of the adjective '**adenoid**' in the name of these tumours. If the cystic spaces are large and numerous, the term '**cribriform carcinoma**' is applied. Epithelial cells of duct origin appear here and there within the masses of myoepithelial cells, and are easily recognizable because of their eosinophilic cytoplasm.

In some parts of the tumour, the cribriform pattern is replaced, either by cells arranged in solid clumps or by a tubular pattern in which, because ducts can be cut in various planes, the appearances are complex. The microscopic patterns have a bearing on prognosis.

Tumours with a predominantly solid pattern have the worst prognosis (5-year survival rate 50%); those with a mainly tubular pattern have the best (5-year survival rate more than 90%), while cribriform tumours are intermediate in their behaviour.

The islands of tumour cells are surrounded by a sheath consisting of hyaline connective tissue or mucoid material. This cylinder-like sheath is derived from basement membrane and is synthesized by the myoepithelial cells.

Natural History
Spread occurs either directly through connective tissue or via perineural spaces, for which this tumour shows a marked predilection. Bone may also be permeated insidiously by columns of tumour cells so that the tumour may penetrate through to the nose or antrum. This insidious pattern of invasion makes it extremely difficult to eradicate the tumour surgically and local recurrence is very common, despite the fact that the tumour is both well differentiated and slow growing. Distant metastases may occur at a fairly late stage, the lungs being the most frequent site for secondary deposits.

Acinic Cell Carcinoma
Acinic cell carcinoma is rare, accounting for only 2–3% of tumours of the parotid, in which almost all such tumours occur. Occurring at any age, the peak incidence is in the fifth decade and there is a slight female preponderance. In the majority of cases, growth is slow and the tumours present as painless enlargement of the parotid. In a few instances, however, growth may be accelerated and patients complain of pain as well as swelling.

Macroscopic Features
The tumours are solid, being slightly firmer in consistency than the surrounding normal gland. They appear well circumscribed in the majority of cases and the cut surface is a pale grey, occasionally showing some yellowish flecks.

Microscopic Features
The constituent cells of acinic cell carcinoma resemble closely the acinar or secretory cells of the parotid, although they are larger than their normal counterparts. The tumour cells are thought to arise from the stem cell compartment (the reserve cells) of the intercalated ducts.

The tumour cell cytoplasm is basophilic and, in most instances, markedly granular. The granules resemble the zymogen granules of the normal parotid acinar epithelium and stain, as they do, with PAS. Other cell types, some of which show ductular differentiation, may be seen, but the presence of some typical granular cells is mandatory for the diagnosis.

The tumour cells may be arranged in a solid acinar pattern or in compact sheets. Fluid, probably derived from secretions, may accumulate between the cells, giving a lattice-like appearance.

Overt evidence of malignancy in the form of cellular pleomorphism and a high mitotic rate is not usually seen.

Natural History
A small proportion (8–10%) of acinic cell carcinomas metastasize and a further 12–20% are associated with a history of local recurrence.

Mucoepidermoid Carcinoma
The defining criterion of this tumour is the presence of both mucin-producing cells and epithelial cells of epidermoid type with typical intercellular bridges.

Mucoepidermoid carcinoma accounts for 3–5% of tumours of the parotid and submandibular glands, but is much commoner in the minor salivary glands where it makes up 15% of all tumours, the palate being particularly likely to be affected. It can occur at any age but peak incidence is in the third and fourth decades.

Most present as slow-growing painless masses and, on naked-eye examination, appear well circumscribed, thus resembling pleomorphic adenoma. This impression is misleading because there is usually infiltrative growth at some point on the periphery of the lesion and thus failure to remove the tumour with an adequate margin of grossly normal gland tissue is likely to be followed by local recurrence. Both macroscopic and microscopic appearances depend on the relative proportions of mucin-secreting and epidermoid cells. If the former predominate, the cut surface of the tumour may show the presence of numerous small cysts.

Microscopic Features
Microscopic examination shows clear, mucin-secreting cells and epidermoid cells in proportions that vary from lesion to lesion and from area to area of the same lesion. In the, usually, rather slow-growing tumour, these two cell populations are present in roughly equal numbers. Mucin-secreting cells are frequently seen lining small cystic cavities but they can also occur in solid clumps.

Natural History
All mucoepidermoid tumours have malignant potential. Only about 10% ever metastasize and these tend to be high-grade tumours showing overt evidence of

malignancy on microscopic examination. The 5-year survival rate is of the order of 90%.

The Oesophagus

NORMAL ANATOMY

The oesophagus is a 25-cm long hollow muscular tube. It extends from the cricopharyngeus muscle lying opposite the sixth cervical vertebra (and which acts as a sphincter between the pharynx and the oesophagus) to the gastric cardia at the level of the 10th or 11th thoracic vertebrae. All but the distal 1.5 cm is intrathoracic, its lowest portion being infradiaphragmatic.

With the exception of its infradiaphragmatic portion, the oesophagus is **lined by non-keratinizing, stratified squamous epithelium**. This epithelium shows a well-marked basal layer, accounting for about 15% of the epithelial thickness. If inflammation due to reflux of gastric contents into the oesophagus occurs, this basal layer becomes thicker.

The lower two-thirds of the oesophagus shows the presence of a thick muscularis mucosae, deep to which lies a wide submucosa containing the oesophageal glands. The glands secrete sulphated acid mucins and vary widely in number from individual to individual.

The propulsive force of the oesophagus is provided by two layers of the **muscularis propria**. The inner layer is arranged in a circular fashion around the lumen; the outer is longitudinally oriented. Unlike the rest of the gut, where all the muscularis propria consists of smooth muscle fibres, in the case of the oesophagus voluntary muscle fibres are present in the upper one-third of the oesophagus. Between the two muscle layers lies the myenteric nerve plexus where preganglionic fibres from the vagus and sympathetic nerves terminate.

The nerve supply is divided into **extrinsic** and **intrinsic** components. The extrinsic supply is derived from the autonomic nervous system and consists of sympathetic and parasympathetic fibres, coming largely from thoracic spinal nerves in the case of the former and from the vagus in the latter. The intrinsic nerve supply comes from the myenteric plexus and the different types of fibre can exert an excitatory or an inhibitory effect, the normal balance of which is vital for normal motor function.

Lastly, the intrathoracic part of the oesophagus is noteworthy for the absence of a serosal layer. The lack of a serosa is believed to play a part in the fairly early spread of malignant neoplasms from the oesophageal wall into the surrounding organs and tissues.

NORMAL FUNCTION

Oesophageal disorders can be understood most easily against the background of normal function, which is more complex than the rather simple anatomy of the part might suggest.

The two basic functions are:
1) Propulsion of food from the mouth and oropharynx to the stomach through the act of swallowing
2) Prevention of reflux of food admixed with acid and peptic gastric secretions from the stomach back into the oesophagus

Propulsion of Food Bolus from Mouth to Stomach
For this to be successful, certain **negative** conditions must be fulfilled:

- **The lumen must be free from mechanical obstructions such as**:
  1) foreign bodies
  2) webs of mucosa-covered tissue protruding into the lumen
  3) abnormal contraction rings usually sited just above the gastric cardia
  4) neoplasms arising from the wall of the oesophagus and protruding into the lumen
- **The motor function of the oesophagus must be normal. This criterion hides a double functional requirement: not only must normal forward propulsion of the food bolus by means of peristalsis take place, but there must be simultaneous relaxation of the functional gastro-oesophageal sphincter.**
- **There must be an absence of scarring and hence of local narrowing.**

Failure to meet any of these conditions will result in dysphagia (difficulty in swallowing).

DISORDERS ASSOCIATED WITH MECHANICAL OBSTRUCTION

DEVELOPMENTAL ABNORMALITIES

Congenital Oesophageal Atresia
The most important developmental abnormality causing obstruction is **atresia** or, less often, **congenital stenosis**. Both are rare in a pure form, being most often associated with **tracheo-oesophageal fistula** (*Fig. 34.2*). This association is not particularly rare (1 in 800–1500 live births). It may occasionally form part of a complex, the VATER syndrome, which gets its name from the following:

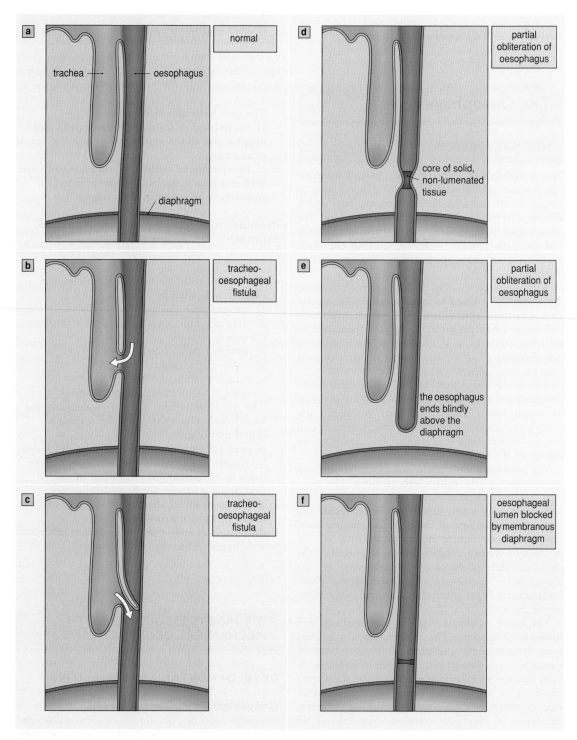

FIGURE 34.2 **a–f** Morphological variants of oesophageal atresia and tracheo-oesophageal fistula.

- **V**ertebral defects (hemivertebrae or bifid vertebrae)
- **A**nal atresia
- **T**racheo–
- **E**sophageal (oesophageal)

- **R**enal dysplasia

The cause of atresia and fistula is not known, although associated maternal hydramnios has been noted in some cases. Several anatomical variants exist (*Fig. 34.2*).

By far commonest (90%) is where the upper end of the oesophagus ends as a blind pouch and the proximal end of the lower portion communicates with the posterior wall of the trachea. In the upper portion, which on occasion is fused with the trachea, all the layers of normal oesophagus are present and the muscularis propria is hypertrophied. There is a distinct gap between the upper and lower portions, which may measure up to 5 cm and, sometimes, may be bridged by a fibrous cord.

In the remaining 10%, the most common anomaly is one in which the upper end of the oesophagus communicates with the trachea while the lower portion, the proximal end of which ends blindly, communicates normally with the stomach. This defect gives rise to a very characteristic clinical picture, in which feeding is followed immediately by severe coughing and choking as the ingested milk is diverted to the trachea.

OTHER CAUSES OF OBSTRUCTION

Oesophageal Webs
These are constrictions appearing most commonly at or near the level of the cricoid cartilage. They consist of a thin fibrous tissue layer covered on both sides by normal epithelium, and may nearly occlude the lumen. This condition is known as the Paterson–Kelly or Plummer–Vinson syndrome, or as **sideropenic dysphagia**. The syndrome consists of:
- iron-deficiency anaemia
- oesophageal web
- achlorhydria
- atrophy of the mucosa of the tongue, pharynx and stomach

It occurs almost exclusively in women and may be associated with **dysplastic changes in the oesophageal epithelium away from the web, and an increased risk of developing carcinoma of the upper part of the oesophagus** (so-called postcricoid carcinoma). Whether the webs are, in fact, responsible for the dysphagia is open to doubt.

Oesophageal Rings (Schatzki's Rings)
Constriction rings at the junction between squamous and columnar epithelium at the lower end of the oesophagus cause dysphagia more commonly than do oesophageal webs. The rings narrow the lumen rather than occlude it. On histological examination they consist of a projection of connective tissue, in which some muscle fibres may be present and may be covered by either squamous or columnar epithelium or, on some occasions, both. The pathogenesis is unknown.

Obstruction due to Foreign Bodies
Obstruction may be caused by foreign bodies:
- found in normal food (e.g. fish or meat bones and fruit stones)
- not associated with food (e.g. coins, toys, broken dentures, etc.)

- inappropriately but deliberately swallowed. This is seen most often in patients who are psychologically disturbed.

Neoplasms Partly Within the Lumen and Partly Within the Wall
For a description of these lesions, see pp 501–502.

Motor Disorders: Dysfunction Caused by Inadequate or Incoordinated Muscular Contraction
Motor disorders may involve disturbances of forward propulsion of the food bolus by waves of peristaltic contraction, or of relaxation of the functional gastro-oesophageal sphincter. Interference with these may result from:
- loss of normal innervation or imbalance between excitor and inhibitor neurones and the transmitters released by them
- damage to the muscle and/or its replacement by fibrous tissue, as, for example, in progressive systemic sclerosis, or by deposition of amyloid

Achalasia
Achalasia literally means **failure of relaxation**. The basal tone of the lower oesophageal sphincter is increased and there is a failure of sphincteric relaxation associated also with significant reduction in the primary and secondary peristaltic contractions that normally propel food along the oesophagus.

The morphological correlate of this failure of peristalsis is an absence of ganglion cells in the myenteric plexus in the body of the oesophagus, and there may also be a loss of ganglion cells from this plexus in relation to the lower oesophageal sphincter. In the latter site, it is likely that the neurones affected are those that contain vasoactive intestinal polypeptide, the inhibitory transmitter for oesophageal smooth muscle.

About 5% of cases occur in childhood and may thus represent a congenital, developmental failure of normal innervation, but most patients are aged over 40 years, the sexes being equally affected. The cause of achalasia is unknown.

With time, the combination of functional defects leads to a grossly dilated oesophagus which may contain more than 1 litre of food and fluid; this dilatation is well seen on barium swallow.

Patients complain of **dyspepsia, regurgitation of food and pain** over a long period, but more sinister is the occurrence of bouts of regurgitation associated with **aspiration of the oesophageal contents into the airways**, resulting in inhalation pneumonia. Secondary oesophagitis may also develop and this can occasionally lead to ulceration and bleeding. Some controversy exists as to whether there is an increased risk of squamous carcinoma in the affected part of the oesophagus.

Diffuse Muscle Spasm

This disorder of oesophageal motility is associated with substernal pain occurring either at rest, even waking patients, or immediately after swallowing very hot or very cold liquids. In the latter case, quite severe pain may be associated with dysphagia.

This syndrome results from a motor abnormality in which peristaltic contractions appear to involve only the upper one-third of the oesophagus. From this point down, muscle contractions are totally irregular and uncoordinated, mirrored by an exaggeratedly saccular pattern on barium swallow which has been likened to a corkscrew. The cause is unknown. The morphological correlate is hypertrophy of the smooth muscle, which may be either focal or diffuse, the thickness of the muscle layer reaching up to 1 cm in severe cases.

Neuropathies Associated with Systemic Disorders

Patients with diabetes mellitus or amyloidosis may show impaired oesophageal motor function as a result of an autonomic neuropathy. Long-standing overingestion of alcohol is also associated, in some patients, with impairment of primary peristalsis and this may be accompanied by lower than normal resting pressure in the sphincter at the lower end of the oesophagus.

Motor Dysfunction due to Scleroderma (Progressive Systemic Sclerosis)

Scleroderma is the commonest connective tissue disease affecting the motor functions of the oesophagus, although disturbances may also occur in patients with dermatomyositis–polymyositis, systemic lupus erythematosus and other mixed connective tissue disorders. Some 75% of patients with scleroderma show impairment of oesophageal function. The basic pathological lesion is **progressive atrophy of the smooth muscle**, the lost muscle being replaced by scar tissue. It is most likely that this muscle loss is due to ischaemia resulting from the characteristic vascular changes of scleroderma.

Scleroderma affects both peristalsis in the lower two-thirds of the oesophagus and the functional integrity of the lower oesophageal sphincter, the result of the latter being reflux of acid and pepsin-containing gastric juice.

Pharyngeal and Oesophageal Diverticula

A diverticulum is a localized outpouching of the wall of a hollow muscular organ. Diverticula in which all the layers of the normal viscus are present are called true diverticula, and those in which the muscularis propria is lacking are called false.

Pharyngeal Pouch

The commonest diverticulum in the upper gastro-intestinal tract is a pharyngeal diverticulum occurring on the posterior aspect of the pharynx (pouch). This is believed to be due to incoordination in the contraction of the inferior constrictor of the pharynx. Oesophageal mucosa herniates through a potential gap between the horizontal fibres of the inferior constrictor and the oblique thyropharyngeal fibres.

These pouches gradually enlarge, producing increasingly severe dysphagia by pressing on the oesophagus from behind. A characteristic clinical feature is a gurgling sound heard on swallowing or with pressure applied to the neck. An aesthetically unpleasing feature is regurgitation of undigested food from the pouch, usually some hours after a meal. Some patients complain of nocturnal cough due to inhaling small amounts of regurgitated food during sleep. Males are affected three times as frequently as females and the condition becomes more common with increasing age; it is uncommon below the age of 50 years.

Traction Diverticula

So-called 'traction' diverticula affect the middle and lower thirds of the oesophagus. They are associated with inflammation in mediastinal lymph nodes, most commonly tuberculous, and appear to be related to the presence of fibrous adhesions between the wall of the oesophagus and affected nodes. They have a wide neck in relation to their size and thus food does not tend to collect within them.

Epiphrenic Diverticula

As their name implies, these diverticula occur just above the diaphragm. They are true diverticula and are believed to be associated with motor dysfunction in which luminal pressure may be markedly raised. The diverticula are lined by squamous epithelium and are often inflamed. Food and secretions collect in the sacs; nocturnal regurgitation is a frequent complaint.

Diffuse Intramural Oesophageal Diverticulosis

This is a rare condition in which many small (1–3 mm) flask-shaped diverticula are found **within the wall** of the oesophagus, most commonly in the upper third. A short stricture is usually present in the region where these small outpouchings form and dysphagia is the usual presenting symptom. It has been suggested that these lesions are not true diverticula but instead represent cystically dilated submucosal gland ducts.

Disorders Associated with Gastro-oesophageal Reflux

The lower oesophageal sphincter is a segment of smooth muscle in the oesophageal wall. It is 2–4-cm long and is sited just above the gastro-oesophageal junction. The normal resting pressure in this segment is 10–30 mmHg above the intragastric pressure, and the pressure difference constitutes a barrier to reflux of gastric contents. As intragastric and intra-abdominal pressure rises, so does that of the lower oesophageal sphincter. It is clearly necessary that the sphincter should relax in order to allow the food bolus to enter the stomach, and this occurs more or less simultaneously with the commencement of peristalsis.

Factors that lower sphincter pressure and thus increase the chances of reflux are listed in *Table 34.4*.

Aetiology

Gastro-oesophageal reflux occurs when the pressure of the sphincter falls below a critical level, an event that is usually episodic rather than continuous. The pressure fall may be associated with a diagnosable disorder such as scleroderma, and it is also a common event in the obese, in pregnancy and in women taking oral contraceptives. In many instances it is not possible to pinpoint the cause of the reflux. However, factors that promote reflux include lying flat after meals, bending over, lifting heavy weights, or wearing tight garments or corsets that compress the abdomen.

Effects of Reflux

Whatever the underlying cause, gastro-oesophageal reflux manifests with 'heartburn', an often wave-like, burning, substernal pain, and 'water brash', the awareness of acid gastric juice in the oesophagus.

The morphological effects in the early stages are a combination of **acute inflammation**, in the form of a neutrophil and eosinophil infiltrate, and **epithelial proliferation**, the fraction of the squamous lining made up of basal cells increasing significantly. The connective tissue papillae become hypertrophic and show the presence of prominent blood vessels.

Persistent reflux may lead to ulceration. Such ulcers are usually superficial but, in some instances, chronic ulceration may develop, the lesions closely resembling the chronic peptic ulcers seen most commonly in the stomach and duodenum. Deep chronic ulcers are associated with scarring in the affected segment of the wall, leading ultimately to stricture formation.

Barrett's Oesophagus

Definition

Barrett's oesophagus is defined as the occurrence of columnar epithelium lining a segment of distal oesophagus that is normally lined by squamous epithelium. It is generally held that the diagnosis should not be made unless this change involves 3 cm or more of the length of the distal oesophagus.

Pathogenesis

There has been a prolonged and sterile debate as to whether this abnormality is congenital or acquired. Most pathologists now accept the view that this is an acquired change and represents **metaplasia of the lining of the distal part of the oesophagus following reflux oesophagitis** and ulceration in most instances, although there have been reports of Barrett's oesophagus occurring in children as a complication of chemotherapy for leukaemia.

Microscopic Features

Three forms may be seen:
1) intestinal metaplasia with villi, crypts and a mixed population of cells such as is seen in the **small intestine**
2) mucosa resembling the **fundus of the stomach** with parietal and chief cells
3) mucosa resembling that of the **cardia of the stomach** showing the presence of many mucous glands

Dysplasia and Carcinoma Complicating Barrett's Oesophagus

Carcinoma of the oesophagus is an important complication of Barrett's oesophagus. It is nearly always an **adenocarcinoma** and is generally preceded by and associated with dysplasia of the columnar epithelium. The risk for developing carcinoma has been said by some to be 30–40 times greater than in the general population, and adenocarcinoma associated with Barrett's oesophagus is thought to account for 5–10% of all oesophageal cancers.

Hiatus Hernia

Hiatus hernia is a diagnosis made quite frequently by radiologists but which causes symptoms in only a small minority (approximately 10%) of affected individuals.

Definition

It is the condition in which **the gastro-oesophageal junction and/or a variable amount of the upper part of the stomach lie within the thorax instead of within the abdomen.**

Table 34.4 Factors Affecting Sphincter Pressure

Hormones
    Oestrogen and progesterone
    Glucagon
    Secretin
    Cholecystokinin
    Prostaglandin E_2

Drugs
    Atropine
    Theophylline
    Meperidine

Dietary and other habits
    High fat intake
    Smoking
    Alcohol
    Chocolate

There are two anatomical types:

1) **Sliding hernia** (*Fig. 34.3a*). This is by far the most common (90% of cases). Here the infradiaphragmatic portion of the oesophagus and part of the stomach move up through the hiatus in the diaphragm through which the oesophagus normally passes, thus forming a roughly bell-shaped dilatation just above the diaphragm.

Sliding hernias may be congenital, as a result of a short oesophagus, and in some cases may be familial. In other instances factors playing a role in gastro-oesophageal reflux are thought to contribute to the formation of this type of hernia.

In patients whose sliding hernia causes symptoms, reflux oesophagitis, heartburn and water brash are found.

2) **'Rolling' or paraoesophageal hernia** (*Fig. 34.3b*). In this type, a portion of the stomach herniates through the diaphragmatic hiatus alongside the oesophagus, carrying with it a sac of peritoneum. In most instances the cardia lies in a normal position and reflux does not occur because the normal angulation at the gastro-oesophageal junction is preserved.

With the passage of time, the defect at the connective tissue margin of the hiatus may increase in size and more of the stomach may herniate through into the thorax.

In a small number of cases where the hernia is very large, there may be interference with lung expansion and, even more rarely, the intrathoracic portion of the stomach may twist ('volvulus'), thus causing ischaemic necrosis of the portion of the stomach distal to the volvulus.

Infective Oesophagitis

The most frequently encountered infective variants are:
- herpes simplex oesophagitis
- oesophagitis due to *Candida* infections

Herpes Simplex Oesophagitis

The oesophagus is a common visceral site for infection with herpes simplex virus; up to 25% of oesophageal ulcers as seen at post-mortem examination are said to be caused by this virus. Herpes infection at this site is particularly likely to occur in patients with leukaemia or malignant lymphoma, but may also be seen in individuals with no obvious predisposing cause.

The lesions begin as small vesicles which later break down to form small ulcers. On histological examination the herpetic nature of the ulcers is suggested by the presence in the oesophageal epithelium of multinucleated giant cells with intranuclear viral inclusion bodies.

Another cause of viral oesophagitis is **cytomegalovirus** (human herpesvirus 5), which is particularly likely to occur in patients with depressed cell-mediated immunity such as those with acquired immune deficiency syndrome (AIDS) or treated with immunosuppressive agents.

Candida Oesophagitis

Oesophageal candidiasis is also associated with AIDS and immunosuppressive drugs but may also be seen in patients treated with broad-spectrum antibiotics or steroids.

The oesophageal mucosa may show the presence of

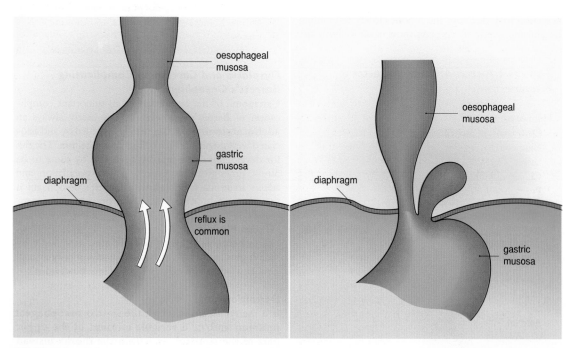

FIGURE 34.3 **a** Sliding oesophageal hernia. **b** Rolling oesophageal hernia.

whitish plaque-like areas which represent colonies of the fungus, or there may be slightly raised ulcerated areas in which the fungi may be seen.

Non-Infective Oesophagitis

Causes include:

1) ingestion of corrosive chemical such as strong acid or alkali

2) irradiation of the thorax

Both of these may lead to the formation of ulcers and tight strictures of the oesophagus, which require frequent dilatation.

3) graft versus host disease

4) presence of a nasogastric tube

5) certain associated conditions such as pemphigoid, epidermolysis bullosa and uraemia

OESOPHAGEAL TUMOURS

Benign tumours are rare. Most are connective tissue lesions, leiomyoma being the commonest, but haemangiomas, lipomas and nerve sheath tumours may be seen on occasion. Benign epithelial tumours in the form of small warty lesions; **squamous papillomas** do occur but are very rare.

Carcinoma of the Oesophagus

Most (90%) carcinomas of the oesophagus are, not surprisingly, **squamous** in type. Such adenocarcinomas as do occur are found almost exclusively in the lower one-third of the oesophagus.

Epidemiology

In the UK and USA the overall incidence of all forms of oesophageal cancer is reported as ranging from 5.2 to 10.4 per 100 000 population annually; this tumour is responsible for between 2% and 5% of deaths from malignant disease in these countries.

The frequency of oesophageal carcinoma shows striking variations in relation to different geographical locations. Countries with a high incidence include China, Japan, Finland, France and certain parts of Iran and South Africa. **Within single countries, marked variations in incidence also exist, suggesting that environmental rather than genetic factors are responsible for the observed differences**. For example, in the parts of Iran that border on the eastern shores of the Caspian Sea, the incidence of oesophageal cancer is **140 per 100 000** annually, whereas in the south of the country the frequency is much lower. Similarly in parts of northern China, oesophageal cancer occurs 70 times more frequently than in the USA, although in other parts the incidence is comparable with that found in North America. Within the USA it is noteworthy that Afro-Americans have a higher risk of developing carcinoma of the oesophagus than Caucasians.

Aetiology

Factors that may contribute to the geographical differences include:

- low concentrations of certain trace metals, notably molybdenum, in the soil of high incidence areas
- dietary habit. Among the associations that have been described are:
  a) a high consumption of very hot beverages
  b) a high intake of pickled vegetables that may contain nitrosamines
  c) a low intake of fresh fruit and vegetables

In developed countries the most important risk factors appear to be tobacco and alcohol. The tobacco-associated risk holds good for all forms of tobacco exposure, including cigarette and pipe smoking and also the chewing of tobacco. Excess ingestion of alcohol also appears to be a potent risk factor, **spirits** rather than wine or beer, being especially associated with the risk of cancer. The combination of heavy smoking and high alcohol intake appears to be particularly baneful.

An increased risk of oesophageal cancer is also said to be associated with chronic oesophagitis, as seen, for example, in achalasia.

Cytological studies carried out in high-incidence areas of China suggest that **there is a sequence of epithelial changes leading to full-blown cancer, analogous with what is seen in the uterine cervix. This starts with mild dysplasia and progresses through severe dysplasia to invasive cancer.**

The hallmark of dysplasia is an abnormal (dyskaryotic) nucleus which is enlarged and darkly staining. In mild dysplasia these nuclei are confined to the basal layer. As the dysplasia worsens, so the proportion of epithelium showing dysplastic change increases until, eventually, the entire thickness of the lining epithelium is replaced by abnormal cells. Severe dysplasia is associated with some degree of naked-eye change in the mucosal surface, manifesting either as a white plaque or an erosion.

Pathological Features

Most squamous carcinomas arise in the middle third (50%) or the lower third (30%) of the oesophagus, only 20% being found in the upper third. Three main macroscopic varieties are seen (*Figs 34.4* and *34.5*):

1) **Crateriform.** These tumours have everted edges raised above the level of the surrounding oesophageal mucosa. The surface is pinkish-grey and is ulcerated, granular and friable. In some instances the ulcer floor lies below the level of the uninvolved mucosa and the edges are vertical or undermined.

2) **Polypoid or fungating.** Here the neoplasm forms a soft bulky mass, protruding into the oesophageal lumen, which it may fill and even distend.

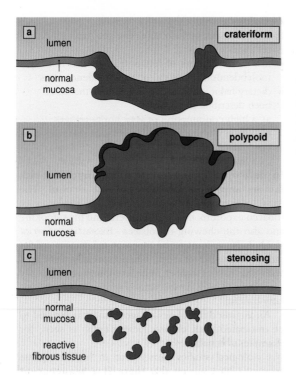

FIGURE 34.4 Principal morphological variants of oesophageal cancer.

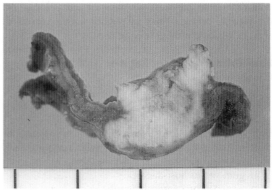

FIGURE 34.5 Large crateriform carcinoma of oesophagus. Note how deeply the white tumour tissue has infiltrated the oesophageal wall.

3) **Stenosing.** In this variety the tumour infiltrates the oesophageal wall extensively. The cells elicit a marked fibrous tissue response which produces a segment of puckering and narrowing.

Microscopic Features
These tumours may show all grades of differentiation from those in which there is obvious keratinization associated with well-formed cell nests, to very poorly differentiated examples in which keratin is absent and it is difficult to find recognizable prickles. There is a marked tendency for these lesions to spread submucosally and, in the case of surgically removed specimens, the whole circumference of the resection lines should be examined histologically to ensure complete removal of the tumour.

Adenocarcinoma of the Oesophagus
About 5–10% of oesophageal cancers are adenocarcinomas. The majority of these arise from metaplastic columnar epithelium (Barrett's oesophagus) but a small proportion are believed to originate from the submucosal glands of the oesophagus. It is by no means always easy to distinguish primary adenocarcinoma of the oesophagus from tumours arising within the stomach itself and spreading upwards into the oesophagus. **However, the presence of normal or dysplastic** columnar epithelium in the vicinity of the tumour strongly supports a local origin within a Barrett's oesophagus.

Patterns of Spread of Oesophageal Carcinoma

Direct Spread
Spread within the wall of the oesophagus is conspicuous, and is particularly marked in relation to the submucosa and submucosal lymphatics. Once the tumour has breached the muscularis propria, it commonly spreads to involve the trachea or main bronchi, the lung parenchyma and the structures in the superior or posterior mediastinum. Less commonly the aorta may be invaded directly and, more rarely still, the pericardium, heart and recurrent laryngeal nerves may be involved.

Metastatic Spread
Spread well beyond the confines of the oesophagus has already occurred in the majority of cases by the time a clinical diagnosis of carcinoma is established.

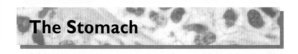

The Stomach

NORMAL ANATOMY

The stomach is a J-shaped hollow muscular organ with a normal volume of 1.2–1.5 litres. It is divided into **four** zones:

1) the **cardia**, occupying a small area distal to the gastro-oesophageal junction
2) the **fundus**, lying above an imaginary line drawn horizontally through the gastro-oesophageal junction

3) the **body**, representing about two-thirds of the remaining gastric area, is the area in which most gastric acid and pepsin secretion occurs

4) the **pyloric antrum**, occupying the remaining one-third of the stomach and leading into the pyloric sphincter

Gastric Mucosa

The mucosa is the site of the commonest and most important disorders affecting the stomach. **Its microscopic features are non-uniform, the differences corresponding roughly with the anatomical divisions mentioned above.** Both fundus and body mucosa show essentially the same appearances and these areas are, therefore, considered together.

On its deep aspect, the lining mucosa is delimited by the **muscularis mucosa**. In general terms, the mucosa consists of glands of varying type embedded in a delicate meshwork of well-vascularized connective tissue. These glands lead into straight-sided pits (**crypts or foveolae**), some of which fuse, whereas others drain directly into the gastric lumen.

The entire mucosal surface consists of a single layer of tall, mucin-secreting columnar cells with basal nuclei, and this epithelium continues downwards to form the pit lining. The secretion of mucus, sodium and bicarbonate by these cells contributes to the defence of the mucosa against acid and pepsin attack.

The different areas of mucosa are classified on the basis of two sets of histological criteria:

1) **the proportion of the mucosal thickness occupied by the crypts**
2) **the types of epithelial cells lining the glands in the different areas**

Cardiac Mucosa

The cardiac mucosa stretches down from the gastro-oesophageal junction for 0.5–3.5 cm. **The crypts occupy about half the thickness of the mucosa** and lead into glands lined by **mucin-secreting cells**, although occasional acid- or pepsin-secreting cells may also be seen and endocrine cells are quite common. Glands are often separated into lobules by strands of smooth muscle derived from the muscularis mucosae.

Body Mucosa

It is here that most acid and pepsin secretion occurs. **The crypts occupy only a quarter of the mucosal thickness**, the remainder being composed of tightly packed, straight-sided glands; a normal stomach contains 35 million body-type glands.

The two main secretory cell types are:

- **parietal cells, which are the source of acid, intrinsic factor and blood group substances**
- **chief cells, from which pepsinogen and other proteolytic enzymes are derived**

Parietal cells occur chiefly in the upper parts of the glands; the nucleus is central and cytoplasm is bright red in haematoxylin and eosin-stained sections. Maximal acid output correlates with the parietal cell mass and is normally 20–25 mmol per hour. Gastric mucosa maintains an enormous concentration gradient of hydrogen ions, H^+ concentrations in the gastric lumen being 2–3 million times greater than in blood or tissues.

Chief cells are concentrated in the deeper parts of the glands. Their nuclei are basal and the cytoplasm is basophilic, reflecting active protein synthesis. As the pyloric region is approached, the number of chief cells decreases and that of parietal cells increases.

Antral Mucosa

The antral mucosa occupies a roughly triangular area in the distal third of the stomach. **The gastric pits penetrate more deeply than in the body mucosa, occupying about half the mucosal thickness.** Glands are fewer than in the body and, hence, less tightly packed. They are lined chiefly by mucin-secreting cells with a basal nucleus, although some parietal cells may also be seen.

Gastric Neuroendocrine Cells

Neuroendocrine cells occur in all parts of the gastric mucosa and are recognized in conventionally stained sections by their clear cytoplasm. Some are foregut-derived, others from the mid-gut; most stain black with silver salts after exposure to reducing agents (**argyrophilia**). A minority are **argentaffin** (stain with silver salts in the absence of a reducing agent) but all can be identified easily with antibodies against the enzyme neurone-specific enolase. Gastric neuroendocrine cells produce a large number of products including **gastrin (G cells), somatostatin, serotonin, vasoactive intestinal peptide, bombesin (gastrin-releasing peptide) and pancreatic polypeptide.**

DEVELOPMENTAL DISORDERS

Congenital Hypertrophic Pyloric Stenosis

This occurs in about **1 in 400 live births**. It is commonest in first-born children and affects males much more frequently than females (M : F ratio 4 : 1). There appears to be a **polygenic pattern of inheritance**, siblings and offspring of affected individuals being at increased risk. It may uncommonly be associated with other congenital abnormalities in the gut such as **imperforate anus and duodenal or oesophageal atresia**. It is probably a motor disorder, analogous to oesophageal achalasia; indeed, there is a paucity of ganglion cells relating to the circular muscle layer in the pylorus.

Clinical presentation, characterized by projectile vomiting, usually occurs at the age of 2–4 weeks.

The main pathological feature is hypertrophy of the circular layer of the muscularis propria which is increased in thickness by a factor of two to four. This mass of hypertrophied muscle stretches up from the pylorus for about 2 cm. It is often possible to feel the hypertrophied pylorus on abdominal palpation just after the infant has fed. Loss of H^+ and Cl^- in the vomitus leads to **hypochloraemic alkalosis**. The infants fail to thrive and become severely malnourished. Incision through the hypertrophied muscle usually produces complete relief of the obstruction.

GASTRITIS AND PEPTIC ULCERATION

This is a set of disorders ranging from acute, relatively mild, inflammation in gastric or duodenal mucosa to chronic, deeply penetrating, ulcers. These disorders are considered as separate entities, but it is important to appreciate that **all represent an imbalance between factors, chiefly acid and pepsin, that are liable to damage the mucosa and those that defend the mucosa** (*Fig. 34.6*). **Thus disease may occur in this context, either as a result of an increase in aggressive factors (e.g. increased acid secretion) or a decrease in the strength of the defence mechanisms.**

Factors Likely to Damage the Gastric and Duodenal Mucosa

These factors are:

- **high acid secretion**★
- **high pepsin secretion**★

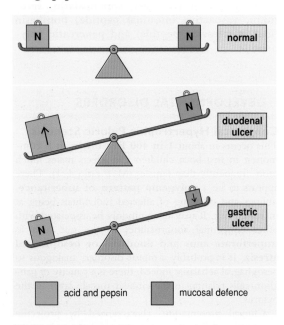

FIGURE 34.6 *Injury and defence in peptic ulcer formation.*

- **reflux of duodenal contents into the stomach**★
- **organ-specific autoimmune mechanisms** are associated with one type of chronic gastritis
- **infections with *Helicobacter pylori*★**
- **mucosal ischaemia**

The asterisked factors are thought to play a pathogenetic role in peptic ulceration.

Acid Secretion

Gastric acid is secreted by the parietal cells. Stimulation of these cells causes changes in the cytoskeleton, increasing the area of intracytoplasmic membrane in contact with luminal surface membrane.

Secretion of hydrogen ions into the gland lumen is accomplished by the action of a proton pump acting as an exchanger of protons for extracellular K^+ in the gastric lumen. This pump is H^+, K^+, adenosine 5′-triphosphatase, which after parietal cell stimulation is translocated from tubulovesicles into a compartment linked with the apical membrane of the cell. Inhibitors of this pump (substituted benzimidazoles) have been used in the treatment of peptic ulcer.

Control of Acid Secretion

Parietal cell acid secretion is regulated by the binding of extracellular signals to specific plasma membrane receptors. These signals may be either **stimulatory** or **inhibitory** and reach the parietal cells via a number of pathways:

- **Endocrine.** The hormone circulating in the blood that stimulates the production of acid is **gastrin** released from the G cells, which constitute a major proportion of the gastric neuroendocrine cell population. They are concentrated in the antral mucosa. **Release of gastrin is triggered by both nervous and chemical stimuli.** The mechanisms for the first of these is **gastrin-releasing peptide**, liberated from the mucosal nerve endings, and showing homology with **bombesin**. The main intraluminal chemical agents stimulating gastrin release are breakdown products of protein digestion.

  Both gastrin and acid secretion are inhibited by **somatostatin**, which acts on the parietal and G cells in a paracrine fashion. Somatostatin release is mediated by β-adrenergic stimuli, cholecystokinin, acidification of the luminal contents and, weakly, by gastrin itself. Release of acid is also inhibited by locally synthesized prostaglandins.

- **Nervous, involving release of acetylcholine from mucosal nerve endings.** This acetylcholine binds to a receptor on the parietal cell.

- **Paracrine chemical signals released from cells in the neighbourhood of the parietal cells.** The chief paracrine stimulus to acid secretion is **histamine** released from mucosal mast cells. Blockage of histamine receptors on the parietal cells by drugs such as ranitidine reduces basal secretion of acid and lowers the effects of physiological stimulation of gastric secretion and of gastrin on the parietal cell.

Pepsin Secretion

The acid protease pepsin is produced from two inactive precursors, pepsinogens I and II, which occur in five sites:

- the chief and neck cells in the fundus and body, which produce both varieties of pepsinogen
- the cardiac glands, the glands of the antral mucosa and Brunner's glands in the duodenum (type II only)

Secretion is stimulated by a vagal cholinergic pathway and also by secretin and vasoactive intestinal polypeptide.

Pepsin is an important potential noxa in the stomach and duodenum because it can digest the surface mucus layer.

Helicobacter Pylori *Infection, Gastritis and Peptic Ulcer*

Helicobacter is a Gram-negative curved bacillus found in gastric mucosal biopsies from patients with chronic gastritis and peptic ulcer. It was originally named *Campylobacter pylori*, but differs in many ways from true campylobacters, one of the most noteworthy being its powerful **urease** activity. Thus it was assigned a new name – *Helicobacter pylori* – in 1989. The urease leads to an increase in local pH and this may enable the organism to survive in what is normally a hostile acid environment. In addition, *H. pylori* also produces enzymes and an exotoxin, some of which may injure the surface epithelium of the antral mucosa, which is preferentially colonized.

H. pylori is found in humans **only in association with gastric epithelium** or with metaplastic gastric epithelium in the duodenum or oesophagus and, rarely, in heterotopic gastric epithelium in Meckel's diverticulum or the rectum. It is not found in the blood.

The organism is commonly found on microscopic examination of gastric biopsies from patients with dyspepsia of varying degrees of severity. It does not penetrate the mucosa nor is it found in mucosal surface cells. It is not difficult to see on haematoxylin and eosin-stained sections but is rendered much more obvious if the Giemsa stain or silver stains (Warthin–Starry) are used. It can be cultured from biopsy material.

A non-invasive diagnosis can be made by means of the **urea breath test**. The patients ingest ^{14}C-labelled urea. If sufficient *H. pylori*-derived urease is present in the stomach, labelled carbon dioxide is split from the urea, absorbed into the blood and then expired in the breath, where it can be detected readily.

H. pylori is present on the gastric mucosa in a proportion of apparently healthy individuals, this proportion increasing with age. About 10% of those younger than 30 years have *H. pylori* infections, whereas the

prevalence rate in healthy 60 year olds is 60%. Being Afro-American, socioeconomically deprived, and/or in jail all increase the chances of infection. Transmission is believed to be from person to person; no exogenous source such as food or water has yet been identified. In the duodenum the presence of the organism is noted only in patients with duodenitis associated with gastric metaplasia or duodenal ulcer.

There is a strong association between *H. pylori* infection and gastroduodenal disorders.

- Virtually all patients with duodenal ulcer show evidence of infection, as do about 80% of those with gastric ulcer and 60% with non-autoimmune chronic gastritis.
- The gastritis associated with *H. pylori* infection shows, in addition to the presence of chronic inflammatory cells through the whole thickness of the mucosa, a superficial infiltration by neutrophils. **The presence of intramucosal lymphoid follicles is strongly associated with the presence of *Helicobacter* and, when seen, should prompt a careful search for the organisms.** Intramucosal lymphoid follicles are not present in the normal stomach; thus there is no normal cell population from which gastric lymphoma can arise. The fact that low-grade B-cell gastric lymphomas occur, and that they show morphological features of antigen responsiveness, has suggested an association between *H. pylori* infection and such mucosa-associated lymphoid tissue tumours (**MALT lymphomas**).

  Recently, it has been shown that neoplastic B cells from gastric MALT lymphomas and non-neoplastic T cells respond to *H. pylori* by **proliferating**, by **secreting more interleukin (IL) 2** and by **expressing the IL-2 receptor** to a greater degree. In several cases of *H. pylori*-associated gastric lymphoma, eradication of the organisms led to regression of the lymphoma.

- Evidence exists to suggest that *H. pylori* is the cause rather than merely an association of one form of gastritis. Voluntary ingestion of *H. pylori* leads to achlorhydric gastritis, which can progress to chronic gastritis. Elimination of the organism by bismuth compounds, metronidazole and antibiotics in patients with gastritis has been followed by histological improvement. An aetiological role for *H. pylori* in ulcer disease is less clear. **Recent studies have shown that *H. pylori* infection of antral mucosa is associated with increased gastrin production, and thus with increased postprandial acid secretion.** It has been stated also that patients with peptic ulcer who have been treated both with drugs that reduce acid secretion (e.g. H_2-receptor antagonists) and with those that may eliminate *H. pylori* have a lower prevalence of ulcer recurrence than patients who have been treated with H_2-receptor antagonists alone.
- It is now accepted that, in addition to its

pathogenetic role in peptic ulceration, *H. pylori* also acts as a carcinogen in relation to the gastric mucosa. Gastric cancer is believed to occur in 1% of those infected with *H. pylori*, whereas the risk of duodenal ulceration is about 20%. Thus a paradox exists in relation to *H. pylori* infection, because normally the risk for gastric cancer is inversely related to the existence of a duodenal ulcer. It seems likely that factors additional to *H. pylori* infection must operate in the pathogenesis of duodenal ulceration and gastric cancer, and that these sets of factors must be different for each of these two disorders.

Gastric cancer is commonest in countries of the developing world where *H. pylori* infection is most likely to occur during early childhood. Such early infections lead to multiple foci of atrophic gastritis which predispose affected individuals to both gastric ulcer and gastric cancer. In developed countries, the prevalence of *H. pylori* infection is decreasing and, in any event, occurs later in life. Thus gastric cancer is not commonly a sequel of *H. pylori* infection, and duodenal ulceration is commoner than in the developing world.

Factors Believed to Defend the Gastric and Duodenal Mucosa

Mucus and Bicarbonate Secretion
A surface layer of mucus admixed with bicarbonate is an important barrier to the back-diffusion of acid (*Fig. 34.7*). The mucus may provide a zone of limited mixing, allowing maintenance of an alkaline pH at the gastric surface. This mucus allows the formation of diffusion gradients of bicarbonate from mucosa to lumen, and of acid from lumen to mucosa. Thus the pH at the luminal aspect is 1–2, whereas at the epithelial side it reaches 7.

The effectiveness of this barrier depends on four interacting factors:
1) the rate of mucus **secretion**
2) the rate of mucus **breakdown**, occurring partly from acid–pepsin digestion and partly as a result of mechanical shearing stresses on the surface of the mucous layer
3) the rate of **bicarbonate secretion** at the epithelial surface. This is stimulated by glucagon, gastric inhibitory polypeptide, noradrenaline and prostaglandins of the E type. Acidification of the fundus promotes bicarbonate secretion from the fundus but not from the duodenum, whereas acidification of the duodenum promotes bicarbonate release from both sites
4) the rate of **penetration** of the mucus layer by intraluminal acid

Prevention of Back-Diffusion of Hydrogen Ions
Secretion of mucus and bicarbonate protects surface epithelium from the effects of acid and pepsin, but does not explain how acid-secreting glandular epithelium is protected from acid that passes over it during secretion.

Glandular epithelial cells form high-resistance intercellular junctions of approximately 2000 ohms/cm² (at pH 3.5–6.5). If the pH is decreased to 2, resistance is increased by a factor of nearly three. This barrier function is a property of apical cell membranes, and is absent from basal and lateral aspects; it is disrupted by aspirin, which may adversely affect the mucosal milieu in different ways.

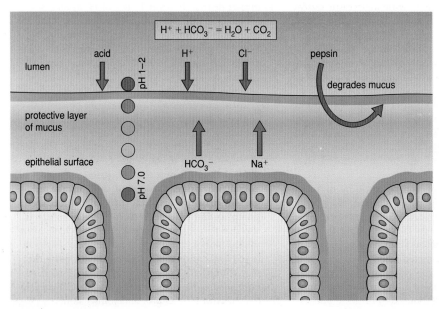

FIGURE 34.7 *Mucus and bicarbonate secretion as defence mechanisms against acid and pepsin.*

Local Production of Prostaglandins Chiefly of the E Type

Prostaglandins exert a cytoprotective effect on both gastric and duodenal mucosa; a decline in local production of prostaglandins decreases bicarbonate production by gastric and duodenal mucosal cells. This may be the basis of aspirin-associated gastritis as aspirin inhibits the cyclo-oxygenase pathway and thus blocks prostaglandin production.

GASTRITIS

The term gastritis covers many conditions in which the only common feature is the presence of mucosal inflammation. Biopsy of gastric mucosa at fibreoptic endoscopy has allowed more precise definition in terms of morphology and function.

Acute Gastritis (Acute Erosive Gastropathy)

Definition

In this condition, the mucosa is hyperaemic and, in severe cases, there may be evidence of bleeding and/or mucosal erosions (by definition not involving the whole thickness of the mucosa) (*Fig. 34.8*).

Associations

Acute gastritis has been associated with many potentially mucosa-damaging situations such as overindulgence in alcohol and cigarettes, treatment with corticosteroids, aspirin and non-steroidal anti-inflammatory drugs like phenylbutazone, strong acids and alkalis, bile reflux, certain chemotherapeutic agents and some systemic infections.

In addition a similar picture may be seen in seriously ill patients suffering the effects of trauma, burns, sepsis or hypothermia, and in these cases mucosal ischaemia has been invoked as the responsible mechanism. Erosions associated with aspirin toxicity and excess alcohol can be found anywhere on the gastric mucosa, whereas those accompanying trauma or sepsis tend to be localized on the antral portion of the lesser curve. Endoscopy shows erosive lesions are common in patients who have been 'stressed' in the ways mentioned above (erosions present in 86% of patients with major burns, and 75% in cases of serious head injury).

> ### Microscopic Features
>
> The correlate of the naked-eye picture is **hyperaemia, oedema and focal haemorrhage** within the upper part of the interglandular connective tissue. If erosions are present, there is obvious focal necrosis of surface epithelium with a fibrin-rich slough covering the denuded areas. If the circumstances causing the gastritis are removed or reversed, the mucosa regenerates within a few days.

Chronic Gastritis

Chronic gastritis is a set of mucosal inflammatory disorders with different histological appearances, aetiologies and natural histories. Some are associated with intestinal type metaplasia, an increased risk of peptic ulcer disease and carcinoma of the stomach.

Chronic gastritis may be classified on the basis **of either the histological appearances or the aetiological and pathogenetic mechanisms believed to be involved**.

Classification

Histological classification is based on four criteria, the use of which shows two basic histological types as summarized in *Table 34.5*.

Gastric Atrophy

This is the most severe form of chronic gastritis and is characterized by mucosa that is much thinner than normal. Very few specialized glands survive and intestinal metaplasia is a prominent feature (*Figs 34.9* and *34.10*).

The inflammatory infiltrate has usually regressed by this stage, although lymphoid aggregates may still be present. The long-term risk for gastric cancer is 2–4%.

Aetiological and Pathogenetic Classification of Chronic Gastritis

When the correlations between histological appearances and functional changes are studied in patients with chronic gastritis, it is clear that there are two major types, known as **types A and B**, the features of which are summarized in *Table 34.6*.

Type B gastritis can be further subdivided in an attempt to delineate the factors responsible and the likely natural history. Two groups have been described: hypersecretory and environmental gastritis.

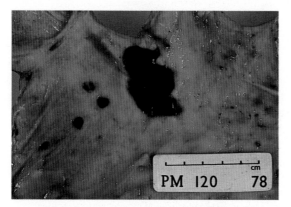

FIGURE 34.8 Acute gastric erosions in a patient dying from hypothermia.

Table 34.5 Criteria for the Histological Classification of Chronic Gastritis

Disorder	Chronic superficial gastritis	Atrophic gastritis
Type of mucosa	Any area	Body and antral mucosa
Level of involvement (superficial or deep)	Superficial: glandular elements spared	All layers of mucosa involved, resulting in glandular atrophy and loss of specialized cells. If associated with pernicious anaemia, gastrin-producing cells in the antrum become hyperplastic
Inflammatory infiltrate	Plasma cells, lymphocytes and some neutrophils. Cells may invade glandular epithelium. Aggregates of lymphoid cells may be present, especially if caused by *H. pylori* infection	Similar to superficial variety but more extensive and severe
Presence of intestinal metaplasia (transformation of part of gastric mucosa into structures resembling small or large intestine)	No	Two types are seen: 1) **Complete**, showing both mucin-secreting goblet cells and absorptive cells with a brush border 2) **Incomplete**, showing mucin-producing cells only. Either sialomucins or sulphated mucins produced by goblet cells. Only 12% of patients produce sulphated mucins but 90% of these develop carcinoma. This finding on biopsy demands surveillance of the patient.

Hypersecretory Gastritis

In this variant there is increased secretion of both acid and pepsin. This exceeds the protective powers of the mucus–bicarbonate layer, and first gastritis and then ulceration may result. Such ulcers are usually found in the duodenum or just proximal to the pylorus. Intestinal metaplasia is not a prominent feature and there is no increased risk of developing gastric carcinoma.

Environmental Gastritis

The prevalence of this type shows considerable geographical variation: prevalence rates are highest in parts of the world where there is a high frequency of gastric cancer. In Japan, gastric cancer is very common, and a strong association exists between increasing age and the risk of chronic atrophic gastritis of this type. Fewer than 10% of Japanese people aged above 60 years have a normal gastric mucosa. The geographical variation suggests

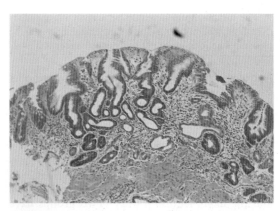

FIGURE 34.9 Gastric atrophy. The mucosa is thinner than normal and there is a paucity of specialized glands.

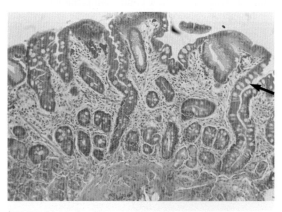

FIGURE 34.10 Another case of atrophic gastritis showing intestinal metaplasia; numerous goblet cells (arrow) are seen in some glands.

Table 34.6 Aetiological and Pathogenetic Classification of Chronic Gastritis

Type A	Type B
Affects mainly body mucosa	Chiefly involves antrum. Either no or slight patchy involvement of body
Associated with low or absent acid secretion (achlorhydria)	Associated with high or normal gastric acid secretion
Associated with high plasma gastrin levels	High frequency of *H. pylori* infection
Decreased secretion of pepsinogen	Normal or high levels of pepsinogen secretion
Often associated with antiparietal cell antibodies (50–90% in patients with pernicious anaemia; 20–40% in those with type A gastritis without pernicious anaemia)	Not associated with antiparietal cell antibodies
Believed to be an organ-specific autoimmune disease. Immunoglobulin G antibodies bind to the gastrin receptor on parietal cells. Other antibodies react with intrinsic factor (see pp 880–882)	

that environmental factors, probably dietary in nature, are responsible. Acid and pepsin secretion are not increased in amount.

The inflammation usually starts at or near the junction between the antrum and the body, in the form of multiple small foci, and then spreads along the lesser curvature in both proximal and distal directions. Intestinal metaplasia is commonly found.

Associations with Chronic Gastritis

Gastric Ulcer

There is a strong association between chronic gastritis and gastric ulcer; the more proximal the ulcer, the more extensive is the gastritis and the greater the likelihood of intestinal metaplasia. Healing of the gastric ulcer is not usually accompanied by regression of the gastritis. It has been suggested that a likely sequence of events is **biliary reflux** leading to gastritis, leading to gastric ulcer. The gastritis is of the type B variety.

Iron Deficiency Anaemia

Of patients with iron deficiency anaemia, in whom no other cause has been demonstrated, about 40% have chronic gastritis. The anaemia may be due to occult bleeding from tiny erosions in the gastric mucosa or may be due to failure to absorb non-haem iron, for which gastric acid is necessary.

Gastric Carcinoma

There is a greater risk of cancer occurring in association with chronic atrophic gastritis than in a matched population without gastritis. A Finnish study showed a 10% prevalence of gastric cancer, over a 20-year follow-up period, in patients whose biopsy showed chronic gastritis. Of individuals with a normal biopsy, 0.6% developed cancer over the same follow-up period. This increased risk appears to be related chiefly to type B gastritis, the link being the development of type 2 intestinal metaplasia-associated production of sulphated mucins.

PEPTIC ULCER

Definition

Peptic ulcer is a set of disorders characterized by **well-circumscribed mucosal defects, found only in portions of the gastrointestinal tract that are exposed to the acid and pepsin components of gastric juice**. Thus, although most ulcers occur in the stomach and the first part of the duodenum, they may also be seen in:

    a) the oesophagus as a result of reflux of gastric contents
    b) at the sites of gastrojejunal anastomosis
    c) in and adjacent to a Meckel's diverticulum, should this contain ectopic gastric mucosa
    d) in the second, third and fourth parts of the duodenum and, occasionally, in the upper jejunum in patients with a gastrin-secreting pancreatic islet cell tumour (the Zollinger–Ellison syndrome)

Classification

Peptic ulcers may be classified as **acute** or **chronic**; acute lesions are further subdivided into erosions and acute ulcers. These categories refer to the depth of penetration within the gut wall and the presence or absence of scarring at the ulcer base.

- **Erosions** are lesions in which the focal loss of mucosa **does not involve the full thickness of the mucosal layer, found in association with acute gastritis due to a variety of causes**.
- **Acute ulcers** are lesions **involving the full thickness of the mucosa**. They may or may not penetrate to the deeper layers of the gastric or duodenal wall, and **are not associated with the presence of scarring at the base**.
- **Chronic ulcers** are lesions in which the depth of penetration varies, although the **muscularis**

mucosae is always breached. Scarring is always present at the ulcer base.

Epidemiology

The prevalence of peptic ulcer is difficult to determine accurately, but ulcer constitutes a major cause of ill health. The prevalence of gastric and duodenal ulcers differs sharply, reinforcing the view that different pathogenetic mechanisms operate in these two disorders.

In men in the USA and UK, the frequency of duodenal ulcer ranges from 1 to 3.5 per 1000 per year and that of gastric ulcer is about 0.5 per 1000 per year. Males are more often affected than females, the male : female ratio in duodenal ulcer being about 4 : 1, whereas for gastric ulcer this ratio falls to about 1.5 : 1. Gastric and duodenal ulceration tend to occur at different ages, the peak incidence of duodenal ulcer being in the thirties, whereas gastric ulcer is a disorder of much older people, with a peak incidence in the fifties. Peptic ulceration is rare in children but may be seen from time to time, such ulcers carrying with them a high risk of perforation.

Sites of Ulcer Formation within Stomach and Duodenum

Within the stomach and duodenum chronic peptic ulcers are found in a fairly restricted area. **In the stomach, ulcers occur chiefly along the lesser curvature just distal to the transition zone between the acid-secreting body mucosa and the non-acid-secreting antral mucosa.** The localization of gastric ulcers to the antral mucosa may well reflect the predilection for reflux-mediated gastritis to affect this area, but relative ischaemia of the mucosa due to contraction of prominent muscle bundles may also play a part.

In the duodenum, the ulcers are concentrated in an area about 1 cm distal to the pylorus, usually in the anterior or posterior aspect of the duodenal bulb.

Pathogenesis

Peptic ulcer disease represents a **disturbance in the normal equilibrium existing between factors likely to injure the mucosa and those defending it from such injury.** Such a disturbance can be brought about in several ways and, thus, not only are there striking pathogenetic differences between gastric and duodenal ulcers, but even the single entity, duodenal ulcer, may be simply a common pathological endpoint with different pathogenetic routes.

Pathophysiology

Gastric Ulcer

Gastric ulcer is associated with an increased frequency of antral gastritis and intestinal metaplasia. A major causal factor is duodenogastric reflux. The refluxing duodenal contents contain sodium taurocholate derived from the bile. This decreases bicarbonate secretion and thus diminishes the pH gradient across the mucous layer, an effect also produced by aspirin (see p 506).

The tendency for reflux to occur is enhanced by any reduction in pyloric sphincter tone. Interestingly, in view of the association of cigarette smoking with ulcer, such tone is decreased following smoking.

Both maximal acid secretion and pepsinogen secretion are within normal limits or slightly lower than normal. Lower than normal acid secretion causes an increase in plasma gastrin levels as a result of a reduced negative feedback effect on the G cells.

Duodenal Ulcer

In terms of pathogenesis, duodenal ulcer shows a remarkable degree of **heterogeneity. Many pathophysiological abnormalities have been described in association with duodenal ulceration but none of these appears to be present in more than 20–50% of patients with duodenal ulcer.** To a much greater extent than gastric ulcer, duodenal ulcer seems to result from interactions between factors altering the microenvironment of the duodenal mucosa and certain inherited characteristics. In general terms, aggressive mechanisms (i.e. acid and pepsin secretion) seem to play a more important role than in gastric ulcer, but this may simply be a reflection of relative ignorance about mucosal defence mechanisms in the duodenum.

Genetic Considerations

- There is an increased risk of duodenal and prepyloric ulcers, and of combined gastroduodenal ulcers, in individuals of blood group O. This association does not exist in respect of ulcers of the fundus or body of the stomach.
- A fairly high degree of concordance is observed for the risk of duodenal ulcer in monozygotic twins and, in certain inbred strains of mice, virtually 100% of the animals develop duodenal ulcers.
- Some increase occurs in the prevalence of HLA-B5 in patients with duodenal ulcer, compared with the general population.
- Certain rare, genetically determined, syndromes are associated with a high risk of duodenal ulcer. These include:
  1) **Zollinger–Ellison syndrome**, when it occurs as part of the multiple endocrine neoplasia syndrome (type 1). About 60% of cases of Zollinger–Ellison syndrome are now believed to be determined genetically. The pancreatic adenomas in this disorder secrete large amounts of gastrin, which sharply increases gastric acid secretion and also the growth of acid- and pepsin-secreting cells.
  2) **Systemic mastocytosis.** This is a rare inherited condition in which there is diffuse

hyperplasia of mast cells which release their contents thus eliciting skin rashes, flushing, abdominal pain and, in about 30% of cases, duodenal ulcer. The release of histamine from the mast cells is presumably the cause of acid hypersecretion.

3) A familial syndrome has been reported of tremor, nystagmus and narcolepsy in which 50% of affected members of the kindred developed duodenal ulcer. The mechanism operating here is quite unknown.

4) A familial form of hyperpepsinogenaemia I has also been identified. Blood levels of pepsinogen I are raised in about half the patients with duodenal ulcer, and, because pepsinogen secretion correlates positively with maximal acid output, these patients also have hypersecretion of gastric acid.

Pathophysiology

Gastric Acid Secretion
About one-third of patients with duodenal ulcer show increased maximal gastric acid secretion; higher than normal basal acid secretion rates are found in a similar fraction. It seems likely that this is not due simply to an increase in parietal cell mass but also reflects an increased sensitivity of the parietal cells to gastrin.

Pepsinogen Secretion
Maximal pepsinogen secretion correlates with maximal acid secretion, and intragastric proteolytic activity is higher in patients with duodenal ulcer than in matched controls, especially with respect to pepsinogen I, which appears to have greater mucolytic properties than other forms of pepsin.

Gastrin Secretion
Basal secretion of gastrin is not raised in patients with duodenal ulcer, but plasma levels of gastrin after feeding are greater than in matched controls. This food-stimulated release of gastrin probably plays a significant part in promoting the increased gastric acid secretion in patients with duodenal ulcer.

Gastric Emptying
In a proportion of patients with duodenal ulcer, gastric emptying is abnormally fast, thus the duodenal mucosa is exposed to an acid load not yet buffered by ingested food. Acidification of the duodenal contents normally delays gastric emptying but this mechanism seems to be impaired in patients with an ulcer.

Associations with Duodenal Ulcer
Associations reported between certain systemic diseases and duodenal ulceration include:
- chronic obstructive airway disease
- hyperparathyroidism
- cirrhosis of the liver
- chronic renal failure
- α_1-antitrypsin deficiency

Pathology of Peptic Ulcer

Macroscopic Features
Active lesions have well-demarcated margins and are usually round or oval, although occasionally a linear outline is present (*Fig. 34.11*). The ulcers are usually single, being multiple in only 5% of cases. Most are less than 3 cm in diameter, although much smaller ones also occur.

The edges are well defined; the proximal margin often has an overhanging edge, whereas that of the distal margin is usually sloping.

In an active ulcer the floor is covered by a greyish-white exudate and the base is firm as a result of the replacement of muscle by scar tissue.

On the mucosal aspect of the stomach, there is some flattening of the immediately adjacent mucosa; beyond this zone the mucosal folds appear to radiate out from the ulcerated area.

Occasionally a very large ulcer may be present; at one time this was thought to be suspicious of malignancy but this is no longer believed to be the case.

Microscopic Features
All active chronic peptic ulcers have a similar histological appearance, with four zones (Askanazy's zones) being distinguishable. These reflect the overlapping processes that occur in chronic inflammation from whatever cause:
- a) cell and tissue injury and destruction
- b) the resulting inflammatory response
- c) demolition of exudate and dead tissue by macrophages
- d) attempted healing represented by granulation tissue and scar tissue formation

From the mucosal surface outwards one sees:-

1) A thin layer of exudate composed of a fibrin meshwork containing acute inflammatory cells, and some remnants of dead cells.

2) A layer of necrotic tissue appearing as an amorphous eosinophilic layer containing the bluish remains of nuclei of destroyed cells, and a moderate number of leucocytes.

3) A layer of inflammatory granulation tissue containing numerous large capillaries and a mixed inflammatory infiltrate.

4) A layer of dense fibrous tissue replacing the muscularis propria to varying depths. Embedded within this scar tissue are blood vessels showing fibromuscular intimal thickening, presumably due to the paracrine effects of growth factors. The fact that these vessels are surrounded by dense scar tissue is believed to contribute to the severe bleeding that occurs if they are eroded by inflammation. They are thought to be unable to contract or retract normally.

At the margins of the ulcer bed, fusion between the muscularis mucosae and the surviving muscularis propria on each side is common. This is a useful histological sign as it is absolutely characteristic of chronic peptic ulceration and is *not* seen in cases of carcinoma of the stomach where the tumour has ulcerated.

The adjacent mucosa, in gastric ulcers, is usually of the antral type and shows the presence of chronic gastritis and intestinal metaplasia. If healing has commenced, the epithelium at the ulcer edges starts to regenerate and this proliferating epithelium may, in some cases, be mistaken by the inexperienced for malignant transformation.

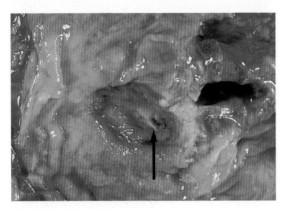

FIGURE 34.11 An active, deeply penetrating, duodenal ulcer with a bleeding point (arrow) in the ulcer floor.

Complications of Peptic Ulceration

Haemorrhage

This occurs in 15–20% of patients with a chronic ulcer. Ulcers in the postbulbar region of the duodenum and stomal ulcers are especially likely to bleed. Chronic small-scale bleeding manifests as iron-deficiency anaemia, the haemorrhage being diagnosed by the presence of 'occult' blood in the stools.

The clinical presentation of a large bleed may be the vomiting of fresh or altered blood (haematemesis) or the passing of stools admixed with large amounts of blood, which causes the stools to become black and shiny ('tarry' stools). An acute large bleed should always be regarded as a serious, indeed a potentially life-threatening event, the mortality rate being about 5%.

Perforation

Perforation complicates less than 10% of peptic ulcers. Perforation is most frequently seen in ulcers on the anterior aspect of either the gastric antrum or the first part of the duodenum. Escape of gastric or duodenal contents into the peritoneal cavity is classically associated with the sudden onset of very severe pain and the rapid development of board-like rigidity of the abdomen due to peritoneal irritation. However, especially in the elderly, unsuspected perforated ulcers may be found at post-mortem examination, the usual clinical features having been absent.

The perforation can be recognized as a sharply punched-out hole in the serosal surface of the anterior wall of the stomach or duodenum, the surrounding serosa showing a loss of its normal glistening appearance as a result of the deposition of fibrin in the inflamed area.

Penetration

A deeply penetrating ulcer is often associated with an inflammatory reaction on the serosa and this may lead to the affected area of the stomach or duodenum becoming adherent to an adjacent organ. This most frequently involves the pancreas, the substance of which can become eroded by the active ulcer. Localized inflammation within the pancreas develops and is often associated with intractable pain radiating to the back.

Erosion of blood vessels within the pancreatic bed with resulting haemorrhage and/or acute haemorrhagic pancreatitis can occur, but is distinctly rare.

Occasionally the ulcer-bearing area of the stomach becomes adherent to the serosal surface of the transverse colon. If the ulcer penetrates the entire thickness of the stomach wall, a channel may be formed between the stomach and the colon (gastrocolic fistula).

Obstruction due to Scarring

Chronicity in inflammatory disorders is associated with scarring, and the stomach and duodenum are no exceptions. If the ulcer is in the prepyloric region, severe scarring may lead to pyloric stenosis and, thus, obstruction. If such scarring occurs in relation to an ulcer in the middle of the stomach, a curious deformation, rather appropriately called an 'hour-glass stomach' can develop and, once this has occurred, the only rational form of treatment is gastrectomy.

Malignant Transformation

This is very rare, the term 'ulcer cancer' being used for a carcinoma that has developed at the margins of a pre-existing chronic peptic ulcer. If strict microscopic criteria are observed, probably less than 1% of chronic ulcers are complicated by carcinoma.

Before a histological diagnosis of ulcer cancer is made, the following criteria must be satisfied:
1) **There must be basal scarring which interrupts the muscularis propria**, and malignant cells must not be present in this scarred area, which is never invaded in true ulcer cancers.
2) **Fusion of the main muscle layers with the muscularis mucosae** must be present.
3) **There must be undoubted malignancy at the ulcer margins.**

TUMOURS AND TUMOUR-LIKE LESIONS

GASTRIC CARCINOMA

Epidemiology

At the beginning of the twentieth century, the leading cause of death from malignancy was carcinoma of the stomach. However, the incidence of gastric cancer has been decreasing steadily over the past three decades, although in the USA it is still the third commonest malignancy of the gastrointestinal tract.

The geographical variation in incidence is even more marked than for oesophageal cancer. For example, the prevalence rates in Japan for both males and females are eight times higher than those in the USA. Other countries in which there is a higher risk of gastric cancer include China, Chile, Brazil, Columbia, Iceland, Yugoslavia and Spain. Even within single countries, there appear to be regional and racial differences in risk. Thus, in the USA, Afro-Americans and native Americans have a higher incidence of gastric cancer than Caucasians.

These data suggest that environmental factors play a significant part in the genesis of gastric cancer, and consideration of the fate of migrant populations suggests further that these factors influence the target populations relatively early in life. Thus adults who migrate from high-risk to low-risk countries maintain their high level of risk, although their children and grandchildren show a lower risk of developing gastric cancer.

A clear relationship exists between the geographical distribution of gastric cancer and the actual type of carcinoma, leading some to conclude that gastric carcinoma is not one but two separate disorders. Carcinoma of the stomach found in 'high-risk' areas is chiefly of the so-called **'intestinal'** variety, whereas the **'diffuse'** type shows no geographically determined differences in frequency.

Aetiology and Pathogenesis

Possible Hereditary Factors

- **Familial clustering of gastric cancer occurs.** For example, in China the risk of gastric cancer in blood relatives of patients is nearly eight times higher than that of controls.
- **Blood group A is linked with the risk of developing the 'diffuse' type of gastric cancer.** Some 38% of the population have blood group A and 50% of patients with gastric cancer belong to this group.
- **Inheritance of the phenotype for secretion of one type of pepsinogen rather than another** carries with it an eightfold increase in risk.

Possible Environmental Factors

Carcinogens or precarcinogens may be encountered in the diet and are worthy of consideration in relation to the epidemiology of this tumour.

Nitrosamines and the Diet

Nitrosamines are well recognized as carcinogens in various animal models. Are they present or formed in human diets and, if so, does their presence correlate with observed geographical variations in cancer incidence? **The answer to both these questions is a qualified yes.**

In China, the regions of highest risk for gastric cancer are those where the level of nitrites and nitrates in drinking water and in vegetables is also highest. In Columbia, another high-risk country, patients with atrophic gastritis have high nitrite levels in the gastric juice.

Nitrates, whether derived from food or water, can be converted in the stomach to **nitrites** by nitrate reductase-synthesizing bacteria. The proliferation of such bacteria is aided by a pH of 5 or more, which may reflect atrophy of acid-producing gastric glands as a result of atrophic gastritis.

When amines and amides from food breakdown react with this endogenously produced nitrite, potentially carcinogenic N-nitroso compounds are formed. Thiocyanate, which is present in cigarette smoke, catalyses the formation of such compounds, whereas the antioxidants vitamins C and E inhibit nitrosation.

Potentially carcinogenic nitroso compounds may be present, ready formed, in certain foods. These include nitrite-cured meats, smoked and salted fish, beer and some cheeses.

In Japan and Iceland, large amounts of salted fish and pickled vegetables, which contain nitrosamines, and smoked fish containing benz(a)pyrene are eaten. In Columbia and Chile, foods containing large amounts of nitrates are common items in the diet, consumption of the fava bean in Columbia correlating strongly with the risk of gastric cancer.

As a result of the known effects in animal models of N-nitroso compounds, some interest has been expressed in the possibility that certain H_2 antagonists such as cimetidine may be potentially carcinogenic because they increase nitrite and N-nitrosamine levels in humans. The data are still equivocal.

In summary, a dietary pattern that, epidemiologically, appears to correlate positively with the risk of developing gastric cancer is characterized by the following:

- a **high** nitrate intake
- a **low** intake of green and yellow vegetables, salads and fresh fruit (antioxidants)
- a **low** intake of animal protein and fat
- a **high** salt intake
- a **high** intake of complex carbohydrates

Pathological Features

Precancerous Conditions and Precancerous Lesions

It is important to distinguish between precancerous **conditions** and precancerous **lesions**. The first is a pathophysiological state increasing the risk of cancer developing at the affected site; the second is a set of microscopic characteristics indicating that cancer is more likely to occur than if these characteristics were not present.

Pernicious Anaemia   Pernicious anaemia increases the risk of both adenomatous polyps and carcinoma of the stomach, the incremental factor for cancer being about three to four times.

Presence of a Gastric 'Stump'   There is still controversy as to the importance of a gastric stump following partial gastrectomy in the genesis of gastric cancer. The reported frequency of such 'stump' carcinomas varies greatly, ranging from 0.4 to 8.7%, and the increased risk has been estimated as being from three-to sixfold. The risk reaches a peak 20–30 years after surgery. Those who do not believe that a gastric stump increases the risk of cancer point out that the true risk of such a tumour developing has to be compared with the risk of gastric cancer in the **local** population and that, when this is done, there is no increase in risk.

Intestinal Metaplasia   The most important precancerous histological change (in terms of populations) appears to be incomplete intestinal metaplasia (see p 508), which develops almost exclusively in relation to type B (chronic atrophic) gastritis.

Epithelial Dysplasia   For the individual patient, **dysplasia** seen in biopsies is the most worrying single factor. Its presence should stimulate a search for a coexisting carcinoma. If this is absent, the patient should be followed carefully so that any subsequent neoplasm may be diagnosed and treated at an early stage. The difference in survival following treatment of patients with 'early' cancer and those with 'advanced' gastric cancer makes the advantages of such practice very clear.

Microscopic Features
Gastric dysplasia is defined by the presence of three features.

Cellular Atypia
This is recognized by an increased nuclear : cytoplasmic ratio, nuclear pleomorphism, increased nuclear staining intensity and irregular nuclear arrangement giving the epithelium a pseudostratified appearance.

Abnormal Differentiation
This is recognized by a decrease in the number of secretory granules, atrophy of normal glands leading to intestinal metaplasia, loss or irregular distribution of Paneth

---

cells where intestinal metaplasia is present, and disappearance of maturing surface cells.

Disorganized Mucosal Architecture
This is shown by glandular or tubular irregularities, irregularities of the muscularis mucosae and cystic dilatation of glands.

Classification
Dysplasia is classified as being mild, moderate or severe. Mild and moderate forms are reversible, but severe dysplasia, although not an indication for immediate surgery, requires endoscopic follow-up at frequent intervals.

The transition from severe dysplasia to intramucosal carcinoma may not be easy to identify. Carcinoma is characterized by the appearance of pleomorphic cells with large, darkly stained, nuclei and abnormal mitoses. The distinction between carcinoma *in situ* and invasive carcinoma, where single cells trail off through the gland basement membrane into the lamina propria, is much more difficult than in the case of a multilayered epithelium such as that of the uterine cervix. For this reason, it is probably wise to use the term **intramucosal carcinoma** to cover both carcinoma *in situ* and cases where invasion of the lamina propria by malignant cells has already occurred.

Early Gastric Cancer

Definition
Early gastric cancer is defined **in terms of the depth of invasion of the stomach wall**, tumour being limited either to the mucosa alone or to the mucosa plus the submucosa. The distinction from more deeply invasive lesions is important **because the prognosis of early gastric cancer is so much better than that of carcinoma that has invaded the muscularis propria at the time of diagnosis. The overall outlook for a patient with gastric cancer is dismal, with a 5-year survival rate of about 12%. In contrast, 5-year survival rates reported for patients with early cancer are excellent, ranging from 80 to 100%.**

The term **early cancer** implies a recent origin and that it represents the initial phases of a continuum leading inevitably to deep invasion. This may well be a total misconception, 'early cancer' instead representing a type of tumour that tends to grow **laterally** rather than **vertically** for much of its natural history. Most patients with early gastric cancer are asymptomatic and diagnosis is made in the course of screening programmes.

Frequency of Early Gastric Cancer
The frequency of this diagnosis has increased greatly in the past 20 years owing to the introduction of screening

for this form of cancer. In Japan the proportion of cases of gastric cancer classed as 'early' has increased from just under 4% to over 30%. About 30% of gastrectomies performed for cancer in Japan are in patients with early gastric cancer. In other countries, the order of magnitude of these increases is much lower, the proportion of all cases of gastric cancer in Britain diagnosed as 'early' being about 10% (1978 figures).

Morphology and Classification

The classification of early gastric cancers is based largely on their **macroscopic appearances**, seen either at endoscopy or in gastrectomy specimens. There are three main types, one of which has three subtypes (see *Table 34.7*).

Combinations of these three patterns are seen more often than the pure forms, the dominant pattern being cited first. Thus an individual lesion might be classified as I + II(c).

It is not known how long early gastric cancer remains confined to the mucosa or to the mucosa and submucosa, although tumours are believed to remain intramucosal until they attain a diameter of at least 3 mm.

Invasion of the submucosa takes place through breaches in the muscularis mucosae associated with lymphoid aggregates. Once within the submucosa, rapid expansion occurs, the submucosal portion of the lesion having a much greater diameter than the intramucosal portion.

Lymph node metastases are not incompatible with the diagnosis, their frequency correlating with the depth of invasion. Thus, 4.2% of intramucosal tumours show lymph node deposits, in contrast to 16.8% in those where submucosal spread has occurred. This difference may be explained by the paucity of lymphatics in the gastric mucosa compared with the submucosa.

Table 34.7 Types of Early Macroscopic Gastric Carcinoma

Type	Features
I (protruded)	Tumour projects into gastric lumen
II (superficial)	The mucosal surface is slightly uneven and there is no evidence of protrusion or ulceration. This variety is further subdivided into: a) elevated b) flat c) depressed
III (excavated)	This type is associated with ulceration, the ulcers extending for variable distances into the mucosa and submucosa

Advanced Gastric Cancer

Definition

The defining criterion of advanced gastric cancer is extension into or beyond the muscularis propria. More than 80% of patients with gastric cancer in the UK or USA fall, alas, into this category; in Japan, advanced cancer accounts for 50–65% of patients with cancer of the stomach.

The distribution of advanced gastric carcinoma follows that of pyloric-type mucosa, being most common in the prepyloric region, the pyloric antrum and on the lesser curve.

Classification

The tumours are classified on the basis of:
- **macroscopic appearance**
- **pattern of infiltration**
- **extent**
- **histological type**

Macroscopic Features

Advanced gastric carcinoma may be **ulcerating, nodular or fungating**, or **infiltrating**.

Ulcerating gastric carcinoma is commonest and is usually found in the antrum or on the lesser curve. The ulcers show several differences from benign peptic ulcer:
- The margins are irregular, the edges being raised and often everted. The surrounding tissue is much firmer than normal and the mucosal surface appears uneven.
- Mucosal folds radiating from the ulcer are much thicker than those seen in inflammatory lesions and are often fused. In many instances, however, the radiating pattern of the mucosa round the ulcer is lost.
- The ulcers occurring in cancer tend to be much larger than their benign counterparts.

These criteria are simply guidelines and some ulcerating cancers do not show these features. Thus, all ulcerating lesions seen on endoscopy should be biopsied, even if they appear benign and seem to be healing.

Nodular or fungating carcinomas consist of masses of friable tissue projecting from a broad base out into the lumen. They are found in the body or fundus and, not infrequently, along the greater curve. They are often quite large at the time of diagnosis and may draw attention to themselves as a result of ulceration and consequent bleeding.

Infiltrating carcinoma may spread superficially within the mucosa, giving rise to a flat, plaque-like thickening, loss of normal mucosa folds being a striking feature. More commonly, the tumour involves the **entire thickness of the stomach wall, causing the thickening and increased firmness that has been called 'linitis plastica' or 'leather bottle stomach'** (*Fig. 34.12*).

Of these three macroscopic variants, infiltrating carcinoma carries the worst prognosis.

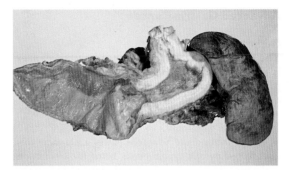

FIGURE 34.12 Carcinoma of the stomach (infiltrating type). The wall of the proximal part of the stomach is grossly thickened by white tumour tissue.

Pattern of Infiltration

A classification of advanced gastric cancer is currently based on microscopic patterns of infiltration. In this system, gastric cancers are divided into two types:

1) expanding
2) infiltrative

The expanding pattern is found in about two-thirds of gastric cancers and is characterized by well-defined tumour nodules, often composed of well-differentiated glands. The infiltrative type, which accounts for the remainder, shows diffuse infiltration by individual tumour cells without glands being formed.

Extent of Tumour (Staging)

The classification based on this criterion is the well-known TNM system (T = tumour; N = node metastases; M = distant metastases), which was introduced in 1978 by the American Joint Committee for Cancer Staging and End Results Reporting.

Histological Type

The most widely used classification is that of Laurén, who divided gastric cancers into two types which he called either **intestinal** or **diffuse** (signet-ring or mucous cell cancer).

The intestinal type is the most frequent in countries where there is a high risk of gastric cancer and appears to be related to environmental risk factors. As these factors have declined in the West, so intestinal-type cancer has decreased in frequency (rather than the diffuse variety). Diffuse cancers account for a disproportionately high proportion of gastric cancers in the young, and show no evidence of a decrease in frequency.

Microscopic Features

In general, **intestinal-type cancers have a glandular structure somewhat resembling the glandular pattern of the intestine**, although some solid or papillary areas are often present (Fig. 34.13).

Diffuse type carcinomas are made up either of separated single cells or of small aggregates of malignant cells; glandular structures may be seen but are distinctly uncommon. The individual cells are small and uniform with small dark nuclei in which mitoses are relatively infrequent. Mucin secretion is a prominent feature, the intracellular mucin accumulation tending to push the nucleus against the plasma membrane, thus giving a 'signet-ring' appearance.

These rather bland-looking mucin-producing cells may be confused with mucin-laden macrophages, seen in certain non-malignant conditions. This trap may be avoided by using immunohistochemical markers for epithelial cells, an especially useful manoeuvre in examining endoscopic biopsies.

Intramucosal spread is more extensive in diffuse carcinomas, and these lesions tend also to elicit a more marked fibrous tissue response than do intestinal-type tumours. Intestinal metaplasia is more common in association with intestinal-type than with diffuse carcinomas, which is not surprising in view of the association between the former and chronic atrophic gastritis.

Other differences between these two variants have been noted. The male : female ratio in cases of intestinal-type cancer is 2 : 1, whereas that for diffuse cancer is 1 : 1. The mean age of patients with intestinal-type tumours is 55.4 years, and that for diffuse-type tumours is 47.7 years. Survival rates for diffuse tumours are somewhat lower than those for intestinal-type tumours.

These differences have led to the suggestion that these two types might also differ with regard to cause and pathogenesis. This view is an attractive one, but there are some problems with this classification. Some tumours show features of both types and Laurén himself was unable to classify 14% of the tumours in his series as being either intestinal or diffuse.

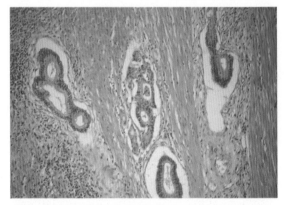

FIGURE 34.13 Intestinal-type gastric carcinoma. Note the comparatively well-formed glands which have infiltrated deeply to involve the main muscle layer.

Other Rare Types
Some of these have a natural history which differs from that of the more common forms.

Tumours Showing Evidence of Neuroendocrine Differentiation
Such tumours occur in the stomach in a number of different guises. The spectrum includes:

1) **Typical, well-differentiated and slow-growing carcinoid tumours which may consist of any of the endocrine cells normally found in the gastric mucosa.** These tumours tend to be small and well defined, and may present, macroscopically, as small polyps. On histological examination the cells are small and uniform in size and appearance. They are arranged in either trabecular or ribbon-like pattern, or in the form of small glands. They contain low molecular weight cytokeratins and also markers of neuroendocrine differentiation such as neurone-specific enolase and chromogranin. Electron microscopy shows dense-core secretory granules within the cytoplasm. These lesions produce a wide range of peptide secretion products. Two well-defined subtypes are:

- G-cell (gastrin-secreting cell) tumours, which are usually single and situated within the antrum.
- Carcinoids composed of enterochromaffin cells which are strongly argyrophilic but not argentaffin. Unlike the G-cell tumour, no gastro-duodenal hormones are detected in the tumour cells. These lesions are usually multiple, often polypoid, and are found most frequently in the fundus. They are usually associated with chronic atrophic gastritis and intestinal metaplasia. Pernicious anaemia may be present but is not a mandatory part of the syndrome.

2) **Atypical carcinoids.** These show obvious morphological signs of neuroendocrine differentiation, but also evidence of invasiveness, an increased degree of mitotic activity and necrosis. The prognosis is better than that for adenocarcinoma but worse than that of typical carcinoid.

3) Tumours that are the morphological homologues of **small cell carcinoma** of the lung may occur in the stomach. Like the lung tumour, their clinical behaviour is very aggressive.

4) Many otherwise perfectly typical adenocarcinomas of the stomach show the presence, focally, of cells with evidence of neuroendocrine differentiation. The presence of these cells has no effect on the biological behaviour of the carcinoma.

Mucoid Adenocarcinoma
This is a rare tumour in which there is abundant mucin secretion, much of the mucin being extracellular. This mucin accumulates in large pools in which there are islands of tumour cells. The mucin accumulation may be so great as to give the tumours a glistening or 'colloid' appearance on naked-eye examination. These tumours pursue a rather indolent course; mean survival rates of 9 years have been reported.

Hepatoid Adenocarcinoma
This is a recently described variant in which there is an admixture of cells, some clearly glandular in type, whereas others are large, eosinophilic and polygonal, somewhat resembling liver cells. The suggestion of a degree of hepatocellular differentiation is strengthened by the finding that these cells synthesize α-fetoprotein and α_1-antitrypsin.

Choriocarcinoma
Choriocarcinoma may occur rarely, either in association with adenocarcinoma or in a pure form. The tumours are large, fleshy and often haemorrhagic, and may show extensive areas of necrosis. Microscopic examination shows the presence of large bizarre cells resembling syncytiotrophoblasts, an impression strengthened by the finding of the β subunit of human chorionic gonadotrophin in these cells.

Clinical Features
The onset of symptoms of advanced gastric cancer is, unfortunately, often insidious and the symptoms are non-specific. Thus many patients are diagnosed relatively late. Common symptoms are given in *Table 34.8*.

Non-metastatic Systemic Manifestations
The formation of immune complexes with tumour antigens may lead to microangiopathic haemolytic anaemia, glomerular lesions associated with the nephrotic syndrome or, rarely, neurological abnormalities.

There may be **secretion of growth-stimulating factors** believed to be implicated in the pathogenesis of the filiform and papular pigmented skin lesions known as **acanthosis nigricans**. These tend to occur particularly in the body folds and around the mouth and anus. The appearance of a striking rise in the neutrophil count is similarly attributed to secretion by the tumour cells of granulocyte-stimulating factor.

Table 34.8 Common Symptoms of Advanced Gastric Cancer

Clinical feature	Frequency (%)
Abdominal pain	66
Weight loss	50
Nausea and vomiting	32
Anorexia	25
Dysphagia	23
Bleeding	23

Spread of Gastric Cancer

In addition to the classical pathways of spread – **direct, lymphatic permeation** and via **blood vessels** – gastric cancer also spreads by means of **peritoneal dissemination**.

Local Extension

This involves the duodenum in about 50% of cases. A roughly similar proportion of proximally situated carcinomas spreads upwards to involve the oesophagus. This spread may occur directly through the submucosa or via permeation of intramural lymphatics and is difficult to identify with the naked eye at surgery.

Tumours on the greater curve may extend into the mesocolon or transverse colon and, on occasion, may produce gastrocolic fistulae; gastrojejunal fistulae can also occur, but only rarely. Large lesions that have undergone ulceration may extend directly to involve the pancreas or spleen.

Lymphatic Spread

Of patients coming to post-mortem examination, lymph node deposits can be found in about 85%. In surgical specimens the frequency varies depending on the depth of invasion and the histological type of tumour. In intestinal-type tumours that have reached the serosa at the time of operation, lymph node metastases are present in nearly 90%, whereas the proportion falls to 71% in the case of diffuse-type tumours. In both cases, invasion beyond the confines of the muscularis propria and the subserosa is associated with a sharp increase in the frequency of lymph node deposits. Lymph node deposits can also be seen in mediastinal nodes (about 30% in post-mortem cases) and occasionally in cervical nodes.

Distant Metastases

Spread to distant sites can occur via both lymphatics and blood vessels. The commonest sites are the **liver, lungs, adrenals and ovaries**. Diffuse-type carcinomas have a predilection for involvement of the lungs and ovary, whereas intestinal-type tumours tend particularly to involve the liver.

Peritoneal Dissemination

This is seen in about 25% of cases of advanced gastric cancer. The vast majority of these patients will have involvement of the gastric serosa by tumour. From these serosal deposits, free tumour cells will be released which subsequently become implanted on the peritoneal surface. Bilateral ovarian metastases are often encountered (**Krukenberg tumours**). Involvement of the peritoneum appears to occur more frequently in patients with diffuse-type tumours than in those with lesions of intestinal type.

CONNECTIVE TISSUE NEOPLASMS

Connective tissue neoplasms large enough to cause clinical disturbances are uncommon in the stomach. Most (70%) are smooth muscle tumours, and most of the remainder are nerve sheath tumours.

Small smooth muscle tumours are quite common at post-mortem examination, but most are symptomless throughout their natural history. Larger tumours, which show a predilection for adult males, commonly present with gastric bleeding as a result of ulceration of the mucosa overlying the tumour. Such bleeding may be chronic, leading to iron-deficiency anaemia, or acute, massive transfusiuon sometimes being required.

Macroscopic Features

The tumours are well circumscribed and have a tan, grey or pink colour and a firm, rather rubbery, consistency. They arise within the muscle coat of the stomach but, if they attain a large size, may project into the gastric lumen or from the serosal surface.

Microscopic Features

On **microscopic examination**, the pathologist is faced with two tasks. The first is identification of the tumour as showing smooth muscle differentiation and the second, which is often more difficult, is to decide whether it is benign or malignant.

Well-differentiated Leiomyoma

In this, the commonest pattern, the tumour is composed of bundles of easily recognized smooth muscle cells which have elongated, blunt-ended nuclei and brightly eosinophilic cytoplasm. Individual nuclei may show bizarre degenerative changes and care should be taken not to overdiagnose malignancy on this ground alone.

Epithelioid Leiomyoma

Some smooth muscle cell tumours have an 'epithelioid' appearance. The cells in this variant are large and either rounded or polygonal. The nucleus is situated centrally and there is abundant, faintly eosinophilic, cytoplasm which, in sections from fixed, paraffin-embedded material may show vacuolation. This last feature is an artefact of fixation. The epithelioid pattern *per se* has no implications as to the behaviour of the tumour, and histological evaluation of a lesion's malignant potential must be made on other grounds.

Immunohistochemistry

Where difficulties exist in identifying tumour cells as showing smooth muscle differentiation, the use of immunohistochemical methods to identify characteristic smooth muscle cell antigens may be helpful.

The characteristic antigens found in smooth muscle are the intermediate filament protein **desmin** and **smooth muscle actin**. About 50% of gastrointestinal stromal tumours show cells that bind antibodies against desmin.

Smooth muscle actin is a more sensitive but less specific marker than desmin, being found in many non-muscle tumours. The epithelioid variant tends as a rule not to bind antibodies raised against desmin, but about 40% show the presence of smooth muscle cell actin.

Assessing the Malignant Potential of Smooth Muscle Tumours

In the gastrointestinal tract, as at other sites, features associated with malignancy include (*Fig. 34.14*):

- **Tumour size.** Lesions larger than 5 cm in diameter tend to behave in an aggressive fashion.
- **Mitotic rate.** Tumours in which more than five mitoses per ten high-power fields are seen are likely to be malignant. As low a rate as one mitosis per ten high-power fields may be considered malignant if this finding is present consistently in samples examined from a single lesion.
- **The presence of marked pleomorphism and areas of necrosis** are indicative of malignancy even if the mitotic rate is less than five mitoses per high-power field.

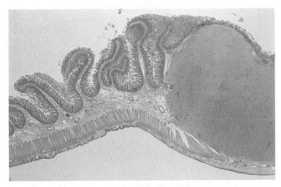

FIGURE 34.14 *Leiomyosarcoma of the stomach. Note the well-defined margin of the tumour and the way in which the gastric mucosa is stretched over it. At this magnification it is possible to ascertain only that the general features are those of a connective tissue neoplasm.*

The Small Intestine

NORMAL ANATOMY AND FUNCTION

The small intestine commences at the pylorus and terminates at the ileocaecal valve. It ranges in length from 3.5 to 6 m, the first 20–25 cm constituting the duodenum. This is at once the widest and the most fixed part. Of the remainder, the jejunum occupies about 40% and the ileum the remaining 60%, although there is no sharp distinction between ileum and jejunum.

The main functions are:
1) **Completion of the process of digestion begun in the stomach.** This involves breakdown of food components by pancreatic enzymes and solubilization of fat, to which bile salts make a major contribution.
2) **Absorption of digested and solubilized food components.** This depends on:
   - **a normal absorptive area** – any significant loss of the surface epithelium can lead to a serious failure of absorption
   - **normal transport mechanisms** across the gut wall, failure of which affects absorption of specific classes of food
3) **Transport of non-absorbed luminal material to the colon, from which it ultimately makes its exit.** This function depends, in part, on **normal motility**, which may be disturbed in a number of disorders resulting in either diarrhoea or constipation. In addition, an important contribution to normal transport comes from **transport of water and electrolytes across the mucosal surface**. Water and solutes are both absorbed and secreted across the mucosa–lumen boundary; any disturbance in these two pathways may result in profound diarrhoea.
4) **Immunological surveillance of the very large number of environmental antigens to which the epithelial surface of the small gut is exposed.** These include dietary antigens, pathogenic microorganisms and normal microbial inhabitants of the gut lumen.

In many ways the microanatomy of the small intestine reflects these functions.

Small Gut Mucosa

The mucosal lining presents an enormous absorptive surface in proportion to the length of the small gut. This is because, on a macroscopic level, the mucosa, freely moveable over the deeper layers of the gut wall, is thrown into a series of folds, the **valvulae conniventes**, which are largest in the upper jejunum.

Villi

Microscopic examination shows the mucosal lining to be arranged characteristically in a series of processes or villi which can be seen clearly with a dissecting microscope. This configuration vastly increases the absorptive surface. In the duodenum the villi have a rather leaf-like appearance which changes more distally to a finger-like appearance. In Caucasians, the finger-like form predominates, while broader, more leaf-like, villi are found in larger numbers in Asians. Normal villi are 320–570 μm in height and 85–140 μm in width. The covering columnar epithelial cells are involved in absorption and possess a microvillous brush border, visible only on electron microscopy. In addition to absorptive columnar cells, the covering of the villus includes a few mucin-secreting cells and neuro-endocrine cells.

Crypts

Between each pair of villi lies a crypt with a depth roughly equal to one-third of the height of the adjacent villi. New epithelial cells arise from stem cells at the crypt base; these migrate upwards to cover the villi, maturing in the process, and eventually being shed from the villus surface. This cycle takes 2–4 days. Increased epithelial cell loss leads to increased size of the basal zone of the crypt and increased mitotic activity.

In addition to the stem cells, crypts contain Paneth cells with large brightly eosinophilic granules; their function is still unknown but it is suggested that they regulate the intestinal microflora. The crypt lining also contains undifferentiated cells, in which conjugation of immunoglobulin (Ig) A with its secretory component is carried out, and neuroendocrine cells.

Mucosa-associated Lymphoid Tissue

Unlike the stomach, the small intestine contains abundant lymphoid tissue which is involved in the generation of mucosal antibody, largely IgA.

The highest concentration of lymphoid tissue is found in Peyer's patches of the terminal ileum. These constitute the **gut-associated lymphoid tissue (GALT)**. They are in close contact with the overlying epithelium, known as the 'dome' epithelium, and consist of B-cell follicles with areas of T cells between the B-cell follicles and the underlying muscularis mucosae. The germinal centre of the Peyer patch is surrounded by a mantle of small lymphocytes merging with a broader band of B cells extending up to the dome epithelium. These more superficially placed B cells express IgM or IgA, but no IgD, in contrast with mantle zone cells. These cells have some of the morphological features of **centrocytes** (see p 961) and some are invariably present within the dome epithelium. These are not the only lymphocytes to be found within the epithelium: T cells form the greater part of the intraepithelial lymphocyte population.

Antigens from the gut lumen are transported across the 'dome' epithelium via specialized cells which present them to appropriate cells in the lymphoid nodules. The B cells, activated by antigen exposure, leave the follicles via the efferent lymphatics, eventually reaching the bloodstream via the mesenteric nodes and the thoracic duct. Once in the blood these B cells 'home' back to the intestinal mucosa in which they appear in the form of plasma cells. Most of these secrete dimeric IgA which, in conjunction with the 'secretory piece', is transported to the mucosal surface.

CONGENITAL ABNORMALITIES

Meckel's Diverticulum

Meckel's diverticulum occurs in about 2% of the population and is by far the commonest congenital abnormality of the gastrointestinal tract. It represents **the remains of the vitellointestinal duct** (*Fig. 34.15*) and is found on the antimesenteric border of the small gut about 1 m proximal to the ileocaecal valve.

In adults, it varies in length from 2 to 12 cm and usually has about the same calibre as the bowel from which it arises. In most instances the blind end is free, but in a small minority it is linked to the umbilicus by a fibrous cord-like structure representing the obliterated remainder of the vitellointestinal duct. It is a true diverticulum in that all the layers normally found in the small gut wall are present.

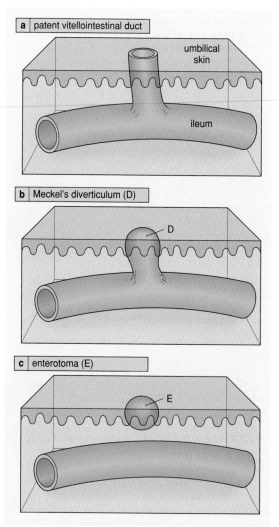

FIGURE 34.15 Principal congenital anomalies associated with persistence of the vitellointestinal duct.

In many instances Meckel's diverticulum is without clinical significance. In about 50% of cases, however, the diverticulum is lined partly by gastric mucosa, and peptic ulceration may occur in the adjacent small-intestinal mucosa. Such an ulcer may perforate or bleed, haemorrhage being particularly common in children.

As in any blind sac, acute inflammation may occur, the clinical picture being very similar to that seen in acute appendicitis. Heterotopic pancreas may also be found in Meckel's diverticulum and, although these nodules of pancreas may be subject to any of the pathological conditions found in the normally sited pancreas, they are not usually associated with any functional disturbance.

Acquired Diverticula

Solitary acquired diverticula may occur in any part of the small gut but are commonest in the duodenum. Multiple acquired diverticula are seen mostly in the elderly and represent herniations of mucosa through the muscularis at points where blood vessels enter the gut along the mesenteric border. They are most commonly found in the jejunum and ileum (*Fig. 34.16*). They may function as 'blind' loops and thus be associated with alterations in bacterial flora and the consequences this brings (see pp 524–525).

Atresia or Stenosis of the Small Bowel

Congenital atresia (absence of the lumen) or stenosis (narrowing of the lumen) may occur in any part of the small gut but is commonest in the second part of the duodenum and in the ileum. The lesions are usually solitary.

Experimental occlusion of portions of the blood supply to the small gut in embryos causes segmental atresia or stenosis, and localized vascular insufficiency during fetal life may be responsible for these lesions. The 'blind' portions of the small gut may be connected by a fibrous cord or may be completely separate, and occasionally the atretic portion is represented by a membrane stretching transversely across the gut lumen.

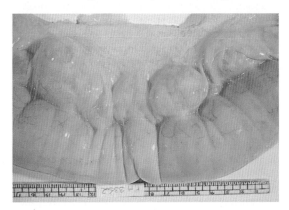

FIGURE 34.16 Congenital jejunal diverticula on the antimesenteric border of the gut.

Small bowel atresia causes acute intestinal obstruction in the first few days of life and requires urgent corrective surgery.

Failure to Complete Physiological Rotation of the Gut: Exomphalos

Normally, the mid-gut herniates into the umbilical cord at about the fifth week of fetal life and, during this time, rotation of this portion of the gut commences, the mid-gut returning to the abdominal cavity at about the tenth week. Portions of this mid-gut may either adhere to the hernial sac or fail to return to the abdominal cavity because the neck of the hernial sac is too narrow.

Other failures of rotation exist in the form of:
- the caecum, appendix and ascending colon being placed on the left side with displacement of the small gut to the right
- abnormal mobility of the caecum as a result of persistence of the right mesocolon
- failure of the caecum to descend to its normal position in the right iliac fossa
- retrocaecal and thus extraperitoneal displacement of the appendix

These abnormalities are important for two reasons. Firstly, the abnormal mobility of parts of the mid-gut resulting from these malrotations increases the risk of volvulus and thus of acute intestinal obstruction and localized gut ischaemia. Secondly, inflammatory or other disorders occurring in misplaced segments of gut may give rise to misleading clinical signs and thus make accurate clinical diagnosis difficult.

Duplication

Duplication of small gut segments is distinctly rare, but occurs more often in this location than in other parts of the gastrointestinal tract. The duplicated segments may be tubular or spherical and may, in some cases, communicate with the small bowel. In other instances the duplicated segments are free from any communication with other parts of the gut and have their own mesenteries. The commonest complication is the occurrence of inflammation in the duplications, but well-authenticated cases of malignant neoplasm occurring in these duplicated segments exist.

THE MALABSORPTION SYNDROME AND ITS CAUSES

The malabsorption syndrome results from deficiencies in a number of physiological processes:
- **Failure to absorb fat and fat-soluble vitamins and other nutrients of all classes.** This results in excess faecal fat loss (steatorrhoea) and the resulting extraintestinal effects, such as osteomalacia due to defective absorption of calcium and vitamin D.

This may be due to a **reduction in the mucosal area available for absorption**, as seen in patients wih coeliac sprue or after extensive surgical small bowel resection. In some patients the area of mucosa available for absorption is normal but there is, instead, **a failure to transport certain specific classes of nutrients across the gut wall**, for example in Hartnup disease, where there is a failure in tryptophan metabolism, or in disaccharidase deficiency, where there is a failure to absorb certain sugars.

- **Failure to digest foodstuffs adequately within the small gut lumen and thus render them suitable for transport across the intestinal mucosa.** This may occur in patients with primary or secondary deficiencies of the exocrine secretions of the pancreas, in cases where there is a deficiency of conjugated bile salts, and in those in whom bile salts are deconjugated as a result of bacterial overgrowth within the gut lumen.

A large number of causes of the malabsorption syndrome have been described, of which the commonest are: **coeliac sprue, Crohn's disease and pancreatic insufficiency due to chronic pancreatitis.**

Coeliac Sprue (Coeliac Disease; Gluten-associated Enteropathy)

Coeliac sprue is a chronic disorder occurring at any age and characterized by differing degrees of villous atrophy in the small bowel mucosa. This is associated with malabsorption of varying grades of severity and is caused by an abnormal reaction to the ingestion of wheat gliadins (the alcohol-soluble fraction of wheat protein or gluten) or to their homologues in barley, rye and oats, known as prolamins. If these protein fractions are removed from the diet there is prompt improvement in the malabsorption and slow reversal of the mucosal lesions with, ultimately, a return to normal. Cases with mucosal lesions confined to the proximal small gut are very mild and may never be diagnosed; existing prevalence rates may represent an underestimate of the frequency of this disorder.

Coeliac disease also occurs in association with other disorders. There are well-recognized associations with **insulin-dependent diabetes mellitus, selective IgA deficiency and the inflammatory skin disease dermatitis herpetiformis**. The latter is characterized by an intensely itchy, patchy, blistering skin eruption associated, in most patients, with IgA deposits, in either a granular or linear pattern, at the dermoepidermal junction. The granular pattern of IgA deposition shows strong correlation with histological changes in the small gut, identical with those of coeliac disease. Withdrawal of gluten from the diet of patients with coincident dermatitis herpetiformis and coeliac disease results in an improvement in both skin and gut lesions.

Epidemiology

Coeliac sprue is found predominantly among Caucasians. Although cases have been reported from the Indian subcontinent, the disease is very rare among Chinese, Japanese and the indigenous population of Africa. In Europe the highest rates are found in the west of Ireland (1 in 300) with an average prevalence of 1 in 1000–1200 in the rest of the continent.

Pathogenesis

Clearly, coeliac sprue must be the result of an interaction between wheat gliadins or prolamins and host factors. What the latter are is still unclear. Mechanisms that have been proposed include:

1) The existence of an **enzyme deficiency** leading to accumulation of toxic peptides as a result of incomplete digestion. Such defects in digestion as have been found are reversed after gluten withdrawal and are, thus, more likely to be the result rather than the cause of coeliac sprue.

2) **Abnormal glycosylation of cell membrane glycoproteins resulting in a lectin-like interaction between gluten and the absorptive cells of the villus.** Certain plant lectins certainly can damage small intestinal mucosa, but there is no convincing evidence that this occurs in patients with coeliac sprue.

3) **Abundant evidence exists for a genetic component** in this disorder. Concordance rates in identical twins reach 70% and there are many recorded instances of multiple cases in single families as well as a prevalence for first-degree relatives of patients ranging from 8 to 12%.

Some striking human leucocyte antigen (HLA) associations have emerged, particularly in relation to MHC class II-coded antigens. In 70–90% of northern European patients, HLA-DR3 is found and HLA-DQw2 occurs in more than 90%. In southern Europe the HLA-DR3 association is less marked but the same HLA-DQ α–β heterodimer is found. This suggests that this heterodimer may play a significant part in determining which individuals are likely to be susceptible. An association with HLA-B8 has also been recorded. These haplotypes are by no means confined to sufferers from coeliac disease and some additional susceptibility gene or genes must be postulated.

4) **Immune mechanisms.** There have been many suggestions that abnormal immune reactions to gliadins and prolamins cause coeliac sprue.

So far as **humoral** responses are concerned, organ cultures of mucosa from patients with coeliac disease produce more IgA and IgM antibodies to gliadin than do those taken from control subjects, and the number of antibody-producing B cells in the mucosa of patients is also much greater than that in controls. However, antibodies to gliadin may be found in patients with other types of bowel disease and even in some controls, and some patients with coeliac disease lack circulating antibodies to gliadin.

Other circulating antibodies have been identified in coeliac disease and have been used as part of the diagnostic investigation of patients suspected of having coeliac disease. They include an antibody against **endomysium**, the matrix substance surrounding primate smooth muscle cells. This finding is said to show a high degree of both sensitivity and specificity. Why an antibody against a connective tissue antigen should appear in this condition remains a mystery. In 1990, yet another antibody, an IgA antibody that binds *in vitro* to human jejunum (JAB), was identified in patients with untreated coeliac disease. The withdrawal of gluten from the diet is associated with disappearance of the antibody from the patient's serum. The sensitivity of this test appears to be substantially lower in infants and children aged less than 2 years than in older patients. Tissue absorption studies have shown that the antijejunal antibody differs from antigliadin antibodies, but that it is probably closely related, if not identical, to the anti-endomysial antibody.

A role for **cell-mediated immunity** in the pathogenesis of coeliac disease has also been suggested. There is a considerable increase in the total number of T cells in the mucosal epithelium. The composition of this T-cell population in patients with coeliac disease also differs from normal in that there is a marked increase in the number of CD8+ T cells expressing the γ–δ receptor rather than the more usual α–β receptor and also a significant increase in the number of T cells expressing CD45RO (an indicator of T-cell priming).

A close degree of homology exists between a gliadin fragment and part of the E1b protein of type 12 adenovirus. It has been suggested that infection with this virus may, through the operation of molecular mimicry, sensitize genetically appropriate hosts against this part of the gliadin molecule. Controversy exists as to whether serological evidence of infection by this virus is commoner in coeliac patients than in controls.

Mucosal Pathology

Biopsy of the small intestinal mucosa remains the gold standard for the diagnosis of coeliac disease.

Microscopic Features

Under the dissecting microscope, the mucosa appears flat, an impression confirmed in histological sections. The flattening is due to **total or subtotal villous atrophy**. This is accompanied by **crypt hyperplasia** associated with increased mitotic activity in crypt epithelium, so that the overall thickness of the mucosa is not diminished (*Figs 34.17* and *34.18*).

There is an **increase in the concentration of intraepithelial lymphocytes** and a similarly marked increase within the lamina propria, where neutrophils and increased numbers of eosinophils and mast cells may also be noted. In some patients lymphocytes may be seen within the epithelium and the lamina propria of both the gastric and colonic mucosae, and it has been reported that enemas containing gliadin can elicit an inflammatory response in the rectal mucosa of patients suffering from coeliac disease.

It is important to understand that, although these histological appearances are characteristic of coeliac disease, they are **not specific** for it, as the same histological

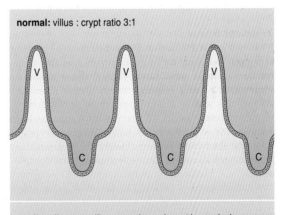

normal: villus : crypt ratio 3:1

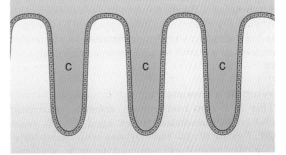

coeliac disease: villous atrophy and crypt hyperplasia

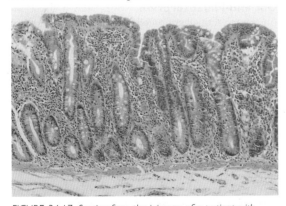

FIGURE 34.17 *Section from the jejunum of a patient with severe malabsorption due to coeliac disease. There is virtually total villous atrophy; the crypts, however, are hyperplastic, the normal villus:crypt ratio being grossly disturbed. Note also the heavy inflammatory cell infiltrate in the lamina propria.*

FIGURE 34.18 *Villus:crypt ratios in normal small gut and in coeliac disease.*

picture may be seen in a number of other intestinal disorders, including **tropical sprue, various intestinal infections and gastric hypersecretion resulting from the presence of a gastrin-secreting tumour**. Thus an **unequivocal** diagnosis of coeliac disease cannot be made unless there is both a clinical and histological improvement following the withdrawal of dietary gluten.

Coeliac Disease and Malignant Disease in the Alimentary Canal

The long-term prognosis in patients suffering from coeliac disease is dominated by an increased risk (some 10–15% of all patients) of developing malignant gastrointestinal neoplasms. Most of these are lymphomas, now recognized as arising from **T lymphocytes**.

The frequency with which lymphomas complicate coeliac disease is difficult to assess because it seems clear that a number of patients diagnosed as having experienced this sequence may have had lymphoma from the start, the mucosal changes being secondary to the lymphoma.

Coeliac disease is also associated with an increased risk of malignant lymphoma occurring **outside** the intestine, and carcinomas of the oropharynx, breast, oesophagus and small intestine also appear to occur more frequently in these patients.

Tropical Sprue

This is a coeliac disease-like syndrome occurring amongst inhabitants of certain parts of the tropics or in those who have visited these areas. In some patients small intestinal biopsy shows a virtually normal appearance, but in others there is villous atrophy of differing grades of severity associated with an inflammatory cell infiltrate in both the mucosal epithelium and the lamina propria. Unlike the inflammatory reaction seen in coeliac disease, eosinophils are conspicuous.

This syndrome is believed to be of infective origin and is associated particularly with certain toxin-producing strains of *Escherichia coli*. It is endemic in the Caribbean (but not in Jamaica), the northern part of South America, Puerto Rico, India, parts of South-East Asia and the Philippines. Gluten appears to be unrelated to the pathogenesis of this condition, which is treated most effectively with broad-spectrum antibiotics.

Whipple's Disease

This is a rare multisystem disorder occurring chiefly in Caucasian males aged 30–40 years (M : F ratio 10 : 1). Steatorrhoea with malabsorption, abdominal cramps and fever is a classic mode of presentation, but the patients may also have a flitting polyarthritis, increased skin pig- mentation, generalized lymph node enlargement, inflammatory changes affecting serosal membranes and heart valves, evidence of central nervous system involvement and amyloidosis of the reactive systemic type. Indeed, in some patients the presentation is entirely extraintestinal.

Microscopic Features

Pathological changes in the small intestinal mucosa are highly characteristic, consisting essentially of **large numbers of macrophages within the lamina propria. These are distended by material that stains with periodic acid–Schiff (PAS) stain, this indicating 1–2 glycol groups as found in glycoproteins, glycolipids, neutral mucins and glycogen. On electron microscopy, this PAS-positive material is seen to consist of densely packed masses of what appear to be bacilli.** Identical macrophages are seen in lymphatics draining the small gut and in mesenteric lymph nodes.

Attempts to culture the intracellular organisms have so far failed and immunohistochemical studies have yielded conflicting and inconstant data. However, the fact that patients improve clinically, and that the number of bacilliform structures diminishes after treatment with tetracyclines, provides support for an infective origin for Whipple's disease. Recently tissues from a small number of patients with Whipple's disease have been shown to contain a unique bacterial RNA sequence, which is believed to be characteristic of a **Gram-positive actinomycete** not closely related to any known genus. The organism has been provisionally named *Tropheryma whippelii* (Gk. *trophe* nourishment; *eryma* barrier).

Abnormal Growth of Bacteria in the Small Gut and Malabsorption

An abnormal small gut bacterial flora can cause a severe malabsorption syndrome characterized by steatorrhoea, diarrhoea and protein malnutrition.

Bacteria are normally present in the upper part of the small gut, but the size of this population and its composition are tightly regulated. Fluid aspirated from the duodenum and jejunum usually contains 10^3–10^4 organisms per millilitre; these are normally acid-resistant Gram-positive organisms. A few coliform organisms may also be present but strict anaerobes are not found. In the lower part of the ileum, coliforms and anaerobes are present in considerable numbers.

The bacterial population of the small gut depends on:

- **the rate of entry of organisms into the gut,** which correlates with the degree of contamination of food and the destruction of organisms normally occurring within the stomach

- **the rate of proliferation of organisms** within the gut
- **the rate of clearance of organisms** from the gut

Regulatory factors include:

1) **The mechanical cleaning action of small gut peristalsis.** Any disorder that interferes with normal motility is likely to be associated with bacterial overgrowth, even in the absence of an anatomical lesion such as a blind loop, causing stasis of the luminal contents of the small gut. Thus, the syndrome may be seen in patients with an autonomic neuropathy affecting innervation of the small gut, and in those in whom systemic sclerosis, amyloidosis or postsurgical denervation of the gut is present.

2) **Gastric acidity normally destroys most organisms in food before they reach the small gut**; thus any condition leading to reduced or absent secretion of acid by the stomach increases the risk of the bacterial overgrowth syndrome.

3) **Normal concentrations of bile salts** in the small gut lumen are said to discourage bacterial proliferation, especially in relation to anaerobes.

4) **Secretion of immunoglobulins** into the gut lumen.

In addition to failure of one or more of the above, the **establishment of segmental stasis in the course of formation of a blind loop surgically, in the presence of distal obstruction of the small gut from any cause, or a gastrocolic or enterocolic fistula**, the full-blown picture of bacterial overgrowth is likely to develop.

The Adverse Effects of Bacterial Overgrowth are Multifactorial

Several different mechanisms have been canvassed as being responsible for the structural and functional disturbances seen in the bacterial overgrowth syndrome. These include:

- **inhibition of brush–border enzymes** such as sucrase and maltase by proteases secreted by some species of *Bacteroides*
- **damage to the mucosa produced by secondary bile acids** (deoxycholic and lithocholic acids) formed as a result of hydroxylation of primary bile acids by bacteria
- **breakage of the amide bonds linking bile acids and the glycine or taurine with which they are conjugated.** Only conjugated bile acids can form the micelles that are necessary for fat absorption.

The diagnostic gold standard is provided by culture of aspirated small intestinal juice. However, non-invasive 'breath' tests may provide useful information. For example, deconjugation of bile acids can be demonstrated by giving the patients a small dose of ^{14}C-labelled glycine. Bacterial deconjugation leads to splitting of the glycine from bile acid, and the former is metabolized and excreted in the breath in the form of radioactive carbon dioxide which can be measured. Unfortunately there is a false-negative rate of about 30%. However, if this test is combined with one to measure the amount of hydrogen in the breath (hydrogen derived from bacterial fermentation of carbohydrate in the small gut), the false-negative rate is decreased greatly.

Abetalipoproteinaemia

This is a **rare autosomal recessive inherited disorder presenting in infancy with steatorrhoea and failure to thrive**. The functional defect is failure to synthesize the carrier protein apoprotein B48 within the enterocyte; as a result chylomicrons cannot be assembled within the small bowel wall and dietary fat accumulates in the form of intracytoplasmic droplets of triglyceride.

In addition to the steatorrhoea, malabsorption of dietary lipid and fatty change in the liver, changes develop subsequently in the eye and central nervous system, presumably because of a shortage of lipids required for cell membrane synthesis. In the eye, an atypical form of retinitis pigmentosa involving the macula is seen and the infants may also develop an ataxic neuropathy owing to degeneration in the posterior columns of the spinal cord and in the pyramidal and cerebellar pathways in the brain. 'Burr'-type red blood cells (acanthocytes) are seen in blood films.

Congenital Lymphangiectasia

This is a rare condition characterized by abnormal development of the intestinal and, often, the limb lymphatics. Functionally it is dominated by protein loss from the gut leading to hypoproteinaemia, and there is also failure to absorb fat, which is usually less severe than the protein loss.

The small intestinal villi are thickened; the outstanding histological abnormality is gross dilatation of the lymphatic channels within the villi. The small intestinal lining epithelium and the lamina propria usually contain fat droplets, this being the morphological correlate of inability to transport fat from the gut wall.

If the lymphatics in the lower limbs are also affected, the most striking clinical feature is lower limb oedema, caused partly by the abnormal lymphatic drainage and partly by hypoproteinaemia. Ascites and pleural effusions may be seen and, in this case, the fluid that accumulates is chylous.

OBSTRUCTION OF THE SMALL INTESTINE

One of the important functions of the small gut is the transport of non-absorbable luminal contents onwards to the colon. Any condition that interferes with this transport is classified as **obstructive**.

Obstruction may be complete or incomplete, the onset of clinical features being sudden or gradual. The causes of intestinal obstruction may be classified as **mechanical, neural or vascular**.

Mechanical obstruction may be due to causes arising:

- **within the lumen**; for example, foreign bodies, gallstones, food, tumours and, in the neonatal period, blockage of the lumen by abnormally viscid mucus and epithelial debris (meconium ileus). The last named is especially likely to occur in association with cystic fibrosis.
- **within the gut wall**; for example, fibrosis secondary to inflammation such as is seen in Crohn's disease or in the annular ulceration of the ileum or lower jejunum associated with taking 'enteric-coated' tablets of potassium chloride; congenital atresia or stenosis; strictures following ischaemic necrosis of part of the thickness of the gut wall.
- **outside the gut wall** as a result of external compression.

ISCHAEMIC DISEASE

The small gut receives its blood supply from two main sources:

1) The **coeliac artery** supplying the stomach, duodenum, pancreas and liver.

2) The **superior mesenteric artery** supplying the jejunum and ileum. The major branches of this vessel are linked by an extensive collateral circulation, arterial arcades seen near the border between the mesentery and the intestinal wall. Thus **the presence of severe underperfusion implies, for the most part, either occlusion of the main superior mesenteric artery or one or more of its major branches or severe vasoconstriction affecting a substantial amount of the superior mesenteric bed**.

Ischaemia may be acute or chronic, and the degree of underperfusion and the speed with which this develops determine the pathophysiological results:

- **Pain** that occurs about 30 minutes after eating, as a result of increased oxygen demands in the gut wall, and which may last for hours. This is known as **'intestinal angina'** and is a purely functional disturbance associated with chronic stenosis of the supplying arteries. There is *no* evidence of any significant degree of tissue necrosis, the condition being a homologue of stable angina pectoris.
- **Localized fibrosis due to chronic ischaemia** of a rather more severe degree than described above.
- **Ischaemic necrosis confined to the mucosa and submucosa, presenting clinically with abdominal pain and bloody diarrhoea** (*Fig. 34.19*). Necrosis affecting the cells lining the tips of

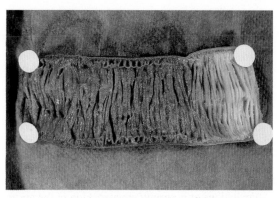

FIGURE 34.19 *Ischaemic necrosis of the small gut involving the mucosa and submucosa. The affected portion of the mucosa is a deep plum colour; there is clear demarcation between ischaemic and non-ischaemic bowel.*

the villi is the earliest morphological change seen and, depending on the severity of the underperfusion, the necrotizing process may extend more deeply to involve the full thickness of the mucosa and submucosa. The presence of necrotic mucosa is marked by the appearance of a **pseudomembrane**, composed in part of the necrotic mucosal tissue and in part of inflammatory exudate. If perfusion is restored to normal, regeneration of the ulcerated areas of mucosa may occur which, in some instances, is associated with pseudopyloric metaplasia. The submucosa is often the seat of formation of granulation tissue in which haemosiderin-laden macrophages may be seen.

- **Full-thickness ischaemic necrosis of the bowel wall (transmural infarction, gangrene). This reflects an acute and severe decrease in perfusion of the affected segment, and occurs most often as a result of thrombotic or embolic occlusion of the superior mesenteric artery (50% of cases) occurring against a background of atherosclerotic narrowing.** Other causes of occlusion of the superior mesenteric artery include **immune-mediated inflammatory disorders, such as polyarteritis nodosa, and fibromuscular dysplasia** of the superior mesenteric artery.

Approximately 25% of cases of transmural infarction occur in the absence of superior mesenteric artery occlusion; underperfusion of the gut is the result of **prolonged vasoconstriction** of the splanchnic vessels such as can occur in cardiogenic or hypovolaemic shock.

The remaining cases of acute small intestinal ischaemia are due to mesenteric **vein** occlusion, which is most often caused by thrombosis. This can occur in patients who are suffering from an endogenous hypercoagulable state such as **polycythaemia rubra vera** or in whom hypercoagulability has occurred for some other reason such as taking oral contraceptives with a high oestrogen content. Venous thrombosis in the mesenteric drainage may also occur if the veins are infiltrated by a malignant neoplasm.

Macroscopic Features

Acute transmural infarction of the gut is always associated with gut wall haemorrhage, and thus infarcted bowel has a dark reddish-purple colour. The serosal surface of the non-viable segments of intestine lose the normal shiny appearance and appears **matt** as a result of a fibrin-rich exudate on the serosa. When the affected segment is opened, the mucosa shows patchy ischaemic ulceration, and **perforation** of the intestine with soiling of the peritoneal cavity is by no means an uncommon event. Even in the absence of such perforation, endotoxin in large amounts may be released into the venous drainage and the patient's already parlous state made worse by the distributive shock characteristic of endotoxaemia.

Acute transmural infarction occurs most often in the middle aged and elderly. It is a very serious development (50–75% of treated patients die, and, if untreated, the mortality rate is 100%). Early and accurate diagnosis and prompt resection of the affected bowel are required because regeneration is not possible. The patients present with the abrupt onset of severe abdominal pain associated with vomiting, fever and distension of the abdomen. There is associated failure of peristalsis, giving rise to a functional intestinal obstruction characterized by absence of bowel sounds when the patient's abdomen is auscultated.

HAMARTOMAS OF THE SMALL GUT

Definition
A hamartoma is a non-neoplastic error in the development of an organ or tissue characterized by an abnormally assembled mixture of elements native to that organ or tissue. Hamartomas may be present at birth or may appear later in life.

Peutz–Jeghers Syndrome
This is defined as hamartomatous gastrointestinal polyposis associated with mucosal and cutaneous pigmentation. It is an autosomal dominant syndrome, characterized externally by excessive melanin pigmentation in the oral mucosa and in the vermilion area of the lips, and, more rarely, in the skin of the fingers and toes. Polyps are found most commonly in the jejunum, ileum and stomach, and rather more rarely in the colon.

Macroscopic Features
Peutz–Jeghers lesions do not differ from adenomatous polyps; they vary in size from a few millimetres to 5 cm in diameter (*Fig. 34.20*).

Microscopic Features
The polyps show a highly characteristic appearance in which there is a branching arrangement of muscularis mucosae, along which the surface epithelium and glands native to that portion of the gut are arranged. On occasions, the glands are misplaced to the deeper layers of the gut wall and this appearance has given rise to mistaken diagnoses of malignancy.

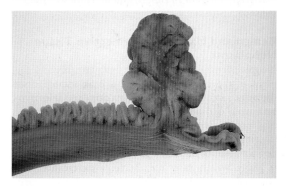

FIGURE 34.20 A hamartomatous polyp in the small gut of a patient with Peutz–Jeghers syndrome.

Natural History
Carcinoma very occasionally develops in relation to these hamartomatous polyps and, in addition, positive correlations appear to exist between the Peutz–Jeghers syndrome and the risk of developing ovarian sex cord neoplasms and carcinoma of the breast.

The most common complications of the Peutz–Jeghers syndrome are recurrent bouts of **intussusception** leading to intestinal obstruction, frank intestinal bleeding and iron-deficiency anaemia due to long-continued occult bleeding.

Brunner's Gland Hamartoma
These rare lesions resemble the polyps of Peutz–Jeghers syndrome, in that they show the same abnormal, branched arrangement of muscle fibres derived from the muscularis mucosae. They arise in relation to Brunner's glands and are thus found, exclusively, in the first and second parts of the duodenum. Patients with such lesions occasionally present with gastrointestinal bleeding and, rarely, duodenal obstruction may occur.

The Cronkhite–Canada Syndrome
This is characterized by polypoid changes rather than individual polyps occurring in the stomach, small gut and colon. The resulting functional abnormality is

excessive protein loss from the gut wall leading, ultimately, to hypoproteinaemia. Abnormalities may also occur in the skin (hyperpigmentation), hair (baldness) and nails (atrophy).

TUMOURS AND TUMOUR-LIKE LESIONS

Benign Epithelial Neoplasms (Adenomas)

With the exception of the ampulla of Vater, adenomas of the small gut are very rare. They may undergo malignant transformation in the same way as their counterparts in the large bowel. Like large bowel polyps they may have the form of tubular, tubulovillous or frankly villous adenomas.

Benign and Malignant Connective Tissue Neoplasms

Neoplasms may arise in the gut from virtually any element of the connective tissue, such as adipose tissue (**lipoma**), smooth muscle (**leiomyoma** and **leiomyosarcoma**) and nerve sheath (**schwannoma**). Patients may present with severe gastrointestinal bleeding and the tumours may function as the starting point for the development of intussusception.

Many writers now use the term **gastrointestinal stromal tumour** for these connective tissue neoplasms. This is because, in some cases, it is difficult to distinguish between lesions showing smooth muscle differentiation (leiomyoma or its malignant counterpart, leiomyosarcoma), those resembling nerve sheath tumours and those that show no differentiation pattern at all. The problems of identifying neoplastic smooth muscle cells have been discussed elsewhere (see pp 518–519).

Malignant Epithelial Neoplasms (Adenocarcinoma)

Adenocarcinoma occurs in the small gut some 40 to 60 times less frequently than in the colon and rectum. It has been suggested that this may be related to the much greater speed with which the luminal contents pass through the small gut and to dilution of potential carcinogens by the small intestinal and pancreatic secretions. The tumours may develop in any part of the small bowel but are most common in the upper part, about 40% being found in the duodenum. Most of these are related to the ampulla of Vater. Small bowel adenocarcinomas in other parts may arise as a complication of Crohn's disease or, rarely, of the Peutz–Jeghers syndrome.

Macroscopic Features

Lesions arising in the region of the ampulla have a papillary appearance; adenocarcinomas of the small gut occurring more distally tend to elicit a marked fibrous tissue response and thus to cause local areas of stenosis involving the whole circumference of the gut wall, giving a so-called 'napkin ring' appearance.

Microscopic Features

The majority are moderately well-differentiated adenocarcinomas, most of which produce mucin and carcinoembryonic antigen. In some instances the tumour cells also express muramidase, suggesting that some degree of differentiation towards the Paneth cell may be taking place.

Other histological variants have been described. These include the **small cell carcinoma ('oat cell')**, which is the morphological homologue of small cell carcinoma of the lung. Electron microscopic examination of the small, round or oval, darkly staining cells shows the presence of neurosecretory granules in which various peptide products can be identified. These tumours, which are worth distinguishing from other intestinal neuroendocrine neoplasms such as carcinoid tumours, are happily rare as they carry a very poor prognosis owing to their propensity to invade deeply and to metastasize.

Carcinoid Tumours

These are tumours with a wide spectrum of biological behaviour arising from cells of the diffuse neuroendocrine system in all parts of the body.

In the gut **the cells of origin are either the Kulchitsky (enterochromaffin) cells, which are found within the crypts, or sub epithelial neuroendocrine cells (argentaffin or argyrophil cells)** (see p 520).

Carcinoid tumours can arise anywhere in the gut:
- 60–80% in the appendix and ileum (**mid-gut origin**). These account for about one-third of all neoplasms in the small gut.
- 10–20% in the large bowel, especially the rectum (**hind-gut origin**)
- the remainder in the proximal part of the small intestine, the stomach and oesophagus (**fore-gut origin**)

Anatomical location is significant in relation to the biological behaviour of carcinoids. **Carcinoids in the appendix and rectum rarely behave in an aggressive fashion, whereas those in the ileum, colon and stomach are often malignant and show a definite tendency towards early metastasis.** In 15–35% of cases of carcinoid of the small intestine, the tumours are multiple and the finding of a carcinoid in this location during surgery suggests that the rest of the gut should be examined carefully.

Mid-gut Carcinoids

The appendix is the commonest site for mid-gut carcinoids but these appendicular neoplasms are usually without clinical significance; they are most often an incidental finding in appendices removed for some other reason.

Apart from the appendix, the commonest site for mid-gut carcinoids to occur is the ileum, the most frequent variant here being known as the 'classical' or insular carcinoid.

Macroscopic Features

The lesion presents as a nodule, usually covered by intact mucosa. Invasion of the underlying mucosa and the resulting fibrosis cause a localized 'buckling' of the bowel wall. **After formaldehyde fixation the tumour often acquires a bright yellow colour.** The size of the neoplasm at the time of resection gives useful prognostic information. Lesions with a diameter of less than 1 cm have a less than 1 in 20 chance of having metastasized; two-thirds of those with a diameter greater than 2 cm have already metastasized.

Microscopic Features

Classical carcinoid shows the presence of solid islands (hence the adjective **insular**) of rather uniform tumour cells with scanty, pale pink, granular cytoplasm, round to oval nuclei and inconspicuous nucleoli with a slightly stippled chromatin pattern (*Fig. 34.21*). The cells at the periphery of each of the islands are smaller and more darkly staining, and are arranged in a palisaded pattern, rather like basal cell carcinoma in the skin. The mitotic rate is usually low.

In the appendix and stomach a variant characterized by the presence of numerous mucin-producing cells of characteristic 'signet-ring' morphology may occur. These are known as 'goblet cell' carcinoids or 'crypt cell carcinomas'. Other variants have been described based on the presence or absence of a 'ribbon-like' pattern of architecture, the presence of a tubuloacinar appearance with extracellular lakes of neutral mucin, and lack of staining wih silver salts which may be seen in an undifferentiated small cell type.

The introduction of immunohistochemistry has increased the ease and accuracy of microscopic diagnosis and has largely obviated the need for the traditional silver staining methods. **Carcinoids show evidence of both epithelial and neuroendocrine differentiation**: first, by their ability to bind antibodies that react with low molecular weight cytokeratins, and second, by their ability to bind such 'pan-endocrine' antibodies as those raised against **chromogranin, neurone-specific enolase, serotonin and synaptophysin**. Many different peptide hormones have been identified in these tumours. These include **gastrin, somatostatin, glucagon, bombesin (gastrin-releasing hormone) and growth hormone-releasing peptide. Peptide YY is consistently found in rectal carcinoids** and only rarely in relation to mid-gut tumours.

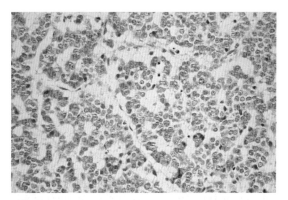

FIGURE 34.21 Mid-gut carcinoid showing the typical arrangement of rather uniform tumour cells in islands and ribbons.

Biological Behaviour of Carcinoid Tumours

The 'Carcinoid Syndrome'

Classical carcinoid tumours have a slow growth rate but they are also highly invasive and tend to metastasize (with the exception, as already stated, of those in the appendix and rectum).

Regional lymph nodes and the liver are the most frequent targets, and secondary tumours in the latter site may be associated with what is known as the 'carcinoid syndrome', a multisystem disturbance caused by the release of large amounts of pharmacologically active compounds from the tumour cells into the hepatic veins.

KEY POINTS: Carcinoid Syndrome

The syndrome is characterized by:
- **flushing and cyanosis** affecting predominantly the face and anterior surface of the chest wall
- episodes of **asthma-like wheezing**
- severe **watery diarrhoea**
- episodic periods of **hypertension and palpitations**
- **right-sided cardiac failure** due to fibrous scarring of the tricuspid and pulmonary valves, associated with the presence of subendocardial fibrous plaques affecting the right atrium and ventricle. Such subendothelial scarring may also be seen in mesenteric blood vessels, where, if it is severe, ischaemic necrosis of the small bowel may result.

Originally it was assumed that this syndrome was due to the release of large amounts of **5-hydroxytryptamine** (5-HT, serotonin), an indolamine that is one of the prominent secretion products of the tumour cells. This can be detected in the urine as 5-hydroxyindole acetic acid by a simple chemical test. The severity and, indeed, the presence of the carcinoid syndrome do not correlate well with the presence and concentration of 5-HT in the blood of affected patients, and other tumour cell secretion products may also contribute.

In more proximal parts of the small bowel, especially in the duodenum, classical carcinoid is rarely found and many of the tumours in this site are composed either of cells that secrete large amounts of gastrin (G cells) or of cells secreting somatostatin (D cells). There is an association between the D cells (which are usually 'silent' in endocrinological terms) and neurofibromatosis.

MALT Lymphoma

The distinctive features of **mucosa-associated lymphoid tissue** (MALT) have already been described (see pp 98, 101) and are reflected in the characteristic malignant lymphomas found in the gut. Geographical factors appear to have a striking effect on the incidence of primary gut lymphoma, this group of disorders being much commoner in the Middle East than in the West. These mucosa-associated lymphomas include:

1) **A primary B-cell lymphoma in which follicles, centrocyte-like cells and plasma cells may be seen.** The tumour cells characteristically invade the epithelial lining of the crypts and the surface epithelium. This is the commonest form of gut lymphoma both in the West, where it is seen most commonly in the stomach, and in Middle Eastern countries, where it most frequently presents as a small gut tumour.

2) **Mediterranean lymphoma, a small gut B-cell lymphoma frequently associated with abnormal immunoglobulin α-chain synthesis (α-chain disease).** It appears to have a different pathogenesis from primary B-cell lymphoma as described above. Mediterranean lymphoma is believed to represent the malignant phase of the disorder called **immunoproliferative small intestinal disease**, which starts as a benign-looking infiltrate of plasma cells or lymphoplasmacytic cells within the mucosa and draining lymph nodes. These plasma cells synthesize (although they do not always secrete) an abnormal α-immunoglobulin heavy chain. The lymphoid and plasma cell infiltrate is monoclonal, as expected in a neoplastic lymphoid proliferation, but nevertheless the disorder responds at this stage to broad-spectrum antibiotics. Removal of an abnormal bacterial population by antibiotics at a stage when the disease is still premalignant could remove a stimulus that is causing the B cells to divide. In this way, the development of full-blown lymphoma could be aborted.

3) **Malignant histiocytosis of the intestine. This term is a misnomer because it is now realized that the small intestinal tumour originally thought to be of monocyte–macrophage (histiocyte) origin is in fact a T-cell lymphoma (enteropathy-associated T-cell lymphoma).** It occurs most commonly in late middle age (50–70 years) and affected patients usually have a history of coeliac disease or of a disorder that mimics coeliac disease. Not all patients have antibodies to gliadin and this has led to the suggestion that the disorder represents a specific T-cell abnormality that may have induced malabsorption. The cells share markers with intraepithelial T cells and it is believed that the tumour arises from this cell population.

4) **Burkitt's lymphoma or a Burkitt-like lymphoma** (see pp 968–969) is also common in the Middle East. Children are chiefly affected and the ileocaecal region appears to be the site of predilection.

5) **Multiple lymphomatous polyposis is a B-cell lymphoma usually arising in the ileocaecal region. Unlike other B-cell tumours in the gut, early spread to extra-abdominal sites is a characteristic feature and thus the prognosis is worse than for other MALT-associated B-cell tumours.** The tumour cells resemble centrocytes morphologically, but differ phenotypically from these cells.

The Appendix

NORMAL ANATOMY

In embryological terms **the appendix is a diverticulum of the caecum**. In adults its length ranges from 4 to 20 cm (mean 7 cm). Variations in the anatomical relationship of the appendix to the ascending colon and terminal ileum are not without interest because they influence the clinical picture seen in acute appendicitis.

The mucosal lining of the appendix is similar to that of large bowel, the non-branching crypts being lined by absorptive and mucin-secreting cells. At the crypt bases, between the epithelium and the basement membranes, are **neuroendocrine cells** containing various peptides. Neuroendocrine cells occur also in the lamina propria of the mucosa and these, which contain serotonin, are associated closely with a delicate network of nerve fibres permeating the mucosa.

DISORDERS OF THE APPENDIX

Acute Appendicitis

Acute appendicitis, although less common than previously, is still the cause of many emergency laparotomies in the UK. The term appendicitis was introduced by Bostonian, R.H. Fitz, who first identified the appendix as the seat of right-sided intra-abdominal sepsis in 1886. It was an attack of acute appendicitis needing surgery that delayed the coronation of Edward VII in 1902. In view of the late king's comfortable shape (he was called 'tummy' by his intimates, although presumably not to his face) and the chronic bronchitis that went with his being a heavy smoker, the operation, not forgetting the anaesthetic, must have been a fairly demanding occasion.

Epidemiology

Acute appendicitis is still quite common in western Europe and North America but rare in Africa, except among the white communities of South Africa, and Asia. It is uncommon in children below the age of 5 years, the peak incidence being in the second and third decades, although ·it is by no means limited to this period. These data may be the expression of:

- dietary differences between populations with a high and low prevalence, the African diet, for instance, containing a small proportion of meat and a large proportion of fibre
- a difference in the time at which various gut pathogens are encountered, this occurring much earlier in African and Asian populations

Pathogenesis

Most cases arise from the interaction of two processes: obstruction and infection.

Obstruction

Obstruction of the appendix lumen may result from processes occurring within the lumen or the wall. Luminal blockage may be due to inspissated faecal material which may have a foreign body at its centre (faecolith). These have been reported in a high proportion of surgically removed inflamed appendices. When faecoliths are associated with acute appendicitis, the inflammation is **distal to the faecolith**, a finding that supports the view that luminal obstruction is an important pathogenetic factor.

Another postulated cause of obstruction is hyperplasia of the lymphoid follicles. Such hyperplasia may result from bacterial or viral infection, and is most prominent in the immediate prepubertal period.

Morphological evidence of obstruction is not always present. It is suggested that obstruction has occurred on a functional basis due either to abnormal contraction of muscle at the base of the appendix, or as a result of abnormally forceful contraction of the main muscle coat along the length of the appendix. Such events are said to be more likely in association with low-fibre diets.

Infection

The immediate pathophysiological effect of luminal obstruction is a rise in pressure within the lumen (up to 90 mmHg in some cases). The increased intraluminal pressure causes an increased pressure within the appendix wall, resulting in mucosal ischaemia and focal loss of the mucosal lining. **Thus a portal for the entry of microorganisms is pro-** **vided and inflammation results, starting within the wall and then spreading back into the lumen and outwards towards the serosa.**

A wide variety of microorganisms may be associated with acute appendicitis, but some specific aetiological agents are worthy of attention.

For example, the appendix is not infrequently involved in *Yersinia* infections, although this species more commonly produces inflammatory changes in the terminal ileum and mesenteric nodes. The microscopic picture may, in some cases, be indistinguishable from that of any other acute appendicitis, but in others characteristic microabscesses within lymphoid follicles are present.

Actinomycosis may also be associated with acute appendicitis. This is not an easy condition to diagnose for the mere presence of the actinomyces in the appendix lumen, even if the appendix is inflamed, does not necessarily indicate that this is the cause of the appendicitis. The presence of the actinomyces **within inflamed tissue** is said to be an unequivocal indicator of actinomycotic appendicitis. It is important that such cases be identified so that appropriate systemic treatment can be given.

Viral infections may also manifest within the appendix. In some instances, **measles** may cause the syndrome of acute appendicitis, probably due to marked hyperplasia of the lymphoid follicles. A confident microscopic diagnosis may be made by identifying the characteristic multinucleated giant cells of measles (Warthin–Finkeldy giant cells). Marked lymphoid hyperplasia may also occur in patients with **adenovirus** infection.

Macroscopic Features

What the pathologist or surgeon sees depends on how advanced the process is at the time of appendicectomy:

- In the early stages the appendix is mildly to moderately swollen and the serosal surface is hyperaemic. Section of the appendix at this stage shows some dilatation of the lumen and there may be a little thin pus within the lumen.
- As the inflammatory process becomes more advanced the swelling increases and the normally translucent serosal surface becomes opaque as a result of the presence of a fibrinous or fibrinopurulent exudate.
- With further progression, the affected part of the appendix becomes soft in consistency and sections made into the appendix wall show the presence of abscesses. This stage is given the name gangrenous appendicitis. This extensive destructive inflammation within the appendix wall is the prelude to rupture.

Consequences of Acute Appendicitis

These depend largely on whether or not perforation has occurred. **If perforation is present the consequences may be:**

- **Generalized peritoneal soiling** leading to generalized peritonitis. This carries with it the risk of development of septic shock as a result of the release of endotoxin into the bloodstream. Even though the peritoneal cavity may be diffusely involved by the inflammatory process, pus tends to collect in certain areas, most notably in the pelvic cavity and subdiaphragmatically.
- **Localized collections of pus in the region of the appendix: appendix abscess.** If leakage of pus from the perforated appendix has been slow and, especially, if the appendix is situated behind the caecum, the extra-appendicular collection of pus remains localized, its limits being formed by the serosal exudate that causes the appendix to adhere to surrounding structures. In some cases the localized periappendicular inflammatory process is followed by the formation of a mass of fibrous tissue which, clinically, may simulate a neoplasm.

In both the presence and absence of perforation:

- **Thrombosis may occur in the small veins of the mesoappendix.** These thrombi are infective and occasionally may extend into larger draining vessels. Rarely, portions of these thrombi may become dislodged and travel in the portal circulation until they impact at some point in the portal venous system within the liver. These emboli give rise to multiple abscesses within the liver parenchyma, the condition being termed **suppurative pylephlebitis**.
- **Adhesions may form** if the exudate fails to be lysed. Such adhesions may lead to subacute or chronic intestinal obstruction.
- The exudate within the lumen of the appendix may become **replaced by fibrous tissue**. If this involves the distal portion of the appendix, that portion may become converted to something resembling a fibrous cord. If intraluminal scarring takes place in the proximal portion of the organ, the mucinous secretions of the crypts may become dammed up and the distal portion of the appendix becomes distended with mucus. This is known as a **mucocele** of the appendix. Very rarely, such a mucocele may rupture and discharge epithelial cells and mucus into the peritoneal cavity; this is known as **pseudomyxoma peritonei**. The extra-appendicular collections of mucus in this event are usually localized, and it must be remembered that there are other causes of pseudomyxoma.

Chronic Non-specific Appendicitis: Does it Exist?

A proportion of the appendices removed from patients complaining of right iliac fossa pain, on microscopic examination, shows no evidence of active inflammation, despite the fact that the pain disappears after removal. Some cynical pathologists have called this condition **'chronic remunerative appendicitis'**.

It has been suggested that this syndrome is due to hyperplasia of the small nerve bundles within the appendix wall. A recent study has shown that there is, in fact, no increase in the number of small nerve fibres compared with control appendices (appendices removed in the course of some other surgical procedure). In the appendices derived from patients complaining of abdominal pain, staining for serotonin was significantly decreased compared with the control group. It has been suggested that this appearance is the expression of discharge of serotonin stores, which could be responsible for the pain.

Specific Forms of Chronic Inflammation do Occur within the Appendix

The appendix may be the seat of some specific chronic inflammatory disorders:

- **tuberculosis**, which is associated in most instances with ileocaecal involvement
- **Crohn's disease**, appendiceal involvement being common when the terminal ileum is involved
- **schistosomiasis**

Tumours and Tumour-like Lesions of the Appendix

Carcinoid

By far the commonest neoplasm of the appendix is carcinoid tumour, which accounts for 80% of appendicular neoplasms. It is said that 0.3% of surgically removed appendices contain such a tumour. Carcinoids of the mid-gut type (composed of argentaffin cells) are the commonest variety but hind-gut-type carcinoids (composed of argyrophil cells) also occur. The microscopic appearances and biological behaviour of carcinoid, including appendicular carcinoid, are described elsewhere (see pp 528–529).

Polyps

The appendix, not surprisingly, shows the presence of a similar range of polyps as seen in the large gut. These include:

- **metaplastic** polyps
- **hamartomatous** polyps of both the Peutz–Jeghers and juvenile types
- **adenomas**

The adenomas, which must be regarded as true neoplasms, differ from those so commonly encountered in the colon and rectum in that the **commonest morphological type seen in the appendix is a diffuse papillary lesion** with a sessile base occupying extensive areas of the mucosa. These lesions, like their counterparts in the large gut, represent an incomplete phenotypic expression of malignancy and always show some histological evidence of epithelial dysplasia.

If the tumour cells secrete large amounts of mucus into the appendix lumen, the latter becomes distended (mucocele) and may in some instances become a large cystic mass (cystadenoma). Occasionally, rupture of the distended appendix occurs, with the production of pseudomyxoma peritonei.

Adenocarcinoma

This is rare and usually arises from a pre-existing adenoma. It may present clinically in the form of a right iliac fossa mass or as acute appendicitis resulting from luminal obstruction by the tumour.

Microscopic diagnosis requires the identification of **true invasion of the appendix wall by neoplastic epithelium**. At the time of diagnosis about 25% of affected individuals have regional nodal metastases. Curative surgical treatment involves right hemicolectomy and, as for other tumours of large gut origin, grading of the tumour and Dukes' classification influence the prognosis considerably. The overall 5-year survival rate is approximately 60%.

Infectious and Inflammatory Bowel Disease

Disorders of the gastrointestinal tract have, so far, been considered on an anatomical basis. However, **many diseases, some associated with inflammation, can affect either the small and large gut, presenting with the same pathophysiological disturbance: diarrhoea**. These disorders are therefore discussed together, emphasizing anatomical considerations where appropriate.

Diarrhoeal diseases of the small and large intestine may be classified, in terms both of their pathology and of their clinical presentation, as **acute** or **chronic**. Most are infective in origin; the aetiology of the two major chronic inflammatory bowel diseases, Crohn's disease and ulcerative colitis, remains unknown, although there have been repeated but unproven suggestions that infectious agents are involved.

ACUTE INFECTIOUS ENTEROCOLITIS

The acute infectious enterocolitides are diarrhoeal illnesses with an incidence that is affected profoundly by adverse socioeconomic conditions. They are the leading cause of death among children in the Third World; it is estimated that each year between 4.5 and 6 million children in Africa, Asia and South America die from such illnesses. In addition these disorders are associated with much morbidity: in the USA the mean incidence is 1.5–1.9 attacks per person per year. In some underprivileged communities, the frequency among children is ten times as great.

Aetiology

Intestinal infections may be caused by **bacteria, viruses** or **protozoa**, which elicit their effects by:

1) **release of toxins within the gut lumen without invasion of the gut wall by the responsible organisms.** Toxins may also be released into food that is contaminated by organisms and thus infection by living microorganisms may not be necessary for acute diarrhoeal illness. The usual target in such infections is the upper part of the small gut. Where no invasion of the gut wall and no damage to the lining epithelium occur, as in **cholera** or *Escherichia coli*-related 'travellers' diarrhoea', no inflammatory reaction takes place. Certain toxins, however, most notably those of *Clostridium difficile* or, much more rarely, *Staphylococcus aureus* cause patchy necrosis of surface epithelium in the colon leading to a pseudomembranous inflammation.

2) **invading the gut wall, damaging the lining epithelium and causing an associated inflammatory reaction.** This may occur in the course of the viral gastroenteritides (e.g. **rotavirus** infection). The infection is restricted to the mature epithelial cells at the tips of the villi. Viral infection causes cell lysis and the villi may become shortened, associated with a mild lymphocytic infiltrate in the lamina propria.

Several bacteria invade the gut wall and produce necrotizing lesions affecting surface epithelium. These include a number of *Shigella* species, some invasive strains of *E. coli, Campylobacter* and certain protozoa such as *Entamoeba histolytica*.

The release of exotoxins plays a significant part in the pathogenesis of invasive bacterial infections. For example, a severe, often fatal, necrotizing enteritis has been described in children in New Guinea who have eaten large quantities of undercooked pork. This disorder, known as 'pig-bel' is due to infections by certain strains of *Clostridium perfringens* which release a β toxin responsible for the cytotoxicity. In very severe cases there may be part or full-thickness gut infarction, and healing of the severely affected areas is accompanied by scarring.

3) **invasion of the gut wall and localization in Peyer's patches, such as occurs in typhoid fever caused by *Salmonella typhi*.** In the lymphoid tissue an immunological response takes place before the organisms invade the bloodstream, usually at the end of a 10–14-day symptom-free period. Multiplication occurs in the blood and is associated with a toxaemic state characterized by fever, headache and a peculiar 'clouded' mental state. Some of the organisms within the blood return to the gut lumen via the bile and in this phase highly characteristic ulceration localized to the sensitized Peyer's patches may occur. Organisms may spread via the bloodstream to colonize a wide

variety of other organs and tissues including the heart, kidneys, liver, bone, meninges and lungs. Other microorganisms that can behave in this way include other *Salmonella* species such as *paratyphi* A and B, *Yersinia* and *Campylobacter fetus*.

The occurrence and severity of any infective diarrhoeal illness depend on interactions between:

- **the dose and virulence of the infecting microorganism**
- **local and systemic defence mechanisms of the patient**

Dose and Virulence

The importance of personal and food hygiene is very great, as each organism has a **minimal infective dose (MID)**, which in some instances may be quite small; in the case of *Shigella* the MID is 10^3 organisms, whereas most enteric bacteria cause clinical effects only **at doses of 10^5–10^8 organisms**.

Organisms also vary greatly in their **virulence**. For example, *E. coli* may be a normal component of the bacterial flora of the gut; it may produce an exotoxin which, like cholera toxin, produces functional alterations in the small gut epithelium associated with a watery non-inflammatory diarrhoea; or it may behave as an invasive organism causing a necrotizing enteritis associated with the synthesis and secretion of a Shiga-like toxin (**verotoxin**) which halts protein synthesis in target cells.

No less important than toxin production is the ability of enteropathogenic organisms to **colonize** the bowel by a variety of adhesion molecules and to **invade** the surface epithelium, which may involve attachment to transmembrane glycoproteins of the epithelium.

Host Defences

Several **host** factors may influence the likelihood of a diarrhoeal illness following infection:

1) **The normal gastric acid barrier.** Antacids or the achlorhydria associated with *Helicobacter pylori* infections increase the chances of postinfective diarrhoea, as does gastrectomy in which much of the acid-producing gastric mucosa is removed.

2) **Gastrointestinal motility.** Impairment leads to increased susceptibility to invasive microorganisms.

3) **Normal bacterial flora.** This appears to have a protective effect. *C. difficile*-associated pseudomembranous enterocolitis is more likely following the use of certain antibiotics such as clindamycin that alter the normal gut flora.

4) **The immune status of the host.** In infants **passive immunity** conferred by antibodies and other protective molecules in breast milk is important in preventing enteric infections. The importance of **active** immunity is shown by the frequent diarrhoeal disorders in patients with acquired immune deficiency syndrome (AIDS).

Cell-mediated Immunity in the Gut

The lymphocyte population in the gut is divided, topographically, into three compartments:

1) Peyer's patches
2) the lymphocytes scattered within the lamina propria
3) intraepithelial lymphocytes

Antigens are transported across the mucosa by the specialized M (microfold) cells which present antigen to lymphocytes in Peyer's patches. These M cells also serve as a route for the invasion of the gut wall by certain bacteria and for the transport of certain parasites that do not normally invade tissues such as *Cryptosporidium*, a well-recognized cause of diarrhoea in patients with AIDS.

Immunoglobulin (Ig) A binds to bacterial antigens and prevents their attachment to the mucosal surface. Secretion of IgA requires synthesis within the gut epithelium of a secretory component; this synthesis is stimulated by interferon γ and tumour necrosis factor α. A selective failure to produce the secretory component is associated with an increased risk of intestinal **candidiasis**.

A high proportion of patients with AIDS have diarrhoea. In Zaire, 84% of patients with diarrhoea of more than 1 month's duration were found to be positive to human immunodeficiency virus, and 40% of patients with AIDS present with persistent diarrhoea. **The commonest pathogens causing diarrhoea in patients with AIDS are cytomegalovirus, *Cryptosporidium* and Microsporidia.** Other pathogens can also be involved. *Salmonella* infections occur 20 times as frequently in patients with AIDS and are five times more likely to be associated with bacteraemia than in HIV-negative individuals.

IMPORTANT EXAMPLES OF INTESTINAL INFECTION

BACTERIAL DISORDERS

Cholera

Cholera results from colonization of the small intestine by the comma-shaped bacillus *Vibrio cholerae*, one of the commonest contaminants of surface waters in the Third World. The organism neither invades the gut wall nor causes epithelial necrosis. The characteristic, profuse, watery diarrhoea is life threatening because of severe dehydration and loss of electrolytes. It is caused by a subunit of the bacterial exotoxin.

Cholera toxin belongs to the group that enter target cells and produce their effects by acting as intracellular enzymes. How this toxin acts is described in the section on cell injury (see pp 17–19).

Toxins of Escherichia Coli

The mechanism described above also causes many cases of 'travellers' diarrhoea'. One of its important causes is a **heat-labile** toxin of certain strains of *E. coli*. This toxin acts in exactly the same way as cholera toxin, sharing antigenic determinants with the latter.

Some strains of *E. coli* produce a **heat-stable** toxin which activates guanylate cyclase in small gut epithelium. This also stimulates fluid secretion from the gut wall into the lumen. A second heat-stable toxin can also stimulate such fluid secretion, but does this by a cyclic nucleotide-independent mechanism.

Some strains produce a toxin known as **verotoxin because of its cytotoxic effect on Vero** cells, a line of African green monkey kidney cells. Verotoxin-producing *E. coli* invade the gut wall, producing haemorrhagic enterocolitis of a similar kind to that produced by *Shigella* toxin; indeed, the two toxins share a number of properties. In some instances the diarrhoeal illness is followed by the appearance of the **haemolytic-uraemic syndrome** (see p 695) a triad of:

- acute renal failure
- low platelet count
- haemolytic anaemia

Diffuse microvascular thrombosis is the characteristic pathological feature. The kidneys show involvement of glomeruli and arterioles; in some very severe cases extensive necrosis of the renal cortices occurs. Urinary levels of platelet-activating factor (PAF) are increased during the acute phases and PAF secretion by glomerular endothelial or mesangial cells may play a significant pathogenetic role in this syndrome.

Bacillary Dysentery and the Shigellae

Shigellae are slender Gram-negative bacilli whose natural habitat is the primate gut. Infections are transmitted by 'food, fingers, faeces and flies' and are confined for the most part to the gut, resulting in **bacillary dysentery**. Shigellae are highly infective, the MID usually being less than 10^3. The four main pathogenic species are:

- *S. dysenteriae*
- *S. flexneri*
- *S. boydi*
- *S. sonnei*

Pathogenesis involves invasion of the mucosal epithelium, followed by the formation of small abscesses in the wall of the colon and the terminal ileum. This leads to stripping of parts of the mucosal lining, bleeding, and the formation of a pseudomembrane consisting of fibrin, cell debris, portions of necrotic mucosa, acute inflammatory cells and bacteria.

As well as endotoxin (lipopolysaccharide) derived from its cell wall, *S. dysenteriae* produces a **heat-labile exotoxin** that affects both gut and central nervous system. This disorder is characterized by the sudden onset of abdominal pain, fever and watery diarrhoea. Within a few days the stool becomes less fluid and shows mucus and blood. In some cases, the organisms persist in the gut and the mucosal ulcers fail to heal.

Most of the ulcers are superficial; deep ulcers occasionally occur and mucous retention cysts in the submucosa (so-called colitis cystica profunda) mark their sites after healing.

Campylobacter Infections

Campylobacter are motile, comma-shaped Gram-negative bacilli. One, *C. jejuni*, is as common a cause of infectious diarrhoea as *Salmonella* and *Shigella* species.

Infections are acquired orally from food, drink, infected animals or some recherché varieties of oral sexual activity. Organisms multiply in the small intestine, invade the gut wall and produce acute inflammation. Patients present with fever, abdominal pain and bloody diarrhoea. *C. jejuni* infections are not confined to the small bowel: involvement of the appendix, colon and rectum is now well recognized. In some instances, bacteraemia may be present and a clinical picture resembling typhoid fever develops.

Clostridium Difficile and Pseudomembranous Colitis

C. difficile is part of the normal gastrointestinal flora in 2–10% of humans and is resistant to a wide variety of commonly used antibiotics. Antibiotics such as lincomycin, clindamycin and ampicillin suppress the normal bacterial flora and, as a result, *C. difficile* multiplies to excess. The risk of colitis caused by toxin-producing *C. difficile* is greatest in the elderly.

C. difficile produces two toxins. The first, which has a similar effect to cholera toxin and is also cytotoxic for gut epithelium, binds to brush-border receptors on epithelium. The second is cytotoxic; its binding site is unknown.

In severe cases, the rectum is often involved; sigmoidoscopy shows the presence of pale, yellowish-grey plaques of membrane adhering to the mucosal surface. The plaques vary in size from a few millimetres to 15–20 cm. Microscopic examination shows that the lesions start as focal areas of mucosal necrosis overlain by tufts of fibrin, admixed with mucus and acute inflammatory cells which seem to 'mushroom' out directly from the necrotic foci (*Fig. 34.22*). These are known as 'summit lesions'.

Diagnosis is established by identifying the presence of toxin in the stool.

Outside the acute hospital situation, *C. difficile* infections are becoming a growing problem in residential homes for the elderly.

Yersinia Enterocolitis

Yersinia are short, rather pleomorphic, Gram-negative rods. Species implicated in human disease are *Y. enterocolitica* and *Y. pseudotuberculosis*.

Y. enterocolitica, has been isolated from domestic animals, rodents and also the waters contaminated by these species. Humans become infected from food or drink contaminated by the faeces of infected animals. A large

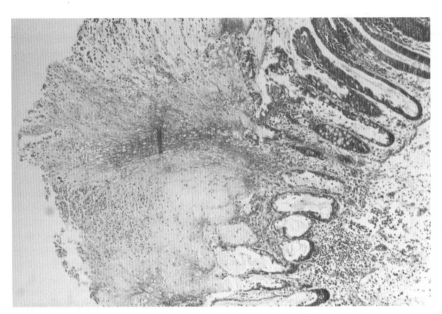

FIGURE 34.22 *Pseudomembranous enterocolitis due to* Clostridium difficile *infection. Note the necrotic mucosa on the left and the mushroom-like mass of fibrin appearing to erupt from the mucosa.*

dose (10^8–10^9 organisms) must be ingested if infection is to occur. In young infants, *Yersinia* infections may present as acute gastroenteritis, whereas in older children the clinical syndrome may resemble acute appendicitis.

During the 5–10-day incubation period, the organisms multiply intramucosally, particularly in the ileum. This elicits acute inflammation associated with ulceration and intramucosal microabscesses, involving especially the gut lymphoid tissue and mesenteric nodes. Macrophages tend to cluster around the margins of the microabscesses. True granuloma formation is rare in infections with *Y. enterocolitica* but is not uncommon if the responsible organism is *Y. pseudotuberculosis*. The microscopic picture in the latter may be mistaken for Crohn's disease.

Most infections are self-limiting, although on occasion gut infection may be followed by pneumonia or meningitis.

Salmonella Infections

Salmonellae are motile Gram-negative bacilli that are oral pathogens both for humans and animals. Classification of the Salmonellae is complex and is based on analysis of the bacterial antigens.

Three of the Salmonellae primarily infect humans:

- *S. typhi*
- *S. paratyphi* A
- *S. schottmülleri* (formerly *S. paratyphi* B)

Isolation of these from patients indicates that the source of the infection was another human. In respect of other *Salmonella* infections, a wide variety of animal species, including pigs, poultry, cattle, rats, mice and domestic pets, constitutes the reservoir for human infections. Infection is by the oral route and due to:

- faecally contaminated water, milk and other dairy products
- shellfish, meats and meat products derived from infected animals (chiefly poultry) or contaminated by infected faeces
- infected dried or frozen egg

The MID for most of the Salmonellae is 10^5–10^8 organisms, but with *S. typhi* a dose as low as 10^3 may be sufficient to cause typhoid fever.

Host factors contributing to resistance include gastric acidity, normal intestinal bacterial flora and local gut immunity. Individuals suffering from **sickle cell disease** are more susceptible to *Salmonella* infections and are particularly at risk of developing *Salmonella*-related osteomyelitis.

In humans, *Salmonella* infections produce three principal types of disease:

1) **enterocolitis**, which is the commonest clinical manifestation of *Salmonella* infection
2) **bacteraemia with focal lesions**, many of which occur outside the gastrointestinal tract
3) **typhoid fever** ('enteric fever')

Salmonella **enterocolitis** may be caused by many different *Salmonella* serotypes, *S. typhimurium* being a frequent offender. Ingestion of infected food or drink is followed in 8–48 hours by nausea, fever, headache, vomiting and profuse diarrhoea. Most episodes resolve within 2–3 days; antibiotic treatment is not indicated. Indeed, antibiotics may lead to a prolongation of both the clinical features and *Salmonella* excretion in stools.

Macroscopic Features

Both mucosa and serosa show hyperaemia, and Peyer's patches are enlarged. Shallow ulcers may be present on the mucosal surface in both the small gut and colon. In the latter the appearances resemble those of bacillary dysentery.

Bacteraemia associated with focal tissue lesions is commonly but by no means exclusively caused by *S. enterica*. Following oral infection, the organisms rapidly gain access to the bloodstream and focal necrosis may occur in the liver, heart, bones, joints and meninges.

Typhoid Fever ('The Enteric Fevers')

These are caused by *S. typhi*, *S. paratyphi* A and *S. schottmülleri*, the first two usually causing more severe disease. These infections follow a classical sequence:

1) **The organisms are invasive, localizing within Peyer's patches** where, in non-immune individuals, they cause a primary immune response. Infected macrophages carry some of the organisms to regional lymph nodes, and during the incubation period (7–20 days) the organisms multiply within macrophages in the gut-associated lymphoid tissue and in regional nodes. Peyer's patches become hyperplastic, the swollen lymphoid nodules projecting into the gut lumen as submucosal elevations.

2) **The organisms then reach the bloodstream where they go on multiplying and from which they can be isolated during the first 1–2 weeks of the clinical illness.** In the first week, the rate of isolation is about 90%, falling to about 50% in the third week. The bloodborne organisms are phagocytosed by fixed tissue macrophages in the liver sinusoids and spleen, and proliferation of immunologically competent cells in these sites follows. Thus a moderate splenomegaly and some degree of liver enlargement are quite common in this phase.

This bacteraemic phase is characterized by fever (with characteristic afternoon spikes), malaise, headache, myalgia, mental clouding and a bradycardia which appears inappropriate for the degree of fever. At this stage, the patient often complains of constipation. The white cell count is normal or low. Many of these features can be ascribed to cytokine release due to interactions between endotoxin and fixed tissue macrophages. The fever often reaches a plateau during the second week and starts to decline during the third and fourth weeks. In the second week, a maculopapular rash ('rose spots'), which fades on pressure, appears on the thorax and upper abdomen but is usually present for only a few days.

Towards the end of the first week of illness, specific agglutinating antibodies make their appearance in the patients' serum, their titre rising to a peak in the third week of illness.

3) **Some circulating organisms are excreted in the bile and thus can reach the gallbladder (where they can cause cholecystitis) and make a second appearance in the gut lumen.** At this time, many other tissues, including the bone marrow, can also be colonized by the organisms. In the small gut the organisms encounter specific IgA on the mucosal surface and in sensitized gut-associated lymphoid tissue. **This is associated with characteristic ulcers in Peyer's patches. The lesions are oval lesions, their long axes oriented along the long axis of the gut, in contrast to the tuberculous ulcers that encircle the gut wall in a 'napkin-ring' fashion.**

Microscopic Features

The ulcers are characterized by large numbers of rounded macrophages with abundant opaque cytoplasm. Neutrophils are alleged to be absent but may certainly be seen in some cases. The macrophage response is also seen in typhoid lesions in tissues outside the gastrointestinal system such as the liver. Recovery is accompanied by mucosal regeneration from the ulcer edges; little or no scarring is apparent. At this stage, diarrhoea may be a prominent feature and it is usually possible to culture the offending organisms from the stool, although, because they are also excreted in the urine, urine culture may be a useful diagnostic adjunct.

Complications

Complications are most frequent in the third and fourth weeks of illness. The most important gut-related ones are haemorrhage and perforation.

Other less common complications are:
1) acute cholecystitis which may be followed by chronic inflammation of the gallbladder and a carrier state. Cholecystectomy may be required to bring the bacterial shedding to an end.
2) paralytic ileus
3) myocarditis
4) focal necrosis in organs such as the liver and kidneys
5) Zenker's degeneration of abdominal muscle. The affected fibres have a pale, waxy appearance and show segmental necrosis. The pathogenesis is not understood.

Tuberculosis of the Gut

Gut involvement by tuberculosis is not infrequently seen in Third World countries where tuberculosis is still common.

The infection may be **primary** as a result of drinking milk infected by *Mycobacterium bovis*. Culling of infected dairy cattle following tuberculin testing and pasteurization of milk have largely eliminated *M. bovis* infections in developed countries.

Secondary tuberculous infection in the gut occurs as a result of swallowing infected sputum in patients with pulmonary tuberculosis. Tuberculosis most commonly affects the jejunum and ileum, and may occur also in the appendix, colon, rectum and duodenum, in descending order of frequency. Oesophageal, gastric and anorectal tuberculosis is very rare.

Macroscopic Features

Two types of lesions may be seen. The first is ulceration, usually involving the whole circumference of the affected segments of bowel wall. Healing is associated with scarring, leading to a circumferential stricture of the gut.

In other instances the inflammatory process extends right through the entire thickness of the bowel wall, forming a mass of inflamed fibrous tissue. Adhesions between adjacent segments of bowel or between the bowel, the mesentery and involved lymph nodes may form masses mimicking carcinoma and other conditions such as Crohn's disease. Microscopic distinction of tuberculosis from the latter may be very difficult.

In both the ulcerative and hypertrophic forms of the disease, small 'tubercles' may be seen on the mucosal and serosal surfaces of the affected gut.

AIDS *and* Mycobacterium Avium Intracellulare *(MAI)*

Patients with AIDS are prone to infection by **MAI**. In the absence of adequate cell-mediated immunity, well-formed granulomata are not seen; instead the lamina propria is infiltrated by many large granular macrophages, resembling those seen in Whipple's disease (see p 524). Appropriate special stains show the presence of very large numbers of acid-fast bacilli in the macrophage cytoplasm.

Intestinal Spirochaetosis

This is due to infestation of the colorectal and appendiceal epithelium by numerous spirochaetes of the genus *Borrelia*. In haematoxylin and eosin-stained sections, the spirochaetes appear as an intense blue fringe on the mucosal surface. Electron microscopy shows many spiral microorganisms attached to the surfaces of both absorptive and goblet cells and, occasionally, within the cytoplasm of the epithelial cells. It is not clear whether these spirochaetes are pathogenic and cause diarrhoea in humans, although similar organisms cause a dysenteric illness in pigs.

Chlamydial Infections

Chlamydiae are small, obligate, intracellular parasites occupying a taxonomic position between viruses and bacteria. *Chlamydia trachomatis* includes the agents responsible for the disease **lymphogranuloma venereum**, which occurs most commonly in tropical and subtropical regions. Infection occurs as a result of sexual contact, and anal intercourse is associated with rectal involvement. In females rectal involvement may be due to spread from vaginal lesions.

Chlamydial proctitis, due to other species of *Chlamydia*, causes anal pain and tenesmus accompanied by the passage of blood and mucus from the anus. Sigmoidoscopy shows a reddened, friable and ulcerated mucosa, resembling the appearance of ulcerative colitis. Perianal abscesses and fistulae may occur and granulomas may be found in the rectal tissues and in draining inguinal nodes.

Scarring is common and the rectal wall may become very thick, stiff and severely ulcerated. The microscopic picture is that of florid, non-specific inflammation associated with much fibrosis. Carcinoma has been described in relation to some cases of lymphogranulomatous stricture.

VIRAL DISORDERS

The importance of viral infections in connection with diarrhoeal disorders is very great. Rotavirus is the commonest cause of severe diarrhoea in infants and young children, accounting for 3.5 million cases each year in the USA alone.

Five major human gastroenteritis viruses have been defined:

- **rotavirus**
- **Norwalk virus**
- **enteric adenovirus**
- **calicivirus**
- **astrovirus**

Rotavirus

This is one of the Reoviridae. The virion is made up of four major structural proteins which form a three-layered, wheel-like (hence 'rota') viral capsid. VP4, one of the two proteins of the outer layer of the capsid, forms spike-like projections that stick out for more than 10 nm from the viral surface. This protein is a haemagglutinin and an important determinant of viral pathogenicity.

Rotavirus accounts for a median of 34% of all episodes of hospitalization required in children under 2 years of age. In developing countries, it is said to cause 125 million cases of diarrhoea every year. Some 18 million of these are severe and, of these, 800 000–900 000 are fatal. Infections are transmitted via the faecal–oral route, although it is suggested that respiratory transmission may also occur.

The diagnosis of rotavirus infection is simple: the virus is excreted in very large amounts in the patient's faeces, and kits (both sensitive and specific) are available for the detection of rotaviral antigens. The virus can also be seen in the stools on electron microscopy.

The severe diarrhoea is caused by one of the viral

proteins, NSP4, which acts as a 'viral exotoxin' causing severe fluid loss from infected enterocytes, the mechanism for this being changes in calcium concentration. Antibodies against another viral protein, VP6, prevents infection and it is likely that vaccines based on this protein will soon be available for clinical trials.

Norwalk Virus

This causes diarrhoea in adults and school-age children. It is an important cause (40% of cases) of epidemic gastroenteritis in such environments as camps, cruise ships, college hostels, etc. Infection results from drinking infected water or eating poorly cooked shellfish from infected waters. Norwalk virus cannot be cultured in cells, nor does it produce any disease in animals.

The virion contains a single structural protein, the characteristics of which suggest that this virus should be classified as a **calicivirus**. One of its effects is to delay gastric emptying, and this probably explains the nausea and vomiting that characteristically occur.

Enteric Adenoviruses

These are the adenoviral serotypes producing gastroenteritis (group F, serotypes 40 and 41). Unlike most adenoviruses they do not affect the respiratory tract or the eye. Adenoviral diarrhoea occurs mainly in children under the age of 2 years and accounts for about 20% of cases of infectious diarrhoea in this age group. The infection causes a watery diarrhoea which may be followed by vomiting. It tends to be more long-lasting than any other form of viral diarrhoea (5–12 days).

Caliciviruses

These are small round viruses, which until recently could be diagnosed only by examining faeces with the electron microscope, although immunoassays are now available. They usually cause a fairly mild diarrhoeal illness in infants and young children which, although it occurs in the general paediatric population, seems especially to affect groups such as children in schools, day nurseries or orphanages.

Astroviruses

Astroviruses are small round viruses with a single-stranded RNA genome. They are structurally and immunologically distinct from the caliciviruses. Children aged 1–7 years are most commonly affected. These viruses produce a watery diarrhoea, which is usually less severe than in rotaviral infections. These infections must be common as, by the age of 4 years, 70% of British children have antibodies against astrovirus. Because outbreaks of astroviral disease have been reported only in children and, occasionally, among the elderly, it seems likely that these antibodies exert a protective effect.

Viral Infections in Immunosuppressed Patients

Patients immunosuppressed for whatever reason are at risk of developing herpes simplex virus colitis or cytomegalovirus gut infections. Herpes simplex virus infections may produce mucosal inflammation and erosions resembling ulcerative colitis. The diagnosis is made by finding the typical multinucleated giant cells and also the characteristic intranuclear inclusions in biopsy material.

Cytomegalovirus infection is especially likely to be seen in patients following renal transplant. The typical cytomegalic inclusions are usually found in this situation within endothelial cells, fibroblasts and macrophages, the epithelial cells usually being spared.

PROTOZOAL DISORDERS

Giardiasis

Giardia lamblia is one of the commonest protozoa infecting the human small gut. Its prevalence is greatest in areas where standards of sanitation and hygiene are poor; infection is usually acquired by **drinking contaminated water**. In areas where *Giardia* is prevalent, substantial numbers of the indigenous population are infected, but only a small proportion of these develop *Giardia*-related illness. This contrasts with travellers, many of whom develop diarrhoea, abdominal pain and, in some instances, steatorrhoea. The risk of *Giardia* infection is increased in subjects who have low serum IgA concentrations and also in children in day nurseries or orphanages.

Microscopic Features

Infection may produce no significant microscopic abnormalities. In other instances lymphocytes, both within the surface epithelium and in the lamina propria, are increased. Some degree of villous atrophy may be present, and is most marked in patients with evidence of malabsorption.

The trophozoite form of the *Giardia*, which has a pear-shaped, binuclear structure with four pairs of flagella, is found near or attached to the mucosa of the duodenum or jejunum.

On electron microscopy, trophozoites can be seen to have a sickle shape, the concave side of this sickle being a 'sucker' which attaches the parasite to the enterocytes. Under most circumstances, the trophozoites do not pass out with the faeces except during the acute diarrhoeal illness. In water and in chronic carriers, infection is transmitted by the encysted form of the parasite. The most reliable diagnostic method is examination of duodenal aspirate.

Intestinal Apicomplexa Infections

Cryptosporidium *and* Isospora

The phylum Apicomplexa comprises a large number of organisms that have in common the possession of a set of ultrastructural organelles is known as the apical complex. This is located at the anterior end of the parasites.

This phylum includes important pathogenic genera such as the *Plasmodia*, which cause malaria, and *Toxoplasma*, which causes toxoplasmosis, but it is only recently with the emergence of AIDS that other genera such as *Cryptosporidium* and *Isospora* have emerged as fairly important human gut pathogens. The acute self-limiting diarrhoeas caused by these parasites also occur frequently in immunologically competent individuals.

***Cryptosporidium* infection is due to ingesting mature oocysts in water or food.** In the small intestine the oocysts release sporozoites, which become attached to the brush border of the small intestinal epithelium. They then enter the cells and undergo asexual development, releasing merozoites which can invade other cells in the vicinity.

The clinical effects depend on the immunological status of the host. In immunologically competent persons, a watery diarrhoea with cramping abdominal pain and loss of appetite occurs, the illness lasting between 5 days and 2 weeks. In immunologically suppressed hosts, the clinical picture is more severe and can last for months or even years. *Cryptosporidium* is recorded as being found in 14–26% of patients with AIDS and diarrhoea.

Microscopic Features

The morphological appearances of affected small gut range from normal to an inflamed mucosa in which crypt abscesses may be present and where there is blunting, shortening and destruction of small intestinal villi. The parasites can be seen in the brush border. They are small, basophilic bodies, 3–4 μm in diameter, which are arranged in clusters or short rows. They are acid fast and are most easily seen, on light microscopy, when stained with Ziehl–Neelsen carbolfuchsin.

Isospora Belli

Isospora belli is another acid-fast protozoon that can cause diarrhoea and malabsorption. Its habitat is the small gut epithelium. Infection is transmitted by oocysts ingested in contaminated water or food; sporozoites released from the cysts in the small gut lumen enter the epithelium.

In immune-suppressed hosts, *I. belli* causes a chronic illness characterized by diarrhoea, cramping abdominal pain, nausea and weight loss. Most cases show a striking increase in blood eosinophil concentration. Some 2–6% of patients with AIDS and diarrhoea are infected by *I. belli*.

Microscopic Features

The small gut mucosa shows differing degrees of villous atrophy and a moderately intense inflammatory cell infil-trate consisting of lymphocytes and plasma cells. The parasites, at different stages of their development, may be seen in the cytoplasm of epithelial cells.

Amoebic Dysentery

This disorder affecting the colon is caused by the protozoon *Entamoeba histolytica*. Amoebiasis has a worldwide distribution but is most prevalent in the tropics. Entamoeba can exist in two forms:

1) an **active motile vegetative form** found in the stools of patients during the acute dysenteric illness
2) a **cystic form** passed in the stools, which is swallowed in contaminated water or food, its wall dissolving in the intestinal lumen

In its motile form the parasite is rounded with a small nucleus and a very small, centrally placed, karyosome. It has a glycogen-rich cytoplasm with a peripheral clear zone from which the pseudopodia mediating its movement project. The amoeba is phagocytic and ingested red cells can often be seen in its cytoplasm. The parasite produces its ulcerogenic effect on the colonic wall by means of the proteolytic enzymes that it secretes (hence the name *E. histolytica*) and penetrates through the lamina propria to reach the submucosa.

Patients usually present with a moderately severe diarrhoea characterized by blood and mucus in the stools.

Small amoebic ulcers are most commonly seen in the caecum and rectum but may occur anywhere in the large gut. They are oval in shape and tend to lie with their long axes at right angles to the long axis of the colon.

Microscopic Features

On section the ulcers can be seen to have a narrow neck and a much broader base; the lesion thus has a flask-shaped appearance. The amoebae are usually found on or just below the ulcer surface. They are usually not difficult to see in surgical specimens but are rendered more distinct by the periodic acid–Schiff method, in which they appear as moderately large red bodies.

Occasionally an overwhelming diffuse colitis with a fulminant clinical picture may occur, particularly in undernourished Africans.

Complications

Perforation of the affected colon may occur with soiling of the peritoneal cavity. This is usually fatal and is, happily, rare. A not uncommon complication is the development of an **amoeboma**, which is a mass of inflammatory granulation tissue that can readily be mistaken for carcinoma or diverticular disease. These lesions are commonest in the caecum and rectum and may be difficult to diagnose clinically, radiologically and histologically, because amoebae may be very scanty at this stage. In a substantial proportion of cases, the amoebae penetrate the small vessels of the submucosa and travel in the portal vein radicles to reach the liver. Once established in the liver they can cause **abscesses**, which may be single or, more rarely, multiple, or what has been termed **amoebic hepatitis**.

In amoebic abscess, the parasites cause small zones of liquefactive necrosis that coalesce to form large cavities filled with brownish-red, semifluid, sterile pus ('anchovy sauce' pus). Such abscesses are associated with intense pain and tenderness. They may become chronic, being encapsulated by a thick fibrous tissue layer, or may rupture through:

1) the diaphragm into the lung
2) the diaphragm into the pleural cavity causing an amoebic empyema
3) the liver capsule into the peritoneal cavity
4) the diaphragm into the pericardium

Infected material may also gain access to small hepatic venules and produce metastatic lesions in various tissues.

CHRONIC INFLAMMATORY BOWEL DISEASE OF UNKNOWN AETIOLOGY AND PATHOGENESIS

Most cases falling under this rubric are either **Crohn's disease or ulcerative colitis**. It is usually possible, on clinical and pathological grounds, to make a clear distinction between these two entities, but **in some cases it is not possible to differentiate between them**. This has led some workers to question whether these two named diseases are, in fact, separate entities. There is an obvious familial tendency in both conditions: first-degree relatives of patients with Crohn's disease may develop either Crohn's disease or ulcerative colitis, and the identical situation has been recorded in first-degree relatives of patients with ulcerative colitis. Because the aetiology of both these conditions is still unknown, it is simpler to treat them as if they are indeed distinct until such time as the nature of their relationship, if any, becomes clearer.

CROHN'S DISEASE

Crohn's disease can be defined, and thus to a considerable extent differentiated, from ulcerative colitis, in terms of its topographical distribution (*Fig. 34.23*) **and morphological features**.

It is a **chronic inflammatory disease which, in about 60% of cases, shows a granulomatous pattern**. In terms of the **sites affected** it:

- **can occur anywhere in the gastrointestinal tract from the mouth to the anus (small gut in 66% of cases, large gut in 17%, and both small and large gut in 17%). The lesions are**

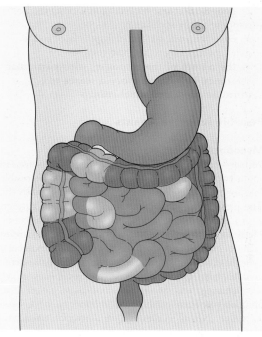

FIGURE 34.23 *Crohn's disease of the large and small gut, as shown here, is typically discontinuous, with 'skip' areas of unaffected bowel between affected areas.*

  characteristically discontinuous, with segments of normal bowel between affected areas.
- **involves the entire thickness of the gut wall** (i.e. the inflammation is **transmural** in distribution)
- **may involve sites outside the gut** such as the **skin**, especially round ileostomy or colostomy stomas, **vulva, bone and joints**.

Epidemiology

Crohn's disease is most common in temperate climates and amongst those of European origin. Jews are relatively more frequently affected than non-Jews and, in both the USA and Israel, Ashkenazy Jews are more at risk than Sephardic ones. While the incidence of ulcerative colitis has remained steady since the 1960s, the frequency of Crohn's disease increased until about 1980, at which time it seemed to plateau with an annual incidence of 2–5 per 100 000 population and a prevalence of about 30–75 per 100 000. There appear to be three age peaks for the development of the disease: 20–29, 50–59 and 70–79 years, the highest of these being the earliest.

Aetiology and Pathogenesis

The cause of Crohn's disease is still unknown. A theoretical model could be constructed using a number of rubrics, including:

1) an **exogenous injurious agent such as a microorganism**

2) **genetic factors**, which might modify the host's response to any such injury

3) environmental factors, perhaps related to life style, contributing to the host response

4) **the nature of the response, with particular reference in inflammatory diseases to immune-mediated mechanisms**

Possible Infective Agents

Mycobacteria

Perhaps because of the granulomatous response in about two-thirds of Crohn's disease lesions, a possible role for mycobacteria has been canvassed extensively. The presence of mycobacteria in tissues from patients with Crohn's disease has been reported several times. Methods employed for identification of these organisms include culture, electron microscopy and molecular hybridization. Most commonly, potentially pathogenic mycobacterial species such as *Mycobacterium kansasii, M. paratuberculosis* and *M. avium intracellulare*, rather than obligate pathogens such as *M. tuberculosis*, have been identified. Not all studies support a mycobacterial aetiology and at present a 'not proven' verdict seems appropriate.

Other Pathogens

Ultrafiltrates of affected gut tissue have been shown to cause granulomatous inflammation when injected into small animals and also to have a cytopathic effect on mucosal epithelial cells in culture. These results have been interpreted as indicating a viral origin for the disease and a number of viruses including rotavirus and, most recently, measles virus have been suggested as being likely candidates. Again, proof is lacking.

Genetic Factors

Familial clustering occurs in Crohn's disease and, to a lesser extent, in ulcerative colitis. Monozygotic twins with Crohn's disease show a very high degree of concordance (58%) and a single instance has been reported of monozygotic triplets all developing Crohn's disease. Some minor alterations in risk are found in respect of certain HLA antigens: an increase in risk with HLA-A2 and a decrease with HLA-A11. A complex segregational analysis involving 265 patients with Crohn's disease and 5387 of their relatives has suggested that the risk of Crohn's disease may be conferred by the presence of a recessive gene with incomplete penetrance.

Additional Exogenous Factors

The most significant of these so far identified is cigarette smoking, which doubles the risk of Crohn's disease independent of dose. Interestingly, case-control studies have shown that there is a **decreased risk for ulcerative colitis in smokers**. When heavy smokers stop smoking, the risk of developing ulcerative colitis increases quite sharply.

A positive association with risk for Crohn's disease has also been observed in respect of the dietary intake of refined sugars. Smoking and high intake of refined sugars do not appear to act synergistically. This has been interpreted as suggesting that they operate via the same unknown mechanism.

Immune-mediated Mechanisms

Data implicating the immune system include:

1) increased concentrations of antigen-presenting cells, notably macrophages, in the affected areas of the mucosa

2) activated lymphocytes, both in the affected portions of mucosa and in draining nodes

3) decreased natural killer cell activity and decreased antibody-dependent cytotoxicity

Despite these, there is still no proof that an altered immune state plays a pathogenic role in Crohn's disease.

Pathological Features

Macroscopic Features

The site of the lesions affects the morphological features of Crohn's disease far less than does the stage of development.

Early phases are characterized by small superficial ulcers which coalesce and become serpiginous. The combination of the ulcers with oedema and lymphoid hyperplasia gives the mucosal surface a 'cobblestone' appearance. The submucosa and muscularis propria become oedematous and thickened. Inflammation may involve the serosa as well, and, in some instances, the affected serosa may adhere to the serosa of other loops of gut or to the peritoneal lining of the abdominal wall. Lesions occur most commonly in the distal ileum (hence Crohn's original name for this disease – 'terminal ileitis') but may occur anywhere in the gastrointestinal tract. Multiple discontinuous or 'skip' lesions may be present at this stage.

With disease progression, some ulcers form deep fissures which plunge down through the entire thickness of the bowel wall. The combination of the serosal adhesions mentioned above and the transmural fissures form the basis for **fistula** formation. Fistulae may occur:

● **between adjacent loops of bowel**
● **between affected loops of bowel and the skin of the abdominal wall**
● **between affected loops of bowel and other hollow viscera such as the urinary bladder**
● **anal fistulae.** Rectal and anal fistulae are found in about one-third of patients with Crohn's disease. These fistulae are distinctive because they are not continuous with lesions in the gut and may precede the appearance of lesions within the gastrointestinal tract by years in some cases.

At the same time as fissure development, the lymphoedema affecting the submucosa and muscle becomes more pronounced and this, with associated fibrosis, confer on the affected segment of bowel **a rigid 'hose-pipe'-like appearance**. These areas, described by some as resembling an 'eel in rigor mortis' are the sites of severe luminal narrowing and the cause of the intestinal obstruction with which some patients present (*Fig. 34.24*). They are the morphological correlate of the 'string sign' seen on barium studies. The peri-intestinal adipose tissue may also be thickened and scarred, and there is often obvious enlargement of draining nodes. The adjacent mesentery shows a similar appearance.

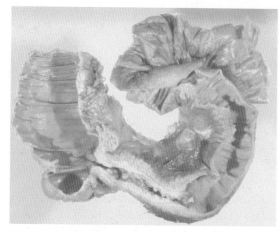

FIGURE 34.24 *Crohn's disease of the terminal ileum showing the characteristic thickening of the wall and narrowing of the lumen.*

In about 10–20% of cases of colitis, it is not possible on morphological grounds to distinguish between Crohn's disease and other forms of colitis. Macroscopic features of most value in making a diagnosis of Crohn's disease are:

- **the discontinuous nature of the gut involvement ('skip' lesions)**
- **the thickening of the bowel wall**
- **the long, deep and narrow ulcers**

Microscopic Features

Principal features serving to distinguish Crohn's disease from other chronic inflammatory bowel disorders are (*Figs 34.25* and *34.26*):

- **the transmural distribution of the inflammatory process**, all layers from the mucosa to the serosa being affected
- **marked oedema of the submucosa leading to a striking degree of thickening of the affected segment**

- **the presence of foci of lymphoid cells, often with a well-marked follicular arrangement, distributed transmurally.** This is often so conspicuous that a working histological diagnosis can be made, often merely by naked-eye inspection of sections stained with haematoxylin and eosin, when the lymphoid aggregates show up as blue spots against the pink background of the rest of the section.
- **patchy ulceration of the mucosa, often in the form of fissures**
- **the presence of non-caseating tuberculoid granulomata at any level within the thickness of the bowel wall and in the draining lymph nodes.** These are highly characteristic of Crohn's disease but are found in only 50–60% of cases. The granulomata are often rather poorly formed and may be difficult to see.

Other changes seen in the gut in Crohn's disease are less characteristic. They include:

1) the presence of **metaplasia of some of the mucosal glands** that have an appearance resembling those of the pylorus
2) **thickening of nerve fibres** with an increased content of vasoactive intestinal polypeptide
3) **marked thickening of the muscularis mucosae**
4) a variety of **changes in blood vessels**

Clinical Features

The clinical features may vary considerably from patient to patient and may be so subtle as to defy diagnosis for considerable periods. Principal features of uncomplicated Crohn's disease are:

- **mild to moderate diarrhoea, present in 80% of cases. If the colon is involved this diarrhoea may be associated with blood in the stools.**
- **fever**
- **abdominal pain**, experienced most commonly in the lower part of the abdomen. In about 20% of cases, the onset is abrupt with severe, localized abdominal pain suggesting an intra-abdominal emergency such as acute appendicitis or gut perforation.

Features relating directly to the bowel involvement tend to reflect the site and type of that involvement. **Thus the formation of strictures is mirrored by clinical features of chronic or subacute intestinal obstruction.** Fistula formation between segments of large and small gut alter the bacterial flora of the latter and the resulting bacterial overgrowth leads to the development of malabsorption (see pp 524–525). Malabsorption may also develop if the distal part of the ileum is severely affected, and **a protein-losing state** ensues. Similarly, **pernicious anaemia may develop as a result of specific malabsorption of vitamin B_{12}.**

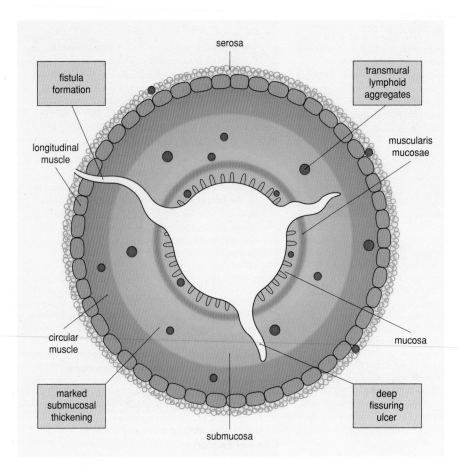

FIGURE 34.25 *The pattern of bowel wall involvement seen in Crohn's disease.*

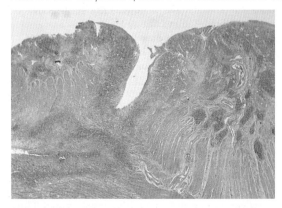

FIGURE 34.26 *Crohn's disease of the colon showing deep fissuring, marked submucosal oedema and many lymphoid aggregates.*

Gut Malignancy in Crohn's Disease

Patients with Crohn's disease have an increased risk of developing carcinoma as a late complication. The neoplasms occur in either the small or large bowel and have been recorded also in affected segments of small bowel that have been 'bypassed' surgically. About 3% of patients with Crohn's disease are affected by such intestinal cancer.

Extraintestinal Complications of Crohn's Disease

Patients with Crohn's disease may present with a variety of disorders outside the gastrointestinal tract. The sites most commonly affected are:

- **The eye.** Some 4% of patients experience inflammatory diseases such as conjunctivitis, episcleritis or, most seriously, inflammation of the uveal tissues.
- **The joints.** About 15% of patients suffer from either sacroileitis or a monoarticular arthritis. Ankylosing spondylitis is found in association with Crohn's disease in 2–6% of cases.
- **The liver.** Fatty change is found commonly in the liver of patients with Crohn's disease, as is an inflammatory reaction around the intrahepatic bile ducts. Fibrous obliteration of the small intrahepatic bile ducts (**sclerosing cholangitis**) is rare in Crohn's disease (less than 1%), but is found in 12% of sufferers from ulcerative colitis.
- **The skin. Erythema nodosum** occurs in 5–10% of patients with Crohn's disease. **Pyoderma**

gangrenosum, an ulcerating and necrotizing process associated with a brisk neutrophilic reaction but no obvious infection, occurs in about 1% of patients with Crohn's disease.

- **Renal and gallbladder calculi** are seen in about 30% of patients with Crohn's disease. **Reactive systemic amyloidosis**, with deposition of amyloid fibrils of the amyloid protein A type, also occurs but is an uncommon complication.

ULCERATIVE COLITIS

Ulcerative colitis is an inflammatory condition of unknown cause, affecting primarily the large intestinal mucosa. It starts in the rectum and spreads proximally in continuity to involve other parts of the colon (*Fig. 34.27*). **In some instances the entire colon may be involved, with some involvement of the terminal ileum ('backwash ileitis').** The appendix is involved in about half the cases.

The disease pursues a chronic course, often for more than 20 years, punctuated by episodes of relapse and remission.

Epidemiology

Ulcerative colitis is somewhat more common than Crohn's disease; its annual incidence in Europe and the USA is 8–11 per 100 000 population, with a prevalence of 80–120 per 100 000. As with Crohn's disease, Caucasians are more commonly affected than Afro-Americans, and Jews relatively more often than non-

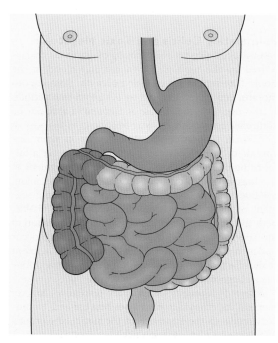

FIGURE 34.27 *Ulcerative colitis characteristically begins in the rectum and spreads proximally in continuity.*

Jews. Women are more often affected than men. Over the past 25 years the incidence of this disorder has remained static, with the exception of the Faroe islands where there has been a sixfold increase.

Aetiology and Pathogenesis

The aetiology and pathogenesis of this condition are still not known. It may conveniently be considered under the same rubrics as those used for Crohn's disease (see pp 541–542).

Possible Infective Agents

No infectious agent has been identified, although serum antibodies that bind both to colonic epithelial antigens and to some strains of *E. coli* are present in some cases.

Genetic Factors

Epidemiological data suggest that some genetic component exists. No markers have yet been identified. There is a strong positive association between HLA-B27 and ankylosing spondylitis and ulcerative colitis, but this association is almost certainly based on the presence of the former rather than the latter disease.

Additional Exogenous Factors

The only relevant factor is cigarette smoking, which has a negative association with the risk of ulcerative colitis.

Immune-mediated Mechanisms

Much effort has been expended in this field and, although many data relating to the immune response have been accrued, no clear answer has yet emerged.

1) There is evidence of **increased number of antibody-producing cells in affected areas of mucosa** and the appearance of these cells may antedate by several weeks the appearance of an inflammatory reaction. Unlike what occurs in Crohn's disease, most of these cells produce IgG, some of which binds to antigens on anaerobic gut bacteria.

2) **Type 1 hypersensitivity (atopy) appears to be increased in frequency in patients with ulcerative colitis.** IgE-producing cells can be identified in the mucosa in some cases, and there is evidence of an increased mucosal histamine content in some patients. These data appear to be most relevant in respect of infantile ulcerative colitis, where IgE-producing cells and eosinophils are prominent in the mucosa and where some clinical improvement may follow withdrawal of certain foodstuffs.

3) Antibodies have been demonstrated in the serum of patients with either ulcerative colitis or Crohn's disease which react with colonic epithelial mucins. These antibodies also cross-react with proliferating bile ductules in the liver, an interesting finding in view of the frequency with which sclerosing

cholangitis complicates ulcerative colitis (12% of cases).

4) **Circulating immune complexes** can be found in the serum of patients in both ulcerative colitis and Crohn's disease. The concentrations of these complexes correlate with the severity of the disease and with the presence of extraintestinal manifestations such as iritis, liver disease or arthritis.

5) Both in Crohn's disease and ulcerative colitis, **the inflamed mucosa contains a larger than normal population of T lymphocytes**. In addition mononuclear cells isolated from the blood of patients with active inflammatory bowel disease are cytotoxic for colonic epithelial cells in culture. These cytotoxic cells are lymphocytes which carry neither T- nor B-cell markers but do have Fc receptors. Their relationship to natural killer cells is not clear.

6) Recently an association has been reported between ulcerative colitis and the presence of an antibody directed against some component of the cytoplasm of neutrophils. In 70% of cases, sera from patients suffering from ulcerative colitis was found to bind to the perinuclear zone of the neutrophil cytoplasm. This antibody is said to be quite distinct from the antineutrophilic cytoplasmic antibody common in Wegener's granulomatosis (see pp 406–408) and is also seen in some patients with microscopic polyarteritis nodosa (see pp 405–406). Interestingly, the same antibody has been found in patients with sclerosing cholangitis.

Pathological Features

The main features of ulcerative colitis that serve to distinguish it from colonic involvement by Crohn's disease are:

1) its confinement to the large gut (with the exception of the 'backwash' ileitis)
2) the fact that it always involves the rectum and spreads proximally
3) the continuity with which the spread occurs, with none of the discontinuous 'skip' lesions so characteristic of Crohn's disease

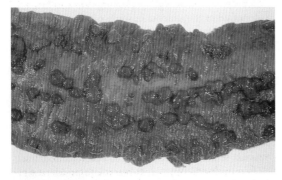

FIGURE 34.28 *Colon showing numerous small ulcers in a case of ulcerative colitis.*

4) its confinement to the mucosa in most instances, in marked contrast to the transmural pattern of involvement seen in Crohn's disease

Macroscopic Features

The affected mucosa is reddened and has a roughened, rather velvety, appearance. It is clearly more fragile than normal as it bleeds easily when touched with a swab or instrument. Later, small superficial ulcers appear (*Fig. 34.28*) and these may coalesce to form large irregular ulcerated areas. The non-ulcerated surviving mucosa is swollen and oedematous. Occasionally the ulcers extend as 'tunnels' under the adjacent mucosa and in this way relatively large areas of mucosa may strip away from the underlying bowel wall.

A polypoid appearance of the mucosal surface is quite common. The polyps are not neoplastic and consist of islands of inflamed and swollen mucosa standing proud of the adjacent ulcerated surface. These inflammatory polyps assume bizarre shapes and can be very numerous. They are seen more commonly in the colon than in the rectum.

In surgically resected material where colectomy has been performed either because of continuing disease activity or because of the detection of dysplasia, the serosa is seen to be normal and the bowel is shortened. This shortening is always greatest in relation to the rectum and distal colon, and is not caused by fibrous scarring, which is usually, either inconspicuous or entirely lacking.

Fulminating Colitis and Toxic Megacolon

Most patients present complaining of diarrhoea characterized by the presence of mucus and blood in the stools. The attacks are variable in length, from days to months, and are punctuated by symptom-free periods. In the majority, the disease is fairly mild and can be controlled adequately by drug treatment.

A small proportion (5–10%), either in their first episode or in the course of a relapse, experience a fulminating diarrhoeal illness during which a segment of the large bowel, most frequently the transverse colon, becomes acutely dilated. The wall of this dilated segment of bowel is markedly thinned and very friable, with the texture of 'wet blotting paper'. Perforation of the affected bowel with peritoneal soiling may occur under these circumstances. Peristaltic activity is absent in the affected segment; water and electrolytes accumulate in large amounts within the lumen.

Affected segments show very extensive loss of mucosa; the stripping off of both mucosa and submucosa results in the exposure of the muscularis propria which can be seen easily on naked-eye examination. A plain radiograph of the abdomen shows a dilated thin-walled colon with a diameter greater than 5 cm in which the surviving mucosal islands can be very clearly seen, projecting into the gas and fluid-filled lumen. The presence of such mucosal islands correlates with a high risk of perforation and is regarded by some as an indication for emergency colectomy. If perforation does occur, the mortality rate is high.

Microscopic Features

Inflammatory Changes

In actively inflamed mucosa, there is a marked degree of hyperaemia with dilatation of the thin-walled vessels in the mucosa. The lamina propria shows an inflammatory infiltrate in which plasma cells, eosinophils and neutrophils are prominent. Neutrophils also appear in the lumina of the crypts of Lieberkühn and destroy part or all of the crypt wall; the exudate within the crypt becomes co-terminous with that in the lamina propria (*Figs 34.29* and *34.30*). This process is probably the major factor in stripping of mucosa away from the underlying surface. These lesions are known as **crypt abscesses** and are characteristic, although not pathognomonic, for ulcerative colitis because they may also occur in infective colitis, acute appendicitis and Crohn's disease.

The mucosal surface shows the presence of pus and there is loss of surface epithelium, varying in severity from case to case.

Loss of Crypt Goblet Cells

Active inflammation is paralleled by loss of much of the goblet cell population lining the surviving crypts; the goblet cells are replaced by simple cuboidal epithelium. Resolution of the inflammatory process is characterized by restoration of the goblet cell population and, indeed, there may be epithelial hyperplasia at the crypt bases during this phase.

Regeneration and Mucosal Atrophy

In the course of resolution, restoration of crypts that have been damaged or lost is associated with the appearance of new crypts, which may show branching or other irregularities. If the mucosal loss has been severe, the new tubules will grow down towards the muscularis mucosae for only a relatively short distance, and a permanent gap will exist between the bases of these new crypts and the muscularis mucosae. In uninflamed mucosa this is a useful sign of previous damage and consequent mucosal atrophy. The muscularis mucosae itself in these instances is often thickened and shows splaying out of its fibres. The presence of **Paneth cell metaplasia in the crypts** and of endocrine cell hyperplasia or of adipose tissue in the mucosa are all signs of long-standing disease.

Dysplasia and Malignancy in Ulcerative Colitis

There is general agreement that long-standing and extensive ulcerative colitis carries with it an increased

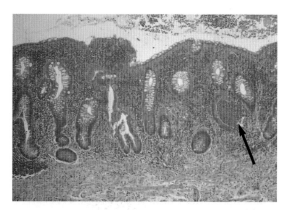

FIGURE 34.29 Ulcerative colitis showing severe inflammation in the lamina propria and crypt abscess formation (arrow).

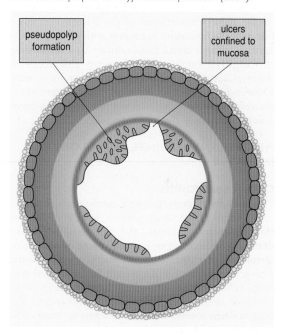

FIGURE 34.30 Unlike what is seen in Crohn's disease, the inflammation in ulcerative colitis is confined to the mucosa.

risk for carcinoma of the large bowel. Some differences exist, however, as to the magnitude of this risk. A multicentre cohort study (1988) suggested a colorectal cancer risk of 7.2% after 20 years of disease in patients with total or extensive colitis. After 30 years, this rises to 16.5%. An earlier study (1977) suggested that after 10–20 years the risk of cancer developing in patients with extensive disease is 23 times as great as that expected in the general population.

Cancers arising in patients who have had ulcerative colitis are often **multiple, flat and diffusely infiltrative**. These tumours are most likely to arise in patients in whom colonoscopy has shown the presence of **dysplasia**. This might be interpreted as indicating that patients with extensive and long-standing disease should undergo regular colonoscopy to evaluate the colorectal mucosa for epithelial dysplasia. However, histological recognition of premalignant mucosal changes in patients with ulcerative colitis is not always easy. If cytological or glandular atypia is accompanied by active inflammation, it is unwise to label these changes as being premalignant. The main cytological features suggesting dysplasia are:

1) nuclear pleomorphism
2) an increase in the nuclear : cytoplasmic ratio
3) increased mitotic activity
4) loss of normal nuclear polarity

Extra-intestinal Manifestations in Ulcerative Colitis

Ulcerative colitis shows the same spectrum of changes in organs and tissues outwith the gut as does Crohn's disease. However, **cirrhosis of the liver** occurs more than twice as frequently in patients with ulcerative colitis than in those with Crohn's disease, and **sclerosing cholangitis** is found in 12% of patients with ulcerative colitis as compared with less than 1% of those with Crohn's disease. An association between ulcerative colitis and ankylosing spondylitis is well recognized; these patients often show the haplotype HLA-B27.

MISCELLANEOUS INFLAMMATORY DISEASES

Collagenous Colitis

This term describes the principal histological abnormality in some middle-aged women who complain of chronic watery diarrhoea. **An abnormally thick, dense layer of collagen is present just beneath the basement membrane of the surface epithelium.** This is most obvious in the rectum and in the left side of the colon, and may be patchily distributed. A mild to moderate non-specific inflammatory infiltrate in the mucosa often accompanies the collagenous band. The cause is unknown and collagenous colitis may well represent an abnormal reaction to various mucosal insults.

Colitis in Graft Versus Host Disease

Patients who have had allogeneic bone marrow transplants not infrequently develop colonic inflammation. This may be due to one or a combination of a number of factors, including pretransplant chemotherapy, radiation and opportunistic infections, and the **graft versus host reaction** itself.

The latter causes focal apoptosis in crypt epithelium which may be associated with crypt abscess formation and some atypia of the nuclei of the lining epithelium. Ultimately the major portion of the epithelial cell population of the affected crypts may be lost, although neuroendocrine cells at the crypt base tend to survive.

Radiation Colitis

Radiation damage to the large gut is most likely to occur in cases of carcinoma of the uterine cervix treated with radiotherapy. Acute damage is accompanied by diarrhoea, colicky abdominal pain and tenesmus. Histological examination of rectal or colonic biopsies at this stage shows a picture characterized by:

- loss of surface epithelium and damage to the crypt epithelium
- infiltration of the lamina propria and crypt epithelium by eosinophils

Not infrequently, patients treated by pelvic radiotherapy may manifest colonic symptoms months or years later. Chronic radiation damage is characterized by:

1) scarring within the affected segments of gut wall
2) connective tissue changes including:
- oedema
- homogenization of collagen fibres
- the presence of large, darkly staining, atypical fibroblasts
- vascular changes including fibrinoid necrosis of small vessels, endothelial cell swelling, subendothelial accumulations of lipid-laden macrophages and thrombosis

This combination of changes results in a scarred and ulcerated segment of large bowel, which may cause chronic obstruction.

Solitary Rectal Ulcer Syndrome (Mucosal Prolapse)

Solitary rectal ulcer syndrome is something of a misnomer; it would be more appropriately called the mucosal prolapse syndrome. The term is applied to a syndrome found most commonly in young adults complaining of rectal bleeding, pain and the passage of mucus in the stools. Sigmoidoscopy commonly but by no means always shows an ulcer on the anterior or anterolateral wall of the rectum.

Histological examination shows a highly characteristic appearance with evidence of some scarring in the lamina propria, and splitting and arborization of the muscularis mucosae with muscle fibres sweeping up into the mucosa. The crypts are hyperplastic and there is depletion of the mucin-secreting goblet cell population.

These changes are due to prolapse of the rectal mucosa, perhaps associated with faulty motility of the affected segment of bowel and resultant straining at stool. Identical histological changes may be seen in other situations where mucosal prolapse has occurred, such as in the tips of colostomies, at the apices of prolapsing haemorrhoids and in relation to complete prolapse of the rectum. In all these situations, ischaemia of the mucosa may be the common pathogenetic factor.

The Colon and Rectum

NORMAL ANATOMY

The large gut extends from the ileocaecal valve to the rectum. It is about 1.5 metres long and is divided into six regions: caecum, ascending colon, transverse colon, descending colon, sigmoid colon, and rectum.

The caecum and transverse colon are completely surrounded by peritoneum, apart from their mesenteric attachments. The ascending and descending colon are invested by peritoneum only on their anterior aspects. The upper one-third of the rectum is covered by peritoneum on its anterior and lateral aspects; the middle third has a peritoneal covering on its anterior aspect only, and the lowest third of the rectum lies below the peritoneal reflection.

The Mucosa

The large bowel mucosa has no villi; the bulk of the epithelium is arranged in the form of **non-branching crypts** lying at right angles to the mucosal surface, roughly parallel to one another. Both surface epithelium and crypt lining are one cell thick, four principal cell types being present.

Microscopic Features

- **Mature columnar cells** which absorb water and electrolytes and also secrete glycocalyceal material and brush-border enzymes and transport immunoglobulin (Ig) A into the lumen. These are the major epithelial cell components, outnumbering goblet cells by 4–5 : 1.
- **Goblet cells**, mainly secreting acid mucins.
- **Endocrine cells**, located chiefly in the left side of the colon in the lowest part of the crypts. These cells contain small subnuclear granules and secrete a range of peptides including a vasoactive intestinal peptide-like product, somatostatin, 5-hydroxytryptamine and glucagon.
- **Undifferentiated stem cells** from which the other cell types originate. These are situated in the lowest portions of the crypts; daughter cells move up the crypts towards the mucosal surface, this taking 3–7 days.

The crypts are surrounded by the lamina propria, demarcated from the epithelium by a basement membrane and a thin collagenous plate about 7-μm thick. The lamina propria is well vascularized and contains IgA-secreting plasma cells, fibroblasts, mast cells, eosinophils, macrophages and non-myelinated nerve fibres.

Submucosa and Muscularis Propria

The colonic **submucosa** does not differ from that in other parts of the gut, but the muscularis propria is arranged in a markedly different pattern from that of the small intestine. The inner layer consists of circularly arranged fibres forming a continuous sheath, whereas the outer layer of longitudinally arranged fibres, although also a continuous layer, is concentrated into three linear bands: the **taeniae coli**. These muscle bands are slightly shorter than the length of colon that they invest, and the extra length of bowel is taken up by outpouchings known as haustra.

Blood Supply

The right side of the colon and half the transverse colon receive their blood supply from branches of the superior mesenteric artery; the left side of the colon and the rectum are supplied by the inferior mesenteric artery. **The 'watershed' between these two sources of perfusion is in the region of the splenic flexure and it is thus not surprising that this region is particularly at risk for developing ischaemic lesions of differing grades of severity.** The arterial branches are accompanied by veins, nerves and lymphatics. A well-formed plexus of veins is present in the submucosa and a rather less well-developed one in the serosa. Veins drain into the portal system and portal–systemic anastomoses are present where the superior rectal veins communicate with veins draining into the internal iliac and internal pudendal veins.

Lymphatic Drainage

Lymphatic channels drain either into nodes following blood vessels or into nodes lying close to the gut wall ('pararectal' nodes). Lymphatics draining the lowest part of the rectum feed mainly into the internal iliac nodes and to some extent into the inguinal nodes.

Nerve Supply

The colon and rectum are supplied by the two arms of the autonomic nervous system. Parasympathetic fibres are derived from the vagus and sacral spinal nerves, and their preganglionic fibres terminate in the myenteric (Auerbach's) plexus that lies between the two layers of the muscularis propria. The sympathetic supply is derived from lower thoracic and lumbar spinal nerves, the preganglionic fibres terminating in the superior and inferior mesenteric ganglia. The postganglionic sympathetic fibres terminate in either the myenteric plexus (Auerbach) or Meissner's plexus, which is situated in the submucosa. These two complexes form a network of communicating ganglia, each ganglion showing the presence of nerve cells, glia and nerve processes. The two complexes may have either an excitatory or inhibitory effect on the smooth muscle of the gut and **normal peristalsis depends on coordination of these**.

HIRSCHSPRUNG'S DISEASE (CONGENITAL MEGACOLON) AND RELATED DISORDERS

Definition

Megacolon is gross dilatation of the colon usually associated with a severe degree of constipation. Hirschsprung described such a situation, present **from birth** and due to defective migration of cells from the neural crest. This results in **absence of ganglion cells in the submucosal and myenteric plexuses, usually in the anorectal region**. This defective innervation leads to a failure of normal peristalsis in the affected segment and thus to the development of a **functional obstruction to the passage of faeces**. The cause of this failure of innervation is not known, but **congenital megacolon occurs ten times as commonly in infants with Down's syndrome as in non-Down's infants; 2% of infants suffering from Down's syndrome have congenital megacolon**.

Frequency and Genomic Abnormalities

Hirschsprung's disease affects about 1 in every 5000 individuals. An autosomally inherited gene mapping to chromosome 10 has recently been implicated in the genesis of this disorder. The genetic defect is a mutation in the proto-oncogene *ret* coding normally for a cell surface tyrosine kinase receptor. 'Knock out' of the tyrosine kinase domain of this gene in mouse embryos results in the birth of mice with absence of intestinal ganglia, similar to that seen in human Hirschsprung's disease.

Pathological Features

The gut lacking ganglion cells is narrowed, whereas gut proximal to this segment is **grossly dilated**, shows a considerable degree of **smooth muscle hypertrophy** owing to the increased workload, and contains **normal numbers of ganglion cells**. In most cases (82%) the aganglionic segment is short and does not extend above the junction of the descending and sigmoid colons. In 13%, the whole colon is involved.

Microscopic Features

Diagnosis is established by demonstrating the absence of ganglion cells in a transmural biopsy. In addition a marked degree of hypertrophy of nerve fibres is seen; these contain large amounts of cholinesterase, a finding absent in normal large gut. This is particularly useful because it obviates the need to take full-thickness biopsies. In cases where the aganglionic segment is being removed surgically, it is important to be sure that the lines of section contain normal numbers of ganglion cells; otherwise, functional obstruction will recur.

The disorder may make its presence known by the development of severe constipation any time from within days of birth to adult life. In some instances a diffuse enterocolitis may develop, and may present a serious threat to life.

There are patients who present with a clinical and radiological picture identical to that in Hirschsprung's disease but in whom normal numbers of ganglion cells are seen on transmural biopsy. Two such syndromes have been described:

1) **Neuronal intestinal dysplasia**, characterized by abnormalities of the parasympathetic innervation affecting the large gut in a localized or diffuse pattern. These abnormalities include:
- hyperplasia of nerve fibres in the myenteric plexus
- an increase in acetylcholinesterase activity
- the formation of giant ganglion cells

2) **Adynamic bowel syndrome**, which shows deficiencies in some of the cholinergic fibres.

Ganglioneuromatosis

In some patients suffering from the multiple endocrine neoplasia syndrome type IIb, characterized by the presence of **medullary carcinoma of the thyroid and phaeochromocytoma**, multiple ganglioneuromata (consisting of nodular masses of nerve fibres and large numbers of ganglion cells) of the intestinal nerve plexuses occur; this is associated with severe chronic constipation in childhood.

Acquired Megacolon

Disorders of large gut motility associated with colonic or rectal dilatation are not always congenital and may have many causes including:
- **obstruction** as a result of intraluminal neoplasm or stricture, which may be postinflammatory or due to a connective tissue response to malignant neoplasms
- **endocrine disorders** such as hypothyroidism
- **destruction of ganglion cells** in the gut wall, as may occasionally be seen in Chagas' disease caused by infection with *Trypanosoma cruzi*, which is common in parts of South America, most notably Brazil
- certain **central nervous system disorders** such as Parkinson's disease and various paraplegic disorders
- **drugs** that may have a toxic effect on gut innervation
- certain **psychogenic disorders**

DIVERTICULAR DISEASE

Diverticular disease is the term used to cover two pathological situations:

1) **diverticulosis** – the presence of colonic diverticula **(outpouchings of mucosa which extend through the muscular part of the gut wall to reach the serosal tissues)**

2) **diverticulitis** – the condition in which one or more diverticula are inflamed

The diverticula are 'pulsion' diverticula ('pushed out' rather than 'pulled out', as is the case with traction diverticula).

Diverticulosis

This affects the sigmoid colon predominantly; the rectum is never involved. It increases in prevalence with advancing age: about two-thirds of individuals in Western communities who reach the age of 80 years are affected.

Striking geographical variations in prevalence exist; the lesion is rare where the diet is predominantly vegetarian and high in fibre (e.g. rural Africa). High-fibre diets cause bulky stools, the reverse being true for low-fibre diets. Low-fibre diets are associated with an **exaggeration of normal peristalsis**, leading in time to muscle hypertrophy associated with some degree of bowel shortening. The latter may be due to deposition of elastin between the smooth muscle cells of the thickened taeniae coli. There is no hard evidence of either increased intraluminal pressure within the colon (although zones of high pressure may exist locally) or prolonged spasm of colonic muscle, two theories that have been canvassed extensively.

Macroscopic Features

The muscle changes are associated with a peculiar concertina-like or corrugated appearance of the mucosal aspect of the affected colon. The diverticula themselves can be seen as rounded sacs at the apex of the sacculations formed by the corrugated circular muscle. They protrude through potential defects in the circular muscle coat (*Fig. 34.31*) which exist at the points where the blood vessels that supply the colonic wall pass through the muscle, lying in rows between the mesenteric taenia and the two antimesenteric taeniae.

The diverticula are situated within either the serosa or pericolic adipose tissue, and may be surrounded by a thin layer of longitudinal muscle fibres.

Diverticulitis

Whereas diverticulosis is a common finding at postmortem examination in the elderly, only a small proportion of affected individuals develop symptoms related to the lesions. **These occur as a result of inflammation within one or more diverticula (diverticulitis).**

The inflammation results initially from erosion of the mucosal lining of the diverticula by dry, hard, faecal material. Faecal material in the sigmoid colon has a low fluid content and, once within the diverticulum, can be discharged only with difficulty through the narrow neck of the diverticulum back into the colonic lumen. Mucosal erosion provides a channel through which infected material from the colon may reach the peri-

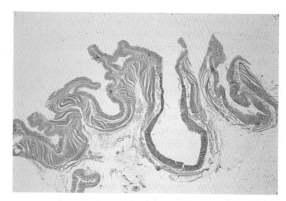

FIGURE 34.31 *Small pulsion diverticulum in the large gut.*

colic tissues, and an acute inflammatory process that may be associated with suppuration and abscess formation can result. Patients complain of lower left-sided abdominal pain, tenderness in the left lower quadrant, fever and, possibly, signs of peritoneal irritation.

The pattern of clinical disease is characteristically intermittent with episodes of remission and exacerbation. The repeated inflammatory episodes lead to oedema and scarring of the pericolic tissue. This, together with the grossly thickened muscle, may form a firm mass, which may be mistaken for a neoplasm at laparotomy.

Once diverticulitis has supervened, the microscopic appearances are those of small abscesses present in the pericolic tissues. The presence of foreign body-type giant cells and easily recognized fragments of vegetable material provide evidence of the entry of colonic contents through the diverticulum into the pericolic adipose tissue.

Rare complications include:

- perforation
- haemorrhage
- fistula formation, fistulous tracks between the colon and bladder being the commonest
- low colonic obstruction

VASCULAR DISORDERS OF THE LARGE GUT

Ischaemia

As in other organs and tissues (see pp 218–222), underperfusion of sufficient severity to cause structural damage results from the interaction of:

- **defective perfusion drive**, such as is seen in patients with episodes of severe hypotension as may occur in cardiogenic shock or hypovolaemia
- **stenosis or occlusion of large supplying vessels** associated with atherosclerosis, thrombosis or embolism
- **spasm in arteries** supplying one or other region of

the gut, the risk of which appears to be increased in patients who have been digitalized

- disorders, often mediated by immune mechanisms, that affect small intramural blood vessels (**vasculitides**) (see pp 402–410)

The ischaemic damage may be aggravated when reperfusion occurs. Such reperfusion injury is mediated, at least in part, by the generation of cytotoxic free radicals.

The morphological correlates of colonic underperfusion do not differ significantly from those described in the small gut, being expressed as:

- **full-thickness (gangrenous) necrosis**
- **ischaemic enterocolitis.** If the changes are confined to the mucosa, complete resolution may occur. More commonly, fairly large areas of ulceration may be seen and scar tissue will form in these areas
- **ischaemic stricture**, which occurs as the result of fibrous tissue repair of necrotic segments. This particularly likely to occur in the splenic flexure

Necrotizing Enterocolitis in the Neonatal Period

This is a rare, often fatal, form of ischaemic bowel disease affecting premature infants. The clinical picture is that of abdominal distension, bloody diarrhoea and vomiting. Both small and large bowel may be affected. Patchy necrosis of mucosa and submucosa is present and full-thickness necrosis with perforation may be seen in some cases. Submucosal gas-filled cysts, termed 'pneumatosis intestinalis', are quite common. The pathogenesis is not well understood.

Vascular Anomalies Associated with Haemorrhage

Several blood vessel abnormalities associated with abnormal dilatation and a high risk of gastrointestinal bleeding have been described. Most of these are rare, with the exception of **angioectasia (angiodysplasia)** and **cavernous haemangioma**.

Angioectasia (Angiodysplasia)

This disorder, of unknown aetiology and pathogenesis, chiefly affects elderly patients, who may present with severe iron-deficiency anaemia resulting from chronic blood loss or, more rarely, with acute massive colonic haemorrhage.

The lesion itself consists of groups of thin-walled, dilated blood vessels in the mucosa and submucosa, seen most commonly in the right side of the colon opposite the ileocaecal valve.

Diagnosis may be made by angiography or fibreoptic colonoscopy.

In some instances angioectasia may occur in association with one of a number of inherited syndromes. These include von Willebrand's disease, hereditary

haemorrhagic telangiectasia (Rendu–Osler–Weber syndrome), Turner's syndrome and a number of others.

Cavernous Haemangioma

This is a vascular hamartoma which tends to increase in size as the colon grows during childhood and adolescence. It is most often found in the rectum or sigmoid colon, and patients usually present complaining of rectal bleeding.

Macroscopic Features

The affected mucosa appears plum-coloured and, as a rule, no mass is obvious, although occasional polypoid haemangiomas may occur.

Microscopic Features

Many tortuous, dilated vessels, some of which contain thrombi of differing ages, may be seen.

MASS LESIONS: NEOPLASMS AND HAMARTOMAS

POLYPS

Definition

A polyp is a lesion, arising from the mucosal epithelium (adenomas and hyperplastic polyps) or from submucosal connective tissue, that protrudes into the gut lumen.

In pathogenetic terms polyps may be divided into two major groups: **non-neoplastic** and **neoplastic polyps**.

Non-neoplastic Polyps

Hyperplastic Polyps

Hyperplastic polyps occur only in the colon and appendix, where they are common (present in 30–50% of adults). They are small (up to 5 mm in diameter), pale, mucosal nodules which are usually sessile; they may be present in large numbers.

Microscopic Features

There is no increase in crypt **number**, but the lower one-third of the crypt, lined predominantly by goblet cells, may show some dilatation. The upper part shows an irregular 'saw-tooth' outline, the cell lining being made up of hyperplastic, mucin-secreting, columnar cells. The crypt basement membrane is often thickened and Paneth cell metaplasia is seen in some cases. The lesion is *not* premalignant but can occur in association with neoplastic adenomatous polyps.

Retention Polyps

These are the commonest colonic polyps in children; two-thirds of these polyps occur in childhood, the commonest presentation being rectal bleeding. In some instances the polyp may be sloughed off from the surface of the bowel wall and passed in the stool.

Macroscopic Features

The juvenile retention polyp is often single but multiple examples occur, most commonly in the sigmoid colon. The polyp surface is red and granular, and the cut surface characteristically shows the presence of numerous mucin-filled cavities.

Microscopic Features

The cavities are seen to be cystically dilated crypts, distended by mucus and separated from each other by inflamed and oedematous lamina propria. Retention polyps are probably hamartomatous in nature and do not undergo malignant transformation. Morphologically similar lesions may be seen occasionally in patients who have undergone ureterosigmoidostomy.

Rarely, retention polyps may be present in large numbers throughout the bowel. This condition is termed **multiple juvenile polyposis**; it may be associated with the development of adenocarcinoma anywhere in the large bowel or pancreas. Multiple retention polyps are seen also in the Cronkhite–Canada syndrome (see pp 527–528). As in the case of multiple juvenile polyposis, adenomatous polyp formation and adenocarcinoma may supervene.

Other Hamartomatous Polyps

- **Peutz–Jeghers syndrome** (see p 527)
- **Cowden's syndrome**, which is inherited in an autosomal dominant fashion: it is characterized by an association between hamartomatous colorectal polyps, and involves disorganization and proliferation of the muscularis mucosae are seen, tumours and tumour-like lesions of skin and mucosal surfaces, and an increased incidence of malignancy in various sites.

Neoplastic Polyps

Adenoma

An adenoma is a polypoid lesion representing a focus of intraepithelial neoplasia within the gut mucosa. It is monoclonal, arising from the stem cell compartment of a single crypt. Adenomas may be single or multiple. Some 40% are sited within the right side of the colon, 40% in the left and 20% in the rectum. In an adult post-mortem population, the prevalence is about 30%, frequency increasing with increasing age. Most uncomplicated adenomas are asymptomatic but they may ulcerate, causing the passage of blood in the stools.

Macroscopic Features

An adenoma, in its early stages, is often sessile but, with increasing growth, may become pedunculated with a knob-like lesion projecting into the bowel lumen from a submucosal stalk, lined on each side by normal mucosa (*Fig. 34.32*). Some adenomata remain sessile but with surface epithelium thrown into many complex finger-like folds, which gives the lesion a velvety macroscopic appearance (**villous adenomas**) (*Fig. 34.33*).

Microscopic Features

Adenomas consist of a rather crowded mass of branching epithelium-lined tubules which may appear well differentiated or show dysplasia of differing degrees of severity .

These lesions are known as **tubular adenomas**. About one-third show a papillary configuration, a feature that is commoner in lesions greater than 1 cm in diameter. If the papillary or villous component is roughly equal to the tubular component, the term **tubulovillous adenoma** is used.

The relatively uncommon **villous adenoma** is usually a single lesion in the sigmoid colon or rectum of older subjects; 90% are sessile. Some lesions may be associated with a marked fluid and electrolyte loss into the lumen with the development in some cases of muscle weakness due to potassium loss. All adenomas have malignant potential, but villous adenoma has a particularly high risk of carcinoma, the recorded incidence ranging from 30 to 70%.

Polyps and Colorectal Cancer

The relationship between adenoma and colorectal carcinoma is discussed in the following section, as are the series of genomic alterations believed to occur in the **sequential transformation of colonic epithelium from normal, through adenomas of increasing size and atypia to the fully malignant phenotype of invasive carcinoma.**

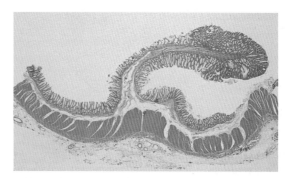

FIGURE 34.32 *Tubulovillous adenoma protruding from the colonic wall. Note that the stalk is lined by normal-looking mucosa.*

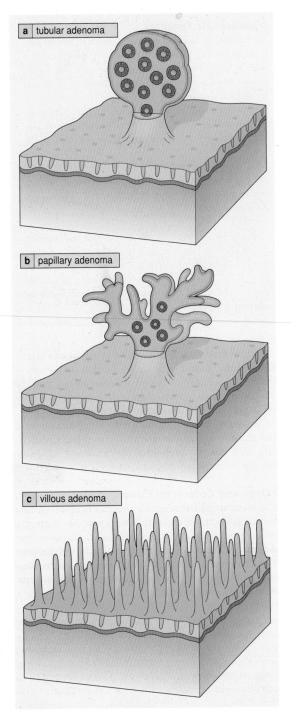

a | tubular adenoma

b | papillary adenoma

c | villous adenoma

FIGURE 34.33 Principal morphological variants of polyps.

COLORECTAL CARCINOMA

Colorectal cancer is one of the commonest neoplasms in the West. It causes 19 000 deaths annually in the UK and, if skin tumours are excluded, is the second most frequent malignant lesion in the USA.

Epidemiology

Environmental Factors

The prevalence of colorectal carcinoma shows considerable geographical variation. It is commonest in populations with high living standards (Europe, North America and Australia) and correspondingly rare in Africa, South America and Asia. This suggests that environmental factors are important in the aetiology, a view supported by the known positive correlation between risk and high levels of dietary consumption of meat, and the increasing incidence of colorectal cancer in previously low-risk populations whose lifestyle has become more affluent. **Meat consumption correlates with a high intake of saturated fatty acids and a correspondingly high output of bile acids in the faeces. In this connection, it is interesting that the use of agents such as clofibrate, which increases bile acid output, to decrease coronary heart disease risk is associated with an increased incidence of colorectal cancer.**

Any consideration of 'high-risk' diets in colorectal cancer should be concerned not only with high intakes of potentially risk-increasing foodstuffs, such as meat, but also with low intakes of potentially protective fibre-containing foods. The latter feature prominently in the diets of low-risk populations.

Genetic Factors

There is almost certainly an interaction between inherited and environmental factors. Indeed there are **well-defined inherited syndromes characterized by excess risk of colorectal cancer**. These may be divided into two classes: multiple familial polyposis syndromes and hereditary non-polyposis colorectal cancer (HNPCC).

Multiple Familial Polyposis Syndromes

These syndromes are inherited in an autosomal dominant fashion: if the aberrant gene is expressed, cancer is almost inevitable. These syndromes include, **familial adenomatous polyposis coli, Gardner's syndrome** and **Turcot's syndrome**; their molecular genetics are discussed below.

The hereditary polyposis-related colorectal cancers account for about 1% of all colonic cancers. Familial adenomatous polyposis coli (APC) itself is thought to occur in 1 in 8000–29 000 individuals and, of these, new mutations in germline cells make up between one-quarter and one-third of cases. **The defining criterion of the APC phenotype is the presence of 100 or more polyps in the large bowel** showing no structural difference from common sporadic polyps.

Polyps are not present at birth and may appear at any time from 4 to 70 years of age (mean 35 years). The average number of polyps is 100, although some individuals have as many as 5000. Two patterns of distribution are seen:

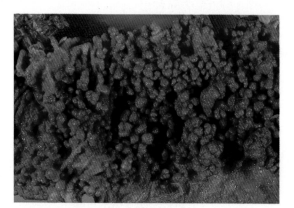

FIGURE 34.34 Large bowel from a patient with familial adenomatous polyposis coli. The mucosal surface is completely 'carpeted' with small polyps.

- a 'carpet'-like pattern with numerous tiny polyps covering large areas of mucosa (*Fig. 34.34*)
- the number of polyps is smaller but individual lesions are larger

Once multiple polyps are present, carcinoma is virtually **inevitable**, unless prophylactic colectomy is undertaken. Colorectal cancer in patients with APC presents at a mean age of 39 years and the average life expectancy of patients with APC who do not have prophylactic colectomy is 42 years.

After colorectal cancer, the most common cause of death in APC is carcinoma of the upper gastrointestinal tract. This may be because there is a high prevalence of polyps in the duodenum in APC (almost 90%), especially in the region of the ampulla of Vater. Hyperplastic gastric polyps occur in 30–50% of patients with APC, although true gastric adenomas are much rarer. Other extra-colonic neoplasms include:
- papillary carcinoma of the thyroid
- carcinoid tumours of the ileum
- a higher than expected number of brain tumours. The association of brain tumours with polyposis in some families has led to the view that Turcot's syndrome is a recessive form of APC

Hereditary Non-polyposis Colorectal Cancer

This is divided into two types:
1) an excess of cancer **affecting the colon and rectum only**. This is known as **Lynch syndrome I**.
2) an excess of cancer of the colon and rectum associated with an increased risk of cancers of the endometrium, ovary and pancreas. This is known as **Lynch syndrome II**.

In both, the excess in cancer of the large gut affects the proximal portion of the colon particularly, and the inheritance pattern is of the autosomal dominant type.

Molecular Genetics of Carcinoma of the Large Bowel

Evidence, some cited in the Key Points box below, strongly suggests that **most carcinomas of the colon and rectum arise from pre-existing benign tumours (adenomas)**.

KEY POINTS: Genetics of Colorectal Cancer

- The prevalence of adenomas is high in populations with a high risk of colonic carcinoma and low in those with a low cancer risk.
- The average age at which adenomas develop is lower than that for carcinoma.
- Small areas of cancer (less than 5 mm in diameter) are often found in adenomas, whereas it is extremely rare to find lesions of this size malignant *ab initio*.
- The risk of carcinoma developing is positively correlated with both the size and number of adenomas.
- Both adenomas and carcinomas are **monoclonal**, unlike normal colonic epithelium which is polyclonal. They often show similar types of genomic alteration and may represent **different stages in tumorigenesis** rather than being intrinsically different lesions.

Genomic events occurring in carcinogenesis of the large bowel consist of both **mutational activation of at least one proto-oncogene and mutational inactivation of more than one tumour suppressor gene**. Both changes provide affected stem cells with a selective growth advantage and thus the clone derived from it will expand and, ultimately, form the neoplasm.

Activation of the ras Oncogene

The only somatic proto-oncogene mutation that occurs commonly in colorectal neoplasms is mutation of the *ras* gene, the Ki-*ras* gene being affected in about 80% of these mutations. About 50% of all colorectal cancers show *ras* mutations, as do a similar proportion of adenomas of 1 cm or more in size. Mutations in Ki-*ras* can also be **detected in stool samples by extracting the DNA contained in about 100 mg of stool and using a polymerase chain reaction to amplify the relevant exons of the *ras* gene**. In small adenomas (1 cm or less in size) the prevalence of *ras* mutations is less than 10%. These data can be interpreted in at least two ways:
1) *ras* gene mutations may be the initiating event in some colorectal tumours and these may be more likely to progress and acquire a malignant phenotype than those without *ras* mutations.
2) *ras* gene mutations may not be the initiating event in colorectal neoplasia and may instead be a

later step responsible for the conversion of a small adenoma to a larger one more likely to progress to carcinoma.

Inactivation or Loss of Tumour Suppressor Genes

Colorectal cancers frequently show **loss** of certain specific chromosomal regions. These regions are the locations of tumour suppressor genes, the gene products of which normally act to restrain unbridled growth.

5q15–22

Familial APC is a syndrome in which two-thirds of the patients will have carcinoma by the age of 35 years (see pp 284, 554–555). Other inherited multiple polyp syndromes are Gardner's and Turcot's syndromes. Gardner's syndrome, also inherited in an autosomal dominant fashion, is associated with connective tissue lesions such as fibromatosis of the abdominal wall, osteomas of the skull and mandible, cysts in the skin, and many other extracolonic manifestations. Turcot's syndrome is inherited in an autosomal recessive pattern and here the adenomatous polyps, which are fewer in number than in the other two syndromes, are associated with malignant tumours of the central nervous system.

In both Gardner's and Turcot's syndromes the risk of carcinoma is of the same order as in familial APC, and they may represent variations on a single theme: adenomatous polyposis.

Linkage analysis has shown an association between APC and a region on the long arm of chromosome 5 (5q15–22). Deletions in this region are found both in Gardner's syndrome and APC, and the responsible gene, *APC*, was cloned in 1991. Allelic losses on the long arm of chromosome 5 have been recorded in 20–50% of colorectal cancers and in about 30% of adenomas. It is suggested that the *APC* gene is involved directly in the widespread epithelial hyperproliferation that comes before adenomatous polyps formation.

It is believed the *apc* gene product ensures that cell division is balanced by programmed cell death (**apoptosis**). This is particularly important in relation to epithelial cells which acquire mutations; most of such cells are removed by apoptosis. In colorectal cancer cells containing a defective *APC* gene, apoptosis can be induced by transfection of a normal 'wild type' *apc* gene into the cell line.

In mice which carry a defective *apc* gene, the number of adenomas which develop varies by up to ninefold depending on other genetic factors. For example, a gene on chromosome 4 at a locus originally designated *Mom1* accounts for about 50% of the variation in risk. It is believed that this gene encodes secretory phospholipase A2 (sPLA2) which is involved in the release of arachidonic acid (the substrate for prostaglandin production) from cell phospholipid.

The importance of lipid metabolism in relation to carcinogenesis in the colon and rectum is further emphasized by the discovery that disruption of the gene, *COX-2* encoding prostaglandin endoperoxide synthase-2) reduces the number of tumours occurring in mice with a defective *apc* gene by more than sixfold, and treatment of such mice with drugs selectively inhibiting *COX-2* also reduces tumour incidence.

In man, regular use of non-steroidal anti-inflammatory drugs reduces the risk of colorectal cancer, while the *COX-2* gene is expressed at high levels in 85% of colorectal cancers. Thus the degree of expression of *COX-2* may play a part in determining whether progression from adenoma to carcinoma takes place.

18q Deletions and the *DCC* Gene

The second commonest region of allelic loss in colorectal tumours is the long arm of chromosome 18. Loss of material in the q21–22 region is found in 70% of these carcinomas and in almost 50% of large (and presumably late) adenomas. A candidate tumour suppressor gene has been identified in this region and been given the name **DCC (deleted in colonic cancer)**. Deletion in 18q has prognostic implications, being associated with a marked decrease in the 5-year survival rate of patients with stage II (TNM) colorectal cancer.

The gene product of *DCC* is homologous to cell surface adhesion molecules such as neural cell adhesion molecule and contactin. Reduction of the expression of the *DCC* gene in colonic epithelial cells could lead to decreased adhesion, and thus to a decrease in the growth-restraining signals associated with normal cell–cell adhesion.

17p Deletions and the *p53* Gene in Colorectal Cancer

The loss of a portion of the short arm of chromosome 17 (17p) has been reported in more than 75% of colorectal carcinomas. This appears to be a relatively late event associated with the **progression from adenoma to carcinoma**, as it occurs in relatively few adenomas. 17p deletions occur also in a number of other very common adult neoplasms, such as those of the **breast, lung, ovary, bladder and brain**.

The site of loss of chromosomal material contains the ***p53* gene**. The normal or wild-type *p53* gene product functions as a suppressor of abnormal growth and promotes apoptosis of cells containing aberrant DNA. It is not necessary that the *p53* gene should be deleted: **the presence of a mutation in one of the *p53* alleles can affect cell growth even though the other *p53* allele is of the wild-type**. Thus, a mutated *p53* gene may act in a dominant negative fashion and not as a recessive gene would normally be expected to do. The subsequent loss of the remaining normal or wild-type allele amplifies the growth advantage conferred by the original mutation and is probably associated with the progression from adenoma to cancer.

Other Allelic Losses in Carcinoma of the Colon and Rectum

These genomic alterations are the commonest found in association with colorectal tumours, but many others have been described. Deletions have been recorded in relation to chromosomes 1q, 4p, 6p, 6q, 8p, 9q and 22q, and when losses from the chromosomes of individual tumours are considered it becomes clear that the median number of chromosomes showing deletions in any one tumour is 4–5. **Tumours in which the number of deletions is greater than median are associated with a worse prognosis, even though the size and clinical stage of these lesions does not differ materially from those in which a smaller number of deletions is present. Thus it seems probable that malignant transformation in colonic epithelium requires several genomic alterations for the full phenotypic expression of cancer and that it is the total number of events rather than any specific sequence of such events that is important.**

Genomic Instability and HNPCC

Two large kindreds with this syndrome have shown linkage to a region on the short arm of chromosome 2. One gene on chromosome 2 that is abnormal in HNPCC is known as *hMSH2*, the human homologue of a prokaryotic gene known to be involved in the **repair of DNA mismatches**. A variety of mutations in this gene has been detected in affected members of families with HNPCC. Two other genes also believed to be involved in DNA mismatch repair – *hMLH1* on chromosome 3 and *hPMS2* on chromosome 2 – have also been found to be mutated in the germ cell line of individuals with HNPCC.

Other Somatic Alterations of Functional Significance in Large Bowel Neoplasms

At an early stage of colorectal tumour development, a decrease in the number of methyl groups in the tumour cell DNA is seen. Loss of methyl groups from DNA contributes to genomic instability in both adenomas and carcinomas because it leads to inhibition of chromosome condensation and thus to possible mitotic non-disjunction. Similarly, most colonic carcinomas show an increased expression of the proto-oncogene c-*myc* but it is not clear whether this is implicated in tumour causation or results from the presence of such a tumour. Colorectal tumours also show loss of major histocompatibility antigens and it has been suggested that this loss of antigens, important in the presentation of antigens to the immune system, may confer a growth advantage on tumour cells, which may express specific tumour antigens but be shielded from antitumour lymphocyte attack by an inability to present the antigens.

Pathological Features

About 50% of carcinomas of the large gut occur in the rectum and rectosigmoid. The caecum and lower part of the ascending colon account for further 15% and the remainder are distributed more or less evenly in the transverse and descending colon.

The **macroscopic appearances**, the **mode of presentation** and, to a certain extent, the **prognosis** depend on the interplay of a number of factors:

- **whether the growth pattern is predominantly exophytic (i.e. protruding into the gut lumen) or endophytic (infiltrating deeply into the bowel wall)**
- **how much of the circumference of the bowel is involved**
- **the degree of fibrous tissue response to the presence of tumour**
- **the presence or absence of ulceration**
- **the amount of mucin production**

Macroscopic Features

1) **Protuberant masses with a polypoid surface usually involving only part of the circumference of the bowel wall.** These occur most commonly in the caecum and ascending colon. Because this part of the large gut has the greatest luminal diameter, obstruction is a late event and the lesions remain 'silent' for a long time. Chronic oozing of blood from the surface of the tumour and a resulting iron-deficiency anaemia are common. It is the weakness and easy fatiguability caused by this anaemia that are the predominant presenting symptoms. This highlights the importance of examining the stools of patients with iron-deficiency anaemia for the presence of 'occult' blood; indeed, there is a strong case for using this simple procedure as a regular screening method for the detection of early carcinoma of the colon in asymptomatic individuals in middle and old age.

2) **Plaque-like lesions that undergo ulceration, the ulcers having a rolled and everted edge** (*Fig. 34.35*). This is most commonly seen in the rectum and rectosigmoid region, and is often associated with the passage of fresh blood admixed with the stool.

3) **Lesions that infiltrate deeply and involve the whole of the circumference of the gut wall. If there is a marked fibrous tissue response to the presence of tumour cells, a 'napkin-ring'-like constriction is produced.** Such lesions may be associated with symptoms and signs of chronic obstruction, although if they occur proximally in the descending colon where the faeces are still liquid, evidence of obstruction may be lacking.

4) **Lesions in which large amounts of epithelial mucin have been secreted into the matrix surrounding the tumour cells are known as**

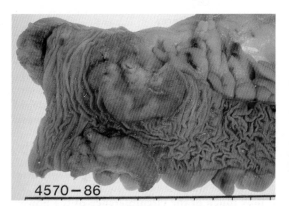

FIGURE 34.35 Ulcerated carcinoma of the sigmoid colon. Note the typical rolled and everted edges of the lesion.

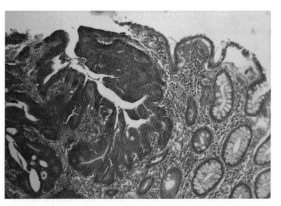

FIGURE 34.36 This section shows the junction between normal colonic mucosa on the right and invasive carcinoma on the left. The tumour shows grossly atypical glands lined by darkly staining epithelium.

colloid carcinomas. On naked-eye examination, these tumours have a gelatinous appearance. This is mirrored on histological examination when small groups of tumour cells may be seen apparently 'floating' in pools of mucin.

Microscopic Features

Most colorectal carcinomas are clearly adenocarcinomas showing a tubular pattern and some mucin secretion (*Fig. 34.36*). Mucin secretion dominates the histological picture in 10–15% of lesions. In some cases this is manifested in the form of glands, the lumina of which are filled with mucin; in others there are clumps of mucin-secreting cells with a 'signet-ring' appearance owing to the nucleus being compressed against the plasma membrane by accumulated intracellular mucin. These cells are themselves surrounded by large amounts of extracellular mucin. Tumours with an exclusively signet-ring cell population carry the worst prognosis of all the histological variants.

Grading and Prognosis of Colorectal Cancer

The degree of differentiation of colorectal carcinoma gives valuable prognostic information, as shown in *Table 34.9*.

Spread of Colorectal Cancer: Staging and Prognosis

Colorectal carcinoma may spread via a number of routes:

1) **By direct invasive growth through the wall of the gut.** Spread through the relatively open connective tissue network of the submucosa presents few problems, but the muscle layer does present a tough barrier to infiltrating cells and thus the usual path through the muscularis propria is **between** the muscle fibres rather than **through** them. Poorly differentiated tumours tend to spread distally within the submucosa and this has implications for the choice of surgical procedure because anterior resection may not succeed in clearing the distal margin of the tumour. **The extent of direct spread through the gut wall carries very significant prognostic implications** (*Fig. 34.37*). Lesions confined to the mucosa at the time of excision are unlikely to spread to lymph nodes. If the tumour has not penetrated the muscularis propria to reach the serosa and there are no deposits in lymph nodes (**Dukes stage A**), surgical excision

Table 34.9 Grading and Survival in Colorectal Cancer

Grade	Frequency (%)	5-year survival rate (%)
Well differentiated: well-formed tubules; nuclei uniform in size and appearance	20	80
Moderately differentiated: glands still recognizable although the outline is irregular and tumour cell nuclei show variation in size and staining	60	60
Poorly differentiated: gland formation scanty or absent	20	25

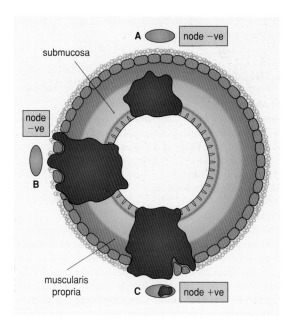

FIGURE 34.37 Staging of colorectal carcinoma with Dukes' system for assessing local invasion.

should be curative in almost all cases. Unfortunately only about 15% of operable cancers of the large bowel fall into this category. If the tumour has spread into the pericolic or perirectal soft tissues and there are no lymph node deposits, it is classified as a **Dukes stage B** lesion and these tumours (which account for 35% of operable cancers) have a 70% chance of cure.

2) **Via lymphatics.** The presence of lymph node deposits is found in about 50% of colorectal carcinomas, which are classified as **Dukes stage C**. This finding alters the prognosis considerably: the 5-year survival rate is reduced to 30–35%. The greater the number of tumour-containing nodes identified, the worse is the prognosis, presumably because this correlates with an increased chance of occult metastasis in sites such as the liver.

3) **Via blood vessels.** If large veins outside the colonic wall are invaded, the 5-year survival rate drops, although, interestingly, the presence of tumour cells in small veins **within** the bowel wall does not appear to affect the prognosis materially.

4) Once having penetrated the peritoneal covering (in parts of the large bowel where it is present), tumour cells may spread **through the peritoneal cavity** and, especially with poorly differentiated carcinomas, cause multiple deposits in the peritoneum.

The St Mark's Prognostic Classification
This is based on four variables:
1) **the number of lymph nodes containing**

tumour deposits (no involvement, 0; one to four nodes involved, 1; more then four nodes involved, 2)

2) **the character of the invasive margin** ('expanding', 0; 'infiltrative', 1).

3) **the presence or absence of a lymphocytic infiltrate** at the tumour margins (no infiltrate, 1; conspicuous infiltrate, 0)

4) **the degree of local spread, expressed in terms of only two categories:**
- **tumour confined within the bowel wall (0)**
- **tumour spread through the bowel wall** to reach the perirectal or pericolonic tissues (1)

Thus each case can be scored as being between 0 and 5: (see *Table 34.10*)

The survival values for these new prognostic groups are similar to those obtained with the Dukes staging system. However, this new prognostic classification places twice as many patients into groups, providing a confident prediction of clinical outcome, and may be of value in selecting patients (group IV) who might benefit most from adjuvant treatment aimed at eradicating occult metastases.

Table 34.10 The St Mark's Prognostic Classification

Group	Score	Survival rate (%)
I	0–1	91
II	2	67
III	3	42
IV	4–5	24

Tumour Markers and Colorectal Carcinoma
Colorectal cancers produce a variety of oncofetal antigens. The one most extensively studied is carcinoembryonic antigen (CEA). The serum concentrations of this epithelium-derived glycoprotein correlate positively with the size and extent of spread of colorectal carcinomas.

The presence of increased serum concentrations of CEA is not diagnostic of colonic carcinoma because such increases may be seen in association both with other neoplasms (cancer of the breast, ovary, lung, prostate and bladder) and with certain non-neoplastic disorders.

However, measurement of CEA concentrations can be useful in monitoring the progress of patients with colorectal carcinoma in the period that follows primary excision of the tumour. In a patient with raised preoperative levels of CEA, surgical removal should be followed by the disappearance of CEA from the patient's blood. If raised CEA concentrations reappear, this constitutes good evidence of recurrence and a surgical 'second look' may be indicated.

The Anus

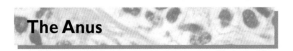

NORMAL ANATOMY

The anus is the segment of intestine connecting the perineal skin to the lower end of the rectum. It is 3–4 cm long and is demarcated by the proximal and distal margins of the internal sphincter.

The junction of the anal canal with the perineal skin is marked by the appearance of skin adnexal structures in the latter. From this junction the anal canal is lined for approximately half its length by squamous epithelium. Above this, it is lined by mucosa identical to that of the rectum. The junction between these two types of epithelial lining is marked by the anal valves, which collectively form what is known as the **pectinate line**. The anal valves form the inner boundary of small pits, the anal crypts. The latter are branching ducts that pass into the submucosa. They are important because they act as channels for infection to reach the perianal tissues.

Immediately above the pectinate line there is a narrow zone, about 0.3–1.0 cm in length, which is known as the transitional or cloacogenic zone. It represents the junction point between the endodermally derived rectal type mucosa and the ectodermally derived squamous epithelium of the lower portion of the anal canal. The epithelial lining here resembles to some extent the urothelial lining of the bladder.

CONGENITAL DISORDERS

The only relatively common congenital abnormalities affecting the anus are atresia or stenosis. About 1 in 5000 liveborn children are affected by one or other. Atresia is by far the commoner of the two, outnumbering stenosis by 9 to 1.

Most cases of atresia are characterized by a large gap between the blind end of the rectum and the perineal skin. In some instances the anus is represented by a small dimple in the perineum, in others (about 10%) the anal canal is normally developed but ends well short of the rectal stump. Atresias in which the rectal stump ends above the puborectalis component of the levator ani muscle (40% of cases) have a serious prognosis because they are associated with:

- a severe degree of obstruction
- other congenital abnormalities affecting the vertebrae and lower urinary tract
- defective innervation of pelvic floor muscles.

In these proximal atresias a fistula connecting the rectum to the urinary bladder, urethra or vagina is not infrequently seen.

In cases of atresia in which the anomaly is more distal, obstruction is rarely severe, and pelvic muscle innervation is normal. Quite simple surgery is usually curative in these children.

INFLAMMATORY DISORDERS

Fissure

Anal fissure is a primarily mucosal lesion, commonest on the posterior aspect of the lower anal canal. It is usually triangular in shape and causes severe pain associated with defecation. Its pathogenesis is not clear. Histological examination shows features of chronic non-specific inflammation.

Fistula

The defining criterion of an anal fistula is the presence of an abnormal track opening into the anal canal usually at the level of the pectinate line. The track may pursue a course through the perianal tissues and open on the skin surface, or it may end blindly within perianal soft tissues. Several anatomical variants of anal fistula have been described, but these are beyond the scope of this text.

All begin with sepsis in the anal crypts and their underlying ducts. The anatomical varieties are a reflection of the patterns of branching of the ducts. It has been suggested that the chronicity of inflammation, which such a marked feature of this condition, is due to the persistence of epithelium within the tracks, this being said to interfere with closure of these structures in the course of healing.

> ### Microscopic Features
> In most cases there is a mixed acute and chronic inflammatory cell infiltrate.
>
> Multinucleated, macrophage-derived giant cells are present in many cases. They have the haphazard arrangement of nuclei characteristic of so-called 'foreign body' giant cells, and are, presumably, elicited by the presence of faecal material. Care should be taken not to misinterpret the presence of these giant cells as indicating a specific granulomatous process such as Crohn's disease or tuberculosis. These disorders should not be diagnosed in the absence of aggregates of activated macrophages (epithelioid cells).
>
> In some cases, a reaction to fat droplets is present, indicating that the latter are exogenous in origin. This is probably due to the use of Vaseline-impregnated gauze or liquid paraffin, which is sometimes used to soften stools.

SOME SPECIFIC INFLAMMATORY CONDITIONS

Crohn's Disease

The anus is affected in 25% of cases of Crohn's disease involving the small gut and in 75% of those in which the large intestine is the seat of the lesions. In the anal region, Crohn's disease may manifest as:

- chronic anal fissure
- anal fistula
- perianal oedema associated with a dusky-blue discolouration

The clinical diagnosis can be confirmed by the identification of sarcoid-like granulomatous lesions in anal and perianal biopsies. It must be remembered, however, that only about 60% of cases show the presence of typical granulomas and, thus, false-negative reports will inevitably occur. It is not possible on histological grounds alone to make an absolute distinction between Crohn's disease of the anal region, sarcoid and tuberculosis. The presence of caseation, if obvious, favours a diagnosis of tuberculosis but this feature may not be present, and examination of sections stained to show acid-fast bacilli often yields false-negative results. Culture of a portion of the specimen removed is necessary in many cases of tuberculosis.

Anorectal tuberculosis is very uncommon in the West but, in countries where the prevalence of tuberculosis is still high, anorectal manifestations of the disease are far from rare. In patients who have active pulmonary tuberculosis, anal ulcers may be seen in which mycobacteria can usually be demonstrated. Other patients may present with a past history of tuberculosis but no currently active systemic disease and yet still have tuberculous fissures or fistulae. In these individuals, histological diagnosis and, in particular, the distinction between tuberculosis and Crohn's disease can be very difficult, but is obviously important from the point of view of instituting appropriate treatment.

Sexually Transmitted Disorders Affecting the Anus

Anal intercourse is associated with a number of local infections including:

- syphilis
- herpes simplex infections
- lymphogranuloma venereum due to infection by *Chlamydia*
- granuloma inguinale caused by *Calymmatobacterium granulomatis*
- chancroid caused by *Haemophilus ducreyi*

The pathological features of these conditions is discussed in the section dealing with the penis and scrotum on pp 737–739.

Pilonidal Sinus

The defining event in the pathogenesis of pilonidal sinus is the penetration of the skin of the natal cleft by hair shafts. Outside their normal microenvironment, hair shafts are recognized as 'foreign' and elicit a striking chronic inflammatory reaction associated with multinucleated 'foreign body' giant cells.

The lesion associated with these events is a sinus track that opens on to the skin of the natal cleft and penetrates down into the subcutaneous tissues. It may have a complex branching pattern, which makes complete excision difficult in some instances. Microscopic examination shows the presence of sinus tracks lined partly by squamous epithelium and partly by inflamed granulation tissue. Hair shafts that are intensely birefringent when examined in polarized light are usually, but not always, seen within the inflammatory infiltrate.

Similar lesions may occur in other areas such as the axilla, umbilicus and the webs between the fingers of barbers, the pathogenesis presumably being the same as in pilonidal sinus.

Pilonidal sinus is much more common in males than in females, and hirsutism and obesity appear to be significant incremental risk factors.

Haemorrhoids

At the anorectal junction in the left lateral, right anterior and right posterior aspects of the canal are structures known as **vascular cushions**. These are complexes consisting of arterioles, arteriovenous communications and venules. Haemorrhoids or 'piles' are believed to represent prolapses of one or more of these cushions. Such prolapse is thought to be associated with straining at stool.

Prolapse of vascular cushions interferes with their venous drainage, and the increased hydrostatic pressure resulting from this causes further engorgement and enlargement of the haemorrhoids. The most frequent complication of this engorgement is bleeding. This is rarely massive in amount but may be chronic or repetitive and cause iron deficiency anaemia. Thrombosis within the dilated vessels of the haemorrhoids or even strangulation may occur.

Microscopic examination shows the presence of dilated vessels with a rather thick muscle layer. Evidence of current or past thrombosis may be present and the overlying epithelium is somewhat thicker than normal.

ANAL TUMOURS AND TUMOUR-LIKE LESIONS

It is important to distinguish between neoplasms in the anal canal and those at the anal margin. The latter are tumours of skin and their natural history is characteristic of such tumours.

Human Papillomavirus and Anal Neoplasia

As is the case with surface epithelia in other anatomical situations, most notably the penile and vulvar skin and the epithelium of the cervix uteri, there is a spectrum of change in anal epithelium which appears to be caused by sexually transmitted infections with certain strains of human papillomavirus (HPV).

Such infections may be associated with the appearance of exophytic, papillary lesions starting with the, alas only too familiar, viral warts (**condylomata acuminata**), passing through the giant condyloma (Buschke–Lowenstein tumour), which appears histologically benign and does not metastasize but can erode deeply into the underlying tissues, and then to the verrucous carcinoma, which some regard as being synonymous with the Buschke–Lowenstein lesion. In other instances, a series of intraepithelial changes of differing degrees of severity occurs, in the absence of the formation of papillary lesions, known as intraepithelial neoplasia. The more severe grades of intraepithelial neoplasia are associated with a significant increase in the risk of frankly invasive carcinoma.

These entities are discussed in some detail in Chapters 38 and 39 and will not be pursued further here.

Perianal Paget's Disease

Paget's disease is rare, and is found most often in the elderly. It presents as a perianal, red, scaly area. Examination of biopsy material shows appearances identical with those seen in Paget's disease of the nipple. The epidermis is infiltrated by large vacuolated cells, believed to originate within apocrine ducts. The vacuoles can be shown to contain mucin in appropriately stained sections. Extramammary Paget's disease of this type is thought to represent extension from low-grade adenocarcinoma of the apocrine gland ducts. There is often a very long preinvasive phase and identification of the underlying tumour is not always easy. Rarely, the perianal skin may be infiltrated by cells from the, very uncommon, primary adenocarcinoma of the anal canal.

Anal Carcinoma

By far the commonest malignant neoplasms involving the anal canal or perianal skin are squamous carcinomas. Anal carcinoma is fortunately rare in the UK. There is persuasive evidence of an increased risk of anal carcinoma in passive male homosexuals, this resumably being associated with the increased risk of HPV infection: evidence of type 16 HPV infection has been found in a number of anal tumours. Apart from this risk factor, anal carcinoma tends to occur more frequently in areas where there is extreme poverty and associated poor standards of hygiene. Carcinoma of the anal canal tends to occur more frequently in females than in males, but perianal carcinoma shows a fairly strong predilection for males.

Clinical Features

The common clinical presentations are shown in *Table 34.11.*

Table 34.11   Clinical Presentations of Anal Carcinoma

Clinical presentation	Frequency (%)
Rectal bleeding	50
Pain	40
Local mass	25
Pruritus	15
Asymptomatic	25

Carcinoma occurring in the anal canal is three times as common as in the perianal skin; many of these tumours arise just proximal to the pectinate line. Tumours occurring in this site tend to spread proximally into the rectum or laterally into the perianal tissues, rather than distally into the lower part of the anal canal.

Pathological Features

Microscopic Features

Anal canal carcinomas are squamous cell tumours, although there is considerable variation in their degree of differentiation. About 20% of the tumours show the presence of solid nests of rather small cells. These nests of tumour cells have a palisaded arrangement at their margins reminiscent of basal cell carcinoma of the skin and the well-demarcated keratin plugs seen in basal cell carcinoma may also be present. This **basaloid** variant, which has sometimes been termed a **cloacogenic carcinoma**, is believed to arise from the transitional epithelial zone just above the pectinate line. Its behaviour does not differ significantly from that of other histological variants of anal canal carcinoma and, indeed, the determining histological factor in prognosis, apart from the degree of spread, is **grade** rather than histological subtype.

Spread

Tumours in the anal canal tend to invade lymphatics draining into the superior haemorrhoidal lymph nodes (these nodes are involved in more than 40% of the cases of anal canal carcinoma coming to surgery at St Mark's Hospital) and also to nodes on the lateral walls of the pelvic cavity. Involvement of the inguinal nodes occurs in a significant number of cases but seems to be a later event than haemorrhoidal node spread.

Carcinoma of the anal margin tends to spread principally to inguinal nodes.

CHAPTER 35

The Liver, Biliary System and Exocrine Pancreas

Disorders of the Liver

NORMAL STRUCTURE AND FUNCTION

The liver consists of **three principal, functional, anatomical compartments**. These constitute a convenient framework for considering liver disease and are:

1) The **parenchyma**, consisting predominantly of specialized liver cells (hepatocytes). Most parenchymal disorders are due to conditions in which there is **loss of hepatocytes** and, thus, a decrease in the liver cell mass. In other parenchymal diseases, there is a **decline in liver cell function** rather than in **number**, either because of cell injury or some inborn defect.

2) The **vasculature**. Hepatic vascular abnormalities are expressed chiefly as **disturbances of flow** leading, on the one hand, to abnormally high pressures in the portal system (**portal hypertension**) and, on the other, to failure of blood to be exposed to the metabolic and detoxifying actions of the hepatocytes (**shunting**).

3) The **biliary drainage system**. Abnormalities affecting this compartment lead to **bile stasis** and a consequent increase in the concentration of bile constituents in the blood. The chief clinical expressions are **jaundice** (due to an increase in bile pigments) and **itch** (due to an increased blood concentration of bile salts).

Most of the groups of diseases discussed in this chapter affect, principally, one or other of these compartments. In some cases, most notably in cirrhosis, abnormalities of structure and function may involve more than one.

Normal Microanatomy of the Parenchyma

The **basic functional unit of the liver is the acinus.** This can be defined as **that part of the liver cell mass dependent for perfusion on blood derived from the vessels in a single terminal portal tract**. The portal vein and hepatic artery branches in such a portal tract divide into sinusoids which supply blood to the hepatocytes and then drain into terminal hepatic venules (central veins) that receive blood from more than one acinus.

Each acinus is divided into three zones on the basis of distance from its terminal portal tract (*Fig. 35.1*). Those that are nearest are said to be in zone 1, those that are furthest away are in zone 3, and those that are intermediate in position are in zone 2. Zone 1 liver cells express the greatest degree of metabolic activity, probably because the blood they receive has the highest concentration of oxygen, amino acids, insulin and glucagon. This zonal arrangement accounts for the fact that anoxia, for example, affects the cells of zone 3 more severely than those of zone 1.

The distribution of functions within the acinus is not entirely dependent on the proximity of the liver cells to the blood vessels in the portal tract. For example, mixed-function oxidases are found predominantly in zone 3 (the perivenular part of the acinus) and this remains so even if the direction of perfusion of the liver is reversed.

The liver cells radiate from the portal tracts towards the terminal hepatic venules. They are arranged in columns **one cell thick**, a sinusoid being present between each of these columns (liver cell plates). The liver cell plates are two cells thick in babies and small children but by the age of 5 years the normal one-cell-thick pattern is established.

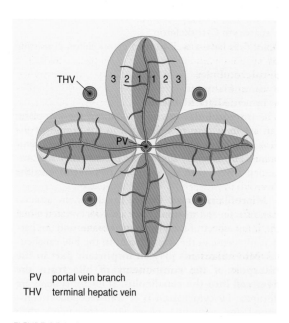

PV   portal vein branch
THV   terminal hepatic vein

FIGURE 35.1 Acinar structure of the liver. Zone 1, which is closest to the portal veins, receives the most oxygen and nutrients, whereas zone 3 receives the least.

The portal tract itself is surrounded by a concentric layer of liver cells which is not continuous, being breached by the sinusoids. This portal tract–hepatic parenchyma interface is known as the **'limiting plate'** and, in many instances, is a target for chronic liver cell damage.

The Liver Cell

The liver cell (hepatocyte) is large, its longest axis measuring 20–30 μm. The nucleus is round and in most cases has finely dispersed chromatin and a single large nucleolus. Most of the cells are diploid but, with increasing age and in the course of regeneration, the proportion of tetraploid and polyploid cells increases.

Vacuoles that appear to be intranuclear are not uncommon, especially in diabetic patients and in those with Wilson's disease. They are, in fact, not intranuclear but represent instead invaginations of endoplasmic reticulum. Electron microscopy shows large amounts of **glycogen** associated with these invaginations.

Hepatocyte Plasma Membranes

Liver cell plasma membranes facing either the blood-containing sinusoid or the bile-draining canaliculus show many microvilli, which add considerably to the surface area of these membranes. Many proteins bind to specific receptors on the sinusoidal plasma membrane being endocytosed in vesicles, some of which (as in the case of the low density lipoprotein receptor) are coated by **clathrin**. The other four sides of the cell are linked by tight junctions which prevent communication between the bile canaliculi and the subendothelial space on the sinusoidal aspect.

Hepatocyte Cytoskeleton

Liver cells have a well-formed cytoskeleton consisting of

- **microtubules**
- **microfilaments**
- **intermediate filaments**

The **microtubules** extend throughout the cytoplasm but are most densely aggregated in the region of the Golgi apparatus and along the sinusoidal plasma membrane. This is highly appropriate because they are concerned chiefly with the secretion of proteins into the sinusoids.

Microfilaments are formed largely by the association of actin and myosin. They are concentrated along the inner aspect of the plasma membrane, and are particularly dense in the area adjacent to the bile canaliculus. **Microfilaments play an important part in the transport of the components of bile from the liver cell into the canaliculus.** If microfilaments are disrupted by cytochalasin B (a well-recognized compound for inhibiting phagocyte movement) then cholestasis results.

Intermediate filaments are cytokeratins and, in normal liver, cytokeratins 8 and 18 predominate,

although other types are sometimes expressed following injury. The intermediate filaments are responsible for the spatial organization of the liver cells and are arranged in an irregular meshwork extending from the plasma membranes to the perinuclear regions.

Organelles

As might be expected in a cell so active metabolically, the liver cell contains numerous organelles. There is well-developed rough endoplasmic reticulum and a prominent Golgi apparatus. **Smooth endoplasmic reticulum** (SER) is also present, being particularly marked in hepatocytes from zone 3. This is interesting because the mixed function oxidases, responsible for the formation of free radicals from compounds such as carbon tetrachloride, are found chiefly in the SER. This could account for the predilection for toxic damage by such compounds to affect zone 3 cells rather than those in zone 1 or 2.

Each liver cell contains about 800 **mitochondria**. Another type of organelle involved in oxidative reactions, the **peroxisome**, is present within the liver cell in the ratio of one peroxisome for every four mitochondria. The peroxisome is a single-membrane-bound particle, measuring about 0.5 μm. Peroxisomes receive this name because they usually contain one or more enzymes that use molecular oxygen to remove hydrogen atoms from organic substrates in an oxidative reaction leading to the production of hydrogen peroxide. The excess hydrogen peroxide is destroyed by catalase within the peroxisome. Like mitochondria, peroxisomes are thought to be self-replicating but contain no DNA or ribosomes. They are believed to contain a unique membrane receptor which allows them to import all their proteins by selective transfer from the cytosol of the cells they inhabit. They take part in the metabolism of long-chain fatty acids, purines and alcohols, in the oxidation of nicotinamide adenine dinucleotide (NAD) and in gluconeogenesis. They increase in number in the liver after administration of salicylates.

Both primary and secondary **lysosomes** are also present in the liver cell. Their number increases in anoxic injury, viral hepatitis and cholestasis. In infants born with a deficiency of the enzyme α_{1-4}-glucosidase (type II glycogen storage disease), there are large glycogen deposits within these lysosomes.

Tests for Liver Cell Function

Liver cells have many functions, but those that are usually tested in clinical practice relate to:

- **protein synthesis**
- **bile secretion**
- **maintenance of the integrity of plasma membranes**

Defects in protein synthesis (*Fig. 35.2*) may be viewed in **two** ways:

1) A general decline in the synthetic functions of the liver cell mass, as is seen in chronic and acute

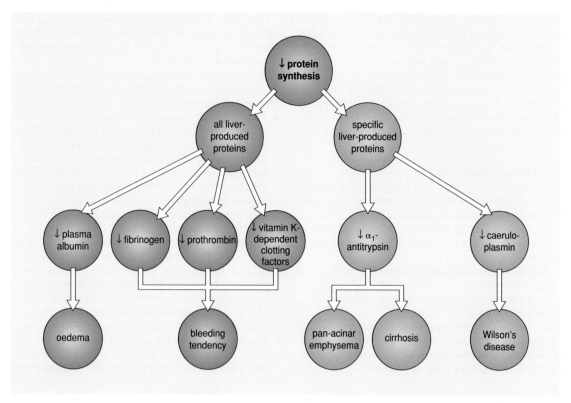

FIGURE 35.2 *Defects in protein synthesis occurring in liver disease.*

liver failure, leading to a lowered plasma concentration of proteins such as **albumin, components of the clotting system such as prothrombin and fibrinogen and some of the components of the complement system**. In acute liver failure, a severe decrease in the ability to synthesize clotting proteins carries an ominous prognosis.

2) Inability to produce certain specific proteins, for example:

- α_1-**antitrypsin deficiency**, in which the liver is able to synthesize only a molecular form of the protein, which cannot be secreted from the liver cell.
- **Wilson's disease**, where there is a relative decline in the ability of the cells to synthesize and secrete **caeruloplasmin**, the copper-transporting protein.

Defects in biliary secretion are considered in the section on bile drainage (see pp 567–571).

Loss of integrity of liver cell plasma membranes occurs when the degree of cell injury to the cells is sufficiently severe as to cause cell death. **Water-soluble enzymes such as lactic dehydrogenase and the mitochondrial and cytosol-associated enzymes aspartate aminotransferase (ASAT) and alanine aminotransferase (ALAT) leak from these fatally damaged cells and their concentration in the plasma are thus raised.** The degree to which such increases occur, as in the case of myocardial infarction, correlates approximately with the extent of cell loss.

Normal Liver Vasculature

The liver receives its blood supply from two sources:

1) **The portal vein**, which supplies about 75% of the blood reaching the liver and which is formed by the joining of the splenic and superior mesenteric veins. Normally, portal vein pressure is between 5–10 mmHg. If there is an increase in resistance to flow within the hepatic venous drainage, within the liver itself or within the portal vein, this pressure will rise and a collateral circulation will develop between the portal and systemic venous systems.

2) **The hepatic artery**, which carries only 25–30% of the liver's blood supply but furnishes about half the oxygen delivered to the liver. Hepatic artery occlusion does not usually lead to necrosis within the liver, except in transplanted livers.

At the hilum of the liver, both these vessels divide into a major right and left branch supplying the corresponding sides of the liver. The right and left branches then divide progressively throughout the liver, and are sheathed by fibrous tissue trabeculae derived in the first instance from the fibrous capsule surrounding the liver. The branches of the portal vein and hepatic artery, as separately identifiable vessels, terminate in the portal tracts, which are cores of connective tissue in which the smallest bile ducts, nerves and lymphatics are also present. Small branches then lead from these blood vessels into the sinusoids, which eventually drain into the terminal hepatic veins.

The Hepatic Sinusoids

The sinusoids (*Fig. 35.3*) are fairly wide endothelial cell-lined spaces separating the columns of liver cells. Sinusoidal endothelium is unusual in three respects:

1) There are no tight junctions between adjacent endothelial cells as there are in most other vascular beds.

2) The cytoplasm of some of the cells contains holes (fenestrae).

3) There is no basement membrane under the endothelium.

This anatomical arrangement allows free access of plasma from sinusoidal blood to liver cell, thus facilitating the two-way exchange of molecules between liver cells and blood.

The endothelium is separated from underlying liver cells by the **space of Disse**, which contains collagen fibres of various types (type III predominating), proteoglycans and some fibronectin.

There is a distinct cell population associated with the sinusoids apart, of course, from the endothelial lining. On the luminal aspect there are:

- **Kupffer cells**, which are attached to the endothelium. These cells function as fixed tissue macrophages and have an important role in phagocytosing effete blood cells and gut-derived bacteria. Like macrophages in other situations these cells have many secretory products that play an important pathogenetic role, for example in endotoxin-related shock. The Kupffer cell population is greatest in zone 1 of the liver cell acinus.
- **'Pit' cells.** These curiously named cells are large granular lymphocytes that are believed to function as natural killer cells. They are much fewer in number than Kupffer cells (1 : 10) and may play a part in defence against viral infections in the liver.

Within the space of Disse are cells that are known as:

- **Perisinusoidal or Ito cells.** These cells are in close contact with the liver cells and may extend into small recesses between liver cells. Most of them

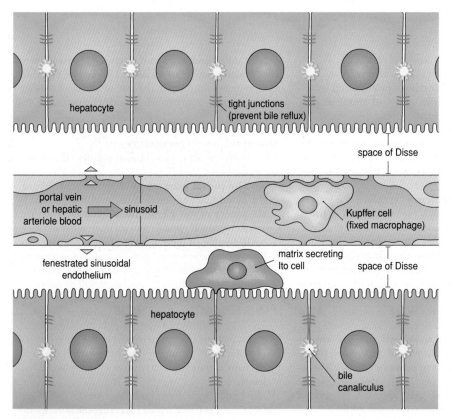

FIGURE 35.3 The hepatic sinusoid and perisinusoidal space.

contain vitamin A and many contain other lipids as well. They are believed to belong to the fibromyoblast family and, apart from any possible storage role, they are thought to synthesize extracellular matrix proteins.

Bile Drainage

The Duct System

Liver cells secrete bile into the canaliculi, through which the bile flows in a direction opposite to that of blood. The canalicular microvilli are surrounded by a meshwork of contractile protein which, presumably, maintains tone within the canalicular system. From the canaliculi, the bile flows into the preductules or canals of Hering, which are lined by both liver cells and bile ductular epithelium. These drain into the bile ductules entirely lined by cuboidal epithelial cells and lying at the periphery of the portal tracts. From these, bile flows into the interlobular bile ducts situated in the portal tracts with hepatic artery branches on either side, and which have a diameter of less than 100 μm. The union of two interlobular ducts constitutes a septal duct and these then fuse to form segmental ducts.

Bile secretion enables excretion of:

1) **endogenous compounds** such as cholesterol, bilirubin and effete proteins

2) **exogenous compounds** such as a variety of drugs

In addition, bile:

- helps to maintain the ionic environment in the duodenum, as bile is rich in bicarbonate.
- plays a role in mucosal immunity via the immunoglobulin (Ig) A secreted in bile.

Bilirubin

Bilirubin is the catabolic product of haem. Its relatively low concentration in human plasma reflects the fact that **there is a balance between the rate of production of bilirubin and its secretion in the bile**. Thus **hyperbilirubinaemia may arise because of**:

- **an increase in the rate of bilirubin production**
- **some defect in bilirubin handling within the liver cell**
- **some defect in bilirubin transport within the intrahepatic or extrahepatic biliary system**

The chief precursor of bilirubin is the haemoglobin of effete red cells broken down at the end of their 120-day lifespan. This accounts for 70% of the 250–300 mg bilirubin normally excreted daily. Obviously, if there is inappropriate destruction of red cells, as in intravascular haemolysis, the amount of bilirubin formed will be greatly increased and this will be reflected clinically by the appearance of a yellow discoloration of the sclerae and skin (**jaundice**).

A small amount of bilirubin is formed from the destruction of immature red cells in the bone marrow (so-called 'ineffective erythropoiesis').

The remaining bilirubin is derived from breakdown of haem-containing proteins other than haemoglobin. These include cytochrome P450, catalase and various other oxidizing enzymes. Normally these proteins are the source for about 30% of the daily bilirubin excretion.

The sequence of events from the release of haem to the secretion of bile into the canaliculi is outlined below.

Bile Formation

The first step (*Figs 35.4* and *35.5*) is removal of the haem prosthetic group from haemoglobin. The haem is then oxidized by a microsomal enzyme (**haem**

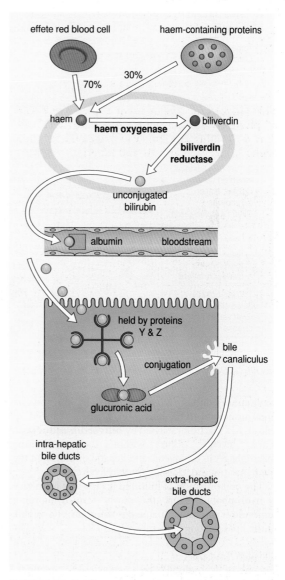

FIGURE 35.4 The formation, metabolism and excretion of bilirubin.

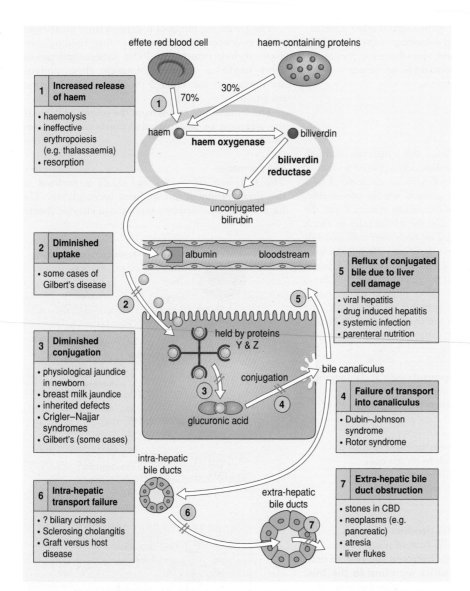

FIGURE 35.5 *The causes of jaundice. Any of the steps in bilirubin formation, metabolism and excretion may go wrong.*

oxygenase) with the release of biliverdin, iron and carbon monoxide. The biliverdin is then reduced to bilirubin, a reaction catalysed by **biliverdin reductase**. These events occur within the fixed-tissue macrophages in the splenic and hepatic sinusoids, in the bone marrow and, possibly, within liver cells.

The conformation of bilirubin is such that its surface is hydrophobic. Thus, the newly formed bilirubin molecule is insoluble in aqueous solutions but soluble in the lipid regions of membranes.

Bilirubin Transport
Because of its insolubility in aqueous media, unconjugated bilirubin is transported in plasma reversibly bound to plasma albumin. Only a very small fraction of

the bilirubin remains unbound in the plasma, and accurate measurement of this free bilirubin is very difficult. This fraction is important because free lipid-soluble bilirubin can cross cell membranes such as the blood–brain barrier. It has been calculated that the amount of free bilirubin in adult plasma is about 0.12 nmol/l; in neonates, the safe upper limit of free bilirubin is about 50 nmol/l, a concentration that is reached when about 80% of the high-affinity binding sites on albumin are occupied by bilirubin.

Long-chain fatty acids, such as are found in high concentration in breast milk, can compete with bilirubin for the binding sites. In some breastfed infants the 'physiological' jaundice so often seen in the neonatal period (when plasma albumin concentration may be rather low and there is accelerated breakdown of red cells), may be prolonged considerably. Many drugs also compete for the bilirubin-binding site on albumin and, if given to lactating mothers or to neonates, may increase the risk of bilirubin toxicity to brain tissue.

Uptake of Unconjugated Bilirubin by Liver Cells

Because of the fenestrated endothelium in the liver sinusoids, the albumin-bound bilirubin easily reaches the space of Disse, coming into close contact with the plasma membrane of the liver cells. It is not clear whether dissociation of bilirubin from albumin occurs in the plasma or whether there is binding of the albumin–bilirubin complex with subsequent dissociation at the cellular level. Whatever the case may be, bilirubin uptake seems to depend on the existence of carrier proteins that bind both bilirubin and other molecules such as bromsulphthalein (BSP) as well.

Once within the cell, bilirubin binds to proteins known as **ligandin** (protein Y, glutathione-S-transferase B) and **protein Z** (fatty acid-binding protein). Protein Z has a lower **affinity** than protein Y for bilirubin, but a greater **capacity** for bilirubin.

The precise role of protein Z in bilirubin transport within the liver cell is still not proven and it may have a more important part to play in the binding of fatty acids. In quantitative terms, ligandin is an important protein, accounting for 5% of the soluble protein content of the liver.

Competition for the binding sites on these proteins occurs with certain drugs, and jaundice, for example, is seen in some patients treated with the antituberculous agent rifampicin, which binds to ligandin. Once treatment has been discontinued, the plasma bilirubin concentration returns to normal.

Conjugation of Bilirubin

The amount of bilirubin that can be stored complexed with ligandin and protein Z is limited, and the chief process involved in clearance of bilirubin from the blood is secretion into the bile canaliculus. This cannot be accomplished without making the bilirubin **soluble in aqueous solutions**, and is achieved by the addition of glucuronic acid to one or both of the propionic acid groups of the bilirubin. This process, known as conjugation, is catalysed by the enzyme **uridyl-1-phosphate glucuronyl transferase**. The addition of the bulky glucuronic acid forces open the folded structure of the bilirubin molecule, allowing hydrophilic residues to interact with water; this renders the bilirubin–glucuronide complex water-soluble.

Absent or reduced glucuronyl transferase activity leads to an increase in the plasma concentration of unconjugated bilirubin, seen in its most severe form in the autosomally recessive, inherited, metabolic defect known as **Crigler–Najjar syndrome type 1**.

In **Crigler–Najjar syndrome type 1**, severe unconjugated hyperbilirubinaemia is recognized within the first few days of life, and severe brain damage due to the deposition of free bilirubin occurs. In some cases the onset of clinical evidence of such brain damage has been delayed until adolescence but, in most, such damage makes itself apparent within the first 18 months of life.

A second type of Crigler–Najjar syndrome (type 2) has been described. This is believed to be inherited as an autosomal dominant abnormality with variable penetrance. Glucuronyl transferase activity is not as severely decreased as in the type 1 syndrome and the degree of unconjugated hyperbilirubinaemia and resulting risk of brain damage are both lower.

Both variants of the Crigler–Najjar syndrome are rare, but this is not the case with another disorder in which there is reduced activity of glucuronyl transferase: **Gilbert's syndrome**. This is a disorder characterized by mild unconjugated hyperbilirubinaemia presenting with intermittent episodes of jaundice. The actual prevalence is not easy to determine but Gilbert's syndrome may affect 3–7% of the general population, with a distinct preponderance in males.

The clinical features usually appear for the first time during the second or third decades of life. This may be due to hormone-related changes in glucuronyl transferase activity following puberty. Mild intermittent jaundice, often precipitated by a decrease in food intake, is the sole abnormality in about one-third of affected individuals. In the remainder there may be vague symptoms such as abdominal discomfort and excessive fatigue. There are no structural abnormalities in the liver and the prognosis is excellent. There is no mutation in the gene for glucuronyl transferase, but mutations have been described in the promoter region of this gene.

Secretion of Bile into the Canaliculus

The secretion of bile into the bile drainage system involves much more than the transport of conjugated bilirubin from the liver cell into the canaliculus.

Bile formation is the means for excretion of:
- conjugated bilirubin
- a number of detoxified chemical compounds
- cholesterol
- bile salts which, when they reach the lumen of the small intestine, mediate the absorption of dietary fat

There appear to be at least two pathways for the secretion of bile:
1) **bile acid dependent**
2) **bile acid independent**

There is active secretion of bile salts via a 100-kDa carrier protein, and of sodium from the liver cell into the canaliculus. This creates an osmotic gradient and water then flows passively in the same direction as the bile salts and sodium. The greater the active secretion of bile salts, the greater the passive flow of water.

However, biliary water can be formed in the absence of bile salts (the bile acid-independent fraction) and this is thought to be the result of adenosine 5'-triphosphatase (ATPase) activity, whereby sodium is pumped from the liver cell into the canaliculus. Certain drugs, such as chlorpromazine, appear to affect ATPase activity in an idiosyncratic fashion and may cause cholestasis. It is not certain whether secretion of bilirubin–glucuronide is coupled with bile salt secretion.

There are two inherited disorders, the **Dubin–Johnson syndrome** and **Rotor's syndrome**, in which there is failure to transport conjugated bilirubin from the liver cell into the canaliculus. As a result there is an increase in plasma concentration of conjugated bilirubin and the patient becomes jaundiced. This failure to transport the bilirubin is *not* accompanied by a similar failure to transport bile salts.

Both the Dubin–Johnson and Rotor's syndromes are inherited in an autosomal recessive fashion. In the former, the conjugated hyperbilirubinaemia usually appears in early adult life, whereas in the latter, jaundice usually appears in childhood. Histologically, Dubin–Johnson syndrome differs from Rotor's syndrome in that the liver cells in the former show the presence of coarse granular brown pigment, which is probably a lipofuscin and derived from incomplete oxidation of lipids within lysosomes. It is believed that this pigment is the result rather than the cause of the functional defect.

Cholestasis

It is important to realize that failure to drain bile must lead to the appearance in the plasma of increased concentrations of all the constituents of bile, and not only of conjugated bilirubin. Thus, there will be increased plasma concentrations of alkaline phosphatase, IgA and, less often, cholesterol. The causes of cholestasis are listed in *Table 35.1*.

Morphological Changes in Cholestasis

The morphological picture of cholestasis can be considered most conveniently under two headings: evidence of the existence of cholestasis and secondary changes in the liver.

Evidence of the Existence of Cholestasis in the Affected Liver

The presence of cholestasis is marked by the accumulations of brownish-yellow bile within dilated canaliculi and within some of the hepatocytes. The masses of bile pigment within the canaliculi are known as **bile plugs**. Ultrastructural studies of liver biopsies in cases of cholestasis show blunting of the microvillous processes on the canalicular aspects of the liver cells, and the liver cell cytoplasm in the pericanalicular zone is wider than normal. This feature is due to an increase in the number of microfilaments. In the early stages of cholestasis, the bile plugs are found in zone 3; with chronic obstruction to bile flow, plugs appear also in zones 2 and 1, and their presence in these locations is an indicator of chronicity.

Secondary Changes Resulting from Cholestasis

Such secondary changes include:

- Scattered necrotic liver cells. These have, presumably, succumbed because of high intracytoplasmic concentrations of bile.
- Accumulation of bile pigment and cellular debris within the resident macrophage population.
- Periportal fibrosis and proliferation of bile ductules. This finding is non-specific and occurs in other types of continuing liver cell injury.
- 'Feathery degeneration' of liver cells, in which the cells become swollen because of the accumulation of water, the cytoplasm assumes a reticulated pattern, and there is intracellular accumulation of bile pigment.
- Formation of 'bile lakes'. These are areas in which

Table 35.1 Causes of Cholestasis

Type of cholestasis	Causes
Extrahepatic mechanical obstruction	Gallstones, neoplasms of bile duct or papilla of Vater, sclerosing cholangitis, pancreatic disorders including inflammation or neoplasia
Intrahepatic mechanical obstruction	Granulomas, metastatic neoplasms, cystic fibrosis in infancy in which mucous plugs are seen in small bile ducts
Mechanical obstruction in infancy	Extrahepatic or intrahepatic bile duct atresia
Intrahepatic cholestasis without obstruction	Certain infections, α_1-antitrypsin deficiency, as part of a paraneoplastic syndrome (e.g. in renal carcinoma), pregnancy in some individuals, viral hepatitis, drugs, idiopathic recurrent cholestasis, familial progressive cholestasis (Byler's disease), early stages of primary biliary cirrhosis, cirrhosis of other types

groups of liver cells have become necrotic. Extravasated bile pigment collects in these areas to form brownish-yellow masses admixed with cellular debris.

The last two features are associated with long-standing cholestasis.

DISORDERS AFFECTING PRINCIPALLY THE LIVER PARENCHYMA

ACUTE VIRAL HEPATITIS

The liver may be affected by many viruses, some of which, such as herpesvirus or cytomegalovirus, also affect other organs. However, where the liver is the sole target, the responsible agents are known as hepatitis viruses of which five are now recognized and characterized.

Infection with these hepatotropic viruses may produce an acute clinical illness of varying grades of severity, ranging from an episode associated with mild jaundice, nausea and anorexia to a fulminating illness leading to acute liver failure and death.

In many instances, the initial effects of the viral infection may be clinically silent and thus pass unnoticed. However, some subclinical infections progress to chronic liver disease in which continuing necrosis of liver cells is associated with fibrosis and loss of normal liver architecture (cirrhosis) and in which there is an increased risk of liver cell cancer. **Chronicity of the inflammatory process and its attendant risks are particularly associated with infections by hepatitis viruses B, C and D.** The hepatitis viruses are listed in *Table 35.2*.

Pathological Changes in Acute Viral Hepatitis

The patterns of reaction to injury in the liver are limited and thus acute viral hepatitides tend to show similar morphology irrespective of their precise aetiology. The mechanisms likely to be involved in causing damage to the liver parenchyma are twofold:

1) The viruses may have a direct cytopathic effect.
2) The virally infected liver cells express viral neoantigens in association with major histocompatibility complex (MHC) class I-coded proteins, leading to an attack on these cells by cytotoxic T and K cells. Thus the actual process of virus elimination by the immune system may be responsible for a significant part of the liver cell injury.

Macroscopic Features

In viral hepatitis, naked-eye examination is undertaken only when the process has been fulminating and has led to fatal acute liver failure. In these circumstances the liver may be much reduced in weight because necrotic liver cells are autolysed rapidly and removed. **The presence of wrinkling of the liver capsule bears obvious testimony to the rapid decrease in liver cell mass.**

The cut surface of such a liver may show a uniformly

Table 35.2 The Hepatitis Viruses

Virus	Genome, genus and family	Transmission
Hepatitis A	RNA, **picornavirus** family, enterovirus genus	Chiefly faecal–oral route
Hepatitis B	DNA **hepadna** virus; newly classified group affecting humans and a number of other species	Parenteral, via blood, sexual transmission, perinatal ('vertical') transmission
Hepatitis C	Single-stranded RNA; related to **flavivirus** family	Major cause of post-transfusion, non-A, non-B hepatitis, antibodies present in blood of 60–90% of haemophiliacs and intravenous drug abusers; some evidence of low-efficiency sexual transmission; vertical transmission also documented
Hepatitis D (the δ agent)	**Defective** RNA virus which requires the presence of hepatitis B virus for infection to occur; the latter provides the outer coat of the infecting agent	Usually parenteral but some evidence of sexual transmission also. Acute co-infections with hepatitis B virus common in drug addicts in the UK
Hepatitis E	Single-stranded RNA virus related to **caliciviruses**	Transmission chiefly by faecal–oral route, especially faecally contaminated drinking water; disease may occur in epidemics, small outbreaks or as sporadic cases

red appearance. In some instances, there is evidence of commencing regeneration in the form of rounded yellowish areas scattered against the red background of necrotic liver.

Microscopic Features

Structural changes in acute hepatitis (*Fig. 35.6*) include:
- evidence of liver cell damage or death
- inflammatory reactions within the liver acini
- inflammatory reactions within the portal tract connective tissue
- changes to the connective tissue framework of the liver; these usually occur only with extensive and severe loss of parenchymal cells

Liver Cell Changes

Evidence of cell damage is present throughout the liver cell acinus but is most severe in zone 3. The two patterns most commonly seen are:

1) **'Ballooning degeneration'**, characterized by the cells being swollen to twice their normal size. Nuclei are surrounded by a cuff of granular cytoplasm from which strands stretch to the plasma membrane. The cytoplasm between these strands does not bind eosin and thus much of the cytoplasm appears to be 'empty'. These appearances are the correlate of intracellular oedema and consequent dilatation of the endoplasmic reticulum, loss of ribosomes and swelling of the mitochondria. Ballooning degeneration may affect many cells and, while some of the affected cells undergo **lysis**, this is not inevitable, the effects of cell injury being reversible in some instances.

2) **Acidophilic degeneration**, which indicates **irreversible** cell damage. Some cells show increased eosinophilia and condensation of the cytoplasm, whereas others in which the process has advanced consist simply of balls of eosinophilic material. These are known as Councilman bodies and represent the end result of apoptosis.

Intra-acinar Inflammatory Response

A diffuse cell infiltrate may be seen within the acinus. This is made up of lymphocytes, macrophages and plasma cells and, like the liver cell damage, is most severe in the perivenular region of acinar zone 3.

Portal Tract Inflammatory Response

The portal tract is also the site of an inflammatory reaction, again consisting predominantly of lymphocytes, plasma cells and macrophages. The presence of a few neutrophils and eosinophils is not uncommon.

Changes in the Connective Tissue Framework

In most cases, there is insufficient liver cell necrosis to cause any significant alteration in the architectural arrangement of liver cell plates. In more severe cases there may be extensive liver cell death (*Fig. 35.7*) with conflu-ent loss of liver cells bridging the area between a terminal hepatic venule and a portal tract. This is known as **bridging necrosis** and is associated with collapse of the reticulin fibre framework in this area. It is a serious development because this is one of the factors increasing the risk of subsequent cirrhosis.

Hepatitis A

The Virus and its Transmission

Hepatitis A (HAV) is caused by an RNA enterovirus of the Picornaviridae group. Picornaviridae infect by attaching to receptors on target cells. In the case of HAV, the sole target for such attachment appears to be the liver; viral replication occurs **only** in liver cells. There is only one antigenic type of HAV.

Anti-HAV IgG antibodies, which may persist for years in the plasma of blood donors, indicate past infection and this enables regional differences in the prevalence of hepatitis A to be recorded. Such studies show infection to be a relatively common event, anti-HAV antibodies being found in 29% of Swiss blood donors and in 90% of those in Israel and the former Yugoslavia.

Antibody positivity rises with increasing age and it is clear that many HAV infections must be subclinical. Transmission is via the faecal–oral route. Some edible shellfish appear to concentrate the virus and are not infrequently the source of infection. HAV infection, although not classified as a sexually transmitted disorder, is seen quite commonly in homosexuals practising oral–anal contact.

Clinical Features

The incubation period ranges from 3 to 7 weeks. The early phase of the clinical picture is dominated by the abrupt onset of malaise, nausea and anorexia, sometimes associated with fever. At this stage there is already clear evidence of damage to liver cells in the form of raised plasma concentrations of ALAT, and faecal shedding of the virus (excreted from the liver in the bile) occurs.

After about 10 days the raised enzyme levels start to decline and it is at this point that the patient becomes jaundiced. The jaundice usually clears within about 10 days, by which time plasma concentrations of liver cell enzymes have returned to their preinfection levels. Only a tiny fraction of patients with this form of hepatitis develop fulminant hepatitis; mortality rates are lower than 0.1%.

Three important points to remember are:
1) Chronic hepatitis never occurs.
2) Infection with HAV confers lifelong immunity.
3) Viral elimination is total: there is no carrier state.

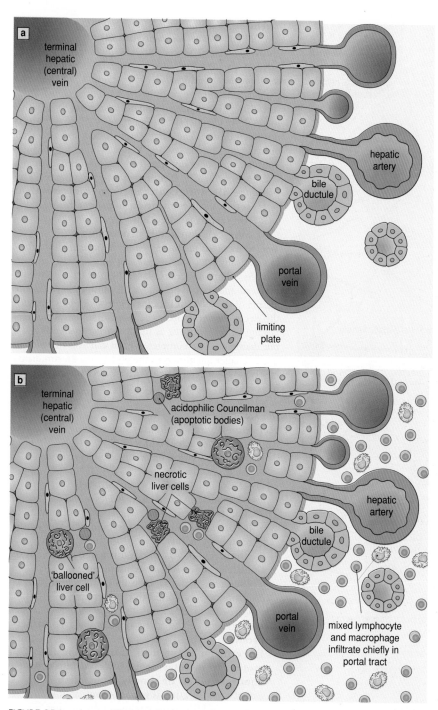

FIGURE 35.6 **a** A normal liver acinus showing parenchyma and portal tract. **b** Morphological features of acute hepatitis.

Microscopic Features

The general features are as described in the previous section on acute viral hepatitis. Cholestasis is, however, more prominent than in other forms of hepatitis and the main target for cell damage appears to be the periportal region.

The spread of HAV in a community can be reduced by such public health measures as prevent faecal contamination of water supplies. At the individual level, prophylactic administration of pooled normal human immune serum immunoglobulin can prevent HAV infection in travellers going to high-risk areas.

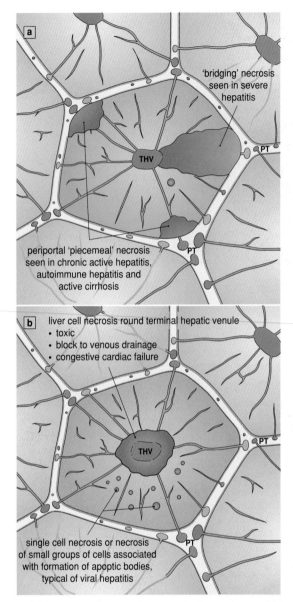

FIGURE 35.7 **a** and **b** Patterns of parenchymal necrosis in liver disease.

Hepatitis B

The Virus and its Transmission

Hepatitis B is caused by a member of an unusual group of viruses known as the hepadnaviridae (*hepa*totropic *DNA* viruses). All members of this small group are hepatotropic; other species affected include the woodchuck, the ground squirrel and certain strains of duck. The small number of susceptible species reflects the lack, in most species, of cell surface receptors reacting with hepatitis B virus (HBV) envelope proteins.

The DNA of the virus is arranged in a peculiar fashion. There is one long circular strand in which the entire genome is present and an incomplete complementary strand comprising about 50–70% of the content of the complete circular strand. The genome consists of four open reading frames. Three code for the surface and core viral antigens and for DNA polymerase; the product of the fourth open reading frame is not yet known. The viral core, in addition to DNA polymerase, contains two antigenically distinct products known as the core antigen (HBcAg) and the e antigen (HBeAg), which is related to the core antigen. **The presence of e antigen in the serum indicates that:**
  1) **active viral replication is proceeding**
  2) **the serum is infective**
  3) **liver cell damage is proceeding**

The viral core is enclosed in a lipid, protein and carbohydrate surface coat expressing a surface antigen (HBsAg). This surface coat is synthesized separately from the core and may appear in excess amounts within the plasma of the affected patients. Here it can be seen with the electron microscope either as small spherical particles (20 nm in diameter) or as tubular structures with a 20-nm diameter. The complete virion can also be seen (in much smaller quantities) in the plasma as a 43-nm diameter double-shelled particle with an electron-dense core. This is known as the Dane particle (*Fig. 35.8*).

Replication

Hepatitis B virus replicates in a unique way, seen only in the hepadnaviridae.
  1) The intact virion enters the host liver cells, where it uncoats.
  2) The viral DNA is processed in a series of steps to form covalently closed circular DNA.
  3) This DNA acts as the template for the formation of RNA, which is termed 'pregenomic'. This name is given because this RNA forms the template for the formation of viral DNA through the medium of a virally encoded reverse transcriptase.
  4) Negative-strand DNA is transcribed from the pregenomic RNA and this then replicates to form positive-strand DNA.

Transmission of the virus occurs via two principal routes:
  1) **Perinatal or 'vertical' transmission from mother to infant as from infected blood or liquor amnii at, or shortly after, birth.** The risk of such infection is strongly correlated with the presence of HBe antigenaemia in the mother, which in some populations is very prevalent.
  2) **'Horizontal'** transmission may occur in childhood in high-risk populations, although the actual mode of such transmission is not clear.

In adults, horizontal transmission occurs parenterally following exposure to infected blood or blood products (*Fig. 35.9*). Such infections may occur as a result of:

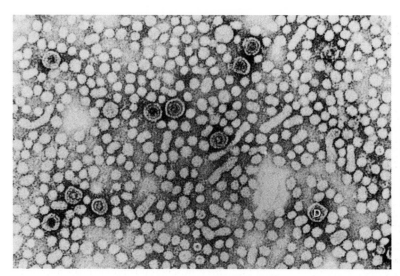

FIGURE 35.8 *Hepatitis B virus. This concentrated preparation shows the three morphological forms in which the virus may be seen in the serum of infected individuals: (1) the Dane particle or complete virion (D); (2) small spherical particles composed of the same lipid and protein that constitutes the outer shell of the complete virion; (3) long particles that represent aggregates of the spherical particles.*

- the use of infected needles by drug abusers
- the process of tattooing
- the use of infected blood in transfusion

This last circumstance accounts for less than 1% of HBV infections in the UK as blood for transfusion is screened for the presence of HBsAg, although occasional examples of infection have occurred after transfusion of blood negative for surface antigen.

Cases of hepatitis B have also been reported after administration of infected plasma protein products such as clotting factors and vaccines stabilized with human serum.

There is a distinct danger of infection in haemodialysis units, a danger that is greater for attending staff than for patients. Cross-infection within such units is the chief means of keeping the infection going, and, certainly, dialysis patients who are positive for HBsAg have a high chance of also having the infective e antigen and viral DNA polymerase in their plasma.

Sexual transmission of HBV is quite important, especially in populations where the prevalence of infection is low. The infection may be acquired by either heterosexual or homosexual contact and it is worth remembering that body fluids such as saliva and semen may be infective as well as blood. Another fact worth remembering is that only synthetic (non-rubber) condoms are impermeable to the virus. Rarely, infections have occurred after artificial insemination, and screening of semen donors for surface antigen is probably a wise precaution.

Laboratory Diagnosis

Methods now exist for the detection of: **HBsAg, HBeAg, HBcAg, HBV DNA and the antibodies** **corresponding to these viral antigens**. These enable the detection of the intrahepatic events that occur in the course of HBV infection and, equally, some of the responses of the immune system.

Sequence of Serological Events in Acute Hepatitis B

1) **The first marker to appear in the serum of an infected patient is HBsAg.** This may be detectable between 1 week and 2 months after exposure, or anywhere from 2 weeks to 2 months before the appearance of clinical symptoms. It disappears from the blood during the convalescent phase.

2) **The second marker to appear is HBeAg.** As already stated, its presence is correlated with a period of maximal infectivity and intense viral replication. As with HBsAg, it appears before the onset of clinical symptoms and usually disappears from the serum in about 2 weeks. As the e antigen is cleared from the blood, antibody to e usually makes its appearance, but there may be a gap between disappearance of the antigen and detection of the antibody.

3) **With the onset of the clinical illness anti-HBc usually appears in the serum (both IgG and IgM)**. Anti-HBc remains present, at a low titre, for life but does not appear to play a significant role in viral elimination and serves rather as a marker for infection.

4) **The last marker to appear in serum is anti-HBs.** Its appearance in measurable amounts indicates that antibody excess is present. Until this point is reached, the antibody forms immune complexes with the circulating HBsAg and these

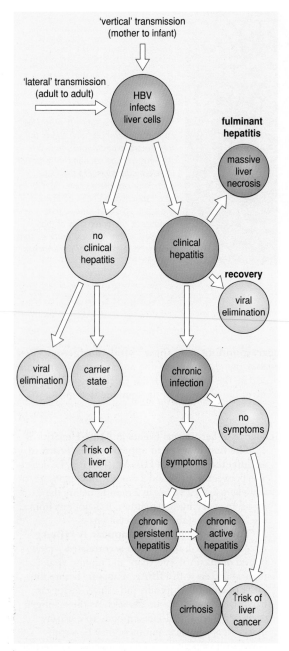

FIGURE 35.9 The range of natural histories occurring as a result of hepatitis B infection.

Failure to clear HBsAg from the serum after 6 months is the hallmark of chronicity in respect of hepatitis B infection. It occurs in only a small minority of patients (probably less than 5%). The presence of HBeAg, HBV DNA or DNA polymerase in the serum either singly or together indicates that active viral replication is occurring. In cases where there is no viral replication, the continuing secretion of HBsAg into the blood is believed to be the correlate of integration of the viral genome into the genome of the host liver cell.

These events are summarized in Table 35.3.

Epidemiology

While hepatitis B occurs worldwide, there are marked differences in its prevalence. It is believed that between 300 and 400 million people have chronic HBV infection and that 250 000 deaths are caused annually by the combined effects of acute and chronic HBV infection.

On the basis of prevalence, the world can be divided roughly into three zones:

1) **High risk**: 8–15% of the population show the presence of HBsAg in their serum and more than 60% show some serological marker of HBV infection (South-East Asia, China, Phillipines, Indonesia, Middle East (excluding Israel), Africa, Pacific islands, Arctic Eskimo, Amazon Basin).

2) **Intermediate risk**: 2–7% of the population show the presence of HBsAg in their serum and 20–60% show some serological marker of HBV infection (eastern and southern Europe, the former USSR, Central Asia, Japan, Israel, the northern part of South America).

3) **Low risk**: less than 2% of the population show the presence of HbsAg in their serum and less than 20% show some serological marker of HBV infection (North America, western Europe, New Zealand, Australia, southern part of South America).

Hepatitis C

The Virus and its Transmission

With the development of reliable serological methods for identifying HAV or HBV infection, it became apparent that a substantial number of cases of hepatitis, some related to blood transfusion, were not due to either HAV or HBV. This type of hepatitis, originally defined by exclusion was termed non-A, non-B hepatitis (NANBH).

NANBH is both common and significant; the Center for Disease Control in the USA estimates that about 150 000 cases occur annually in that country and that only 5–10% result from blood transfusion. **About 50% of affected individuals go on to develop biochemical evidence of chronic liver disease and 10% develop chronic active hepatitis or cirrhosis.**

Blood from patients with NANBH can infect chimpanzees, this infectivity being associated with:

complexes may produce a number of complications outside the liver such as glomerulonephritis, necrotizing vasculitis and a serum sickness-like syndrome. The antibody to HBsAg may well be an important factor in viral elimination and in clearing HBsAg from the serum. Not infrequently there is a 'window' between the disappearance of HBsAg from the serum and the appearance of the corresponding antibody.

Table 35.3 Serological Events in HBV Infection

HBsAg	HBeAg	Anti-HBe	Anti-HBc	Anti-HBc IgM	Anti-HBs	Significance
+	+/−	+/−	+	+	−	Acute HBV infection
+	+	−	+	− or weak +	−	HBV carrier (high infectivity)
+	−	+	+	−	−	HBV carrier (low infectivity)
−	−	+/−	+	−	+	Past HBV infection
−	−	−	−	−	+	Past HBV immunization

- tubular structures seen on electron microscopy of affected liver cells
- abolition of infectivity passing the blood through a filter with a pore size of 80 nm
- abolition of infectivity by treating infective samples with organic solvents

These findings suggested that the hepatitis was due to a small enveloped virus. A breakthrough came when Choo and colleagues were able to clone and sequence the genome of the responsible virus, which has been called hepatitis C virus (HCV). Following this came the detection of an antibody in the serum of patients with NANBH that reacted specifically to a product of the cloned HBC genome. This antibody binds to a non-structural HBC protein known as NS4; its presence in serum is currently the 'gold standard' for the diagnosis of hepatitis C in both acute and chronic forms.

The virus is a small single-stranded RNA virus distantly related to the flavivirus and pestivirus family. It has no homology with any other hepatitis virus and is present in the serum only in low titre.

Transmission

While NANBH was first recognized in the context of post-transfusion hepatitis, it is now clear that only 5–10% of HBC sufferers have a history of blood transfusion:

- At least 40% of patients have a history of parenteral drug abuse.
- In less than 5% of cases has there been occupational exposure to blood.
- In 10% of cases the only identifiable source of infection is heterosexual contact (usually with multiple partners).

This leaves about 40% of patients with no history of possible parenteral infection. Thus, screening blood donors for antibody to HCV is likely to have only a small effect on the incidence of hepatitis C.

Clinical Features

Most infections are subclinical and, when an acute illness develops, it is usually mild. Only 25% at most of the patients become jaundiced. A very characteristic feature is fluctuation of serum transaminase concentra-

tion, which may vary by as much as 10–15-fold from week to week. Between exacerbations the transaminase concentration may return to normal. Seroconversion is slow and antibodies may not be detected for 3 months or more from the onset of clinical illness.

Half the patients will show evidence of chronicity and 20% of these will develop cirrhosis. Carriers of HCV also have a greatly enhanced risk of developing primary liver cell carcinoma.

Microscopic Features

In addition to the features common to viral hepatitis, HCV infection may produce:

1) **'Cytopathic' changes in the liver cells.** All liver biopsies from patients with hepatitis C show scattered liver cells with an intense degree of eosinophilia. It is thought that these cells have been damaged by the virus. No inflammatory reaction is noted in relation to these cells.

2) **The presence of inflammatory cells within the sinusoids.** The sinusoids are infiltrated by large numbers of lymphocytes and macrophages. The intensity of inflammation seems to be out of proportion to the relatively small amount of liver cell damage. Lymphocytes also infiltrate the portal tracts, in which they sometimes form well-organized follicles with germinal centres.

3) **Evidence of intrahepatic bile duct damage.** Bile duct damage in the form of lymphocyte infiltration of the epithelium of intrahepatic bile ducts is seen in about 30% of biopsies from patients with NANBH.

4) **Sublethal liver cell injury in the form of small-droplet fatty change.**

Hepatitis D

The Virus and its Transmission

An additional infective agent causing hepatitis was discovered in 1977. Liver biopsy material from HBsAg-positive patients, when treated with fluorescein-labelled anti-HBcAg, showed nuclear fluorescence. These fluorescing nuclei showed **no core particles on**

electron microscopy. The antigen was named the δ **agent** and is now known as hepatitis D virus (HDV). **This virus is found only in the liver cells of patients who are positive for HBsAg and its presence, and that of HBcAg, are mutually exclusive.**

HDV is a defective agent which, for infectivity, needs to be encapsidated by pre-surface and surface antigens of HBV. It is the smallest animal virus thus far discovered and is the only defective RNA virus capable of infecting animal cells. The genome consists of single-stranded RNA which replicates only inside liver cells. The presence of infection can be established by detection of either the appropriate antigen or antibody in the serum.

Hepatitis D has worldwide distribution but the populations of some geographical locations appear to be particularly at risk. These high-risk areas include southern Italy, Venezuela, Colombia, the Amazon Basin and western parts of Asia.

In other areas where the risk appears to be lower, there is a strong positive association between the risk of acquiring hepatitis D, parenteral drug abuse and haemophilia (as a result of infection via dried plasma products).

The disease may be acquired by one of two means:
1) **Co-infection,** i.e. simultaneous infection with both HBV and HDV.
2) **Superinfection**: infection by HDV of a carrier of HBV, who may be clinically healthy or who may suffer from chronic liver disease.

The results of these differing modes of infection are summarized in *Table 35.4*. Both co-infection and superinfection may be followed by acute hepatitis. In co-infection the serum of the patients will show both HDV markers and IgM anti-HBc antibodies. In patients who have acquired HDV as a result of superinfection, the acute hepatitis will *not* be accompanied by the appearance of anti-HBc IgM in the serum. By and large, superinfection is associated with a worse natural history (see *Table 35.4*) than co-infection.

Hepatitis E

The Virus and its Transmission

Another form of NANBH that differs markedly in respect of its epidemiology from hepatitis C is hepatitis E. **This disorder is characterized by faecal–oral transmission and is endemic in areas where there is the unhealthy combination of an undernourished population and low standards of sanitation.** Massive outbreaks involving tens of thousands of individuals have occurred, especially in the Indian subcontinent (29 000 cases in Delhi in 1955, and 79 000 in Kunpur in 1991), and smaller outbreaks and sporadic cases are also seen in the areas where the disease is endemic. Not surprisingly, the main agent for viral transmission is faecally contaminated drinking water.

Serum obtained from convalescent patients was found to aggregate virus-like particles from stool samples gathered from patients during a hepatitis outbreak, and this allowed the virus to be characterized morphologically by electron microscopy.

Hepatitis E virus (HEV) has now been cloned and sequenced. It is a single-stranded, spherically shaped, non-enveloped RNA virus. It is believed to be related to the **caliciviruses**, which are known to cause gastroenteritis especially in children.

Clinical Features

The incubation period is 3–9 weeks, the average being 6 weeks. The population particularly at risk in epidemics appears to be adolescents and young adults, in whom the attack rate can be as high as 2.9%.

In most instances, hepatitis E is an acute self-limiting disease, clinically not unlike hepatitis A, and most patients make a full recovery. Fulminant hepatitis with acute liver failure occurs in 0.5–3% of patients. A most curious feature of the natural history of this disease is the fact that, of women infected during the third trimester of pregnancy, 20% develop fulminant hepatitis and die from acute liver failure. This is as yet totally unexplained.

OTHER VIRAL INFECTIONS AFFECTING THE LIVER

Many other viruses affect the liver. The hepatitis they cause occurs either as:
- part of a systemic illness
- the result of an immunocompromised host acquiring an opportunistic infection

Such viruses are listed in *Table 35.5*.

Table 35.4 Co-infection and Superinfection in Relation to Differing Natural Histories of Hepatitis D

	Co-infection	Superinfection
Status of patient before infection	Normal	HBV carrier
Risk of developing fulminant hepatitis	Greater than with HBV alone; approximately 3–4%	Greater than with co-infection; approximately 7–10%
Risk of developing chronic liver disease	Very small; chronic liver disease rare	Much greater; 10–40% develop chronic hepatitis which may progress to cirrhosis

Table 35.5 Other Viral Infections of the Liver

Virus group	Disease or virus involved
Flaviviruses	Yellow fever
	West Nile fever
	Dengue
Adenoviruses	
Herpesviruses	Epstein–Barr virus
	Cytomegalovirus
	Herpes simplex
	Zoster or varicella
Arenaviruses	Lassa fever
	Argentinian and Bolivian
	haemorrhagic fevers
Filoviruses	Marburg virus
	Ebola virus

Yellow Fever

The yellow fever virus is an RNA virus transmitted via mosquito bites. It is endemic among primates in the Central African and Central and South American jungles, and replicates in both its hosts and the vector. In the jungle type, the vector is usually a mosquito of the *Haemogogus* variety, whereas in urban yellow fever, in which the cycle is primarily between humans and mosquitos, the vector is the mosquito *Aëdes aegyptii*.

Many infections are clinically inapparent. In patients with clinical disease, the usual presenting features are **fever, headache, nausea and vomiting. Jaundice** is present in more severe cases.

Microscopic Features

Liver abnormalities are most prominent in zone 2 of the acinus; the most striking of these is the acidophil change in liver cells associated with apoptosis (Councilman bodies). In addition, ballooning degeneration and fatty change may be seen in other hepatocytes. Kupffer cells also show acidophil change; this occurs a few days before the hepatocytes are affected. This acidophil change correlates with the presence of virus in these cells.

Herpesvirus Infections

The Epstein–Barr Virus

The commonest consequence of infection with the Epstein–Barr virus is infectious mononucleosis (glandular fever). This is characterized by fever, malaise, sore throat and lymph node swelling, chiefly in young adults and adolescents. About 15% of these individuals have associated hepatitis, and raised aminotransferase concentrations are found in most patients.

Epstein–Barr virus-induced hepatitis also occurs in recipients of liver transplants.

Microscopic Features

Histological examination of liver biopsies shows little evidence of liver cell injury and death, but there is usually a fairly marked degree of regenerative activity (characterized by the presence of many mitoses). The most striking change is a florid lymphocytic infiltrate, which may be so pronounced as to give rise to suspicion of malignant lymphoma.

Cytomegalovirus

Infections with this virus are common, the peak prevalence being in early adult life. The virus can also be transmitted transplacentally.

In adult life, infections usually present as febrile illnesses, often associated with hepatitis and sometimes with acute polyneuropathy of the Guillain–Barré type. Immunosuppression puts individuals at much greater risk and post-transplant patients on immunosuppressive treatment frequently suffer from cytomegalovirus infections.

The pathological changes in the liver are similar to those of acute viral hepatitis, although, occasionally, granulomas may be seen in the portal tracts. Characteristic viral inclusions in either the liver cells or the vascular endothelium are seen in only about 20% of cases.

Herpes Simplex

The herpes simplex virus causes a disseminated infection, either in neonatal life or in adults who are immunosuppressed as a result of therapy against graft rejection or because of a disorder such as Hodgkin's disease or ulcerative colitis.

The liver shows foci of rather haemorrhagic necrosis, which can be seen on naked-eye examination in fatal cases. On histological examination the liver cells surrounding the necrotic foci are usually seen to contain viral inclusions and the lesion elicits a mononuclear cell reaction.

Arenavirus Infection

Lassa Fever

Lassa fever is endemic in certain parts of West Africa such as Sierra Leone, where it is responsible for many hospital admissions and deaths (one-sixth of all admissions and up to 30% of adult inpatient deaths in some hospitals). It is caused by an **arenavirus** transmitted to humans from a rodent host *Mastomys natalensis*.

The clinical picture is that of a multisystem disease in which myocarditis, encephalitis, myositis and an abnormal bleeding tendency may be present. The more pronounced the bleeding tendency, the greater is the death rate; infection during pregnancy carries an especially ominous prognosis.

> ### *Microscopic Features*
> Liver samples show focal areas of necrosis and evidence of damage to individual liver cells, as well as extensive acidophil change. The lesions are particularly marked in zone 3 and elicit a macrophage response. Viral particles can be seen on electron microscopy.

Filovirus Infections

Marburg Virus
In 1967, 27 individuals who had been working with African Green monkeys in Marburg, Frankfurt and Belgrade became very seriously ill with fever, conjunctivitis, hepatitis, diarrhoea, renal abnormalities and a bleeding tendency. Five of the 27 died. Subsequently it was shown that the illness had been caused by a virus, for which monkeys were the reservoir. This virus has a tubular structure with a hollow core.

Histological examination of liver from infected humans shows focal necrosis, beginning with acidophil changes in the liver cells. Only a mild inflammatory reaction occurs in relation to these necrotic foci.

Ebola Virus
This is another filovirus causing a severe haemorrhagic fever associated with a 70% mortality rate. Antibodies to this virus are present in 12.4% of the population of six African countries, including the Sudan and Zaire, indicating that the disease is endemic there. The virus is very similar to the Marburg virus and causes numerous areas of focal necrosis within the liver.

CHRONIC HEPATITIS
The term chronic hepatitis is defined as a chronic inflammatory process that may be associated with continuing liver cell necrosis and which lasts for more than 6 months. It may follow an attack of acute viral hepatitis or, instead, may have a much more insidious onset with no history of an antecedent attack of acute hepatitis.

Clinical Features
In many, the disease may be asymptomatic, being detected only as a result of screening. In others, the principal complaint is of **fatigue** or epigastric discomfort.

Chronic hepatitis may result from infection with one of the hepatitis viruses, most notably hepatitis B, C and D. It may also be seen in:
- **reactions to certain drugs** including α-methyldopa, oxyphenisatin, halothane, isoniazid, nitrofurantoin
- **autoimmune disorders**
- **Wilson's disease**
- **α_1-antitrypsin deficiency**

There is a spectrum of changes, the extremes being:
- **chronic persistent hepatitis**
- **chronic active (or aggressive) hepatitis**

Originally, these were regarded as distinct entities with different natural histories. Many now believe that they represent different points in the spectrum of a single disease. Thus, some cases of chronic persistent hepatitis may progress to the chronic active form and, indeed, go on to frank cirrhosis, whereas other cases of chronic active hepatitis may regress to the persistent form.

Chronic Persistent Hepatitis
This is defined on histological criteria (*Fig. 35.10*), shown in the box.

> ### *Microscopic Features*
> These are a combination of:
> - **a brisk mononuclear cell infiltrate of the portal tract connective tissue.** This infiltrate consists of lymphocytes, macrophages and plasma cells, and normally does not transgress the boundary between the portal tract and the liver parenchyma (the so-called 'limiting plate').
> - **preservation of the normal acinar architecture** of the liver.
> - **an absence of patchy hepatocyte death in the part of the acinus that abuts on the portal tract connective tissue** (so-called 'piece-meal necrosis').

Chronic lobular hepatitis is regarded by some as a variant of the chronic persistent form (see below).

> ### *Microscopic Features*
> In chronic lobular hepatitis there is:
> - **preservation of the acinar architecture** for the most part, although there may be some collapse of the reticulin framework in the region of the terminal hepatic venules and some clustering of Kupffer cells containing ceroid pigment (partly oxidized lipid). These findings indicate that loss of hepatocytes has occurred.
> - **evidence of patchy liver cell damage**, expressed chiefly in the form of ballooning degeneration and acidophil change.

Chronic Active Hepatitis
This is, without doubt, the most serious form of chronic hepatitis and that in which cirrhosis is most likely to supervene.

> ### *Microscopic Features*
> - The pathological benchmark that serves to distinguish chronic active hepatitis from other forms of chronic

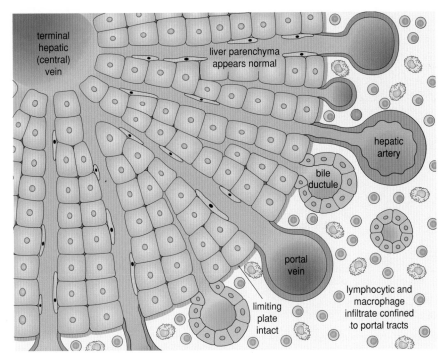

terminal hepatic (central) vein

liver parenchyma appears normal

hepatic artery

bile ductule

portal vein

limiting plate intact

lymphocytic and macrophage infiltrate confined to portal tracts

FIGURE 35.10 Morphological features of chronic persistent hepatitis.

hepatitis is **'piecemeal necrosis'** (*Figs 35.11* and *35.12*). This is defined as destruction of hepatocytes at the parenchyma–portal tract interface, the destruction being carried out chiefly by immunologically competent cells transgressing the limiting plate in significant numbers. In very severe cases there is bridging necrosis, which can connect vascular structures by a thick band of collapsed reticulin.

- In addition to the **portal tract inflammation which is similar to that seen in chronic persistent hepatitis, there is obvious activation of both Kupffer cells and connective tissue matrix-producing cells**. Evidence of the latter is seen in the form of collagenous septa extending from the periphery of the portal triads out into the liver parenchyma. These divide the acini into abnormal nodules of different sizes.

- **Evidence of regeneration is a prominent feature.** This is expressed by the formation of liver cell plates two cells thick or by the formation of rosettes (groups of liver cells, usually up to eight in number, surrounding a small, centrally placed, bile canaliculus). Additional evidence is present in the form of a marked variation in nuclear size; giant multinucleated hepatocytes are often seen.

- **Segmental bile duct lesions may be present.** Both large and small interlobular ducts are affected, the basic change being epithelial hyperplasia leading to narrowing or occlusion.

Hepatitis B in Relation to Chronic Hepatitis

More than 250 million people are believed to suffer from chronic HBV infection. Of these, most live in China and the Far East generally (70–90% of the population of Taiwan show serological markers of HBV infection); chronic hepatitis due to HBV is distinctly uncommon in western Europe and North America. The great prevalence of chronic HBV infection in Asia correlates positively with the high risk of liver cancer in this part of the world.

Why Should this Epidemiological Pattern Be?

Chronicity represents a failure of viral elimination by the infected host, this elimination being mediated via a combination of cellular and humoral immunity and the action of interferons.

The age at which infection occurs appears to have an important bearing on the efficacy of viral elimination. Most adults who become infected succeed in eliminating the virus and thus do not become carriers or develop chronic hepatitis. Indeed, only 1–5% of this group (mostly males) develop chronic infection. In areas of high prevalence such as China, vertical transmission (from mother to infant) plays a very much larger role than in areas of low prevalence; more than 90% of babies infected in this way will become chronic carriers of HBV.

Apart from the effects of age and sex, chronicity is more likely to develop in those in whom cell-mediated immunity is suppressed, for whatever reason.

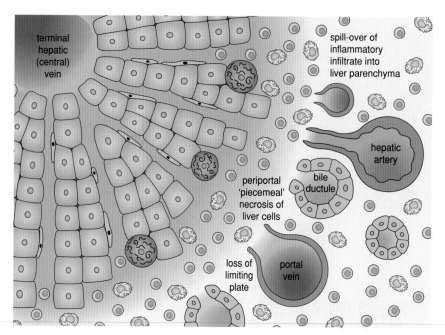

FIGURE 35.11 Morphological features of chronic active (aggressive) hepatitis.

The effects of chronic HBV infection depend on whether or not viral replication is occurring. Thus, in serological terms, patients may be:

1) HBsAg positive, HBeAg positive, HBV DNA positive
2) HBsAg positive, HBeAg negative, HBV DNA positive
3) HBsAg positive, HBeAg negative, HBV DNA negative

The first *two* of these combinations indicate that viral replication is proceeding and these patients are likely to have chronic hepatitis of greater or lesser degrees of severity. The third combination represents individuals who are chronic carriers of HBV but in whom viral replication is not occurring. Serum transaminase levels in this last group are usually normal and, if liver biopsy is performed, the liver shows no evidence of inflammation, although **'ground glass' hepatocytes** may be seen (*Fig. 35.13*).

These are liver cells in which the cytoplasm has a pale, homogeneous appearance, owing to the presence of hypertrophied endoplasmic reticulum. The appearance is associated with HBsAg, which can be identified immunohistochemically. 'Sanded' nuclei may be seen in patients in whom viral replication is proceeding. These are liver cell nuclei in which the chromatin is arranged peripherally, the centre of the nucleus being occupied by granular eosinophilic material. This appearance is due to the accumulation within the nucleus of large numbers of HB core particles.

The continuing expression of HBsAg in carriers in whom there is no viral replication is believed to be due to integration of the HBV genome into the genome of the host cells and subsequent transcription **of only the HBs gene.**

Chronic Autoimmune Hepatitis ('Lupoid' Hepatitis)

This type of chronic liver disease occurs chiefly in young women and is characterized by **jaundice, acne, amenorrhoea, enlargement of liver and spleen, and high plasma immunoglobulin concentrations.**

A pathogenetic role for immune-mediated mechanisms is suggested by:

- a positive LE (lupus erythematosus) cell phenomenon (10% of patients)
- antinuclear antibodies in the plasma of patients (more than 50% of patients)
- a heavy plasma cell infiltrate in the liver
- smooth muscle antibodies in the plasma (40–60% of patients)
- an autoantibody binding specifically to a receptor on liver cell membranes
- an autoantibody reacting with microsomes, distinct from the antimitochondrial antibody found in patients with primary biliary cirrhosis
- a reduction in the number and functional ability of suppressor T cells
- a rapid response to treatment with immunosuppressive agents

Evidence of multisystem disease is suggested by the additional presence of:

- Sjögren's syndrome

a

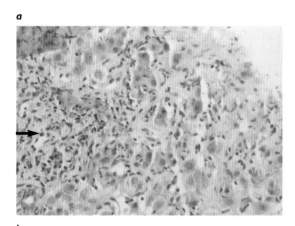

b

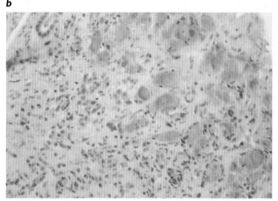

FIGURE 35.12 Chronic active hepatitis. **a** *The portal tract (arrowed) is inflamed and on the left-hand side, the normal clear demarcation between parenchyma and portal tract connective tissue is lost.* **b** *This section has been treated with an antibody against hepatitis B surface antigen, which shows brown staining in cells undergoing piecemeal necrosis.*

- ulcerative colitis
- arthritis
- thyroid disease
- fibrosing alveolitis

Such multisystem disease is found in about 14% of patients and constitutes further support for an autoimmune pathogenesis. The aetiology is less clear. There is a strong association between chronic autoimmune hepatitis and HLA-B8 and HLA-DR3, suggesting a disturbance in immune regulation. In this connection it is interesting that HLA-DR3 may be linked with a regulator gene for suppressor cells.

Antibodies against a number of bacterial and viral species are present in high titre in patients with autoimmune hepatitis. These include enterobacteria, measles, rubella and cytomegalovirus.

Chronic autoimmune hepatitis, if untreated, is associated with a poor prognosis; death is usually due to liver failure.

Autoantibodies are found in many liver diseases, as shown in *Table 35.6*.

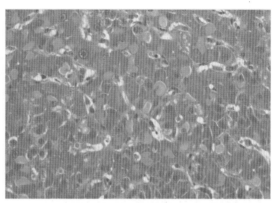

FIGURE 35.13 Chronic active hepatitis. Haematoxylin and eosin-section showing 'ground-glass' liver cells infected by hepatitis B virus.

Some histological clues to the aetiology of chronic hepatitis are shown in *Table 35.7*.

Cirrhosis

Cirrhosis is the final stage of several pathogenetic mechanisms operating either alone or in concert to produce a liver diffusely involved by:

- **fibrosis**
- **the formation of structurally abnormal parenchymal nodules**

Both of these structural changes must be present for a diagnosis of true cirrhosis (*Fig. 35.15*). Fibrosis may occur alone, as in hepatic schistosomiasis, and diffuse nodularity can also be present alone, as in nodular regenerative hyperplasia; neither constitutes true cirrhosis.

The distinction between fibrosis and cirrhosis is worth making because the clinical features and natural histories of these entities differ, as shown in *Table 35.8*.

Aetiology and Pathogenesis

The main pathogenetic pathways leading to cirrhosis are:

1) chronic active hepatitis
2) steatohepatitis (fatty change with evidence of liver cell damage and inflammation)
3) portal fibrosis
4) fibrosis occurring in acinar zone 3

Each of these pathogenetic pathways may be brought about by a number of different causal agents. The first two listed account for most cases of cirrhosis; alcohol-induced steatohepatitis accounts for more than 60% of cases of cirrhosis in Western communities.

Table 35.6 Autoantibodies In Liver Disease

Antibody	Disease	Frequency (%)
Antimitochondrial antibody	Primary biliary cirrhosis	80–95
	Chronic active hepatitis	10–25
Anti-smooth muscle antibody	Chronic active hepatitis	20–60
	Primary biliary cirrhosis	10–30
	Viral hepatitis	50–80
	Alcoholic liver disease	10–15
Antinuclear antibody	Chronic active hepatitis	20–50
	Primary biliary cirrhosis	15–40
	Drug-associated chronic active hepatitis	10–30
Anti-DNA antibody	All types of liver disease	30–60
Liver cell membrane antibody	HBsAg-negative acute hepatitis	15
	Chronic active hepatitis	40
	Cirrhosis	60
Bile canalicular antibody	Chronic active hepatitis or primary biliary cirrhosis	20–40

Table 35.7 Histological Findings in Chronic Hepatitis

Types of hepatitis	Histological finding
Chronic hepatitis B	Ground-glass hepatocytes; sanded nuclei
Chronic hepatitis C	Mild fatty change; numerous acidophil (Councilman) bodies; heavy intra-acinar lymphocytic infiltration; parenchymal giant cells; heavy portal tract lymphocytic infiltration with, in some cases, follicle formation
Chronic hepatitis D	Very severe inflammatory changes; immunohistochemical identification of δ agent
Drug-related chronic hepatitis	Presence of eosinophils in portal inflammatory infiltrate; evidence of cholestasis; granulomas sometimes present
Autoimmune chronic hepatitis	Active parenchymal inflammation; large numbers of plasma cells in infiltrate
Wilson's disease	Chronic hepatitis and fatty change in liver cells; liver cell nuclei vacuolated; Mallory bodies present in cytoplasm; stainable copper present in liver cells
α_1-antitrypsin deficiency	Presence of eosinophilic inclusions in liver cells, staining red with periodic acid–Schiff (PAS) stain. The PAS positivity is resistant to diastase (*Fig. 35.14*), indicating that the inclusions do not consist of glycogen. The inclusions bind antibody raised against α_1-antitrypsin.

From Triger and Wright (1992).

Chronic Active Hepatitis

In cirrhosis that occurs on the basis of chronic hepatitis, the chief processes involved are:

- **regeneration occurring on a substrate of continuing necrosis of liver cells**
- **inflammation in both the portal tract and the liver acini**

The pathological picture of chronic active hepatitis is *not* necessarily synonymous with a chronic viral infection, being seen also in Wilson's disease, chronic autoimmune hepatitis, α_1-antitrypsin deficiency and certain drug-related conditions.

It was originally thought that piecemeal necrosis of liver cells in the region of the parenchyma–portal tract

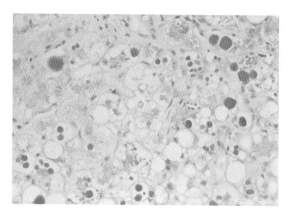

FIGURE 35.14 α$_1$-Antitrypsin deficiency. This liver biopsy has been stained by the periodic acid–Schiff method and subjected to diastase digestion. Note the magenta-coloured bodies in the liver cell cytoplasm.

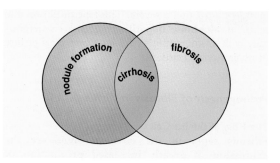

FIGURE 35.15 Two processes are involved in true cirrhosis.

interface was the principal mechanism, but that bridging necrosis (see pp 572 and 574) and intra-acinar necrosis are now believed to be more important.

Steatohepatitis

This is defined in terms of a set of microscopic features, shown in the box. **This picture is seen particularly in alcohol abusers** but may also occur in very obese individuals and in the cirrhosis sometimes caused by the antiarrhythmic agent **amiodarone**.

> ### Microscopic Features
> - a variable degree of **large droplet-type fatty change** in liver cells
> - ballooning degeneration of liver cells, most severe in zone 3 of the acinus
> - **an inflammatory cell reaction** composed of **neutrophils** as well as lymphocytes
> - **new collagen fibres around the affected liver cells**
> - in some instances, **Mallory bodies** in some liver cells. These are amphophilic intracytoplasmic masses (i.e. they bind both haematoxylin and eosin) (see p 589)

Portal Fibrosis

Cirrhosis arising on the basis of portal fibrosis occurs in patients with genetically determined haemochromatosis and in those with chronic biliary obstruction. It is characterized by scarring of the portal tracts, which eventually link up. At this stage, the criteria for cirrhosis (i.e. the combination of fibrosis and nodule formation) are not met, but, with time, true cirrhosis ultimately develops. The parenchymal nodules in this type tend to have an **irregular outline rather than the rounded shape characteristic of the two previously described types of cirrhosis**.

In some instances, cirrhosis may develop via more than one of the pathogenetic pathways listed (see pp 590–594). This is seen especially in two disorders involving intrahepatic bile ducts: **primary biliary cirrhosis and sclerosing cholangitis**, in both of which there is evidence of both portal scarring and ongoing liver cell injury.

Fibrosis in Acinar Zone 3 (Centrilobular Fibrosis)

Here the target zone for scarring is that part of the acinus surrounding the terminal hepatic venules (central veins). These areas of scar tissue become linked up to zone 3 in a mirror image of portal fibrosis. This is most often the result of chronic hepatic venous outflow obstruction. Such obstruction can occur at any level of the venous drainage, ranging from occlusion of the small hepatic venules, as occurs in alkaloid-induced veno-occlusive disease, to chronic cardiac tamponade, as seen in constrictive pericarditis.

Acinar fibrosis in its pure form is fibrosis rather than cirrhosis, but true cirrhosis may develop in time if the

Table 35.8 Features of Fibrosis Compared With Those of Cirrhosis

Feature	Fibrosis	Cirrhosis
Portal hypertension	+++	+
Intrahepatic shunts contributing to portal-systemic encephalopathy	0	+
Impaired liver cell function	0	+
Increased risk of liver cell cancer	0	+

outflow obstruction is severe. This type of fibrosis also occurs in **alcoholic hepatitis** and can act synergistically with steatohepatitis to produce the typical picture of alcohol-related cirrhosis.

Pathogenesis of Fibrosis in Cirrhosis

The Role of the Ito Cell
Fibrous septa in the cirrhotic liver are the expression of greatly increased production of collagen and other matrix proteins. At one time, it was held that such fibrosis resulted from collapse of the existing connective tissue scaffolding following large-scale necrosis of liver cells.

Active growth of connective tissue matrix in the liver requires cells capable of being stimulated to produce connective tissue matrix proteins. Because much of the new matrix in cirrhosis is found in relation to the liver cell plates and the spaces of Disse, it seems reasonable that the candidate cell for the production of matrix proteins should be found in this region. **This cell is the Ito cell, or lipocyte.** The production of fibrous tissue matrix by these cells has been demonstrated in a number of ways, and there is convincing morphological evidence that fibrogenesis in the liver is accompanied by the appearance of the Ito cell changing towards that of a myofibroblast.

A wide variety of chemical signals in culture systems stimulates both proliferation of Ito cells and the production by them of connective tissue matrix proteins. Two important factors are transforming growth factor β (TGF-β) and platelet-derived growth factor (PDGF), which appear to act on the Ito cell in a sequential fashion as the unstimulated Ito cell does not express receptors for PDGF. TGF-β, released by Kupffer cells, appears to have a 'priming' effect on the Ito cell in that exposure causes these cells to express PDGF receptors, but this is unlikely to be its only effect.

Morphological Classification
Attempts to classify cases of cirrhosis morphologically rest on some not very firm supports:
1) **the size and uniformity of the nodules**
2) **the width of the connective tissue septa separating them**
3) **special histological features suggesting one or other specific cause**

Using the first two criteria, cirrhosis has been classified as:
- **Micronodular.** The nodules are uniform in size and small (less than 3 mm in diameter). The fibrous septa are thin and also rather uniform in thickness (*Fig. 35.16*).
- **Macronodular.** The nodules vary in size and are larger than those seen in the micronodular type, ranging in diameter from 3–4 mm to more than

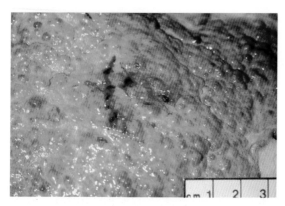

FIGURE 35.16 *The capsular surface of the liver in micronodular cirrhosis showing rather uniform, small nodules.*

1 cm. The fibrous tissue septa vary in thickness and some may be several millimetres in width.
- **Mixed.** There is a wide variation in nodule size, ranging from small to large.

Such a classification is valuable only if it gives reliable aetiological or pathogenetic information. On these criteria this system fails on a number of counts. It is true that some forms of cirrhosis are predominantly micronodular (e.g. alcoholic cirrhosis in its earlier stages), but nodule size *per se* does not give many aetiological clues and other data must be factored in, as shown in *Tables 35.9* and *35.14*. In addition, cirrhosis that starts as a micronodular process can become either macronodular or mixed if the patient survives long enough for large regenerating nodules to develop.

Another unhelpful feature is that it is not possible to make a diagnosis of macronodular cirrhosis on a needle biopsy because the diameter of the usual biopsy needle falls well short of that of a 'macronodule'. One useful piece of information, however, that can be obtained from assessing nodule size is that micronodular cirrhosis tends to occur in cases in which the injury (e.g. alcohol abuse) is long continued.

Basic Microscopic Features of Cirrhosis
- **Fibrous septa** of differing widths often containing blood vessels (both venous radicles and small arteries), small bile ducts and bile ductules.
- **Regeneration nodules** recognizable by their being surrounded by fibrous tissue septa. Within these nodules, normally situated terminal hepatic venules and portal tracts are not seen; this disturbance of the normal vascular architecture is very striking. Liver cell regeneration is shown by the presence of liver cell columns which, for the most part, are two cells thick instead of just one as normal. Some care must be taken in interpreting this feature should the biopsy

come from a child, because the presence of liver cell plates that are two cells thick is perfectly normal from birth until about 6 years of age.

- In addition, there may be evidence of continuing liver cell injury and its associated inflammatory reaction in the form of **piecemeal necrosis**. Another non-specific feature, regarded by some as evidence of 'activity' of the cirrhotic process, is the presence within the fibrous tissue of relatively large numbers of proliferated bile ductules.

Other histological features that may provide clues as to aetiology are discussed in the appropriate sections or shown in *Tables 35.9* and *35.14*.

MICRONODULAR CIRRHOSIS

ALCOHOLIC LIVER DISEASE

The association between liver disease and alcohol abuse has been known for more than 2000 years. At one time, it was believed that alcohol affected the liver indirectly, the liver damage being mediated via alcohol-related malnutrition. It is now accepted that alcohol is indeed a hepatotoxin and, in Europe and North America, the frequency of chronic liver disease mirrors trends in alcohol intake. The mortality rate from cirrhosis increases during periods of increased alcohol consumption and decreases with decreased alcohol intake.

The majority of heavy drinkers develop fatty change in the liver cells, associated with an increase in the size of the liver. Evidence of more severe alcohol-related damage is seen in 20–35% of such drinkers and full-blown cirrhosis as diagnosed on liver biopsy affects 17–30% of heavy drinkers.

The 'average' daily alcohol intake in cirrhotics has been estimated as being 180 g over a period of 25 years. There is a continuum of risk, as shown in data relating to males (see *Table 35.10*)

Several studies have shown that both the average intake required to produce cirrhosis and the 'threshold' intake are lower in women than in men. The type of alcoholic beverage and the drinking pattern – 'bingeing versus soaking' – do not seem to be responsible for any variations in the risk, of developing chronic liver disease.

Table 35.10 Daily Intake of Alcohol and Risk of Cirrhosis in Men

Daily intake (g)	Relative risk of cirrhosis
0.2	1
40–60	6
60–80	14

Table 35.9 Micronodular Cirrhosis

Frequency	Aetiology	Typical microscopic features
60–70%	Alcohol	Fatty change and/or ballooning degeneration of liver cells; neutrophils in inflammatory cell infiltrate; Mallory bodies in liver cells; may be haemosiderin in liver cells
5%	'Primary' biliary cirrhosis	In early stages heavy lymphocyte infiltrate in portal tracts; presence of epithelioid cell portal tract granulomas; destruction of medium-sized bile ducts; cholestasis in zone 1 (periportal); high levels of copper in liver cells (intralysosomal and apparently non-toxic); presence of Mallory bodies in some cases
<5%	Large bile duct obstruction	Severe degree of cholestasis; marked bile ductule proliferation; irregular outline of nodules
5%	Haemochromatosis	Large amounts of haemosiderin in liver cells, Kupffer cells and ductular epithelium
Rare	Intestinal bypass	Marked fatty change in liver cells; Mallory bodies present in some cases
Rare	Cystic fibrosis	Periodic acid–Schiff-positive material in proliferated ductules in portal tracts
Rare	Indian childhood cirrhosis	Mallory bodies

Metabolic Pathways for Alcohol within the Liver

Three major steps are involved in the metabolism of alcohol by liver cells:

1) **Oxidation of alcohol to acetaldehyde.** This takes place within the liver cell cytosol.
2) **Conversion of acetaldehyde to acetate**, occurring within the mitochondria.
3) **Release of acetate from the liver cell into the blood**, where it is utilized by peripheral tissues in which final oxidation to fatty acids, water and carbon dioxide takes place.

The major pathway for oxidation of alcohol is catalysed by the enzyme **alcohol dehydrogenase**, coded for on the long arm of chromosome 4 and existing in a number of variant forms.

$$CH_3CH_2OH + NAD = CH_3CHO + NADH + H^+$$

Conversion of alcohol to acetaldehyde requires nicotinamide adenine dinucleotide (NAD), which is reduced to NADH. An increase in the ratio of NADH to NAD results in a reduction in the redox state of the liver cells. It is this change that is associated with most of the main acute metabolic effects of alcohol, including:

- **inhibition of gluconeogenesis**, leading to hypoglycaemia
- **impairment of fatty acid oxidation**, which, together with a decreased synthesis of carrier proteins necessary for triglyceride transport from liver cell to the blood, leads to increased amounts of fat accumulating within the liver cells
- **a decrease in the activity of the citric acid cycle**

Acetaldehyde itself has a number of potentially deleterious effects on the liver:

- It forms adducts with proteins which then act as new antigens and elicit the formation of, possibly, cell-damaging antibodies.
- It inactivates certain enzymes.
- It causes a decrease in the repair of damaged DNA.
- It produces alterations in microtubules, mitochondria and plasma membranes.
- It causes depletion of the major intracellular scavenger systems based on reduced glutathione, and thus promotes free radical-mediated damage.

A second pathway for the oxidation of ethanol exists within the microsomes and is known as the **microsomal ethanol-oxidizing system (MEOS)**. Increased activation of MEOS produces increased amounts of acetaldehyde but, in addition, oxygen free radicals are formed and these may cause damage to hepatocytes via a number of different pathways.

Induction of these microsomal enzymes is believed to account for the increased susceptibility, seen in heavy drinkers, to the hepatotoxic effects of industrial solvents, anaesthetics, chemical carcinogens and drugs such as paracetamol and isoniazid.

Most studies show that chronic alcohol ingestion increases the elimination of alcohol by the liver as a result of adaptive changes, not yet clearly understood, in the metabolic pathways involved in alcohol oxidation. If, however, there is existing liver damage, or if the person is suffering from restricted food intake, this increase in alcohol elimination does not occur.

Pathological Features

Three sets of pathological changes, either isolated or coexisting, occur in the livers of alcohol abusers. In order of increasing severity these are:

1) alcoholic fatty liver
2) steatohepatitis
3) cirrhosis

Alcoholic Fatty Liver

This is both the most frequent and the earliest morphological liver change to occur as a result of excess alcohol intake. It is also the only alcohol-related lesion that can be expected to resolve if excess alcohol intake is stopped. There is good evidence that alcoholic fatty liver is almost certainly the result of a direct toxic effect on the liver and is not related to malnutrition.

Macroscopic Features

The liver may be grossly enlarged from a normal weight of 1.5 kg to 2.0–2.5 kg. It is pale yellow and feels greasy. In extreme cases, the accumulation of fat may be so great that the organ floats in water.

Microscopic Features

Conventionally prepared paraffin sections, treated with lipid solvents, show accumulated fat, chiefly as large clear vacuoles within the liver cell cytoplasm (*Fig. 35.17*). The nucleus and other cell components are compressed against the plasma membrane.

Occasionally, a different pattern of intrahepatocyte fatty change is seen, the large vacuoles being replaced by small droplets such as are more commonly seen in the fatty liver of Reye's syndrome and fatty liver of pregnancy. From time to time, cell membranes between adjacent fat-loaded liver cells rupture, forming very large intrahepatic spaces called '**fat cysts**'. Usually there is no evidence of either cell necrosis or an inflammatory reaction, but occasionally these may be seen, the resulting lesion being termed a **lipogranuloma**.

This pathological picture is reversible but, in some cases, a more menacing feature makes its appearance in the form of fibrosis around the terminal hepatic venules; this may be accompanied by some pericellular scarring in zone 3. Such fibrosis is a marker of increased risk of alcoholic cirrhosis.

Steatohepatitis (Alcoholic Hepatitis)

Alcoholic hepatitis is much less common than alcoholic fatty liver. Its defining criteria are shown in the box.

Microscopic Features

The defining criteria of alcoholic hepatitis are:

1) Hepatocytes showing 'ballooning' degeneration, especially in acinar zone 3. This feature is very suggestive of alcoholic liver disease.

2) Fatty change of the large droplet type in many liver cells.

3) Focal necrosis of liver cells eliciting a **neutrophil** response.

4) Mallory's hyaline bodies in some liver cells, very frequently those that show 'ballooning'. The Mallory body is an irregularly shaped, rather coarse, clump of material that has a reddish blue colour in haematoxylin and eosin-stained sections (*Fig. 35.18*). These bodies represent a derangement of the cytoskeleton of the liver cell and consist of twisted meshworks of fibrils believed to be derived from the prekeratin, intermediate, filaments of the cell. **In the context of the other morphological changes described here, the presence of Mallory bodies strongly suggests that alcohol is the responsible aetiological agent.** They may occur, however, in association with a number of other pathological states in the liver and, **by themselves**, must not be regarded as being pathognomonic of alcohol-related damage.

5) Grossly enlarged mitochondria may be seen in the form of large granules that stain red with trichrome methods. They are held to indicate that heavy drinking has occurred recently and may disappear after several weeks' abstinence.

6) In some cases, evidence of cholestasis, in the form of small plugs of inspissated bile in the canaliculi, may be present.

7) Some degree of fibrosis in relation to the terminal hepatic venules and to the liver cells in zone 3 is almost always present. These changes may be very severe, and, in some cases, there may be a linkage between the fibrous tissue around the terminal hepatic venules and the connective tissue of the portal tract. This is accompanied by extensive loss of liver cells in the affected acini. The term **central hyaline sclerosis** has been applied to this striking morphological feature. It carries an ominous prognostic significance.

Clinical Features

Patients with alcoholic hepatitis may be symptom-free, although hepatomegaly is usually found on examination. They may complain of vague abdominal discomfort and a few have a frankly hepatitic illness associated with jaundice, fever, nausea, abdominal pain and a neutrophil leucocytosis.

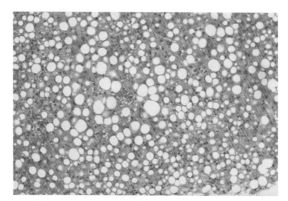

FIGURE 35.17 Fatty liver in an alcoholic. The paraffin-embedded, haematoxylin and eosin-stained section shows numerous large clear vacuoles occupying most of the cytoplasm of the affected cells.

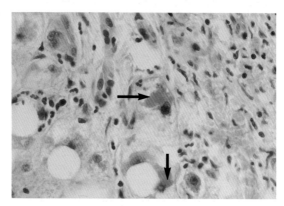

FIGURE 35.18 Alcoholic liver disease. Note the reddish-blue Mallory bodies in ballooned hepatocytes (arrows).

In the long term, **the incidence of full-blown cirrhosis is nine times higher in patients with steatohepatitis than those with alcoholic fatty liver**. Much depends on whether the patient can be persuaded to abstain from alcohol. Of those who persist in alcohol abuse, about one-third will develop cirrhosis within 2 years. Resolution of the pathological changes can occur in those who stop drinking alcohol.

Alcoholic Cirrhosis

Cirrhosis is the final stage in the development of alcoholic liver disease. The morphological features depend on the stage at which the liver is examined.

Macroscopic Features

The early cirrhotic liver is usually enlarged, mostly because of the large amounts of intracellular fat. The liver is a pale yellowish-brown; both the capsular and cut surfaces show a fine, uniform nodularity, the nodules being separated by narrow fibrous septa (*Fig. 35.19*).

With longer duration of the cirrhosis, the micronodular pattern alters. The uniformity of the nodules is lost and some large nodules develop, presumably as the result of differential degrees of regeneration in different areas. Fat becomes a less conspicuous component and the colour changes to brown.

As a consequence of the disappearance of the fat loading in the liver cells, the size of the organ decreases and in the final stages the liver may have shrunken to a weight well below normal.

Microscopic Features

In the early stages, the fine nodularity seen on naked-eye examination correlates with fine fibrous septa connecting portal tract connective tissue with the terminal hepatic venules. These septa may either enclose individual lobules or, as is more common, subdivide the lobules so that the normal relationship between portal tracts and terminal hepatic venules is lost. This architectural abnormality is compounded by regeneration of the parenchyma.

The portal tract connective tissue may show the presence of a chronic inflammatory cell infiltrate, and bile ductule proliferation may also be present (*Fig. 35.20*). In addition the abnormalities seen in alcoholic hepatitis may also be present. Another, not uncommon, feature is stainable iron in the form of haemosiderin, which stains blue in sections treated with potassium ferrocyanide at acid pH. This iron overload may be due to increased absorption from the gut and this may be associated with increased intake of liquors that are rich in iron, such as red wine and some of the home-brewed beers consumed in large quantities in certain parts of Africa.

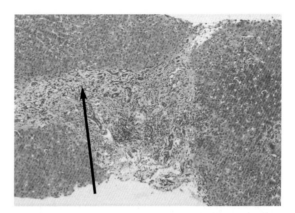

FIGURE 35.20 *Alcoholic cirrhosis. This low-power view shows nodules separated by fibrous septa (arrowed) in which numerous proliferated ductules are present.*

intimal lining of hepatic veins and the fibrosis occurring in relation to terminal hepatic venules will tend to impede the **outflow** of blood from the liver. In addition, there may be compression of hepatic veins by regenerating nodules and this also contributes to the genesis of **postsinusoidal portal hypertension**.

Equally important from the metabolic viewpoint, the effective circulation in the liver parenchyma is decreased, partly as a result of the vascular channels that appear in the fibrous septa and which constitute small portal–systemic shunts. In addition, intra-acinar fibrosis in the spaces of Disse will still further isolate liver cells from the blood flowing into the liver from the hepatic artery and portal vein.

Prognosis in Alcoholic Cirrhosis

The survival rate for patients with histologically proven cirrhosis depends on two factors:

1) whether diagnosis is followed by abstinence from alcohol
2) whether jaundice, ascites or haematemesis has supervened

The importance of these factors is emphasized in *Table 35.11*.

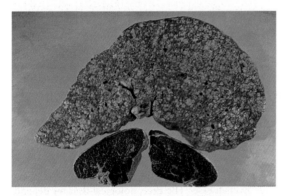

FIGURE 35.19 *Alcoholic cirrhosis. The liver shows diffuse nodularity; the presence of portal hypertension can be inferred by the increased size of the spleen shown below the liver.*

Effects of Cirrhosis on Blood Flow Patterns in the Liver

The combination of fibrosis and regeneration has major effects on blood flow in the liver. Thickening of the

Table 35.11 Five-year Survival Rates in Patients with Alcoholic Cirrhosis

| | 5-year survival rate (%) | |
	abstainers	continuing drinkers
No jaundice, No ascites, No haematemesis	88.9	62.8
Jaundice	57.5	33.3
Ascites	52.4	32.7
Haematemesis	35	21

OTHER FORMS OF MICRONODULAR CIRRHOSIS

Primary Biliary Cirrhosis

The term **primary biliary cirrhosis** is something of a misnomer because only comparatively late in its natural history does true cirrhosis develop. A name more accurately describing the pathology of this condition is **chronic, non-suppurative, destructive cholangitis**.

The disease starts with inflammation and destruction of small septal and interlobular bile ducts (35–75 μm in diameter), and only later proceeds to fibrosis and to the formation of abnormal parenchymal nodules. The cells mediating this bile duct injury are almost certainly cytotoxic T lymphocytes, and primary biliary cirrhosis can, with justice, be regarded as an autoimmune disease.

Epidemiology

Primary biliary cirrhosis shows a marked predilection for middle-aged women: 90% of patients are female and 75% of these are aged 40–59 years. The reason for this marked skewing of the female : male ratio is unknown. The disorder is fairly rare (estimated prevalence 3.7–14.4 cases per 100 000 population; estimated incidence 5.8–15 per million population per annum; proportion of deaths due to cirrhosis 0.6–2%).

Clinical Features

Clinical presentation may be in one of two forms:
1) **Symptomatic.** Here the principal clinical features are:
- pruritus (itch)
- slowly progressive jaundice

2) **Asymptomatic.** These cases are identified by the finding of:
- unexplained enlargement of the liver
- raised serum alkaline phosphatase concentrations, coupled with increased concentrations of γ-glutamyl transpeptidase.

Important for diagnosis is the finding of high titres of antimitochondrial antibodies in the plasma of patients suspected of having the disease. Such antibodies are present in 95% of patients with primary biliary cirrhosis. It is not without interest that there are resemblances between mammalian and bacterial mitochondria. Serum from patients with primary biliary cirrhosis binds not only to the mitochondrial antigens mentioned but also to antigens of a similar molecular weight derived from Enterobacteriaceae. It has been suggested, therefore, that the mitochondrial antibody response in these patients might be elicited by bacterial antigens. There is as yet no supporting evidence for this intriguing idea.

Aetiology

The presence of a large number of associated immunological abnormalities in primary biliary cirrhosis, as shown in *Table 35.12*, strongly suggests that immune regulation is seriously disturbed.

Macroscopic Features

At post-mortem examination in long-standing cases, the liver is enlarged and a rather dark green in colour because of the severe and prolonged cholestasis (*Fig. 35.22*). The lymph nodes in the portal hepatis are enlarged.

Microscopic Features

The appearances seen on histological examination of liver samples from patients with primary biliary cirrhosis depend on the stage of the disease at the time of examination.

1) In the early stages the **only pathognomonic lesion is inflammatory destruction of interlobular or septal bile ducts** (not often seen in needle biopsies). There is a florid lymphocyte and plasma cell infiltrate, even in portal tracts where no bile ducts can be seen, and some of the lymphocytes are arranged in a follicular pattern. Damaged bile ducts show swelling of the lining epithelium and focal breaks in the basement membrane. The end result of this process is disappearance of the affected bile duct segments.

2) In some affected portal tracts, **epithelioid granulomas** may be seen. Their presence, in association with the features just described, is strongly suggestive of primary biliary cirrhosis.

3) With disease progression a number of other features may be seen. These include **cholestasis** in the form of numerous bile plugs in canaliculi in acinar zone 1 (the periportal zone), **widening of the portal tracts as the result of fibrosis**, and **proliferation of bile ductules**, which may be very striking.

4) Extension of the inflammatory process to involve the parenchyma in zone 1 of the acinus is often seen. The 'limiting plate', which normally constitutes a boundary between the portal tract and the liver parenchyma, becomes blurred and piecemeal necrosis as described in chronic hepatitis is seen. It may be difficult at this stage to differentiate between primary biliary cirrhosis and chronic active hepatitis.

5) This distinction is helped by identifying a set of changes in the liver cells in zone 1 resulting from long-continued cholestasis. These changes ('cholate stasis') consist of swelling and pallor of the liver cells; the accumulation of coarse granules (lysosomes that have accumulated copper and copper-binding protein); and the presence, in some cases, of Mallory bodies. It has been suggested that these changes are due to a detergent effect of accumulated bile salts, hence the term cholate stasis.

Table 35.12 Immune Abnormalities in Primary Biliary Cirrhosis

Abnormality	Comment
Increased levels of serum immunoglobulins	This applies particularly to IgM. This IgM is very immunoreactive and can spontaneously convert C3 to C3b via the classical pathway.
Presence of circulating autoantibodies	Many autoantibodies, apart from the very common antimitochondrial antibody are found. Antigens recognized include epitopes on nuclear membranes, thyroid, lymphocytes, acetylcholine receptors and RNA.
Skin anergy	Patients have negative skin reactions when tested with such antigens as tuberculin or DNCB.
Presence of granulomas	Granulomas are found not only in the inflamed portal tracts (*Fig. 35.21*) during the early stages of the disease but also in lymph nodes draining the liver, lung (where it may be associated with interstitial scarring) and bone marrow.
Decreased suppressor T-cell function	There is a decreased number of T cells in the blood, associated with decreased T suppressor cell function *in vitro*. There is no evidence that this plays a pathogenetic role. Some 25% of healthy first-degree relatives also show depressed suppressor cell function *in vitro*.
Resemblance of lesions to those of graft versus host reaction	
Association with other diseases believed to have an autoimmune basis	Non-hepatic disorders are associated with primary biliary cirrhosis in at least 70% of cases. These include Sjögren's syndrome, scleroderma, the full-blown **CREST** syndrome (**calcinosis cutis, Raynaud's phenomenon, oesophageal dysfunction, sclerodactyly, telangiectasia**), autoimmune thyroiditis and interstitial fibrosis in the lung associated with granuloma formation. Curiously, though, autoimmune mechanisms cannot be invoked here; patients with primary biliary cirrhosis also show an increased risk of breast carcinoma.
Chronic activation of the complement system	The rate of C3 turnover is markedly increased as a result of activation of the classical pathway of complement activation.

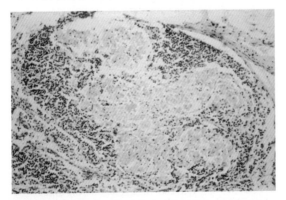

FIGURE 35.21 *Primary biliary cirrhosis: portal tract showing lymphocytic infiltration and epithelioid cell granuloma formation.*

Continuing liver cell injury is followed by nodular regeneration and thus by the development of true cirrhosis. These patients may develop most of the complications to which any cirrhotic patient is at risk, but there are some special features that arise from prolonged cholestasis:

1) **The development of xanthomata as a result of increased in serum lipid concentrations.** Bile acid excretion is an important pathway for the control of blood cholesterol levels, and if this is interfered with, secondary hyperlipidaemia develops. There is a marked increase in the serum concentration of lipoprotein X. This is due to reflux of biliary lecithin into the plasma. This lecithin interacts with free cholesterol, albumin and apoprotein C. If the rate at which this reaction

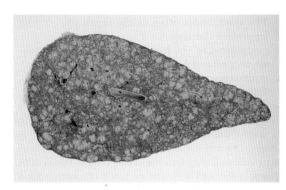

FIGURE 35.22 *Primary biliary cirrhosis. Note the dark green colour of this diffusely nodular liver.*

occurs exceeds the ability of lecithin cholesterol acyltransferase to esterify the cholesterol, lipoprotein X is formed. The occurrence of skin xanthomata around the eyes, on the upper lid and in the palmar creases is *not* associated with accelerated atherogenesis. Sometimes the hyperlipidaemia may be associated with a xanthomatous neuropathy, manifested clinically as pain in the fingers (experienced particularly when opening doors) and in the toes.

2) **An increased risk for developing duodenal ulcer.** This is believed to be due to the decreased amounts of **alkaline** bile present in the duodenum.

3) **A marked risk of developing the disorders of bone remodelling: osteomalacia and osteoporosis.** Osteomalacia is associated with vitamin D deficiency due partly to bile salt lack and steatorrhoea and partly to increased loss of vitamin D in the urine. The mechanisms leading to osteoporosis are unknown.

Prognosis

This is extremely variable. Now that it is possible to diagnose primary biliary cirrhosis in the prejaundice stage, it is clear that the duration of the illness may be very long. Serum bilirubin levels are the best indicator of prognosis. These may rise very little during the first few years of jaundice. A steep rise, however, suggests that the patient may die within the next 2 years. Obviously signs of liver failure such as ascites, oedema, decreased concentrations of serum albumin and an increased prothrombin time also carry an ominous prognostic significance.

An association with other autoimmune disorders such as Sjögren's syndrome usually indicates a poor prognosis, as does the presence of bridging necrosis, cholestasis and piecemeal necrosis on biopsy of the liver.

Sclerosing Cholangitis

Sclerosing cholangitis is a progressive and incurable disorder of unknown aetiology. It is characterized by irregular periductal fibrosis affecting both extrahepatic and intrahepatic bile ducts, although in some cases only intrahepatic ducts are affected. The scarring process causes focal stenosis in the affected ducts. On cholangiography this is expressed in the form of a highly characteristic 'beaded' appearance of the ducts.

Scarring of bile ducts can, of course, occur in association with stones, tumour or bacterial infection, but the sclerosing process discussed here is not associated with any of these and is designated as primary sclerosing cholangitis.

Aetiology

Although the cause of sclerosing cholangitis is not known, there are some well-recognized associations. These include:

- Some 50–70% of cases of sclerosing cholangitis occur in patients with chronic inflammatory bowel disease, the vast majority of whom have ulcerative colitis. Occasionally sclerosing cholangitis is found in patients with retroperitoneal fibrosis, mediastinal fibrosis and chronic pancreatitis. Of patients with chronic inflammatory bowel disease, 4–5% also suffer from sclerosing cholangitis. Inflammatory bowel disease affecting the colon proximal to the splenic flexure is more likely to be associated with sclerosing cholangitis than that in which the distal colon is the principal target for the inflammatory process.
- Sclerosing cholangitis and the major histocompatibility antigens B8 and DR3. These data have been adduced as suggesting an autoimmune origin, although there is also some evidence, principally from animal experiments, that toxin-mediated damage associated with the inflammatory bowel disease may be responsible.

Clinical Features and Epidemiology

There is a striking male predominance with the male : female ratio being 2 : 1. The commonest age at which patients present is between the third and fifth decades of life. As in the case of primary biliary cirrhosis, the diagnosis of sclerosing cholangitis may be made in either the **symptomatic** or the **asymptomatic** phase. In the first case, patients are most likely to present complaining of the insidious onset of **jaundice, fatigue and itch.** Asymptomatic cases are usually identified because of the discovery of a **raised serum alkaline phosphatase** concentration.

The signs on physical examination depend on the stage of the disease. In long-established cases there may be a combination of hepatomegaly, splenomegaly and jaundice.

Diagnosis is established on the basis of a combination of biochemical, radiological and histological criteria.

Biochemical Features

The chief biochemical abnormality, as already pointed out, is an increase in the plasma concentration of alkaline phosphatase. Frequently, abnormalities of copper metabolism are noted. These are seen in all types of biliary cirrhosis and are most likely to be the result of long-term cholestasis.

Radiological Features

Retrograde cholangiography shows:
1) diffusely distributed annular strictures which are multifocal; intervening segments of the bile ducts appear normal
2) short band-like strictures
3) sac-like outpouchings

All three features combine to give a characteristic beaded appearance to the intrahepatic bile ducts.

Histological Features

The tissue diagnosis of sclerosing cholangitis is not easy because the characteristic changes are not usually seen in needle biopsies of the liver, although they are visible on wedge biopsies.

Macroscopic Features

Extrahepatic duct segments which are involved show obliteration of their lumina by scar tissue and have the appearance of fibrous cords.

Microscopic Features

The most characteristic feature is concentric layering of fibrous tissue around the duct lumina, associated with atrophy of the epithelial lining. The duct lumina become filled with fibrous tissue and eventually the smaller ducts within portal tracts disappear, leaving fibrous scars behind. In the early stages of the disease there is a brisk inflammatory reaction within the portal tracts and this may make the histological distinction between sclerosing cholangitis and primary biliary cirrhosis difficult.

The later stages of sclerosing cholangitis follow much the same path as described in relation to primary biliary cirrhosis (i.e. the development of cholate stasis, portal fibrosis and eventually true cirrhosis).

Complications

These are the same as those of primary biliary cirrhosis. In addition, patients suffering from sclerosing cholangitis have an increased risk of:
1) gallstones
2) recurrent episodes of acute duct inflammation (cholangitis)
3) carcinoma of the gallbladder

Secondary Biliary Cirrhosis

Secondary biliary cirrhosis is the consequence of long-standing, unrelieved, extrahepatic bile duct obstruction. The causes of such obstruction include:
- **postinflammatory stricture of the common bile duct, most often as the result of operative damage**
- **neoplasms of the bile duct, head of pancreas or ampulla of Vater**
- **impaction of gallstones in the extrahepatic biliary system**
- **congenital biliary atresia**

Bile stasis is a prominent and early feature in the natural history of this disorder and bile may be seen within the lumina of interlobular bile ducts as well as in canaliculi, liver cells and Kupffer cells. This retained bile is commonly associated with the presence of neutrophils in and around the duct lumina. This inspissated bile damages the lining of the bile ducts and canaliculi, and areas of bile staining of the parenchyma associated with necrosis of the liver cells develop. These are known as **bile infarcts**. In some instances central liquefaction develops in such lesions, producing what is called a **bile lake**. In due time, adjacent portal tracts become connected by septa of fibrous tissue and eventually true cirrhosis develops.

HAEMOCHROMATOSIS AND OTHER IRON STORAGE DISORDERS AFFECTING THE LIVER

Results of Iron Overload: Haemosiderosis and Haemochromatosis

The patterns of disease are determined largely by the **site of excess iron deposition**. In turn, the site of iron deposition is determined largely by plasma iron concentrations.

Where plasma iron concentrations are high and the degree of transferrin saturation is greater than 60% (as in genetically determined haemochromatosis), iron tends to be deposited in parenchymal cells, in which considerable damage may be produced. It is the degree of parenchymal iron overload that determines the severity of the disease rather than the total body iron content. In iron overload states in which plasma iron concentrations are not high (as in overload from repeated blood transfusions), the iron is stored principally in cells of the reticuloendothelial system. This is associated with very little tissue injury or scarring. The term **haemosiderosis** is used in this situation and need not imply an increase in the total iron content of the body.

In contrast, the term **haemochromatosis** is applied to a situation in which there is:
1) deposition of excess iron in the parenchymal cells of the liver and of a number of other organs, this deposition leading to cell damage, scarring and eventually dysfunction of the affected organs
2) an increase in total body iron content due to an inappropriately high level of iron absorption.

The toxicity of excess intraparenchymal iron is believed to be due to the generation of reactive oxygen species (oxygen free radicals) within the affected cells, resulting in increased demands on the antioxidant defences and eventual membrane damage as a result of lipid peroxidation.

Haemochromatosis is an inherited disorder of iron metabolism. It is characterized by defective regulation of iron absorption across the small intestinal epithelium and, consequently, a marked increase in the body's total iron content. This excess iron is stored in the parenchymal cells of a number of different organs and tissues, the pathophysiological effects being related to these storage sites.

Epidemiology

Haemochromatosis is one of the commonest genetic disorders in the Western world, and is inherited in an autosomal recessive pattern. The defective gene is known to be tightly linked to the A genes of the major histocompatibility complex on the short arm of chromosome 6. A candidate gene called *HLA-H*, encoding an HLA class I-like molecule, has been identified and cloned. In haemochromatosis there is a characteristic point mutation leading to the substitution of tyrosine for cysteine at position 282. The vast majority of patients with haemochromatosis are homozygous for this mutation.

There is some controversy as to the A3 gene frequency with which the risk of haemochromatosis has been linked. Homozygosity in respect of this gene occurs in 3–5 per 1000 individuals of European descent. There is a carrier frequency ranging from 1 in 10 to 1 in 15. Thus, in a city the size of London (approximately 10 million inhabitants), 30 000 people should have the disease. The gene frequency in the general population cannot be the only determining factor because **haemochromatosis occurs five times as commonly in males as in females** even though the frequency of homozygosity for the abnormal gene is equal for both sexes. The diagnosis must often be a presumptive one, because there is no phenotypic marker for the disease other than the presence of iron overload.

Clinical Features

Haemochromatosis was first recognized in 1865, the defining criteria being **hepatomegaly, skin pigmentation and diabetes mellitus**. It is now realized that the manifestations of haemochromatosis are at once more protean and more subtle than the triad described above, and the frequency with which the diagnosis is made has increased greatly.

Pathogenesis

Iron Metabolism

The pathogenesis of haemochromatosis cannot be appreciated other than against the background of normal iron metabolism. A normal man has a total iron content of 4–5 g.

Iron in the Tissues

Half of the iron in the tissues is accounted for by haemoglobin, about a quarter is stored (chiefly in the cells of the reticuloendothelial system) and the remainder is located in other body cells. Normally, most stored iron is bound to the protein **apoferritin**, which can absorb several hundred atoms of iron. A small amount of ferritin circulates in the plasma and an increase in circulating ferritin levels indicates an excess of stored iron.

Iron in the Plasma

This is transported bound to the protein, **transferrin**. Circulating transferrin is usually only about one-third saturated and there is sufficient of this protein in the plasma to transport 300 μg iron per 100 ml blood.

Iron Absorption from the Gut

The absorption of dietary iron is regulated in the small gut wall by mechanisms still poorly understood. Depletion of the body's iron stores, (e.g. in chronic bleeding) leads to increased iron absorption; conversely, if iron stores are increased, absorption decreases.

Iron Excretion

Although there is no specific excretory pathway, iron loss does occur. In males, daily loss is about 1 mg. About 65% of iron loss occurs from the gut; the remainder is lost in the urine and sweat. Obviously, females lose additional iron in the course of menstruation; about 15–30 mg iron is lost per cycle. This is compensated for by additional iron absorption from the gut. Pregnancy brings with it additional needs for iron, and this too is provided for by increases in absorption.

Disorders Associated with Iron Overload

A number of different mechanisms may account for increases in total body iron content:

1) Where the genetic abnormality specific for haemochromatosis exists, there is **a much higher than normal level of iron absorption, unrelated to the body's needs for iron**. Over a period of 25–50 years, as much as 15–50 g iron may be stored in the tissues.

2) Certain **disorders of red cell formation can be associated with increased absorption of iron**. The most significant examples are those in which red cell formation is ineffective, such as **thalassaemia major** and **hereditary sideroblastic anaemia** (see pp 888–889).

3) Certain types of **liver disease**, most notably alcohol-related cirrhosis, may be complicated by iron overload. In the alcoholic most of the iron deposited in the liver is present in the Kupffer cells rather than in the liver parenchyma, and the total amount of iron stored rarely exceeds 2 g. In practice, the distinction between pure alcoholic liver disease and haemochromatosis may be difficult

because there is a high prevalence of alcoholism in patients with true haemochromatosis. Indeed, it has been suggested that alcohol may increase the expression of the gene for haemochromatosis.

4) **A great deal of debate has occurred over the** proposition that iron overload can occur in metabolically normal people as a result of **prolonged oral ingestion of large amounts of iron, usually in alcoholic beverages** (see p 590).

5) Iron overload can also occur as a result of **parenteral administration of iron**. The chief route is by repeated blood transfusions in patients with chronic anaemia not treatable by other means.

Pathological Features

In established cases of haemochromatosis, the total iron content ranges between 15 and 50 g. The organs most severely affected are the liver and the pancreas, in which the iron content may be 50–100 times as great as normal. Other sites of predilection for iron deposition are cardiac muscle, skin and other endocrine glands, with the curious exception of the testis where

the iron content is not significantly raised despite the fact that hypogonadism is a characteristic clinical feature which often occurs early in the course of the disease. This hypogonadism, which is accompanied by testicular atrophy, sterility and decreased body hair, is probably of pituitary origin and, indeed, large amounts of iron are deposited in the pituitary in haemochromatosis.

The morphological changes occurring in some of the most severely affected organs and tissues are shown in *Fig. 35.23* and *Table 35.13*.

MACRONODULAR CIRRHOSIS

The macronodular cirrhoses are characterized by:

1) a lack of uniformity in nodule size

2) large regeneration nodules measuring 1 cm or more in diameter

3) separation of these nodules by coarse, irregular scars

The causes and typical features are shown in *Table 35.14*.

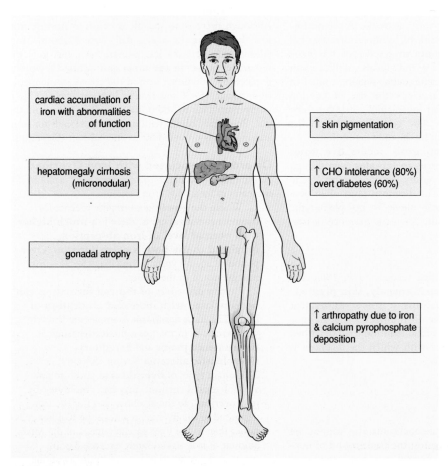

FIGURE 35.23 Features of haemochromatosis.

Table 35.13 Pathological Features of Haemochromatosis

Organ	Pathological features
Liver	The liver is greatly enlarged, often weighing more than 2 kg. It is firmer than normal and has a striking **reddish-brown colour**. This can be shown to be due to haemosiderin deposition by immersing a small portion of the tissue in a mixture of potassium ferrocyanide and dilute hydrochloric acid. The presence of iron is shown by the development of a turquoise blue colour, known as the Prussian blue or Perl's reaction (*Fig. 35.24*). The increased firmness of the tissue is due to **fibrosis**. The fibrous tissue septa, which extend out from the portal triads, form a network surrounding groups of liver cell acini. In the early stages of the disease iron-deposition is confined to the liver cells but, with time, the bile duct epithelium and the Kupffer cells also become sites for haemosiderin deposition. The full picture of cirrhosis with nodular regeneration of liver cells develops only comparatively late in the disease. In patients in whom advanced cirrhosis due to iron deposition has occurred, there is a high risk (8–22%) for the subsequent development of hepatocellular carcinoma. If it is accepted that the iron deposition is the pathogenetic agent for the development of cirrhosis, then it is important that the disease be diagnosed as early as possible because treatment of the disease either by bleeding or by the use of iron-chelating agents both prolongs life and may delay or prevent the development of morphological changes, such as cirrhosis, that are largely irreversible. A useful screening method is the measurement of serum iron concentrations. If serum iron levels are increased, then serum ferritin concentrations and the degree of saturation of transferrin should be measured.
Pancreas	The pancreas is often a deep brown colour. On histological examination, haemosiderin deposition can be seen to affect the acinar and ductal epithelium, the islets of Langerhans and the interstitial connective tissue. Some degree of carbohydrate intolerance occurs in 80% of patients, and overt diabetes mellitus affects about 60%. The diabetes is probably multifactorial in origin but, to some extent, the intensity of the haemosiderin deposition parallels the severity of the diabetes.
Heart	Most cases show the presence of haemosiderin in the cardiac muscle fibres and atrioventricular node involvement is quite common. About 15% of patients show some abnormality of cardiac function, the commonest of which are arrhythmias or progressive cardiac failure, which may develop quite rapidly.
Skin	Skin pigmentation giving a metallic grey colour to the skin is one of the characteristic signs of haemochromatosis. Most of this colour change is due to the presence of excess amounts of melanin in the basal layer of the epidermis. Haemosiderin deposition does occur to some extent but tends to be concentrated in the connective tissue surrounding the sweat glands.
Joints	Some 25–50% of patients show the presence of an arthropathy characterized by the deposition of both iron and calcium pyrophosphate in the synovium (chondrocalcinosis). Both small and large joints may be involved and the patients complain of pain, swelling and stiffness of the affected joints. The relationship of the iron deposition to the arthropathy is not clear: increased iron loading does not make the joint problems worse and treating the patients by bleeding them does not improve the clinical picture of the arthropathy.

The commonest varieties classified under this rubric are:
- postviral hepatitis cirrhosis
- 'cryptogenic' cirrhosis; no cause identified

Chronic viral hepatitis and its pathological features have been discussed in a previous section and will not be dealt with further here.

Wilson's Disease (Hepatolenticular Degeneration)

Wilson's disease is defined as a defect in copper metab-olism; it has a worldwide prevalence of about 1 in 30 000. It is inherited in autosomal recessive fashion; the defect is expressed when there is a pair of abnormal recessive genes localized to the long arm of chromosome 13. **The functional defect results in deposition of large amounts of copper in liver, brain, eye, kidney, skeleton** and a number of other tissues.

Normally copper balance is zero throughout life. In Wilson's disease, however, there is a small net positive balance from birth onwards and this leads eventually to the accumulation of large amounts of copper. Copper is

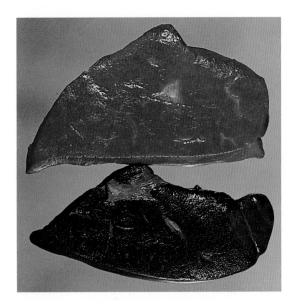

FIGURE 35.24 Haemochromatosis. Two slices of liver are shown: the upper shows the characteristic brown colour of iron deposition; the lower (treated by the Perl method, which demonstrates ferric iron) is a deep turquoise.

- An abnormally high copper content in the liver.

Each of these defects may occur singly in a number of other conditions but the combination occurs only in Wilson's disease. In these patients:

- total serum copper is lower than normal
- excess amounts of urinary copper are present
- concentrations of copper in the bile are low

The handling of copper by the liver is defective and the hepatic lysosomes contain more than 40 times more copper than those of normal liver. These data have been interpreted as suggesting that the accumulation of excess copper in the liver in Wilson's disease is due to defective excretion of copper from the lysosomes.

Although the accumulation of excess copper in the tissue begins at birth, or even *in utero*, the disease rarely surfaces above the clinical horizon before the age of 5 years and clinical manifestations related to the liver occur before those related to copper deposition in other organs.

Neurological disturbances, most often due to basal ganglia disease, usually appear during adolescence, and deposits of copper in Descemet's membrane of the cornea (Kayser–Fleischer ring) also occur later than liver disease.

normally absorbed from the gut and transported to the liver, where excretion into the bile takes place.

The primary and defining biochemical defects in Wilson's disease are:

- **A deficiency of the copper-transporting plasma protein, caeruloplasmin.** This protein, synthesized in the liver, is present in the plasma of normal people at a concentration of 200–400 mg/l. Some 95% of patients with Wilson's disease have low serum levels of this protein.

Microscopic Features

In the early stage, before cirrhosis develops, the liver cells show large droplet-type fatty change. The nuclei are enlarged and appear 'empty' because of large amounts of glycogen. Electron microscopy at this stage shows marked pleomorphism of mitochondria, and the peroxisomes are enlarged and misshapen.

The rate of progress, in untreated patients, is variable. In some, there is a mild focal mononuclear cell infiltrate

Table 35.14 Macronodular Cirrhosis

Frequency	Aetiology	Typical microscopic features
10–20%	Chronic viral hepatitis	'Ground glass' hepatocytes; identification of viral antigens by immunohistochemistry
Rare	Wilson's disease	Excess copper in liver cells shown by staining with rubeanic acid; fatty change in liver cells; glycogen vacuoles in nuclei; Mallory bodies sometimes present in liver cells
Rare	α_1-Antitrypsin deficiency	Periodic acid–Schiff stain-positive and diastase-resistant globules and granules in liver cell cytoplasm. These react with antibodies raised against α_1-anti-trypsin
Rare	Various drugs and toxins	
Rare	Hereditary haemorrhagic telangiectasia	Large dilated vessels in fibrous septa
Common	Cryptogenic cirrhosis	Macronodular cirrhosis with no aetiological clues

and this may be followed by fibrosis. In others, the picture of chronic active hepatitis develops and this can, in a few instances, be complicated by the appearances of fulminant hepatitis with subacute necrosis of the liver.

Ultimately, macronodular cirrhosis develops. The excess copper at different stages of the disease can be demonstrated by special stains such as rubeanic acid.

Prognosis

A diagnosis of Wilson's disease before 1951 meant a relentless downhill course, ending with premature death. This has been changed drastically by the introduction of effective chelating agents such as dimercaprol, D-penicillamine (the drug of choice) and trientine. These agents greatly increase the excretion of copper in the urine and can reverse the clinical abnormalities in most patients. Thus, the earlier the diagnosis is established, the better the prognosis for the affected individual.

α_1-Antitrypsin Deficiency

α_1-Antitrypsin deficiency is a genetically determined disorder which may cause either **pan-acinar pulmonary emphysema, chronic liver disease** in both children and adults, or **both** of these conditions.

α_1-Antitrypsin acts as a powerful antiprotease with a particularly important role in inhibiting the tissue-damaging effects of neutrophil-derived elastase. It is coded for on the long arm of chromosome 14 and the gene locus shows marked polymorphism: more than 70 different alleles have been identified. Thus there is considerable variation in the final protein product. These variants have been separated on the basis of their electrophoretic mobility. The commonest (present in more than 80% of the general population) is the M variant. The genotype for someone homozygous in respect of the allele producing this form is PiMM (Pi = protease inhibitor).

A variant associated with seriously abnormal biological function is the Z form, which may be inherited in either homozygous, heterozygous or hemizygous (PiZ–) patterns. The Z variant differs from the common M form by the substitution of lysine for glutamic acid at position 342. Normally the glutamic acid at position 342 forms a salt bridge with lysine at position 290. The substitution disrupts this bridge, with resulting changes in molecular folding. Thus the Z form cannot be secreted normally from liver cells and accumulates within them in the form of eosinophilic globules, concentrated in zone 1 liver cells (see *Fig. 35.14*). These globules stain strongly with the periodic acid–Schiff stain and resist digestion with diastase. This indicates that they are glycoprotein in nature.

Liver Disease in α_1-Antitrypsin Deficiency

Characteristics of liver disease in patients developing α_1-antitrypsin deficiency at different ages are shown in *Table 35.15*.

Hepatic Tumours

PRIMARY MALIGNANT TUMOURS

HEPATOCELLULAR CARCINOMA

Epidemiology

On a worldwide basis, primary liver cell carcinoma is one of the commonest malignant neoplasms (annual incidence 250 000 cases).

There is a marked geographical variation in its frequency. In the UK, the annual incidence is 1–2 per 100 000 population. A much higher incidence is found in South-East Asia and sub-Saharan Africa, reaching a peak in Mozambique, of 104 per 100 000 males and 31 per 100 000 females. This suggests that a significant environmental factor is implicated in the cause (*Fig. 35.25*).

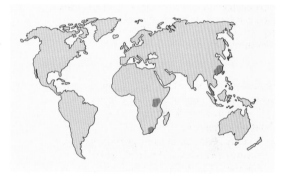

FIGURE 35.25 The geographical distribution of liver cell cancer.

Aetiology

The likeliest candidate for such an environmental factor is hepatitis B virus (HBV) infection. The evidence favouring this hypothesis is as follows:

- **A high degree of positive correlation between the frequency of HBV infection and that of liver cell cancer.** In areas where the carrier rate for HBV is very high, such as Taiwan, primary carcinoma of the liver is one of the most common causes of death in adults. In Taiwan, as many as 98% of patients with liver cell cancer have serological evidence of HBV infection. A patient who develops chronic hepatitis following HBV infection has a lifetime risk of developing liver cell cancer of 40–59%. An increased risk of liver cell cancer is also associated with hepatitis C virus (HCV) infections, but this has not yet been quantified accurately.

  It is important to realize that **hepatocellular carcinoma associated with HBV infection can occur in the absence of a clinically recognizable hepatitic illness**. This applies with particular force in **vertically transmitted**

Table 35.15 Liver Disease in Patients with α_1-Antitrypsin Deficiency

Age	Disease type	Characteristics
Infancy and childhood	Neonatal hepatitis	Infants may present with cholestatic jaundice. Microscopy shows marked cholestasis, liver cell necrosis, a mononuclear cell infiltrate, portal fibrosis and proliferation of bile ductules. The globules of α_1-antitrypsin described above are not easily demonstrable by conventional histological methods before 6 months have passed, but can be seen either on electron microscopy or by using antibodies to α_1-antitrypsin. Between 5 and 17% of children with the PiZZ genotype are said to develop this syndrome.
	Childhood cirrhosis	If jaundice lasts for more than 6 months, cirrhosis is very likely. In contrast to the neonatal hepatitis syndrome in which recovery is quite common, the development of the picture of chronic hepatitis and subsequent progression to cirrhosis is irreversible.
Adult life	Macronodular cirrhosis	Chronic liver disease due to α_1-antitrypsin deficiency is usually not associated with lung disease. It tends to appear in middle age (sixth and seventh decades) as a macronodular cirrhosis in which it is usually possible to identify the cytoplasmic globules of the abnormal protein.
	Hepatocellular carcinoma	There is a considerably increased risk of developing liver cell cancer or cancer of small intrahepatic bile ducts (cholangiocellular) in men but not in women. In one report from Sweden, 14 cases of liver cell cancer occurred in a group of 35 patients with the PiZZ genotype and established cirrhosis.

infections where the virus is passed on from an infected mother to her children. It is not without interest that the greater the incidence of infection in a given population, the younger is the peak age of incidence of hepatocellular carcinoma.

- **A positive correlation between HBV infection and the presence of dysplasia of the liver cells.** Such dysplasia is regarded as premalignant.
- **HBV antigens in the cells of hepatocellular carcinomas.**
- **Hybridization studies show the presence of part of the HBV genome in the cells of some primary liver cancers.** It is not yet known how such insertion exerts an oncogenic effect. The virus itself has not yet been shown to have a **direct** oncogenic effect, such as might occur if it possessed a viral oncogene. Interesting results have come from studies of transgenic mice in whose genome regions of the HBV genome have been incorporated. These mice express hepatitis B surface antigen (HBsAg) and develop morphological changes in the liver similar to those seen in humans with chronic HBV infection. Some of these animals develop liver cell adenomas and eventually carcinoma.

- **A hepadna virus similar to HBV affects woodchucks and causes hepatitis in them. Some of these animals develop chronic hepatitis, cirrhosis and liver cell carcinoma.**

Thus a strong presumptive case exists for a causal role for HBV in primary hepatocellular carcinoma, but absolute proof is still lacking and there is still no agreement as to the transforming mechanisms that might be activated by HBV or HBC infection.

Other Possible Aetiological Factors

Cirrhosis

Cirrhosis from whatever cause increases the risk of the development of primary liver cell cancer. Cirrhosis alone operates less powerfully than does the presence of HBV or HCV infection combined with cirrhosis. For example, of Japanese cirrhotics who had evidence of chronic HBV infections, 59% developed liver cell cancer; in those with a history of post-transfusion hepatitis (presumably related to HCV infection), 53% developed liver cell cancer, whereas of those whose cirrhosis was ascribed to alcohol 22% subsequently developed liver cell cancer.

The risk appears to be much lower in patients with primary biliary cirrhosis, sclerosing cholangitis or cirrhosis related to autoimmune disease. It has been suggested that the increased cell turnover associated with the formation of regenerating nodules increases the chances of random mutations occurring in the liver cells and, hence, the chance of developing hepatocellular carcinoma.

Metabolic Disorders

Some inherited metabolic diseases carry an increased risk of hepatocellular carcinoma. Of these, the most important are:

- Haemochromatosis (see pp 594–596)
- Homozygous α_1-antitrypsin deficiency (see pp 599–600)
- Tyrosinaemia. This rare disease (1 per 100 000 live births) is inherited in an autosomal recessive pattern. The biochemical defect in the type 1 form (affecting the liver and kidneys) is a **deficiency in the enzyme fumaryl acetoacetate hydrolase**. This leads to a build-up of tyrosine precursors in affected organs. It is expressed in the form of renal tubular abnormalities and disturbances in liver function.

  Macronodular cirrhosis is a common occurrence in children who survive infancy, and a significant proportion of these (about one-third) develop liver cell cancer at quite a young age. Most of the affected children die before the age of 10 years.
- Glycogen storage disease type 1 (von Gierke's disease). This also is a rare disease (1 per 100 000–500 000), inherited in an autosomal recessive pattern. There are two types, of which the first is characterized by an **absence of the enzyme glucose-6-phosphatase**. The liver, kidneys and gut accumulate glycogen, leading to enlargement and pallor. Microscopic examination of the liver shows a marked degree of swelling of the liver cells, the cytoplasm of which looks clear in conventionally processed sections. The use of special stains, such as the periodic acid–Schiff method, shows that the cells are distended by glycogen.

  Among many other problems, these children show a tendency to develop multiple hepatic adenomas and malignant transformation has been reported in some of these.

Aflatoxins

These are produced by the fungus *Aspergillus flavus*, a contaminant of cereal and groundnut crops in Africa and Asia. Aflatoxins at high dose levels cause liver cell necrosis in poultry, and at lower doses they cause liver cell carcinoma. There is positive epidemiological correlation between the frequency of human liver cell cancer and cereal crop contamination by aflatoxin. The magnitude of its contribution to the total burden of liver cell cancer is hard to assess because the populations likely to be affected by the toxin also show a high prevalence of HBV infection. A possible mechanism for an oncogenic effect of the toxin has been identified; aflatoxin produces a point mutation in codon 249 of the important tumour suppressor gene *p53* (see pp 285–286).

Drugs and Toxins

The compound for which the most direct evidence exists for a causal link with hepatocellular carcinoma is Thorotrast. This was a radiological contrast agent used in the 1930s and 1940s, and there are reports of the development of a number of different types of liver tumour (liver cell cancer, angiosarcoma and bile duct cancer) following its use.

An association between taking androgens and the subsequent development of liver cell cancer has also been reported. In this connection, it is not without interest that liver cell cancer is predominantly a tumour that occurs in males. Messenger RNA for androgen receptors has been shown to be present both in samples of human liver cell cancer and in cultured cell lines established from such tumours.

Cigarette Smoking

Cigarette smoking is associated with an increased risk for the development of liver cell cancer. This is most obvious when the cohort studied consists entirely of individuals negative for HBsAg. In such people the risk ratio (risk in smokers : non-smokers) is between 7 and 8.

Clinical Features

Patients with hepatocellular carcinoma show a wide spectrum of clinical features. The most frequent complaint is of abdominal pain or discomfort, which in advanced cases may be acute. Loss of appetite, weight loss, fever and jaundice are other common complaints. In patients known to have chronic liver disease, any sudden clinical worsening in the condition is a warning sign that carcinoma may have supervened.

The commonest clinical sign is hepatomegaly. Establishing that such enlargement is due to the presence of carcinoma has been eased greatly by the introduction of real-time ultrasonography, which makes it possible to identify quite small masses (less than 3 cm in diameter) at a time when they are likely to be surgically resectable.

Use of 'Tumour Markers' in the Diagnosis of Liver Cell Cancer

Liver cell tumours produce a wide range of proteins, some normal, some variant forms of normal proteins, and some **proteins that are normally expressed only in fetal life (onco–fetal antigens)**.

The most useful of the latter in the context of liver cell cancer is **α-fetoprotein (AFP)**. This an α_1-globulin produced in the first trimester of pregnancy by the yolk sac, fetal liver and gut, and not normally present in the blood in postembryonic life. Many patients with liver cell cancer show raised plasma concentrations of this protein. Sustained rises above 500 µg/l are, for all practical purposes, seen only in patients with liver cell cancers, malignant liver cell tumours of childhood (hepatoblastoma), and malignant gonadal and extra-gonadal teratomas. Lower levels may be found in patients with chronic liver disease but with no evidence of carcinoma, but if the diagnostic level is set at 500 µg/l then the **specificity** of the test is very high. Unfortunately the **sensitivity** of AFP in the diagnosis of liver cell cancer is lower than its specificity, perhaps because some variants of liver cell cancer (fibrolamellar cancer, minute cancer and pedunculated cancer) produce much lower levels of AFP.

An increase in the plasma concentration of the β sub-unit of human chorionic gonadotrophin has also been reported in some patients with either liver cell cancer or hepatoblastoma. In young prepubertal patients, this has, in some instances, caused precocious sexual development.

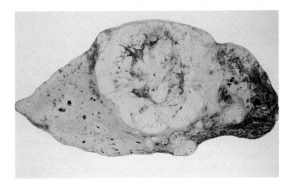

FIGURE 35.26 Liver cell cancer: a large expansile mass in a non-cirrhotic liver.

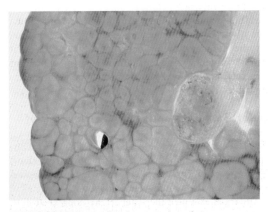

FIGURE 35.27 Liver cell cancer: an expansile tumour associated with hepatic cirrhosis.

Macroscopic Features

A number of macroscopic variants exist.
- a large, apparently **single and expansile mass** (*Figs 35.26* and *35.27*)
- **infiltrative**
- **multifocal** with numerous tumour nodules that may be confused with metastases. The absence of central umbilication in the nodules is a useful pointer to their primary nature.

These tumours can spread extensively throughout the portal vein and hepatic artery branches. It is not uncommon to find macroscopic evidence of portal vein spread with large tumour nodules within the vascular channels. This is often associated with thrombosis and will either cause portal hypertension or exacerbate it if already present as a result of cirrhosis. If the main hepatic veins are involved, they may become occluded, with the production of acute congestion and necrosis in the liver (Budd–Chiari syndrome).

Liver cell carcinoma is usually rather soft in consistency and its cut surface may show focal areas of necrosis and haemorrhage. If the tumour is well differentiated and is secreting bile, the lesions will have a greenish colour.

Less common variants are minute carcinomas and pedunculated carcinomas.

Minute carcinomas, most common in Japanese people, are small tumour nodules occurring against a background of a cirrhotic liver; they are identifiable because they are firmer and paler than the surrounding liver tissue. Histological examination shows the characteristics of malignancy.

Pedunculated carcinomas, as the name implies, are tumours protruding from the capsular surface of the liver. They show little invasion of the substance of the underlying liver. These anatomical features make them relatively easy to resect in their entirety and patients have a better prognosis than the majority of those with hepatocellular carcinomas.

Microscopic Features

The histological appearances of any individual liver cell cancer derive from the interaction of:
- the degree of cellular differentiation
- the architectural arrangement of the tumour cells

In some instances the tumour cells are well differentiated and show a close resemblance to non-neoplastic liver cells. In such cases, bile secretion may be a feature and, if present, obviously constitutes strong support for the diagnosis of liver cell carcinoma. Such bile secretion is found in about 10% of cases.

In other cases, the degree of differentiation is much less. Aneuploid giant cells may be present in large numbers and one variant is made up of spindle-shaped cells, giving the tumour a resemblance to a sarcoma. Mallory's hyaline is seen occasionally, as may be α_1-antitrypsin, and

AFP can be demonstrated immunohistochemically in 60–80% of the tumours.

The commonest architectural arrangement is one in which the cells are arranged in a trabecular pattern with cords of cells, two to five cells thick, bordered by a sinusoidal type of blood supply (*Fig. 35.28*).

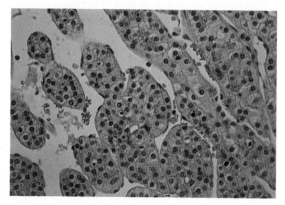

FIGURE 35.28 *Liver cell cancer: the tumour cells are arranged in a characteristic trabecular pattern.*

Fibrolamellar Carcinoma

An important variant is **fibrolamellar carcinoma**. This tumour occurs at a much younger age than is usual for liver cell cancers: more than 90% of cases are in persons less than 25 years old and in populations in whom the carrier rates for HBV are low. There is no associated liver disease and females are quite often affected. These tumours are also unusual in that about 65% arise in the left lobe of the liver.

The microscopic pattern is quite characteristic, with islands and columns of eosinophilic and rather granular tumour cells separated from one another by broad bands of collagen. AFP is not usually present in the tumour cells, but tumour cells in all cases of this variant contain the neural antigen PGP 9.5.

Liver cell carcinomas, as a group, carry a very bleak prognosis, but the fibrolamellar variant can sometimes be resected in its entirety and has a better prognosis than the more usual type of tumour, the 5-year survival rate being 60%.

CHOLANGIOCARCINOMA

Cholangiocarcinoma arises either from extrahepatic bile ducts or from bile ductules within the liver. Here, only the latter is considered. Cholangiocarcinoma is far less common than liver cell carcinoma, accounting for only 6–7% of primary liver cancers, and tends to occur fairly late in life, with a peak incidence in the sixth decade.

Aetiology

Unlike liver cell cancer, cholangiocarcinoma shows no correlation with hepatitis virus infections, and cirrhosis is absent in virtually all cases. Some cases occur in association with sclerosing cholangitis (see pp 593–594), but rarely. In the Far East there is a clear association with infestation by liver flukes (*Opisthorchis sinensis* in China and *O. viverrini* in Malaysia and Thailand). The flukes are found in both extrahepatic and intrahepatic bile ducts, and deposit their ova at these sites. It appears to be the ova that elicit an inflammatory reaction followed by scarring, this being the prelude to malignant transformation of the bile ductular epithelium.

Other factors that have been implicated include the contrast agent Thorotrast, which is, however, more commonly associated with an increased risk of liver cell carcinoma. As with a number of other adenocarcinomas of endodermal origin, mutations in the *ras* oncogene (not seen in association with liver cell cancer) have been described in cholangiocarcinoma.

> ### Microscopic Features
>
> Most intrahepatic cholangiocarcinomas are well differentiated, mucin-secreting adenocarcinomas which elicit a striking fibrous tissue response. Unlike liver cell cancers, they never secrete bile.
>
> Intrahepatic blood vessel invasion is a less well-marked feature than in liver cell cancer, malignant cells tending to spread along the walls of affected blood vessels rather than forming solid intravascular cores.
>
> Curiously, distant blood-borne metastases to sites such as the skeleton, brain, adrenals and lung are more common in the case of cholangiocarcinoma than in liver cell cancer, in which venous involvement is such a prominent feature.

HEPATOBLASTOMA

This is an embryonal tumour found most commonly in infants of up to 3 years of age, males being affected more often than females. While rare in absolute terms, it is the commonest primary malignant tumour of the liver in children.

Clinical Features

Affected children usually present with fairly marked constitutional symptoms including anorexia, nausea, abdominal pain and vomiting. When the abdomen is palpated, an enlarged liver is usually found. A number of congenital abnormalities has been reported in association with hepatoblastoma, but such abnormalities are by no means always present in children with this tumour. Serum AFP levels are usually raised.

> ### Microscopic Features
>
> Two types of hepatoblastoma have been described:
>   1) The **epithelioid type** is made up of cells resembling fetal liver cells; in the better-differentiated examples, they are arranged in columns separated by sinusoidal blood vessels. In addition there is a second

population of smaller and more darkly staining (embryonal) cells arranged in rosettes and primitive acini.

2) The **mixed type**, in which a primitive mesenchymal stroma separates the fetal and embryonal liver cells. This stroma may show focal evidence of differentiation into various forms of connective tissue such as cartilage, osteoid or muscle.

BENIGN EPITHELIAL TUMOURS AND TUMOUR-LIKE LESIONS

Understanding this group of lesions is not made easier by the rather confusing nomenclature. The lesions considered here under this rubric are:

- **hepatic adenoma** (which can be regarded as a true neoplasm)
- **focal nodular hyperplasia** (the nature of which is uncertain but which may be a hyperplastic response to the presence of a pre-existing vascular anomaly)
- **partial nodular transformation** (a rare regenerative phenomenon in which multiple nodules in the liver occur in association with one of a number of systemic disorders including rheumatoid disease, systemic lupus erythematosus, infective endocarditis and various extrahepatic malignancies)

Hepatic Adenoma

Hepatic adenoma is, in most cases, solitary, ranging from 2 to 20 cm in diameter. Some 90% occur in women of childbearing age and there is a strong positive association between this lesion and taking oral contraceptives. It is not clear which hormonal component of the contraceptives is responsible.

The commonest clinical presentation is acute abdominal pain. This is due either to rupture of the tumour into the peritoneal cavity, this being associated with haemorrhage, or to haemorrhage within the tumour itself.

Macroscopic Features

Hepatic adenoma is usually a single nodule. In almost half the cases, the diameter of the lesion is greater than 10 cm. The tumour is not always encapsulated but it can be identified on naked-eye examination by its pallor, compared with the surrounding liver tissue.

Microscopic Features

The most striking feature is the **absence of normal acinar structure and of portal tracts and bile ducts**.

Some hepatic adenomas undergo malignant transformation, a frequency of up to 10% being quoted by some.

Focal Nodular Hyperplasia

Focal nodular hyperplasia is expressed in the form of well-demarcated masses within the liver. They are only partly, if at all, encapsulated and are both firmer and paler than the surrounding liver tissue. In some instances, focal nodular hyperplasia is associated with the presence of vascular anomalies or with tumours expressing neuroendocrine differentiation.

This type of hyperplasia is more common in women than in men, but **there is no association with oral contraceptive** use and the lesions may occur at any age. Most cases are discovered incidentally, the majority of patients remaining asymptomatic.

The chief clinical problem is distinguishing between this lesion and benign hepatic adenoma, because the natural history is so different. To make this distinction, it is often deemed necessary to resect the nodule so that detailed pathological examination may be carried out.

Macroscopic Features

The lesions are tan-coloured and usually have a much more irregular margin than is the case with hepatic adenoma; the cut surface shows fibrous septa which divide the lesion into lobules. These septa radiate from a central scar which, in large lesions, tends to be stellate in shape (*Fig. 35.29*).

Microscopic Features

The nodules are made up of liver cells arranged in columns that are thicker than normal. These columns are separated by sinusoids but the normal vascular relationships characteristic of liver acini are lost. The scarred areas show the presence of thick-walled blood vessels, and duct-like structures may also be present.

The pathogenesis is unknown but it has been suggested that focal nodular hyperplasia may represent a response of the liver tissue to a pre-existing vascular anomaly. There is no risk of malignant transformation.

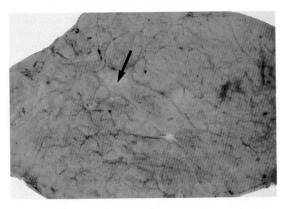

FIGURE 35.29 Focal nodular hyperplasia. Note the central scar (arrowed) from which fibrous septa radiate.

Nodular Transformation

This term describes an entity in which multiple nodules are present within the liver parenchyma. It is seen in several different systemic disorders including connective tissue diseases such as systemic lupus erythematosus or rheumatoid disease.

Microscopic Features

The essential pathological features are a combination of:
- liver cell plates that are more than one cell thick but with preservation of normal vascular relationships
- small rounded nodules of liver cells in which no hepatic vein radicles are present

The pathological picture can be distinguished from micronodular cirrhosis as there are no fibrous tissue septa between the nodules.

The principal pathophysiological effect is portal hypertension and clinical presentation is related to complications of the latter, for example bleeding from oesophageal varices.

BENIGN VASCULAR TUMOURS

Benign Cavernous Haemangioma

This is the commonest benign neoplasm in the liver, present in almost 1% of all autopsies (100 times more frequent than benign hepatic adenoma). It can occur at any age but the peak incidence appears to be between the third and fifth decades. Most of the lesions are small and affected individuals are usually symptom-free.

In some cases, the lesions are larger (more than 4 cm in diameter) and these patients may develop a consumptive coagulopathy (with a low platelet count and low plasma fibrinogen concentrations), possibly due to thrombosis occurring within the abnormal vascular channels of the haemangiomas.

Infantile Haemangioendothelioma

This is a highly cellular variant of haemangioma which may be solitary or multicentric. It is not infrequently associated with vascular lesions in other sites such as skin, bone or lung. It occurs almost exclusively in infants aged less than 6 months.

Macroscopically the lesions appear as reddish brown, spongy areas in which focal calcification may develop. On histological examination the vascular spaces that make up the lesion are seen to be lined by plump endothelial cells which may, in some instances, form solid masses within the vascular channels.

Despite the fact that the tumours are benign, in that they neither invade nor metastasize, the mortality rate is high. Death is due either to liver failure or high-output cardiac failure.

MALIGNANT CONNECTIVE TISSUE TUMOURS

Sarcomas of the liver are very rare. Of these, the commonest is **angiosarcoma**, characterized by the presence of numerous, anastomosing abnormal vascular channels. Most examples are found in adults, males being affected more frequently. Associations believed to have causal significance include:
- **cirrhosis**
- **exposure to vinyl chloride monomer** in the course of the manufacture of polyvinyl chloride, which is an important component of many plastic materials
- **exposure to the contrast medium Thorotrast** (see also p 601); the latent period from exposure to diagnosis of the tumour ranges from 20 to 40 years
- **prolonged ingestion of therapeutic doses of arsenic**

Macroscopic Features

The liver, which is usually much enlarged, shows numerous dark reddish-brown nodules or, in some cases, cystic spaces filled with blood.

Microscopic Features

On microscopic examination the tumour cells are seen to be spindle shaped. They may line vascular channels or may be arranged in the form of solid masses. Extramedullary haemopoiesis is a common associated finding. Unless the tumour is extremely poorly differentiated, it is usually possible to demonstrate the endothelial nature of the tumour cells by the use of appropriate antibodies (e.g. against Factor VIII or the CD34 component of endothelium QB-END/10).

Spread is usually rapid and can involve lymph nodes in the porta hepatis, spleen and lungs. The prognosis is poor: survival time after clinical presentation is usually about 1 year.

Other Malignant Connective Tissue Tumours

These include:
- embryonal rhabdomyosarcoma
- leiomyosarcoma
- fibrosarcoma
- malignant mesenchymoma

Malignant lymphoreticular disorders frequently involve the liver. In most instances, this represents spread from the primary site, but in a small proportion of cases the liver may be the primary site of the lymphoma.

SECONDARY MALIGNANT TUMOURS IN THE LIVER

Despite all the foregoing material, the commonest neoplasms in the liver are metastatic. Such metastases may be present in almost 40% of adults with malignant disease.

The liver may be involved by direct spread from malignant tumours in the vicinity, such as those of the pancreas, extrahepatic bile ducts, stomach and gallbladder.

Other common sites from which hepatic metastases are derived include carcinoma of the large gut, lung, breast, kidney and stomach, and malignant melanoma (*Fig. 35.30*). The finding of metastases **confined to the liver** is more probable in association with tumours drained via the portal vein.

The secondary deposits are frequently visible on the capsular surface of the liver; they appear typically as nodules of differing sizes which are centrally umbilicated; a result of central necrosis. Occasionally the metastases are concealed within the substance of the liver and the capsular surface is uninvolved.

The presence of space-occupying metastatic masses in the liver is suggested by finding an unexplained increase in the serum concentration of alkaline phosphatase. At a later stage jaundice may appear, which can be due either to extensive destruction of liver parenchyma or to intrahepatic bile duct obstruction.

In untreated patients the median survival time for those with hepatic metastases varies between 4 and 15 months, although occasional examples of much longer survival times are recorded. The longer survival times tend to be noted in patients in whom a solitary metastasis is present. If resection of the metastases is undertaken in this highly selected group, then 3-year survival may be obtained in up to 40%.

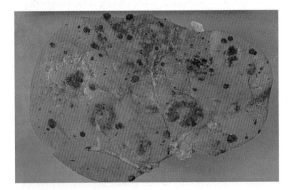

FIGURE 35.30 *Secondary deposits from a malignant melanoma. The pigmentation of the tumour nodules makes the diagnosis obvious.*

Liver Disease in Infancy and Childhood

This section covers aspects of liver disease in infancy and childhood that are not considered elsewhere. Only the most important are discussed.

KEY POINTS: *Liver Disorder in Childhood*

The chief clinical and pathological expressions of liver disorder in childhood are:

- **jaundice** (in the form of unconjugated or conjugated hyperbilirubinaemia)
- **Reye's syndrome**
- **autoimmune chronic liver disease**
- **hepatic and biliary lesions of cystic fibrosis**
- **Indian childhood cirrhosis**
- **glycogen storage disease**
- **various lysosomal storage disorders**
- **polycystic disease**
- **congenital hepatic fibrosis**

JAUNDICE

In addition to physiological jaundice and inherited anomalies discussed earlier (see pp 567–570), there are many other causes of increased serum concentrations of unconjugated bilirubin.

These include such entities as **haemolytic disease of the newborn** (due mainly to rhesus incompatibility), **bacterial infections, hypoglycaemia** and the **inherited metabolic abnormalities galactosaemia and fructosaemia**. It is important that the cause of such hyperbilirubinaemia be identified as soon as possible and the hyperbilirubinaemia treated to prevent the irreversible damage associated with **kernicterus**.

If hyperbilirubinaemia is due to a rise in the level of **conjugated bilirubin**, the jaundice can **never** be regarded as 'physiological'. There are many causes of conjugated hyperbilirubinaemia in infancy, shown in *Table 35.16*.

GALACTOSAEMIA AND FRUCTOSAEMIA

It is vital that galactosaemia and fructosaemia be recognized as promptly as possible in a jaundiced child because their effects may be avoided completely by eliminating the responsible sugar from the child's diet.

Galactosaemia

Galactosaemia, inherited in an autosomal recessive pattern, is characterized by **low levels of the enzyme galactose-1-phosphate uridyltransferase** in the liver and blood cells. Excessive amounts of galactose, galactose-1-phosphate and galactitol accumulate within the tissues.

Table 35.16 Jaundice Due to Raised Levels of Conjugated Bilirubin

Anatomical site	Type of process	Examples
Hepatocellular	Infection	**Bacterial** (e.g. *Escherichia coli*); **viral** (e.g. rubella, cytomegalovirus, herpes simplex virus, adenovirus, coxsackie B); **protozoal** (malaria, toxoplasmosis)
	Inherited metabolic disorders	Galactosaemia★, fructosaemia★, tyrosinaemia, α_1-antitrypsin deficiency★, Gaucher's disease, etc. Familial disorders such as arteriohepatic dysplasia (Alagille's syndrome)★, familial recurrent cholestasis, progressive familial cholestasis (Byler's disease), trisomies 13 and 18
	Toxic or deficiency disorders	Liver changes associated with total parenteral nutrition★
	Endocrine	Some cases of hypothyroidism, hypoadrenalism and hypopituitarism
	?Idiopathic	Neonatal hepatitis syndrome
Bile duct abnormalities		Extrahepatic biliary atresia★, choledochal cyst★, spontaneous perforation of bile duct★, biliary hypoplasia
Vascular		Veno-occlusive disease, lymphatic defects

★ Indicates a condition discussed in the text.

The liver is affected within 2 weeks of birth as all types of milk contain lactose. Fat accumulates in the liver cells and there is proliferation of bile ductules, a curious pseudoacinar transformation of the liver cell plates and iron deposition. Occasional necrotic liver cells and some multinucleated giant forms may be seen. Cirrhosis may well have developed by the time the infant is 3 months old. Cataract formation is a characteristic feature and brain damage leading to mental retardation occurs. Much of the malign effect of the enzyme defect can be avoided if the disease is recognized early and the child put on a galactose-free diet.

Fructosaemia

Fructosaemia sufficiently severe to cause tissue damage arises on the basis of:

- an inherited absence of the enzyme **fructose-1-phosphate aldolase**, normally present in the liver, kidney and intestinal mucosa. Absence of the enzyme leads to impaired uptake of dietary fructose by the liver. In addition there is inhibition of the breakdown of hepatic glycogen and decreased gluconeogenesis, both of which lead to profound hypoglycaemia.
- an inherited absence of the enzyme **fructose-1-6-diphosphatase**, which is essential for gluconeogenesis; thus, hypoglycaemia is a prominent feature.

The first biochemical defect leads to a more severe clin-ical and pathological picture; symptoms appear as soon as fructose is introduced into the diet, usually at about the time of weaning. The children eat poorly, fail to thrive and vomit frequently. On examination, the liver is generally found to be enlarged. In due time, drowsiness and coma may supervene.

Microscopic Features

The liver shows a marked degree of fatty change and, as is the case with galactosaemia, there may be liver cell necrosis associated with the appearance of multinucleated giant liver cells. Fibrous tissue is laid down in the portal tracts and, if the offending fructose is not removed from the diet, cirrhosis ultimately develops.

Alagille's Syndrome (Arteriohepatic Dysplasia)

Children with this disorder have a characteristic facies with:

- prominence of the forehead
- a straight nose which, when seen in profile, is in the same plane as the forehead
- deep-set eyes

Cardiovascular abnormalities, of which the commonest is pulmonary stenosis, are generally present.

Hypoplasia of the intrahepatic bile ducts is present by the time the child reaches the age of 1 year and is associated with itch (generally a prominent feature) and jaundice of differing grades of severity. The jaundice may clear within 1–2 years, and death from liver disease is uncommon. The disorder is inherited as an autosomal dominant defect.

Liver Changes in Association with Total Parenteral Nutrition

Prolonged intravenous nutrition without oral feeding in early infancy may cause bile stasis and injury to liver cells sufficiently severe as to cause cirrhosis and even liver cell cancer. The cause of this series of developments is unknown.

Examination of liver biopsies shows expansion of the portal tract connective tissue with proliferation of bile ductules in a manner similar to what is seen in biliary obstruction. Withdrawal of the intravenous feeding and substitution of oral feeds causes the jaundice to fade and eventually disappear. However, the abnormal histological features in the liver may persist for up to 1 year.

SURGICALLY CORRECTABLE CAUSES OF JAUNDICE IN INFANCY

Extrahepatic Biliary Atresia

Biliary atresia is characterized by postinflammatory fibrous obliteration of a segment of the extrahepatic biliary system. It is one of the commonest causes of prolonged cholestatic jaundice in infants; its frequency has been estimated as about 1 per 14 000 live births.

Microscopic Features

The histological picture seen on liver biopsy is characterized by:

- oedema and fibrosis of the portal tracts
- bile duct reduplication in all portal tracts, leading to tortuous, proliferated ductules
- giant cells in about half the cases

If the obstruction to bile drainage is not relieved, a secondary biliary cirrhosis develops and death occurs by the age of 1–2 years.

Choledochal Cyst

Choledochal cyst is one of the forms of congenital dilatation of the bile ducts. It may involve both the extrahepatic and intrahepatic portions of the biliary tree and, for unknown reasons, shows a marked female preponderance.

Functionally, it is associated with reduced flow of bile and histological changes within the liver closely resembling those of biliary atresia. If normal bile drainage is not established, secondary biliary cirrhosis develops.

The clinical picture depends on the age at which symptoms first appear. In infants there may be prolongation of physiological jaundice, as seen in cases of biliary atresia, or a hepatitic picture may be present. In older children the complaint may be of recurrent upper abdominal pain and jaundice. In these cases, a palpable mass may be present in the right upper quadrant of the abdomen.

Choledochal cyst is the basis for a number of serious complications. The cyst, which may contain up to 10 litres of bile, readily becomes infected and this may lead to an ascending inflammatory process involving the biliary system (ascending cholangitis). The cyst may rupture, leading to bile peritonitis, stones may form within its lumen, there may be episodes of acute pancreatitis and, rarely, malignant transformation may occur in the epithelial lining of the cyst wall.

Spontaneous Perforation of the Bile Duct

This sometimes occurs at the junction of the cystic duct and the common hepatic duct in infants who seem to have a distal obstruction within the bile duct system. A cyst may form around the bile duct and the chief dangers to affected infants are severe malnutrition or infection.

REYE'S SYNDROME

Reye's syndrome is an acute disorder in which more than 90% of the patients are children. They present with severe vomiting associated with marked irritability and disturbances of consciousness ranging from agitated delirium to frank coma and death. Mortality rates are high (up to 40–50%) and survivors may show evidence of brain damage.

This encephalopathy, characterized by cerebral oedema with no evidence of associated inflammation, is accompanied by severe small droplet-form fatty change in the liver and some milder fatty changes in other viscera.

Typically there is a history of a mild viral illness starting 2–5 days before the onset of the vomiting and cerebral symptoms. About 95% of affected children have been given aspirin to relieve the symptoms of the viral febricula, and it has been suggested that the syndrome may represent some genetically determined abnormal response to the aspirin. Biochemical investigations usually show an increase in serum transaminase concentration (despite the fact that there is no histological evidence of cell death) and an increase in plasma ammonia concentration.

Electron microscopy consistently shows mitochondrial abnormalities. The mitochondria are swollen, their matrices are expanded, and dense material is deposited within the matrices.

INDIAN CHILDHOOD CIRRHOSIS

This is an apparently unique form of liver disease confined to the Indian subcontinent, Sri Lanka, Burma and

Malaysia. It is far from rare, being reported as the fourth most common cause of death in young children in certain centres in India. Presentation occurs most commonly between the ages of 6 months and 4 years.

Microscopic Features

In the earliest phase of the disease there is patchy necrosis of liver cells with an associated focal inflammatory response. Mallory's hyaline appears in many liver cells and fibrous septa divide the parenchyma into small nodules, although there is a striking lack of regenerative activity. The copper content of the liver is very high (10–60 times normal), even exceeding that found in patients with Wilson's disease.

Two principal clinical forms are recognized:
1) There is a phase of anorexia, nausea and irritability, followed by abdominal distension and enlargement of the liver. Over the next few months, signs of portal hypertension appear, the liver becoming even larger and very hard on palpation. The final picture may be a combination of the effects of portal hypertension and liver failure.
2) In about one-quarter of cases the clinical picture is dominated by a hepatitis-like syndrome and death occurs 3–4 months after onset of the illness.

The cause of this unique disorder is not really understood but it is thought to be due to the accumulation of very large amounts of copper in the liver. This is, in part, environmental and appears to be associated with the drinking of boiled buffalo's milk stored in vessels made from a copper-containing alloy. Whether there are genetic or other environmental factors that play a part is not yet known. The pathogenetic role of copper accumulation is emphasized by the fact that treatment of these children with copper-chelating agents, at a stage before either ascites or jaundice has appeared, leads to survival in 50% of affected children.

CONGENITAL HEPATIC FIBROSIS

Congenital hepatic fibrosis is an autosomal recessive disorder. It is characterized by linkage of portal tracts by bands of fibrous tissue in which elongated or cystic spaces lined by bile duct epithelium are present. These spaces resemble the earliest forms of bile ducts, known as ductal plates. It has been suggested, therefore, that failure of normal involution of the embryonal ductal plate may contribute to the genesis of congenital hepatic fibrosis. There is usually *no* evidence of hepatocellular disease in the form of inflammation, necrosis or regeneration.

Affected children have an enlarged and very firm liver (*Fig. 35.31*) and may show signs of portal hypertension, which constitutes the chief clinical problem.

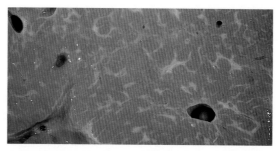

FIGURE 35.31 *Congenital hepatic fibrosis showing well-defined, stellate, fibrous tissue septa on the cut surface of the liver.*

Congenital hepatic fibrosis is a member of a set of congenital abnormalities involving the biliary tree, termed the **fibropolycystic disorders**; these are shown in *Table 35.17*.

Vascular Disorders of the Liver

In this section, vascular disorders other than portal hypertension are discussed, although some of the entities described here cause portal hypertension.

Functionally, vascular pathology in the liver can be conveniently classified as shown in *Table 35.18*.

IMPAIRMENT OF HEPATIC VENOUS DRAINAGE

Chronic Venous Congestion

Chronic venous congestion is a common finding in the liver at post-mortem examination. This because the agonal phase in most patients is associated with some degree of cardiac failure, Severe chronic venous congestion is most often seen in association with chronic heart failure, especially involving the right side of the heart and also in patients with constrictive pericarditis.

The hepatic venous radicles and the sinusoids in zone 3 of the hepatic acinus are dilated and congested. The increase in sinusoidal pressure in zone 3, together with the fact that this part of the liver acinus is most likely to suffer if there is any element of hypoperfusion, leads initially to fatty change and later to atrophy of the zone 3 hepatocytes. Hypoperfusion is almost certainly an important contributor to the pathological picture of chronic venous congestion, a view supported by the more or less identical morphological changes in the liver of patients with shock.

Table 35.17 Fibropolycystic Disorders

Disorder	Features
Congenital hepatic fibrosis	See text
Caroli's disease	Congenital dilatation of intrahepatic bile ducts either alone or combined with congenital hepatic fibrosis. Associated risk of ascending bacterial infection
Choledochal cyst	See text
Microhamartoma (von Meyenburg complex)	These are rounded nodules of fibrous tissue containing multiple biliary channels lined by normal bile duct epithelium (*Fig. 35.32*), usually found incidentally at surgery and normally of no clinical significance. Occasional cases of carcinoma have been reported in association with multiple microhamartomas
'Infantile' (autosomal recessive) polycystic disease	Associated with polycystic disease of kidneys. If the kidneys are severely affected, there is usually minimal hepatic involvement. Liver changes resemble those of congenital hepatic fibrosis
'Adult' (autosomal dominant) polycystic disease	Cystic disease of liver found in 16–21% of cases of the dominant form of polycystic renal disease. Liver diffusely cystic with cysts ranging in diameter from a few millimetres to more than 10 cm. The cysts do not communicate with the biliary system. von Meyenburg complexes are often found in association

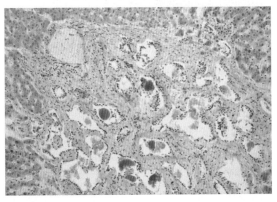

FIGURE 35.32 *von Meyenburg complex in the liver. Numerous small spaces lined by bile duct epithelium are seen.*

Macroscopic Features

The liver has a variegated red and yellow appearance which has been likened to the surface of a **nutmeg** (*Fig. 35.33*).

Microscopic Features

The dark areas of the nutmeg are represented by the dilated and congested venous radicles and zone 3 sinusoids, and the pale areas are represented by the hypoxic and fat-laden hepatocytes (*Fig. 35.34*). In more severe cases, necrosis of these hepatocytes occurs and macrophages laden with iron pigment or with ceroid (incompletely oxidized lipid) appear in these areas. A small proportion of cases show bile stasis within canaliculi.

In cases where the congestion has been both chronic and severe, as, for example, in patients with incompetence of the tricuspid valve, fibrous tissue may become laid down in the perivenular area. Bridges of fibrous tissue link these perivenular scarred areas with others in the vicinity.

Because of these changes, the acinar pattern becomes exaggerated and a false impression may be gained that the portal tract lies at the centre of the acinus surrounded by a cuff of zone 1 and 2 hepatocytes. This appearance is termed by some writers 'reverse lobulation'. This post-congestion fibrosis may produce a liver that appears very finely nodular, and this is sometimes called 'cardiac cirrhosis' although it is clear that the defining criteria for cirrhosis are not met.

Occlusion of Hepatic Veins (Budd–Chiari Syndrome)

Occlusion of the hepatic veins at their ostia, or of the inferior vena cava distal to its junction with the hepatic veins, constitutes the Budd–Chiari syndrome.

This condition may develop acutely or may be insidious in its origin. It is usually due to thrombosis or to invasion of the main hepatic veins by tumour; liver cell carcinoma and renal cell carcinoma are the two that behave most frequently in this way.

Aetiology of Large Hepatic Vein Thrombosis

- primary myeloproliferative disorders such as polycythaemia rubra vera
- paroxysmal nocturnal haemoglobinuria

Table 35.18 Classification of Vascular Pathology in the Liver

Mechanism	Causes
Conditions with impairment or failure of hepatic drainage	Chronic venous congestion associated with right-sided cardiac failure or constrictive pericarditis Occlusion of hepatic veins either at their ostia or outside the liver by thrombi or, more rarely, by fibrous septa (Budd–Chiari syndrome) Occlusion of intrahepatic venous radicles as a result of poisoning by plant alkaloids or as a long-term effect of irradiation (veno-occlusive disease)
Conditions with impairment of arterial perfusion	Left-sided cardiac failure Shock Arteritis affecting the liver vascular bed
Miscellaneous	Hereditary haemorrhagic telangiectasia (see pp 911–912) Peliosis hepatis, characterized by blood-filled cysts in the liver parenchyma (see p 613)

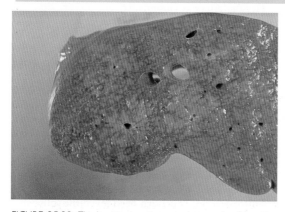

FIGURE 35.33 The liver in chronic venous congestion. Note the alternating red (congested) and yellow (showing fatty change) areas which have given this condition the name 'nutmeg liver'.

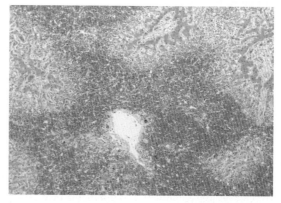

FIGURE 35.34 'Nutmeg' liver showing severe congestion of the liver in zone 3 of the liver acinus.

Other conditions or factors that have been implicated include:
- the presence in the patient's plasma of an antiphospholipid autoantibody known as the 'lupus anticoagulant'. Such antibodies may be found in association with multisystem connective tissue disorders such as systemic lupus erythematosus, but may also occur independently
- Behçet's disease
- oral contraceptives
- allergic vasculitis
- pregnancy and the postpartum state

In about 10% of cases no precipitating cause can be found.

Clinical Features

The clinical picture of the Budd–Chiari syndrome is the expression of a rapid and very marked increase in intrasinusoidal pressure resulting from obstruction to hepatic venous outflow.

The clinical features and their frequency, as reported in one series, are shown in *Table 35.19*.

On microscopic examination of the liver, the greater part of each acinus is replaced by blood, leaving only a rim of zone 1 hepatocytes surviving.

Occlusion of Intrahepatic Venous Radicles (Veno-occlusive Disease)

Veno-occlusive disease is characterized by non-thrombotic luminal narrowing affecting the hepatic vein radicles and sublobular veins. **This narrowing is due to the growth of a new layer of subendothelial connective tissue,** usually preceded by a phase in which there is severe subendothelial oedema with, in some cases, entrapment of red blood cells in the oedematous areas.

Table 35.19 Clinical Features and their Frequency in Budd–Chiari Syndrome

Clinical manifestation	Frequency (%)
Ascites	96
Enlargement of the liver	90
Abdominal pain	80
Enlargement of the spleen	64
Oedema	46
Jaundice	44
Fever	40
Hepatic encephalopathy	22
Gastrointestinal bleeding	14

Aetiology

This condition has been reported as occurring in association with:

- poisoning with pyrrolizidine alkaloids, either as a result of contamination of flour or by ingestion of 'teas' derived from alkaloid-containing plants. *Crotalaria* and *Senecio* species have been particularly implicated
- irradiation of the liver. Sensitivity to liver irradiation appears to vary from patient to patient. No reason for this variation has yet been found but it may represent variations in the antioxidant status of liver cells
- treatment with certain antitumour drugs
- 'conditioning' for bone marrow transplantation. This is now regarded as a major cause of hepatic veno-occlusive disease. Conditioning involves treating the patient with cyclophosphamide and total body irradiation. Veno-occlusive disease makes its appearance within about 4 weeks of transplantation and may complicate 13–20% of such transplantations
- graft versus host reaction

The clinical picture is very much the same as seen in the Budd–Chiari syndrome, with abdominal pain, ascites, and enlargement of the liver and spleen.

IMPAIRMENT OF ARTERIAL PERFUSION

Underperfusion of the liver may occur on either a **functional** or a **structural** basis.

Functional Underperfusion

The first of these is most frequently exemplified in patients with low-output cardiac failure. The pathological picture resembles that seen in chronic venous congestion in that there is either fatty change or atrophy of the hepatocytes in zone 3 of the liver acini.

Sinusoidal dilatation is also present but, unless there is an increase in venous pressure, the congestion seen in chronic venous congestion is not present. In some cases of heart failure the degree of liver cell necrosis is so great that a clinical picture is found similar to that in viral hepatitis.

Underperfusion of the liver also occurs in shock of all types. Again, the chief parenchymal targets are the liver cells in zone 3. In some cases, however, there is evidence of cholestasis in canaliculi adjacent to the portal tracts. The reason for this is still not known.

Structural Underperfusion

The hepatic artery and its branches can and do show the same spectrum of pathological change as is seen in other medium-sized vessels, with the exception of atherosclerosis which seems to spare this vessel. Polyarteritis nodosa (see pp 405–406) not infrequently involves the territory of the hepatic artery and may cause areas of infarction.

Hepatic artery occlusion may also occur, although rarely, as a result of impaction of an embolus or invasion by a malignant neoplasm. Ligation of the artery in the course of surgery may cause underperfusion but this is likely to be associated with infarction only if the artery is ligated at a certain level.

Infarction in the liver is rare, no doubt because of the double blood supply via the hepatic artery and portal vein. Infarcts in the liver, when they do occur, differ in no essential respect from those in other sites, with the affected liver cells undergoing coagulative necrosis.

Occlusion of branches of the portal vein within the liver give rise to a curious, well-demarcated area of dark red discoloration, which has been given the somewhat unfortunate name of a Zahn infarct (*Fig. 35.35*). This lesion is not a true infarct and there is no evidence of ischaemic necrosis of liver cells. Histologically these areas show the presence of a marked degree of sinusoidal dilatation and congestion, associated with some atrophy of the liver cell plates.

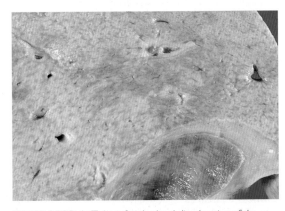

FIGURE 35.35 A 'Zahn infarct' – local discoloration of the parenchyma as a result of congestion.

MISCELLANEOUS INTRAHEPATIC VASCULAR CONDITIONS

Peliosis Hepatis

This is a very rare condition, of uncertain pathogenesis, characterized by blood-filled cystic spaces partly lined by endothelial cells within the liver parenchyma. These lesions were originally described in patients with wasting diseases such as tuberculosis and the cachexia associated with malignant disease, but are now known to develop also in patients treated with oral contraceptives or anabolic steroids. Peliosis has also been recorded in renal transplant patients in whom rejection is being held in check by treatment with azathioprine.

The patients usually have an enlarged liver and may in some instances become jaundiced. Microscopic examination shows the presence of 'lakes' of blood, these spaces existing in continuity with the sinusoids.

Congenital Haemorrhagic Telangiectasia (Rendu–Osler–Weber Disease)

This is a rare disorder inherited in an autosomal dominant pattern. It is characterized by the presence of numerous cavernous blood-filled spaces which affect many tissues (see pp 911–912).

Pathophysiology of Liver Disease

PORTAL HYPERTENSION

Portal blood flow is of the order of 1–1.2 l/min and normal portal vein blood pressure is about 7 mmHg. As in any other vascular bed, this pressure results from the **interaction between the amount of blood flowing through the system and the resistance to that flow.**

Thus, portal hypertension may arise on the basis of:

- **increased resistance to blood flow anywhere in the portal system**
- **increased blood flow through the system; or**
- **both of these acting in concert**

Under **normal** circumstances, the major physiological component of portal blood pressure is flow, which is directly dependent on splanchnic blood flow. A number of stimuli, such as the ingestion of food and exercise, can alter splanchnic blood flow and thus homoeostatic mechanisms must exist that alter the resistance to portal venous inflow to the liver so that portal venous pressure can be kept within narrow limits. The presence of portal hypertension is the expression of *failure* to alter either portal venous inflow to the liver or resistance to that inflow. **In the vast majority of** cases it is increased resistance in the prehepatic, hepatic or posthepatic vascular tree that is responsible.

Portal hypertension leads to a significant diversion of blood from the portal circulation into the systemic venous circulation.

The chief functional effect of portal hypertension is the development of a high-pressure collateral circulation from which serious bleeding may occur. The development of this collateral circulation starts once the portal blood pressure rises above 10 mmHg. Blood is diverted from the now high-pressure portal circulation into low-pressure systemic veins. The magnitude of this diversion of portal blood can be appreciated from the fact that, under normal circumstances, nearly 100% of portal blood is recoverable from the hepatic veins. In patients with cirrhosis who develop severe portal hypertension, this falls to as little as 13%.

Principal Sites for Development of Collateral Vessels

Oesophageal and Gastric Veins

At the cardia of the stomach and lower end of the oesophagus, anastomoses form between the left gastric vein, the posterior gastric vein and the short gastric veins of the portal system and veins draining into the caval system, such as the azygos vein, the diaphragmo-oesophageal veins and intercostal veins. The veins in the submucosa of the gastric fundus and of the lowest few centimetres of the oesophagus become tortuous and dilated **varices** (*Fig. 35.36*). In the oesophagus this is associated with atrophy of the muscularis mucosae and, as a result, the dilated submucosal veins come to lie very close to the mucosal surface. This closeness of the dilated oesophageal veins to the luminal surface plays a significant part in the frequency of varix rupture occurring at this site.

The oesophageal varices can be seen on upper gastrointestinal tract endoscopy and are graded as to their severity on the basis of endoscopic appearances. Thus:

- **Grade 1:** the varices can be depressed by pressure from the endoscope

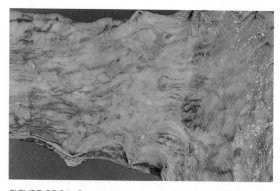

FIGURE 35.36 *Oesophageal varices in portal hypertension.*

- **Grade 2:** the varices cannot be depressed by the endoscope
- **Grade 3:** the varices are confluent and extend round the whole circumference of the oesophageal lumen

Anterior Abdominal Wall

The umbilical vein remnants of the fetal circulation lying in the falciform ligament can become an anastomotic link between the main left portal vein and the epigastric veins of the anterior abdominal wall. The presence of such dilated and tortuous veins in the anterior abdominal wall is termed a **'caput medusae'** (the gorgon Medusa had a rather unusual coiffure in the form of a mass of writhing snakes).

Submucosa of the Rectum

The superior and middle haemorrhoidal veins form part of the portal venous drainage, whereas the inferior haemorrhoidal vein drains into the vena cava. Anastomoses forming between these two systems lead to the development of rectal varices, from which bleeding may occur.

Left Renal Vein

Shunting of blood from the portal to the left renal vein may occur, either directly from the splenic vein or from pancreatic or gastric veins.

Portal–portal Anastomoses

When the obstruction to blood flow is within the main extrahepatic part of the portal vein, additional collaterals form, which re-enter the portal vein beyond the site of blockage.

The development of collaterals should decompress the portal circulation. In fact, despite the development of collateral vessels, the portal blood pressure usually remains raised in affected individuals. This is because a hyperdynamic splanchnic and systemic circulation develops, so that portal vein flow does not decrease.

Morphological Correlates of Portal Hypertension

The two chief morphological consequences of portal hypertension are:

1) the presence of varices
2) congestive splenomegaly

At post-mortem examination the dilated collateral vessels are by no means easy to see, because they collapse after death. The spleen is considerably enlarged. Its congested nature is shown by the dark red colour and the fact that blood oozes from the cut surface. The white malpighian corpuscles are inconspicuous. In some instances brown, iron-laden, fibrous nodules may be seen.

On microscopic examination, the sinusoids are, as expected, very dilated. They are lined by endothelial cells that are more prominent than normal. Macrophages are prominent and many contain haemosiderin granules. In some areas where small haemorrhages may have occurred, there are small scars in which much iron pigment is deposited.

Classification

At a functional level, portal hypertension may be divided into three main groups (*Fig. 35.37*) (see *Table 35.20*):

- **postsinusoidal**, due to pathology in the heart, inferior vena cava or hepatic veins
- **sinusoidal**, usually associated with hepatic parenchymal disease

Table 35.20 Classification of Portal Hypertension

Type	Site and cause
Postsinusoidal	
Extrahepatic	**Heart:** increased atrial pressure as in constrictive pericarditis **Inferior vena cava:** fibrous tissue webs, thrombosis, tumour invasion **Large hepatic veins:** thrombosis, tumour invasion, fibrous webs
Intrahepatic	**Small hepatic veins:** veno-occlusive disease, alcoholic central hyaline sclerosis
Sinusoidal	
Intrahepatic	Cirrhosis (most common), non-cirrhotic nodules, acute alcoholic hepatitis, cytotoxic drugs (methotrexate), vitamin A intoxication (reversible)
Presinusoidal	
Intrahepatic	**Mainly portal tract lesions:** schistosomiasis, early primary biliary cirrhosis, congenital hepatic fibrosis, chronic active hepatitis, toxins (vinyl chloride, arsenic, copper), sarcoidosis, 'idiopathic'
Extrahepatic	**Portal vein:** thrombosis, congenital, tumour invasion or compression **Splenic vein:** thrombosis, tumour invasion or compression **Increased portal blood flow:** idiopathic tropical splenomegaly, arteriovenous fistula

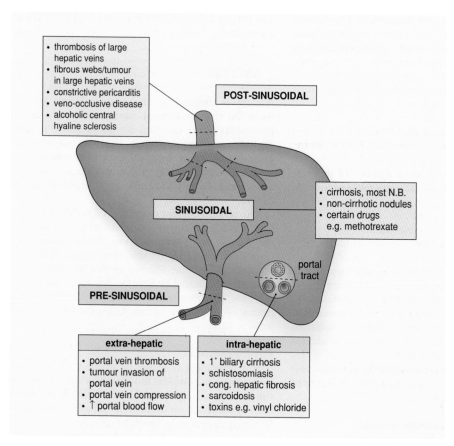

FIGURE 35.37 *Sites and causes of portal hypertension.*

- **presinusoidal**, which may be extrahepatic or intrahepatic. In presinusoidal portal hypertension, **the wedged hepatic vein pressure is normal even though portal vein pressure is raised**. This contrasts with sinusoidal and postsinusoidal portal hypertension, where the resistance to flow extends from the central hepatic veins through the sinusoids to the portal veins, and thus **the portal vein pressure and the wedged hepatic vein pressure are both raised to the same degree**. **Patients with presinusoidal portal hypertension usually have normal liver cell function. If they have an episode of bleeding from one of the varices, this is not, as a rule, followed by liver failure. In contrast, patients with sinusoidal portal hypertension, such as cirrhotics, frequently have liver failure following a variceal bleed.**

Extrahepatic Portal Vein Obstruction
Thrombosis in the portal vein is the principal pathological cause. In young children, in particular, this may be due to infection. In neonates, such infection may spread along the umbilical vein to reach the left portal vein, whereas in older children intra-

abdominal sepsis such as appendicitis may be responsible.

Portal vein thrombosis among children appears to be especially common in India, and variceal bleeding is not at all uncommon in this age group. Probable contributory factors are dehydration associated with gastroenteritis and infection.

Chronic inflammatory bowel disease such as ulcerative colitis and Crohn's disease may occasionally be complicated by portal vein thrombosis, as may sclerosing cholangitis.

Postoperative portal vein thrombosis may occur in some circumstances. It may be due to trauma as a consequence of surgery of the liver or biliary tract, but as a postoperative event is more commonly associated with the postsplenectomy state, especially in patients in whom the platelet count rises after operation. Similarly, hypercoagulable states are not uncommon causes of portal vein thrombosis, as, indeed, they are in the case of hepatic vein thrombosis. Such hypercoagulability is quite often a manifestation of a myeloproliferative disorder.

Tumour invasion may cause portal vein obstruction, the presence of intraluminal tumour frequently being associated with thrombosis. The tumour most commonly involved in this way is **hepatocellular carcinoma**, although occasionally pancreatic carcinomas may cause portal vein obstruction.

A number of other associations has been recorded, but in about half the cases of portal vein block no causal association can be identified.

Extrahepatic Presinusoidal Portal Hypertension in the Absence of Portal Vein Obstruction

This situation has been given a number of different names, including non-cirrhotic portal hypertension. It is characterized by:

- splenomegaly
- functional evidence of hypersplenism
- no occlusion of extrahepatic portions of the portal vein or its tributaries

Despite the absence of obvious liver pathology such as cirrhosis, it is clear that the portal blood pressure rises because of increased hepatic resistance to portal blood inflow, and it is believed that injury to the endothelial lining of intrahepatic portal vein radicles and sinusoids is the common denominator. The aetiology is unclear but geographical differences in the prevalence of this condition (it is commonest in middle-aged Japanese women and young Indian men) suggest the influence of some environmental factor(s).

Intrahepatic Presinusoidal Portal Hypertension

The pathological common denominator for this form of portal hypertension is a disorder affecting the portal tracts.

Hepatic schistosomiasis is a good example of this group of processes; in areas, where schistosomiasis is endemic, such as Egypt, this variety of portal hypertension is common in both relative and absolute terms. The schistosome ova are deposited in the portal tracts and elicit scarring, which is, presumably, the cause of the presinusoidal block.

Intrahepatic Sinusoidal Portal Hypertension

In Europe and North America this is the commonest form of portal hypertension. In these areas, 90% of patients presenting with bleeding from oesophageal varices have cirrhosis.

The causes of the resistance to portal blood flow in cirrhosis are complex, and probably include:

- fibrous tissue formation in the space of Disse, leading to sinusoidal narrowing
- compression of hepatic venous radicles by regeneration nodules
- action of contractile myofibroblasts in the space of Disse
- swelling of liver cells, such as may occur in alcoholic hepatitis and severe fatty change due to other causes

The principal clinical features of portal hypertension are shown in *Fig 35.38*.

ASCITES

Ascites is defined as the accumulation of free fluid in the peritoneal cavity. It is not usually possible to detect less than 500 ml of ascitic fluid by clinical examination, other than by sophisticated imaging techniques. In practice, patients with decompensated cirrhosis may accumulate many litres of ascitic fluid, causing gross distension of the abdominal cavity.

The protein content of the fluid is usually fairly low (about 1–2 g per 100 ml); most ascites in liver disease is the expression of **transudation**. Protein concentrations significantly higher than this suggest either that the fluid has become infected or that the cirrhosis has become complicated by hepatocellular carcinoma. The presence of blood-stained ascites, in the absence of a history of recent paracentesis, makes the latter possibility very likely.

Pathogenesis

The development of ascites in a patient with chronic liver disease is complex and there are aspects that are still difficult to understand. Defects in the liver relating both to the functions of the liver cell and to the vascular system appear to be involved (*Fig. 35.39*).

- In most patients with ascites there is **raised pressure at the venous end of the splanchnic capillaries** and this favours transudation of fluid from the vascular to the extravascular compartment. This situation is particularly likely to arise in the presence of sinusoidal portal hypertension where there is collagenization in the space of Disse.
- Sinusoidal portal hypertension is associated with **a marked increase in the formation of hepatic lymph**. Lymphatics at the hilum of the liver are distended and the flow of lymph in the thoracic duct is increased (in some patients up to 20 l/day). It is likely that the 'weeping' of lymph from the liver surface occurs only when the capacity of the thoracic duct is exceeded. Support for this view comes from the fact that, in some patients, thoracic duct drainage can lessen the amount of ascitic fluid.
- Chronic decompensation in the liver is characterized by decreased protein synthesis by liver cells. This results in a **decreased plasma albumin concentration associated with a lowered plasma oncotic pressure** and a consequent reduction in fluid reabsorption at the venous end of the splanchnic and other capillaries.
- Patients with ascites due to cirrhosis **retain large amounts of sodium and consequently large amounts of water** as well. Mechanisms underlying this are complex:

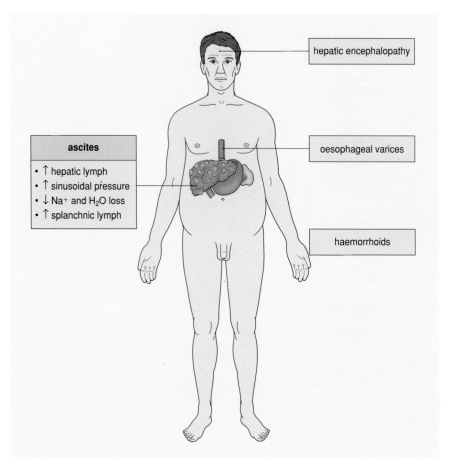

FIGURE 35.38 *Clinical features of portal hypertension.*

1) Sodium retention can be demonstrated **before** ascitic fluid begins to accumulate. Thus, it may act as a causal factor in the formation of ascitic fluid and is not, as previously thought, merely a consequence of ascites. This 'primary' retention of sodium and water is thought to lead to expansion of the plasma volume and overflow into the extravascular compartment. It constitutes the **'overfill'** theory of the origin of ascites and is likely to be important in the early stages of ascites development. Some support for this view comes from the fact that ascites can be induced in cirrhotic patients by expanding the extracellular fluid by administering mineralocorticoids. In addition, if portal venous pressure is reduced by portosystemic shunting, ascites may disappear and be replaced by generalized oedema.

2) The traditional view of the cause of sodium retention has been that it is a consequence of ascites formation. The combination of hypoalbuminaemia, high portal vein pressure, and dilatation of splanchnic and systemic capillaries contributes to a situation in which fluid is sequestered away from the central arterial system. The effective circulating plasma volume falls and the consequent underperfusion of the renal cortex leads to increases in the output of renin and hence of angiotensin. This results in a rise in aldosterone production and increased renal tubular absorption of sodium. There is also an increase in sympathetic activity and a rise in the renal production of prostaglandin E_2. This is known as the **'underfill'** theory, and appears to operate in about one-third of cirrhotic patients with ascites. This pattern, with stimulation of the renin–angiotensin–aldosterone axis, is particularly likely to occur in patients with advanced disease.

HEPATIC ENCEPHALOPATHY

Patients with liver disease may show a spectrum of neuropsychiatric disturbances known as **hepatic encephalopathy**. This may occur against a background of chronic liver disease such as cirrhosis or in association with fulminant necrotizing processes giving rise to acute liver failure.

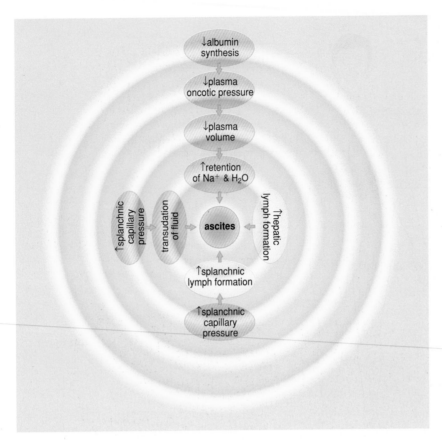

FIGURE 35.39 Pathogenesis of ascites in liver disease.

Acute Liver Failure

In patients with acute liver failure due to fulminant hepatitis or drug-related necrosis, the onset of hepatic encephalopathy tends to be rapid, the degree of disturbance severe and the prognosis poor. The clinical features are shown below:

- Onset is rapid with a short prodrome.
- The patient becomes drowsy and this may be followed by delirium and fits.
- In some cases decerebrate rigidity develops.
- The patient may become unresponsive and lapse into deep coma.

This sequence of events may take as little as 24 hours.

Chronic Liver Disease

In patients with chronic liver disease, the clinical pattern is quite different. The natural history of the encephalopathy may be an episodic one, the episodes being precipitated by some identifiable cause which may be reversible, such as a gastrointestinal tract haemorrhage. In the intervals between such episodes, the patient's neurological and psychiatric status may appear quite normal. The prodrome in these patients may be very gradual, and the type and degree of disturbance rather subtle, although in many cases the end result is coma.

- The onset is gradual and the initial changes affect the patient's mood, either euphoria or depression being present. Judgement may be impaired and the patient appears tired and withdrawn. Disturbances in sleep patterns are common, with patients being wakeful at night and sleepy during the day.
- As the syndrome progresses, patients become slow to respond and may be confused in respect of place, time and person. The handwriting often deteriorates and the patients are unable to copy simple shapes such as a star (**constructional apraxia**).
- At this stage rather typical electroencephalographic (EEG) changes are often present. These take the form of slowing of the EEG involving slow waves of the δ type.
- A striking feature is the presence of a 'flapping tremor' (**asterixis**). This is characteristic of hepatic encephalopathy but not pathognomonic, because it may also be seen in uraemia, respiratory failure, cardiac failure and hypoglycaemia.

KEY POINTS: Hepatic Encephalopathy

Patients with hepatic encephalopathy may have a variety of biochemical abnormalities associated with the liver disease, but there are only a few more or less specifically related to the presence of the encephalopathy.

- **An increase in the concentration of ammonia in the blood.** This is the most widely performed investigation in hepatic encephalopathy. It is not, however, an absolutely reliable indicator, because some patients with unequivocal hepatic coma have normal blood ammonia levels.
- **Glutamine levels in the cerebrospinal fluid (CSF) are usually raised in patients with hepatic encephalopathy.** Some state that measurement of CSF glutamine levels is the most accurate and useful test in this disorder. There is also an increase in the CSF concentrations of certain aromatic amino acids, most notably methionine, phenylalanine, tyrosine and tryptophan.

Macroscopic Features

The brain may appear entirely normal. In about half the cases **cerebral oedema** is present. This finding is commonest in young patients with fulminant hepatitis, who have been in deep coma for some days.

Microscopic Features

Early

The most striking early change is an **increase in the number and size of protoplasmic astrocytes in the deeper layers of the cortex, the basal ganglia and the dentate nucleus in the cerebellum**. The commonest cytological change in these astrocytes is an enlarged, pale and sometimes lobulated nucleus. Such altered astrocytes are called Alzheimer type II cells.

Late

In patients in whom there have been many episodes of hepatic encephalopathy extending over a considerable time, the cerebral cortex becomes thinned and there is irreversible loss of both neurones and fibres. Demyelination is an occasional feature and this may affect the spinal tracts, producing spastic paraplegia.

Pathogenesis

Central to the development of hepatic encephalopathy is the fact that **portal blood is shunted to the systemic circulation without being exposed to the metabolic functions of liver cells** (*Fig. 35.40*).

In patients with massive liver necrosis, resulting from fulminant or toxic damage, this shunting is purely **functional** in that the liver cells are unable

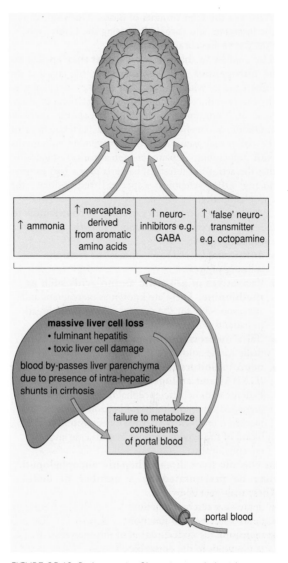

FIGURE 35.40 Pathogenesis of hepatic encephalopathy.

adequately to metabolize the constituents of the portal blood. In the case of cirrhosis, shunting is **anatomically based**. The portal blood bypasses the liver cells to a very considerable extent via the collateral vessels and via the anastomotic channels between the portal vein branches and the hepatic vein radicles in the fibrous septa separating the nodules of liver parenchyma.

Support for the importance of portosystemic shunting comes from observations that hepatic encephalopathy may complicate portocaval anastomoses carried out in patients with portal hypertension, and that portosystemic anastomoses (Eck fistulae) in normal dogs cause acute neuropsychiatric disturbances if the dogs are fed a high protein diet.

What are the Constituents of Blood, Derived from the Intestine, and Largely Bypassing the Liver Cells, that Cause Cerebral Intoxication?

The answer to this question is that they appear to be nitrogenous, a view supported by the fact that, in some patients with chronic liver disease, encephalopathy can be induced by high protein diets, urea, methionine and ammonium chloride. Measures, such as antibiotic treatment, that reduce the bacterial flora of the colon may cause clinical improvement in patients with impending hepatic encephalopathy, suggesting that the actions of intestinal bacteria play a part in producing the chemical species responsible for encephalopathy.

Among the compounds canvassed as contributors to the altered cerebral metabolic activity in hepatic encephalopathy are:

- **ammonia** derived from amines and from the splitting of urea
- **derivatives of aromatic amino acids such as methionine.** These are known as mercaptans and are responsible for the curious odour of the breath in patients with liver failure (**fetor hepaticus**)
- **'false' neurotransmitters such as octopamine** made in the colon as a result of bacterial action
- **neuroinhibitors such as γ-aminobutyric acid (GABA) and endogenous benzodiazepines.** Patients with hepatic encephalopathy show increased cerebral binding of benzodiazepines, and increased levels of GABA have been found in the blood of those with chronic liver disease and encephalopathy.

In chronic liver disease, hepatic encephalopathy may be precipitated by a number of factors. These may operate by:

- depressing cerebral function
- depressing liver cell function
- increasing the concentration of nitrogenous compounds in the portal blood
- increasing the degree of portal–systemic shunting

The events that may induce encephalopathy are shown in *Table 35.21*.

OTHER MANIFESTATIONS OF LIVER FAILURE

In addition to the foregoing, liver failure due to chronic liver disease can adversely affect many other physiological systems (*Fig. 35.41*). In some instances this is a reflection of failure of:

- the **synthetic functions** of the liver cell mass (as in the decreased concentration of many coagulation factors)
- **the hepatic clearance of active chemical species** from the blood

Table 35.21 Triggers of Hepatic Encephalopathy

Mechanism	Examples
Infection	'Spontaneous' bacterial peritonitis Urinary tract infection Chest infection
Haemorrhage	From oesophageal and gastric varices From gastroduodenal erosions or peptic ulcer From tears in the oesophagus precipitated by vomiting (Mallory–Weiss syndrome)
Electrolyte disturbances	Diuretics Diarrhoea Vomiting
Drugs and toxins	Morphia, benzodiazepines, barbiturates, alcohol

Effect of Liver Disease on the Cardiovascular System

Patients with chronic liver disease may have a hyperkinetic circulation with high cardiac output and decreased peripheral vascular resistance associated with vasodilatation. This state appears to be related to the severity of the liver disease and improves if liver function improves.

The reason for the vasodilatation is not known. It is likely to be due to the action of a number of compounds with vasodilator activity. Candidates include GABA, formed both by the intestinal mucosa and by the action of gut bacteria, and there is some evidence that increased amounts of vasodilator prostaglandins are released into the portal circulation in chronic liver disease.

Effects of Liver Disease on the Lungs and Pulmonary Vascular System

A number of respiratory disturbances can occur in chronic liver disease. These include:

- **Reduced arterial oxygen saturation.** This may be due, in part, to a shift of the oxygen dissociation curve of haemoglobin to the right because of increased concentrations of 2,3-diphosphoglycerate in the red blood cells of these patients. Another contributor to hypoxia may be the presence of microscopic arteriovenous shunts within the lungs, as demonstrated both functionally and following injection studies of lung tissue from affected patients.
- **Pulmonary vasodilatation that fails to respond to hypoxia.** This, combined with the shunts

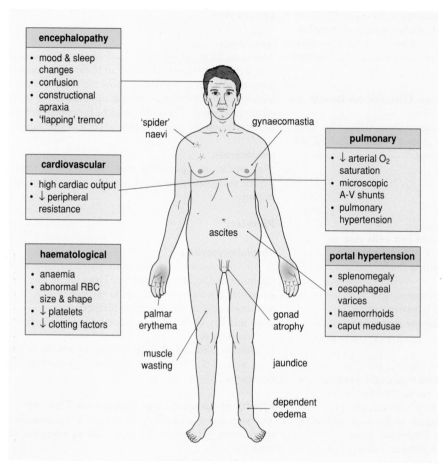

encephalopathy
- mood & sleep changes
- confusion
- constructional apraxia
- 'flapping' tremor

'spider' naevi

gynaecomastia

pulmonary
- ↓ arterial O$_2$ saturation
- microscopic A-V shunts
- pulmonary hypertension

cardiovascular
- high cardiac output
- ↓ peripheral resistance

ascites

haematological
- anaemia
- abnormal RBC size & shape
- ↓ platelets
- ↓ clotting factors

portal hypertension
- splenomegaly
- oesophageal varices
- haemorrhoids
- caput medusae

palmar erythema

gonad atrophy

muscle wasting

jaundice

dependent oedema

FIGURE 35.41 Manifestations of liver failure.

referred to above, leads to some degree of mismatch between ventilation and perfusion, and thus tends to worsen the degree of hypoxia. Chronic hypoxia is associated with finger clubbing.

- **Pulmonary hypertension** can occur both in patients with hepatocellular disease and those with extrahepatic portal hypertension in whom portal–systemic shunting is present. The causes are not well understood. In a minority of cases there may be evidence of recurrent thromboembolism in the pulmonary circulation; in others it is suggested that the increase in pulmonary blood pressure may be due to vasoconstrictor compounds that are not deactivated by the liver.

Effects of Liver Disease on the Endocrine System

The chief, though by no means the only, endocrine effects of chronic liver disease are on **gonadal function**, the paradigm being a syndrome consisting of **cirrhosis, gynaecomastia and hypogonadism** in the male.

It is too simplistic to regard these changes as being entirely due to failure of the liver cells to inactivate steroid hormones such as oestrogen. This may well be important but other factors that should be taken into account are:

- the degree of portal–systemic shunting present
- the rate of secretion of the hormone
- the concentration of hormone-binding proteins in the plasma
- the degree of receptor-mediated sensitivity of the target organ concerned

Most studies of sexual dysfunction in patients with chronic liver disease have been carried out in men. In its fully developed form **the syndrome is characterized by gynaecomastia and testicular atrophy**, the latter being associated with loss of libido, impotence and a decrease in body hair. The last-named features are interesting in view of the fact that the testis shows atrophy of the seminiferous tubules and not of the testosterone-producing Leydig cells. This suggests a role for decreased sensitivity of the receptors binding testosterone.

Hypogonadism and feminization are especially likely to occur in patients with alcoholic cirrhosis. Alcoholism itself may be a pathogenetic factor, oestradiol concentrations being higher in patients with alcohol-related liver disease.

Effects of Chronic Liver Disease on Blood Cells

A wide range of haematological abnormalities has been reported in chronic liver disease. These affect all the formed elements of the blood.

Red Cells

Anaemia

This may be the result of:

- **increased destruction of red cells due to hypersplenism**
- **increased plasma volume** due to sodium and water retention
- **recurrent bleeding** associated with varix formation due to portal hypertension
- **failure of normal marrow responses** due to general ill-health

Changes in Red Cell Size

Red cells may be normocytic, macrocytic or microcytic:

- **Macrocytosis** may be due to disturbances in vitamin B_{12} and folate metabolism, leading to megalopoiesis, or to changes in the lipid content of the red cell membranes, leading to 'thin' macrocytosis where the diameter but not the volume of the red cells is increased.
- **Microcytosis** is associated with recurrent haemorrhages, and the red cells will also be hypochromic.
- In most cases red cells will be **normocytic**.

Changes in Red Cell Shape

- **Formation of target cells.** Target cells are red cells that have assumed a saucer or bowl shape which, in conventional blood films, looks like a target with a central dark area. It is associated with increased amounts of cholesterol or of cholesterol plus phospholipid in the red cell membranes.
- **Formation of 'echinocytes'.** Echinocytes are red cells that appear 'spiky' when seen in wet films or are examined by scanning electron microscopy. They result from the binding of an abnormal high density lipoprotein to the red cell surface.
- **Formation of acanthocytes.** These are bizarre cells with many projections on their surfaces. The mechanism involved in their formation is not known; they reflect severe liver disease.

Erythrocytosis

Nearly 25% of patients with liver cell cancer have a raised erythropoietin level and between 3 and 12% have a raised red cell count.

Leucocytes

Leucopenia

This tends to occur especially in alcoholic cirrhosis and may be due to hypersplenism or to toxic effects on the bone marrow. It is difficult to know the relative contributions of the liver disease itself as opposed to the toxic effects of alcohol. There appear to be functional defects in the response of the white cells to chemotactic signals.

Leucocytosis

This occurs in association with fulminant hepatitis, hepatic malignancy, ascending cholangitis and alcoholic hepatitis.

Platelets

Thrombocytopenia

A mild to moderate decrease in platelet numbers is common in chronic liver disease. This may be due to:

- increased pooling of platelets in the spleen
- a shortening in the life of the platelets
- an inability of the marrow to compensate fully for these defects

In addition, although the platelet membranes are richer than normal in cholesterol, platelet aggregatibility is decreased.

Effects of Chronic Liver Disease on Clotting

The well-recognized effects of chronic liver disease on coagulation of blood may come about in a number of ways:

1) **a decrease in the synthesis of proteins,** including:
   - clotting factors and their substrates
   - naturally occurring anticoagulants such as proteins C and S and antithrombin III
   - profibrinolytic proteins such as plasminogen
   - antifibrinolytic proteins such as plasminogen activator inhibitors
2) **synthesis of abnormal forms of proteins**:
   - fibrinogen
   - Factor VIII and von Willebrand factor
   - vitamin K-dependent factors
3) **a decrease in clearance function involving**:
   - activated clotting factors
   - plasminogen activators synthesized by endothelium
   - thrombin–antithrombin III complexes

With all these different defects, it is not surprising that several functional bleeding disturbances may be seen. Affected patients have a prolonged one-stage prothrombin time and also show accelerated fibrinolysis. In some patients, disseminated intravascular coagulation occurs.

Effects of Chronic Liver Disease on the Skin

Apart from such expected phenomena as jaundice, the most striking effects of liver disease on skin are those that affect the skin blood vessels. Characteristic lesions are:

- **Spider naevi.** These are lesions consisting of a central dilated arteriole from which numerous small vessels radiate. Pressure on the central arteriole causes blanching of the lesion. What is extremely odd is that spider naevi are very rarely found below an imaginary line joining the nipples. If the liver disease becomes worse, more spider lesions appear, and the converse is true if the liver pathology improves.
- **Palmar erythema.** Patients with chronic liver disease frequently have warm red palms, with the thenar and hypothenar eminences especially affected. 'Liver' palms may appear independently of spider naevi, and presumably a different mechanism is responsible for their genesis.

Drugs and the Liver

More than 600 different drugs have been implicated in liver damage. The importance of drug-related liver injury is shown by the fact that **2% of cases of jaundice and 25% of cases of fulminant acute liver failure** are believed to be caused by drugs.

Drug reactions can mimic virtually every form of 'spontaneous' liver disease and, therefore, a detailed drug history forms an essential part of the investigation of patients with liver disease.

In simple terms, the liver-damaging activity of any individual compound may be:

- **predictable**: the damage is related to the **dose** of the compound
- **unpredictable**: occurs because the intracellular defences of an individual may be inadequate (as in conditions where there is depletion of intracellular reduced glutathione (GSH)) or where an unusual immune response has taken place, as is believed to occur in halothane-related liver damage

REACTIVE METABOLITES IN THE CAUSATION OF LIVER DAMAGE

Some drugs may damage the liver directly, but many others require prior metabolism with the formation of reactive metabolites before liver damage can occur.

Most drugs reaching the liver are lipid soluble and must be converted to water-soluble metabolites before they are excreted in the urine or bile. In most instances two steps are required for the conversion of these lipophilic compounds:

1) **Oxidation of the compound by cytochrome P450**, which exists in several isoenzymic forms. Genetic differences in the catalytic activity of the P450 enzymes may well be responsible for some of the unexpected or 'idiosyncratic' reactions to drugs. In addition, certain compounds (e.g. phenobarbitone, alcohol) will induce P450 enzymes, rendering the patient more likely to sustain liver damage from some other compound.

2) **The conjugation of the compound** with a polar, water-soluble group such as glucuronic acid.

The activation of cytochrome P450 by reduced nicotinamide adenine dinucleotide phosphate (NADPH)–cytochrome P450 reductase and the resulting oxidizing effects of the P450 are central to this theme and lead to the formation of:

- highly reactive electrophilic compounds
- semiquinone free radicals which may have a fairly long half-life and from which reactive oxygen species are generated
- free radicals derived from haloalkanes such as carbon tetrachloride

The cell damage resulting from these reactive metabolites is mediated via:

- **Covalent binding of electrophilic compounds to nucleic acid** resulting in either cell death or mutagenesis.
- **Lipid peroxidation of unsaturated fatty acids in plasma membranes** leading to disruption of the cytoskeleton and to abnormal permeability of the plasma membranes. Calcium accumulates in large amounts within the damaged cells and is a powerful mechanism in causing cell death.
- **Depletion of the powerful antioxidant GSH.** A decline in the intracellular concentrations of GSH enhances the severity of the two processes listed above and also leads to the oxidation of intracellular thiols, with deleterious effects on a number of cellular functions.

IMMUNOALLERGIC MECHANISMS IN DRUG-RELATED LIVER DAMAGE

Halothane-induced Hepatitis

In some instances reactive metabolites may cause liver damage via an immune-mediated reaction. One particularly striking example is the hepatitis-like injury that occurs in some patients after anaesthesia has been induced with halothane.

In affected individuals, liver cell plasma membranes are trifluoroacetylated by a reactive product of halothane. The altered plasma membrane proteins act as new antigens, eliciting the formation of a cytotoxic antibody. Reactive metabolites of halothane are probably formed in all individuals and the alteration of plasma membranes is also believed to be very common. Only a small proportion, however, become immunized against the altered proteins. This increased susceptibility for the formation of antibodies is thought to be due to genetic factors not yet understood. With each succeeding halothane induction, the consequences in susceptible individuals are likely to be more severe, as would be expected with an immunologically based reaction.

A similar mechanism is believed to be operating in the causation of liver damage due to a number of other drugs including imipramine, erythromycin and α-methyldopa.

MORPHOLOGICAL CHANGES ASSOCIATED WITH DRUG-MEDIATED LIVER DAMAGE

These may affect one or more of the following:
- liver cells
- bile ductules and ducts
- blood vessels
- mononuclear phagocytes

Lesions that occur in the first two categories are listed in *Tables 35.22* and *35.23*.

The Extrahepatic Biliary System: The Gallbladder

Normal Anatomy

The gallbladder is a pear-shaped sac between 7 and 10 cm long with **a capacity of about 50 ml**. It lies in the gallbladder fossa, a shallow depression between the quadrate and right lobes of the liver. The liver secretes 0.5−1 litres of rather watery bile per day. Most of this is stored in the gallbladder which can concentrate bile by a factor of between five and ten. In addition, **the gallbladder secretes mucins derived from glands in its neck into its lumen**.

The gallbladder mucosa is thrown into many folds (thus increasing the absorptive surface) and is lined by tall columnar epithelium. There is no muscularis mucosae but there is muscularis propria which is, for the most part, composed of longitudinally oriented fibres admixed with collagen and elastic tissue.

Table 35.22 Lesions Affecting the Liver Cells

Lesion	Mechanism	Examples of responsible drug
Coagulative necrosis showing ghost outlines of eosinophilic liver cells. This may be focal or confluent. Toxic hepatic necrosis is usually most severe in zone 3 liver cells where the concentration of cytochromes is greatest	Reactive metabolites	Paracetamol poisoning, associated with depletion of GSH as a result of binding of electrophilic metabolites. Also seen in poisoning by the mushroom, *Amanita phalloides*, and carbon tetrachloride
Cytolytic necrosis. Usually focal ('spotty' necrosis) and elicits an intralobular inflammatory reaction, similar to that of acute hepatitis	Damage by reactive metabolites or immunoallergic damage due to the formation of neoantigens as a result of linkage of haptens with liver cell proteins	Halothane, erythromycin, isoniazid, α-methyldopa (*Fig. 35.42*)
Acute hepatitis-like picture associated with evidence of cholestasis	? Immunoallergic reaction to reactive metabolite	Phenothiazines, sulphonylureas, tricyclic antidepressants
Chronic hepatitis-like picture. May culminate in cirrhosis	Probably an immunoallergic reaction	α-Methyldopa, nitrofurantoin, oxyphenisatin, methotrexate
Large-droplet fatty change with nucleus pushed to side by single large accumulation of intracellular fat. So-called macrovesicular variety	Failure to export triglyceride in form of very low density lipoprotein. Probably due to decreased protein synthesis with lack of apoprotein B_{100}. May also be associated with structural damage to endoplasmic reticulum, Golgi apparatus or plasma membrane of liver cell	Alcohol, methotrexate

Table 35.22 Lesions Affecting the Liver Cells—*continued*

Lesion	Mechanism	Examples of responsible drug
Small-droplet fatty change (microvesicular variety). Nucleus remains centrally placed and cytoplasm contains very numerous small droplets of fat	Reflects impaired mitochondrial oxidation of fatty acids	Tetracyclines and valproic acid, an anticonvulsant. Also in Jamaica in patients poisoned by the unripe ackee fruit, and in Reye's syndrome
Phospholipidosis. Accumulation of phospholipid in lysosomes. Lysosomes are increased in size and number and contain lamellar bodies	Drugs form complexes with phospholipids and inhibit the action of lysosomal phospholipases	Amiodarone, perhexiline maleate and 4,4′-diethylaminoethoxyhexestrol. In some patients on these drugs there is a microscopic picture resembling alcoholic hepatitis, and cirrhosis occasionally occurs
Granulomatous hepatitis with small rounded foci of epithelioid cells in the portal tracts. Occasional multinucleate giant cells seen	Cell-mediated immune reaction	Sulphonamides, allopurinol, carbamazepine, phenylbutazone, quinine
Neoplasms: hepatic adenoma, hepatocellular carcinoma, angiosarcoma	?	Oestrogens, Thorotrast, anabolic steroids

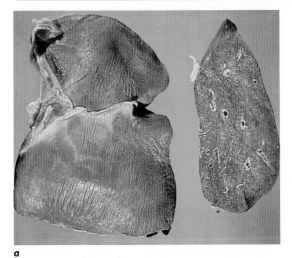

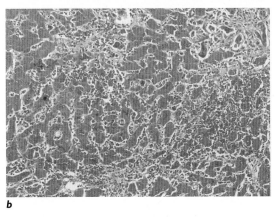

FIGURE 35.42 **a** *Massive necrosis of the liver. Note wrinkling of the capsule due to rapid autolysis of the dead liver cells – a useful sign of massive or submassive necrosis.* **b** *Submassive necrosis of the liver; most cells have lost their nuclei and some liver cell cords are broken up.*

Function

The gallbladder **concentrates, stores** and **releases bile** (*Fig 35.44*). The **release of stored bile from the gallbladder** is associated with taking of fatty food. This requires coordinated contraction of the gallbladder muscle and relaxation of the sphincter of Oddi at the distal end of the common bile duct where it enters the duodenum. These functions are mediated by **increased plasma concentrations of cholecystokinin**, which follow the entry of fatty food into the duodenum.

GALLSTONES (CHOLELITHIASIS)

Gallstones are very common, affecting 10–20% of the adult population in Europe and the United States. An important risk factor is **female sex, the female:male**

Table 35.23 Lesions Affecting the Bile Ducts

Lesion	Mechanism	Examples of responsible drug
Acute bland cholestasis. No inflammation or necrosis associated	(a) Increase of permeability in canaliculi leading to increase in back–diffusion of bile constituents; (b) decreases in membrane fluidity with inhibition of Na^+ and K^+ adenosine triphosphatase activity; (c) formation by oestrogens of 17β-glucuronides, which are potent cholestatic agents	Oral contraceptives; anabolic and androgenic steroids
Prolonged cholestasis due to rarefaction of bile ducts. Starts with a cholestatic hepatitis-like picture followed by gradual destruction of small bile ducts. The bile duct lesions continue to become more severe long after the drug has been eliminated. Associated with eosinophilia and the presence of circulating immune complexes	Probably an immune-mediated reaction with haptens binding to proteins of bile duct epithelium	Chlorpromazine (*Fig. 35.43*), paraquat poisoning, some arsenical derivatives
Lesions resembling sclerosing cholangitis with multiple and seg-mental strictures that may affect both intrahepatic and extrahepatic bile ducts	?	Infusion of floxuridine into hepatic artery in the treatment of liver metastases from colorectal carcinoma

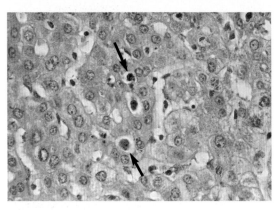

FIGURE 35.43 *Cholestasis in chlorpromazine jaundice. Note the green bile plugs (arrowed).*

ratio being roughly 2:1. Female preponderance is presumably linked with hormonal influences: evidence suggests that oral contraceptives can increase the level of biliary cholesterol and that males treated with oestrogens show an increased risk of developing gallstones. **Obesity** and **diabetes** are also common associations.

MAJOR TYPES OF GALLSTONES
The vast majority of human gallstones can be classified into *two* groups: **cholesterol** and **pigment** stones.

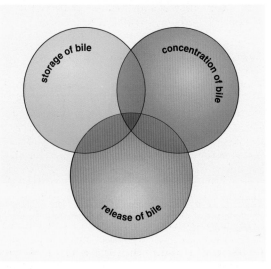

FIGURE 35.44 *Functions of the gallbladder.*

Cholesterol Stones
In Western countries more than 75% of stones contain significant amounts of cholesterol. This category can be subdivided into:
- **Pure cholesterol** stones, in which 90% of the content is cholesterol. They are usually single, large

(greater than 2.5 cm in diameter) and white or pale yellow in colour. Their consistency is soft, and they are easily cut, the cut surface having a radiating structure made up of cholesterol crystals.

- **Mixed stones.** Some 50% of the content is cholesterol, the rest being made up of mucoprotein, calcium and bilirubin. They are smaller than the pure cholesterol stones (0.5–2.5 cm in diameter) and are usually multiple. This multiplicity leads to their having a highly characteristic **faceted appearance**.

Pigment Stones

Pigment stones account for only 10% of cases of gallstones in Western countries but are rather more common in Asia. They are subdivided into two main categories:

- **Black pigment stones** which contain large amounts of a polymerized degradation product of oxidized bilirubin. This is the commonest form of pigment stone. They are found worldwide and occur most frequently in association with haemolysis and cirrhosis. **They are virtually confined to the gallbladder and the bile is usually sterile.**
- **Brown pigment stones** which contain mainly calcium bilirubinate. They are soft and have a laminated cut surface. They are found chiefly in the Far East, especially in patients with bile duct infections or helminth infestations. **They may occur in either the gallbladder or the bile ducts; the bile is usually infected.**

Composition of Bile and its Relation to Cholesterol Gallstone Formation

Some 97% of hepatic bile is water and only 3% is made up of solutes. **The relative proportions of these solutes are, however, very important in the pathogenesis of gallstones.** In normal bile, solutes are present in the proportions listed in *Table 35.24*.

Bile is the chief pathway for eliminating cholesterol in the form of bile salts and free cholesterol. Free cholesterol, although it makes up only 4% of the total solute fraction of bile, is of great importance in the pathogenesis of gallstones, because it is **insoluble in aqueous solutions**. In bile, cholesterol is made soluble by its association with bile salts and phospholipid. **Stones tend to form when the cholesterol concentration in the bile exceeds the ability of the bile salts and phospholipid to hold the cholesterol in solution, that is when the bile is supersaturated with cholesterol.** Such bile is termed 'lithogenic' bile and results from the mechanisms listed in *Table 35.25*.

The relative contributions of cholesterol, phospholipid and bile acids to the solute fraction of bile may be examined in the form of a triangular diagram in which each coordinate represents one of these solute constituents. Cholesterol appears to be most soluble in a mixture that, in molar terms, contains at least 50% bile acids and about 30% phospholipid.

Table 35.24 Bile Solutes

Solute	Percentage present in total solute
Cholesterol	4
Bile salts (derived from cholic acid, chenodeoxycholic acid and deoxycholic acid). The bile acids are derived from the catabolism of cholesterol and are linked with taurine or glycine to form the bile salts	67
Phospholipids (mainly lecithin)	22
Protein	4.5
Bilirubin	0.3

Table 35.25 Causes of Disturbances of Molar Ratios of Cholesterol and Bile Acids in Bile

Mechanism	Associations
Increased output of cholesterol in hepatic bile	Increasing age Obesity Geographical factors (e.g. common in Scandinavia) Oestrogen treatment in men Lipid-lowering drugs such as clofibrate, colestipol and cholestyramine
Decreased concentrations of bile acids in bile	Disorders causing decreased absorption of bile salts from small gut (e.g. chronic inflammatory bowel disease, extensive bowel resection, prolonged fasting) Impaired regulation of bile acid synthesis in liver
A combination of the above	Genetic; common in North American Indians Oestrogen treatment in women Female sex

Supersaturation of bile with cholesterol is, by itself, not sufficient to explain cholesterol gallstone formation. For a given degree of cholesterol supersaturation, bile from patients with gallstones forms stones much more rapidly than does bile from those without gallstones. Stone formation begins with the formation of tiny crystals of cholesterol. This process is called **nucleation** and leads to the formation of 'sludge', which consists of mucoprotein containing small, entrapped cholesterol crystals and bilirubin. The presence of sludge may be asymptomatic but, in some cases, there may be gallbladder colic, inflammation of the gallbladder and acute pancreatitis. Factors promoting sludge formation include **pregnancy, prolonged total parenteral nutrition, starvation or rapid weight loss due to dieting.** The antibiotic ceftriaxone may also precipitate in the gallbladder as sludge.

Other intrabiliary factors include the **pH and concentration of calcium in the bile**. Many patients with gallstones have increased bile concentrations of calcium. Solubilization of calcium is enhanced by **acidification** of the bile, and it has been suggested that, in patients with calcium-containing stones, this acidification is impaired.

Lastly, **stasis** of the gallbladder with impaired emptying is a risk factor for the development of stones (*Fig. 35.45*). Stasis is associated, in females, with pregnancy and oral contraceptive use. Prolonged total parenteral alimentation also causes severe gallbladder stasis.

CLINICAL EFFECTS OF GALLSTONES

- **Most patients with gallstones have no symptoms** referable to the stones, these being an incidental finding.
- **In patients in whom the gallstones cause symptoms, the cause of the latter is usually impaction, the site of such impaction dictating the clinical and pathological effects** (*Fig. 35.46*).
- **Most patients with symptoms referable to gallstones complain of abdominal pain, most commonly localized to the epigastrium or right upper quadrant.** Despite this being called **'biliary colic'**, the pain is steady rather than intermittent and usually lasts for several hours. The commonest pathological correlate is **impaction of a stone in the cystic duct.**

Acute Cholecystitis

Some patients present with symptoms related to acute cholecystitis, i.e. with severe abdominal pain, nausea, vomiting, fever and a raised neutrophil count. Most cases of acute cholecystitis are thought to be due to bile stasis associated with impaction of a stone in the cystic duct. Only 10% of all patients with acute cholecystitis have no gallstones.

It is not clear why and how cystic duct obstruction should lead to acute inflammation. It may be due to chemical injury caused by increased concentrations of

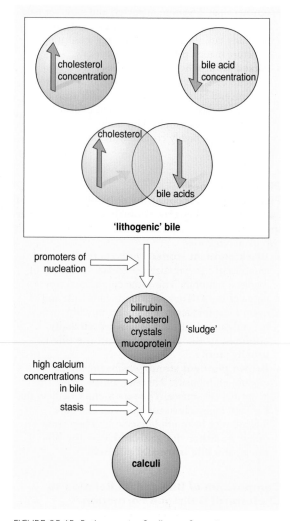

FIGURE 35.45 *Pathogenesis of gallstone formation.*

cholesterol, bile salts or lysolecithin. Alternatively, the presence of the gallstones themselves may cause mucosal injury. In general, cholecystitis does not seem to be **primarily** infective, although proliferating pyogenic organisms are found in the bile in about 20% of cases. This may be associated with suppuration leading to:

- a gallbladder distended with pus (**empyema**)
- focal necrosis of the gallbladder wall with perforation and peritonitis

In 10% of cases, acute cholecystitis occurs in the absence of stones. This may be associated with conditions in which the **normal filling and emptying of the gallbladder is defective**, and may be seen in patients suddenly immobilized by acute trauma, burns or cardiovascular problems, especially if nutrition is parenteral. Rare cases of cholecystitis in the absence of stones may occur also as a result of infection, most

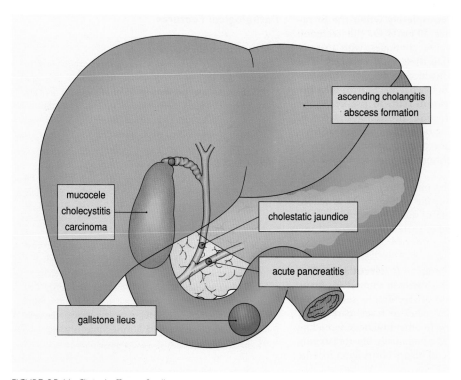

FIGURE 35.46 Clinical effects of gallstones.

notably that caused by *Salmonella* species, and, rarely, from ischaemia in cases of acute vasculitis affecting gallbladder wall blood vessels.

Acute cholecystitis without stone is more serious than the commoner variant associated with stone impaction. **This is due to a greater tendency for suppurative and necrotizing inflammation of the gallbladder wall to develop with resulting empyema of the gallbladder, perforation and biliary peritonitis.** Fortunately, generalized bile peritonitis occurs infrequently; it carries a mortality rate of approximately 30%. Unlike calculous cholecystitis, men are affected more commonly than women (male:female ratio 2:1).

Pathological Features

Macroscopic Features

In acute cholecystitis the gallbladder is enlarged and shows the typical features of acute inflammation: marked hyperaemia and oedema, the wall appearing reddened and feeling 'boggy' and thickened. The cystic duct is often blocked by a stone. The contents of the gallbladder vary, depending on whether infection is present or not. In the former case the lumen may contain frank pus. Microscopic examination shows features of acute inflammation, ranging from oedema and vasodilatation associated with a mild neutrophilic infiltrate, to extensive wall necrosis associated with haemorrhage.

In some patients, where cystic duct obstruction is complete, the bile becomes resorbed and the lumen of the organ is instead filled with mucous gland secretions. When the contents are watery, this is spoken of as **hydrops of the gallbladder**. In due time, however, the concentration of mucins in the by now considerably distended gallbladder increases, and the contents become sticky. This is termed a **mucocele of the gallbladder**.

Gallstones may pass from the gallbladder into the common bile duct, in which they can impact and obstruct the flow of bile into the duodenum. Most ductal stones originate in the gallbladder but a few form within the common bile duct. About 40% of such 'primary' ductal stones are brown pigment stones. Bile duct obstruction can lead to:

- jaundice
- ascending infection (cholangitis), which may end in the formation of hepatic abscesses
- secondary biliary cirrhosis (see p 594)
- pruritus

The normal pressure within the common bile duct is 10–15 cmH$_2$O and, when this is exceeded, bile

flow slows, stopping completely when the intra-ductal pressure reaches 30 cmH$_2$O. Bile secretion into the canaliculi, however, continues, with a rise in hydrostatic pressure within these small channels. This leads to changes in the junctional complexes between liver cells and backflow of bile occurs. **Serum alkaline phosphatase concentration** starts to rise very soon after the onset of obstruction, preceding any rise in serum bilirubin levels. The **bilirubin concentration** is proportional to the degree of obstruction, but there is no such quantitative relationship with serum alkaline phosphatase levels.

If the static bile becomes infected, ascending cholangitis supervenes on the picture of obstruction. The clinical manifestations of such cholangitis are:
- fever and chills (related to bacteraemia)
- pain
- jaundice

This classical symptom complex (**Charcot's triad**) is not seen in all cases: fever is absent in about 20%. Acute cholangitis may present as recurrent, self-limiting episodes characterized by spikes of fever, dark urine, rigors and abdominal pain. In other instances, ascending cholangitis may present as a potentially life-threatening septicaemia and evidence of biliary obstruction may be inconspicuous.

Stones passing through the common bile duct may provoke acute pancreatitis. They do this by transiently obstructing the main pancreatic duct, which may open into the duodenum at the ampulla of Vater. This allows a reflux of bile into the pancreatic duct with resulting activation of pancreatic proenzymes such as trypsin and various lipases. Sludge and microscopic stones may also be involved in the pathogenesis of acute pancreatitis and it is for this reason that cholecystec-tomy or treatment with bile acids may decrease the risk of relapse of acute pancreatitis.

In some instances an inflamed gallbladder may form serosal adhesions between itself and some neighbouring viscus, most commonly a loop of small bowel. Erosion of the walls of the gallbladder and intestine may occur and the stone may pass into the lumen of the intestine. If large enough it may block the gut lumen, causing acute intestinal obstruction, this being known as **'gallstone ileus'**.

Chronic Cholecystitis

This is more common than the acute form. It may fol-low recurrent episodes of acute cholecystitis, but this is rare; most cases have no past history of acute cholecys-titis. Because of its strong association with gallstones, chronic cholecystitis is roughly three times as common in females as in males. Its pathogenesis and natural his-tory are poorly understood.

The common clinical presentation is that of rather vague, right-sided, upper abdominal pain, dyspepsia, flatulence and intolerance of fatty foods.

Pathological Features

Macroscopic Features

A wide range of pathological appearances may be seen in chronic cholecystitis.

Gallstones are present in 95% of cases. These are usually multiple and of the **mixed** variety. The gallblad-der may be shrunken and scarred, or enlarged. The wall may be either thickened or atrophic.

Microscopic Features

The microscopic appearances also vary. The wall may be strikingly thickened, in part due to scarring and in part to muscle hypertrophy. Bile pigment may be present in the wall and this may be associated with cholesterol crystals, which elicit a lipid-laden macrophage reaction. Outpouchings of gallbladder mucosa (termed **Rokitansky–Aschoff sinuses**) extending through the muscularis are often seen and focal dystrophic calcifica-tion sometimes occurs. The chronic inflammatory cell reaction differs in severity from case to case. It is predom-inantly lymphocytic in nature; in some instances, the cells assume a follicular pattern ('follicular cholecystitis').

CHOLESTEROLOSIS OF THE GALLBLADDER

This common condition is characterized by the pres-ence of **focal aggregates of macrophages laden with esterified cholesterol in the gallbladder mucosa**. It is present in 25% of gallbladders removed surgically, and in approximately 12% at autopsy. There is marked predilection for middle-aged females. Its clinical significance, if any, is not known.

Macroscopic Features

On naked-eye examination the lesion is recognized by the presence of bright yellow flecks which appear to be projected slightly above the surrounding mucosa. When the mucosa is diffusely involved, the rather inappropriate term **'strawberry'** gallbladder is applied.

Microscopic Features

On microscopic examination the diagnostic feature is the presence of foamy macrophage aggregates within the mucosa.

TUMOURS AND TUMOUR-LIKE LESIONS OF THE GALLBLADDER

As in any other location, tumours of the gallbladder may be **benign** or **malignant**, and may arise from any of the tissue elements present in the organ. Thus a number of benign connective tissue tumours occur rarely in the gallbladder. These include **paraganglioma, leiomyoma, granular cell tumour and lipoma**.

Tumour-like lesions that are not true neoplasms include:

- **Cholesterol polyps** which are lobulated, yellow, submucosal masses composed of large aggregates of lipid-laden macrophages lying under an intact mucosa. It is possible that they represent a variant of cholesterolosis.
- **Adenomyoma.** These are focal mass lesions characterized by the presence of proliferating tubular glands and smooth muscle cells within the gallbladder wall.

Benign Epithelial Tumours

Adenoma of the gallbladder resembles its analogues in the large gut, being either pedunculated or sessile. Like colonic polyps, their growth pattern may be entirely tubular, tubulovillous or entirely villous. Some degree of atypia may be found and can be sufficiently severe as to amount to carcinoma *in situ*.

Carcinoma of the Gallbladder

Carcinoma of the gallbladder is rare. The female : male ratio is 3–4 : 1. More than 90% of cases occur in people older than 50 years, the peak incidence being 60–70 years. In the USA, the incidence is highest in North American Indians and in those of Hispanic origin, lower in Caucasians of European extraction and very rare indeed amongst Afro-Americans.

An epidemiological association exists between gallstones and carcinoma of the gallbladder in that more than 75% of cases of carcinoma occur in patients with gallstones. The degree of risk conferred by gallstones cannot be very high because gallbladder cancer develops in only 0.5% of patients with gallstones. Other reported associations of gallbladder carcinoma include fistulae between the gallbladder and the gut, extensive calcification in the gallbladder (**porcelain gallbladder**), sclerosing cholangitis, ulcerative colitis, the hereditary polyposis syndromes of the large gut and anomalous connections between the common bile and pancreatic ducts.

Pathological Features

Macroscopic Features

Two macroscopic growth patterns of gallbladder cancer exist:

- a **diffuse** pattern, found in 70% of cases
- a **polypoid** pattern, present in the remainder

Diffuse carcinoma usually elicits a marked fibrous tissue response in the surrounding tissue (i.e. it is a scirrhous tumour) and feels gritty when it is cut into. Polypoid carcinomas appear as cauliflower-like masses protruding into the gallbladder lumen. As with polypoid malignant tumours at other sites, necrosis and haemorrhage of the surface is often noted.

Microscopic Features

The vast majority of gallbladder cancers are **adenocarcinomas** which vary in their degree of differentiation. The glands appear to be well formed in an architectural sense and are surrounded by abundant, rather cellular, fibrous stroma. They are lined by one or more rows of cuboidal epithelium which shows a high degree of cytological atypia.

Evidence of spread at the time of cholecystectomy is very common indeed, only 10% of tumours being confined to the gallbladder. The tumour has a marked tendency to invade the liver directly, as well as the stomach and duodenum. Metastases also involve the liver, lymph nodes in the lesser omentum and lymph nodes posterior to the first part of the duodenum.

As with adenocarcinomas of the large gut, the prognosis for the individual patient is influenced by the extent to which the tumour has spread (**staging**) (*Table 35.26*).

Unfortunately, by the time carcinoma of the gallbladder is diagnosed, most of the tumours will be of stage IV or V, and the prognosis for this lesion is bleak.

Carcinoma of the Extrahepatic Bile Ducts

Unlike gallbladder cancer, cancer of the extrahepatic bile ducts has an equal sex incidence, implying that different aetiological factors may be operating. This view is strengthened by the fact that the association between gallstones and carcinoma of the extrahepatic bile ducts is much weaker than that which obtains between gallstones and gallbladder cancer.

An increased incidence of bile duct carcinoma has been reported in patients with **ulcerative colitis, sclerosing cholangitis, infestations with the liver fluke *Clonorchis sinensis* and in a variety of congenital cystic disorders of the biliary system**.

The tumours may occur at any point in the system, the anatomical distribution, excluding tumours of the ampulla of Vater, being as follows, the upper one-third being the most frequent site. As with carcinoma of the gallbladder, different growth patterns may be seen. These are:

- **a diffuse, sclerosing variety.** This occurs most commonly in the proximal part of the extrahepatic biliary system. It causes ill-defined thickening of the duct wall and may spread proximally to involve the intrahepatic bile ducts, a development that renders the tumour irresectable.
- **a nodular variant**, which occurs most often in the middle one-third of the bile duct system.
- **a papillary variant**, found most often in the distal one-third of the common bile duct and often involving the ampulla of Vater (*Fig. 35.47*).

Table 35.26 Staging of Gallbladder Carcinoma

Stage	Extent of spread	Prognosis
I	Intramucosal	Cured by cholecystectomy
II	Mucosa and muscularis involved	Cured by cholecystectomy
III	All three layers of gallbladder wall involved	5-year survival rate of about 11%
IV	All three layers and cystic lymph node involved	5-year survival rate of about 11%
V	Liver or other organs involved	Uniformly fatal

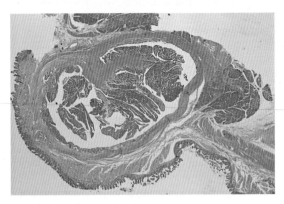

FIGURE 35.47 *Papillary carcinoma of the common bile duct.*

Spread occurs mainly by direct extension, growth along perineural spaces being prominent. Prognosis is poor with an overall 5-year survival rate of about 10%. The chances of survival are improved in tumours located in the lower one-third (5-year survival rate 25%).

The Exocrine Pancreas

The anatomical situation of the pancreas, lying retroperitoneally on the posterior wall of the abdomen, coupled with its large reserve capacity for exocrine function means that in many instances pancreatic disease may exist for a considerable time before the onset of symptoms elicits attention.

Until recently, the pancreas was difficult to image satisfactorily and virtually impossible to biopsy without major surgical exploration. These two problems have been largely solved through the introduction of ultrasonography and computed tomography on the one hand, and of needle-core biopsies on the other; it is now possible to obtain reliable tissue diagnosis in chronic pancreatitis or carcinoma of the pancreas without laparotomy.

NORMAL DEVELOPMENT

The pancreas develops from two gut-derived buds: a dorsal one and a ventral one. The ventral bud rotates to the left and then fuses with the dorsal bud, which ultimately forms most of the **body** and **tail** of the gland. The original dorsal duct (Santorini's duct) anastomoses with the ventral duct (Wirsung's duct) to form the main pancreatic duct, draining into the common bile duct just proximal to the papilla of Vater in 60% of people. The remnant of Santorini's duct drains into the duodenum by a separate accessory papilla.

DEVELOPMENTAL ABNORMALITIES

Pancreas Divisum
An important developmental abnormality occurring in 5% of the population is failure of the two duct systems to anastomose. This is known as **pancreas divisum**. In this case the main pancreatic duct is derived from Santorini's duct, and a rudimentary Wirsung's duct drains part of the head of the pancreas. Some patients develop, in later life, a segmental chronic pancreatitis more common in the dorsally than in the ventrally derived pancreas. It seems likely that the factor operating in these patients is **obstruction** in the region of the accessory papilla.

Annular Pancreas
In annular pancreas there is a ring of pancreatic tissue encircling the descending duodenum or, more rarely, the junction of the first and second parts of the duodenum. This anomaly probably arises from failure of the ventral bud to migrate to its normal posterior position. The endocrine component of the annular pancreas is identical with that of the posterior–inferior portion of the pancreatic head, containing cells with a very high pancreatic polypeptide concentration.

Most cases of annular pancreas are observed in newborns and infants (male:female ratio 3:1). It may be associated with other gut malformations (e.g. duodenal atresia, oesophageal atresia, Meckel's diverticulum) and about one-third of the affected infants have **trisomy 21**.

In infants, the clinical expression of annular pancreas is persistent vomiting due to the duodenal narrowing, although it is not clear whether the narrowing is due to the annular pancreas or merely **associated** with it. In adult cases, the presenting symptoms are also referrable to duodenal stenosis (as a result of chronic inflammation causing fibrosis in the annular segment).

Ectopic Pancreas

Pancreatic ectopia is found in about 2% of autopsies. It results from displacement of parts of the pancreas along the intestine, either before or during rotation of the ventral anlage. The commonest sites are shown in *Table 35.27*.

Grossly, the ectopic pancreas appears as a small, firm, rounded and lobular mass lying in the:

● submucosa (50%)
● muscularis (25%)
● serosa (10%)

Histologically the tissue may consist of one of the following:

● **well-formed pancreas with acini, ducts and islets of Langerhans**
● **mainly of ducts with only a few acini**
● **proliferating ducts only**

Ectopic pancreas may cause no functional disturbances but there have been reports of mucosal ulceration over nodules of pancreatic tissue and occasional cases of obstruction.

Table 35.27 Common Sites of Ectopic Pancreas

Site	Frequency (%)
Duodenum	27.7
Stomach	25
Jejunum	16
Meckel's diverticulum	6

INFLAMMATION: ACUTE PANCREATITIS

Acute pancreatitis is the expression of sudden enzymatic destruction of pancreatic parenchyma caused by the escape of activated pancreatic enzymes into the glandular and periglandular tissue. This may lead to:

● the formation of areas of fat necrosis in and around the pancreas and in the abdominal cavity (due to the action of lipases)
● rupture of pancreatic blood vessels with resulting haemorrhage due to the activation of elastases (*Fig. 35.48*)
● necrosis

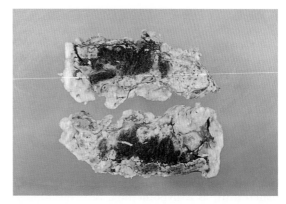

FIGURE 35.48 *Acute haemorrhagic pancreatitis.*

Acute pancreatitis usually affects adults between the ages of 30 and 70 years, although it may be seen in children with type 1 hyperlipidaemia (see pp 340–341); the annual incidence is about 50–100 per million.

Clinical Features

Patients usually present with acute and severe abdominal pain associated with **an increase in the concentrations of pancreatic enzymes in the blood**. For this increase to reach **diagnostic** significance, there must be an increase in the concentration of at least two pancreatic enzymes to a level greater than five times the upper limit of normal.

The other definitive diagnostic criterion is evidence of typical morphological changes in the pancreas. Such evidence may be obtained by imaging techniques (such as ultrasonography), at surgery or at autopsy.

Aetiology

The aetiology of acute pancreatitis is not well understood but some associated factors have been identified, largely as a result of epidemiological studies. These may be divided into *four* main groups:

1) **Biliary tract disease especially associated with stone formation.** In gallstone-associated pancreatitis, a stone impacted in the distal portion of the common bile duct can obstruct the main pancreatic duct as it enters the duodenum at the ampulla of Vater. The obstruction appears to be temporary in that the proportion of cases in which impacted stones are found on surgical exploration decreases sharply if such exploration is carried out more than 48 hours after the onset of symptoms. Cases of pancreatitis of this variety are associated with inflammation in the ducts and periductal connective tissue.

   The pathogenic mechanism in these patients is likely to be reflux of bile into the obstructed main pancreatic duct. Reflux of normal bile into the duct does not produce ductal damage, but if the bile is infected (a common finding in gallstone-associated pancreatitis) or contains secondary bile salts due to the action of trypsin, then duct damage does occur.

2) **Chronic alcoholism.** As in gallstone-associated pancreatitis, the ducts and periductal connective tissue are the chief targets for injury; the mechanism is not known.

3) **Idiopathic**

4) **Other factors** (shown in *Table 35.28*) (*Fig.35.49*).

Ischaemia

Ischaemia is a well-recognized cause of acute pancreatitis, as is hypothermia. Ischaemic damage may be due to generalized poor perfusion coupled with activation of platelets and the coagulation system, but may also occur in patients on cardiopulmonary bypass. About 25% of patients undergoing cardiac surgery with bypass show biochemical evidence (raised levels of pancreatic enzymes) of acute pancreatic damage. More than one-quarter of these have symptoms and signs of

Table 35.28 Other Factors Implicated in Acute Pancreatitis

Factor	Associations
Mechanical	Pancreatic duct stenosis
Infection	Mumps Coxsackie virus Hepatitis
Toxic	Diuretics α-Methyldopa
Endocrine	Hyperparathyroidism Steroids
Metabolic	Hyperlipidaemia (types I and V)
Vascular	Ischaemia (as in shock)
Traumatic	

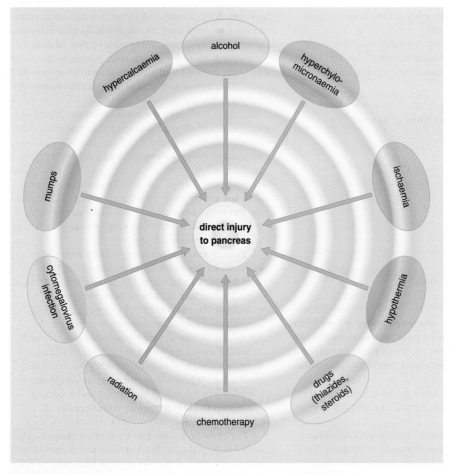

FIGURE 35.49 Causes of pancreatic injury implicated in acute pancreatitis.

pancreatitis and a few develop severe acute pancreatitis, resulting in death.

The location of the pathological changes in post-ischaemic pancreatitis differs from that described above in relation to the gallstone-associated disease. Because each pancreatic lobule is supplied by a single artery, poor perfusion affects that part of the lobule furthest from the arterial inflow, i.e. the periphery of the lobule.

The strength of these associations differs between different populations. For example, in South Africa alcoholism is associated with acute pancreatitis in 60% of cases and biliary tract disease in 16%. In Europe biliary tract disease is found in patients with acute pancreatitis in 53% of cases and alcohol in only 6%.

Pathogenesis

Normally the pancreatic parenchyma is protected from enzymatic 'self-digestion' by a number of factors:

- Pancreatic enzymes are secreted in an inactive or 'proenzyme' form known as **zymogens**.
- The zymogens are separated from other cell proteins by being enveloped within storage granules.
- Pancreatic secretions and pancreatic tissue contain inhibitors of enzyme activity.
- Pancreatic ducts are normally impermeable to the enzymes that pass through them on their way to the duodenum.

Three main questions arising from this are:

1) What initiates the **intrapancreatic** activation of pancreatic proenzymes?
2) What allows these activated enzymes to gain access to the pancreatic parenchyma?
3) What mechanism determines that the early oedematous form of acute pancreatitis should progress to the haemorrhagic and necrotic form?

In experimental models acute pancreatitis can be induced by perfusing the pancreatic ducts with activated pancreatic enzymes. In animals, duct permeability can be increased by a number of manoeuvres, including:

- exposure of the duct epithelium to bile salts
- increase in intraductal pressure
- ingestion of ethanol
- increase in plasma calcium concentrations

All these are of clinical relevance because each may be found in association with some cases of acute pancreatitis in humans. Although these models explain how pancreatic enzymes may reach the interstitium of the pancreas where the inflammatory process appears to begin in most cases, it does not explain how the normally inactive pancreatic enzymes become activated.

As mentioned above, normally there are mechanisms operating to prevent the activation of proenzymes within the acinar cells. Both the digestive pancreatic enzymes and the pancreatic lysosomal hydrolases are synthesized in the rough endoplasmic reticulum. They are then transported to the Golgi complex where post-translational modification takes place and where the

digestive enzymes are separated from the lysosomal ones by being stored in zymogen granules. This strict separation of the two classes of enzyme is of fundamental importance in preventing activation of the zymogens, most particularly trypsinogen. Manoeuvres in small animals that lead to failure of segregation of digestive and lysosomal enzymes cause acute pancreatitis.

In such models zymogens and lysosomal enzymes such as cathepsin B, a known activator of trypsinogen, are mixed and the activated zymogens are extruded from the acinar cells into the periacinar connective tissue.

The pivotal activation event in acute pancreatitis is the cleavage of trypsinogen. The key role in the genesis of acute pancreatitis is probably played by trypsin, which has the ability to activate the majority of the enzymes instrumental in causing pancreatic necrosis (*Fig. 35.50*).

Activation of trypsinogen thus appears to be a fundamental step in the cascade of events embodied in acute pancreatitis. How this comes about cannot be stated with any degree of certainty. In many cases it is suggested that reflux of bile may activate trypsinogen, such reflux being particularly liable to occur in patients with gallstones. In one series of cases of acute pancreatitis associated with biliary tract disease, nearly all showed the presence of gallstones in the faeces, implying movement of the stones within the biliary passages, in contrast to the findings in patients with pure biliary tract disease (including colic and obstructive jaundice), only very few of whom had stones in the faeces.

The morphological changes in acute pancreatitis mirror the enzymic activities outlined above. Thus we see:

- **proteolytic digestion of tissues due to trypsin activation**
- **necrosis of vessels leading to haemorrhage as a result of elastase activation**
- **fat necrosis due to lipase activation**
- **accompanying inflammatory reaction due to tissue injury**

Macroscopic Features

The extent and severity of such features depend on the duration and degree of the enzyme action. In the most severe cases the pancreas may be converted into little more than a mass of blood clot.

The main diagnostic marker is fat necrosis in the form of chalky white patches within the pancreas, the peripancreatic adipose tissue and the omentum. In very rare instances there may be foci of fat necrosis in subcutaneous adipose tissue.

In fat necrosois, neutral stored fats within the adipocytes are broken down with subsequent resorption of the glycerol. The remaining fatty acids combine with calcium salts in the extracellular fluid to form calcium soaps, accounting for the white flecks.

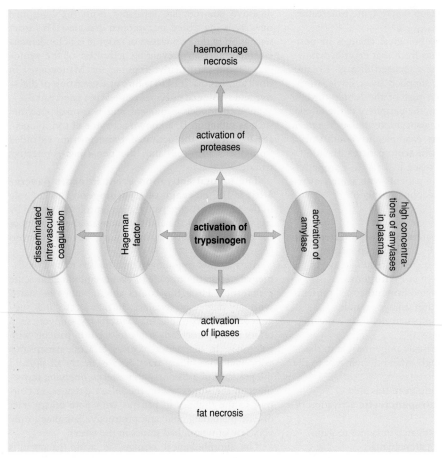

FIGURE 35.50 Activation of pancreatic enzymes and its effects in acute pancreatitis.

In more severe cases, coagulation necrosis of the acinar elements develops and the pancreas now shows a variegated appearance with red friable areas of tissue breakdown intermingled with grey ischaemic areas and areas of haemorrhage. It is likely that this necrotizing process is due to the action of activated elastase on the blood vessels with resulting thrombosis.

Frank haemorrhage may occur from disrupted blood vessels both within the gland and in the peripancreatic tissues. Some of this blood may track along tissue planes and present as areas of bluish discoloration in the costovertebral angles or round the umbilicus.

Microscopic Features

Initially there is only a mild white cell reaction but in some cases secondary infection supervenes and abscess formation may come to dominate the pathological picture. If the patient survives, reparative fibrosis occurs and any foci that have already undergone liquefactive necrosis are walled off, thus forming **pseudocysts** which contain tissue debris, blood pancreatic juice and droplets of fat.

These pseudocysts may resorb spontaneously but, if they are related to a damaged pancreatic duct, may persist for long periods.

The early stages of acute pancreatitis are characterized by the presence of perilobular fat necrosis extending along the interstitial septa. Associated with this is a mild, acute, inflammatory cell infiltrate. The acinar cells that border on these areas of perilobular fat necrosis show flattening and depletion of their content of zymogen granules. These changes are termed **acute oedematous pancreatitis**.

In addition to the obvious local and systemic effects of acute pancreatitis listed above, a number of other pathophysiological disturbances may be seen. These are considered in *Table 35.29*.

CHRONIC PANCREATITIS

There have been a number of attempts in the past few years to find an appropriate definition of chronic pan-

Table 35.29 Pathophysiological Disturbances Seen in Acute Pancreatitis

Disturbance	Mechanisms
Shock	Shock occurs for a number of reasons. There is release of the vasoactive amines kallidin and bradykinin from the pancreas. These are cleaved from kininogens as a result of the action of kallikrein. Kallikrein is normally present in the pancreas, salivary glands and plasma in an inactive form, activated by trypsin. The kinins cause vasodilatation and increased vascular permeability, contributing to shock. In addition, hypovolaemia may occur due to plasma exudation in the retroperitoneal space, vomiting, haemorrhage and the collection of fluid in the lumen of an atonic gut. Shock occurs in about 40% of patients with acute pancreatitis.
Hypocalcaemia	About 33% of patients develop transient hypocalcaemia in the course of acute pancreatitis, although this is rarely severe enough to cause tetany. A number of factors may mediate this: <ul><li>sequestration of calcium in calcium soaps in the areas of fat necrosis</li><li>a decline in calcium-binding plasma proteins</li></ul>
Hyperglycaemia	Mild, transient hyperglycaemia occurs in about 15–25% of patients, associated with high levels of glucagon and low levels of insulin.
Impaired lung function	Some arterial hypoxia develops in most patients with acute pancreatitis. The cause of this is the development of intrapulmonary right to left shunts, the cause of which is not clear. In a small minority of patients, respiratory distress syndrome (ARDS) develops. The chances of this occurring increases with the severity of the pancreatitis.
Renal impairment	This results from the combination of hypovolaemia and declining plasma protein concentrations. The alteration in function may be mild or may be so severe as to render the patient anuric.

creatitis. The revised Marseilles classification defines the disorder in clinical terms (*Fig. 35.51*) as being characterized by:

- **recurrent or persistent abdominal pain**
- **evidence of exocrine or endocrine pancreatic insufficiency (e.g. steatorrhoea, diabetes). In some patients this may occur in the absence of abdominal pain.**

Microscopic Features

In **morphological terms** the defining criteria are (*Fig. 35.52*):

- irregular scarring of the pancreas with patchy loss of exocrine tissue
- patchy chronic inflammation
- focal strictures and segmental dilatation of the pancreatic ducts
- intraductal protein-rich plugs and calculi

Aetiology and Pathogenesis

Chronic pancreatitis is more often associated with chronic alcoholism than with biliary tract disease. Alcoholism accounts for 60–85% of cases of chronic pancreatitis in Western countries. Non-alcohol-related chronic pancreatitis is common in tropical countries, where it has been suggested that it is associated with protein undernutrition. In some patients (the reported frequency ranges from 9 to 40%), no predisposing factors are found. The disorder affects males more frequently than females.

The pathogenesis of chronic pancreatitis is no better understood than that of acute pancreatitis, although in cases where alcoholism is implicated, it has been suggested that **secretin-mediated excess secretion of high protein fluid could lead to plugging of the pancreatic ductules** and thus contribute to the obstructive features of the disease. The protein content of secretin-stimulated pancreatic juice is certainly higher in alcoholics than in non-alcoholics, and it has been suggested that there is a deficiency in a particular protein which serves to keep calcium in solution and that this deficiency is responsible for the extensive calculus formation.

A subset of chronic pancreatitis exists in which the principal pathogenetic factor is obstruction of the main ducts. In morphological terms this obstruction is expressed in the form of diffuse, rather uniform, involvement of the gland, in contrast to the patchy distribution of lesions seen in the alcohol-related form of the disease. In the obstructive type of chronic pancreatitis, removal of the cause of the obstruction can lead to relief of symptoms. In patients with pancreas divisum (see p 632), where most of the pancreatic juice drains via the accessory duct, a segmental type of chronic pancreatitis may occasionally occur.

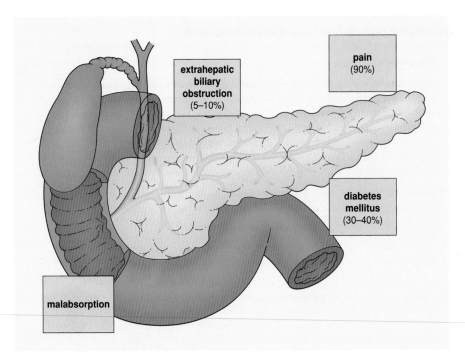

FIGURE 35.51 Clinical features of chronic pancreatitis.

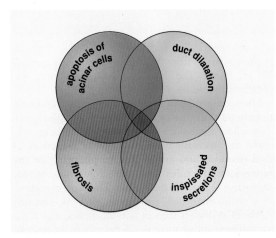

FIGURE 35.52 Morphological features of chronic pancreatitis.

Microscopic Features

The most prominent features are loss of acinar tissue and its replacement by chronically inflamed scar tissue.

The endocrine component usually is not affected and often appears more prominent than normal.

Especially in cases associated with alcoholism, the duct system shows plugging either by inspissated protein-rich secretions or by calcified material, which can be present in large amounts.

The duct system distal to these stones is dilated and pseudocysts are often found in such instances. In contrast to cases associated with obstruction in the terminal portion of the duct system in the region of the ampulla, such pancreatic duct calculi are found only rarely, and the inflammation and fibrosis affect mainly the head of the pancreas.

Pathophysiological Disturbances in Chronic Pancreatitis

These are shown in *Table 35.30.*

PANCREATIC TUMOURS AND TUMOUR-LIKE LESIONS

Epithelial tumours account for the vast majority of non-endocrine pancreatic neoplasms; more than 90% are adenocarcinomas. Some benign epithelial tumours do arise within the pancreas, and connective tissue neoplasms are seen occasionally. More common epithelial lesions are listed in *Table 35.31.*

Carcinoma of the Exocrine Pancreas

Epidemiology

The incidence of carcinoma of the pancreas has been rising steadily over the past 30 years and it is now the fourth most common cause of death from cancer in men (exceeded by carcinoma of the lung, large bowel and prostate) and the fifth most common cause of death

Table 35.30 Pathophysiological Disturbances Seen in Chronic Pancreatitis

Disturbance	Mechanisms or association
Pain	Pain may be chronic or associated with attacks of acute pancreatitis occurring in a chronically damaged gland. Such attacks of acute inflammation occur in about 50% of patients. In most of the others, pain is either continuous or intermittent. About 10% of patients are pain-free; their pancreatitis is expressed in the form of malabsorption or obstructive jaundice.
Malabsorption	A decrease in secretion of pancreatic enzymes is found in most cases but failure to absorb fat and protein does not occur until about 90% of the exocrine tissue has been destroyed (by no means an uncommon event). Lipase secretion declines more rapidly than that of proteases and thus steatorrhoea tends to precede the development of protein loss.
Diabetes mellitus	Despite the fact that, on histological examination, islets of Langerhans appear to survive in chronic pancreatitis, diabetes is common, with a prevalence of 30–40%. The diabetes is usually mild and the vascular complications that are so prominent in other types of diabetes are rare. Neuropathies are common, perhaps because of the associated high intake of alcohol.
Extrahepatic biliary obstruction	This occurs in 5–10% of patients with chronic pancreatitis. Fibrosis of the head of the pancreas causing a long tapered stricture of the common bile duct is the commonest mechanism.

Table 35.31 Epithelial Pancreatic Lesions

Benign

Papillary adenoma
An uncommon tumour with an equal incidence in males and females and a peak age for presentation of 50–70 years. They resemble tubulovillous adenomas of the colon and tend to obstruct the lumen of the pancreatic duct. They may show a considerable degree of atypia, which can make the distinction from adenocarcinoma difficult.

Serous cystadenoma
An uncommon tumour composed of multiple cysts lined by cuboidal epithelium. It tends to occur in elderly women. Most cases are sporadic, but similar lesions occasionally occur in association with von Hippel–Lindau syndrome. The tumours are quite large (6–10 cm in diameter) and their cut surfaces show the presence of many small cysts.

Solid and cystic tumour
This tumour occurs chiefly in young females (10–35 years). They form large rounded masses (9–10 cm) and their cut surfaces may be partly solid and partly cystic. Microscopic examination shows solid sheets of cells somewhat resembling islet cells. Tumour breakdown is common and this leads to the formation of a focal pseudo-papillary pattern and small cysts.

Malignant

Adenocarcinoma
- common ductal type
- acinar cell type
- adenosquamous carcinoma
- giant cell-type carcinoma
- mixed cell carcinoma

Squamous cell carcinoma

Small cell anaplastic carcinoma

Cystadenocarcinoma

Pancreaticoblastoma

Osteoclast-like tumour

from cancer in women (exceeded by cancer of the breast, large bowel, lung, and ovary and/or uterus). Excess alcohol consumption, high fat diets and cigarette smoking have all been suggested as being causally related but the evidence is not strong. Even in the case of cigarette smoking, the strength of the association is much weaker in pancreatic cancer than in lung cancer. Mutations in the Ki-*ras* proto-oncogene are present in about 90% of cases.

Natural History

The vast majority of carcinomas arise from ductal epithelium and about two-thirds of them arise in the head of the pancreas. They may grow silently for a long time and have a very low cure rate after resection (5-year survival rate approximately 2%).

Microscopic Features

Most pancreatic carcinomas are fairly well-differentiated adenocarcinomas (*Fig. 35.53*) which tend to elicit a marked fibrous tissue response. Occasionally much more anaplastic tumours may occur, including one in which large numbers of multinucleated giant cells resembling osteoclasts may be seen. This tumour carries a somewhat better prognosis than the common ductal carcinoma.

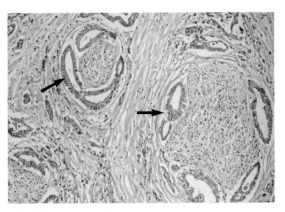

FIGURE 35.53 *Well-differentiated adenocarcinoma of the pancreas infiltrating along the perineural spaces (arrow).*

Clinical Features

Carcinomas of the head of the pancreas tend to be small but, because of the proximity of the common bile duct and ampulla, commonly draw attention to themselves in the form of relatively painless jaundice. If the patient has not had any previous inflammatory episodes affecting the gallbladder and leading to fibrous thickening of the gallbladder wall, the gallbladder can become

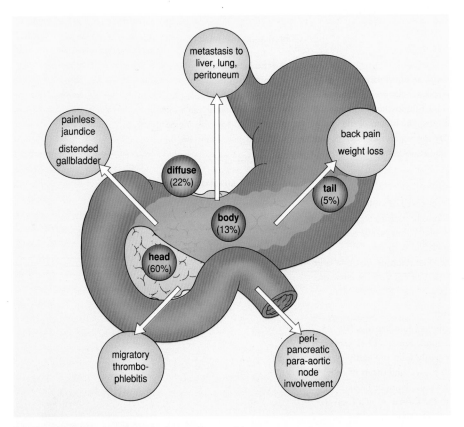

FIGURE 35.54 *Features of ductal adenocarcinoma of the pancreas.*

distended as a result of the obstruction in the common bile duct and may thus be palpable on examination of the abdomen (Courvoisier's sign). A rather curious clinical feature, sometimes occurring in association with pancreatic cancer, is migratory thrombophlebitis (see pp 641, 926) (*Fig. 35.54*).

Carcinomas of the body and tail tend to be larger than those of the head by the time a diagnosis is made, because they do not, as a rule, interfere with biliary drainage and thus are diagnosed later. Often they cause clinical effects as a result of infiltration of neighbouring structures such as the vertebral column, stomach and colon. By the time the lesion has been detected, most patients show extensive spread of tumour to regional lymph nodes, or involvement of the liver as a result of invasion of the splenic vein radicles by malignant cells.

CYSTIC FIBROSIS (MUCOVISCIDOSIS) AND THE PANCREAS

Cystic fibrosis is a disorder of exocrine glands throughout the body affecting both mucus-secreting glands and eccrine sweat glands. The secretions are abnormally viscid leading, in the context of the pancreas, to obstruction in the duct system and consequent dilatation. It is this dilatation of ducts, and the postobstructive atrophy and fibrosis within the exocrine tissue that are its natural consequences, that led to the name '**cystic fibrosis** of the pancreas' being coined.

Clinical Features

Such obstruction in affected organs leads to the chief clinical features of the disease (*Fig. 35.55*):

- **pancreatic insufficiency**
- **steatorrhoea**
- **malnutrition**
- **chronic pulmonary disease with bronchiectasis and recurrent infection**
- **cirrhosis of the liver**
- **intestinal obstruction**

Aetiology

Cystic fibrosis is the commonest of all inherited disorders, occurring in about 1 in 2500 live births. Its inheritance pattern is archetypal for an **autosomally**

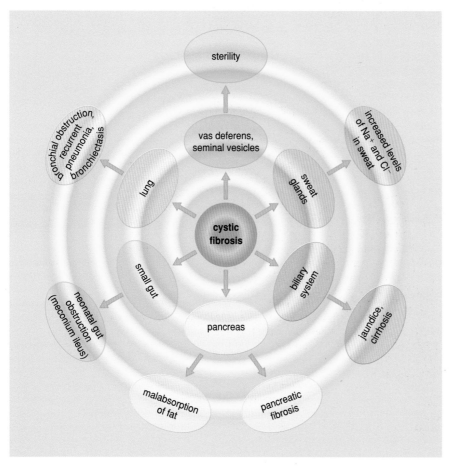

FIGURE 35.55 Effects of cystic fibrosis.

recessive defect; the gene frequency is about 1 in 25 of the population. The only consistent biochemical abnormality related to a putative gland abnormality is **an abnormally high concentration of chloride and sodium in the sweat**. It has also been suggested that there are low molecular weight glycoproteins in the serum of patients with cystic fibrosis which have an inhibitory effect on ciliary activity.

The genomic abnormality in cystic fibrosis is a mutation of a gene on the long arm of chromosome 7 (7q31). This gene normally encodes a chloride transporter called the cystic fibrosis transmembrane conductance regulator (CFTR) and mutations interfere with the normal reabsorption of chloride by certain cells, such as those of the sweat duct; hence the abnormally high concentration of chloride in secretions such as sweat. In the lungs, the epithelial cells cannot transport the chloride outwards, and this results in decreased transport of cell water leading to abnormally viscid bronchial mucus. A number of different mutations exists. The commonest of these is known as ΔF508 and antenatal screening for this can be undertaken. The frequency of this mutation (a deletion of the codon for phenylalanine at position 508) varies between different populations. In Italy the frequency is approximately 50%, whereas in Denmark it is much greater (90%).

Macroscopic Features

At birth the pancreas usually appears macroscopically normal, except for a somewhat increased firmness in consistency. Soon after, the lesions start to develop and by the age of 2 years the pancreas appears lobulated and is markedly firmer than normal; this change is due to fibrosis. The cut surface may show the presence of numerous cystic spaces containing a cloudy fluid.

Microscopic Features

Histologically the pancreatic ducts and ductules are dilated, containing inspissated periodic acid–Schiff-positive glycoprotein secretions. In the advanced form of the disease these appearances are very marked and are associated with acinar atrophy similar to that seen in post-obstructive chronic pancreatitis.

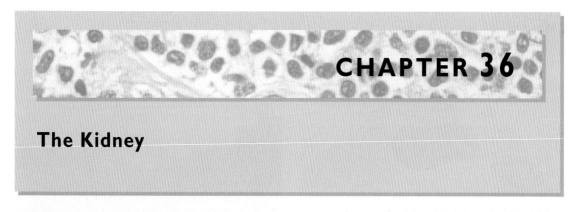

Disorders of the Kidney

NORMAL ANATOMY

Each adult kidney weighs approximately 150 g and has a medial hilum where the renal artery enters the kidney and the main renal vein and the ureter leave it.

The cut surface shows an outer **cortex**, 4–6 mm in thickness, and an inner **medulla**. The latter consists of 12 roughly wedge-shaped **pyramids**, the bases of which constitute the corticomedullary junction, the apices draining into minor calyces via renal **papillae**. Between each two pyramids is a prolongation of the cortex known as the column of Bertin.

Blood Supply
The kidney filters 150 litres of blood per day (25% of the cardiac output). Its vascular anatomy is, not surprisingly, complex in view of the kidney's principal excretory functions:

- **ultrafiltration of blood across the glomerular capillary wall**
- **reabsorption of many chemical species from the glomerular filtrate within the renal tubules**

Arterial Supply
This is derived from the main **renal artery**, arising from the abdominal aorta. It divides at the hilum into anterior and posterior branches. These then divide again into five **segmental arteries**, each supplying a specific area of renal parenchyma. No collaterals exist between these segmental vessels, an anatomical arrangement with considerable functional implications should one of them become blocked.

At the junction between cortex and medulla, a series of arteries, the **arcuate arteries**, arise from the segmental vessels. The arcuate vessels curve round the outer surface of the medullary pyramids, and give rise to the **interlobular arteries** running more or less perpendicular to the arcuate arteries out into the cortex.

From the interlobular vessels are derived **afferent arteriole**s which divide into the **glomerular capillaries**; a single afferent arteriole serves each glomerulus. These capillaries fuse forming an **efferent arteriole** which is much smaller than the afferent vessel. Efferent

arterioles subdivide into a network of capillaries running close to the renal tubules.

Venous Drainage
This is in most ways a mirror image of the arterial supply. Peritubular capillaries drain into interlobular veins, which empty into arcuate veins. These then drain into segmental veins, which eventually fuse at the hilum to form the main renal vein.

Vascular arrangements in the **renal papillae** are somewhat different; the papillae are supplied by vessels known as **arteriolae rectae spuriae**, derived from efferent arterioles leaving the glomeruli in the juxtamedullary zone.

In addition, the medulla also receives some blood from a series of vessels arising directly from the interlobular arteries and which are known as the **arteriolae rectae verae**. These last two sets of vessels constitute the system known as the **vasa recta**. Blood from these vessels drains back into the arcuate veins via series of loops.

Viewed functionally, the cortex consists of both glomeruli and tubules; the medulla contains no glomeruli and is the site of the collecting tubules of each nephron.

THE GLOMERULUS
Much of renal pathology relates to disordered structure and function of the glomerulus. The abnormalities that occur in this structure are best appreciated in the context of normal microanatomy (*Fig. 36.1*).

Glomerular Capillary Tuft
The glomerulus is a tuft of capillaries which, like all capillaries, are lined by a single layer of endothelium. This differs from most other capillaries in being **fenestrated**.

The endothelium rests on basement membrane which is incomplete; thus the part of the capillary lumen that faces the mesangium has no basement membrane and is separated from mesangial cells only by thin endothelial cytoplasm.

Glomerular Basement Membrane
This is about 300 nm thick and consists of three layers. The central layer (**lamina densa**) is the most electron dense and lies between two less dense zones called **lamina rara interna** and **lamina rara externa**

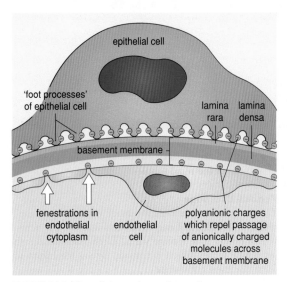

FIGURE 36.1 Normal glomerular capillary wall.

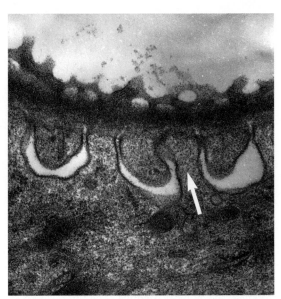

FIGURE 36.2 Transmission electron micrograph of glomerular capillary wall showing foot processes of epithelial cells (large arrow).

respectively. Because the endothelium is fenestrated, the lamina rara interna is, in places, in direct contact with the blood. Apart from its complement of connective tissue components, the glomerular basement membrane is also the site of two antigens important in certain specific types of renal disease:

1) **Amyloid P component**, a member of a family of pentameric glycoproteins known as the pentraxins. Amyloid P is widely distributed in the body, chiefly in relation to connective tissue fibrillar proteins, and it binds strongly to amyloid proteins.

2) **The Goodpasture antigen**, which is intimately associated with type IV procollagen in the lamina densa of the glomerular capillary basement membrane.

The outer surface of the basement membrane is covered by **epithelial cells** which, on electron microscopy, can be seen to have **foot processes** (*Figs 36.2* and *36.3*) resting on the basement membrane surface. These processes are separated from each other by a narrow space measuring 20–50 nm. This is the **filtration slit** and is covered by a delicate membrane called the slit diaphragm.

Apart from their role in controlling filtration through the capillary wall, epithelial cells have important functions related to **protein synthesis** and **signal reception**. They synthesize and secrete the basement membrane components, **type IV collagen, laminin** and **heparan sulphate**.

Glomerular Polyanion

The glomerular basement membrane and the sides of the epithelial foot processes are coated with strongly negatively charged polyanion, rich in sialic acid. The polyanion plays an important part in regulating clearance of molecules from the glomerular

capillary blood and in preventing the escape of major plasma proteins (which are negatively charged) into the urinary space. Because of the negative charge of the polyanion, cationic molecules tend to pass through the basement membrane, whereas anionic ones tend to be held back. The presence of this negatively charged layer on the epithelial cell surface mediates normal separation of the foot processes via mutual repulsion of adjacent negatively charged surfaces.

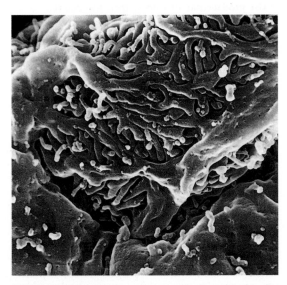

FIGURE 36.3 Scanning electron micrograph of an epithelial cell showing how the glomerular basement membrane is covered by many branching processes.

The Mesangium

The area between glomerular capillaries is the **mesangium**. It is of considerable functional significance. The mesangium is populated by *two* cell types:

- intrinsic mesangial cells
- mononuclear phagocytes

These are surrounded by connective tissue matrix containing collagen, fibronectin, laminin and entactin.

Because of the intimate focal relationship between mesangium and capillary endothelium, under normal circumstances, some plasma reaches the mesangium directly through endothelial fenestrations. Large molecules become trapped between the closely aggregated matrix fibrils, some of these being endocytosed by mesangial cells whereas others are engulfed by mononuclear phagocytes. Plasma within the mesangium can leave it again via a number of routes, one of which is through the epithelial cells into the urinary space. Thus macromolecules leaving the mesangium may become trapped against the basement membrane, a common location for the impaction of immune complexes.

Intrinsic Mesangial Cell

This cell shows ultrastructural resemblances to smooth muscle cells. It is capable of contractile activity, thus contributing to modulation of glomerular blood flow. In addition, the intrinsic mesangial cell has both receptor and synthesizing functions, the former for angiotensin II, a potent vasoconstrictor, and atrial natriuretic peptide.

The cell's chief product is **interleukin 1**, a mediator that not only has a powerful regulatory role in inflammation and the immune response, but which, in the mesangium, acts as an **autocrine growth factor**, stimulating proliferation of the intrinsic mesangial cells. It is suggested that release of interleukin 1 may play a part in controlling the cell proliferation and matrix production seen in various glomerular diseases.

Intrinsic mesangial cells *cannot* phagocytose material such as immune complexes, although they can endocytose proteins. Neither can they present antigen, as HLA-DR-coded proteins are not expressed.

Mesangial Mononuclear Phagocytes

These cells show all the characteristics of monocyte-derived macrophages; under normal circumstances, they are present only in very small numbers.

The Juxtaglomerular Apparatus

This consists of three elements, all associated with sympathetic nerve endings:

1) **Granular cells**, which are modified smooth muscle cells found in the terminal part of the afferent arteriole. The granules contain active renin and angiotensin II.

2) **Lacis cells**, which lie in the V formed at the glomerular hilus by afferent and efferent arterioles. They resemble intrinsic mesangial cells.

3) **The macula densa**, part of the wall of the distal convoluted tubule lying nearest to the glomerular hilum and in close apposition to the lacis cells. The epithelial cells of the macula densa are narrower and taller than those in the rest of the distal convoluted tubule.

The juxtaglomerular apparatus is the chief source for the formation and release of **renin**. Renin may be released into the blood in an active or inactive form, the latter usually predominating. Renin release is stimulated by:

- a fall in blood pressure within the afferent arteriole
- a decrease in the concentration of sodium and chloride in the macula densa
- sympathetic discharge via the small nerve endings related to the juxtaglomerular apparatus

Renin is released into the interstitium, gains access to the blood via peritubular capillaries and initiates the following sequence:

1) It cleaves angiotensinogen, yielding angiotensin I.

2) Angiotensin I is cleaved by angiotensin-converting enzyme (ACE) to produce angiotensin II, a potent vasoconstrictor and stimulus for aldosterone secretion.

3) Aldosterone triggers sodium reabsorption from the distal nephron.

Thus renin release causes both vasoconstriction and expansion of plasma volume.

While being morphologically inconspicuous, the juxtaglomerular apparatus plays a vital role in:

- sodium and water regulation
- control of arterial blood pressure

NORMAL KIDNEY DEVELOPMENT

Normal kidney development depends on the integrity of two primitive forms:

1) The **pronephros** originates from a mass of mesodermal cells (**nephrogenic cord**) lying on the ventral surface of the 21-day embryo. The pronephros starts to degenerate almost as soon as it

is formed, but gives rise to the second primitive kidney or **mesonephros**.

2) The **mesonephros (wolffian duct)** rises from the caudal end of the pronephros. Some differentiation into glomeruli and tubules takes place at this stage and urine is excreted from this primitive kidney until the end of the fourth month of gestation.

A **ureteric bud** then arises from the posteromedial aspect of the mesonephric duct near the cloaca after the degeneration of the mesonephros. From this and from the primitive cells of the metanephric blastema arises the **metanephros**, from which the mature kidney is formed.

The ureteric bud is the source of the ureter, renal pelvis, calyces and connecting tubules. It grows upwards into the metanephric blastema dividing dichotomously, although not always symmetrically, when it encounters the blastema. The bud has an anterior growing end, the **ampulla**, of great importance in kidney development, being responsible for:

• outward extension of the bud
• cell division
• induction of nephron formation by the blastema
• establishment of communication between the bud and the more proximal portion of the nephrons

ABNORMALITIES OF RENAL DEVELOPMENT

Bilateral Agenesis

This results either from failure of the mesonephric duct to give rise to the bud or from absence of the lower half of the mesonephric duct itself. Because the fetus then cannot excrete urine, oligohydramnios results. Bilateral agenesis is incompatible with more than a few hours of life; indeed many of the affected children are stillborn. The male : female ratio is 2 : 1. Associated abnormalities include:

• pulmonary hypoplasia
• absence or deformity of the lower limbs
• the Potter facies (named after Edith Potter, the well-known paediatric pathologist who described it), which consists of **low-set ears, a receding chin, a widened and flattened, rather beaked, nose, and wide-set eyes with a prominent inner canthus** (*Fig. 36.4*).

Unilateral Agenesis

Unilateral agenesis is found in approximately 1 in 500 post-mortem examinations on stillborn infants and neonates, males being more frequently affected than females. The single kidney is hypertrophied. A single kidney is certainly compatible with normal life but these children often have other congenital defects.

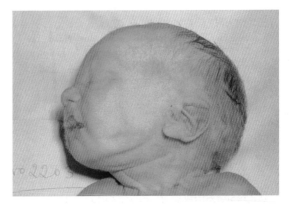

FIGURE 36.4 *Facies of an infant with bilateral renal agenesis (Potter facies). Note the low-set ears and receding chin.*

Renal Aplasia

In this condition a ureter is present but there is no functioning kidney tissue. This is caused by a defect either in the metanephric blastema or in the stimulatory activity of the ureteric bud on the blastema.

Horseshoe Kidney

In early embryonic life the lower poles of the kidneys are closer together than the upper poles. This may occasionally lead to fusion if both metanephric ducts move medially. When horseshoe kidney is found in stillborns or neonates, other abnormalities are present in 75% of cases. Horseshoe kidney may also sometimes occur in association with trisomy 18.

Renal Dysplasia

The term **renal dysplasia** covers a spectrum of abnormalities ranging from massive polycystic kidney on the one hand (*Fig. 36.5*) to a small irregularly shaped organ on the other. It is a developmental abnormality resulting from anomalous differentiation of the metanephric blastema. It is nearly always associated with other abnormalities of the urinary tract such as duplication of the ureters, ureteral ectopia and posterior urethral valves which cause obstruction.

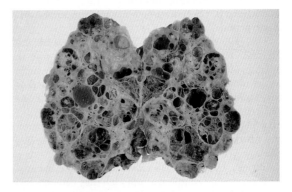

FIGURE 36.5 *Renal dysplasia. Both kidneys are grossly polycystic.*

A diagnosis of dysplasia can be established only if there is microscopic evidence of aberrant differentiation. Expression of this maldifferentiation includes:

- primitive ducts lined by columnar or occasionally by ciliated epithelium. These may be surrounded by a mantle zone of primitive mesenchymal cells.
- portions of metaplastic cartilage
- immature-looking glomeruli
- multiple fibrous-walled cysts. In some instances these dominate the pathological picture producing an enormously enlarged polycystic kidney, presenting clinically as an intra-abdominal mass. **In such cases it is important to establish the diagnosis of renal dysplasia (which is not inherited) because of the genetic implications of other multicystic conditions affecting the kidney.**

Renal dysplasia may also occur as part of various familial syndromes that are autosomally recessively inherited. In these, the renal abnormality is usually bilateral and is not associated with other malformations of the urinary tract.

Renal Cystic Disease

A spectrum of renal cystic disease exists, as shown in *Table 36.1* and *Fig. 36.6*.

Mechanisms of Renal Cyst Development

Mechanisms suggested as underlying renal cyst formation include **intratubular obstruction, increased basement membrane** and **hyperplasia of renal tubular epithelium**. Of these, the third seems most likely.

Cellular Hyperplasia

In renal cysts the size of the epithelial cells remains nearly normal, so it has been suggested that epithelial hyperplasia and formation of new basement membrane must occur as cysts form and grow. This view is supported by the frequent presence of mitoses in the epithelium of genetically determined renal cysts, and their rarity in normal tubular epithelium.

Cystic kidney epithelial cells in mice show increased expression of the proto-oncogene c-*myc*, and the insertion of activated c-*myc* into a transgenic mouse results in the formation of polycystic kidney. Transgenic mice expressing either transforming growth factor α or the **large-T antigen of the SV40 virus** have also been reported as developing polycystic kidney.

Subsequent accumulation of fluid is an essential part of the cyst formation; this fluid is probably secreted by the epithelium. The abnormal fluid secretion is associated with a curious mislocation of $Na^+ K^+$ adenosine triphosphatase which, instead of being basally and laterally located, is found at the apices of the cells lining the cysts.

Polycystic Renal Disease

Autosomal Dominant Type (ADPKD-1)

This disorder presents for the most part in **adult** life, thus being termed adult polycystic kidney disease, although cases occur in infants and young children. In most, the disease is inherited in an **autosomal dominant pattern** but some arise as a result of spontaneous mutations. It is one of the commonest inherited disorders, exceeding in frequency sickle cell disease, haemophilia and cystic fibrosis. In the USA there are 500 000 patients with this disorder and 6000 new cases occur annually. It accounts for 10% of all cases of chronic renal failure.

Some 85% of cases of ADPKD-1 are associated with a mutant gene found on the short arm of chromosome 16, closely linked with locus for α-haemoglobin. Penetrance is virtually complete but gene expression varies considerably. It is suggested that the gene product of the normal *PDK-1* gene has a role either in cell–cell interaction or in interactions between cells and extracellular matrices.

Some patients with inherited disease do not have a mutant gene on the short arm of chromosome 16. These patients, who are less severely affected, have an abnormality on the long arm of chromosome 4 (4q13–q23).

Progressive renal failure develops in 50% of those who inherit the mutant gene and dialysis or transplantation are required eventually. The clinical features and their relative frequency are shown in *Table 36.2*.

Macroscopic Features

In autosomal dominant-type polycystic disease both kidneys are grossly enlarged and diffusely cystic with **marked irregularity of the subcapsular surface** (*Fig. 36.7*). Cysts are present, in both the cortex and medulla. Some

Table 36.1 Renal Cysts

Condition	Cause or associated disease
Polycystic kidney	Autosomal dominant
	Autosomal recessive
Medullary cysts	Medullary cystic disease
	Juvenile nephronophthisis
	Medullary sponge kidney
Simple cysts	
Acquired cystic disease	Associated with chronic renal failure
Cysts associated with hereditary syndromes	
Renal dysplasia	

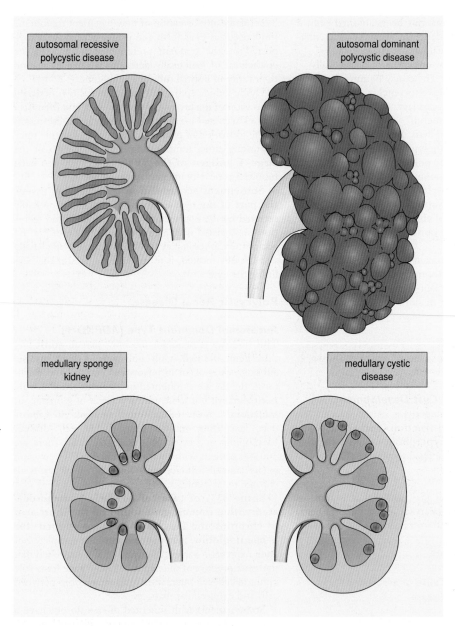

FIGURE 36.6 *Variants of congenital renal cystic disease.*

cysts communicate with the renal tubules and are lined by normal-looking tubular epithelium. Cysts originating from the proximal tubules contain fluid that resembles glomerular filtrate; the urea, creatinine and electrolyte content is similar to that of plasma. Cysts arising from the distal tubules contain fluid with concentrations of sodium and chloride that are lower than those in plasma, and concentrations of potassium, hydrogen ions, urea and creatinine that are higher than those found in plasma.

Liver cysts are found in 30−40% of patients with this type of polycystic disease, and **cerebral aneurysms affecting the circle of Willis** are present in 10−20%. **Other extrarenal manifestations include:**

- aortic aneurysm
- colonic diverticula
- ovarian cysts
- heart valve defects including floppy mitral valve

Table 36.2 Clinical Features of Autosomal Dominant Polycystic Kidney Disease

Clinical feature	Frequency (%)
Flank pain; dull and aching (probably represents stretching of the renal capsule); relieved by decompression of the cysts	60
Haematuria	60
Nocturia (reduced concentration capacity)	
Hypertension (believed to be associated with increased renin secretion by the kidney)	50
Urinary tract infections	
Stone formation	10–20

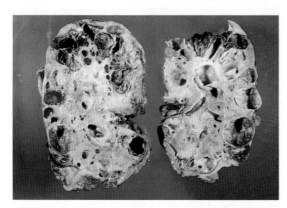

FIGURE 36.7 *Autosomal dominant-type polycystic disease showing marked irregularity of the cortical outline.*

Pathogenesis

The cysts originate from small groups of cells that proliferate abnormally, thus extending the wall of the affected tubule with undifferentiated epithelium, accompanied by expansion of underlying extracellular matrix. Abnormal transepithelial secretion of fluid contributes to cyst growth, and the expanding cyst compresses the surrounding normal parenchyma.

Only 50% of affected individuals go on to develop chronic renal failure, suggesting that factors other than the physical presence of cysts cause the decline in renal function. One suggestion is that macrophage-mediated scarring is responsible, whereas other studies suggest that renal failure is due to accelerated apoptosis (programmed cell death) in the non-cystic parenchyma.

Autosomal Recessive Type

This is rare, being found in 1 in 16 000 live births. Although often termed infantile type polycystic disease, it may occasionally manifest in adult life.

Patients present most commonly with bilateral loin masses, which may be palpable at birth. The kidneys are considerably enlarged but, **in contrast with the autosomal dominant type, the capsular surfaces are smooth**.

The cut surface shows many small cysts (1–2 mm in diameter) in the cortex. These connect with radially oriented, dilated channels derived from collecting duct epithelium, where cyst development appears to start. Interstitial fibrosis and nephron atrophy are common and it is characteristic for significant renal dysfunction to be present **early** in the course of the disorder.

Associated hepatic fibrosis of unknown pathogenesis may lead to presinusoidal portal hypertension. This association with liver disease is said to be present in all cases of autosomal recessive polycystic kidney.

If the disorder is fully developed at birth, death in early infancy from renal failure is the usual outcome. If the condition is mild, hepatic changes may come to dominate the clinical picture. Parents of an affected child should be advised that there is a one in four chance that succeeding children will inherit the condition.

Cystic Disease Affecting the Renal Medulla

This group contains three major entities, all characterized by cystic dilatation of distal and collecting tubules associated with interstitial fibrosis.

Juvenile Nephronophthisis

This is an **autosomal recessive** disorder which progresses to renal failure in childhood or adolescence. Juvenile nephronophthisis presents with:

- anaemia
- growth retardation
- chronic azotaemia associated with polyuria and salt wasting

End-stage renal disease by the age of 20 years is the rule.

Medullary Cystic Disease

This is inherited in an **autosomal dominant** fashion and renal failure generally occurs in adult life.

In juvenile nephronophthisis and medullary cystic disease, the kidneys are small and fibrotic. The cut surfaces show the presence of numerous small cysts in the **corticomedullary** region. Glomerular scarring and interstitial fibrosis are characteristic accompaniments.

Patients with medullary cystic disease are generally diagnosed in adulthood and most have a family history of renal failure consistent with an autosomal dominant inheritance.

Medullary Sponge Kidney

This presents typically in adult life and is characterized by marked irregular dilatations of the medullary and papillary collecting ducts (*Fig. 36.8*). The lesions are usually bilateral and diffuse, but may sometimes be restricted to only a few papillae. No genetic factors have been implicated and the disorder affects approximately 1 in 5000 people.

The presenting clinical features are usually:

● haematuria
● renal stone formation

Diagnosis is made by intravenous urography; pooling of contrast medium in the ectatic papillary ducts is seen.

Simple Cysts

These are the most common renal cysts but have the least clinical significance. Their incidence increases with age; 50% of people over the age of 50 years have at least one simple cyst. The cysts may be single or multiple, unilateral or bilateral. They occur typically in the cortex, but the deeper portions of the medulla may also be affected. Most are less than 1 cm in diameter but 3–4-cm examples may occur. The cysts are derived from local outpouchings or diverticula of distal tubules or collecting ducts. Most are clinically silent but a minority may be associated with:

● flank pain
● haematuria
● urinary tract infections
● hypertension

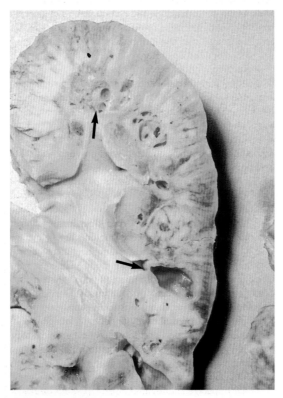

FIGURE 36.8 Medullary sponge kidney. Note the gross dilatation of ducts in the region of the papillae (arrows).

Acquired Renal Cystic Disease

This is a recently recognized entity confined to patients who have **advanced chronic renal failure, especially those on dialysis for end-stage renal disease**. Some 30–50% of patients on chronic dialysis suffer from this disorder, the risk becoming significant from about the third year of dialysis. This risk appears to be related to prolonged chronic renal failure rather than to dialysis itself.

The condition is characterized by the presence of multiple small cysts (5 mm in diameter) distributed throughout a shrunken end-stage kidney. The cysts originate from tubules and are found in both the cortex and medulla. They are lined by flattened cuboidal epithelium and contain clear, or sometimes haemorrhagic, fluid. Atypical hyperplasia of cyst wall epithelium is frequent and may be striking in degree. This may account for the high prevalence of neoplasms within the cysts.

Neoplastic lesions are found in 25% of affected patients. Most of the tumours are benign adenomas but about 15% are renal cell carcinomas. The incidence of renal carcinoma in patients with end-stage kidney failure is many times higher than that in the general population, and virtually all of these are associated with acquired renal cystic disease. The tumours in this group tend to be relatively slow growing and to have a low potential for metastasis, although this may occur.

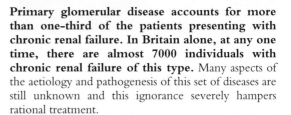

Glomerular Disease

Primary glomerular disease accounts for more than one-third of the patients presenting with chronic renal failure. In Britain alone, at any one time, there are almost 7000 individuals with chronic renal failure of this type. Many aspects of the aetiology and pathogenesis of this set of diseases are still unknown and this ignorance severely hampers rational treatment.

Pathophysiological Effects

Injury of the glomerulus may present with one or more **functional disturbances**, which include:

● **Disturbance of sieving functions** so that the glomerular ultrafiltrate contains large molecules, normally not passing the glomerular barrier. This results in **proteinuria**.
● **Disturbance of the regulatory functions in respect of sodium and water.** Abnormal retention of these must lead to expansion of the plasma volume, expressed in the form of **oedema**, **hypertension** or both of these.
● **An inability to keep all the red cells within the capillary lumen and the consequent**

development of haematuria. The red cells that make their way into the urinary space are usually distorted and damaged. It is not clear what the structural basis is for this leakage of red cells from the glomerular capillaries (see sections on immunoglobulin (Ig) A and thin basement membrane nephropathy).

- **A decline in the glomerular filtration rate (GFR).** This may be of rapid onset or may develop insidiously and become chronic. In the latter case obliteration of the glomerular capillary tuft by scarring is the usual mechanism.

CLINICAL PRESENTATION

These functional abnormalities of the glomeruli express themselves in a number of **different clinical patterns**:

- **the nephritic syndrome**
- **proteinuria and the nephrotic syndrome**
- **haematuria and an abnormal urinary sediment**
- **rapidly progressive renal failure**
- **chronic renal failure**

The Nephritic Syndrome

This is characterized by:

- some reduction in urinary volume
- mild to moderate proteinuria
- hypertension
- retention of sodium and water
- some expansion of the intravascular volume
- haematuria (macroscopic or microscopic)

Proteinuria and the Nephrotic Syndrome

The defining characteristics of the **nephrotic syndrome** are:

- massive protein loss in the urine (greater than 3.5 g per day)
- hypoalbuminaemia
- oedema

It may be complicated by:

- **Thrombosis**, particularly affecting the renal veins and their tributaries. Nearly half the patients with the nephrotic syndrome due to membranous glomerulonephritis have angiographically detectable renal vein thrombi and, in adults so affected, it is by no means uncommon to find venous thrombosis in other parts of the body.

  Children with the nephrotic syndrome are liable to develop thrombi in the arterial side of the circulation, and thrombi within the chambers of the heart or within the pulmonary arterial bed are quite common.

- **Infections**, especially with *Streptococcus pneumoniae*. Such infections present not uncommonly in the form of peritonitis without any evidence of inflammation or perforation of intra-abdominal viscera.

Proteinuria

Protein loss in the urine greater than 150 mg per day is abnormal and proteinuria exceeding 1 g per day almost certainly indicates glomerular as well as tubular damage.

Proteinuria is described as being either **selective** or **non-selective**. 'Selective proteinuria' implies the clearance of proteins of lower molecular weight such as albumin or transferrin, whereas 'non-selective proteinuria' involves clearance of proteins of higher molecular weight, such as IgG and IgM, as well.

Protein loss in the urine greater than 3.5 g per 24 hours exceeds the liver's ability to synthesize protein. This leads to hypoalbuminaemia and a lowering of plasma oncotic pressure, and thus to oedema (*Fig. 36.9*). The reduction in intravascular volume which this implies causes secondary hyperaldosteronism, resulting in sodium retention and some worsening, therefore, of the oedema. The hypoalbuminaemia also leads to a general increase in protein synthesis by the liver. This includes an increase in the output of apoproteins, the carrier proteins for lipids, which is believed to account for the hyperlipidaemia seen in some patients with the nephrotic syndrome.

Haematuria and an Abnormal Urinary Sediment

Haematuria in glomerular disease may be gross, or detectable only by microscopy. The presence of red cell casts in urine strongly suggests active glomerular disease. Recurrent haematuria occurs in focal proliferative glomerulonephritis and in some forms of mesangio-capillary glomerulonephritis.

Rapidly Progressive Renal Failure

'Rapid' in this context means severe deterioration in renal function **over a period of weeks or months**, usually *not* accompanied by hypertension. This clinical picture has a strong association with 'crescentic' forms of glomerulonephritis.

Unfortunately there is no 'one-for-one' correlation between these syndromes and the various microscopic patterns. Thus, several different pathological conditions may be present with a single clinical syndrome. For example, the **nephrotic syndrome** may be caused by:

- minimal change disease
- membranous glomerulonephritis
- focal segmental glomerulosclerosis
- reactive systemic amyloidosis
- diabetes mellitus
- some cases of mesangiocapillary (membranoproliferative) glomerulonephritis
- some cases of systemic lupus erythematosus (SLE)

Similarly a single pathological entity may present with different clinical syndromes.

To compound the difficulties, many different disorders may give rise to a **single morphological picture**, as in **'crescentic' glomerulonephritis**, which may be seen in:

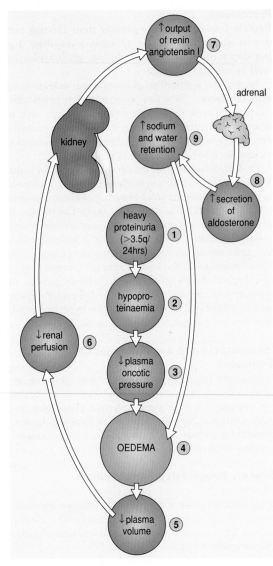

FIGURE 36.9 Pathogenesis of oedema in the nephrotic syndrome.

- anti-glomerular basement membrane disease
- post-infective glomerulonephritis
- Henoch–Schönlein disease
- SLE
- mesangiocapillary glomerulonephritis
- mixed cryoglobulinaemia
- vasculitis
- 'idiopathic' crescentic glomerulonephritis

MECHANISMS OF GLOMERULAR INJURY

Immunological Mechanisms
Glomerular injury may occur as a result of:

- deposition of preformed immune complexes
- formation of immune complexes *in situ* (as in the active form of experimental Heymann nephritis)
- by the alternate pathway of complement activation
- by nephrotoxic antibody binding to glomerular basement membrane antigens

Approximately 45% of cases of human glomerulonephritis show immune complex deposition in affected glomeruli; a much smaller proportion (5%) is due to the effects of a nephrotoxic antibody directed against **glomerular basement membrane** antigens.

Some of these processes can be illustrated in animal models.

Experimental Glomerulonephritis

Immune Complex-mediated Glomerulonephritis

'Single-Shot' Serum Sickness   Injection of a single large dose of a foreign serum protein in rabbits is followed in 5–14 days by an acute self-limiting glomerulonephritis due to trapping in glomeruli of soluble immune complexes formed in the blood, in the zone of antigen excess. In humans this occurs in 'serum sickness' following the administration of large doses of, for example, tetanus antitoxin prepared by immunizing horses against the toxin.

Multiple Injections of Foreign Protein   Injection of multiple small doses of foreign protein causes a progressive glomerulonephritis in rabbits. If small immune complexes are deposited at a slow rate, the animal develops glomerular disease analogous with membranous glomerulonephropathy in humans. If the antibody response is quantitatively greater, proliferative glomerulonephritis is found.

In Situ Formation of Immune Complexes   Injection of rat kidney together with adjuvant into susceptible strains of rat, leads to formation of an antibody against a lipoprotein present in the brush border of the proximal tubule and also on the foot processes of the epithelial cells. A chronic glomerulonephritis develops which, in morphological terms, resembles human membranous glomerulonephritis. This model is known as **active Heymann nephritis**. Passive Heymann nephritis may be induced with a single intravenous injection of heterologous anti-brush border antibody and bears a much less close resemblance to human membranous nephropathy.

Nephrotoxic Glomerulonephritis (Anti-glomerular Basement Membrane Disease)
Injection of kidney (rabbit) into a different species (guinea-pig) produces antibodies. If these antibodies are injected into rabbits, a progressive glomerulonephritis results.

Two phases of glomerular damage exist in this model. In the first, or **heterologous**, phase the guinea-pig antibody binds to rabbit glomerular **basement membrane antigen**. The rabbit then produces antibody against the bound foreign protein and this rabbit antibody then binds to the guinea-pig globulin within the kidney (the **autologous** phase). In the absence of this second phase, the glomerulitis is self-limiting. In humans anti–glomerular basement membrane disease can cause Goodpasture's syndrome and some cases of crescentic glomerulonephritis.

Common modes of immune-mediated injury are depicted in *Figs 36.10* and *36.11*.

Non-immunological Mechanisms

Of these, **hyperfiltration** appears to be the most important.

Non-immune-mediated glomerular injury has been studied adequately only in animal models, in which five-sixths of the kidney substance has been removed. This leads to **hypertension, proteinuria and renal failure** associated with glomerular injury in the form of thickening of the capillary loops, the formation of adhesions between Bowman's capsule and the glomeruli, swelling of the epithelial cells and patchy fibrinoid necrosis.

The abnormalities are believed to be due to increased plasma flow through the glomerulus and an increase in GFR. Injury can be inhibited by heparin, which also lowers the blood pressure in these animals and prevents the development of renal failure.

Factors that are believed to be significant in this model are:

1) **increased glomerular plasma flow**
2) **increased glomerular capillary pressure**, associated with a decreased resistance in the afferent arteriole. Systemic hypertension injures glomeruli only when afferent arteriolar resistance is decreased. In this context angiotensin-converting enzyme (ACE) inhibitors have a greater effect in inhibiting glomerular injury than do diuretics, because the former lower the resistance in the **efferent** arterioles and thus reduce the glomerular capillary pressure.

The relationship of this model to human disease is not clear but these mechanisms may determine the **rate of progression to end-stage renal disease** once a critical number of nephrons has been lost as a result of primary glomerular pathology.

Human Glomerular Diseases

We are still ignorant about many aspects of this set of disorders. This makes it difficult to classify glomerular diseases on an aetiological or pathogenetic basis, and current classifications are based on the microscopic patterns.

Such classifications, although far from perfect, give a reasonable amount of information as to natural history and prognosis. Many find morphological classifications difficult to understand and remember, largely because of the nomenclature used. The number of morphological responses to injury in the glomerulus is remarkably small and it is possible to build on this to create a better understanding.

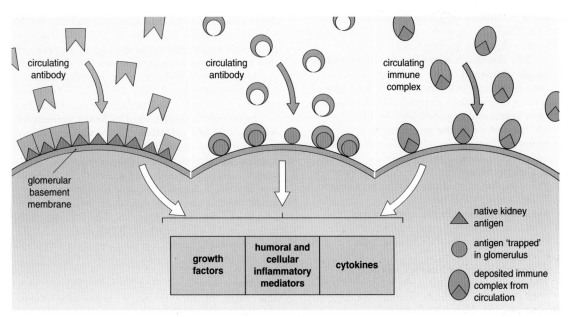

FIGURE 36.10 Common modes of immune-mediated glomerular injury.

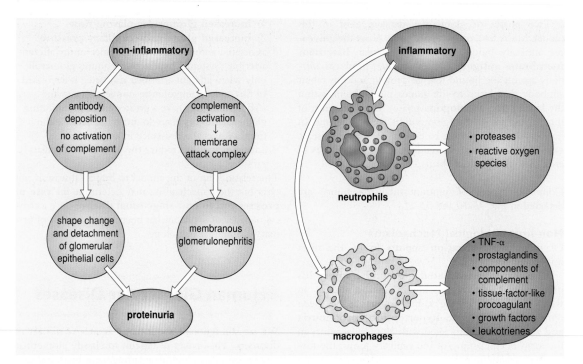

FIGURE 36.11 Immune-mediated injury may or may not elicit an inflammatory reaction.

PRIMARY GLOMERULAR DISORDERS

A Basis for Morphological Classification

This rests on the foundations of three sets of criteria:

1) **The distribution of abnormal glomeruli within the kidney.** If more than 70% of the glomeruli in a given section are affected, the disease is termed **diffuse**. The term **focal** is applied to cases where the proportion of affected glomeruli is smaller (Fig. 36.12).

2) **The distribution of abnormalities within single glomeruli.** If the whole of a single glomerulus shows abnormalities, the term **global** is used. If only part of a glomerulus is affected, the term **segmental** is applied (Fig. 36.13).

3) **The nature of the glomerular abnormalities.** These can be categorized on the basis of the following abnormalities:

- **Cell proliferation.** This may involve the endothelial or mesangial cells, or may indicate an inflammatory cell infiltrate.
- **Basement membrane appearances.** The basement membrane may be normal or may show diffuse or focal thickening, splitting or be abnormally thin.
- **The presence or absence of immune complex deposition** or the binding of antibody to glomerular structures. Immune complex may be seen on electron microscopic examination of renal biopsies or by the use of immunohistology

at the light microscopic level. If present, immune complexes may be located in subepithelial, subendothelial, intramesangial or intrabasement membrane positions.

Minimal Change Glomerular Disease (Epithelial Cell Disease)

This is the commonest cause of the **nephrotic syndrome in childhood, most cases appearing by the age of 6 years. More than 75% of cases of nephrotic syndrome up to the age of 16 years are due to minimal change disease.** This disorder also accounts for 18–25% of the cases of this syndrome in adults. In children a male : female ratio of 2 : 1 is noted; this difference tends to disappear after the age of 15 years.

The disorder is characterized by **heavy proteinuria which is highly selective.** This is the only urinary abnormality and other aspects of renal function are unimpaired. However, in adults protein loss is not selective and some evidence of impaired renal function may be seen. A dramatic response to steroids is characteristic of minimal change disease and provides the best clinical criterion for its diagnosis. The majority of the patients make a full recovery. Relapses are not infrequent but most of these children retain a favourable response to steroids.

Aetiology

The cause of the disease is unknown. Immune complexes are not found in the glomeruli, although **non-complement-binding complexes, the signi-**

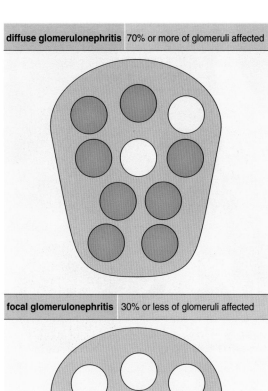

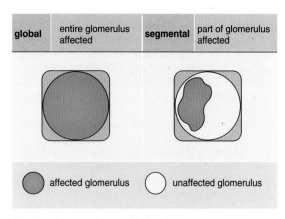

FIGURE 36.13 *Concept of global and segmental glomerular involvement.*

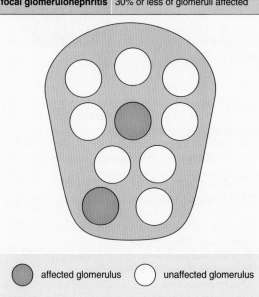

FIGURE 36.12 *Focal and diffuse glomerular injury.*

ficance of which is not known, may be found in the plasma. An association exists between the presence of atopy and also of Hodgkin's disease and an increased risk of minimal change disease; there is also some evidence of T-cell dysfunction. Possible links with disturbances of the immune system are strengthened by the facts that:

1) measles, known to have a suppressive effect on T-cell function, may induce remission.
2) patients with minimal change disease have an increased susceptibility to pneumococcal infections.
3) there is an increased frequency of HLA-DR7 in children with minimal change disease.

Morphological Features (*Table 36.3*)

Table 36.3 Morphological Features in Minimal Change Disease

Cell proliferation	Absent
Basement membrane alteration	Absent
Immune complex deposition	Absent
Other	Withdrawal of foot processes due to loss of glomerular polyanion seen on electron microscopy

Macroscopic Features

In the rare fatal cases, the kidneys are enlarged and have rather pale cortices, very clearly demarcated from the medulla.

Microscopic Features

Glomeruli appear quite normal in most cases, although in some instances there may be slightly increased cellularity of the mesangium. Tubular epithelium may show intracellular lipid, believed to be a reflection of the hyperlipidaemia associated with the nephrotic syndrome.

Immunohistology

Immunohistological studies show a complete absence, in most cases, of any localization of immunoglobulins, complement or fibrin.

Electron Microscopic Features

In **morphological** terms a positive diagnosis can be made only on the basis of electron microscopy, the characteristic feature being **fusion or withdrawal of the epithelial cell foot processes** (*Figs 36.14* and *36.15*). The epithelial changes are due to retraction of the foot processes into the epithelial cell bodies and represent the result of loss of the glomerular polyanion. Identical ultrastructural changes can be produced in experimental animals by injecting the aminonucleoside puromycin, which causes loss of the polyanion. Spontaneous clinical recovery is accompanied by a full return to normal morphology of the foot processes. If steroid therapy is required, the recovery of normal foot process appearances is only partial.

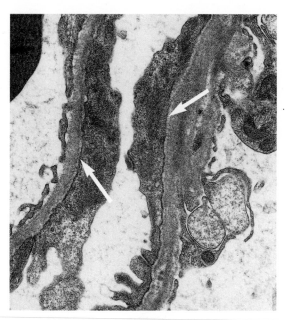

FIGURE 36.15 *Transmission electron micrograph showing epithelial cell foot process fusion in minimal change disease (arrows).*

Some cases of minimal change disease are complicated by the later development of focal glomerular sclerosis (see pp 658–659). This is most likely to occur if the affected patient has had several relapses. Focal glomerular sclerosis is a serious complication which is likely, in about 50% of cases, to cause chronic renal failure.

Membranous Glomerulonephritis

Membranous glomerulonephritis accounts for about 30% of cases of the nephrotic syndrome in adults. In the West, it is most commonly **idiopathic**, no cause being identified in about 70% of cases. Recognized associations include:

- **Neoplasms** (approximately 10% of cases). The association appears to be strongest in relation to carcinoma of the bronchus and of the large bowel, although many others have been reported.
- **Heavy metal toxicity** (e.g. gold therapy in rheumatoid disease and mercury poisoning; mercury was once used by some individuals to lighten their skin colour).
- **Penicillamine**, also used in rheumatoid disease.
- **Persistent hepatitis B infection**
- **Quartan malaria.** This is particularly important in some parts of Africa. A study from Nigeria reported 28% of children with the nephrotic syndrome to be infected with *Plasmodium malariae* (infection rate in controls 6%) and a further 60% had a mixed infection with *P. malariae* and *P. falciparum* (15–18% in controls).
- Some cases of SLE
- **Syphilis** in both its congenital and acquired secondary forms can be complicated by glomerulonephritis. The most common form of renal disease in this setting is membranous glomerulonephritis. This usually responds to appropriate antibiotic treatment.

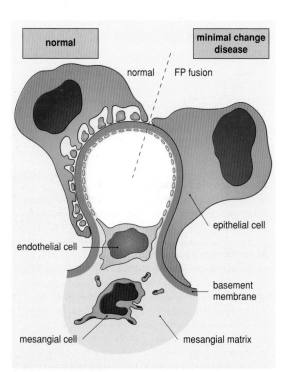

FIGURE 36.14 *Diagrammatic representation of the epithelial cell changes in minimal change disease as compared with the normal.*

Clinical Features

The onset is insidious; common presentations are either the nephrotic syndrome or asymptomatic proteinuria.

Table 36.4 Morphological Features in Membranous Glomerulonephritis

Cell proliferation	Absent
Basement membrane alterations	**Uniform thickening of the basement membrane.** Spikes of new basement membrane material protrude from the epithelial aspect of the membrane between subepithelial immune complexes; these spikes eventually enclose the remains of the complexes within basement membrane substance.
Immune complex deposition	Early in the course of the disease, small **subepithelial complexes** are deposited along the basement membrane. These increase in number and grow larger.

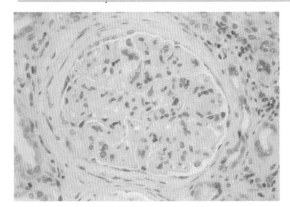

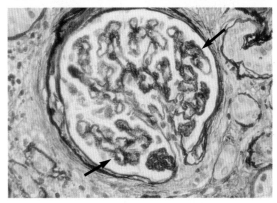

FIGURE 36.16 Membranous glomerulonephritis: The glomerular tuft is swollen and the pink basement membrane is uniformly thickened; there is no increase in cellularity of the tuft.

FIGURE 36.17 Membranous glomerulonephritis. This glomerulus has been stained with a silver salt which shows the basement membrane as black. Note the numerous tiny spikes on the abluminal surface of the basement membrane (arrows).

This proteinuria is characteristically **non-selective**. Serum complement levels are normal, although immunoglobulin concentrations may be reduced because of urinary loss of IgG. Circulating immune complexes are, as a rule, not present. There is a strong association with the haplotype HLA-DR3.

Natural History

Spontaneous remission occurs in about 25% of the patients. A further 25% continue to show proteinuria over many years with no significant loss of renal function, and the remainder ultimately develop renal failure because of progressive scarring of the glomeruli.

Morphological Features (Table 36.4)

Microscopic Features

Light microscopy of established cases shows **diffuse thickening of the capillary basement membrane in the glomerular tuft.** There is no evidence of cell proliferation (*Figs 36.16* and *36.17*).

Immunohistology

Immunohistological studies show **granular deposits of IgG and C3 along the basement membrane** (IgG in virtually all cases; C3 in about one-third).

Electron Microscopy

The electron microscopic appearances depend on the stage of evolution of the disease (*Fig. 36.18*).

- **Stage 1:** The earliest event is the accumulation of small electron-dense deposits on the **epithelial** side of the basement membrane. At this stage, fusion of the foot processes is already seen. The light microscopic appearances of the glomeruli are normal.
- **Stage 2:** Basement membrane substance increases and protrudes between the immune complexes to give the characteristic 'spiked' appearance which can be seen well on light microscopy in sections stained with methenamine (hexamine) silver.
- **Stage 3:** The spikes of basement membrane now fuse and thus enclose the deposits. Some of the deposits become much less electron-dense and appear to fade into the basement membrane substance.
- **Stage 4:** Glomeruli collapse and fibrosis is found on light microscopy, while on electron microscopy it may be difficult to distinguish the enclosed deposits from the surrounding basement membrane, so similar

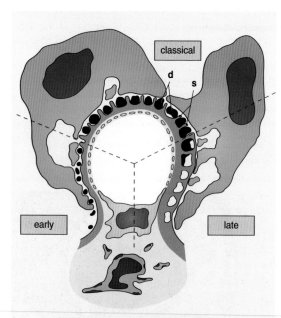

d subepithelial deposit of immune complex

s spikes of basement membrane material between
deposits as seen in classical phase of
membranous glomerulonephritis

FIGURE 36.18 Membranous glomerulonephritis. Morphological
evolution of the disease.

ally, but not always, **non-selective**. Some 50–75% of
patients also have some degree of **haematuria**, usually
microscopic. Hypertension and renal failure tend to
occur late in the disease, most often in adult patients,
but the ultimate prognosis is bad.

Morphological Features (Table 36.5)

**Table 36.5 Morphological Features of Focal
Segmental Glomerulosclerosis**

Cell proliferation	Very mild increase in number of mesangial cells
Basement membrane alterations	Thickening and wrinkling of basement membrane
Immune complex deposition	Absent
Other features	Early stages marked by the presence of foam cells in glomerular capillaries and focal adhesions to Bowman's capsule. Acellular, hyaline, periodic acid–Schiff (PAS)-positive material distributed segmentally. Affected segments eventually collapse and hyaline masses enlarge. Retraction of foot processes of epithelial cells

have their electron densities become. The development of chronic renal failure in some patients reflects
obliteration of glomeruli by hyaline fibrous tissue
with consequent loss of nephrons. It is still not
known what determines whether the process will
remit or progress to scarring.

Focal Segmental Glomerulosclerosis

**This accounts for 10–20% of cases of the
nephrotic syndrome in adults and about 10% in
children.** It affects mainly the juxtamedullary
glomeruli and, unless renal biopsies include this part,
the diagnosis can be missed. There is some controversy
as to whether this pathological variant should be classified as a separate disorder: some regard it as part of the
spectrum of changes seen in minimal change disease,
whereas others maintain that the pathological picture
may be seen in many different disorders of the kidney.

Clinical Features

In children, who are frequently affected, most cases
occur before the age of 6 years. In most there is no history of a preceding infective illness and the presenting
features are usually those of the nephrotic syndrome,
preceded by heavy proteinuria. The proteinuria is usu-

Microscopic Features

Light microscopic appearances are characteristic, provided the biopsy includes both cortex and medulla.
Typically involved glomeruli show a **segmental** and
non-proliferative sclerosis or hyalinization, often accompanied by adhesions between the glomerular tuft and
Bowman's capsule. Eosinophilic hyaline droplets may be
seen in the glomerulus and large lipid-laden cells may be
present in the mesangium. PAS-positive material may
accumulate within the lesions, this being a useful point
for distinguishing the lesions of focal segmental glomerulosclerosis from other forms of postnephritic scarring.

Immunohistology

On immunohistological examination segmental trapping
of IgM or C3 has been reported, but this is not believed
to be significant in pathogenetic terms.

Electron Microscopy

This shows typical thickening and wrinkling of the basement membrane, which may also show evidence of splitting. Obvious fusion of the foot processes is another

characteristic feature. Foot process fusion may also be seen in cortical glomeruli, even though these may appear normal on light microscopy.

PROLIFERATIVE GLOMERULONEPHRITIDES

Anti-glomerular Basement Membrane Disease

Anti-glomerular basement membrane disease is the human homologue of experimental nephrotoxic nephritis. This is shown by induction of glomerulonephritis by injecting IgG eluted from the kidneys of patients with anti-glomerular basement membrane disease into primates. It usually complicates one of a variety of systemic diseases. Most involve immune-mediated vascular injury (vasculitis) but in 20–30% of cases no precipitating factor can be found. The defining characteristics are:

- **focal, segmental, necrotizing glomerulonephritis**
- **circulating anti-basement membrane antibodies** in the plasma of affected individuals
- **deposition of IgG on the glomerular capillary basement membrane** in a characteristic **linear fashion**

Anti-glomerular basement membrane disease accounts for about 5% of all cases of glomerulonephritis. It is commonest in young adults, especially males, but is by no means restricted to this age group. There is a major genetic component in that about 90% of those affected possess the HLA-DR2 antigen. Susceptibility to experimental anti-glomerular basement membrane disease in animals also appears to be, at least in part, determined genetically.

Clinical Features

These may take the form of one of some distinct but pathogenetically related syndromes:

- severe, rapid progressive, glomerulonephritis
- acute pulmonary haemorrhage associated with glomerulonephritis (Goodpasture's syndrome)
- pulmonary haemorrhage alone

Patients with glomerular involvement often develop rapidly progressive renal failure. If dialysis is required, as it is in about 70% of sufferers, the outlook is very bleak: few, if any, recover.

Serological Features

The plasma in all cases contains IgG antibodies that react with an antigen in the globular non-collagen domain of type IV procollagen (the Goodpasture antigen). These antibodies do not bind exclusively to glomerular basement membranes but also to basement membranes in the lung alveoli and in the choroid of the eye. More than 50% of the patients with anti-glomerular basement membrane antibodies also have circulating antibodies that react with renal tubular basement membranes.

Other antibodies may also be found. In 30% of cases these are antineutrophilic cytoplasmic antibodies (**ANCAs**) which are often present in polyarteritis nodosa or other types of systemic vasculitis (see pp 400–401). IgA and IgM antibodies are seen occasionally but their pathogenetic significance, if any, is not known.

Morphological Features (*Table 36.6*)

Microscopic Features

Characteristically **crescents** (proliferations of cells partly or totally obliterating the space between the glomerular tuft and Bowman's capsule) are present. Crescent formation is usually extensive, involving up to 95% of the glomeruli in some cases.

The crescent is the histological correlate of severe, acute and progressive glomerular damage and **appears to be causally linked to the escape of fibrin from the damaged glomerulus into Bowman's space.** Crescent formation was thought to be a reactive proliferation of the **epithelial cells** lining Bowman's capsule; immunohistological studies show that **macrophages** form a significant part of the cell population of the crescent (*Figs 36.19* and *36.20*).

Some glomeruli show focal necrosis of part of the tuft, destruction of capillaries being associated with fibrin accumulation. Affected glomeruli may be infiltrated by neutrophils and there is some increase in the mesangial cell population.

Immunohistology

The single most important diagnostic feature of anti-glomerular basement membrane disease is the presence of IgG (or, less frequently, IgM or IgA) distributed in a **linear**, non-granular fashion which outlines the capillary walls with striking clarity, even in the few glomeruli that appear normal on light microscopy. In about 50%, C3 can also be identified, bound to basement membrane.

Goodpasture's Syndrome

This syndrome, first described during the great influenza pandemic in 1918, is a variant of anti-glomerular basement membrane disease in which pulmonary haemorrhage is present as well as the nephritic picture described above. It is, fortunately, uncommon.

Clinical Features

Haemoptysis of varying degrees of severity is the outstanding clinical feature; the pulmonary haemorrhage is severe enough to cause anaemia in some cases. Chest

Table 36.6 Morphological Features of Anti-basement Membrane Disease

Cell proliferation	Some increase in mesangial cells and infiltration of neutrophils into affected glomerular segments
Basement membrane alterations	Some irregularity and thickening of the basement membrane but this is not a characteristic feature
Immune complex deposition or antibody binding	Deposition of IgG along the basement membrane in a very characteristic linear fashion. This feature is present in more than 90% of cases
Other features	Some 80% of cases show the presence of 'crescents' wholly or partially obliterating the urinary space

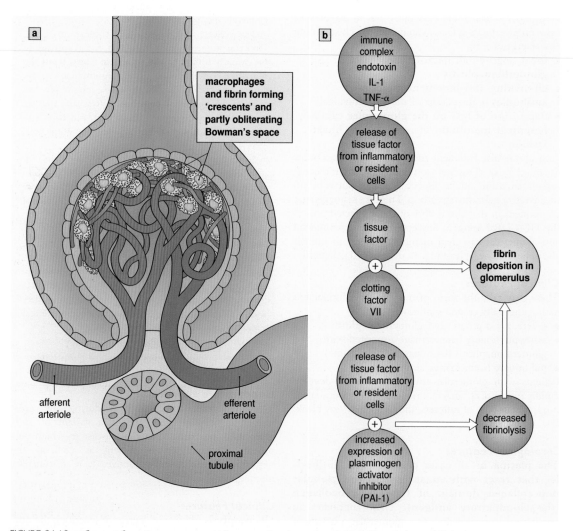

FIGURE 36.19 *a* Crescent formation as seen in rapidly progressive glomerulonephritis. *b* Coagulation and fibrinolysis in glomerulonephritis.

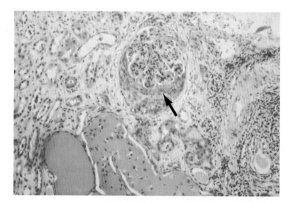

FIGURE 36.20 *The kidney in rapidly progressive glomerulonephritis showing 'epithelial' crescent formation (arrow).*

radiography reveals bilateral shadowing, which may fluctuate in intensity during the course of the illness. Associated **haematuria** is common (more than 90% of patients) and granular casts are found in the urine in more than 50%.

Pathological Features

The renal abnormalities are the same as those seen in anti-glomerular basement membrane disease *not* associated with lung haemorrhage. The lungs, when seen at necropsy, are bulky, firm and congested owing to the presence of intra-alveolar haemorrhage. On microscopic examination the alveolar septa are thickened and some show evidence of disintegration or rupture, somewhat similar to what is seen in idiopathic pulmonary haemosiderosis.

Immunohistological studies show linear deposits of IgG and complement along the pulmonary basement membranes, in a fashion identical to that seen in the glomeruli. Antibody eluted from the lung cross-reacts with kidney basement membranes and, similarly, antibody eluted from the kidney cross-reacts with pulmonary basement membranes.

Pathogenesis

Tissue damage is clearly antibody mediated but what initiates antibody formation in this disorder is much less well understood. Possibilities that have been canvassed include:

1) cross-reaction of antiviral antibodies with glomerular basement membrane
2) a possible alteration of the patient's own tissues so as to render them immunogenic as, for example, when anti-glomerular basement membrane disease develops after the inhalation of hydrocarbon solvents
3) other events related to environmental factors that might expose sequestered basement membrane antigens

Other Causes of Crescentic Glomerulonephritis

Isolated crescentic glomerulonephritis is most commonly the correlate of anti-glomerular basement membrane disease but may occur in other disorders. Some of these are **multisystem diseases** such as:

- SLE
- mixed cryoglobulinaemia
- Henoch–Schönlein disease
- polyarteritis nodosa
- Wegener's granulomatosis
- malignant hypertension
- haemolytic–uraemic syndrome

Other instances of crescent formation may occur in association with postinfective glomerulonephritis or membranoproliferative (mesangiocapillary) disease. Occasionally crescentic glomerulonephritis may occur in an 'idiopathic' form in which no evidence of an immune-mediated mechanism is found. The aetiology and pathogenesis of this variant are quite unknown.

Idiopathic diffuse crescentic glomerulonephritis is, fortunately, a rare disease, commonest in middle-aged and elderly individuals and showing a predilection for males.

Clinical and Serological Features

Patients present either in **acute renal failure** or with **rapidly progressive renal failure** associated with moderate to heavy proteinuria. Haematuria is uniformly present, at least at the microscopic level.

Anti-glomerular basement membrane antibodies are not found in the plasma but ANCAs are present in the majority (as in most cases of microscopic polyarteritis nodosa). The renal abnormalities in microscopic polyarteritis nodosa and diffuse crescentic glomerulonephritis are identical; the two disorders are probably closely related.

Acute Diffuse Proliferative Glomerulonephritis (Acute Diffuse Endocapillary Glomerulonephritis, Postinfectious Glomerulonephritis)

One of the commoner presentations of glomerular disease in the preantibiotic era was an **acute nephritic syndrome** following streptococcal pharyngitis. The histological correlate is **diffuse** glomerular involvement with **cell proliferation** distributed **globally** within the glomerulus.

Renal symptoms appear 10–18 days after the infection and appear homologous with those of experimental serum sickness (see p 652). The organisms are all Group A β-haemolytic streptococci; certain types, most notably types 12, 49, 55, 57 and 60, appear to be most nephritogenic. Pharyngitis is the most frequent antecedent of the poststreptococcal form of acute glomerulonephritis, but some cases are known to occur following infection of the skin and middle ear.

Today, poststreptococcal glomerulonephritis is rare in the UK; most patients presenting with the acute nephritic syndrome do not have a history of a preceding streptococcal infection. Instead numerous other types of infection have been implicated. These include bacterial, viral and parasitic diseases. In other parts of the world, however, such as Africa, the Middle East, India, many other parts of Asia, South America and the Caribbean, poststreptococcal glomerulonephritis is still common.

Clinical Features

Following a latent period after the infection, onset of the nephritic syndrome is usually abrupt. The syndrome is characterized by:

- oedema of the face, giving a puffy appearance below the eyes
- increase in blood pressure
- a decline in urine output
- biochemical findings indicating a decline in the GFR. In some cases this may be so severe as to cause acute renal failure.

Examination of the urine shows:

- moderate proteinuria (usually less than 5 g per 24 hours)
- haematuria, which may be sufficiently severe as to make the urine brownish in colour
- neutrophils and a variety of casts

The combination of blood, white cells and casts leads to the presence of some sediment, which gives the urine a 'smoky' appearance when shaken.

In a few patients, this form of glomerulonephritis is expressed in the form of the nephrotic syndrome.

It is important to realize that presentation with an acute nephritic syndrome can occur in association with other forms of glomerular disease; acute diffuse endocapillary glomerulonephritis is not the only cause.

Serological Features

There is usually an early decline in the plasma concentration of C3, a finding suggesting that complement activation is involved in glomerular injury. C3 levels usually return to normal in 6–8 weeks.

Circulating antibodies that react with several glomerular basement membrane antigens are usually present, but probably are not involved in the pathogenesis.

Although circulating immune complexes are commonly found, it is believed that the glomerular damage is initiated by immune complexes, formed *in situ* within the glomeruli as a result of localization of streptococcal antigen on the glomerular basement membrane.

Morphological Features (*Table 36.7*)

Macroscopic Features

Death during the acute nephritic stage of acute proliferative glomerulonephritis is uncommon. In such rare instances, the kidneys are slightly enlarged with a smooth greyish surface which may be punctuated by petechial haemorrhages. The swollen glomeruli may be seen quite easily as grey dots on the cut surface.

Microscopic Features

Chief features of acute diffuse endocapillary glomerulonephritis are:

- a diffuse involvement of glomeruli
- an increase in the cellularity of the tufts
- neutrophils within the tufts
- in some cases, fibrin in Bowman's space
- occasional foci of glomerular necrosis

The increase in the cell population of the glomeruli is due, in part, to **proliferation of mesangial cells** and, in part, to **infiltration of neutrophils and macrophages**.

Clinically, the presence of fibrin in Bowman's space can be inferred by the detection of fibrin degradation products in urine; this indicates a very active process.

Immunohistology

This characteristically shows the presence of **IgG and C3** distributed in a **granular** or 'lumpy-bumpy' pattern along the basement membrane.

Electron Microscopy

The outstanding feature is the presence of large, dome-shaped, subepithelial, electron-dense deposits called **'humps'**. These are variable in number and are often related to enlarged or fused epithelial foot processes. Immuno-electron microscopy shows these deposits to correspond with the immune complexes seen on immunohistology (*Fig. 36.21*). Some deposits may also be seen in the mesangium and beneath the endothelium. These are usually smaller and vary in shape.

Natural History

Until fairly recently the prognosis has been regarded as uniformly good, complete recovery being the usual outcome in most patients. However, some recent studies suggest that up to half the patients show **morphological** evidence of chronicity in the form of sclerosed glomeruli. Poor prognostic indicators in biopsy material include tubular atrophy, interstitial fibrosis and large, confluent, electron-dense deposits, particularly when these are associated with a marked degree of cellular proliferation.

Mesangiocapillary (Membranoproliferative) Glomerulonephritis

These names imply, quite correctly, that in this form **both proliferation of mesangial cells and**

Table 36.7 Morphological Features of Acute Diffuse Proliferative Glomerulonephritis

Cellular proliferation	All the glomeruli are hypercellular. This is due partly to proliferation of mesangial cells and partly to the presence of neutrophils and monocytes in both the mesangium and the capillary lumen. The endothelial cells do not proliferate but are swollen.
Basement membrane alterations	The basement membrane is not thickened.
Immune complex deposition	Large electron-dense deposits are frequently present on the epithelial side of the basement membrane. They have a characteristic 'dome' shape. There may also be small deposits of variable shape in other locations.
Other features	Occasionally, capsular crescents may be seen.

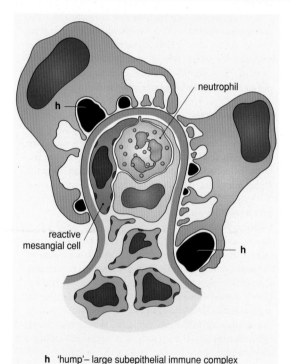

h 'hump'– large subepithelial immune complex

FIGURE 36.21 Morphological features of diffuse (endocapillary) glomerulonephritis.

glomerular capillary basement membrane abnormalities are present. Some cases are associated with:
- SLE
- malaria
- ventriculoatrial shunts
- persistent hepatitis B infection
- chronic renal allograft rejection
- some cases of liver cirrhosis associated with α_1-antitrypsin deficiency
- infective endocarditis
- deficiencies in the complement system
- both epithelial and lymphoreticular neoplasms

In the majority of cases there is no identifiable cause.

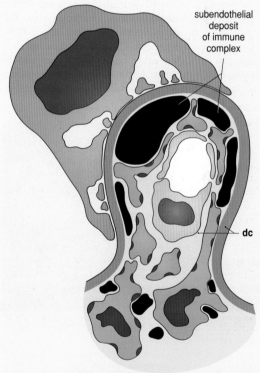

dc double contour appearance of basement membrane and new mesangial matrix as seen on silver staining

FIGURE 36.22 Mesangiocapillary glomerulonephritis: type I disease.

Two main forms of the disease exist. The distinction between them is made on the basis of immunohistological and electron microscopic features:
- **Type I disease shows deposits in the mesangium and in the subendothelial space**; the majority of 'idiopathic' cases fall into this group (*Fig. 36.22*).
- **Type II, or 'linear dense deposit disease', is characterized by the presence of electron-dense material arranged in a curious ribbon-**

like pattern within the capillary basement membrane. Unlike what is seen in type I disease, this material does not appear to represent immune complex.

Type I Disease

This occurs most commonly in the age group 8–16 years, females being more commonly affected than males. Clinical presentations vary from case to case. Some patients show features of the **nephrotic syndrome**; others present with elements of the **nephritic syndrome** or with **recurrent haematuria**. Most patients have at least microscopic haematuria, and hypertension is present in about one-third at the time of presentation. Chronic renal failure develops in most patients but this may be delayed for 10 years or more. In one large series the 10-year survival rate was 49%.

Hypocomplementaemia is characteristic, but is not seen in all patients. Approximately 50% of patients have a depressed C3 plasma concentration when first seen, but other components may also be depressed. C3 nephritic factor (**C3nef**), an immunoglobulin which stabilizes the C3bBb convertase of the

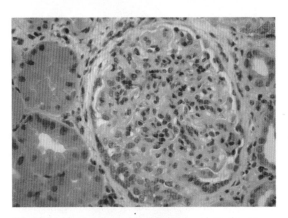

FIGURE 36.23 *Mesangiocapillary glomerulonephritis showing marked hypercellularity of the tuft.*

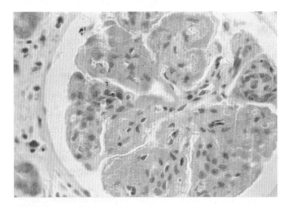

FIGURE 36.24 *Mesangiocapillary glomerulonephritis showing lobulation of the affected glomerulonephritis.*

alternate pathway of complement activation, and thus promotes alternate pathway complement activation, may be found in up to 30% of patients. The relationship between complement and this group of disorders is discussed further in the section on type II disease below.

Microscopic Features

The glomeruli are enlarged and hypercellular (*Fig. 36.23*), and tend to be lobulated (*Fig. 36.24*). There is an increase in mesangial matrix, which may obliterate part of the glomerular tuft and which is responsible for the lobulation.

The mesangial cell population is increased. The glomerular capillary wall is thickened and silver staining shows a typical double contour, which electron microscopy has shown to be due to the interposition of mesangial matrix and mesangial cell cytoplasm between the endothelium and the basement membrane.

Immunohistology

Irregular, granular deposition of C3 is found at the periphery of the lobules and in the mesangium. Less commonly C1q and C4 may be found. IgM and IgG are frequently found in the same distribution as the complement, but IgA is not usually seen.

Electron Microscopy

Ultrastructural examination confirms the presence of mesangial cell proliferation and an increase in mesangial matrix. A most striking feature is the interposition of mesangial cell cytoplasm and matrix between the capillary basement membrane and the endothelial cells. There is loss of epithelial foot processes. Electron-dense deposits are found characteristically in the subendothelial position. The thickening of the capillary walls, sometimes seen on light microscopy, is due partly to the presence of these deposits and partly to intrusion of the mesangial cytoplasm into the subendothelial space.

Type II Disease

The clinical pictures of types I and II disease are essentially similar but a few helpful distinguishing features exist. The sexes are equally affected; the age at onset tends to be younger in type II than in type I disease. The most frequent clinical presentations are of the **nephritic syndrome** or of the **nephrotic syndrome associated with macroscopic haematuria**. Hypertension is a frequent finding. Some patients show partial lipodystrophy with absence of subcutaneous fat over the trunk, which may precede the clinical onset of the glomerulonephritis by a considerable time.

Table 36.8 Morphological Features of Type I Disease

Cellular proliferation	Marked increase in the number of mesangial cells and in the bulk of the mesangial matrix. This latter feature leads to lobulation of the glomerular tufts and, sometimes, to the presence of nodules of mesangial tissue. Small numbers of neutrophils may also be present.
Basement membrane alterations	On light microscopy the walls of the capillaries are thickened and, when silver stains are used, the basement membranes appear split giving a 'tramline' or double-contour effect. Positive histological diagnosis requires this change to be present in 80% of the glomeruli. This is due partly to the presence of complement deposits, partly to the presence of mesangial cell cytoplasm and matrix, and partly to the formation of new basement membrane matrix just beneath the endothelial cells.
Immune complex deposition and antibody binding	Electron-dense deposits are present in the subendothelial layer of mesangium and in the new basement membrane described above. Some of these deposits are large and elongated and, because of their shape, have been called 'slugs'. Subepithelial deposits are present in 15–20% of cases. All deposits consist principally of C3.
Other features	If proteinuria is heavy, the foot processes of the epithelial cells may be retracted.

Microscopic features

In many cases it is impossible to distinguish between type I and type II disease on light microscopy, although the ribbon-like deposits characteristic of the latter may sometimes be seen in thin sections.

Crescents, while not numerous, are not unusual. In later stages tubular atrophy and interstitial fibrosis are common and marked features.

Immunohistology

Immunohistological studies in type II disease usually show C3 **alone** in the glomeruli, although some properdin may occasionally be present.

Electron Microscopy

This shows extremely electron-dense deposits (hence the name **linear dense deposit disease**) **within** the lamina densa of the basement membrane and this causes marked thickening of the capillary wall (*Fig. 36.25*). Dense deposits can also be seen round the tubular basement membranes and in the mesangium. The epithelial cell foot processes are fused and there is an increase in the mesangial cell population and in the amount of mesangial matrix.

Complement and Type II Disease

Inappropriate activation of complement plays an important, although probably not exclusive, role in the pathogenesis.

Serum complement shows a distinctive pattern of alteration in this disorder. Levels of the components involved in the classical pathway of complement activation (C1q, C4 and C2) are usually normal, whereas that of C3 is greatly decreased. It is believed that this isolated C3 depression is brought about, at least in part, by inappropriate C3 activation via the alternate pathway.

A second element in the depression of serum levels of C3 is a reduction in C3 synthesis, the origin of which is not understood.

Alternate pathway activation of complement is brought about by the production of a convertase (C3bBb) originating from C3 and Factor B. This convertase is produced in very small amounts under normal circumstances, by a 'tick-over' mechanism controlled by the action of two naturally occurring **inhibitors**: C3b inactivator I and β_1-H-globulin.

A reduction in the concentration of either of these leads to uncontrolled activation of C3 because the small amounts of C3bBb generated become stabilized and thus split more C3, generating more C3bBb *ad infinitum* until the system becomes exhausted. C3 nephritic factor (C3neF) has a similar effect on the C3bBb complex and renders it resistant to both the C3b inactivator and β_1-H-globulin. C3neF is an immunoglobulin directed against certain epitopes on the C3bBb convertase, to which it binds by its Fab portion.

Its role in the pathogenesis of mesangiocapillary glomerulonephritis is still obscure. Stimulating the alternate pathway of complement activation in animals does not produce glomerulonephritis, and patients with lipodystrophy may have C3neF in the plasma without

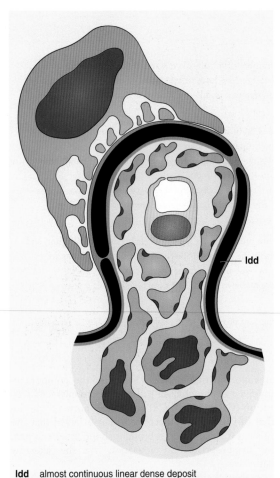

Idd —

Idd   almost continuous linear dense deposit
within the basement membrane

note: mesangial cell cytoplasm (green) interposed between
the basement membrane and the endothelial cell,
which results in marked narrowing of the capillary lumen

*FIGURE 36.25 Mesangiocapillary glomerulonephritis: type II
(linear dense deposit disease).*

Mesangial proliferative glomerulonephritis may be
found in:
- the recurrent haematuria syndrome (IgA
nephropathy)
- Henoch–Schönlein disease
- infective endocarditis
- SLE (mesangial proliferative glomerulonephritis is
the most common renal expression of this disorder)
- some instances of Goodpasture's syndrome
- Alport's syndrome (a hereditary form of
glomerulonephritis associated with nerve deafness)

Recurrent Haematuria Syndrome (IgA Nephropathy, Berger's Disease)

The defining criteria of this disorder are:
- **deposits of IgA and usually also C3 in the
mesangium** of most glomeruli
- **haematuria**, which may be gross or so mild that it
is picked up only on microscopic screening

Clinical Features

Patients with the recurrent haematuria syndrome are
most commonly children or young adults (patients
older than 40 years account for only 15% of cases) **who
present with haematuria**. The haematuria is often
associated with acute infections such as those of the respiratory tract, but may also be associated with trauma or
even with periods of vigorous exercise. Mild proteinuria may be present but there is no hypertension or any
other manifestation of renal impairment.

Epidemiology

Striking geographical variations exist; the countries in
which prevalence is greatest are France (where it accounts
for 20% of cases of nephritis), Italy, Japan, Singapore,
South Korea and Australia. In these locations it is the
commonest form of glomerular disease, IgA nephropathy being found in more than 40% of renal biopsies carried out for primary glomerular disease in Japan; in Britain
the prevalence in biopsy material is only 10%.

developing glomerulonephritis. However, patients
with genetically determined C3 deficiencies are prone
both to infection and to glomerulonephritis, and it is
possible that C3neF-driven C3 deficiency may have a
similar effect.

Mesangial Proliferative Glomerulonephritis

This term is applied to an inflammatory disorder of the
glomeruli characterized by:
- an increase in the number of mesangial cells
- an increase in the amount of mesangial matrix

These changes usually involve about 80% of the
glomeruli and may be quite subtle. It is essential that
thin sections of renal biopsies be examined, or mild
degrees of mesangial change may be missed.

Microscopic Features

The changes seen on light microscopy in biopsy samples
may be subtle. There is some localized crowding of nuclei
within the glomerular tuft, associated with an absence of
visible capillary lumina in these areas. Tuft necrosis may
be seen but is not common. In older lesions adhesions
between the capillary tuft and Bowman's capsule may be
present. The lesion progresses to segmental hyaline scarring. A small number of crescents may be seen but diffuse
crescentic forms of this disease are rare.

Immunohistology

The **immunohistological pattern** is very characteristic.
IgA is consistently deposited in the glomeruli (*Fig.*

36.26), the secretory piece being absent, and some IgG and C3 may be seen. The components for classical pathway activation of complement are not present and this suggests that activation of the alternate pathway plays a pathogenetic role.

Electron Microscopy

This confirms mild mesangial cell proliferation. Electron-dense deposits are localized to the mesangium, usually in the part of the mesangium related to that portion of capillary wall furthest from the urinary space (*Fig. 36.27*). Sometimes the deposits may extend into the subendothelial or subepithelial position.

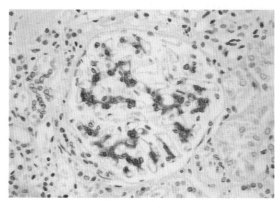

FIGURE 36.26 *Recurrent haematuria syndrome (Berger's disease). The section has been treated with a anti-IgA antibody; sites of antibody binding within the glomerulus are shown by the brown staining.*

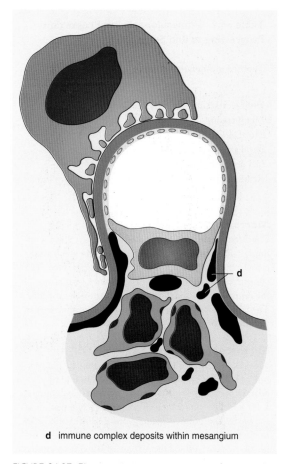

d   immune complex deposits within mesangium

FIGURE 36.27 *Electron microscopic appearance of mesangial proliferative glomerulonephritis.*

Although originally viewed as a benign disease, only 50% of the patients are alive with good renal function 20 years from the time of diagnosis.

Thin Basement Membrane Nephropathy with Persistent Haematuria of Renal Origin

Although IgA nephropathy is probably the most important cause of recurrent haematuria of renal origin, a group of patients with haematuria has been delineated in whom light microscopic appearances are normal and in whom the only ultrastructural abnormality is an abnormally **thin** glomerular capillary basement membrane (mean 191 nm ± 28; normal 350 nm ± 43). This feature appears to be seen particularly in those with macroscopic haematuria. It is difficult to be sure that the basement membrane abnormality is the **cause** of the haematuria, because thin basement membranes may occur in the general population in the absence of haematuria.

The disorder can be inherited as an **autosomal**

dominant condition or may occur sporadically, in which case clinical presentation is more likely to occur in adult life.

CHRONIC GLOMERULONEPHRITIS

The End-stage Kidney

Many of the types of glomerular disease described in the previous section progress at different rates to cause chronic renal failure.

The morphological correlate of chronic renal failure due to glomerular disease is called **chronic glomerulonephritis**. It is important to realize that this term represents a common destination or end stage, which may be reached via several different aetiological and pathogenetic pathways. It is not usually possible on histological examination to identify the initial type of glomerular injury; the chances of progression to the chronic stage differ from one type to another, as seen in *Table 36.9*.

Table 36.9 Glomerulonephritis: Proportion Progressing to End Stage

Type of glomerular disease	Frequency of progression (%)
Diffuse crescentic	90
Membranous	50
Mesangiocapillary	50
Focal glomerulosclerosis	50–80
IgA nephropathy	30–50
Acute diffuse endocapillary	1–2

Macroscopic Features

The kidneys are usually reduced in size by about one-third. The capsules are often difficult to strip and the sub-capsular surfaces show a finely granular appearance. The cut surface shows thinning of the cortex and blurring of the normal clear distinction between cortex and medulla. The renal atrophy is often accompanied by an increase in the amount of peripelvic adipose tissue.

Microscopic Features

Many of the glomeruli show partial or complete obliteration of both the capillary tuft and the mesangium by acellular, rather featureless, connective tissue in which there is a considerable amount of glycoprotein accumulation as shown by the positive staining obtained with the PAS method. Concentrically arranged rings of connective tissue may be seen around the margins of Bowman's capsule in the affected glomeruli (**periglomerular fibrosis**). Because of the failure of blood to flow between afferent and efferent arterioles in affected glomeruli, the remainder of the nephron undergoes ischaemic atrophy of differing degrees of severity, the tubules being shrunken or even absent. In nephrons in which the glomeruli are relatively unaffected, the tubules may hypertrophy so that alternating zones of large hypertrophic tubules and shrunken, atrophic ones may be seen.

There is an increase in interstitial connective tissue and a moderate lymphocytic infiltrate may be seen in some instances.

Because the blood pressure usually rises in association with chronic ischaemia of the kidneys, changes due to this hypertension are seen in the renal vasculature. At the arteriolar level this takes the form of thickening of the vessel walls and some loss of structure, especially of smooth muscle cells. The arteriolar wall has an eosinophilic and rather featureless appearance (hyaline).

Chronic Renal Failure

In the clinical sense, loss of nephrons over a long period is a silent process and the clinical features of chronic renal failure will not appear until the greater part of the functional nephron population has been lost. It is worth remembering that the **adaptive changes occurring in surviving glomeruli may themselves ultimately contribute to a worsening of the situation**. These adaptations consist essentially of increased glomerular blood flow and increased glomerular filtration, which can lead to both functional and structural injury.

Monitoring of Deteriorating Renal Function

Progression on the path to chronic renal failure may be monitored in relation to decreases or loss of a variety of normal kidney functions. These include:

- **a decreased ability to excrete nitrogenous waste products such as urea and creatinine.** Creatinine concentrations in the plasma are correlated with glomerular filtration and measurements of creatinine clearance from the blood give a fairly accurate measurement of GFR.
- **changes in the regulation of electrolytes and water**
- **changes in acid–base regulation, leading to metabolic acidosis**
- **changes in the renal handling of calcium and phosphorus**
- **changes in the production of renal hormones such as erythropoietin, renin and prostaglandins**

It is these changes in renal function, together with the retention in the plasma of dialysable toxic substances, that constitute the pathophysiological basis of chronic renal failure.

The first stage on the path to full-blown chronic renal failure is:

- **Diminished renal reserve.** Although GFR is decreased and there may be a loss of up to 50% of nephrons, normal excretory and regulatory functions are still well maintained. Additional stresses such as severe dehydrating episodes or the administration of catabolic drugs can alter this precarious state.
- **Renal insufficiency.** Here the patients show some increased retention of nitrogenous waste products; there is impaired concentration of urine, which may result in nocturia. Some degree of normocytic normochromic anaemia may be present.
- **Renal failure.** In addition to the above, there is:
  1) increasingly severe anaemia
  2) increased phosphate and decreased calcium levels in plasma
  3) metabolic acidosis
  4) fixed urinary specific gravity
- **Uraemia.** In addition to these biochemical abnormalities, there may now be clinical evidence of abnormalities affecting:
  1) the cardiovascular system
  2) the gastrointestinal tract
  3) the nervous system
  4) the skin
  5) the locomotor system

Pathophysiology

Handling of Sodium and Water
Normally a fall in GFR should lead to a fall in the filtered load of sodium. If sodium levels in blood are to remain normal, then more of the filtered sodium must be excreted and tubular reabsorption of sodium must fall. Fractional excretion of sodium rises significantly in chronic renal failure. The underlying mechanisms are complex and may include an inhibitor of $Na^+ K^+$ adenosine triphosphatase and high levels of atrial natriuretic peptide in the blood. Renal tubules are working at near capacity so far as sodium excretion is concerned. Any increase in dietary sodium intake will lead to sodium retention and expansion of the extracellular fluid volume.

A similar situation arises when GFR falls below 10–20 ml/min. Even with a stable sodium intake, sodium, and consequently water, will be retained and there will be expansion of the plasma volume, contributing to the hypertension shown by these patients.

Potassium
The most common problem related to potassium metabolism in patients with chronic, or indeed acute, renal failure, is **hyperkalaemia**, although some patients may show potassium wasting as a result of increased tubular epithelial excretion.

Hyperkalaemia in the context of chronic renal failure usually results from **impaired tubular secretion** and may be precipitated by abrupt increases in potassium intake, the development of metabolic acidosis (which shifts cellular potassium into the extracellular space) or episodes of dehydration.

The tubular dysfunction may result from:
- increased sodium reabsorption in the proximal tubule leading to insufficient **distal** tubule sodium absorption to permit potassium secretion
- damage to the distal tubular epithelium resulting from interstitial nephritis

Acid–Base Changes
Metabolic acidosis may occur as a result of chronic renal failure. Mechanisms involved include:
- a reduced tubular capacity to produce ammonia
- an inability to increase titratable acid excretion
- a decrease in the ability to reabsorb bicarbonate via the renal tubules

The retention of H^+ ion is partly countered by the buffering effect of bone minerals; this is believed to contribute to the demineralization of bone seen in renal osteodystrophy.

Calcium, Phosphorus and Vitamin D
In chronic renal failure, phosphate is retained to an abnormal degree and there is a corresponding fall in plasma ionizable calcium levels.

The fall in calcium stimulates secretion of parathyroid hormone (PTH). This acts on the renal tubules, increasing calcium reabsorption and phosphate excretion. In addition PTH stimulates osteoclast activity, thus releasing calcium from bone. Serum calcium levels tend to rise and phosphate levels to fall. In this way calcium and phosphate concentrations are kept more or less within normal limits until the GFR falls to about 20% of normal.

Maintenance of reasonably normal serum calcium and phosphate levels has a price. This is the development of **bone disease characterized morphologically by changes consistent with both osteomalacia and the resorptive features of hyperparathyroidism**.

Nephron loss itself leads to a **decrease in the output of the active form of vitamin D from the renal tubules**. As the plasma levels of this vitamin fall, absorption of calcium from the gut decreases. This will lead to a further decline in serum calcium concentration and still further stimulation of the parathyroid (see also pp 1045, 1050).

Uraemic Toxins
Some manifestations of chronic renal failure are believed to be due to the **retention of 'dialysable toxic' substances**. Catabolic states worsen some of the clinical features of uraemia, whereas protein restriction has the opposite effect; it is likely, therefore, that these putative toxic substances are nitrogenous.

While an increasing plasma urea concentration indicates declining renal function, urea itself does not cause the clinical features of uraemia. The addition of urea to the fluids used in renal dialysis has no effect on clinical manifestations such as drowsiness, asterixis and muscle twitching, and there must, therefore, be other causes.

Current evidence suggests that a group of molecules with molecular weight of 300–1500 Da is responsible for some of the troublesome manifestations of uraemia. These **'middle'** (middle-sized) **molecules** are polypeptides and addition of them to dialysates produces uraemic symptoms. Absolute proof of their role in uraemia is still lacking.

Carbohydrate Intolerance in Renal Failure
Most patients with untreated uraemia have impaired glucose tolerance. This is believed to be due to:
- increased resistance of the peripheral tissues to insulin; this is improved by dialysis
- increased plasma concentrations of glucagon

Hyperlipidaemia and Atherosclerosis
Patients with chronic renal failure have a very high incidence of coronary artery disease and myocardial infarction. These risks are *not* lessened by dialysis. These patients are often hyperlipidaemic, the major lipid class affected being triglyceride. The likely metabolic defect is a failure of post-hepatic lipoprotein lipase. The effects of the hyperlipidaemia on the artery wall are aggravated

by hypertension, which may be due to high levels of renin secretion and/or hypervolaemia.

Other Endocrine Abnormalities

Endocrine abnormalities in association with renal failure may be due to:

- **overproduction of a normal hormone** as a response to the biochemical disturbances caused by renal disease. This is seen in secondary hyperparathyroidism.
- **blunting of a hormone effect due to relative failures of ligand–receptor binding**, such as occurs in the increased peripheral resistance to insulin.
- **diminished catabolism of a hormone normally carried out in the kidney** and consequent accumulation of the hormone in the blood (e.g. growth hormone).
- **failure of secretion of a hormone in adequate amounts by the kidney.** Chronic renal failure is associated with a decline in the renal production of **erythropoietin** and this leads to the occurrence of normocytic normochromic anaemia.

Pathological Features (*Table 36.10* and *Fig. 36.28*)

Tubulointerstitial Disease

This term describes a group of disorders with the common feature of predominant localization of the lesions to the renal interstitial tissue and to the tubules.

In general the affected kidneys show:

- an inflammatory cell infiltrate in the interstitium
- oedema of the interstitial tissue
- scarring
- atrophy or necrosis of some of the tubules

Injury to the tubulointerstitial compartment of the kidney may be produced by mechanisms as diverse as:

- **infection**
- **drugs**
- **immune reactions**
- **obstruction to the urinary tract (with or without infection)**
- **necrosis of the renal papillae**
- **heavy metal poisoning**
- **acute toxic injury**
- **metabolic disorders (hereditary or acquired)**
- **hereditary tubular diseases**

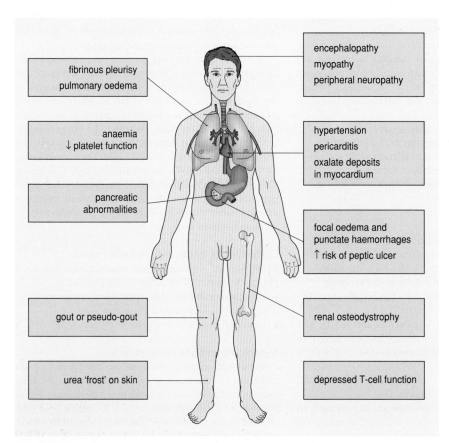

FIGURE 36.28 Clinical features occurring in uraemia.

Table 36.10 Organ and System Pathology in Chronic Renal Failure: a Summary

System	Abnormalities	Possible mechanisms
Cardiovascular system	Hypertension	Combination of increased plasma volume and increased renin secretion
	Serofibrinous pericarditis	?Uraemic toxins
	Myocardial oxalate deposition	Increased plasma oxalate concentrations
Lungs	Fibrinous pleurisy	?Uraemic toxins
	Pulmonary oedema with high protein concentration of oedema fluid. Marked tendency to organization of intra-alveolar fluid and formation of hyaline membranes in alveolar ducts	High central hydrostatic pressure and increased permeability of alveolar capillaries
	Intrapulmonary calcification	??
Gastrointestinal tract	Focal oedema and punctate haemorrhages in gut from oesophagus to colon. Bleeding leads to bacterial invasion and development of ulcers with necrotic bases.	?Uraemic toxins
	Increased risk of peptic ulceration	Increased gastrin secretion
Pancreas	Dilatation of acini, flattening of acinar epithelium and damming back of secretions with inspissation	?
	May have episodes of pancreatitis with pain, nausea and vomiting	?
Haemopoietic	Anaemia: usually normocytic and normochromic	Decline in renal production of erythropoietin
	Abnormal bleeding due to platelet dysfunction	?Uraemic toxins
Bone	Osteodystrophy: morphological picture is a combination of parathyroid bone disease and osteomalacia	Due to retention of phosphate and loss of calcium via tubules; also to impairment of formation of active form of vitamin D due to nephron loss
Joints	May have attacks of arthritis as a result of true gout or pseudogout	In true gout there is excess deposition of urate, in pseudogout excess deposition of pyrophosphate in the synovium
Nervous	May have encephalopathy associated with degeneration of neurones, myopathy affecting quadriceps and flexors of hip or shoulder girdle muscles, and peripheral neuropathy	?Uraemic toxins
Immunological	Decline in various T-cell functions	?Uraemic toxins
Skin	Curious pigmentation, itch and whitish deposit known as 'urea frost'	?

- **neoplasms**
- **glomerular disorders**
- **miscellaneous**

Each of these categories has many causes. It is well to remember, however, that in **more than 30% of patients with acute, and in a rather smaller percentage of those with chronic, tubulointerstitial disease, no cause can be identified.**

Clinical and Pathological Features

In the **acute** form onset is sudden and the pathological picture is characterized by:

- interstitial oedema
- an inflammatory infiltrate dominated by lymphocytes, plasma cells and macrophages, although neutrophils and eosinophils are often present.

The most common acute tubulointerstitial disorders are:

- acute bacterial pyelonephritis
- acute hypersensitivity nephritis induced by drugs

Chronic tubulointerstitial disease may cause no symptoms until late in its natural history; many affected individuals present for the first time with chronic renal failure.

The **pathological** picture is characterized by:

- interstitial fibrosis
- tubule atrophy
- an interstitial lymphocyte–macrophage infiltrate

Common causes of chronic tubulointerstitial disease include:

- chronic pyelonephritis
- analgesic nephropathy
- chronic potassium deficiency
- ischaemia

FUNCTIONAL EFFECTS OF TUBULOINTERSTITIAL DISEASE

This is best viewed against the background of the normal functions of the tubules (*Figs 36.29* and *36.30*). **Medullary function** is the chief physiological target, manifested as:

- **inability to concentrate the urine**, leading to polyuria and nocturia. The term **nephrogenic diabetes insipidus** is applied to this functional defect when it is very severe.
- **reduced ability to excrete hydrogen ions**, leading to **metabolic acidosis**
- **decrease in the tubular reabsorption of sodium and other solutes.** This 'salt-losing' nephropathy can lead to severe hyponatraemia with resulting hypotension and vascular collapse.

In **acute diffuse tubulointerstitial disease** the pathophysiological picture may be dominated by a **reduction in the glomerular filtration rate** accompanied by oliguria, proteinuria, haematuria and raised blood pressure.

The general pattern of tubular dysfunction is modified depending on where the damage is predominantly located. Principal targets are **the proximal tubule, the distal tubule and the medulla**.

Proximal tubule damage occurs in:

- heavy metal poisoning
- multiple myeloma

- paroxysmal nocturnal haemoglobinuria

It is characterized by **proximal tubular acidosis** in which there is:

- **loss of bicarbonate leading to acidaemia**
- **a reduction of extracellular volume**
- **a consequent stimulus for aldosterone production leading to potassium loss and hypokalaemia**

Distal tubule damage occurs in:

- methicillin nephritis
- hypercalcaemia
- chronic obstruction to urine outflow
- renal transplantation
- granulomatous inflammation
- Balkan nephropathy (an unusual form of chronic renal disease found near the River Danube in adjacent areas of Roumania, former Yugoslavia and Bulgaria. The cause is unknown).

The principal functional defect in these disorders is **distal tubular acidosis characterized by**:

1) a defect in hydrogen ion secretion such that the urine cannot be acidified maximally no matter how acidaemic the patient becomes

2) associated salt wasting, hyperkalaemia and decrease in the ability to concentrate the urine

Medullary damage occurs in:

- analgesic nephropathy
- acute pyelonephritis
- sickle cell disease
- hyperuricaemia
- hyperoxalaemia
- polycystic disease of the kidney
- sarcoidosis

The pathophysiological correlate of medullary damage is inability adequately to concentrate the urine.

Chemical Injury in Tubulointerstitial Disease

The kidney is particularly liable to suffer from chemical injury because of:

- the large blood supply of the metabolically active renal cortex
- increases in local levels of certain chemical species either because of increased absorption via the proximal tubules or as a result of concentration in the medulla
- precipitation of certain compounds, such as urates, at acid pH in the distal tubules. This may give rise to obstruction of the tubules.

Potentially damaging chemicals produce injury in a number of different ways:

1) by a **direct chemical effect** which may be severe and acute (e.g. mercuric chloride poisoning)

2) as a result of **hypersensitivity**

3) by mild, recurrent injury leading to a cumulative effect sufficient to cause chronic renal failure

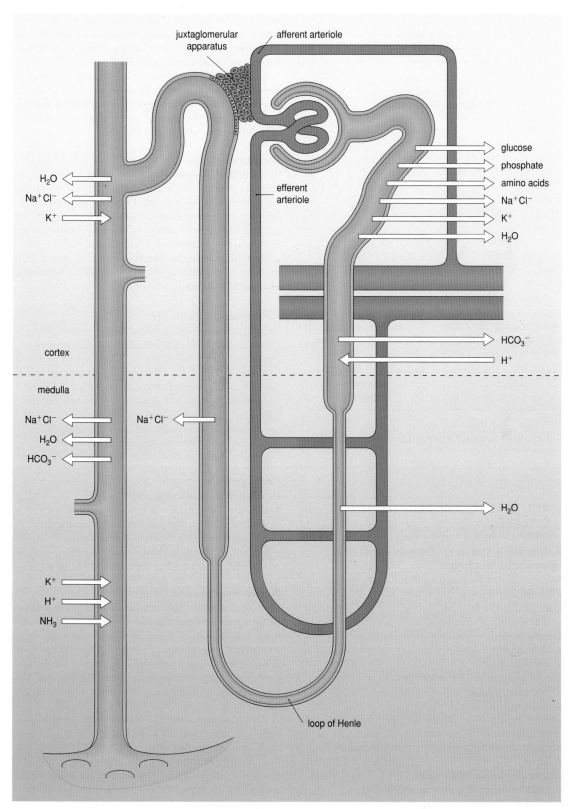

FIGURE 36.29 *Functions of different parts of the renal tubular system.*

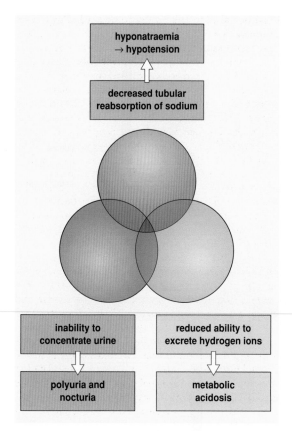

FIGURE 36.30 Functional effects of tubulointerstitial disease in general.

ACUTE TUBULOINTERSTITIAL DISEASE

Acute Drug-induced (Hypersensitivity) Interstitial Nephritis

Many drugs can cause acute interstitial nephritis:

- methicillin
- ampicillin
- rifampicin
- cephaloxin
- allopurinol
- phenytoin
- non-steroidal anti-inflammatory drugs
- ?thiazide diuretics
- ?frusemide

Patients present clinically, for the most part, with **acute renal failure** with or without oliguria. The acute decline in renal function is often accompanied by:

- **fever**
- **maculopapular skin rash**
- **high eosinophil count in the blood**
- **painful joints**

The existence of a latent period between starting the drug and the onset of renal dysfunction, together with lack of correlation between the drug dose and the risk of developing renal failure, suggests that an immunologically mediated mechanism is responsible.

Early recognition of renal involvement is important because most patients will recover quickly if the responsible drug is stopped. However, if renal damage is severe and prolonged, more than one-third of affected patients will require dialysis.

Diagnosis

The **clinical diagnosis** may be difficult because the clinical picture of acute drug-induced interstitial nephritis may be seen in other types of acute renal failure (e.g. tubular necrosis). Gallium scanning may be helpful; radioactive gallium is taken up avidly by the kidney in acute interstitial nephritis, and hardly at all in acute tubular necrosis. Absence of oliguria and a short duration of impairment of renal function are favourable prognostic indicators.

Microscopic Features

On light microscopy glomeruli appear normal. There may be a florid interstitial cell infiltrate consisting of lymphocytes, plasma cells, eosinophils and, less frequently, neutrophils. The distal tubules show evidence of focal epithelial cell necrosis, and hyaline droplet change in the renal tubular epithelium may be a prominent feature. Multinucleated epithelial cells are sometimes seen.

On electron microscopy fusion of epithelial cell foot processes may be seen in some glomeruli (10–20%).

Pathogenesis

Possible mechanisms include:

- the effect of anti-tubular basement membrane antibodies elicited by alteration of the normally non-immunogenic basement membrane
- a possible cell-mediated immune reaction
- a possible immunoglobulin E-mediated reaction

Acute Pyelonephritis

One of the most important and frequent causes of tubulointerstitial disease is infection of the urinary tract. This is normally sterile, although some commensal organisms may occur in the distal urethra. Women are far more susceptible to urinary tract infection than men (female : male ratio 20 : 1), and this epidemiological difference is probably anatomically based.

There are *two* routes by which pathogenic microorganisms may reach the kidney:

1) via the **bloodstream**
2) by **ascent** from the lower urinary tract

Bacterial infection of the kidney is most often ascending in type (*Fig. 36.31*). Successful colonization of the kidney requires a series of events that allows pathogenic organisms to:

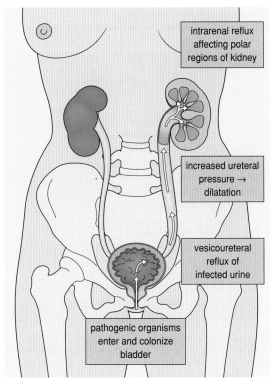

intrarenal reflux affecting polar regions of kidney

increased ureteral pressure → dilatation

vesicoureteral reflux of infected urine

pathogenic organisms enter and colonize bladder

FIGURE 36.31 *Pathogenetic events in ascending acute pyelonephritis.*

1) **gain entry to**
2) **survive in**
3) **multiply within**

the successive compartments of the urinary tract.

Factors involved in these events include the intrinsic properties of:

- the offending microorganisms
- the host (principally anatomical in nature)

Microorganisms in Acute Pyelonephritis

The offending organisms are derived from the lower part of the gastrointestinal tract and are part of the normal faecal flora. Thus, in most cases, acute pyelonephritis is an autoinfection.

The organism most commonly involved is *Escherichia coli*, although *Enterobacter*, *Proteus* species, *Klebsiella* species or *Staphylococcus albus* may be responsible. *Enterobacter* species and *Klebsiella* infections occur most frequently in neonates; *S. albus* is the responsible organism in many cases of acute pyelonephritis in adolescent girls.

Certain serotypes of *E. coli* **frequently cause urinary tract infections.** About 5% of the different serotypes cause about 75% of the infections. These successful strains:

- have a **short generation time** in the urine
- **resist the antibacterial properties** of urinary epithelium

- **adhere firmly to urinary tract epithelium.** This appears to be of especial importance in individuals with anatomically normal urinary tracts. Adhesion is achieved by binding of a molecule known as an **adhesin**, situated at the tip of certain types of fimbriae (stiff, proteinaceous, rod-like structures protruding from the bacterial surface). In strains of *E. coli* with the type called P fimbriae, **the adhesin recognizes a carbohydrate receptor on the urothelial cell surface**, which is related to the blood group P antigen system. In individuals with positive secretor status (i.e. they express blood group antigens of the A and B system on their cell surfaces), the adhesin receptors are obscured and the likelihood of *E. coli* infection is therefore reduced. Women especially prone to recurrent attacks of acute pyelonephritis are usually non-secretors of blood group antigens.

Organisms gain access to the bladder after first colonizing the perineum, vagina and urethra. Once within the urethra, the organisms are more likely to survive and multiply in **females** because they lack the **antibacterial action of prostatic secretions**.

The **entry** of bacteria to the **bladder** may be related to trauma (e.g. instrumentation, mild trauma as in so-called 'honeymoon cystitis') but is usually not related to any obvious event. **In females entry to the bladder is facilitated by their short urethra.**

Survival and **multiplication** of organisms within the bladder is favoured by:

- an increase in residual urine
- pregnancy, which is associated with a decrease in the tone of the detrusor muscle resulting from progesterone secretion
- diabetes mellitus (glycosuria favours bacterial growth)

Entry of organisms to the ureter is favoured by **vesicoureteric reflux**; this may result from the angle of insertion of the ureter into the bladder. This angle is normally steep and thus the distal portion of the ureter has a fairly long course within the bladder wall between the bladder mucosa and the muscularis. With contraction of the detrusor muscle during micturition, the resulting increase in wall pressure compresses and occludes the intravesical part of the ureter; this prevents reflux of urine into the ureter caused by a rise in intravesical pressure.

In some, the angle of insertion of the ureter is much less steep and the course of the distal ureter through the bladder wall is short. Thus, when intravesical pressure rises during micturition, urine refluxes into the ureter with considerable force. This increases the risk of acute pyelonephritis.

The ascent of organisms within the ureters is favoured by the antiperistaltic effects produced by the organisms, which are particularly marked in the case of Gram-negative bacteria.

Entry of organisms from the calyces to the

renal parenchyma is modulated partly by the anatomy of the renal papillae. The papillae related to the central calyces are convex, almost conical, in shape and do not readily admit refluxing urine. Those at the poles of the kidney, the so-called 'compound' papillae, are concave and admit refluxed urine much more readily.

Survival and multiplication of the organisms within the medulla, which is much more susceptible to infection than the cortex, is facilitated by the relatively poor blood supply (compared with that of the cortex) of the former. In addition, the fairly high concentrations of ammonia normally present in the medulla inhibit activation of C4 and thus interfere with the classical pathway of complement activation. The acute inflammatory response elicited by infection within the medulla is also much more sluggish than in other parts of the kidney.

Clinical Features

The commonest presenting syndrome is:

- lumbar pain and tenderness, the onset of which is usually sudden
- fever and rigors
- malaise

Diagnosis

This depends on isolating the responsible organism from the urine. It is important to be sure that such isolation represents urinary tract infection and not merely contamination of the specimen of urine.

If organisms are present in numbers greater than 10^5 per ml, then it is almost certain that the patient has a urinary tract infection. Where the bacterial count is less than this, about one-third of the patients will still have a renal infection.

Asymptomatic bacteriuria may occur in both children and adults. It is seen in about 1% of girls, who, although they have no symptoms referable to the bacteriuria, tend to have a higher frequency of renal

scarring in later life. Asymptomatic bacteriuria in adults seldom leads to significant kidney damage.

Macroscopic Features

The kidney is slightly enlarged and reddened, and there may be small abscesses on the subcapsular surface (*Fig. 36.32*). The cut surface shows yellowish streaks of pus in the medullary rays. If obstruction has been present, the pelvis and calyces may be dilated and there may be deformation of the renal papillae.

When small abscesses are diffusely distributed throughout the kidney, the origin of the acute pyelonephritis is more likely to have been a blood-borne infection, occurring as a result of infective endocarditis or septicaemia.

Microscopic Features

Sections show interstitial oedema and a florid intratubular and interstitial acute inflammatory cell infiltrate, which may be associated with some necrosis of tubular epithelium. In severe cases there may be some necrosis of the tips of the papillae (see section on papillary necrosis).

A rare variant is emphysematous pyelonephritis in which there is frank necrosis of the kidney tissue, accompanied by gas formation. This type is most commonly seen in elderly, diabetic women.

CHRONIC TUBULOINTERSTITIAL DISEASE

Chronic Pyelonephritis

Chronic pyelonephritis is common, accounting for 15% of adults requiring dialysis and/or renal transplantation and 25% of children and young adults. It is best defined in morphological terms because its aetiology and pathogenesis are still matters of debate.

Definition

A chronic disorder characterized by coarse asymmetric scarring affecting principally the renal pelves, tubules and interstitium. **The scars overlie dilated calyces with distorted pyramids** (*Figs 36.33* and *36.34*). This association of calyceal deformity with scarring of the area of the parenchyma drained by the affected pyramid is important in establishing the diagnosis, because other conditions giving rise to coarse parenchymal scarring show microscopic features difficult to distinguish from those of chronic pyelonephritis.

Role of Infection in Chronic Pyelonephritis

Whether infection of the urinary tract is **necessary** for the development of chronic pyelonephritis is not entirely clear. Certainly patients who have had many, well-documented, recurrent episodes of urinary tract

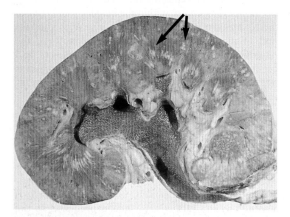

FIGURE 36.32 Acute ascending pyelonephritis. Note the reddening of the pelvis and calyces and the numerous small subcortical abscesses (arrow).

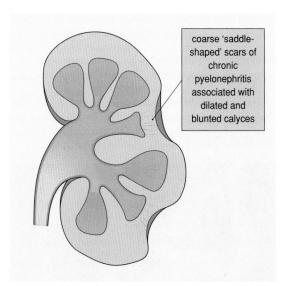

coarse 'saddle-shaped' scars of chronic pyelonephritis associated with dilated and blunted calyces

FIGURE 36.33 Morphological features of chronic pyelonephritis. Note the relationship of the saddle-shaped scars with distortion of the calyces.

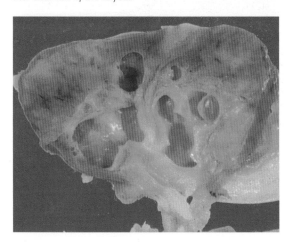

FIGURE 36.34 Chronic pyelonephritis showing marked distortion of the calyceal system and scarring, which has caused blurring of the corticomedullary junction.

infection need not develop pyelonephritic scarring; similarly, some patients develop chronic pyelonephritis in the absence of a history of urinary tract infection and in the absence of bacteriuria.

Kidney tissue from patients with chronic pyelonephritis seldom shows pathogenic microorganisms. However, in some studies, immunohistological methods have identified **bacterial antigens** in apparently sterile pyelonephritic scars.

Failure to culture organisms from pyelonephritic kidneys may well be due to their absence from the affected tissue, but it is possible that another explanation exists: the bacteria responsible for the inflammatory reaction may have lost their capsules and become trans-

formed into **protoplasts or L forms**. Such variants can reproduce themselves by budding and are antibiotic resistant.

Mechanical Factors in the Pathogenesis of Chronic Pyelonephritis

Obstruction

Obstruction to urinary outflow is associated, in some instances, with chronic pyelonephritis; the production of experimental unilateral ureteral obstruction in animals causes **intravenously** injected microorganisms to localize within the kidney with impaired urine drainage.

In chronic pyelonephritis associated with obstruction, the ureter and pelvis are dilated and the high pressure resulting from obstruction within the system usually affects all the calyces.

Vesicoureteric Reflux

Vesicoureteric reflux of urine, in both humans and animal experiments, is associated with the development of pyelonephritic scars, and is probably the most important pathogenetic factor in human chronic pyelonephritis. Such scars are situated for the most part at the poles of the kidneys. This localization of the lesions appears to be due to the nature of the papillae:

- The central papillae are simple conical structures with slit-like orifices through which reflux of urine does not occur readily unless intracalyceal pressures are very high, as is the case in obstruction.
- At the poles of the kidney, however, some of the papillae have a flat, concave, or even deeply indented, surface and their orifices are wide open. It has been suggested that **intrarenal** reflux of urine with possible entry of pathogenic microorganisms into the renal parenchyma occurs via such papillae, and that this accounts for the polar localization of pyelonephritic scars.

Vesicoureteric reflux in childhood may well lay the foundations of future chronic pyelonephritis. Improvement and gradual disappearance of reflux in later childhood or adolescence has been well documented and thus it is possible that adults may present with clinical features of chronic pyelonephritis largely due to reflux, and yet show no evidence of reflux at the time of presentation.

Macroscopic Features

Appearances differ depending on whether obstruction has been present or not. In the former case, especially where both infection and high intracalyceal pressures have been present, there is **dilatation of the renal pelvis** and **many or all of the calyces are deformed and dilated**. Frequently both kidneys are involved, although in an asymmetrical fashion. Coarse, often rather flat, scars alternate with areas of grossly normal kidney. It used to be said that the scars of chronic pyelonephritis are U-shaped whereas those due to ischaemia are V-shaped, but this is a gross oversimplification and the character of the scars is not a reliable diagnostic criterion. What is valuable is the invariable relationship between a parenchymal scar and an underlying dilated calyx with a deformed pyramid.

If vesicoureteric reflux has been present, the scars, as already stated, tend to be polar in distribution.

Microscopic Features
The macroscopic features are mirrored in the histological appearances, where areas of normal parenchyma may be juxtaposed with grossly abnormal ones.

The primary target is the tubulointerstitial compartment. Interstitial tissue is increased in amount and obviously scarred, and there is a patchy infiltrate of lymphocytes and plasma cells. The tubules may be either collapsed and atrophic with abnormally thick basement membranes (the most common picture) or greatly distended by featureless eosinophilic material and lined by flattened epithelium. This appearance is often referred to as 'thyroidization' because of the superficial resemblance of these tubules to thyroid acini filled with colloid.

The glomeruli present variable appearances. In some areas they appear quite normal, whereas in others periglomerular fibrosis (concentric layers of fibrous tissue laid down outside Bowman's capsule) is a prominent feature.

The medulla and, in particular, the pyramids show areas of scarring surrounded by atrophic collecting tubules. The pelvic epithelium may be normal but there may also be subepithelial oedema associated with dilatation of small blood vessels and a chronic inflammatory cell infiltrate.

Where the disease is due to obstruction, areas of squamous metaplasia of the transitional epithelium of the pelvis and ulceration of the epithelium may be seen.

Changes in the renal blood vessels are frequent but inconstant. In some instances the arcuate and interlobular arteries may show quite severe intimal fibrosis leading to narrowing of their lumina, whereas in others the vessels appear quite normal.

A serious complication may arise once extensive damage has occurred, in the form of focal segmental glomerulosclerosis in the surviving renal parenchyma. The pathogenesis is not completely understood but it has been suggested that this may be due to hyperfiltration damage to the surviving glomeruli.

Variants of Chronic Pyelonephritis

Xanthogranulomatous Pyelonephritis
This descriptive name is derived from Greek (*xanthos* yellow) and is so called because of the accumulation of many lipid-laden macrophages within the interstitial

tissue. These are present in such profusion that yellow areas on the cut surface of the affected kidney may be seen with the naked eye. This occurs most often in association with obstruction to the urinary tract; such obstruction is due, in most instances, to a stone in the renal pelvis or ureter (*Fig. 36.35*).

This rare condition is usually unilateral and, although the basic pathology is inflammatory destruction of the renal parenchyma, the lipid-laden macrophage infiltration may extend outwards into the perirenal fat.

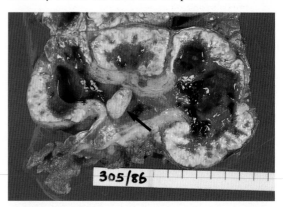

FIGURE 36.35 *Xanthogranulomatous pyelonephritis. Note the calculus at the pelviureteric junction (arrow). The calyces are grossly dilated and reddened, and the renal tissue is yellow due to the presence of large numbers of lipid-laden macrophages in the interstitial tissue.*

Renal Botryomycosis
This describes a condition in which chronic, suppurative, bacterial infection is associated with pus in which granules composed of masses of bacteria can be seen with the naked eye. These granules resemble somewhat those seen in actinomycosis. The organism most commonly, but by no means exclusively, involved is *Staphylococcus aureus*.

RENAL PAPILLARY NECROSIS

Necrosis of the renal papillae occurs most commonly under one of four sets of circumstances:
   1) **chronic analgesic abuse**
   2) **acute pyogenic infection of the urinary tract, often associated with diabetes mellitus**
   3) **hypotensive shock, especially in the neonate**
   4) **sickle cell disease**

Chronic Analgesic-related Nephropathy
Chronic overconsumption of analgesics can produce necrosis of the renal papillae without any accompanying inflammatory reaction at the junction between viable kidney and the necrotic papilla.

This disorder may well have been underdiagnosed in

the past. In former West Germany, for example, 16.8% of patients with end-stage renal disease had analgesic-associated nephropathy, and in Australia, until the 1980s when analgesic mixtures were made 'prescription-only' drugs, analgesic abuse has been estimated to cause 20–25% of cases of end-stage renal failure.

Women are more often affected by analgesic-associated nephropathy than men (F:M ratio 4 : 1); the peak incidence is in the fifth decade. These patients may have had one or other of a number of 'chronic pain' syndromes; peptic ulcer and low back pain are among the most common triggers for daily consumption of analgesics.

The resulting defects in renal function relate especially to the **medulla** and **patients show deficits related to urinary concentration, urinary acidification and sodium conservation**. These may lead to **metabolic acidosis** and **volume depletion**, aggravated during periods of hot weather or fluid deprivation. On the other hand, many cases have been reported from countries such as Switzerland, Finland and Sweden suggesting that climatic conditions constitute only a supplementary factor in the pathogenesis of this condition.

What Drugs are Responsible and in What Amounts?

The strongest relationship has been with analgesic mixtures containing phenacetin, which has now been withdrawn from the market. Aspirin by itself has, in some experimental studies, been reported to cause papillary necrosis, and necropsy studies have shown an increased frequency of papillary necrosis and interstitial nephritis in patients with rheumatoid disease who consume aspirin and other non-steroidal anti-inflammatory drugs over a long period.

Acetaminophen, the major metabolite of phenacetin, has replaced phenacetin in many combination analgesic preparations and a recent study from the USA suggests that there is an increased risk of developing chronic renal disease in daily users of these compounds.

Fairly large cumulative doses of analgesics seem to be needed for renal papillary necrosis to occur. A large German study of more than 500 cases of end-stage renal disease revealed a dose-dependent increase in risk with the cumulative use of more than 1 kg of analgesic mixture, although others have suggested that the minimal requirement is 2–3 kg taken over a period of 3 years.

Pathogenesis

The biochemical mechanisms mediating analgesic-related papillary necrosis are not clear. Phenacetin is metabolized in the liver with the formation of acetaminophen, which accumulates in the renal medulla especially during antidiuresis.

Acetaminophen can either be:

- conjugated to a non-toxic form

- co-oxidized with arachidonic acid by cyclo-oxygenase and prostaglandin hydroperoxidase in the inner part of the renal medulla. When acetaminophen is present in high concentrations, this second pathway is emphasized.

The reactive intermediate products yielded by these reactions can bind to macromolecules within tubular epithelial cells and produce cell damage. This effect is augmented if intracellular reduced glutathione (GSH) is decreased (which can happen as a result of salicylate administration). Salicylates also inhibit the formation of prostaglandins and this tends to decrease the flow of blood to the inner medulla and thus increases the risk of tissue damage. Caffeine, because of its action as an adenosine antagonist, may increase transport-associated respiratory activity in the thick ascending limb of the loop of Henle and thus, by stimulating cell activity in the face of relative hypoxia, may also play some part in the pathogenesis of analgesic-related nephropathy.

Macroscopic Features

The kidneys are bilaterally and equally contracted, being reduced in weight to 45–65 g each. The subcapsular surfaces are usually scarred, the scars being related to necrotic papillae. The papillae themselves show a spectrum of abnormality ranging from normal or near normal, through minute areas of necrosis near the tip of the pyramid, pallor, shrinkage associated with brown discoloration, to partial or complete detachment of the necrotic papillae.

Microscopic Features

The earliest lesions are found adjacent to the tip of the papilla and in the loops of Henle, where foci of necrotic epithelial cells can be seen. Evidence of epithelial cell regeneration is also present.

The necrosis in the loops of Henle then becomes more pronounced and extensive. Many tubules appear as 'ghost' outlines and there may be necrosis in the endothelium of adjacent capillaries. The extreme tip of the pyramid often remains viable because its blood supply remains separate from that of the rest of the papilla via vessels derived from the minor calyces. The necrotic papillary tissue fails to elicit any acute inflammatory reaction at the boundary zone between viable and non-viable tissue, and this is a useful distinguishing feature from the papillary necrosis that may occur in diabetics with acute pyogenic infections of the upper urinary tract.

In the late stages, a clear demarcation zone may be seen between viable and non-viable tissue, and focal areas of dystrophic calcification may be present. When sloughing and detachment of the papilla have taken place, the edges of the calyx appear ragged and the tissue proximal to this is scarred and shows a chronic inflammatory reaction in the interstitium.

Renal Papillary Necrosis Complicating Acute Urinary Tract Infections and Diabetes Mellitus

Urinary tract infections are common in diabetics, and especially, although not exclusively, in patients suffering from some degree of obstruction to urine outflow, papillary necrosis is a fairly common complication. In most cases both kidneys are affected and the condition is often fatal.

In these fatal cases the kidneys show markedly inflamed pelves which may be filled with purulent debris. Abscesses may be present both in the medulla and cortex, and some or all of the papillae are frankly necrotic. As with analgesic-related disease, detachment of the necrotic papillae may take place, leaving a ragged edge to the affected calyx.

Microscopic examination may show complete necrosis, although the 'ghost' outlines of collecting tubules may still be seen. Unlike what is seen in analgesic-related nephropathy, there is a brisk acute inflammatory cell infiltrate in the demarcation zone and the tubules in the adjacent viable tissue may contain pus cells. The diagnosis of acute papillary necrosis may sometimes be made during life in those cases in which papillae are passed in the patient's urine.

Pathogenesis

The mechanism of papillary necrosis under these circumstances is largely obscure. The relatively poor blood supply of the medulla may be further compromised in the face of diabetic microvascular disease. The importance of papillary underperfusion is emphasized by the fact that papillary necrosis can occur purely as a result of hypotension and shock. The upper urinary tract infection so often found in acute papillary necrosis, coupled with relative ischaemia and poor local tissue defences, probably accounts for most of the cases.

Acute Renal Papillary Necrosis in Infancy

This occurs, fortunately only rarely, in infants with shock secondary to severe dehydration following gastroenteritis. This form of papillary necrosis may give rise to subsequent deformities of the renal parenchyma associated with maldevelopment, and the resulting scarring may be difficult to distinguish from that of chronic pyelonephritis.

Sickle Cell Disease

Papillary necrosis is not an uncommon complication of sickle cell disease. In one study 65% of patients with clinical evidence of sickle cell disease showed urographic changes suggestive of papillary necrosis, although by no means all the patients had urinary tract symptoms.

It has been suggested that the renal medulla is a favourable environment in which 'sickling' of red cells can occur, because its osmolality is high and pH relatively low. These factors lead to:

- an increase in blood viscosity
- an increased risk of microthrombus formation in the vasa recta
- ischaemic damage to the papilla

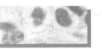

Acute Renal Failure

Acute renal failure is loosely defined as a syndrome characterized by a significant decline in renal function over a period of hours or days. Unlike chronic renal failure, where there is irreversible damage to many nephrons, acute renal failure has a significant functional component and a chance of recovery that in otherwise healthy individuals may be substantial.

Acute renal failure is usually classified under three main rubrics:

1) **prerenal**
2) **renal**
3) **postrenal**, which effectively equates with acute obstruction to urinary outflow

PRERENAL CAUSES OF ACUTE RENAL FAILURE

In functional terms the causes classified under this heading are those resulting in **underperfusion of the kidney**. This may occur if there is:

1) **Pump failure**, as in cardiogenic shock after a myocardial infarction
2) **A decrease in circulatory volume**, which can occur as a result of:
- blood loss
- plasma loss (as in patients with extensive burns)
- loss of salt and water, as in patients with severe diarrhoea or vomiting
3) **Microvascular dilatation and damage**, as seen in septicaemic shock

These causes of underperfusion can be modulated by vasoactive substances that alter renal blood flow and, in particular, glomerular blood flow by acting on the afferent or efferent arterioles (see *Table 36.11*).

Renal function in these patients, if they are treated promptly and appropriately, improves rapidly after renal perfusion is normalized, and many regard this sequence of events as a defining criterion of prerenal acute renal failure.

Anuria or oliguria are characteristic during the acute phase and **urine** examination shows a combination of:
- low sodium concentrations (less than 20 mmol/l)
- high osmolality (urine : plasma osmolality greater than 1.5 : 1)
- high urea and creatinine concentrations (urine : plasma urea concentration greater than 10 : 1)

There is a considerable degree of overlap between this

Table 36.11 Vasoactive Substances Acting on the Kidney

Vasoconstrictors	Vasodilators
Angiotensin II	Prostaglandins E_2 and I_2
Catecholamines	Atrial natriuretic peptide
Vasopressin	Bradykinin
Signals from nerves	Glucagon
Thromboxanes	Vasoactive intestinal
Leukotrienes	peptide
Adenosine	

renal underperfusion syndrome and a more severe form of acute renal failure, classified under 'renal' causes, which has the – not altogether accurate – name of acute tubular necrosis.

RENAL CAUSES OF ACUTE RENAL FAILURE

Acute renal failure due to pathological changes within the kidney may be associated with **acute tubular necrosis**. This, the commonest form of 'renal' acute renal failure, has **two** pathogenetic bases:

1) **Ischaemia**, which is associated with the factors outlined for prerenal failure with, in addition, extensive, crushing trauma to soft tissues especially muscle.

2) **Toxic damage** to renal tubules. This may occur in:
- heavy metal poisoning
- organic solvent poisoning
- antibiotic-mediated damage (both polyene and aminoglycoside antibiotics)
- snake venoms
- tubular deposition of Bence–Jones proteins

Other renal causes of acute renal failure are shown in *Table 36.12*.

The natural history and the urinary findings show some important differences from those of prerenal acute renal failure. These include:
- Reversing the underperfused state of the kidney (e.g. by correcting hypovolaemia) does not improve renal function rapidly as it does in the prerenal type.
- In civilian practice, acute tubular necrosis most commonly occurs against a background of an established illness. In war, trauma is usually sufficiently severe as to cause acute renal failure in previously healthy individals. Thus, surgical complications are responsible for about 50% of cases, extensive traumatic or atraumatic destruction of muscle for a further 25%, obstetric disorders, such as severe postpartum haemorrhage or sepsis following abortion, for about 5%, and miscellaneous disorders including intravascular haemolysis for 5%.
- The findings in the urine suggest tubular dysfunction.

KEY POINTS: Acute Tubular Necrosis
- Acute tubular necrosis is not associated with anuria; in some cases, polyuria may be present.
- Sodium reabsorption is impaired and the urine sodium concentration is therefore high (greater than 40 mmol/l).
- Urine concentration is decreased, the osmolality of the urine approximating to that of plasma (urine : plasma osmolality less than 1.1 : 1).
- Numerous granular and cellular casts are present, as may be isolated epithelial cells.

Macroscopic Features
In fatal cases of acute tubular necrosis, the kidneys are enlarged and somewhat swollen. As one cuts through the capsule and into the cortex, the latter bulges slightly. The

Table 36.12 Renal Causes of Acute Renal Failure, other than Acute Tubular Necrosis

Anatomical target	Disorder
Blood vessels within the kidney	Persisting intrarenal vasoconstriction
	Occlusion of renal artery
	Microvascular disorders such as thrombotic thrombocytopenic purpura
	Malignant hypertension
	Bilateral cortical necrosis associated with separation of the placenta
Glomeruli	Various forms of glomerulonephritis, especially crescentic types
Interstitium	Acute interstitial nephritis of various types
Tubular lumen	Crystal deposition (e.g. oxalates, sulphonamides)

cut surface usually shows a marked degree of cortical pallor, contrasting strikingly with the much darker medulla (*Fig. 36.36*).

Microscopic Features

The main changes are seen in the renal tubules, most particularly in the distal convoluted tubules (*Fig. 36.37*). Despite the name – acute tubular necrosis – evidence of such necrosis may be inconspicuous. Once focal necrosis of epithelial cells occurs, the affected cells tend to separate from the underlying basement membrane, leaving small segments of tubular basement membrane which are 'bare'. In a very small proportion of cases (about 5%), there are breaks in the tubular basement membrane itself (**tubulorrhexis**) and these basement membrane lesions may be associated either with local inflammation or with the formation of communications between the affected tubule and the peritubular venules.

Casts of various types are commonly seen in the affected distal tubule. In the case of crush injury involving muscle, they are composed of myoglobin; in cases of acute tubular necrosis due to intravascular haemolysis (e.g. in incompatible blood transfusion), the principal component is haemoglobin.

In some instances the presence of tubular epithelial necrosis must be **inferred** from changes characteristic of **regeneration**. The affected tubules show epithelial flattening, and basophilia and occasional mitoses are present. All these regenerative changes are more common in the distal tubules but one interesting morphological change is often seen in the proximal tubule: thinning or loss of the brush border of epithelial cells. This presumably also reflects regeneration, with imperfect formation of tubular epithelial microvilli.

Light microscopic examination probably leads to underestimation of the extent and severity of tubular lesions in acute tubular necrosis because of the sampling error involved. In fatal cases, complete nephrons can be dissected out and these show the presence of lesions patchily distributed along the course of the tubular part of the nephron.

Secondary effects are seen in the glomeruli and interstitium. While the glomerular capillary tufts appear normal, there is often swelling of the epithelial cells lining Bowman's capsule and the juxtaglomerular apparatus quite often appears to be hyperplastic. The interstitium is oedematous and contains a moderate mixed inflammatory cell infiltrate.

Pathogenesis

There is clearly an ischaemic background to the majority of cases of acute tubular necrosis (other than those caused by drugs and poisons), but the complex interrelated mechanisms causing both lesions and clinical disturbances are still not understood. Mechanisms additional to the ischaemia, which have been suggested, include:

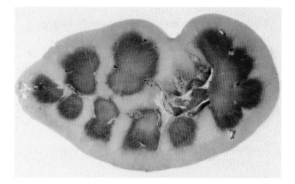

FIGURE 36.36 Acute tubular necrosis. Note the extreme pallor of the cortex and how it contrasts with the much darker medulla.

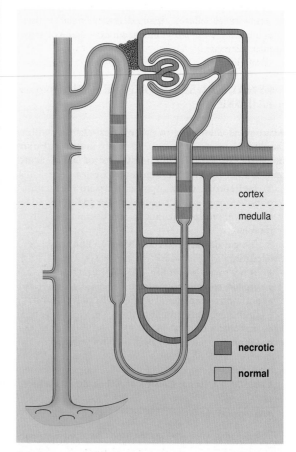

cortex
medulla

■ necrotic
□ normal

FIGURE 36.37 Location of tubular lesions in ischaemic tubular damage.

- **prolonged vasoconstriction of intrarenal vessels, especially afferent arterioles.** This would cause diminished glomerular filtration and, thus, oliguria. Renal blood flow is certainly decreased both in human acute tubular necrosis and ischaemic animal models, and there is a marked rise in plasma renin concentrations during the acute phase and a fall in the recovery phase. This suggests that the level of angiotensin II may be increased during the acute phase and may be responsible for intrarenal vasoconstriction.

- **leakage of tubular fluid across the tubular basement membrane.** In animal models of ischaemic acute tubular necrosis, only about half the inulin injected into the proximal tubule is recovered in the urine.
- **obstruction of the tubules by casts** made up partly of necrotic cells and partly of precipitated protein
- **secondary changes in glomerular flow.** These might occur if there is inadequate tubular reabsorption of sodium and chloride in the proximal tubule. This increased concentration is sensed by the macula densa, causing increased production and release of renin. This sequence of events has been called **tubuloglomerular feedback**.

It seems likely that inappropriate constriction of intrarenal vessels is the strongest candidate, but absolute proof is lacking.

Acute Tubular Necrosis due to Drugs and Poisons

Many ingested, inhaled and cutaneously absorbed drugs and chemicals have been reported as causing acute tubular necrosis, for example aminoglycosides such as gentamicin, amphotericin B, methoxyflurane, ethylene glycol (antifreeze) and mercury.

The striking difference between this form of acute tubular necrosis and that associated with ischaemia is the fact that the necrosis of tubular epithelium is both obvious and widespread on light microscopic examination. Tubulorrhexis is not seen and the proximal tubule is the principal target in most instances (*Fig. 36.38*). Within the proximal tubule certain segments appear to be particularly affected by certain kidney toxins. For example, mercuric chloride affects the straight and convoluted parts of the proximal tubule. The severity of the tubular lesions correlates with the dose of noxious agent.

Systemic Hypertension

In any given population, systemic blood pressure has a unimodal distribution curve, somewhat skewed to the right. Thus, the distinction between high blood pressure (hypertension) and normal blood pressure is more or less arbitrary. There is no doubt, however, that within the curve of distribution there is a direct correlation between the magnitude of the blood pressure and

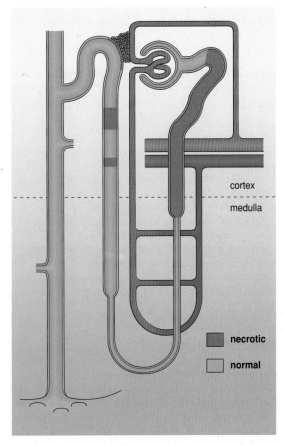

FIGURE 36.38 *Location of tubular lesions in toxic tubular damage.*

the risk of death or disability from cardiovascular disease, most particularly:

- stroke
- coronary heart disease and other atherosclerosis-related syndromes
- left ventricular cardiac failure
- renal failure (in patients with accelerated or malignant phase of hypertension)

Despite this continuum of risk, some arbitrary distinctions are necessary to enable decisions to be taken as to whether to treat individuals with blood pressure-lowering drugs or not. The World Health Organization (WHO) suggests the pressures shown in *Table 36.13*.

If the borderline level is used to categorize individuals as hypertensive, about 25% of the population would fall into this bracket. If the higher WHO level is used as the breakpoint, about 18% of the adult population would be regarded as being hypertensive. These values have important implications in relation to the blood pressure levels at which decisions to treat should be made. Females are more at risk than males, and Afro-Caribbeans more so than Caucasians.

Table 36.13 WHO Levels for Hypertension

	Hypertension	Borderline hypertension
Systolic pressure	160 mmHg or more	140–160 mmHg
Diastolic pressure	95 mmHg or more	90–95 mmHg

Classification

Systemic hypertension is classified under *two* major rubrics:

- **Essential hypertension** (95% of cases), in which the mechanisms are ill understood and are probably multiple.
- **Secondary hypertension** (5% of all cases), in which the increase in blood pressure is due to some recognizable disease state such as chronic renal parenchymal disease, renal vascular disease or an aldosterone-secreting adrenal tumour.

Despite the relatively small chances of an individual patient having one of the secondary forms of hypertension, it is worth excluding these (*Table 36.14*), especially as some are curable.

Essential Hypertension

Aetiology and Pathogenesis

Arterial blood pressure is the product of **cardiac output** and **peripheral vascular resistance**; blood pressure will rise if either of these is increased. There is evidence that both these factors are involved in the pathogenesis of the sustained increase in blood pressure in essential hypertension:

- Cardiac output will increase if there is an increase in fluid volume.

- Fluid volume will increase if there is decreased sodium excretion via the kidney.

In the early stages of essential hypertension in some patients and in rats that have been made hypertensive by removal of one kidney and partially occluding the renal artery on the other side, there is an increase in cardiac output. Once the high blood pressure is established in both humans and rats, the cardiac output becomes normal. **Thus the maintenance of raised blood pressure must be due to increased tone in the resistance vessels of the arterial tree – the small arteries and arterioles, the smallest vessels with smooth muscle cells in their walls.**

Increased Tone in Peripheral Vessels

Epidemiological Considerations

There is still no complete explanation as to why the peripheral resistance vessels increase their tone in hypertensives. Any explanation must take account of certain epidemiological facts:

- **The prevalence of essential hypertension correlates positively with the dietary intake of sodium.** Experiments with animals have also shown that hypertension can be induced in a number of species by a high salt intake.

Table 36.14 Causes of Secondary Hypertension

Organ involved	Diseases
Kidney	Parenchymal diseases affecting either glomeruli or tubules and interstitium; chronic glomerulonephritis, chronic pyelonephritis Disorders affecting large or small vessels of renal vasculature (see also section on vasculitides, pp 396–410)
Adrenal	Cortex: aldosterone-secreting adenoma (Conn's syndrome); cortisol-secreting adenoma or carcinoma (Cushing's syndrome); congenital adrenal hyperplasia Medulla: phaeochromocytoma
Other endocrine organs	Pituitary: acromegaly Thyroid: thyrotoxicosis Parathyroid: hyperparathyroidism
Other diseases or lifestyle factors	Renin-secreting tumour Pre-eclampsia and eclampsia Excessive alcohol intake

- A normal kidney exposed to high arterial pressure responds by excreting extra sodium and water. **This relationship between pressure and natriuresis seems to be reset in hypertensive patients** as a result of increased resistance in the efferent arterioles of the glomeruli. This results in an inappropriately high plasma volume for the particular level of blood pressure.

Mechanisms for Increased Tone

Genetic factors play a part in the variations in susceptibility to a high salt intake. This susceptibility appears to be related to a renal factor and can be transferred between animals by renal transplantation. The suggestion that nature as well as nurture plays a part in the genesis of hypertension is supported by the marked racial differences that exist in relation to the risk of hypertension in adult populations.

So far as the resistance vessels themselves are concerned, a number of possible abnormalities have been canvassed as being related to the increased tone:

- **Abnormalities of sodium and potassium transport across cell membranes.** This can result in an increased calcium content within cells. In vascular smooth muscle cells, increased calcium levels lead to an increase in tone of up to 50%. Some support for this view comes from the fact that compounds that block the entry of calcium into cells via the slow calcium channel are very effective in lowering high blood pressure.
- **An increase in vasoconstrictor signals.** These may be derived from without or within the vessel walls. For example, activity of the sympathetic nervous system could modify vascular tone by:
  1) acting upon the juxtaglomerular apparatus to cause the secretion of more renin. About 15% of patients with essential hypertension have raised plasma concentrations of renin and it seems unlikely that the renin–angiotensin system is an important factor in the genesis of essential hypertension.
  2) having a direct vasoconstrictor effect on the resistance vessels.
- Vasoconstriction could occur also as a result of the **release of compounds synthesized within the vessel wall, such as endothelins, or a decrease in the synthesis and release of nitric oxide.**

Thus the aetiology and pathogenesis of essential hypertension are still far from clear. Currently, it seems that **a combination of genetic factors and high salt intake are the most important factors.**

Natural History

In addition to the aetiological classification which divides hypertension into essential and secondary types, **hypertension may also be classified on the basis of its natural history into benign and malignant** forms.

Benign hypertension is associated with a long clinical course and, certainly in its early stages, with little clinical effect. In contrast, **malignant hypertension is characterized by a rapidly rising blood pressure** with severe effects on the vascular system and kidneys. When no effective treatment for high blood pressure existed, the onset of the malignant phase of hypertension was frequently followed by death within a year. Fortunately this form of hypertension is relatively uncommon (about 5% of patients with raised blood pressure). It tends to occur more commonly in the young, in males and in Afro-Caribbeans.

Patients with malignant hypertension have a very high diastolic pressure (greater than 130 mmHg) and renal failure was the commonest (90%) cause of death in these patients. The malignant phase of hypertension is also associated with increases in intracranial pressure and the clinical presentation may be related to this. Thus, patients may complain of:

- headache
- nausea and vomiting
- visual disturbances
- rarely there may be fits and disturbances of consciousness ('hypertensive encephalopathy')

The correlate of these symptoms, on clinical examination, is papilloedema and small retinal haemorrhages.

Pathological Features

The increased pressure within the systemic arterial circulation exerts powerful effects on the heart, arteries and arterioles.

The Heart

> **KEY POINTS: Effects on the Heart**
> The principal effects on the heart are:
> - **left ventricular hypertrophy of high pressure overload type**
> - **decreased diastolic compliance of left ventricle**
> - **greater thickness of left ventricular wall leading to decreased perfusion of subendocardial region of the myocardium**

Left Ventricular Hypertrophy

Increased resistance in the arterial systemic arterial bed leads to an increased workload on the left ventricle. This is of the high pressure type and is characterized by the development of a **concentric form of hypertrophy in the presence of a normal or slightly small left ventricular cavity.** Although this is the general cardiac response to hypertension, a considerable degree of variation exists and there is no linear relationship between the magnitude of the blood pressure and the degree of increase in left ventricular muscle mass. If the increased pressure is not reduced by treatment, the ultimate result is left ventricular failure.

The functional effects of the hypertrophy itself are:

- a decrease in left ventricular diastolic compliance as a result of the increased stiffness of the ventricle wall. This leads to suboptimal filling of the left ventricle during diastole.
- decreased perfusion of the subendocardial region of the myocardium during diastole and thus a greater liability to subendocardial ischaemia.

The Arteries

> ### KEY POINTS: Effects on the Arteries
> The chief effects on arteries are:
> - **increased atherogenesis and increased risk of coronary heart disease**
> - **decreased arterial compliance**
> - **increased shearing stresses leading to increased risk of aortic dissection**
> - **microaneurysm formation in small penetrating arteries within the brain (Charcot–Bouchard aneurysms)**

Increased Atherogenesis

In large elastic and muscular arteries, the chief effect of hypertension is to increase and accelerate atherogenesis. In most populations studied, the presence of systemic hypertension is associated with a greater extent and severity of involvement of these vessels by mature fibrolipid plaques (see p 338).

In Western countries, where there is a high background level of both atherosclerosis and ischaemic heart disease, hypertension is a potent incremental factor and many more hypertensive patients die with one of the manifestations of myocardial ischaemia than with left ventricular failure secondary to the long continued presence of raised blood pressure.

Loss of Arterial Compliance and Increased Risk of Aortic Dissection

In the arterial media, the principal effect of hypertension is smooth muscle cell hypertrophy, which is most evident in the small resistance vessels. In due time, some of this smooth muscle is replaced by fibrous tissue and the affected artery tends to dilate; the dilatation is accompanied by loss of arterial compliance.

High arterial blood pressure is associated with high shearing stresses on the arterial intima and superficial part of the media, and this explains the increased risk of aortic dissection that is associated with high blood pressure. In small intrarenal arteries such as the interlobular arteries, some intimal thickening is noted, associated with reduplication of the internal elastic laminae.

Microaneurysm Formation

In the cerebral circulation, hypertension is one of the most potent factors in the formation of small aneurysms of the penetrating arteries of the brain. These are known as Charcot–Bouchard aneurysms (see p 1149). They are multiple and increase in number both with age and with degree of hypertension. Rupture of these aneurysms is the cause of hypertensive intracerebral haemorrhage. In patients who have congenital aneurysms affecting the arteries of the circle of Willis, hypertension is a potent risk factor for rupture leading to subarachnoid haemorrhage.

Arterioles

> ### KEY POINTS: Effects on Arterioles
> The chief effects on these small resistance vessels are:
> - hyaline arteriolosclerosis
> - fibrinoid necrosis (in patients with malignant hypertension)

Hyaline Arteriolosclerosis

Arteriolosclerosis is the term applied to thickening of the arteriolar walls with replacement of smooth muscle cells by rather featureless, eosinophilic material ('hyaline') (*Fig. 36.39*). On light microscopy, this hyaline change resembles that seen in diabetes mellitus and amyloidosis.

In benign hypertension and diabetes mellitus, immunohistological examination shows the presence of plasma proteins, most notably fibrinogen and low density lipoprotein, in this hyaline material. It has, therefore, been suggested that hyaline change is due, in part, to **an increase in the inflow of plasma across the arteriolar wall** and **an accumulation within the arteriolar wall of these high molecular weight proteins**. The term 'plasmatic vasculosis' has been coined to cover these twin processes.

In certain vascular beds, hyaline arteriolosclerosis is a normal accompaniment of ageing. The best example of this is the spleen, in which about 90% of the arterioles that lie in the malpighian corpuscles show this change

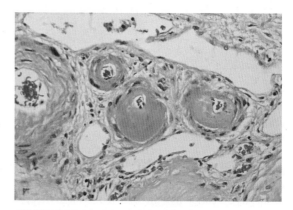

FIGURE 36.39 *Arterioles in the kidney of a hypertensive individual. The vessel walls show marked thickening by structureless, eosinophilic material (so-called 'hyaline').*

by the time individuals have reached middle age. In benign hypertension, the renal arterioles are most severely affected but hyaline change is also seen in the arterioles of the retina, adrenal capsule and abdominal viscera.

In the kidneys the appearances caused by these vascular lesions are collectively termed **benign nephrosclerosis**.

Benign Nephrosclerosis

Macroscopic Features

A kidney with benign nephrosclerosis may be normal or moderately reduced in size. The subcapsular surface is typically finely granular due to small scars related to ischaemia brought about by the small vessel disease. The cut surface shows thinning of the cortex in kidneys in which there has been a reduction in parenchymal mass, and there is an apparent increase in the hilar adipose tissue.

Microscopic Features

In addition to the arteriolar hyalinization already described, the glomeruli show ischaemic changes in the form of:

- collapse and shrinkage of part of the capillary tuft, combined with a decline in the cell population of the glomerulus
- obliteration of the lumina of the glomerular capillaries
- the laying down of collagen fibres on the inner aspect of Bowman's capsule

Ultimately these glomerular changes culminate in complete sclerosis of affected glomeruli and their conversion to relatively acellular masses of hyaline fibrous tissue. The tubules related to the sclerosed glomeruli become atrophic and eventually disappear. Tubules related to intact nephrons become hypertrophied and this alternate scarring and hypertrophy of nephrons is responsible for the finely granular subcapsular surface.

Changes in Small Arteries and Arterioles in Malignant Hypertension (Fibrinoid Necrosis)

The archetypal lesion of malignant hypertension, **fibrinoid necrosis**, affects small arteries and arterioles.

On light microscopy this is characterized by a smudgy, intensely eosinophilic, change in the vessel wall (*Fig. 36.40*). Immunohistology shows fibrin and certain other plasma proteins. **This insudation of plasma-derived molecules is associated with necrosis of the arteriolar smooth muscle cells** and there may, in some instances, be extravasated red cells within the thickened arteriolar wall. If this change affects the afferent arteriole of the glomerulus, the fibrinoid necrosis may extend to involve the glomerular capillaries which, in addition, may become thrombosed.

Fibrinoid arterial and arteriolar necrosis, in the context of hypertension, is associated with rapidly rising intraluminal pressure, which is high enough to over-

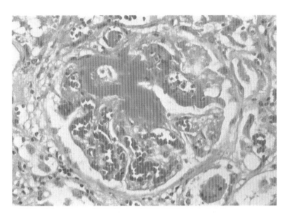

FIGURE 36.40 Deeply eosinophilic fibrinoid necrosis in the glomerular capillary tuft in a patient with malignant hypertension.

come the normal autoregulatory vasoconstriction. With increased flow in the affected segment, dilatation is likely to occur; this leads to increased tension in the vessel wall and damage to its cellular elements. In the presence of such glomerular abnormalities, it is not surprising that many of these patients show proteinuria and microscopic haematuria.

In small arteries such as the **interlobular arteries** in the kidney, a characteristic change known as **proliferative endarteritis** occurs. This is a thickening of the innermost layer of tunica intima, characterized by concentrically arranged layers of smooth muscle cells between which lie fine layers of collagen. This layered appearance is spoken of as 'onion skin' endarteritis and causes marked thinning of the vessel lumen and atrophy of the underlying medial smooth muscle cells.

The renal vascular changes and their consequences are subsumed in the term **malignant nephrosclerosis**.

Malignant Nephrosclerosis

Macroscopic Features

The size of kidneys in patients dying from malignant hypertension depends on the duration of the hypertension. If the malignant phase has supervened on a long period of benign hypertension, the macroscopic appearances are very similar to those of benign hypertension. If an accelerated type of hypertension has been present from the start of the illness, the kidneys are likely to be normal in size and to have smooth unscarred subcapsular surfaces showing small petechial haemorrhages.

Microscopic Features

The essential features have been described above. Similar changes may be seen in some types of the haemolytic-uraemic syndrome (see p 695) and the microscopic form of polyarteritis nodosa (see pp 405–406).

Hypertension Due to Disorders of the Renal Vasculature

Diseases affecting either the renal parenchyma or the renal vasculature account for the vast majority of cases of **secondary hypertension**. Renal parenchymal diseases have been considered previously, as have disorders of the small blood vessels associated with hypertension (see p 668). This section, therefore, describes conditions affecting larger renal vessels.

Renovascular hypertension appears to be associated with underperfusion of one kidney. In larger renal vessels, such underperfusion is the functional correlate of **unilateral renal artery stenosis**.

The causes of such stenosis are:

- **narrowing or occlusion of the renal artery ostium on one side as the result of the presence of a large atherosclerotic plaque.** This accounts for about 70% of cases of renal artery stenosis. The renal artery is usually relatively free from atherosclerosis, other than in diabetics, and diabetes mellitus is a definite risk factor for such stenosis.

- **fibromuscular dysplasia of the renal artery.** This is a set of disorders, commoner in females, in which renal artery stenosis is produced by fibrous or fibromuscular thickening of the vessel wall. This thickening may occur in relation to any of the three layers of the arterial wall, but most commonly the intima or the media is affected. Thus we have:

  1) **Intimal fibroplasia in which there is non-atherosclerotic thickening of the innermost layer or tunica intima.** This is a rare form of dysplasia of the artery.

  2) **Medial dysplasia. This may occur in association with aneurysms of the renal artery and tends to affect the distal part of the artery.** There is alternating segmental stenosis and dilatation of the vessel, the stenotic areas being produced by accumulations of fibromuscular tissue which replace both the intima and the normally muscle-rich media. This segmental pattern is expressed in the form of a beaded pattern on angiographic examination of the affected renal artery. This is the commonest variant of renal artery dysplasia.

     Pure medial hyperplasia with a marked increase in the number of medial smooth muscle cells does sometimes occur, but is relatively uncommon. Slightly more common is so-called **perimedial fibroplasia** in which the outer half to two-thirds of the media is replaced by fibrous tissue, which shows segmental variation in thickness.

Whatever the cause, significant degrees of renal artery stenosis lead to ischaemic atrophy of the kidney. There is:

- diminished renal blood flow

- decreased glomerular filtration rate, expressed in the form of a delayed appearance of contrast medium in the affected kidney when angiography is undertaken.

The renin–angiotensin system appears to play a significant role in the pathogenesis of renovascular hypertension. The secretion of increased amounts of renin and thus an increase in plasma concentrations of angiotensin II affects the control of blood pressure in more than one way:

- **Angiotensin II causes increased peripheral resistance via a direct effect on the smooth muscle of resistance vessels.** In addition, angiotensin II can act as growth factor for smooth muscle and the secondary medial hypertrophy in the resistance vessels will help to maintain raised blood pressure.

- **Increased plasma concentrations of angiotensin II lead to an increased output of aldosterone** and thus to an increased reabsorption of sodium in the distal tubules. This in turn causes an increase in plasma volume.

Glomerular Disorders Secondary to Systemic Disease

Glomerular damage occurs as part of many systemic disorders. Some of the latter have already been discussed in other sections. These include infective endocarditis (pp 366–369), the renal lesions of diabetes mellitus (pp 853–854) and Henoch–Schönlein disease (pp 409–410).

Foremost among conditions that have not yet been considered are a number of immunologically mediated diseases which are termed collectively, and rather inaccurately, the 'collagen diseases'. These include such entities as:

- systemic lupus erythematosus (SLE)
- rheumatoid disease
- progressive systemic sclerosis
- ankylosing spondylitis
- Sjögren's disease

SYSTEMIC LUPUS ERYTHEMATOSUS

SLE is an autoimmune disease characterized by the formation of antibodies directed chiefly against 'self' **nuclear antigens**. The continued production of these autoantibodies leads to the formation of circulating immune complexes which may be deposited in a variety of anatomical situations where they trigger inflammatory tissue-damaging events. **The sites of immune complex deposition predicate the pathological and clinical manifestations of the disease.** Many systems may be involved, and the clinical picture varies considerably from case to case. Indeed, SLE may mimic many other disorders.

In SLE, the chief sites of complex deposition are (*Fig. 36.41*):

- **small vessels**, leading to vasculitis
- **glomeruli**, leading to glomerulonephritis. About 40% of patients with SLE have disturbances of renal function at the time of presentation and in the course of the disease this increases to about 75%. Renal biopsy shows the presence of immune complexes even when there is no clinical evidence of renal disease.
- **synovium**, leading to an arthritis principally affecting the small joints of the fingers, wrists and

knees. The symptoms are often much more severe than the degree of joint dysfunction and, unlike rheumatoid arthritis, pannus formation with erosion of the underlying articular surface is not a feature of SLE.

- **skin**, leading to a highly characteristic eruption over the 'butterfly area' of the face. The dermatological features are described in Chapter 43. The effects of complex deposition on small blood vessels are often manifested in the skin in the form of pain and tenderness in the fingers and toes, dilatation of capillaries at the base of the nails, and small 'splinter' haemorrhages. Patchy areas of baldness not associated with scarring are quite common (20–50% of cases).
- **brain**, leading to a variety of neurological and psychiatric disturbances. These include migraine and grand mal epileptic seizures. The latter may be the presenting feature in a small proportion of patients, but eventually occur in about 20% of sufferers from SLE.
- **lung and pleura**, leading to dyspnoea and pleural effusions. Pleuritic pain is by far the commonest manifestation of lung involvement and is found in 40–60% of affected individuals. Pleural effusions, which are generally not very large, occur in 20–30% of cases, as do interstitial fibrosis, interstitial pneumonitis and pulmonary vasculitis.
- **heart.** Pericarditis is common. A significant number of patients with evidence of pericardial involvement, on either echocardiographic or post-mortem examination, show no **clinical** evidence of pericardial disease. One of the classic morphological features of SLE in the heart is the so-called Libman–Sacks endocarditis, which is found in approximately half the cases coming to autopsy. This type of heart valve involvement is expressed in the form of small warty vegetations, most commonly on the aortic and mitral valves. The vegetations consist partly of platelets and fibrin and partly of degenerating valve tissue. These lesions may be identified on echocardiography, but they do not cause significant functional disturbances.

SLE is not uncommon, the prevalence in the USA being about 0.02% of the population. It is much commoner in females especially Afro-Caribbean females, than in males (F:M ratio 9:1) and this ratio rises to 15:1 during childbearing years. Renal involvement is manifested initially as:

- **Proteinuria.** In about 50% of the patients this will be sufficiently severe as to produce the nephrotic syndrome.
- **Microscopic haematuria** associated with the presence in the urine of hyaline and red cell casts.
- **Hypertension**, usually mild, is seen in about 25% of patients at clinical presentation.

A remarkably wide range of antibodies is seen in SLE, as shown in *Table 36.15* and *Fig. 36.42*.

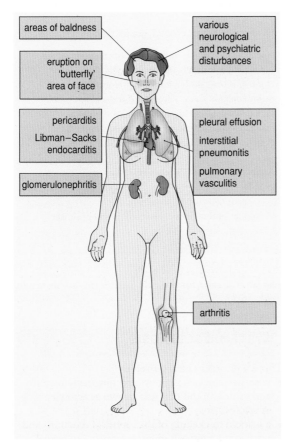

areas of baldness

eruption on 'butterfly' area of face

pericarditis
Libman–Sacks endocarditis

glomerulonephritis

various neurological and psychiatric disturbances

pleural effusion

interstitial pneumonitis

pulmonary vasculitis

arthritis

FIGURE 36.41 *Clinical features in systemic lupus erythematosus.*

Table 36.15 Antibodies Seen in SLE

Antigen group	Antigen	Function
Nuclear antigens	Double-stranded DNA	Positive in more than 60% of cases of SLE. Highly specific for the disease and thus very useful in diagnosis
	Single-stranded DNA	Non-specific as found in many autoimmune diseases. However, they do provide a useful measure of the activity of SLE as the concentration increases with increasing severity of the disease
	Histones	Present in both 'spontaneously' occurring and drug-induced SLE
	Smith (Sm) antigen	This antigen is an extractable nuclear antigen. Antibody found in about 30% of Afro-Caribbean and Chinese patients with SLE but in only 7% of Caucasian patients
	Ribonucleoprotein (RNP)	Positive in about one-quarter of patients with SLE. Presence associated with Raynaud's phenomenon
	Ro (another small ribonucleoprotein)	Positive in 24% of patients with SLE. May be present in the absence of anti-DNA antibodies. Presence in pregnant patients with SLE is associated with development of congenital heart block in offspring
Phospholipid	Cardiolipin	Gives a false-positive VDRL test for syphilis
	A phospholipid, the antibody to which is known as the **lupus anticoagulant**	Is neither specific for SLE nor an anticoagulant in that it does not specifically inactivate any of the known clotting factors, although it does prolong the partial thromboplastin time. Thrombosis is the major problem in patients with the lupus anticoagulant. It is also associated with a high risk of recurrent abortion. Positive in 30–40% of patients with SLE
Immunoglobulins	Altered immunoglobulin G	Antibodies known as **rheumatoid factors**. Common in SLE
Blood cells	Lymphocytes and neutrophils	Cytotoxic antibodies for these cells found in almost 50% of patients with SLE

Renal Pathology In SLE

SLE is the great mimic in so far as the glomerular changes that it may cause are concerned. Almost any morphological variant can be found and none is specific for SLE. The classification given here is that published by the World Health Organization (WHO) in 1982, in which **six** classes of glomerular change are specified (*Table 36.16*).

Prognosis

Renal failure is responsible for the death of about one in five patients with SLE. The most serious of the different forms of SLE-associated renal disease described above is the diffuse proliferative form. Five-year survival rates for these different forms are shown in *Table 36.17*.

SYSTEMIC SCLEROSIS

This is a disorder characterized by:
- excessive collagen deposits affecting many organs and tissues. In the skin it is known as acrosclerosis or scleroderma.
- a marked thickening of the intima of medium- and small-sized arteries leading, eventually, to virtual obliteration of their lumina

Progressive systemic sclerosis occurs more commonly

Table 36.16 WHO Classification of Glomerular Lesions in SLE

Class	Disorder	Pathological features
I	Minor abnormalities	Normal on light microscopy; complexes seen on electron microscopy or on immunohistology. Accounts for about 16% of cases
II	Mesangial changes	Increase in number of mesangial cells and mesangial matrix, affecting most of glomeruli. Seen in about 16% of biopsies from patients with SLE. Usually correlates with mild clinical disease or periods of remission
III	Focal segmental glomerulonephritis	Segmental distribution of mesangial cell proliferation, inflammation, fibrinoid necrosis associated with capillary thrombosis, or scarring. Often seen with class II lesions associated. This picture is seen in about 20% of biopsies
IV	Diffuse proliferative glomerulonephritis	Histological patterns seen under this rubric include: • A mesangial proliferative glomerulonephritis in which there is mesangial cell proliferation associated with necrosis and scarring. Some segments of the glomerular capillary wall are thickened and eosinophilic, an appearance that is termed **'wire looping'**. The thickening of the vessel wall is due to the presence of immune complexes. In necrotic areas nuclear debris may be seen in the form of portions of material that stain a lilac colour with haematoxylin. These are known as haematoxyphil bodies • diffuse endocapillary proliferative glomerulonephritis. This resembles poststreptococcal glomerulonephritis but other changes suggestive of SLE such as wire loops, focal necrosis or small intracapillary thrombi may be seen • diffuse mesangiocapillary glomerulonephritis • diffuse crescentic glomerulonephritis These four types of proliferative glomerulonephritis are found in just under 40% of renal biopsies from patients with SLE
V	Diffuse membranous glomerulonephritis	This may occur in a pure form in which case it is indistinguishable from primary membranous glomerulonephritis. It may, however, be mixed with other morphological changes of SLE such as have been described above. About 10% of renal biopsies from SLE patients show this picture
VI	Sclerosing glomerulonephritis	As the proliferative forms of SLE-associated renal disease progress, the glomeruli become scarred and many may be completely replaced by fibrous tissue

in females than in males; the peak incidence is between the ages of 20 and 50 years. On the basis of the clinical presentation the disorder may be divided into two major classes: **acrosclerosis** and **diffuse or progressive systemic sclerosis**.

In **acrosclerosis**, the commoner of the two forms, the skin is the chief target organ. Skin of the fingers and the face becomes scarred and atrophic after an initial period of oedema.

Table 36.17 Survival in Patients with SLE

Class	5-year survival rate (%)
II	100
III	73
IV	60
V	90

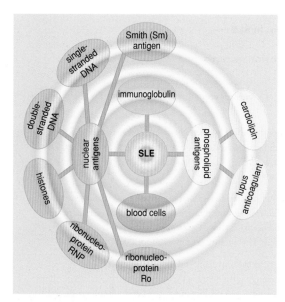

FIGURE 36.42 Autoantibodies in systemic lupus erythematosus.

This form of systemic sclerosis is often associated with what is known as the **CREST** syndrome. CREST is an acronym of:

- *c*alcinosis
- *R*aynaud's phenomenon
- *e*sophageal dysfunction
- *s*clerodactyly
- *t*elangiectasia

This form of the disease tends to pursue a slow course and renal involvement is uncommon.

Diffuse or progressive systemic sclerosis, the less common form of systemic sclerosis, shows extensive skin lesions and early involvement of viscera; the organs affected principally are the:

- kidneys
- heart
- lungs
- gut
- musculoskeletal system

A genetic factor is clearly involved in the aetiology of systemic sclerosis because there is an increased incidence of HLA-DR5 and HLA-DRw8 in patients than in the general population. There is a decline in the number of circulating T lymphocytes, CD8 (cytotoxic suppressor) cells being particularly affected.

Evidence of autoimmune reactions is present in the form of antinuclear antibodies. Two of these appear to be found only in systemic sclerosis. They are:

1) an antibody reacting with a nuclear enzyme, DNA topoisomerase 1. This antibody is known as Scl–70 and is present in the serum of 30–40% of patients with progressive systemic sclerosis.
2) an antibody reacting with centromeres. This is

found in 50–70% of patients with the CREST syndrome.

Other expressions of immune disturbances are:

- hypergammaglobulinaemia, which is present in 50% of patients
- the presence of rheumatoid factors in 25% of patients
- increased plasma concentrations of the complement fragments C3d and C4d in about 50% of patients. The presence of increased levels of these fragments is an expression of complement activation.

Clinical Presentation

- The majority of patients first complain of **Raynaud's phenomenon**, followed soon afterwards by thickening of the skin of the fingers and hands and difficulty in moving the joints in affected areas.
- **Muscular weakness and difficulty in swallowing** follow and there may be other manifestations of problems with gastrointestinal motility.
- If the **lung** is involved, the patients may complain of **cough and dyspnoea**.
- **Myocardial fibrosis** is the cause of **arrhythmias and conduction defects**, and patients may also experience anginal pain.
- **Renal involvement is the manifestation of systemic sclerosis most likely to prove fatal.** About 50% of patients develop high blood pressure and a quarter of these have malignant-phase hypertension which leads to the appearance of renal and cardiac failure, possibly associated with fits (hypertensive encephalopathy). About 25% of patients with renal involvement go on to develop chronic renal failure.

Pathological Changes in the Kidney

Macroscopic features
In fatal cases, naked-eye examination may show the presence of many, very small, cortical infarcts.

Microscopic Features
The principal light microscopic change is to be found in the interlobular arteries. These show a marked degree of intimal thickening in which the cells in the neointima are arranged in concentric layers. The fibres of this thickened intima tend to be rather loosely arranged, because of the presence of large amounts of connective tissue mucins.

In the media there is some reduplication of the internal elastic lamina and the media itself shows some degree of atrophy.

In patients who have an acute clinical course associated with the development of malignant hypertension, the main vascular targets are the small arteries and arterioles. The afferent arterioles show fibrinoid necrosis and this may extend into the glomerular tuft in a manner analogous to that seen in any case of malignant hypertension. The affected glomeruli develop ischaemic changes with collapse and wrinkling of their basement membranes. In these patients, who run a rapidly progressive course, thrombi in the small arteries and arterioles are common.

Other Renal Vascular Disorders

Many of the small vessel diseases that affect the kidney have already been considered. There are, however, some conditions affecting both large and small vessels that have not been dealt with in other sections, and these are described briefly here.

RENAL INFARCTION

Renal infarcts are fairly common, most being due to impaction of systemic emboli in the main renal artery or its branches. Because so great a proportion of the blood volume passes through the kidney, when emboli are present in the circulating blood, it is not surprising that the kidney is often affected.

Systemic emboli most commonly arise from intracardiac thrombi. They may occur in the left ventricle:

- as a consequence of previous myocardial infarction
- because of abnormal haemodynamics within the ventricular cavity such as are seen in cases of dilated cardiomyopathy

Intracardiac thrombi occur on damaged valves, whether or not this is associated with infective endocarditis, and thrombi are often seen in the atria in association with atrial fibrillation from whatever cause.

Occasionally renal embolization may occur because atheromatous debris enters the systemic circulation as a result of plaque ulceration. Such emboli are easily recognized on microscopic examination because they almost always contain crystalline cholesterol, which appears in paraffin sections as 'cigar'-shaped spaces where the lipid has been dissolved out.

Clinical Features

Unless large, most infarcts in the kidney are clinically silent and go undetected. Patients who have large infarcts complain of the sudden onset of loin pain, followed by haematuria and proteinuria. In the uncommon event of both renal arteries being occluded, acute renal failure develops.

Macroscopic Features

The appearances of any infarct depend on the size of the occluded vessel (the larger the vessel, the larger the infarct), and the stage in its natural history at which it is seen.

Most renal infarcts measure 1–3 cm along their longest axis, although much larger ones may be seen. They have a typical wedge shape, the base of the wedge being on the subcapsular surface (see *Fig. 19.4*). In the first few hours the infarcted area is red because of the escape of red blood cells from damaged vessels within the infarct. It is firm and swollen, because the oncotic pressure within the necrotic tissue is higher than that in the surrounding tissue. As intracellular and intercellular oedema develop, so the infarcted area becomes paler, and within a few days it has a typical yellowish-grey colour such as is seen in infarcts occurring in most solid viscera. At this stage the infarct shows a narrow red zone representing dilated vessels at the junction with normal tissue.

The peripheral hyperaemia and the swelling gradually diminish and within 7–10 days the infarct is depressed below the level of the surrounding subcapsular surface. In the case of small infarcts, scarring develops rapidly and within as little as a month the site of infarction may be represented by a deep V-shaped scar. This bears no constant relationship to the calyces, as is the case with pyelonephritic scars.

This description applies only to infarcts caused by sterile emboli. If the emboli are infected, the centre of the ischaemic area breaks down to form an abscess.

Microscopic Features

Renal infarcts show essentially the same features as those occurring in other solid viscera. In order of occurrence:

- the red blood cells in the capillaries become sludged and lose their haemoglobin content
- tubular epithelial nuclei start to condense (pyknosis)
- the dead tissue triggers the release of inflammatory mediators, and neutrophils are attracted to the periphery of the infarct
- tubular epithelial cell and mesangial cell nuclei either break up or are lysed but the basement membranes of Bowman's capsule and the tubular basement membranes persist, giving a ghost-like picture of the renal architecture
- fibrous tissue eventually replaces most or all of the infarcted area

Renal Cortical Necrosis

Most renal infarcts result from intraluminal obstruction of vessel lumina by thrombus or embolus. One rare form of extensive ischaemic damage to the kidney, renal cortical necrosis, appears to be associated, instead, with widespread spasm of vessels supplying the kidneys.

Renal cortical necrosis is usually bilateral and causes

acute renal failure; the clinical picture is associated with a profound degree of oliguria. As its name implies, the essential pathological feature is ischaemic necrosis of most of the renal cortex, with sparing of the medulla, a thin rim of cortex just under the capsule and the juxtamedullary zone of the cortex. About half the patients will have sufficient functioning kidney left to avoid the need for chronic dialysis. Even in patients who regain function after a period of oliguria, there is a high risk of a decline into chronic renal failure as a result of hyperfiltration damage to the surviving glomeruli.

KEY POINTS: Renal Cortical Necrosis

The aetiological and pathogenetic associations of bilateral renal cortical necrosis are:

- **accidental haemorrhage of pregnancy, most notably associated with separation of the placenta, abortion or placenta praevia.** This accounts for more than 50% of all cases of bilateral renal cortical necrosis
- **septicaemia with endotoxic shock** accounts for a further 30–40%
- **any severe dehydrating illness** associated with profuse diarrhoea and vomiting

The acute and severe underperfusion responsible for bilateral renal cortical necrosis is considered to be due to spasm of the feeding blood vessels, which may last for many hours. The mechanism(s) responsible for the spasm are unknown. Vessels distal to the sites of spasm often show thrombosis, no doubt because of haemodynamic abnormalities.

Macroscopic Features

Kidneys with cortical necrosis are somewhat enlarged. Virtually the whole of the cortex shows a marked degree of pallor, associated with a yellow coloration of the affected areas. The renal parenchyma immediately beneath the capsule and in the juxtamedullary region are much darker in colour, a reflection of their being spared by the ischaemia.

Microscopic Features

There is extensive coagulative necrosis and thrombi may be seen in small blood vessels. In some instances the necrosis appears patchy and there are islands in which surviving nephrons are present.

Renal Vein Thrombosis

About half the cases of this rare event occur in infants and neonates, producing haemorrhagic infarction. Thrombosis usually complicates some severely dehydrating illness such as gastroenteritis.

Affected children present with:

- acute loin swelling on the affected side
- haematuria

- a non-functioning or poorly functioning kidney

Diagnostically useful features, which suggest thrombosis, include:

- a low platelet count
- the presence in some instances of fibrin degradation products in the urine

As might be expected, the degree of damage correlates with the size and/or number of veins that are occluded. If the main renal vein is blocked, the affected kidney will be swollen and darkly congested on naked-eye examination. Microscopic examination shows the features of haemorrhagic infarction.

The condition carries a mortality rate of more than 60%. In those who survive, hypertension, the nephrotic syndrome and evidence of tubular dysfunction are among the reported consequences.

In adults and older children, renal vein thrombosis occurs principally as a complication of the nephrotic syndrome. This is particularly likely to occur in association with membranous glomerulonephritis. Some reports claim that one in five patients with the nephrotic syndrome develop renal vein thrombosis and that 50% of patients with membranous glomerulonephritis are likely to have an episode of renal vein thrombosis at some time in the course of the disease.

In renal biopsy material, diagnosis depends on finding organized or partly organized thrombi in veins of different sizes. In addition, there may be a greater degree of tubule atrophy than might be expected for the stage of the primary disease, but this is rather subtle. The result is a mild additional decline in renal function.

Pathogenesis

As in other cases of venous thrombosis, there must be an imbalance between procoagulant and anticoagulant factors. Increases in certain coagulant factors certainly do occur in patients with the nephrotic syndrome, but in this respect there is little to distinguish patients who develop renal vein thrombi from those who do not. The strong association between membranous glomerulonephritis and renal vein thrombosis also remains a puzzle.

SMALL VESSEL DISEASE

Polyarteritis, Wegener's granulomatosis, Churg–Strauss syndrome, Henoch–Schönlein disease and cryoglobulinaemia have been described (see pp 405–411). This section describes a group of diseases presenting with:

- microangiopathic haemolytic anaemia (haemolysis secondary to small vessel disease). Fragmented and deformed red cells are present in the blood
- acute renal failure
- a low platelet count
- evidence of intravascular clotting
- damage to small vessel endothelium

- activation of platelets and clotting pathways

The diseases classified under this rubric are:

- **the various types of haemolytic uraemic syndrome**
- **thrombotic thrombocytopenic purpura (TTP)**
- **disseminated intravascular coagulation**
- **progressive systemic sclerosis**

Haemolytic Uraemic Syndrome

Childhood Form

Haemolytic uraemic syndrome occurs more commonly in infancy and childhood than in adult life and **is the commonest cause of acquired acute renal failure in children**. Its occurrence may be sporadic, endemic or epidemic. In a small proportion of cases (approximately 3%), haemolytic uraemic syndrome is familial. This form usually presents insidiously in older children. In the acute form, the affected children present, usually after a gastrointestinal or respiratory tract infection, with:

- severe oliguric renal failure
- bleeding, most commonly from the gastrointestinal tract
- haematuria
- haemolytic anaemia
- thrombocytopenia
- hypertension (in about half the cases)

The prodromal illness may be due to infection by a strain of *Escherichia coli* which produces a powerful exotoxin known as **verotoxin** (the toxin kills cells from a line of cultured kidney cells derived from a monkey called Vero) (see p 535). Verotoxins are also cytotoxic for endothelial cells and are likely to be the cause of the microvascular damage in some cases.

The morphological changes seen in the kidney in fatal cases are those of patchy ischaemic necrosis, which may be extensive, amounting to cortical necrosis.

Microscopic Features

On light and electron microscopy, the small vessels of the kidney show:

- fibrin and red cells within the walls of the interlobular arteries, arterioles and glomerular capillaries (fibrinoid necrosis)
- thrombosis in these vessels
- mucoid intimal thickening of the affected vessels
- subendothelial and mesangial accumulation of electron-lucent material in the glomeruli

Adult Form

In adults, haemolytic uraemic syndrome is much less frequently the sequel of an infectious illness. The circumstances under which it may occur include:

- **pregnancy**, especially in the event of some complication such as accidental haemorrhage
- **in the postpartum period** as a complication of normal pregnancy and delivery
- **the use of contraceptive compounds.** The mechanism underlying this association is unknown
- **in infections including *E. coli* septicaemia**, in which presumably both the verotoxin and endotoxin may play a part

There are no significant differences between the adult and childhood forms in respect of the clinical or morphological features. The prognosis, in adults, however, is significantly worse than that in children.

Thrombotic Thrombocytopenic Purpura
(see also p 915)

This is an uncommon disorder, sharing some of the clinical and pathological features of haemolytic uraemic syndrome. It is commoner in females than in males (F:M ratio 3:2); the peak incidence is in the fourth decade.

The characteristic lesions are platelet-rich thrombi occurring in arterioles and capillaries; the clinical picture depends on the location of the occluded microvessels. In addition to the presence of the thrombi there are subendothelial deposits in both capillaries and arterioles, and microaneurysm formation may be noted. The lesions of TTP are seen most commonly in the:

- brain
- abdominal viscera
- heart

but they can occur anywhere in the body. Accurate diagnosis requires the finding of capillary thrombi in biopsy material derived from the skin, muscle or gums, but the false-negative rate is high and it may be impossible to obtain a definite tissue-based diagnosis.

There are five main features in the clinical presentation, not all of which are present in every case. These are:

1) microangiopathic haemolytic anaemia
2) thrombocytopenia
3) neurological symptoms
4) fever
5) renal dysfunction

The principal clinical distinction from haemolytic uraemic syndrome is **the predominance of neurological effects, which are present in 92% of cases**. Neurological symptoms include headache, confusion, stupor, coma, hemiparesis, cranial nerve palsies and fits.

Aetiology and Pathogenesis

Both the aetiology and pathogenesis of this disease are enigmas. The clinical observation that there is marked improvement following exchange plasmapheresis suggests two possibilities, which are by no means mutually exclusive:

1) there is some abnormal chemical species in the plasma of patients with TTP which is responsible for producing the pathophysiological picture

2) there is some chemical species missing from the plasma of sufferers, the absence of which is responsible

A number of possibilities that are consistent with this model have been examined. These include:

- **Abnormalities in circulating von Willebrand's factor (vWF).** vWF is normally secreted by endothelial cells in the form of large multimers, which are broken down into smaller molecules by a depolymerase in the plasma. It has been suggested that there is an abnormal inhibitor of this depolymerase in the plasma of patients with TTP. The presence of abnormally large multimers of vWF in the plasma promotes intravascular platelet clumping and adhesion of the platelet clumps to the microvessel walls.
- A relative deficiency of prostaglandin I$_2$ (prostacyclin). Prostaglandin I$_2$ acts as a powerful antiaggregatory compound so far as platelets are concerned. It has been suggested that many, although not all, patients with TTP show a variety of abnormalities related to the secretion and metabolism of prostaglandin I$_2$.
- A relative deficiency of an inhibitor of platelet-activating factor. This permits the latter to act in an uncontrolled way and thus promotes the inappropriate aggregation of platelets within the microvessels.
- It has also been suggested that TTP is, in essence, an immunologically mediated vasculitis, but there is no hard evidence to support this view.

Renal Stones

In the industrialized West, renal stones, or **calculi**, are very common, constituting the third most common renal disease. In developing countries, kidney stones are comparatively rare, although, curiously, bladder stones, especially in children, are common.

KEY POINTS: Composition of Renal Stones
Renal stones consist of two main elements:
1) a small amount (about 3–5%) of a mucoprotein matrix
2) aggregated crystalline material derived from the precipitation of urine solutes, which constitutes 95–98% of the stone mass

Ureteric colic due to stone is common in the UK. It has been estimated that, on a cumulative basis, 12% of men and 5% of women will have had an attack of stone-associated colic by the time they reach the age of 70 years.

Table 36.18 Main Types of Renal Stone

Stone type	Percentage of stones
Calcium oxalate and mixed calcium oxalate–calcium phosphate	75%
Magnesium ammonium phosphate (struvite)	Approximately 15%
Uric acid	6–7%
Cystine	3–4%
Other	Very rare

The main types of renal stone and their relative frequencies are listed in *Table 36.18*.

Calcium Oxalate and Mixed Calcium Oxalate–Calcium Phosphate Stones
These are the commonest of all renal stones. They occur most frequently in males (M : F ratio 4 : 1)

These stones tend to be a yellowish-brown colour and they may have a dark surface as a result of the deposition of altered blood. The shape depends on whether calcium oxalate predominates. Oxalate-predominant stones tend to be nodular with spikes protruding from the surface; this shape is responsible for the common term 'mulberry' stone. If considerable amounts of calcium phosphate are present, the stones have a smooth surface.

Clinical Features
The commonest presentation is ureteric colic which appears when the stones start to pass down the ureter and become impacted. These episodes are associated with very severe pain indeed. Obviously, only small stones will pass from the renal pelvis into the ureter, and large stones may remain clinically silent for long periods.

The complications are those of obstruction to the outflow of urine from the affected kidney to the bladder and are, therefore:

- pyelonephritis, which may be acute or chronic
- dilatation of the ureter proximal to the impacted stone and consequent dilatation of the renal pelvis with, eventually, atrophy of renal parenchyma – (hydronephrosis)

Factors Promoting the Formation of Calcium Oxalate Stones
Normal urine is supersaturated with calcium oxalate and it is, in fact, surprising that oxalate stones are not even more common. Increases in the urinary concen-

tration of either calcium or oxalate are potent factors in causing stone formation and concentrations may rise in three ways:

1) **an increase in calcium excretion in the urine (hypercalciuria).** This is present in 70% of individuals who form this type of stone.

2) **an increase in the urinary output of oxalate.** This is seen in about 5% of cases of calcium oxalate stone formation.

3) a decrease in the urinary volume with a resulting increase in concentration of solutes.

In about one-quarter of cases of calcium oxalate or mixed stone, no obvious predisposing cause can be found.

Hypercalciuria may occur in the presence or absence of hypercalcaemia (see *Table 36.19*).

Hyperoxaluria accounts for only 5% of cases of oxalate or mixed oxalate–phosphate stones. Hyperoxaluria may be:

- **Primary – an inherited disorder of metabolism is responsible.** This arises from a deficiency in one or other of two enzymes. Both forms of primary hyperoxaluria are rare and account for only 1% of patients who form this type of stone.

- **Secondary.** This accounts for 4% of this type of stone and can occur under two sets of circumstances:

1) Intestinal diseases of a number of different types, all of which result in a relative failure to absorb bile acids in the small gut. As a result, the concentration of these acids in the large gut is higher than normal and this leads to increased permeability of the bowel wall to oxalates. The disorders of the small gut are, therefore, those associated with malabsorption, such as coeliac disease, small bowel diverticula in which overgrowth of bacterial flora may occur, extensive small bowel resection and chronic pancreatitis.

2) Excessive oxalate intake, from such foods as rhubarb, spinach, strawberries, beetroot, tea, cocoa, peanuts and orange, lemon and grapefruit juice.

Magnesium Ammonium Phosphate (Struvite) Stones

These account for 15% of all renal stones. They occur as a result of the action of urease produced by certain bacteria that may infect the urinary tract, most notably *Proteus* species. The urease splits urea, producing ammonia and hydroxyl (OH) ions, both of which make the urine alkaline. The increase in pH leads to a state of supersaturation of the urine with the constituents of the struvite stones. The matrix that binds the crystals is composed partly of normal urinary mucoproteins and partly of a carbohydrate-rich glycocalyx secreted by the urease-producing bacteria.

Clinical Features

Struvite stones occur twice as commonly in females as in males. This is almost certainly due to the increased liability of females to suffer from urinary tract infections. The importance of this factor is emphasized by the fact that males who, for any reason, have an increased risk of urinary tract infection, also have an increased risk of developing struvite calculi.

The effects arising directly from the presence of the stones are often combined with evidence of infection and it is as important to treat the infection and, if

---

Table 36.19 Causes of Hypercalciuria

Hypercalcaemia present	Hypercalcaemia absent
Primary hyperparathyroidism Neoplasm associated hypercalcaemia which may be humoral due to release of osteoclast-stimulating factors or the presence of osteolytic secondary deposits in bone Sarcoidosis Excessive intake of calcium and the 'milk alkali' syndrome Prolonged immobilization	'Idiopathic' hypercalciuria. This is the commonest cause of this form of stone (50%). May be due to increased absorption of calcium from the gut lumen Medullary sponge kidney Renal tubular acidosis (type 1), in which the distal tubules cannot establish an adequate hydrogen ion gradient between the urine in the tubule and the blood in the peritubular veins. It may be inherited (autosomal dominant transmission) or may be secondary to a number of other diseases such as Sjögren's syndrome, Wilson's disease, systemic lupus erythematosus, primary biliary cirrhosis. It may also occur in patients treated with carbonic anhydrase inhibitors for glaucoma, about 10% of whom develop stones Cadmium poisoning. Stones occur in 40% of those exposed to cadmium in the course of their work ? Diets high in protein

possible, its underlying causes as it is to treat the stone itself.

The stones are whitish or grey in colour and may be very large. Some have an irregular shape, often filling the pelvis and calyces (the so-called 'stag-horn calculus'). The combination of infection and interference with urine outflow from the kidney may lead to abscess formation within the kidney parenchyma or to a dilated pelvicalyceal system, which may be filled with pus (pyonephrosis). If the calculus is not removed, there is a substantial chance that the affected kidney will lose most if not all of its function.

Prognosis in the absence of adequate treatment is serious. Failure to remove the unilateral struvite calculi completely will result in 60% of patients dying within 15 years. Failed removal in the case of bilateral struvite calculi results in 50% of patients dying within 5 years.

Uric Acid Stones

Uric acid stones occur much more frequently in males than in females (M : F ratio 9 : 1). In the UK, uric acid stones account for about 5% of all renal calculi, and 10% of patients known to have gout develop renal colic. In Israel, however, 40% of renal stones are uric acid calculi and 75% of patients with gout develop stones. Climatic factors may account for these geographically determined prevalence patterns.

The chief pathogenetic factors are:
- increased concentration of uric acid in the urine
- persistently low pH in the urine
- low urinary volumes

A minority of the patients (25%) have true gout and thus have hyperuricaemia, but in most cases there appears to be no systemic metabolic cause for the stone formation. Treatment for true gout involves, of course, the use of compounds that will increase urinary output of uric acid. Care must, therefore, be taken to keep the urine volume up by increasing fluid intake and to maintain an alkaline urinary pH.

If there is an increase in purine breakdown, as may occur in myeloproliferative disorders, especially following treatment with chemotherapy or radiotherapy, uric acid production is greatly increased and this is reflected in increased urinary output of uric acid.

Increases in blood levels of uric acid are also seen in certain rare inherited metabolic disorders:
- **Deficiency of the enzyme hypoxanthine guanine phosphoribosyl transferase.** This X-linked condition is associated with an inability to salvage purine bases and thus with raised uric acid levels in the blood as a result of the breakdown of these bases. In its most severe form, this disorder is expressed as the Lesch–Nyhan syndrome (gout, choreoathetoid movements, spasticity, self-mutilation and mental disability). Uric acid stone formation often occurs in these unfortunate people and, when bilateral, may block both ureters, leading to acute renal failure.

- **Increase in activity of 5-phosphoribosyl pyrophosphate.** This leads to increased production of purines and thus to increased blood levels of uric acid.
- **The von Gierke type of glycogen storage disease (glucose-6-phosphatase deficiency).** Hyperuricaemia is common in these patients, who frequently develop clinical features of gout associated with an increased risk for the formation of uric acid stones.

In patients in whom the uric acid levels in the plasma are not raised, the chief pathogenetic factor appears to be an acid urine. Why some individuals should produce urine of a persistently low pH is not known. In a few patients who have severe diarrhoea, or who lose excess fluid and bicarbonate via an ileostomy, there is both a low urinary pH and a low urine volume, and the risk of uric acid stone formation in these patients is high.

Uric acid stones are hard, yellowish-brown in colour and have a smooth outer surface. They rarely reach a very large size, few of them being more than about 2 cm in diameter. They are frequently multiple. Their clinical effects are basically similar to those of other types of stone.

Cystine Stones

Cystine stones, which account for about 3% of all stones, occur only in patients suffering from the autosomal recessive disorder, **primary cystinuria. This is characterized by inability to reabsorb cystine, lysine, ornithine and arginine from the filtrate in the proximal renal tubule**, or from the lumen of the small intestine. The disorder is rare, occurring in about 1 in 20 000 individuals in a homozygous form. The increased amounts of cystine in the urine of these patients is associated with stone formation in about two-thirds.

The stones are yellowish-white and waxy in appearance. They are usually multiple and, although most are small round stones, in a few instances they may increase in size and fill the pelvicalyceal system, forming 'stag-horn' calculi.

The clinical effects do not differ from those described in relation to other stones.

Renal Tumours and Tumour-like Lesions

BENIGN NEOPLASMS

Cortical Adenoma

The commonest benign tumour is **cortical adenoma**. Adenomas are usually small (less than 2 cm in diameter, often much smaller) and appear as discrete yellowish-grey nodules in the renal cortex.

Microscopic Features

Adenomas are composed of rather uniform, cuboidal, epithelial cells, presumably derived from renal tubules. Many contain abundant lipid or abundant glycogen, closely resembling the cells of renal adenocarcinoma.

The lesions may show a number of different **architectural patterns**. Some exhibit a papillary growth pattern, whereas in others the cells grow in a solid alveolar pattern, in tubules or well-formed glands. **Histological** distinction of these tumours from well-differentiated adenocarcinoma is not always easy. By convention, lesions less than 3 cm in diameter are classified as adenomas and do not, for the most part, behave in an aggressive fashion, whereas those with dimensions greater than this are classified as carcinomas. Obviously this is a somewhat crude oversimplification and there must be a rather fuzzy border zone between adenoma and carcinoma.

Table 36.20 Primary Malignant Renal Tumours

Age	Site	Tumour type
Adult life	Parenchyma	Renal cell carcinoma; oncocytoma
	Pelvis	Transitional cell carcinoma
Childhood	Parenchyma	Wilms' tumour; rhabdoid tumour; clear cell sarcoma

Angiomyolipoma

This is probably not a true neoplasm and is best classified as a **hamartoma**. These lesions, which usually present clinically in adult life, are composed of an admixture of well-differentiated smooth muscle, adipose tissue and thick-walled blood vessels. This lesion has a strong association with tuberous sclerosis. This is an autosomally dominant, inherited disorder in which there are:

- lesions of the cerebral cortex causing epilepsy and mental disability
- peculiar skin lesions (adenoma sebaceum of Pringle)
- sometimes visceral lesions such as rhabdomyoma of the heart and pancreatic cysts; 40% of patients with angiomyolipoma are so affected

The renal lesion usually does not cause symptoms, although if there is haemorrhage into the mass, the patient may experience pain.

Other benign tumours of connective tissue are seen from time to time (e.g. fibroma, haemangioma and leiomyoma). They are usually small but of no clinical significance.

MALIGNANT NEOPLASMS

Primary malignant renal tumours constitute 2.5% of all malignancies. These are listed in *Table 36.20*.

Renal Cell Carcinoma (Renal Adenocarcinoma, Hypernephroma)

Renal adenocarcinoma accounts for about 1–3% of all visceral malignancies and for approximately 85% of primary malignant disease of the kidney in adult life. It occurs in middle and later life with a peak incidence in the seventh and eighth decades, and there is a male:female predominance (2:1). There is an increased risk in smokers and in patients with the rare, inherited von Hippel–Lindau syndrome. This is an autosomal dominant disorder characterized by the presence of a variety of benign and malignant neoplasms in a number of different tissues (e.g. retinal haemangioblastoma, renal cell carcinoma and cerebellar haemangioblastoma).

Predisposing conditions are shown in *Table 36.21*.

Incidence

Renal cell carcinoma shows geographical variation in incidence, as indicated in *Table 36.22*.

Clinical Features

The 'classical' diagnostic features of renal adenocarcinoma are:

- **flank pain**
- **a mass in the loin**
- **haematuria**

Haematuria is the most reliable sign, occurring in about 60% of cases, but unfortunately it is not always gross enough to be detected by the patient, so clinical presentation may occur late in the natural history of the disease when distant spread has already occurred (radiological evidence of metastases is present in about 25% of patients at diagnosis of the renal tumour). The clinical picture may be dominated by the symptoms and signs caused by these metastases.

The clinical picture may be further complicated by the fact that renal adenocarcinoma frequently produces systemic manifestations in no way linked to the presence of metastatic deposits. These are listed in *Table 36.23* and *Fig. 36.43*.

Table 36.21 Factors Predisposing Towards Renal Cell Carcinoma

Risk factor	Findings
Von Hippel–Lindau disease (congenital cystic disease)	In this disorder the incidence of renal cell carcinoma is 28%. The locus for von Hippel–Lindau disease is close to that of the oncogene *raf-1* on chromosome 3p25. The normal gene presumably acts as a tumour-suppressor gene.
Acquired cystic disease	Associated with dialysis for chronic renal failure. Some 10–20% of cases of acquired cystic disease have microscopic adenomas after 3 years' dialysis and a further 3–6% have carcinoma after 5 years' dialysis. Acquired dialysis-related cystic disease is associated with a 50-fold increase in the risk of renal cell carcinoma.
Cigarette smoking	This doubles the risk and appears to be associated in about one-third of all cases.
Obesity	This risk factor operates especially in women in whom there is a direct relationship between increasing body-weight and risk.
Inherited predisposition	Associated with a 3,8 or 3,11 translocation. Breakpoint is at the proximal end of 3p. Cumulative risk at age 59 years is 87%. The loss of one allele from the short arm of chromosome 3 occurs in 96% of sporadic renal cell carcinomas and is not confined to hereditary cases.

Table 36.22 Influence of Location on Incidence of Renal Cell Carcinoma

Location	Incidence (per 100 000 per year)
Iceland	12.2
UK	3.5
Africa, South America, Spain, Asia	Less than 3.0

Table 36.23 Systemic Manifestations of Renal Cell Carcinoma

Clinical feature	Mechanism
Fever	? Prostaglandins
Hypercalcaemia	Parathyroid hormone-related peptide production
Erythrocytosis (4% of patients)	Increased production of erythropoietin
Amyloidosis (3% of patients)	Stimulation of serum amyloid (SAA) production by liver cells
Hypertension (rare)	Increased renin production
Galactorrhoea	Ectopic production of prolactin
Gynaecomastia	?

Macroscopic Features

Renal adenocarcinomas may arise in any part of the kidney but are found most commonly at the poles, with a slight predilection for the upper pole. They form roughly spherical masses, ranging in size from about 3 to 15 cm. The cut surface shows a rather heterogeneous appearance with areas of yellow lipid-rich tumour juxtaposed with areas of necrosis and haemorrhage (*Fig. 36.44*).

As the tumour grows it may bulge into the calyces and renal pelvis; not infrequently, ulceration occurs with shedding of the tumour cells and, of course, there is haematuria. There is a marked tendency for venous invasion to take place and sometimes a solid cord of tumour may grow along the renal vein and up into and along the vena cava. The lesion is very vascular; this is useful diagnostically because angiography shows up the rich vascular pattern and thus delineates the tumour.

Microscopic Features

A number of different architectural patterns may be seen. The tumour cells may be arranged in tubules, in a solid alveolar pattern or in a papillary one, and in any single tumour all of these may be seen.

The most common cell type is a rounded polygonal cell which has a rather **clear** cytoplasm, due to the presence of glycogen (which is largely removed during processing of the tissue) and lipid (*Fig. 36.45*). About 14% of the tumours consist of spindle-shaped cells, somewhat resembling those found in connective tissue neoplasms, and a further 12% have a granular cytoplasm. The degree of nuclear atypia and of mitotic activity is very variable

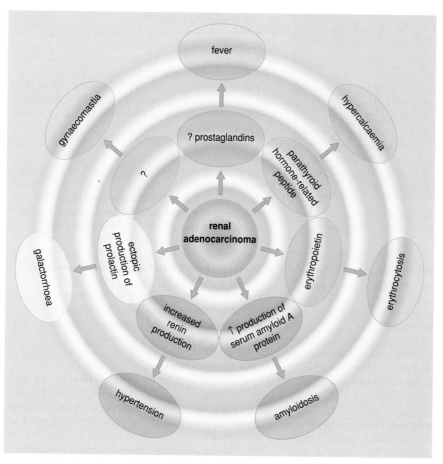

FIGURE 36.43 *Systemic non-metastatic manifestations of renal cell carcinoma.*

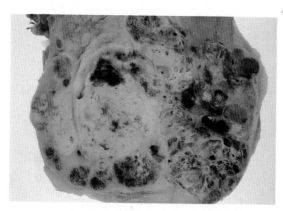

FIGURE 36.44 *Renal cell carcinoma at the lower pole of the kidney. Note the characteristically variegated appearance of the cut surface.*

and there is some correlation between this and the prognosis: tumours showing a marked degree of nuclear atypia have the worst outlook.

A number of variant forms exist. These include **papillary renal carcinoma** and **sarcomatoid renal cell carcinoma**.

Papillary Renal Carcinoma

This is not associated with any abnormalities of the short arm of chromosome 3. Trisomy of chromosomes 7 and 17, and loss of the Y chromosome, which are not seen in non-papillary tumours are, however, present. These tumours tend to undergo a much greater degree of necrosis than is usually seen in renal cell carcinoma and have a somewhat **better** prognosis, probably because they tend to spread more slowly.

On microscopic examination most of the structure of these lesions is clearly papillary, the papillae consisting of stalks of vascularized connective tissue covered by tubular epithelium. The connective tissue stalks often show the presence of large numbers of lipid–laden macrophages. The immunohistochemical profile suggests an origin from the distal tubule.

Sarcomatoid Renal Cell Carcinoma

This accounts for about 2% of renal cell carcinomas.

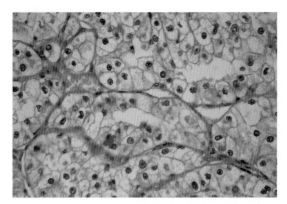

FIGURE 36.45 Renal cell carcinoma. This section shows the typical clear cell appearance of many renal cell carcinomas.

These tumours consist largely of malignant spindle cells in which many mitoses may be present. Some part of the papillary tumours usually shows the presence of ordinary clear cell or granular cell epithelium. The prognosis for this variant is very poor.

It has been suggested that differentiation between the various types of renal epithelial tumour may be made purely by using genetic criteria referred to above.

Staging

Staging of renal cell carcinoma gives more prognostic information than any other single criterion. A number of different systems are employed, one of which is illustrated in *Table 36.24*. **The single most important prognostic factor in staging is whether the tumour has invaded the perinephric tissues or not.**

Spread

The most common sites for metastasis are the:
- **lungs** (30%)
- **bone** (35%)

- **regional lymph nodes**
- **liver**
- **adrenals**
- **brain**

However, virtually **any** tissue may be involved.

The average 5-year survival rate is 45%: 70% in those with no evidence of metastasis and only 10–15% in patients with evidence of renal vein invasion or direct spread into the perinephric fat.

Complications

Apart from the systemic manifestations of renal carcinoma listed above, and the effects related to metastases, patients with renal carcinoma may develop:
- **Reactive systemic amyloidosis.** This occurs in about 3% of cases. This incidence is strikingly greater than is the case with other cancers, where this complication is seen in only 0.1–0.4%.
- **Mesangial proliferative glomerulonephritis.** This is seen fairly often in the uninvolved part of the kidney in nephrectomy specimens from patients with renal carcinoma. A mild proteinuria may be present; more often the glomerular changes are not associated with clinical abnormality.

Renal Oncocytoma

The term oncocyte is applied to a tumour cell with large amounts of eosinophilic, finely granular cytoplasm; the granules are mitochondria. A renal tumour composed predominantly of such cells is termed an **oncocytoma**.

Oncocytomas are three times as common in males as in females and generally behave in a benign fashion. There are no diagnostic cytogenetic changes.

> ### Macroscopic Features
> The tumours are well circumscribed and tan coloured. The cut surface often shows a central area of scarring and dilated vessels are seen at the periphery.

TABLE 36.24 Staging of Renal Cell Carcinoma: Robson's Method

Stage	Spread	5-year survival rate (%)	10-year survival rate (%)
I	Confined to kidney	65	56
II	Through renal capsule but not through renal fascia (Gerota's fascia)	47	20
III	Into regional lymph nodes or renal vein or both without involvement of perinephric fat	51	37
IV	Distant site metastases or through Gerota's fascia to involve neighbouring structures	8	7

Microscopic Features

Microscopic examination shows sheets and islands of large cells, with central nuclei and abundant granular cytoplasm (*Fig. 36.46*). Electron microscopy shows the granules to be abnormally large mitochondria, present in very large numbers.

In most instances, the distinction between oncocytoma and renal cell carcinoma is made relatively easily on microscopic examination. Because the natural history of these two tumours is very different, this distinction is important. Apart from electron microscopy, immunocytochemistry may be of help. Most renal cell carcinomas express vimentin, whereas oncocytomas express only cytokeratins.

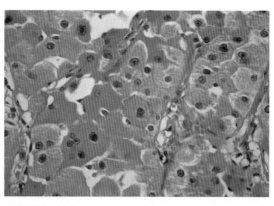

FIGURE 36.46 Renal oncocytoma. The cells are large, eosinophilic and granular. This last feature is due to the presence of many mitochondria.

Nephroblastoma (Wilms' Tumour)

Nephroblastoma is the commonest renal tumour of childhood and constitutes 6% of all malignancies in children between the ages of 0 and 14 years. Peak incidence is 1–4 years, but occasionally adults are affected.

Some children with nephroblastoma show other abnormalities such as aniridia (absence of the iris) (1%) and genitourinary abnormalities (5%).

Predisposing Factors

Some conditions associated with Wilms' tumour are shown in *Table 36.25*.

Cytogenetic Features

A number of chromosome abnormalities has been described in these children. One of the most interesting is a deletion of material in the short arm of chromosome 11 (11p13). This deletion, like that described in association with retinoblastoma on the long arm of chromosome 13, is believed to be associated with loss of tumour suppressor gene activity. Cell lines cultured from nephroblastomas are tumorigenic when injected into congenitally immunodeficient mice ('nude mice'). Cell lines transfected with DNA prepared from the short arms of normal chromosome 11 lose their tumorigenicity.

Table 36.25 Conditions Associated with Wilms' Tumour

Condition	Finding
Aniridia	Absence of iris may be complete or partial
Hemihypertrophy	Increase in size of whole of one side of body or part of one side
Pseudohermaphroditism and Drash syndrome	Male pseudohermaphroditism Diffuse mesangial scarring leading to the nephrotic syndrome
Beckwith–Wiedemann syndrome	Trisomy 11 Exomphalos (defect of anterior abdominal wall in region of umbilicus) Macroglossia Hydramnios Prematurity Gigantism
Familial Wilms' tumour	Anomalies of chromosome 11p
Nephroblastomatosis	Abnormal persistence in kidney of renal blastemal cells with neoplastic potential. This is found at post-mortem examination in 1% of infants dying before the age of 3 months. It is present in 20–40% of kidneys with Wilms' tumours.

Clinical Features

Affected children usually present with an **abdominal mass, fever** and **abdominal pain**; the commonest of these is an abdominal mass. In many patients there are already detectable pulmonary metastases at the time of presentation. Until fairly recently the prognosis was poor (5-year survival rate 10–40%) but the introduction of combined surgery, radiotherapy and chemotherapy has produced strikingly better results (see *Table 36.26*).

Macroscopic Features

Lesions are large greyish-white masses which grow in an expansile fashion, becoming so large in some cases as to exceed greatly the size of the kidney from which they arise. They are usually unilateral but a small proportion (5–10%) are bilateral.

Microscopic Features

The classical or triphasic nephroblastoma has three components: **blastema, stroma** and **epithelium** (*Fig. 36.47*). Within this pattern there is considerable variation. The stroma may show evidence of connective tissue differentiation in the form of **striated muscle, cartilage, bone** or **adipose tissue**, and the epithelial component is represented by primitive tubules set in a spindle-cell background. Occasionally poorly formed glomeruli may be seen. **Marked atypia in the stromal elements and extension through the kidney capsule are features that indicate a poorer than usual prognosis.**

Some variations of nephroblastoma have been described and there are also renal tumours of childhood arising from mesenchyme rather than nephrogenic blastema, described below.

Congenital Mesoblastic Nephroma

This is a rare tumour (3% of renal tumours in childhood) that tends to occur in the first few months of life. Affected children usually present with a large intra-abdominal mass, which may be present at birth.

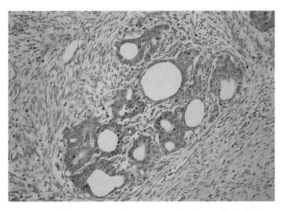

FIGURE 36.47 *Wilms' tumour (nephroblastoma). The section shows ill-formed tubules set against the background of a very cellular, primitive-looking, connective tissue stroma.*

The tumour consists of spindle cells arranged in sheets, between which collagen fibres are present. Most of the tumour cells are fibroblasts but some evidence of smooth muscle differentiation may be seen.

Prognosis is good if the tumour is removed with a rim of normal kidney.

Rhabdoid Tumour of the Kidney

This, too, is a rare lesion (2% of renal tumours in childhood). It occurs early in life (within the first year) and, unlike Wilms' tumour, is highly malignant, carrying a very poor prognosis. More than 75% of affected children die within 2 years. It may in some instances be associated with a coincident medulloblastoma of the cerebellum. Males are more often affected than females.

The tumour is composed of cells that have abundant cytoplasm, often containing hyaline inclusions. Electron microscopy shows these to consist of twisted bundles of intermediate cytoskeletal filaments. Despite the name 'rhabdoid', which suggests muscle differentiation, there is no immunohistochemical or electron microscopic evidence of this.

Table 36.26 Staging of Nephroblastoma. National Wilms' Tumour Study (USA)

Stage	Extent of spread	4-year survival rate (%)
I	Confined to kidney and excised completely	96.5
II	Tumour extends through renal capsule, with or without invasion of renal vein or involvement of periaortic nodes. No residual tumour after resection	92.2
III	Residual tumour confined to abdomen. No evidence of blood spread	86.9
IV	Blood-borne metastases present	73
V	Bilateral kidney tumours	76 (3-year survival rate)

Clear Cell Sarcoma of the Kidney

This tumour accounts for 4% of primary renal tumours in childhood. On microscopic examination, the tumour cell population is seen to be composed of islands of polygonal cells with small rounded nuclei and rather vacuolated cytoplasm with indistinct boundaries between the cells.

Characteristically, this tumour spreads widely via both the bloodstream and the lymphatics, and metastases to bone are frequent, unlike nephroblastoma. This has led to use of the synonym 'bone-metastasizing renal tumour of childhood'.

Urothelial Tumours of the Pelvis and Ureter

Approximately 5–10% of renal tumours arise from the transitional epithelium of the pelvis. These lesions are more or less identical with the much more common urothelial tumours of the bladder, and span the same gamut of appearances:

- papillary or solid
- well, moderately or poorly differentiated
- invasive or non-invasive

Associated aetiological factors are the same as for bladder cancer, with the exception of a marked increase in risk associated with analgesic-related nephropathy and so-called Balkan nephropathy (see p 672).

geneic kidney grafts are the morphological expression of one or more of the factors shown in the box.

> **KEY POINTS: Findings in Patients with Allogeneic Kidney Grafts**
>
> - presence or absence of **signs of immunological rejection** of the graft
> - **changes that may have occurred in the kidney before it was transplanted.** These are usually the result of ischaemia, the morphological correlate of which is tubular necrosis
> - **changes due to the immunosuppressive drugs used to inhibit rejection**
> - changes **associated with any pre-existing disease in the donor kidney**
> - **changes associated with the development in the donor kidney of a pre-existing disease in the recipient.** Thus, various forms of glomerulonephritis may be transmitted to the donor kidney, the most common of these, in descending order, being linear dense deposit disease, immunoglobulin A nephropathy, mesangiocapillary (type I), and focal segmental glomerulosclerosis. If the transplantation was carried out because of renal failure due to amyloidosis, amyloid may be deposited in the donor kidney
> - **changes associated with the development of a new disease in the donor kidney after transplantation**

Pathology of Renal Transplantation

Many, if not most, patients with chronic renal failure are suitable for renal transplantation, the greatest limiting factor being the shortage of donor kidneys.

In a small number of cases, the donors and recipients are identical twins. Under these circumstances, the grafts are known as **syngeneic** or **isografts** because the donor and recipient are identical in their genetic make-up.

The donors, in the vast majority of renal transplants, are to some extent genetically distinct from the recipients and, in this instance, the grafts are called **allogeneic** or **allografts**. It is inevitable that allografts will elicit an immune response on the part of the recipient and this response, if severe, will lead to the destruction of the transplanted kidney as a functioning organ (**rejection**). Rejection may be rapid or may occur over months or even years, and for a transplanted kidney to continue functioning efficiently the recipient will require continuing treatment with one or a combination of immunosuppressive drugs, the most widely used of which is cyclosporin A.

The histological changes seen in biopsies of allo-

REJECTION

The basis of rejection is the recognition by the recipient's immune system of a group of glycoprotein antigens on the surface of the donor cells known as **histocompatibility antigens**. In some ways, this is a misleading name because it obscures the fact that these antigens play a vital role in the regulation of immune responses in general.

The principal histocompatibility antigens are governed by a set of genes known as the **major histocompatibility complex (MHC)**, located on the short arm of chromosome 6.

The MHC complex encodes three major sets of molecules, known as class I, II and III antigens.

Class I antigens are present on the surface of most nucleated cells and there are three loci, A, B and C, at which these antigens are coded. The A and B gene products act as cell-surface recognition markers for cytotoxic T cells. They usually present viral antigen on the surface of infected cells, thus enabling the cytotoxic T cells (CD8) to eliminate the virus by destroying the infected cells. In kidney grafts, class I antigens are present on the vascular endothelium, on tubular epithelium and on interstitial and mesangial cells.

Human **class II antigens** are classified into three

subgroups related to specific regions on the chromosome. These are DP, DQ and DR. The antigens themselves are normally displayed on antigen-presenting cells. In renal transplantation, it is more important in the avoidance of graft rejection to match class II antigens as closely as possible between donor and recipient than it is to have a close match in respect of class I antigens. In the kidney, class II antigens are expressed on capillary endothelium, on mesangial cells, on proximal tubular epithelium in about 70% of the population, and on dendritic cells within the interstitial tissue.

The MHC is not the only antigen-encoding system that is important in determining whether a renal graft survives or is rejected. **The ABO red cell antigen system** acts in a similar way, as does a non-human leucocyte antigen (HLA)-encoded system on human endothelial cells, and there are probably many histocompatibility antigens that are yet to be discovered.

The products of the MHC show a marked degree of polymorphism and it is virtually impossible, other than in the identical twin donor–recipient situation, to obtain a complete match of the MHC-encoded antigens. Nevertheless, the closer the match in respect of the histocompatibility antigens, the greater the chances of long survival of the graft.

Before the introduction of cyclosporin A for the suppression of graft rejection, it was noted that the chances of graft survival were increased if the recipient had had several blood transfusions before transplantation took place. The mechanism for this is not understood, although it is likely that the repeated transfusions induced a degree of immunological unresponsiveness. Now that cyclosporin A is so widely used in the treatment of graft recipients, the differences between transfused and non-transfused patients in respect of graft survival appear to be insignificant.

PATTERNS OF REJECTION
Rejection is usually classified on the basis of the length of time that passes before the transplanted kidney shows evidence of dysfunction.

Thus rejection may be:
- **hyperacute**, in which the graft may be rejected within minutes or hours
- **acute**, usually occurring within the first few weeks of the life of the graft
- **chronic**, usually manifesting some months or even years after transplantation. It may follow several episodes of acute rejection or may appear as an insidious decline in the function of the transplanted kidney with no history of acute rejection episodes.

Hyperacute Rejection
Hyperacute rejection is fortunately rare (0.5% of all rejections). It reflects the presence, at the time of transplantation, of circulating antibodies within the plasma of the recipient which bind to antigens on the endothelial cells of vessels in the donor kidney. Such antibodies may be due to:
- ABO incompatibility
- previous loss of a renal allograft by rejection
- immunization by blood transfusion of a woman during a previous pregnancy

Binding of the recipient antibodies to donor endothelium activates complement and this in turn activates platelets and the clotting system, leading to occlusion of the vessels in the transplanted kidney and to ischaemic cortical necrosis. The process is irreversible and the failed graft must be removed.

The events of hyperacute rejection are, in morphological terms, quite spectacular. The donor kidney, instead of being pink and firm as it is perfused by the recipient's blood, becomes blue, mottled and flabby. Angiography shows occlusion of the intrarenal small vessels and, over the next day or so, complete cortical necrosis develops.

Light microscopic examination of biopsy specimens shows extensive occlusion of the small vessels by fibrin and platelets, this process extending into the glomeruli. Immunohistology shows immunoglobulin (Ig) G and C3 bound to the endothelial surfaces of the small blood vessels.

Acute Rejection
Acute rejection is common. A kidney showing acute rejection is not necessarily doomed to fail and many patients have one or more acute rejection episodes during the first few weeks after transplantation.

Acute rejection manifests in a number of ways. These include:
- oliguria
- a rise in serum creatinine concentration (which may be the only evidence of rejection)
- fever
- some swelling and tenderness of the kidney
- the presence in the urine of protein, lymphocytes, tubular epithelial cells and interleukin (IL) 2.

Unlike hyperacute rejection, which is entirely antibody mediated, the mechanisms involved in acute rejection are diverse and renal biopsy can be a helpful guide both to the pathogenesis and the progress of the kidney following treatment for the rejection. Thus, acute rejection can be the result of:
- **a cellular response mediated via recipient T cells.** The principal targets for such a reaction are the tubules and the interstitial tissues. Light microscopic examination of renal biopsies shows severe oedema of the interstitial tissue, associated with a dense mononuclear cell infiltrate. Many grafts that are not undergoing rejection show some cells in the interstitium, but the infiltrate seen in rejection episodes is much more extensive and severe. The T lymphocytes and macrophages that make up the infiltrate are often seen to be invading

the walls of the tubules and evidence of tubular necrosis (see pp 681–683) is frequently present. Immunohistological examination shows the T cells to be activated and to be producing IL-2 as well as other activation and proliferation markers.

The reaction occurs because of a reaction on the part of the recipient's T cells to antigens presented on donor vascular endothelium and on dendritic cells present in the donor kidney interstitium. There is no evidence of binding of either IgG or C3. Recognition of donor antigens by recipient T helper cells is followed by the release of a number of lymphokines including IL-2. IL-2 is not synthesized by cytotoxic T cells and, therefore, a cytotoxic T-cell response in acute rejection depends on IL-2 synthesis by the B cells. In this connection, it is not without interest that the most effective immunosuppressive drug in common use, cyclosporin A, inhibits the synthesis of IL-2 and the expression of HLA class II antigens (see p 146).

- **an acute vascular response mediated by antibody.** The clinical and laboratory findings are, for the most part, identical with those of acute cellular rejection, but an additional feature, seen in some instances, is platelet sequestration within the transplanted kidney.

Cell infiltration in this type of rejection, is concentrated on and between the vascular endothelial cells of the donor kidney. In severe cases, small blood vessels show fibrinoid necrosis extending into glomerular capillary tufts with resulting thrombosis. IgG and IgM antibodies are often found to be bound to the donor endothelium, as are C1q and C3 components of complement. **The presence of the former suggests classical pathway activation of the complement system.**

While it is clear that an antibody-mediated reaction with subsequent complement activation occurs, it is likely that T cells are also involved (CD8 cells are found in relation to the damaged endothelium). Once there is evidence of fibrinoid necrosis and/or thrombosis in the small blood vessels and glomerular capillaries, the outlook for long-term survival of the graft is bleak.

- **acute transplant glomerulopathy.** About 4–10% of allogeneic kidney transplants develop a rather characteristic lesion in the glomeruli of the donor kidney. Clinically, the patient presents with evidence of an acute rejection episode, no different from any other.

The affected glomeruli show occlusion of the capillary lumina by swollen endothelial cells and mononuclear inflammatory cells. This glomerular lesion is often accompanied by evidence of tubulointerstitial rejection or, in a minority of cases, by signs of vascular rejection. The pathogenesis is not known.

Chronic Rejection

Chronic rejection is responsible for about 8% of the kidneys rejected in the first year after transplantation and for the vast majority of those rejected at a later stage. Because it is basically ischaemic in nature, it is not surprising that most of the affected patients become hypertensive.

Macroscopic and Microscopic Features

The archetypal pathological changes are:
- thickening of the intima of the intrarenal arteries with eventual obliteration of their lumina; and/or
- thickening of the walls of the glomerular capillaries

Arterial Changes in Chronic Vascular Rejection

The arteries most commonly affected are the arcuate and interlobular arteries. The intima is grossly thickened, the whole circumference of the vessel wall being involved. The intimal thickening is due partly to the presence of cells and partly to connective tissue, which is rich in mucins. Lipid-laden macrophages are also present.

As the lesion ages, so the amount of collagen in the intima increases and the vessels become stiff and non-compliant. The pathogenesis of this arterial lesion is unclear. There is no direct evidence for the involvement of immune mechanisms but, equally, there is no doubt that the closer the match between donor and recipient in terms of histocompatibility antigens, the lower is the risk of chronic vascular rejection.

Serial renal biopsies have shown that development of the intimal thickening of chronic vascular rejection is associated with the presence of mural thrombi on the endothelial surface of the affected vessels. This tells us two things:

1) The chronic vascular changes are likely to be due to continuing or recurrent endothelial injury leading to the formation of these thrombi in the affected vessels.
2) The intimal thickening itself is likely to be mediated by growth factors released from the thrombi.

Glomerular Changes in Chronic Rejection

Glomerular damage as part of chronic transplant rejection occurs in about 4% of all grafted kidneys. Clinically, it is expressed in the form of a moderately heavy proteinuria (greater than 1 g per day) and the loss of protein may be so great as to lead to the nephrotic syndrome.

On light microscopy of renal biopsy material, the walls of the glomerular capillaries are seen to be thickened, due in part to widening of the subendothelial region with interposition of mesangial cell cytoplasm. This results in a double-contour basement membrane similar to that of mesangiocapillary glomerulonephritis.

In addition, there is some increase in the mesangial matrix and mesangial cell population.

Effects of Immunosuppressive Treatment

The survival of renal allografts depends, in the vast majority of cases, on adequate immunosuppression. Such immunosuppression is not without problems, which may be caused in a number of ways and have a number of effects.

Nephrotoxicity

There may be a direct nephrotoxic effect of the immunosuppressive agent. Cyclosporin A, for example, can cause acute nephrotoxicity at high dose levels. In such cases there may be vacuole formation in the cells of the proximal tubules and hyalinization of arterioles.

Chronic nephrotoxicity can also occur as a result of cyclosporin treatment. This takes the form of interstitial fibrosis and tubular atrophy. The fibrosis shows a peculiar 'striped' pattern, focal in distribution.

The use of antilymphocyte globulin to combat rejection occasionally leads to serum sickness associated with a diffuse endocapillary proliferative glomerulonephritis similar to that which can occur after streptococcal infection.

Infection

Immunosuppression must increase the risk of infection. Any variety of infectious agent may be involved. Viral inclusions may be seen, the commonest of these being the result of cytomegalovirus infections.

Hypertension

Hypertension is quite common in postrenal transplant patients, being seen in about 50%. It has been suggested that cyclosporin may contribute to this. The vasoconstriction associated with cyclosporin does not appear to be due to action by the renin–angiotensin system and is responsive to restriction of the patient's sodium intake.

Hyperlipidaemia

Hyperlipidaemia is seen in about 60% of post-transplant patients. The hyperlipidaemia is of the combined type: both cholesterol and triglyceride are increased.

Because post-transplant patients have both hyperlipidaemia and high blood pressure, it is not surprising that they show an increased risk of cardiovascular events; such events are responsible for 30% of the deaths that occur in these patients.

Post-Transplant Neoplasia

The concept that immunosurveillance may play a role in inhibiting the development of malignant neoplasms gains some support from the fact that post-transplant patients have an increased incidence of such tumours. In order of frequency, the tumours that complicate renal transplantation are:

1) squamous carcinoma of the skin
2) B-cell lymphomas, especially those associated with infection by the Epstein–Barr virus
3) Kaposi's sarcoma
4) cancer of the cervix uteri

CHAPTER 37

The Lower Urinary Tract

The Urinary Bladder

NORMAL ANATOMY

The bladder is a largely extraperitoneal organ, chiefly endodermal in origin. Its lining is a specialized type of transitional epithelium, the **urothelium**.

The Urothelium

The urothelium consists of three layers:

1) A superficial layer composed of large flat cells which cover a considerable area of the underlying epithelium and are known as **umbrella cells**.

2) An intermediate zone which may be up to four cells thick when the bladder is contracted. The cells have their long axes perpendicular to the basement membrane of the urothelium in the contracted bladder but flatten out on distension.

3) A basal layer made up of cuboidal cells, which become flattened and difficult to see when the bladder is distended.

Some Common Urothelial Variants

Morphological variation is common (*Fig. 37.1*):

- **Brunn's nests.** These are invaginations of the urothelium into the underlying connective tissue. They begin as little areas of budding from the basal layer. Loss of continuity with the surface epithelium leads to their appearing as epithelial islands in the lamina propria.

- **Cystitis cystica.** Breakdown of the centres of the solid Brunn's nests may occur with resulting cyst formation. This histological picture is known as **cystitis cystica**.

- **Cystitis glandularis.** Epithelial metaplasia can occur in foci of cystitis cystica. The cells become cuboidal or columnar and some undergo goblet cell change and secrete mucin. These spaces resemble large intestinal crypts, the condition being termed **intestinal metaplasia** or **cystitis glandularis**.

- **Squamous metaplasia.** Squamous metaplasia is common especially in the region of the trigone in women. It is believed to be related to levels of oestrogen. Squamous metaplasia, associated with keratinization, can also occur as a result of chronic irritation.

- **Adenomatous metaplasia (also known as nephrogenic adenoma).** This is most often found in patients with recurrent inflammation, bladder stones or repeated catheterization. Cystoscopy shows small, sometimes polypoid, nodules. Microscopy shows solid clusters of cells or small gland-like spaces within the lamina propria. The lesion is not neoplastic and behaves benignly. It is important that it is not misdiagnosed as carcinoma.

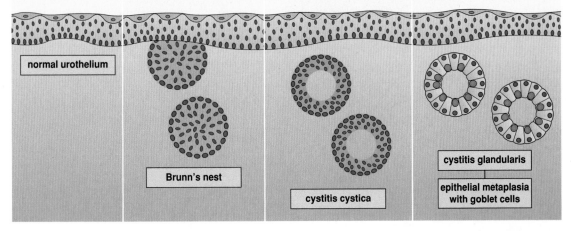

FIGURE 37.1 Common urothelial variants in the bladder.

The Lamina Propria

Beneath the urothelium is a well-vascularized connective tissue zone, the lamina propria. Its connective tissue fibres are loosely arranged, allowing folding of the urothelium when the bladder is relaxed and empty. Some smooth muscle fibres are often present and, in some instances, these form a continuous layer, constituting a muscularis mucosae.

Muscularis Propria

Apart from the bladder neck, where it is possible to discern three layers of muscle – an inner and outer longitudinal layer and a central circular layer – the muscle layers mix freely and have no definite orientation. They are separated from each other by well-vascularized connective tissue. The muscle fibres make up the detrusor muscle, reflex contraction of which, combined with relaxation of the outlet sphincters, is essential for normal micturition. In various neurological disorders, the detrusor–sphincter coordination is lost. The bladder becomes over-distended and overflow incontinence and incomplete emptying results. **The presence of a substantial volume of residual urine after micturition is a major risk factor for infection of both the lower and upper parts of the urinary tract.**

OBSTRUCTION TO THE OUTFLOW OF URINE FROM THE BLADDER

This serious disturbance of normal function may be due to:

- **some morphologically identifiable abnormality which may be congenital or acquired** (*Fig. 37.2*)**. Such lesions include:**

  1) **prostate enlargement** (*Fig. 37.3*) in middle-aged and elderly men
  2) **an acquired urethral stricture** due to previous inflammation
  3) **congenital urethral valves** in children

- **functional causes of obstruction related to the nervous system and including such entities as:**

  1) **spina bifida**
  2) **degenerative disorders such as multiple sclerosis** and tabes dorsalis
  3) **spinal cord damage** associated with tumour or trauma

Bladder Changes Resulting From Obstruction

In the short term, outflow obstruction causes bladder dilatation. Later, a combination of muscle hypertrophy and an increase in interstitial fibrous tissue is seen. Because of the arrangement of the muscle fibres, this hypertrophy causes the bladder lining to appear trabeculated, and diverticula may develop between these trabeculae (*Fig 37.4*).

In the still longer term, as a result of the sustained high intravesical pressure, decompensation occurs and the bladder dilates again. This may extend to involve the ureters as well (**hydroureter**). Reflux of urine into the ureters may occur, with a consequent risk of infection.

DEVELOPMENTAL ABNORMALITIES

Several congenital anomalies have been described, the most important of which are **exstrophy of the bladder** and **congenital abnormality of the urachus**.

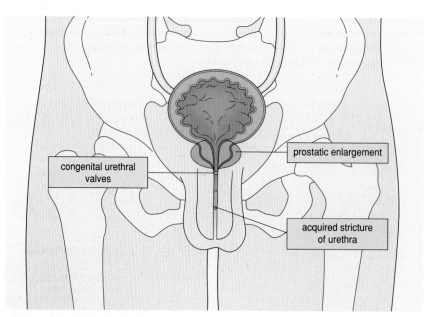

FIGURE 37.2 Structural causes of obstruction to urine outflow from the bladder.

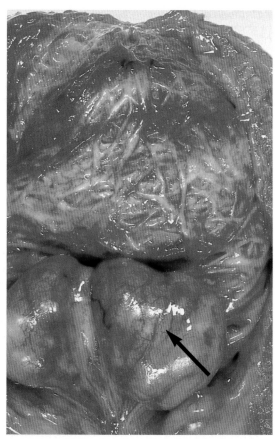

FIGURE 37.3 *Obstruction caused by markedly enlarged prostate (arrow). Note the trabeculated appearance of the bladder wall caused by hypertrophy of the detrusor muscle.*

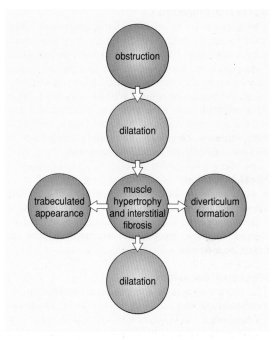

FIGURE 37.4 *Sequence of changes in the bladder, resulting from obstruction.*

Exstrophy of the Bladder

Exstrophy is defined as a set of conditions that arise from a failure of the mesoderm to migrate normally into the cloacal membrane to reach the midline. The anterior wall of the bladder and that part of the anterior abdominal wall lying below the umbilicus fail to develop. It is rare, occurring in 1 in 20 000–40 000 live births. It is commoner in males than in females, the male : female ratio being 2 : 1.

In its most severe form, the bladder, lacking its anterior wall, presents as a reddened mass on the anterior abdominal wall with the trigone and ureteric orifices occupying the lower part of the exposed surface. In males, the penis also shows anomalies, often being very small and being open on the anterior surface (**epispadias**). In females, the clitoris shows analogous abnormalities. In both sexes there is failure in normal development of the symphysis pubis and the resulting separation of the pubes leads to an abnormal 'waddling' type of gait.

The mucosa is exposed to recurrent trauma and infection, and inflammation is always present with consequent squamous or glandular metaplasia of the surface epithelium. Infection may extend to involve the upper urinary tract and this is an important cause of death in untreated patients.

In those who survive into adult life, carcinoma may supervene. This is most often adenocarcinoma rather than the usual transitional cell variety.

Abnormalities Related to the Urachus

In embryonic life the urachus connects the urogenital sinus to the allantois via the umbilicus. In adults, the urachus persists as a midline fibrous band stretching between the apex of the bladder and the umbilicus. Urachal abnormalities are of two types:

- **persistence of part or all of the urachal lumen.** If the whole length of the urachus is patent, urine will leak from the umbilicus. Patency at the umbilical end leads to the formation of a urachal sinus, whereas patency at the bladder end gives rise to a diverticulum projecting from the bladder. Patency of the central part constitutes only a urachal cyst.
- **tumour formation.** Tumours arise from the epithelial lining of the urachus and may be benign (adenoma) or malignant (adenocarcinoma).

INFLAMMATORY DISORDERS OF THE BLADDER: CYSTITIS

Inflammation in the bladder may be acute or chronic and can be caused by infection or other agents such as chemicals or trauma.

Bacterial Infection

This is common: about 20–30% of women will have acute bacterial cystitis at some time. Urine is normally sterile and the bladder is resistant to infection. Pathogenic organisms within the bladder are usually derived from the urethra, which becomes contaminated by faecal organisms. Women are much more often affected than men, owing to anatomical factors such as the close relationship of the female urethra to the perineum. Organisms commonly implicated are *Escherichia coli*, *Proteus* and *Klebsiella* species.

Viral Infection

A number of viruses can cause cystitis. These include **adenovirus type II**, which has been reported in patients with bone marrow transplants, and, in children, **herpes simplex, herpes zoster, papovavirus** and **cytomegalovirus**.

Metazoal Parasites

The most important of these is infestation by **Schistosome** ova. In the urinary tract *Schistosoma haematobium* is most common.

S. haematobium is found in the Nile and many other African rivers in which the host for the asexual cycle of *Schistosoma* is a freshwater snail, *Bulinus contortus*. The asexual cycle within the snail culminates in the release of large numbers of motile larvae known as **cercariae** into the water. These secrete a cytolytic compound which allows them to penetrate the epidermis of humans who walk or swim in the infested water. Maturation takes place in the portal circulation. From here, the schistosomes migrate in the systemic circulation. The adult worms themselves do not injure the host tissues, but their ova elicit a florid granulomatous reaction.

Cystoscopy shows a granular bladder mucosa. Microscopic examination shows the presence of numerous granulomas and an infiltrate in which eosinophils are prominent. The diagnosis is made by seeing the ova in the lamina propria. They are elliptical in shape and *S. haematobium* has a characteristic terminal spine.

An important late complication of schistosomiasis of the bladder is carcinoma, which is extremely common in areas in which schistosomiasis is endemic, such as Egypt. The tumours appear at an earlier age than do the transitional bladder cancers seen in the West, and are usually well-differentiated squamous carcinomas. There is no evidence that either the worms or the ova exert a direct oncogenic effect on the bladder. Schistosomiasis tends to be associated with chronic bacterial cystitis, and urinalysis shows the presence of potentially carcinogenic nitrosamines derived from breakdown of nitrites and nitrates in the urine by bacteria.

Non-infective Cystitis

This may be caused by chemical irritants, drugs (such as cyclophosphamide), irradiation and trauma.

Pathological Features

In **acute cystitis** the mucosa appears red and velvety. Biopsies show the expected features of acute inflammation (i.e. oedema, dilatation of blood vessels and an acute inflammatory infiltrate in which neutrophils are most prominent).

In more severe cases, the epithelium may show areas of ulceration and the acute inflammatory reaction may spread to involve the muscle layer.

In **chronic cystitis** due to either persistent or recurrent infections, the urothelium is thickened and may have undergone squamous metaplasia. The underlying lamina propria shows scarring and is infiltrated by a mixed chronic inflammatory cell infiltrate.

Some variants of chronic cystitis have been described:

- **follicular cystitis**, characterized by the presence of aggregates of lymphoid cells in the lamina propria, some of which show germinal centres
- **haemorrhagic cystitis**, seen most commonly after treatment with the antitumour agent, cyclophosphamide
- **eosinophilic cystitis**, a rare condition occurring in children and young adults in the context of allergy and accompanied by a high blood eosinophil count. It occurs occasionally in elderly males with a history of prostatic disease.
- **malakoplakia** (Gk. *malakos* soft; *plakia* plaque), a curious chronic granulomatous disease occurring most commonly in the bladder, but also in the upper urinary tract, retroperitoneal tissues, genitalia and gastrointestinal tract. Peak incidence is in the sixth decade and there is a marked predilection for females (F:M ratio 4 : 1). Soft yellowish-brown mucosal plaques are present.

  On microscopy the lamina propria is seen to be infiltrated by large eosinophilic macrophages. Small, target-shaped, bluish, concentric bodies are found both within the macrophages and extracellularly. These contain iron and calcium and periodic acid–Schiff-positive material indicating the presence of 1 : 2 glycol groups. These characteristic bodies are known as **Michaelis–Gutmann bodies** and are thought to represent partially degraded bacteria in phagolysosomes. The pathogenesis of this unusual tissue response is not known.
- **interstitial cystitis**, a chronic inflammatory disorder of the bladder, affecting chiefly middle-aged and elderly women. Clinical features are:
  1) frequency of micturition
  2) suprapubic discomfort
  3) pain which may be pelvic, suprapubic or perineal
  4) dyspareunia

  Two forms of interstitial cystitis are now recognized:
  1) **an ulcerated form known as Hunner's ulcer** in which the urothelium shows the presence

of ulcers from which bleeding occurs when the bladder is distended. This form accounts for about 10% of cases.

2) **a non-ulcerated variety in which there is marked scarring, associated with a mixed inflammatory cell infiltrate in which mast cells are prominent.**

There is no agreement as to the cause or causes of this distressing condition.

CANCER OF THE BLADDER

More than 95% of bladder tumours are epithelial, arising from the urothelium. Of these, **the commonest by far is transitional cell carcinoma of the bladder,** although several other tumour types are recognized (see *Table 37.1*). As the urothelium lines not only the bladder but also the ureters, renal pelves and part of the urethra, what is described here in relation to the bladder applies equally to urothelial tumours in these other sites.

Prevalence and Incidence

In the UK, bladder cancer accounts for 4–7% of malignant tumours in males and for 2–3% of those occurring in females. In Egypt, bladder cancer (mostly squamous cell carcinoma) accounts for 11% of all cases of malignant disease, this being related to the high prevalence of schistosomiasis (see p 712). Apart from countries where schistosomiasis is endemic, bladder cancer is rare in the first five decades of life, but after this age the incidence rises steeply. Bladder cancer may be compatible with long survival, and only about 50% of patients with bladder cancer die from their disease.

The natural history of transitional cell cancer suggests that it is not a single disease; there appear to be two groups of patients, with distinct natural histories. These are:

Table 37.1 World Health Organization Classification of Bladder Tumours

Epithelial tumours
  Transitional cell papilloma
  Inverted type of transitional cell papilloma
  Transitional cell carcinoma
  Transitional cell carcinoma with glandular or
  squamous elements
  Squamous cell carcinoma
  Adenocarcinoma
  Undifferentiated carcinoma

Non-epithelial tumours
  Benign: leiomyoma, neurofibroma, haemangioma
  Malignant: rhabdomyosarcoma, etc.

- patients with superficial patterns of growth
- patients with tumours that invade deeply into muscle

Superficial Disease

Some 70% of patients with bladder cancer present with superficial papillary tumours. Of these, 80% will experience recurrence of tumour after treatment, but only 10–30% will develop deeply invasive tumours and very few will die from metastatic disease. Patients with initially superficial tumours who go on to develop deeply invasive tumours (*Fig. 37.5*) have:

- high-grade carcinomas from the start
- early invasion of the lamina propria
- areas of carcinoma *in situ* associated with papillary tumours

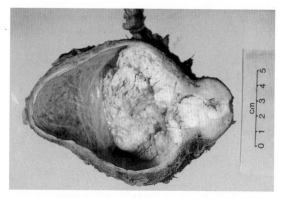

FIGURE 37.5 Large carcinoma of the bladder involving a substantial proportion of the urothelial surface.

Deeply Invasive Tumours

These account for the remaining 30% of patients. Of these, 80% have *no* previous history of superficial papillary lesions.

The tumours are very aggressive and invade deeply into the muscle. If left untreated, death may occur within 2 years and, irrespective of treatment, at least 50% of these patients eventually die as a result of metastases.

Natural History

Despite being confined to the surface urothelium, carcinoma *in situ* has a worse prognosis than superficial papillary carcinoma. The mucosa in carcinoma *in situ* is macroscopically normal. Without treatment muscle invasion will occur in up to 80% of cases, although there are patients with carcinoma *in situ* whose disease remains stable.

The existence of different behaviour patterns suggests that different molecular genetic events may be involved in pathogenesis, and that different combinations and permutations of these may influence biological behaviour.

Chromosomal Changes in Bladder Cancer

Several non-random chromosomal abnormalities have been described in bladder cancer. They may be the expression of activation of oncogenes or inactivation of suppressor genes. They are summarized in *Table 37.2*.

Table 37.2 Chromosome Abnormalities in Bladder Cancer

Chromosome	Abnormality
1	Several abnormalities have been described. It is believed that they are not of primary importance in tumorigenesis and may represent a secondary change.
5	Isochromosome formation affecting the short arm (p) has been reported in 40% of transitional bladder cancers and also in cancers of the cervix, ovary and lung. Isochromosomes arise from transverse division of the centromere during meiosis instead of the normal longitudinal division.
9	Monosomy in respect of this chromosome has been reported in about 50% of superficial papillary tumours. 9q deletions appear to be common in advanced bladder cancer (67%). This deletion has *not* been reported in any other solid tumour to date.
11	Deletions from the short arm (p) of this chromosome have been reported in about 40% of bladder cancers. It is considered by some to represent a secondary change related to **invasiveness**.
17	17p deletions probably related to the *p53* tumour suppressor gene have been reported in 63% of bladder cancers. In bladder cancer, 17p deletions seem to be particularly associated with **invasiveness**.
7	Trisomy of chromosome 7 in a few cases. The c-*erb* gene, which encodes the **receptor for epidermal growth factor**, is sited on this chromosome and **this receptor is expressed in over 80% of invasive bladder cancers and in only 29% of superficial tumours**.

Aetiology

The aetiological factors in the microenvironment relating to bladder cancer can be considered under two headings:

1) the action of some specific chemical carcinogen
2) the effects of chronic inflammation and resulting metaplasia

Chemical Carcinogenesis in Relation to the Urothelium

Occupational Risks

Bladder cancer was one of the first neoplastic diseases in which an industrial association was noted as a result of the high risk of bladder cancer seen in workers in the aniline dye industry. The responsible chemical species is β**-naphthylamine**. This compound is **a remote carcinogen, i.e. it requires to be metabolized before it can exert its effect on target tissues** and, if instilled into the bladder in susceptible species, does not produce tumours. In the liver, the β–naphthylamine is converted to 2-amino-1-naphthol, which is oncogenic, and this is conjugated with glucuronic acid to form a harmless glucuronide. The glucuronide is excreted in the urine, and in the bladder is cleaved by a urothelial glucuronidase, allowing the urothelium to be exposed to the carcinogen.

Other occupations implicated in naphthylamine-mediated bladder cancer include the rubber and cable industries, gas-retort-house working and the chemical industry. It has been estimated that in the USA and the UK up to 20% of bladder cancers may be related to occupation.

Several other chemicals such as methylnitrosourea and *N*-butyl-nitrosamine are bladder carcinogens in animal models, but it is not known whether they cause human disease.

Cigarette Smoking

There is good epidemiological evidence that cigarette smoking is a risk factor for bladder cancer; smokers are 1.5−4 times as liable as non-smokers to develop bladder cancer.

Cyclophosphamide

This is an alkylating agent used in the treatment of certain tumours and also, in some cases, as an immunosuppressive agent. It causes haemorrhagic cystitis (see p 712) and in the long term is associated with an increased risk of bladder cancer.

Analgesics

There is an increased risk of transitional cell carcinoma of the renal pelvis in patients who have taken large amounts of analgesics with a resulting analgesic nephropathy.

Chronic Inflammation

The role of vesical schistosomiasis in relation to the risk of bladder cancer has already been discussed. There is also some increase in risk in patients who have diverticula of the bladder or who have had operations that divert the flow of urine from the bladder to the colon by ureteric transplantation.

Morphological Features of Transitional Cell Carcinoma of the Bladder

Three basic patterns are seen (*Fig. 37.6*):

- **papillary** tumours, which are largely non-invasive
- **solid, non-papillary** tumours, which are generally invasive
- **flat *in-situ*** tumours

Any combination of these three may occur.

Papillary tumours vary in size from small, delicately fronded, lesions to much larger ones with thick papillae. Solid tumours are nodular infiltrative lesions which are often associated with ulceration. In combined papillary and solid tumours, the bladder wall usually shows evidence of infiltration in the region of the tumour stalk. *In situ* tumours appear as localized reddened patches on the bladder mucosa but occur also in macroscopically normal areas.

Pathological examination is aimed at determining the prognosis and best treatment options for an individual patient, and to this end the tumours are **staged** (*Table 37.3* and *Fig. 37.7*) and **graded**.

There are *three* grades of bladder cancer if true papil-

Table 37.3 Staging of Urothelial Cancer

Stage	Finding
P_{is}	Flat preinvasive carcinoma; carcinoma *in situ*
P_a	Papillary non-invasive carcinoma
P_{1a}	Invasion limited to core of papilla
P_{1b}	Invasion of lamina propria
P_2	Superficial muscle invasion
P_{3a}	Deep muscle invasion
P_{3b}	Invasion of tissues around bladder
P_{4a}	Invasion of prostate, uterus or vagina
P_{4b}	Invasion of pelvic or abdominal wall

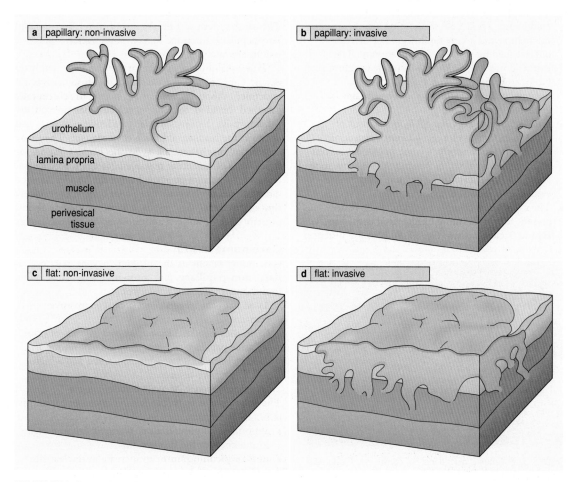

FIGURE 37.6 *Principal morphological variants in bladder cancer.*

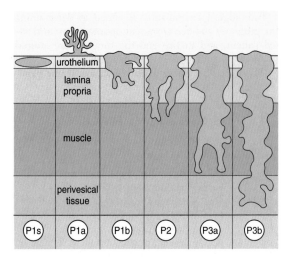

FIGURE 37.7 Local staging of bladder cancer.

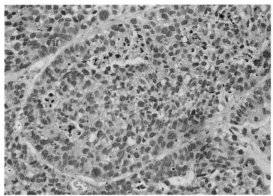

FIGURE 37.9 Poorly differentiated grade 3 carcinoma of the bladder.

lomas, the existence of which is a controversial issue, are excluded:

- **Grade 1 papillary tumours** show an increase in the number of layers of cells in the surface epithelium. These cells show some loss in orientation and a very mild degree of increase in nuclear staining. Mitotic figures are rare. The epithelium is still clearly recognizable as transitional. No invasive foci are seen and, although these tumours may recur, they do not invade the underlying bladder wall.

- **Grade 2 tumours** (*Fig. 37.8*) also consist of epithelium that can be recognized as transitional. Cell proliferation is greater than in grade 1 lesions and there is more loss of normal cell polarity, more variation in nuclear size and staining, and more evidence of mitotic activity.

- The cytological changes mentioned above are present to a much more exaggerated degree in **Grade 3 carcinoma** (*Fig. 37.9*). In some instances

it is no longer possible to recognize the epithelium as being of transitional type. In the superficial layers of the neoplastic urothelium, adhesion between cells is lessened and abnormal cells are exfoliated into the urine, where they may be found on cytological examination.

The same system can be employed in relation to solid non-papillary tumours but, in this variety, grade 1 lesions are rarely encountered.

True squamous carcinomas of the bladder certainly do occur. They are rare in areas where schistosomiasis is not endemic, although they may occur in chronically inflamed bladders. Squamous carcinomas are usually solid invasive lesions. Similarly, adenocarcinomas can occur in the bladder, although they are rare. They may arise from urachal remnants in the bladder fundus or from areas of glandular metaplasia at the bladder base. Such adenocarcinomas at the base of the bladder must be distinguished from invasive prostatic cancer. Fortunately this is relatively easy with antibodies raised against prostate-specific antigen and prostatic acid phosphatase.

Carcinoma *in situ*

Carcinoma *in situ* in the bladder may be regarded as **flat, non-papillary** and **non-invasive**. It may be found under three circumstances:

1) in flat bladder mucosa adjacent to invasive transitional cell carcinoma

2) in the 'normal' bladder mucosa in cases of non-invasive papillary tumour. This is an ominous finding because it presages recurrence and a high risk of invasive disease

3) in the absence of overt bladder cancer

The microscopic features resemble those of carcinoma *in situ* in other sites:

- abnormal cell proliferation, as shown by an increase in thickness of the urothelium

- nuclear pleomorphism, an increase in nuclear size and staining and an increased nuclear : cytoplasmic ratio

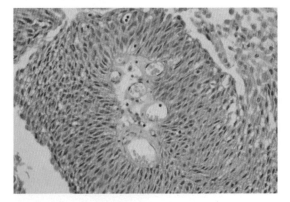

FIGURE 37.8 Grade 2 transitional cell carcinoma. The tumour is moderately well differentiated and still recognizable as transitional epithelium.

- the presence of numerous mitoses

Invasion occurs in 55–80% of cases within 5 years of diagnosis, but some patients survive, apparently well, for 10 years or more.

Disorders of the Urethra

CONGENITAL DISORDERS

Posterior Urethral Valves

This anomaly is the commonest cause of urinary obstruction in infancy and childhood. It occurs almost exclusively in males. In the normal male urethra, the inferior urethral crest represents a continuation in the midline of the verumontanum. This crest ends in two folds near the lower limits of the prostatic urethra. These two folds diverge laterally and anteriorly in the membranous urethra; when they are abnormally large, they balloon forward during the passage of urine, constituting a valvular obstruction.

Clinical Features

The time and type of clinical presentation depend on the severity of the obstruction. Some 50% of affected individuals present within the first year of life, many in the neonatal period. As might be expected, it is these very young children who are most severely affected.

The clinical features include:
- failure to thrive
- vomiting
- easily palpable kidneys and bladder, the bladder, ureters and the pelvicalyceal system being grossly dilated
- retention of urine
- urinary tract infection
- evidence of chronic renal failure

In some very severely affected infants, disruption of the urinary tract with leakage of urine either within the capsule of the kidney or in the retroperitoneal space may occur. The commonest sites for this disastrous complication are:
- at the junction between the renal pelvis and the ureter
- at the junction between the ureter and the bladder

Diagnosis may be most effectively established by a micturating cystogram, which demonstrates the level of obstruction to urine outflow and reflux from the bladder into the ureters. Early diagnosis is important as methods of treatment have improved so much as to lower the mortality rate from this condition from 10–40% overall (50–78% in neonates) to 0–3%.

In older children, the presentation is less severe and more variable; it is usually expressed by problems in voiding urine.

Another type of valve-related obstruction may occur if there is an abnormal concentric diaphragm within the prostatic urethra, but this is rare.

INFLAMMATORY DISORDERS

Gonococcal Urethritis

Urethritis is the earliest manifestation of gonorrhoea, infection with *Neisseria gonorrhoeae* accounting for about one-third of all cases of urethritis.

Adherence of the bacteria to the epithelial surface of the urethra is pivotal for the development of infection. This is accomplished largely through the medium of filamentous appendages (pili) extending from the bacterial surface and binding to sugars in cell surface glycoproteins. Following bacterial attachment, some organisms enter the epithelial cells where they multiply before being released into the subepithelial tissues; others enter the subepithelial tissues directly. Once there, an acute inflammatory reaction is elicited and acute inflammatory cells, fluid exudate and desquamated epithelial cells form the characteristic yellow discharge.

The inflammatory process spreads in the first instance to periurethral glands and may then involve the corpora spongiosa and cavernosa, seminal vesicles, prostate, Cowper's gland, penile lymphatics, inguinal nodes and prepuce.

In the preantibiotic era, the damaged surface epithelium was replaced by stratified squamous epithelium, and the acute inflammatory reaction within the subepithelial space became chronic and eventually scarred leading to urethral **stricture**. Such strictures occurred most commonly in the bulbous urethra, possibly because this is the site of the greatest concentration of periurethral glands, and presented clinically years, even decades, after the original gonococcal infection.

Non-gonococcal Urethritis

Non-gonococcal urethritis (NGU) presents clinically much less dramatically than does gonorrhoea. The patients, usually young men, complain of:
- mild dysuria and frequency of gradual onset
- a clear mucoid urethral discharge

The commonest infective causes of NGU are shown in *Table 37.4*.

Chlamydia trachomatis is isolated from the urethra in 25–58% of cases of NGU, although it is also present in a small proportion of control subjects. Its pathogenic role in NGU is supported by the observation that intraurethral inoculation of the organism in non-human primates causes urethritis.

The diagnosis may be established by cytological examination of urethral smears. The organisms proliferating inside host cells form paranuclear crescent-shaped inclusions known as **elementary bodies**, which stain purple with Giemsa stain. The formation of these

Table 37.4 Infective Causes of Non-gonococcal Urethritis

Responsible organism	Frequency (percentage of cases)
Chlamydia trachomatis	30–50%
Ureaplasma urealyticum (a mycoplasma)	Approximately 30%
Trichomonas vaginalis	Rare
Yeasts	Rare
Herpes simplex	Rare
Unknown	20%

Clinical outcomes of Reiter's syndrome are shown in *Table 37.5.*

Table 37.5 Clinical Outcome of Patients with Reiter's Syndrome

Outcome	Frequency %
Complete recovery	25
Occasional recrudescence affecting one or more of the sites mentioned above	50
Recurrent chronic manifestations	25

inclusions takes about 48 hours from the time of infection of the host cells.

Both sensitivity and specificity of cytological diagnosis may be improved by using fluorescein-linked monoclonal antibodies raised against the chief membrane proteins of the chlamydia.

Little is known about the morphological appearances in chlamydial urethritis; most existing knowledge has been gained from animal models. The chief microscopic change is a subepithelial lymphocytic infiltrate, which persists even after the organisms have been eliminated. The overlying epithelium appears undamaged. A similar subepithelial lymphoid infiltrate is seen in the cervix uteri of women who have had chlamydial genital infections, a condition termed **follicular cervicitis.**

Reiter's Syndrome

Reiter's syndrome is defined largely by a triad of clinical features:
- urethritis
- conjunctivitis
- arthritis involving particularly weight-bearing joints such as the sacroiliac (see p 1083).

There is a strong association with the human leucocyte antigen (HLA)-B27 locus (the B27 phenotype confers a 37-fold increased risk of developing Reiter's syndrome).

Reiter's syndrome commonly follows an infection of either the gut or the genital tract and shows a marked male predominance. Occurrence is most frequent between the ages of 18 and 40 years. The earliest manifestation is urethritis associated with large numbers of neutrophils in the urine. Few data exist regarding the pathological changes, but a subepithelial mixed inflammatory cell infiltrate may be expected to be present. Most patients show symptoms of prostatitis and about 20% also have haemorrhagic cystitis.

Urethral Caruncle

This is a polypoid lesion occurring exclusively in the female urethra, usually in the postmenopausal period. There may be no symptoms associated with caruncle but some patients present complaining of dysuria or mild bleeding.

Microscopic Features

Three basic histological patterns exist which can show some degree of overlap:
- a **papillomatous** variety in which the irregular and clefted surface of the lesion is covered by thickened transitional or squamous epithelium
- an **angiomatous** variant in which there are numerous cavernous vascular spaces in the subepithelial tissue
- a **granulomatous** variant in which the surface epithelium is thinned and the subepithelial connective tissue shows a florid inflammatory infiltrate and numerous granulation tissue-type capillaries

NEOPLASTIC DISEASE

Urethral Carcinoma

The urethra is an uncommon site for malignancy and most of the patients are elderly. The commonest tumour site is in the anterior portion at the junction between the squamous epithelium at the meatus and the transitional epithelium lining the rest of the urethra. Most are squamous carcinomas but transitional carcinomas and adenocarcinomas have also been described.

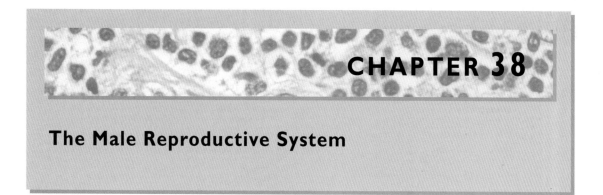

CHAPTER 38

The Male Reproductive System

The Testis and Epididymis

NORMAL ANATOMY AND HISTOLOGY

The adult testes weigh 15–19 g each; the right testis is usually about 10% heavier than the left. Each is covered by a fibrous tissue capsule, the **tunica albuginea**. From this are derived many fibrous septa, separating the parenchyma into about 250 lobules. Each lobule contains from two to four seminiferous tubules in which germ cell development leading to sperm formation occurs. Groups of seminiferous tubules merge to form about six efferent ductules; these drain into a series of straight tubules connecting with the epididymis.

The Epididymis

This lies on the posterior and lateral surfaces of the testis. It is a complex coiled tubular structure, classically divided into three regions: the head, body and tail. It is responsible for:

- **sperm transport** mediated by contraction of a thick muscular layer surrounding the epididymal tubules
- **part of the process of sperm maturation**, including the sperm becoming motile
- **concentration of sperm**
- **storage of sperm.** This takes place mainly in the tail of the epididymis, where maturation also takes place. The stored sperm leave the tail of the epididymis at ejaculation and the vas deferens along which they pass originates from the epididymal tail. All in all, the sperm spend about 12 days in the epididymis.

In fetal life, the testis develops from a urogenital ridge on the posterior wall of the abdomen. At about the 28th week of gestation it descends into the scrotum, bringing with it an investment of peritoneum, the **tunica vaginalis**. This covers most of the testis: only an area on the posterior surface where vascular structures enter and leave the testis is uncovered.

In about 10% of boys the testes have not descended into the scrotum at the time of birth but in the vast majority this will occur within the first year of life.

Seminiferous Tubules

The seminiferous tubules are coiled, closed loops that ultimately drain into the efferent ductules. The total length of the roughly 1000 tubules within the testis can be as much as 980 m (average more than 500 m), giving some idea of how densely they are packed.

Each tubule wall is composed of a limiting membrane made up of basement membrane glycoprotein, collagen and some cells resembling smooth muscle. The cellular lining consists of germ cells in different stages of development and Sertoli cells; the ratio of germ cells : Sertoli cells is 13 : 1.

Sertoli Cells

In the normal adult testis, the Sertoli cells do not divide. They are tall columnar cells sited on the tubular basement membrane, and they have cytoplasmic extensions investing the developing germ cells. The nuclei have a prominent nucleolus, which makes it easy to distinguish Sertoli cells from germ cells. The cytoplasm usually contains phagocytosed material derived either from residual bodies of spermatids or from degenerating germ cells. They also contain rather characteristic crystalloid bodies consisting of bundles of filaments. These are easy to see on electron microscopy and can sometimes be seen on light microscopic examination as well.

The functions of the Sertoli cells appear to be related to the age and sexual maturity of the individual (*Fig. 38.1*):

- In embryonic life the Sertoli cell secretes a steroid **müllerian-inhibiting factor** which causes the müllerian duct system to regress.
- In the prepubertal period, the Sertoli cell secretes a product that inhibits the meiotic division of spermatocytes.
- In adult life the Sertoli cells:
  1) regulate germ cell movement in the tubule
  2) have a phagocytic function
  3) secrete many proteins including transferrin, caeruloplasmin, a growth factor and inhibin, a peptide modulating the communications between the hypothalamus and the anterior pituitary.

Germ Cells

The germ cells originate in the yolk sac, migrating in early fetal life to the gonadal ridge on the posterior abdominal wall. In the adult testis they make up the bulk of the cell population of the seminiferous tubules;

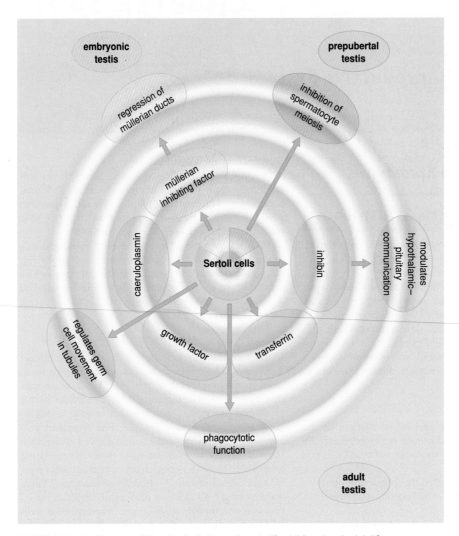

FIGURE 38.1 *The functions of Sertoli cells during embryonic life, childhood and adult life.*

their maturation takes about 10 weeks. The sequence of events is:

1) The undifferentiated **spermatogonium** lying in the basal compartment of the tubules proliferates; some of the offspring give rise to **primary spermatocytes**.

2) The spermatocytes move out of the basal compartment; a maturation cycle follows, the stages of which correlate with changes in the nuclear chromatin pattern. This stage takes about 24 days.

3) The first meiotic (reduction) division occurs, with formation of **secondary spermatocytes**. These have a short life and soon undergo further meiotic division to form **spermatids**.

4) The spermatids mature, this culminating in the shedding of excess cytoplasm in the form of residual bodies, which are then phagocytosed by Sertoli cells.

5) Until spermatozoa are formed, all the progeny of a single spermatogonium are connected to each other by cytoplasmic bridges. Failure of these to break leads to the formation of either multinucleated spermatids or multiheaded spermatozoa.

In normal healthy tubules, where spermatogenesis is proceeding in an orderly fashion, about half the germ cells should be in the spermatid stage and there should be, on average, no more than about 12 Sertoli cells in a tubule cross-section.

Leydig Cells

Leydig cells, which secrete testosterone under the influence of luteinizing hormone derived from the pituitary, occupy part of the interstitium between the tubules. They occur either in groups or singly, usually set in close proximity to capillaries. Leydig cells are present in large numbers in the 1–20-week fetal testis. After this their numbers decline sharply, although some Leydig

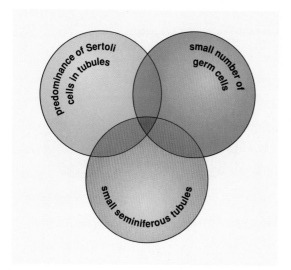

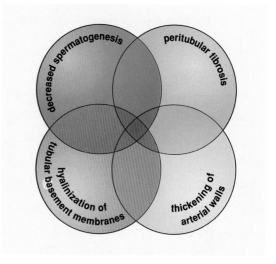

FIGURE 38.2 *Morphological features of the prepubertal testis.*

FIGURE 38.3 *Morphological features of the ageing testis.*

cell precursors are present in the infant testis. At about the age of 7 years the Leydig cell precursors start to differentiate and mature Leydig cells may be seen at the time of puberty.

These mature Leydig cells have abundant intensely eosinophilic cytoplasm. Lipid droplets and lipofuscin pigment are usually present, the amount of pigment increasing with age. Some Leydig cells contain curious crystalloid bodies known as Reinke's crystalloids. Curiously they are seen only in humans and wild bush rats.

The Prepubertal Testis

The testis in infancy and childhood (*Fig. 38.2*) is characterized by:

- **small seminiferous tubules**, with a diameter at birth of about 50 μm; this increases slowly so that at the age of 12 years the average diameter of the tubules is about 65 μm.
- **a predominance of Sertoli cells in the tubules.** These decrease by about two-thirds between childhood and adult life. The decrease in number is associated with a steady increase in the **cell volume**, which increases by a factor of five between birth and adult life.
- **a small number of germ cells.** At birth, spermatogonia and their precursors, gonocytes, are seen at the periphery of the tubules. The gonocytes disappear by 5 years of age and some early forms of primary spermatocytes can now be seen. The germ cell population increases strikingly at the time of puberty.

The Ageing Testis

There is no doubt that a decline in testicular function occurs with ageing. This is mirrored by certain morphological changes (*Fig. 38.3*) including:

- a decrease in spermatogenesis
- a degree of peritubular fibrosis
- some hyalinization of the tubular basement membranes
- some thickening of the arterial walls and an apparent decrease in the capillary bed, these vascular changes being, perhaps, responsible for the peritubular fibrosis.

DEVELOPMENTAL DISORDERS

Cryptorchidism

By the age of 1 year, 99% of testes have descended into the inguinal canal. **Arrest of a testis somewhere along the path of normal descent is termed cryptorchidism.** Common sites of such arrest (*Fig. 38.4*) are:

- **the inguinal canal.** When in this position, care must be taken not to confuse an abnormally retractile testis with a truly undescended one.
- **superficially in the inguinal region**
- **within the abdomen**

Effects of Maldescent

Failure to correct the position of an undescended testis has two major effects (*Fig. 38.5*). These are:

1) **Decreased fertility** if the maldescent is bilateral.

2) **The most serious risk is of developing a malignant germ cell tumour of the testis. Compared with intrascrotal testes, the increased risk is of the order of 30–50 times, and is greatest in patients in whom the undescended testis has been intra-abdominal.**

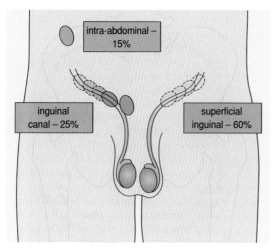

FIGURE 38.4 Sites of arrest in testicular maldescent.

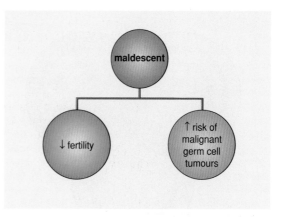

FIGURE 38.5 Complications of testicular maldescent.

This highlights the importance of surgical correction if descent is not complete by the age of 2–3 years.

Even if the maldescent is corrected surgically, some increase in risk persists. This applies particularly when surgical correction takes place **after the age of 6 years**. In addition, the normally placed testis in a patient with one undescended testis has a greater chance of developing a malignant germ cell tumour than is the case when both testes are normally sited.

Macroscopic Features
In adults, undescended testes are smaller than normal and have a brown colour on section.

Microscopic Features
- The seminiferous tubules are smaller than normal and are separated from one another by increased amounts of fibrous tissue.
- There is a decrease in the number of germ cells and, sometimes, atypical germ cells may be seen on or near the basement membranes.
- The tubular basement membranes are thickened and hyalinized.
- Sertoli cells are relatively greater in number than normal and nodules of immature Sertoli cells called 'congeries' may be seen in some tubules. If the changes are severe, Sertoli cells constitute the whole cell population of some tubules.
- Leydig cells appear more prominent than normal. This may be because of the shrinkage of the tubular mass.

Ectopic Testis
The defining criterion of testicular ectopia is a site away from both the scrotum and the normal pathway of descent.

The commonest site of ectopic testis is in the perineum, but testes have also been identified in the thigh, the pelvis and the root of the penis.

THE PATHOLOGY OF MALE INFERTILITY

Infertility leads one in six married couples to seek medical help. Of these, about 40% will be discovered to have a problem involving the fertility of the male partner.

'Normal male fertility starts in the head.' This is a frivolous way of emphasizing that the ejaculation of normal numbers of normally active spermatozoa is the final objective of a sequence of events that starts with the synthesis of gonadotrophin–releasing hormones in the hypothalamus. At any point in this sequence, something may go wrong, resulting in infertility. Thus, the causes of male infertility may be most easily and logically considered against a background of the normal sequence of events.

Inadequate Follicle-stimulating Hormone
Germ cell development requires adequate concentrations of the gonadotrophin, follicle-stimulating hormone (FSH), and testosterone secretion by Leydig cells requires adequate concentrations of luteinizing hormone (LH). Normal concentrations of these hormones depend on:

1) secretion of normal amounts of gonadotrophin-releasing substances by the hypothalamus
2) the ability of these releasing hormones to travel down the pituitary stalk to reach the anterior pituitary
3) the secretion of normal amounts of the gonadotrophic hormones FSH and LH in a biologically active form by the anterior pituitary

If any of these steps is interfered with, then the syndrome of **hypogonadotrophic hypogonadism** results (*Fig. 38.6*). In an average male 'fertility' clinic,

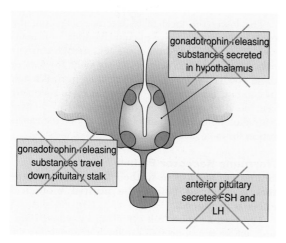

FIGURE 38.6 *The causes of hypogonadotrophic hypogonadism viewed against the background of the mechanisms involved in gonadotrophin production.*

this will account for about 1% of cases of male infertility. The plasma concentrations of FSH and LH will both be low.

The pathological causes of this syndrome vary somewhat with the age of the patient (*Fig. 38.7*).

- In childhood, the likeliest causes are **craniopharyngioma** abutting on the anterior pituitary or, rarely, birth trauma.
- In the hypothalamus, there may be anomalies in the gene coding for the releasing hormone; in adult life, the problem may be due to involvement of the hypothalamus or pituitary stalk by granulomatous inflammation such as sarcoidosis (which is commonest in the UK) or tuberculosis. Kallman's syndrome is characterized by failure of gonadotrophin-releasing hormone (GRH)-secreting neurones to migrate from the olfactory placode.
- In adult life, the pituitary is most commonly affected by pituitary tumours, chromophobe adenoma being the one most frequently associated with hypogonadotrophic hypogonadism.
- Gonadotrophin secretion may also be impaired in serious systemic disorders such as chronic renal failure or severe inflammatory bowel disease; if an

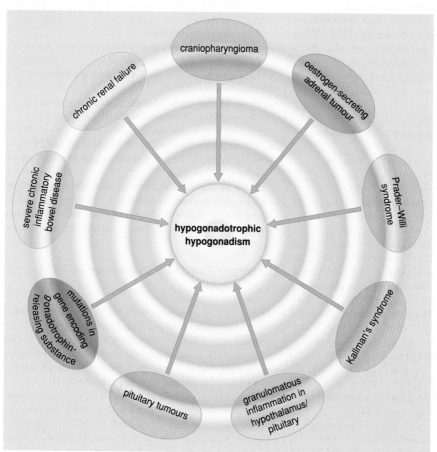

FIGURE 38.7 *Pathological causes of hypogonadotrophic hypogonadism.*

oestrogen–secreting adrenal tumour is present, gonadotrophin secretion will be suppressed.

- The Prader–Willi syndrome is another cause of such hypogonadism. This consists of:
  a) short stature
  b) hypotonic muscles
  c) small hands and feet
  d) hypogonadism

Testicular pathology depends on whether the absence of gonadotrophic stimuli occurs in the prepubertal or postpubertal period.

- If the former is the case, then the testicular morphology will be identical with that of a normal prepubertal testis: the tubules are lined principally by Sertoli cells and Leydig cells are scanty or absent. These patients, of course, show other evidence of hypogonadism in the form of an undersized phallus, small prostate, high-pitched voice, and scanty or absent growth of pubic and axillary hair.
- In adult patients who have testes that were previously normal, the failure of a gonadotrophic drive results in atrophic changes that affect especially the germinal epithelium.

Inadequate Testosterone Secretion

Successful germ cell growth and maturation requires testosterone in addition to FSH. Thus failures in Leydig cell function may also be a cause of infertility. The great majority of patients who are infertile because of failure to secrete sufficient androgen fall into the group labelled as Klinefelter's syndrome, characterized by:

- eunuchoidism which may be severe, slight or absent. Gynaecomastia is present in 50% of cases
- small firm testes
- complete absence of sperm from the ejaculate
- raised basal levels of FSH
- mental dullness; an unusually high number of patients with Klinefelter's syndrome are found in institutions catering for males with learning disabilities.

Klinefelter's syndrome occurs in about 1 in 1400 live births, making a significant contribution to male infertility. The clinical syndrome is ascribed to the presence of an extra X chromosome in a phenotypic male (the classic karyotype being 47XXY). In such patients Barr bodies are found in exfoliated epithelial cells.

Microscopic Features

- The tubules are small.
- Germ cells are rare.
- Tubule basement membranes are hyalinized and some of the tubules are completely hyalinized.
- Leydig cells appear prominent. Their volume may be normal, decreased or increased. Light microscopy shows them to be deficient in Reinke's crystalloids.

On electron microscopy they show a number of abnormalities consistent with their very limited capacity to secrete testosterone.

The lower the level of testosterone secretion, the more severe is the degree of eunuchoidism. In patients with Klinefelter's syndrome, the testosterone concentrations in spermatic vein blood are only 35–45% of those obtained from the blood draining normal testes. In contrast, the oestradiol concentrations in spermatic vein blood are normal. Thus these patients have a raised oestradiol : testosterone ratio and this may be the explanation for the gynaecomastia.

Hormone Receptor Failure

Binding of androgens to their appropriate receptors is required before the normal biological effect is produced.

Testosterone enters cell cytoplasm by passive diffusion, where it is converted to dihydrotestosterone; the reduction that this requires is catalysed by the enzyme 5α-reductase. The altered steroid binds to a high-affinity receptor and the hormone–receptor complex enters the cell nucleus where it exerts its androgenic effect.

Dihydrotestosterone:
- **mediates normal embryological development of the male external genitalia**
- **is responsible for virilization at puberty**

Testosterone:
- **induces the embryological development of the wolffian duct derivatives** (i.e. seminal vesicles and ductus deferens)
- **exerts negative feedback control of GRH**
- **takes part in the stimulation and regulation of spermatogenesis**

Failure of androgens to bind to their appropriate receptors can lead to failures in each of the functions listed above and to the various syndromes subsumed under the term androgen resistance (*Fig. 38.8*).

Androgen Resistance Syndromes

Testicular Feminization

This term is synonymous with male pseudohermaphroditism in which there is a contradiction between gonadal and phenotypic sexual differentiation. It is due to **a mutation in the gene coding for androgen receptors**, and in its complete form the patients appear to be **phenotypically normal females**.

They have, however, a normal 46XY karyotype and testes are always present, although they are usually either inguinal or intra-abdominal in position. Testosterone levels are normal and the administration of extra testosterone is quite without effect. Studies carried out using skin fibroblasts from these patients in cul-

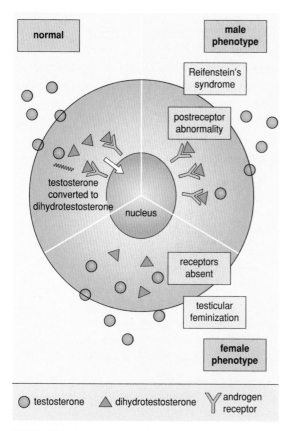

FIGURE 38.8 *Androgen resistance syndromes.*

ture show that the dihydrotestosterone receptor is either completely absent or functionally defective.

Incomplete forms of this syndrome also occur. In these the external genitalia may be ambiguous.

Reifenstein's Syndrome

Here patients are phenotypic males with a 46XY karyotype. They show:

- gynaecomastia
- deficient virilization
- cryptorchidism
- complete absence or severely reduced numbers of sperm in the ejaculate
- a severe degree of penile abnormality in the form of hypospadias

Binding of androgen to cellular receptors is normal but the expected biological effects are absent and this must represent some postreceptor failure.

These endocrine abnormalities account for only a small proportion of infertile males. Many more cases are due to either complete or partial failure of the germinal epithelium.

Lack of Testicular Tissue

Atrophy or destruction of testicular tissue (*Fig. 38.9*) may be due to:

1) **inflammatory diseases**, such as orchitis associated with mumps, mycobacterial infection, infection with pyogenic bacteria or 'granulomatous' orchitis. Following mumps orchitis, there is usually complete ablation of sperm production. The microscopic appearances in the testis resemble those of Klinefelter's syndrome.

2) **radiation**, sometimes accidental but more commonly therapeutic

3) **chemotherapy** for malignant disease, cyclophosphamide being especially implicated

4) severe **trauma**

5) **increased plasma concentrations of oestrogen**, such as may be seen in hepatic cirrhosis and in patients treated with oestrogens or GRH analogues for prostatic cancer

6) **an intrinsic failure in spermatogenesis**, the causes of which are not well understood. In the absence of the causes listed above, infertile male testes may totally lack sperm in the ejaculate (azoospermia). Their testes may show a variety of patterns including:

- **germ cell aplasia.** Here the tubules are lined with Sertoli cells only. Of the intrinsic causes of azoospermia, this is the commonest. Its aetiology is unknown and it cannot be treated successfully.
- **an arrest of maturation**, usually at the stage of the primary spermatocyte
- **generalized fibrosis**
- **obstruction within the efferent ductules in the testis itself or more distally.** For azoospermia to occur, such obstruction would have to affect both testes.

Post-testicular Causes

Finally, even if the endocrine pathways are normal and normal spermatogenesis is present, there is a last stage that must be completed successfully: the delivery of normal, active sperm into the ejaculate. Two types of post-testicular pathology may be encountered:

- **obstruction**, which may be congenital, postinflammatory or postsurgical
- faults in the last stages of sperm **maturation** within the epididymis or in the **storage of sperm** in this site. These are believed to be the mechanisms responsible for impaired motility of the spermatozoa.

INFLAMMATORY DISEASES OF THE TESTIS (ORCHITIS)

INFECTIVE ORCHITIS

Many infective agents can cause orchitis (*Fig. 38.10*). These include bacteria (usually of the types implicated

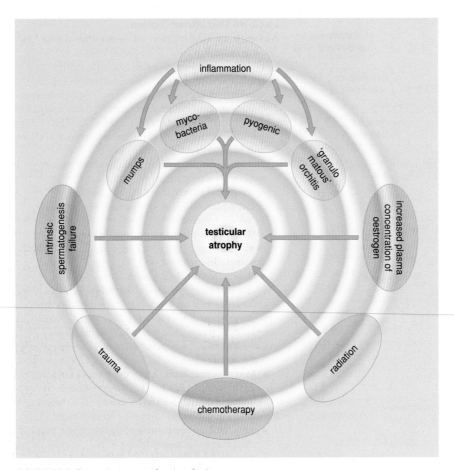

FIGURE 38.9 Testicular causes of male infertility.

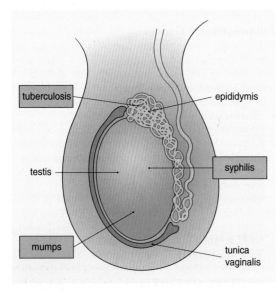

FIGURE 38.10 Some targets for infection in inflammation in the testis.

in urinary tract infections), viruses, fungi and parasites. Only a few of these are discussed here.

In some instances, infective orchitis occurs as **extension from epididymitis**. This is likely to be the case both in non-sexually transmitted infections such as are caused by *Escherichia coli*, *Pseudomonas* species and *Brucella*, and in sexually transmitted infections like gonorrhoea and chlamydial infections.

In the epididymis and testis, infections cause an acute, non-specific acute inflammatory reaction. Initially confined to the interstitial tissues, this spreads to involve the tubules and tissue breakdown with pus formation may occur. Both the testis and epididymis are enlarged, tense and painful due to the inflammatory oedema. This oedema, occurring as it does in an organ enclosed in the tough fibrous tunica albuginea, leads to a steep rise in intratesticular pressure resulting in ischaemic damage.

The common endpoint of many of these infections is scarring leading to sterility (see above).

Tuberculosis

The epididymis is the primary target of tuberculous infections of the intrascrotal contents but extension to involve the testis can occur. In most instances genital tract tuberculosis is a reflection of haematogenous dissemination of organisms and is usually associated with pulmonary disease.

The pathological changes within the epididymis are in no way different from what is seen in tuberculous involvement of other organs. Caseation necrosis is usually extensive and severe. The testis, in comparison with the epididymis, is relatively resistant to involvement by the tuberculous process, but in some instances extension does occur, although it is not clear whether this represents direct spread in continuity with the epididymal lesions or spread via lymphatic channels.

Syphilis

Involvement of the testis is a late manifestation of syphilis and is now rare. Two types of lesion may be found:

1) The first is one of the hallmarks of tertiary syphilis, a **gumma**, an area of coagulative necrosis associated with a macrophage and plasma cell reaction. The necrotic areas still show the 'ghost' outlines of the tissue architecture, unlike what is seen in caseation necrosis where this feature is lost.

2) In other cases the syphilitic infection is manifest in the form of a diffuse plasma cell infiltrate associated with the characteristic vascular lesions of syphilis, **obliterative endarteritis**, in which there is marked intimal thickening with reduction of the lumina of the small blood vessels.

In either case, the end result is scarring of the testicular parenchyma leading to sterility. Leydig cells appear to resist the process and sexual potency is preserved.

Mumps

Mumps is an acute contagious illness caused by a **paramyxovirus**. Clinically, it is most commonly expressed as a non-suppurative inflammation of one or both parotid glands (see p 490).

Involvement of other organs can occur and **an orchitis develops in about 20% of male patients over the age of 13 years who acquire the infection**. In the majority of cases (85%) the orchitis is unilateral but bilateral orchitis can and does occur. Classically, the orchitis makes its appearance at a time when the parotid enlargement is subsiding. Patients complain of intense pain related to the enlarged testis, due to a severe grade of oedema raising the intratesticular pressure steeply and causing considerable stretching of the tunica albuginea.

The inflammatory process starts in the interstitium with a mild neutrophil infiltrate but then spreads to involve the seminiferous tubules. The interstitial infiltrate becomes predominantly lymphocytic and the tubules show neutrophils and macrophages admixed with necrotic germ cells.

In due time, the inflammation resolves, although some residual scarring may be seen. In almost half the patients, testicular atrophy results; the microscopic appearances are the same as with any other type of atrophy occurring in the postpubertal testis.

NON-INFECTIVE ORCHITIS

Granulomatous Orchitis

Chronic granulomatous orchitis occurs predominantly in middle-aged patients. Its origin is unclear. A history of preceding trauma is often obtained but it is not known whether this is causally related to the testicular inflammation.

It is characterized by a nodular, often quite painless, enlargement of the testis, which feels very firm. For these reasons it may give rise to clinical suspicions of testicular malignancy.

> ### *Macroscopic Features*
> The testis is enlarged and feels firm and rubbery. The tunica vaginalis is thickened and the cut surface of the testis is lobulated and greyish-white in colour.
>
> ### *Microscopic Features*
> Many epithelioid cell granulomas, which appear to have seminiferous tubules at their centres, are present. There is no necrosis as such, but degeneration of the germ cells is a prominent feature.

TUMOURS OF THE TESTIS

More than 90% of testicular neoplasms arise from germ cells and almost all of these show metastatic potential. They account for just over 1% of all malignancies in males; excluding leukaemia and lymphoma, they are the commonest malignant disorder in men aged 15–34 years.

Epidemiology

Epidemiological studies show quite gross geographical differences in incidence. For example, the incidence of germ cell tumours is eight times higher in Denmark than in Japan. In the USA, Caucasians are affected about four times as often as black-skinned individuals.

Clinical Features

Most germ cell tumours call attention to themselves as a result of increasing painless enlargement of the testis. Occasionally the initial clinical presentation may be due to metastatic deposits, for example in the lung or mediastinum, and a small testicular primary may be found only at this rather late stage.

Manifestations of some endocrine disturbance may be present; the most frequent is **gynaecomastia**. Most germ cell tumours are unilateral but a small proportion (1–2.5%) involve both testes. If the germ cell tumour occurs against a background of bilateral undescended testes, the chances of bilaterality increase to about 15%.

Classification

Testicular neoplasms as a whole may be divided into five broad categories:

1) **germ cell tumours** (90% of all testicular neoplasms). These arise from the germ cells lining the seminiferous tubules.

2) **sex cord–stromal tumours** (about 2% of all testicular neoplasms)

3) **mixed germ cell–sex cord–stromal tumours**

4) **primary tumours found also in sites other than the testis**

5) **secondary deposits** from other primary sites

GERM CELL TUMOURS

Classification

Many classifications exist for **germ cell tumours**. At the simplest level they can be divided into three groups:

1) **seminomas**
2) **non-seminomatous germ cell tumours**
3) **a combination of the above**

The common cell of origin for both seminomatous and non-seminomatous groups is the germ cell (*Fig. 38.11*); different types of non-seminomatous

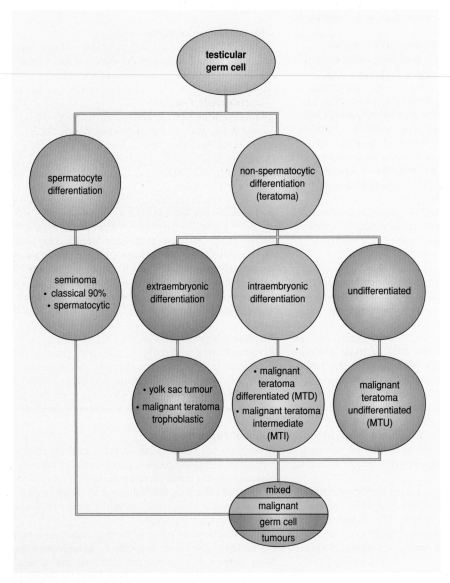

FIGURE 38.11 Classification and lineage of testicular germ cell tumours.

germ cell tumours mirror embryogenesis histologically. In simple terms, their differentiation patterns resemble components of the embryo and associated extraembryonic structures such as the placenta and yolk sac.

Two systems of classification of germ cell tumours are commonly used, as shown in *Table 38.1*. **The chief confusing factor in comparing these relates to the use of the term teratoma, which has a less aggressive connotation in the World Health Organization (WHO) classification than in the British one.**

Precursor Lesions: The Origins of Germ Cell Tumours – Intratubular Germ Cell Neoplasia

With the sole exception of spermatocytic seminoma, it is believed that there is a precursor lesion for most invasive germ cell tumours. This lesion is termed intratubular germ cell neoplasia (ITGCN). The defining feature is the replacement of normal germ cells with large vacuolated cells with irregular nuclei and prominent nucleoli. These cells have many morphological and histochemical features in common with the primordial germ cells or gonocytes originating in the yolk sac region and later migrating to the gonad. **Tubules in which ITGCN is present do not show normal spermatogenesis.** The gonocyte-like cells synthesize the enzyme **placental alkaline phosphatase (PLAP)** and the extent of tubular involvement can be shown immunohistochemically by using monoclonal antibodies to PLAP.

Support for a premalignant role for ITGCN comes from the observations that:

- ITGCN is found in tubules adjacent to germ cell tumours in most instances.
- There is a strong positive association between the risk of developing a germ cell tumour and the presence in a cryptorchid testis of ITGCN. The same applies when this finding is made in biopsies of the testes from infertile men.
- Continuities are found between areas of ITGCN and frankly invasive germ cell tumours.
- Patients in whom ITGCN has been found on biopsy have a 50% chance of developing a germ cell tumour in the next 5 years.

Seminoma

Seminomas, in a pure form, account for about 40% of germ cell tumours. They can be divided into two basic groups (*Table 38.1*)**:**

1) **classical or typical**, a group in which a number of morphological variants exists
2) **spermatocytic**

Classical (Typical) Seminoma

This accounts for over 90% of seminomas. They have a rather broad curve of age incidence, the peak being 30–50 years.

Macroscopic Features

Seminomas are well-defined masses with a greyish-white cut surface in which occasional areas of necrosis may be present (*Fig. 38.12*).

Microscopic Features

Tumours consist of sheets of primitive-looking germ cells divided characteristically into lobules by fine bands of connective tissue (*Fig. 38.13*). In about 80% of cases the connective tissue septa are infiltrated by lymphocytes and plasma cells; this may be an immune reaction to the tumour. Epithelioid cell granulomas with occasional Langhans-type giant cells are also seen in some cases and this granuloma formation may be so marked as to obscure the neoplastic nature of the whole lesion.

Table 38.1 Classification of Germ Cell Tumours of the Testis

British Testicular Tumour Panel	World Health Organization
Seminoma	Seminoma
Classical	Typical
Spermatocytic	Spermatocytic
Malignant teratoma, undifferentiated	Embryonal carcinoma
Malignant teratoma, intermediate (i.e. with some differentiated or organoid elements)	Embryonal carcinoma with teratoma
Teratoma, differentiated	Teratoma mature
Malignant teratoma, trophoblastic	Choriocarcinoma
Yolk sac tumour	Yolk sac tumour

The tumour cells are large and have abundant, rather clear, cytoplasm with very well-defined plasma membranes. The nuclei are centrally placed and show one or two nucleoli and a somewhat clumped chromatin pattern.

Immunohistochemical examination shows no evidence of epithelial differentiation (the cells do not bind antibodies against cytokeratins) **but the cells do synthesize placental alkaline phosphatase, angiotensin-converting enzyme, ferritin and vimentin**. In about 40% of cases, the serum placental alkaline phosphatase concentrations are raised. This can be very useful, both for diagnosis and, perhaps more importantly, for monitoring the patient's progress after removal of the primary tumour.

Occasionally (in 10% of cases) very large multinucleated giant cells, which morphologically resemble cells of the syncytiotrophoblast, are noted. These produce large amounts of the β subunit of **human chorionic gonadotrophin**, which is released in measurable quantities into the bloodstream. Such tumours do not behave differently from typical seminoma in which no such cells are present.

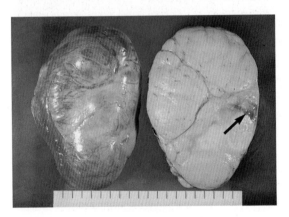

FIGURE 38.12 A seminoma arising in an undescended testis. Note the bulging, rather uniform, cut surface with an occasional area of necrosis (arrow).

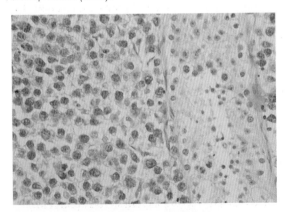

FIGURE 38.13 The typical cells of a 'classical' seminoma with centrally placed round nuclei and rather clear cytoplasm.

Spermatocytic Seminoma

Spermatocytic seminoma (about 5%) differs both morphologically and biologically from classical seminoma. It is suggested that these differences reflect an origin from spermatocytes rather than from gonocytes.

Spermatocytic seminoma:
- **occurs at an older age than classical seminoma,** the median age being 55 years.
- **behaves in a much less aggressive fashion**; metastases are rare. The prognosis after orchidectomy is excellent and no further treatment is required after tumour removal in most cases.
- **always occurs in a pure form**, unlike classical seminoma which is often seen as part of a combined germ cell tumour.

Macroscopic Features

The lesions tend to be very large and rather gelatinous in consistency.

Microscopic Features

There is marked variation in the size and appearance of the tumour cells.

The tumour cells are arranged in sheets and the lymphocyte-infiltrated connective tissue septa, so typical of classical seminoma, are usually not present. The tumour cells have very characteristic nuclear appearances. In well-preserved sections a thread-like chromatin pattern can be seen, resembling what is seen in a spermatocyte undergoing meiosis. Many tumour cells have cytoplasm similar to that of plasma cells and multinucleated cells with two to four nuclei are quite common. Mitoses are frequent. The tumour cells do *not* produce placental alkaline phosphatase.

Spermatocytic seminoma is *not* associated with ITGCN in the neighbouring tubules.

Anaplastic Seminoma

Basically these are seminomas of classical type. Their defining criterion is three or more mitoses per high-power field on microscopic examination. In addition, there is more nuclear and cellular pleomorphism and more necrosis than in classical variants. It is not clear whether anaplastic seminoma has a more aggressive behaviour than classical seminoma. It is true that the anaplastic variant seems to present clinically at a more advanced stage than does classical seminoma, but stage for stage a prognostic difference between the two entities is not proven.

Teratoma

The term teratoma is used in Britain to describe a group of neoplasms derived from germ cells which have the potential to differentiate into cells or tissues of ectodermal, mesodermal or endodermal types. In the USA, use of the word teratoma is confined to tumours in which such differentiation has actually occurred.

Teratomas may be gonadal or extragonadal. Ovarian teratomas are usually well differentiated and benign (see pp 782–783). In the testis such well-differentiated teratomas account for only 5–10% of germ cell tumours, and even they may metastasize.

Malignant Teratoma Differentiated (MTD)
(WHO classification: teratoma)

This variant accounts for about 3% of testicular teratomas but is **the commonest type in childhood**. Its defining characteristic is differentiation into cell types reflecting more than one embryonic differentiation pattern, i.e. ectoderm, endoderm and mesoderm (*Figs 38.14* and *38.15*). Thus a single tumour may contain epithelial structures such as skin, sweat and sebaceous glands, structures reminiscent of bronchus, gut, brain, retina, muscle and cartilage. Small cysts are present in many instances.

MTD of childhood usually shows a high degree of differentiation, and its potential for spread is low. In adults, however, this relatively benign behaviour cannot be relied on. This may be because the adult tumours contain small foci of frankly malignant tumour tissue which sampling has failed to reveal.

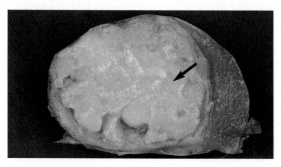

FIGURE 38.14 *Well-differentiated teratoma (MTD) in a child. The cut surface shows cystic spaces and some cartilage-like area (arrow).*

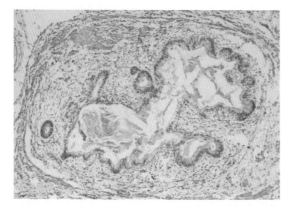

FIGURE 38.15 *Well-differentiated teratoma (MTD) showing a cystic space lined by well-differentiated columnar epithelium.*

Metastases often show the same tendency to differentiate as do primary lesions. For example, there may be secondary deposits in the lung that are polycystic and contain islands of cartilage and bone. Very rarely, malignant transformation may occur, affecting one of the differentiated components exclusively; thus a squamous carcinoma may occur in a mature teratoma.

Malignant Teratoma Undifferentiated (MTU)
(WHO classification: embryonal carcinoma)

This tumour shows **little or no evidence of differentiation**. In pure form, undifferentiated teratomas account for about 10% of testicular neoplasms. The peak age for the occurrence of this tumour is 20–30 years, some 10 years less than is the case for seminoma.

Macroscopic Features
The cut surface of this tumour shows a much more variegated appearance than is seen in seminoma, with focal areas of haemorrhage and necrosis which may be extensive.

Microscopic Features
There are sheets of undifferentiated cells which show a considerable degree of variation in size and shape; mitoses are frequent. In some examples there appear to be attempts at differentiation in the form of tubular or papillary structures.

Immunohistochemical examination shows that the tumour cells express cytokeratins, in marked contrast to seminomas. Some cells may bind antibodies to human chorionic gonadotrophin and α-fetoprotein (AFP), but this appears to have no bearing on the biological behaviour, which is highly aggressive.

Malignant Teratoma Intermediate (MTI)
(WHO classification: embryonal carcinoma with teratoma)

This is the commonest variety of testicular teratoma. It shows features of both MTU and MTD. The appearances depend on the relative proportions of differentiated and undifferentiated elements. There is, therefore, a wide range of microscopic appearances. In general, the greater the amount of undifferentiated tumour, the more aggressive the behaviour of the tumour.

Malignant Teratoma Trophoblastic (MTT)
(WHO classification: choriocarcinoma)

Trophoblastic differentiation in germ cell tumours occurs in three principal forms:

1) **Isolated syncytiotrophoblastic giant cells without any accompanying cytotrophoblast.** This occurs in association with seminoma (see above), yolk sac tumours and undifferentiated

teratomas (MTUs). The presence of these cells may be associated with raised serum concentrations of the β subunit of human chorionic gonadotrophin, and the hormone can be found within the tumour cells (*Fig. 38.16*).

2) Syncytiotrophoblast accompanied by cytotrophoblast. This is the defining criterion of choriocarcinoma in the WHO classification. In a pure form it is very rare.

3) Syncytiotrophoblast and cytotrophoblast arranged in a papillary pattern with the syncytial tissue forming a surface layer over the trophoblast. This papillary pattern is mandatory for classification as MTT. The tumours are usually haemorrhagic and show foci of necrosis. Like the WHO 'choriocarcinoma', MTT is very rare in pure form, although areas of MTT may be seen admixed with other germ cell tumour elements.

Choriocarcinoma and MTT are aggressive in their biological behaviour, showing a marked tendency to metastasize early via the bloodstream. This is not surprising because the chief functional characteristic of normal syncytiotrophoblastic cells is the erosion of uterine blood vessels in the course of placentation.

Yolk Sac Tumour

Yolk sac tumour has been given a number of names, including endodermal sinus tumour and, in infants, orchioblastoma. It reflects an **extraembryonic differentiation pattern** resulting in tissue resembling normal human yolk sac both morphologically and functionally.

Yolk sac differentiation may be seen in two forms:

1) In a pure form occurring in infancy and early childhood (less than 2 years of age). Patients with this tumour have an excellent prognosis.

2) As part of a mixed germ cell tumour in adults. Controversy exists as to its frequency but some workers maintain that yolk sac differentiation occurs in 65–75% of adult teratomas. Controversy also exists as to the prognostic significance of yolk sac differentiation in adult teratoma or combined germ cell tumours. It has been held generally that prognosis is no better and may, in fact, be worse as a result of the presence of yolk sac elements. A Medical Research Council (MRC) study published in 1987 found that the presence of yolk sac tumour areas was an indicator of a more favourable outcome in terms of a lower incidence of relapse after treatment.

Macroscopic Features
Pure yolk sac tumour occurring in infancy is a soft white or yellowish mass, often with small cystic spaces on its cut surface.

Microscopic Features
The tumour resembles adenocarcinoma, the cells forming tubular or papillary structures lined by cuboidal or columnar cells. The most reliable diagnostic feature is the presence of *Schiller–Duval bodies*. These are formed from one or more layers of tumour cells surrounding a central blood vessel (*Fig. 38.17*).

The yolk sac normally produces AFP in the embryo, as does the fetal liver. AFP production can be demonstrated in the cells of yolk sac tumour or area of yolk sac differentiation by immunohistochemical methods. The serum levels of this oncofetal antigen may also be raised and the view has been expressed that raised concentrations of AFP in patients with a germ cell tumour always indicates a non-seminomatous component.

Spread of Germ Cell Tumours
Germ cell tumours spread in a rather predictable fashion. The first groups of lymph nodes to be involved are the iliac and periaortic nodes and, later, supradiaphragmatic nodes become involved. In most cases, the nodal

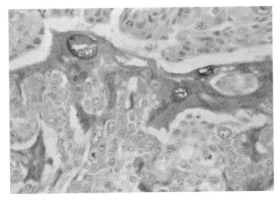

FIGURE 38.16 *Syncytiotrophoblastic giant cells in a malignant teratoma treated with an antibody to the β subunit of human chorionic gonadotrophin. The sites of antigen binding stain brown.*

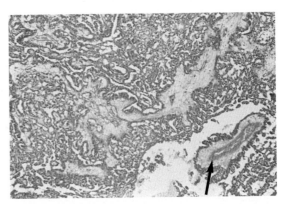

FIGURE 38.17 *Yolk sac differentiation in a testicular teratoma. Note the Schiller–Duval body (arrowed), which consists of a vascular core surrounded by tumour cells.*

deposits occur on the same side as the tumour but in about 15% there is bilateral node involvement.

Distant blood-borne metastases are found most often in the lungs, liver, brain and bones. The skeleton is particularly likely to be affected in cases of seminoma that have disseminated, and choriocarcinoma shows a tendency to metastasize to the brain.

Prognosis

The introduction of cisplatin as a chemotherapeutic agent has revolutionized the outlook for patients with testicular germ cell tumours; a majority of such patients, with the exception of those with trophoblastic tumours, can now be cured. Nevertheless it would be wrong to regard all testicular germ cell tumours as having the same natural history.

Factors that influence the prognosis include:
- **the nature of the tumour.** Patients with pure seminomas, especially spermatocytic seminomas, and differentiated teratomas have a good prognosis. Similarly, pure yolk sac tumours in infants hardly ever metastasize. Seminomas that are combined with teratomatous elements have a somewhat worse prognosis, and undifferentiated teratomas and especially choriocarcinomas behave in an even more aggressive fashion.
- **Stage of the tumour at the time of diagnosis.** In Britain, testicular germ cell tumours are staged with the Royal Marsden Hospital system shown in *Table 38.2.*
- **Concentration of tumour markers in the serum.** Very high serum concentrations of AFP (1000 ng/ml) or of human chorionic gonadotrophin (above 50 000 IU/l) are associated with a worse prognosis.
- **Microscopic features in stage I tumours.** According to an MRC working party report, a score of 1 is given to each of the following features:
  - a) the presence of undifferentiated teratoma in the tumour
  - b) the absence of yolk sac tumour
  - c) the presence of blood vessel invasion
  - d) the presence of lymphatic invasion

A score of 0 is given when any of these features is not present. Thus any stage I tumour can be graded from 0–4. The chance of recurrence after surgical removal of the tumours was found to be greater in those with higher scores. The practical importance of these data is that they provide a basis on which to select patients in whom primary tumour resection should be followed by immediate chemotherapy or radiation therapy.

LEYDIG CELL TUMOUR

Leydig cell tumours account for 1–3% of all testicular neoplasms, and occur at any age. The most common clinical manifestations are:
- testicular swelling
- gynaecomastia (in 30% of patients). Of those who show this feature, about 25% also have a decline in libido and/or potency
- In prepubertal patients, sexual pseudoprecocity develops. The term pseudoprecocity is used because the growth in pubic hair and enlargement of the penis are unaccompanied by any maturation of spermatocytes. About 10% of these children with precocious sexual development also have gynaecomastia.

Macroscopic Features

Most Leydig cell tumours are unilateral. The tumours are well circumscribed and have a characteristic brownish colour, presumably due to lipofuscin within tumour cells.

Microscopic Features

The tumour cells resemble normal Leydig cells. They are arranged either in a diffuse sheet-like fashion or in trabeculae. The Reinke crystalloids, typical of Leydig cells, are found in about one-third of the cells.

Natural History

About 10% of Leydig cell tumours show malignant behaviour, with metastases appearing up to 9 years after removal of the affected testis. These malignant examples occur in older age groups and there is no record of a prepubertal Leydig cell tumour behaving in a malignant fashion.

SEX CORD–STROMAL TUMOURS

These rare neoplasms are composed of Sertoli cells and gonadal stromal elements. The relative proportions of these two major components differ from case to case.

Tumours can occur at any age but are especially likely in children, who account for almost 40% of the reported cases. Two important behavioural characteristics are:

1) The frequent occurrence of gynaecomastia in prepubertal patients and in those more than 50 years old. The incidence of gynaecomastia is increased if the tumours are clinically malignant.

Table 38.2 Staging of Testicular Tumours

Stage	Criteria
I	Tumour confined to the testis
II	Lymph nodes below the diaphragm involved
III	Lymph nodes above and below diaphragm involved
IV	Extranodal metastases

2) The high frequency of malignant behaviour (almost 40%) in relation to sex cord–stromal tumour occurring in patients older than 10 years at the time of clinical presentation.

The appearances of these lesions cover a wide spectrum, which includes:

- **tumours resembling granulosa cell tumours of the ovary.** These tend to occur in infants less than 6 months old and are the commonest testicular tumours in this age group.
- **Sertoli cell tumours** of various types, one of which is a large-celled lesion characteristically undergoing calcification. This variety is often bilateral and may be multiple.

These lesions are often associated with endocrine disturbances and may, in some instances, also be associated with the Peutz–Jeghers syndrome (see p 527). They may also occur as part of a syndrome that includes cardiac myxomas and spotty cutaneous pigmentation.

MIXED GERM CELL–SEX CORD–STROMAL TUMOURS

The best known example of this group is the **gonadoblastoma**. This is a complex lesion in which there is a combination of germ cell tumour resembling seminoma and immature sex cord components showing either Sertoli cell- or granulosa cell-type differentiation. These cellular elements are arranged in discrete packets separated by stroma. In about 50% of cases, the germ elements invade the stroma and the lesion becomes converted to a seminoma or (in the ovary) its homologue, dysgerminoma.

Only about 20% of these tumours arise in the testis (the remainder are ovarian). The affected males are almost all young (under 20 years of age), usually have bilateral cryptorchidism and almost always have hypospadias owing to failure of fusion of the urethral folds over the urogenital sinus. In addition, these patients often have a uterus. Most have underlying pseudohermaphroditism or mixed gonadal dysgenesis.

MALIGNANT LYMPHOMA

Malignant lymphoma accounts for only about 5% of neoplasms arising within the testis but is the commonest testicular malignancy in men aged more than 55 years. Nearly all of these are non-Hodgkin's lymphomas of B-cell origin.

The patients present with testicular enlargement; the cut surface of the testis shows infiltration by whitish tumour tissue (*Fig. 38 18*).

Microscopic Features
There is infiltration of the testis by the malignant lymphoid cells that surround and infiltrate the seminiferous tubules. The differential diagnosis on microscopic examination includes spermatocytic seminoma and anaplastic seminoma. The use of monoclonal antibodies raised against leucocyte antigens as immunohistochemical reagents is of great help in making this distinction.

About 40% of patients are found to have bilateral testicular involvement and a considerable proportion have systemic dissemination at the time of diagnosis.

The testis is also often involved in leukaemia. This occurs more commonly with lymphocytic than with myeloid leukaemia.

Adenomatoid Tumour

This rather common lesion affects the epididymis rather than the testis, occurring most commonly in men aged 30–40 years.

The patients present with a small firm lump, which may be painful, just above the superior pole of the testis.

Macroscopic Features
Adenomatoid tumour appears as a greyish-white nodule measuring 1–2 cm in most cases. The cut surface may show some small cystic spaces.

Microscopic Features
Proliferating cells are arranged either in solid cords or as a lining for channels which may resemble vascular spaces. The cells are, in fact, neither epithelial nor endothelial in derivation and their immunohistochemical and ultrastructural features suggest they are mesothelial.

Natural History
Occasionally, adenomatoid tumour may extend into the adjacent testis and it may also be found in the spermatic cord and tunica vaginalis. In all these sites, however, its behaviour is completely benign.

VASCULAR DISTURBANCES IN THE TESTIS AND ITS ADNEXAE

Testicular Ischaemia and Infarction due to Torsion of the Spermatic Cord
Twisting of the spermatic cord is the commonest cause of testicular ischaemia. It occurs for the most part

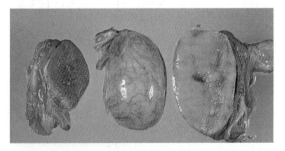

FIGURE 38.18 Normal testis (left) contrasted with enlarged infiltrated testis in a case of non-Hodgkin's lymphoma.

within the first year of life and in the immediate prepubertal stage; the main predisposing factor is abnormal mobility of the testis within the tunica vaginalis. This may be due to:

- absence of scrotal ligaments
- absence of the gubernaculum testis
- incomplete descent of the testis into the scrotum
- an abnormally high attachment of the tunica vaginalis around the spermatic cord, the so-called 'bell-clapper' deformity

There is often a history of trauma shortly before the onset of symptoms.

The clinical picture is characterized by the rapid onset of severe pain and swelling of the testis, and these may be accompanied by nausea, vomiting and abdominal pain.

Twisting of the cord is followed, in the first instance, by cutting off the venous drainage of the testis at a time when the arterial supply remains patent. Thus the testis becomes intensely congested.

The natural history depends on the amount of time elapsing between the torsion occurring and surgical treatment. If more than 10 hours has passed since the onset of symptoms then irreversible ischaemic necrosis of the germ cells is likely to have occurred; complete coagulative necrosis (infarction) may be seen in patients in whom treatment has been delayed beyond this point.

Twisting of small vestigial remnants of ducts (of either wolffian or müllerian origin), in the form of small cysts attached to the superior pole of the testis and to the epididymis, may also occur. This causes a clinical syndrome out of proportion to the size of these structures. The patients present complaining of severe scrotal pain which may be associated with scrotal oedema. The severe ischaemic consequences following spermatic cord torsion do not occur here.

Varicocele

This term is applied to a situation in which the veins of the pampiniform plexus are abnormally dilated and tortuous. This plexus, which runs within the spermatic cord, drains into the internal spermatic veins; varicocele results from incompetence of the valves in the internal spermatic vein leading to reflux of blood into the plexus.

Varicocele is quite common, being present in 15–20% of the male population. It is somewhat more common than this in men seeking advice for infertility and, curiously enough, its frequency is also increased in smokers.

In most instances (85%) varicocele is unilateral, the left side being affected far more often than the right. It is suggested that this is because the internal spermatic vein on the left side drains more or less at a right angle into the left renal vein, whereas on the right side the spermatic vein drains obliquely into the inferior vena cava.

The chief clinical effect of varicocele appears to be on fertility. Analysis of semen specimens shows a diminished number of sperm, a reduction in sperm motility and increased numbers of morphologically abnormal sperm. This is believed to occur because of alterations in testicular blood flow affecting not only the testis on the same side as the varicocele but the contralateral one as well.

SPERM GRANULOMA

This is a non-infective chronic inflammatory lesion that most commonly affects the epididymis and the spermatic cord, but which may also, although rarely, affect the testis.

The majority of cases occur in men who have undergone vasectomy and about one-third of cases of vasitis nodosa are associated with a sperm granuloma. Vasitis nodosa is a condition that may follow vasectomy and is characterized by scarring in the vas deferens together with proliferation of small tubules lined by epithelium. It is a reactive, not a neoplastic, process and causes thickening of the vas either uniformly or in a nodular fashion.

The principal pathogenetic step in sperm granuloma formation is disruption of the tubular basement membranes leading to the release of spermatozoa into the interstitial tissue. This causes an acute inflammatory reaction followed by a granulomatous response in which numerous macrophages are mixed with sperm, some of which are engulfed by these macrophages. In due time scarring occurs at the site of the granulomas. It is of interest that the extravasation of sperm into the interstitial tissues is not inevitably followed by an inflammatory response. It has been suggested that the inflammation is related to the presence of partly oxidized lipid (ceroid) in some of the sperm.

Patients complain of pain and some degree of swelling in the epididymis; on exploration, the lesion appears as a firm yellowish nodule which may measure up to 3 cm in diameter.

The Penis and Scrotum

Most disorders affecting the penis relate to two anatomical considerations:

1) **The penis is a skin-covered organ.** Thus many skin disorders occur, only a few of which affect particularly the penile or scrotal skin.

2) **The most distal portion of the urethra passes through it.** In the same way the penile urethra may show pathological changes identical with those seen in other urothelium-lined sites.

In addition, for obvious reasons, the risk of sexually transmitted infections is very high.

CONGENITAL DISORDERS

These are expressed as:
- abnormalities of **size**
- abnormalities of penile and penile urethral **development**
- abnormalities in **number**
- abnormalities of **lymphatic drainage**
- complete **absence** of the penis. This is extremely rare, occurring in only 1 in 30 million live births.

Abnormalities of Size
In this group the most striking abnormality is **micropenis** (abnormally short penis, defined as one more than 2.5 standard deviations shorter than the mean).

The mechanisms involved are much the same as those operating in congenital hypogonadism:
- pituitary or hypothalamic failures
- failure to secrete sufficient testosterone during fetal development
- resistance to the effect of androgens at the level of the end-organ

Abnormalities of Penile and Urethral Development

Hypospadias
The defining criterion is that the urethra opens either on to the ventral surface of the penile shaft, or, more rarely, the perineum (*Fig. 38.19*). The term is derived from the Greek word '*spadon*' meaning a 'rent' or 'tear'. It represents failure of closure of urethral folds over the urogenital sinus and is often associated with defective production of androgens in fetal life.

Hypospadias occurs in roughly 1 in 300 live births. Common associations are undescended testis and inguinal hernia. Especially in cases where the urethral meatus is situated on the **ventral** aspect of the penile shaft, there is an abnormal curvature of the penis, often causing lateral deviation. This is termed '**chordee**'. It is suggested that this is due to fibrous tissue replacement of part of the normally elastic urethral plate.

More severe hypospadias may be associated with intersex disorders including male pseudohermaphroditism, mixed gonadal dysgenesis, true hermaphroditism and Klinefelter's syndrome.

Epispadias
This is characterized by the urethral meatus opening on to the **dorsal** surface of the penis. It develops as a result of the failure of the precursors of the genital tubercle to meet dorsally in the midline. The penile corpora are

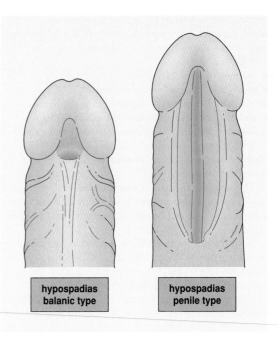

FIGURE 38.19 *Variants of hypospadias involving either the glans or the penile shaft.*

often abnormally short and curved, causing chordee to develop, the curvature being directed dorsally. Occasionally, epispadias may be associated with exstrophy of the urinary bladder.

Abnormalities of Number

Diphallus
Double penis (diphallus) is very rare. It may occur in three forms, listed below in increasing order of severity:
1) a bifid glans penis
2) partial separation involving the whole glans and much of the penile shaft
3) complete separation with two penises, both of which may be malformed

Abnormalities of Lymphatic Drainage
Congenital lymphoedema may occur as part of a syndrome comprising lymphoedema of both lower limbs as well as the external genitalia, or may affect the penis and scrotum alone. Penile swelling may cause compression of the urethra and obstruct urinary outflow.

Acquired lymphoedema may, of course, also occur in patients with tropical elephantiasis due to infection by the microfilariae of the nematode worm *Wuchereria bancrofti*. These block lymphatics causing a spectacular lymphoedema. Non-tropical acquired lymphoedema usually occurs as a result of surgical dissection in the area or of recurrent inflammation with scarring of the lymphatics.

INFLAMMATORY DISORDERS

The penis and scrotum may be the site of many inflammatory dermatoses such as **lichen planus, psoriasis and pityriasis rosea** (see pp 990–994, 1004–1005, 1006–1007).

SPECIFICALLY PENILE INFLAMMATORY DISORDERS

Non-infective Inflammation

Balanoposthitis

This term is used to delineate non-infective inflammation of the glans (**balanitis**) and prepuce (**posthitis**).

The inflammatory process may be **non-specific**, occurring in non-circumcised men who are careless in matters of penile hygiene and in whom smegma accumulates between the prepuce and the glans.

Specific variants exist in the form of:
- balanitis xerotica obliterans
- balanitis of Zoon

Balanitis Xerotica Obliterans

This is a chronic disorder affecting the surface of the glans and the mucosal aspect of the prepuce. It is the male homologue of the vulval lesion occurring in middle-aged and elderly women known as **chronic vulvar dystrophy** or **lichen sclerosus et atrophicus**.

On clinical examination the lesions appear as white plaques which give the glans and prepuce a mottled appearance.

Microscopic Features
Biopsies show a rather characteristic picture:
- hyperkeratosis, which is probably responsible for the white appearance
- thinning of the epidermis with atrophy of the rete pegs
- a curious homogenized appearance of the dermal collagen which forms an oedematous, eosinophilic and relatively cell-free band beneath the epidermis
- some dilatation of capillaries and a mild chronic inflammatory cell infiltrate beneath this zone of altered dermis

There has been considerable controversy as to whether this condition has neoplastic potential, but there is no convincing evidence of an increased risk of developing squamous carcinoma. However, the condition is not clinically trivial: wrinkling and retraction of tissues may occur and the prepuce may become adherent to the glans (phimosis).

Balanitis of Zoon

This is an inflammatory lesion of unknown aetiology characterized by **shiny, sometimes velvety, patches on the glans and prepuce.**

Microscopic Features
The epidermis is slightly thinned and there is loss of both the rete ridges and the granular layer. The epidermal cells have a very characteristic appearance. Their long axis lies parallel to the skin surface and the cells themselves become diamond shaped and tend to be separated one from another by oedema. The dermis is the site of a dense plasma cell infiltrate and dermal capillaries are dilated.

Behçet's Syndrome

This is a curious multisystem syndrome characterized by:
- recurring mouth ulcers
- recurring ulcers on the penis and scrotum (vulva and vagina in women)
- an acute, usually self-limiting, arthritis somewhat resembling rheumatoid arthritis
- cutaneous vasculitis

The aetiology is unknown and there is no evidence of immune complex deposition in the lesions. There may be increased concentrations of C9 in the serum and a decrease in the secretory component of immunoglobulin A. Young adult males are the most common victims and the disorder occurs more frequently in the Middle East than in western Europe.

The penile ulcers range in size from 2 to 10 mm and are usually painful. Within 2 weeks they heal spontaneously but may reappear.

Microscopic Features
In the early stages there is a marked perivascular chronic inflammatory infiltrate consisting of lymphocytes and macrophages. The endothelial cells of the affected vessels swell and fibrinoid necrosis is seen, the picture of a local vasculitis. This leads to ischaemic necrosis of the overlying epidermis and, thus, to ulcer formation.

Infective Inflammation
This is of three types:
- bacterial
- viral
- fungal

Bacterial Infections

Syphilis
The vast majority of cases of syphilis are sexually transmitted, being caused by the spirochaete *Treponema pallidum*. The natural history of this disease falls into three distinct phases, known as:
- primary
- secondary
- tertiary

The penis is affected principally in the primary stage. In males, apart from those who indulge in the less usual forms of sexual congress, the site for primary lesions to occur is the penis. The lesion, known as the **chancre**, is a small nodular lesion that appears usually about 3 weeks after infection. Within a few days the nodule ulcerates and a thin serous fluid exudes from the surface. This fluid contains large numbers of spirochaetes and is highly infective.

Classically, the chancre is described as being painless but many atypical forms can occur and some of these are very painful. It is important to be aware of this, as an erroneous clinical diagnosis of genital herpes simplex infection may be made because of the pain, and the chance of diagnosing syphilis at this early stage, before systemic dissemination of the organism has occurred, may be missed.

The chancre normally heals without treatment in about 3–6 weeks, leaving a small scar.

Microscopic Features

Chancres show thinning of the epidermis with central erosion. The dermal capillaries show a marked degree of swelling of the endothelial cells, and these vessels are surrounded by a dense inflammatory cell infiltrate consisting of lymphocytes and plasma cells. Organisms may be demonstrated in the tissues by means of special staining methods such as the Warthin–Starry stain in which the spirochaetes appear black. This is not altogether a reliable method and a higher proportion of positive results comes from examining the fluid from chancres by dark-field illumination.

The penis may also be involved in the secondary stage of syphilis, the glans being covered by flat papules. These lesions are known as mucous patches.

Microscopic Features

Biopsies show some thickening of the epidermis and a florid dermal infiltrate in which large numbers of plasma cells are present. As in the chancre, there is a marked degree of endothelial cell swelling in the small dermal blood vessels. Large numbers of organisms are present in these lesions, which are highly infective.

Chancroid

This is another sexually transmitted disorder commonly involving the penis. It is caused by a Gram-negative bacillus known as *Haemophilus ducreyi*.

The incubation period is about 5 days, after which a small pustule appears which breaks down to form a painful ulcer. This small lesion may heal leaving a scar, but in some patients there is more destructive inflammation; this is associated with enlargement of the inguinal lymph nodes, which become tender and matted together. The skin overlying the enlarged lymph nodes may break down.

Microscopic Features

The appearance of chancroid is rather distinctive, with a multilayered character.
- The surface of the ulcer shows necrotic tissue admixed with fibrin and a neutrophil infiltrate. The organisms, if still present, will be in this most superficial area.
- Deep to this is a zone in which large numbers of new capillaries can be seen, growing in a 'palisaded' fashion in relation to the ulcer floor.
- The deepest layer shows a striking chronic inflammatory cell infiltrate in which lymphocytes and plasma cells are prominent.

Granuloma Inguinale

This a venereal disease caused by a Gram-negative bacillus of the *Klebsiella* family known as *Calymmatobacterium granulomatis* (Donovan bodies).

The initial lesion appears either on the glans or the prepuce as a raised ulcer with an irregular margin. The ulcers are usually painless and may bleed from time to time. They tend to heal with a considerable degree of scarring.

Microscopic Features

- thickening of the epidermis at the margins of the ulcer
- a macrophage and plasma cell infiltrate in the upper dermis
- Donovan bodies in the cytoplasm of some of the macrophages. The organisms appear as small 'safety-pin'-like structures which are revealed by silver staining of tissue sections.

Lymphogranuloma Venereum

This is a sexually transmitted disease caused by *Chlamydia trachomatis*, an obligate intracellular parasite closely related to Gram-negative bacteria. This organism also causes non-specific urethritis (see pp 717–718) but in this case the serotypes concerned are different, lymphogranuloma being caused by serotypes L1–L3. Both males and females may act as asymptomatic carriers of this disorder, the frequency of the carrier state being almost 11% in sexually active heterosexual males.

In clinically apparent infections, the initial lesion is a small red papule usually sited on the coronal sulcus of the penis. Like the chancre, this lesion may be easily missed by the patients and heals spontaneously within a short period and without scarring.

The next stage is the development of enlargement of inguinal nodes, which soften and become attached to the overlying skin. Multiple sinuses then form. The intranodal inflammation is destructive and may, in females and in male homosexuals who practise anal intercourse, extend to involve the rectum with the subsequent development of low rectal strictures and rectal fistulae.

Microscopic Features

- The ulcer floor shows necrotic debris infiltrated by neutrophils.
- Deep to this there is a chronic inflammatory infiltrate in which macrophages can be seen to be invading small blood vessels. These cells aggregate to form granulomas which obliterate the affected vessels leading to local ischaemia and necrosis. The necrotic areas become infiltrated by acute inflammatory cells.
- A similar process is seen in the inguinal nodes, necrosis in the cortex leading to the formation of large stellate abscesses. These soft fluctuant abscesses drain via the multiple sinuses referred to above.

Viral Infections

The most important viral infections at this site are those with herpesvirus, and one or other strain of human papillomavirus (HPV). HPV infections are discussed in the section dealing with tumours of the penis and scrotum.

Herpes Simplex Virus

Genital herpes simplex virus (HSV) infections constitute a major problem: they are very common, very painful and liable to recurrence. HSV infection is, arguably, the commonest sexually transmitted disorder.

The production of skin lesions involves:

- proliferation of epidermal cells
- ballooning degeneration of the cells
- the formation of intranuclear inclusions. In the early stages, the inclusion is rich in DNA and almost fills the nucleus. Later, much of this DNA is lost and the inclusion becomes separated from the nuclear chromatin by a clear halo.

Clinically, the initial lesions are painful blisters that rupture and become even more painful. The extent to which the penile skin is affected varies from case to case. In immunosuppressed patients, vesicles may not be present. In addition to the pain, fever, dysuria and enlargement of inguinal nodes may occur. A primary infection of this type usually lasts for 2–3 weeks.

Recurrence in the absence of new infection is a major problem and is more likely in patients infected with HSV-2 than in those infected with HSV-1. Recurrence occurs in nearly 90% of HSV-2 infections and in about 50% of HSV-1 infections. This difference may relate to the high frequency with which HSV-2 remains latent in the sacral sensory ganglia, which it reaches via sensory nerves in the skin.

Microscopic Features

The most characteristic feature is intraepithelial vesicles. These occur because of marked cytoplasmic swelling of infected cells leading to loss of the normal intercellular bridges so that the affected cells separate from one another.

The cells surrounding the vesicle usually contain intranuclear inclusions. These appear as round structures that stain intensely with eosin and that have a clear halo. A few multinucleate giant cells may also be present. The underlying dermis is the seat of an inflammatory reaction in which both acute and chronic inflammatory cells may be seen.

Electron microscopy shows the presence of large, spherical virus particles. The whole virion has a diameter of 100–120 nm; this includes the 'envelope', which is derived from the nuclear membrane of the infected cell.

Spontaneous recovery is due to cell-mediated immune mechanisms, although high titres of antibody also develop. The importance of this cell-mediated response is shown by the development of devastating disseminated herpesvirus infections in patients with defective T-cell function.

TUMOURS AND TUMOUR-LIKE LESIONS

Condyloma Acuminata

This increasingly common lesion, called by some a 'venereal wart', is a sexually transmissible disorder with an incubation period of 1–2 months. It is caused by an infection with a papillomavirus that has a circular genome composed of double-stranded DNA. **This virus has a particular tropism for surface epithelia such as skin, vagina and cervix.** HPV causes several different types of wart, of which condyloma acuminata is but one. There are more than 50 types of HPV; types 6 and 11 are most frequently related to anogenital condylomas.

It is widely agreed there is a spectrum of disease related to this virus, ranging from lesions of low malignant potential through grades of intraepithelial neoplasia to frankly invasive carcinomas involving surface epithelia. In penile skin showing intraepithelial neoplasia, evidence of papillomavirus infection is found in most cases, but here the virus type is most often 16 or 33.

In the sexual partners of those who have either condylomas or areas of intraepithelial neoplasia there is a remarkable concordance in respect of:

- the presence of lesions
- the histological type of lesions
- the presence of papillomaviruses of certain types

Macroscopic Features

The lesions are most common on the glans but may involve the shaft as well. The commonest sites are at the penile meatus or in the fossa navicularis. They are reddish and have a cauliflower-like appearance. The infection may be expressed in the form of a single lesion but multiple warts are not infrequent and these may coalesce to cover quite large areas of penile skin.

Microscopic Features

- marked thickening of the squamous epithelium (acanthosis), which is arranged in a papillary fashion
- a lack of atypia in the squamous epithelial cells
- clearing of the cytoplasm in the epithelial cells in the upper layers of the surface covering associated with shrinkage of the nucleus (**koilocytosis**)
- the presence of the virus shown either by immunohistochemical techniques or by *in situ* hybridization

Intraepithelial Neoplasia

The term intraepithelial neoplasia used in relation to penile lesions covers three named entities:

- **erythroplasia of Queyrat**
- **Bowen's disease**
- **bowenoid papulosis**

With respect to the first two of these, there has been a long-standing controversy regarding their relationship and the malignant potential they possess.

Both entities have the same basic nature, showing the histological and behavioural features of intraepithelial neoplasia; what separates them is simply their location:

- **Bowen's disease occurs on the true skin of the penile shaft or scrotum.**
- **Erythroplasia of Queyrat affects the glans or prepuce.**

In view of this, one might legitimately wonder whether the use of either of these eponyms is any longer justified.

Clinically the appearances of these lesions are modified by their site. The lesions of Bowen's disease are well demarcated, rather scaly, red plaques on the skin of the penile shaft. Queyrat's erythroplasia appears as red velvety patches on the surface of the glans or the inner aspect of the prepuce.

Microscopic Features

Changes of intraepithelial neoplasia involve the full thickness of the surface epithelium in the form of:

- large hyperchromatic nuclei
- individual cell keratinization (dyskeratosis)
- a greater than normal number of mitoses
- abnormal mitoses

In about 5% of cases, these changes progress to invasive squamous carcinoma.

Bowenoid Papulosis

This is a disorder of the surface epithelium of the penis (both shaft and glans). Microscopically it somewhat resembles intraepithelial neoplasia, although the degree of epithelial disturbance is less marked than in Bowen's disease. Bowenoid papulosis tends to occur in younger men than Bowen's disease or erythroplasia of Queyrat, and the majority of cases have been reported as showing evidence of infection by HPV type 16.

Clinically the lesions appear as fleshy, usually pigmented, nodules, occurring more commonly on the shaft than on the glans. They may resolve spontaneously in some instances; in others, conservative local surgery usually suffices. The lesions are, in any event, most unlikely to progress to invasive carcinoma.

Invasive Neoplasms

For all practical purposes, invasive neoplasms of the penis are squamous carcinomas. They are relatively rare tumours in Western countries but in some locations, most notably parts of Asia, Africa and Latin America, the lesions are much more common (10–18% of all cancers). Patients range in age from 40 to 70 years.

The risk of developing penile carcinoma is inversely correlated with circumcision, particularly if this operation is carried out in early life. Whether the low risk of developing penile carcinoma is related to the circumcision itself or to the sexual mores of groups in whom the young are circumcised is not clear.

The effects of circumcision on the risk of penile carcinoma is well shown in India where 98% of penile carcinomas occur in Hindus who are not circumcised, whereas only 2% occur in Moslems, circumcised between the ages of 4 and 9 years. The presence of phimosis (a state in which the foreskin cannot be retracted because of the presence of postinflammatory scarring) is a strong additional risk factor.

There is a strong association between penile cancer and HPV infection. DNA sequences of the papillomavirus are integrated into the host cell genome, type 16 sequences being found in almost half the cases and type 18 in just under 10%. The same situation exists in relation to squamous carcinoma of genital surface epithelia in women, especially cervical carcinoma.

Macroscopic Features

Two macroscopic growth patterns can be detected on clinical examination of patients with this tumour. These are:

- a papillary mass growing outwards from the glans or prepuce
- an ulcerating tumour which tends to infiltrate. This variety is more common in tumours arising from the prepuce, whereas the papillary type is more common in those derived from the glans.

Microscopic Features

The papillary tumours tend to be well-differentiated keratinizing squamous carcinomas, whereas the ulcerating variety are poorly differentiated and highly invasive. Spread occurs predominantly via lymphatics; nodal metastases are present in about 15% of cases. Because the tumours frequently become infected, reactive lymph node enlargement is common and this makes clinical staging of the lesions difficult.

Verrucous Carcinoma

Verrucous carcinoma is now believed to be identical with the lesion formerly known as the giant condyloma of Buschke and Lowenstein, and is believed to be of viral (HPV) origin.

This tumour, which accounts for about 5% of penile carcinomas, presents as a bulky cauliflower-like growth with an unpleasant smell.

Microscopic Features

Verrucous carcinoma is well-differentiated *throughout*, which helps to distinguish it from the more usual type of invasive squamous carcinoma. The individual cells are extremely large in size, which is another helpful diagnostic feature. The rete pegs of the enormously thickened squamous epithelium grow down in a characteristically bulbous pattern and true invasion of the underlying stroma appears only at a relatively late stage in the natural history.

Although it has a papillary appearance, the connective tissue cores present in the papillae of a true condyloma are not seen here. If only biopsies, rather than resection specimens, are available for microscopic examination, a correct diagnosis may be difficult to make, because of the well-differentiated nature of the proliferated epithelium. It is important, therefore, that the pathologist should be aware of the naked-eye appearances of the lesion from which the biopsy has been derived.

Other neoplasms affecting the penis are rare. They include malignant melanoma, various connective tissue tumours and extramammary Paget's disease.

OTHER DISORDERS OF THE PENIS AND SCROTUM

Fournier's Gangrene

Fournier's gangrene is a type of necrotizing fasciitis in which the scrotal and, sometimes, the penile skin becomes necrotic and sloughs away. It was originally said to occur predominantly in young males but may, in fact, be seen in all age groups.

Clinically, the patients complain of pain in the genital area and there may be an accompanying fever. The skin of the scrotum becomes blackened and sloughs; microscopic examination shows extensive necrosis associated with bacterial invasion of small blood vessels and consequent thrombosis leading to ischaemic necrosis of the parts they normally perfuse.

Infection is clearly present in most cases, the commonest infecting organisms being *Pseudomonas* species and β-haemolytic streptococci, although many others can be identified. A significant proportion of patients who develop Fournier's gangrene have urological disorders of various kinds and the presence of diabetes mellitus also appears to confer increased risk. It has been suggested that the scrotal skin may easily become dry and excoriated, which allows invasion by the mixed bacterial flora normally resident in the perineum.

Peyronie's Disease

This is a progressive scarring process involving the corpora cavernosa, principally in middle-aged men. It manifests as:
- curvature of the erect penis
- pain on erection

The lesions may be so severe as to render normal sexual activity impossible.

On clinical examination a mass may be felt, usually on the dorsal aspect of the penile shaft.

Microscopic examination shows scarring in the zone between the corpora cavernosa and the tunica albuginea. This is associated with a chronic inflammatory cell infiltrate and, in a few patients, metaplastic bone formation.

The cause is unknown, although it is not without interest that a few cases have been associated with Dupuytren's contracture. It is possible that repeated mild trauma in individuals predisposed to fibrosis may be the cause of this lesion, which is difficult to treat and which can cause much distress.

The Prostate

NORMAL ANATOMY AND DEVELOPMENT

The prostate, a composite organ made up of glandular and non-glandular components, is the largest accessory sex organ in the male, weighing about 20 g in young males. Prostatic weight remains fairly constant unless nodular hyperplasia develops. The function of the gland is still unknown.

The most significant reference point is the **prostatic urethra**. This is divided into two parts of roughly equal length by an abrupt anterior angulation of about 35°, situated about half way between the bladder neck and the apex of the prostate itself. The verumontanum arises at this point, protruding from the posterior wall of the distal prostatic urethra into the lumen. Both the ejaculatory ducts and most of the ducts arising from the glandular element of the prostate enter this distal portion of the urethra.

Coronal sections through the prostate, along the course of the ejaculatory ducts and the distal urethral segment, show the different functional zones of the prostate and their relationships (*Fig. 38.20*):

- **The central zone** accounting for about 25% of the gland volume. Its duct exits from the verumontanum in close relation to the orifices of the ejaculatory ducts.
- **The peripheral zone** comprising about 70% of the gland volume. The ducts from this region exit from the posterior wall of the distal prostatic urethra, along which they are arranged in a double row.
- **The transitional zone** accounting for about 5% of the gland volume. This lies lateral to the lower end of the preprostatic sphincter, a sleeve of smooth muscle surrounding the proximal segment of the urethra.

The glands in these three zones show both morphological and functional differences (*Table 38.3*)

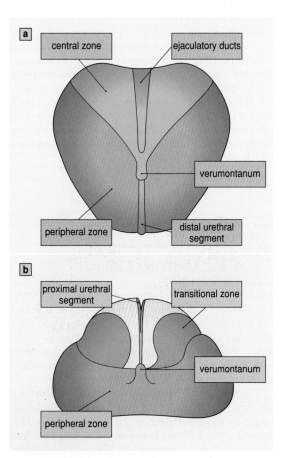

FIGURE 38.20 Zones of the prostate.

and they are believed to arise from different sites in the embryo. The peripheral and transitional zones are thought to stem from the urogenital sinus, whereas the central zone glands are thought to be derived from the wolffian duct. These differences are significant because different prostatic disorders show definite predilections for one or other of these zones.

Prostatic Biopsy

Tissue sampling may be carried out in two ways:
1) by **needle biopsy** via the perineum or transrectally
2) in the course of **transurethral resection**

Most **needle biopsy specimens** consist chiefly of tissue from the **peripheral zone**, whereas **transurethral specimens** consist of tissue from the **transition zone, the urethra, periurethral tissues, bladder neck and anterior fibromuscular stroma** (see below). As shown in *Table 38.3* the diagnostic information obtained from biopsies must depend heavily on the region sampled. Thus well-differentiated carcinoma found in transurethral specimens usually represents cancer that has arisen in the transition zone, whereas poorly differentiated tumour probably represents spread from the peripheral zone. Nodular hyperplasia is unlikely to be seen on needle biopsy because this approach does not, as a rule, yield any transition zone material.

Prostatic Stroma

The prostate functions by slowly accumulating small amounts of fluid secretion which is expelled only occasionally and, then, rapidly. This pattern of behaviour is indicative of the fact that the major component of the prostatic stroma is muscle, which is arranged in four principal anatomical areas:

- **the preprostatic sphincter**, probably functioning during ejaculation to prevent backflow of seminal fluid from the distal segment of the urethra
- **a striated muscle fibre sphincter**, extending from the base of the verumontanum to the apex of the prostate
- **an anterior fibromuscular stroma**, a sheet of tissue extending downwards from the bladder neck over the anterior surface of the prostate and blending at its lateral margins with the prostatic capsule
- **the prostatic capsule**, enclosing most of the surface of the gland. It consists of an inner layer of mainly transversely oriented smooth muscle fibres and an outer layer of collagen fibres. The relative proportion of these two elements varies in different parts of the prostatic surface, as does capsular thickness. In assessing invasion of the capsule in patients with carcinoma of the prostate, only complete penetration of the tumour through the capsule appears to have any prognostic significance.

Table 38.3 Anatomical and Functional Zones of the Prostate

	Characteristics		
	Central	Transitional	Peripheral
Glands	Complex, large, polygonal glands with intraluminal ridges	Simple, small, rounded glands	Simple, small, rounded glands
Stroma	Dense	Dense	Loose, open
Pepsinogen II production	+	0	0
Tissue plasminogen activator production	+	0	0
Binding of the lectins, *Ulex europaeus*, pea nut lectin, succinyl wheatgerm agglutinin	+	Not known	0
Nodular hyperplasia	Rare	Common	Rare
Inflammation	Rare	Variable	Common
Cancer	Rare (5% of prostatic cancers)	Moderately common (25% of prostatic cancers)	Common (70% of prostatic cancers)

Disorders of the Prostate

NODULAR HYPERPLASIA

Epidemiology

Nodular hyperplasia is extremely common. It seldom causes clinical symptoms before the age of 50 years but there is some evidence that nodule development starts much earlier. By the age of 50 years, morphological evidence of nodular hyperplasia is present in 50% of males; this proportion increases with advancing age, to reach 75% or more in the eighth decade. There are no obvious predisposing factors, nor any protective ones – if the rather drastic step of submitting to castration at a relatively early age is excluded. It is clearly of considerable clinical and economic importance because, in the USA alone, some 400 000 prostatectomies are performed annually.

Aetiology and Pathogenesis

Of all mammalian species studied, only humans and dogs develop nodular hyperplasia of the prostate. Thus, much of what we know of the causes and development of this hyperplasia is derived from studies in the dog.

Prostatic hyperplasia does not occur in either species in the absence of intact testes. This suggests a local tissue role for androgens, which, in the form of

dihydrotestosterone, are increased in concentration in hyperplastic prostatic tissue. The conversion of testosterone to the dihydro- form is catalysed by the enzyme 5α-reductase. Men born without this enzyme have small or absent prostates but retain potency and the ability to ejaculate (*Fig. 38.21*).

This view of a causal role for dihydrotestosterone is

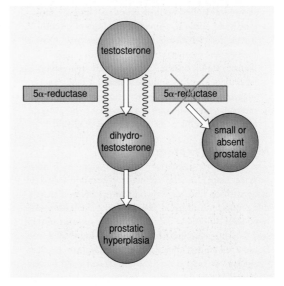

FIGURE 38.21 Role of dihydrotestosterone in prostatic hyperplasia.

supported by the fact that administration of androgens to castrated dogs leads to prostatic hyperplasia. This is aggravated if, at the same time, 17β-oestradiol is also administered. The oestrogen appears to increase the expression of androgen receptors in that part of the prostate affected by nodular hyperplasia. A counterpart of this model exists in human males who tend to increase their adrenal secretion of oestrogens with ageing.

Macroscopic Features

Nodular hyperplasia is confined to the transition and periurethral zones, peripheral zone tissue being compressed as the nodules expand. This suggests that there is greater expression of appropriate receptors for dihydrotestosterone in these areas. Certainly, the concentrations of this androgen in nodular prostates are highest in the affected areas.

The gland may be considerably enlarged. Specimens removed by retropubic prostatectomy are found often to weigh as much as 100–200 g, and hyperplastic prostates weighing up to 800 g have been recorded.

The enlarged glands may be nodular or smooth. The appearances of the cut surfaces are greatly influenced by whether the hyperplasia affects principally glandular or stromal components:

- If the **glands are chiefly involved**, many nodules are seen on the cut surface, each surrounded by fibromuscular stroma. Often the nodules show a 'honeycomb' appearance and milky fluid can be squeezed from the cystic spaces. Larger cysts may also be present and some of these may show calculi or yellow casts of glycoprotein, known as **corpora amylacea**.
- If the hyperplasia is mainly **stromal**, the cut surface shows a much less nodular appearance and is rather glossy and uniform. Sometimes nodules of smooth muscle cells are seen in the peri-urethral area. On microscopic examination these look not unlike benign smooth muscle tumours but the temptation to label them as such should be resisted. It has been suggested that the formation of fibromuscular nodules represents the earliest phase of nodular hyperplasia and that this induces the proliferation of glands.

Microscopic Features

The hyperplastic nodules are seen to contain both fibromuscular and glandular elements. These are called by some workers fibroadenomyomatous nodules. The relative proportions of gland and muscle differ from nodule to nodule. Within individual nodules the number of acini may be strikingly increased in both number and size. Because of the hyperplasia, some glands show papillary infoldings, whereas others are dilated and lined by flattened epithelium. In all these hyperplastic glands it should be possible to detect a second layer of darkly staining, small basal cells situated just above the basement membrane of each gland.

Secondary Changes Within The Hyperplastic Nodules

Inflammatory Changes Focal aggregates of chronic inflammatory cells are commonly seen within the hyperplastic nodules. These may be related to dilated ducts which are filled with inspissated secretions.

Infarcts Infarction occurs in about a quarter of hyperplastic prostates. As the prostate expands within its capsule, it is not surprising that interstitial pressure, especially within the peripheral zone, rises; this may compress the vascular supply to the nodules derived from vessels passing through the peripheral zone.

Infarcts are speckled, greyish yellow areas, often with haemorrhagic centres. They range in diameter from a few millimetres to several centimetres. They may bulge above the cut surface of the rest of the gland.

On microscopic examination they show coagulative necrosis involving both glandular and stromal elements. Infarcts quite commonly elicit squamous metaplasia in the ducts at their periphery. This must not be mistaken for squamous carcinoma, which, in any event, is very rare in the prostate.

Functional Effects of Prostatic Hyperplasia

The effects of prostatic enlargement are due, in the first instance, to distortion and compression of the prostatic urethra and interference with sphincter function. The symptoms that arise from prostatic hyperplasia have been classified into two main groups: **'obstructive'** and **'irritative'** symptoms.

'Obstructive' Symptoms

These symptoms involve:

- **weakening of the urinary stream.** In a patient complaining of this, an objective assessment should be made of the actual flow rate.
- **terminal dribbling.** This results from a fall in detrusor pressure occurring towards the end of micturition.
- **hesitancy** (i.e. an increased time lapse between initiating micturition and actual commencement of flow of urine)
- **a sense of incomplete emptying** of the bladder

Prostatic outflow obstruction is normally followed by an increase in the contraction (pressure) of the detrusor muscle and this may be sufficient to maintain urine flow at normal levels for a long time. With more severe obstruction, the rise in detrusor muscle voiding pressure is insufficient to overcome this and flow rates will fall. In patients with **chronic** retention of urine secondary to prostatic obstruction, detrusor muscle pressure falls giving a combination of **low voiding pressure and low urine flow**.

'Irritative' Symptoms

These symptoms include:

- **nocturia** (i.e. being awakened from sleep by the desire to micturate)
- **frequency** (i.e. voiding urine more than seven times during the daytime). This can have many causes. In the context of prostatic hyperplasia it is probably due to either chronic retention of urine or detrusor muscle instability.
- **urgency**
- **incontinence**

Acute and Chronic Urine Retention

Roughly 20% of patients with prostatic outflow problems will present at some point with **acute** retention of urine. Often, these patients do not have a long-standing history of significant obstructive or irritative symptoms. It is not uncommon for acute retention to develop in older males following a surgical procedure not associated with the urinary tract. It is suggested that this retention is precipitated by the anticholinergic effects of premedication and anaesthesia.

The defining criterion for **chronic retention** is the habitual presence of more than 50 ml of urine in the bladder immediately after micturition. The presence of even a relatively small amount of residual urine in the bladder is a risk factor for infection, usually by *Escherichia coli*, and the resulting cystitis is expressed as:

- pain on passing urine
- frequency
- macroscopic haematuria

Pathophysiology

Chronically raised levels of detrusor muscle tone and large volumes of residual urine might be expected to have an effect on the ureters and kidneys. Indeed, this can occur, but it is relatively infrequent: only 5–10% of patients with prostatic outflow symptoms show evidence of ureteric or renal pelvic dilatation on pretreatment radiological investigation. Nevertheless it is important to identify this subgroup of patients who, if left untreated, will develop potentially life-threatening chronic renal failure.

In terms of bladder function, patients who are most likely to develop dilatation of the upper urinary tract and renal failure are those who have what is termed 'high pressure chronic retention'.

The retention of large amounts of residual urine in the bladder may lead to one of two morphological consequences in respect of the bladder wall. These are:

1) a bladder that is dilated and has **a thin, almost transparent, wall**
2) a bladder containing large amounts of residual urine but with **an abnormally thick wall with marked detrusor muscle hypertrophy**

It is the second of these that is associated with dilatation of the upper parts of the urinary tract and the risk of renal failure. In functional terms its defining characteristic is **a raised intrinsic detrusor pressure during the filling phase of micturition**.

Clinically these patients have:

- **late-onset enuresis** (i.e. a small leakage of urine occurring shortly after falling asleep)
- **a tense, palpable bladder which is painless.** Patients are usually unaware of the bladder distension; the higher centres in the nervous system seem unable to sense the presence of an overfull bladder
- **high blood pressure**
- **bilateral dilatation of the ureters and renal pelves** leading to progressive renal failure

Radiological examination of the urinary tract shows varying degrees of dilatation of both ureters and renal pelves. When postmicturition pressure within the bladder is measured, it is found to be raised in all these patients.

INFLAMMATORY DISORDERS

The term prostatitis implies an inflammatory process affecting the prostate. **Its use should be reserved for those cases in which the clinical features encountered are due to the presence of the inflammation rather than for prostatic tissue in which a few aggregates of inflammatory cells are seen**, something that is very common in nodular hyperplasia.

Acute Prostatitis

Acute inflammation in the prostate may be **bacterial** or **abacterial** in type.

Clinically, patients present with a syndrome characterized by:

- fever and rigor
- pain in the lower back, rectum and perineum
- discomfort on passing urine

On rectal examination, the prostate is felt to be enlarged, tender, warm and rather firmer than normal.

Microscopic Features

If material is available for microscopic examination, an acute inflammatory cell infiltrate is seen to be present in and around the ducts, the intraductal component being mixed with the debris of epithelial cells shed from the duct walls.

Diagnosis can be established, in the case of acute bacterial prostatitis, by culture of prostatic secretions obtained by prostatic massage. **Massage of an infected prostate is by no means a risk-free procedure because it may lead to bacteraemia.** For this reason it is usually sufficient to rely on urine culture instead. The bacteria associated with acute prostatitis are much the same as those responsible for urinary tract infections, such as *E. coli* (found in 80% of cases) and other enterobacteria, *Pseudomonas, Serratia* and *Klebsiella* (10–15%) and enterococci (5–10%). Gonococcal prostatitis was common before antibiotic treatment was introduced, but is now rare.

Abscess formation may occur and this may be diagnosed and localized by ultrasonography. This makes drainage of the abscesses much easier and efficient.

Effect of Immunodeficiency

Being immunocompromised, especially if this is associated with acquired immune deficiency syndrome (AIDS), is a risk factor for infectious prostatitis, and almost one in six patients with AIDS will suffer from acute bacterial prostatitis. In these patients a wider range of microorganisms causes the inflammation than is the case in individuals who are immunologically competent.

Chronic Prostatitis

The groups of disorders falling under this rubric include:

- non-specific, chronic, bacterial inflammation
- non-specific, chronic, abacterial inflammation
- granulomatous prostatitis due to many different causes

Chronic Bacterial Prostatitis

Chronic bacterial prostatitis is the commonest cause of recurrent urinary infection in men who have no evidence of urinary outflow obstruction. Diagnosis can be made by culturing urine voided after prostatic massage.

Most cases are due to infections with *E. coli*, and small calculi within prostatic ducts often serve as nidi for infection. The secretions of inflamed prostatic ducts are alkaline and the high pH of the prostatic tissue makes it difficult for antibiotics to diffuse through the inflamed tissues.

Chronic Abacterial Prostatitis

This is commoner than chronic bacterial inflammation of the prostate. The patients may complain of pain on ejaculation and both culture and Gram stain examination of prostatic secretions fail to show any bacteria. An aetiological role for *Chlamydia trachomatis* and *Ureaplasma urealyticum* has been proposed, but this question is unresolved.

Chronic Granulomatous Prostatitis

The defining criterion for granulomatous prostatitis is a prominent macrophage infiltration associated with the presence in some instances of multinucleated giant cells of the Langhans type seen in many granulomatous disorders. Prostatitis of this type accounts for about 1% of prostatic inflammations. It causes the prostate to become very firm and nodular, and this may give rise to clinical suspicions of carcinoma, from which it must be distinguished.

The classification of granulomatous prostatitis is difficult and somewhat controversial, because it appears to be the common endpoint of many widely different conditions (*Table 38.4*).

CARCINOMA OF THE PROSTATE

Epidemiology

Cancer of the prostate is extremely common, being the second most common cause of death from cancer in males in the USA (18% of all cancer deaths in males). In the USA the incidence of prostatic cancer is 50% higher in Afro-Americans than in Caucasians, and the lifetime risk for death from prostatic cancer is twice as high. This ethnic difference is interesting because the incidence in Afro-Americans is very high (greater than 70 per 100 000), whereas it is only 10 and 4.3 per 100 000 in Africans in Nigeria and Senegal respectively.

On a worldwide basis, considerable differences in prostatic cancer incidence exist. The highest incidence is found in North America and the Caribbean, and the lowest in China and Japan.

Aetiology

The cause of prostatic cancer is unknown. There are data suggesting that androgen interactions with the prostate play a part:

- Carcinoma of the prostate is very rare in eunuchs.
- Carcinoma of the prostate is very rare in patients with Klinefelter's syndrome (phenotypic males who have two X chromosomes instead of the normal one).
- Orchidectomy causes regression of prostatic cancer.
- Treatment with oestrogen similarly tends to cause tumour regression.
- Testosterone appears to stimulate the activity of the tumour cells.
- The incidence is low in patients with high oestrogen levels associated with cirrhosis of the liver.

There is obviously an age effect because the incidence rates rise steadily after the age of 50 years, as shown in *Table 38.5*.

Pathology and Biological Behaviour

The vast majority of prostatic cancers arise within the peripheral zone. A small minority of tumours derive from the larger ducts in the transitional and central zones.

Prostatic cancers can be divided into four categories on the basis of their natural history and presentation:

- **Latent carcinomas.** These are carcinomas found at autopsy in 25–37% of males and which have been entirely unsuspected during life. The prevalence of small latent carcinomas shows no geographical variation; larger latent tumours are found most frequently where the mortality rates from prostatic cancer are highest.

Table 38.4 Classification of Granulomatous Prostatitis

Group	Cause	Features
Idiopathic		Accounts for nearly 70% of cases. Believed to be caused by blockage of ducts and stasis of secretions. Secretions escape into the stroma and elicit the granulomatous response.
Infections	Bacterial Fungal Parasitic	Tuberculosis now rare. Shows presence of caseating granulomas. Brucellosis can mimic tuberculosis. Fungal infections do occur but not as primary infections; they are associated with systemic dissemination of the fungi. Prostatic involvement by platyhelminths such as *Schistosoma* is a common association of bladder schistosomiasis.
Iatrogenic	Postsurgery Postirradiation Following BCG treatment for bladder cancer	Both transurethral prostate resection and needle biopsies of the prostate may result in granulomas which resemble the necrotizing lesions seen in rheumatoid disease. These lesions are usually focal in contrast to the diffuse distribution of other forms.
Other non-infective	Malakoplakia Allergic prostatitis	Granulomatous lesions due to defective intralysosomal digestion of bacteria. Most commonly found in bladder (see p 712). Causes obstructive symptoms and fever. Found in association with asthma and eosinophilia (Churg–Strauss syndrome). Shows granulomatous lesions in which eosinophils are prominent and there may also be evidence of vasculitis.

Table 38.5 Annual Age-related Incidence Rates in North American Caucasians

Age group	Incidence (per 100 000 per year)
50–54	19
55–59	61
60–64	154
65–69	303
70–74	487
75–79	705
80–87	944

- **Incidental carcinomas.** These are tumours found in 6–20% of samples of prostatic tissue removed surgically from patients with urinary outflow tract obstruction, thought on clinical grounds to be due to benign prostatic hyperplasia.

- **Occult carcinomas.** The defining criterion here is that the patient presents with symptoms and signs of metastatic disease due to cancer of the prostate but has no symptoms referable to the urinary outflow tract.
- **Clinical carcinomas.** This term applies to patients whose tumours have caused prostatism and in whom the finding of a hard nodular prostate on rectal examination has aroused the suspicion of carcinoma.

This range is the expression of a spectrum of biological behaviour. **It is clear that some prostatic cancers progress very slowly, if at all. They may cause no clinical disturbance nor contribute in any way to shortening the patient's life. At the other extreme there are tumours that can grow rapidly and cause death.** Fortunately, **grading** of prostatic cancers provides valuable prognostic information, and is discussed in more detail on pp 748–750.

Macroscopic Features

Cancer may or may not be associated with prostatic enlargement. Areas of tumour infiltration may be difficult to see on the cut surface and are grey or yellowish, poorly demarcated, usually firmer than the surrounding prostatic tissue. The distribution of cancer within the prostate can be seen well in specimens removed at radical prostatectomy. Sections across the entire area of the prostate can be prepared and stained; the tumour-infiltrated areas can be seen either with the naked eye or with the help of a hand lens.

Microscopic Features

The tumours are principally **adenocarcinomas** showing considerable variation in the appearances of individual tumour cells and in gland architecture. In some instances, the carcinoma is very well differentiated (*Figs 38.22* and *38.23*) and may be difficult to diagnose. In such cases, evidence of stromal invasion must be relied upon; the finding of acini on or within muscle bundles is very helpful in this regard.

Four major patterns have been described; these may be present alone or in combination:

- a **cribriform pattern** which is predominantly intraductal
- a **diffuse infiltrating pattern** in which the cells are poorly differentiated and stream out individually into the stroma
- a carcinoma consisting of medium-sized glands in which cytological changes suggestive of malignancy are often not present. The architectural pattern, especially in relation to muscle bundles, is important here, as is the presence of nucleoli in glandular epithelium. The cytoplasm of the malignant glandular epithelium is usually finely granular but may sometimes have a foamy appearance due to the accumulation of neutral fat. In contrast to normal prostatic epithelium in which neutral mucins are secreted, about two-thirds of the tumours secrete acid mucins, which can be detected by appropriate staining
- a **carcinoma consisting of small glands in which cellular atypia is a prominent feature.** Mitoses are rarely present

Immunohistochemical Features

The tumour cells mark with two monoclonal antibodies reacting homospecifically with:

- **prostate-specific antigen (PSA)**, a glycoprotein localized to the endoplasmic reticulum, but which is also found within gland lumina
- **prostate-specific acid phosphatase**, which is normally localized to the lysosomes

The chief usefulness of these immunohistochemical methods is in the cases of biopsies from metastatic tumours in which the site of the primary has not been established. Within the prostate itself, immunohistochemistry is used to help in the dis-

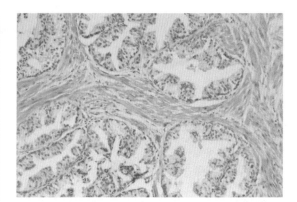

FIGURE 38.22 *Histological features of the normal prostate.*

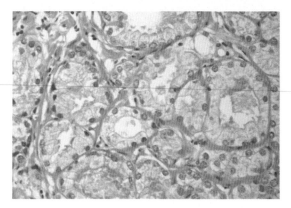

FIGURE 38.23 *Well-differentiated prostatic carcinoma with well-formed glandular spaces.*

tinction of poorly differentiated prostatic carcinoma from poorly differentiated bladder cancers invading the prostate.

These tumour markers may also be present in **serum**:

- About 60% of localized prostatic cancers and 80% of those with bony metastases show raised levels of **prostatic acid phosphatase**.
- Serum levels of **PSA** may also be raised in prostatic cancer and, in view of the high prevalence of this tumour, it has been suggested that serum PSA measurement might be employed as a screening procedure. The normal concentration of PSA is less than 4 ng/ml. Increases above this level are found in 40–60% of patients with localized cancer of the prostate. Unfortunately, similar increases may be found in 30–40% of patients with nodular hyperplasia of the prostate. Thus the PSA concentration in serum is neither very sensitive nor specific and its usefulness as a screening test for prostatic cancer is controversial.

Microscopic Grading of Prostatic Cancer

There have been many reports of a strong positive correlation between the microscopic appearances of the tumours and their degree of

aggressiveness. Poorly differentiated prostatic cancers (*Fig. 38.24*) **progress rapidly, whereas the reverse is true for well-differentiated ones.**

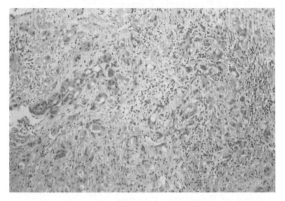

FIGURE 38.24 *Poorly differentiated carcinoma of the prostate with ill-formed glands and marked cellular pleomorphism.*

Grading is extremely important in forecasting the behaviour of prostate cancers because accurate pathological staging can be carried out only in the minority of cases where radical prostatectomy has been performed.

The Gleason Grading System

The grading system most widely used was devised by Gleason. It assigns the histological patterns seen into five groups, each group being delineated by:

- the degree of glandular differentiation
- the pattern of infiltration in the stroma

Because more than one pattern may be found within a single tumour, scoring is done by assigning a grade to both the predominant pattern (by area) and to the pattern that occupies the second greatest area of the tumour. Thus an individual tumour might, for example, be graded as Gleason 3/2.

Follow-up studies show that biological behaviour is

'Gleason grading' for prostate cancer. Numbers and sub-letters refer to the standardizing drawing

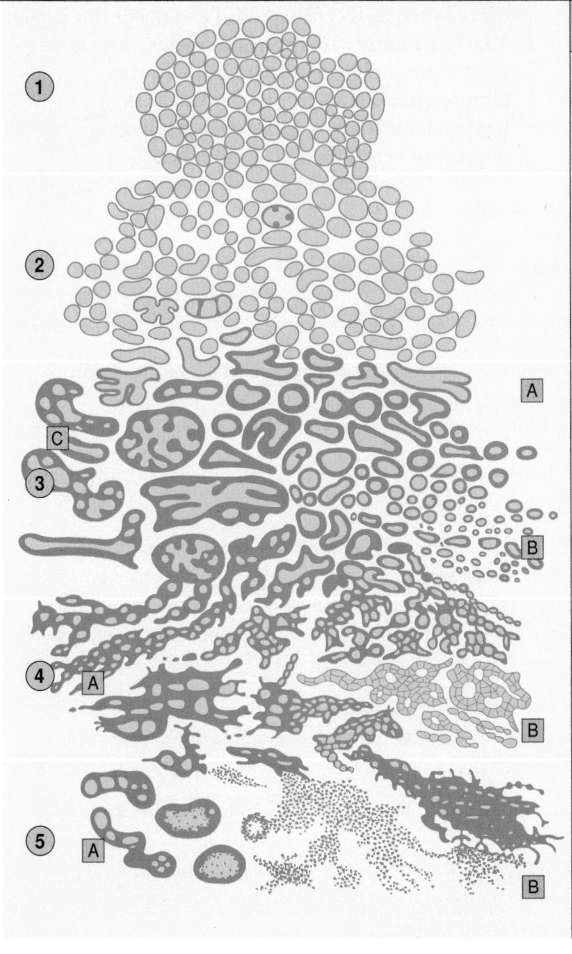

	Gland differentiation	Gland distribution
1	**1.** 'Round', lined by single layer of rectangular cells.	Close packed in rounded masses, definite edge.
2	**2.** Slightly more variable in size and shape.	Separated up to one gland diameter, 'loose' edge.
3	**3A.** Definitely irregular in shape. Variable medium to large size	Irregularly spaced apart, poorly defined 'edge'. Surround normal structures.
	3B. Small to very small glands, not fused or 'chained'.	Very irregular spacing and distribution. No 'edge'. Surround normal structures.
	3C. Masses of cribriform and/or papillary epithelium with smooth outer surfaces.	Very irregular spacing and distribution. No 'edge'. Surround normal structures.
4	**4A.** Raggedly outlined masses of fused glandular epithelium. 'Bare' tumour cells in stroma.	Ragged infiltrating masses. Overrun normal structures. Loss of ability to form smooth surfaces against stroma.
	4B. Same as 4A, large clear cells.	Same as 4A.
5	**5A.** Smooth, cribriform to solid masses, often central necrosis. 'Comedocarcinoma'.	Ragged infiltrating masses. No definable 'edge'.
	5B. Anaplastic carcinoma with just enough vacuoles and glands to suggest adenocarcinoma.	Ragged infiltrating masses. Infiltrate stromal fibres. No definable 'edge'.

FIGURE 38.25

Table 38.6 Cancer Mortality Rates in Relation to Histological Grade, Expressed as Deaths per Patient-year

Grade	Deaths per patient-year
2	0
5	0.02
6	0.05
7	0.07
8	0.13
9	0.2
10	0.25

more closely related to the **average** of the two grades given than to the worse of the two grades. This has led to the suggestion that each prostatic cancer be scored by adding together the two grades. If only one type of pattern is present, the grade is multiplied by 2. This provides a grading system ranging from 2 to 10. Thus a 3/2 carcinoma would have a total score of 5.

Both cancer and all-cause mortality correlate with increasing tumour grades, as shown in *Table 38.6.*

The histological patterns used for assigning grades have been 'frozen' (Gleason, 1990) into a simplified drawing, so as to assist pathologists in maintaining standardized criteria in their assessment of prostatic cancer (*Fig. 38.25*).

An abbreviated and simplified account of the histological criteria used is given in *Table 38.7*.

Staging of Prostatic Cancer

Staging of prostatic cancer can be done using one of two systems:

- a clinical staging system devised in the USA (*Table 38.8*)
- the tumour node metastasis (TNM) system recommended by the International Union against Cancer (UICC).

Some correlations between clinical and pathological staging are shown in *Table 38.9.*

Accurate pathological staging is possible only when the whole prostate has been removed by radical prostatectomy.

Spread of Prostatic Cancer

Like most neoplasms prostatic cancers may spread:

- **Directly** through the prostatic tissue and capsule into surrounding structures such as the seminal vesicles, prostatic urethra, bladder and periprostatic connective tissue, to all of which the prostate can become fixed. Rectal invasion can occur but is rare.
- **Via lymphatics to regional nodes.** The nodes most commonly affected are those in the periprostatic connective tissue. Bilateral lymphadenectomy is performed as a staging procedure before undertaking radical prostatectomy; this gives some idea of the frequency

Table 38.7 Histological Criteria of the Gleason System

Grade	Histological pattern
1	Closely packed, uniform, simple glands lined by a single layer of rectangular epithelial cells. The glands form a mass with a 'pushing' edge. The presence of at least a few epithelial cells with nucleoli is a 'must' for diagnosing cancer rather than atypical hyperplasia.
2	Some degree of separation of the glands from each other (usually by a distance no greater than the diameter of one gland) plus a mild degree of variation in the size and shape of the glands.
3	A higher degree of variation in size and shape of glands and much wider separation of the individual glands. The glands extend irregularly into the stroma and the tumour appears to have what Gleason has called a 'ragged' edge. Some morphological forms, included by Gleason in grade 3, consist of tumours with papillary and/or cribriform patterns. For this type to retain its place in grade 3, the edge of the tumour mass should be smooth and rounded.
4	The tumour may be either papillary, cribriform or microacinar but the tumour areas here have a characteristic ragged and infiltrating edge. Fusion of some of the glands occurs with tumour cells joining up to form cords.
5	Two patterns are included under this rubric: 1) highly undifferentiated with only an occasional gland lumen. It is said by Gleason to resemble small cell carcinoma of the lung. 2) a mass of closely packed papillary or cribriform cylindrical masses which show the presence of focal central necrosis rather like what is seen in comedocarcinoma of the breast. Gleason states that any necrosis of the tumour epithelium automatically assigns a tumour to grade 5.

Table 38.8 Clinical Staging System for Prostatic Cancer

Stage	Extent of involvement and clinical features
A	Clinically inapparent
A1	Focal
A2	Diffuse
B	Palpable on rectal examination
B1N	Focal: a solitary nodule less than 1.5 cm in diameter and confined to one lobe of prostate
B1	Focal: an area of palpable induration more than 1.5 cm in diameter but involving less than one lobe of prostate
B2	Diffuse
C	Local spread beyond prostatic capsule
C1	With no seminal vesicle invasion
C2a	With seminal vesicle invasion
C2b	With fixation to wall of pelvis
D	Metastatic spread

Table 38.9 Correlation between Clinical and Pathological Staging

Clinical stage	Percentage of cases confined to prostate
A2	81
B1N	79
B1	38

of regional nodal involvement, estimated as being about 40% at the time of diagnosis. From the pelvic node deposits further spread takes place to involve the periaortic nodes. In addition, lymph nodes above the diaphragm may be affected, some patients with prostatic cancer presenting initially with enlarged supraclavicular or mediastinal nodes.

- **Via the bloodstream.** Bloodstream spread is expressed most frequently in the form of bony metastases. These occur in about 70% of cases of metastatic prostate cancer. The pelvis and the lumbar spine are the most frequent sites to be involved, but any bone may be affected.

  The route by which tumour cells reach the skeleton is controversial. Two possibilities exist, which are not mutually exclusive:

    1) Spread via the systemic venous drainage to the lungs with some tumour cells passing through the pulmonary capillary bed and gaining access to the systemic arterial circulation.
    2) By retrograde spread from the periprostatic venous plexus into the vertebral venous plexus. Reversal of flow through these veins is said to occur as a result of the frequent changes that occur in intra-abdominal pressure.

The tumour deposits elicit, in many instances, new bone formation and are thus termed **osteosclerotic**. Associated osteoblastic activation results in an increase in the serum alkaline phosphatase concentration.

CHAPTER 39

The Female Reproductive System

Disorders of the Female Genital Tract

NORMAL DEVELOPMENT

The Ovary

Every journey starts with a single step. In ovarian development that step is the appearance of primitive germ cells within the yolk sac wall at about the fourth week of gestation. These cells migrate at about 6 weeks to gonadal ridges formed by proliferation of coelomic epithelium and by condensation of the mesenchymal tissue lying just below and lateral to the developing mesonephros.

The primitive gonad is neither ovary nor testis, **gonadal sex being determined by chromosomal sex. Unless a Y chromosome encoding a testis-determining factor is present, the indifferent gonad will inevitably become an ovary.** The mesodermal cells of the gonadal ridge proliferate, as do the germ cells, the latter being incorporated into the former from which are derived both the ovarian stroma and the ovarian surface epithelium.

The Genital Tract

At about the sixth week of gestation, there develop on the anterolateral aspect of the gonadal ridges, two ducts each lying lateral to the mesonephric duct. These are the müllerian ducts, which grow down towards the urogenital sinus, undergoing three important developments:

1) **As they extend caudally, the ducts grow towards the midline with two contiguous portions being separated by a septum.**
2) **This septum must then break down with fusion of the distal portions of the müllerian ducts, leading to formation of the uterine canal.** The fused müllerian ducts continue to grow caudally until they reach the urogenital sinus. The unfused cephalad portions of the ducts remain separate and ultimately become the fallopian tubes.
3) **The vagina grows down initially from the fused portions of the müllerian ducts as a solid cylindrical mass of cells (the vaginal plate), which becomes cavitated by an ingrowth of cells from the urogenital sinus.**

Anatomical abnormalities of the genital tract encountered in females who have neither gonadal nor endocrine disorders can be related directly to failure of different degrees of severity in these three processes (*Fig. 39.1*):

1) **Failure of the müllerian ducts to come together as they grow caudally may result** in the following anomalies, listed in decreasing order of severity:
   - two uterine bodies, two cervices and two vaginas. This is known as **uterus didelphys**
   - two uterine bodies, two cervices and one vagina (**uterus bicornis bicollis**)
   - two uterine bodies, one cervix and one vagina (**uterus bicornis unicollis**)
   - a uterus in which the fundus is deeply notched in the midline (**arcuate uterus**)
2) **Failure of the septum to break down**, resulting in a uterine cavity divided into two by a septum. Failure in septum breakdown may affect the vagina as well, but this is probably due to failure of septum breakdown between the two arms of the urogenital sinus.
3) **Anomalies of the müllerian duct system and of the development of the distal portion of the vagina.** These are surprisingly common, being found in 0.25–0.5% of females. Not all anomalies are severe, but women with fusion defects have a high incidence of problems associated with pregnancy such as abortion, premature onset of labour, abnormal presentation of the fetus and uterine rupture during labour. Dysfunctional uterine bleeding, dysmenorrhoea and infertility are also associated with defects in müllerian duct fusion.

ANOMALIES IN SEXUAL DEVELOPMENT

Chromosomal sex (i.e. the presence or absence of a Y chromosome) determines gonadal sex. The type of gonad in its turn is the principal factor in determining whether an individual has a male or female phenotype. Thus abnormalities of sexual development can be considered at three levels.

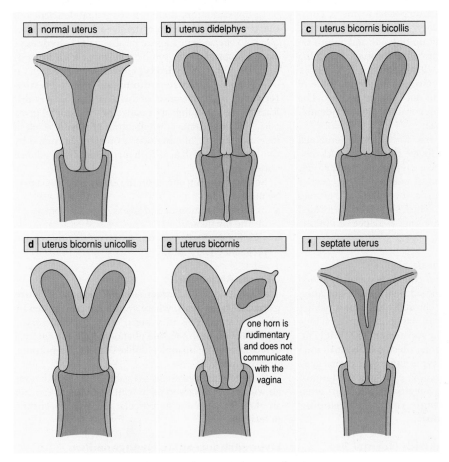

| a | normal uterus | b | uterus didelphys | c | uterus bicornis bicollis |

| d | uterus bicornis unicollis | e | uterus bicornis | f | septate uterus |

one horn is
rudimentary
and does not
communicate
with the
vagina

FIGURE 39.1 **a–f** *Congenital anomalies of the uterus, cervix and vagina.*

Anomalies Associated with Abnormal Sex Chromosomes

There are *four* principal syndromes associated with such abnormalities:

1) Turner's syndrome
2) Klinefelter's syndrome (see p 724)
3) true hermaphroditism
4) mixed gonadal dysgenesis

Turner's Syndrome

Turner's syndrome results from **absence of the whole or part of one X chromosome**. It occurs in about 1 in 3500 live births but also contributes to fetal loss; early abortion is common where there is monosomy for the X chromosome in female embryos.

In most live-born cases, the karyotype is 45X0. Most of the remainder show deletion of the short arm of the X chromosome, which in some cases is only partial. In the latter circumstance physical appearance may be virtually normal and the presenting abnormality is primary amenorrhoea, of which Turner's syndrome is a most important and common cause. A small minority show X0 mosaicism (e.g. 45X0/46XX).

Ovarian development in early embryonic life is normal. However, the fall in oöcyte numbers starting in intrauterine life and continuing normally throughout childhood, adolescence and reproductive life is grossly accelerated in Turner's syndrome. By the age of 2 years, the oöcytes have dwindled to virtually nil, a sequence of events described as 'the menopause occurring before the menarche'. **At this stage the ovary is reduced to a fibrous streak.** In cases where Turner's syndrome is the result of mosaicism, a few ova may persist into adult life, and menstruation and even pregnancy may occur in a few patients.

The characteristics are discussed in Chapter 30 (see pp 312–313) and *Figs 30.6* and *30.7*.

True Hermaphroditism

The defining criterion is the presence of both ovarian and testicular tissue. It is primarily a disorder of gonadal rather than of chromosomal sex, 60% of the patients having a normal 46XX karyotype. The remainder show various mosaicisms involving the sex chromosomes, such as 46XX/46XY or 45X0/46XY. With the 46XX karyotype, it is possible that translocation of part of the Y chromosome to the X chromosome may have occurred.

An ovary may be present on one side and a testis on the other, although a single 'mixed' gonad containing both ovarian and testicular elements is not uncommon. In most cases a uterus is present, although evidence of both wolffian and müllerian duct systems persists. The external genitalia are ambiguous and gender identity may be either male or female.

There is an increased risk for gonadal germ cell tumours, although this is lower than in gonadal dysgenesis. Because testicular tissue is present, virilization is likely to occur at the time of puberty. If the gender identity of the patient is female, then clearly the correct treatment is gonadectomy, which should be performed before the onset of puberty brings evidence of virilization in its trail.

Mixed Gonadal Dysgenesis

Gonadal development in this condition is usually asymmetrical, with a testis on one side and a streak gonad on the other. A number of chromosomal abnormalities may occur in association with this gonadal maldevelopment, the commonest being mosaicism (45X0/46XY).

Despite the Y chromosome, affected individuals usually show a **female phenotype**, although external genitalia may show masculinization, chiefly in the form of clitoral hypertrophy. At puberty, virilization often occurs and **there is a high risk of developing gonadal germ cell tumours**.

Anomalies Associated with Normal Sex Chromosomes

The disorders falling under this rubric fall into two major groups:
- those in which the gonads are macroscopically **normal**
- those in which the gonads are macroscopically **abnormal**

Gonads Normal

Such disorders result in **pseudohermaphroditism**, which may be defined as the condition in which the gonads and genotype are of one sex type whereas the external genitalia are more appropriate for the opposite sex. This may be seen in individuals with either a 46XX or a 46XY karyotype. Male pseudohermaphroditism is discussed in the chapter on testicular disorders (see p 724) and will not be further considered here.

The basic mechanism underlying female pseudohermaphroditism is the exposure of a fetus with a 46XX karyotype to a virilizing influence during embryonic life. The commonest cause of this is **congenital adrenal hyperplasia** (see pp 240, 839).

In this condition, there is a congenital deficiency of one or other of the enzymes involved in the synthesis of cortisol. The enzyme most often absent is **21-hydroxylase**. This block in the synthetic pathway leads to accumulation of **17-hydroxyprogesterone**, which is converted to **androstenedione** and then to **testosterone**. It is the operation of this alternate pathway that leads to the masculine appearance of the external genitalia. The low plasma concentrations of cortisol result in increased output of adrenocorticotrophic hormone by the pituitary, and hence to hyperplasia of the adrenal cortex.

Similar virilizing effects on the external genitalia may be produced by:
- maternal ingestion of androgens or progestogens during pregnancy
- a virilizing ovarian tumour in the mother during pregnancy (very rare)

Gonads Abnormal

The commonest disorder in this group is **pure gonadal dysgenesis**, where gonads are represented by fibrous streaks. This may occur with a 46XX karyotype. Patients have a female phenotype but the external genitalia remain infantile; unlike Turner's syndrome, stature is normal.

Pure gonadal dysgenesis may also occur in individuals with a 46XY karyotype in which the 'streak' gonads are thought to be due to testicular regression occurring in fetal life.

Hypogonadotrophic Hypogonadism

Just as in the case of the testis (see pp 722–724), hypogonadism in the female may result from a failure of ovarian stimulation by gonadotrophic hormones. An interesting example is **Kallman's syndrome**, resulting from an isolated deficiency in gonadotrophin-releasing hormone (GnRH) secretion. This syndrome may be inherited as an X-linked defect or an autosomal one.

Clinical Features

Clinical features include:
- hypogonadism
- hyposmia (inability to smell)
- colour blindness in some cases

Other associated abnormalities can include:
- unilateral renal agenesis
- disorders of movement

Kallman's syndrome is thought to arise from failure of the migration during embryonic life of both olfactory neurones and GnRH-synthesizing nerve cells from the anlage of the olfactory lobe into the hypothalamus.

The Endometrium

NORMAL ANATOMY AND FUNCTION

The endometrium lines the uterine cavity, acting as a substrate for fertilized ovum implantation. It consists of tubular glands in a well-vascularized stroma, both of which undergo many changes, some associated with maturation and ageing and others with cyclic fluctuations in the hormones involved in development and maturation of the ovum and preparation for blastocyst implantation.

The normal menstrual cycle lasts 21–34 days and menstruation itself takes up to 5 days. Cycle events are timed **from the onset of menstruation**, termed day 1, and are described in *Table 39.1 (Fig. 39.2)*.

If a fertilized ovum has been implanted, then menstruation does not occur and a different set of changes termed **gestational hyperplasia** follows, which includes:

- the continuing presence of predecidual cells
- the reappearance of secretion by the endometrial glands
- the reappearance of stromal oedema

The Arias–Stella Phenomenon

In some instances conception is followed by the Arias–Stella phenomenon, characterized by:

- hypersecretion by the endometrial glands
- vacuolation of the cytoplasm of the gland epithelium

Table 39.1 Cyclic Changes in the Endometrium

Phase	Morphology
Menstrual phase (days 1–5): This is due to a sharp drop in oestrogen and progesterone secretion, occurring when the corpus luteum degenerates (about 14 days after ovulation).	Necrosis of the endometrium associated with haemorrhage.
Proliferative phase (days 6–21): This phase corresponds with follicular secretion of large amounts of oestrogen under the influence of follicle-stimulating hormone (FSH) and precedes ovulation.	Endometrial glands increase in length becoming tortuous. Mitoses appear within the glandular epithelium and in the stromal cells and, in the later stages, pseudostratification of the epithelial nuclei is noted. During this phase, progesterone receptors are expressed on the endometrial cells.
Early secretory phase (lasts on average for 4–5 days after ovulation): In the average cycle, ovulation occurs on or about the 14th day and this ushers in a stage characterized by glandular secretion and differentiation of stromal cells. Once the ovum leaves the follicle, the latter becomes converted to a corpus luteum, which is stimulated by luteinizing hormone (LH) to secrete oestrogen and progesterone.	The features of this phase develop about 24–36 hours from the time of ovulation. The most characteristic is the appearance of glycogen-containing vacuoles beneath the nuclei of the glandular epithelial cells. If all the cells of about 50% of the endometrial glands show this vacuolation, it is safe to assume that ovulation has occurred.
Mid-secretory phase (lasts from about the fifth to the ninth postovulatory day).	The vacuoles move to the supranuclear part of the cytoplasm and discharge some or all of their contents into the gland lumina. The glands are now dilated and tortuous and the stroma begins to show oedema.
Late secretory phase (begins on or about the tenth postovulatory day).	Tortuosity of gland outlines is now very marked, the epithelial lining being thrown into folds. Glandular secretion lessens and stromal cells start to differentiate into 'predecidual' cells (plump cells with rounded nuclei and abundant granular and eosinophilic cytoplasm). This change occurs first round spiral arterioles. By about the 26th day, neutrophils start to appear in the endometrium, as do granular lymphocytes (K cells), and these cells are the harbinger of focal necrosis and haemorrhage, marking the early phases of menstruation.

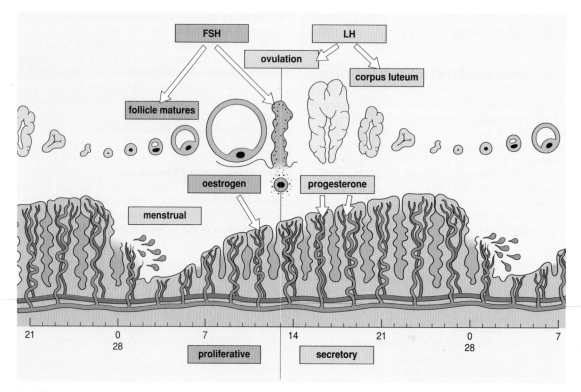

FIGURE 39.2 Events of the menstrual cycle and the hormonal changes that mediate them.

- the presence of enlarged, darkly staining and pleomorphic epithelial cell nuclei

These features, often focal, may occur whenever implantation has taken place, irrespective of the site. Thus it may be seen in ectopic pregnancies as well as in aborted intrauterine pregnancies.

Effects of Hormonal Disturbances on the Endometrium

Because the endometrium during reproductive life is regulated by absolute and relative concentrations of oestrogen and progesterone, it is not surprising that abnormalities in their concentrations lead to abnormalities in endometrial morphology and to functional disturbances in the menstrual cycle.

Low Oestrogen Concentrations

Oestrogen depends on normal development of ovarian follicles. Failure of follicle development must be the correlate of one of the following (Fig. 39.3):

- **absence of functioning tissue**, as in streak gonads where no follicles are present
- **absence of hormonal drive**, as in absent or inadequate secretion of FSH by the pituitary
- **increased resistance to FSH drive**

Ovarian follicle failure leads to a reduced or absent oestrogen drive on the endometrium. The endometrium is much thinner than normal and

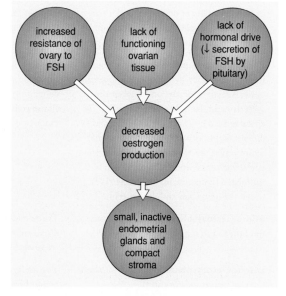

FIGURE 39.3 Basic causes of hypo-oestrogenism and its effects on the endometrium.

contains the **small inactive glands and compact stroma** normally seen in the non-functioning basal layer and similar to those in the postmenopausal endometrium.

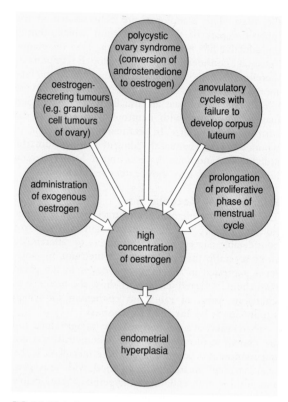

FIGURE 39.4 *Causes of an increased oestrogen drive on the endometrium.*

Increased Oestrogen Concentrations

Increased oestrogen concentrations (*Fig. 39.4*) may occur in:

- **anovulatory cycles** in which follicle maturation occurs but no ovum is released, resulting in failure of corpus luteum development and thus unopposed and continuing oestrogen stimulus on the endometrium, which becomes hyperplastic. Anovulatory cycles and, thus, this type of hyperplasia occur most frequently around the time of the menarche and the menopause; patients complain of heavy, irregular or prolonged periods. Both functional and morphological features revert to normal if progesterone is administered or ovulation resumes
- **the administration of oestrogen** for therapeutic purposes
- **the presence of an oestrogen-secreting ovarian tumour** such as a **granulosa cell tumour** or a **thecoma**
- **the polycystic ovary syndrome** in which there is excess production of androgen by both the ovary and adrenal. Conversion of excess androstenedione to oestrogen leads to chronically raised concentrations of the latter.
- **longer than normal proliferative phases.**

Sometimes the proliferative phase may last more than 21 days. Oestrogen concentrations do not increase, but the endometrium is subjected to its growth-promoting effects for longer than normal; the glands show multilayering of their epithelial lining and the amount of functioning endometrium is mildly increased.

Low Progesterone Concentrations

Low postovulatory concentrations of progesterone indicate a failure of development or function of the **corpus luteum** due to:

- inadequate follicle development
- inadequate concentrations of LH or too short a peak of LH secretion immediately before ovulation occurs
- raised prolactin levels which suppress progesterone production (but may also occur in women who ovulate normally)

Low progesterone concentrations lead to abnormalities in the cyclic endometrial pattern, which include:

- delay in the morphological evolution of both glands and stroma during the secretory phase
- loss of the normal coupling between gland and stromal maturation, the latter appearing more mature than the former
- loss of the synchronous maturation of the glands so that in one biopsy one might find glands showing different stages of the secretory phase (**irregular ripening**).

Clinical correlates of luteal insufficiency are:

- small amounts of bleeding occurring before the time of menstruation
- infertility
- a risk of early abortion
- prolonged menstruation

High Progesterone Concentrations

These are due to treatment with exogenous progestogens for contraceptive or therapeutic purposes. The initial effect is to induce secretory phase changes in endometrium primed by oestrogen from the follicles. In addition, endogenous oestrogen secretion is inhibited and **regression and atrophy of the glands results, as does a marked pseudodecidual change in the stroma**.

Effects of Age on the Endometrium: the Menopause

In the perimenopausal period, anovulatory cycles are quite common; for this reason, simple endometrial hyperplasia is often encountered during this time. The menopausal decline in oestrogen secretion means that there is an abrupt withdrawal of growth-promoting stimuli and the endometrium becomes atrophic, showing thinning, small and inactive glands and a compact spindle-cell stroma. The speed with which this occurs varies but **it is a good working rule that mitoses in the endometrium 3 years or more after the** menopause imply either an abnormal source of endogenous oestrogen (such as an oestrogen-secreting tumour) or that the patient has been given exogenous oestrogen.

Postmenopausal endometrium often shows cystic dilatation of the atrophic glands. This may be diffuse or focal and is believed to be due to blockage of gland outlets during atrophy.

ENDOMETRIAL INFLAMMATION (ENDOMETRITIS)

Unlike most other tissues, some neutrophils in the endometrium are perfectly normal, **provided only that their appearance is restricted to the time of menstruation**. Neutrophils at other times constitute evidence of acute inflammation as do **plasma cells, granulomas, lymphoid aggregates with germinal centres** or **other inflammatory cells**.

Acute Infective Endometritis

This is comparatively rare because:

1) **endometrial infection is inhibited by a cervical mucus barrier** which tends to prevent the ascent of organisms from the vagina.
2) endometrial shedding, occurring at the times of the menses, serves as a drainage mechanism for the uterine cavity.

The effectiveness of these protective mechanisms may be diminished. Any condition interfering with uterine drainage, such as polyps or tumours within the cavity, or scarring of the cervix, will increase the chances of endometritis, as will circumstances such as cervical infection that interfere with the cervical mucus barrier.

The commonest cause of acute endometritis is **postabortal retention of products of conception**. Sexually transmitted infections with *Neisseria gonorrhoeae* are still fairly common and also cause an acute, rather short-lived, endometritis.

Chronic Endometritis

Chronic non-granulomatous endometritis is characterized by **plasma cells and macrophages in the endometrium**. Intrauterine contraceptive devices (IUCDs) constitute a well-recognized cause, as does long-continued retention of products of conception.

Recent abortion is suggested by **hyalinized stromal blood vessels**. While **plasma cells are the hallmark of chronic endometritis**, in some cases, particularly where there is cervical obstruction, the inflammatory process is dominated by foamy macrophages. This is termed **xanthomatous endometritis** because of the resemblance of the macrophages to those in xanthomas associated with hyperlipidaemia.

Chronic granulomatous endometritis is almost always due to **tuberculosis** spreading from the fallopian tube to the endometrium. It is now seldom seen in the West. The granulomas are concentrated in the superficial part of the endometrium which, during reproductive life, is shed each month. Thus the granulomas take considerable time to develop. It is important, therefore, to take endometrial biopsies during the **late secretory phase**, as otherwise false-negative results are likely. The granulomas are usually non-caseating and may be associated with neutrophils in some of the adjacent gland lumina. In postmenopausal women, in whom there is no regular shedding of endometrium, the individual granulomas have a much longer natural history and, thus, may show extensive caseation.

Endometrial Metaplasia

The tissues of the female genital tract, with the exception of the ovary, are müllerian in origin and retain to a considerable degree, müllerian capacity to differentiate along several pathways. In the endometrium, metaplasia is expressed in the form of changes in the gland epithelium. Affected glands may show the presence of squamous, tubal or mucinous epithelium, of which **squamous is by far the commonest**.

The clusters of squamous cells are intraglandular and are known as morules. Chronic endometritis is a not uncommon association and squamous metaplasia is also seen in patients treated for long periods with oestrogens and in those with endometrial hyperplasia (presumably oestrogen related). Squamous metaplasia within the endometrium has no clinical significance.

Endometrial Hyperplasia

Endometrial hyperplasia can be classified as:

1) **simple hyperplasia**
2) **complex hyperplasia**
3) **atypical hyperplasia**

The histological distinction between the first two and the last is important because only atypical hyperplasia carries an increased risk of endometrial adenocarcinoma.

Simple Hyperplasia

Endometrial growth is mediated by oestrogen and thus hyperplasia occurs when the oestrogenic stimulus is inappropriately great. Both simple and complex hyperplasia occur in women with high oestrogen concentrations for any reason (see pp 756–757).

> ### *Microscopic Features*
> - In the **simple** form, hyperplasia affects both glands and stroma, so preserving a normal gland : stroma ratio with no 'crowding' of glands as in other forms of endometrial hyperplasia.
> - The glands vary in size: some are small whereas others show cystic dilatation.
> - The gland outline is mostly smooth and regular, although some outpouchings into the surrounding stroma may be seen.

- The gland epithelium may show some evidence of multilayering but the cells are well differentiated and show no atypia.
- Mitoses are, not surprisingly, present both in the gland epithelium and the stroma, just as they are in the proliferative phase of the normal cycle. Atypical mitoses are, however, not seen.

Clinical presentation usually takes the form of irregular, prolonged and heavy bleeding. Because repeated anovulatory cycling is the commonest cause of simple hyperplasia, presentation usually occurs either around the time of the menarche or in the perimenopausal period.

Natural History

It is important to remember that simple hyperplasia:
- does not develop into atypical hyperplasia
- carries *no* increase in the risk of endometrial carcinoma
- regresses if a progestogen is given or, in the case of anovulatory cycles, if ovulation commences

The features of simple endometrial hyperplasia are summarized in *Fig. 39.5*.

Complex Hyperplasia

Complex hyperplasia occurs for the same reasons as simple hyperplasia but may also be seen in some patients with normal cycles.

Microscopic Features
- Unlike simple hyperplasia, this is usually **focal**.
- Only glands are affected. **The gland : stroma ratio is therefore greater than normal and the glands are crowded together.**
- Glands are larger than normal but still vary in size. Their outlines are more irregular and there are finger-like outpouchings into both the surrounding stroma and the gland lumina.
- Gland epithelium shows no evidence of atypia.

As in the case of simple hyperplasia there is *no* evidence of an increased risk of endometrial carcinoma.

Atypical Hyperplasia

While atypical hyperplasia may develop under the hyperoestrogenic circumstances listed above, **there is no doubt that it is associated with a substantially increased risk for endometrial adenocarcinoma**. The size of this risk is difficult to measure but follow-up studies suggest that 14–25% of patients with atypical hyperplasia develop carcinoma.

As all three forms of hyperplasia may occur in hyperoestrogenism, it is difficult to see why only one, atypical hyperplasia, carries an increased risk of malignancy.

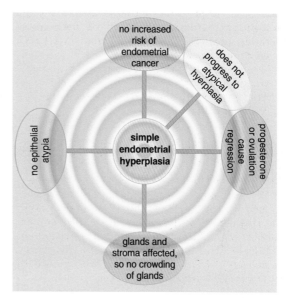

FIGURE 39.5 *Features of simple endometrial hyperplasia.*

It is possible that, in atypical hyperplasia, some genomic alteration has occurred previously in some of the endometrial epithelial cells and that increased oestrogen activity acts as a promoter for the phenotypic expression of malignancy. As in other types of endometrial hyperplasia, administration of progestogens causes regression of this lesion.

Microscopic Features
- Only the glands are affected. The gland : stroma ratio is increased and thus the glands are crowded together. So marked may this be in some areas, that the glands are seen to lie 'back to back' with hardly any intervening connective tissue stroma.
- The condition tends to be focal rather than diffuse.
- Gland size is variable and the gland outlines are markedly irregular showing infoldings within the lumina of the glands and complex outpouchings into the stroma.
- Gland epithelium shows atypia of differing degrees of severity, with an increase in nuclear : cytoplasmic ratio, loss of normal nuclear polarity and the presence of mitoses.

The features of atypical endometrial hyperplasia are summarized in *Fig. 39.6*.

ENDOMETRIAL CARCINOMA

This is one of the commonest **invasive** gynaecological malignancies; 80% of the patients are post-menopausal, when diagnosed, peak incidence being 55–65 years.

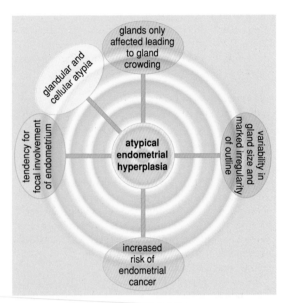

FIGURE 39.6 Features of atypical endometrial hyperplasia.

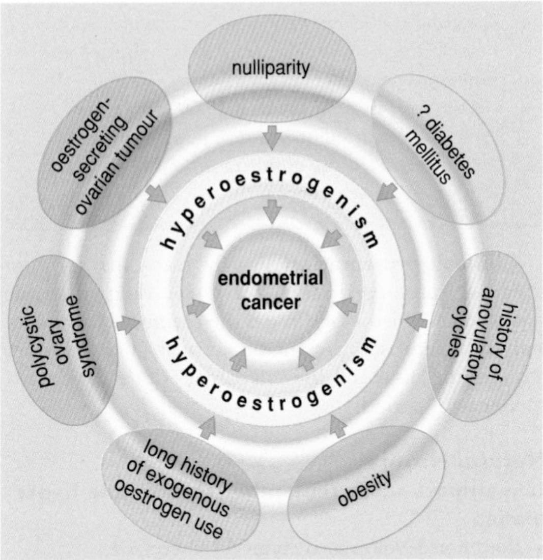

FIGURE 39.7 Risk factors for endometrial cancer.

Risk Factors

- **nulliparity**
- **obesity** (in which there is an increased conversion of Δ4 androstenedione to oestrone, this reaction occurring in adipocytes)
- **diabetes mellitus.** There is some doubt as to the validity of this link with endometrial carcinoma.
- **a history of anovulatory cycles** with dysfunctional uterine bleeding
- **a long history of exogenous oestrogen use** (as for postmenopausal hormone replacement or in the treatment of gonadal dysgenesis)
- **the presence of an oestrogen-secreting ovarian tumour** (granulosa cell tumour or thecoma)
- **polycystic ovary syndrome**, in which there is gross overproduction of androstenedione

The unifying feature in all of these is the presence of excess oestrogenic stimulation of the endometrium (*Fig. 39.7*), **although it must be emphasized that not all endometrial carcinomas are associated with hyperoestrogenism.**

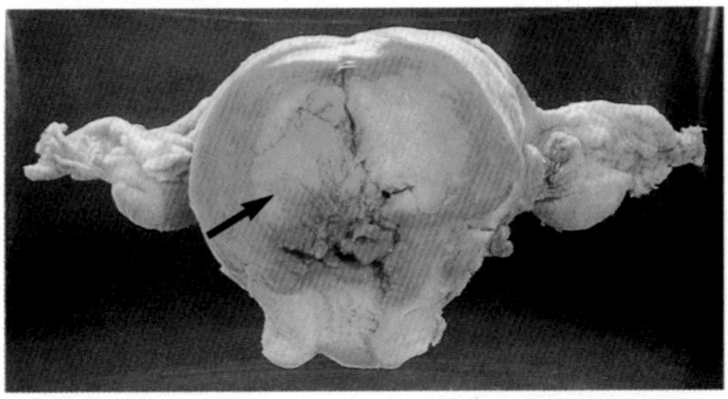

Macroscopic Features

The lesion may be:

- a broad-based polypoid mass, usually in the fundus
- a diffuse lesion infiltrating deeply into the myometrium (*Fig. 39.8*) and/or growing into the uterine cavity, almost filling it

Microscopic Features

Most endometrial adenocarcinomas (about 80%) bear some resemblance to normal endometrium, thus being termed **endometrioid**.

FIGURE 39.8 Adenocarcinoma of the endometrium. Note the white tumour tissue (arrowed) extending deeply into the uterine wall.

- The neoplastic glands are irregular in shape and variable in size. Intraluminal epithelial tufts are common and there may be a cribriform pattern of epithelial proliferation within gland lumina.
- The epithelium shows atypia of varying degrees of severity. Focal epithelial multilayering, nuclei varying in size and staining, and mitoses, some atypical, are present.
- Stroma is scanty, many of the glands being arranged in a 'back to back' pattern. Necrosis, haemorrhage and acute inflammation may be present, and collections of lipid-laden stromal cells are common, being regarded by some as a reliable 'marker' of carcinoma.

Histological Grading

This is based on a combination of the **growth pattern** (**acinar**, compared with **solid sheets** of tumour cells (*Fig. 39.9*)) and the degree of **epithelial atypia**:

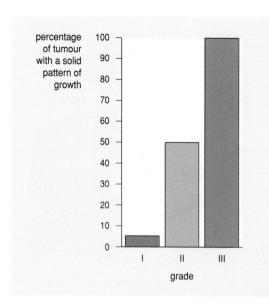

FIGURE 39.9 *The percentage of an endometrial carcinoma showing a solid pattern of growth rather than an acinar one determines its grade.*

- **Grade I** (about 50% of endometrioid carcinomas): 5% or less of the tumour mass consists of tumour with a solid rather than an acinar growth pattern
- **Grade II** (35% of endometrioid carcinomas): 5–50% of the tumour grows in a solid pattern
- **Grade III** (15% of endometrioid carcinoma): 50% or more of the tumour has a solid appearance

This grading is modified by the degree of atypia present. If atypia is very prominent, then tumours graded as I or II are raised a grade.

Variants of endometrioid carcinoma are:

- those characterized by extensive squamous metaplasia. This variant, which occurs in 10–20% of endometrioid tumours, is called by some **adenoacanthoma**, but this pattern seems to have no prognostic implications.
- those with a papillary pattern

Non-endometrioid Variants of Endometrial Carcinoma

Serous Papillary Carcinoma

These tumours appear identical with papillary serous carcinoma of the ovary. There is a complex papillary growth pattern, marked cellular atypia, numerous mitoses, psammoma bodies (calcified, laminated spheres) and patchy necrosis. Papillary serous endometrial carcinoma behaves aggressively; deep invasion of the myometrium is a prominent feature.

Clear Cell Carcinoma

This is composed of large, clear, glycogen-filled cells with well-marked plasma membranes. A papillary arrangement is quite common and cells with a 'hob-

nail' appearance may be seen. This led to the tumour being called 'mesonephroid carcinoma'; it is now recognized that this appearance is as characteristic of müllerian-derived tissue origin as it is of those derived from the mesonephros.

Adenosquamous Carcinoma

Both **adenocarcinoma** and invasive **squamous carcinoma** are present. It occurs in older women than does endometrioid carcinoma and pursues an aggressive course (5-year survival rate 40% or less).

Spread of Endometrial Carcinoma

Direct spread occurs into the myometrium and cervix. Well-differentiated tumours remain within the uterus for a long period. Non-endometrioid variants tend to penetrate rapidly through the uterine wall. Once the tumour has invaded right through the uterine wall, deposits may be found on:

- the serosal surface of the uterus
- the pelvic peritoneum and in the pouch of Douglas
- the broad ligament and in the parametrial tissues

Tumours arising in the uterine cornu may spread along the fallopian tube, giving rise to ovarian deposits.

Spread via lymphatics usually involves **para-aortic** and **pelvic nodes**.

Blood spread tends to be a late event. The commonest sites in which secondary deposits of tumour are found are the **lungs, liver, adrenals** and **bones**.

Prognosis and Staging

Prognosis depends largely on the extent of spread (expressed as the tumour stage, shown in *Table 39.2* and *Fig. 39.10*) and histological grade.

Table 39.2 Staging of Endometrial Cancer according to the International Federation of Gynaecology and Obstetrics (FIGO), 1989

Stage	Degree of spread
Ia	Tumour confined to the endometrium
Ib	Tumour involvement of less than half the depth of the myometrium
Ic	Tumour involves more than half of the depth of the myometrium
IIa	Additional involvement of the endocervical glands
IIb	Cervical stroma invaded
IIIa	Serosal and/or adnexal involvement and/or malignant cells found on peritoneal cytology
IIIb	Vaginal metastases present
IIIc	Pelvic and/or para-aortic node deposits
IVa	Invasion of bladder and/or bowel mucosa
IVb	Distant metastases including inguinal and abdominal node deposits

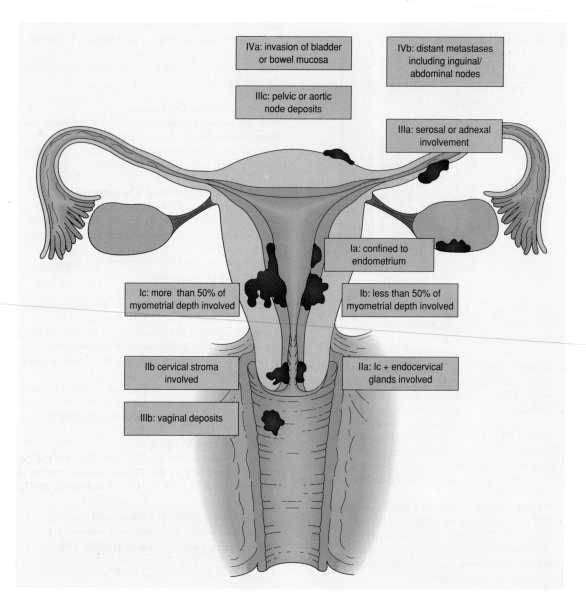

FIGURE 39.10 Staging of endometrial cancer (FIGO system).

Other factors indicating a worse prognosis include:

- **tumour type**: serous papillary and clear cell variants of endometrial carcinoma carry a worse prognosis than does endometrioid carcinoma
- **absence of steroid hormone receptors** on tumour cells
- **the presence of tumour cells in capillary spaces**
- **loss of a diploid pattern in the tumour cells**

This staging scheme is too recent for any corresponding survival figures to be available. The previous FIGO system (only four stages) shows the overall 5-year survival rate to be about 65%. The relation of survival to staging is shown in *Table 39.3*.

ENDOMETRIAL STROMAL NEOPLASMS

Low-grade Stromal Sarcoma

The defining criterion of a low-grade stromal sarcoma is a mitotic rate of ten or fewer mitoses per ten high-power fields.

Low-grade tumours infiltrate extensively via myometrial blood vessels and lymphatics. This gives them a rather characteristic naked-eye appearance in which cords of tumour within vascular channels protrude as 'worm-like' masses from the myometrial cut surface.

The microscopic features are those of spindle cell

Table 39.3 Survival according to FIGO Stage	
Stage	5-year survival rate (%)
I	72.3
II	56.4
III	31.5
IV	10.5

masses, the cells resembling normal, proliferative, stromal cells. The tumours run a long indolent course, although invasion of the parametrial tissues can occur, as can (rarely) metastasis to sites such as the lung. About 20% of the patients die from their tumour, although the clinical course may last for 20 years or more.

High-Grade Stromal Sarcoma
High-grade stromal sarcomas tend to grow out into the uterine cavity as soft fleshy masses. They appear less invasive than low-grade tumours but the cells are much more pleomorphic and mitoses are frequent. Rapid spread to both neighbouring and distant sites is common. The 5-year survival rate is about 15–25%.

Mixed Müllerian Tumours
Müllerian cells can differentiate into both endometrial glands and endometrial stroma, endometrial carcinomas and endometrial sarcomas being the respective expressions of malignancy. **An endometrial neoplasm showing evidence of both epithelial and mesenchymal differentiation is termed a mixed müllerian tumour.**

The nomenclature for this group depends on the degree of malignancy of each element involved (*Table 39.4*).

These, fortunately rare, tumours tend to occur in the elderly. Bulky masses protrude into the uterine cavity and often extend into the endocervical canal. Carcinosarcomas behave in a very aggressive fashion. At the time of diagnosis, the tumours have often spread beyond the uterus and blood-borne metastases are common.

Endometrial Polyps
These are defined as non-neoplastic lesions, most common in the perimenopausal period, protruding into the uterine cavity either as sessile nodules or as pedunculated polyps (*Fig. 39.11*). They consist of both glands and stroma, and represent local overgrowths, perhaps arising from areas of the endometrium not shed at menstruation. Such areas of unshed endometrium receive a recurrent growth stimulus with each proliferative phase and gradually increase in size.

Table 39.4 Nomenclature for Mixed Müllerian Tumours	
Tumour	Degree of benignancy or malignancy of epithelial and mesenchymal elements
Adenofibroma	Both epithelial and mesenchymal elements appear benign
Adenosarcoma	Epithelium appears benign but stroma shows histological evidence of malignancy
Carcinosarcoma	Both epithelium and stroma are malignant. The stroma may be homologous (i.e. it contains connective tissue elements normally present in the uterus) or heterologous (i.e. contains elements such as cartilage, bone or striated muscle not normally present). The presence of heterologous elements has no prognostic significance.

Macroscopic Features
Polyps may be single or multiple and vary in size, the larger ones measuring 2 cm or more along their longest axes. The superficial parts of such large lesions may show haemorrhage and necrosis, accounting for the uterine bleeding.

Microscopic Features
Polyps may consist of:
- inactive basal endometrium

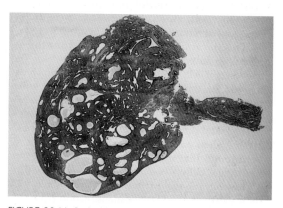

FIGURE 39.11 *Pedunculated endometrial polyp. Note the cystic dilatation of glands.*

- functional endometrium which appears out of phase with the rest of the corporeal endometrium
- hyperplastic endometrium with cystic dilatation of the glands
- senile endometrium with cystic dilatation of glands in postmenopausal women

These lesions are benign but may be associated with haemorrhage and, rarely, torsion with resulting infarction.

ENDOMETRIOSIS

The defining criterion of endometriosis is **the presence of endometrial glands and stroma outside the uterus**. Ectopic endometrium within the myometrium constitutes **adenomyosis**, believed to have a different pathogenesis from endometriosis.

Epidemiology
Endometriosis is common: about 10% of women of reproductive age are affected. Mean age at diagnosis is 25–29 years. It may also occur in adolescence, endometriosis being found in 45–60% of women aged under 20 years with chronic pelvic pain or dyspareunia.

Pathogenesis
Several theories are canvassed:
1) **Metaplasia of the pelvic peritoneum. Both endometrium and peritoneum originate from the same precursors – the lining cells of the coelomic cavity.** However, endometriosis occurs exclusively in females, with the exception of some males with prostatic cancer treated with high doses of oestrogen. Some role for oestrogens is suggested by the fact that endometriosis is confined largely to premenopausal women. Against this is the observation that endometriosis is uncommon in association with anovulatory menstrual cycles and high concentrations of circulating oestrogen.
2) **Translocation of endometrium from the uterus to an ectopic situation.** Viable endometrial cells can be found within the lumen of the fallopian tube and in the peritoneal cavity, but there is still no direct evidence that implantation of such cells on serosal surfaces leads to endometriosis.
3) The third theory combines elements of theories 1 and 2: **shed endometrial cells release some compound that induces metaplasia of peritoneal cells.**
4) **Retrograde menstruation.** Many women show evidence of retrograde menstruation (75–90% in some studies). It is certainly true that the smaller the number of cycles, the less the risk of

endometriosis. Some evidence suggests that reflux of glands and stroma occurs more often and to a greater extent in women with endometriosis than in those with no endometriosis. In addition, endometriosis is more common in women who have abnormalities of müllerian duct development leading to outflow obstruction and, hence, increased risk of retrograde menstruation.

Endometrial tissue implanted on serosal surfaces will grow only if stimulated; paracrine signals via growth factors are probably involved. Both normally sited and endometriotic endometrium secrete epidermal growth factor, transforming growth factor α and epidermal growth factor receptors. In cell culture, platelet-derived growth factor and another macrophage-derived growth factor stimulate growth of endometrial stroma. The maximal effect on cultured endometrium is seen with a combination of oestrogen and growth factors.

Clinical Presentation
Although some cases may be asymptomatic, endometriosis may present with a wide range of clinical disturbances:
- **infertility**, occurring in 14–30% of women with endometriosis
- **pelvic pain**, worse at the time of menstruation. Foci in the rectovaginal septum are associated with rectal discomfort.
- symptoms and signs related to the presence of endometriosis outside the pelvis (e.g. in the lung or in the brain)
- clinical features associated with endometriosis in the skin or subcutaneous tissue. Such foci are especially likely to occur in relation to surgical scars and to the umbilicus, and draw attention to themselves by swelling, pain and tenderness at the time of menstruation.

Pathological Features
The main diagnostic criterion is the finding of ectopic endometrial glands and stroma (*Fig. 39.12*). In some instances this shows cyclical changes similar to those in the uterine endometrium; in others the ectopic endometrium is inactive. Bleeding within foci of endometriosis is a common event and this may destroy the endometrial glands which constitute the only 'hard' evidence, leaving only haemosiderin-impregnated fibrous tissue behind.

Macroscopic Features
Early endometriotic foci are bluish-grey serosal nodules ranging from a few millimetres to 2 cm or more in diameter. In the ovary, lesions are often cystic and the cyst lumina, as a result of haemorrhage, contain rather sticky

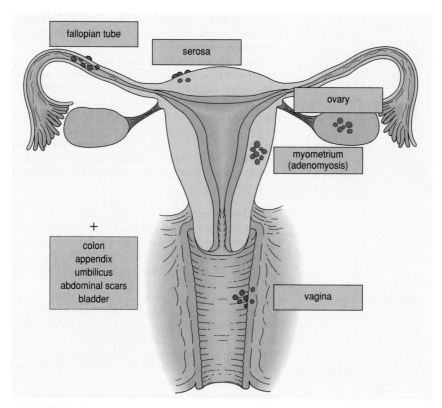

FIGURE 39.12 Sites at which foci of endometriosis may occur.

brown fluid ('chocolate' cysts). Local scarring and adhesion formation due to leakage of blood into the tissue around the cyst is quite common, as is the case with extraovarian foci of endometriosis. Such adhesions may lead to the mistaken diagnosis of pelvic inflammatory disease due to salpingitis.

Not uncommonly, the endometrial lining of such an ovarian cyst is destroyed by recurrent bleeding, the cyst wall showing large numbers of iron-laden macrophages.

Because ectopic and normal endometrium may be affected by the same factors, it is not surprising that foci of endometriosis may be the seat of:
- hyperplasia
- glandular atypia
- malignancy, of which **endometrioid carcinoma of the ovary** is the most common form (see p 778)

Adenomyosis
This condition, tending to occur in the latter part of reproductive life, is defined as the ectopic presence of benign endometrial tissue deep within the myometrium. The word 'deep' is open to a number of different interpretations. Some suggest that the diagnosis should not be made unless the ectopic endometrium

is at a distance from the endometrial–myometrial junction of not less than a quarter of the full thickness of the uterine wall.

The ectopic foci may be either focally or diffusely distributed with the myometrium, their presence being associated with marked hypertrophy of the uterine smooth muscle. This gives the cut surface of affected areas a coarse trabeculated appearance (*Fig. 39.13*). In cases where adenomyosis is diffuse, the uterus is globally enlarged. Less commonly, where the adenomyosis is focal, there may be a poorly demarcated, nodular thickening of the uterine wall (adenomyoma).

Microscopic Features
Both glands and stroma are present. More often than not, the glands are inactive, resembling those seen in the basal layer of the endometrium. In some cases the glands respond to oestrogenic stimuli but not to progestational ones and may thus show the features of simple hyperplasia or, more rarely, of atypical hyperplasia.

Pathogenesis
Ectopic endometrial foci within the myometrium are believed to be due to downgrowth of both glands and

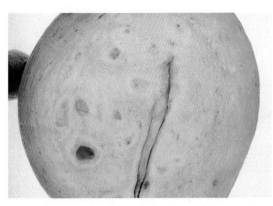

FIGURE 39.13 *Adenomyosis. Note the thickening of the uterine wall and the focal deposits (one of which shows haemorrhage) of endometrium deep within the uterine wall.*

stroma, but why this should occur is a mystery; there is no association between adenomyosis and endometriosis.

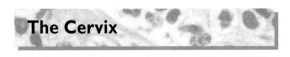

The Cervix

NORMAL ANATOMY AND DEVELOPMENT

The most distal part of the uterus is the cervix. The outer surface of its intravaginal portion is the **ectocervix, this being covered by stratified squamous epithelium which differs from epidermis** in that the cells do not express high molecular weight cytoker-

atins. Leading to the body of the uterus is the **endocervical canal**, lined chiefly by **mucin-secreting columnar epithelium**.

The endocervical canal terminates distally at the **external os**, and proximally at the **internal os**. The latter is not a distinct orifice, but instead a widening of the canal characterized by a change from mucinous lining epithelium to endometrium. Distally, the columnar epithelium of the canal changes to the squamous epithelium of the ectocervix at the **squamocolumnar junction**. The location of this junction differs with age; during reproductive life it is ectocervical, well away from the canal.

Transformation Zone

In 65% of female infants, endocervical mucosa is present at the ectocervix. Soon after birth, this mucosa retreats into the canal until puberty (*Fig. 39.14*). At the menarche, the endocervical mucosa again moves out on to the ectocervix (*Fig. 39.14*).

This results from hormone-induced swelling of cervical connective tissues which causes the cervical lips to 'roll' outwards, pulling endocervical mucosa outwards on to the ectocervix. Endocervical mucosa, pulled out in this way, is redder than the surrounding ectocervical tissue. This reddened area has been incorrectly called an **'erosion'** implying ulceration when, in fact, it represents a normal eversion of the endocervical mucosa.

During reproductive life the everted endocervical mucosa is gradually replaced by squamous epithelium (*Fig. 39.14*). The area where glandular tissue is replaced by squamous epithelium is the **transformation zone**. This is the site of predilection for neoplastic transformation in the cervix and is thus of great importance.

The transformation zone can be viewed on colposcopy and thus, the macroscopic features of cervical intraepithelial neoplasia can be identi-

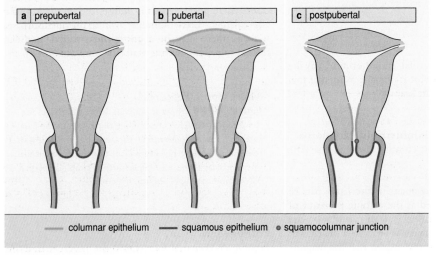

| a | prepubertal | b | pubertal | c | postpubertal |

—— columnar epithelium   —— squamous epithelium   • squamocolumnar junction

FIGURE 39.14 *Age- and hormone-related changes at the squamocolumnar junction.*

fied and monitored. **This accessibility also makes it possible easily to obtain material for cytological and histological examination.**

In later reproductive life, the squamocolumnar junction moves back towards the endocervical canal, so that by the time of the menopause the junction is likely to be concealed within the canal.

Two mechanisms are thought to create the transformation zone:

1) A direct 'pushing' form of growth of mature squamous epithelium under the glandular epithelium with resulting sloughing of the latter. Often, this results in the squamous epithelium covering the orifices of mucus-secreting endocervical glands. Secretion may continue in these glands resulting in small cysts (nabothian cysts) containing inspissated mucus.

2) A metaplastic conversion of endocervical mucosa to squamous epithelium. This entails proliferation of small inconspicuous basal cells known as **reserve cells** which differentiate into squamous cells.

CERVICAL CANCER

- Worldwide, cervical cancer is the second most common malignancy in women after breast cancer.
- Major differences in the incidence of cervical cancer appear to be the expression of both different levels of sexual activity and differences in screening policies for cervical pathology.
- In some countries mass screening for cervical intraepithelial neoplasia has produced striking decreases (60% or more) in both cervical cancer deaths and disease incidence. Screening every 3 years produces a reduction in the cumulative risk of developing cervical cancer between the ages of 35 and 64 years of the order of 90%; annual screening has a comparatively small incremental effect.

Aetiology

Sexual History
There is a well-recognized association between certain aspects of sexual history and cervical cancer risk. Two correlates of such increased risk are:

1) **Age at first intercourse.** First intercourse before the age of 18 years produces a 2.5-fold increase in risk compared with first intercourse after the age of 21 years.

2) **Number of sexual partners.** The relative risk of cervical cancer in a woman who has had five or more sexual partners compared with a woman who has had only one is 2.8. There is also an increased risk with only one sexual partner if that partner has been sexually promiscuous.

These data suggest the involvement of a sexually transmitted agent in the causation of cervical cancer.

Human Papillomaviruses and Cervical Neoplasia
There are about 50 different types of the DNA virus, human papillomavirus (HPV); at least nine infect the female genital tract. The infection is sexually transmitted with a remarkable concordance between the HPV types found in couples (see section on penile tumours). HPV infections of the cervix fall into two groups, as shown in *Table 39.5*.

Table 39.5 Infections of the Cervix

HPV type	Associations
6, 11, 31, 35, 42, 50	Condyloma acuminata Low-grade, non-progressive cervical intraepithelial neoplasia (CIN) Very rarely associated with invasive carcinoma
16, 18	Low-grade progressive CIN Advanced CIN (grade 3) Invasive tumours

HPV types 16 and 18 are oncogenic; they can transform cells in culture and the transformed cells form tumours when injected into susceptible animals. This transforming ability seems to reside in two viral proteins, E6 and E7.

E7 protein shows considerable homologies with two other transforming proteins, large T antigen of the SV40 virus and the E1A protein of adenoviruses. **All three bind the gene product of the retinoblastoma (RB1) gene**, a tumour suppressor gene with a powerful controlling function in relation to the cell cycle. **Its functional inactivation by viral protein binding is likely to explain the transforming activity of the latter.** The E6 protein inactivates the product of the tumour suppressor gene *p53* (see pp 285–286).

Most frank cervical cancers show integration of HPV sequences into host DNA, this being rare in normal cervical tissue.

It seems, however, unlikely that HPV infection is the sole cause of cervical cancer. Use of sensitive polymerase chain reaction methods show that the prevalence of infections with HPV type 16 in women with *normal* cervical cytology is high. **Thus, there must be other factors promoting expression of the malignant phenotype.**

Cigarette Smoking
Strong correlations exist between cigarette smoking and cervical cancer risk. Some maintain that they are

the expression of a different sexual lifestyle in cigarette smokers and that the smoking itself is not an aetiological factor. Others maintain that cigarette smoking plays a causal role; certainly, nicotine and its breakdown product cotinine occur in the cervical mucus of smokers.

Oral Contraceptives

There is no clear association between taking oral contraceptives and cervical cancer risk once studies have been controlled adequately for the sexual histories of the women involved . Barrier methods for contraception are associated with diminished risk, again suggesting that a transmissible agent is involved.

Cervical Intraepithelial Neoplasia

The natural history of most cervical cancer involves a **preinvasive period** characterized by increasingly extensive and severe epithelial changes. **This set of morphological changes is termed cervical intraepithelial neoplasia (CIN)**; its recognition allows cervical cancer to be treated effectively **before it becomes invasive**.

We owe this advance to the ability to:
- **examine cells exfoliated from the cervical epithelium** (cytological screening)
- **look at the cervix with the colposcope**, which provides a magnified view of the area. Application of acetic acid to the cervix results in dysplastic epithelium turning white; this helps to select areas for biopsy.

Squamous Intraepithelial Neoplasia

This term covers a spectrum of morphological changes beginning with a mild dysplastic process (**CIN I**), which can progress through moderate dysplasia (**CIN II**) to **CIN III**, the correlate of **severe dysplasia** or **carcinoma *in situ***. Once CIN III is present, **failure to treat will lead to invasive cancer in more than one-third of affected women in the 20 years following the diagnosis**.

CIN is virtually always found in the transformation zone. While CIN affects mostly squamous epithelium, *in situ* carcinomas may also occur in columnar cells. These are rarer, being recognized by cellular and glandular atypia in the endocervical canal.

Criteria for histological diagnosis include:
- **changes within individual cells** which include:
  a) darkly staining nuclei
  b) an increased nuclear : cytoplasmic ratio
  c) variations in nuclear size and shape
  d) mitoses in suprabasal cells
  e) abnormal mitoses
- **abnormalities of cellular organization** including:
  a) loss of polarity (the normal relationship of the epithelial cells one to another)
  b) absence of normal stratification

These changes are seen in *Fig. 39.15*.

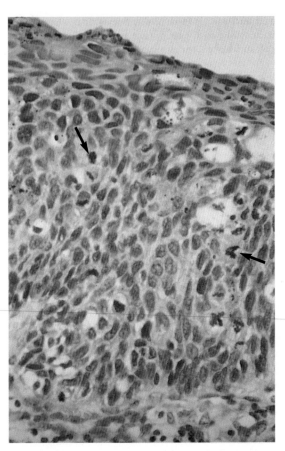

FIGURE 39.15 *Severe cervical intraepithelial neoplasia (CIN III). Both the individual cells and the architectural pattern are disturbed. Note the many mitoses including (arrowed) some abnormal ones.*

Grading

CIN is **graded** by determining the abnormal fraction of the epithelium (in terms of its thickness). (*Table 39.6*).

In CIN I and CIN II, microscopic evidence of HPV infection is common. This takes the form of

Table 39.6 Grading of Cervical Intraepithelial Neoplasia

Grade	Extent of involvement
CIN I	Involves one-third or less of the cervical squamous epithelium
CIN II	Involves one- to two-thirds of the cervical squamous epithelium
CIN III	Involves more than two-thirds of the cervical squamous epithelium

koilocytosis (perinuclear vacuolization of epithelial cells associated with a peculiar prune-like wrinkling of the nuclei), multinucleation of some cells, and individual cell keratinization. **This is less common in CIN III, where, presumably, there has been full integration of HPV sequences into the host cell genome.**

Microinvasive Squamous Carcinoma
Once tumour cells breach the basement membrane, the lesion must be regarded as invasive. In cervical squamous carcinoma, **a minimally invasive phase** is recognized in which the tumour behaves biologically as if it were still completely intraepithelial. **The depth of invasion in these lesions is 5 mm or less.** Diagnosis of microinvasive carcinoma depends on being able to examine the **whole cervical lesion**.

Invasive Cervical Carcinoma
Most invasive cervical carcinomas of the cervix have been regarded, almost by default, as being squamous. This is incorrect: only about 70% of such invasive tumours are purely squamous. This change of view results from the application of simple methods for identifying epithelial mucins, the **hallmark of secretory epithelium**. The fact that about 30% of tumours, previously classified as squamous carcinomas, must be relabelled as either adenosquamous tumours or poorly differentiated adenocarcinomas has clinical significance, because some state that mucus-secreting neoplasms morphologically resembling squamous carcinoma are more aggressive and have a worse prognosis than pure squamous carcinomas.

Invasive carcinoma of the cervix can, therefore, be classified under a number of histological rubrics, each of which can be further subdivided (the histological details of all of these is beyond the scope of a general text):

- squamous carcinoma
- adenocarcinoma
- mixed tumours
- small cell carcinoma
- undifferentiated carcinoma
- secondary tumours

The site of development of invasive, as of intraepithelial, cancer depends on the site of the transformation zone. Thus, in young women, tumours usually present on the ectocervix, whereas in older women they are usually within the endocervical canal.

> ### Macroscopic Features
> Ectocervical tumours usually show an **exophytic growth pattern**, presenting either as a bulky friable mass which may appear polypoid, and have a papillary surface, or as a typical cancerous ulcer with firm, raised edges (*Fig. 39.16*).
>
> Endocervical canal tumours tend to expand the cervix, forming a firm cylindrical mass.

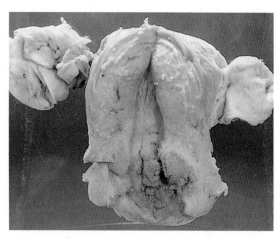

FIGURE 39.16 *Ulcerating carcinoma of the cervix extending downwards to involve the vagina.*

Squamous carcinomas can be further divided on the basis of their cell size and the presence or extent of keratinization, an important marker of differentiation (*Table 39.7*).

Natural History
The outcome in invasive cervical cancer depends chiefly on two factors:

1) the extent of local disease
2) the presence or absence of tumour deposits in draining lymph nodes

Direct Spread
The extent of the local disease reflects the proportion of the cervix involved and the extent of invasion. The smaller the amount of cervix involved by tumour, the better the prognosis. Involvement of 20% or less carries a 5-year survival rate of 70%; if 60% or more is involved, the survival rate drops to 54%.

Spread occurs directly through natural tissue planes and via perineurial and perivascular spaces. The directions of such spread are:

- upwards into the body of the uterus
- downwards into the vagina
- laterally into the parametrial soft tissues
- posterolaterally into the sacrouterine ligaments
- anteriorly into the urinary bladder
- posteriorly into the rectum

Direct spread may eventually involve the wall of the pelvis with compression of the ureters, causing hydroureter and hydronephrosis.

Lymph Node Deposits
These affect first the external iliac, hypogastric and obturator nodes. This is followed later, and rather less commonly, by involvement of sacral, aortic and inguinal nodes.

Table 39.7 Squamous Carcinoma of the Cervix

Microscopic features	Frequency (%)	Appearance
Well–differentiated, large cell, keratinizing tumours	20	Islands of cells with obvious squamous differentiation (intercellular bridges) and numerous concentric whorls of keratin in the centres of the cellular islands.
Moderately differentiated tumours (large cell, focally keratinizing type)	60	Cells appear squamous but intercellular bridges are scanty and the epithelial cells show more atypia than those of well-differentiated tumours. Well-formed whorls of keratin are not seen.
Poorly differentiated (large cell, non-keratinizing) or small cell, non-keratinizing	20	Sheets of uniform large cells or small cells with darkly staining nuclei. No evidence of keratin. The presence of mucin should be excluded before a diagnosis of poorly differentiated squamous carcinoma is made.

Blood-borne metastases occur, affecting principally the lungs, liver and bone, but this is usually a late manifestation.

Staging

A simplified version of the International Federation of Gynaecology and Obstetrics (FIGO) scheme is given in *Table 39.8*.

The overall 5-year survival rate is about 55%.

Other Factors of Prognostic Significance

Histological Type

In most series, cervical **adenocarcinomas** have a poorer survival rate than purely squamous tumours.

Tumour Grade

Grading of squamous tumours appears to have little effect on prognosis. Small cell tumours, however, in which there is no evidence of intercellular bridges or keratin formation, appear to behave more aggressively than pure squamous tumours.

Permeation by Tumour Cells of Lymphatics or Blood Vessels

Evidence of vascular permeation is an ominous sign because it correlates strongly with the presence of nodal tumour deposits.

NON-NEOPLASTIC DISORDERS OF THE CERVIX

Chronic Cervicitis

Chronic cervicitis is greatly overdiagnosed; its presence is often inferred by a few lymphocytes and plasma cells at the squamocolumnar junction, although their presence is without significance. Nevertheless true inflammatory reactions do occur in the cervix:

- **Non-infective**, such as the reactions following surgical or obstetric trauma, diathermy or the use of intrauterine contraceptive devices.
- **Infective**, resulting from infection with:

Table 39.8 Staging of Cervical Cancer according to the FIGO Classification

Stage	Extent of spread	5-year survival rate (%)
I	Invasive carcinoma confined to cervix	85–90%
II	Cancer extends beyond cervix but has not involved pelvic wall; vaginal involvement limited to upper two-thirds	70–75%
III	Cancer extends to either lateral pelvic wall and/or the lower third of the vagina	30–35%
IV	Involvement of urinary bladder and/or rectum or extension beyond the true pelvis	10%

a) **Viruses**, such as herpesvirus which causes an ulcerating lesion. HPV is an important cervical pathogen in another context (see p 767).

b) **Bacteria**, such as *Neisseria gonorrhoeae* which, because of the relatively high resistance of the ectocervical squamous epithelium, tends to affect the endocervix.

c) **Chlamydia**, causing either a destructive lesion associated with much scarring or a non-specific inflammation in which a follicular lymphocytic reaction may be seen.

d) **Spirochaetal** infections; nearly half the primary lesions of genitally acquired syphilis occur in the cervix.

e) **Protozoal** infections. Infections by *Tricho-monas vaginalis* often involve the cervix. In the acute stages the cervix is markedly reddened as a result of dilatation of capillaries in subepithelial papillae. The squamous epithelium shows infiltration by acute inflammatory cells and some of the superficial layers appear degenerate.

f) **Helminth** infestations. In areas where the worms are endemic, **schistosomiasis** of the cervix is common. The connective tissue response to the presence of the schistosome ova leads to an overgrowth of scar tissue and considerable distortion of the cervix, which can lead to an erroneous clinical diagnosis of carcinoma.

Cervical Polyp

The word polyp is used here in a purely **descriptive** sense; these lesions are *not* neoplastic and probably result from chronic inflammation.

They are usually small but occasionally may measure several centimetres along their longest axis. Microscopic examination reveals dilated endocervical glands set in an inflamed and oedematous stroma. In some instances the surface epithelium shows the presence of squamous metaplasia.

Microglandular Hyperplasia of the Endocervical Epithelium

This is a microscopic diagnosis characterized by a complex proliferation of small glands lined by rather flat epithelium. If the change is extensive, the affected area may project from the cervical surface in a polypoid fashion. It is seen most often in association with oral contraceptives and pregnancy.

Decidual Reaction in the Cervical Stroma

During pregnancy, cervical stromal cells may show changes identical with those of decidua at the implantation site. The lesions may be small and multiple, in the form of small yellowish or red nodules on the cervical mucosa. In a few instances, there may be large single nodules in which such decidual changes have occurred.

They are quite harmless and would be unimportant but for the fact that they may be misdiagnosed clinically.

Tumours of the Myometrium

Nearly all tumours of the myometrium arise from uterine smooth muscle. Most are benign, some have an intermediate and others a frankly malignant behaviour.

BENIGN NEOPLASMS

Leiomyoma

This is the commonest of all uterine tumours and is found in 20% of women aged more than 35 years. The neoplastic element consists entirely of smooth muscle cells but fibrous tissue is also present, leading to the inaccurate term **'fibroids'**.

It is suggested that oestrogen binding to the uterine smooth muscle cells plays a part in tumour genesis. This is supported by the facts that leiomyomas:

- occur most commonly during reproductive life
- tend to enlarge during pregnancy
- tend to regress during the menopause
- decrease in size when antagonists of luteinizing hormone releasing hormone (LHRH) (which downregulates ovarian function) are given

Leiomyomas are frequently multiple. They vary considerably in size, ranging from less than 1 cm to more than 20 cm. Each leiomyoma is monoclonal. This has been elegantly demonstrated in Negro females heterozygous in respect of glucose-6-phosphate dehydrogenase. Their normal myometrium, because of random X-chromosome inactivation, contain both isoforms of the enzyme. Cells of a leiomyoma contain only one isoform, indicating monoclonality.

Macroscopic Features

The tumours have a classically expansile growth pattern with a well-defined edge and a pseudocapsule composed of compressed myometrium (*Fig. 39.17*). This enables them to be shelled out should it be decided not to perform a hysterectomy as, for example, in a woman who wishes to bear more children.

The cut surface of the leiomyoma has a characteristic whorled appearance which has been likened to that of watered silk.

Leiomyomas may be situated (*Fig. 39.18*):
- entirely within the myometrium ('intramural')
- immediately beneath the endometrium (submucosal). These tumours bulge into and distort the uterine cavity, being covered by a 'cap' of thinned

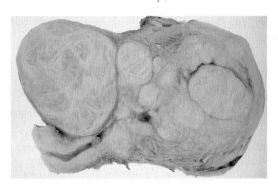

FIGURE 39.17 Several large leiomyomas of the uterus showing the typical whorled cut surface and causing marked distortion of the uterus.

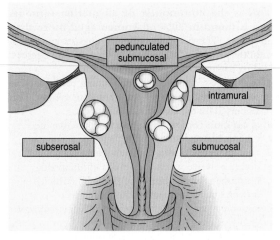

FIGURE 39.18 Sites of leiomyoma formation within the uterus.

endometrium. In some instances they may extend into the endocervical canal.

- beneath the peritoneal covering of the uterine body (subserosal). These tumours bulge outwards from the uterus and may become attached to neighbouring structures, such as the omentum, and detached from the uterus. Leiomyomas that have acquired a new blood supply from the vessels in their new lodging are termed parasitic.

Microscopic Features

The tumours are composed of smooth muscle cells arranged, for the most part, in interlacing bundles separated from each other by well-vascularized fibrous tissue. The smooth muscle cells are elongated and their nuclei spindle-shaped. The degree of cellularity differs between tumours but is not of prognostic significance.

In some cases, the smooth muscle cells have a rounded or polygonal shape with clear cytoplasm and centrally placed nuclei (epithelioid). They are termed by some

writers as leiomyoblastomas, an inappropriate term because they are not precursor forms of smooth muscle cells. They do not differ in behaviour from the more usual variety.

Some tumours show large bizarre cells, some of which may be multinucleated. Their nuclei vary in size and shape, and some are markedly hyperchromatic. Mitoses are, however, not seen. Despite these alarming appearances, this variant (atypical or pleomorphic leiomyoma) does not behave aggressively. Care must be taken, therefore, not to misdiagnose it as a malignant tumour of smooth muscle.

Natural History

In the course of the natural history of these lesions a number of changes occur, some of which can be appreciated best with the naked eye. Roughly two-thirds of leiomyomas undergo one or other of these (*Table 39.9*).

Table 39.9 Changes in the Leiomyoma

Type of change	Frequency (%)
Hyaline change	63
Mucoid or myxomatous change	19
Calcification	8
Cystic change	4
Fatty change	3
'Red' degeneration	3

All these changes are ascribed to chronic ischaemia; it is suggested that the lesions have 'outgrown' their blood supply. Whether this is really true remains to be seen. Red degeneration occurs particularly in pregnant women. The cut surface of the affected tumour has a dull red appearance and a somewhat fishy smell. It is believed that this change represents haemorrhagic infarction in which much of the tumour has already been replaced by hyaline fibrous tissue. It may be associated with abdominal pain and fever.

Malignant transformation is very rare. However, there are some behavioural variants that pursue a course somewhere between that of clearly benign and frankly malignant tumours.

Intravenous Leiomyomatosis

Here, cords of neoplastic smooth muscle extend into veins within the uterine wall and in the connective tissue adjacent to the uterus. 'Ordinary' leiomyomas are often found in association with this lesion. The cords of tumour cells that distend the affected veins may, on occasion, grow as far as the inferior vena cava.

The cut surface of a uterus affected in this way may show worm-like casts of tumour in the distended veins, giving an appearance resembling some cases of low-grade endometrial sarcoma. Despite the alarming growth pattern, distant metastases are very rare.

Benign Metastasizing Leiomyoma

In this rare condition leiomyomas with 'benign' histology are found in both the uterus and the lung. It is suggested that some of these cases are due to the simultaneous development of uterine and pulmonary smooth muscle tumours. In other cases, especially where there has been a history of curettage of the uterus, it is believed that the pulmonary lesions are due to dissemination of the uterine tumours during surgical trauma.

Disseminated Peritoneal Leiomyomatosis

This is a rare **benign** condition in which typical uterine smooth muscle tumours are associated with the presence of many small nodules of smooth muscle in the omentum and peritoneum. It has been suggested that this condition is not due to dissemination of neoplastic smooth muscle from the uterus, but represents instead an *in situ* change in the connective tissue of the peritoneum. There is a strong association between disseminated peritoneal leiomyomatosis and pregnancy; steroid receptors have been detected in the nodules of smooth muscle.

Other Benign Myometrial Tumours

A variety of other benign connective tissue neoplasms can occur in the myometrium but most are very rare. One moderately common entity is the **adenomatoid tumour**, occurring in about 1% of uteri.

They are usually small (mean diameter 2 cm), ill-defined lesions that tend to be situated subserosally in the cornual region of the uterus.

These tumours are mesothelial in origin and consist of complex spaces lined either by flattened cells or by low cuboidal epithelium. Between these spaces is a fibromuscular stroma, which can contain abundant smooth muscle. The behaviour of these lesions is entirely benign.

MALIGNANT NEOPLASMS

Leiomyosarcoma

Malignant connective tissue neoplasms of the uterus are uncommon, accounting for about 2% of malignant uterine tumours. Of these, leiomyosarcoma constitutes about 50%.

It tends to occur in older women than does leiomyoma (mean age 54 years) and its relation with leiomyoma is not clear. Theoretically, sarcoma of smooth muscle could arise as a result of malignant transformation of a benign counterpart or *de novo*. Benign leiomyomas are commonly multiple, and leiomyosarcoma is single in about two-thirds of cases; thus a *de novo* origin seems likely but remains unproven.

Macroscopic Features

Some sarcomas resemble ordinary benign leiomyoma; most are soft fleshy lesions with evidence of haemorrhage and necrosis and which, grossly, appear invasive.

Microscopic Features

Lesions are hypercellular, showing a greater or lesser degree of resemblance to smooth muscle. Even in poorly differentiated examples, actin and myosin are present in the tumour cells. The main difficulties in diagnosis arise in connection with relatively well-differentiated tumours. **Here, the frequency with which mitoses are found assumes the greatest importance and there is universal agreement that the greater the number of mitoses, the greater is the chance of frankly malignant behaviour.** There is no consensus as to how individual tumours should be classified (see *Tables 39.10* (UK) and *39.11* (USA)).

Table 39.10 Classification of Myometrial Tumours in the UK according to Mitotic Rate

Mitotic rate	Type of tumour
15 or fewer mitoses per 10 high-power fields and a bland cellular appearance	Leiomyoma
More than 15 mitoses per 10 high-power fields and a bland cellular appearance	Smooth muscle tumour of uncertain malignant potential
Two to four mitoses per 10 high-power fields and a significant degree of pleomorphism	Smooth muscle tumour of uncertain malignant potential
More than four mitoses per 10 high-power fields and cellular pleomorphism	Best regarded as leiomyosarcoma

Uterine leiomyosarcomas invade the pelvic organs locally but also show a marked tendency for haematogenous dissemination. Pulmonary metastases are common and the 5-year survival rate is 20–30%; the outlook is worse if the tumour occurs during the premenopausal period.

Table 39.11 Classification of Myometrial Tumours in the USA according to Mitotic Rate

Mitotic rate	Type of tumour
Fewer than five mitoses per 10 high-power fields, even in the presence of cellular pleomorphism	Practically always behave in a benign fashion
Five to nine mitoses per 10 high-power fields	Smooth muscle tumour of uncertain malignant potential
Ten or more mitoses per 10 high-power fields, even if atypia is minimal	Behave, for the most part, in a malignant fashion

Disorders of the Ovary

OVARIAN FAILURE

It is normal for ovarian failure to occur at the time of the menopause, when it is due to atresia leading to depletion of oöcytes and ovarian follicles at about the age of 50 years. If atresia proceeds significantly faster than normal, depletion of oöcytes and follicles must occur **earlier** than normal; the syndrome of premature ovarian failure.

Oöcytes within the ovary do not divide and, thus, **the ovary has a finite number of germ cells**. Only a few hundred oöcytes are involved in ovulation. Most atresia occurs during fetal life and, in some circumstances, for example in Turner's syndrome, intrauterine germ cell loss is greatly increased (see pp 312–313, 753).

Postnatal causes of premature ovarian failure include:
- irradiation involving the ovaries
- certain forms of cancer chemotherapy
- viral infections such as mumps oöphoritis
- the accumulation of certain toxic metabolites such as occurs in galactosaemia
- associations with certain autoimmune diseases such as autoimmune thyroiditis, adrenalitis and insulin-dependent diabetes mellitus. Antibodies against thyroid and adrenal glands are present in almost 80% of patients with premature ovarian failure, once chromosomal abnormalities have been excluded.
- the presence in ovarian follicle fluid of congeners of nicotine such as cotinine. This may explain the earlier menopause that occurs in cigarette smokers.

Clinical features of premature ovarian failure are a combination of **infertility** and **oestrogen deficiency**.

THE POLYCYSTIC OVARY SYNDROME

The polycystic ovary syndrome may be defined in either morphological or clinical (*Fig. 39.19*) terms.

In terms of **morphological abnormality**, ovaries are enlarged (usually about three times as large as normal) and contain many small peripheral cysts (6–8 mm in diameter). Microscopically, these are seen to be cystic follicles showing luteinization of the theca interna cells. The ovary is covered by a thick fibrous capsule.

The patients, usually in their late teens or early twenties, complain of a combination of:
- the effects of **hyperandrogenization** (e.g. hirsutism)
- **menstrual disturbance** (amenorrhoea or oligomenorrhoea)
- **infertility** (due to failure of ovulation and hypersecretion of luteinizing hormone)
- **obesity**, often characterized by an increase in the waist : hip ratio

The patients who have amenorrhoea are not oestrogen deficient. Indeed, oestrogen levels may be so high as to cause a florid degree of endometrial hyperplasia recognizable on ultrasonography; this may require treatment with cyclical administration of progestogens or curettage.

Endocrine Features
The classical endocrine profile is:

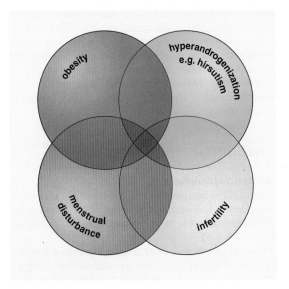

FIGURE 39.19 *Clinical features of the polycystic ovary syndrome.*

- hypersecretion of luteinizing hormone (LH)
- normal concentrations of follicle-stimulating hormone (FSH), prolactin and thyroxine
- in some, raised testosterone levels

High levels of LH appear to be related to infertility and those of testosterone to hirsutism.

The nature of the primary disturbance in polycystic ovary syndrome is not known.

Clearly a pivotal defect is the failure of the ovary to convert androgens (secreted in excessive amounts by the stroma and cells of the theca interna) into oestrogen.

Many patients respond favourably to wedge resection of the ovary or to treatment with clomiphene, which stimulates ovulation.

Ovarian Tumours and Tumour-like Lesions

A wide variety of ovarian neoplasms exists. These may be **primary** or **secondary** and either specific to the ovary or non-specific. Ovarian cancer is responsible for about 4000 deaths annually in the UK. There has been no decrease in the mortality rate from ovarian cancer; it is now the fifth commonest cause of cancer deaths among women, causing more deaths than any other gynaecological malignancy. By the time it is diagnosed, the disease is usually far advanced. The search for a means of earlier diagnosis which is sensitive, specific and affordable is a major challenge.

The nomenclature of **primary tumours specific for the ovary** may confuse non-specialists. The easiest approach is based on the fact that ovarian tumours may arise from any tissue elements **normally present** (*Fig. 39.20*). These include:

- **The surface or germinal epithelium. This is the commonest site of origin; 65% of all ovarian neoplasms and 95% of malignant ovarian neoplasms originate from the surface epithelium.** The latter is derived from coelomic mesothelium covering the ovary and **retains the ability to differentiate into any müllerian tract elements**. Thus the morphological patterns that tumours from this source assume can imitate endometrium (**endometrioid** tumours), tubal epithelium (**serous** tumours) and endocervical epithelium (**mucinous** tumours).
- **Germ cells.** These cells originate from the endoderm of the yolk sac and migrate into the ovary.
- **The sex cords**, which first appear in the genital ridge as a collection of cells just beneath the surface epithelium, and the **specialized ovarian stroma**. The granulosa cells, and Sertoli and Leydig cells, are derived from these two elements; the relative

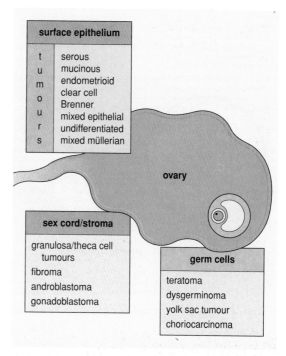

FIGURE 39.20 *Sites from which ovarian neoplasms arise.*

contribution of each is not yet known. For this reason, sex cord and stroma are regarded as a single compartment for the origin of tumours.

TUMOURS ARISING FROM THE SURFACE EPITHELIUM

In general terms, common morphological features that tend to be found in this group are:

- **the presence of a cystic component** with either a single or multiple cavities
- **the presence of a fibrous tissue stroma**
- **the presence of a papillary pattern in the epithelial component**

These tumours show a spectrum of behaviour that correlates well with their microscopic appearances which are, therefore, categorized as being:

- **benign**
- **borderline (of low malignant potential)**
- **malignant**

These correlations are shown in *Table 39.12* and *Fig. 39.21*, and the named morphological entities and their frequency are listed in *Table 39.13*.

Serous Tumours

Serous tumours show differentiation towards the epithelial pattern seen in the fallopian tube. They are the commonest of all ovarian neoplasms and cover a range of histological appearances and biological behav-

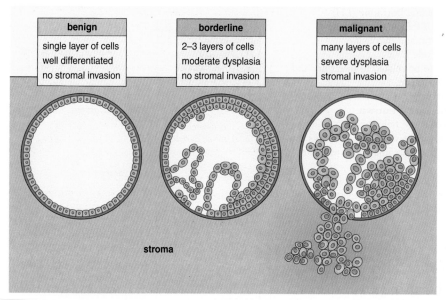

FIGURE 39.21 *Benign, borderline and malignant ovarian tumours derived from surface epithelium.*

Table 39.12 Morphological and Behavioural Features in Ovarian Tumours Derived from Surface Epithelium

Biological behaviour	General morphology
Benign	Lined by a single layer of well-differentiated and normally oriented epithelial cells. If papillary projections are present, these consist of well-vascularized fibrous stroma covered by a single layer of the same cells.
Borderline	These are highly proliferative neoplasms in which the epithelium may be two or three cells thick and in which the papillary pattern, if present, may be very complex. The epithelial cells show only a moderate degree of dysplasia. The most important defining criterion for this group is the **absence of stromal invasion**. As a group these lesions have a better prognosis than do frankly malignant tumours of this type. There is a 5-year survival rate of 90% and a 15-year survival rate of 70%. With unilateral borderline tumours, there is about a 15% chance that another tumour will appear in the contralateral ovary in the following 5–7 years.
Malignant	These tumours have an anaplastic epithelial component **which invades both the stroma of the tumour and neighbouring structures**. The tumour cells are poorly differentiated and are often many layers thick. The prognosis is very bleak with only about 15% of the patients surviving for more than 5 years.

iour extending from benign serous cystadenoma to frank carcinoma. In between a third and a half of the cases, the tumours are bilateral.

Macroscopic Features

The macroscopic appearances of serous ovarian tumours depend on the relative contributions of:

- cyst formation
- papilla formation
- fibrous stroma formation

Thus serous tumours may be large thin-walled cysts with few or no papillae, cysts in which there are few or many papillae both on the internal and external aspects (*Fig. 39.22*), or firm lobulated fibrous tissue masses with or without associated cysts.

Table 39.13 Morphological Types of Surface Epithelial Tumours

Morphological type	Frequency
Serous tumours	40% of ovarian cancers
Mucinous tumours	10%
Endometrioid tumours	20%
Clear cell tumours	5%
Brenner tumours	
Mixed epithelial	
Undifferentiated	10%
Mixed müllerian tumours	

Microscopic Features

Tumours at the benign end of the spectrum are usually cystic. The cysts are usually unilocular and contain clear fluid which may be either watery or viscid. This serous fluid contains mucins but the lining epithelial cells that secrete it are of low columnar type and lack mucin vacuoles. Papillary processes are common and although these are seen, for the most part, to project into the cyst cavities, they may be present on the external surface as well.

The covering epithelium mimics quite closely the appearances of ciliated tubal epithelium. About 30% of all serous tumours, irrespective of their biological behaviour, contain calcified spherical bodies with a concentrically laminated structure (**psammoma bodies**). A fibrous stroma is always present, sometimes in large amounts. Such lesions will have plump papillae and large fibrous areas. This variant is termed a serous **cystadenofibroma**. Most of these are benign but borderline and malignant examples may be seen occasionally.

Borderline tumours (about 15% of serous tumours), are often multilocular. They have a more complex and closely packed papillary pattern, the papillae being covered by two or three layers of epithelial

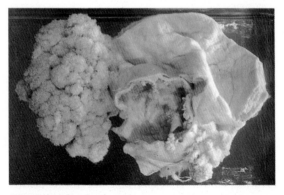

FIGURE 39.22 A partly cystic and partly solid papillary serous carcinoma of the ovary.

cells showing varying degrees of cellular atypia. **Their defining criterion is a negative one: absence of stromal invasion.**

Frankly malignant serous tumours (serous cystadenocarcinomas) are defined by the **presence of stromal invasion**. In addition, these tumours show multilayering of the epithelial component, a marked degree of cellular atypia and a complex glandular and papillary pattern. They are usually partly cystic and partly solid; the solid areas are composed of closely packed papillae.

Mucinous Tumours

Mucinous tumours, **which represent differentiation towards an endocervical pattern**, are less common than serous tumours. They constitute 10–20% of ovarian neoplasms. They tend to be much larger than serous tumours: diameters of 15–30 cm are common. At the benign end of the spectrum, mucinous tumours are predominantly cystic; the cysts are usually multilocular and filled with clear mucoid material.

Microscopic Features

The epithelial component consists of tall columnar cells with basally situated nuclei and prominent supranuclear mucin vacuoles. These cells resemble those normally seen lining endocervical glands.

In some instances, the lining cells have a more intestinal appearance and both Paneth cells and neuroendocrine cells may be present. Gastrointestinal peptide hormones may be found in these cells and hypergastrinaemia of sufficient degree as to cause a Zollinger–Ellison syndrome has been described.

As with serous neoplasms, there is a spectrum of behaviour from benign mucinous cystadenoma through borderline tumours to frankly malignant mucinous cystadenocarcinomas. The latter tumours show solid areas in which foci of necrosis and haemorrhage may be present.

Stromal invasion is, once again, the hallmark of malignancy, although both architectural and cellular atypia may be prominent. Stromal invasion is not easy to assess in mucinous tumours and labelling an individual mucinous tumour as borderline may be very difficult. If invasion is equivocal, some workers recommend that tumours be categorized as malignant if the epithelial lining is more than four cells thick.

Pseudomyxoma Peritonei

Spillage of cyst contents following perforation may lead to **pseudomyxoma peritonei**, in which large amounts of mucoid material accumulate within the abdomen. Cytological examination of this material shows the presence of small groups of mucin-secreting cells. It is not certain as to whether this condition arises as a result of peritoneal implantation of cells derived from the ovarian tumour or whether it represents mucinous metaplasia of the serosal cells lining the peritoneum. An identical condition is associated with cyst-adenocarcinoma of the appendix.

Endometrioid Tumours

Endometrioid carcinomas, **so named because their differentiation pattern closely resembles that of endometrial adenocarcinoma**, constitute 10–25% of primary ovarian cancers. Benign and borderline examples of this type are rare. In a proportion of cases (10–20%), endometriosis is present in the same ovary but pre-existing endometriosis is not a prerequisite for endometrioid carcinoma, which can arise *de novo* from surface epithelium.

Macroscopic Features

The tumours are of moderate size and show the presence of partly cystic and partly solid areas. The cyst fluid is often brown or frankly bloodstained. Unlike what obtains with serous and mucinous carcinomas, papillae are not conspicuous and may be absent.

Microscopic Features

There is a close resemblance to endometrial adenocarcinoma, which is best appreciated in well-differentiated examples. **Focal squamous metaplasia is present in about 50% of these tumours.** In most cases this squamous component is benign, but in a few instances an adenosquamous carcinoma similar to its homologue in the uterus may develop.

The overall prognosis in endometrioid carcinoma is twice as good as that in serous and mucinous carcinoma. This is due partly to the fact that a significant proportion of endometrioid cancers are well differentiated and partly because diagnosis tends to be made before extensive spread has occurred. **Coexistence of endometrioid cancer of the ovary and endometrial cancer of the uterine body is quite common.** It is currently believed that each represents an independent primary neoplasm rather than indicating that metastatic spread has occurred.

Clear Cell Carcinoma ('Mesonephroid' Carcinoma)

Microscopic Features

Clear cell carcinoma shows a spongy, partly cystic, naked-eye appearance. The epithelial component is arranged in the form of:

- tubules and small cysts
- papillary projections
- solid sheets

The epithelial cells have **abundant clear cytoplasm** as a result of intracellular glycogen, although mucin and fat are seen in some examples. In some areas the nuclei may protrude into the tubule lumen giving a characteristic **'hobnail'** appearance.

Because of these histological features, these tumours were originally called **mesonephroid**, arising from mesonephric 'rests'. Most would now regard this tumour as being of surface epithelial origin, in fact closely related to endometrioid carcinoma.

Pelvic endometriosis quite often coexists with clear cell carcinoma; the association is six times as common as with other ovarian cancers. Transition from endometriotic lesions can be seen in some cases, tumour cells showing electron microscopic resemblances to endometrial epithelium. Fewer than 10% of these lesions are bilateral and most are malignant.

Brenner Tumour

Brenner tumours are uncommon (1–2% of ovarian neoplasms). Unlike surface epithelium-derived ovarian tumours considered so far, **most Brenner tumours are benign**. Most patients with Brenner tumours are over 40 years old at clinical presentation. In some cases, this presentation is expressed in the form of post-menopausal uterine bleeding as Brenner tumours may cause endometrial hyperplasia.

Macroscopic Features

The vast majority are quite small, less than 2 cm in diameter. The tumours are firm and fibrous, the cut surfaces showing a greyish, rather whorled, appearance.

Microscopic Features

The distinguishing feature of benign Brenner tumours is the presence of sharply demarcated nests of epithelial cells set in a fibrous stroma. The cells are round or ovoid and have clear cytoplasm and nuclei with a characteristic longitudinal groove. These cell nests resemble urothelium. In roughly one-third of the tumours, small mucin-filled cysts are found in the epithelial nests, about 20% of Brenner tumours being associated with mucinous cyst-adenoma.

The origin appears to be from the surface epithelium of the ovary. Three-dimensional reconstructions from serial sections show that the nests are really anastomosing cords of epithelium connected to the surface epithelium. Borderline and malignant forms do exist but are rare.

OVARIAN CANCER

Epidemiology

Ovarian cancer is responsible for more deaths annually than all other gynaecological malignancies put together.

The cause is still unknown. Most cases are sporadic but a minority of patients inherit a predisposition for ovarian cancer.

In general terms, ovarian cancer of the types discussed in the foregoing section appears to be associated with (*Fig. 39.23*):
- nulliparity
- an early menarche
- a late menopause

There appears to be a **decreased risk** in women who:
- have had many children
- have had their first child before the age of 25 years
- have taken oral contraceptives

These epidemiological data suggest that the greater the number of ovulations during reproductive life, and the fewer interruptions to those ovulations, the greater is the risk of developing ovarian cancer.

Familial Ovarian Cancer

About 1% of patients with ovarian cancer have two or more close relatives who have had the disease, and preliminary analysis suggests that the lifetime risk of death from ovarian cancer in a woman with affected relatives is significantly increased (*Table 39.14*).

Table 39.14 Risk of Ovarian Cancer in Women with Affected Relatives

No. of affected close relatives	Lifetime risk of ovarian cancer
0	1 in 120
1	1 in 40
2	1 in 3

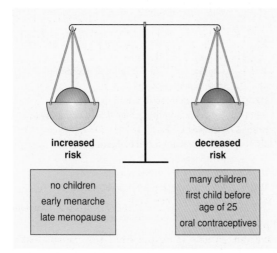

FIGURE 39.23 *Risk factors in ovarian cancer.*

These data suggest that predisposition for ovarian cancer may be conferred by a single autosomal dominant gene.

Hereditary ovarian cancer may occur as part of three inherited disorders:
1) hereditary site-specific ovarian cancer
2) with hereditary non-polyposis rectal cancer and endometrial cancer (Lynch syndrome type II)
3) hereditary breast and ovarian cancer syndrome

Women with a strong family history should be screened regularly.

Cytogenetic Changes in Ovarian Cancer

The genetic alterations associated with ovarian cancer are not yet understood. Allele loss, possibly associated with loss or inactivation of suppressor genes, appears particularly to affect **3p, 6q, 11p and 17q.**

The gene involved on chromosome 17 may be the *BRCA-1* gene discussed previously in relation to breast cancer (see pp 289, 815). Studies are still in a comparatively early stage and we are still some way off from being able to construct a hypothesis as to what is happening at a molecular level in the development of ovarian cancer.

Some ovarian cancers overexpress the proto-oncogene *HER-2/neu* (*c-erbB2*), this being associated with lower survival times. Close homologies exist between the epidermal growth factor (EGF) receptor and the product of *HER-2/neu*; advanced and aggressive ovarian cancers, like some aggressive breast cancers, express large amounts of the EGF receptor. Like many other cancers, ovarian epithelial malignancies show mutations or deletions of the *p53* gene in about 50% of cases.

Clinical Features

It is a tragic fact that the clinical presentation of ovarian cancer is often related to its extension beyond the pelvis. The commonest symptom is abdominal discomfort and fullness, and diagnostic investigation for gastrointestinal disease often precedes recognition of pelvic disease. These symptoms are due either to involvement of the omentum, accumulation ascites, or both. Disease limited to the pelvis is often symptomless. Occasionally, the first sign of ovarian cancer may be the appearance of a secondary deposit in the umbilicus (a 'Sister Mary-Joseph nodule').

Non-metastatic systemic manifestations include:
- **humoral hypercalcaemia of malignancy** (see p 1051)
- **cerebellar degeneration**
- **recurrent arterial and/or venous thrombosis** (see p 209)
- **the appearance of basal cell papillomas** (seborrhoeic keratoses)

Screening for Ovarian Cancer

Screening for the presence of ovarian cancer is currently undertaken in two ways:

1) **transvaginal ultrasonographic examination of the pelvis**

2) **measurement of certain putative 'markers' of ovarian malignancy**

Tumour Markers in Ovarian Cancer

CA-125 Antigen

CA-125 is a high molecular weight glycoprotein expressed by müllerian epithelium. Its plasma concentration is increased before operation in 80–85% of women with epithelial ovarian malignancy.

Unfortunately, the finding of raised concentrations of CA-125 lacks specificity, because this may also occur in pregnancy, in non-neoplastic disorders such as endometriosis, pelvic infections and liver failure, and in association with other neoplasms such as endometrial, breast and colonic cancers. Diagnostic accuracy can be improved if measurement of CA-125 levels is combined with pelvic ultrasonography.

Measurement of CA-125 also lacks **sensitivity**. In about 50% of early stage ovarian cancer, CA-125 levels are normal.

Serum Inhibin Concentrations

A recent study showed that 82% of postmenopausal women with either malignant or borderline **mucinous** tumours had raised serum concentrations of inhibin. Only 17% of those with **serous** tumours showed a similar increase. Unfortunately 27% of women with non-neoplastic ovarian disease also show raised inhibin levels.

Inhibin is a glycoprotein secreted in the ovary by granulosa cells. Its major activity is inhibition of FSH secretion. Whether measurement of FSH levels will be useful for ovarian cancer screening will become apparent in time.

Prognosis

The most important prognostic factors are:

- **the extent of spread of the disease (stage)** (*Fig. 39.24*)
- **the degree of differentiation, which appears to be more important than cell type**, although, stage for stage, clear cell and mucinous tumours behave more aggressively.

The commonly used International Federation of Gynaecology and Obstetrics (FIGO) staging system is shown in *Table 39.15*.

Other adverse factors include:

- older age
- a high grade of tumour
- the presence of residual tumour after primary surgery: **the greater the bulk of such residual disease, the shorter the survival time is** likely to be
- the presence of tumour of clear cell or mucinous type

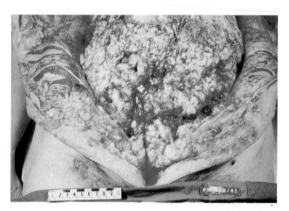

FIGURE 39.24 *Extensive peritoneal involvement by ovarian cancer.*

- overexpression of the EGF receptor
- overexpression of the *HER-2/neu* proto-oncogene

GERM CELL TUMOURS

About 20% of ovarian neoplasms are of germ cell origin. As in the testis, ovarian germ cells give rise to a variety of tumours, many reproducing the pattern of their testicular homologues, though they may have different names (*Fig. 39.25*). Ovarian germ cell neoplasms are distinguished from their testicular counterparts by the fact that **95% of ovarian germ cell neoplasms**

Table 39.15 Staging of Ovarian Cancer according to the FIGO System

Stage	Features
IA	One ovary involved; capsule intact; no ascites
IB	Both ovaries involved; capsules intact; no ascites
IC	Capsule involved or ruptured; malignant cells in peritoneal fluid
IIA	Pelvic extension to uterus or tubes
IIB	Extension to other pelvic organs (e.g. bladder)
IIC	Pelvic extension and malignant cells in peritoneal fluid
IIIA	Microscopic seeding outside pelvis
IIIB	Macroscopic deposits less than 2 cm in diameter
IIIC	Macroscopic deposits greater than 2 cm in diameter or nodal involvement
IV	Involvement of distant organs

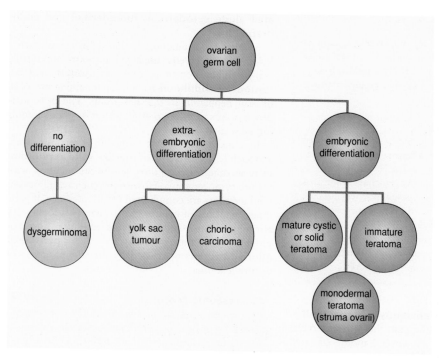

FIGURE 39.25 Ovarian neoplasms of germ cell origin.

are benign cystic teratomas, whereas only a small proportion of testicular germ cell lesions are of this type.

Germ Cell Tumours Showing No Evidence of Differentiation

Dysgerminoma

Dysgerminoma is the ovarian homologue of seminoma of the testis and is an **undifferentiated germ cell tumour.** It accounts for about 1% of all ovarian neoplasms and about 5% of the malignant ones. It is a tumour of young women (more than 80% occur in women aged 30 years or less). The right ovary is more often affected than the left, and in about 15% of cases the lesion is bilateral.

In some instances **microscopic foci** of tumour may be present in a contralateral ovary, which appears normal at the time of surgery. For this reason it is wise to take a sample of such a normal-looking ovary for frozen-section examination. About 5% of dysgerminomas arise in a previously abnormal gonad.

Macroscopic Features

Dysgerminoma is a fairly large tumour (mean diameter about 15 cm). The fleshy grey-white cut surface shows occasional haemorrhagic or necrotic foci.

Microscopic Features

These closely resemble those of seminoma. The tumour cells are large, rounded or ovoid, with well-defined plasma membranes and central nuclei. These cells are arranged in islands separated from each other by fine fibrous tissue septa usually containing a lymphocytic infiltrate. Sarcoid-like granulomas, similar to those seen in testicular seminoma, may be present, as are occasional multinucleated giant cells containing human chorionic gonadotrophin (HCG). Their presence does not alter the prognosis which, on the whole, is good. Five-year survival rates are 70–90% and, like seminoma, dysgerminoma is very radiosensitive.

Germ Cell Tumours Showing Evidence of Extra-embryonic Differentiation

Yolk Sac Tumour (Endodermal Sinus Tumour)

This is the homologue of the tumour of the same name occurring in the testis. Its structure shows a close relationship with that of the endodermal sinuses of Duval, formed by invaginations of yolk sac endoderm. This is mirrored functionally by secretion of α-fetoprotein (AFP), the normal product of the yolk sac. It is a tumour of the young (mean age 19 years), almost 25% of the patients being prepubertal.

Macroscopic Features

The naked-eye appearances are rather similar to those of dysgerminoma. They are large, encapsulated and either smooth or nodular. The cut surface is a yellowish-grey, and haemorrhage and necrosis are more prominent than is the case with dysgerminoma.

Microscopic Features

The appearances are variable and complex; specialized texts should be consulted for a description of the variants.

A loose network of microcysts lined by flattened cells is often seen, as are the papillary structures known as **Schiller–Duval** bodies, which have a mesenchymal core containing a small blood vessel, the core being covered by cuboidal or columnar epithelium.. Hyaline periodic acid–Schiff-positive material is usually present both within the cytoplasm of the tumour cells and in the extracellular space, and this can be shown to be AFP.

Yolk sac tumour is inherently a highly malignant neoplasm and, in the past, the 3-year survival rate was about 13%. However, more effective chemotherapeutic treatment has led to a considerable increase in the survival rate. In stage 1 tumours, 5-year survival rate is now about 80%; even patients with more advanced disease have a one in two chance of 5-year survival.

The presence of AFP in the serum provides a tool for monitoring the activity of the disease. Disappearance of this marker from the serum after initial surgery suggests absence of significant residual disease; subsequent reappearance suggests that recurrence has occurred.

Choriocarcinoma

Choriocarcinoma of the ovary may be either **primary** (which is rare) or **secondary** to gestational choriocarcinoma. Primary ovarian choriocarcinoma may occur in a pure form, but is more likely to be seen as a component of a mixed tumour.

These tumours vary in size and show extensive areas of necrosis and haemorrhage. The microscopic appearances are similar to those of the more common gestational choriocarcinoma (see pp 799–800). Because these tumours may produce HCG, examples in prepubertal girls may be associated with precocious sexual development. Unlike gestational choriocarcinoma, the response of primary ovarian choriocarcinoma to chemotherapy is poor.

Germ Cell Tumours Showing Evidence of Embryonic Differentiation

Mature Cystic and Solid Teratoma

A differentiated teratoma is composed of elements that can be recognized to have differenti-ated along ectodermal, mesodermal and endodermal lines.

Mature cystic teratoma is the archetype of such a lesion. These chiefly unilateral tumours are usually benign. They constitute the **commonest ovarian tumour of childhood** accounting for about 50% of all ovarian neoplasms in this age group. The peak incidence occurs from 20 to 40 years but ovarian teratoma can be seen at any age.

In some instances, cyst formation is inconspicuous, and such lesions are termed **mature solid teratomas**. In most other respects these lesions are identical with mature cystic teratoma. However, some cases of mature solid teratoma are complicated by the presence of peritoneal implants of mature glial tissue. This looks very alarming on microscopy, but the condition does not progress and the presence of such **peritoneal gliomatosis** does not materially alter the prognosis of mature teratoma.

Macroscopic Features

The tumours are usually multiloculated. The cyst cavities contain a greasy and unpleasant mixture of hair-containing keratin and sebum (*Fig. 39.26*). These latter are derived from the epidermis and skin adenexae, which are the most prominent differentiated element in many cases. This morphological characteristic led to the term '**dermoid cyst**' being applied to these lesions.

In addition to skin and adnexal structures, other differentiated structures that are commonly seen include adipose tissue, bone, cartilage, neural tissue including glia and neurones, bronchi (in which the changes of asthma have been described), salivary glands, retina, pancreas, smooth muscle, thyroid and teeth (*Fig. 39.27*).

Often, these differentiated structures are contained within a nipple-like nodule (the mamilla), which protrudes from the cyst lining.

In occasional cases, organogenesis may be far advanced so that, for example, a well-formed but miniature cerebellum may be recognized on naked-eye examination of the lesion.

Malignant transformation of one of these elements occurs in about 2% of cases. Any of the

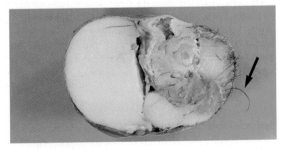

FIGURE 39.26 *Mature ovarian teratoma showing abundant yellowish sebum and some hair (arrowed).*

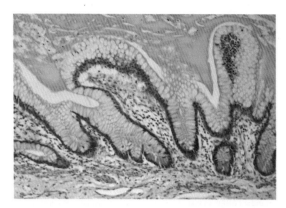

FIGURE 39.27 *Intestinal-type epithelium in a mature ovarian teratoma.*

components may undergo such change but the commonest malignant tumours seen in association with mature cystic teratoma are:

- epidermoid carcinoma, which accounts for 85% of such instances of malignant transformation
- carcinoid tumours
- adenocarcinomas of different types

The clinical presentations are usually those of any intrapelvic mass. Occasionally, torsion of the tumours can occur and this can lead to ischaemic necrosis of the cyst wall, rupture and spillage of the contents of the cyst. Rarely, a patient with a mature teratoma may present with haemolytic anaemia. The mechanism for this is still obscure but it has been suggested that there may be a cross-reaction between tumour and red cell antigens, and that the presentation of such antigens on a new carrier may overcome tolerance.

Immature Teratoma

The term immature is used in this context to indicate the presence of embryonic-type tissue within a teratoma. These rare tumours occur most frequently during the first two decades of life.

They are usually large nodular lesions with a predominantly solid cut surface which may, however, contain some very small cysts.

Microscopic Features of Immature Teratoma

A mixture of immature and well differentiated elements is present. Neural tissue, identified by antibodies reacting with glial fibrillary acid protein (GFAP), is often conspicuous.

Natural History

The prognosis depends on the amount and degree of differentiation of the embryonal components. It is best in lesions in which a neural element predominates.

Until recently, the prognosis was very bleak, 5-year survival rates being less than 20%. With newer chemotherapeutic asgents, the outlook has improved greatly and complete remission can be expected in a significant proportion of cases.

Monodermal Teratoma

These are germ cell tumours that differentiate along only one pathway, or in which one differentiated element may predominate and obliterate evidence of others. The commonest of these is a cyst lined purely by intestinal-type mucinous epithelium. In some cases the dominant differentiated element is thyroid epithelium; this type is known as **struma ovarii.** This thyroid tissue is quite normal in the functional sense and a number of cases of hyperthyroidism associated with ovarian struma have been reported. Struma ovarii is almost always benign but a curious complication: ascites and/or pleural effusion may occur in about 10% of these benign lesions.

Primary carcinoid tumours may also be seen in the ovary, either as part of a teratoma or as a pure primary carcinoid tumour with no teratomatous element. Carcinoids arising in association with a teratoma are usually asymptomatic, but about 30% of the pure primary form produce the carcinoid syndrome (see pp 529–530).

Strumal carcinoid is a rare variant in which carcinoid is combined with struma ovarii (see above).

SEX CORD AND STROMAL TUMOURS

The sex cords first appear as a group of cells just beneath the epithelium of the genital ridge. They migrate to the gonad and arrange themselves in a sheath-like pattern around the oöcyte. In the adult gonad some cells of the sex cord retain the ability to differentiate along either ovarian or testicular lines, and this bigonadal potential accounts for the wide range of differentiation patterns encountered.

The tumours show a variety of differentiation patterns and a wide range of steroid hormone secretions, encompassing those of both ovarian and testicular type. These differentiation patterns include lesions containing granulosa and theca cells, both of which are a normal feature of the ovary, and Sertoli and Leydig cells, both of which are normally found only in the testis. These elements may appear in a pure form or in combination.

Granulosa–Theca Cell Tumours

Adult-type Granulosa Cell Tumour

This accounts for about 1.5% of all ovarian tumours. It is unilateral in more than 90% of cases. **The 20-year survival rate is about 50–60% and it is difficult to label an individual example as being unequivocally benign.** These tumours are most frequent after the menopause but about 33% occur in women during reproductive life and a small proportion (5%) occur in prepubertal girls.

About 75% of granulosa cell tumours produce steroid hormones, usually oestrogen. Very occasionally, a granulosa cell can have a virilizing effect. The effects of the oestrogen depend on the age of the patient. In prepubertal cases, the oestrogen causes precocious sexual development. In postpubertal females, endometrial hyperplasia results, commonly presenting with abnormal uterine bleeding. In a proportion of these cases (6–10%), the endometrial hyperplasia develops into endometrial adenocarcinoma.

Macroscopic Features

Tumours differ markedly in size, ranging from those too small to see with the naked eye to over 40 cm in diameter. The average diameter is 12 cm. The lesions are usually solid, or partly solid and partly cystic, and somewhat rubbery in consistency. The cut surface does not show any specific features but may vary in colour from case to case. Foci of haemorrhage and necrosis are seen commonly.

Microscopic Features

The characteristic cell is rounded or ovoid and the nuclei have a characteristic longitudinal groove giving the nucleus a **'coffee bean-like'** appearance.

A wide range of architectural patterns exists, including:

- a microfollicular pattern in which small rosettes of tumour cells are seen. These rosettes contain eosinophilic material admixed with nuclear debris. These small rosette-like structures are known as **Call–Exner bodies**.
- a large follicle pattern which arises from the development of areas of liquefaction necrosis within masses of granulosa cells. It is these cystic macrofollicular type tumours that are likely to secrete androgens and to produce evidence of virilization.
- a type of follicle that resembles the ovarian follicles seen in newborn infants.

Juvenile Granulosa Cell Tumours

Of the prepubertal granulosa cell tumours, 85% show a rather characteristic microscopic appearance which has been termed juvenile granulosa cell tumour.

The age distribution of juvenile granulosa cell tumours is shown in *Table 39.16.*

Macroscopic Features

The tumours, usually unilateral, are, for the most part, solid.

Microscopic Features

Islands or sometimes diffuse sheets of tumour cells set in a loose and oedematous stroma are seen. The islands of tumour cells contain granulosa cell-lined follicles, and also rather large cystic spaces lined by several layers of granulosa cells. The longitudinal grooving of the nuclei seen in adult-type tumours is not present in this variant and luteinization is often a feature of both tumour and stromal cells.

Table 39.16 Age Distribution of Juvenile Granulosa Cell Tumours

Age range (years)	Frequency (%)
up to 10	45
11–20	32
21–30	20
over 30	3

About 5% of these tumours are malignant. In this group, the indolent behaviour characteristic of the adult type is not seen, and rapid recurrence and metastatic spread are the rule.

Theca Cell Tumours (Thecoma)

Thecomas, which occur about one-third as frequently as granulosa cell tumours, are solid tumours arising from the **ovarian stroma** (*Fig. 39.28*) and consist of interlacing bundles of spindle cells. Some of the spindle cells are

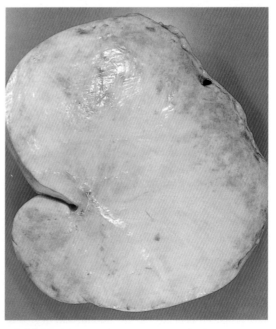

FIGURE 39.28 *Large solid thecoma arising from ovarian stroma.*

plump and contain **lipid which, in their case, is the morphological expression of steroid production**. The presence of this lipid gives the cut surfaces of these tumours a yellow colour on naked-eye examination.

Thecomas are most commonly seen in post-menopausal women. The actively secreting component of the cell population usually produces oestrogen and, thus, they have the same stimulating effect on the endometrium as is seen in oestrogen-producing granulosa cell tumours. Very occasionally, androgen-producing thecomas are encountered. Most thecomas are benign.

Fibroma of Ovary

Large tumours consisting of well-differentiated fibrous tissue are not uncommon in the ovary, accounting for about 5% of all ovarian neoplasms. These have no endocrine effect and invariably behave in a benign fashion. For reasons that are not clear, fibromas may be associated, in some instances, with the presence of ascites and/or a pleural effusion. This condition, known as **Meigs' syndrome**, resolves when the tumour is removed.

Sertoli–Leydig Cell Tumours

Very rare tumours (0.2% of all ovarian neoplasms) are seen in which both Sertoli and Leydig cells are present. It has been suggested that the Leydig cell element is not truly neoplastic but represents a differentiation process in the ovarian stromal cells induced by the Sertoli cell element. These tumours occur for the most part in young women; the mean age at diagnosis is 25 years.

Macroscopic Features

Tumours consisting entirely of Sertoli cells are rare and almost invariably benign. They are usually not very large, with a mean diameter of 9 cm. They are solid tumours and the cut surfaces have a yellow or orange colour. Although they show a differentiation pattern that is characteristic of the testis, Sertoli cell tumours, like all sex cord–stromal neoplasms, show a female karyotype.

Microscopic Features

Most Sertoli cell tumours consist of well-formed tubules, although a trabecular pattern may also be seen. The tubules are lined by a single layer of columnar or cuboidal epithelial cells which, in some instances, contain large amounts of lipid.

Androblastoma (Arrhenoblastoma)

Androblastomas are tumours arising from cells of sex cord origin. **Their defining criterion is the presence of Sertoli cells and Leydig cells, either alone or in combination.** Despite the names androblastoma and arrhenoblastoma, suggesting that all these tumours have a virilizing effect, some androblastomas produce oestrogen and some have no endocrine activity:

- 70% of the tumours have an oestrogenic effect
- 20% have an androgenic effect
- 10% show no signs of endocrine activity

Microscopic Features

These lesions consist essentially of tubular structures with variable numbers of cells resembling Leydig cells present in the intertubular spaces. The tumours are classified on the basis of the degree of differentiation as **well, intermediate** or **poorly** differentiated.

Rare malignant examples are almost always poorly differentiated. Endocrine activity is common and is usually androgenic in type, the clinical picture being dominated by virilization.

Steroid Cell (Lipid Cell) Tumours

Several tumours exist with certain common features:
- an origin from the ovarian stroma (or, rarely, from hilar cells)
- secretion of steroid hormones

The tumour cells may show differentiation into Leydig cells, into cells resembling adrenal cortical cells or into cells that it is possible to classify only as steroidogenic. Most of these lesions are benign and the majority are associated with virilization, although a few cases of Cushing's syndrome have been described as occurring with tumours showing adrenocortical differentiation.

Gonadoblastoma (Mixed Germ Cell–Sex Cord–Stromal Tumour)

This is a rare tumour that tends to arise in dysgenetic gonads. Patients are, for the most part, **phenotypically female** (85%), but the majority are **genotypically male** (they have a Y chromosome).

Microscopic Features

Both immature germ cells and sex cord–stromal cells, which resemble either granulosa or Sertoli cells are present. The sex cord cells tend to be arranged in nests and, in the intervening stroma, Leydig cells are often present. Foci of calcification are common.

Gonadoblastomas themselves are benign, but there is a 50% chance that a malignant germ cell tumour will develop in these lesions. It is this high risk of malignancy at a later date that has led to the recommendation that a dysgenetic gonad in a person with a Y chromosome should be removed prophylactically.

PRIMARY NEOPLASMS NOT SPECIFIC TO THE OVARY

The ovary is frequently involved in patients with disseminated malignant lymphoma. Primary extranodal lymphoma can occur in the ovary but is very rare.

The ovary is a site of predilection for Burkitt's lymphoma, especially but not exclusively the type that is common in sub-Saharan Africa and which is associated with infection by the Epstein–Barr virus. The ovary is involved in 70–80% of female patients with Burkitt's lymphoma, and an ovarian mass may call attention to the existence of this disease in a significant number of female sufferers.

METASTATIC TUMOURS

Nearly three-quarters of women dying from malignant disease can be found at autopsy to have involvement of the ovaries, and ovarian metastases account for about 7% of all ovarian neoplasms.

The commonest primary sites are the breast, gastrointestinal tract and uterus.

The eponym Krukenberg's tumour frequently surfaces when ovarian metastases are discussed. Using the Humpty Dumpty principle that 'a word means what I choose it to mean', this term has been used in different ways by different people. The consensus seems to be that a Krukenberg tumour is a metastatic, mucin-secreting carcinoma, the cells of which are set in a dense, somewhat hypercellular, stroma, in which some degree of pleomorphism and mitotic activity is often present.

Grossly, these tumours, which are commonly bilateral, are usually solid and have a smooth or nodular external surface. Microscopic examination shows the presence of strands, clumps or sheets of 'signet-ring', mucin-secreting cells set against a background of a very active connective tissue stroma.

The prognosis for patients with metastatic tumour in the ovaries is bleak; the 2-year survival rate is 10% or less.

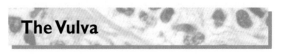

The Vulva

NORMAL ANATOMY

The vulva as an anatomical entity includes the:
- mons pubis
- the labia majora and minora
- the clitoris
- the vestibule of the vagina and its bulb
- the greater vestibular (Bartholin's) glands

Much is covered by skin, some hair-bearing and some containing sebaceous glands. Pathological changes occurring in this site are, at least in part, dictated by these tissue components. Thus the vulva may be affected by **dermatological disorders** occurring also in other sites (see pp 988–1034).

DISORDERS OF THE VULVAR SKIN AND MUCOSA

Itching of the vulva is a common and distressing symptom. It may have a recognizable cause such as allergy, chemical irritation or infection, but in many cases there is no obvious cause. Itching may be associated with hyperkeratosis in the form of white patches on the affected vulval skin (**leucoplakia**). This is a purely descriptive term with no implications for either its microscopic features or natural history.

In 1961 the term **vulvar dystrophy** was introduced for these disorders of vulvar squamous epithelium. This term encompassed benign disorders as well as those with malignant potential, an unsatisfactory solution. Thus, the blanket term 'dystrophy' has been abandoned and a root and branch reclassification of vulvar epithelial disorders undertaken.

It is recommended that vulvar skin and mucosal disorders be divided into two main groups (see *Table 39.17*).

This classification presents some difficulties in practice. Some 10–15% of affected women have a **combined** condition with both a non-neoplastic and a neoplastic disorder of the vulva, and 2–4% of women with lichen sclerosus (a non-neoplastic condition) ultimately develop carcinoma of the vulva, although not necessarily in the area affected by the lichen sclerosus.

Non-neoplastic Dermatoses

Lichen Sclerosus

This is the commonest cause of vulvar itching in elderly females. It occurs occasionally in younger women and even in children. The cause is not known; a little under 10% of the patients have thyroid disease, pernicious

Table 39.17 Disorders of Vulvar Skin and Mucosa

Group	Disorders
Non-neoplastic	Lichen sclerosus Squamous cell hyperplasia (formerly called hypertrophic dystrophy) Other dermatoses
Vulvar intraepithelial neoplasia(VIN)	Squamous VIN VIN I (mild dysplasia) VIN II (moderate dysplasia) VIN III (severe dysplasia, carcinoma *in situ*) Non-squamous VIN Paget's disease

anaemia or diabetes, associations that suggest a possible autoimmune mechanism.

The lesion is white (because of the hyperkeratosis) and the skin looks thin and wrinkly unless the patient has been rubbing the affected area, in which case it may become thickened (**lichenified**).

Microscopic Features

Defining criteria include:
- hyperkeratosis
- atrophy of the epithelium with variable loss of rete ridges
- liquefaction degeneration of the basal layer of the epidermis (frequent but not invariable)
- hyalinization or oedema of the underlying papillary and reticular dermis giving a curiously featureless and 'homogenized' appearance
- a band-like, non-specific, chronic inflammatory cell infiltrate at the deep margin of the abnormal dermis

Immunohistochemical studies show that, with the exception of the basal layer, the full thickness of the epidermis in lichen sclerosus contains **involucrin**, a marker of late keratinocyte differentiation, normally found only in superficial epidermal cells. Premature maturation of epidermal cells may, therefore, be part of the natural history.

Squamous Hyperplasia

Microscopic Features

Squamous epithelial hyperplasia is characterized by:
- epithelial proliferation involving the malpighian layer of the epidermis (**acanthosis**), with no evidence of atypia
- elongation of rete ridges
- hyperkeratosis
- a chronic inflammatory cell infiltrate within the dermis

It may be the expression of a dermatosis such as lichen simplex, psoriasis or a *Candida* infection. If no cause can be identified, the lesion is classified as 'squamous hyperplasia'. It may be seen in conjunction with lichen sclerosus.

Other Dermatoses

Many other dermatoses occur on the vulva. Their clinical appearance may be somewhat altered by the local conditions obtaining in this area but essentially they do not differ from what is seen in other parts of the body. Such conditions include:
- **allergic or irritant dermatitis**
- **psoriasis**
- **intertrigo** (inflammation occurring in moist folds of skin) and often complicated by secondary

infections most notably fungal infections (*Candida albicans*). Such lesions are especially likely to occur in obese diabetics
- **lichen planus**, presenting either with reddish-purple plaques or in an erosive form characterized by pain, itching and, in some cases, bleeding

Ulcers of the Vulva

Several conditions are associated with vulval ulceration. These include:
- **infection with herpesvirus.** Herpes genitalis causes very painful ulceration, sometimes associated with features such as fever and inguinal lymph node enlargement.
- **syphilis in its primary phase**
- **Crohn's disease.** The vulva or perineum are affected in about 25–30% of patients with Crohn's disease.
- **Behçet's syndrome.** This is described in the section on the penis (see p 737).
- **aphthous ulceration.** Small, painful ulcers with a yellow base occur from time to time on the vulva. They appear to be the homologue of aphthous ulceration in the mouth (see pp 485–486).
- **Lipschütz ulcers.** These acute and painful ulcers affect the labia minora and are associated with enlargement of the inguinal nodes and fever. Their histological features are entirely non-specific and their cause is unknown. Healing occurs spontaneously.

VULVAR TUMOURS AND TUMOUR-LIKE LESIONS

Vulvar Intraepithelial Neoplasia (VIN)

The condition may present as pruritus vulvae but, in many cases, is asymptomatic being found in the course of gynaecological examination. The lesions may be multicentric; their appearance depends on the degree of keratinization. As in cervical intraepithelial neoplasia (CIN), recognition is helped by the application of 5% acetic acid to the vulval skin. After 2–3 minutes, any areas of VIN show up as white patches.

Microscopic Features

VIN shows abnormalities in:
- **the stratification pattern of epithelial cells**
- **maturation of the cells**

Two forms have been described:
1) where basal or parabasal cells extend upwards through the epidermis
2) the bowenoid form, in which there is premature maturation of the cells with individual cell keratinization, koilocytes and abnormal mitoses (similar to Bowen's disease of the skin in other sites)

Grading of VIN is carried out in the same way as for CIN (see pp 768–769).

Aetiology

Epidemiological data suggest involvement of a sexually transmitted agent; about 25% of patients with VIN suffer or will suffer from CIN. A significant proportion of women with VIN also have other sexually transmitted diseases. As with CIN, an association has been demonstrated between VIN and infections with human papillomavirus (HPV) type 16.

Infections with other types of papillomavirus may cause genital warts or condylomata acuminata just as in the cervix. These are papillomatous lesions in which the cytological changes of HPV infection (koilocytosis) can be seen.

Natural History

VIN runs a rather variable course; it is impossible to predict the course in an individual patient. Factors that appear to increase the risk of invasive cancer include:

- an immunocompromised state
- the presence of a basaloid rather than a bowenoid pattern

It is clear that VIN runs a much more benign course than CIN. Only about 5% of cases progress to invasive squamous carcinoma and a roughly equal proportion regress spontaneously.

Paget's Disease of the Vulva

Paget's disease of the vulva is the expression of an adenocarcinoma *in situ*. In most cases the process is purely intraepidermal; only in a minority (20–30%) are adnexal structures such as sweat glands or ducts, Bartholin's glands, the urinary tract or the anorectal area involved. This contrasts with Paget's disease of the nipple, usually associated with an underlying intraductal carcinoma.

Different views exist as to the origin of the Paget cells. Some regard Paget's cells as being abnormally differentiated, multipotent, basal cells of the epidermis, whereas others suggest they are derived from the intraepidermal portion of sweat ducts.

Macroscopic Features

The lesions present as crusting, red, scaly areas on the labia or perineal skin.

Microscopic Features

The defining feature is the large, round or oval **Paget's cell which has large amounts of pale cytoplasm**. In most cases, this cytoplasm stains positively for mucin, another difference from Paget's disease of the nipple. Cells may be arranged singly, or in nests or clumps within the epidermis. When mucin is absent or present in only very small amounts, it may be difficult to distinguish Paget's cells from those of intraepidermal melanoma or

the bowenoid type of VIN. The fact that the Paget cells bind antibodies to 54-kD cytokeratins, whereas the others mentioned do not, may be useful in making this distinction.

Invasive Carcinoma of the Vulva

The annual incidence of invasive cancer of the vulva in England and Wales is about 3 per 100 000 (750 new cases each year). This tumour accounts for about 5% of gynaecological malignancies; almost 90% are squamous in type.

It is a disease predominantly of late middle age (peak incidence 63–65 years). In countries with a high prevalence of sexually transmitted, vulval, chronic inflammatory diseases, carcinoma tends to appear in a younger age group.

Aetiology and Pathogenesis

Some cancers of the vulva develop from VIN, but in a considerable proportion of cases VIN does not precede vulvar cancer. A wide range of sexually transmitted chronic inflammatory diseases is reported as increasing vulvar cancer risk. These include syphilis, lymphogranuloma venereum and granuloma inguinale. A positive association has also been reported between cigarette smoking and the risk of vulvar cancer; it is suggested that this is mediated via potentially carcinogenic metabolites of smoke in urine.

Clinical Features

Common presenting features are shown in *Table 39.18*.

Invasive cancer affects the labia majora in two-thirds of cases. The clitoris is the second commonest site, followed by the labia minora, posterior fourchette and perineum. Lymph from these areas drains to the inguinal glands on both sides and thence to the femoral and external iliac glands. The bilaterality of lymph drainage means that bilateral inguinal node dissection should be undertaken at the time of excision. In about 25% of cases, nodal deposits, if present, affect the nodes on both sides.

Table 39.18 Presenting Features of Vulvar Cancer

Symptom	Frequency (%)
Itching or irritation of the vulva	71
Local mass or ulcer	57
Bleeding	28
Discharge	23

Macroscopic Features

The lesion may appear as an intact plaque or mass but more often is ulcerated, the ulcer having raised and indurated edges.

Microscopic Features

Most cases are well-differentiated squamous carcinoma with many keratinous 'pearls'.

Natural History

The most important factor is the extent of spread at the time of primary excision. Vulvar cancer is staged by the International Federation of Gynaecology and Obstetrics (FIGO) system, as shown in *Table 39.19*.

Table 39.19 Staging of Vulvar Cancer according to the FIGO System

Stage	Extent of spread
I	Maximum diameter 2 cm or less. Confined to vulva and/or perineum. Groin nodes not palpable
II	As above, but lesion more than 2 cm in diameter
III	Lesion extends beyond the vulva with no palpable nodes; lesion of any size with unilateral nodal metastases
IVa	Involves mucosa of rectum or bladder, upper urethra or pelvic bones and/ or bilateral nodal metastases
IVb	Distant metastases including pelvic nodal involvement

The overall 5-year survival rate is about 70%. If nodes are not involved, this figure rises to 90%; if spread to pelvic nodes has occurred, the rate drops to 25%.

Other Less Common Vulvar Tumours

Verrucous Carcinoma

This is a slow-growing squamous tumour whose distinction from condyloma is difficult in biopsy material. It is the precise homologue of verrucous tumours occurring on penile skin (see p 741).

Malignant Melanoma

The second commonest primary malignant neoplasm occurring on the vulva is malignant melanoma; about 5% of all malignant melanomas in women occur at this site. In view of the known correlation between expo-sure of the skin to excessive amounts of sunlight and the risk of developing malignant melanoma, the relative frequency with which the vulva is involved is puzzling. The tumour spreads early to inguinal nodes and the overall prognosis is poor, the 5-year survival rate being about 30–40%.

Other Rare Malignant Tumours of the Vulva

- basal cell carcinoma
- tumours of skin appendages
- Bartholin's gland cancer (usually an adenocarcinoma which occurs in a younger age group and which spreads early to lymph nodes)
- connective tissue tumours
- secondary tumours

Benign Neoplasms

The benign neoplasms found in the vulva are the counterparts of those in other areas of the skin, which are discussed in the section dealing with skin tumours (see pp 1021–1022). They include lesions derived from surface epithelium, such as squamous papilloma and basal cell papilloma, and from the epithelium of adnexal structures, such as sweat glands and ducts. Benign connective tissue tumours also occur. These are often polypoid and tend to become pedunculated.

NON-NEOPLASTIC CYSTS OF THE VULVA

The non-neoplastic cystic lesions found in the vulva fall into two principal groups:

1) **cysts occurring in hair-bearing skin in any part of the body**, such as epidermoid cysts which are lined by well-differentiated squamous epithelium and are filled with keratin. Rupture of such a lesion with the release of keratin into the surrounding connective tissue can elicit a florid inflammatory response in which foreign-body giant cells are prominent.

2) **cysts occurring in structures specific to the vulva.** These include:

- **cysts arising from developmental remnants (mesonephric or peritoneal residua).** Mesonephric remnant cysts usually occur in the posterior part of the labia majora; those thought to have arisen from peritoneal remnants carried to the vulva by the round ligament (cysts of the canal of Nuck) tend to occur in the anterior part of the vulva.

- **cysts arising from obstruction to mucus-secreting vulval glands.** These glands include the lesser vestibular glands, Skene's glands and the greater vestibular glands (Bartholin's glands).

  Bartholin's glands lie in the subcutaneous tissue in the posterior third of the vulva. Ductal blockage leads to retention of the secretions and a tense cyst forms. Cyst formation is often followed by infection and the patient presents with a painful tense swelling which must be treated by being laid open and drained if a chronic inflammatory process is to be avoided.

The Vagina

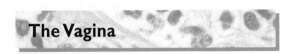

NORMAL ANATOMY

The vagina forms the conduit between the vestibule of the vulva and the uterus. Its long axis forms an angle of more than 90° with the uterus. Its ventral wall is approximately 8 cm long and the dorsal wall 11 cm.

The wall is a three-layered structure:
- a lining epithelium
- a muscular coat
- an adventitia composed of connective tissue

Vaginal Epithelium
The non-keratinizing, stratified, squamous epithelium has a folded pattern. As with the cervix, vaginal epithelium is very responsive to oestrogenic stimulation and, with the menopause, it atrophies. This atrophic epithelium is much more likely to be the seat of infection than is the vaginal epithelium during reproductive life.

Maturation of vaginal epithelium mediated by oestrogen is associated with large amounts of glycogen in the superficial epithelial cells. This glycogen is a substrate for the organism, *Lactobacillus vaginalis*, normally present in the vagina. The lactic acid produced from the glycogen results in a low pH (between 4 and 5) and this is said to be an effective barrier against many infections.

INFLAMMATORY DISORDERS (VAGINITIS)

It is unusual to find **isolated** inflammation of the vagina; associated cervicitis or vulvitis are very common.

Vaginal inflammation may be infective or non-infective, the latter resulting from causes such as trauma, irradiation, surgery, the application of certain chemical compounds or the use of a pessary.

Infective Vaginitis
The vagina may become infected by:
- **bacteria**
- **viruses** (most notably herpes)
- **fungi** (most commonly *Candida albicans*, associated in most instances with a fungal vulvitis)
- **protozoa.** One of the commonest causes of

vaginitis during reproductive life is *Trichomonas vaginalis*, a flagellate protozoon which is transmitted sexually. In the acute phase, patients present clinically with a rather 'frothy' discharge, and examination of the vagina shows it to be granular and hyperaemic.

Microscopic examination shows a mixed inflammatory infiltrate consisting of lymphocytes and plasma cells. This may extend upwards to involve the epithelium. Not infrequently the process may become chronic. In some patients the inflammatory process dies down but the patients remain asymptomatic carriers.

The chief clinical expression of vaginitis is a vaginal discharge which frequently has an unpleasant smell and which may cause vulvar itching.

Most infections are sexually transmitted but the ability of organisms introduced in this way to establish themselves depends in part on the normal vaginal bacterial flora, which is related to oestrogen and progesterone levels. Excess amounts of progesterone act in the opposite way to oestrogen and thus tend to promote infection.

Some cases of vaginitis occur in the prepubertal or perimenopausal period; these have been termed nonspecific. The greater number of these are due to infection. Prominent amongst the responsible organisms is the Gram-negative bacillus *Gardnerella vaginalis*, which may be solely responsible or act in concert with anaerobic organisms. *Gardnerella* adheres to the epithelial surface and does not penetrate into the subepithelial tissues.

Vaginal Adenosis
This term is defined as the presence of glandular structures derived from müllerian epithelium within the vaginal wall. These remnants represent a partial failure of the orderly replacement of müllerian structures by squamous epithelium derived from the urogenital sinus.

The condition may be asymptomatic or associated with rather mucoid vaginal discharge. On examination the anterior wall of the vagina shows patchy red areas which appear roughened. Microscopic examination shows the presence within the vaginal wall of glandular structures, usually lined by mucus-secreting epithelium. In some instances other forms of müllerian differentiation are expressed. Not infrequently squamous metaplasia occurs in the epithelial lining of the glandular spaces; this may lead to the erroneous diagnosis of squamous carcinoma of the vagina.

There is a strong association between the presence of vaginal adenosis and a history of the patient's mother having been treated with diethylstilboestrol before the eighth week of gestation in an attempt to ward off a threatened spontaneous abortion. This manoeuvre, quite common in the 1940s and early 1950s, produced vaginal adenosis in

70% of the female children resulting from these pregnancies.

Vaginal adenosis is important because it is a precursor lesion for vaginal adenocarcinoma.

VAGINAL TUMOURS AND TUMOUR-LIKE LESIONS

Vaginal Intraepithelial Neoplasia

As with all squamous epithelium–lined surfaces in the lower female genital tract, the vaginal lining can be the seat of intraepithelial neoplasia, known as vaginal introepithelial neoplasia (VAIN).

On examination, the lesions of VAIN appear as reddish or sometimes whitish patches on the vaginal epithelium. Many affected women have been treated previously for intraepithelial or frank invasive neoplasia of the cervix. It is likely that the aetiological factors are the same (see pp 767–768).

Microscopic examination shows changes more or less identical to those seen in cervical intraepithelial neoplasia (CIN). Grading of the changes is performed in the same way as with CIN (*Table 39.20*).

The natural history of VAIN has been studied less than that of CIN. Some suggest that 20% of cases of VAIN III may progress to invasive squamous carcinoma.

Invasive Carcinoma of the Vagina

Most cases of vaginal cancer represent spread from cervical cancers: primary carcinoma of the vagina is a rare lesion, representing only about 1% of gynaecological malignancies.

Some 95% of primary vaginal cancers are squamous in type and they occur most frequently in elderly women.

The site of predilection is the upper part of the vagina and there is debate as to whether the posterior or the anterior and lateral walls are more frequently involved.

The lesions are usually nodular and may be missed easily on vaginal examination during the early stages of development.

Table 39.20 Grading of Vaginal Intraepithelial Neoplasia

Grade	Proportion of thickness of epithelium involved
I	Lower third
II	Lower and middle thirds
III	Process extends into upper third or involves full thickness of epithelium

Microscopic Features

Most are well or moderately differentiated squamous carcinomas, although occasionally the tumours may be spindle-shaped, giving a false impression of a sarcomatous pattern.

Direct extension dominates the patterns of spread. The tumour may spread **laterally** to involve the paravaginal connective tissue, **upwards** to involve the bladder and **posteriorly** to involve the rectovaginal septum and rectum. Tumours in the lower part of the vagina may spread to involve inguinal lymph nodes; those situated higher in the vagina tend to involve the pelvic nodes. Spread via the bloodstream can occur but is a late event. If it does occur, the deposits are most commonly seen in the bones and lungs.

The International Federation of Gynaecology and Obstetrics (FIGO) system for staging vaginal cancers is shown in *Table 39.21*.

Adenocarcinoma of the Vagina

Five varieties of vaginal adenocarcinoma are described but only one of these, **clear cell adenocarcinoma**, is discussed here.

Clear cell adenocarcinoma is one of the very rare malignant tumours of the lower female genital tract occurring at a young age. The average age at diagnosis is 17 years. It is very rare before the age of 12 years and after 30 years of age. **In two-thirds of patients there is a history of the girl's mother having been treated in the early part of pregnancy with diethylstilboestrol.** As stated above there is a strong association with the presence of vaginal

Table 39.21 Staging of Vaginal Cancer according to the FIGO System

Stage	Extent of spread	5-year survival rate (%)
I	Tumour limited to the vaginal wall	70
II	Tumour involves subvaginal tissue but has not spread to pelvic wall	30–60
III	Tumour has extended to pelvic wall	24–35
IV	Tumour has extended beyond the true pelvis or involves the mucosa of the bladder or rectum	Virtually no 5-year survival

adenosis. Approximately 1 in 1000 girls exposed to the synthetic oestrogen *in utero* will develop this tumour.

Macroscopic Features

The tumour generally develops on the anterior wall of the vagina in its upper part. Its growth pattern tends to be exophytic and by the time of diagnosis it may be a bulky mass filling much of the vagina.

Microscopic Features

The lesions characteristically show tubules and cysts lined by clear cells, these spaces being admixed with more solid epithelial areas and with papillary structures. The individual tumour cells have abundant clear cytoplasm due to glycogen and some fat. Mucin is not present. Some of the cells have a 'hobnail' appearance with large nuclei and relatively little cytoplasm, projecting into the lumina of the glandular spaces.

Natural History

The prognosis is relatively good, provided the diagnosis is made when the tumour is still confined to the vagina. If extension has occurred, the survival rate falls steeply, as shown in *Table 39.22*.

Table 39.22 Survival of Patients with Clear Cell Adenocarcinoma of the Vagina

Stage	5-year survival rate (%)
I	80
II	17
III	few or no survivors
IV	few or no survivors

Embryonal Rhabdomyosarcoma (Sarcoma Botryoides)

This is a rare invasive tumour occurring in infants and young children. About 90% of the cases occur before the age of 5 years and 65% occur before the age of 2 years.

Macroscopic Features

The tumour arises from the anterior vaginal wall and consists of a conglomerate of several soft, polypoid masses, thought by some to resemble a bunch of grapes; hence the use of the word **botryoides** (grape-like).

Microscopic Features

The polypoid masses are covered by normal epithelium. The underlying tissue consists of a myxoid stroma in which round or spindle-shaped cells are present. A very characteristic feature is the tendency for the tumour cell to be concentrated in a dense layer under the surface epithelium.

Some cells have abundant granular cytoplasm, producing a racquet- or strap-like shape. The cytoplasm stains strongly with eosin. These features are thought to indicate differentiation towards rhabdomyoblasts.

Natural History

Sarcoma botryoides tends to invade locally and to recur after excision. Death is usually due to local extension within the pelvis.

The Fallopian Tube

NORMAL ANATOMY

The uterus is covered on its anterior and posterior aspects by a reflection of the pelvic peritoneum; this continues laterally on both sides to form the leaves of the broad ligaments, in which uterine blood vessels, efferent lymphatics draining the uterus and the **fallopian tubes** are situated.

The tubes are 11–12 cm long. They are hollow muscular structures lined by epithelium. The fallopian tube has four main anatomical divisions:

1) an **intramural segment** about 8 mm in length running within the uterine wall

2) a thick-walled narrow-calibre segment 2–3 cm in length, known as the **isthmic segment**

3) a thin-walled expanded area, known as the **ampulla**

4) a trumpet-shaped segment known as the **infundibulum**, the mouth of which opens on to the peritoneal cavity. This mouth is fringed by about 25 fimbriae, one of which is attached to the ovary. At the time of ovulation, the fimbriae sweep over the surface of the ovary, capturing the ovum.

The tubal epithelial lining is thrown into a series of folds (**plicae**), becoming more complex from the isthmus towards the infundibulum. It shows three cell types:

- **Ciliated cells**, which play an important part in ovum transport, are present in greatest numbers at the infundibular end; as one might expect, they increase in number at around the time of ovulation.

- **Secretory cells** are most prominent at the uterine end of the tube; their secretion contains amylase.

- **Intercalated cells**, the role of which is not clear.

INFLAMMATORY DISEASE OF THE TUBES

Acute Salpingitis

Most significant tubal inflammatory disorders are infective in origin. The main routes by which pathogenic organisms reach the tubes are:

- **by direct ascent from the vagina**, through the endocervix and uterine cavity, and then into the mural segment of the tube. Infections acquired via this route tend especially to produce mucosal inflammation; this type of reaction is known as **endosalpingitis**. It is the commonest variety of tubal inflammation. *Chlamydia trachomatis* is a frequently implicated organism and *Neisseria gonorrhoeae* remains another significant cause.
- **via the lymphatics** draining the cervix. The resulting inflammation affects principally the submucosal wall, and is known as **interstitial salpingitis**.

Macroscopic Features

In the early stages of endosalpingitis, as seen on laparoscopic examination, the tube is congested and oedematous. The mucosa, if it can be seen, is also swollen and hyperaemic.

Microscopic Features

There may be focal loss of tubal epithelium, the plicae tend to be adherent and the subepithelial tissues are infiltrated by an acute inflammatory cell infiltrate. Acute inflammatory cells admixed with amorphous debris and fibrin are present in the tubal lumen.

At a later stage, and in severe cases, inflammation spreads to the deeper parts of the wall as evidenced by fibrinous exudate on the external surface. This local serosal reaction may lead to adhesions between tube and ovary, and spread of inflammation to the ovary with the formation of a tubo-ovarian abscess. Leakage of pus from the fimbrial end of the tube may lead to generalized or localized intraperitoneal inflammation.

Obstruction of the fimbrial end may occur and the tube may become distended with pus (**pyosalpinx**).

Natural History

The outcome of acute salpingitis depends largely on the severity of the initial acute inflammation and the associated epithelial necrosis:

- If these are mild, more or less complete resolution can occur.
- If resolution does not occur, the inflammatory process becomes chronic and scarring takes place, because the acute inflammatory exudate is not demolished.
- Scarring may cause folds of epithelium to become densely adherent to each other; this produces a complicated multicystic lumen, exaggerated by continued secretion by the epithelium. This pattern has been termed **follicular salpingitis**.
- Follicular salpingitis is associated in some cases with diverticulum formation in the isthmic segment (**salpingitis isthmica nodosa**). Microscopic examination shows epithelium-lined channels within the tube wall, each surrounded by prominent bundles of smooth muscle. The risk of ectopic pregnancy is increased in both follicular salpingitis and salpingitis isthmica nodosa. Some suggest that salpingitis isthmica nodosa is not due to previous inflammation and may be the fallopian tube homologue of uterine adenomyosis.
- In some cases the tube is distended by watery fluid, the plicae flattened and the wall thinned and translucent (*Fig. 39.29*). This is known as **hydrosalpinx**. There is some doubt as to whether hydrosalpinx is a consequence of acute salpingitis because, in many instances, there is no antecedent history of pelvic inflammation.

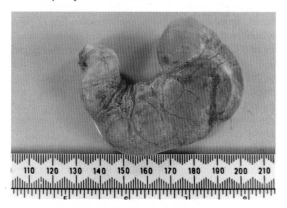

FIGURE 39.29 Hydrosalpinx. The fallopian tube is grossly distended by watery fluid.

Chronic Granulomatous Salpingitis

Granulomatous salpingitis occurs significantly only in geographical locations where chronic, infective, granulomatous disease is endemic. The two commonest and most important forms are **tuberculous** and **schistosomal** salpingitis. Both may cause sterility or increase the risk of tubal pregnancy.

Tuberculous Salpingitis

This arises secondary to tuberculosis elsewhere in the body. Infection is commonly haematogenous but may also occur via lymphatics draining a focus in the gastrointestinal tract.

About 20% of fatal cases of tuberculosis in women show tuberculous salpingitis and about half of these also have tuberculous endometritis.

In severe cases, the tubes are distorted and may be distended by caseous material. In less severe examples, the tubal wall shows nodular focal thickening and there may be tubo-ovarian adhesions.

In earlier stages the mucosa shows the presence of abundant epithelioid cell granulomata in which caseation is not necessarily present. The mucosal inflammatory process extends into the wall and the end result may be a tuberculous pyosalpinx in which the mucosa has been largely destroyed and the wall of the tube is lined by granulation tissue in which only a few recognizable granulomata may be seen. The damaged wall is often the seat of dystrophic calcification.

The presence of tuberculous salpingitis is often associated with a marked degree of epithelial hyperplasia, which must not be confused with adenocarcinoma of the tube, a distinction that is not always easy or straightforward. The most common gynaecological consequence of tuberculous salpingitis is sterility.

BENIGN CYSTS OF THE FALLOPIAN TUBES

Small translucent cysts of paramesonephric origin related to the fimbrial ends of the tubes are quite common. They are known as **hydatid cysts of Morgagni** and contain clear watery fluid (hence the use of the term hydatid). The cyst has a tubal type of epithelial lining, ciliated cells usually being prominent. Rarely, the tubes may become twisted and produce quite severe abdominal pain; for the most part the cysts remain asymptomatic.

Occasionally, small inclusion cysts derived from the serosal covering of the tube may undergo transitional cell metaplasia. These are known as **cystic Walthard cell nests** and appear as minute white nodules on the serosal surface of the tube. They are entirely without significance.

TUMOURS AND TUMOUR-LIKE LESIONS OF THE FALLOPIAN TUBE

Benign Neoplasms

Benign tubal neoplasms are very rare. The commonest is the mesothelium-derived **adenomatoid tumour**. Adenomatoid tumour of the tube is the homologue of the tumour of the same name that is found in the epididymis (see p 734). It is usually quite small (1–2 cm in diameter) and is situated on the serosal surface of the tube, where it appears as a firm yellowish-white nodule.

The next most common benign tumour is the **leiomyoma**, although this lesion occurs far less frequently in this site than it does in the myometrium of the uterus.

Malignant Neoplasms

Primary malignant tumours of the tube are also rare, accounting for only 0.3% of gynaecological malignan-

cies. They are almost exclusively adenocarcinomas. Their cause is unknown, although they do tend to occur somewhat more frequently in nulliparous women or in women who have had only one child than in multiparous women. These tumours tend to be found in women aged 40–60 years, the peak incidence being in the early fifties.

The clinical presentation consists of one or more of:
- cramp-like attacks of pain in the iliac fossa
- abnormal vaginal bleeding
- a vaginal discharge, which, on occasions may be profuse

Macroscopic Features

By the time exploration is undertaken, growth of tumour within the tubal lumen is usually extensive and the lumen is distended by greyish-white, friable tumour tissue.

Microscopic Features

In most cases the tumour is a well-differentiated papillary adenocarcinoma. The appearances closely mimic those of a serous carcinoma of the ovary.

Spread may occur **directly**:
- through the fimbrial ostium to involve peritoneum or ovary
- through the uterine ostium into the uterus
- through the tube wall to involve neighbouring structures

or **via lymphatics** to the:
- iliac, lumbar and para-aortic nodes.

Staging

The (FIGO) staging system with survival rates, is shown in *Table 39.23*.

Table 39.23 Staging of Malignant Tumours of the Fallopian Tubes according to the FIGO System, with Survival Rates

Stage	5-year survival rate (%)	Extent of spread
I	> 50	Tumour confined to the tube; no penetration of serosa
II	16	Tumour involves the serosal surface of the tube
III	10	Involvement of the ovary or uterus
IV	< 10	Extension of the tumour to involve extragenital structures

The overall survival rate is only about 25%, probably reflecting late diagnosis rather than inherent aggressiveness.

Disorders Associated with Pregnancy

ECTOPIC PREGNANCY

In ectopic pregnancy, implantation of the fertilized ovum takes place in a site other than the uterine cavity. It is not uncommon, occurring in about 1% of all recognized pregnancies. In most ectopic sites, an adequate environment for the continued growth of the embryo cannot develop. Thus, with few exceptions, **ectopic pregnancies are non-viable**.

Some 95% of all ectopic pregnancies occur in the fallopian tube. Other rarer sites for ectopic implantation include ovary, peritoneal cavity, broad ligament and abnormal intrauterine sites such as the cervix or myometrium.

Aetiology
For normal intrauterine implantation to occur, **the fertilized embryo must arrive in the uterine cavity at the optimal time for implantation**. Any factor or combination of factors delaying this arrival increases the risk of tubal implantation. Normal tubal transport depends on:
- **a normal fallopian tube lumen**
- **normal ciliary activity by the tubal epithelium**
- **normal smooth muscle function in the tubal wall**

These are disturbed in several tubal disorders, of which **the commonest by far is postinfective, chronic, non-specific salpingitis**. In this disorder, transport is impaired by loss of ciliary activity and damage to smooth muscle. Other tubal conditions causing impaired transport of the fertilized ovum are:
- congenital deformities
- deformities following failed reconstructive surgery or failed tubal sterilization
- certain specific chronic inflammatory disorders such as tuberculosis or schistosomiasis (see pp 157–165)
- salpingitis isthmica nodosa (see p 793)

Functional transport failures may also occur in women on low-dose progestogen-only contraceptives.

Local tubal pathology accounts for 35–50% of tubal pregnancies. In the remainder, the tube appears normal. It is suggested that tubal implantation in these cases is due to delayed ovulation. By the time the fertilized ovum reaches the uterus, the concentration of human chorionic gonadotrophin (hCG) produced by the conceptus is insufficient to prevent corpus luteum decay, and thus menstruation occurs. This can lead to the fertilized ovum being swept back by refluxing menstrual blood into the tube, where it then implants.

Failure of tubal pregnancy is due to:
- inability of the tubal wall to develop an adequate decidua
- the thinness of the tube wall
- the relative non-distensibility of the tube wall

Rupture occurs in at least 50% of tubal pregnancies. This is an acute event associated with life-threatening intra-abdominal haemorrhage (*Fig. 39.30*). It presents with severe abdominal pain and a sharp fall in blood pressure. The pregnancy may also end as a result of:
- complete or partial separation of placenta with the formation of a large haematoma in which portions of decidua and/or occasional chorionic villi may be seen
- abortion into either the uterine or peritoneal cavity

Early diagnosis is highly desirable because, although tubal pregnancies can be treated effectively by surgery, this usually involves sacrifice of the affected tube. If diagnosis is established before tubal rupture has occurred, the conceptus can be removed by laparoscopic salpingostomy.

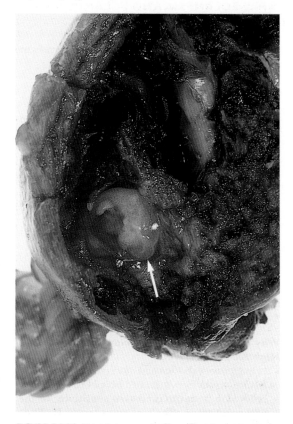

FIGURE 39.30 *Ectopic pregnancy. The affected tube is grossly distended and shows the presence of abundant blood clot. The intratubal embryo (arrowed) is easily seen.*

Successful early diagnosis depends, in the first instance, on defining the group at risk. This includes **patients with a history of pelvic inflammatory disease, tubal disease, tubal surgery or previous ectopic pregnancy**.

In early pregnancy women at risk should be screened by measuring their serum progesterone concentrations, as these reflect the activity of a corpus luteum stimulated by a viable pregnancy:

- A serum progesterone level of 79.5 nmol/l or greater indicates a viable pregnancy with a sensitivity of 97.5%.
- A serum progesterone level of 15.9 nmol/l or less indicates a non-viable pregnancy in 100% of cases.

In a non-viable pregnancy the distinction between a spontaneous abortion and an ectopic pregnancy must be made, either by transvaginal ultrasonography and/or diagnostic uterine curettage. **The presence of chorionic villi in curettings excludes ectopic pregnancy.** If chorionic villi are absent, the β-hCG level should be monitored. If β-hCG levels do not fall within 12–15 hours of curettage, then trophoblastic tissue and, by implication, ectopic pregnancy must exist.

PRE-ECLAMPSIA AND ECLAMPSIA (TOXAEMIA OF PREGNANCY)

Pre-eclampsia is a pregnancy-dependent syndrome characterized by:

- hypertension
- proteinuria
- oedema

It is more common in first than in subsequent pregnancies, clinical presentation usually occurring in the third trimester. It appears to be trophoblast rather than embryo-dependent because it can occur in association with **hydatiform mole, in which no fetus is present**.

Pre-eclampsia may terminate in a life-threatening syndrome known as **eclampsia**, which includes:

- convulsions
- cerebral oedema
- cerebral haemorrhage
- pulmonary and laryngeal oedema
- disseminated intravascular coagulation
- renal cortical necrosis
- retinal detachment

Why do Women with Pre-eclampsia Develop High Blood Pressure?

- Hypertension, the first and most characteristic feature, results from increased peripheral resistance, believed to be due to **increased sensitivity to the vasoconstrictor effects of angiotensin II. The increased response to angiotensin II** is thought to result from decreased placental prostaglandin secretion.

- Decreased prostaglandin secretion is thought to be due to placental ischaemia.
- Placental ischaemia may be caused by changes in the intramyometrial portions of the **spiral arteries**, the end-arteries supplying the placental intervillous space.
- Two principal changes occur in the spiral arteries in pre-eclampsia:
  1) **failure of placental trophoblastic cells to infiltrate the walls of spiral arteries during placentation.** This infiltration normally occurs between 8 and 18 weeks of pregnancy and is believed to be an essential step for spiral artery dilatation to accommodate the increased blood flow from uterus to placenta in the second half of pregnancy.
  2) **accumulation of lipid-laden macrophages associated with fibrin and platelets in both the walls and lumina of the spiral arteries** (acute atherosis), which can partially or completely block the affected portions of the spiral arteries. It bears a strong morphological resemblance to the arterial lesions seen during rejection of renal transplants.

Systemic Changes in Pre-eclampsia and Eclampsia

Many maternal tissues can be affected and the fetus may show growth retardation and die *in utero* or perinatally.

Maternal tissues principally affected include the liver, kidneys and central nervous system

The Liver

Macroscopic Features

The appearances are striking: the liver is pale yellow owing to fatty change and numerous focal haemorrhages stand out against the pale background.

Microscopic Features

The earliest change is fibrin deposition in the sinusoids, especially in zone 1 (the periportal region). Haemorrhages may occur here, and differing grades of ischaemic damage, ranging from severe fatty change to extensive infarction, may be seen.

The haemorrhages arise from small portal tract vessels, which usually contain small fibrin thrombi.

The patients may complain of epigastric pain and vomiting and, in very severe cases, jaundice and hepatic encephalopathy can occur.

Liver damage is likely to be associated with disseminated intravascular coagulation and, in some instances, microangiopathic haemolysis may also be present (see pp 695–696). This triad has been termed the **HELLP** syndrome: *H*aemolysis, *E*levated *L*iver enzymes, *L*ow *P*latelet count.

Kidneys

Macroscopic Features
In the fortunately rare fatal cases, the kidneys show the presence of subcapsular petechial haemorrhages and a pale, yellowish cortex.

Microscopic Features
Glomeruli appear swollen and bloodless; this is attributed to endothelial cell swelling and to an increase in the volume of the mesangium. Electron microscopy shows:
- marked swelling of the cytoplasm of the glomerular endothelial cells (so-called endotheliosis)
- an amorphous deposit, part of which is fibrin, between the endothelial cells and the basement membrane
- an increase in mesangial cells, which contributes to narrowing of the glomerular capillaries

These changes regress, in many cases, after pregnancy ends. If eclampsia supervenes, acute renal failure arising from renal cortical necrosis or acute tubular necrosis may occur (see pp 693–694).

Central Nervous System
Involvement of the nervous system in eclampsia is heralded by the onset of convulsions.

Microscopic Features
Changes seen in the brain in fatal cases consist of:
- arteriolar thrombosis
- arteriolar fibrinoid necrosis
- petechial haemorrhages
- diffuse microinfarcts

Placental Changes in Pre-eclampsia

Macroscopic Features
The placenta is smaller than normal, although this decrease in size is not marked. Placental infarction is increased significantly in incidence and in extent. Evidence of retroplacental haematoma is also found more frequently than normal.

Microscopic Features
On microscopic examination, the chief features are:
- increased thickness of the trophoblast basement membrane
- proliferation of cells of the cytotrophoblast
- villi that are smaller than normal and rather poorly vascularized; these may show the presence of syncytial knots (multinucleated protrusions from the villus surface)

All these changes are regarded as being due to underperfusion of the placenta as a result of abnormalities in the uteroplacental circulation.

TROPHOBLASTIC DISEASE

The term trophoblastic disease encompasses several entities:
- hydatidiform mole (complete or partial)
- invasive mole
- choriocarcinoma
- placental site trophoblastic tumour
- persistent trophoblastic disease. This term is used in certain circumstances. Strictly, it is defined as the situation that obtains when, after a mole has been removed from the uterus, serum hCG levels remain raised or increase further. It does not imply the existence of any specific histopathological entity and may be the expression of:
  1) an exuberant placental site reaction
  2) invasive mole
  3) choriocarcinoma

Hydatidiform Mole
This curious term is derived from the Greek word *hydatis* (a drop of water) and the Latin word *mola* (a mass). It derives from the outstanding macroscopic feature: **grape-like clusters of swollen, watery chorionic villi** (*Fig. 39.31*). Hydatidiform moles are classified as being either **complete** or **incomplete**.

The **defining criteria of complete mole** (*Fig. 39.32*) **are:**
- an abnormal conceptus **without an embryo**. This is due to fertilization of an ovum lacking a nucleus
- gross, hydropic swelling of the placental villi
- proliferation of the trophoblast; both cytotrophoblast and syncytiotrophoblast are involved

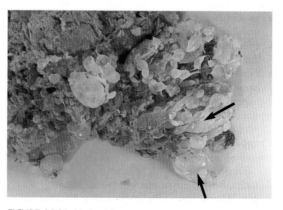

FIGURE 39.31 *Hydatidiform mole showing typical grape-like structures (arrowed).*

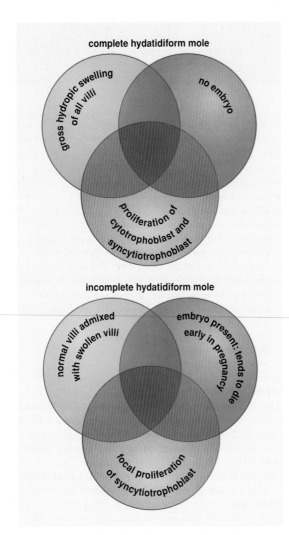

complete hydatidiform mole

gross hydropic swelling of all villi

no embryo

proliferation of cytotrophoblast and syncytiotrophoblast

incomplete hydatidiform mole

normal villi admixed with swollen villi

embryo present: tends to die early in pregnancy

focal proliferation of syncytiotrophoblast

FIGURE 39.32 Characteristics of complete and incomplete hydatidiform mole.

An incomplete mole (*Fig. 39.32*) **shows:**
- an abnormal conceptus with an embryo that tends to die early
- a placenta in which focal villous swelling occurs, the abnormal villi being admixed with normal ones
- a degree of trophoblastic hyperplasia which usually involves the syncytiotrophoblast and in which the hyperplasia affects the villi focally rather than in a circumferential pattern

Complete Mole

The condition occurs in about 1 in 1500 pregnancies in the UK and USA. In parts of Asia, Africa and Latin America, for unknown reasons, the incidence is much higher. Women under 20 years or over 40 years old at the time of pregnancy are at greater risk of hydatidiform mole.

The Origin of Complete Mole

Complete mole arises from the fertilization of an ovum from which the nucleus has been lost or inactivated. In 90% of cases the karyotype is 46XX, both X chromosomes being paternal in origin. The presence of the two X chromosomes is the result of duplication of a haploid sperm; such a mole is termed monospermic or homozygous. In the remaining cases, the karyotype is 46XY. This results from the fertilization of an 'empty' ovum by two haploid sperm which fuse and reduplicate. These moles are termed dispermic or heterozygous.

Macroscopic Features

The appearances of complete mole are characteristic, the uterine cavity being filled by a mass of grape-like vesicular villi. The volume of this mass is much greater than that of a normal placenta of the same gestational age; there is no recognizable normal placenta.

Microscopic Features

The outstanding feature is distension of individual villi, the entire villous population being involved to a greater or lesser extent. The swollen villi are usually rounded and often have central cavities. Fetal vessels within the abnormal villi are generally absent.

Trophoblastic hyperplasia is the defining histological criterion for the diagnosis of complete mole. Most villi are affected and hyperplasia involving the whole villous circumference is very characteristic. Some atypia of the trophoblast is often present but this does not usually exceed that seen in the first trimester of pregnancy.

Clinical Presentation and Natural History

Most cases are diagnosed between the 8th and 24th week of pregnancy, the peak time being at about the 14th week. The commonest presenting feature is vaginal bleeding and, in many cases, molar tissue may be present admixed with the blood. On examination, the uterus appears 'large for dates' in about 50% of cases.

The hyperplastic trophoblast of the mole secretes large amounts of hCG, with two interesting side-effects:
- Bilateral ovarian theca lutein cysts may be present in many cases. The cysts may be associated with abdominal pain due to rupture or torsion, and generally take a few months to resolve after the mole has been evacuated.
- Because hCG has a mild thyroid-stimulating effect, evidence of hyperthyroidism may occasionally be present.

About 10% of cases will develop persistent trophoblastic disease and 3–5% will develop choriocarcinoma. This degree of risk for subsequent choriocarcinoma, although not great in absolute terms, is estimated to be about 1000-fold greater than is the case for a woman who has just completed a normal pregnancy. Follow-up is essential for women who have had a molar pregnancy in order to detect cases of invasive mole or choriocarcinoma, because such women require chemotherapy.

This follow-up depends on measurement of the concentration of hCG in serum or urine, and should be rigorous. Measurements should be continued for at least 6 months after hCG has become undetectable in the serum, and further pregnancy should not be started until hCG has been undetectable for 6 months.

Incomplete (Partial) Mole

Macroscopic Features
In the formation of a partial mole, only some of the placental villi are affected and thus the macroscopic appearances are of an essentially normal placenta of normal size for the period of gestation, in which scattered swollen villi are present.

Microscopic Features
Vesicular villi are seen to be admixed with normal ones. The affected villi tend to be smaller than those of complete mole and often have an irregular indented shape, rather than the rounded shape characteristic of complete mole.

A degree of trophoblastic proliferation is always present but, again, this is less marked than in complete mole and is focal rather than circumferential.

Most partial moles have a triploid karyotype, 69XXY being the commonest. Triploidy *per se* is not always associated with partial mole formation and it has been suggested that, if the extra chromosome is derived from the father, then partial mole formation will result.

Natural History
Persistent trophoblastic disease follows partial mole as frequently as complete mole, and these patients should be followed in the same way. There is, however, *no* increased risk of choriocarcinoma.

Invasive Hydatidiform Mole
The defining criterion is penetration into the myometrium and its blood vessels by abnormal villi of either complete or partial hydatidiform mole.

Invasive moles call attention to themselves usually some weeks after a mole has been evacuated, the commonest presenting features being vaginal bleeding or a brownish vaginal discharge. The degree of invasion varies greatly: some lesions are associated with large, deeply penetrating and haemorrhagic cavities within the myometrium, whereas others are inconspicuous.

Histological diagnosis depends on finding abnormal, molar villi within the myometrium or its blood vessels and, thus, on having a hysterectomy specimen to examine. Before the introduction of effective chemotherapy for persistent trophoblastic disease, invasive moles could cause death, as a result of either perforation of the uterus or torrential uterine haemorrhage. Invasive mole is currently treated as persistent trophoblastic disease and a tissue diagnosis is no longer made or required.

The abnormal molar tissue may be transported within the bloodstream and impact within certain small blood vessels, most notably in the lungs and vagina. These impacted trophoblastic emboli may then grow in the same way as do emboli derived from malignant neoplasms, presenting in the vagina as haemorrhagic nodules. Their origin is revealed on histological examination, when **abnormal placental villi** are found; this observation totally rules out a diagnosis of choriocarcinoma. The lung lesions may be asymptomatic or may, in some instances, cause haemoptysis.

Choriocarcinoma

Definition
Choriocarcinoma is a highly malignant neoplasm that is composed **entirely** of syncytiotrophoblast and cytotrophoblast; **the presence of placental villi excludes the diagnosis**.

Epidemiology
In Western countries, choriocarcinoma is uncommon, with an incidence of about 1 in 50 000 gestations. Its associations with different types of pregnancy are shown in *Table 39.24*.

The length of time between the pregnancy and clinical presentation of the tumour varies considerably, ranging from a few weeks or months to as long as 15 years, but the majority occur within 1 year of gestation.

Table 39.24 Association of Choriocarcinoma with Different Types of Pregnancy

Type of preceding gestation	Percentage
Molar pregnancy	50
Spontaneous abortion	30
Normal pregnancy	20

Macroscopic Features
Choriocarcinoma appears as single or multiple, soft, dark red, rounded, haemorrhagic nodules.

Microscopic Features

The tumour consists of clusters of cytotrophoblastic cells covered by a peripheral rim of syncytiotrophoblast. The degree of atypia and mitotic activity do not, in general, exceed that of a normal implanting blastocyst. **No villi are present.** Haemorrhage and necrosis are prominent features but have no particular diagnostic significance.

Microscopic grading is of little value but it is noteworthy that there appears to be an improved prognosis in tumours that have an intense lymphocytic infiltrate at the interface between tumour cells and stroma.

Malignant trophoblastic cells show a marked propensity to invade blood vessels; this explains the fact that spread occurs predominantly via the bloodstream. The principal targets for metastases are the lungs, liver, brain, kidneys and gut, but virtually any tissue may be the site of secondary deposits.

Effects of hCG Secretion by Malignant Trophoblast

Choriocarcinoma secretes large amounts of hCG, leading to morphological and functional changes in different tissues (*Fig. 39.33*):
- endometrial gland hyperplasia
- a decidual reaction in the endometrium and in ectopic sites
- bilateral ovarian enlargement as a result of the formation of theca lutein cysts
- hyperplasia of breast lobules

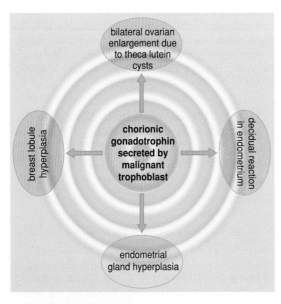

FIGURE 39.33 *Effects of human chorionic gonadotrophin (hCG) secretion by malignant trophoblastic cells.*

Natural History

Formerly, choriocarcinoma was regarded, quite correctly, as one of the most malignant and aggressive neoplasms. Survival rates before the introduction of chemotherapy ranged from 10 to 20% and, in many patients, death occurred in months rather than years. This bleak outlook has been transformed by the introduction of appropriate and effective chemotherapy and, in those in whom the disease is confined to the uterus, the survival rate approaches 100%. In patients with metastatic disease at the time of diagnosis, the survival rate falls to about 80%.

Factors associated with a worse prognosis include:
- age greater than 39 years at the time of diagnosis
- a longer interval between the antecedent pregnancy and the time of starting treatment
- high concentrations of hCG in the serum
- increasing tumour size (the larger the tumour, the worse the prognosis)
- the site of metastases, those in the brain carrying the worst prognosis
- the number of metastases, patients with more than eight having the worst outlook for survival
- the patient having had previous chemotherapy

On the basis of these criteria, patients may be stratified into **high**, **middle** and **low** risk groups. The prognostic implications of such stratification are shown in *Table 39.25.*

The drugs that are most effective against trophoblastic tumours are methotrexate, actinomycin D and etoposide. In low-risk patients, single drug regimens, usually employing methotrexate, are effective. In high-risk patients, multiagent regimens are needed if the patients are to be rescued.

Table 39.25 Mortality of Patients with Choriocarcinoma according to Risk Group

Risk group	Mortality rate (5 years) (%)
High	47
Middle	1.3
Low	0.25

Placental Site Trophoblastic Tumour

This is a rare lesion; for every 100 cases of invasive mole or of choriocarcinoma only one of these tumours is seen. Most occur after a normal full-term pregnancy, although a very small proportion (5%) follow a pregnancy associated with hydatidiform mole formation. The tumour arises from the extravillous trophoblastic cells of the placental bed.

The clinical presentation is varied. Some patients present with amenorrhoea and, because the uterus is enlarged and about one-third of patients have a positive pregnancy test, it is not surprising that an incorrect diagnosis of pregnancy may be made. Other patients present with irregular vaginal bleeding.

Macroscopic Features
The tumour presents as a mass within the myometrium which may project into the uterine cavity in some instances.

Microscopic Features
There is infiltration of the myometrium by cytotrophoblastic cells together with multinucleated cells resembling those seen at the normal implantation site. The two-layered structure of a choriocarcinoma in which clumps of cytotrophoblastic cells are covered by syncytiotrophoblast is not seen. Similarly, although myometrial invasion is a feature, the haemorrhage and necrosis that tend to occur in association with choriocarcinoma are not present.

In biopsy material, the distinction between an exuberant placental site reaction and a placental site trophoblastic tumour is not easy. Even when a confident diagnosis of the latter has been made, the assessment as to whether the lesion is likely to behave in a malignant fashion or not is difficult. Some 10–15% of placental site trophoblastic tumours are aggressive. A high mitotic count suggests malignancy but a low one is no guarantee of benign behaviour.

Natural History
Unlike choriocarcinoma or invasive mole, placental site trophoblastic tumour does not respond well to chemotherapy. Progress after surgery may be monitored by regular measurement of the principal tumour cell product, **placental lactogenic hormone**, which is normally produced by extravillous trophoblast.

The Breast

Among disease-prone organs, the breast is unique because it is affected by only one life-threatening disease: **cancer**, which, in the UK, kills 28 per 100 000 women annually. Thus, the material in this section relates mainly to cancer and, to a lesser extent, those conditions believed to increase the risk of subsequent cancer or, clinically, to mimic cancer.

The breast is no exception to the general principle that pathology is best understood in the context of normal anatomy and physiology. The latter includes profound changes, partly related to ageing and partly to cyclical hormonal influences associated with the menstrual cycle and pregnancy, during which the breast is prepared for its functional role of **lactation**.

NORMAL ANATOMY

The breast is often described as a modified sweat gland, but this laconic term fails to communicate the complexities of breast structure outlined below (*Fig. 39.34*).

Breast Lobules
The functional unit of the breast is the terminal duct lobular unit (*Fig. 39.35*). This consists of a number of small luminated structures called acini, encased in a sheath of loose connective tissue lacking elastic fibres. These acini, of which there are about 30 in each lobule at the menarche, drain into a duct (the intralobular portion of the terminal duct), which passes across the border of the lobular connective tissue to become the extralobular portion of the terminal duct. In the resting state the units measure about 1 mm in diameter and there are thousands of them in the female breast. The terminal duct lobular unit is the principal site for important pathological conditions in the breast (*Fig. 39.36*) including:
- so-called 'fibrocystic change'
- epithelial hyperplasia
- most carcinomas

Both acini and terminal ducts are lined by a double cell layer. The inner layer is composed of secretory epithelium beneath which lie **myoepithelial cells** containing contractile protein filaments (actin). The function of myoepithelial cells is to squeeze acinar secretions into the duct system (*Fig. 39.37*).

The Extralobular Duct System
The **extralobular terminal duct** joins up with others in the same region to form a **subsegmental duct**. These then join to form **segmental ducts**, of which there are about 20, draining into large **lactiferous ducts** that exit at the nipple. The lactiferous ducts show segmental dilatation just below the nipple; these segments are known as **collecting sinuses**, in which milk is held before suckling. The connective tissue in which the ducts are embedded is denser than the delicate intralobular connective tissue and contains elastic fibres running alongside the ducts. The extralobular duct system is the seat of:
- most solitary large papillomas
- duct ectasia (abnormal duct dilatation often associated with the presence of inspissated secretions)

BREAST DEVELOPMENT

The breast develops from the milk streaks; bilateral ridges appear between the upper and lower limb buds at about the sixth week of fetal life. Localized thickenings appear along these ridges, from which the nipples develop. The remainder of the milk streaks atrophy. Cords of cells

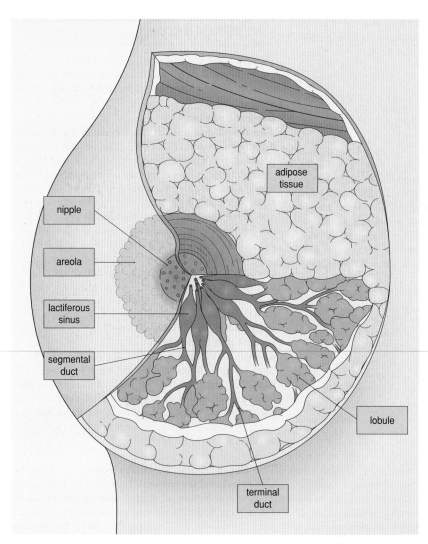

FIGURE 39.34 General structure of the breast.

grow downwards from the basal layer of these epithelial thickenings and each bud of cells acquires a lumen and constitutes part of the first generation of the breast ducts.

In the prepubertal stage, the ducts elongate and branch, a process greatly enhanced by puberty and the onset of the menarche. It is at this time that the terminal duct lobular unit forms. There is coincident growth of the periductal connective tissue sheaths and a marked increase in adipose tissue, which makes up most of the bulk of the breast. The adult breast undergoes cyclical hormonal changes, described in *Table 39.26*.

INFLAMMATORY DISORDERS

Mammary Ectasia
This affects extralobular ducts and is characterized by **abnormal duct dilatation**.

Macroscopic Features
Excised areas of mammary duct ectasia show the presence of dilated spaces filled with whitish material, probably derived from inspissated colostrum.

Microscopic Features
Microscopic examination confirms the presence of obstruction and periductal inflammation and scarring. **There is no hyperplasia of the duct-lining epithelium and the condition has no implications whatever for the future development of carcinoma.**

Clinically, severe ectasia may give rise to suspicions of cancer because the scarring associated with the periductal inflammation may cause retraction or inversion of the nipple; about one in five of patients com-

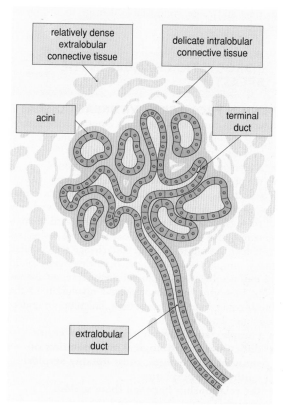

FIGURE 39.35 *The terminal duct lobule surrounded by a sheath of delicate connective tissue.*

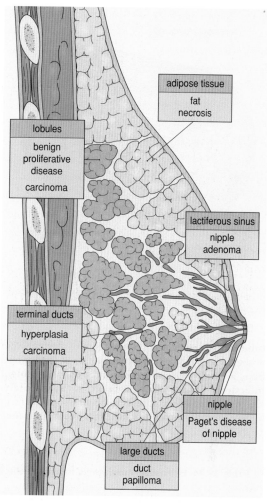

FIGURE 39.36 *Sites of origin within the breast for different pathological processes.*

plain of nipple discharge. Dystrophic calcification may be seen on mammography as linear opacities outlining the walls of the affected ducts. Some disagreement exists as to the peak age of presentation, with some authorities maintaining that it is a disorder found chiefly in premenopausal parous women, whereas others state that it is most common in the postmenopausal period.

Fat Necrosis

True fat necrosis affects subcutaneous adipose tissue rather than breast tissue itself. It presents clinically as a discrete lump in the breast.

Trauma is the likeliest cause, although a definite history of such trauma is obtained in only about half the cases. A few cases are associated with therapeutic radiation of the breast, and fat necrosis may also occur occasionally as part of Weber–Christian disease, an inflammatory condition affecting adipose tissue.

The process starts with rupture of the fat cell plasma membranes and discharge of their contents into the extracellular milieu. This elicits a macrophage response: the macrophages engulf large amounts of lipid and thus acquire a foamy appearance. Fusion of macrophages to form foreign-body giant cells may occur. The injury elicits a chronic inflammatory reaction, which, like other non-specific inflammatory reactions, is characterized by attempts at healing in the form of scarring.

The cut surface of an area of fat necrosis is usually an orange colour owing to the deposition of iron pigment released from red blood cells at the time of trauma. It feels firm but droplets of liquid fat may ooze from the surface and this makes the preparation of frozen sections of good quality rather difficult.

Breast Abscess

This is most common during lactation and results from rupture of one of the mammary ducts and subsequent infection. The lesion consists of a central pus-filled cavity, surrounded by a zone of inflamed breast tissue, which ultimately becomes scarred.

Granulomatous Inflammation

A variety of granulomatous lesions may occur in the breast but all are rare. The most important clinically is

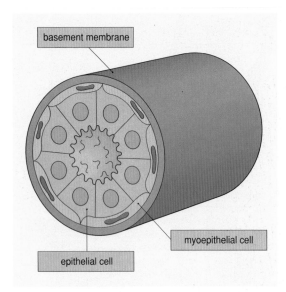

FIGURE 39.37 Structure of terminal ducts characterized by a double cell lining.

tuberculosis, which may be the result of dissemination of the organisms via the bloodstream or of local spread from a nearby lesion. **Actinomycosis and fungal infections** may also affect the breast, as can **sarcoidosis**. In addition, there appears to be an idiopathic form of granulomatous mastitis which may recur from time to time and cause considerable damage to the breast tissue.

FIBROCYSTIC CHANGES IN THE BREAST

BENIGN PROLIFERATIVE BREAST DISEASE
Fibrocystic changes in the breast constitute the pathological correlate of clinical syndromes that include:
- cyclical pain in the breast
- nodularity of the breast tissue on palpation
- the presence of discrete well-defined lumps

These changes are also found at post-mortem examination in many women who have *not* presented with any of these clinical features; some workers regard them as so common as to be within the spectrum of normality.

Under the rubric of fibrocystic change are classified many morphological changes, occurring singly or in various combinations. Many of them represent aberrations in normal development and involution of the breast tissue, but they still present difficulties in understanding, which relate to:
- **complex and inappropriate nomenclature**
- **difficulties in histological interpretation of some of the changes, most notably atypical epithelial hyperplasias**
- **the relationship between these various morphological changes and the risk of subsequent development of cancer**

Table 39.26 Hormone-mediated Changes in the Breast

Physiological state	Changes
Menstrual cycle	**Both epithelium and lobular stroma are affected:** • During the secretory phase of the cycle following ovulation, the stroma becomes oedematous; this reaches a peak a few days before the commencement of menstrual bleeding. • Ductal and ductular cells proliferate from early in the proliferative phase of the cycle, whereas the terminal duct lobular unit structures proliferate late in the secretory cycle. • When the plasma concentrations of oestrogen and progesterone fall at the time of menstruation, programmed cell death or apoptosis affects the proliferated epithelial cells and there is desquamation of the apoptotic bodies from the duct, ductular and acinar linings.
Pregnancy	During pregnancy the number of acini in each lobule increases markedly and the size of each lobule increases. The secretory glands become lined by cuboidal epithelium and, in the later stages of pregnancy, show the presence of secretory granules consisting of both lipid and proteins (most notably casein). Oestrogen, progesterone and prolactin all influence these breast changes but once delivery has occurred it is prolactin that plays the major role in initiating and maintaining lactation.
Involution	When lactation ceases, the secretory acini and ducts atrophy. With the menopause, still further atrophy takes place, the intralobular acini being particularly affected. Basement membranes thicken and the intralobular myxoid stroma becomes condensed.

Microscopic Features

The changes, all of which affect the terminal duct lobular unit, include (*Figs 39.38* and *39.39*):

- **fibrosis**, involving both intralobular and interlobular stroma
- **adenosis** (an increase in the number and size of glandular elements in the breast)
- **cyst** formation
- **papilloma** formation
- **apocrine metaplasia** of lining epithelium
- **sclerosing adenosis**
- **fibroadenomatoid hyperplasia and fibroadenoma** formation
- **epithelial hyperplasia**. This is divided into two classes – **'usual'** and **atypical** – and two cytological types – **ductal** and **lobular** hyperplasia. The distinction between usual and atypical variants is clinically significant because **atypical hyperplasia, unlike the seven other morphological changes listed above, is associated with an increased risk of subsequent breast cancer four to five times that in the general female population.**

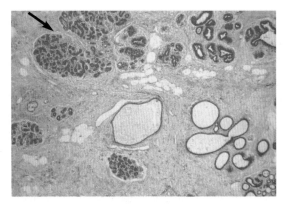

FIGURE 39.38 *Hyperplastic changes in the breast showing cystic dilatation of some ducts and adenosis (arrowed).*

Fibrosis

Fibrosis of the extralobular stroma is common. It may be a reaction to rupture of cysts, but this is probably an oversimplification. Hyperplasia of the delicate, rather myxoid, stroma of the lobule itself is also quite frequent, especially in the involuting postmenopausal breast. It may occur also in association with an increase in the number of acinar structures, producing the appearance known as **sclerosing adenosis**.

Cyst Formation

Cyst formation is probably due to duct obstruction. The cysts differ in size from microscopic to macroscopic (1–5 cm in diameter). They usually contain cloudy yellow fluid, but sometimes this is much darker because of previous haemorrhage. Some of the larger cysts appear bluish when intact ('Bloodgood's blue-domed cysts').

Microscopically, large cysts are lined by a single layer of flattened epithelium, but in some instances no epithelial lining can be seen.

Adenosis ('Blunt Duct Adenosis')

If this term is not qualified by any other description, it refers to a condition in which there is **an increase in**

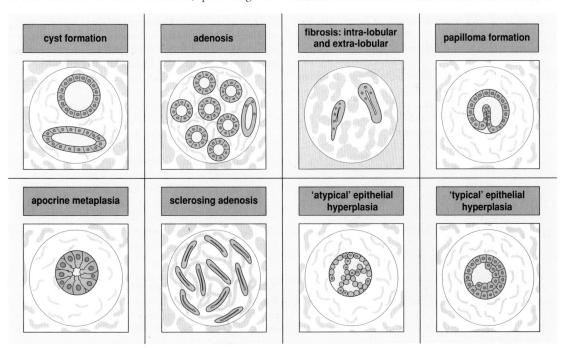

FIGURE 39.39 *Spectrum of morphological changes in fibrocystic disease of the breast.*

the number of acini within individual lobules with some resulting enlargement of the lobule. In pure adenosis, there is no proliferation of the epithelial lining of the affected acini.

Sclerosing Adenosis

This is the morphological appearance that results from a **combination of an increase in the number of intralobular acini and intralobular fibrosis** (*Fig. 39.40*), the latter causing marked distortion of the acini. Many believe that it has no particular clinical significance but there are some data suggesting an increase in cancer risk. The most important diagnostic feature of sclerosing adenosis on microscopy is best seen at low magnifications. It is the **preservation of a normal lobular pattern in the affected portion of breast tissue.** The acini, which are compressed by fibrous tissue, appear elongated and distorted but still preserve the normal two-layered pattern of epithelial and myoepithelial cells. The myoepithelial cells tend to proliferate to a greater extent than the secretory epithelium. Occasionally, the compressed and distorted acini may be seen within perineural spaces and this appearance must not be interpreted as malignancy. Other lesions exist in which there is both sclerosis and proliferation of epithelial structure (see below).

Microglandular Adenosis

This is a rare form of adenosis in which the proliferated acini are not distributed within the lobules but appear instead either within the extralobular connective tissue or in the adipose tissue. The acini are lined, in most instances by only one layer of cells, the myoepithelial cells being absent. At present there is no convincing evidence that this type of adenosis is associated with an increased risk of cancer. Its chief importance is that it may be mistaken on histological examination for a well-differentiated tubular carcinoma.

Radial Scars and Complex Sclerosing Lesions

These two names refer essentially to the same process. Many reserve the term **radial scar** for lesions that are 10 mm or less in diameter and call lesions larger than this **complex sclerosing lesions**.

These lesions show the general features of:

- a stellate shape
- a central fibrous area in which elastic fibres may also be present
- a variable degree of epithelial distortion and proliferation

These sclerosing lesions are usually found in association with other features of benign proliferative breast conditions. The small ductal spaces that are present within the fibrosed area have a normal two-layer cell lining and must not be mistaken for tubular carcinoma. Most believe that these sclerosing lesions do not increase the risk of breast cancer.

Apocrine Metaplasia

This is a common appearance, seen most often in cysts but which can occur in normal-sized ducts and ductules as well. **The cells lining the lumina are tall and columnar with granular, very pink, cytoplasm and a typical apical 'snout'. This is identical with the appearance of the lining epithelium of apocrine sweat glands, such as those in the axilla.** The mechanism underlying this change is not known. There is no increased risk of developing breast cancer; indeed, its presence is often interpreted as supporting the diagnosis of a **benign** proliferative process.

Epithelial Hyperplasia

This represents one of the most difficult areas in the recognition and interpretation of proliferative conditions of the breast. **It is also the most important because it is the one variety of so-called 'benign' proliferative breast disease that confers an increased risk for the subsequent development of breast cancer.**

In the context of the terminal duct lobular unit, epithelial hyperplasia is defined as a condition in which there are more than two cell layers above the acinar or ductular basement membrane.

As stated above, epithelial hyperplasia may be classified in two ways:

1) **Type** – either **'usual'** or **atypical** varieties. Atypical hyperplasia, according to some large studies, is found in about 4–5% of biopsies in which benign proliferative conditions are present.
2) **Site** – **ductal** or **lobular** hyperplasia. Both of these occur in the terminal duct lobular unit but show somewhat different differentiation patterns.

In relation to the increased risk of cancer associated with epithelial hyperplasia, the College of American Pathologists has suggested that patients with benign proliferative breast disease should be classified as shown in *Table 39.27*.

'Usual' Epithelial Hyperplasia (i.e. without Atypia)

Ductal epithelial hyperplasia is regarded as mild when there are only three or four cell layers lining the affected acini. More severe grades are classified as being moderate to florid. The terms **papillomatosis**

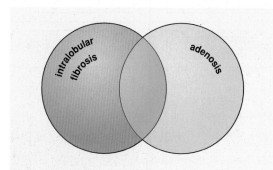

FIGURE 39.40 Sclerosing adenosis involves an increase in the number of intralobular ducts and intralobular fibrosis.

Table 39.27 Effect of Epithelial Hyperplasia on Breast Cancer Risk

Hyperplasia (presence or absence, degree and type)	Risk for subsequent invasive carcinoma compared with the general female population
No or mild hyperplasia	No increased risk
Moderate or florid hyperplasia without atypia	1.5–2-fold risk
Atypical ductal or lobular hyperplasia	**4–5-fold risk**

KEY POINTS: Benign Proliferative Breast Disease

- Only a small minority of all breast cancers occur in women with a previous history of biopsy-proven proliferative breast disease.
- Only a small proportion of women with biopsy-proven proliferative changes in the breast subsequently develop breast cancer, although there is some increase in risk (see above).
- The risk of subsequent breast cancer after a unilateral biopsy showing proliferative changes affects both breasts.
- Only about a third of women with breast cancer have a known risk factor.
- A history of breast cancer in a first-degree relative is a very strong additive risk factor in a woman who has atypical hyperplasia.

and **epitheliosis** have also been used in this context of usual hyperplasia but do not add to our understanding. Certainly, infolding and projections of proliferated epithelium into the lumina of the affected ductules are seen, but these are not true papillomas in that they neither branch nor possess a connective tissue core.

Atypical Hyperplasia

Atypical hyperplasia is recognized because of its resemblance to ductal or lobular carcinoma *in situ*. The affected epithelial cells show cytological abnormalities suggestive of neoplastic transformation, and architectural ones with loss of the normal orderly pattern of growth. The severity of the changes seen in atypical hyperplasia is, almost by definition, less severe than that in carcinoma *in situ*.

Ductal carcinoma *in situ* is characterized by:
- a uniform cell population which occupies the whole of the duct space bounded by the basement membrane
- the presence of 'punched out', neatly rounded spaces or well-defined papillary fronds
- the presence of round, hyperchromatic, randomly placed nuclei

Atypical ductal hyperplasia differs from the above in that the cell population of the affected ducts has a residuum of normal epithelial cells which rest on a basement membrane and which are normally oriented with their long axes pointing towards the lumen.

Atypical lobular hyperplasia also resembles carcinoma *in situ*, although in this case it is of the lobular variety in which the acini are grossly distended by a uniform population of cells which appear to have lost their cohesion and which have rather clear cytoplasm. Again the degree of change in hyperplasia falls short of that seen in carcinoma *in situ*. The distinction between the two, on microscopic examination, is not always easy.

BENIGN TUMOURS AND TUMOUR-LIKE LESIONS

FIBROADENOMA

Fibroadenoma is the commonest lesion presenting as a breast lump in a women aged 20–35 years. Many texts classify this lesion as a benign neoplasm but there is evidence suggesting that it is, in fact, a localized form of nodular hyperplasia involving both epithelial and stromal elements of the breast lobule.

Clinically, fibroadenomas present as mobile, firm masses with well-defined edges. In 80% of cases they are single. They increase in size with pregnancy and tend to regress with advancing age.

Macroscopic Features

Fibroadenomas are firm, rubbery masses with a sharply demarcated edge. This is so marked that it is possible to enucleate the lesions by blunt dissection from the surrounding tissue. They are seldom larger than 3 cm along the longest axis.

The cut surface is a greyish-white colour showing a characteristic whorled appearance in which slit-like spaces can be seen.

Microscopic Features

As both lobular stroma and epithelium are involved, the appearances vary depending on which of these elements shows the greater degree of overgrowth.

Typically one sees an increased number of acini, with a normal two-layered structure, separated by large amounts of loose myxoid stroma. In some instances the acini are compressed by stroma which appears to invaginate into them (*Fig. 39.41*). In other areas the acini retain their luminated structure. The first of these appearances is called **intracanalicular** and the second **pericanalicular**. The distinction is not significant.

The stroma lacks any elastic tissue (a feature that reinforces the view that the lesion arises from the terminal duct lobular unit). Variations in stromal cellularity occur and this may give rise to the suspicion that the lesion may be a phyllodes tumour (see pp 817–818). Phyllodes tumour occurs only rarely in the age group in which fibroadenoma is common and this fact helps in assessing fibroadenomas with hypercellular stroma.

On occasion, the margins of the lesion are ill defined and appear to blend with breast tissue showing fibrocystic changes. This variant – **fibroadenomatoid hyperplasia** – suggests a common pathogenetic pathway for both fibroadenoma and fibrocystic change.

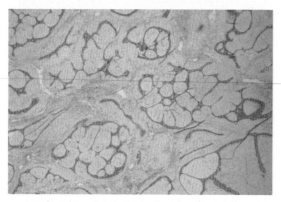

FIGURE 39.41 *Fibroadenoma, predominantly of the intracanalicular variety, with compression of ducts by exuberant fibrous tissue.*

Natural History
Most fibroadenomas behave in an entirely benign fashion. Malignant change occurs in about 0.1% of the lesions. In most cases it is the epithelial component that undergoes transformation and the commonest change is to lobular carcinoma *in situ.* If the carcinoma is confined to the limits of the original fibroadenoma, the prognosis following resection is excellent.

Malignant change in the stroma with the development of sarcoma is very rare.

Juvenile Fibroadenoma
As its name implies, this variant tends to occur in adolescent girls, especially in those of African or West Indian origin. It grows rapidly and reaches a large size: tumours of 10 cm or more in diameter are not uncommon. Microscopic examination shows hypercellularity, which may affect the acinar or the stromal element. The combination of large size and hypercellularity may give rise to fears of a phyllodes tumour (see pp 817–818), but the latter hardly ever occurs in this age group and the stroma of juvenile fibroadenoma does not show the atypia that occurs in phyllodes tumour.

ADENOMA
The term adenoma is applied to a small number of lesions, some of which are hyperplastic rather than neoplastic.

Tubular Adenoma
This presents mainly in young adults as a solitary well-circumscribed lump with a tan-coloured cut surface.

Microscopic examination shows the presence of closely packed well-formed small tubules with both epithelial and myoepithelial layers.

Lactating Adenoma
This is a hyperplastic rather than a neoplastic lesion, occurring during pregnancy or the puerperium. Despite its hyperplastic nature, the lesion is well demarcated from the surrounding breast tissue.

Microscopy shows slightly dilated tubules, lined by actively secreting epithelium closely packed together in a 'back to back' fashion.

Nipple Adenoma
This occurs in the subareolar ducts of women aged between 30 and 50 years. The commonest presentation is of a bloody discharge from the nipple. Occasionally the overlying nipple epithelium is ulcerated and this may give rise to a misdiagnosis of Paget's disease of the nipple.

Microscopy shows a complex glandular pattern, due partly to a florid degree of papillomatous change within the affected ducts and partly to scarring.

INTRADUCTAL PAPILLOMA
Unlike fibroadenoma, papilloma is most commonly a lesion of middle age, the mean age being 48 years. It may affect large or small ducts. In the former, the commonest presentation is of a blood-stained nipple discharge; indeed, intraductal papilloma is the commonest cause of such a discharge. This clinical feature results from the soft, friable nature of large duct papillomas.

Macroscopic Features
The lesions are usually solitary (about 90% of cases) and distend the ducts in which they are sited. Benign papilloma seldom exceeds 3 cm in diameter; papillary tumours significantly larger than this should arouse suspicions of papillary carcinoma, and the cytological appearances must be evaluated carefully.

Microscopic Features
There is a typical complex, branched appearance with central cores of fibrous tissue well supplied with small blood vessels. The surfaces of these cores are covered, in most instances, by well-differentiated epithelium (*Fig. 39.42*); some myoepithelial cells are also present.

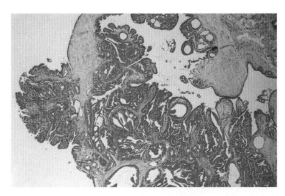

FIGURE 39.42 *Duct papilloma showing a complex pattern of fibrovascular cores covered by well-differentiated ductal epithelium.*

Carcinoma of the Breast

Breast cancer imposes a tremendous burden of suffering and loss of life in the West. **It was until recently the commonest malignant disease in women; approximately 1 in every 11 women will suffer from breast cancer.** It is responsible for 20% of all cancer-related deaths in women.

The most important morphological determinant of the natural history of breast cancer is whether, at the time of primary excision, the tumour is:

- **non-invasive – confined within the ducts or acini in which the tumour cells originate.**
  Non-invasive carcinomas may certainly progress to invasion, but it is important to realize that this progression is *not* inevitable.

or

- **invasive – the tumour cells have infiltrated through ductal or acinar basement membranes to reach the connective tissue.**

NON-INVASIVE CARCINOMA (CARCINOMA *IN SITU*)

Non-invasive and invasive cancers are of one of two basic morphological types:

- **ductal carcinoma**
- **lobular carcinoma**

Both arise from the terminal duct lobular unit but their cytological features and natural history are distinct.

Ductal Carcinoma *in situ* (DCIS)

The advent of mammography has increased greatly the frequency of this diagnosis. Mammograms can show small lesions that are not clinically obvious, and many of these are found to be DCIS.

Morphologically distinct variants of DCIS occur. These are discussed below.

Comedo Carcinoma

Comedo carcinomas are so called **because the tumour tissue in the expanded ducts undergoes central necrosis**. Pressure on the tumour-bearing area of an excised specimen squeezes plugs of necrotic tumour tissue from the ducts in a manner similar to that which occurs when a skin comedo is squeezed.

They reach quite a large size, about 50% being greater than 2 cm in diameter, although there is no direct correlation between tumour size and the likelihood of invasion. About a third of the lesions are multicentric.

Macroscopic Features

The cut surfaces of these lesions show the presence of closely packed, thick-walled ducts interspersed with normal breast tissue.

Microscopic Features

The ducts are packed with a mass of pleomorphic tumour cells with large, darkly staining nuclei in which mitoses are common. There is very little visible connective tissue stroma. **The most characteristic, indeed the defining, feature is the presence of central necrosis**, in which deposits of calcium are quite common.

Solid Non-comedo Carcinoma in situ

In this variant, central necrosis is lacking and the cell population is far more uniform than that found in comedo carcinoma. Important diagnostic clues are the pallor of the cytoplasm of the tumour cells and their sharply demarcated plasma membranes.

Cribriform Carcinoma

The intraductal tumour cell masses show the presence of well-demarcated, 'punched out', round spaces, giving a sieve-like appearance. The regularity in size and shape of these spaces contrasts markedly with the non-uniform appearance of the spaces seen in ducts affected by 'usual' epithelial hyperplasia, and is a useful diagnostic clue. The presence of spaces may be associated with two other morphological features suggestive of intraductal malignancy:

- **'trabecular bars'.** These are rather rigid-looking rows of cells that cross the spaces and have their cells arranged roughly perpendicular to the long axis of the cell row.
- **'Roman bridges'.** These are curved bars connecting two portions of the lining epithelium.

Micropapillary Carcinoma

This variant shows long epithelial projections extending into the lumen of the affected ducts. Although the term 'papillary' is used, these projections have no supporting fibrovascular core and tend not to branch.

Papillary Carcinoma in situ

Most intraductal papillary lesions are benign, but a small number of papillary carcinomas do occur. These may be localized within a duct segment or may spread intra-ductally to involve part or all of a breast segment. The histological distinction between these lesions and benign papillomas is not always easy. Features suggesting malignancy in a given papillary lesion include:

- uniformity of size and shape of the tumour cells
- the presence of one cell type only, myoepithelial cells being absent
- the presence of large, darkly staining nuclei
- the presence of many mitoses
- the absence of associated benign proliferative breast disease
- the absence of obvious fibrovascular connective tissue cores in relation to the papillae

Natural History

The natural history of DCIS has not been easy to determine because mastectomy was for a long time the treatment of choice for these patients. In one small series of patients with non-comedo carcinoma *in situ*, in whom only biopsy had been performed, 7 of 25 patients developed invasive carcinoma in the same breast within 3 years. In mastectomy specimens from patients who had had a diagnosis of carcinoma *in situ* 6 months previously, the prevalence of invasive carcinoma ranged from 6 to 18%.

Lobular Carcinoma *in situ* (LCIS)

LCIS does not usually present as a breast lump and is often discovered in breast tissue removed for some other clinically apparent lesion. Thus the diagnosis is made only as a result of microscopic examination. In about 70% of cases it is multicentric, and bilateral breast involvement is present in about 30–40%. These two facts obviously have significant implications for treatment of affected women.

Microscopic Features

The area of the affected lobules is increased in LCIS and the acini are filled, indeed distended, by tumour cells.

The cell population consists of uniform, small to medium, round cells with rounded, usually normochromatic, nuclei (*Fig. 39.43*). The cytoplasm is characteristically clear and the cells often appear non-cohesive. 'Signet ring' change, due to accumulation of mucin within the tumour cells and resulting displacement of the nuclei, is fairly common.

Similar cells may be present in the extralobular terminal ducts, often lying under the existing epithelial lining. This pattern has been described as 'pagetoid'.

Natural History

The natural history of LCIS is associated with the following:

- **About 25–30% of patients with a diagnosis of LCIS will develop invasive carcinoma.**

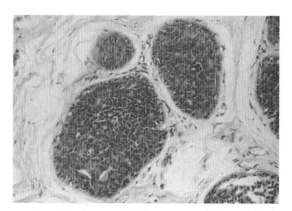

FIGURE 39.43 *Lobular carcinoma invading ducts.*

- **The increased risk operates in respect of both breasts**, although it is somewhat greater on the side from which the positive biopsy was derived.
- The invasive tumour that develops is not necessarily an invasive **lobular** carcinoma. **Both ductal and lobular invasive cancers may develop after a diagnosis of LCIS.**
- The **extent of involvement** by LCIS **does not correlate with the risk of subsequent development of invasive carcinoma**.

INVASIVE CARCINOMA

The vast majority (85%) of invasive carcinomas are ductal in type. Invasive ductal carcinoma is divided into a number of morphological types. This classification is based on:

1) **the architectural pattern of the tumour**
2) **the patterns of spread within the breast**

ARCHITECTURAL PATTERNS

Invasive ductal carcinoma (NOS)

The acronym NOS means 'not otherwise specified'. This by far the commonest variety of invasive breast cancer (greater than 80% of cases).

Macroscopic Features

These depend to a considerable extent on the relative proportions of tumour cells and stroma in the individual lesion. Very often the tumour is associated with a striking degree of fibrous and elastic tissue response, which makes it very hard, as is appreciated both on clinical palpation and when the resected specimen is cut. The old term applied to such a cancer is **scirrhous** (a Greek adjective meaning 'hard').

Characteristically, such a tumour is very hard, sometimes retracted below the cut surface of the whole specimen and with an ill-defined, usually infiltrating, edge.

The lesion is a grey-white colour, often with streaks of chalky-white material running through it, these representing areas in which elastin is abundant. Often there is a grating sound as the tumour is cut, somewhat like that of cutting an 'unripe pear'.

In other instances the fibrous tissue formation is less in amount and the lesions appear softer.

Microscopic Features

Tumours show a wide range of appearances. **The cancer cells may grow in diffuse sheets, in solid islands, in the form of more or less well-differentiated glandular spaces, in infiltrating cords and as individual cells.**

Just as the **architectural** appearance of the tumours **varies**, so does the **appearance of their constituent cells**. On the whole, they are larger and more pleomorphic than the cells of a lobular carcinoma. The nuclear appearances vary from one lesion to another, and even from one area of a single lesion to another, and mitoses are present in most instances, although, again, the numbers vary from case to case.

As stated above, the fibrous tissue response varies from case to case. Masses of elastic tissue are present in about 90% of cases and focal calcification is seen in about 60%. A chronic inflammatory cell infiltrate is present to some degree at the interface between the tumour cells and stroma, but this too varies greatly in intensity.

The tumour cells bear a number of **immunohistological markers**. Some of these are the same as those seen in many other adenocarcinomas, but others are more clearly breast-associated. The latter include:
- **low molecular weight cytokeratins**
- **epithelial membrane antigen**
- **a milk-fat globule membrane**
- **lactalbumin (about 70% of cases)**

Spread within preformed vascular channels within the breast, especially lymphatics, can be seen in many cases. It is not always easy to be sure that this is present as retraction of cells from their surrounding stroma may give a false impression of lymphatic permeation. Confirmation of vascular permeation can be obtained by using antibodies that mark vascular endothelium.

Tubular Carcinoma

This accounts for about 2% of invasive carcinomas. The prognosis is much better than that with the much commoner invasive ductal carcinoma (NOS).

Macroscopic Features

Tubular carcinomas are usually quite small (about 1 cm in diameter) and have a gritty cut surface and an ill-defined edge.

Microscopic Features

The diagnosis may be quite difficult because the malignant glands are so well differentiated and are associated with such a brisk fibroelastic tissue response that a misdiagnosis of complex sclerosing lesion or radial scar may be made (see above). The diagnostic clues are:
- the presence of a single layer of cells in the tubules
- the haphazard arrangement of the tubules
- the lack of a basement membrane in relation to the tubules
- the frequent invasion of adipose tissue at the periphery of the lesion
- the frequent association of intraductal carcinoma *in situ* in other portions of the material sampled

The prognosis in patients with tubular carcinoma is excellent. In one large study only 4% of patients developed metastatic or recurrent tumour in a 7-year follow-up period. It is important to recognize that, in some cases of invasive ductal carcinoma (NOS), areas of tubular carcinoma may be seen. The natural history in these cases is that of the invasive ductal carcinoma and not that of tubular carcinoma.

Mucinous Carcinoma ('Colloid Carcinoma')

These tumours, which usually occur in postmenopausal women, have a well-defined edge and consist of a jelly-like mass of mucin in which islands of tumour cells float. They constitute about 2–3% of breast cancers and have a much better prognosis than invasive ductal carcinoma (NOS), probably because of the very low prevalence of nodal metastases found on examination of surgically·removed specimens.

Microscopic Features

The characteristic feature is the presence of large lakes of extracellular mucin in which groups of tumour cells can be seen. The malignant cells make up only a small proportion of the volume of the lesion, this being dominated by the mucin. About 25% of the tumour cells show some evidence of neuroendocrine differentiation in the form of dense-core secretory granules seen on electron microscopy.

Medullary Carcinoma

This variant accounts for about 1% of all breast cancers.

Macroscopic Features

Medullary carcinoma tends to have a well-defined edge, an impression that is reinforced by seeing a **'pushing'** rather than an infiltrative margin on histological examination. The cut surface is characteristically fleshy, grey and soft, and foci of haemorrhage and necrosis may be present.

Microscopic Features

The growth pattern of the tumour cells tends to be confluent with little or no stroma between them; indeed, there may be a syncytial pattern similar to that seen in some germ cell tumours of the gonads. They show the same epithelial markers on immunohistological examination as do invasive ductal tumours of other types but, in addition, mark with antibodies to the neural marker S-100.

The striking fibrous tissue response so often seen in cases of invasive ductal carcinoma (NOS) is never present. The tumour cells themselves are large and pleomorphic and have large nuclei with prominent nucleoli. Mitoses are common. There is no evidence of glandular differentiation. Extensive necrosis, highly atypical tumour giant cells and focal dystrophic calcification are also common features.

A highly characteristic microscopic feature of medullary cancer is the presence of a prominent infiltration of lymphocytes and plasma cells at the periphery of the lesion.

Despite these unpromising histological appearances, the prognosis in medullary carcinoma is better than that for the more common invasive ductal carcinoma (NOS). In one series the 10-year survival rate for patients with medullary carcinoma was 84%, compared with 63% for those with ordinary invasive ductal carcinoma.

PATTERNS OF SPREAD

Paget's Disease of the Nipple

The classical clinical presentation is that of a red, eczematous lesion affecting the nipple. Its significance is that, in virtually all instances, **the nipple changes are associated with the presence of an underlying intraductal carcinoma which may have already spread to involve the stroma**. The presence of a palpable breast mass is a strong indicator of invasion having taken place.

The nipple lesion itself is the expression of invasion of the epidermis by cancer cells that have spread up the duct system. Histological examination shows this in the form of the presence of large cells with atypical nuclei which largely replace the basal layer of the epidermis and spread upwards into the malpighian layer. This invasion of the epidermis must be distinguished from malignant melanoma or intraepithelial squamous carcinoma (Bowen's disease), both of which can involve the nipple. In a small number of cases, Paget's disease of the nipple may occur in the absence of underlying breast cancer and it has been suggested that in these cases an *in situ* malignant transformation of basal epidermal cells has taken place, this being associated with glandular differentiation of the transformed cells.

Inflammatory Carcinoma

The term inflammatory carcinoma is applied to a breast cancer in which there is diffuse or local swelling, redness and heat – the classical signs of inflammation.

Its most common association is carcinoma in which extensive permeation of dermal lymphatic channels is present. The breast cancers themselves may be of diverse appearance but are most commonly poorly differentiated. The prognosis is poor and it is fortunate that less than 1% of breast cancers present in this way. Blockage of lymphatics within the breast, as a result of permeation of tumour, may give rise to the clinical sign known as *peau d'orange* (orange skin), which is the result of localized lymphoedema.

Invasive Lobular Carcinoma

Invasive lobular carcinoma probably accounts for about 10% of invasive breast cancers. The marked tendency for these tumours to be multicentric and bilateral has already been mentioned, in the section on the *in situ* variant of lobular carcinoma.

Recognition of these tumours, which may occur in the absence of an *in situ* component, is based on:

- **the appearance of the cells.** These are smaller than those of a ductal carcinoma, more uniform, and show less evidence of atypia. As with the *in situ* variant of lobular carcinoma, decreased cell cohesiveness is a prominent feature. 'Signet ring' change in the tumour cells, due to the intracellular accumulation of mucin, is a fairly common event in infiltrating lobular carcinoma.
- **the pattern of infiltration of the breast tissue.** The characteristic appearance is that of individual tumour cells infiltrating the breast tissue in an 'Indian file' fashion. It is interesting to observe how often these tumour cells infiltrate around normal large ducts.

The frequency of different morphological types of breast cancer is shown in *Fig. 39.44*.

GRADING AND STAGING IN CARCINOMA OF THE BREAST

Grading in relation to breast cancer in the UK is most commonly done by using a modification of the system first described by Bloom and Richardson in 1957. The modified system analyses breast cancers in terms of three morphological parameters (*Fig. 39.45*). These are:

1) **The degree of tubule formation.** A tumour in which there is extensive tubule formation is graded as 1; one with no well-formed tubules is graded as 3.
2) **The degree of nuclear atypia.** Using a scale

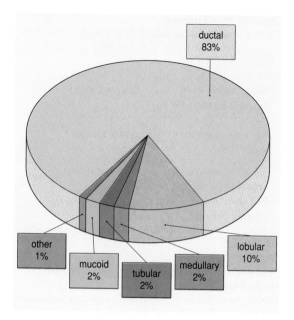

FIGURE 39.44 *Frequency of distribution of different morphological types of breast cancer.*

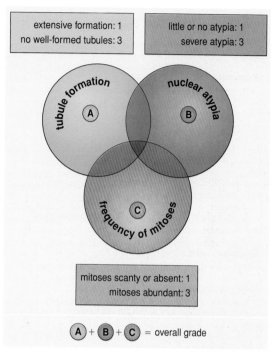

FIGURE 39.45 *Grading of breast cancer is based on three sets of criteria.*

between 1 and 3, the greater the degree of nuclear atypia, the higher the score.

3) **The frequency of mitoses.** Again using a scale of 1–3, the greater the number of mitoses, the higher the score assigned.

These three scores are added together to obtain the grade. Thus:

- a score of 3–5 = grade 1
- a score of 6–7 = grade 2
- a score of 8–9 = grade 3

The higher the grade, the worse the clinical behaviour of the lesion is likely to be, but there are other prognostic factors that must be considered.

A number of systems of **staging** exists. These are based on:

- **tumour size**
- **the presence or absence of lymph node metastasis**
- **the presence or absence of extension to neighbouring structures such as the chest wall or overlying skin**
- **the presence or absence of evidence of distant metastasis**

Probably the most commonly used system is that recommended by the International Union Against Cancer (UICC), which again is based on tumour size, nodal status and the presence or absence of distant metastases. The nomenclature used is the familiar TNM system in which **T refers to the primary tumour, N to the regional nodes, and M to the presence or absence of distant metastasis.** This is basically a clinical rather than a pathological system (*Table 39.28*).

PROGNOSTIC FACTORS IN BREAST CANCER

To assess the effects of various factors on prognosis in breast cancer, one must have some idea of the natural history of the disease in a sufficiently large sample.

If the disease is localized at the time of treatment (i.e. no involvement of skin or pectoralis muscle, no lymph node involvement and no evidence of metastasis), the 5-year survival rate is about 73% and the proportion of the cohort with no cancer obviously present at this 5-year point will be about 60%.

If regional disease is present (i.e. involvement of nodes or of adjacent structures such as skin or muscle), the 5-year survival rate is about 49% and the proportion of these patients with no evidence of cancer will be about 34%.

It is against this background that other factors of prognostic significance should be studied.

Presence or Absence of Invasiveness

This is the single most important prognostic factor in breast cancer. Non-invasive cancer is curable, although, because *in situ* lesions are often multicentric, the most appropriate treatment may be mastectomy.

Table 39.28 The UICC Staging System

Stage Description

Tumour

T₁   Less than 2 cm along longest axis; T_{1a}, no fixation to pectoral muscle or fascia; T_{1b}, fixation to these structures

T₂   More than 2 cm but less than 5 cm along longest axis; T_{2a} and T_{2b} as for above

T₃   More than 5 cm along longest axis; T_{3a} and T_{3b} as for T_{1a} and T_{1b}

T₄   Tumour of any size with direct extension to chest wall or skin

Regional nodes

N_0 No palpable nodes on same side as tumour

N_1 Palpable, mobile nodes

N_2 Palpable, fixed nodes on same side as tumour

N_3 Palpable, supraclavicular nodes or oedema of arm on side of tumour

Distant metastasis

M_0 No evidence of distant metastasis

M_1 Evidence of distant metastasis

TNM stage

I	T_{1a} or T_{1b}	N_0 or N_{1a}	M_0
II	T_0, T_{1a} or T_{1b}	N_{1b}	M_0
II	T_{2a} or T_{2b}	N_0, N_{1a} or N_{1b}	M_0
III	T_{1a} or T_{1b}; T_{2a} or T_{2b}	N_2	M_0
III	T_{3a} or T_{3b}	N_0, N_1 or N_2	M_0
IV	T_4	Any N	Any M
IV	Any T	N_3	Any M
IV	Any T	Any N	M_1

Size of the Primary Tumour

The diameter of the breast cancer correlates with the likelihood of node involvement. Similarly there is a correlation between tumour size and survival. The proportion of patients surviving for 5 years and clinically free from cancer at the 5-year point falls steadily with increasing tumour diameter whether or not the patients are node-negative or node-positive. It is worth remembering, however, that even amongst the smallest primary tumours lymph node spread occurs in about 25% of patients.

Type of the Tumour

The influence of morphology (e.g. tubular, mucinous) on prognosis is shown in *Table 39.29*.

Table 39.29 Prognosis in Breast Cancer with Respect to Morphology

More favourable prognosis	Less favourable prognosis
Tubular carcinoma	Signet-ring invasive
Medullary carcinoma	carcinoma
Pure mucinous carcinoma	'Inflammatory' carcinoma
Papillary carcinoma	

Presence or Absence of Axillary Lymph Node Metastasis

This is one of the most important prognostic indicators.

There is a significant decrease both in cancer-free and non-cancer-free survival if regional lymph nodes are found to contain tumour. In one study the 5-year cancer-free survival rate in node-negative patients was 85%. In patients in whom one to three axillary nodes were found to be involved by tumour, this value fell to 60%.

Prognosis appears to be related not only to the presence of node positivity but also to the number of nodes affected and the extent of involvement within individual nodes. Thus, the disease-free survival rate fell progressively with an increase in the number of affected axillary nodes (*Table 39.30*).

Characteristics of the Tumour

- **The degree of differentiation.**
- **The character of the tumour margin:** either 'pushing', which has the better prognosis, or 'infiltrative'.

Table 39.30 Influence of Nodal Involvement on Disease-free Survival in Breast Cancer

No. of positive nodes	Disease-free survival rate (%)
0	85
1–3	60
4	40
> 4	30.5
7–12	28
> 13	16.4

- **The expression of oestrogen receptors in the nuclei of the tumour cells.** It is believed that the presence of these receptors in breast cancer cells indicates the likelihood of a good response to endocrine treatment with antioestrogens. In fact only about half the tumours that express receptors for oestrogen respond to such treatment. The presence and extent of distribution of oestrogen receptors can be visualized by using monoclonal antibodies raised against the receptors.

- **The expression of epidermal growth factor (EGF) receptors on the tumour cell membranes.** Binding of an appropriate ligand (either EGF or transforming growth factor α) to the receptor produces a conformational change which makes the intracytoplasmic part of the receptor act as a tyrosine kinase, and this is followed by rapid triggering of the proto-oncogenes c-*myc* and c-*fos*. The gene products of these are DNA-binding proteins and are important in initiating transcription of DNA and, ultimately, cell division. It is not without interest that there appears to be an inverse relationship between the presence of EGF receptors in tumour cells and the presence of oestrogen receptors.

  There is good epidemiological evidence of a poorer prognosis in patients whose tumours express large amounts of EGF receptor. In patients without evidence of nodal deposits, EGF receptor expression is associated with a fall in the 5-year survival rate. In one such study 50% of the patients whose tumours showed EGF receptors died; the mortality rate in patients without EGF receptors in their tumour cells was 26%.

- **Expression of the gene product of the proto-oncogene c-*erb*-B2.** c-*erb*-B2 (also known as HER-2 or *neu*) encodes a transmembrane protein known as p185 which shows homology with the EGF receptor. Amplification of this gene has been found in 15–40% of primary breast cancers and this results in increased expression of the p185 protein. In about 10% of cases of overexpression of this protein in breast cancers, there is no evidence of amplification of the gene, and it is likely that these cases are due to increased transcription. Amplification of the oncogene is associated with a poorer prognosis than in patients with comparable tumours in which there is no such amplification or overexpression of the gene product.

- **Ploidy of the tumour cell population.** The introduction of flow cytometry enables the identification of the fractions of a cell population that are diploid, tetraploid and aneuploid. In breast cancer, evidence suggests that those with aneuploid cell populations behave in a more aggressive manner than those with diploid characteristics. The potential of this method for providing accurate prognostic information is still uncertain, and flow cytometry is not widely used at present.

RISK FACTORS IN RELATION TO BREAST CANCER

The risk factors are summarized in *Fig. 39.46*.

Female Sex

This seems almost too obvious to be stated, but breast cancer does occur in the male breast (see p 819), although with only about 1% of the frequency with which it is found in the female. The differential risk between the sexes is constant all over the world in both high- and low-risk populations.

Genetic Factors

It has been known for a long time that the first-degree female relatives of a woman with breast cancer have an increased risk of developing breast cancer themselves. Thus, for example, a woman whose mother and sister both had breast cancer has a fivefold increase in risk. In addition, families can be identified in which there is a high risk of both breast and ovarian cancers (*Fig. 39.47*).

In 1990 an abnormal gene was discovered which appears to be associated with the risk of familial and early-onset breast cancer. This gene, which has been called **BRCA1**, is believed to be responsible for about 2% of all breast cancers, although in women who develop breast cancer before the age of 30 years the frequency of involvement of the *BRCA1* gene may be as high as 8%. Studies by the Breast Cancer Linkage Consortium have shown that *BRCA1* is implicated in about 50% of families with at least four cases of breast cancer in·women aged under 60 years and in over 80% of families with histories of both breast and ovarian cancer. An additional breast cancer susceptibility gene, *BRCA2*, has been described but not yet cloned. It is situated on chromosome 13 (see p 289).

The *BRCA1* gene maps to the long arm of chromosome 17 (17q21). The mutated gene appears to be inherited in an autosomal dominant pattern. The frequency of *BRCA1* mutations is much higher in Ashkenazi Jewesses; 20% of such women who develop breast cancer under the age of 40 years carry a specific *BRCA1* mutation.

It is interesting that the first breast cancer susceptibility gene should be located on chromosome 17, because other genes that may be implicated in breast pathology are also situated on this chromosome. These include:

- the *neu* (*erb*-B2) oncogene, which codes for a truncated version of the EGF receptor and which is amplified in many breast cancers
- the gene for oestradiol 17β-dehydrogenase, an enzyme that codes for the conversion of oestrone to oestradiol in breast tissue
- the *NM23* gene, **lack** of whose gene product is correlated positively with the likelihood of nodal metastasis

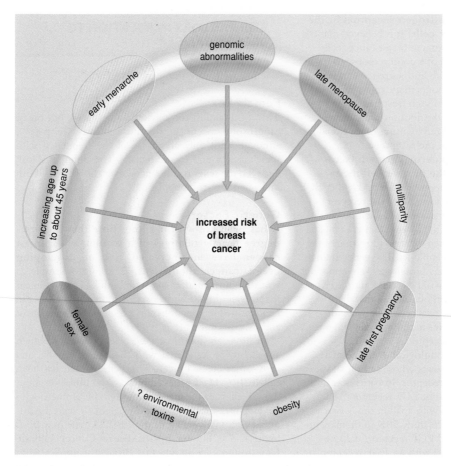

FIGURE 39.46 Risk factors in breast cancer.

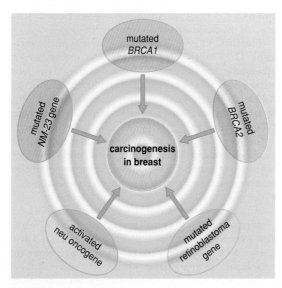

FIGURE 39.47 Genomic abnormalities that may contribute to carcinogenesis in the breast.

- the gene for the retinoic acid receptor, which some believe is anticarcinogenic
- the gene *WNT3*, which is the human counterpart of an integration site for the mouse mammary tumour virus

The Retinoblastoma Gene (Rb)

In as many as 25% of breast cancers, there is homozygous deletion of part or all of the retinoblastoma gene. Whether these patients have loss or alteration of one allele for this gene in the germ cell line (as is the case in familial retinoblastoma) is not known, and the role of *Rb* gene alteration in relation to breast cancer is also unknown at present.

Factors Likely to be Associated with Prolonged Exposure to Ovarian Hormones

Age at Menarche and Menopause

Women who start to menstruate at a relatively early age show an increased risk for developing breast cancer. A similar increment of risk is associated with a late menopause: the risk of breast cancer is doubled in a woman who has her menopause at the age of 55 years compared with one whose menopause occurs 10 years earlier.

Protective Effects of Childbirth at a Young Age

Of all the biological events in a woman's life, childbirth has one of the strongest effects on the chances of developing breast cancer in later life. Nulliparous women have a greater risk of developing breast cancer than parous women, provided the time of first pregnancy in the latter occurs before the middle of the fourth decade. In women who have their first child after the age of 35 years, the protective effects of pregnancy appear to be lost.

These data suggest that it is prolonged overstimulation with oestrogen and relative underexposure to progesterone that is the operative mechanism.

Geographical Factors

It is clear from studying standardized breast cancer mortality rates that there are marked differences in risk in different populations. For example, the UK has the highest mortality rate from breast cancer (28 per 100 000 women per year), whereas at the other end of the spectrum the rate in Japan is only 5.8 per 100 000 women annually. In general terms, women in western Europe and North America are most commonly affected, whereas those living in Asia, Africa and South America are relatively spared.

Some evidence suggests that these differences are environmentally determined. For example, the daughters of Japanese immigrants to the USA have a higher incidence of breast cancer than their mothers, and the grand-daughters have a still higher incidence. This change does not appear to be associated with any significant degree of intermarriage.

Further support comes from studies of single, non-migrant populations whose way of life may have changed significantly. For example, the change in Iceland between 1920 and 1960 from a predominantly rural and fishing economy to a more industrialized one was accompanied by a steep rise in the incidence of breast cancer.

What the environmental factors concerned are, is still unknown. Well-nourished and, in particular, obese women are more at risk than poorly nourished ones and it has been suggested that diets high in fat may play a part. There is some epidemiological support for this, and it has been found that diets high in fat increase the incidence of breast cancer in rats. Obesity is associated with an increased tendency for $\Delta 4$-androstenedione to be converted to oestrone and this may be the basis for the increased risk.

Recently it has been suggested that the association between breast cancer risk and industrialization may be related to atmospheric pollution by polychlorinated biphenyls which are stored in adipose tissue and which, it is hypothesized, may have an oestrogen-like effect on breast epithelium.

PATTERNS OF SPREAD IN BREAST CANCER

As with other tumours, spread from breast cancer may be:

1) **Direct**, involving neighbouring structures such as the skin, the pectoral fascia and the pectoral muscles

2) **Via lymphatics.** The lymph nodes most often involved, in order of frequency, are:

- **the axillary nodes.** Spread to these nodes has already occurred in about 50% of patients with breast cancer at the time of primary excision.
- **internal mammary nodes.** These nodes are related to the internal mammary artery. They are particularly likely to be involved in patients whose tumour is located in the upper inner quadrant of the breast.
- **supraclavicular nodes**
- **nodes within the abdomen**

3) **Via the bloodstream.** Distant spread of breast cancer is the event most likely to lead to death of the patient from the tumour. The **lungs, liver, bones and adrenals** are particularly likely to be involved by bloodborne metastases, but secondary deposits are by no means confined to these sites.

OTHER TUMOURS OF THE BREAST

STROMAL TUMOURS

Phyllodes Tumour

This tumour was originally called '**cystosarcoma phyllodes**', a term that has now been abandoned because it has sinister prognostic implications that are not completely accurate. The name **phyllodes** is derived from the fact that the cut surface of the tumour characteristically shows the presence of cleft-like spaces, giving an impression of leaves protruding into a cystic cavity (Gk. *phyllos* leaf). **It exhibits a range of behavioural patterns. Some of the tumours are cured by excision, some recur and a small proportion (3–12%) metastasize.** The type of behaviour seems to be predicated on the nature of the connective tissue stroma but it is not always possible, on the basis of the microscopic appearances, to predict whether an individual phyllodes tumour will behave in a benign or malignant fashion.

The mean age at presentation for phyllodes tumours is 45 years. This is much older than the usual age for fibroadenoma, and the age of the patient can thus be a useful pointer in distinguishing phyllodes tumours from large, rather cellular, fibroadenomas.

Phyllodes tumours can be very large in some instances: diameters of 45 cm have been recorded. Size itself, however, is not a reliable diagnostic indicator because some phyllodes tumours are as small as 2 cm in diameter, and the diagnosis must be made on microscopic criteria.

Macroscopic Features

Phyllodes tumours tend to be well demarcated from the surrounding breast tissue and it is easy in many cases, if perhaps not wise, to 'shell' them out from the breast (*Fig. 39.48*).

Microscopic Features

Like the fibroadenoma, phyllodes tumour involves both the fibrous and epithelial elements of the breast. Where it differs from the fibroadenoma is in the nature of the connective tissue stroma. At the 'benign' end of the spectrum, the fibroblastic stroma, although much more cellular than in the case of fibroadenoma, lacks atypia and does not show the presence of large numbers of mitotic figures. Occasional foci of mature adipose tissue can be seen within the substance of the tumour.

Phyllodes tumours that are regarded as being histologically malignant show marked nuclear atypia and many mitoses. A striking feature is the loss of normal relationship between ducts and stroma so that some microscopic fields may consist purely of this atypical stroma. In some instances the malignant-looking stroma may be very pleomorphic and can show, in addition, the presence of metaplastic bone or cartilage. Interestingly, the stromal cells may have receptors for progesterone but not for oestrogen. The common sites for distant spread, should this occur, are bone and lung, and, not surprisingly, it is only the stromal element that is seen in the metastases.

Angiosarcoma

Angiosarcoma in the breast is rare and occurs most commonly in young women.

The tumour consists characteristically of anastomosing vascular channels lined by plump, atypical, endothelial cells. A papillary appearance is present in some areas and, in some cases, the tumour is so poorly

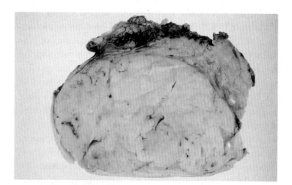

FIGURE 39.48 Phyllodes tumour: a large, well-defined, rather lobulated mass.

differentiated that the vascular nature of the lesion is difficult to appreciate.

Angiosarcoma carries a very poor prognosis. In various series, the average time from appearance of the tumour to death has ranged between 1.6 and 2.6 years.

Lymphangiosarcoma can develop in the soft tissues of the arm in patients who have had long-standing lymphoedema as a result of mastectomy.

Stromal Sarcoma

This term is given to malignant breast tumours that are thought to derive from the specialized stroma of the breast but which lack the epithelial component seen in phyllodes tumours. Most of these lesions are fibrosarcomatous in appearance, but foci of metaplastic bone may be seen.

Malignant Lymphoma

Malignant lymphomas in the breast may be part of a generalized disease or may be primary in this site, in which case the tumour is usually a non-Hodgkin's lymphoma. In some instances, the lymphoma belongs to the rather specialized group in which the cells are believed to arise from mucosa-associated lymphoid tissue (MALT).

OTHER TUMOURS

It is well to remember that the breast consists not only of specialized breast tissue but also contains many other elements such as skin, adipose tissue, sweat and sebaceous glands. A number of neoplastic and hamartomatous lesions can arise from these elements.

DISORDERS OF THE MALE BREAST

The chief structural difference between the female and male breasts is the **absence of acini in the latter**. Microscopic examination shows the presence of comparatively scanty ducts and the appearances resemble those seen in the prepubertal female.

The principal diseases of the male breast are **gynaecomastia** and **carcinoma**.

Gynaecomastia

This is a **benign** condition defined as **enlargement of the male breast due to hypertrophy and hyperplasia of both ductal and stromal elements**. In the majority of cases the enlargement is unilateral but about 25% of patients show bilateral involvement.

Gynaecomastia occurs under two basic sets of circumstances:

1) **In the absence of any disease or drug known to affect the breast in this way.** In this first instance, gynaecomastia appears to have two peaks of incidence. The first is during adolescence and the second in elderly men. The responsible mechanism is likely to be either an increase in

oestrogen secretion or a relative decline in androgen production.

2) **As a result of some disorder outside the breast or because of the administration of certain drugs that can cause breast enlargement.** Such disorders include:

- **endocrine disorders** such as hyperthyroidism and pituitary disorders
- **hormone-secreting neoplasms**, such as Leydig cell tumours of the testis, germ cell tumours secreting human chorionic gonadotrophin and certain small cell carcinomas of the lung which secrete ectopic hormones
- **cirrhosis of the liver** from whatever cause
- **certain drugs**, including chlorpromazine, reserpine, digitalis, spironolactone and epanutin
- after **treatment of prostatic carcinoma with oestrogen**

Clinically, the patients may present with a generally enlarged breast not greatly different from that of a young female, or with a well-defined disc of rather firm breast tissue centrally placed under the nipple.

Microscopic Features

Ducts commonly show some degree of epithelial hyperplasia, but there is no atypia. The stroma is abundant and, especially in the adolescent form of the disorder, appears oedematous because it contains large amounts of acid mucopolysaccharides, giving it an appearance similar to that seen in fibroadenoma. In long-standing cases, this oedematous stroma tends to be replaced by one in which fibrosis is more prominent.

Carcinoma

Carcinoma of the male breast is rare, accounting for only 1% of all breast cancers in the USA. In some countries, however, cancer of the male breast is more common. An example of this is Egypt, where almost 10% of breast cancers occur in males. This much higher risk among Egyptian males is associated with a relatively high frequency of gynaecomastia, which has been ascribed to the frequent occurrence of cirrhosis of the liver caused by schistosomiasis. An increased risk of developing cancer of the male breast in also seen in patients with Klinefelter's syndrome (defined as the presence in a phenotypic male of at least two X chromosomes in association with a Y chromosome).

The clinical presentation is most commonly that of a breast lump which may, in some cases, be associated with a discharge from the nipple.

Microscopic Features

The same spectrum of histological types seen in the female breast is present. Of these, invasive lobular carcinoma is the rarest variety in the male. No doubt because of the much smaller size of the male breast, Paget-type involvement of the nipple and tethering of the skin occur at an earlier stage in males than in females.

Prognosis

It is usually stated that the prognosis for males with breast cancer is worse than that for females similarly placed. More recent studies suggest that, for tumours of the same stage and grade, there is little or no significant difference between the natural history in the two sexes.

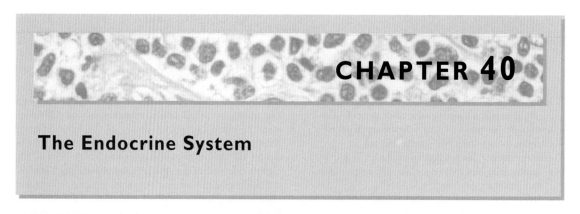

CHAPTER 40

The Endocrine System

The Pituitary

Functionally, the hypothalamus and the pituitary form a unit, in which there is a blurring of the boundaries between the nervous and endocrine systems.

NORMAL ANATOMY AND DEVELOPMENT

The pituitary consists of two portions that are embryologically, histologically and functionally quite distinct. These are:

- **the anterior pituitary** or **adenohypophysis**
- **the posterior pituitary** or **neurohypophysis**

The anterior pituitary is derived from an outpouching of the fetal buccal cavity known as **Rathke's pouch.** This grows dorsally towards the forebrain, eventually coming to lie in a hollow within the sphenoid (the **sella turcica**) and losing its connection with the buccal cavity at about the 11th week of gestation. Residual cells of the connection between the buccal cavity and the adenohypophysis may persist in various sites along the pathway of the original connection (or craniopharyngeal duct) and, possibly, give rise to the benign neoplasm, craniopharyngioma.

The posterior pituitary is derived from a diverticulum in the floor of the third ventricle of the brain; it grows downwards towards the sella and comes into contact with the primitive anterior pituitary at about the eighth week of gestation.

The pituitary is a bean-shaped organ with an average weight of 0.6 g. This increases considerably during pregnancy and diminishes with the advance of old age. The anterior portion makes up about 80% of the gland. Macroscopically the anterior and posterior portions can be readily distinguished by their colours. The anterior pituitary is a reddish-brown colour, whereas the posterior is grey. The pituitary is covered by the dura mater lining the sella and extending over the top of the sella as a firm sheet through which the pituitary stalk penetrates.

Cell Population of the Anterior Pituitary

Before the advent of immunohistochemistry, the cells of the anterior pituitary were classified on the basis of their staining characteristics in haematoxylin and eosin-stained sections. There are three groups known as:

- acidophil (red)
- basophil (bluish)
- chromophobe (no staining)

Functioning tumours (adenomas) of the anterior pituitary, which cause most cases of pituitary hyperfunction, were classified on the basis of the staining characteristics of their main cell types (e.g. basophil adenoma or chromophobe adenoma). On this basis, attempts were made to correlate the staining patterns with function. For example, growth hormone-producing tumours are usually acidophil in type.

Because there are only three staining reactions and six hormones derived from the anterior pituitary, only a very crude structure–function correlation can be drawn from haematoxylin and eosin-stained material. The introduction of stains based on the Mallory trichrome method provided more information than could be obtained from sections stained with haematoxylin and eosin. In one form – the periodic acid–Schiff–Orange G stain – acidophils stain orange and basophils pink.

The introduction of immunohistochemistry has greatly improved our knowledge of pituitary cytology and it is now recognized that there are **five cell types** responsible for the **six anterior pituitary hormones.** Attribution of the function of chromophobe cells has been less easy. Their cytoplasm does not stain because it contains many fewer secretory granules than acidophil or basophil cells. Nevertheless, electron microscopy shows that they do contain some granules and they have other fine structural features enabling us to determine their function. The cell types and their products are shown in *Table 40.1*.

The Hypothalamic–Pituitary Axis

The hypothalamus has a pivotal role in controlling secretion of the anterior pituitary hormones, as shown in *Table 40.2*.

The hypothalamus is divided longitudinally into a midline zone immediately adjacent to the third ventricle, two medial zones flanking this, and two lateral zones. The use of antibodies raised against the hypothalamic peptide hormones enables mapping of the principal collections of functioning cells. Thus, for example, the cells secreting gonadotropin-releasing hormone are situated in the preoptic area whereas

Table 40.1 Cells of the Anterior Pituitary

Cell type	Hormone	Staining	Location
Somatotropes	Growth hormone	Acidophil	Mainly in the lateral wings of the adenohypophysis. Account for about 50% of the cell population
Lactotropes	Prolactin	Acidophil or chromophobe	Random distribution but with some concentration in the posterolateral region. Account for 15–20% of the cell population
Corticotropes	ACTH and other fragments of POMC	Basophil	Mainly in the central wedge of the anterior pituitary. Account for 15–20% of the cell population
Thyrotropes	TSH	Basophil	Mainly in the anteromedial portion of the central wedge. Account for about 5% of the cell population
Gonadotropes	FSH and LH	Basophil	Many are found in the central wedge but some are distributed in the lateral wings close to the prolactin-producing cells. Account for about 10% of the cell population

ACTH, adrenocorticotropic hormone; TSH, thyroid-stimulating hormone (thyrotropin); POMC, pro-opiomelanocortin; FSH, follicle-stimulating hormone; LH, luteinizing hormone.

growth hormone-releasing hormone (GHRH) is found in the highest concentration in nerve cells in the median eminence and the pituitary stalk.

In addition to the chemical signals controlling the release of anterior pituitary hormones, the hypothalamus is also rich in biogenic amines and in a number of other neurotransmitters. These include dopamine, believed to be important in the regulation of pituitary function, especially in relation to prolactin release.

Vascular Supply to the Hypothalamus and its Interconnections with the Anterior Pituitary

The hypothalamus receives its blood supply from the arteries that make up the circle of Willis; the posterior pituitary is supplied by the inferior hypophysial artery. The vascularization of the anterior pituitary is more complex. Apart from the most superficial layers of the gland, supplied by small arteries that penetrate the

Table 40.2 Control of Anterior Pituitary Hormone Secretion by the Hypothalamus

Anterior pituitary hormone	Controlling hypothalamic hormone
Growth hormone (GH)	a) Growth hormone-releasing hormone (GHRH) b) Somatostatin, which inhibits the release of GH
Follicle-stimulating and luteinizing hormones (FSH, LH)	Gonadotropin-releasing hormone (GnRH)
Thyrotropin (TSH)	Thyrotropin-releasing hormone (TRH)
Pro-opiomelanocortin (POMC) (from which ACTH and a number of other compounds are released)	Corticotropin-releasing hormone (CRH)
Prolactin (PRL)	Probably: a) TRH b) Vasoactive intestinal polypeptide (VIP)

capsule, the bulk of the anterior pituitary has no direct arterial supply. Instead it receives 70–90% of its blood supply via a system of long portal vessels derived from the capillary network in the median eminence (*Fig. 40.1*). These long portal vessels extend downwards in the pituitary stalk and break up into a capillary network within the anterior pituitary. The blood within them is rich in hypothalamic secretions.

The remaining blood supply comes from another portal system made up of short portal vessels that originate in the distal part of the stalk and in the posterior pituitary. This neat vascular arrangement means that the hypothalamic chemical signals stimulating anterior pituitary function are directed in high concentration via the portal vessels to their targets in the anterior pituitary.

Pituitary Disorders

Disorders of the pituitary may be expressed in *two* main ways:

1) **Quantitative disturbances in endocrine function:**
   - **hyperpituitarism**, usually due to the presence of a functioning neoplasm arising from one of the cell types of the anterior pituitary
   - **hypopituitarism**, most commonly due to destruction of functional pituitary tissue; the most common causes are the presence of a non-hormone-secreting neoplasm, postpartum pituitary infarction (Sheehan's syndrome) and pressure atrophy of the anterior pituitary associated with a defect in the sheet of connective tissue that covers the sella (the 'empty sella syndrome')

2) **Local manifestations of a space-occupying intracranial lesion.** These most often arise from functional changes in the optic chiasma. The clinical features most often include:
   - visual defects, of which bitemporal hemianopia is the classic example
   - headache
   - diplopia which is not due to paralysis of ocular muscles
   - pallor of the optic discs

HYPOPITUITARISM

In any endocrine organ, hypofunction may be the result of:
- **lack of adequate amounts of functioning tissue**
- **lack of drive**
- **lack of substrate**
- **lack of enzymes involved in biosynthetic pathways**

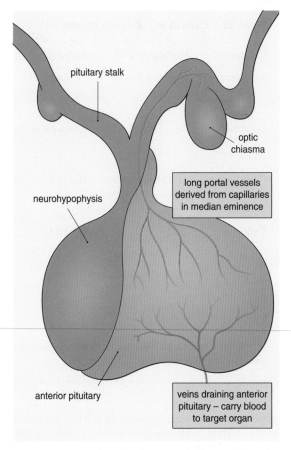

FIGURE 40.1 *Vascular supply of the anterior pituitary.*

In the pituitary, only the first two of these are involved in hypofunction; lack of sufficient functioning tissue is by far the most important (*Fig. 40.2*).

Hypopituitarism due to Lack of Sufficient Functioning Tissue

A lack of functioning tissue (*Fig. 40.3*), in any anatomical situation, may result from:
- failure of the organ to develop adequately in the first place
- destruction of part or whole of a normally developed organ

Failure of the Anterior Pituitary to Develop
Developmental failure may occur in two ways:

1) **because of defective formation of its anlage, Rathke's pouch.** This is a rare abnormality associated with differing degrees of hypopituitarism.

2) **in embryos with anencephaly.** This is because of absence of the hypothalamus and, thus, of any neurohormonal regulation. A posterior lobe may or may not be present and, within the anterior pituitary, the corticotropes are affected most severely.

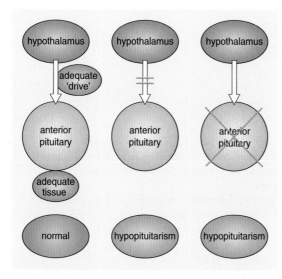

FIGURE 40.2 *Basic mechanisms leading to hypopituitarism.*

Destruction of Pituitary Tissue

The causes of destructive hypopituitarism are shown in *Table 40.3*. Only the most common of these (marked with an asterisk) are discussed. **Pituitary and parapituitary tumours constitute the commonest single cause, accounting for more than half the cases.** Of the tumours in and around the pituitary, adenomas within the gland make up the majority. Such adenomas may be **secretory** or **nonsecretory**. In the former, the clinical picture may be dominated by overproduction of one or other pituitary hormone, but it is worth remembering that the expansile growth pattern of the tumour may lead to atrophy of the non-involved portion of the gland and, thus, to hypopituitarism.

Pituitary and Parapituitary Tumours Causing Hypopituitarism

Non-secreting Pituitary Adenoma

Adenomas in the pituitary are divided into two classes based on size:

* **microadenoma** less than 10 mm in diameter
* **macroadenoma** greater than 10 mm in diameter

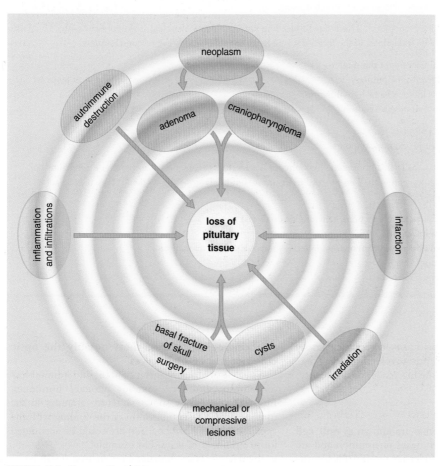

FIGURE 40.3 *Causes of loss of functioning pituitary tissue.*

Table 40.3 Destructive Lesions Causing Hypopituitarism

Basic pathology	Circumstances under which the lesion occurs
Neoplasms	**Pituitary adenoma*** **Craniopharyngioma*** Other parasellar primary tumours such as meningioma Metastatic tumour
Infarction	**Sheehan's syndrome.** This results from severe ischaemic necrosis of the pituitary, most commonly following a severe fall of blood pressure during the late stages of pregnancy or in the course of parturition. Such falls in blood pressure are commonly associated with serious haemorrhage at or around the time of delivery. During pregnancy, a marked degree of pituitary enlargement occurs, the gland reaching a size of almost twice normal. This increase in bulk also affects the sinusoidal vessels, which become compressed. These developments make the gland vulnerable to any drop in perfusion pressure. It has been suggested that disseminated intravascular coagulation may also play a part in the genesis of this ischaemic necrosis. The major presenting features are: • hypoprolactinaemia with inability to lactate postpartum • hypothyroidism • hypoadrenalism Rarely, Sheehan's syndrome may occur in non-pregnant females or in males. Such patients have a compromised pituitary perfusion due to such conditions as diabetes mellitus with severe small vessel disease or sickle cell disease. Pituitary 'apoplexy'. This is due to bleeding into a pituitary adenoma. It may present with extreme suddenness in the form of severe headache followed by loss of consciousness.
Other mechanical or compressive lesions	Basal fractures of the skull Surgery to the pituitary Cysts in the sella or hypothalamus The 'empty sella syndrome'. This is a rare cause of hypofunction
Irradiation	For a pituitary lesion For head and neck tumours
Autoimmune	Occasionally an autoimmune hypophysitis is seen that is analogous to autoimmune adrenalitis but much less common. This process occurs most commonly in young women, often in association with pregnancy.
Inflammation and infiltrations	Acute bacterial infections – meningitis or abscess Viral infections Granulomatous inflammation, especially sarcoidosis and tuberculosis Histiocytosis X Haemochromatosis

Non-functioning adenomas cause hypopituitarism by producing atrophy of the non-involved gland. These fall, most frequently, into the macroadenoma category.

Null Cell Adenoma

Most non-secreting adenomas are known as **null cell tumours**. They are by no means uncommon and are found more commonly in older age groups. Their principal clinical features relate to **pressure effects on surrounding structures, most notably the optic chiasma and cranial nerves**.

The cells are usually chromophobic and immunohistochemistry shows no anterior pituitary hormones. Electron microscopy shows secretory granules in the tumour cells. The combination of this finding with the apparent lack of hormonal activity could be accounted for in a number of ways. For example:

• the rate of normal hormone production might be too low to have any biological effect

- the granule contents might represent biologically inactive hormones
- the granule contents might represent precursor molecules only
- the granule contents might be products which, thus far, have been neither identified nor characterized

Oncocytic Adenoma

This is a variant of null cell adenoma in which the number of mitochondria is greatly increased, giving the tumour cells a granular appearance. In some cases these tumours are very large and are associated with slight increases in prolactin levels. This is not due to synthesis of prolactin by the tumour cells, but to **interference with the passage of dopamine from the hypothalamus** to the pituitary down the portal vessels in the stalk. Dopamine normally inhibits the release of prolactin from the lactotropes and, in its absence, more hormone is released.

Silent Adenoma

Occasionally, adenomas occur in which the majority of the tumour cells show immunoreactivity for one or other pituitary hormone, most frequently adrenocorticotropic hormone (ACTH) or other portions of the pro-opiomelanocortin molecule (POMC). Despite this, the affected patients show no evidence of hyperfunction of the pituitary. These tumours are known as 'silent adenomas'. The reason for this discrepancy between morphology and function is unknown. It may be that the hormones secreted by the tumour cells are biologically inactive or that there may be some block to the release of the hormones from the tumour cells.

Lesions of the Parasellar Region

The commonest of these is craniopharyngioma.

Craniopharyngioma

Craniopharyngioma occurs most commonly in children, accounting for 5–10% of all brain tumours in children. It also occurs in adults; about 25% are found in patients aged over 40 years at the time of presentation. It has been suggested that the tumour arises from squamous cell rests representing the remains of Rathke's pouch.

Most are suprasellar, although occasional intrasellar examples occur. The majority are histologically benign, but infiltration into surrounding tissues is sometimes seen.

> ### Macroscopic Features
>
> Craniopharyngiomas are usually 3–4 cm in diameter and may be solid or cystic; the cyst contents often contain large amounts of crystalline cholesterol. Focal calcification is an extremely common finding, present in 75% or more of these lesions, often to a degree that is obvious on skull radiography.

> ### Microscopic Features
>
> The microscopic appearances resemble those seen in the epithelial tumour of the jaw known as **ameloblastoma**. Solid tumour consists of islands of epithelial cells. These tend to be interlinked and show a **palisaded outer layer and an inner zone composed of cells with a stellate appearance.** These last two features are very helpful in diagnostic terms. Foci of squamous cells and areas of degeneration and calcification are quite common.

Clinical Features

The clinical presentations of craniopharyngioma fall into three groups (*Fig. 40.4*):

1) **visual symptoms and signs** including loss of visual acuity and the development of visual field defects. The commonest of these is bitemporal hemianopia.
2) **evidence of endocrine dysfunction**
3) **evidence of increased intracranial pressure** due to interference with the normal flow of the cerebrospinal fluid (hydrocephalus). This tends to occur particularly in children with craniopharyngioma, about 80% showing signs of increased intracranial pressure in the form of headache, vomiting and papilloedema.

Endocrine Dysfunction

In craniopharyngioma, disturbances may be seen in relation to:

- **Growth.** In childhood cases, the majority of the patients show some deficiencies in growth hormone secretion and up to 40% are of short stature showing retarded bone growth on radiological examination.
- **Adrenotropic function.** Pituitary adrenal dysfunction may be present in 50% of patients.

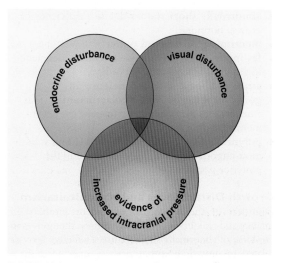

FIGURE 40.4 Pathophysiological effects of craniopharyngioma.

- **Gonadotropic function.** This is very common among adult patients, with complaints of loss of libido, menstrual irregularities or impotence being the most common.
- **Diabetes insipidus** is quite a common occurrence and obesity, sleepiness and disturbances in temperature regulation may also be seen, indicating a disturbance in hypothalamic function.
- **Thyrotropic function.** Low serum thyroxine levels are common and some patients have an inadequate thyroid-stimulating hormone (TSH; thyrotropin) response to administration of thyrotropin-releasing hormone.

CLINICAL FEATURES OF HYPOPITUITARISM

The clinical features of hypopituitarism reflect reduced or absent secretion of one of the hormones produced by the gland. In cases due to tissue loss, about 75% of the functioning tissue needs to be lost before manifestations of reduced function are noted.

Rarely, the clinical syndrome will reflect diminished secretion of *all* pituitary hormones (so-called **panhypopituitarism**), but more often the production of one hormone appears to be particularly affected (selective hypopituitarism). Selective hypopituitarism most commonly affects the production of growth hormone and the gonadotropic hormones. If the hypopituitarism results from the presence of a non-secreting pituitary adenoma, TSH, ACTH and antidiuretic hormone (ADH) secretions are the last to be lost.

In general terms, hypopituitarism is expressed in the form of:

- **deficiency in the secretion of one or more 'target' endocrine glands** such as the thyroid or adrenal. If this is accompanied by a low plasma concentration of the appropriate pituitary hormone, then either pituitary or hypothalamic dysfunction should be suspected (*Table 40.4* and *Fig. 40.5*).
- **abnormally short stature** due to a deficiency of growth hormone
- **incomplete or delayed puberty**
- **fasting hypoglycaemia** due to either a deficiency in growth hormone, ACTH or both
- **amenorrhoea due to a deficiency in gonadotropins or hyperprolactinaemia.** This amenorrhoea may be primary (patient has never menstruated) or secondary.
- **polyuria** due to a deficiency in ADH. This is the most important sign of loss of function in the posterior pituitary.

Growth Disturbances and Hypopituitarism

Disorders of the hypothalamus and/or pituitary in infancy and childhood commonly express themselves in the form of abnormally short stature. Defective growth related to growth hormone activity may occur in a number of different ways (*Fig. 40.6*):

Table 40.4 Expressions of Endocrine Target Gland Deficiencies in Hypopituitarism

Gland	Symptoms
Thyroid	Intolerance to cold, drowsiness, fatigability, constipation
Adrenal	Fatigue, weakness, weight loss, nausea and vomiting, hypoglycaemia
Gonads	Decrease in libido, alterations in menstruation, infertility, impotence, small prostate, soft testes, breast atrophy, atrophy of vagina and labia, 'eunuchoidal' habitus if hypopituitarism was prepubertal
Prolactin deficiency	Failure to lactate postpartum
Growth hormone deficiency	May be no symptoms in adults other than sometimes fasting hypoglycaemia. Various growth defects in children
Antidiuretic hormone deficiency	Nocturia, polyuria, increased thirst

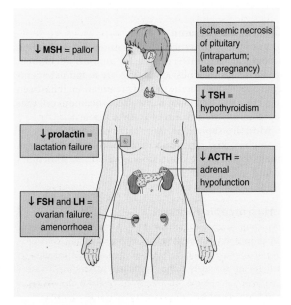

FIGURE 40.5 *Target organ failure in Sheehan's syndrome.*

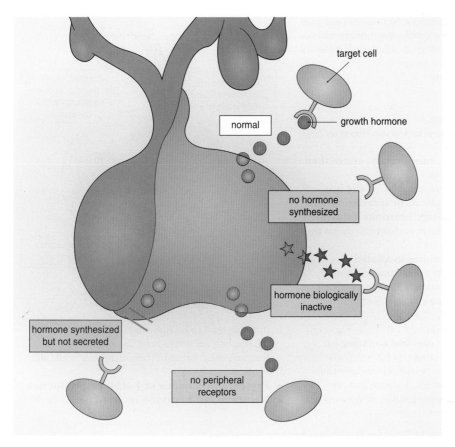

FIGURE 40.6 *Failures of growth may derive from a number of abnormalities involving pituitary secretions.*

- **There is an absolute deficiency of growth hormone synthesis by the adenohypophysis.** This may be inherited (there are several different inheritance patterns) and may be expressed either as isolated growth hormone deficiency or as multiple hormone deficiencies.

  Any trauma or disease process that affects the hypothalamopituitary axis in infancy and childhood may produce the same effect. Gliomas arising in the region of the optic chiasma in young infants may cause the diencephalic syndrome in which the affected children show severe emaciation, few, if any, neurological disturbances, and are alert and happy.
- **The rate of secretion of growth hormone is normal but the molecule is biologically inactive.**
- **The rate of secretion of growth hormone is normal and the hormone is biologically active, but there is a lack of growth-hormone binding receptors in the liver. The liver therefore fails to respond to growth hormone by making the ultimate effector molecule, insulin-like growth factor 1 (IGF-1;** somatomedin C).** This condition is known as Laron dwarfism.
- **The growth hormone is synthesized normally and is biologically active but there is a defect in secretion of the peptide into the blood.** Normal children usually have more than six episodes of growth hormone secretion per day. In the case of growth hormone 'neurosecretory dysfunction', the number of secretory episodes is usually fewer than four.

HYPERPITUITARISM

While hyperpituitarism can occur as a result of an increased drive by hormone-releasing signals to the pituitary, by far the commonest cause of pituitary hyperfunction is a secreting tumour of the anterior pituitary.

PITUITARY ADENOMAS

Pituitary adenomas are benign epithelial neoplasms arising from one or other of the cell components of the anterior pituitary. In neurosurgical practice they constitute 10–15% of all intracranial tumours and may be found in 6–24% of unselected post-mortem examinations. The pathophysiological effects of pituitary tumours fall into two major classes:

- **endocrine dysfunction**
- **local pressure effects**

Endocrine Dysfunction

Pituitary adenoma may cause endocrine effects by (*Fig. 40.7*):

- **oversecreting one or, more rarely, more than one pituitary hormone**
- **causing either pressure atrophy of the non-involved part of the gland, or interfering with the discharge of pituitary hormone-releasing factors**, derived from the hypothalamus, down the stalk
- **interfering with dopamine-mediated inhibition of prolactin secretion**, and thus causing hyperprolactinaemia. This, too, is related to interference with the pituitary stalk (see p 825).

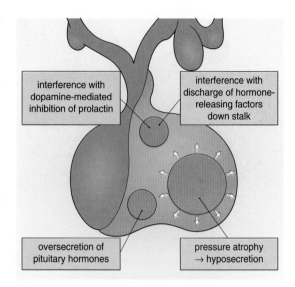

FIGURE 40.7 *Pituitary adenomas can cause endocrine disturbances in a number of ways.*

Classification

Pituitary adenomas may be classified according to:

- **Size** (see p 823). Large tumours (*Fig. 40.8*) are more difficult to remove completely and are thus more likely to recur than small lesions that are entirely within the sella turcica. The larger pituitary tumours tend to be non-functioning; the functioning adenomas tend to call attention to themselves by virtue of their secretions while still small.
- **Presence or absence of hormone production**
- **Nature of the hormone secreted** (see *Table 40.5*)

Table 40.5 Classification of Pituitary Adenomas by their Secretions

Cell type	Product	Percentage of cases	Syndrome
Lactotropic cells	Prolactin	26	Hyperprolactinaemia, amenorrhoea, galactorrhoea, infertility, decreased libido, impotence
Null cells	0	17	Pressure effects
Somatotropic cells	Growth hormone	14	Acromegaly or gigantism
Corticotropic cells	ACTH and other cleavage products of POMC	15	Cushing's disease; the tumours are usually microadenomas
Plurihormonal adenoma. May be made up of one cell type producing two hormones or of two cell types, each producing one hormone	Most often growth hormone and prolactin; other combinations may be seen	13	Acromegaly and mild hyperprolactinaemia
Gonadotropic cells	FSH and LH	8	
Oncocytic non-secreting cells	0	6	Pressure effects
Thyrotropic cells	TSH	1	Hyperthyroidism if thyroid is normal and can respond to the increased TSH level

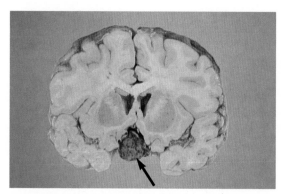

FIGURE 40.8 A large pituitary adenoma showing haemorrhage (arrowed).

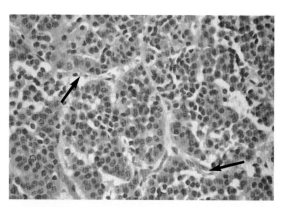

FIGURE 40.9 Chromophobe adenoma of the pituitary, stained with haematoxylin and eosin. Note the ribbon-like pattern of the tumour cells and the sinusoidal blood supply (arrows).

- **Growth pattern of the tumour.** Pituitary tumours may have either an expansile growth pattern or, more rarely, an invasive one. They may be confined within the boundaries of the sella or extend into the surrounding tissues. **Those with an expansile growth pattern generally grow slowly and have well-defined margins** marked by condensed reticulin fibres and by the compressed cells of the surrounding normal pituitary tissue. Some intrasellar adenomas have a **diffuse growth pattern** and fill the sella, on occasion, eroding its wall.

    Invasive adenomas grow faster than those with an expansile growth pattern. They usually erode the wall of the sella and spread to involve such structures as the sphenoid bone, the cavernous sinus and the posterior pituitary and hypophysial stalk. In addition to causing local effects because of pressure on the optic chiasma and cranial nerves, they may involve the brain substance including, of course, the hypothalamus.

    True carcinomas of the anterior pituitary do exist, although they are very uncommon. They behave in a frankly malignant fashion and can give rise to metastases at distant sites. In some instances these malignant tumours show the expected histological signs of malignancy such as nuclear pleomorphism, abundant and atypical mitoses, and focal necrosis. In others, the tumours behave in a malignant way but do not show morphological evidence of malignancy; and examples have also been described in which there is histological evidence of malignancy but the tumours do not give rise to distant metastases.

Prolactin-producing Adenoma

This is the commonest of the secreting pituitary adenomas. It can occur at any age but is most often seen in young women. On haematoxylin and eosin staining, the tumour cells are chromophobes (*Fig. 40.9*) in most instances, but the use of antibodies raised against prolactin provides histological confirmation of

the diagnosis. Amyloid deposition in the stroma of the tumour is a fairly common finding. It has no diagnostic significance as it may be seen in other types of pituitary adenoma from time to time.

Prolactin secretion differs from that of other hormones of the adenohypophysis in that it is under tonic inhibitory control by the hypothalamus, mediated by dopamine. This has important implications for treatment. If the prolactin-secreting tumour is a microadenoma, then the use of a dopamine agonist such as bromocriptine can effectively restore blood prolactin levels to normal. In the case of macroadenomas, functional normality is achieved much less often, but the use of bromocriptine can produce significant shrinkage of the tumour.

The clinical effects of prolactinaemia are summarized in *Fig. 40.10*.

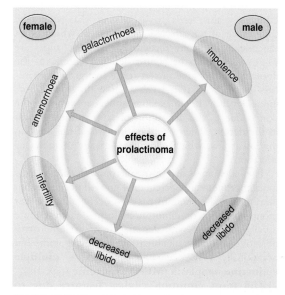

FIGURE 40.10 The clinical effects of prolactinaemia in males and females.

Growth Hormone-secreting Adenomas

Adenomas consisting of somatotropic cells secrete large amounts of growth hormone and are associated with:

- **gigantism, if epiphysial union has not occurred in the skeleton**
- **acromegaly, if epiphysial union has occurred**

Occasionally these syndromes may be due to ectopic production of either growth hormone or GHRH by a tumour outside the pituitary.

Microscopic Features

The tumour cells are either acidophilic or chromophobe. Electron microscopy shows the acidophilic tumours to be densely granulated, whereas chromophobe cell adenomas usually contain few granules. This is significant as densely granulated tumours tend to grow slowly, are more easily removed at surgery and recur less often than do the sparsely granulated adenomas. The electron-dense granules in somatotropic cell tumours tend to be uniform in size, whereas those in prolactinoma tend to be variable in both size and shape.

Clinical Features

The principal biological effect of growth hormone is to increase protein secretion. **This effect is mediated to a very considerable extent via insulin-like growth factors (IGFs; somatomedins)**; it should be remembered that deficiencies in growth may arise because of a lack of either growth hormone or IGF.

Acromegaly

In adults excess growth hormone secretion leads to acromegaly, a disorder in which there is marked overgrowth of bone and connective tissue. Ultimately this leads to a striking change in the appearance of the affected individual, at which point the disease is usually recognized. These changes are so common as to be almost defining criteria of the disorder. The degree of soft tissue overgrowth correlates better with IGF levels than with growth hormone levels. The thickening and coarsening of the skin is due to the deposition of glycosoaminoglycans in the dermis. There is excess growth of the bone in the lower jaw, which contributes greatly to the facial alterations.

The adenomas that cause acromegaly are usually monomorphous and secrete only growth hormone, but plurihormonal adenomas do occur (in either monomorphous or dimorphous forms) and these are usually associated with acromegaly as well. Growth hormone-secreting adenomas are usually sporadic but occasionally may occur as part of the **multiple endocrine neoplasia (MEN) syndrome** (type I).

The most common clinical features due to excess growth hormone secretion are shown in *Table 40.6* **and** *Fig. 40.11*:

Table 40.6 Clinical Features of Acromegaly

Clinical feature	Frequency (%)
Acral (limbs, fingers and toes) growth causing enlargement of the hands and feet, and **skin changes**	98
Oligomenorrhoea or amenorrhoea in females	72
Excessive sweating	64
Headaches	55
Paraesthesia or carpal tunnel syndrome, which is associated with thickening of the peripheral nerves and eventual nerve compression	40
Impotence	36
Carbohydrate intolerance. This ranges from abnormal glucose tolerance to overt diabetes, which is found in 10–25% of acromegalic patients	50
Hypertension	25–35

The Cardiovascular System in Acromegaly Cardiac disease is present in about a third of acromegalic patients and is a major contributor to the increased mortality associated with this disorder. In addition to high blood pressure, many patients show concentric thickening of the wall of the left ventricle (not surprising in hypertension), asymmetric septal hypertrophy and a reduced systolic ejection fraction. Myocardial ischaemia, congestive cardiac failure and arrhythmias are all rather common events in acromegalic patients. Cardiac muscle changes can occur in the absence of hypertension or stenosing coronary artery atherosclerosis; thus excess growth hormone may have a direct effect on cardiac muscle in some cases.

Rheumatological Changes in Acromegaly Symptoms and signs referable to joints occur in 50–75% of patients with acromegaly. Most of the joint abnormalities are degenerative in nature. The knee is the peripheral joint most commonly involved, followed, in decreasing order of frequency, by the shoulder, hip, ankle, elbow and joints of the hand. Pain at rest is not uncommon, and swelling and stiffness of the affected joints are also frequently seen. Pain in the spine occurs in about 50%

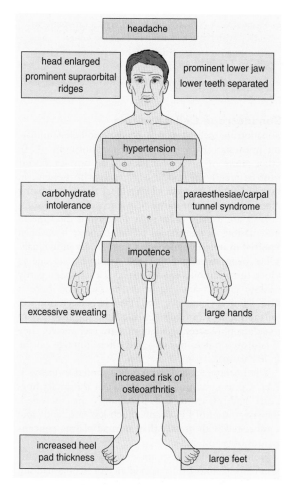

headache

head enlarged
prominent supraorbital
ridges

prominent lower jaw
lower teeth separated

hypertension

carbohydrate
intolerance

paraesthesiae/carpal
tunnel syndrome

impotence

excessive sweating

large hands

increased risk of
osteoarthritis

increased heel
pad thickness

large feet

FIGURE 40.11 *Clinical features of acromegaly.*

of acromegalics and appears to be related to the formation of new bony processes (osteophytes) and to widening of the disc spaces.

The changes in the joints seen in acromegaly are due to the increases in local and circulating concentrations of IGF-1 that result from excess secretion of growth hormone. IGF-1 binds to receptors on the cartilage cells and causes these cells both to increase in number and to secrete more cartilage matrix. The resulting cartilage thickening leads to widening of the joint spaces and to changes in the normal geometry of the affected joints. In addition there is an increase in the growth of periarticular structures such as ligaments, which tend to become laxer than normal. This laxity of the ligaments increases the uneven mechanical loading of the joint. As a result, the cartilage wears unevenly and fissures in the same way as in osteoarthritis, to which the final joint appearances in acromegaly bear a strong resemblance.

Aetiology

There is controversy as to whether growth hormone-producing adenomas arise *de novo* in the adenohypophysis or are the result of excess stimulus from the hypothalamus. If excess hypothalamic drive were the only, or even the principal, cause, evidence of hyperplasia of somatotropes would be expected in that part of the anterior pituitary not involved by tumour. No such evidence is present, pointing to an intrinsic pituitary origin for the adenomas. This view finds support from the fact that the lesions appear to be monoclonal, arising, therefore, from a single precursor cell that has been altered genomically.

Genomic Alterations in Growth Hormone-producing Adenoma

At the molecular level in any tissue, neoplastic transformation may occur either because:
- **a dominant mutation leads to excessive growth promotion**
- **there has been a deletion or mutation of a growth-inhibiting gene (a tumour suppressor gene)**

Both of these may operate in relation to growth hormone-producing adenomas.

When GHRH, derived from the hypothalamus, binds to the somatotropic cells it activates a stimulating G protein. These G proteins transduce the signals generated as a result of ligand–receptor binding, by activating the adenylate cyclase system. Two groups of growth hormone-producing adenomas have been identified in respect of this G protein – cyclic 5′-adenosine monophosphate (cAMP) coupling:

1) The first of these has a normal adenylate cyclase response to GHRH and normal basal levels of intracellular cAMP.

2) The second has raised basal levels of cAMP which do not rise further as a result of GHRH stimulation. The basal level of cAMP is 24 times as great as in the type I tumours, and the basal rate of growth hormone secretion is five times as great as in type I tumours. **Thus, in the type II tumour, the stimulating G protein appears to be constitutively 'switched on' in the absence of ligand–receptor binding**. This appears to be due to the presence of point mutations in the α chains of the G protein, which prevent it from exerting its guanosine triphosphatase function. This tumour-associated mutation has been termed *gsp* and may result either from arginine at position 201 being replaced by cysteine or histidine, or from glutamine at position 227 being replaced by arginine.

Deletion of suppressor genes appears to be involved in the pituitary adenomas forming part of the MEN type I syndrome (parathyroid, pancreatic and pituitary tumours). The MEN-I susceptibility locus maps to **chromosome 11q13** and may undergo recessive mutations in affected individuals.

Pituitary Gigantism

If excess growth hormone is present in the blood during childhood or adolescence, affected individuals become extremely tall. The syndrome is known as **pituitary gigantism** and is very rare. The most common cause is a pituitary adenoma arising from somatotropes; occasionally this syndrome may develop either because of excess GHRH secretion, or because there is an ectopic source of growth hormone from an extrapituitary tumour such as, for example, a pancreatic islet tumour.

Corticotrope Cell (ACTH-secreting) Adenomas

Corticotrope cell adenomas produce excess ACTH and other cleavage products of the POMC molecule. They are responsible for about 70% of cases of Cushing's syndrome in adults (see pp 840–842) and are associated with Nelson's syndrome.

Nelson's syndrome is the term used to describe the growth of an ACTH-secreting adenoma in the pituitary following bilateral adrenalectomy in a patient with Cushing's disease. It almost certainly represents progression of a pre-existing microadenoma arising from corticotropes. This progression is due to the removal of the inhibiting influence of the previously high plasma cortisol levels as a result of the adrenalectomy; the very high ACTH levels that occur in Nelson's syndrome can be suppressed with large doses of cortisol.

Following bilateral adrenalectomy for Cushing's disease:

- 30% of the patients develop classical Nelson's syndrome with high ACTH levels and progressive hyperpigmentation. This hyperpigmentation is due to the increased secretion of melanocyte-stimulating hormone (MSH), which is the inevitable consequence of high secretion rates of POMC, of which MSH is a cleavage product.
- 50% show evidence of a microadenoma that does not progress
- 20% do not develop a pituitary adenoma

The tumours associated with Nelson's syndrome tend to be fast growing and thus these patients tend to present with both hyperpigmentation and clinical symptoms and signs due to the local space-occupying effects of the adenoma.

Microscopic Features

The adenomas responsible for Cushing's disease are most commonly microadenomas. In conventionally stained material, they are most often basophilic, although occasionally chromophobe adenomas cause Cushing's disease. Immunohistochemical staining shows ACTH and other cleavage fragments of POMC within the tumour cells. On electron microscopy, bundles of microfilaments are often seen within the cells. In the adenomas associated with Nelson's syndrome, which otherwise are identical with those occurring in Cushing's disease, these microfilaments are not present. The reason for this is not known.

Gonadotrope Cell Adenoma

Gonadotrope cell adenomas produce follicle-stimulating hormone (FSH) and luteinizing hormone (LH), either alone or in combination. The tumour occurs most frequently in middle-aged men who present, in most instances, because of the local space-occupying effects of the tumour rather than for endocrine reasons. Patients are usually older than 40 years at the time of presentation, but examples of this tumour have been reported in much younger and much older individuals. It has been suggested that the relatively late age at which these tumours are diagnosed is a reflection partly of slow growth and partly of the fact that there is little clinical evidence of the hypersecretion of gonadotropins. Certainly, by the time the majority of gonadotropin-secreting adenomas are recognized, they have grown out of the sella and often impinge on the optic chiasma.

The hormone most commonly secreted to excess is FSH. Concentrations in the plasma of the intact hormone and of its α and β subunits are increased. Hypersecretion of LH occurs much less frequently and is associated with greater than normal plasma concentrations of testosterone.

From the endocrine point of view, the most common clinical abnormality is evidence of hypogonadism. Decreased libido and impotence are relatively frequent findings.

Microscopic Features

In conventionally stained material most gonadotrope adenomas are chromophobe, but the function of these cells can be established by the use of appropriate immunostaining.

Thyrotrope Adenomas

Thyrotropin-secreting adenomas are rare. **They occur most commonly in individuals who have primary hypothyroidism.** The assumption is that low levels of thyroid hormone cause large amounts of thyrotropin-releasing hormone to be secreted from the hypothalamus and that the chronic stimulatory 'drive' on the thyrotropes leads first to hyperplasia and later to adenoma formation. Despite the fact that normal thyrotropes stain basophilically in haematoxylin and eosin-stained sections, most thyrotrope cell adenomas are chromophobic.

More rarely a thyrotrope cell adenoma arises *de novo* in the pituitary in an individual whose thyroid function is normal. **In these patients hyperthyroidism may be the consequence of the excess TSH secreted by the pituitary adenoma.**

DISORDERS OF THE NEUROHYPOPHYSIS

Normal Structure and Function

The neurohypophysis (posterior lobe of the pituitary) is an extension of the ventral portion of the hypothalamus. It is attached to the dorsal and caudal surface of the adenohypophysis (anterior lobe of the pituitary). It is divided by the diaphragm of the sella into an upper portion known as the median eminence or infundibulum, and a lower portion known as the pars nervosa.

The cellular components of the neurohypophysis consist of:

- **unmyelinated axons originating from the supraoptic and paraventricular nuclei of the hypothalamus** and, to a lesser extent, from its cholinergic neurones.
- **specialized glial cells known as pituicytes.** In the same way as astrocytes, the pituicytes react with antibodies raised against glial fibrillary acidic protein (GFAP). The secretion products of the posterior pituitary – oxytocin and vasopressin – accumulate within the axons. There appear to be two types of neurosecretory axon:
  1) Type A, the more numerous, contains relatively large (300 nm in diameter) granules in which oxytocin and vasopressin are stored.
  2) Type B axons contain smaller granules (50–100 nm in diameter) in which, it is believed, amines are stored.

Biological Functions of Neurohypophysial Secretions

Vasopressin (ADH)

Vasopressin conserves body water by reducing urine output. This antidiuretic effect is achieved by the reabsorption of solute-free water from the distal and collecting tubules in the kidney, the membranes of which are rendered more permeable to water by the vasopressin.

Oxytocin

The principal biological function of oxytocin is in relation to breastfeeding. The hormone causes the ejection of milk from the ducts by causing contraction of the myoepithelial cells that lie peripheral to the breast duct epithelium.

Deficiency in Vasopressin Secretion

The commonest and most important disorder of the neurohypophysis is a deficiency in vasopressin secretion. This produces the syndrome known as diabetes insipidus, characterized by:

- **polyuria** (due to failure to reabsorb adequate amounts of water from the glomerular filtrate)
- **hyperosmolarity** of the blood

Diabetes insipidus may occur because of:

- **a deficiency of vasopressin secretion – hypothalamic diabetes insipidus**
- **decreased sensitivity to normal vasopressin concentrations by the renal tubular cells – nephrogenic diabetes insipidus**
- **ingestion of excessive volumes of fluids leading to vasopressin suppression and polyuria – primary polydipsia**

Most cases of hypothalamic diabetes insipidus are due to damage to either the neurohypophysis or the hypothalamus itself. The disorders encountered in this region may be familial (rarely) or acquired as shown in *Table 40.7*.

Inappropriate or Excessive Antidiuresis

Just as polyuria and plasma hyperosmolality may develop in the absence of adequate secretion of

Table 40.7 Causes of Hypothalamic Diabetes Insipidus

Type	Causes
Familial	Hereditary: X-linked recessive or autosomal dominant '**DIDMOAD**' an association of *d*iabetes *i*nsipidus with *d*iabetes *m*ellitus, *o*ptic *a*trophy, nerve *d*eafness and atonia of the bladder and ureters
Acquired	Trauma, including neurosurgical trauma Tumours in the parasellar and suprasellar region. These include primary lesions such as craniopharyngioma and germ cell tumours as well as metastatic deposits in the hypothalamus or posterior pituitary, most commonly from carcinoma of the breast or bronchus Granulomatous disorders such as tuberculosis or sarcoidosis Infiltrations such as histiocytosis X Acute infections, both viral and bacterial Ischaemic necrosis Circulating antibodies to vasopressin-producing cells in the hypothalamus

vasopressin, so may the reverse occur if there is inappropriate secretion of this hormone. **The syndrome of inappropriate secretion of ADH is the commonest cause of hypo-osmolality in the presence of a normal plasma volume; indeed, it is the commonest cause of all varieties of hypo-osmolality (less than 275 mOsm per kg water), accounting for 30–40% of all hypo-osmolar patients.**

Disorders that cause inappropriate antidiuresis due to raised plasma levels of vasopressin may do so in one of two ways:
- the excess vasopressin secretion may be **ectopic** (i.e. it is not secreted by the neurohypophysis but in some other tissue – most frequently a tumour outside the central nervous system (CNS))
- the excess vasopressin is derived from the pituitary. There is evidence that, in some cases, this increased secretion is due to stimulation of the neurohypophysis by some product of an unrelated tumour.

Causes of inappropriate ADH (vasopressin) secretion include:
- **Tumours.** The most common cause for inappropriate vasopressin secretion is a tumour. Small-celled bronchogenic carcinoma is characteristically associated with the syndrome, although ectopic ADH secretion has been described, rarely, in association with squamous carcinoma of the bronchus. The syndrome has also been reported in association with some other intrathoracic tumours, such as thymoma, mesothelioma and Hodgkin's disease. Extrathoracic associations include carcinoma of the pancreas, duodenum, uterus and prostate.
- **Disorders of the CNS.** A variety of disorders of the CNS can cause inappropriate secretion of ADH. The neurones that produce vasopressin receive input from a number of sources including the osmoreceptor cells of the anterior hypothalamus and centres in the brainstem. **Some of these inputs are believed to be inhibitory and it has been suggested that interruption of such inhibitory pathways may lead to increased secretion of ADH.** Pathways leading from the brainstem to the hypothalamus are long and probably contain many synapses. Any diffuse disorder of the CNS may be able to disrupt these pathways at some point and thus remove the restraint on overproduction of ADH.
- **Drugs.** Administration of certain compounds can cause hypo-osmolality. A number of different mechanisms may be involved, including:
    a) a direct stimulating effect on the posterior pituitary
    b) direct activation of vasopressin receptors in the kidney by the drug with a resulting antidiuretic effect
    c) upregulating the effect of normal concentrations of vasopressin on the kidney

- **Disorders of the lung.** Inappropriate secretion of vasopressin can occur in patients with non-neoplastic lung disorders. In most of these the hypo-osmolality has developed against a background of acute respiratory failure in which hypoxia and/or hypercapnia are present. It is of considerable interest that mechanical ventilation can itself cause inappropriate secretion of vasopressin and can worsen such inappropriate secretion if present.

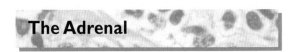

The Adrenal

NORMAL ANATOMY AND DEVELOPMENT

The adrenals are paired organs, each normally weighing 4–5 g. Each consists of two portions – the **cortex** and **medulla – which are histologically, functionally and embryologically distinct.**

During fetal life the cortex is divided into two zones:
- a large, central zone known as the **fetal cortex**, which starts to disappear after birth
- a thin outer layer, the **definitive cortex**, which survives and becomes divided into three functional areas during early childhood, described below in the section on the cortex

Cortical growth during gestation depends on stimulation from the pituitary, **and thus anencephaly is associated with adrenal hypoplasia.**

The **adrenal medulla** arises from primitive cells of the sympathetic nervous system known as **sympathogonia**. These differentiate into:
- **neuroblasts**, which form the sympathetic ganglia lying on either side of the vertebrae and anterior to the aorta
- **phaeochromoblasts**, which differentiate into adrenal medullary cells. These secrete catecholamines, which bind chrome salts. It is this that has led to their being called **chromaffin cells**. After birth most of the chromaffin cell accumulations outside the adrenal involute, but some persist and account for the occurrence of extra-adrenal catecholamine-secreting tumours (**phaeochromocytomas**).

The Cortex
The adult cortex constitutes the peripheral 80% of the adrenal plus a cuff of cortical tissue surrounding the central vein. There are three functional zones:
1) **The zona glomerulosa (5–10%)** secretes **aldosterone**. It is a discontinuous layer of small cells with large nuclei and relatively little cytoplasmic lipid.

2) **The zona fasciculata** (80%) and the **zona reticularis** produce the same hormones (**cortisol** and **androgens**), but differ histologically. The zona fasciculata consists of cells arranged in columns two cells thick, bounded on each side by capillaries and perpendicular to the capsule. The cells are large and contain abundant cholesterol. In histological material treated with lipid solvents, they appear clear. Electron microscopy shows a well-developed Golgi apparatus because the steroid hormones are not stored.

3) **The zona reticularis** (5–10%) consists of anastomosing columns, one cell thick. In general, cells are smaller than those in the fasciculata and contain little lipid. These appearances have led to the term **compact cells** being applied.

Age and Stress-related Changes in the Adrenal Cortex

With ageing, small nodules appear in many adrenals and, as they grow larger, may compress surrounding tissue. They are more frequent in hypertensive and/or diabetic individuals.

At autopsy, especially after long illnesses, the adrenals often weigh significantly more than normal. **This is believed to be a response to stress** mediated via increased adrenocorticotropic hormone (ACTH) secretion by the anterior pituitary. The fasciculata cells lose their lipid content, resembling the compact cells of the reticularis.

The Medulla

The medulla, usually not more than 2 mm thick, occupies the central portion of the head and body of the gland and accounts for about 10% of adrenal weight. There is a single cell type, the **phaeochromocyte** (chromaffin cell). In material treated with chrome salts, these cells stain brown because of an oxidizing effect of adrenaline on these salts.

On electron microscopy the defining criterion is the presence of neurosecretory granules, the majority of which contain adrenaline (epinephrine), but noradrenaline-containing granules are also present.

HORMONES OF THE ADRENAL CORTEX

The adrenal cortex synthesizes and secretes about 50 different steroids in three main functional groups. **The commonest and most important diseases affecting the adrenal are expressed in terms of changes in one or more of these.** Disturbances that can result in either lack of hormones or their overproduction are best understood against a background of the normal state.

Three major groups of hormones are produced by the cortex; the production of each is related to a particular zone of the cortex (*Table 40.8*).

Table 40.8 Hormones Produced by the Adrenal Cortex

Hormone group	Principal site of production
Mineralocorticoids	Zona glomerulosa
Glucocorticoids	Zona fasciculata
Sex steroids	Zona reticularis

All these hormones share a common precursor, **cholesterol**, most of which is derived from low density lipoprotein.

Actions of Adrenal Steroids: Some General Principles

Adrenal steroids diffuse through target cell plasma membranes, bind to intracellular receptor proteins and cause selective upregulation or downregulation of gene transcription.

Six classes of receptor exist, each of which corresponds to a biological action of the steroid hormones:
- mineralocorticoid
- glucocorticoid
- progesterone
- oestrogen
- androgen
- vitamin D

The thyroid hormone receptor shows some degree of structural homology with the steroid receptors and belongs to the same gene family. It is important to remember that some steroids exert more than one effect in a given tissue because they may bind with more than one receptor. The biological effects of a steroid hormone depend on its binding affinities; thus, although cortisol binds to both glucocorticoid and mineralocorticoid receptors, its binding affinity for the former is much greater than for the latter. Thus cortisol exerts a powerful glucocorticoid effect and a relatively weak mineralocorticoid one. The principal actions of glucocorticoids are shown in *Table 40.9*.

Principal Actions of Mineralocorticoids

The chief members of the mineralocorticoid group are **aldosterone**, which is responsible for about 50% of mineralocorticoid activity, **11-deoxycorticosterone (DOC)** and **18-oxocortisol**.

Glucocorticoids show some mineralocorticoid activity but aldosterone is about 400 times as active as cortisol in this respect.

Mineralocorticoids **maintain a normal intravascular volume** by retention of sodium and elimination of potassium and hydrogen ions.

Target organs for mineralocorticoids include the kidney (the collecting tubules in particular), gut,

Table 40.9 Principal Actions of Glucocorticoids

Target process	Effects
Metabolism	**Carbohydrate** Inhibits action of insulin ↑ Blood sugar ↑ Gluconeogenesis ↓ Glucose uptake in tissues **Lipid** ↑ Lipolysis. Fat cells in different sites differently affected. Glucocorticoid causes fat loss from the extremities but accumulation in the trunk, neck and face **Protein** ↑ Protein breakdown
Immune system	↓ Circulating lymphocytes (T cells more than B cells) ↓ Antibody formation Causes thymic and lymphoid tissue atrophy ↓ Cell-mediated responses ↓ Resistance to infection ↓ Vascular events in acute inflammation ↓ Chemotaxis and phagocytosis
Connective tissue	↓ Collagen formation and impairs wound healing
Calcium and bone	↓ Serum calcium levels ↑ Osteoporosis
Circulatory system	Positive inotropic effect ↑ Cardiac output ↑ Sensitivity to catecholamines and in excess leads to hypertension
Kidney	↑ Renal blood flow and glomerular filtration rate ↑ Free water clearance ↓ Action of vasopressin ↑ Excretion of potassium and H^+. In excess leads to hypokalaemic alkalosis
Central nervous system	↓ Cerebral oedema ↓ Libido Causes mood lability and may produce psychosis in some patients
Growth	In pharmacological doses may inhibit bone growth In the fetus, important for development of the liver and gut, and for the production of surfactant in the lungs
Endocrine	↓ Response to thyroid-stimulating hormone ↓ Response to growth hormone-releasing hormone ↓ Secretion of gonadotropins These actions cause decreased production of gonadal steroids

salivary glands, sweat glands, vascular endothelium and brain.

A **deficiency of mineralocorticoids causes**:
- weight loss

- hypotension
- hyperkalaemia

A **mineralocorticoid** excess leads to:
- mild oedema

- hypertension
- hypokalaemia
- metabolic alkalosis

Principal Actions of Adrenal Androgens

The adrenal androgens are converted to active androgens such as testosterone, and to active oestrogens such as oestrone and oestradiol, and exert their effects via these products. In males less than 2% of androgens are derived from the adrenal but in females this rises to 50%. Normally adrenal androgens play a role in the development of pubic and axillary hair during puberty. In adrenal disease, they make significant contributions to the clinical picture in such disorders as:

- congenital adrenal hyperplasia
- functioning adrenal tumours
- Cushing's syndrome
- premature adrenarche (maturation in the adrenal which leads to increased androgen production between the ages of 6 and 16 years). The histological correlate of this is the appearance and development of the zona reticularis.

Regulation of Adrenal Steroid Secretion

Cortisol secretion is regulated by ACTH, a 39-amino-acid peptide produced by the anterior pituitary. ACTH is cleaved from a larger precursor molecule known as **pro-opiomelanocortin (POMC)**, which is the source of both ACTH and β-lipotropin. Both these molecules are further cleaved to yield α- and β-melanocyte-stimulating hormone (**MSH**), β- and γ-endorphins and enkephalin. ACTH binding in the adrenal activates adenylate cyclase, leading to an increase in the concentration of cyclic 5′-adenosine monophosphate (cAMP). The cAMP activates a protein kinase that ultimately triggers **the first step in steroidogenesis – the conversion of cholesterol to pregnenolone.**

ACTH production is stimulated by hypothalamic release of corticotropin-releasing hormone (**CRH**). Vasopressin has a similar action and can act synergistically with CRH.

The release of both CRH and ACTH is mediated by the negative feedback effect of blood levels of cortisol that is exerted at both the hypothalamic and pituitary level.

Disorders of the Adrenal

HYPOFUNCTION OF THE ADRENAL CORTEX

The causes of adrenal cortical hypofunction can be summed up as follows:

- **lack of tissue**
- **lack of drive**
- **lack of enzymes**

LACK OF TISSUE

Hypofunction due to lack of functioning cortical tissue may occur as a **chronic** disorder, as in Addison's disease, as an **acute phase** in patients with Addison's disease or in those on long-term steroid treatment in whom sudden steroid withdrawal occurs, and as a **hyperacute phenomenon associated with haemorrhagic necrosis of the cortex**, such as occurs in the **Waterhouse–Friedrichsen syndrome** associated with meningococcal septicaemia.

The two main causes of Addison's disease are **autoimmune adrenal destruction** and **tuberculosis** (*Fig. 40.12*).

In the West, autoimmune adrenalitis accounts for about 70% of cases of adrenal hypofunction caused by loss of cortical tissue. In economically and socially deprived populations, the commonest cause of adrenal cortical destruction is still tuberculosis.

The belief that adrenal destruction can be an autoimmune phenomenon is supported by a number of observations:

- **Antibodies directed against adrenal cortical antigens are found in about 65% of cases.** Similar antibodies are *not* present in adrenal cortical destruction from other causes.
- **Autoimmune Addison's disease is associated with a high prevalence of other organ-specific antibodies** such as react with thyroid, parathyroid, ovary, gastric mucosa and pancreatic islets.
- **Autoimmune Addison's disease tends to cluster in families. Increased prevalence of the major histocompatibility complex-coded antigens B8 and DR3 is noted** in patients, compared with that in control populations.
- **The microscopic appearances** resemble those seen in other autoimmune processes.
- **Immunization of certain strains of rats with homogenates of adrenal cortex and adjuvants**

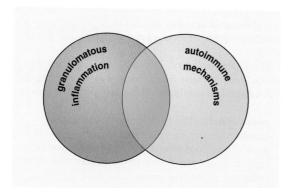

FIGURE 40.12 Causes of Addison's disease.

leads to an adrenalitis transferable by lymphoid cells.

About 40% of cases of autoimmune Addison's disease may be part of **polyglandular autoimmune deficiency syndromes**, as shown in *Table 40.10*.

Table 40.10 Polyglandular Autoimmune Deficiency Syndrome

Type	Combination
I	Addison's disease, hypoparathyroidism, mucocutaneous candidiasis (at least two of three are present)
II	Addison's disease, autoimmune thyroiditis and/or insulin-dependent diabetes mellitus
IIIa	Thyroid autoimmune disease and insulin-dependent diabetes mellitus
IIIb	Thyroid autoimmune disease and pernicious anaemia
IIIc	Thyroid autoimmune disease and vitiligo and/or alopecia and/or other organ-specific disorders

Type I, the commonest, is principally a disorder of childhood, the mean age of onset being 12 years. Type II tends to occur in young adults.

In Addison's disease due to tuberculosis, virtually the entire cortex is destroyed by caseating granulomas. Other important infective causes of Addison's disease include fungi, of which *Histoplasma capsulatum* is the most common.

The clinical features of chronic adrenal hypofunction are shown in *Table 40.11*.

Table 40.11 Clinical Features of Chronic Adrenal Hypofunction

Symptoms	Signs
Weakness, fatiguability, nausea, abdominal pain, diarrhoea and, occasionally, orthostatic hypotension. Some patients may complain of a craving for salt	Weight loss and hyperpigmentation of the skin, believed to be due to excess amounts of MSH, derived from cleavage of ACTH and β-lipotropin, which are secreted in large amounts as a result of the feedback effects of low plasma cortisol levels

Laboratory Findings

- **The commonest finding is a low plasma sodium concentration**, present in 90% of patients. High serum potassium levels occur in about 65% of patients. If the patient has been eating poorly, hypoglycaemia may occur.
- **Plasma cortisol levels are low.** In accordance with this, the urinary products of steroid metabolism, such as 17-oxogenic steroids, are similarly decreased.
- **If the adrenal insufficiency is due to destruction of tissue (so-called primary adrenal insufficiency), the plasma ACTH levels are likely to be higher than normal.** An ACTH infusion over a 2-day period, which normally increases urinary steroid excretion quite markedly, is without effect in adrenal hypofunction due to loss of tissue, and the plasma cortisol fails to rise after injection of ACTH or a synthetic product, Synacthen, which comprises the biologically active fragment of the molecule.

Acute Adrenal Failure and the Waterhouse–Friedrichsen Syndrome

The clinical hallmarks of acute adrenal failure are **hypotension and peripheral vasoconstriction** occurring in an individual with chronic adrenal insufficiency or in a child with meningococcal meningitis.

The Waterhouse–Friderichsen syndrome comprises:
- profound and often irreversible peripheral circulatory collapse
- cutaneous petechial haemorrhages
- massive adrenal haemorrhage
- the finding of the haematological and morphological features of disseminated intravascular coagulation

The commonest association is **meningococcal septicaemia**. Meningitis may be clinically obvious at the time, but in some cases the first evidence of disease is the appearance of the Waterhouse–Friedrichsen syndrome. **In pathogenetic terms, this syndrome is an expression of endotoxic shock**, and the adrenal failure secondary to haemorrhagic necrosis aggravates this. This syndrome can also occur in association with infection with *Enterobacteriaceae* and *Pseudomonas* species.

Rarer examples of lack of sufficient functional adrenal cortical tissue are the various forms of **congenital adrenal hypoplasia**. These may occur in association with:
- **anencephaly.** The fetus is usually stillborn and characteristically has either no pituitary or a very poorly developed pituitary. The adrenals may be very small or even absent. In the former case, there is absence of the fetal cortex.
- **pituitary hypoplasia**
- **hypothalamic malformations**

In these three rare entities, the lack of adrenal tissue is a reflection of a **lack of normal drive** during fetal life.
- **so-called idiopathic hypoplasias, where the pituitary is normal.**

LACK OF DRIVE

Lack of CRH or ACTH due to hypothalamic or pituitary pathology interrupts the normal negative feedback pathway regulated by plasma cortisol concentrations. This may be due to virtually any lesion at these sites. Such lesions include:

- **local space-occupying lesions**, such as craniopharyngioma, pituitary adenoma or secondary deposits from tumours in other sites
- **inflammatory lesions**, such as sarcoidosis, tuberculosis or fungal infection
- **trauma to the pituitary stalk** or interruption to the blood supply of the pituitary

Loss of drive and, thus, adrenal suppression occurs most commonly, however, as a result of **prolonged treatment with glucocorticoids for inflammatory disorders of various kinds**. This rarely occurs unless the daily dose of hydrocortisone or an equivalent exceeds 15 mg/m^2.

Similarly, adrenal suppression can occur in the presence of an extra-adrenal tumour that secretes glucocorticoids ectopically.

LACK OF ENZYMES

Congenital Adrenal Hyperplasia

Congenital adrenal hyperplasia (CAH) is a set of genetically determined disorders that are due to enzymatic defects in cortisol synthetic pathways. The resulting low plasma cortisol levels lead to a compensatory overproduction of CRH and ACTH, and thus to hyperplasia of the adrenal cortex. Absence of any one of the five enzymes involved may cause such hyperplasia.

The clinical effects vary with the enzyme defect. Virilization is common because the block in cortisol synthesis leads to excess adrenal androgen secretion. In the commonest forms of CAH, virilization is evident in the female at birth, whereas in genotypic males it appears during childhood.

In enzyme defects occurring early in the chain (e.g. the catalysis of cholesterol's conversion to pregnenolone), both cortisol and sex steroid production will be deficient. The latter causes failure of the male to 'masculinize' adequately.

Defects in the synthesis and secretion of **aldosterone** with resulting **hyponatraemia and hyperkalaemia** may occur. Infants with CAH are very likely to develop salt loss, because sodium reabsorption mechanisms in the proximal renal tubule are somewhat immature and the demand for aldosterone may be greater than can be met.

The commonest enzyme deficiency is that of **21α-hydroxylase**, accounting for more than 90% of cases of CAH and most cases of female pseudohermaphroditism. The enzyme catalyses:
- the conversion of progesterone to 11-deoxycorticosterone
- the conversion of 17-hydroxyprogesterone to 11-deoxycortisol

A mild deficiency is not uncommon and may produce hirsutism, oligomenorrhoea and infertility in women. The prevalence of CAH due to this enzyme defect in white populations has been estimated to be 1 in 5000, although in a non-classical form it is much commoner. In general, the carrier rate for the recessive abnormality is estimated to be 1 in 35.

Virilization is the chief expression in mild cases. In severe cases, there is salt wasting as well.

Adrenoleukodystrophy

This is a syndrome characterized by a combination of:
- **chronic adrenal insufficiency due to atrophy of the cortex**
- **diffuse demyelination of cerebral white matter**

It is a genetically determined failure in peroxisomal function, resulting in accumulation of very long chain fatty acids within the affected cells and in the blood. There is deficient activity of the enzyme, **very long chain acyl-coenzyme A (CoA) ligase**, which normally converts free fatty acid to its acyl-CoA ester before oxidative breakdown occurs. The defect does not appear to reside within the enzyme itself but in a transport protein required for its importation into peroxisomes. The genomic abnormality is related to a mutated gene on the long arm of the X chromosome.

The disorder may present as:
- an X-linked recessive disease presenting at 5–10 years of age and characterized by rapid deterioration of cerebral function and death, usually within 3 years. This is the commonest form (50% of cases).
- an autosomal recessive disorder that may be present at birth
- an X-linked recessive disorder that presents in early adult life and in which gonadal failure and severe spastic paraparesis, sensory disturbances in the lower limbs and disturbances of sphincter function may occur. This variety has been called **adrenomyeloneuropathy** (25% of cases).

Microscopic Features

In the brain there is progressive destruction of myelin with sparing of the axons and a sparse macrophage infiltrate. Some of these macrophages contain periodic acid–Schiff-positive material, whereas others contain stainable lipid.

The adrenal changes, centred on the inner part of the zona fasciculata and the zona reticularis, are due to accumulation of very long chain fatty acids, which show up as striations within the affected cortical cells.

Attempts have been made to restrict the accumulation of the very long chain fatty acids by administering derivatives of erucic acid, an inhibitor of very long chain fatty acid synthesis, but this appears to have little effect.

HYPERFUNCTION OF THE ADRENAL CORTEX

The clinical syndromes of adrenal cortical hyperfunction are due to overproduction of adrenal steroids. The features will depend on which of the steroid groups is dominant. Thus, there may be an excess of **gluco-corticoids (Cushing's syndrome), aldosterone (Conn's syndrome) or adrenal androgens, which produce virilization**.

GLUCOCORTICOID OVER-SECRETION

Cushing's Syndrome
This syndrome was first recognized by Harvey Cushing in 1910 while he was still a student at Johns Hopkins School of Medicine. The patient, who was a 23-year-old woman with an adrenal tumour, had (*Fig. 40.13*):

- centripetal obesity (affecting the central part of the body)
- high blood pressure
- weakness affecting proximal muscles
- abdominal striae
- hirsutism
- thinning of the scalp hair
- backache
- purpura
- insomnia

Cushing also described the association of this syndrome with tumours arising from the basophil cells of the anterior pituitary. Thus were laid the foundations for the classification of Cushing's syndrome.

Cushing's syndrome can be due to increased drive (75% of cases of endogenous Cushing's syndrome) (i.e. it is dependent on excessive stimulus to the adrenal cortex by ACTH) or it can be independent of ACTH (*Fig. 40.14*).

ACTH-independent hypercortisolism may be:

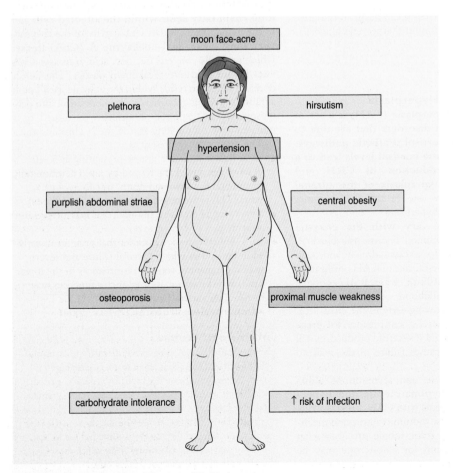

FIGURE 40.13 Common clinical features of Cushing's syndrome.

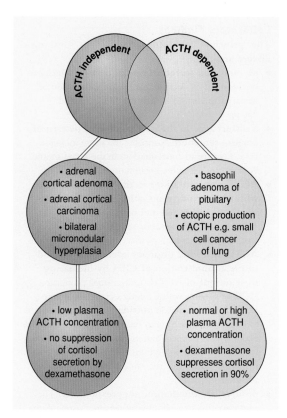

FIGURE 40.14 Causes and features of Cushing's syndrome.

• **exogenous, due to large doses of glucocorticoids** in the treatment of certain inflammatory and/or autoimmune disorders. This exogenous Cushing's syndrome is the commonest type.
• **endogenous due to:**
  a) adrenal carcinoma
  b) adrenal adenoma
  c) micronodular adrenal disease

Endogenous ACTH-independent Cushing's Syndrome

The chief causes are:

• **cortisol-producing adrenal cortical adenomas, which are usually unilateral**
• **cortisol-producing adrenal carcinomas**
• **bilateral, micronodular, adrenal hyperplasia, which in pathogenetic terms** is probably a set of disorders

In biochemical terms, the defining criteria are:

• **a low plasma ACTH concentration** – the pituitary responds normally to the feedback effect of high plasma cortisol levels
• **failure of suppression of cortisol secretion by dexamethasone**

Primary Adrenal Neoplasms

Primary adrenal neoplasms may be **benign (adenoma) or malignant (carcinoma)**.

Macroscopic Features

Adenomas are usually rounded, well-defined, encapsulated lesions. They average about 5 cm in diameter and are usually yellow in colour (*Fig. 40.15*), although some may be blackish because of the accumulation of lipofuscin within the tumour cells.

Microscopic Features

Microscopic examination shows the adenomas to consist of a mixture of clear and compact cells, arranged in well-formed nests and clusters. The part of the adrenal cortex that is not involved by the adenoma is suppressed and therefore atrophic.

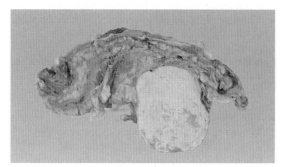

FIGURE 40.15 Adrenal cortical adenoma presenting as a well-defined yellow nodule.

Adrenal cortical carcinomas may be functioning or non-functioning. There are no recognized morphological differences between these two classes of tumour other than the **presence of suppression-related atrophy in the non-involved part of the adrenal cortex or in the contralateral adrenal in cases of functioning tumour.**

Macroscopic Features

Adrenal carcinomas causing Cushing's syndrome are usually large, weighing more than 1 kg. This suggests that cortisol secretion rates by tumour cells are not great. The cut surfaces of the lesions are usually yellow, but focal areas of haemorrhage and necrosis are often seen.

Microscopic Features

Microscopy shows the tumour cells to contain less lipid than their normal counterparts and to be arranged in cords and solid alveoli. Cellular and nuclear pleomorphism are present and nucleoli may be prominent. Histological recognition of malignancy is not always easy.

The prognostic outlook for patients with adrenal cortical carcinoma is bleak: most patients die within 3 years of presentation. Spread may occur locally or to distant sites; the lungs and liver are most frequently involved.

Fortunately these tumours are rare; the prevalence in the USA is about two per million population. Peak incidence is between the ages of 30 and 50 years. Functioning tumours are more common in women, and non-functioning ones are commoner in men.

Bilateral Nodular Adrenal Hyperplasia

Some patients with normal ACTH secretion develop nodular hyperplasia of the adrenals and evidence of hypercortisolism. This is due to **abnormal sensitivity of the adrenal cortical cells to ACTH**. There are other patients whose excess secretion of cortisol is truly independent of ACTH stimulus and in whom there is no adrenal cortical neoplasm. A number of different syndromes with different underlying mechanisms fall into this group of cases of Cushing's syndrome:

- **The Carney complex** – primary nodular dysplasia of the adrenal cortex associated with myxomas, peripheral nerve tumours, pigmented skin lesions and various endocrine tumours. This is inherited as an autosomal dominant disorder. Immunoglobulins that have a stimulating effect on the adrenal cortex have been found in the serum of these patients.
- **The McCune–Albright syndrome.** Here, nodule formation and hyperfunction may occur in the adrenal, pituitary, thyroid and gonads. The syndrome is due to a mutation occurring during embryonic life that affects the α subunit of the stimulatory G protein activating adenylate cyclase. Affected individuals are mosaics in respect of this protein. In the cells that contain the mutant protein, the G protein is permanently 'switched on' and thus the production of cAMP and steroidogenesis are constitutively increased.
- **Rare cases of ACTH-independent Cushing's syndrome occur in which it has been suggested that the adrenal cortex is stimulated by some factor that is not ACTH.** Intake of food appears to stimulate cortisol production in these patients. **The stimulating factor may be gastric inhibitory polypeptide (GIP)**, cortical cells being abnormally sensitive to normal postprandial increases in GIP. This abnormal sensitivity appears to be the expression of GIP-binding receptors on the plasma membranes of cortical cells.

ACTH-dependent Cushing's Syndrome

This commonest cause is **a pituitary adenoma involving the basophil cells of the anterior pituitary. This variety of the syndrome has been called Cushing's disease.** The pituitary tumours are usually small (1–9 mm in diameter) and the adrenals show bilateral nodular hyperplasia.

Laboratory Findings

The **principal laboratory findings in Cushing's disease** are:

- **an increased secretion rate of cortisol** which can be measured by determining the daily excretion of urinary free cortisol, which should not exceed 250 µg.
- **a disturbance in the normal diurnal pattern of cortisol secretion**. Normally, the mean midnight value for cortisol concentrations in the blood should be less than half of the mean morning value.
- **ACTH concentrations in the blood of patients with pituitary-driven Cushing's syndrome should be either normal or raised** because ACTH-secreting adenomas resist the normal feedback effect of high plasma cortisol concentrations.
- **ACTH-secreting pituitary adenomas respond to the administration of CRH by increasing their output of ACTH.** Only a small proportion (10%) of patients with Cushing's syndrome due to excess ACTH secretion **outside** the pituitary respond to CRH administration in this way. Raised or normal plasma ACTH concentrations and a positive response to CRH in Cushing's syndrome indicates a greater than 95% chance that the cause is a pituitary adenoma.
- **positive dexamethasone suppression test.** The administration of high doses of dexamethasone (8 mg per day) to patients with pituitary-driven Cushing's syndrome decreases cortisol secretion in 90% of cases.

Other causes of ACTH-dependent Cushing's syndrome are:
- **the ectopic production of ACTH by a neoplasm outside the adrenal.** This accounts for about 15% of cases. The most common cause of ectopic ACTH production is **small cell carcinoma of the lung**. Other tumours that can behave in this way include **thymoma, islet cell tumours of the pancreas, bronchial carcinoid, medullary carcinoma of the thyroid and certain gonadal tumours**.
- very rare tumours that produce ectopic CRH.

ALDOSTERONE OVERSECRETION

Hyperaldosteronism is usually expressed in the form of:
- **hypertension**
- **hypokalaemia**
- **alkalosis**

It may be either **primary**, the commonest cause being a benign adrenal cortical tumour (adenoma), or **secondary**, arising from any situation associated with **high plasma renin levels** (e.g. in patients with renal ischaemia, oedema from a variety of causes or renin-producing tumours). Plasma renin levels in patients with primary hyperaldosteronism are usually low.

Primary Hyperaldosteronism

Primary hypersecretion of aldosterone (Conn's syndrome) accounts for about 2% of all cases of hypertension. Four pathological conditions may produce Conn's syndrome; it is important to differentiate among these if appropriate treatment is to be given. They are:

- an aldosterone-producing adrenal cortical adenoma
- idiopathic hyperaldosteronism associated with bilateral adrenal cortical hyperplasia
- dexamethasone-suppressible hyperaldosteronism
- an aldosterone-producing adrenal cortical carcinoma. This is very rare.

Aldosterone-producing Adenoma

Macroscopic Features

These adenomas are usually single, unilateral and fairly small, rarely exceeding 2.5 cm in diameter. Peak incidence occurs between the ages of 20 and 40 years.

Grossly, the adenomas are characteristically bright yellow and do not appear to be encapsulated.

Microscopic Features

Microscopic examination shows them to consist of cell nests and columns that resemble the zona fasciculata rather than the glomerulosa (*Fig. 40.16*).

Clinical Features

The symptoms complained of most frequently are **headache, fatiguability** and **muscle weakness**, the last two being related to hypokalaemia. High blood pressure may be the only manifestation.

Laboratory Findings

The classical findings of hyperaldosteronism are:

- high plasma and urinary aldosterone levels
- hypokalaemia
- low plasma renin concentrations

Unfortunately 'life is rarely pure and never simple' and values for the chemical species listed above may be intermediate. A suspected diagnosis may be confirmed by measuring the plasma aldosterone : renin ratio after giving 25–50 mg captopril, an angiotensin-converting enzyme inhibitor. In virtually all cases there is a considerable degree of separation between the values obtained in patients with primary hyperaldosteronism and those in patients with essential hypertension.

Idiopathic Hyperaldosteronism

This variety of primary hypersecretion of aldosterone is due to bilateral adrenal cortical hyperplasia involving the zona glomerulosa. This may be due to abnormal stimulation of the zona glomerulosa by a circulating peptide derived from the pituitary.

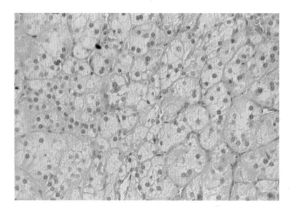

FIGURE 40.16 *Aldosterone-producing adenoma in a case of Conn's syndrome. Note the clear cytoplasm of the tumour cells, which resemble the zona fasciculata more closely than the zona glomerulosa.*

Dexamethasone-suppressible Hyperaldosteronism

This is an inherited autosomal dominant disorder. Its clinical features are the same as those encountered in other forms of primary hyperaldosteronism.

In normal subjects ACTH treatment leads to a transient increase in aldosterone production. In patients with dexamethasone-suppressible hyperaldosteronism, ACTH causes a prolonged period of aldosterone oversecretion. Increased secretion of 18-oxocortisol also occurs and this may account for the very high levels of blood pressure seen in these patients, as 18-oxocortisol also has some mineralocorticoid effect.

Another feature of this syndrome is the fast and striking degree of suppression of aldosterone production that occurs when dexamethasone is given. Treatment with either dexamethasone or a potassium-sparing diuretic is very effective.

ANDROGEN OVERSECRETION

This is expressed clinically in the form of abnormalities of sexual differentiation, known collectively as **adrenogenital syndrome**.

The commonest cause is congenital hyperplasia of the adrenal cortex due to an enzyme deficiency related to glucocorticoid synthesis. The commonest of these are 21-hydroxylase and 11β-hydroxylase deficiencies, which have been alluded to previously.

Disorders of sexual differentiation may occur also as a result of the presence of adrenal cortical neoplasms which produce excess amounts of sex steroids, chiefly androgens. The clinical effects of these lesions depend largely on whether they occur in childhood (which is more common) or in adult life (*Table 40.12*).

These rare neoplasms may be benign or malignant, the latter tending to be larger than the former. There are no microscopic features that distinguish virilizing

Table 40.12 Effects of Androgen Oversecretion

Age	Males	Females
Adult life	No obvious signs	Hirsutism Oligomenorrhoea Increased muscular development
Childhood	Precocious puberty	Enlargement of clitoris Hirsutism

adrenal tumours from those that produce Cushing's syndrome. The atrophy of the non-involved portion of the cortex, which is a prominent feature in patients with cortisol-producing tumours, is *not* seen in the adrenals of patients with virilizing tumours, because the excess androgens do not suppress cortisol production.

Feminizing adrenal cortical neoplasms do occur but are very rare. They occur more commonly in males than in females and the chief clinical manifestation is bilateral gynaecomastia.

THE ADRENAL MEDULLA

The single cell type of the medulla, the chromaffin cell, shares an embryological origin with the ganglia of the sympathetic nervous system (*Fig. 40.17*). **The principal biological function of these cells is to synthe-**

size and store the catecholamines adrenaline and noradrenaline. The clinical features of the most common pathological entity affecting the adrenal medulla – phaeochromocytoma – are due to excess secretion of catecholamine. Most chromaffin cells are found in the adrenal medulla but they may also occur in other sites in which phaeochromocytomas can arise.

Catecholamines are characterized by the presence of a catechol nucleus (3,4-dihydroxyphenyl) and are synthesized from tyrosine. They are released as a result of the release of acetylcholine from preganglionic neurones. Secretion of the stored catecholamines occurs by exocytosis, with the membranes of the storage vesicles fusing with the plasma membrane of the chromaffin cell.

Phaeochromocytoma

This is the commonest and most important condition affecting the adrenal medulla. Its hallmark is hypertension due to excess catecholamine release. Phaeochromocytomas cause about 0.2% of cases of hypertension. About 10% of these tumours are extra-adrenal. The peak incidence is between the ages of 30 and 50 years.

About 10–20% of these tumours are familial, half of which are bilateral. A number of hereditary patterns exists, as shown in *Table 40.13.*

Clinical Features

The defining clinical criterion of phaeochromocytoma is **hypertension**. This may be:

- paroxysmal
- sustained but with paroxysmal increases
- sustained

Paroxysms are characterized by:

- a sudden, **severe increase in blood pressure**
- **severe, throbbing headache**★
- **sweating**, which is most severe over the trunk★
- **anxiety**, which may be associated with a feeling of impending doom
- **nausea**, which may be associated with vomiting
- **palpitations with or without tachycardia**★
- **pallor**
- **abdominal pain**

When all three features marked with an asterisk (headache, sweating and palpitations) are present in a patient with hypertension, they indicate a diagnosis of phaeochromocytoma with a specificity of almost 94% and a sensitivity of almost 91%.

Laboratory Diagnosis

This depends on demonstrating the presence of raised concentrations of catecholamines or their metabolic products in blood or urine.

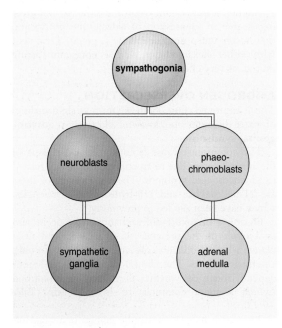

FIGURE 40.17 Relationship between the adrenal medulla and the sympathetic nervous system.

Table 40.13 Familial Phaeochromocytoma

Syndrome	Characteristics
Familial phaeochromocytoma	No associated pathology; inherited as an autosomal dominant trait; tends to occur in childhood
As part of multiple endocrine neoplasia syndrome type IIa	Associated with medullary carcinoma of thyroid and parathyroid adenoma or hyperplasia; transmitted in an autosomal dominant fashion
As part of multiple endocrine neoplasia syndrome type IIb	Associated with medullary carcinoma of thyroid, mucosal neuromas, intestinal ganglioneuroma and, rarely, hyperparathyroidism. Patients may appear 'marfanoid'
Associated with neurofibromatosis; 1% of patients with this disorder also have a phaeochromocytoma and 5% of patients with a phaeochromocytoma have neurofibromatosis	Central and/or peripheral neurofibromas present
Associated with von Hippel–Lindau disease; up to 10% of patients with this disorder have a phaeochromocytoma	Retinal and cerebellar haemangioblastomas present
As part of tuberous sclerosis	Associated with sebaceous adenoma (Pringle), mental deficiency, astrocytoma
As part of the Sturge–Weber syndrome	Associated with haemangiomas

In urine one can measure 24-hour output of:
- adrenaline or noradrenaline
- 3-hydroxy-4-methoxymandelic acid

Raised adrenaline levels suggest an adrenal phaeochromocytoma as the enzyme converting noradrenaline to adrenaline occurs only in the adrenal.

Note that urinary levels of catecholamines and their metabolites may be increased by compounds such as amphetamines, methyldopa and nalidixic acid, and by clonidine withdrawal.

Phentolamine, a short-acting α-adrenergic antagonist, can be used in the diagnosis of phaeochromocytoma. If the patient's blood pressure falls by more than 35 mmHg systolic and 25 mmHg diastolic after an intravenous dose of 1–5 mg phentolamine, the test is regarded as positive for phaeochromocytoma.

Macroscopic Features

The tumours vary greatly in size, ranging from as little as 1 g to as much as 4 kg in weight. The average weight is about 100 g.

The cut surface has a greyish-brown appearance. If a fixative containing dichromate is used, the tumour turns a deep brown colour owing to the presence of stored catecholamine (*Fig. 40.18*).

Microscopic Features

Small tumour cell nests or larger trabeculae with a sinusoidal blood supply are characteristic. The cells resemble those of normal adrenal medulla, being large and having abundant rather basophilic cytoplasm. If the material has been chrome-fixed, brown 'chromaffin' granules are seen within the cytoplasm. The quantity of granules has no implications for function.

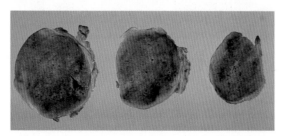

FIGURE 40.18 Phaeochromocytoma. Note the dark brown colour which develops after treatment with potassium dichromate.

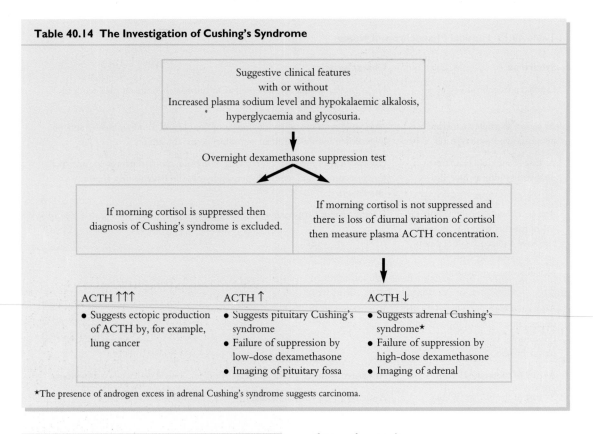

Table 40.14 The Investigation of Cushing's Syndrome

Suggestive clinical features
with or without
Increased plasma sodium level and hypokalaemic alkalosis,
hyperglycaemia and glycosuria.

↓

Overnight dexamethasone suppression test

↙   ↘

| If morning cortisol is suppressed then diagnosis of Cushing's syndrome is excluded. | If morning cortisol is not suppressed and there is loss of diurnal variation of cortisol then measure plasma ACTH concentration. |

↓

ACTH ↑↑↑	ACTH ↑	ACTH ↓
• Suggests ectopic production of ACTH by, for example, lung cancer	• Suggests pituitary Cushing's syndrome • Failure of suppression by low-dose dexamethasone • Imaging of pituitary fossa	• Suggests adrenal Cushing's syndrome★ • Failure of suppression by high-dose dexamethasone • Imaging of adrenal

★The presence of androgen excess in adrenal Cushing's syndrome suggests carcinoma.

Both benign and malignant phaeochromocytoma may have identical microscopic appearances. The defining criterion of malignancy is behavioural: a tumour that metastasizes is malignant; one that does not must be regarded as benign. The overall frequency of malignancy among phaeochromocytomas is approximately 10%.

THE INVESTIGATION OF CUSHING'S SYNDROME

See *Table 40.14.*

The Endocrine Pancreas

DIABETES MELLITUS

Definition

Diabetes mellitus is a **set** of disorders characterized by either an **absolute or a relative deficiency of insulin and/or insulin resistance**. This results in abnormalities of carbohydrate, fat and protein metabolism, expressed primarily as:

- **hyperglucaemia**
- **glycosuria**

Failure of insulin-mediated transport of glucose into cells results in a loss of essential fuels. Alternative oxidizable fuels are therefore needed, and are provided by ketone bodies derived from fat.

Formerly, the clinical picture of diabetes mellitus was dominated by metabolic abnormalities which could lead to **ketoacidosis with dehydration, coma and death**. This syndrome has declined greatly in frequency as a result of the use of insulin; the current long-term dangers of diabetes arise from (*Fig. 40.19*):

1) **a marked incremental effect on atherogenesis and a resulting increase in the risk of major arterial catastrophes such as acute coronary heart disease, stroke and lower limb ischaemia**
2) **structural and functional changes in the microvasculature, principally in the retina, kidney, peripheral and autonomic nerves. These are associated with blindness, renal failure and neurological deficits.**

Classification

At the simplest level diabetes may be divided into **primary** and **secondary** varieties. In the first of these, the **diabetes exists as an independent entity**, whereas in the second **diabetes is part of another disease (e.g. haemochromatosis)**.

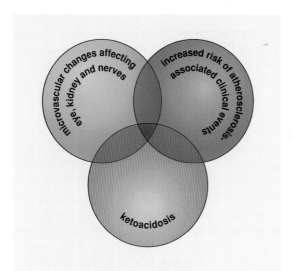

FIGURE 40.19 *Major effects of diabetes mellitus.*

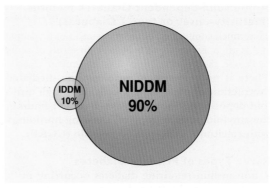

FIGURE 40.20 *Insulin-dependent and non-insulin-dependent diabetes mellitus. Relative frequency 1 : 9.*

PRIMARY DIABETES

Two main types of primary diabetes are recognized (*Fig. 40.20*). These are:

1) **insulin-dependent diabetes mellitus (IDDM)**
2) **non-insulin-dependent diabetes mellitus (NIDDM)**

Insulin-dependent Diabetes Mellitus (Juvenile Onset or type I Diabetes)

This accounts for about 10% of all cases. It occurs mainly, although not exclusively, in young people (peak onset about 12 years). In the preinsulin era, IDDM was often rapidly progressive and caused many premature deaths (*Table 40.15*).

The disease is characterized by autoimmune destruction of the β cells in the islets of Langerhans, this being associated with the presence of antibodies directed against these cells and against insulin (*Figs 40.21* and *40.22*).

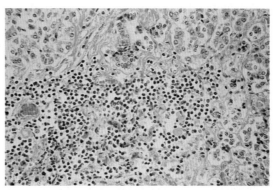

FIGURE 40.21 *Autoimmune destruction of islet cells in diabetes mellitus. Pancreas from a child with IDDM. An islet of Langerhans occupies the centre of the field and is infiltrated by numerous lymphocytes.*

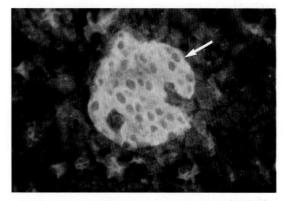

FIGURE 40.22 *Autoantibodies in insulin-dependent diabetes mellitus. The section shows a normal islet (arrowed) in the centre of the field, treated with serum from a patient with IDDM and then with fluorescein-linked antihuman globulin. The islet is brilliantly fluorescent, indicating the presence of bound anti-islet cell antibody.*

Table 40.15 Mortality from IDDM	
Period	Annual mortality rate (%)
1897–1914	82.4
1914–1922 (insulin discovered in 1922)	38.6
1926–1929	1.9
1950–1961	0.1

Non-insulin-dependent Diabetes Mellitus (Maturity-onset or type 2 Diabetes)

This, much commoner, disorder occurs in older people and is often associated with obesity. In terms of acute metabolic disturbances, it is a much milder disease. **There is no evidence of autoimmune-mediated destruction of pancreatic β cells, although amyloid deposition in the islets is a frequent finding, the amyloid protein (amylin) showing homology with calcitonin gene-related peptide (CGRP).**

Rarer Types of Primary Diabetes

- non-insulin-requiring diabetes occurring in the young and inherited as an autosomal dominant or maturity-onset diabetes in the young (MODY)
- a syndrome of 'impaired glucose tolerance' in which there is a 20–60% chance of developing diabetes over a 10-year period
- gestational diabetes mellitus

Genetics of Diabetes

Primary IDDM and NIDDM are genetically, as well as clinically, distinct:

- Both are familial diseases, but it is uncommon for both types to occur in the same family.
- Concordance rates for diabetes mellitus in monozygotic twins differ sharply in the two groups. In NIDDM, the concordance rate is nearly 100%, in IDDM 20–50%.
- Only in IDDM is there an association between diabetes and other autoimmune endocrine disorders.

Genetic Component in IDDM

Histocompatibility Antigens
The **major histocompatibility complex (MHC) haplotype, particularly genes coding for so-called class II proteins**, plays a major role in IDDM susceptibility. Normally the chance of any two siblings inheriting the same haplotype is 25%. However, if both have IDDM, identity between haplotypes occurs in 55–60% of cases.

The part of the MHC associated with IDDM susceptibility in Caucasians appears to be the D region. **Some 95% of patients with IDDM inherit either the human leucocyte antigen (HLA)-DR3 or DR4 allele, or both of these.** In the latter case, the risk of developing IDDM is greater than if only one of these alleles is inherited. This suggests some degree of synergism between the DR3 and DR4 alleles in conferring increased IDDM risk (*Fig. 40.23*). The presence in a haplotype, of **HLA-DR2 appears to protect against IDDM**; this has been interpreted as indicating that a third MHC gene is concerned with susceptibility to IDDM.

Current data suggest that it is the DQ gene, coding for the β chain of the dimeric protein, that is significant in

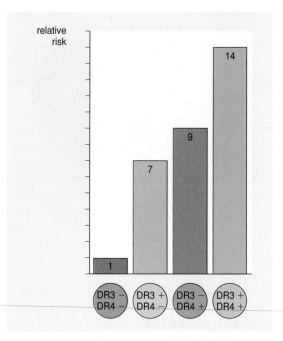

FIGURE 40.23 *Relative risks of diabetes mellitus in relation to HLA-DR3 and HLA-DR4.*

this respect, the **presence of aspartate at the 57 position of the DQ β chain conferring resistance to IDDM.** Substitution of another amino acid for aspartate at this position has the opposite effect. In some studies, the influence of variation in the DQ β-chain gene appears to be much greater than that of the two DR genes.

Inheritance of either DR3 and/or DR4 does not mean that IDDM is inevitable, as 40% of the general population falls into this category. The relative risk for developing IDDM in an individual with HLA-DR3 is 7, with HLA-DR4 it is 9, and with both it is 14 times greater than that of someone with neither of these alleles.

Interestingly, IDDM cases associated with DR3 show some **phenotypic** differences from those seen in association with DR4 (*Table 40.16*).

Table 40.16 Antibodies in DR3-positive or DR4-positive IDDM

Allele	Insulin antibodies	Islet cell antibodies
DR3	– or + in low titre	Antibodies persist
DR4	+ in high titre	Antibodies disappear quickly

Non-MHC Susceptibility Genes
Some evidence exists suggesting that genes outside the MHC also contribute to IDDM susceptibility:

- the variable DNA region near the insulin gene on the short arm of chromosome 11 where a number of DNA polymorphisms has been described in IDDM
- the gene coding for the constant region of the β chain of the T-cell receptor in which polymorphisms associated with IDDM risk have been described
- the non-obese diabetic mouse spontaneously develops IDDM closely resembling the human disease, although IDDM in this mouse occurs twice as frequently in females as in males (sex incidence is equal in humans). Recently two genes influencing IDDM in the mouse have been described. These, named *Idd-3* and *Idd-4*, are located on chromosomes 3 and 11. These genes clearly lie outwith the MHC (on chromosome 17 in mice). On the basis of comparative maps of mouse and human genomes, it has been suggested that homologues of these two genes may be present in humans, that of *Idd-3* on chromosome 1 and that of *Idd-4* on chromosome 17.

Genetic Component in NIDDM

NIDDM is well known to occur in familial clusters. In certain rather inbred populations, the prevalence of NIDDM is very high (*Table 40.17*).

In these populations glucose tolerance is distributed in a bimodal fashion, suggesting that a single major gene is involved, but the nature of this gene remains a mystery.

No reliable genetic marker for NIDDM susceptibility has yet been identified, although some weak associations have been noted in respect of certain candidate loci such as the insulin receptor gene and the glucose transporter gene. A specific mutation in the β_3-adrenergic receptor gene appears to be associated with central abdominal obesity and early onset of NIDDM in susceptible populations such as the Pima Indians. It does not, however, seem to be a deciding factor for the presence of NIDDM.

Table 40.17 Prevalence of NIDDM in Inbred Populations

Population	Age (years)	Prevalence of NIDDM (%)
Pima Indians in Arizona	25+	25.5
Pure-bred Nauruans	60+	80
Non-pure-bred Nauruans	60+	17

Non-genetic Factors in IDDM

The comparatively low concordance rate in monozygotic twins and the modest increment of risk conferred by certain class II MHC genes suggests that **part of the cause of IDDM is encompassed by non-genetically determined factors**. These might be environmental, or random somatic mutations.

Support for an environmental contribution to IDDM derives from the following:

1) **There is considerable geographical variation in the incidence of IDDM.** Generally, the further from the equator, the greater is the risk of IDDM; populations near the equator have a tenfold lower incidence of IDDM than those near the Arctic or Antarctic. Incidence by country of origin and residence also varies. For instance, a Finnish child has 35 times the risk of IDDM that a Japanese child has, although there are genetic as well as geographical differences. The interaction between genetic inheritance and environment is striking, and is shown in the differences in the incidence of diabetes in different parts of Italy. In Sardinia, the annual incidence of childhood-onset IDDM is 30.2 per 100 000; in Lazio, in mainland Italy, the incidence is only 6.5 per 100 000. While this might suggest the importance of environmental circumstances in Sardinia, in fact the incidence of IDDM in Lazio is four times higher in children of Sardinian parents than in those of mainland parents.

2) **Some changes in IDDM incidence have been too rapid to be accounted for by genetic variation.** For instance, in Finland, IDDM incidence inreased from 13 to 33 per 100 000 in the 1980s.

3) **Migrants with a low risk of IDDM acquire a higher risk when they move to a higher-risk country.** This has been seen on a number of occasions; for example, Japanese children moving to Hawaii almost quadruple their IDDM risk.

4) **Certain environmental agents can cause IDDM.** For instance, congenital rubella is associated with a 20% chance of developing IDDM later in life and there is also a high risk of thyroiditis and other immune-mediated disorders in these patients. Other viral infections have also been suggested as triggering factors. There are well-known models of chemically induced IDDM in small laboratory animals (alloxan, streptozotocin).

The interaction between environmental and genetically determined factors results in autoimmune destruction of the insulin-secreting β cells of the pancreatic islets and in IDDM. At the time of diagnosis, about four-fifths of the islets will no longer contain β cells and the islets may be heavily infiltrated by lymphocytes. Islet cells that secrete other peptide hormones are unaffected.

In the period before diabetes presents clinically, both cellular and humoral arms of the immune system are activated. The former manifests by an increased number of T cells expressing HLA-DR on their surface, and alterations in the number and function of immunoregulatory T cells. The latter is shown by the presence of **islet cell antibodies**, which may precede overt clinical features by months or even years. Anticytoplasmic islet cell antibodies and an antibody reacting with a 64-kDa islet cell protein are found in 70% of cases. In contrast, anti-insulin antibodies are found in only 30% of cases. The process appears to be antigen dependent because once the majority of the β cells have been destroyed the titre of islet cell antibodies drops.

What is the Initial Target that Drives the Autoimmune Response in IDDM?

Several other autoantibodies have been identified in IDDM. These include an antibody directed against the enzyme **glutamic acid decarboxylase** (GAD), which is active in the synthesis of GABA (γ-aminobutyric acid) the chief inhibitory neurotransmitter in the brain and a paracrine signal in pancreatic β cells. GAD antibodies appear first in IDDM. It is suggested that loss of tolerance to GAD is an early and necessary step in the development of diabetes in non-obese diabetic mice, a T-cell response developing in the course of the pathogenesis.

Non-genetic Factors in NIDDM

Age

In all populations the incidence of NIDDM increases with age. The age of onset is lowest in communities in which the prevalence of NIDDM is highest. In the UK, NIDDM is rare in patients under 35 years of age, although in some other populations there are significant numbers of such patients. NIDDM is certainly not a 'normal' component of ageing; elderly members of low-prevalence communities have a low prevalence of diabetes, whereas the opposite is true of high-prevalence populations.

Obesity

Obesity does appear to be a factor in the development of NIDDM. In the UK, the diabetic population is very little heavier than the non-diabetic population, and is not especially obese either. The distribution of obesity seems to have some relevance: **abdominal obesity** is more closely correlated with the risk of NIDDM (and with mutations in the β_3-adrenergic receptor gene) than generalized fatness.

Physical Inactivity

In two population studies physical inactivity was found to influence the risk of NIDDM independently. Presumably this relates to insulin sensitivity, which is known to be increased by exercise.

Biochemical Mechanisms Involved in the Development of NIDDM

Diminished Insulin Secretion

The question of whether or not NIDDM is associated with a diminution of insulin secretion has long been controversial. It is true that **absolute** levels of insulin secretion are increased in patients with NIDDM who

are **obese**. If, however, the levels are compared with those in **obese non-diabetic subjects**, the latter show much **higher** insulin levels.

In NIDDM the following sequence of events has been suggested:

1) Basal insulin secretion is adequate to maintain normal glucose concentrations, but the response to feeding is inadequate so that there is hyperglycaemia after meals with a slow return to normal blood glucose levels.

2) Basal insulin secretion then decreases. Blood glucose concentrations rise and stimulate insulin secretion; a new steady state is achieved in which both blood glucose and insulin levels are increased. The increase in insulin concentration is, however, insufficient to restore glucose concentrations to normal.

Several different defects in insulin secretion exist; the key defect is **a selective defect in the acute response to glucose**. The presence of amyloid in the islets of the majority of patients with NIDDM may not be without relevance. The amyloid protein (amylin) is closely related to CGRP, and its precursor is detectable in β cells. CGRP inhibits insulin secretion and it has been suggested that the amyloid protein may do the same. This amyloid protein has also been shown to cause insulin resistance in rats, although not, so far, in humans.

Insulin Resistance

Many patients with NIDDM show insulin insensitivity, much of this in the past being attributed to obesity. Obesity in the absence of NIDDM certainly is associated with insulin resistance but in NIDDM most of the resistance appears to be correlated directly with the diabetic state itself. The insulin resistance found in these patients often appears early; a study of individuals both of whose parents had NIDDM showed that a low glucose disappearance value in the presence of normal insulin secretion was a good predictor for future development of diabetes.

Possible Cellular Mechanisms of Insulin Resistance

Peripheral cell insensitivity to insulin may result from failure in two possible phases:

1) **Binding of insulin to its two-unit glycoprotein receptor**; a deficiency in either receptor number or function would lead to insulin resistance

2) **A post-binding stage** in which the following occur:

   a) second messenger generation

   b) activation of intracellular effector systems such as the synthesis of glucose-transporting molecules, or other insulin-mediated intracellular events

In rare instances circulating antibodies to insulin may play a part in resistance, as may the even rarer situation where antibodies bind to receptors and block the binding of insulin.

Biochemical and Clinical Features of Established IDDM

Typically, patients with IDDM present complaining of:
- **polyuria**
- **polydipsia**
- **tiredness**
- **loss of appetite**
- **loss of weight**

This clinical picture is, not infrequently, complicated by recurrent infections.

The polyuria and polydipsia are due to loss of glucose in the urine, causing an osmotic diuresis. The loss of weight and the fatiguability are, in part, due to loss of protein and electrolytes.

The severity of the metabolic abnormalities in respect of glucose regulation and of fat and protein metabolism are a reflection of the deficiency of insulin. Where this is mild, the chief effect is a failure to store body fuels; in major deficiencies of insulin, not only is the fuel storage in the fed state affected, but there is mobilization of endogenous fuels through the mechanisms of increased hepatic glucose production and an increase in catabolic processes such as lipolysis and proteolysis.

Effects on Fat Metabolism

In untreated diabetics significant changes in fat metabolism occur. Plasma free fatty acids (FFAs), triglycerides and, usually, cholesterol are present in the plasma in increased concentrations. The rise in plasma FFA concentration reflects an increased flow of fatty acids from adipose tissue stores to the liver. This is due to an increase in lipolysis resulting from **loss of the normal inhibitory effect of insulin on a lipase in adipose tissue**. The mechanism responsible for the increase in triglyceride is unclear.

Effects on Amino Acid and Protein Metabolism

Severe insulin deficiency is accompanied by negative nitrogen balance and marked protein wasting. This is not surprising because insulin:
- **stimulates protein synthesis** and uptake of amino acids
- **inhibits protein catabolism** and the release of amino acids from muscle

In addition, the gluconeogenesis resulting from carbohydrate wasting depends, in part, on increased use of protein-derived precursors.

Diabetic Ketoacidosis

The most severe metabolic and clinical manifestation of insulin lack is **ketoacidosis** (*Fig. 40.24*). Despite its decreased frequency since the introduction of insulin treatment for IDDM, ketoacidosis may still be encountered and is an acute, life-threatening, medical emergency.

The most serious pathophysiological abnormalities in this condition are:
- **Metabolic acidosis**, due to accumulation of ketones in body fluids. Ketone accumulation, most

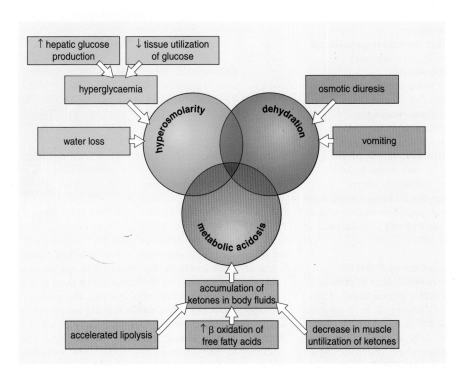

FIGURE 40.24 Mechanisms and features in diabetic ketoacidosis.

notably of β–hydroxybutyric acid and acetoacetic acid, is the result of three distinct metabolic events:

1) **Accelerated lipolysis** due to the lack of insulin, leading to a markedly increased flux of fatty acids to the liver

2) **Increased β oxidation** of FFAs in mitochondria as a result of an increased transfer of FFAs across the mitochondrial membrane. The increase in β oxidation of fatty acids leads to an increase in acetylcoenzyme A (CoA). When the concentration of acetylCoA exceeds the capacity for oxidation to carbon dioxide via the Krebs cycle, the acetylCoA molecules condense to form ketone acids.

3) In addition to overproduction of ketones in uncontrolled diabetics, a contribution is made to the hyperketonaemia by **decreased utilization** of these organic acids in muscle tissue.

- **Hyperosmolarity** due to hyperglycaemia and water loss. Hyperglycaemia results from decreased tissue utilization of glucose and increased hepatic glucose production (glucose release from the liver is increased from 150–200 to 400–600 mg/min).
- **Dehydration** due to:
  1) the **osmotic diuresis** accompanying hyperglycaemia
  2) **vomiting**, which is usually associated with severe metabolic acidosis

Metabolic Aspects of the Complications of Diabetes

With the decline in the frequency of ketoacidosis in diabetics, the chief threats to the well-being and survival of these patients come from:

1) **an incremental effect on atherogenesis** and on the risk of the major clinical syndromes associated with atherosclerosis, i.e.:
- coronary heart disease (relative risk 1.9)
- stroke (relative risk 2.5)
- peripheral large vessel disease leading to intermittent claudication and later to diabetic gangrene (relative risk 4.0) (*Figs 40.25* and *40.26*)

2) **Microvascular abnormalities**, the most baneful effects of which are seen in the kidney, retina and peripheral and autonomic nerves

Particularly in the latter case, these changes result from the long-term effects of metabolic abnormalities, most notably **hyperglycaemia**, on a variety of cell types and extracellular matrices.

Non-enzymatic Glycosylation of Proteins

One of the most important consequences of prolonged hyperglycaemia is non-enzymatic glycosylation of proteins. In aqueous solutions, glucose is in a mixture of ring forms and a straight chain aldehyde form, the latter accounting for only a small proportion of the glucose. The straight-chain aldehyde binds **spontaneously and non-enzymatically** to ε amino groups of lysine residues on the amino terminal of pro-

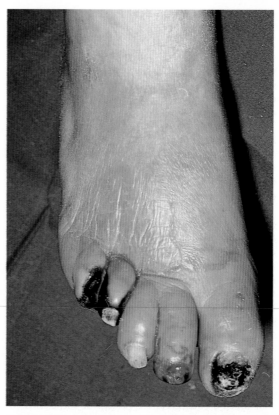

FIGURE 40.25 *Peripheral gangrene in diabetes mellitus.*

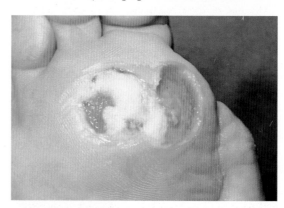

FIGURE 40.26 *Chronic ulceration in diabetes mellitus affecting weight-bearing areas of the foot.*

teins, thus forming compounds known as **Schiff bases**. These are labile and reach equilibrium with the glucose concentration, the rate of formation being equal to the rate of dissociation. Schiff bases can and do, however, undergo a slow but **irreversible** rearrangement into a **ketoamine** configuration; this process is called the Amadori rearrangement, after the chemist who first described it. The sugar–protein adducts are stable but may undergo further modifications if the turnover time of the glycosylated protein is slow. Late glycosylation products formed under these circumstances can be identified as brown pigments and can take part in protein–protein cross-linking. Glycosylation of haemoglobin is a common event, especially if the diabetic control is not efficient. The haemoglobin variant formed is known as HbA1c. **Measurement of the concentrations of glycosylated haemoglobin is an effective means of determining, from a single blood sample, the degree of glycaemic control that has obtained over the last 2–3 months.**

Glycosylation of Serum Proteins
Glycosylated serum proteins, such as **albumin and immunoglobulins**, can form cross-linkages with glycosylated tissue proteins, possibly contributing in this way to capillary basement membrane thickening, the most conspicuous microscopic feature of diabetic microvascular disease.

The role of protein glycosylation in atherogenesis is discussed in Chapter 32 (see pp 337–338).

The Sorbitol Pathway, Myoinositol and Sodium–Potassium ATPase in Diabetic 'Microvascular' Complications

The Sorbitol Pathway
Fructose can be produced from circulating glucose by the 'polyol' pathway. This consists of two steps:

1) glucose + NADPH = sorbitol = NADP$^+$
2) sorbitol + NAD$^+$ = fructose + NADH

The first of these reactions is catalysed by **aldose reductase** and the second by **sorbitol dehydrogenase**. Because aldose reductase has a high Michaelis constant (K_m), sorbitol production is much increased if hyperglycaemia is present. Aldose reductase is found, in particular, in the Schwann cells of peripheral nerves, in the lens and cornea of the eye, in the renal medulla and foot processes of the epithelial cells in the glomeruli, and in the pericytes of the renal capillaries – all sites affected in diabetes.

High levels of intracellular sorbitol are believed to contribute to some diabetic complications as a result of the **increase in tissue osmolality** caused by the sorbitol. Such sites include, perhaps most notably, the **lens**, **cataract** being a well-known complication of diabetes.

Myoinositol Metabolism and Diabetic Peripheral Neuropathy (see p 1175)
Myoinositol is a cyclic hexahydroxyhexanol found in most plant and animal cells in higher concentrations than in the extracellular milieu. It is an essential substrate for forming phosphoinositides, an important intracellular messenger system. The myoinositol molecule resembles D-glucose and enters cells via a transporter system competitively inhibited by high glucose levels. Diabetics lose excessive amounts of myoinositol in the urine and **in experimental diabetes the myoinositol concentration of peripheral nerves is much less than normal and is associated with a reduction in nerve conduction velocity**. In diabetic animals, this can be reversed either by feeding myoinositol or by administering an aldose-reductase inhibitor, although giving myoinositol to human diabetics seems to be without effect.

Morphological Features of Diabetic Complications

Capillary Basement Membrane Thickening
Although the chief targets for diabetic complications are the kidney, the retina, and peripheral and autonomic nerves, the basic pathological feature in all these sites, as well as in many others, is **hyaline thickening of the walls of capillaries and arterioles**. Basement membranes are thickened by structureless and eosinophilic material. This stains strongly with periodic acid–Schiff (PAS) stain, indicating the presence of 1–2 glycol groups characteristically found in glycoproteins and glycolipids. Plasma proteins such as fibrinogen and low density lipoproteins are also present in the thickened basement membranes, probably due to cross-linking of glycosylated plasma and tissue proteins.

Basement membrane thickening is associated with increased vascular permeability. There is a marked decrease in the kidney, of negatively charged proteoglycan component of the basement membrane (the 'glomerular polyanion'). These anionic proteoglycans bind to the extracellular matrices of diabetic patients much less well than normally and this is also seen *in vitro* when matrix proteins containing products of advanced glycosylation are used. In addition, glycosylation of macrophage membranes may lead to synthesis and release of cytokines which may degrade basement membrane proteoglycans.

There have been repeated suggestions that the extent and severity of basement membrane thickening reflects the efficacy of glycaemic control and some studies indicate that meticulous control of blood glucose levels may lead to a considerable degree of inhibition of capillary basement membrane thickening.

The Diabetic Kidney
Renal failure is a frequent complication of diabetes. It may cause death in 30–50% of those who contract diabetes during childhood and also affects a considerable proportion of patients who become diabetic in adult life. The chief clinical presentations of diabetic kidney disease are:

- **glomerular syndromes** – proteinuria, the nephrotic syndrome, chronic renal failure
- **recurrent and chronic pyelonephritis**
- **papillary necrosis**

Diabetic Glomerular Disease
The initial manifestation is proteinuria. This occurs in more than half of patients with IDDM and about one-third of those with NIDDM. The occurrence of proteinuria in a diabetic, although it may be delayed for

10–20 years after the initial diagnosis of diabetes, is ominous in prognostic terms, and renal failure may supervene within 4–5 years.

Microscopic Features

- **Diffuse basement membrane thickening.** This is followed by an increase in the volume of the mesangial matrix, which ultimately obliterates the whole glomerulus converting it to a 'ball' of hyaline material. Both basement membrane and the mesangial deposits stain positively (a magenta colour) with PAS stain. Diffuse basement membrane thickening is *not* diagnostic of diabetes because it may also be seen in membranous glomerulonephritis, but, in functional terms, it is the most threatening of diabetic glomerular lesions. It is associated with hyaline thickening of **both the afferent and efferent arterioles** relating to the vascular stalk of the affected glomerulus, and evidence of immune complex deposition is absent. These two features generally serve to distinguish it from other causes of diffuse basement membrane thickening.
- **Nodular glomerulosclerosis (the Kimmelstiel–Wilson lesion).** This consists of deposition of glycoprotein material in a nodular fashion within the mesangium near the periphery of the glomerular lobules (*Fig. 40.27*). The nodules, which can be single or multiple, may appear laminated and may have a peripheral cuff of mesangial cells around them. Immunohistochemical studies show the presence of fibrin and low density lipoprotein in the deposits. The nodular lesion may be seen by itself or in combination with diffuse basement membrane thickening. It is pathognomonic for diabetes mellitus.
- **Exudative lesions.** These are areas, usually involving the tips of the glomerular capillary loops, that show a rather 'fuzzy', brightly eosinophilic, appearance believed to be due to accumulation of large amounts of plasma protein, most notably fibrin.
- **The capsular 'drop'.** This consists of a small, hyaline, eosinophilic nodule projecting from the capsule into Bowman's space. It stains positively with the PAS method. It is pathognomonic for diabetes but its functional significance, if any, is not known.

Possible Mechanisms Involved in Diabetic Glomerulopathy

Some of these, most notably biochemical changes within the basement membrane and its associated proteoglycans, have already been discussed. However, some other factors need to be taken into consideration.

The first of these is the fact that in early IDDM the **glomerular filtration rate (GFR) is increased**, associated with an increase in kidney size. If a euglycaemic state is attained, for example by continuous subcutaneous infusions of insulin, the GFR can be reduced

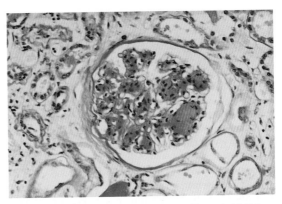

FIGURE 40.27 *Nodular glomerulosclerosis (Kimmelstiel–Wilson lesion). The section has been stained by the PAS method; glycoproteins appear a magenta colour. The nodules so stained are present within the mesangium of the glomerulus. This lesion is characteristic for diabetes mellitus.*

to essentially normal levels but the nephromegaly persists. It has been suggested that the hyperfiltration or, more likely, the haemodynamic circumstances that bring hyperfiltration about, may play a part in producing glomerular damage.

Renal Papillary Necrosis Complicating Urinary Tract Infection

Urinary tract infections are common in diabetics. Especially, although not exclusively, in patients suffering from some degree of obstruction to urinary outflow, acute papillary necrosis may be seen. In most cases both kidneys are affected and the condition is often fatal.

Macroscopic Features

The renal pelves are markedly inflamed and may be filled with purulent debris. Small abscesses may be present in both the cortex and medulla, and some or all of the papillae may be frankly necrotic showing the greyish-yellow appearance of coagulative necrosis. In some instances detachment of the necrotic papillae may occur, leaving a ragged edge to the affected calyx.

Microscopic Features

Microscopic examination usually shows complete necrosis of the affected papillae, although the 'ghost' outlines of collecting tubules may persist. Unlike what is seen in analgesic-mediated nephropathy, there is a heavy acute inflammatory infiltrate in the demarcation zone between the necrotic papilla and the adjacent viable kidney tissue, and the tubules in the viable zone contain pus.

On some occasions a histological diagnosis of acute papillary necrosis may be made during life in cases where a necrotic papilla becomes detached and is passed in the urine. In one study this was recorded with a frequency of 12 of 75 cases.

Possible Pathogenetic Mechanisms

The mechanism responsible for papillary necrosis is obscure. The blood supply of the renal medulla is relatively poor and may be compromised in patients with diabetic small vessel disease affecting the kidney. The importance of papillary underperfusion in this connection is emphasized by the fact that papillary necrosis can occur purely as a result of hypotension and shock. Infection in the upper part of the urinary tract, found so often in patients with acute papillary necrosis, coupled with relative ischaemia and poor local tissue defences, probably accounts for most of the cases.

Diabetic Retinopathy

Every year some 30 000–40 000 people in the UK go blind as a result of diabetic retinopathy. In many countries it is the leading cause of blindness.

The earliest change in the retina of diabetics is loss of retinal capillary pericytes. These cells are thought to have a role both in controlling blood flow through the retinal vessels and in maintaining the stability of these small conduits.

Following this a number of changes now develop which constitute 'background ' diabetic retinopathy. These include:

   a) thickening of the basement membranes of the retinal capillaries

   b) the development of small aneurysms, possibly as a result of the loss of pericytes

   c) the appearance of rather well-defined small yellowish-white patches, which are known as hard exudates and which represent accumulations of lipid

Against this background other changes appear, some of which have an ominous functional significance. These are:

   a) small haemorrhages known as 'dot and blot' haemorrhages

   b) a curious beaded appearance along the course of the vessels

   c) neovascularization, which is elicited by patchy ischaemia of the retina. Ischaemic changes in the retina may also be manifested by the appearance of 'soft' exudates or 'cottonwool' spots, which represent small areas of ischaemic necrosis in the superficial layers of the retina. A more dangerous development is the extension of the new blood vessels into the vitreous, which can be followed by haemorrhages and scarring within the vitreous. The stimulus for the ingrowth of new vessels is ischaemia, associated with the release of an endothelial growth factor from the ischaemic areas.

TUMOURS AND HYPERPLASIA OF THE ISLETS

Islet cell tumours and hyperplasia of the islets are found much more rarely than carcinoma of the exocrine duct epithelium. They may be **benign** (**adenoma**) or **malignant** (**carcinoma**); histological distinction between these two behavioural patterns may be difficult. The tumours occur mainly in adults. They may be silent (in endocrine terms) or characterized by hyperfunction of one or more of the secreting cell types within the islet. In one instance (**pancreatic gastrinoma** – the cause of the Zollinger–Ellison syndrome) there is ectopic hormone secretion; gastrin is not normally secreted by the islets.

Quite commonly islet cell tumours are spoken of as being APUDOMAS. This refers to the concept of the APUD system, put forward by A. Everson Pearse, in which a diffuse set of neuroendocrine cells is believed to be linked by:

   1) **certain common histochemical features** (A, amine; P, precursor; U, uptake; D, decarboxylation)
   2) **a supposed common origin from the neural crest**

There is much to support this view, but it must be remembered that ablation of the neural crest during embryonic life does not lead to failure of development of the pancreatic islets, and that ablation followed by implantation of the neural crest of another species does not lead to the cells of the implanted species being found in the pancreatic islets.

The commonest islet cell tumour is a **β-cell tumour** (**insulinoma**).

These vary in size. In some instances the tumour nodules are tiny, in others large, and some patients have multiple secreting lesions within the pancreas. Histologically insulinomas consist of interlacing cords and ribbons of epithelial cells with a rather sinusoidal type of blood supply not differing significantly from that of other peptide-secreting tumours (*Fig. 40.28*). On electron microscopy the secretory granules show the presence of a rather crystalline core, identical to that seen in the insulin-secreting β cells of the normal pancreas (*Fig. 40.29*). At the light microscopic level, the diagnosis can be confirmed by immunohistochemistry using anti-insulin antibodies.

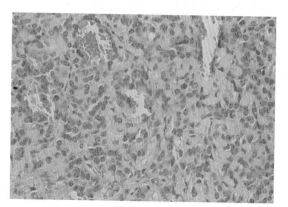

FIGURE 40.28 Islet cell tumour of the pancreas (haematoxylin and eosin staining). Note the typical ribbon-like pattern of the tumour cell arrangement.

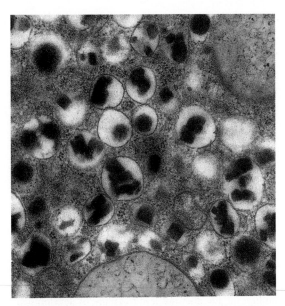

FIGURE 40.29 Crystalline cores in secretory granules of islet cell tumour cells. These are identical with those seen in the insulin-secreting β cells of normal islets of Langerhans.

The clinical features are what would be expected of hyperinsulinism and the resulting hypoglycaemia:

- **confusion**
- **blurred vision**
- **muscle weakness**
- **sweating**
- **palpitations**

Care must be taken not to overlook these features; patients have languished for long periods with a mistaken diagnosis of acute psychological disturbance or drunkenness.

The second commonest islet tumour producing endocrine disturbances is the **pancreatic gastrinoma**. This is the cause of gastric hypersecretion and recurrent peptic ulceration (the Zollinger–Ellison syndrome) and must be regarded as an example of ectopic hormone secretion because gastrin-producing cells have not, thus far, been identified within the normal pancreas. About 60% of these behave in a malignant way, with spread to regional nodes and liver being the commonest expression of this.

α-Cell tumours (glucagonomas) are rare. They occur most frequently in perimenopausal or post-menopausal women, producing a curious syndrome consisting of anaemia, mild diabetes and a migratory erythematous and necrotizing rash mainly over the lower part of the body. More than half the cases reported have behaved in a malignant fashion with involvement of the liver and regional lymph nodes. Preoperative diagnosis depends on the demonstration of raised plasma concentrations of glucagon.

VIPomas arise from the D_1 cells of the islet and secrete large amounts of vasoactive intestinal peptide. Its clinical expression is the Verner–Morrison syndrome, in which patients have profuse watery diarrhoea (sometimes spoken of as pancreatic cholera) accompanied by hypokalaemia and achlorhydria. The diarrhoea is due to the overstimulation of the adenyl cyclase system in the small intestinal epithelial cells, giving rise to excess transport of water, chloride, sodium and potassium from the crypt cell into the gut lumen, and a tendency to block the absorption of water, sodium and chloride from the gut lumen across the villous epithelium. The majority of these rare tumours behave in a benign fashion.

Multiple Endocrine Neoplasia Syndromes and the Pancreas

The term **multiple endocrine neoplasia (MEN)** refers to a number of symptom complexes that arise as a result of either **a tumour or hyperplasia in two or more endocrine organs**. These are classified under three rubrics depending on the combination of endocrine lesions that is present. The only one involving the pancreas is MEN type I (*Table 40.18*). The complex of clinical features **depends on which hormones are secreted by the various lesions**. Thus, for example, a patient suffering from MEN I could present with:

- amenorrhoea and galactorrhoea due to overproduction of prolactin
- hypercalcaemia and its associated clinical complications due to hyperparathyroidism
- the Zollinger–Ellison syndrome

Hyperplasia of the Islets (Nesidioblastosis)

This is a very rare condition, seen mainly in young children. Most of the islets are enlarged and the infant may show a voracious appetite and excessive weight gain. Two basic types of lesion are associated with persistent neonatal hyperinsulinaemic hypoglycaemia. One is diffuse and the other a local form of islet hyperplasia. These two types occur with equal frequency.

Focal hyperplasia is characterized by nodular masses of hyperplastic islets. In some patients only one focus

Table 40.18 MEN Syndromes

Syndrome	Endocrine lesions
MEN I	Parathyroid Pituitary Adrenal cortex Pancreas } tumours or hyperplasia
MEN IIa	Phaeochromocytoma Medullary cancer of the thyroid Parathyroid hyperplasia or adenoma
MEN IIb	Medullary cancer of the thyroid Phaeochromocytoma Mucocutaneous neuromas (skin, eye, bronchus, gut or bladder)

may be present; in others two or three such foci may be found. Diffuse islet hyperplasia involves the whole pancreas. The individual islets are larger than normal, and within these, there is an increase in both size and number of the insulin-producing β cells. In the case of focal nesidioblastosis, partial pancreatectomy effects a cure. If the islet hyperplasia is diffuse, subtotal or total pancreatectomy may be required.

Islet cell hyperplasia is also a striking feature in the pancreas of stillborn infants of mothers who suffer from diabetes mellitus or who show, during pregnancy, minor abnormalities of glucose tolerance that have been given the name of prediabetes. This islet cell hyperplasia, which is characterized by a relative increase in the number of β cells, appears to be a sensitive predictor for the subsequent development of diabetes in the mother. The infants tend to be large, rubicund and rather 'Cushingoid' in appearance, but are in reality very fragile (*Figs 40.30* and *40.31*).

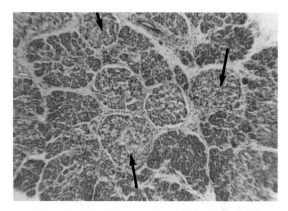

FIGURE 40.31 *Pancreas from the stillborn infant of a diabetic mother. Note how large, prominent and numerous are the islets of Langerhans (arrowed).*

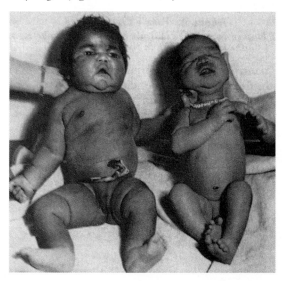

FIGURE 40.30 *The newborn baby on the left of the picture is the child of a multipara who became overtly diabetic 3 years later. The child is large (see the 8 lb baby of a non-diabetic mother on the right) and was rubicund and cushingoid in appearance.*

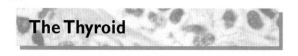

The Thyroid

NORMAL ANATOMY AND DEVELOPMENT

The thyroid, so-called because of its fancied resemblance to a shield (Gr. *thyreos*), consists of two lobes connected by an isthmus. Each lobe is about 4 cm in length and 2–2.5 cm in width.

The normal weight of the thyroid is approximately 14.5 g in women, with some increase during the secretory phase of the menstrual cycle, and 18 g in men.

The medial portion arises from the foramen caecum as a bilobed structure. During development, this anlage is attached to the tongue by the thyroglossal duct. This portion of the gland begins to descend about the fifth week of gestation; during this process, as the thyroid attains its position in the lower portion of the anterior surface of the neck, the thyroglossal duct becomes elongated and in due time atrophies. Persistence of the duct is the basis of **thyroglossal cysts** which, when situated near the base of the tongue, are lined by stratified squamous epithelium; those further down have a pseudostratified lining. Islands of thyroid acini within the cyst wall are diagnostic.

The lateral portion of the thyroid arises from the branchial system, probably from the **ultimobranchial body** situated in the fifth (or possibly in the tail of the fourth) branchial pouch. The **parafollicular** or **C cells** which secrete **thyrocalcitonin** are derived from this body and fuse with the median anlage of the thyroid on its upper and lateral aspects.

Embryological Mishaps

Several anomalies of descent have been described:
- **Non-descent.** Here, thyroid differentiation takes place at the base of the tongue with the production of a **lingual thyroid**.
- **Failure to descend to the normal position low in the neck** leads to the presence of ectopic thyroid tissue anywhere along the normal pathway.
- **Descent to an abnormally low position** can lead to the finding of thyroid tissue in the substernal tissues.
- If the lateral anlage fails to develop normally, there may be failure of fusion of the C-cell portion with the medial anlagen.

Lateral Aberrant Thyroid

This is a controversial term. Lateral aberrant thyroid is defined as **the presence of thyroid tissue lateral to** the jugular vein. If this is *not* within a lymph node, it can be regarded as a developmental anomaly, especially if the gland is itself abnormal or has been the site of previous surgery with possible dislodgement of small portions of thyroid tissue.

If, however, thyroid tissue appears **within lymph nodes** lateral to the jugular veins, it must be regarded as being a secondary deposit from a thyroid cancer.

THYROID HORMONES

Control of Thyroid Hormone Secretion

Control of thyroid hormone secretion is vested in a hypothalamic–pituitary–thyroid axis. This responds to circulating levels of hormone, the system being under 'negative feedback' control (*Fig. 40.32a*).

Thyroid-stimulating hormone (TSH; thyrotropin) synthesis and secretion are controlled by two factors:

- **An inhibitory negative feedback on the anterior pituitary related to circulating levels of thyroid hormone.** Hypothyroidism due to absence of or disease in the thyroid leads to a sustained increase in TSH secretion
- **Stimulation by thyrotropin-releasing hormone (TRH) derived from the hypothalamus.** TRH

is a tripeptide which travels down the nerve endings to the median eminence and then reaches the target cells via the portal capillary system. Tonic stimulation of the anterior pituitary is needed if thyroid hormone secretion is to be maintained.

Thus, severe injury to the hypothalamus or section of the hypothalamo–pituitary stalk is followed by the development of hypothyroidism.

At the level of the thyroid, hormone production is controlled by the binding of TSH to specific membrane receptors on the surface of epithelial cells. This activates intracellular adenylate cyclase, increasing the intracellular concentration of cyclic 5'-adenosine monophosphate (cAMP).

Steps in Hormone Synthesis

These are summarized in *Fig. 40.33*.

Transport of Iodide from Plasma to Follicular Cell

Iodide **'trapping'** is energy dependent; iodide must be transported against a gradient and concentrated 30-fold. This is controlled by TSH and is the rate-limiting step in thyroid hormone secretion. Trapping can be modulated up or down fivefold where there is iodide deficiency or excess. In exactly the same way as with

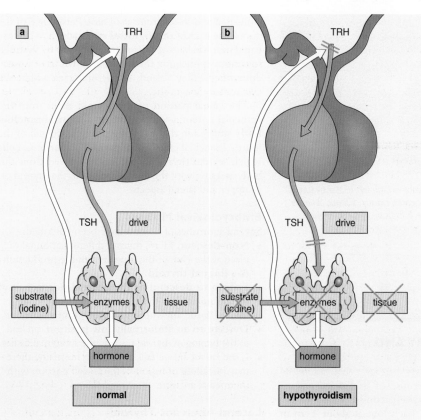

FIGURE 40.32 **a** Normal hypothalamic–pituitary–thyroid axis. **b** Possible basic causes of hypothyroidism.

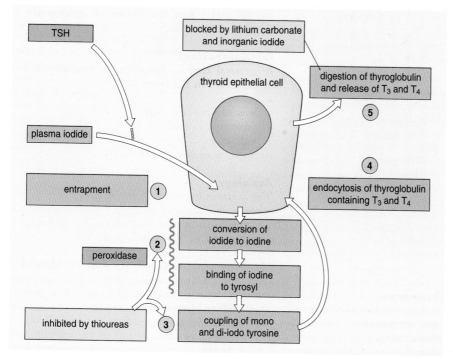

FIGURE 40.33 *Steps in the synthesis of thyroid hormones.*

iodide, the thyroid can clear other monovalent anions such as perchlorate and pertechnetate from the plasma; this can be useful in thyroid imaging.

Synthesis of the thyroid hormones L-thyroxine and L-tri-iodothyronine requires adequate supplies of iodine. For a steady state to be maintained, approximately 80 μg iodide must be transported into the thyroid each day.

Organification

Organification occurs at the apex of the follicular cell; it involves the conversion of iodide to iodine and its binding to tyrosyl residues, which are part of thyroglobulin. This process requires the enzyme **peroxidase**. Congenital absence of the enzyme leads to either cretinism or goitre (thyroid enlargement). Certain drugs used for treating hyperthyroidism, the thioureas such as propylthiouracil, compete with iodide for the peroxidase and inhibit organification.

Coupling

In coupling, either two molecules of **di-iodotyrosine** or one of di-iodotyrosine and one of **mono-iodotyrosine** fuse, forming the **iodothyronines**. Congenital defects in this process have been recognized and, because it is peroxidase dependent, it is also inhibited by thioureas.

Storage and Secretion

Villi from the apical surface of the follicular cell enclose a droplet of thyroglobulin; the latter becomes endocy-

tosed into the cell, lying within a phagosome. As the phagosome moves towards the basal aspect of the cell, thyroglobulin is digested and the freed hormones are secreted across the basal plasma membrane into adjacent capillaries. **This process can be blocked by either lithium carbonate or inorganic iodide.** A small amount of thyroglobulin normally enters the circulation; blood levels are about 5 ng/dl.

> ### KEY POINTS: Requirements For Thyroid Hormone Secretion
> Normal thyroid hormone secretion requires:
> - adequate drive (TSH)
> - adequate amounts of functioning tissue
> - adequate amounts of substrate (iodide)
> - adequate enzymes for organification and coupling
>
> **A deficiency in any one of these will lead to hypofunction of the gland.**

Transport of Thyroid Hormones in the Bloodstream

About 90 μg of T_4 and 30 μg of T_3 are secreted into the blood daily; 99.7% of these two hormones is bound to plasma proteins in the plasma. These include:

- **thyroid-binding globulin (TBG)**, binding 75% of T_4
- **transthyretin** (formerly known as prealbumin), binding about 15% of T_4
- **albumin**, binding the remaining 10% of T_4

Any quantitative change in TBG leads to changes in the amount of circulating free T_4, producing changes in thyroid function test results. Factors affecting TBG levels are shown in *Table 40.19*.

Table 40.19 Factors Affecting TBG Levels	
Factors increasing TBG levels	Factors decreasing TBG levels
Oestrogens	Androgens
Pregnancy	Cirrhosis of the liver
Oral contraceptives	Nephrotic syndrome
Hepatitis	Hereditary
Porphyria	
Hereditary	

Action of Thyroid Hormones

Thyroid hormones affect many systems. The hormone is believed to bind to **nuclear** receptors, which are non-histone proteins bound to nuclear chromatin. Hormone–receptor binding leads to changes in gene expression thought to underlie the functional changes mediated by thyroid hormones. These hormones are extremely important in the development and growth of infants, especially in respect of the differentiation and function of the central nervous system.

Disorders of the Thyroid

Thyroid disease is considered conveniently under a number of rubrics:
- **hypofunction (hypothyroidism)**
- **hyperfunction (hyperthyroidism)**
- **enlargement (goitre). This may be associated with normal function (a euthyroid state), hypothyroidism or hyperthyroidism.**
- **inflammatory disorders, which may or may not be associated with alterations in thyroid function**
- **thyroid neoplasms**

HYPOTHYROIDISM

This term covers a wide spectrum of functional and morphological change. Hypothyroidism in adults ranges from a severe disorder (**myxoedema**) to one that may be much less severe and, not uncommonly, missed. Hypothyroidism is quite common (up to 2% of the population in some studies). It is a disorder of mid-dle age and occurs **ten times as commonly in females as in males**.

Clinical Features
In general terms, symptomatic hypothyroidism is expressed in the form of:
- lethargy
- decreased physical ability
- intolerance to cold

A wide range of organs and systems may be affected clinically, as shown in *Table 40.20*.

Aetiology
The causes of hypothyroidism are many. They may be related conveniently to the major requirements for normal secretion of adequate amounts of thyroid hormone, as shown in *Table 40.21* and *Fig. 40.32b*.

Hypothyroidism in Infancy and Childhood
As with adults, many causes exist for hypothyroidism in infants and young children. Hypothyroidism **present at or before birth** is termed **cretinism** or congenital hypothyroidism. In areas where iodide deficiency is endemic, cretinism may be due to this substrate deficiency. In areas where iodide deficiency goitre is not endemic, the commonest cause of cretinism is **thyroid dysgenesis**, which may range from complete absence of the thyroid to hypoplasia or ectopy.

Hypothyroidism may also occur because of a **lack of appropriate enzymes**. In **Pendred's syndrome**, for example, there is a **peroxidase defect** which may be associated with mild hypothyroidism and nerve deafness.

Clinical Features
The clinical features of children with hypothyroidism differ, depending on the age at which the hypothyroidism appears. Where the thyroid is absent, clinical features may be present at birth, but it is more common for them to develop within the first 2 months of life. As the neonate ages, the facial features become thick and coarse, and linear growth declines during the first month of life. The babies are inactive and it is suggested that any infant who cries seldom and who has to be wakened for feeding should be investigated for hypothyroidism. If the diagnosis is not made early and appropriate replacement therapy instituted, learning disability occurs.

Pathological Features
In general, in those cases where the hypothyroidism is not due to absence of or loss of thyroid tissue or to lack of adequate TSH drive, the thyroid gland shows hyperplasia of the follicular epithelium. This is caused by the secretion of extra TSH in response to the low circulating levels of T_3 and T_4. **Hyperplasia of thyroid follicular epithelium is also seen:**

Table 40.20 Organs and Systems Affected in Hypothyroidism

System	Complaints	Signs
Central nervous system	Lethargy, memory defects, change in personality, poor attention span	Sleepiness, slow speech, may have acute psychotic episodes, defects in hearing and taste, cerebellar ataxia
Nerve and muscle	Weakness, cramps, joint pains	Delayed relaxation of deep tendon reflexes, carpal tunnel syndrome
Gut	Constipation, nausea	Large tongue, occasionally ascites
Skin, hair and nails	Dry rough skin, face puffy, loss of hair, nails brittle	Oedema, which is non-pitting, of ankles, face and hands (myxoedema), pallor, hair coarse, axillae dry
Female genital tract	Decreased libido, menstrual changes, decreased fertility	
Heart, lungs and upper respiratory tract	Decreased exercise tolerance	Hoarse voice, slow pulse rate, mild increase in blood pressure, occasionally pericardial effusion, hyperlipidaemia

Table 40.21 Causes of Hypothyroidism

Deficiency	Cause
Lack of sufficient tissue	Thyroid agenesis Destruction of thyroid by: • surgery • external irradiation • radioactive iodine Autoimmune disease (Hashimoto's thyroiditis) Other forms of thyroiditis (e.g. viral) Systemic diseases infiltrating the thyroid (e.g. sarcoidosis, lymphoma, amyloid) See *Fig. 40.34*
Lack of drive	TSH or TRH deficiency Blocking of TSH receptor
Lack of substrate	Iodide deficiency
Lack of enzymes	Dyshormonogenetic goitre; antithyroid drugs

- **in the presence of hyperfunction of the gland, as in Graves' disease** where there is an abnormal stimulus by a thyroid-stimulating immunoglobulin
- **in euthyroid patients who may be mildly iodide deficient or in those with Graves'** disease who have been rendered euthyroid by antithyroid drugs.

Hashimoto's Thyroiditis
Hashimoto's thyroiditis is the commonest cause of hypothyroidism. It is commonest in middle age, showing a distinct predilection for females. It was the first autoimmune disease to be recognized as such. Its autoimmune nature is expressed in the following ways:
- **Autoantibodies against antigens in thyroglobulin and in thyroid epithelial microsomes are present**, often in high titre, in the blood of patients.
- **It is often associated with other organ-specific autoimmune disorders** such as pernicious anaemia, Addison's disease, myasthenia gravis and diabetes mellitus. This association involves not only patients with Hashimoto's disease but also their relatives.
- **The thyroid tissue shows infiltration by plasma cells and lymphocytes.** The latter are often arranged in a follicular pattern and germinal centres may be seen. This lymphocyte population also contains K (killer) cells, which may have a role in causing the tissue damage.
- **The injection of thyroglobulin together with Freund's adjuvant into rodents produces a thyroiditis resembling Hashimoto's thyroiditis morphologically** and associated with the appearance of circulating antithyroid antibodies.
- **The circulating antibodies marking the presence of the disease may not be the factor that damages the thyroid tissue.** In cell culture

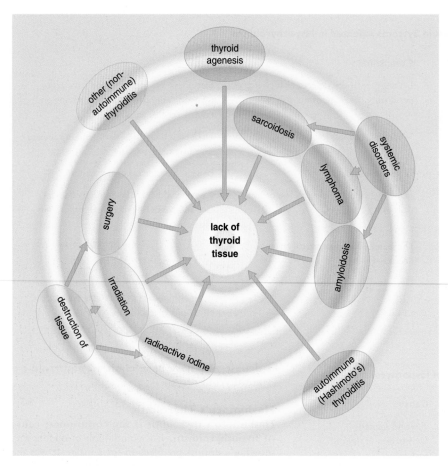

FIGURE 40.34 Causes of lack of thyroid tissue leading to hypothyroidism.

systems, the antimicrosomal antibody is cytotoxic in the presence of complement, but it is not likely that this circulating antibody would gain access to the antigen (which is situated at the apex of the cell in contact with colloid, in the intact host). In addition, in most instances, there is no sign of the disease in infants born to mothers with Hashimoto's thyroiditis (in contrast with Graves' disease).

Clinical Features
Hashimoto's thyroiditis may present in a number of ways:
- with goitre (thyroid enlargement, which may be diffuse or focally nodular). About 75% of these patients are euthyroid when first seen but may become hypothyroid later. The remainder have either clinically overt hypothyroidism or subclinical hypothyroidism, which can be recognized by testing thyroid function.
- hypothyroidism
- as thyrotoxicosis (hyperthyroidism). In this instance it is believed that two diseases are present (Graves' disease and Hashimoto's disease), the resulting

combination being described by some authors as **Hashitoxicosis**).

Laboratory Findings
Confirmation of the diagnosis involves:
- establishing the status of the patient's thyroid function
- immunological diagnosis of Hashimoto's disease by measuring the titres of circulating antibodies to thyroglobulin and to thyroid epithelial microsomes

Aetiology
Hashimoto's thyroiditis is clearly an autoimmune disorder, but its cause and the way in which tissue damage occurs are still unknown.

For some time, it was thought that the thyroid antigens against which autoantibodies appear are 'sequestered' from the immune system and thus tolerance could not occur. Escape of these antigens, in terms of this model, would then lead to an immune reaction against 'self' antigens. Thyroglobulin, however, is certainly not a sequestered antigen and small amounts of thyroglobulin constantly enter the bloodstream. In addition there are B lymphocytes in the bloodstream which have receptors for thyroglobulin.

Alternative possibilities are that:

- There may be abnormal presentation of self-antigens to the T helper cells. Some support for this comes from the fact that the thyroid epithelium in Hashimoto's thyroiditis expresses major histocompatibility complex class II-coded proteins (HLA-DR) on the surface of the epithelial cells.
- There may be a deficiency of T suppressor cells. In general, anything (in animal models of autoimmune disease) that reduces the population of T suppressor cells (for example, neonatal thymectomy) exacerbates the disease. Thus, in the Obese strain of chicken, which spontaneously develops autoimmune thyroiditis, neonatal thymectomy significantly worsens the severity of the disease.
- Strains of animals or birds that spontaneously develop autoimmune thyroiditis exist and multiple cases occur within families. This suggests that genetic factors may be important. The possession of an HLA-DR5 haplotype appears to increase the risk of Hashimoto's thyroiditis, the relative risk being $3.2 : 1$ compared with those individuals without this haplotype.

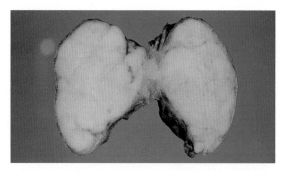

FIGURE 40.35 *Hashimoto's thyroiditis. The thyroid is moderately enlarged, much paler than normal and opaque. The latter features is the correlate of lack of colloid and a heavy infiltrate of lymphocytes and plasma cells.*

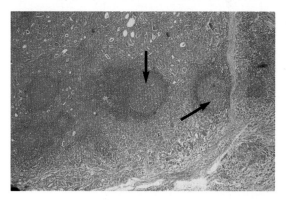

FIGURE 40.36 *Hashimoto's thyroiditis (haematoxylin and eosin stain). The follicles are small; there is very little colloid present and a striking infiltrate of lymphoid cells. Some germinal centres (arrowed) are present.*

Macroscopic Features

The gland may be moderately enlarged and is paler and much more opaque than usual (*Fig. 40.35*). The capsular surface shows, in many instances, a diffuse nodularity and the thyroid can be dissected freely away from the surrounding tissues.

Microscopic Features

- The gland is infiltrated by lymphocytes and plasma cells. The lymphocytes are arranged in follicles in some areas and germinal centres are commonly present (*Fig. 40.36*).
- The thyroid follicles tend to be smaller than normal and contain small amounts of darkly staining colloid. The epithelial cells themselves are cuboidal, eosinophilic and granular; the last feature is due to the presence of large numbers of mitochondria. Cells with this appearance are variously called, **Askanazy cells, oncocytes or Hurthle cells**. The pathogenesis of these epithelial changes is not known.
- In long-standing cases, where severe hypothyroidism is present, the gland is greatly shrunken and may weigh only a few grams. Microscopic examination shows virtually complete loss of recognizable thyroid follicles, these being replaced by fibrous tissue in which a mild to moderate lymphocyte infiltrate is present. This histological picture is the morphological correlate of what used to be called **primary myxoedema**, and is commonest in elderly women.

HYPERTHYROIDISM

Hyperthyroidism results from (*Fig. 40.37*):

1) **autoimmune mechanisms associated with thyroid-stimulating antibodies. This is by far the commonest cause, operating in diffuse hyperplasia associated with hyperthyroidism (Graves' disease) and in so-called 'toxic' nodular goitre. More than 90% of cases of hyperthyroidism fall into this category.**

2) rare causes such as:

- thyroid tumours secreting large amounts of T_3 and T_4
- excessive production of TSH by a pituitary tumour
- administration of thyroid hormones in an inappropriately high dosage
- administration of large doses of iodide
- subacute thyroiditis, which may cause transient hyperactivity
- the mild thyroid-stimulating effect of human chorionic gonadotrophin, as for example in cases of hydatidiform mole

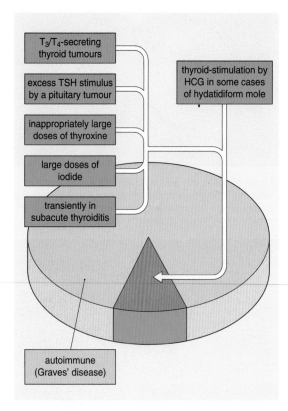

FIGURE 40.37 Causes of hyperthyroidism.

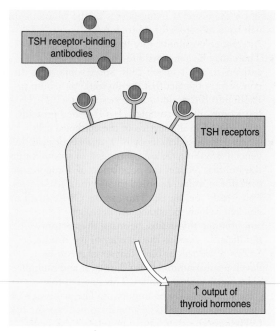

FIGURE 40.38 Autoantibodies that bind to the TSH receptor mediate autoimmune hyperthyroidism.

Autoimmune Thyroid Hyperplasia (Graves' Disease)

Aetiology and Pathogenesis

In about 90% of patients, autoantibodies directed against an epitope on the TSH receptor are present in the serum. The effect on the function of the TSH receptor is the same as that of TSH (i.e. a stimulus for the production of thyroid hormones) (*Fig. 40.38*). Because autoantibody levels are not under negative feedback control, the end result is the production of inappropriately large amounts of thyroid hormones. **The pivotal role of the autoantibodies in this type of hyperthyroidism is demonstrated by the facts that:**

- Congenital, transient thyrotoxicosis can occur in infants as a result of transplacental passage of stimulating antibody derived from the blood of mothers with Graves' disease.
- In cells derived from tissues other than the thyroid transfected with complementary DNA of the TSH receptor, the addition of plasma from a patient with Graves' disease leads to an immediate activation of adenylate cyclase and thus an increase in intracellular cAMP levels.

This autoantibody is not the only one that can stimulate the thyroid. **There exist, in addition, autoantibod-ies stimulating the growth of thyroid epithelium without at the same time increasing hormone production.** Such growth-promoting antibodies are present in about 65% of patients with thyrotoxicosis and may also play a part in the pathogenesis of simple, non-toxic enlargement of the thyroid in cases **where there is no evidence of iodide deficiency and where no goitrogens have been taken.** Where growth-promoting antibodies are present in a significant titre in patients with thyrotoxicosis, the degree of thyroid enlargement is usually great.

Why such antibodies should be formed remains a matter for speculation. Among the mechanisms canvassed are:

- **Genetic factors:**

  a) In about half the cases of thyrotoxicosis here is a family history of the disease.

  b) There is a high prevalence of thyroid autoantibodies (about 30%) in apparently unaffected first-degree relatives of patients with thyrotoxicosis.

  c) Concordance rates for thyrotoxicosis in monozygotic twins are much higher (50%) than in dizygotic twins (5%).

  d) The risks of developing thyrotoxicosis appear to be influenced by haplotype. In Europe and North America, this risk is related to DR3 and B8, the relative risk relating to DR3 being 3.7 : 1.

- **Infections with organisms possessing antigens that cross-react with the TSH receptor.** It has been suggested that antibody formation occurs because of infection with microorganisms that contain antigens very similar to TSH. The organism *Yersinia enterocolitica*, for instance, has a specific TSH binding site and similar receptors have been identified in other organisms.

- **Defects in T suppressor cell activity or abnormal presentation of antigen.** As discussed in the section on Hashimoto's thyroiditis, there may be defects either in T-cell suppression of autoantibody formation or in the presentation of 'self' antigen to T helper cells.

Clinical Features

The disease occurs in both sexes and at any age, but is commonest in women aged 20–40 years. The female : male ratio is about 5 : 1.

Locally, thyrotoxicosis is accompanied by diffuse enlargement of the thyroid. Initially the gland feels soft but with time it becomes firmer. The hyperplastic hyperfunctioning thyroid has a high blood flow and in some instances this may be expressed in the form of a systolic bruit.

The systemic clinical effects are very wide ranging and can involve almost any organ (*Fig. 40.39*). **In general terms the patients usually complain of nervousness, fatigue, inability to concentrate and irritability. Weight loss is very common, as is a fine tremor of the hands.**

Skin

The skin is warm and moist; the patients sweat profusely. In some cases there is connective tissue mucin deposition in the dermis and subcutaneous tissue on the anterior surface of the legs (**pretibial myxoedema**). Similar changes may occur, less commonly, in the arms. Pretibial myxoedema presents as plaque-like, firm swellings in the affected areas.

Some patients show swelling and clubbing of the fingers, associated with periosteal new bone formation (**thyroid acropachy**).

Eyes

Changes in the orbital tissue and eyes occur in 25–50% of thyrotoxic patients. Many patients show lid lag, lid retraction and stare. Those with significant ophthalmopathy typically complain of a gritty sensation in the eyes, blurring of vision, increased sensitivity to light and double vision. On examination, they may show conjunctival oedema (**chemosis**), injection of the scleral vessels and lid oedema. With increasing severity, the eyes appear to bulge from the orbits (**exophthalmos**) and there may be dysfunction of the extraocular muscles and periorbital oedema. Ophthalmopathy is often associated with pretibial myxoedema. About 10% of patients with ophthalmopathy do not have obvious clinical thyrotoxicosis but most show the presence of thyroid-stimulating immunoglobulins.

These clinical features are the expression of an

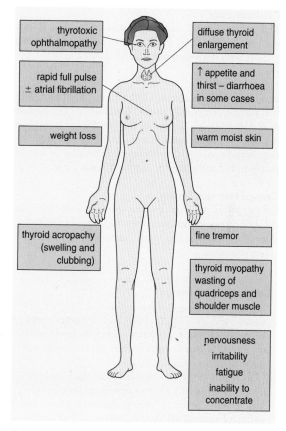

FIGURE 40.39 *Clinical features of thyrotoxicosis.*

increased volume of the intraorbital tissues as a result of accumulation of glycosoaminoglycans in the orbital connective tissue, probably produced by fibroblasts. In addition to the accumulation of this mucoid material, the orbit shows infiltration by lymphocytes, most of which are T cells. These cells express interferon γ, tumour necrosis factor β and interleukin 1α. These cytokines are not seen in normal orbital tissue. It has been suggested that the primary autoimmune target in thyrotoxic ophthalmopathy is the orbital fibroblast; the skin fibroblast is the homologous target in pretibial myxoedema where there is an increase in the volume of the soft tissue of the dermis and subcutis.

The accumulation of connective tissue mucoid substances in the orbit does not seem to be caused directly by TSH receptor-stimulating antibody but rather by T-cell activation. Local release of cytokines may enhance the expression of proteins on the fibroblast surface such as HLA-DR, intercellular adhesion molecule 1 (ICAM-1) and the 72-kDa form of heat shock protein, which modify the immune reaction.

Gastrointestinal Tract

Patients have an increased appetite and increased thirst; diarrhoea is not uncommon.

Cardiovascular

The pulse is rapid and full. Atrial fibrillation is not uncommon and heart block may occur. Some patients present with high-output cardiac failure.

Neuromuscular

In addition to fine tremor of the hands, mild or severe myopathies commonly occur. Weakness of the muscle of the shoulder girdle and of the quadriceps muscle in the thigh is quite common and may be severe. In addition, some patients may experience episodes of flaccid paralysis, the pathogenesis of which is not clear.

Central Nervous System

On occasions, the patients may present with delirium or even manic episodes. Abnormalities of movement sometimes occur, the most common of which is choreoathetosis.

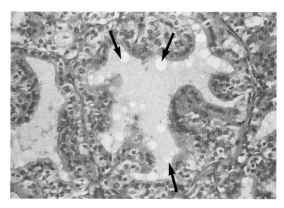

FIGURE 40.40 *Section of thyroid from a patient with thyrotoxicosis. Note the pseudopapillary infolding of the tall epithelial cells and the focal loss of colloid at the epithelial surface (arrowed).*

Laboratory Findings

Diagnosis depends on the demonstration of increased circulating levels of T_3 or T_4. Pure T_3 thyrotoxicosis with normal T_4 levels does occur but is relatively uncommon and tends to be seen in patients whose hyperthyroidism is associated with a toxic nodular goitre.

Occasionally the diagnosis may be difficult to confirm and a TSH stimulation test may then be appropriate. The characteristic response to TRH in thyrotoxicosis is a flat one; an increase in TSH levels of $2-3$ μg/ml excludes the diagnosis of thyrotoxicosis.

If it is deemed necessary to measure TSH receptor antibodies, this can be done either with a bioassay in which the effect of the patient's plasma on intracellular cAMP level in appropriate cell cultures is measured, or by immunological binding assays.

Macroscopic Features

The gland is diffusely enlarged and is often a reddish brown colour because of the increased vascularity. Because there is little stored colloid in the acini, the cut surface is much meatier than normal.

Microscopic Features

The follicles are markedly hyperplastic and the increase in the number of lining cells may be expressed in the form of papillary infolding. Care must be taken not to confuse this hyperplastic process with papillary carcinoma. The lining epithelium consists of tall columnar cells which have a basally situated nucleus and, often, clear cytoplasm in which fat or glycogen may be identified.

The colloid is scanty and stains rather feebly with eosin. Frequently the edge of the colloid has an irregular 'scalloped' appearance where it is normally in contact with apical aspect of the epithelial cells (*Fig. 40.40*).

The stroma contains foci of lymphoid cells and occasional germinal centres may be seen. Most of these are T cells, with the suppressor phenotype predominating.

Toxic Nodular Goitre

Toxic nodular goitre may be defined as nodular enlargement of the thyroid **associated with production of excess amounts of thyroid hormones**. The affected thyroid may show many nodules or, more rarely, there may be a single over-secreting nodule associated with some suppression of the surrounding normal-appearing thyroid tissue. Only a minority of single nodules (about 10–20%) secrete sufficient thyroid hormones to cause clinically overt thyrotoxicosis.

Multinodular goitre associated with overt thyrotoxicosis is usually very large. Such goitres usually occur in an older age group and pretibial myxoedema, eye changes and acropachy are not usually seen. Stimulating TSH receptor antibodies are not usually present but growth-promoting antibodies probably play a part in the genesis of this condition.

NON-TOXIC GOITRE

Non-toxic goitre is defined as thyroid enlargement, **not due to neoplasia or infiltrative diseases and not associated with any evidence of hyperthyroidism**.

Such goitres arise on the basis of a subtle interplay of factors, some environmental (e.g. iodide deficiency) and some intrinsic to the gland or its microenvironment. Such factors include:

- **iodide deficiency**
- **intrinsic defects in hormone synthesis**

Both of these will lead to increased output of TSH and, thus, to hyperplasia of the thyroid. This represents an attempt, usually successful in the case of iodine deficiency, to restore a euthyroid state. Other factors are:

- **growth-promoting immunoglobulins in the plasma**
- **ingestion of large amounts of foodstuffs containing goitrogenic substances.** Members of the brassica family such as cabbage, turnips and kale fall into this category and act by interfering with thyroid hormone synthesis. They are most likely to produce goitre in individuals whose iodide intake is suboptimal.
- **certain drugs that may inhibit iodide uptake, the release of thyroid hormone or one of the steps in hormone synthesis.** Such compounds include excess iodide, thionamides, amiodarone, lithium, fluoride and carbutamide.

Iodide Deficiency Goitre

This disorder may be endemic or sporadic. As the major contribution to dietary intake of iodide comes from sea food, it is not surprising that there is an increased risk of iodide deficiency occurring in areas far from the sea. Mountainous areas such as Switzerland, the Andes and the Himalayas used particularly to be affected. It is still an extremely common condition and, in some areas, affects 10% of the population. The addition of iodide to food, notably salt or flour, prevents this form of goitre. Iodide deficiency goitre may be congenital, but it is more likely to occur at times when there is a greater physiological need for thyroid hormones. Thus, it tends to appear at puberty, during pregnancy and during lactation.

Iodide deficiency goitre may exist in a number of morphological forms.

Diffuse Hyperplastic Goitre

This is dominated by epithelial hyperplasia as a result of the increased output of TSH. Only small amounts of colloid are present and the gland therefore appears fleshy. The follicles are lined by columnar epithelium.

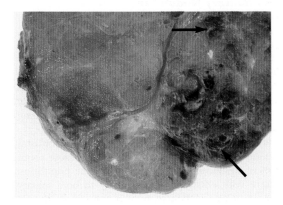

FIGURE 40.41 Multinodular 'colloid' goitre showing focal haemorrhage (arrowed).

The size of the thyroid is not greatly increased and surgery is not usually undertaken at this stage.

Diffuse Colloid Goitre

This is seen particularly in adolescence and during pregnancy. A considerable degree of gland enlargement is present. However, instead of the small follicles lined by hyperplastic epithelium described above, the follicles are enormously distended with colloid and the lining epithelium is flattened. On the basis of experiments in rodents, it has been suggested that this is the morphological correlate of a withdrawal of the extra TSH stimulus and that it may represent a phase of involution.

Nodular Goitre

Macroscopic Features

Here the degree of enlargement can be very great and thyroids weighing up to 2 kg have been reported. The external surface is lumpy and irregular due to nodules ranging in size from a few millimetres to several centimetres. (*Fig. 40.41*). The cut surface confirms the presence of a nodular architectural pattern, the nodules being separated from each other by fibrous tissue bands. The larger nodules show an abundance of pale yellowish colloid but many of the nodules have a grossly altered naked-eye appearance due to combinations and permutations of haemorrhage (old or recent), cystic degeneration and dystrophic calcification.

Microscopic Features

The outstanding feature is the variability and unpredictability of the histological appearances. There is marked variation in the size of the follicles: some are very large and distended with colloid, whereas others are tiny. A similarly wide range of appearances is shown by the epithelium lining the follicles. In some cases the cells are columnar and may protrude into the lumina of the follicles to form papillae. These, however, do not branch as do the papillae of papillary cancer. In other areas the epithelium is cuboidal or, sometimes, flattened. The intervening stroma, which in some areas can be abundant, may show haemosiderin pigmentation and so-called 'cholesterol clefts' (the roughly torpedo-shaped spaces where crystalline cholesterol has been dissolved out by lipid solvents in the course of tissue preparation).

The reasons for the acquisition of a multinodular pattern, very common in areas whereas goitre is endemic, are not clear. It has been suggested that there is a variation in the response of individual areas to TSH stimulation and there may be a similar variation relating to other steps in hormone synthesis. Support for this concept of functional heterogeneity comes from radioactive iodine uptake studies in which some nodules avidly take up the iodine whereas others ('cold' nodules) do not.

THYROIDITIS (EXCLUDING HASHIMOTO'S THYROIDITIS)

Thyroiditis may be considered under the following headings:

- acute bacterial thyroiditis
- subacute thyroiditis (synonyms De Quervain's/granulomatous thyroiditis)
- Riedel's thyroiditis
- atrophic thyroiditis
- silent (painless) thyroiditis

Acute Bacterial Thyroiditis

Acute suppurative thyroiditis occurs as a result of direct spread from an adjacent focus of acute inflammation or of a blood-borne infection. Organisms most commonly involved include *Staphylococcus aureus*, haemolytic streptococci, *Escherichia coli* and pneumococci.

Patients present with severe local pain, tenderness and thyroid enlargement. These features are accompanied in most cases by systemic ones such as fever, rigor and malaise. Histological material is not usually available from affected thyroids because the inflammation generally settles well as a result of antibiotic treatment alone or, if abscess formation occurs, following the use of antibiotics combined with surgical drainage.

Subacute Thyroiditis

Subacute thyroiditis is an inflammatory disorder of the thyroid believed to be viral in origin. The histological appearance is characterized by **granulomas and giant cells**. Such thyroiditis often occurs in the course of a viral infection and is self-limiting; both mumps virus and human syncytial virus have been isolated from thyroid tissue of affected patients.

The clinical picture is a combination of:

- **the pain and swelling related to the inflammatory process within the thyroid**
- **alterations in thyroid function**

Early in the course of the disease, transient **hyperthyroidism** may be present. This is due to leakage of thyroxine into tissue fluid and thence into the bloodstream. Leakage is due to the destruction of follicles in which hormone has been stored in colloid. A euthyroid phase then ensues and this may be followed by a period of **hypothyroidism**. Spontaneous recovery of thyroid function is the rule. The illness may last from 6 weeks to 6 months.

Riedel's Thyroiditis

This is a very rare form of thyroid disease in which the gland is the seat of **extensive scarring**. The thyroid is hard and 'woody' in consistency and is often fixed to surrounding tissue by fibrous adhesions. Indeed, the fibrous tissue often invades the surrounding strap muscles of the neck, making surgical dissection difficult.

The aetiology of this disorder is essentially unknown but there is a resemblance between the pathological picture seen here and that seen in certain other fibrosing disorders such as retroperitoneal fibrosis.

Macroscopic Features

Affected areas of the thyroid are white and stony hard, and there is no evidence of a normal lobular structure.

Microscopic Features

There is extensive replacement of thyroid parenchyma by featureless fibrous tissue, and focal lymphocytic infiltration is present. The surviving thyroid tissue often shows atrophy.

'Silent' Thyroiditis

This is a curious disorder often, but not exclusively, occurring postpartum. Patients often present with the abrupt onset of symptoms and signs of hyperthyroidism, associated with minimal enlargement of the thyroid. This resolves spontaneously over a period of weeks or months. The thyroid enlargement is painless and the gland itself is non-tender. Despite the evidence of thyroid hyperfunction, there is a low uptake of radioactive iodine, a finding that is also present during the early phase of subacute thyroiditis.

Microscopic Features

There is a lymphocyte and plasma cell infiltrate associated with occasional germinal centres. In this respect the histological picture resembles that seen in Hashimoto's thyroiditis but the parenchymal and serological changes of that disorder are not present in silent thyroiditis.

THYROID TUMOURS AND TUMOUR-LIKE LESIONS

The 'Solitary Nodule' and its Relationship to Neoplasia

Malignant thyroid tumours are comparatively rare, accounting for less than 1% of all malignancies. The number of new thyroid malignancies diagnosed annually in the USA is about 10 000 and the number of thyroid cancer-related deaths is 1000 per year. Thus only one death occurs from thyroid cancer for every 50 from breast cancer and for every 130 from lung cancer.

Nevertheless, the diagnosis of thyroid neoplasms presents a considerable clinical problem because about 1.5% of adolescents and 4–7% of the adult population present with what appears **clinically** to be a solitary thyroid nodule. Of these only a very small fraction (perhaps 1–2 per 1000) are thyroid cancers, but it is obviously essential that these should be identified.

Diagnosis

The first step in the diagnostic pathway is to determine, most usefully by ultrasonography, whether a clinically palpable thyroid nodule is in fact **solitary**. At least 50% of such lesions are nodules within a multinodular goitre.

Of the remaining truly solitary nodules, **about 70–80% are benign adenomas of the thyroid**. Only 10–20% of true solitary nodules are **carcinomas**.

Clinical features suggesting that a solitary thyroid nodule may be malignant include:

- **a history of previous irradiation or treatment with radioactive iodine**
- **a family history of phaeochromocytoma, hypercalcaemia or medullary cancer of the thyroid.** These are manifestations of the **multiple endocrine neoplasia (MEN) syndromes (IIa and IIb).**
- **a history of rapid growth, pain or dysphagia**
- **cervical lymph node enlargement**, especially on the same side as the nodule
- any symptoms or signs suggestive of invasion of neighbouring structures (e.g. **Horner's syndrome, hoarseness**)
- **male sex.** A solitary nodule in a male is more likely to be malignant than in a female.
- **young age.** A solitary nodule in a child has a higher index of suspicion for malignancy than in an adult.

Once the presence of a true solitary nodule has been established, the most appropriate step is cytological examination of fine-needle aspirates of the nodule. If the specimen is adequate in amount and quality, it is usually possible to categorize the smears as being:

- **benign**
- **malignant**
- **suspicious**

If all 'suspicious' lesions are followed by surgery, the end results indicate that cytological examination has a sensitivity of 90% and a specificity of about 70% in respect of the diagnosis of thyroid malignancy.

If the lesion is deemed on cytological examination to be a follicular neoplasm, radioactive iodine uptake studies should be performed. If the nodule takes up the iodine (a **hot** nodule) it is unlikely to be malignant. If it does not (a **cold** nodule) then surgical follow-up is probably indicated because 20% of cold nodules are malignant.

BENIGN NEOPLASMS

Although several morphological patterns exist, it seems reasonable to regard all benign neoplasms of the thyroid as being **follicular adenomas**. Histological criteria that must be fulfilled if a follicular nodule is to be regarded as a true neoplasm are:

- **complete encapsulation of the nodule** by fibrous tissue
- the **follicular architecture within the nodule must differ** from that of the surrounding thyroid tissue
- the **surrounding thyroid tissue must show compression atrophy**, indicating an expansile growth pattern within the nodule
- the **lesion must be a true solitary nodule** (i.e. there must be no multinodularity in the rest of the gland

The lesion occurs quite commonly in young adults, and is five times as common in females as in males. The clinical presentation is usually that of a painless lump within the thyroid, although, if haemorrhage occurs into the adenoma, pain may occur.

Macroscopic Features

The lesions are encapsulated, rounded masses measuring up to 10 cm in diameter. They differ in colour and consistency from the surrounding thyroid, because there is usually less colloid within the adenoma than in normal thyroid tissue. This feature will, of course, be modulated by the histological pattern of the adenoma.

Microscopic Features

The follicles are of differing sizes. Lesions are assigned to a particular category according to the dominant pattern:

- **trabecular** (previously referred to as embryonal adenoma)
- **microfollicular** (so-called fetal adenoma), in which follicles are minute and contain very little, if any, colloid
- **normofollicular** or **macrofollicular**, in which the follicles are either normal in size or much larger than normal
- **atypical** adenoma in which cellular pleomorphism may be present. This is not significant unless breaching of the capsule has occurred.
- adenoma in which the cells are enlarged, eosinophilic and granular owing to the large number of mitochondria. These cells are identical with the Askanazy or Hurthle cells described as occurring in Hashimoto's thyroiditis.

None of these patterns has any effect on the natural history of adenoma.

THYROID CARCINOMA

Thyroid cancer is classified under *four* major headings (*Fig. 40.42*):

1. **papillary** carcinoma, accounting for about 70% of all thyroid cancers
2. **follicular** carcinoma (about 15% of thyroid malignancies)
3. **undifferentiated or anaplastic** thyroid carcinoma
4. **medullary** carcinoma, arising from the thyrocalcitonin-secreting parafollicular or C cells

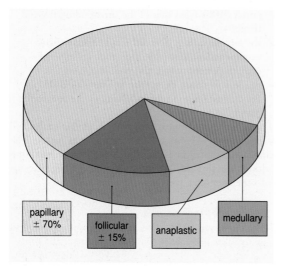

FIGURE 40.42 *Relative frequencies of different histological types of thyroid cancer.*

Papillary Carcinoma

Epidemiology

This is by far the commonest of primary thyroid malignancies. It may be either clinically **overt** or **occult**:

- Occult papillary carcinomas are found in about 10% of autopsies if the thyroid is carefully studied histologically; this prevalence appears to be consistent throughout adult life and affects both sexes equally.
- Clinically overt tumours are much rarer (affecting about 1 in 27 000 people annually), have a peak incidence at 20–50 years and are two to three times as common in females as in males.

Macroscopic Features

The gross pathology varies considerably from case to case. Most of the tumours are well defined but non-encapsulated by fibrous tissue. A small proportion (about 5%) shows total encapsulation and in these metastasis to distant sites is rare and death due to the tumour is almost unknown.

Papillary carcinomas may, in some instances, be very small (less than 1 cm in diameter) and these lesions are star-shaped and show extensive fibrosis. This is the clinically occult variant.

Microscopic Features

The defining criteria for the diagnosis of papillary carcinoma are both cytological and architectural.

Cytological Criteria

The cells are columnar or cuboidal and have characteris-

tic large pale nuclei with an 'empty' appearance. These have been termed 'Orphan Annie' nuclei after the heroine of the comic strip of the same name, whose eyes are drawn as empty circles (*Fig. 40.43*). This nuclear appearance is an important diagnostic criterion because many papillary tumours have a prominent follicular component. It is interesting that this nuclear appearance, so prominent in paraffin-embedded material, is inconspicuous or even absent in frozen sections.

Other nuclear features include pseudo-inclusions and prominent grooving of the nuclei, the grooves being oriented along the long axes of the nuclei. The pseudo-inclusions are sharply demarcated eosinophilic bodies, representing invaginations of the cytoplasm into the nucleus.

Architectural Criteria

There are **papillae** consisting of fibrovascular cores covered with the characteristic epithelial cells. The papillae are complex and branched, and the stroma of the cores may be hyalinized and infiltrated with lymphocytes or lipid-laden macrophages. 'Pure' papillary tumours may occur, although many papillary carcinomas contain follicles, the proportion of the two patterns varying from case to case. The biological behaviour of these 'mixed-pattern' tumours does not differ from that of pure papillary carcinomas.

In addition, **'psammoma bodies'** are found in about 50% of papillary carcinomas. They are spherical, calcified, laminated glycoprotein bodies which may be located either between the tumour cells or in the fibrovascular cores of the papillae. They constitute a virtually pathognomonic indicator of papillary carcinoma as they are exceptionally rare in other thyroid lesions.

Clinically palpable nodal metastases occur in about half the cases and microscopic deposits within lymph nodes are obviously even more common. In some instances, cervical node enlargement is the first

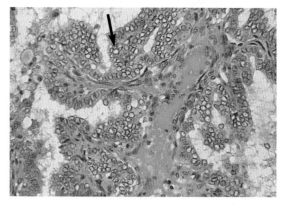

FIGURE 40.43 *Papillary carcinoma. Note the branching papillae and the curious empty-looking 'Orphan Annie' nuclei (arrowed).*

sign of a papillary carcinoma, as the primary tumour may be quite small. Direct extension into the soft tissues of the neck is found in about 25% of cases.

Natural History

The cure rate for papillary carcinoma of the thyroid is high and, even in those who are not cured, the clinical course is likely to be indolent. The 10-year survival rate is over 90%, with 80% surviving 20 years.

Factors suggesting a worse prognosis include:
- occurrence of the tumour at an older age than usual
- direct spread into the extrathyroid soft tissues
- a multicentric origin within the thyroid
- undifferentiated foci within the tumour
- the size of the tumour, larger tumours having a worse prognosis
- blood-borne metastases

Aetiology

The only aetiological factor so far recognized is irradiation. External irradiation during childhood seems to be particularly baneful in this respect. Non-therapeutic irradiation such as occurs in the course of nuclear 'fall out' is a definite risk factor. Nearly 7% of those who survived the nuclear bombing of Hiroshima and Nagasaki subsequently developed thyroid cancer. Most of the tumours associated with irradiation are either papillary or follicular.

Genomic Changes

Transfection of DNA extracted from papillary carcinomas has been shown to cause transformation in cultured murine fibroblasts of the immortalized 3T3 line. The putative oncogene appears to be one not previously recognized, located on chromosome 10 at bands q11–q12 close to the gene for the MEN-IIa syndrome. This oncogene, which has provisionally been called *ptc* (for papillary thyroid carcinoma), arises as a result of fusion between an unknown nucleotide sequence with the tyrosine kinase domain of the proto-oncogene *ret*.

Follicular Carcinoma

This is much rarer than papillary carcinoma, accounting for about 15% of primary thyroid malignancies. It tends to occur later in life, the median age at clinical presentation being 52 years. There is a female preponderance, which has been variously reported as ranging from 2 : 1 to 5 : 1. Unlike papillary carcinoma, follicular carcinoma has not been found as an occult tumour in autopsy material.

Clinical presentation is most commonly in the form of a 'cold' nodule (i.e. one that does not take up radioactive iodine). Clinical involvement of cervical nodes is not often seen at this stage, but about 15% of affected patients show evidence of distant spread at this time; the lung and bones are particularly likely to be involved.

Macroscopic Features

The lesions may appear well encapsulated. It is something of a paradox, bearing in mind the propensity for follicular cancer to spread, that there is often a thicker layer of fibrous tissue around a follicular cancer than is seen in relation to benign adenomas of the thyroid. If the tumour is well differentiated, abundant colloid may be present and it can be difficult to distinguish the tumour from a benign nodule.

Microscopic Features

In well-differentiated tumours, the same difficulties apply in distinguishing microscopically these lesions from benign thyroid nodules. An important practical point is that aspiration cytology is likely to be less helpful in relation to these tumours than is the case with other thyroid cancers.

In these well-differentiated cases, the defining criterion of malignancy is evidence of invasion. Such spread may be expressed in extension of the lesion through the capsule or in the form of blood vessel invasion. Tumour should be sought in small veins, either in the fibrous capsule or just outside it; the criterion for venous invasion should be a clump of tumour cells attached to the wall of the vessel and protruding into its lumen. Such a small mass of tumour may become covered by endothelial cells in a manner analogous to what occurs in mural thrombi.

So far as capsular invasion is concerned, spread of tumour should have occurred right through the entire thickness of the capsule before a diagnosis of malignancy based on this criterion is made.

Other follicular carcinomas are less well differentiated and have a variable growth pattern, which may be microfollicular or trabecular. These histological patterns do not appear to influence the natural history of the disease.

Natural History

For well-differentiated, minimally invasive, follicular tumours the prognosis is good. The overall picture, however, is considerably bleaker than for papillary carcinoma. About 70% of patients die as a result of the tumour in the 10 years following primary treatment.

Factors suggesting a worse prognosis include:
- an older age at diagnosis
- a marked degree of invasiveness
- the presence of metastatic disease at the time of primary treatment
- evidence of aneuploidy of the tumour cells

Genomic Changes

Convincing evidence exists for the existence of transforming *ras* oncogenes in follicular cancers, as judged by the transfection of tumour-derived DNA into murine fibroblasts in culture. In one study, such activated *ras* oncogenes were found in four-fifths of the tumours studied. All three *ras* oncogenes Ha-*ras*, Ki-*ras* and N-*ras* have been identified, and all have shown the presence of point mutations which, no doubt, accounts for their transforming ability.

Anaplastic or Undifferentiated Carcinoma

Anaplastic carcinoma accounts for about 10–15% of primary thyroid malignancies. It is believed to arise from a pre-existing well-differentiated tumour. This view gains some support from the history of an antecedent goitre given by many patients. Anaplastic carcinoma can occur at any age, although its peak incidence is between the ages of 60 and 70 years.

Macroscopic Features

Anaplastic tumours are markedly invasive and by the time the patient presents there is usually extensive infiltration of the thyroid and involvement of the soft tissues around the gland. Necrosis and haemorrhage are frequent findings and are obvious on inspection of the cut surface of the tumour.

Microscopic Features

Histological examination shows a variable pattern. The tumour may consist predominantly of spindle cells (sometimes leading to a mistaken diagnosis of sarcoma), large 'squamoid' epithelial cells and, very strikingly, giant multinucleated cells which morphologically resemble osteoclasts. Frequent and bizarre mitoses are a common finding. In cases resembling sarcoma, the epithelial nature can be established in many cases by the immunohistochemical identification of cytokeratins, which are present in at least 50% of anaplastic carcinomas.

Natural History

Anaplastic carcinoma carries the worst prognosis of all primary thyroid neoplasms. The mean survival time is 6–8 months after presentation. This can be somewhat prolonged if the tumour is diagnosed early and treated with a combination of surgery, external radiation and chemotherapy.

Medullary Carcinoma

Medullary carcinoma arises from the thyrocalcitonin-secreting parafollicular or C cells. It constitutes about 10% of thyroid malignancies. The tumour may occur under various circumstances:

- **Sporadic.** This is by far the commonest; 80–90% of medullary carcinomas are of this type.
- **Hereditary.** Hereditary tumours, inherited in an autosomal dominant fashion, may be:
  1) **part of the MEN syndrome type IIa**, consisting of:
     a) **medullary carcinoma** of the thyroid (more than 90%)
     b) **phaeochromocytoma of the adrenal**

medulla (50%). These tumours may be unilateral or bilateral.
     c) **hyperparathyroidism** (10–20%). Hyperfunction of the parathyroids is most often associated with hyperplasia.
  2) **part of the MEN syndrome type IIb**, consisting of:
     a) **medullary carcinoma** of the thyroid
     b) **phaeochromocytoma**
     c) **ganglioneuromas and neuromas of the tarsal plates, anterior third of the tongue, lips and alimentary tract**
  3) **medullary carcinoma not associated with the MEN syndromes**.

All inherited tumours and also a proportion of patients with sporadic medullary carcinoma show mutations in the *ret* **proto-oncogene**, which normally codes for a tyrosine kinase receptor. Curiously, mutations in the *ret* gene have also been reported as being associated with Hirschsprung's disease, which is characterized by a congenital absence of parasympathetic innervation of the lower part of the large gut. The mutations seen in association with this disorder are different from those encountered in patients with thyroid tumours, but it is still interesting that a single gene defect may be related to different clinical syndromes.

The calcitonin-secreting cells in the thyroid migrate from the neural crest to take up a position at the junction of the upper third and lower two-thirds of the lateral lobes. They fall into that class of neuroendocrine cells termed **APUD** cells, which secrete peptide hormones, take up precursors of amines and contain decarboxylases. **The primary transcript of the gene for calcitonin can be processed in alternative ways to produce either calcitonin, which is the normal product of the thyroid C cells, or calcitonin gene-related peptide, which is normally produced in neural cells and which is a powerful dilator of microvessels as well as inhibiting the secretion of insulin.**

The secretion of calcitonin is regulated principally by serum calcium concentrations but hormone release is also stimulated by pentagastrin. This is useful in the diagnosis of medullary carcinoma because pentagastrin produces an exaggerated rise in serum levels of calcitonin in patients with medullary carcinoma compared with that in normal individuals.

Macroscopic Features

Sporadic tumours are usually single and unilateral, whereas the hereditary ones are frequently bilateral and multifocal, and are often preceded by focal C-cell hyperplasia, which can occur very early in life.

Microscopic Features

The tumour cells, which may be spindle-shaped or rounded, are arranged in sheets or in a nested pattern, which occurs very commonly in endocrine and neuroendocrine neoplasms. **A highly characteristic feature is the presence of amyloid in the tumour stroma**. This is seen both in the primary tumour and in any metastatic deposits that may occur. The polypeptide forming the amyloid is identical with amino acids 9–19 of calcitonin.

Clinical Features

The clinical features seen in patients with medullary carcinoma of the thyroid are the expression of the presence of:

- **tumour within the thyroid.** Thus, many patients are 'picked up' because of a palpable nodule discovered on routine examination.
- **metastases in cervical or mediastinal nodes.** Such deposits are present in about 50% of patients with this tumour.
- **distant metastases.** These occur late in the course of the disease. The principal targets are lung, liver, bone and adrenals.
- **effects mediated by hormones secreted by the tumour cells.** These hormonal effects of the medullary carcinoma itself (excluding any MEN-associated features) include:

  1) **Diarrhoea.** About 30% of patients with widespread tumour have severe diarrhoea. It is not clear which of the secretion products of the tumour (*Table 40.22*) is responsible.
  2) **Cushing's syndrome.** This is a rare complication of medullary carcinoma. It is caused by secretion from the tumour cells of adrenocorticotropic hormone or corticotropin-

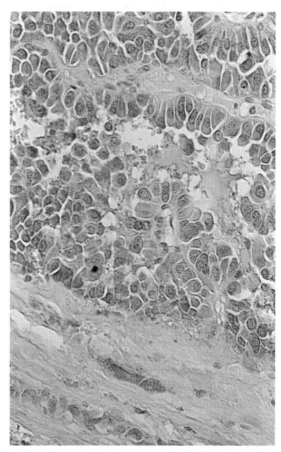

FIGURE 40.44 *Medullary carcinoma of the thyroid, treated with an antibody raised against calcitonin. The presence of brown staining indicates binding of the antibody to tumour cells.*

Table 40.22 Secretion Products of Medullary Carcinoma of the Thyroid

Calcitonin (*Fig. 40.44*)
Calcitonin gene-related peptide
Katacalcin
Adrenocorticotropic hormone
β-Endorphin
β-Melanocyte-stimulating hormone
5-Hydroxytryptamine
Somatostatin
Substance P
DOPA decarboxylase
Neurone-specific enolase
Nerve growth factor
Carcinoembryonic antigen
Synaptophysin

releasing hormone, or by a combination of the two. Removal of the thyroid tumour, in most cases, causes regression of the Cushing's syndrome.

Natural History

Medullary carcinoma behaves in a more aggressive fashion than papillary carcinoma. The overall 10-year survival rate is of the order of 65%.

Factors suggesting a worse prognosis include:
- a sporadic rather than a MEN-IIa-associated tumour
- age greater than 50 years at diagnosis
- the presence of nodal or distant metastases at the time of diagnosis

Early detection and treatment has a significant effect on the natural history of the disease. The appropriate treatment, if the tumour is still confined to the thyroid, is total thyroidectomy, because the tumour is often multicentric.

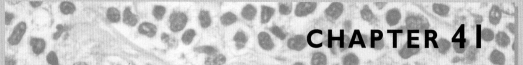

CHAPTER 41

The Haemopoietic System

Haemopoiesis and Disorders of Red Blood Cells

HAEMOPOIESIS

In childhood and adult life blood cells are formed in the bone marrow. However, in fetal life other sites are involved (see *Table 41.1*).

With maturation, active haemopoietic bone marrow is partly replaced by adipose tissue, leaving the axial skeleton (vertebral bodies, ribs, sternum, pelvis) and proximal ends of the femur and humerus as normal sites for haemopoiesis. If haemopoiesis is stimulated by either a normal or an inappropriate drive, the red active marrow spreads down the medullary cavities of the long bones.

Where Does Haemopoiesis Begin?

All the cellular elements of the blood, during both fetal and postnatal life, are derived from a pluripotent stem cell. This gives rise to a series of intermediate progenitors from which the individual haemopoietic cell lineages derive (*Fig. 41.1*).

Growth of the stem cell population is mediated through a ligand–receptor interaction. A local growth factor binds to a tyrosine kinase receptor on the stem cell which is coded for by a cellular proto-oncogene known as *c-kit*. Mutations occur in mice for both the growth factor and the receptor; a deficiency in either leads to defects in stem cell development, pigment-producing epithelial cells and gonadal germ cells.

The Hierarchy of Progenitor Cells in the Bone Marrow

The pluripotent stem cell gives rise to two classes of cell that act as important intermediate progenitors for the further stages of haemopoiesis. These are:

- a common lymphoid cell progenitor
- a cell that, when stimulated appropriately, gives rise to colonies of cells in semisolid agar which show multiple differentiation. This progenitor is called CFU_{GEMM} (colony-forming unit capable of giving rise to cells that differentiate into granulocytes, erythroid cells, monocytes and megakaryocytes). The further differentiation of this progenitor is shown in *Fig 41.1*.

Regulation of Haemopoiesis

This is a complex operation involving at least 14 cytokines and growth factors, the targets and sources of which are shown in *Table 41.2*.

RED CELL FUNCTION

HAEMOGLOBIN

The principal function of red cells is to deliver oxygen to the tissues and to transport carbon dioxide from them to the lung, where much of it is given up in the expired air. These functions are mediated through **haemoglobin**, which makes up the greatest part of the contents of the red cell envelope.

Table 41.1 Sites of Haemopoiesis

Time	Yolk sac	Liver and spleen	Bone marrow
Fetal life			
0–6 weeks	+	–	–
6 weeks to 6–7 months	–	+	–
6–7 months to term	–	+	+
Neonatal period (0–2 weeks)	–	+	+
Childhood and adult life	–	–	+

Table 41.2 Factors Involved in the Regulation of Haemopoiesis

Factor	Cellular target	Source
M-CSF	Monocytes	Endothelial cells Monocytes Fibroblasts
GM-CSF	Granulocytes Megakaryocytes Erythrocytes Stem cells Leukaemic blasts	T cells Endothelial cells Fibroblasts
G-CSF	Granulocytes Endothelial cells Macrophages Fibroblasts Leukaemic blasts	Endothelial cells Placenta Monocytes
IL-3	Granulocytes Red cells and their precursors Multipotent progenitor cells Leukaemic blasts	T cells
IL-4	B and T cells	T cells
IL-5	B cells CFU_{Eo}	T cells
IL-6	B and T cells CFU_{GEMM} CFU_{GM} BFU_E Macrophages Nerve cells Liver cells	Fibroblasts Leucocytes Epithelial cells
IL-7	B cells	Leucocytes
IL-8	T cells and neutrophils	Leucocytes
IL-9	CFU_{GEMM} BFU_E	Lymphocytes
IL-11	B and T cells CFU_{GEMM} Macrophages	Macrophages
Erythropoietin	BFU_E CFU_E	Kidney (90%) Liver (10%)
Stem cell factor (c-*kit* ligand)	Pluripotent stem cells	Bone marrow stromal cells

Interleukin (IL) 1 and tumour necrosis factor (TNF) α stimulate haemopoiesis by stimulating the production of granulocyte–macrophage colony-stimulating factor (GM-CSF), G-CSF, M-CSF and IL-6. BFU, burst-forming unit.

Each haemoglobin molecule consists of four globin chains, each associated with a haem group. In normal adult haemoglobin there are two alpha and two beta chains ($\alpha_2\beta_2$) but during fetal life this is not the case.

In very early fetal life, at the stage when haemopoiesis is occurring extraembryonically (i.e. in the yolk sac), the first haemoglobin synthesized is known as Hb Gower I and this contains two zeta chains

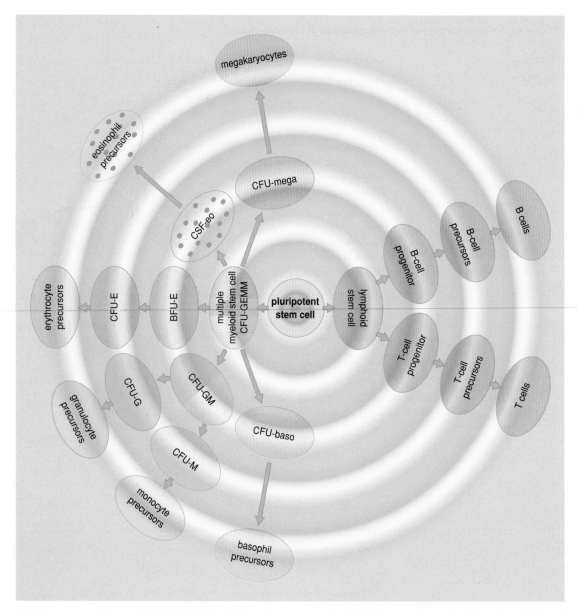

FIGURE 41.1 *Haematopoiesis: Cell lineages developing from the pluripotent stem cell.*

and two epsilon chains ($\zeta_2\epsilon_2$). This is replaced by Hb Gower II and Hb Portland which contain, respectively, two alpha and two epsilon chains ($\alpha_2\epsilon_2$) and two gamma and two zeta chains ($\zeta_2\gamma_2$).

Soon after Hb Gower is detected, synthesis of both α and γ chains begins to increase, forming so-called fetal haemoglobin (HbF) and by 3 months of gestation HbF ($\alpha_2\gamma_2$) accounts for all the red cell haemoglobin. From then until the 35th week of gestation, the proportion of HbF decreases to about 80%, most of the remainder consisting of adult haemoglobin (HbA) ($\alpha_2\beta_2$). Thereafter the proportion of HbF continues to drop at the rate of about 3–4% per week.

The role of haemoglobin in delivering oxygen and in picking up and transporting carbon dioxide is mediated through:
• sliding movements of the β chains relative to each other when oxygen is unloaded
• consequent entry of 2,3-diphosphoglycerate into the molecule, which results in a lower affinity of the haemoglobin molecule for oxygen and thus facilitates the unloading of oxygen. The partial pressure of oxygen at which haemoglobin is 50% saturated with oxygen (the P_{50}) is 26.6 mmHg. If oxygen affinity is increased, this value is decreased (i.e. the haemoglobin–oxygen dissociation curve

shifts to the left); if the affinity for oxygen is decreased, the curve shifts to the right.

Causes of **decreased affinity** of haemoglobin for oxygen include:

- high concentrations of 2,3-diphosphoglycerate
- high concentrations of hydrogen ions
- high concentrations of carbon dioxide
- the presence of certain abnormal haemoglobins such as sickle cell haemoglobin

Causes of **increased affinity** of haemoglobin for oxygen include:

- the presence of large amounts of HbF
- the presence of certain abnormal haemoglobins associated with polycythaemia

DISORDERS OF RED BLOOD CELLS

ANAEMIA

Anaemia is the state in which the haemoglobin concentration in the blood is below normal (i.e. 13.5 g/dl in adult males and 11.5 g/dl in adult females).

Anaemia is not a diagnosis and requires a full diagnostic investigation aimed at establishing its cause. A fall in the haemoglobin concentration is usually associated with a fall in red cell numbers and total red cell mass, but there are exceptions to this as, if there is an increase in plasma volume, the haemoglobin concentration must fall. This is seen in the so-called 'anaemia of pregnancy' and in some cases of splenomegaly; haemodilution occurs in both instances.

Useful diagnostic criteria include red cell size and the content of haemoglobin. These are expressed in the form of:

- **mean corpuscular volume (MCV**; expressed in femtolitres)
- **mean corpuscular haemoglobin (MCH;** expressed in picograms)
- **mean corpuscular haemoglobin concentration (MCHC**; expressed in grams per decilitres (g/dl))

To calculate these it is necessary to determine:

- **the red cell number (per litre)**
- **the haemoglobin concentration (g/l)**
- **the haematocrit (proportion of blood volume occupied by red cell mass) (l/l)**

Thus:

- **the MCV = haematocrit/red cell number (normal range 80–95 fl)**
- **the MCH = haemoglobin concentration/red cell number (normal range 26–33 pg)**
- **the MCHC = haemoglobin concentration/haematocrit (normal range 30–35 g/dl)**

Clinical Features

Anaemias produce their effect by decreasing the oxygen-carrying capacity of the blood. Added to this are special features associated with the underlying cause of the anaemia.

> **KEY POINTS**
>
> **Factors likely to aggravate the clinical effects of anaemia include:**
>
> - **rapid onset**
> - **a severe grade of anaemia**
> - **increasing age** (toleration of anaemia decreases with age)
> - **the character of the haemoglobin–oxygen dissociation curve.** As anaemia develops, **the amount of 2,3-diphosphoglycerate within the red cells increases and, consequently, oxygen affinity falls.** This decrease facilitates the delivery of oxygen to cells and tissues. It has been calculated that this rise in 2,3-diphosphoglycerate concentration may compensate for up to half the expected oxygen deficit for a given grade of anaemia. Thus **failure to increase the intracellular concentration of 2,3-diphosphoglycerate will increase the severity of the clinical picture.**
> - **the capacity of the heart and lungs to compensate for the anaemia**

If haemoglobin concentration drops below 7 g/l, cardiac output increases; an increase in stroke volume, rather than heart rate, plays the dominant role.

The principal cardiovascular symptom is **dyspnoea**, which in severe anaemia may be present at rest. Patients may complain of fatigue, dizziness, weakness and a feeling of faintness especially on standing. Exercise-related increased myocardial oxygen demand may cause ischaemic pain.

Physical Signs of Anaemia

General signs include:

- pallor of skin and mucous membranes
- tachycardia
- a full bounding pulse reflecting high cardiac output
- cardiac enlargement
- pulmonary or apical systolic murmurs due either to increased flow or, in some instances, to functional mitral or tricuspid valve incompetence resulting from cardiac dilatation

Classification

The classification of anaemias may be either kinetic or morphological.

Kinetic

Red cells, which have a high turnover, normally remain fairly constant in number suggesting that **cell production is equal to cell destruction** (*Fig. 41.2*). Consequently, if cell numbers decline this must be due to either:

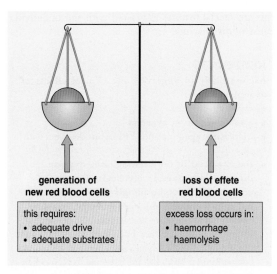

generation of
new red blood cells

this requires:
• adequate drive
• adequate substrates

loss of effete
red blood cells

excess loss occurs in:
• haemorrhage
• haemolysis

FIGURE 41.2 *The stability of the normal red cell mass depends on a dynamic equilibrium between red cell formation and red cell loss, destruction or sequestration.*

• **a decrease in the production of red cells** (*Table 41.3*)
• **an increase in the destruction, loss, 'pooling' or sequestration of red blood cells** (*Table 41.4*)

Morphological

In certain anaemias, the size and haemoglobin content of the red cells are characteristic and are a useful diagnostic guide. Thus, if red cell **numbers** are decreased in relation to **haemoglobin content** and **red cell mass**, then the red cells will be **larger** than normal (**macrocytic anaemia**). If haemoglobin and red cell mass are decreased in relation to the number of red cells, the red cells will be **smaller** than normal and contain less haemoglobin (**microcytic hypochromic anaemia**). If red cell size is unchanged, the anaemia is termed **normocytic**, and if the haemoglobin concentration of each cell is normal the additional term **normochromic** is applied.

The shape of red cells and the presence of certain intracellular features may be useful diagnostically, as, for example, the presence of sickle cells, or Heinz or Howell–Jolly bodies.

Table 41.3 Reasons for Inadequate Production of Red Cells

Process	Circumstance
Deficiency of nutritional substances	Vitamin B_{12} Iron Folic acid Protein Vitamin C Vitamin B_6 Copper
Insufficient erythroblasts	**Atrophy of marrow involving all cell lines** Chemicals and drugs, especially cytotoxic agents Idiopathic Congenital (Fanconi type) **Pure red cell aplasia** Associated with thymoma Congenital (Diamond–Blackfan syndrome) Sometimes in association with autoimmune diseases such as systemic lupus erythematosus
Malignant infiltration of bone marrow	Leukaemia or lymphoma Plasma cell dyscrasias Carcinoma or sarcoma Myelofibrosis
Renal, hepatic or endocrine disease	

Table 41.4 Reasons for Excessive Destruction or Loss of Red Cells

Process	Circumstance
Blood loss	Acute haemorrhage
	Chronic haemorrhage
Haemolysis due to disorders outside the red cell	Antibody mediated
	Infections such as malaria
	Sequestration and destruction of red cells in spleen
	Drugs, chemicals, physical agents
	Disorders such as lymphoma
	Red cell trauma
Haemolysis due to intrinsic red cell disorders	**Hereditary disorders**
	Red cell membrane defects such as spherocytosis
	Synthesis of abnormal haemoglobins such as in sickle cell disease or thalassaemia
	Glucose-6-phosphate dehydrogenase deficiency
	Disorders of carbohydrate metabolism (pyruvate kinase deficiency)
	Acquired disorders
	Paroxysmal nocturnal haemoglobinuria
	Lead poisoning

THE MACROCYTIC ANAEMIAS

KEY POINTS: Features of Macrocytes
A **macrocyte** is a red cell showing:
- an increase in the MCV to more than 100 fl
- an increase in the MCH
- normal MCHC
- In a blood film, such cells are seen to be enlarged, with a diameter exceeding 8.5 μm. They are well filled with haemoglobin and thus the normal central pale zone is absent.

Macrocytic anaemias fall into two main groups: megaloblastic and non-megaloblastic.

MEGALOBLASTIC ANAEMIA
Megaloblastosis is the morphological expression in the bone marrow of **retarded red cell DNA synthesis**. Bone marrow erythroblasts are large (**megaloblasts**) and, although haemoglobin synthesis is normal, the nucleus fails to mature and shows a fine, stippled chromatin pattern characteristic of a much earlier stage of erythropoiesis (*Fig. 41.3*).

These anaemias are characterized by a relative failure of DNA synthesis; the degree of erythroblast nuclear maturation lags behind the accumulation of cytoplasmic haemoglobin. In addition to the nuclear and cytoplasmic asynchrony, there is also an element of

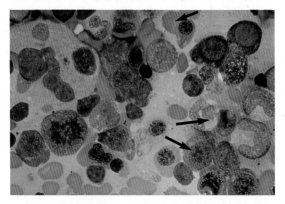

FIGURE 41.3 Bone marrow in pernicious anaemia. The megaloblasts (arrowed) show chromatin deficiency expressed in the form of 'lacy' nuclei. Giant metamyelocytes (arrowed) are characteristic and there is some premature haemoglobinization (arrows) of red cell precursors.

ineffective erythropoiesis, expressed as an increased rate of destruction of erythroblasts within the marrow and a shortened lifespan for the larger than normal red cells that are released from the marrow into the blood.

Aetiology
The causes of megaloblastic anaemia, the commonest of which is a deficiency in either vitamin B$_{12}$ or folate, are listed in *Table 41.5.*

Table 41.5 Causes of Megaloblastic Anaemia

Cause	Clinical context
Vitamin B$_{12}$ deficiency due to lack of intrinsic factor and consequent failure to absorb the vitamin B$_{12}$	Pernicious anaemia
Folate deficiency	Nutritional deficiencies Coeliac sprue and other malabsorption syndromes
Rare inherited disorders of DNA synthesis	Orotic aciduria
Drug-related disorders of DNA synthesis	Anticonvulsants Oral contraceptives

Pernicious Anaemia

This is a chronic disorder resulting from failure of the gastric mucosa to produce sufficient intrinsic factor, a glycoprotein secreted by the parietal cells. Intrinsic factor normally binds to vitamin B$_{12}$. In the absence of such binding, absorption of vitamin B$_{12}$ does not occur and a deficiency develops leading to megaloblastic anaemia.

Vitamin B$_{12}$: Physiological Aspects

Vitamin B$_{12}$ is one of the **cobalamins**. These consist of a corrin ring (similar to the porphyrin ring of haem), which contains a central cobalt atom. A nucleotide is attached to the corrin ring and the cobalt, with either methyl or deoxyadenosyl groups attached. In plasma, most of the vitamin B$_{12}$ is in the form of methylcobalamin.

KEY POINTS

The biochemical role of vitamin B$_{12}$ is to act as a coenzyme in two important reactions:

1) **The methylation of homocysteine to methionine.** The methyl group lost from the vitamin B$_{12}$ is replaced by one derived from methyltetrahydrofolic acid (MTHF) with the release of THF. **This loss of the methyl group from MTHF is a pivotal step in DNA synthesis because, without THF, thymidylate synthesis is inhibited.** Thymidylate synthesis is a rate-limiting step in DNA synthesis in which thymine is synthesized in the form of thymidine monophosphate from deoxyuridine monophosphate. Thus, **vitamin B$_{12}$ deficiency leads to megaloblastic anaemia because of the resulting deficiency in THF**.

2) In the form of deoxyadenosylcobalamin, in the **conversion of methylmalonyl coenzyme A to succinyl coenzyme A**.

---

1) Vitamin B$_{12}$ is found in foods of animal origin such as dairy produce, liver, fish and eggs.
2) In the stomach, the vitamin B$_{12}$ released from food by digestion binds to a protein from which it is later cleaved by pancreatic enzymes in the small gut.
3) Vitamin B$_{12}$ then binds to **intrinsic factor**, secreted by gastric parietal cells. The resulting complex binds to receptors for intrinsic factor in the distal ileum.
4) The vitamin B$_{12}$ is then absorbed, intrinsic factor remaining on the mucosa. The absorbed vitamin B$_{12}$ then binds to two proteins known as transcobalamin I and II (*Fig. 41.4*). Transcobalamin I binds more vitamin B$_{12}$ than transcobalamin II but releases it less readily. Thus most of the vitamin B$_{12}$ delivered to the marrow and other cells is derived from the transcobalamin II-bound fraction.

Body stores of vitamin B$_{12}$ are small (2–3 mg), but so is the daily requirement (1 µg), and a normal diet contains about 20 µg. Thus, there is a long lag phase before impaired vitamin B$_{12}$ absorption becomes apparent clinically.

It should be clear from the foregoing that a vitamin B$_{12}$ deficiency may develop as a result of **deficient intake** or **defective absorption**.

Deficient Intake

Deficient intake of vitamin B$_{12}$ is rare, occurring only in vegans.

Defective Absorption

Of the following causes of defective absorption of vitamin B$_{12}$, pernicious anaemia is by far the commonest:

- **lack of intrinsic factor:**
  1) **pernicious anaemia** in which the gastric mucosa is the site of an autoimmune atrophic gastritis and fails to produce intrinsic factor
  2) a **congenital lack or abnormality** of intrinsic factor
  3) gastrectomy leading to a diminished population of gastric parietal cells
- **lack of a normal absorptive surface in the small gut or competitive binding of vitamin B$_{12}$**
  1) ileal resection or Crohn's disease
  2) chronic sprue
  3) 'blind loop' syndrome with stagnation of gut contents and bacterial overgrowth leading to competition for vitamin B$_{12}$. A similar competitive binding of vitamin B$_{12}$ may occur in individuals infested by *Diphyllobothrium latum,* the fish tapeworm, which

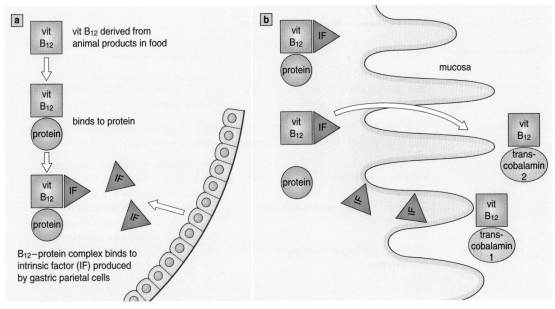

FIGURE 41.4 **a** and **b** *The sequence of events in vitamin B$_{12}$ absorption and action.*

binds vitamin B$_{12}$ firmly and thus prevents its absorption.

Epidemiology

Pernicious anaemia is mainly a disease of late adult life (mean age in Caucasians of 60 years). It occurs occasionally in children, usually due to a congenital (autosomal recessive) failure to produce intrinsic factor from the gastric parietal cells.

To some extent the degree of risk of pernicious anaemia correlates with Scandinavian, Irish or English ancestry, but the disorder is not confined to these groups. In northern Europe the female : male ratio is 1.4 : 1 but in other locations both sexes are equally affected. Other associations include **blue eyes, early greying of hair, blood group A** and an **increased risk of developing gastric cancer** (2–3% of all patients with pernicious anaemia will suffer in this way).

Pathogenesis

Although there may be some genetic contribution, **the pivotal event appears to be the development of severe atrophic gastritis resulting in a deficiency of all secretions, including that of intrinsic factor, from the affected gastric mucosa.**

The development of atrophic gastritis and the resulting anaemia are associated with the appearance of autoantibodies in the plasma. There is also a tendency for pernicious anaemia to be associated with other autoimmune disorders such as thyroiditis, diabetes mellitus and vitiligo. The most relevant antibodies are those that react specifically with **gastric parietal cells and intrinsic factor. The frequency with which these are found in various circumstances is shown in** *Table 41.6.*

Antibody directed against parietal cells is present in most cases, but its presence lacks diagnostic specificity.

Table 41.6 Gastric Antibodies

Group	Parietal cell antibody (%)	Intrinsic factor antibody (%)
Normal females older than 55 years	22.3	≤ 1
Patients with pernicious anaemia	84	56
Relatives of patients with pernicious anaemia	36	6
Patients with gastritis	47	Rare
Patients with thyroiditis	32	—

Table 41.7 Specific Clinical Features in Pernicious Anaemia

Organ or system	Clinical feature	Suggested mechanism
Skin	Pallor Mild jaundice giving lemon-yellow colour	Jaundice is due to increased haemoglobin breakdown due to ineffective erythropoiesis
Gastrointestinal	'Beefy' red sore tongue Mild malabsorption associated with diarrhoea	Due to epithelial abnormalities resulting from abnormalities in DNA synthesis
Nervous system	Paraesthesiae Difficulty in walking Weakness Diminished vibration and position sense Hyperreflexia Syndrome of **subacute combined degeneration**	Degeneration in posterior and lateral columns of spinal cord and in peripheral nerves, probably due to a failure in myelination. **This is believed to be due to a lack of S-adenosylmethionine caused by failure to methylate homocysteine to methionine because of the lack of vitamin B$_{12}$.** Because folate is not involved in this step, subacute combined degeneration is seen **only** in vitamin B$_{12}$ deficiency. In rare, untreated cases, examination of the spinal cord shows severe demyelination of the dorsal and dorsolateral columns

In contrast, antibodies against epitopes on the intrinsic factor molecule are found less often but are much more specific.

Clinical Features

The onset of pernicious anaemia is insidious and the picture is dominated by features common to all anaemias (see p 877). Other interesting clinical features (*Table 41.7*) may be, in part, ascribed to abnormalities of DNA synthesis in cells other than those of the blood and bone marrow.

Laboratory Findings

Blood
- **A variable degree of anaemia.** If symptoms due to anaemia predominate, the haemoglobin concentration is usually about 7–8 g/dl or less.
- **Macrocytosis.** The MCV is more than 100 fl and, in some cases, as high as 160 fl.
- **Decreased platelet count**
- **Morphological findings:**
  1) **hypersegmentation of the granulocyte nuclei.** This is a very sensitive and specific sign of megaloblastic anaemia. A granulocyte nucleus with six or more lobes is rare normally, but common in megaloblastic anaemia (*Fig. 41.5*).
  2) enlarged red cells with a characteristic **oval shape.**

They are well filled with haemoglobin and normal central pallor is diminished or absent (*Fig. 41.6*).

Bone Marrow
- The marrow is hyperplastic, with many erythroid precursors.
- Large numbers of megaloblasts are present. These large cells have nuclei showing a typical stippled chromatin pattern. The cytoplasmic staining depends on whether haemoglobin is present and how much.
- Active, abnormal leucopoiesis is also present. Some cells, especially those of the myeloid series, are much larger than normal, measuring up to 20–30 μm (see *Fig. 41.3*).

Gastric Secretions
The volume of gastric acid secretions is reduced to about 10% of normal; absence of hydrogen ion secretion (**achlorhydria**) occurs in virtually every case. In patients with pernicious anaemia, the rise in hydrogen ion secretion, which occurs normally with histamine stimulation, does not occur. Obviously, little or no intrinsic factor is secreted.

Changes in the Plasma Concentrations of Certain Enzymes
Most patients show a significant rise in the plasma concentration of lactic dehydrogenase, which is about 14

times as great as normal (260 units/ml). This enzyme comes from cells destroyed in the bone marrow because of ineffective erythropoiesis. It is not surprising that increases in the plasma concentration of other red cell enzymes may also occur.

Changes in Plasma Bilirubin Concentrations
There is a slight increase in the plasma level of unconjugated bilirubin, which accounts for increased urobilinogen excretion. It is due to destruction of red cell precursors in the marrow.

Folate Deficiency
- **Folic acid (pteroylglutamic acid)** is synthesized mainly in fruit and vegetables. It is inactivated by cooking; thus **an adequate intake of raw fruit and vegetables is necessary for an adequate (200 μg daily) intake**.
- Dietary folate is absorbed, chiefly in the proximal jejunum, and converted to MTHF.
- THF is released from MTHF by the action of vitamin B_{12}.

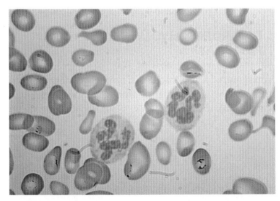

FIGURE 41.5 Blood film in pernicious anaemia. Note the large oval red cells and the hypersegmentation of the neutrophils.

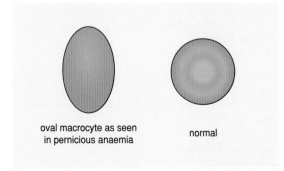

oval macrocyte as seen in pernicious anaemia

normal

FIGURE 41.6 Diagrammatic comparison between normal red cell and oval macrocyte as seen in pernicious anaemia.

Folate deficiency develops under the following circumstances:
- **Deficient dietary intake.** This is common in tropical countries in association with a high starch intake and little fresh fruit or vegetable. Nutritional deficiency is the commonest cause of folate-deficient anaemias.
- **Increased physiological demands**, in pregnancy, in infancy, or in patients with disorders characterized by rapid proliferation of blood cells (e.g. hereditary haemolytic anaemia, leukaemia, myeloma, myelofibrosis).
- **Disordered folate metabolism**, in alcoholism and alcohol-related cirrhosis.
- **Failure of absorption**, in tropical sprue and coeliac disease, and chronic inflammatory bowel disease such as Crohn's disease.
- **Drug related.** This occurs in a small proportion of patients treated with anticonvulsants and folic acid antagonists.

Differential Diagnosis Between Vitamin B_{12} and Folate Deficiency
The distinction between these two deficiency states is helped by determining the vitamin B_{12} and folate concentrations in the serum and in the red blood cells, as shown in *Table 41.8*.

Absorption of Vitamin B_{12}
Absorption of vitamin B_{12} is most commonly measured indirectly by the Schilling urinary excretion test. In this test a small dose of radioactively labelled vitamin B_{12} (0.5–2.0 μg) is given orally. At the same time, or 1–2 hours beforehand, a much larger dose of non-radioactive vitamin B_{12} (1000 μg) is given by intramuscular injection. The purpose of this is to saturate binding sites in the tissue so that none of the radioactive vitamin B_{12} is retained within the tissues. From the time of the administration, *all* urine is collected for a period of 24–72 hours and the radioactivity of the urine measured. In normal subjects, about 9–36% of the radioactive vitamin B_{12} is excreted in the urine. In pernicious anaemia, this is reduced to about 0–1.2%. If intrinsic factor is administered orally at the same time as the radioactive vitamin B_{12}, then excretion rises towards normal levels. If the vitamin B_{12} deficiency is due to a disorder of the small intestine such as coeliac sprue, then the administration of intrinsic factor does not increase the absorption of vitamin B_{12}.

NON-MEGALOBLASTIC ANAEMIA
In the non-megaloblastic anaemias there is **accelerated erythropoiesis with unimpaired DNA synthesis**. As a result:
- Reticulocyte numbers are increased.
- There is premature release of bone marrow reticulocytes; these cells are larger than reticulocytes normally released into the blood when erythropoiesis is increased.

Table 41.8 Vitamin B₁₂ and Folate Levels in Normal and Deficient States

	Serum B$_{12}$	Serum folate	Red cell folate
Normal values*	450 (160–1000) ng/l	10 (6–12) µg/l	316 (166–640) µg/l
Vitamin B$_{12}$ deficiency	Low	Normal or raised	Normal or low
Folate deficiency	Normal	Low	Low

* Values are mean (range).

- Erythropoietin increases the rate of haemoglobin synthesis in red cell precursors without decreasing the interval between cell divisions; this, too, contributes to the increased red cell volume seen in these anaemias.

Hypochromic Microcytic Anaemias

This group of anaemias is defined in terms of two criteria:
1) **a decrease in red cell size**
2) **a decrease in haemoglobin concentration.**
This decrease reflects impaired haemoglobin synthesis, the common functional abnormality in these anaemias.
Thus, the red cells show:

- a lower than normal mean corpuscular volume (MCV)
- a lower than normal mean corpuscular haemoglobin concentration (MCHC); this finding is especially suggestive of iron deficiency anaemia
- a decrease in mean red cell diameter and an increase in the area of central pallor

Normal haemoglobin synthesis requires adequate amounts of iron, protoporphyrin and globin (*Fig. 41.7*). Thus the anaemias in which haemoglobin synthesis is impaired can be divided into three main groups depending on which component is deficient (*Table 41.9*).

DISORDERS INVOLVING THE IRON PATHWAY

Iron required for haemoglobin synthesis is derived from iron carried in plasma by the transporting protein **transferrin**. Normally there is sufficient plasma iron

Table 41.9 Disorders of Impaired Haemoglobin Synthesis

Area of defect	Disorder
Iron metabolism	Iron deficiency anaemia Anaemia of chronic disorders
Globin synthesis	The thalassaemias Haemoglobin E trait and disease Haemoglobin C disease Unstable haemoglobin diseases
Porphyrin and haem synthesis (the sideroblastic anaemias)	Defective synthesis of δ-aminolaevulinic acid (ALA) • vitamin B$_6$ deficiency • drug or toxin-induced defects in metabolism of vitamin B$_6$ • defective ALA synthetase Co-proporphyrinogen oxidase deficiency Haem synthetase deficiency Lead poisoning Unknown

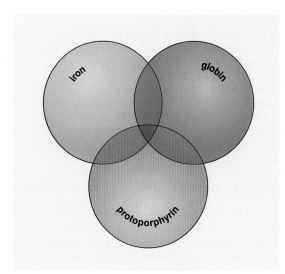

FIGURE 41.7 Requirements for normal synthesis of haemoglobin.

for both normal and accelerated erythropoiesis. If the degree of saturation of transferrin with iron falls to very low levels (less than 16%), the production rate of haemoglobin decreases and a hypochromic microcytic anaemia results.

In anaemias associated with certain chronic disorders, iron is present in macrophages but is not released into the plasma. Thus the iron concentration in plasma falls and iron-deficient erythropoiesis ensues, again resulting in a hypochromic microcytic anaemia.

Iron deficiency anaemias and the anaemias associated with chronic disorders are very common, the former being commonest in children and young women, and the latter in elderly individuals of both sexes.

Some rare or very rare disorders of the iron pathway also exist:

- **atransferrinaemia** in which plasma iron concentrations are reduced because of lack of transporting protein
- **congenital hypochromic microcytic anaemia with iron overload.** Here, transferrin is completely saturated and there is excess iron in the storage pool, but for some reason there is no transfer of iron from transferrin to the developing red cells.
- **the presence of antibodies directed against the cellular receptors for transferrin**

IRON DEFICIENCY ANAEMIA

- About two-thirds of the body iron is contained in haemoglobin. Each day about 6 g haemoglobin are synthesized and this requires about 20 mg iron, much of which is recycled from effete red cells.
- Iron for haemoglobin synthesis is derived from the iron-transporting β-globulin, transferrin; each

molecule of transferrin binds two atoms of iron. Normally, this transferrin is about one-third saturated.

- The transferrin acquires iron from the ferritin and haemosiderin, which are stored within tissue macrophages.
- The erythroblasts and reticulocytes in the bone marrow take iron preferentially from the transferrin because they are richly endowed with specific transferrin receptors.
- Only a proportion of the required iron is derived from the diet and control of iron absorption in the gut is exerted within the mucosa of the duodenum and jejunum where absorption (5–10% of the daily intake) occurs. Excess dietary iron is retained within the mucosal epithelium by forming complexes with the protein apoferritin (ferritin) and is returned to the gut lumen in the course of the normal daily loss of small gut epithelium. In iron deficiency, absorption of dietary iron (derived principally from meat and liver) is increased. **Dietary intake of iron is important and, on a worldwide basis, iron deficiency is the most common form of nutritional deficiency, just as iron deficiency anaemia is the commonest form of anaemia.**

Causes of Iron Deficiency

Iron deficiency arises either because of prolonged negative balance in respect of iron or because stores of iron are inadequate to cope with increased demand (*Fig. 41.8*).

Iron is normally lost in both sexes via the sweat, faeces and urine, this loss amounting to 0.5–1 mg per day. A menstruating female loses a further 0.5–1 mg iron daily.

In childhood and during pregnancy there are increased demands for iron. Thus the groups especially at risk for developing negative iron balance and thus iron deficiency anaemia are children and pregnant or menstruating females, all of whom require a greater daily iron intake than healthy adult males or postmenopausal females. Apart from these factors, **negative iron balance can arise from**:

1) **an inadequate iron intake.** This can result from a **dietary deficiency** or because of **failure to absorb iron** in the duodenum or jejunum.

Defective iron absorption is seen:
- in patients with achlorhydria
- following gastrectomy or vagotomy and gastroenterostomy
- in patents with coeliac disease
- in **pica** (the eating of clay). This is sometimes seen **as a result of iron deficiency but can also cause iron deficiency as substances in the clay act as ion exchangers and interfere with the absorption of iron.**

2) **excessive iron loss.** This is caused in most cases by bleeding:

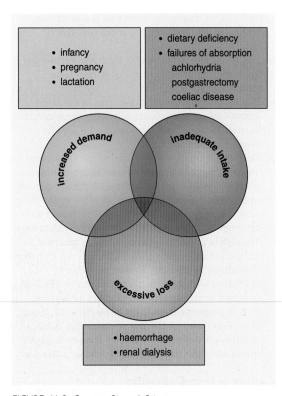

• infancy
• pregnancy
• lactation
	• dietary deficiency
	• failures of absorption
	  achlorhydria
	  postgastrectomy
	  coeliac disease

increased demand

inadequate intake

excessive loss

• haemorrhage
• renal dialysis

FIGURE 41.8 *Causes of iron deficiency.*

• **from the gastrointestinal tract**, as in peptic ulcer, haemorrhoids, oesophageal varices, associated with aspirin or other non-steroidal anti-inflammatory drugs, hiatus hernia, neoplasms of stomach, caecum, colon or rectum, diverticular disease, hookworm infestation (which affects 20% of the world's population) and angiodysplasia.
• **in renal dialysis.** Excess loss of iron also occurs in association with chronic renal failure treated by dialysis; 50% of such patients develop iron deficiency.
• **uterine** – excessive menstrual loss, presence of uterine fibromyomata, etc.
3) **increased demand for iron**, in infancy, in pregnancy and during lactation

Clinical Features

As iron deficiency anaemia has many causes, **the clinical picture is likely to be a compound of the anaemia itself and of the cause of the iron deficiency**. So far as the anaemia itself is concerned, it appears that most patients seek help for the weakness and fatigue that are its typical symptoms at a time when the haemoglobin concentration is 7–8 g/dl. Special features likely to be associated with iron deficiency anaemia are outlined below.

Disturbances of Growth

Normal growth during childhood is impaired by iron deficiency. The growth rate is restored by treatment with iron.

Poor Muscular Performance

Iron deficiency, even without anaemia, appears to impair muscular performance. Decreases are noted in total exercise time and maximal workload, whereas the heart rate and concentration of lactate in the serum increase disproportionately.

Defective Structure and Function in Epithelial Tissues

Nails The nails characteristically show atrophy and flattening. Eventually they develop a concave 'spoon-shaped' appearance known as **koilonychia**. Less specific are increased fragility and brittleness.

Tongue Atrophy of the lingual papillae and a sore, red, smooth tongue occur in about 40% of iron-deficient patients.

Mouth Angular stomatitis (ulcers and fissures at the corners of the mouth) occurs in about 14% of patients with iron deficiency. It is not specific for iron deficiency occurring also in riboflavin and pyridoxine deficiencies.

Hypopharynx and oesophagus A combination of angular stomatitis, tongue abnormalities and dysphagia occurring in patients with iron deficiency anaemia was described in 1919 by Paterson and Kelly, although this syndrome is more commonly known as the Plummer–Vinson syndrome, or **sideropenic dysphagia** (see Chapter 34 on the Oesophagus).

Stomach Gastric biopsies from about 75% of patients with iron deficiency anaemia show a non-specific 'chronic gastritis'. Various degrees of impairment of gastric secretion may be associated with this; achlorhydria occurs in about 16% of cases.

The cause of these epithelial abnormalities is not clear, but the decrease in iron concentration may affect iron-containing enzymes.

Effects of Iron Deficiency on Immunity and Infection

Iron deficiency results in two abnormalities that affect the ability of a host to respond to infection. These are:

1) **a reduction of up to 35% in the number of circulating T cells.** This affects both helper and suppressor T cells. In addition, individuals who are iron deficient do not mount a normal response to certain skin test antigens, such as those from the diphtheria bacillus, various *Candida* species and *Trichophyton*, and, in cell culture, the production of

interleukins 1 and 2 is impaired. These abnormalities are corrected by giving iron.

2) **impaired bacterial killing by phagocytes.** This appears to be related to a decrease in the oxidative burst following phagocytosis, which normally generates bactericidal reactive oxygen species (free radicals).

Laboratory Findings

Degree of Anaemia
If anaemia is the reason for the patient's clinical presentation, the haemoglobin concentration is usually about 7–8 g/dl.

Red Cell Indices
Even before the onset of anaemia the red cell indices are altered. There is a decrease in MCV and mean corpuscular haemoglobin (MCH) in most patients, and, in severe and long-standing cases, the MCHC is reduced as well. Anisocytosis (variation in cell size) is a common finding in iron deficiency anaemia and one that occurs quite early in the course of the disorder.

Morphological Appearances of Red Cells on Blood Film Examination
The most characteristic feature is the decrease in intracorpuscular haemoglobin, expressed in the form of **an increased area of central pallor** (*Figs 41.9* and *41.10*). The more severe the anaemia, the more marked is this change. In addition to the microcytosis and the variation in cell size, there is a considerable degree of poikilocytosis (variation in cell shape); the most common variant is an elongated red cell which is variously described as a 'pencil' or 'cigar' cell.

In patients in whom iron deficiency and folate or vitamin B_{12} deficiency coexist, a dimorphic population of red cells is seen in the blood film; both macrocytosis and microcytosis are present.

Platelet Count
In most cases of iron deficiency anaemia there is a roughly twofold increase in the level of circulating platelets. The reason for this is not clear.

Bone Marrow
The bone marrow shows hyperplasia of the red cell precursors of a mild to moderate degree. Individual normoblasts are smaller than usual and show the presence of scanty cytoplasm which has rather ragged and irregular margins. **Staining by Perls' method for haemosiderin shows that iron is either absent or very much decreased in the bone marrow macrophages, the iron stores in these cells having become exhausted.** This is in marked contrast with the situation in anaemia of chronic disease, in which the macrophage iron stores are quite normal but cannot be released into the serum.

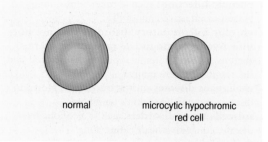

normal   microcytic hypochromic red cell

FIGURE 41.9 *Diagrammatic comparison between a normal red cell and a small cell, with an increase in the diameter of the central pale zone due to relative deficiency of haemoglobin.*

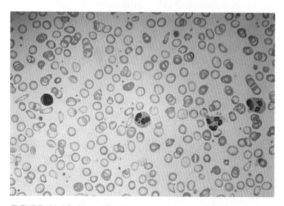

FIGURE 41.10 *Blood film from a patient with iron deficiency anaemia. Note the small size of the red cells and the large, pale, central area.*

Indices of Iron Metabolism
The serum iron concentrations are reduced; the mean value is 28 µg/dl, which is about half of the normal. The total iron-binding capacity (TIBC) usually rises so that the degree of saturation of transferrin is less than 10%. Again, this contrasts with the anaemia of chronic disease, where **both the serum iron level and the iron-binding capacity are decreased**, and other microcytic anaemias, where both these parameters are normal.

The best measure of storage iron is the **serum ferritin concentration**; in iron deficiency this is considerably decreased, the mean value being 12 µg/dl (normal value in adult males 175 µg/dl).

ANAEMIA OF CHRONIC DISORDERS

Anaemia of chronic disorders is common. It is usually mild in degree and appears 1–2 months after the onset of the chronic disease with which it is associated; thereafter it does not appear to increase in severity.

The disorders with which this type of anaemia is most commonly associated are:

- **chronic infections** such as tuberculosis, lung abscess or infective endocarditis
- **chronic inflammatory disorders that are not infective in origin** such as rheumatoid arthritis, rheumatic fever, systemic lupus erythematosus, and the results of severe trauma
- **malignant diseases** such as carcinoma, Hodgkin's disease, and non-Hodgkin's lymphoma
- **miscellaneous disorders** such as alcoholic liver disease, congestive heart failure and thrombophlebitis

Laboratory Findings
- The **anaemia is usually mild** in degree.
- The **red cells are most commonly normochromic and normocytic** but hypochromia and microcytosis may occur, although never with the severity associated with iron deficiency anaemia.
- **Both serum iron concentrations and TIBC are decreased** and saturation of transferrin is below normal. Serum ferritin is either increased or normal, showing that there is no lack of stored iron in the tissues. Iron administration does not improve either the anaemia or the serum iron concentration; for either of these to occur, resolution of the underlying process is required.
- Staining of bone marrow samples to show iron reveals similarly that **there is no lack of iron in macrophages**; indeed, the amount of iron present in these cells appears to be increased.
- Red cell survival studies show **a moderate shortening of red cell lifespan**. Interestingly this is not accompanied by erythroid hyperplasia in the bone marrow or any increase in reticulocyte numbers.

Pathogenesis
The pathogenesis of this type of anaemia is not yet clear. An explanation is needed for the three functional components of the disease, which are:
1) **shortened red cell survival time**
2) **the disturbance in iron metabolism with a failure to transfer iron from macrophage stores to the serum**
3) **impairment in the expected marrow response**

It has been suggested that anaemia of chronic disorders is one of the expressions of the alteration of immune function that occurs with at least some of the disorders with which chronic anaemia is associated. These disorders are associated with macrophage activation and thus increased synthesis and release of the cytokines, interleukin (IL) 1, tumour necrosis factor (TNF) α and IL-6.

IL-1 and TNF-α suppress erythropoiesis in rats and, in humans, the administration of these cytokines inhibits the normal production and release of erythropoietin that follows hypoxia. In addition, there is some evidence that TNF may inhibit cell division in primitive red cell precursors. This view is supported by the observation that macrophages from patients with anaemia of chronic disorders inhibit red cell colony formation in culture systems.

The survival time of labelled red cells from patients with anaemia of chronic disorders is normal when the cells are infused into healthy recipients, suggesting that the typical shortened red cell survival time is due to some cause, as yet unknown but possibly a product of activated macrophages, outside the red cell.

Normal marrow has a reserve capacity, which should make it easy to compensate for the moderate shortening of red cell survival times seen in these anaemias. Why does it fail to do so? Three possibilities have been suggested, none of which excludes the other two. These are:
- a relative failure of erythropoietin secretion
- a relative failure of the marrow to respond to erythropoietin
- a limitation on erythropoiesis imposed by the failure to release iron from the stores in macrophages

THE SIDEROBLASTIC ANAEMIAS

This rather heterogeneous and uncommon group of conditions has as its defining criteria the following features:
- a hypochromic microcytic anaemia indicating impaired production of haemoglobin. In most cases, the anaemia is refractory to treatment other than repeated blood transfusions.
- the presence of amorphous iron deposits in the mitochondria of erythroblasts. These are often arranged in a ring-like fashion around the erythroblast nucleus, and such cells are known as **ring sideroblasts**.
- an increase in total body iron, the transferrin being almost completely saturated. The presence of high concentrations of ferritin in the serum reinforces the picture of a significant increase in body iron stores.
- ineffective erythropoiesis, the reticulocyte count being normal or only very slightly increased
- various forms of impairment of haem synthesis

Classification
The sideroblastic anaemias may be either hereditary or acquired.

Hereditary Forms
These are uncommon and have various inheritance patterns which include X-linked, autosomal dominant and autosomal recessive transmission, as well as some congenital forms in which the inheritance pattern is still unknown.

In the X-linked form the indications are that there is a defect in δ-**aminolaevulinic acid synthetase** underlying the impairment of haem synthesis, but this is certainly not the only defect occurring in this group. Some patients respond to treatment with vitamin B_6 (pyridoxine), but this is very variable.

Acquired Sideroblastic Anaemia

This can occur in a number of different circumstances. These include:

- **an idiopathic form** in which there is **expansion of a single abnormal clone of erythroblasts**. Chromosomal abnormalities at various levels in the hierarchy of haemopoietic cell precursors have been observed in association with this condition. Mutations in the *ras* and *fms* genes have been demonstrated in the blood cells of some patients but the pathogenetic significance of these is not yet understood. Occasional cases have been recorded where the chronic anaemia characteristic of this condition has been followed by marrow failure or leukaemia, but this is rare and the monoclonal expansion should not be regarded as being neoplastic from the start. It seems likely that a second mutation within the altered clone is required before a malignant phenotype develops.
- **sideroblastic anaemias associated with myelodysplasia, haematological malignancies and myeloproliferative disorders.**
- **reversible sideroblastic anaemias.** These occur in association with:

  1) **alcoholism**. Ring sideroblasts are found in about 25% of alcoholics with anaemia. Sideroblastic anaemia is believed to occur only if general malnutrition and folate deficiency are also present. Haem production is impaired by alcohol, which can act at several different steps in the biosynthetic pathway of haem. The haemoglobin concentration is generally between 6 and 10 g/dl and the MCV is usually normal or even somewhat increased. Small granules of iron which show up in the red cells in blood films stained by the Perls' method for haemosiderin (**Pappenheimer bodies**) are seen in about a third of cases. The withdrawal of alcohol is followed by the disappearance of sideroblasts from the marrow within 2 weeks, although recovery from the anaemia takes somewhat longer.

  2) **certain drugs, notably the antituberculous agent, isoniazid, and chloramphenicol.** Isoniazid interferes with **vitamin B_6 metabolism** and there is a resulting **decrease in the synthesis of δ-aminolaevulinic acid**. The risk of severe anaemia occurring as a result of the use of this drug and other antituberculous agents such as pyrazinamide, which may also interfere with vitamin B_6 metabolism, is relatively small. Chloramphenicol both suppresses erythropoiesis and promotes the formation of ring sideroblasts, probably as a result of injury to the mitochondria,

synthesis of certain mitochondrial membrane proteins being inhibited.

ANAEMIA OF LEAD POISONING

This disorder deserves separate consideration because it involves **impairment of haem synthesis without any formation of ring sideroblasts.**

Lead poisoning results from:
- the long-standing presence of lead bullets in the tissues
- inhalation of lead as a result of atmospheric pollution. This may occur either in the course of certain occupations or from inhalation of fumes of petrol to which lead has been added as an anti-'knock' agent
- children licking lead-containing paint from their toys

The anaemia that accompanies lead poisoning is due principally to interference with haem synthesis, which can be affected at several points by lead. In addition, lead affects **globin synthesis** and also interferes with the breakdown of RNA due to interference with pyrimidine 5′ nucleotidase activity. This leads to accumulation of denatured RNA in red cells, which is expressed in the form of **basophilic stippling in the red cell cytoplasm** in blood films stained by one of the Romanowsky methods. In addition, the deficiency in pyrimidine nucleotidase activity causes accumulation of nucleotides which inhibit the pentose phosphate shunt and promote haemolysis of the affected red cells.

- The anaemia is mild to moderate in degree and the red cells are microcytic and hypochromic. If overt haemolysis is present, the reticulocyte count tends to be raised.
- The mean red cell life is shortened.
- Various markers of haem synthesis are affected. For example, there is a decline in the red cell concentration of aminolaevulinic acid dehydratase, the severity of this being proportional to the blood lead levels.

Haemolytic Anaemias

Although haemolysis may occur in many blood diseases, the term **haemolytic anaemias** defines a set of disorders in which there is:
- **accelerated red cell destruction with a marked shortening of red cell survival time**
- **no impairment of the ability of the bone marrow to respond to the extra demands imposed by the haemolytic state**

Clinical Features

The clinical picture has several components (*Fig. 41.11*):

- **Anaemia** resulting from excessive red cell destruction. In certain circumstances, **'crises'** occur in which **the equilibrium between increased red cell destruction and increased red cell production is disturbed**; this can lead to precipitous and severe falls in haemoglobin concentration. The most common type of crisis is due to a transient and acute failure of erythropoiesis. This is termed an **aplastic crisis** and is most frequently associated with infections by the human parvovirus type B19, which normally produces the childhood exanthem, **erythema infectiosum** ('fifth disease'). The P antigen to which the virus binds is expressed on red cell precursors, which are thus targeted for attack by the virus.
- **Effects related to the release of excessive amounts of various red cell components.** For example, the release of excess haemoglobin from red cells destroyed in the liver and spleen leads to increased plasma concentrations of unconjugated bilirubin and, hence, to an increased risk of pigment stones forming in the biliary tract.
- **Effects related to the marked expansion of the marrow compartment**, which can produce a number of characteristic skeletal changes.
- If the cause of the haemolysis is an abnormality of haemoglobin that makes the affected red cells more rigid and, hence, less easily able to pass through small blood vessels, **occlusion of the latter with ischaemic effects on tissues downstream of**

the occlusions occurs. Such changes may play a dominant role in syndromes associated with **sickle cell disease** (see pp 896–899).

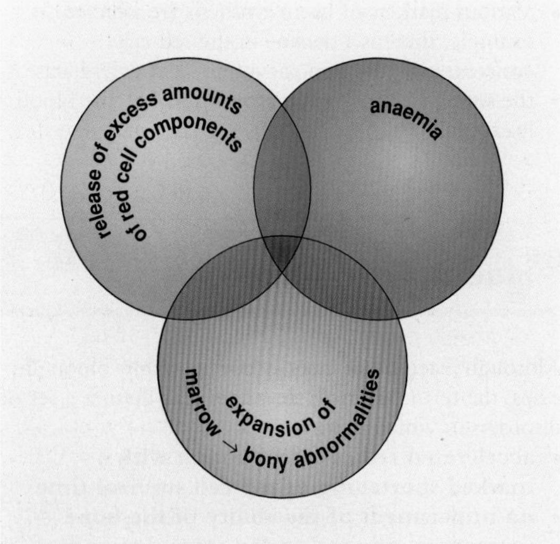

Pathogenesis

The haemolytic disorders occur because of either:

- **some intrinsic abnormality of the red cell which makes it more liable to be destroyed. Normal cells transfused into a patient with such abnormal red cells survive normally.**
- **some factor outside a normal red blood cell which causes sufficient membrane damage to destroy the cell. In this case, normal red cells infused into the patient will have the same shortened life as the patient's own red cells.**

With one exception (**paroxysmal nocturnal haemoglobinuria**) **all the intrinsic red cell abnormalities leading to haemolysis are inherited, whereas disorders in which the injury comes from outside the red cell are acquired.**

The hereditary haemolytic disorders may occur because of abnormalities in a number of red cell compartments or biochemical systems:

- **defects in the red cell membrane:**
  a) hereditary spherocytosis
  b) hereditary elliptocytosis
  c) stomatocytosis
  d) abetalipoproteinaemia
  e) Rh_{null} disease
- **deficiencies in glycolytic enzymes** such as pyruvate kinase in the red cells
- **abnormalities in red cell nucleotide metabolism**
- **deficiencies in enzymes involved in the pentose phosphate pathway and in relation to glutathione metabolism, rendering the red cells more susceptible to oxidant stress:**
  a) glucose-6-phosphate dehydrogenase deficiency
  b) deficiencies in glutathione synthetase or glutathione reductase
- **defects in globin structure or in the regulation of globin synthesis**
  a) sickle cell disease
  b) other homozygous abnormalities of haemoglobin (CC, DD, EE disease)
  c) various forms of thalassaemia
  d) unstable haemoglobin disease. This is rare despite the fact that there are many unstable haemoglobin variants.
  e) doubly heterozygous disorders such as combination of sickle cell and thalassaemia traits or haemoglobin SC disease

Only the commonest of these will be discussed here. For the remainder, reference should be made to specialized texts.

FIGURE 41.11 *Basic clinical effects of haemolysis.*

Congenital Haemolytic Disorders

Clinical Features

Anaemia

The anaemia varies in severity. In some, severe anaemia may be present at birth or occur within the first few months of life. More commonly, the degree of anaemia is mild to moderate because the red cell destruction is counterbalanced by marrow hyperplasia and the resulting increased red cell production. Some patients have no anaemia at all and the diagnosis may go unsuspected until some other manifestations of the haemolytic disorder, such as jaundice, occur.

Jaundice

Different degrees of jaundice may be present. In some neonates there is a severe hyperbilirubinaemia, which may be so intense as to raise suspicions of rhesus incompatibility. In others, jaundice is episodic and mild, often being associated with infections.

The jaundice of haemolysis is **acholuric**, as the excess bilirubin is unconjugated and hence cannot appear in the urine. There is, however, increased production of stercobilinogen and thus stools are dark and urobilinogen is present in the urine.

As a result of the increase in haemoglobin breakdown, gallstone formation is a not uncommon complication of the haemolytic anaemias, and symptoms related to cholelithiasis may call attention for the first time to the underlying blood disorder (see p 627).

Aplastic Crises

The crisis usually begins non-specifically. Changes in the blood picture follow about 4–7 days after the onset of infection, and there may be a fall in haemoglobin concentration of 2–6 g/dl over a comparatively short time. The marrow shows hypoplasia affecting the red cell-forming population and erythroblasts are scanty. Despite the fall in haemoglobin levels there is no corresponding rise in the reticulocyte count during the crisis, although recovery, which usually commences after about 6–8 days, is heralded by an increase in the number of reticulocytes. The duration of a crisis is usually about 10–14 days, although this may be prolonged in cases where immunity is depressed. The parvovirus colonizes dividing cells of the red cell line, thus inhibiting red cell formation at both the colony-forming unit and burst-forming unit stage, but apparently does not affect other cell lines. Viral replication takes place during the S phase of the cell cycle, and the very fact that the marrow is so active in patients with congenital haemolytic disorders may make these individuals more susceptible to viral colonization of the erythroid cell line.

Leg Ulcers

A small proportion of patients with haemolytic anaemias develop chronic leg ulcers. This is most likely

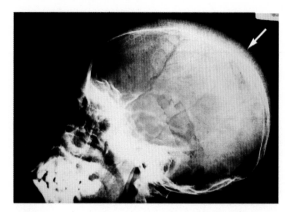

FIGURE 41.12 *Lateral radiograph of the skull in thalassaemia major. Note the 'hair standing on end' appearance of the calvarial bone.*

to be seen in those suffering from **hereditary spherocytosis** or **sickle cell disease**; the prevalence of ulcers in the latter is about 5%. The ulcers are often bilateral and are commonest in relation to the malleoli. They are clearly related to the haemolytic process as, in hereditary spherocytosis, interruption of haemolysis by splenectomy leads to the ulcers healing.

Bony Abnormalities

Severe and chronic haemolysis leads inevitably to expansion of the red marrow. If this occurs during phases of growth and development, skeletal abnormalities occur:

* the development of a tower-shaped skull with thickening and striation of the frontal and parietal bones, the latter feature giving a radiological appearance of 'hairs standing on end' (*Fig. 41.12*).
* prominence of the cheekbone with resulting exposure of the upper teeth. The combination of skull and cheekbone abnormalities causes a characteristic facies known as **'the thalassaemic facies'**, as these abnormalities are often seen in thalassaemia.
* thinning of the bony cortex with increased resorption of bone and decreased bone formation and mineralization. The earliest radiological evidence of this is seen in the hands and feet, where the small bones assume a somewhat rectangular shape associated with a marked degree of trabeculation of the medullary cavity.

Laboratory Findings

Logically, the laboratory findings in haemolytic anaemia can be divided into three groups:

1) correlates of **excessive red cell destruction**
2) correlates of the **compensatory increase in the rate of erythropoiesis**
3) findings related to **specific types of haemolytic anaemia**

Signs of Excessive Red Cell Destruction

Shortened Red Cell Survival Time

On average, red cell survival time is reduced to about half the normal. These tests are time consuming and expensive, and there are simpler ways of demonstrating red cell destruction, such as:

- serial measurements of the degree of anaemia
- the reticulocyte response
- the serum bilirubin concentration

Increased Serum Bilirubin Level

The serum bilirubin concentration is determined by two processes:

- **the rate at which bilirubin is formed from haem**
- **the rate at which it is excreted by the liver**

Thus the serum bilirubin concentration *per se* is not a totally reliable indicator of the degree of red cell breakdown and may, indeed, be within normal limits in some patients with haemolytic anaemia.

Decrease in Plasma Haptoglobin Concentration

When haemoglobin derived from red cell breakdown enters the plasma it complexes with haptoglobin, the resulting complex being removed in the liver. This leads to a decline in plasma haptoglobin levels. Similar decreases in plasma concentration of glycosylated haemoglobin are noted in patients with haemolytic anaemia.

Evidence of Intravascular Haemolysis

Haemoglobin enters the plasma under two circumstances:

- when the **red cell destruction is occurring within the circulation**
- when extravascular destruction of red cells is so gross and so rapid as to exceed the capacity of macrophages to engulf the red cell contents

In either circumstance the following findings occur:

- **haemoglobinaemia**
- **haemoglobinuria**, which occurs when the plasma haemoglobin concentration exceeds the binding capacity of haptoglobins. Urine may range in colour from a pale pink to a deep red. Both haemoglobin and myoglobin in the urine produce a positive result with the benzidine test for occult blood.
- **iron in the urine.** Some of the haemoglobin in the glomerular filtrate is reabsorbed by tubular epithelium and its iron is converted to ferritin and haemosiderin within the epithelial cells. Subsequently, these cells are sloughed into the urine and the haemosiderin may be detected in the sediment.
- **methaemalbuminaemia.** Haemoglobin in the plasma is readily oxidized to methaemoglobin. The haem group detaches from this and becomes bound to albumin, forming methaemalbumin, which gives the serum a coffee colour.

Signs of Compensatory Erythropoiesis

1) **In the blood** there is:
- an increased number of circulating **reticulocytes**
- **macrocytosis** because of the erythropoietin-mediated stimulus to haemoglobin production and also because of the premature release of large reticulocytes
- the occasional **presence of nucleated red cells (erythroblasts) in the blood**. This tends to occur only when haemolysis has been rapid, such as in haemolytic disease of the newborn
- an **increase in the number of neutrophils and platelets**, principally in patients in whom haemolysis has been acute

2) **The bone marrow** shows erythroid hyperplasia.

3) **Iron transport and metabolism:**
- Plasma **iron transport rates** are 2–8 times greater than normal. This is a measure of total erythropoiesis and correlates well with the degree of erythroid hyperplasia.
- The erythrocyte **iron turnover rate** is increased. This is a measure of effective erythropoiesis and correlates with the production of reticulocytes.

4) **Biochemical markers of red cell age.** Red cells are released from the marrow in increased numbers following haemolysis; the circulating red cell population age is therefore reduced compared with normal. The most promising index of red cell age currently under study is the determination of **red cell creatine concentration**, which is higher in young red cells.

Specific Abnormalities that may Indicate the Cause of Haemolysis

Morphological abnormalities detectable on blood films:

- **Spherical red cells** are the defining morphological criterion of **hereditary spherocytosis** but they may also be seen in various types of **acquired** haemolytic anaemia such as that mediated by immune mechanisms.
- Cells with spicules projecting from their plasma membranes and known as **acanthocytes**. These indicate some abnormality in the lipid composition of the red cell membrane which is seen in the rare condition, **abetalipoproteinaemia**, and sometimes in cirrhosis of the liver.
- Red cells with a **central slit or stoma** instead of the normal circular area of central pallor (**stomatocyte**). This is believed to represent a disturbance in red cell

cation metabolism and occurs in rare form of hereditary haemolytic anaemia, **stomatocytosis**.

- **Target cells** are red cells with a central zone of pigment. They occur in:
  1) thalassaemia
  2) homozygous abnormal haemoglobin states
  3) deficiency of the enzyme lecithin–cholesterol acyl transferase
  4) in non-haemolytic states such as cholestatic jaundice and following splenectomy
- **Sickle cells** are found in the anaemia of that name.
- Fragmented red cells (**schistocytes**) suggest that haemolysis has been due to physical trauma.

Other Tests for Red Cell Changes

Changes in Osmotic Fragility of Red Cells

Red cells vary in their resistance to osmotic stress. This resistance is measured by a test in which red cells are exposed to diminishing concentrations of hypotonic saline, and the degree of haemolysis is determined. The osmotic fragility curve is constructed by plotting the percentage of haemolysis on the vertical axis against decreasing concentrations of saline on the horizontal axis. In most individuals a symmetrical sigmoid-shaped curve is obtained.

Increased osmotic fragility occurs typically in hereditary spherocytosis. Conversely, increased red cell resistance to osmotic stress occurs in thalassaemia and sickle cell anaemia.

The Antiglobulin (Coombs') Test

The most widely used test for diagnosis of **immune-mediated haemolytic anaemias** is the direct antiglobulin or Coombs' test. A positive result indicates that the red cells are coated with immunoglobulin (Ig) G (which does not cause spontaneous agglutination) and/or complement. The patient's cells are exposed to serum from rabbits immunized against human serum. If IgG and/or complement are present, the red cells agglutinate.

Heinz Body Formation

In some disorders, haemolysis occurs because of precipitation of haemoglobin with the formation of inclusions known as Heinz bodies, which are then removed in the spleen. They are demonstrated by supravital staining with cresyl violet, the Heinz bodies appearing as deep purple, irregularly shaped inclusions in affected red cells. Heinz bodies are associated with:

- certain red cell enzyme defects, most notably glucose-6-phosphatase dehydrogenase
- the thalassaemias
- unstable haemoglobin disease
- certain types of chemical injury to red cells

DEFECTS IN RED CELL MEMBRANES

Hereditary Spherocytosis

This is the commonest **familial haemolytic disorder** in persons of northern European extraction (USA incidence rate 1 in 5000). Its features are:

- **familial nature**. Inheritance in most cases follows an autosomal dominant pattern
- **anaemia**, which is usually not very severe
- **intermittent jaundice**
- **splenomegaly**
- marked amelioration following **splenectomy**
- a characteristic morphological finding, the **microspherocyte**
- **increased fragility of red cells to osmotic stress**

The plasma membranes of spherocytes show structural and functional abnormalities. These result from an abnormality of the red cell cytoskeleton, **the protein spectrin being either deficient in quantity or defective in function**. Spectrin is attached to the underside of the red cell plasma membrane and maintains the structural integrity of this membrane and the biconcave shape of the red cell.

The shape change is probably due to loss of plasma membrane in areas insufficiently supported by the cytoskeleton. With membrane loss, the ratio of **surface area : volume** decreases and thus the cell becomes more and more spherical (*Fig. 41.13*). Spherocytes are selectively sequestered in the splenic microcirculation and undergo haemolysis there.

In the autosomal dominant form, spectrin is reduced to 60–80% of normal; the lower the spectrin content, the greater the severity of the disease and the greater the red cell osmotic fragility. Spectrin content also predicts the result of therapeutic splenectomy. Patients with spectrin levels greater than 70% of normal usually recover following splenectomy.

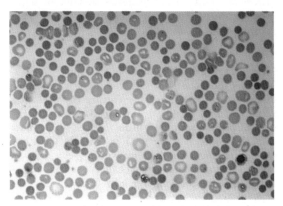

FIGURE 41.13 *Blood film in hereditary spherocytosis. Note the small, round and solid-looking red cells, which are the spherocytes.*

Clinical Features

Cases vary widely in their severity. About 25% of patients show mild disease with fully compensated anaemia and little or no enlargement of the spleen. At the other end of the spectrum, the anaemia and jaundice may be so severe as to require exchange transfusion. In the remainder, there is mild to moderate anaemia, moderate splenic enlargement and intermittent jaundice. Aplastic crises often may occur. Pigment gallstones are very common and may occur in young children.

Laboratory Findings

- anaemia, which is usually mild
- increased reticulocyte count (5–20%)
- increase in mean corpuscular haemoglobin concentration (MCHC), due to red cell water loss
- **spherocytes** which characteristically have **no central area of pallor**. Other morphological changes, related to the increased rate of erythropoiesis, are variations in shape and staining and the occasional presence of nucleated red cells.
- increased osmotic fragility
- increased autohaemolysis when the blood is incubated at 37°C under sterile conditions for 48 hours. This is partly inhibited by glucose and adenosine 5′-triphosphate (ATP)
- intermittent increase in unconjugated bilirubin levels
- negative Coombs' test
- erythroid hyperplasia of the bone marrow

Hereditary spherocytosis is unique among the familial haemolytic disorders in that the anaemia and jaundice can be cured by splenectomy, although red cell survival does not return to normal. This bright picture is somewhat clouded by the fact that splenectomy, especially when carried out early in life, increases the risk of sepsis particularly in relation to infection by *Streptococcus pneumoniae*.

Hereditary Elliptocytosis

This set of genetically determined haemolytic disorders has as its unifying feature the presence of at least 25% of elliptical red cells on examination of peripheral blood films (*Fig. 41.14*). In most cases the disease is either mild or clinically silent but severe haemolytic anaemia may occur, especially in homozygous individuals (elliptocytosis is usually transmitted in an autosomal dominant fashion). In these severe cases, the condition is usually improved by splenectomy.

Hereditary elliptocytosis is worldwide in its distribution and the prevalence is variously estimated as 1 in

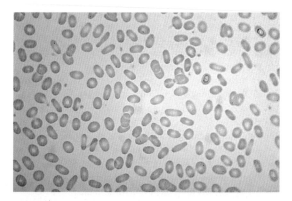

FIGURE 41.14 *Blood film from a patient with hereditary elliptocytosis. Note the numerous elliptical red cells.*

1000 to 1 in 5000. There is some biological advantage in hereditary elliptocytosis in that affected red cells are more resistant to invasion by malarial parasites. This may account for higher than average prevalence of the disorder in some areas, for example in the Malayan jungle.

Hereditary elliptocytosis, like spherocytosis, is due to cytoskeletal abnormalities. Several different abnormalities have been described, affecting different functions of the spectrin molecule.

DEFECTS IN GLYCOLYTIC ENZYMES

Pyruvate Kinase Deficiency

This is the commonest red cell deficiency of the Embden–Meyerhof pathway of anaerobic glycolysis. Pyruvate kinase deficiency is inherited in an autosomal recessive fashion; its principal biochemical consequence is a shortage of ATP because pyruvate kinase takes part in one of the two glycolytic reactions generating ATP. As energy requirements exceed available ATP, membrane pumps concerned with the regulation of cation gradients start to fail. Potassium loss exceeds sodium gain, causing a net loss of water from the affected cells and membrane distortion. The rigidity, distortion and dehydration of the abnormal red cells mark them down for destruction in the reticuloendothelial system.

Clinical Features

There is a wide spectrum of clinical severity, ranging from severe neonatal anaemia and jaundice at one extreme to a fully compensated anaemia at the other. Most cases are diagnosed during infancy, the frequency of neonatal jaundice in this disorder being a little less than 40%. This jaundice is invariably associated with anaemia and splenomegaly. The symptoms related to the anaemia are relatively mild because the oxygen dissociation curve is shifted to the right as a result of an increase in intracellular levels of 2,3-diphosphoglycerate.

Laboratory Findings
- a moderate to severe degree of anaemia (haemoglobin level 6–12 g/dl)
- morphological criteria of accelerated erythropoiesis such as poikilocytosis, polychromasia, anisocytosis and the presence of some nucleated red cells
- normal osmotic fragility
- increased serum concentrations of unconjugated bilirubin
- increased autohaemolysis which, unlike what is seen in hereditary spherocytosis, is not corrected by glucose

None of these is really specific; diagnosis depends on demonstrating the enzyme deficiency. This can be done by a simple 'spot' test. Confirmatory quantitative assays of the enzyme are performed in cases where the spot test is positive.

DEFICIENCIES IN ENZYMES INVOLVED IN THE PENTOSE PHOSPHATE PATHWAY

Glucose-6-phosphate Dehydrogenase (G6PD) Deficiency
G6PD deficiency causes haemolysis because the red cells show a decrease in the intracellular content of reduced glutathione (GSH). GSH and its related enzymes constitute one of the most important cellular defences against oxidative stress and, thus, G6PD-deficient red cells are more liable to membrane damage by reactive oxygen species (free radicals).

The pentose phosphate pathway exists principally to reduce nicotinamide adenine dinucleotide phosphate (NADP) to NADPH. The latter is needed for the regeneration of GSH from the oxidized form of glutathione (GSSG).

The gene coding for G6PD is located on the X chromosome. Thus deficiencies are fully expressed in males, whereas female heterozygotes are clinically 'silent'. Abnormal variants leading to a decline in enzyme activity are associated with an increased resistance to infections by falciparum-type malaria. The parasites that gain access to enzyme-deficient cells are destroyed by oxidant stress.

Epidemiology
G6PD deficiency is by far the commonest red cell metabolic abnormality. Estimates vary but it is likely that between 130 and 200 million individuals are affected. The distribution is a worldwide one but significant variations in frequency occur. The populations most affected are in **west Africa, countries bordering the Mediterranean, the Middle East and South-East Asia.**

Normal G6PD exists in two molecular forms: type A is found predominantly in black Africans and type B in Caucasians. The position with regard to deficiency states is very complicated because there are more than 400 variant forms of the molecule which are deficient either in amount or in function.

Clinical Features
G6PD deficiency may take the following forms:
- **clinically 'silent'**
- **episodic acute, acquired haemolytic anaemia.** Drugs that cause such acute haemolytic episodes include **sulphonamides, antimalarials, sulphones and nitrofurans**. A wide variety of infectious agents, including bacteria and viruses, has also been implicated.
- **congenital non-spherocytic haemolytic anaemia.** Where enzyme activity is extremely low, a life-long haemolytic anaemia may be present.
- **'Favism'** – haemolysis occurring after eating broad beans (*Vicia fava*)

Acute Acquired Haemolysis
The common presentation is jaundice, pallor and dark urine, which may or may not be accompanied by abdominal or back pain.

The laboratory findings are those of:
- intravascular haemolysis
- a sharp fall in haemoglobin concentrations. This fall may be as much as 3–4 g/dl.
- morphological abnormalities of red cells. Some of the cells clearly show small portions of cytoplasm to be missing. Such cells are called 'bite cells' and represent red cells from which Heinz bodies have been removed. In films made from blood that has been supravitally stained, Heinz bodies are seen to be present in some cells.

Congenital Non-spherocytic Haemolytic Anaemia
Anaemia and jaundice in this disorder are usually seen in neonates and the jaundice may be sufficiently severe as to require exchange transfusion. No triggering factor is present in most cases. The severity of the process is due in part to the fact that the neonatal liver cells have distinctly limited antioxidant capacity.

Favism
The fact that eating the broad bean *Vicia fava* is toxic and potentially lethal to some individuals has been known since the time of Pythagoras. The basis for this is, at least in part, a G6PD deficiency. The molecular variant that is most commonly associated with favism is

G6PD Mediterranean and, thus, cases of favism are most often encountered in Greece and Italy. Africans and Americans of African origin who have G6PD deficiency do not suffer from favism.

It occurs most commonly in young children, who present with severe intravascular haemolysis within 5–24 hours of having eaten the beans. Because not all members of a single family who have G6PD deficiency are affected by the fava beans, some other factor must be operating.

DEFECTS IN GLOBIN STRUCTURE OR IN THE REGULATION OF GLOBIN SYNTHESIS

Inherited abnormalities of haemoglobin synthesis may arise in two ways:
- there may be **a structural abnormality in one or more of the globin chains (haemoglobinopathy)**
- one or more of the **normal** chains of haemoglobin **may be synthesized at an abnormally low rate (thalassaemia)**

HAEMOGLOBINOPATHIES
The haemoglobinopathies may be classified on a functional basis into a few groups, as shown below, or on the basis of the structural abnormality. The latter may be a single amino acid substitution (by far the most common), double amino acid substitutions, deletions, and elongations or fusion of polypeptide chains. In the abnormal haemoglobin (HbS) of sickle cell disease, the paradigm of these disorders, the amino acid **valine** is substituted for **glutamic acid** at the sixth position from the amino terminal. Four abnormal haemoglobins, **HbS, HbC, HbD Punjab** and **HbE**, affect millions of individuals and constitute 'the common abnormal haemoglobins'.

> ### KEY POINTS: Functional Variants of Haemoglobin
> - **The haemoglobin may be functionally normal, even though there is a structural abnormality. The condition is, therefore, clinically silent.**
> - **The haemoglobin may, under certain conditions, form polymers (such as happens with HbS) or crystals, as occurs with HbC. In either case, this gives rise to haemolysis.**
> - **The haemoglobin may have a decreased affinity for oxygen, this being associated with cyanosis in the affected individual.**
> - **The haemoglobin may have an increased affinity for oxygen which is associated with erythroid hyperplasia and an increase in the number of circulating red cells.**

> - **The haemoglobin may maintain its iron moiety in the ferric state. This leads to methaemoglobinaemia.**
> - **The haemoglobin may be unstable. This can lead to chronic or episodic haemolysis.**

Haemoglobin S and Sickle Cell Disease
Sickle cell haemoglobin (HbS) is so called because red cells containing appreciable amounts of it undergo a characteristic sickle-shaped deformation in oxygen concentrations below a critical level.

HbS is the commonest abnormal haemoglobin, especially in tropical Africa where, in certain regions, the mutated gene is present in 40–50% of the population. Some 8% of Afro-Americans show the presence of the HbS mutation. **A high prevalence of the HbS gene is found where malaria is endemic.** HbS confers resistance against parasitization by *Plasmodium falciparum*.

Abnormal haemoglobin can be detected in both heterozygotes and homozygotes. Heterozygotes do not normally show any clinically significant phenotypic abnormalities and are said to have the **sickle cell trait**. Homozygotes whose red blood cells contain no normal haemoglobin A show a clinical phenotype (**sickle cell disease**) of differing grades of severity.

Pathophysiology
The sickle cell mutation is characterized by a **substitution of thymine for adenine in the sixth codon of the β-chain gene**. In this way, **valine** is encoded instead of **glutamic acid**. This causes deoxygenated HbS to polymerize and it is this that causes 'sickling'.

Oxygen tension is the most important factor: sickling occurs only when the HbS is deoxygenated.

The functional consequences of irreversible sickling are twofold:

1) **Sickled red blood cells are more adherent to endothelium and macrophages than normal red cells.** This causes more phagocytosis of the abnormal red cells by macrophages and thus contributes to the chronic haemolytic anaemia. Intravascular haemolysis also plays a role and is thought to be due to loss of microfilaments from the red cells and to lysis of irreversibly sickled cells under conditions of high shear.

2) **The flow patterns of sickled red cells are abnormal.** This is partly because of increased intracellular viscosity and partly because of increased rigidity of the red cell membrane, both of which are due to sickling. **The end result is obstruction of small blood vessels, leading to ischaemic tissue damage.**

Clinical Features

> ### KEY POINTS: Haematological Abnormalities
>
> - **A mild anaemia** is usually present by the age of 12 weeks. At all ages, the clinical effects of this are milder than would be suggested by the haemoglobin levels. This is because HbS yields up its content of oxygen more readily than does normal adult haemoglobin (HbA).
> - **Splenomegaly** is usually present by the age of 6 months. So-called **'splenic sequestration crises'** may occur, usually between the ages of 6 months and 2 years. In these, the spleen rapidly increases in size and there is a corresponding drop in the blood volume. This may be so severe as to cause hypovolaemic shock. In fatal cases, the splenic sinuses are seen to be stuffed with sickled cells. Such crises may recur until the age of 5–6 years, at which time the spleen is so fibrotic that it can no longer expand sufficiently to trap large numbers of red cells. In due time, **splenic infarction and marked atrophy** occur as a result of the occlusion of small vessels by the sickled red cells. Loss of splenic function, often starting early in the course of the disease, leads to a marked increase in susceptibility to infection.
> - **Megaloblastic crises** can occur as a result of folate depletion caused by chronic expansion of the erythroid component of the marrow.
> - **Aplastic crises** occur as in other congenital haemolytic disorders.
> - **Haemolytic crises** with a sudden fall in haemoglobin concentration and a rise in the reticulocyte count may also occur.

Ischaemic Manifestations in Sickle Cell Disease

These may be acute or chronic, precipitated by **infection, fever, dehydration, acidosis, hypoxemia and cold**. Such factors should be avoided as far as is possible.

Acute Ischaemic Manifestations

'Hand–foot Syndrome' This term is applied to episodic acute bone ischaemia affecting chiefly the small bones of the hands and feet. It tends to occur fairly early in the course of the disease; in Jamaica, by the age of 2 years, almost 50% of children with sickle cell anaemia have experienced this. The dorsal surfaces of the affected parts become swollen, painful and tender. Within 2–3 weeks of the onset of symptoms, radiological examination shows cortical thinning of the small bones.

Bone and Joint Crises Involving Larger Bones Vascular occlusion in small blood vessels of bones such as the humerus, tibia and femur, rib cage and spine occur after 2–3 years. This causes severe 'gnawing' pain.

Central Nervous System Crises These are the most crippling and life-threatening ischaemic events in sickle cell disease. Stroke affects 6–17% of children and young adults with sickle cell disease. As with stroke in other contexts, it may be thrombotic or haemorrhagic, the latter tending to occur in older children and young adults.

'Acute Chest Syndrome' Pulmonary crises are said to be the single most common manifestation of sickle cell disease requiring hospital admission. They are characterized by:
- fever
- chest pain
- rapid breathing
- a neutrophil leucocytosis
- lung infiltrates seen on radiography
- a sudden decrease in haemoglobin concentration

This acute and dangerous syndrome may in a minority of cases be due to pulmonary infection. Most cases, however, are believed to result from occlusion of small vessels by sickled red cells. This is the commonest cause of death from sickle cell disease.

Abdominal Crises These are characterized by acute attacks of severe abdominal pain with signs of peritoneal irritation. They are believed to be due to small infarcts occurring in the mesentery and abdominal viscera.

Other More Chronic Clinical Features related to Ischaemia

- **destructive changes in bones and joints** leading to such events as collapse of the femoral head
- **chronic ulcers of the lower leg** due to vascular stasis and resulting local ischaemia
- **impairment of growth and maturation**
- **a retinopathy** to which proliferation of new capillaries as a result of retinal ischaemia contributes
- **an increased incidence of pigment gallstones** due to the chronic haemolysis and resulting unconjugated hyperbilirubinaemia
- **haematuria and inability to concentrate the glomerular filtrate normally.** This is due to ischaemic damage to the renal papilla. Occasionally, sickle cell anaemia may be complicated by the nephrotic syndrome. Renal biopsy shows both mesangial and capillary wall changes and immunohistochemical studies show the presence of immune complexes that contain tubular antigen. It has been suggested that ischaemic tubular damage may lead to the release of antigen from the damaged tubules and the resulting formation of immune complexes.

- **priapism.** This may be experienced both in prepubertal and postpubertal males. It is due to episodes of obstruction to venous flow by sickle cells in the corpora cavernosa. Such episodes are usually self-limiting but may occasionally last for some days.

Laboratory Findings

- a decreased haemoglobin concentration (6–9 g/dl)
- the presence of both sickle cells and target cells (*Fig. 41.15*)
- sickling following the addition of sodium metabisulphite or sodium dithionite to blood samples
- absence of an HbA band on haemoglobin electrophoresis; 80–85% of the haemoglobin is HbS, the remainder being fetal haemoglobin (HbF)(*Fig. 41.16*). In the sickle cell trait, about 40% of the haemoglobin is HbS, the remainder being HbA.
- an increased white cell and platelet count
- a low erythrocyte sedimentation rate because sickled red cells fail to form rouleaux

Infection and Sickle Cell Disease

- Infection is a major presenting feature of sickle cell disease in early childhood.
- It is one of the major complications requiring admission to hospital.
- It is a major cause of death in individuals with sickle cell disease.

During the first 5 years of life, the organism most often implicated in serious infections is *Streptococcus pneumoniae*. More than 70% of the cases of childhood meningitis occurring in sickle cell anaemia are due to this organism and these children run a risk of acquiring meningitis said to be more than 300 times greater than that in the general population. After the age of 6 years, the risk of infection starts to diminish and Gram-negative bacteria become the predominant organisms

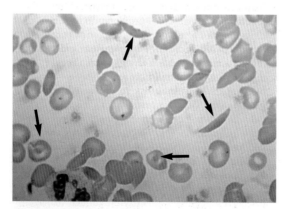

FIGURE 41.15 *Blood film from patients with sickle cell disease. The field shows both typical sickle cells (arrows) and some target cells (arrowed).*

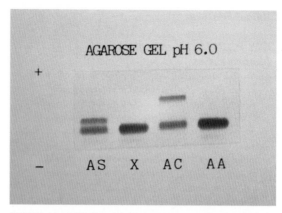

FIGURE 41.16 *Haemoglobin electrophoresis. The lane marked X is from a patient with sickle cell disease. Note the presence of a single band in the S position. This can be seen easily by comparing X with the three known samples.*

responsible for serious infections.

The basis for this increased susceptibility to infection is, in part, the loss of splenic function, which causes a failure of bloodborne antigens to elicit an appropriate antibody response. In the case of the pneumococcus, opsonins are not generated. Other mechanisms that may contribute to the increased liability to infection are:

- comparatively low levels of serum IgM
- defective operation of the alternative complement activation pathway
- deficiency of the phagocytosis-promoting protein 'tuftsin'

The clinical features of sickle cell disease are summarized in *Fig. 41.17*.

Haemoglobin C Disorders

In haemoglobin C, **lysine** replaces **glutamic acid** at the sixth position from the amino terminal. As with HbS, HbC may be found as the HbC trait with only one allele of the β-chain gene affected. In homozygotes virtually all the haemoglobin synthesized is HbC.

Deoxygenated HbC forms intracellular crystals leading to an increase in intracellular viscosity. This renders the red cells less deformable and causes them to fragment easily, to become sequestrated in the spleen and to form small spherocytes.

The resulting anaemia is mild to moderate in degree and reticulocyte counts are raised only slightly. The clinical symptoms of the anaemia are milder than would be suggested by the haemoglobin level because the oxygen dissociation curve is shifted to the right. The presence of **target cells** is a very characteristic feature and such abnormal cells may make up 90% of the red cells. Red blood cell survival is shortened and iron turnover is increased.

Some individuals show the presence of both HbS and HbC. The clinical features in such patients resemble those seen in sickle cell anaemia but, in general, are less severe. The commonest symptom is episodic pain which

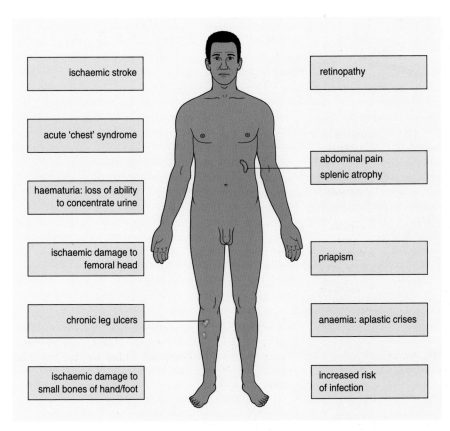

FIGURE 41.17 *Clinical features seen in sickle cell disease.*

may affect the abdomen or the skeleton. Moderate enlargement of the spleen is often present and may persist well into adult life. These patients have an increased risk of venous thrombosis and pulmonary embolism.

Features that serve to distinguish the natural history of HbS/C disease from sickle cell anaemia are:

- a greater incidence of proliferative retinitis
- a greater incidence of aseptic necrosis of the femoral head
- an increased risk of an acute chest syndrome occurring as a result of fat embolism secondary to bone marrow infarcts. This is especially likely to occur during pregnancy.

The Thalassaemias

Quantitative Disorders of Haemoglobin Synthesis

Thalassaemia is a syndrome characterized by:

- **a severe degree of anaemia**
- **enlargement of the spleen**
- **certain bony deformities**

The term thalassaemia encompasses a set of heterogeneous clinical disorders characterized by a deficiency in the synthesis of one or more of the polypeptide chains of haemoglobin. The chains themselves are **normal**. Originally the thalassaemias were classified according to their clinical phenotypes; a patient with severe anaemia was said to have **thalassaemia major**. Now, they are classified according to the deficient globin chain or chains.

On a worldwide basis, thalassaemia is the commonest genetically determined disease. It is distributed with the greatest frequency in a broad belt stretching across the Mediterranean.

THE α-THALASSAEMIAS

The α-thalassaemias are most frequently due to deletions of the genes encoding the α-globin chain; the presence or absence of anaemia and its severity, if present, correlate with the number of genes deleted (*Fig. 41.18*).

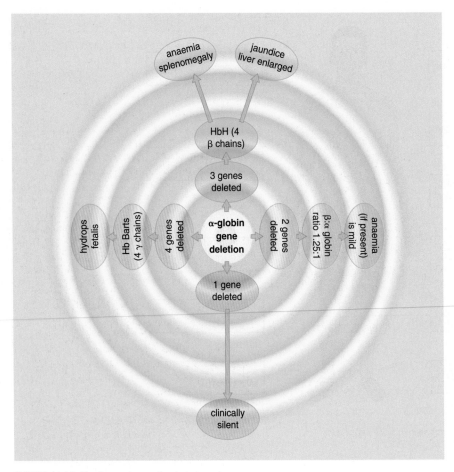

FIGURE 41.18 The four variants of α-thalassaemia.

α-Thalassaemias due to Deletions of the α-Globin Genes

Four α-globin Genes Deleted

No α chain is synthesized. This causes either **hydrops fetalis** or death *in utero*. The haemoglobin consists entirely of **Hb Barts** (tetramers of γ chains). Hb Barts has high oxygen affinity and death, therefore, results from severe hypoxia. Live-born children with hydrops are pale and oedematous, and have obvious cardiorespiratory problems. This devastating syndrome is most common in South-East Asia.

The placenta is enlarged and oedematous and the infant's liver may be grossly enlarged as a result of extramedullary haemopoiesis.

Three α-globin Chains Deleted

This is known as **HbH disease** (HbH consists of tetramers of β-globin chains). It is seen throughout South-East Asia, the Middle East and the islands of the Mediterranean such as Cyprus. It is very rare in Africans.

In terms of clinical phenotype, HbH disease was known as **α-thalassaemia intermedia**.

The affected infants appear normal at birth but by the age of 1 year they have developed **anaemia and splenomegaly; jaundice** and **liver enlargement** occur at a later stage. In most cases compensatory hyperplasia of the red marrow is sufficient to obviate a need for blood transfusion (*Fig. 41.19*). This red marrow hyperplasia, however, causes the **skeletal changes** seen in about 30% of children with HbH disease.

Laboratory Findings

- There is a moderate degree of microcytic hypochromic anaemia (haemoglobin concentration 7–10 g/dl).
- The reticulocyte count is raised (5–10%).
- Some target cells and small distorted red cells are present.
- Incubation of three or four drops of blood with 0.5 ml brilliant cresyl blue at room temperature causes precipitation of HbH. This is expressed in the form of multiple small inclusions in affected red cells.

- Haemoglobin electrophoresis shows HbH to account for 5–40% of the haemoglobin. At birth, 20–40% of the haemoglobin is Hb Barts, this being replaced during the first few months of life by HbH. Acquired HbH disease occurs occasionally in patients with myeloproliferative disorders.

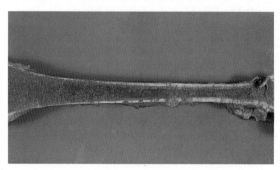

FIGURE 41.19 *Marrow hyperplasia in a case of chronic haemolytic anaemia. Note how the entire femoral shaft shows the presence of red marrow.*

Two α-globin Chains Deleted

The clinical phenotype here is known as **α-thalassaemia minor**. It is essentially a benign disorder in which anaemia, if present, is mild. Haemoglobin concentrations are normal or slightly decreased and there is also some decrease in mean corpuscular volume (MCV) and mean corpuscular haemoblogin (MCH). At birth there is an increase in the amount of Hb Barts but, after the first few months of life, the diagnosis is difficult unless special techniques such as quantitative studies of globin synthesis in reticulocytes or gene mapping are employed. Where this is done, the ratio of β : α globin synthesis is 1.25 : 1 instead of the normal 1 : 1.

One α-globin Gene Deleted

This is associated with a **silent carrier state**; there is neither clinical nor haematological abnormality.

THE β-THALASSAEMIAS

β-Thalassaemia, first recognized by Cooley in 1925, is characterized by relative or absolute failure to synthesize β-globin chains. There is thus a preponderance of α chains and a deficiency in adult haemoglobin (HbA), varying amounts of which are replaced by **fetal haemoglobin (HbF)** and **Hb Lepore** (a hybrid form characterized by δ-globin sequences at the amino end and β-globin sequences at the carboxy end.

Unlike the α-thalassaemias, **this set of disorders is due to point mutations in the genes that encode the β-globin chain**. It is not practical to classify β-thalassaemias on the basis of their genomic abnormalities,

of which more than 100 are recorded. For this reason the **clinical phenotypes** are used as a basis for classification.

KEY POINTS: Clinical Phenotypes of β-Thalassaemia

- **β-Thalassaemia major.** This is the most severe form, characterized by severe anaemia requiring repeated blood transfusions. This leads to a life-threatening iron overload.
- **β-Thalassaemia intermedia.** This shows a less severe degree of anaemia. Repeated blood transfusion with its attendant hazard of iron overload is not required.
- **β-Thalassaemia minor (thalassaemia trait).** This is asymptomatic; there are morphological abnormalities of red cells but no anaemia.

The anaemia of β-thalassaemia has two principal pathophysiological bases:

1) **Subnormal amounts of HbA result in the cells being hypochromic and small.**

2) **The imbalance between α- and β-globin chains leads to formation of α-chain aggregates within the red cells.** These precipitate and form insoluble inclusions, resulting in:

- destruction of red cell precursors within the bone marrow (so-called **ineffective erythropoiesis**). Up to 85% of normoblasts may be destroyed in this way.
- **haemolysis of abnormal red cells**, most of this occurring in the spleen.

KEY POINTS: Genomic Events in β-Thalassaemia

The types of genomic events causing β-thalassaemia include:

- **single base changes**
- **small deletions or insertions of one or two bases.** These can affect introns, exons or promoting regions of the globin gene.
- **deletions of nucleotides or 'frameshifts'** that distort the reading pattern downstream of the DNA abnormality
- **premature chain termination** due to the generation of a translational 'stop' codon
- **abnormalities of splicing**
- **reduction of transcription due to a lesion in the promoter or initiation regions**
- **mutations of the poly(A) addition signal**, resulting in failure of poly(A) addition to occur and thus to the generation of unstable messenger RNA.

Thalassaemia Major

Clinical Features

- **The affected infants appear normal at birth**, showing neither anaemia nor splenomegaly.
- After this time, **progressive pallor develops; the abdominal girth increases because of enlargement of the liver and spleen**, and the child fails to thrive.
- **The haemoglobin concentration falls to between 3 and 5 g/dl** in the absence of blood transfusions.
- **A set of skeletal abnormalities now develops** (see p 891).
- **Growth retardation**, as a result of the severe anaemia, may occur and can be prevented, but not corrected, by blood transfusions. Even when children are optimally transfused in terms of both amount and timing, the normal preadolescent growth spurt is delayed and less in degree than that which is normally seen. This is believed to be due to decreased secretion of somatomedins by the liver, which may have been damaged by iron overload. Puberty is often delayed, either due to a failure in maturation of the hypothalamus or to some defect in pituitary function.
- **Other endocrine abnormalities such as diabetes mellitus, hypothyroidism and hypoparathyroidism** may be seen, usually in patients who have iron overload due to many transfusions.
- **The most common causes of death in patients who have had many transfusions are congestive cardiac failure or the onset of life-threatening cardiac arrhythmias** owing to the deposition of large amounts of iron in the form of haemosiderin in the myocardium. This cardiac damage may be due to free radical generation initiated by free iron. Each unit of blood contains 250 mg iron; clinical abnormalities appear once 50 units have been transfused. The importance of treating these patients with iron-chelating agents should be obvious.
- **Liver enlargement** usually occurs fairly early in life and is probably due to extensive foci of extramedullary haemopoiesis. Later, the iron overload causes hepatic cirrhosis, the appearances of which are similar to those seen in idiopathic haemochromatosis.

These features are summarized in *Fig. 41.20.*

The prognosis is bleak; many affected children do not survive past the age of 5 years. An active policy with regard to blood transfusion may avoid disturbances in growth but brings with it the danger of iron overload to which many succumb.

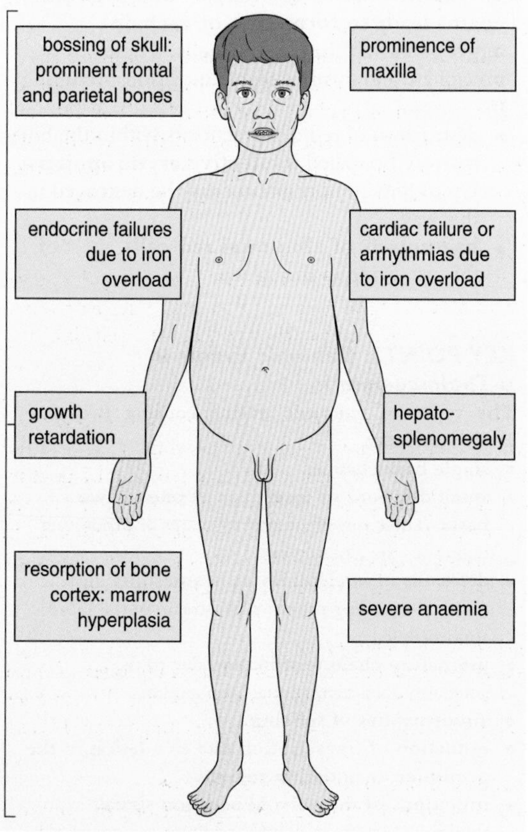

FIGURE 41.20 *Clinical features occurring in children with β-thalassaemia major.*

Laboratory Findings

- **Severe microcytic hypochromic anaemia is** present after the first few months of life.
- There is a striking variation in red cell size (**anisocytosis**). The degree of hypochromia may be so marked that red cells appear to be composed almost entirely of plasma membrane. Target cells are frequent; some of these show a curious appearance with a bridge of pigment joining the central and peripheral zones. Gross distortion of red cell shape may occur and many red cells show basophilic stippling. Nucleated red cells (normoblasts) are usually present in the peripheral blood films.
- **The reticulocyte count is raised to 5–15%** of the circulating red cells. This is lower than would be expected with this degree of anaemia and reflects ineffective erythropoiesis.
- **The osmotic fragility of the red cells is greatly decreased** and some red cells may even resist haemolysis in distilled water.
- In general, **the leucocyte count is raised** but platelet numbers are normal.
- **Electrophoresis of haemoglobin shows that there is either very little or no HbA, most of the haemoglobin being HbF**. Studies of globin chain synthesis in reticulocytes show a marked

increase in the ratio of $\alpha : \beta$ chains; β-chain synthesis is either absent or much reduced. Modern molecular biological methods can be used to identify the allelic defects.

- There is an **increase in serum concentration of unconjugated bilirubin**.

Thalassaemia Intermedia

This syndrome may be due to a wide range of genetic abnormalities.

The anaemia is less severe than that encountered in thalassaemia major: haemoglobin concentrations are generally within the range of 6–9 g/dl. As a result, blood transfusion is not usually required. Retardation of growth rate and pubertal delay are not seen as a rule; the affected individuals usually survive into adult life and, indeed, may have a normal lifespan.

Despite the lack of need for transfusion, many of the affected individuals show evidence of:

- pallor
- intermittent jaundice
- splenomegaly
- the facial and other bony lesions characteristic of expansion of the red marrow
- morphological changes in the red cells identical with those described for the major form of the disorder

Iron overload may occur in these patients despite the fact that they do not receive regular blood transfusions. This appears to be due to an increase in iron absorption related to very active erythropoiesis. Where premature death occurs, it is commonly due to haemosiderin deposition in the myocardium.

Thalassaemia Minor (β-Thalassaemia Trait)

This is extremely common and usually symptomless. Anaemia may be mild or absent, but the morphological features seen in the blood films of more severely affected thalassaemic individuals are also seen here, and the MCV and MCH are low. Haemoglobin electrophoresis may show a number of different patterns, but an increase in HbA_2 is the commonest.

NON-INHERITED ABNORMALITIES OF RED CELLS LEADING TO HAEMOLYSIS

Paroxysmal Nocturnal Haemoglobinuria (PNH)

This is a somewhat misleading term because it describes only one feature of this rare acquired disease. **Its defining criterion is the production of red cells that are abnormally sensitive to lysis by complement.** The disease, which is chronic, begins insidiously and classically is associated with attacks of **intravascular haemolysis occurring mainly at night**. In fact, this occurs in only a minority of patients and the disease complex may include:

- chronic intravascular haemolysis
- pancytopenia
- iron deficiency
- recurrent episodes of thrombosis

Pathophysiology

Red cells from patients with PNH have a shortened survival time whether they are within the circulation of an affected individual or transfused into a normal person. This is due to an **increased sensitivity to complement**.

In a single patient with PNH the red cells vary in their risk of complement-mediated lysis; most patients have red cell populations that respond in three different ways to complement:

- no increased susceptibility (PNH I)
- a three- to fivefold increased susceptibility (PNH II)
- a 15–25-fold increased susceptibility (PNH III)

The severity of the disorder depends on the relative proportions of these functional red cell types. About 80% of patients with PNH show the presence of a mixture of PNH I and PNH III cells.

Red cells in patients with PNH show increased susceptibility to lysis whether complement activation occurs via the alternate or classical pathway.

Membrane abnormalities are due to somatic mutations giving rise to abnormal clones of red cell precursors; it is from these clones that the PNH II and III cells are derived. The mutation(s) must occur at a fairly early stage because neutrophils and platelets also show some of the red cell membrane protein abnormalities.

Clinical Features

PNH starts insidiously and has a prolonged course; mean survival time is about 10 years. The diagnosis is most often made during the third to fifth decades.

Haemoglobinuria

Despite the name paroxysmal nocturnal haemoglobinuria, haemoglobinuria occurs in only about 25% of the patients. Even when it is present, it need not be nocturnal and appears to be associated more closely with sleep than with time of day, as sleep is associated with a fall in plasma pH. Quite small increases in acidity can cause activation of complement via the alternate pathway.

Episodes of Haemolysis

Many patients have irregularly timed episodes of quite severe haemolysis. These may be associated with back or abdominal pain, fever, headache and general malaise.

Aplastic Changes in the Bone Marrow

Marrow aplasia with the development of pancytopenia is not uncommon in PNH. In one series an initial diagnosis of aplastic anaemia was made in more than 25% of patients.

Thrombosis

PNH is associated with a significant increase in the risk of thrombosis, which accounts for 50% of the deaths in this disease. Fatal thrombosis often occurs in relation to the brain and portal system, but no vascular bed is exempt.

Laboratory Findings

- Severe anaemia is present in most patients. The haemoglobin concentration is usually below 6 g/dl and the red cells may appear microcytic and hypochromic.
- A leucopenia, which may be quite severe, is often present.
- The plasma may be golden-brown colour due to excess unconjugated bilirubin, haemoglobin and methaemalbumin. Serum haptoglobin levels are low and serum LDH (lactic dehydrogenase concentration) is high during periods of active haemolysis.
- The urine shows the presence of urobilinogen, haemoglobin and haemosiderin, the latter being due to the accumulation of iron in the tubular epithelial cells.
- The bone marrow shows normoblastic hyperplasia, over 50% of the nucleated cells being normoblasts.
- Addition of acidified human serum to red cells from patients with PNH causes excess lysis. This is known as the Ham test; the optimum pH for lysis to occur is 6.4–6.5. The patient's own serum should not be used for this test. The test depends on activation of the alternate complement pathway.

HAEMOLYSIS DUE TO ABNORMALITIES OUTSIDE THE RED CELLS

These disorders are all acquired and may be mediated by immune or non-immune mechanisms.

IMMUNE HAEMOLYTIC ANAEMIAS

Alloimmune Haemolysis

This term is used when the lytic antibodies are elicited by antigens that are **foreign** to the affected individual, although not to the species. Important examples are:

- **haemolytic transfusion reactions in which the antibodies concerned in the destruction of red cells are, in general, immunoglobulin (Ig) M antibodies** (*Fig. 41.21a*)
- **haemolytic disease of the newborn in which the antibodies are IgG antibodies** (*Fig. 41.21b*). This occurs principally when the fetus is rhesus (Rh) positive and mother Rh negative.

This distinction has some importance because there are substantial differences in the mechanisms of red cell destruction by the two classes of antibody.

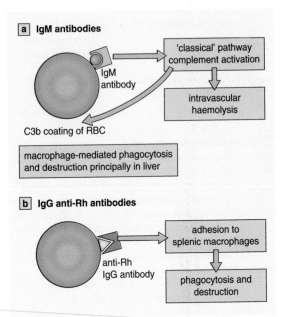

FIGURE 41.21 **a** *Transfusion haemolysis is brought about by the binding of IgM antibodies to the red cell surface, followed by 'classical' complement activation and membrane disruption (intravascular lysis).* **b** *Haemolysis brought about by IgG antibodies such as occur in rhesus incompatibility. The antibody binds to Rh antigen on the red cell surface and then to splenic macrophages so that there is no intravascular lysis.*

IgM Antibodies and Red Cell Destruction

Antibodies elicited by the blood group antigens A, B and H, and also cold agglutinins, are IgM antibodies. They are sometimes termed **'complete antibodies'** in that they can agglutinate red cells suspended in saline.

Red cell destruction is mediated by complement activation via the classical pathway, which starts with the binding of C1q to the immune complex on the cell surface. This has two effects:

- **Red cells coated with C3b adhere to appropriate receptors on macrophages and are phagocytosed by these cells.** In the case of IgM antibody-mediated damage, red cells become sequestrated in the liver and extravascular destruction takes place there.
- **Intravascular lysis takes place through the direct action of the membrane attack complex of complement.**

IgG Antibodies and Red Cell Destruction

In the context of alloimmune haemolysis, the IgG antibodies concerned react specifically with antigens of the Rh system. **In contrast with IgM antibodies, these IgG antibodies do not cause agglutination of red cells suspended in saline and are thus termed 'incomplete antibodies'.** Their failure to agglutinate under these circumstances may be due to:

- a relatively small number of antigenic sites per cell
- the molecular length of the immunoglobulin
- the strength of repulsive forces between red cells such as the negative charges on the cell surfaces

For this reason the presence of incomplete IgG antibodies, whether in serum or bound to red cell surfaces, must be demonstrated by the antiglobulin or Coombs' test. In the **direct antiglobulin test**, red cells, to which either incomplete antibody or complement components are bound, are suspended in serum from rabbits immunized against human serum. If the test red cells are indeed coated with antibody or complement, agglutination occurs.

For the detection of incomplete antibody in **serum**, the **indirect antiglobulin test** is used. In this test, normal red cells are incubated in the patient's serum and, after being washed, are exposed to the rabbit anti-human globulin serum, as in the direct test. Agglutination indicates that the normal red cells have become coated by incomplete antibody or components of complement.

Red cell destruction by anti-Rh IgG antibodies is **never** due to complement-mediated intravascular lysis. The mechanism for destruction is adhesion to and subsequent phagocytosis by mononuclear cells and the presence of bound complement has an incremental effect on this. Sequestration of the antibody and complement-coated red cells takes place largely, sometimes entirely, in the spleen and it is here that the red cells are phagocytosed.

Haemolytic Transfusion Reactions

These almost always involve destruction of donor rather than recipient cells. The degree of severity of the reaction differs from case to case. In ABO incompatibility, rapid intravascular haemolysis develops. In addition, complement activation leads to vascular and other changes mediated via the complement fragments C3a and C5a, and Factor XII cleavage occurs, which can lead both to the generation of kinins and to disseminated intravascular coagulation.

The patients may experience:
- fever
- pain in the back or chest
- shortness of breath

Haemoglobinuria and haemoglobinaemia are present. Complications include:
- shock
- acute renal failure, which probably has an ischaemic basis
- disseminated intravascular coagulation

Haemolytic Disease of the Newborn

The passage of fetal antigens across the placenta leads to the formation of antibodies in the mother **which react with paternal fetal antigens**. Maternofetal incompatibility in respect of the Rh system is by far the commonest cause of haemolytic disease of the newborn and occurs if the mother is Rh negative and the fetal red cells express Rh antigens.

The transplacental passage of small amounts of fetal blood is a common event during pregnancy. Various procedures such as amniocentesis, caesarean section and manual removal of the placenta can lead to the transplacental passage of larger amounts of blood; **the greater the volume of fetal blood that enters the maternal circulation, the greater is the chance of maternal sensitization to the Rh antigens.**

Clinical Features

> **KEY POINTS: Haemolytic Disease of the Newborn**
>
> The most common clinical features of haemolytic disease of the newborn are:
> - anaemia
> - jaundice
> - enlargement of liver and spleen
> - bilirubin encephalopathy (**kernicterus**) in infants with severe jaundice who have not been treated appropriately

If the degree of intrauterine haemolysis has been severe and the resulting anaemia pronounced, the baby may develop ascites and hypoalbuminaemia. The ascites is, at least in part, due to portal hypertension caused by distortion and enlargement of the liver acini by many large islands of extramedullary erythropoiesis. Intrauterine portal hypertension leads to high pressures in the umbilical vein, and placental oedema and hypertrophy of the trophoblast are seen. This clinical syndrome is known as **hydrops fetalis**.

Because of the danger of bilirubin encephalopathy, the serum unconjugated bilirubin concentration must be monitored carefully. At birth, the bilirubin level may not give a true picture of the severity of the process, because bilirubin is so readily transferred across the placenta. After birth, when this can no longer take place, the bilirubin level may rise steeply, due partly to the continuing haemolysis and partly to the immaturity of liver cell enzymes at this age. In most cases the increased bilirubin is all unconjugated but in some infants there may be an increase in conjugated bilirubin as well; this is known as the inspissated bile syndrome.

So far as the central nervous system is concerned **only unconjugated bilirubin is toxic**; indeed, only the fraction of bilirubin that is not bound to albumin is believed to mediate brain damage. Thus low serum albumin concentrations, or acidosis (which displaces bilirubin from albumin), are likely to make the situation worse.

Autoimmune Haemolytic Anaemia

The defining criterion here is that **antibodies are produced against the patient's own red cell antigens**.

This set of disorders is subdivided on the basis of the reactivity of the antibodies in relation to ambient temperature. Thus autoimmune haemolytic anaemia may be due to:

- **warm autoantibodies** – antibodies that bind to red cells most avidly at 37°C
- **cold antibodies**, which bind to the red cells at body temperature but show increasing affinity for their specific antigens as the temperature decreases towards 0°C
- **mixed** warm and cold antibodies. The disease in these patients tends to be severe and chronic; it runs an intermittent course and, in general, is resistant to treatment.

In addition, autoimmune haemolytic anaemias may be induced by treatment with certain drugs. A number of different mechanisms may be involved in these drug-related syndromes and this group of disorders is best considered separately.

Haemolytic Anaemia due to Warm Antibodies

Haemolysis caused by warm-reacting antibodies occurs in association with many different diseases (see box), of which malignant disease of the lymphoreticular system is the most common, accounting for 60% of cases in one large series. The likelihood of autoimmune haemolysis occurring is governed to a considerable extent by genetic factors.

> **KEY POINTS: Associations of Haemolysis due to Warm Reactive Antibodies**
> 1) Primary or idiopathic
> 2) Secondary
> - systemic lupus erythematosus and other autoimmune disorders
> - chronic lymphocytic leukaemia and lymphomas
> - non-haematological neoplasms
> - viral infections such as hepatitis, cytomegalovirus, Epstein–Barr virus, rubella, etc.
> - immune deficiency syndromes

The disorder is not common; the annual incidence is estimated as approximately 1 in 80 000. There is no predilection for any particular race, but there is a tendency for females to be affected more frequently than males, especially with regard to the primary or idiopathic form of warm antibody haemolysis.

Clinical Features

The severity of the haemolysis varies from case to case, ranging from a trivial to a life-threatening state. In general, the most explosive episodes, in terms of severity, appear to be associated with viral infections. The duration of the disease also varies considerably. In some patients it may be short lived, whereas in others it may be chronic and intractable (*Table 41.10*).

As the antibodies coating the red cells are

Table 41.10 Clinical Features of Haemolytic Anaemia due to Warm Antibodies

Symptoms	Signs
Weakness	Splenomegaly (in 80%)
Dizziness	Hepatomegaly (in 45%)
Fever	Lymph node enlargement (in 34%)
	Jaundice (in 21%)

most commonly found to be of the IgG type, red cell destruction takes place mainly in the spleen, as a result of interaction between the red cell-bound antibodies and the Fc receptors on splenic macrophages; intravascular haemolysis does not occur. Portions of red cell membrane are removed as a result and the red cell becomes steadily more spherocyte-like in an attempt to maintain its volume with less membrane.

> **Laboratory Findings**
> - Anaemia. The severity depends on the severity of the haemolysis. Blood films show differing degrees of spherocytosis.
> - The reticulocyte count is raised.
> - The **direct** antiglobulin test will be positive. This test is relatively insensitive, and severe haemolysis may occur in individuals whose red cells fail to yield a positive result. Other, more sensitive, tests have been devised such as radioimmunoassays that employ radiolabelled antihuman IgG.
> - The serum bilirubin concentration is moderately raised.

Haemolysis due to Cold Antibodies

Antibodies that react most strongly with red cell antigens at temperatures below 32°C are known as cold-reactive antibodies. These antibodies may be either **polyclonal** or **monoclonal**. **Monoclonal** cold-reactive antibodies tend to be found in association with the **idiopathic cold agglutinin syndrome** or with **lymphoreticular neoplasms** (*Table 41.11*). **Polyclonal** cold-reactive antibody formation is usually elicited by **infections**, among which *Mycoplasma pneumoniae* is the commonest by far. The mechanism responsible for eliciting the antibody response is not clear but may involve interference with normal suppressor cell function. The antibody is usually IgM and binds to red cells most effectively at 0°C. In most cases the antigen with which the IgM antibody reacts is the 'I' antigen on the red cell surface. In some instances, mostly where the antibody is monoclonal, there may also be reactions with the 'i' antigen on fetal red cells. Most of the red cell destruction associated with cold-

Table 41.11 Disorders Associated with Cold-reactive Antibody Formation

Monoclonal cold antibody	Polyclonal cold antibody
Idiopathic chronic cold agglutinin disease	*Mycoplasma pneumoniae* infections
Lymphomas including Waldenström's macroglobulinaemia	Mumps and cytomegalovirus infections
Chronic lymphocytic leukaemia	Trypanosomiasis
Myeloma	Malaria
Kaposi's sarcoma	Listerial infections
	Infective endocarditis
	Autoimmune diseases involving connective tissue
	Syphilis
	Angioimmunoblastic lymphadenopathy
	Infectious mononucleosis

reactive antibodies is due to C3b-mediated phagocytosis by cells of the reticuloendothelial system.

Chronic Idiopathic Cold Agglutinin Disease

This is a disease of the elderly, the peak incidence being in the seventh and eighth decades. Cold agglutinin disease associated with malignancy has a similar age distribution but, if the syndrome is due to infection, it tends to occur at a much younger age (between the third and fifth decades).

The clinical features are manifestations of two processes:

1) **Vascular disturbances**, which arise on the basis of blockage of blood vessels. As blood flows through the small vessels of the skin and subcutaneous tissue, it is cooled to about 28°C, or even lower. If the antibody binds actively to red cell antigens at this temperature, the cells agglutinate and complement is fixed. The agglutinates occlude the small blood vessels in which they are formed.

The changes seen in the skin are known as **acrocyanosis** and consist of discoloration which has been described as ranging from a white to deep blue-violet. The patients may complain of numbness or pain in these areas and eventually ischaemic tissue damage may become evident. Any part of the skin may be affected but those that are normally most affected by cold, such as the tip of

the nose and the ear lobes, are especially likely to show acrocyanosis. The effect of cold in these patients may be demonstrated very effectively by holding an ice cube to the skin. This is followed by the development of a localized area of acrocyanosis.

2) **The binding of complement may lead either to intravascular haemolysis or to sequestration of C3b-coated red cells within the liver. Chronic haemolysis of moderate severity is usually present**, the degree of haemolysis being controlled to a certain extent by inactivation of the C3b that is bound to the red cells.

Paroxysmal Cold Haemoglobinuria

This is the other principal manifestation of the presence of cold-reactive antibodies that bind to red cell antigens. Its defining characteristic is the **passage of haemoglobin in the urine after the affected individual has been exposed to cold**.

The responsible antibody (the Donath–Landsteiner antibody) is an IgG with a powerful haemolytic effect, exhibited most effectively when a period of cooling is followed by warming. This is because antibody binding is most effective at low temperatures which may not permit complement-mediated lysis.

Originally this syndrome was described in association with tertiary or congenital syphilis but these syndromes are now uncommon and so paroxysmal cold haemoglobinuria is now a rare disorder, occurring most commonly in children with acute viral infections.

Drug-induced Immune Haemolytic Anaemia

Drug-induced immune haemolysis can occur in **three** different ways:

1) **The drug binds to the red cell membrane by covalent bonding and acts as a hapten.** The hapten is now able to elicit IgG antibody, which binds to the hapten. Red cell destruction is usually due to antibody-mediated phagocytosis. Penicillin is characteristically associated with this type of reaction, although tetracyclines and cephalosporins have also been implicated.

2) **The drug binds to a circulating macromolecule such as one of the plasma proteins. Antibody formation is elicited and a large, soluble immune complex is formed, which then becomes deposited on cell surface membranes.** Complement is then bound and the red cell is lysed, having played the role of an 'innocent bystander', although this may well be an oversimplification of the process. The clinical picture is one of **acute intravascular haemolysis** with haemoglobinaemia and haemoglobinuria. The risk of this syndrome being complicated by acute

renal failure is high. Drugs that may be responsible for this type of reaction include para-aminosalicylic acid, quinidine, chlorpromazine, thiazides and fluorouracil.

3) **The drug causes the development of autoantibodies directed against red cell antigens.** The drug classically associated with this type of reaction is **α–methyldopa**. A high proportion of patients treated with this compound develop a positive direct antiglobulin test and some show evidence of haemolysis. The mechanisms responsible for antibody formation being elicited are not known. The antibodies bind specifically with Rh antigens on the surface of the red cells.

NON-IMMUNE HAEMOLYTIC ANAEMIAS

Red Cell Fragmentation Syndromes

These are caused by physical damage to red cells. Such damage may occur in the course of microangiopathic haemolytic anaemias (see pp 695–696) or as a result of interactions between red cells and foreign surfaces such as vascular grafts.

Haemolytic Anaemia due to Direct Injury of Red Cells

KEY POINTS: Infectious Agents that Injure Red Cells

Haemolysis can occur in the course of infections caused by the following:

- **Plasmodia causing malaria.** This is the most prevalent of all serious diseases; the annual mortality rate in Africa alone is 3 million. Anaemia is common in malaria, especially with *Plasmodium falciparum*. The most life-threatening acute syndrome, fortunately rare, is **blackwater fever**, the acute intravascular haemolysis associated with *P. falciparum* malaria. *P. falciparum*, unlike other plasmodia, can parasitize red cells at all stages of their maturation and also parasitizes a much greater proportion of the red cells than other species.
- Other protozoal infections, most notably **trypanosomiasis**
- Infections by the flagellated bacillus *Bartonella bacilliformis*, which produces a severe, acute haemolytic anaemia. The disorder is termed **Oroya fever** and is characterized by malaise, myalgia, fever and rapidly developing anaemia.
- **Clostridial** species, most notably *Cl. perfringens* which produces gas gangrene. Haemolysis is due to secretion of α toxin, a lecithinase which directly attacks the phospholipid membrane of the red cells.
- **Spirochaetes** such as *Borrelia recurrentis* which causes relapsing fever and *Leptospira icterohaemorrhagica* which causes Weil's disease.

Chemical Agents

Chemical agents may directly damage red cells either because of oxidant stress in which haemoglobin is oxidatively denatured or via non-oxidative pathways. Individuals who are deficient in glucose-6-phosphate dehydrogenase are obviously much more at risk from compounds that can induce oxidative stress, but some of these chemicals are powerful enough to damage normal red cells. **Compounds causing haemolysis via oxidative stress include sulphonamides, sulphones, nitrofurans, salicylates, nitrites, chlorates and resorcin.**

Oxidant damage to red cells is expressed by certain highly characteristic morphological changes. These include the presence of:

- **Heinz bodies**, in cases where the anaemia is severe
- **'bite' cells** (see p 895)
- **'hemighosts'** – red cells in which the haemoglobin looks as if it has shifted to one side of the cell leaving the other half clear. The clear area is formed by the bringing together of membrane from two sides of the cells. It usually indicates severe damage oxidative stress.

Chemicals that cause non-oxidative damage to red cells include arsine, copper (in patients with Wilson's disease), lead, glycerol, propylthiouracil, mephenesin and water (as seen in patients whose bladders had been irrigated with water after transurethral prostatic resection). Snake and spider venoms have occasionally been reported to cause haemolytic anaemias, haemolysis due to spider venom being more common.

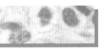

Aplastic Anaemias

The defining criteria of aplastic anaemia are:

- **pancytopenia**
- **decreased production by the marrow of all the cellular elements of the blood** (*Fig. 41.22*)

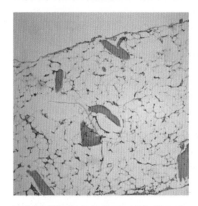

FIGURE 41.22 *Bone marrow trephine from an area normally containing red marrow in a patient with aplastic anaemia. The intertrabecular adipose tissue contains no haemopoietic cells.*

Table 41.12 Causes of Aplastic Anaemia

Familial	Acquired
Fanconi's anaemia	Idiopathic
Pancreatic insufficiency	Chemical and physical agents: • produce aplasia regularly if the dose is sufficient (e.g. benzene) • produce marrow hypoplasia only occasionally (e.g. phenylbutazone, chloramphenicol)
Familial defect in cellular folate uptake	Viral infections (e.g.human immunodeficiency virus, Epstein–Barr virus, hepatitis) Pregnancy Simmonds' disease Sclerosis of thyroid

• **Absence of any primary disease that infiltrates, replaces or suppresses the marrow**

The **causes** of aplastic anaemia are shown in *Table 41.12*.

Familial Aplastic (Fanconi's) Anaemia

Fanconi's anaemia is an autosomal recessively inherited syndrome generally manifesting at the age of 5–10 years. The rather variable clinical picture includes:

• pancytopenia
• bone marrow hypoplasia
• a variety of skeletal abnormalities including absence of the thumbs or radii
• chromosomal fragility with multiple random breaks
• an increased risk of myeloid leukaemia and other neoplasms
• a variety of other features including learning disability, squint, defective development of the genitals, dwarfism and atrophy of the spleen
• patchy brown pigmentation of the skin due to deposition of melanin

Laboratory Findings

• **Anaemia**, which is either normocytic or slightly macrocytic. Target cells may be seen on examination of blood films.
• **The absolute reticulocyte count is reduced**, although the **percentage** of reticulocytes found may be increased.

• **The white cell count is decreased**. Most of this reduction is due to a deficiency of neutrophils, although other white cell lines are also affected.
• **The marrow may be normal or even hypercellular in the early stages of the disease but eventually becomes hypocellular.**
• **Cultured lymphocytes show a high number of chromosomal breaks.**
• **Cultured skin fibroblasts show an increased susceptibility to become transformed by the oncogenic virus SV40**, an interesting finding in view of the increased risk of malignancy associated with Fanconi's anaemia.

Acquired Aplastic Anaemia

Due to Chemical Agents and Drugs

As shown in *Table 41.12*, this form of aplastic anaemia may be either **predictable** or **idiosyncratic**.

In the predictable form, the responsible compounds always induce marrow aplasia so long as the dose of the compound is large enough. Archetypes of this type of reaction are the aplasias associated with **benzene poisoning, ionizing radiation** and with **antitumour chemotherapy** with agents such as:

• sulphur and nitrogen mustards (busulphan, melphalan and cyclophosphamide)
• antimetabolites such as 6-mercaptopurine
• antimitotic compounds such as the vinca alkaloids and colchicine
• anthracycline compounds such as Adriamycin (doxorubicin) and daunorubicin

Benzene has been known to cause marrow aplasia for almost 100 years. It is a common organic solvent with many industrial applications. It is volatile, so that absorption occurs mainly by inhalation.

Idiosyncratic reactions leading to marrow damage occur in association with a very large number of drugs, of which the ones most commonly implicated are shown in *Table 41.13*.

In about 50% of cases of acquired aplastic anaemia, no cause can be identified and these are termed **'idiopathic'**.

Clinical Features

The clinical picture (*Fig. 41.23*) comprises manifestations of:

• **anaemia** due to the deficiency of red cells. The haemoglobin concentration may be as low as 7.0 g/dl at clinical presentation.
• **bleeding** due to thrombocytopenia. Haemorrhage may occur from the nose, mouth, gastrointestinal tract or uterus. Purpura is occasionally seen but is not common. As would be expected in patients with thrombocytopenia, the bleeding time is prolonged.

Table 41.13 Drugs Causing Idiosyncratic Aplastic Anaemia

Type of drug	Examples
Antimicrobials	Chloramphenicol
	Organic arsenicals
	Quinacrine
Anticonvulsants	Mesantoin
	Tridione
Analgesics	Phenylbutazone
Miscellaneous	Gold used in the treatment of rheumatoid arthritis

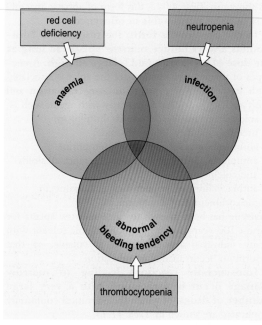

FIGURE 41.23 Clinical features of aplastic anaemia.

- **infection** due to the neutropenia that depresses defence against infection

The pancytopenia is mirrored in the appearances of the bone marrow, which is yellowish-white instead of red. This reflects severe hypoplasia: the marrow, on microscopic examination, is seen to consist largely of adipose tissue, fibrous tissue and lymphocytes. In the early stages in some cases (e.g. in benzene toxicity) the marrow may, however, appear hypercellular.

Features suggesting a particularly poor prognosis include:

- evidence of bleeding at an early stage of the disorder
- the presence of more than 70% non-myeloid cells in the initial bone marrow biopsy
- male rather than female sex
- a low reticulocyte count

'PURE' RED CELL APLASIA

Hypoplasia affecting only the erythropoietic portion of the marrow is referred to as **'pure red cell aplasia'**. The condition may occur in acute or chronic forms and may be congenital or acquired.

Congenital Erythroid Hypoplasia (Diamond–Blackfan Syndrome)

This is characterized by a moderate to severe chronic anaemia beginning in infancy. No erythroblasts can be seen in the marrow and there is an absolute deficiency of reticulocytes. White blood cells and platelets are normal. Fetal haemoglobin levels are higher than would be expected for the child's age. The course is progressive in most cases but about 20% go into remission, induced in some patients by steroid treatment. In those who are steroid resistant, repeated transfusions may be necessary, but these patients face the hazard of transfusion siderosis.

Acute Transient Red Cell Aplasia

This may be seen in a number of circumstances including:

- **aplastic crises due to parvovirus B19 infections** in patients with haemolytic anaemia
- **transient red cell aplasia in children with no obvious underlying disease.** The presence of serum inhibitors of erythropoiesis has been demonstrated in this syndrome
- **acute red cell aplasia in adults in association with hepatitis or other viral infections**, which may be quite trivial
- **acute transient red cell aplasia in association with certain drugs** such as aspirin, heparin, glutethimide, tolbutamide. In most of these complete recovery follows cessation of drug administration.

Chronic Acquired Red Cell Aplasia

This disorder affects adults only. It is believed that *two* forms of the disease exist:

1) cases associated with the presence of a **benign thymoma**
2) cases **not associated with any thymic abnormality**

Thymoma is associated with more than half the cases of chronic acquired red cell aplasia, and, of these, about a sixth show evidence of myasthenia gravis. Despite the association with thymoma, thymectomy produces a haematological improvement in only about 25% and, indeed, some patients in whom thymectomy has been performed for myasthenia gravis have developed red cell aplasia up to 3 years after operation. The mechanisms that underlie chronic acquired red cell aplasia are still obscure.

Haemostasis

Normal function of the body as a whole makes great and, in a sense, conflicting demands on blood vessels, platelets, the clotting system and the fibrinolytic system.

On the one hand, normal flow through the circulatory system demands that the blood remain fluid, and, on the other, survival is possible only if injuries in blood vessel walls are very rapidly plugged by aggregated platelets, these aggregates being stabilized by fibrin.

This normal state of affairs is maintained by a dynamic equilibrium in each of the systems listed. If these equilibria are disturbed, the end result may be either **abnormal bleeding** or an **abnormal tendency for thromboembolic events to occur**. In either event, the disturbances occurring can best be understood and characterized in terms of the normal.

This subject is discussed also in Chapter 18, to which cross-reference should be made, especially in relation to platelet functions.

NORMAL HAEMOSTATIC RESPONSE

Normal haemostasis depends on a series of interlinked responses (*Fig. 41.24*) involving the:
- **blood vessels in the injured area**
- **circulating platelets**
- **clotting factors and the molecules regulating their activity**

BLOOD VESSELS
In injured areas local blood vessels constrict. If the vessels are abnormal or if there are defects in the perivascular connective tissue, this defence mechanism fails and abnormal bleeding occurs. This may be associated with trivial trauma or with no trauma at all, and is most often expressed in the form of **easy bruising, or of small petechial haemorrhages in the skin**.

Blood vessels are not merely more or less passive conduits for flowing blood. The layer in contact with the blood, the lining endothelium, is a versatile tissue, synthesizing and secreting molecules which are:

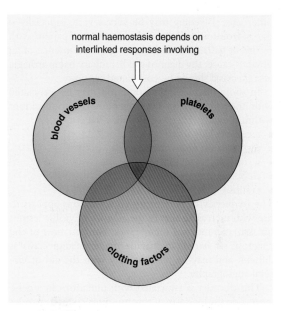

FIGURE 41.24 *Normal haemostasis depends on interlinked responses from three elements, as shown in this Venn diagram. A defect in any one can lead to abnormal bleeding.*

- **procoagulant**
- **anticoagulant**
- **promote the adhesion of platelets**
- **inhibit the adhesion of platelets**

BLEEDING DISORDERS DUE TO ABNORMAL BLOOD VESSELS
Such abnormal bleeding may be **hereditary** or **acquired**.

Hereditary Disorders
The hereditary disorders involve structural malformations of either the blood vessels or the connective tissues that normally support them. The first type is exemplified in hereditary haemorrhagic telangiectasia.

Hereditary Haemorrhagic Telangiectasia (Osler–Weber–Rendu Syndrome)
In this rare autosomal dominant disorder, blood vessels become tortuous and dilated. This is due to the affected segments being abnormally thinned, the walls consisting only of a layer of endothelium. The defect is commonest in venules but can affect other small vessels.

The defect is expressed in the form of **telangiectases**, leashes of abnormally dilated vessels seen most easily in skin and mucous membranes. Lesions usually develop during childhood, although significant bleeding may not manifest until adulthood. The telangiectases range in size from a pinpoint to about 3 mm in diameter, appearing as bright red or purplish dots on the face, ears, lips, tongue, conjunctivae and many other sites. Bleeding may be very severe, especially if the gastrointestinal tract is the site. In any patient with recurrent gastrointestinal bleeding in the absence of an obvious cause, the diagnosis of hereditary haemorrhagic telangiectasia should be considered seriously.

In some instances, the condition may be associated with the presence of arteriovenous communications within the lung. Such patients may have:
- recurrent haemoptysis
- recurrent pulmonary infections
- secondary polycythaemia
- clubbing of fingers
- cyanosis

The frequency of pulmonary complications appears to rise with increasing age. In the absence of visible lesions on skin and mucous membranes, confirmation of the diagnosis of hereditary haemorrhagic telangiectasia is difficult and may be possible only with the aid of visceral angiography.

This disorder is associated with mutations in a gene located on the long arm of chromosome 9 which encodes a protein known as **endoglin**. Endoglin is a membrane glycoprotein which is associated with the receptor for transforming growth factor (TGF) β during binding of the ligand. It has been suggested that the abnormal endoglin is responsible for abnormal signalling and that this leads to abnormal remodelling of blood vessels.

Hereditary Conditions Affecting Supporting Connective Tissue of Blood Vessels

Abnormal bleeding may complicate several inherited connective tissue disorders. These include:
- various forms of the **Ehlers–Danlos syndrome**. The type most likely to be associated with serious bleeding is type IV.
- **osteogenesis imperfecta** (see pp 1036–1037)

- **pseudoxanthoma elasticum**, characterized by an abnormality of the elastic fibres of small blood vessels. The disorder is given this curious name because of the presence of yellowish streaks in the skin (e.g. of the neck and axillae). Microscopic examination of biopsy material shows fragmentation of elastic fibres. Defects in the retinae, so-called 'angioid streaks' are also a characteristic feature.

Acquired Disorders of Blood Vessels Leading to Abnormal Bleeding

These are shown in *Table 41.14*.

PLATELETS AND HAEMOSTASIS

Normal

The contribution of platelets to haemostasis is mediated via a number of steps:
- **adhesion of platelets to the underlying vessel wall**
- **release of pharmacologically active compounds**
- **aggregation (platelet to platelet) to form a plug**
- **provision of co-factors for clotting**

Adhesion

The platelet adheres to damaged endothelial cells or to exposed subendothelial components of the vessel wall. This is mediated through binding of vessel wall-derived ligands to glycoprotein receptors on the platelets. Collagen, which is exposed when a vessel is damaged, binds to a glycoprotein receptor (GP Ia) and von Willebrand's factor (**vWf**), a large multimeric glycoprotein synthesized by the endothelial cells, binds to GP Ib.

Thus either deficient production of vWF (as is seen in von Willebrand's disease) or an absent Ib receptor (Bernard–Soulier syndrome) must lead

---

Table 41.14 Acquired Causes of Abnormal Bleeding

Type	Examples
Autoimmune purpuras	Henoch–Schönlein's disease (see pp 409–410)
Bacterial infections	Meningococcal and other forms of septicaemia Leptospirosis Scarlet fever
Viral and rickettsial infections	Smallpox Rocky mountain spotted fever Typhus
Protozoal infections	Malaria
Acquired abnormalities of connective tissue	Scurvy Cushing's syndrome Senile purpura
Fat embolism	

to defective adhesion of platelets and will be reflected in an abnormally prolonged bleeding time.

Von Willebrand's disease is inherited for the most part as an autosomal dominant trait with variable penetrance. It is characterized by a prolonged bleeding time associated with defective platelet adhesion. vWf also carries Factor VIII in the plasma and prevents its premature degradation. Thus a patient with von Willebrand's disease will show depressed concentrations of Factor VIII in the plasma as well as defective platelet adhesion. The platelets themselves are normal, as are all their postadhesion functions.

Laboratory findings
- prolonged bleeding time
- low plasma concentrations of vWf
- low plasma concentrations of Factor VIII
- defective ristocetin-induced platelet aggregation. Ristocetin is an antibiotic, now withdrawn because it causes thrombocytopenia, which causes aggregation of normal platelets *in vitro*.

Release

Adherent platelets undergo a marked shape change releasing several preformed and newly formed molecules that may affect both the haemostatic process and the metabolism of the underlying vessel wall. Platelets contain two types of storage granules, **α-granules** and **dense bodies**, the latter having a dark electron-dense centre and a less dense peripheral zone. A wide range of active chemical species is released from these (see *Table 41.15*). The release reaction is usually triggered by exposure to collagen or thrombin.

In addition to the release of stored compounds, probably mediated via the activation of protein kinase C, **collagen and thrombin also initiate the release of arachidonate from the platelet membrane, the first step in the synthesis of prostaglandins, including the powerfully antiaggregatory prosta-** cyclin and the equally powerful proaggregatory thromboxane A_2.

Aggregation

This is the adhesion of platelets to other platelets, forming a mass of activated cells. It is accomplished by the formation of fibrinogen bridges between adjacent platelets. The fibrinogen molecule binds to heterodimeric receptors formed by a rearrangement of two platelet surface glycoproteins known as GP IIb and GP IIIa, which are members of the integrin family. This receptor also binds to vWf and may thus make a contribution to platelet adhesion as well. **The stimuli for aggregation are adenosine 5′-diphosphate (ADP) and thromboxane A_2.** These also activate more platelets with the release of more of these two compounds, so that there is a positive feedback effect and a rapid accumulation of platelets at sites of injury.

Provision of Co-factors for Clotting

Platelets also interact with clotting cascade proteins such as Factors V, VIII, IX and X. Once platelets have been activated, phospholipids, normally present on the internal layer of their plasma membranes, are 'flipped' to the external aspect of the cell, playing an important part in the activation of prothrombin by Factor Xa, and in the activation of Factor X by the Factor IXa–VIIa complex.

Normal Size and Number of Platelets

The normal platelet count is $150–450 \times 10^9$/litre. The cells are very small (1–2 μm in diameter) and circulate in the blood in the form of flat discs, not dissimilar to small Scotch pancakes. They are derived from multinucleate cells in the bone marrow – the megakaryocytes. As the megakaryocyte matures, its nuclei divide; when the number of nuclei reaches eight, membrane-bound 'packages' start to form within the cytoplasm and these, the platelets, are released into the circulation. Platelets newly released from the marrow migrate to the spleen, where they usually remain for 1–2 days; indeed, up to a third of the total number of circulating platelets are sequestered within the spleen at any one time.

Table 41.15 Chemical Species Released from Storage Granules

Granule type	Contents
α-Granule	Platelet-derived growth factor, thrombospondin, platelet factor 4, β-thromboglobulin, fibrinogen, fibronectin, vWf, etc.
Dense body	ATP, ADP, GDP, GTP, serotonin, calcium

ABNORMAL BLEEDING DUE TO PLATELET DISORDERS

Failures of normal platelet function are expressed clinically in the form of:
- purpura
- spontaneous haemorrhages
- prolonged bleeding after trauma, surgical or otherwise

Affected individuals will show a prolonged bleeding time.

Such failures may be associated with **quantitative**

abnormalities such as a significant **decrease** in platelet numbers (**thrombocytopenia**), or with **qualitative** defects in which one or more of the functions described previously is impaired. **The distinction between these two groups is made by counting the platelets.**

THROMBOCYTOPENIA

A significant decline in the number of circulating platelets (thrombocytopenia) (*Fig. 41.25*) may be due to:

- deficient production of platelets
- increased platelet destruction or consumption
- abnormal platelet distribution

Failure to Produce Platelets in Adequate Numbers

Decreased platelet production is most often associated with a failure to produce red and white cells as well. Marrow hypoplasia or aplasia may be idiopathic or may be secondary to some well-recognized cause such as the administration of cytotoxic drugs or following irradiation. Generalized bone marrow failure of this type may also occur in patients with leukaemia, with extensive infiltration of the marrow by malignant cells, and with human immunodeficiency virus infection.

Occasionally, the marrow depression may affect platelets in a selective fashion. This is most common as a side-effect of certain drugs such as phenylbutazone (now withdrawn from the market) and penicillamine, and also as a complication of certain viral infections.

A normal number of **megakaryocytes** in the marrow is no guarantee that **platelet** numbers will be normal because, in megaloblastic anaemia, there is ineffective thrombopoiesis despite normal or increased numbers of megakaryocytes.

Platelet production is mediated principally via the binding to megakaryocytes of a regulatory factor known as **thrombopoietin**. Megakarocytes express a growth factor receptor encoded by a gene known as *c-mpl* and **thrombopoietin is the ligand that binds to this receptor**. This *c-mpl* ligand not only causes an increase in megakaryocyte numbers but also promotes maturation of the megakaryocytes with consequent release of increased numbers of platelets. The discovery of the *c-mpl* ligand and the cloning of its gene is a major event, bringing with it the expectation that in the not too distant future an effective treatment will be available for thrombocytopenia.

Increased Destruction or Consumption of Platelets

These lead to stimulation of platelet production and, therefore, to an increase in the number and size of megakaryocytes in the bone marrow. **It is only when the rate of platelet destruction exceeds the capacity for their production that thrombocytopenia develops.** In certain circumstances, increased production matches platelet destruction and, thus, a new balance is established and the platelet count remains normal.

Immune-mediated Thrombocytopenia

Platelets may be destroyed in many cases by immune mechanisms. These may be drug induced, 'idiopathic' (see p 986), or associated with disorders such as systemic lupus erythematosus, various haemolytic anaemias,

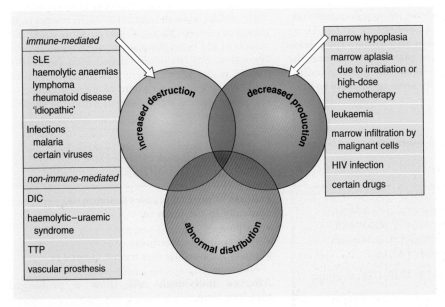

FIGURE 41.25 Causes of thrombocytopenia.

some lymphoreticular diseases, rheumatoid arthritis and hyperthyroidism.

Drug-related thrombocytopenia has been described in association with a number of compounds, including quinine, quinidine, heparin, para-aminosalicylate, sulphonamides, rifampicin and digoxin. The mechanism of platelet damage is the interaction between drug-elicited antibodies and drug bound to the platelet surface, the platelets being in a very real sense 'innocent bystanders'.

Thrombocytopenia may also occur in association with a number of viral and protozoal infections, one of the most important of which is malaria. In malaria the platelet destruction is mediated by the binding of immunoglobulin G antibodies to malarial antigens bound to the platelet surfaces, whereas in viral infections immune complexes are deposited on the platelet surface.

Non-immunological Platelet Destruction or Consumption

This group, defined by a **negative** criterion, the absence of immune-mediated platelet damage, includes:
- **thrombotic thrombocytopenic purpura (TTP)**
- **the haemolytic–uraemic syndrome**
- **disseminated intravascular coagulation (DIC)**
- **contact between flowing blood and artificial or abnormal vascular surfaces**: for example, prosthetic heart valves, synthetic vascular grafts and extracorporeal circulatory pumps

Thrombotic Thrombocytopenic Purpura

TTP is characterized by:
- **widespread thrombosis involving the microcirculation and causing ischaemic damage in many tissues with particular emphasis on the brain and kidney**, with clinical evidence of renal and neurological dysfunction. TTP has common features with the **haemolytic–uraemic syndrome in children** but, in the latter, lesions are confined to the kidney.
- **thrombocytopenia**
- **fever**
- **haemolytic anaemia**

Microscopic Features

Thrombi occur in terminal arterioles and capillaries, and consist of both platelets and fibrin. A highly characteristic feature is the presence of subendothelial hyaline deposits, often associated with endothelial cell proliferation.

Red cells are often damaged as a result of their interaction with the thrombi and this 'microangiopathy' leads to fragmentation haemolysis. The affected vessels show a diminished ability to produce the antiaggregatory compound, prostacyclin.

Aetiology and Pathogenesis

The cause of TTP is not known. The peak incidence is between 30 and 40 years and it is somewhat more common in females than in males. About 85% of cases occur in previously healthy individuals; the remainder are associated with such conditions as systemic lupus erythematosus, immune-mediated vasculitis, graft rejection and various infections (see also pp 695–696).

There is no convincing evidence that TTP is mediated by immune mechanisms. The plasma of patients contains a molecule that is proaggregatory for normal platelets, and some workers have suggested that TTP is due to absence of a normal inhibitor of this aggregating factor. Another suggestion is that, in TTP, the very large multimers of vWF synthesized by the endothelial cells are not cleaved in the plasma, and that their presence in circulating blood has a platelet-activating effect.

Natural History

Before the introduction of plasmapheresis and exchange blood transfusion, more than 80% of the patients died within 3 months and only 10% survived as long as 1 year. Now, about 80% of patients treated with exchange plasmapheresis survive the initial attack and many complete long-term remissions have been recorded.

Disseminated Intravascular Coagulation

DIC may be defined as widespread intravascular deposition of fibrin, associated with consumption of platelets and clotting factors. It is a pathophysiological state which has many causes, listed in *Table 41.16*.

In clinical terms the syndrome may be expressed as:
- abnormal bleeding
- a degree of shock greater than would be expected with this degree of blood loss
- signs of underperfusion of various vascular beds, most notably the kidney, brain, lung and liver

Pathogenesis of DIC

In terms of process, DIC (*Fig. 41.26*) may be the expression of:
- widespread endothelial damage in the microcirculation, as in endotoxaemia and severe burns
- widespread intravascular platelet aggregation
- activation of intrinsic pathways for clotting; for example, the cleavage of Factor XII (Hageman factor) by bacterial endotoxin
- the entry of procoagulant tissue extracts into the blood as, for example, in premature separation of the placenta (abruptio placentae), amniotic fluid embolism, massive trauma and association with mucin-secreting neoplasms. This leads to the formation of large amounts of thrombin.
- the stimulation of fibrinolysis

Activation of these processes is reflected in the laboratory findings shown in *Table 41.17*.

Table 41.16 Causes of DIC

Group of disorders	Examples
Obstetric complications	Amniotic fluid embolism Abruptio placentae Septic abortion Severe eclampsia
Infections	**Viral** (e.g. viral haemorrhagic fevers) **Bacterial** (e.g. meningococcal and Gram-negative septicaemia) **Rickettsial** (e.g. Rocky mountain spotted fever) **Fungal** (e.g. aspergillosis) **Protozoal** (e.g. malaria) **Metazoal** (e.g. heartworm disease in dogs)
Neoplasms	**Carcinoma** of the prostate, pancreas, lung, ovary, etc. Especially likely to be associated with mucin-secreting tumours Disseminated carcinoid, neuroblastoma, others
Blood disorders	Intravascular haemolysis Acute leukaemias Sickle cell disease Fresh water immersion
Vascular malformations associated with increased platelet activation	Giant haemangiomas (Kasabach–Merrit syndrome) Aneurysms Coarctation of the aorta Large prosthetic grafts
Vasculitides	Polyarteritis nodosa Systemic lupus erythematosus
Hypoxia and underperfusion	Myocardial infarction Acute respiratory distress syndrome Various forms of shock
Massive tissue injury	Large traumatic injuries and burns Extensive surgical procedures Fat embolism
Miscellaneous	Acute pancreatitis Hypothermia Graft versus host disease Bites of certain venomous snakes

DIC is a serious state with a reported mortality rate of 54–68%. Because small thrombi are repeatedly being formed and then lysed, it is not always easy to find the thrombi in microscopic examination of post-mortem material, and the clinical disturbances described are often out of proportion to the pathological lesions seen at post-mortem examination. Although many tissues can be involved, the kidney is most frequently affected. Renal lesions vary from patchy tubular necrosis to massive cortical necrosis.

Contact Between Blood and an Abnormal Surface

Even more than red cells, platelets are likely to be damaged by interactions with 'unphysiological' surfaces. The association between atherosclerotic plaques in which injury has occurred to the plaque 'cap' and a markedly increased risk of thrombosis is well known (see pp 335–336).

Modern practice is increasingly associated with the implantation of foreign material within the vascular

Table 41.17 Laboratory Findings in DIC

Laboratory findings	Process involved
Low platelet count	Adhesion of platelets to damaged endothelial surfaces Intravascular platelet aggregation
Low plasma fibrinogen concentration	Consumption of fibrinogen due to increase in thrombin release
Thrombin time prolonged Prothrombin time prolonged Activated partial thromboplastin time prolonged	Consumption of procoagulant factors
Degradation products of fibrin and fibrinogen present in serum and urine	Activation of fibrinolytic system
Fibrin monomer complexes present in blood	Release of thrombin causes formation of fibrin monomers in blood, which form complexes with fibrinogen
Evidence of 'microangiopathy' in the form of haemolysis and fragmented red cells (**schistocytes**) in about 50% of patients	Red cell damage as result of interaction with thrombi

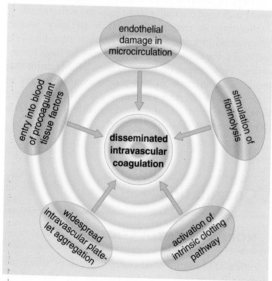

FIGURE 41.26 *Pathogenetic factors in disseminated intravascular coagulation.*

tree, for example prosthetic heart valves, vascular grafts, stents and indwelling catheters. It has not yet been possible to make these from non-thrombogenic materials and varying degrees of platelet activation and consumption occur. In most cases the increased platelet consumption is compensated for by increased platelet production, and thrombocytopenia does not occur in the majority of cases, although it certainly can do so.

ABNORMAL BLEEDING ASSOCIATED WITH QUALITATIVE DISORDERS OF PLATELETS

Hereditary Disorders
- affect only the function of platelets without affecting their number
- affect both the function and, to a limited extent, the number of platelets
- involve cells and tissues other than platelets

Thrombasthenia (Glanzmann's disease)
The defining criteria of this disease, which affects only platelet function, are:
- deficiency in ADP-mediated platelet aggregation
- deficient clot retraction

These deficiencies arise as a result of GP IIb and IIIa surface glycoproteins being either deficient or abnormal as a result of mutation. As a result platelet activation is not followed by rearrangement of these glycoproteins to form the heterodimer to which fibrinogen binds. Thus normal platelet aggregation cannot occur.

Storage Pool Disease
This term defines two disorders in which there is a deficiency either of **α-granules or dense bodies**. The latter situation is more common and is known as δ-storage pool disease. Platelets fail to release adequate amounts of dense granule contents, most notably ADP, and thus the initial stages of aggregation are not amplified by ADP and stable platelet plugs cannot be

formed. This form of storage pool disease may be associated with albinism and an accumulation of ceroid pigment within macrophages; this triad, the **Hermansky–Pudlak syndrome**, is inherited in an autosomal recessive fashion.

A rarer form of storage pool disease is known as the **grey platelet syndrome**, characterized by a deficiency of α-granules. The platelets are enlarged and there may be mild thrombocytopenia. The bleeding time is prolonged, although severe bleeding is not seen usually, and platelet aggregation is usually defective.

Bernard–Soulier Syndrome

This is a rare disorder characterized by:
- giant platelets
- a mild degree of thrombocytopenia
- moderate to severe bleeding expressed in the form of epistaxis, easy bruising and menorrhagia

The platelets show a lack of the surface glycoprotein GP Ib. As a result, the normal interaction between this receptor and vWf does not take place and the crucial early adhesion phase in the formation of a platelet plug is inhibited. The platelet is effectively 'deaf' to the signals sent out by the damaged vascular surface.

Hereditary Afibrinogenaemia

The absence of the substrate of the clotting system is unusual in terms of clotting disorders in that it is expressed in the form of prolonged bleeding time (which normally suggests platelet dysfunction). This is because fibrinogen is required for ADP-induced aggregation of platelets, as described in an earlier section of this chapter.

Acquired Disorders of Platelet Function

Drug-related Changes in Platelet Behaviour

Compounds affecting platelets include a wide range of drugs and also certain substances in the diet, in particular oily fish which contain large amounts of eicosapentaenoic acid. In patients who are uraemic, thrombocytopenic or who have a disturbance of clotting, the administration of drugs affecting platelet function exposes them to the risk of serious bleeding.

One of the most common agents to be implicated in this way is **aspirin**. Aspirin interferes with **cyclo-oxygenase** by acetylation with a resulting deficiency in the production of the cyclo-oxygenase-catalysed metabolic products of arachidonic acid, in particular thromboxane A_2, although prostaglandin production including that of prostaglandin I_2 is also affected but to a lesser degree. Thus, both the aggregation of platelets by collagen and the normal secondary wave of aggregation are inhibited. Because of this disproportionate effect on thromboxane A_2 synthesis, low-dose aspirin therapy is recommended for individuals who have had an episode of coronary thrombosis or who are at high risk of

having one. The effect of aspirin on platelet cyclo-oxygenase is irreversible and operates for the whole lifespan of the affected platelet cohort (7–10 days).

Systemic Disorders Affecting Platelets

Paraproteinaemia

Abnormal bleeding may significantly complicate paraproteinaemias, especially if hyperglobulinaemia is present. The cause of the abnormal bleeding is complicated but there is strong evidence that platelet dysfunction plays a part. Various aspects of platelet activity are disturbed, possibly due to coating of platelet surface membranes with abnormal proteins.

Uraemia

Renal failure from whatever cause may be complicated by abnormal bleeding. The pathogenesis of the bleeding diathesis is complicated and not understood fully. There is, however, strong evidence that platelet dysfunction plays a part, the principal platelet defect being related to the release phase. Abnormalities in prostaglandin production in the form of decreased synthesis have been demonstrated. On the other hand, the rate of production of prostacyclin (prostaglandin I_2) from vessel wall segments of uraemic patients is increased.

Bleeding in these patients may be very severe. Widespread bruising and slow gastrointestinal bleeding are seen quite commonly and there may be large haemorrhages into serous cavities and muscles. Measures that produce an increase in the plasma concentrations of both Factor VIIIc and vWF may shorten the bleeding time and help control the bleeding, although why this should be is not clear.

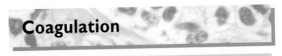

Coagulation

NORMAL COAGULATION

Clotting of blood involves many steps, all of which are **directed towards the formation of thrombin. This cleaves its substrate fibrinogen to produce fibrin, which becomes polymerized and cross-linked to form the basic structure of a clot.**

Basically, coagulation of the blood is a cascade process in which the participant molecules (see *Table 41.18*) act as both substrates and, following their cleavage, as active enzymes. In this model, inactive precursors of blood clotting factors (zymogens) become activated by a process of strictly controlled proteolysis and, with each step, there is a considerable degree of amplification. Thus 1 mol of activated Factor XI may ultimately be responsible for the generation of 2×10^8 mol of fibrin.

Table 41.18 The Clotting Factors

Factor	Name	Cell of origin	Chromosome
I	Fibrinogen	Liver cell	4
II*	Prothrombin	Liver cell	11
III	Tissue factor	Many types	1
IV	Calcium		
V	Labile factor	Liver cell; megakaryocyte	1
VII*	Proconvertin	Liver cell	13
VIII	Antihaemophilic factor	Liver cell	X
	von Willebrand factor	Endothelial cell; megakaryocyte	12
IX*	Christmas factor	Liver cell	X
X*	Stuart–Prower factor	Liver cell	13
XI*	Plasma thromboplastin antecedent	Liver cell	4
XII*	Hageman factor	Liver cell	5
XIII	Fibrin-stabilizing factor	Liver cell	1 and 6

* Serine protease whose activity depends on the presence of serine at the active centre.

Fibrinogen

Fibrinogen is unusual in that each of its three polypeptide chains is coded for by a separate gene, all three of which are located on chromosome 4. Assembly of the three polypeptides occurs in the endoplasmic reticulum of the liver cells.

Clotting Factors that are Dependent on Vitamin K

Six factors, which either take part in the clotting cascade or regulate it, require the presence of vitamin K in order to be activated. They are:

- Factor II (prothrombin)
- Factor VII
- Factor IX
- Factor X
- Protein C
- Protein S

Vitamin K is an 'antibleeding' factor found in several vegetable oils and leafy plants, and also synthesized by certain microorganisms including the normal gut flora.

It exerts its effect by carboxylating certain glutamic acid residues in the clotting factors listed above, activating the enzyme **γ-glutamyl carboxylase**. The modified glutamic acid residues (Gla) bind calcium ions tightly, and these bound calcium ions enable the clotting factors to bind to exposed phospholipid on platelet membranes. Mutations in the genes coding for the vitamin K-dependent clotting factors may affect the Gla regions, leading to incompletely carboxylated forms of the clotting factors. These show decreased function, as for example in the case of Factor IX, where such mutations have caused haemophilia B.

Factors V and VIII

These two proteins, believed to be evolutionary products of a common ancestral gene, act as co-factors for the serine protease vitamin K-dependent factors. Both contain A domains that show homology with caeruloplasmin and that bind calcium, and both have C domains that are homologous with certain lectins and that bind to surface phospholipid on activated platelets. Factor VIII also has a large B domain, the function of which is not known; certainly its absence in genetically engineered Factor VIII does not interfere with the normal procoagulant function.

In the liver cell, Factor VIII undergoes proteolysis into a heavy and a light chain. To exert a procoagulant effect, these chains must be activated; this is carried out by thrombin. Activated Factor VIII takes part in the assembly of Factor IX and calcium close to Factor X. This promotes the activation of Factor X, which is catalysed by activated Factor IX.

Factor V is also activated by thrombin. Its role is to assemble Factor Xa and calcium on platelets so as to promote the conversion of prothrombin to thrombin.

CLOTTING PATHWAYS

In the classical model of coagulation there are two pathways of activation which meet to form a common pathway (see Chapter 18). These are:

1) **the intrinsic pathway** (which is triggered by contact-mediated activation of **Factor XII (Hageman factor)**. In the vascular system, activation of Factor XII is likely to be brought about by exposure of collagen and basement membranes.

   Factor XII, once activated (Factor XIIa), can cleave **Factor XI**. It is not clear how important this first part of the intrinsic pathway is in real life, and it is likely that Factor XI can be cleaved in other ways, most notably by contact with platelets.

The next step is the cleavage of **Factor IX** by activated Factor XI. The activated Factor IX, in conjunction with the co-factor **Factor VIII and calcium**, cleaves **Factor X**. Activation of Factor VIII *in vivo* is the result of cleavage by thrombin. 2) **the extrinsic pathway**, which is triggered by the release of tissue factor which binds to **Factor VII** and, in some hitherto undetermined manner, activates it. The activated Factor VII can activate **Factor X** directly, thus leading to the cleavage of prothrombin. It is now known that **activated Factor VII also activates Factor IX**, which promotes more activation of Factor X. Thus, ultimately, tissue factor makes its effect via both intrinsic and extrinsic pathways. It is believed that the chief effect of activated Factor VII *in vivo* is the activation of Factor IX rather than the direct activation of Factor X. 3) **The common pathway** starts with the assembly of activated Factor X on the platelet phospholipid (**platelet factor 3**) together with **calcium** ions and the co-factor **Factor V**. This complex constitutes a **prothrombinase**, which cleaves **prothrombin** with the formation of **thrombin**. The most obvious function of thrombin is to cleave **fibrinogen**, resulting in the formation of monomeric fibrin. The thrombin cleaves four arginyl–glycine bonds in the fibrinogen with the release of fibrinopeptides A and B. The fibrin monomers then assemble into polymers, which are stabilized by Factor XIII, which is activated by thrombin and calcium.

A model of coagulation which has been recently proposed takes account of all these observations:

- **Clotting is triggered by the action of tissue factor and Factor VII on Factors X and IX, and a small amount of thrombin is generated. This thrombin activates platelets and, through a feedback mechanism, other clotting factors. In this way there is upregulation of the formation of activated X, thrombin and fibrin.**

Commonly Used Tests for Defective Coagulation

Defects in haemostasis are identified by prolongation of the time taken for either *in vivo* haemostasis (**bleeding time**) or **coagulation of plasma** *in vitro* (*Table 41.19*).

Control of Blood Coagulation

Coagulation is a set of processes in which a marked degree of amplification takes place. If this is not to get out of hand and lead to the formation of haemostatic plugs which might compromise the integrity of the vessel lumen, some balancing forces are clearly required. These include:

1) **local processes**, most notably:
- the flow of blood which leads to **dilution of clotting factors** that have been activated at the site of vessel wall injury or abnormality
- **rapid binding of thrombin by fibrin** which has already polymerized at the site of the vessel wall injury. This is referred to as antithrombin I activity, a somewhat confusing term since there is no such molecule as antithrombin I.
2) **Substances that inhibit coagulation:**
- **antithrombin III (AT III).** This plasma protein inactivates serine proteases by forming inert complexes with them which are then cleared from the blood by liver cells. AT III also inactivates activated Factors X, IX and kallikrein, and can be regarded as a broad-spectrum antiprotease.
- **heparin co-factor II.** This is a plasma protein activated by heparin and which shows some degree of homology with AT III. It is a much weaker inhibitor of activated Factor X than AT III.

Table 41.19 Tests for Defective Coagulation

Test	Defect
Bleeding time	A **defect in platelet function** or, rarely, afibrinogenaemia
Prothrombin time (normal 10–14 s)	Deficiency or inhibition of Factors **V, VII, X, II, fibrinogen** Indicates defect in **extrinsic or common pathway**
Activated partial thromboplastin time (normal 30–40 s)	Deficiency or inhibition of Factors **XII, IX, VIII, X, V, II and fibrinogen** Indicates defect in **intrinsic and/or common pathways**. Particularly sensitive for deficiencies in Factors VII and IX
Thrombin clotting time (normal 14–16 s)	A lack of fibrinogen or an inhibitor of thrombin. Useful in differential diagnosis of disseminated intravascular coagulation

- **the protein C–S system.** Protein C acts together with a number of other factors to inhibit coagulation at the interface of the blood and endothelial surface. To be activated protein C requires **thrombin**, a transmembrane protein synthesized by and expressed on the surface of endothelial cells called **thrombomodulin, calcium ions** and **protein S**.

The endothelium-derived thrombomodulin rapidly binds thrombin. This thrombomodulin–thrombin complex then 'captures' protein C. The bound protein C is then activated and binds to protein S on endothelial cells or on platelet surfaces. In this complex, the activated protein C inactivates activated Factors V and VIII, and thus inhibits the generation of more thrombin. Activated protein C also promotes fibrinolysis by splitting tissue plasminogen activator (tPA) from plasminogen activator inhibitor (PAI) 1.

Fibrinolysis

Once fibrin has been formed and polymerized, it can be removed only by the process of fibrinolysis. This results from the conversion of an inert proenzyme in the blood (plasminogen) to an active proteolytic form (plasmin).

Plasminogen is a β globulin with a molecular weight of 88 000. It is a single polypeptide chain with a rather curious structure in that it contains five loop-like structures (**kringles**). These kringle domains are homologous with sequences in the plasminogen activators and **urokinase**, and also with sequences in prothrombin.

Plasminogen Activators

Tissue Plasminogen Activator

tPA is probably the most important activator of the fibrinolytic system. It is synthesized in endothelium, its concentration being greatest in veins and renal blood vessels.

tPA is also secreted by macrophages and by certain malignant cells. Its release from endothelium is stimulated by trauma, exercise, emotional stress, stasis, ischaemia, thrombin, bacterial toxin and many other factors.

tPA binds to fibrin, which is fortunate because cleavage of plasminogen to plasmin is likely, as a result, to be confined to region of the haemostatic plug.

Urokinase

This activator was originally isolated from human urine but can now be prepared from endothelium, kidney cells and certain tumour cells.

Endothelium, Platelets and Coagulation

From the foregoing sections on platelet–vessel wall interactions and the processes involved in coagulation, it is seen that products synthesized by endothelial cells make a significant contribution to both these functional areas. Some of these products and their physiological roles are summarized in *Table 41.20*.

INHERITED DISORDERS OF COAGULATION

Absence or abnormality of a single plasma protein may cause disorders of coagulation; such deficiencies have been described in respect of each of the clotting factors. None is common. More than 90% of inherited disorders associated with abnormal bleeding fall into three classes:

- haemophilia A
- haemophilia B
- von Willebrand's disease (see pp 912–913)

Haemophilia A

This disorder causes a **severe bleeding tendency in the male children** of certain families.

Table 41.20 Effects of Endothelium-derived Products on Coagulation

Product	Effect
Nitric oxide	Inhibits platelet activation
Prostaglandin I$_2$ (prostacyclin)	Inhibits platelet aggregation
Tissue factor	Triggers clotting
von Willebrand factor	Mediates platelet adhesion
Antithrombin III	Inhibits clotting
tPA	Cleaves plasminogen and thus triggers fibrinolysis
PAI-1	Binds to tPA and inhibits its action
Thrombomodulin	Binds thrombin and leads to activation of protein C, which inactivates Factors Va and VIIIa

The disorder, inherited in an **X-linked recessive** fashion, is the expression of either a deficiency or an abnormality of Factor VIII. In males who lack a normal allele for Factor VIII, the genetic abnormality will manifest clinically. Affected males cannot transmit the disorder to their sons but all their daughters will be asymptomatic carriers, as they usually inherit a normal allele from their mothers. However, a substantial proportion of the affected individuals (about one-third) have no family history. In these cases haemophilia must be due to a spontaneous somatic mutation of the gene coding for Factor VIII. This, presumably, is why the disease has not died out. Haemophilia can occur in females but is rare. The most common cause for this is inactivation of their normal X chromosome which may occur at an abnormally early stage of embryogenesis. Another cause is the rare mating of an affected male with a carrier female and, in some instances, haemophilia has been reported in females as the result of a newly mutated gene.

Clinical severity depends on the degree of reduction below the normal plasma concentration of Factor VIII, as shown in *Table 41.21.*

The principal sites of bleeding are the:

- **joints**. Bleeding into the joints (haemarthrosis) is one of the commonest and potentially most crippling manifestations of haemophilia. The bleeding appears often to be unrelated to trauma, although it is possible that some trivial degree of trauma has occurred. The haemorrhage may occur into the joint space or into the neighbouring bone or periarticular soft tissues. Haemorrhage into joints is often recurrent, and the end result is a joint lined

by swollen and thickened synovium in which many vascularized folds and villi are present.

- **muscles**
- **mouth, gums and tongue.** Bleeding after tooth extractions and tonsillectomy may be a serious hazard to the affected individuals.
- **urinary tract**
- **brain**

Tragically, the most common cause of death currently in haemophiliacs is acquired immune deficiency syndrome (AIDS). Some of the concentrates used to treat haemophiliac patients were contaminated with the human immunodeficiency virus (HIV) and it is said that up to 50% of haemophiliacs in the USA and western Europe have antibodies to HIV in their plasma.

Laboratory Findings

These depend on the severity of the Factor VIII deficiency. In severe cases:

- activated partial thromboplastin time is prolonged
- whole blood clotting time may be prolonged
- plasma concentrations of Factor VIIIc are reduced
- bleeding time is normal
- von Willebrand factor concentrations are normal
- Factor IX concentration in plasma is normal

The presence of an abnormal allele on chromosome X can be detected using molecular probes to analyse DNA obtained from chorionic biopsies taken at about 8–10 weeks' gestation. Low levels of Factor VIIIc in affected fetuses can also be measured in blood taken from the umbilical vein at about 18–20 weeks' gestation. Based in these findings, a rational decision can be reached as to whether a fetus should be aborted or not.

Haemophilia B (Christmas Disease, Factor IX Deficiency)

Haemophilia B has clinical features similar to those seen in haemophilia A and a similar inheritance pattern. This is not surprising because the disease is the expression of a deficiency in Factor IX, coded for by a gene near the tip of the long arm of the X chromosome.

Factor XI Deficiency

Deficiency of Factor XI covers a clinical spectrum ranging from the complete absence of any symptoms to trauma-related haemorrhage requiring multiple blood transfusions. Spontaneous bleeding, in contrast to what is seen in haemophilia A and B, rarely occurs.

The deficiency is inherited in an **autosomal recessive** pattern and is relatively common amongst Ashkenazi Jews, the frequency of homozygotes being about 1 in 190. Three independent point mutations have been identified in the gene coding for Factor XI; two of these account for the majority of cases of severe bleeding.

Table 41.21 Clinical Effects of Factor VIII Deficiency

Concentration of Factor VIII	Clinical effect
> 50% of normal	No abnormal bleeding
20–50% of normal	Prolonged bleeding after severe injury or surgery
5–20% of normal	Prolonged bleeding after minor injury or surgery
2–5% of normal	Prolonged injury after trivial injury or surgery; occasional spontaneous bleeding
< 2% of normal	Spontaneous bleeding into joints and muscles; severe bleeding after injury or surgery; increased risk of spontaneous intracerebral bleeding

ACQUIRED DISORDERS OF COAGULATION

Acquired disturbances of coagulation may complicate many diseases (*Table 41.22*). Unlike the inherited disorders, which are expressions of a deficiency in a single clotting factor, the acquired disorders are usually much more complicated and involve several of the contributors to normal haemostasis including platelets. On the whole, bleeding in these hypocoagulable states tends to be less severe than in the hereditary diseases discussed above.

Deficiencies of Vitamin K-dependent Factors

In the absence of vitamin K, carboxylation of Gla regions of vitamin K-dependent factors does not occur and, although the plasma concentration of these coagulation factors is normal, their functions are deficient.

Vitamin K deficiency may occur in both neonatal and adult life. In the former it finds clinical expression in **haemorrhagic disease of the newborn**, which may be due to a combination of factors:

- **immaturity of the liver cells**, thus producing lower levels than normal of Factors II, VII, IX and X
- **delayed colonization of the gut by vitamin K-producing bacteria**

The disorder is now rare because 1 mg vitamin K is given prophylactically to most newborn babies.

Deficiencies of active vitamin K–dependent clotting factors may also be seen in patients with malabsorption due to any cause and in those with biliary obstruction; the deficiency is due to an absence of bile salts in the gut.

Defects in the Clotting Process may be due to the Presence of Pathological Inhibitors of Coagulation in the Plasma

Several 'physiological' inhibitors of coagulation exist which regulate blood clotting. In addition, however, in the plasma of certain individuals there are 'pathological' factors that can inhibit blood coagulation. Most of these are antibodies, such antibodies having been found in relation to Factors VIII, V, IX, XIII and von Willebrand factor.

Antibodies to Factor VIII have been identified in 5–21% of patients with haemophilia A. In these patients the antibodies are probably elicited as a result of the administration of Factor VIII, although the details of this are far from clear.

These antibodies may occur also, for reasons that are not known, in elderly individuals with no obvious associated illness, in the postpartum state (rare), or in patients with chronic inflammatory diseases mediated by immune mechanisms, such as rheumatoid arthritis. Bleeding in these patients may be severe.

Table 41.22 Acquired Disorders Involving Disturbances of Coagulation

Clotting Factor Deficiencies	Causes
Deficiencies of vitamin K–dependent clotting factors	Haemorrhagic disease of the newborn
	Biliary tract obstruction
	Malabsorption of vitamin K
	Nutritional deficiency
	Certain drugs:
	• antagonists of vitamin K (coumarins)
	• broad-spectrum antibiotics that alter gut flora
	• cholestyramine
Liver disease	Deficient or aberrant synthesis of clotting factors
	Impaired clearance of activated clotting factors or plasminogen activator
	Accelerated destruction of clotting factors
Accelerated destruction of clotting factors	Diffuse intravascular coagulation
Presence of pathological inhibitors of clotting	Specific inhibitors such as antibodies reacting with Factor VIII
	Inhibitors of the 'lupus type'
Miscellaneous	After massive transfusion
	After bypass surgery
	Many others
	Overdosage with oral anticoagulants

The 'lupus' anticoagulants are immunoglobulins given this name because they were originally discovered in patients with systemic lupus erythematosus (SLE). It is now known that they can occur in many disparate conditions ranging from prostatic hypertrophy to complications of certain drugs including procainamide, penicillin and chlorpromazine. **Most lupus anticoagulants are believed to be anticardiolipin antibodies** such as are responsible for false-positive serological test results for syphilis in SLE and other connective tissue disorders.

Lupus anticoagulants do not bind to or inhibit any **single** clotting factor. Instead they inhibit a number of steps in both the intrinsic and common pathways, particularly steps that are dependent on phospholipid as, for example, the generation of prothrombinase. Curiously their presence is more likely to be associated with a tendency to thrombosis rather than bleeding; the thrombosis is probably due to the reaction between the antibodies and phospholipid in the plasma membrane of endothelial cells. The commonest site for such thrombi to occur is in the deep veins of the leg, but any part of the vascular system may be affected.

The Hypercoagulable State

The mirror image of abnormal bleeding is an increased risk of thrombosis because of an inherited abnormality or acquired defect.

Definition
A hypercoagulable state is one in which **the normal haemostatic equilibrium is tilted in such a way that thrombosis is favoured.** This may result from the operation of a number of different mechanisms operating singly or in combination.

When the cause of thrombosis is being considered, it is helpful to use Virchow's triad as the frame of reference:
1) **Abnormalities of the blood vessel wall.** These may be expressed, in part, as abnormalities of the blood constituents, as endothelium in atherosclerotic areas will synthesize and secrete less antiaggregatory nitric oxide and prostacyclin than normal endothelium.
2) **Abnormalities in the blood constituents.** These may be due to the absence of a factor such as antithrombin (AT) III, a natural regulator of haemostasis, the presence of an endothelium-damaging molecule not normally present in large amounts, such as homocystine, or a disturbance in the concentration of the normal substrate of the

prothrombinase generated as the final active species in the clotting pathway.
3) **Abnormalities in the blood flow.** These include haemodynamic parameters such as stasis and loss of normal laminar flow patterns.

In terms of the processes involved, an increased risk of thrombosis may therefore be due to:
- **upregulation of platelet–vessel wall interactions.** The most important cause of this is atherosclerosis associated with superficial or deep injury to the plaque cap. The presence of prosthetic heart valves or synthetic grafts also increases platelet reactions with the underlying vascular surface. Thrombosis may also be the consequence of endothelial damage in the rare inherited disorder of metabolism, homocystinaemia.
- **an increase**, which may be general, or, much more frequently, local, **in procoagulant factors**, most notably fibrinogen and Factor VII.
- **a decrease in natural anticoagulant factors** such as antithrombin III or the protein C–S–thrombomodulin system
- **increased viscosity of the blood** as may occur in individuals with raised levels of fibrinogen in the blood or as a result of grossly increased plasma concentrations of immunoglobulins such as may be seen in plasma cell dyscrasias like multiple myeloma. Similar increases in viscosity are seen in patients with polycythaemia.
- **the presence of anticardiolipin antibodies** (lupus anticoagulants)
- **the presence of stasis** in the venous circulation, especially when associated with surgical trauma
- **the release into the blood of procoagulant compounds from malignant tumours** especially adenocarcinomas
- **an increase in the platelet count** (thrombocytosis)
- **an increase in platelet adhesiveness and aggregatability**

Some of these have been discussed already in other sections and will not be considered further here.

INHERITED DISORDERS THAT INCREASE THE RISK OF THROMBOSIS

Abnormalities of Antithrombin III
This disorder is inherited in an autosomal dominant fashion. The majority of affected individuals are heterozygotes whose plasma, therefore, contains 50% of the normal concentration of functional AT III. In patients with a deficiency of normal AT III, there is an increase in the concentration of prothrombin fragments. This gives support to the view that the coagulation system is in a constant state of very low-grade activation, normally regulated and restrained by AT III.

AT III deficiency causes recurrent episodes of mainly venous thrombosis. As is usual with venous thrombi, the leg veins are most frequently affected and complicating pulmonary emboli are common. In women the thrombi are often seen for the first time during pregnancy or in association with the taking of oral contraceptives. In men there is often a history of antecedent injury or surgery. With increasing age, the frequency of the episodes of thrombosis increases.

Protein C deficiency

Protein C deficiency is an autosomal dominant disorder associated with a life-long increased risk of thrombosis. It occurs in two forms. In the first, the **amount** of the protein in the plasma is decreased; the functional deficit is proportional to the reduction of the protein concentration. In the second form, the amount of protein C in the plasma is normal but there is **a gross functional defect**. Levels below 65% of normal are usually associated with an increased incidence of thrombosis.

Clinically affected heterozygotes suffer from thrombosis in the deep leg veins and also have episodes of superficial thrombophlebitis.

Rarely the disorder may occur in a homozygous form. In this case the affected children have a 'devastating thromboembolic diathesis starting in infancy' and involving the renal and mesenteric veins and dural sinuses. The clinical picture may be complicated by purpura fulminans, in which there are widely distributed skin haemorrhages associated with the presence of fibrin plugs occluding small skin vessels.

Protein S deficiency

This disorder presents with much the same clinical picture as protein C deficiency. It is also inherited as an autosomal dominant trait.

Deficiencies in both proteins C and S can occur in association with acquired diseases. Both of these molecules are dependent on vitamin K for their activation and may thus be functionally impaired in patients with vitamin K deficiency from any cause.

Protein C Resistance

A syndrome characterized by recurrent, familial, venous thrombosis has been recognized, in which all the anticoagulant factors are present in normal concentration but **there is abnormal resistance to the normal biological effect of activated protein C**. This phenomenon has been found by one group of workers in about a third of patients referred for evaluation of venous thromboembolism. The abnormality is inherited in an autosomal dominant fashion and confers a sevenfold increase in the risk of developing venous thrombosis. The existence of this disorder implies that there must be a dysfunctional co-factor for activated protein C. This co-factor has been identified as Factor V, which now seems to have an anticoagulant as well as a procoagulant role.

Recently a mutation has been identified in the gene encoding Factor V which correlates with the presence of resistance to activated protein C. It is a single point mutation at nucleotide position 1691, at which there is a G→A substitution. In Holland where this mutation (Factor V Leiden) was identified, the frequency in the population appears to be about 2%, at least tenfold higher than that of all other genetic risk factors for thrombosis together. The combination of this mutation with other risk factors for thrombosis may be very powerful; for example, women with mutated Factor V who take oral contraceptives have a 30-fold increased risk of thrombosis.

Inherited Disorders Affecting the Fibrinolytic Pathways

These are rare and include:
- dysfibrinogenaemia
- dysplasminogenaemia
- defective release of plasminogen activator from the vessel wall

Raised Plasma Fibrinogen and Factor VII$_c$ Concentrations

The Northwick Park Heart Study, a prospective study relating certain factors to coronary heart disease risk, has shown a strong positive association between plasma concentrations of fibrinogen and Factor VII$_c$ and the risk of a first episode of coronary heart disease.

Fibrinogen levels increase with:
- increasing age
- obesity
- the use of oral contraceptives
- the onset of the menopause
- the presence of diabetes
- cigarette smoking

With the exception of smoking, the same factors are associated with increased plasma levels of Factor VII$_c$. In addition, there is a positive association between a diet high in fat, leading to high plasma cholesterol concentrations, and raised plasma levels of Factor VII$_c$. Whether high plasma concentrations of fibrinogen are entirely 'acquired' or whether there is a genetic component is still not known.

ACQUIRED DISORDERS AND ENVIRONMENTAL FACTORS THAT INCREASE THE RISK OF THROMBOSIS

Stasis

Stasis, resulting from impaired venous return, has long been recognized as a major risk factor for venous thrombosis. Prolonged sitting, as occurs in long flights, is associated with an increased risk of leg vein thrombosis, and patients with acute hemiplegia have a four- to ninefold increase in the risk of deep vein thrombosis in the paralysed limb compared with the unaffected limb.

Following surgery, stasis is combined with other risk factors such as old age and obesity, the entry into the circulation of tissue factor and, possibly, endothelial injury. The type of surgery is not without influence on this risk: the highest risk of postoperative venous thrombosis is associated with orthopaedic surgery on the lower limb.

Oral Contraceptives

The introduction of oral contraceptives was followed by the recognition that both arterial and venous thrombosis might complicate their use. Users of 'the pill' had a three- to fivefold increase in the risk of developing a myocardial infarct or stroke, and oral contraceptives appeared to act synergistically with other known risk factors such as cigarette smoking or diabetes mellitus.

This increased risk of thromboembolic disease correlates with the amount of oestrogen in the compound. A decrease in the oestrogen content has been associated with a decrease, but not with abolition, of the increased risk of thrombosis. Contraceptives raise the plasma concentrations of fibrinogen and vitamin K-dependent clotting factors by about 10–20% and there is also a decrease in plasma AT III levels. Factor XII and prekallikrein levels increase, causing an increased contact factor-mediated fibrinolysis potential.

Malignancy

In addition to disseminated intravascular coagulation (see pp 915–916), patients with certain types of malignancy are at increased risk of thromboembolic disease.

It appears that mucin-secreting adenocarcinomas, especially carcinoma of the pancreas, are a risk factor for recurrent episodes of venous thrombosis. There is some evidence that venous thrombosis occurring for no very obvious cause may be followed by the presentation of one of these tumours. Malignant cells may release tissue thromboplastin and there is also evidence that mucins released from certain adenocarcinomas, and proteases released from other tumours, can directly activate Factor X without the extrinsic clotting pathway being involved.

The Nephrotic Syndrome

Venous thrombosis, particularly that involving the renal vein, commonly complicates the nephrotic syndrome (average incidence 35%). Arterial thrombosis has also been recorded as an association but is much rarer.

The cause is not yet clear, although quantitative changes in some clotting and anticlotting factors have been noted. One of the most striking of these is a decline in the plasma concentration of AT III, the levels of which fall proportionally with the decline in serum albumin concentration.

Neoplastic Disorders of White Blood Cells: The Leukaemias

Definition

The leukaemias are neoplastic disorders of the white blood cells. All of them show abnormal monoclonal white cells in the bone marrow. These may replace much of the bone marrow and frequently appear in the circulating blood, where they can be recognized by their morphological abnormalities in stained blood films.

Leukaemias may be defined also in developmental terms as **the uncontrolled proliferation of haemopoietic cells lacking the capacity to differentiate normally to mature blood cells.**

Some haematological disorders are not strictly leukaemias because they display only part of the full leukaemic phenotype – either growth expansion (*myeloproliferative syndromes*) or differentiation block (*myelodysplasia*), yet both of these can proceed to acute leukaemia (*Fig. 41.27*).

Epidemiology

In epidemiological terms, haematological neoplasms in general are common, constituting 7% of male and 6%

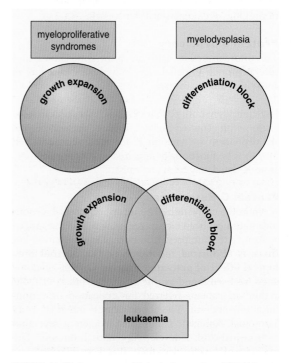

FIGURE 41.27 In contrast with both the myeloproliferative disorders and myelodysplasia, leukaemia involves both a growth expansion and a differentiation block.

of female malignancies. This pales into insignificance when contrasted with the situation in childhood. **Acute lymphoblastic leukaemia (ALL) is the commonest malignant disease in childhood, accounting for almost one-third of all cases of malignancy in this age group.**

Classification

The leukaemias are divided into two major groups: **acute and chronic**. These are not defined in terms of duration but rather **in terms of the proportion of immature or 'blast' cells in the cell population of the marrow.**

Thus acute leukaemias are separated from the chronic forms by the fact that, in the former, more than 50% of the bone marrow cells consist of blast cells. In both acute and chronic leukaemias, further subdivision depends on the cell lineages involved and the degree of differentiation of the neoplastic cells. This aspect is discussed later.

Aetiology and Pathogenesis

As with many other malignant disorders **the pathogenesis of the leukaemias is characterized by several varieties of genomic events such as translocations, mutations and amplifications of proto-oncogenes, and deletion or inactivation of tumour suppressor genes, to be discussed later.** Meanwhile, although the cause of most leukaemias is not known, **there are certain circumstances, some inherited and some acquired, associated with an increased risk.**

Inherited Factors

Down's Syndrome

In children with Down's syndrome there is a 20-fold increase in the risk of developing leukaemia. After the age of 3 years, acute **lymphoblastic** leukaemia (ALL) is commonest, although before this age acute **myeloblastic** leukaemia (AML) is more frequent. It is not known why trisomy 21 confers this increased risk.

Disorders Associated with Increased Fragility of DNA

- ataxia telangiectasia
- Bloom's syndrome
- Fanconi's anaemia

All three disorders are inherited as autosomal recessives. In Bloom's syndrome and ataxia telangiectasia, affected individuals are likely to develop malignant lymphoma or lymphocytic/blastic leukaemia. Children with Fanconi's anaemia are more likely to develop acute myelomonocytic leukaemia.

Other Inherited or Genetically Determined Disorders

- Wiskott–Aldrich syndrome. This is a combination of thrombocytopenia and eczema associated with a

low immunoglobulin M concentration and a poor response to many polysaccharide antigens, and is discussed further in the section on lymphoma. About 25% of the malignancies occurring in this disorder are leukaemias.
- osteogenesis imperfecta
- Klinefelter's syndrome
- leukaemia in a sibling. The risk is heightened further if the sibling is an identical twin.

The inherited risk factors are summarized in *Fig. 41.28.*

Acquired Forms of Increased Risk

Environmental Toxins

An association between exposure to solvents and an increased risk of leukaemia was first noted in Turkey in the 1960s. The responsible chemical was **benzene**, present in quite high concentrations in certain working environments. Within 6 years of the benzene having been replaced in the solvent mixture, the incidence of leukaemia had returned to the baseline level.

Other surveys have confirmed the relationship between chronic benzene exposure, aplastic anaemia and myeloid leukaemia. Benzene is absorbed through the lungs and skin and, because it is lipid soluble, it can be widely distributed in the tissues. A significant source of non-industrial benzene exposure is cigarette smoking. It has been suggested that a typical smoker takes in about 2 mg of benzene daily, in contrast to non-smokers whose intake is only 0.2 mg.

The mechanism of the leukaemogenic effect is not clear. Treating animals with benzene results in the formation of DNA derivatives that are prone to undergo mutations. It is possible that the conversion of benzene to a mutagenic metabolite may be accomplished in the marrow where benzene-derived hydroquinone is converted by haemopoietic enzymes to a mutagen.

Ionizing Radiation

Strong epidemiological evidence exists for an association between exposure to ionizing radiation and an increased risk of leukaemia. One of the most striking demonstrations of this link is the increased incidence of leukaemia found in Hiroshima and Nagasaki in the 20 years following the use of nuclear bombs over these cities in 1945.

Medical use of X-rays is also not without dangers, as was shown by the fact that patients with ankylosing spondylitis treated with a single dose of irradiation to the pelvic region have a fivefold increased incidence of leukaemia compared with non-irradiated age-matched controls.

Even low-level radiation is not free from risk. This is shown by the increased incidence of leukaemia experienced by radiologists in the pioneering days of the specialty. There has been a striking correlation, in terms of time, between nuclear weapon testing in the USA and subsequent waves of myeloid leukaemia in the age

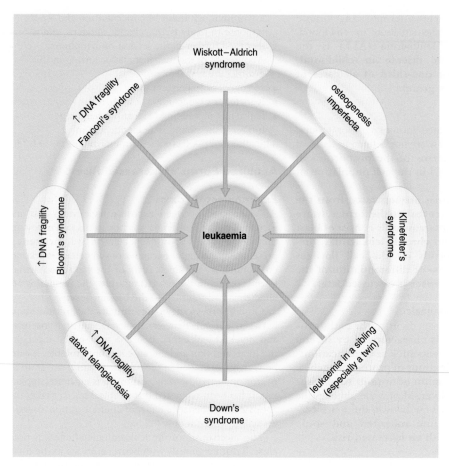

FIGURE 41.28 Inherited risk factors in leukaemia.

group 5–19 years. In these studies the geographical areas in which the concentration of strontium-90 in milk, meat and bones was greatest had the highest incidence of leukaemia.

Non-ionizing Radiation

High-frequency γ- and X-rays are not the only source of exposure to radiation. At the other end of the spectrum are very low frequency long waves emitted from power lines and such mundane objects as electric blankets. Whether such radiation confers an increased risk remains controversial, as does the suggestion that building materials emitting radon gas may convert some homes into leukaemogenic hazards.

Agents Used in the Treatment of Malignant Disease

These may predispose the recipient to develop leukaemia. This applies with particular force to alkylating agents such as chlorambucil and melphalan and to the nitrosoureas such as bis-chloro-ethyl nitroso urea (BCNU).

Viruses

Several viruses cause leukaemias in various non-human species. **There is, however, only one instance in which a causal link has been shown between a viral infection and leukaemia in humans. This is adult T-cell leukaemia/lymphoma caused by the retrovirus, human T-lymphotropic virus (HTLV) 1.**

This virus does not possess a transforming sequence (viral oncogene) in its genome: It does, however, possess the added X region between the *env* gene and the 3′ long terminal repeat which has been called *tax* (transactivator of X), the proteins of which appear to be essential for the virus's oncogenic effect. Possible mechanisms involved in the causation of neoplastic disease by this virus are discussed in the section dealing with viral infection of lymphoid cells (see p 964).

Pre-existing Haematological Disease

Certain haematological diseases are associated with an increased risk of subsequent leukaemia. In some of these it is not surprising that either a frankly neoplastic disorder or an **additional** neoplastic disorder complicates the pre-existing disease, this being especially relevant in the:

- myeloproliferative disorders such as polycythaemia rubra vera and myelofibrosis
- myelodysplasia

In both of these there is **either** growth expansion or a differentiation block. It is perhaps less easy to explain the development of leukaemia against the background of such conditions as:

- paroxysmal nocturnal haemoglobinuria
- aplastic anaemia
- multiple myeloma

Acquired risk factors are summarized in *Fig. 41.29*.

Chromosomal and Molecular Events in Leukaemogenesis

There are many aetiological agents for leukaemia, but the number of final molecular events involved in cell transformation is probably quite small. The machinery for such transformation is believed to be embodied in the protein products of genes which, when activated inappropriately, can confer growth advantages on a clone of cells. These genes are known as **cellular oncogenes**. The actions of these oncogene-derived proteins is opposed by the products of certain recessive genes known as **tumour suppressor genes** or 'antioncogenes'. **Malignant transformation may be the result of an inappropriate degree of activation of one, or more likely several, cellular oncogenes, coupled with the inactivation of suppressor genes.**

Translocations in the Leukaemias

Chronic Myeloid Leukaemia and the Philadelphia Chromosome

Virtually every case of **chronic myeloid leukaemia (CML)** shows a cytogenetic abnormality known as the Philadelphia (Ph) chromosome. This results from a t(9;22) translocation resulting in translocation of the c-*abl* proto-oncogene on chromosome 9 to chromosome 22, where its second exon is fused with 5′ exons of a gene known as *bcr* (breakpoint cluster region) (*Fig. 41.30*).

This hybrid *bcr*–*abl* gene encodes a protein with a molecular weight of 210 kDa (p210), whereas the

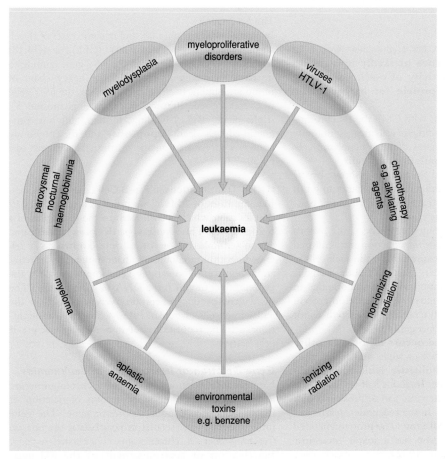

FIGURE 41.29 *Acquired risk factors in leukaemia.*

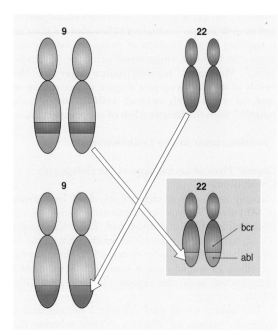

FIGURE 41.30 The 9; 22 translocation which results in the formation of the Philadelphia chromosome.

normal *abl* gene product has a molecular weight of 145 kDa. **The *bcr* sequence markedly upregulates the tyrosine kinase activity of c-*abl*, converting it to a transforming protein for haemopoietic cells.**

Interestingly, in patients with CML the Ph chromosome is found in all haemopoietic cell lineages, not only in myeloid cells; this suggests that the neoplastic cells are derived from **haemopoietic stem cells**.

The power of the fused *bcr–abl* gene is shown by the fact that mice infected with a retrovirus expressing this gene develop leukaemias that may show myeloid, lymphoid or macrophage differentiation.

The growth-stimulating properties of *bcr–abl* depends on the fact that its introduction into cultured haemopoietic cells, or its expression within such cells in the *in vivo* situation, renders these cells both independent of growth factor stimulation and tumorigenic in animals. This ability to remove dependence on growth factors is characteristic of a number of growth factor receptor/tyrosine kinase oncogenes.

The Ph chromosome occurs in diseases other than CML. Some 20–25% of adults and 5% of children with **acute lymphoblastic leukaemia (ALL)** show the Ph chromosome. In about half the cases, the rearrangement involves the same part of the breakpoint cluster region as in CML. In the remainder, rearrangement occurs in the first *bcr* exon. The protein encoded by this variant *bcr–abl* gene has a lower molecular weight (185 kDa instead of 210 kDa) but is much more powerful in terms of its tyrosine kinase activity and in

its transforming potential for both fibroblasts and lymphoid cells.

Retinoic Acid Receptor

A gene whose product is thought to play a part in differentiation is that encoding the retinoic acid receptor (**RAR**). In a form of acute myeloblastic leukaemia known as **promyelocytic leukaemia, a t(15;17) translocation occurs**, disrupting the RAR gene. This translocation results in the formation of a hybrid gene (the carboxy terminus of the RAR gene and the amino-terminal region of a new locus that has been called *myl* (for myelocytic leukaemia)). This discovery is of great interest because:

- **patients with acute promyelocytic leukaemia treated with all-*trans*-retinoic acid can go into complete remission, although maintenance requires the addition of conventional chemotherapy.**
- **cultured leukaemic blast cells from the marrow of patients with acute promyelocytic leukaemia differentiate into mature neutrophils when treated with all-*trans*-retinoic acid.**

The *bcl-2* Gene

In many B-cell lymphomas, and in some cases of B-cell chronic lymphocytic leukaemia (CLL), a t(14;18) translocation takes place, with the *bcl-2* gene coming to lie close to the gene encoding the heavy chain of immunoglobulin. In these circumstances the *bcl-2* gene is overexpressed. Its product, a small guanosine 5′-triphosphate (GTP)-binding protein, inhibits programmed cell death (**apoptosis**) and this obviously confers a survival advantage on the affected cells (see pp 30–32).

t(1;19) Translocations in Pre-B Cell Leukaemias

In some cases of ALL of the pre-B cell type, the 1;19 translocation which is seen leads to the formation of a fusion gene. This consists partly of a translocated amino-terminal region of a gene known as *E2A*, encoding immunoglobulin enhancer-binding proteins, and a homeobox-containing gene known as *PBX*, the gene product of which is a DNA-binding protein. The fused gene product is constitutively expressed in the leukaemic cells, whereas *PBX*, which has transcriptional activity, is not expressed in non-neoplastic pre-B cells.

Gene Deletion or Inactivation in Leukaemias

Non-random deletions of part of a chromosome are usually the morphological expression of deletion or inactivation of a tumour suppressor gene. The gene most frequently inactivated in neoplasia is the one on the long arm of chromosome 17 known as *p53*. **Inactivation or rearrangement of the *p53* gene has been described in AML, in the blast transfor-**

mation phase of patients originally presenting with CML, and in some patients with a myelodysplastic syndrome.

Loss of portions of the **long arms of chromosomes 5 and 7** is often seen in patients with myelodysplastic syndrome and, if present, indicates a high risk of these individuals undergoing transformation to the full leukaemic phenotype.

Gene Mutations in Leukaemias

The family of oncogenes most commonly mutated in neoplasia is *ras*. **Such mutations are seen in 20–30% of cases of AML, 15–20% of cases of ALL, 20–40% of cases of myelodysplastic syndromes and 20% of cases of myeloma**, the oncogene most frequently affected being N-*ras*. The gene product of normal *ras* genes is a G protein and the characteristic mutations inhibit their GTPase activity.

Mutations are also seen in the proto-oncogene c-*fms*. This gene encodes a tyrosine kinase transmembrane receptor normally expressed in monocytes and macrophages. It is the receptor for the **macrophage colony-stimulating factor** (M-CSF). Mutations have been found in the extracellular portion of the *fms*-coded receptor in some patients with AML or myelodysplastic syndromes (about 10% of cases). These mutations probably have the effect of endowing the M-CSF receptor with 'constitutive' tyrosine kinase activity so that it behaves functionally as if it is constantly being activated by its ligand.

THE ACUTE LEUKAEMIAS

Acute leukaemias were defined at the beginning of this chapter in terms of the proportion of the expanded population of bone marrow cells that is immature ('blasts'). **From this definition it can be inferred that the acute leukaemias, whatever the cell lineage involved, are the expression of two processes:**

- **growth expansion**
- **a block to normal differentiation**

Clinical Features

These arise on the basis of:

- lack or dysfunction of normal haemopoietic cells (*Table 41.23*)
- systemic metabolic disturbances such as hypercalcaemia (*Table 41.24*)
- infiltration of organs and tissues producing local effects (*Table 41.25*)

Symptoms referable to organ or tissue infiltration by leukaemic cells reflect the distribution of the infiltrates. Some common sites are listed in *Table 41.25*.

The acute leukaemias fall into two principal groups on the basis of their cell lineage:

Table 41.23 Lack of Normal Haemopoietic Cells

Clinical feature	Possible mechanisms
Increased susceptibility to infection	Neutropenia Decreased production of immunoglobulins Defects in cell-mediated immunity
Haemorrhage	Thrombocytopenia Disseminated intravascular coagulation in some cases Lack of clotting factors if liver severely affected Excess fibrinolytic activity such as occurs in acute promyelocytic leukaemia
Anaemia	Usually of normochromic normocytic type

Table 41.24 Systemic Metabolic Disturbances

Abnormality	Mechanism
Acute tumour lysis syndrome (high plasma levels of potassium, calcium, uric acid, phosphate)	Due to massive breakdown of tumour cells and may be the result of chemotherapy in patients with rapidly proliferating malignancies
High plasma levels of uric acid	Reflects an increased rate of purine metabolism owing to rapid turnover of tumour cells
High plasma levels of calcium	Rare in the leukaemias. Due to the release of factors that stimulate osteoclast-mediated bone resorption (see p 1051)

- **acute lymphoblastic leukaemia** (ALL)
- **acute myeloblastic leukaemia** (AML)

ACUTE LYMPHOBLASTIC LEUKAEMIA

ALL is the commonest malignant disease in childhood (*Fig. 41.31*); 75% of the new cases occurring each year in the USA affect children younger than 15 years. The

Table 41.25 Organ Infiltration in Leukaemia

Site	Clinical effect
Nervous system	Meningeal infiltration leading to features of increased intracranial pressure with headache, lethargy, nausea, vomiting, cranial nerve palsies and neck stiffness. Seen in 26–80% of patients with ALL Visual disturbances Spinal cord compression
Respiratory tract	Infiltration of nasal mucosa leading to nasal blockage Interstitial infiltrates seen on radiography, which may or may not be associated with cough, dyspnoea and haemoptysis
Hepatomegaly and splenomegaly	
Kidney	May show evidence of renal dysfunction which is believed to be associated with infiltration
Bone	Apart from resorption there may be bone pain and cortical thinning due to expansion of bone marrow
Mouth	Gum hypertrophy due to infiltration
Skin	Reddish-brown plaque-like infiltrates may be seen

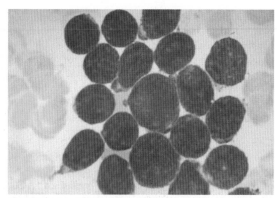

FIGURE 41.31 Marrow aspirate in acute lymphoblastic leukaemia.

Morphological Classification

Acute leukaemias are classified by the modified **FAB system** (French–American–British). This is based on the appearance of blast cells stained with Romanowsky stains, supplemented in some instances by the use of cytochemistry.

In ALL, three subtypes are recognized on the basis of:
- nuclear size and shape
- cell size
- number and prominence of nucleoli
- amount of cytoplasm and its staining characteristics

These subtypes are known as L_1, L_2 and L_3. Their defining features are listed in *Table 41.26*.

This classification has proved to be **prognostically** useful. Patients who fall into the L_1 group have the most favourable prognosis, whereas in the L_3 group remissions are difficult to induce and generally tend to be of short duration.

Use of Immunological Markers in Classifying ALL

On the basis of their antigen expression pattern, ALL may be subclassified into three groups:
- precursor B-cell ALL
- T-cell ALL
- B-cell ALL

In the B-cell subtypes, the immunological classification is best understood against a background of some knowledge of normal B-cell maturation, as shown in *Table 41.27*.

Precursor B-cell ALL

This group contains three subtypes:
- common ALL
- null-type ALL
- pre-B-cell ALL

The antigen expression patterns of these are shown in *Table 41.28*.

T-cell ALL

Here the neoplastic cells express the T-cell markers CD7 and intracytoplasmic CD3. All the nuclei express TdT.

remainder may occur in patients of any age (median age 30–40 years).

Before the introduction of effective chemotherapy, ALL was uniformly fatal. Now 50% of affected children are in remission 5 years after the diagnosis and can probably be considered as being cured. Unfortunately, this is not the case with adult ALL in which the regimens, so successful in children have had little impact on the natural history of the disease.

ALL may be subclassified in a number of different ways, including morphological examination of the blast cells in the marrow and cytogenetic and immunophenotypic characterization.

Table 41.26 Morphological Features in Acute Lymphoblastic Leukaemia

Feature	L_1	L_2	L_3
Cell size	Small	Large	Large
Shape of nucleus	Regular; may be cleaved	Irregular; may be cleaved	Regular, round to oval
Chromatin pattern	Fine or clumped	Fine	Fine
Nucleoli	Usually not seen, but indistinct ones may be present	Large and prominent; may be multiple	Large and prominent; may be multiple
Cytoplasm	Scanty	Moderate	Moderate
Cytoplasmic staining	Slightly basophilic	Slightly basophilic	Deeply basophilic
Vacuoles in cytoplasm	+/−	+/−	++

Table 41.27 Normal B-cell Maturation: Antigenic Expression

Marker	B-cell progenitor	Early pre-B cell	Pre-B cell	B cell	Plasma cell
HLA-DR	+	+	+	+	+
TdT	+	+	−	−	−
CD34	+	+	−	−	−
CD19	−	+	+	+	−
CD24	−	+	+	+	−
CD10 (CALLA)	−	+	+	−	−
CD20	−	−	+	+	−
Cytoplasmic μ chains	−	−	+	−	−
Cytoplasmic immunoglobulin	−	−	−	+	+
CD21	−	−	−	+	−
CD38	−	−	−	−	+

CALLA, common acute lymphoblastic leukaemia antigen.
TdT, terminal deoxynucleotidyl transferase.

Table 41.28 Antigen Expression Patterns of Precursor B ALL Subtypes

Marker	Common ALL	Null-type ALL	Pre-B cell ALL
CD10 (CALLA)	+	−	+/−
CD19	+	+	+
Cytoplasmic CD22	+	+	+
Intracellular μ heavy chains	−	−	+
CD7 (a T-cell marker)	−	−	−
Nuclear TdT expression	+	+	+

B-cell ALL

The distinguishing features of this subtype are:
- **immunoglobulin on the cell membrane**
- **absence of nuclear TdT**

Interestingly, 75% of cases of B-cell ALL fall into the FAB L3 category, indicating that this is a very unfavourable immunophenotype in prognostic terms. In contrast, 90% of the others fall into the L_1 or L_2 categories and have a correspondingly better prognosis.

ACUTE MYELOBLASTIC LEUKAEMIA

AML accounts for only about 10–15% of cases of childhood leukaemia. It is, however, the commonest form of acute leukaemia in adults (*Fig. 41.32*); it is also the one most likely to complicate other haematological disorders, this being particularly relevant in patients with a myelodysplastic syndrome.

Diagnosis

Occasionally there may be difficulty in distinguishing L_2 lymphoblasts from myeloblasts with minimal differentiation. **Myeloblasts show the following:**

- granules staining with Sudan black and with markers for peroxidase
- absence of TdT in most cases
- absence of CD10 (CALLA)
- the presence in most cases of the antigens CD13 and CD33

The FAB system, as applied to AML, subdivides the group into the seven classes shown in *Table 41.29.*

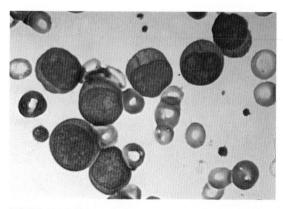

FIGURE 41.32 *Marrow aspirate in acute myeloblastic leukaemia.*

No predisposing cause has been recognized but **more than 95% of patients show the Philadelphia (Ph) chromosome** (see pp 929–930). Whatever the event causing the typical 9;22 translocation, its target appears to be the pluripotent marrow stem cell (the Ph chromosome is found in all haemopoietic cell lineages and not merely in the myeloid line).

In a small proportion of cases, the Ph chromosome is not found. In some of these, despite the absence of the chromosome, there is evidence of the characteristic 9;22 translocation and these patients show features indistinguishable from the Ph-positive form. In the remainder the translocation appears not to have

THE CHRONIC LEUKAEMIAS

CHRONIC MYELOID LEUKAEMIA

CML accounts for a little less than 20% of all leukaemias. It is a disease of adult life, and men are somewhat more likely to be affected than women (M : F ratio 3 : 2).

Table 41.29 The FAB System as Applied to Acute Myeloblastic Leukaemias

Type	Degree or type of differentiation	Morphological features
M_0	AML, undifferentiated	Myeloblasts with no granules, Auer rods, etc.
M_1	AML, minimal differentiation	Scanty granules may be present. MPO or SB +; may be Auer rod and CAE +
M_2	AML, with maturation	Myeloblasts with granules; promyelocytes, few myelocytes
M_3	Acute promyelocytic leukaemia	Promyelocytes with prominent granules; ++ Auer rods; MPO and CAE +
M_4	Acute myelomonocytic (granulocyte and monocyte maturation) leukaemia	More than 20% of cell population is myeloblasts and promyelocytes; more than 20% is promonoblasts and monoblasts. Auer rods +/–; MPO and CAE +
M_5	Acute monoblastic leukaemia	Large monoblasts; Auer rods, MPO and CAE –
M_6	Acute erythroleukaemia	More than 50% megaloblastic erythroid precursors; more than 30% myeloblasts
M_7	Acute megakaryoblastic leukaemia	Megakaryoblasts; no Auer rods or MPO

Auer rods are dysplastic lysosomes that appear as pink intracytoplasmic 'splinters'; MPO, myeloperoxidase; SB, Sudan black; CAE, chloracetate esterase.

occurred; in general these patients have a worse prognosis than those who are Ph chromosome-positive. No chromosomal or molecular disturbances have yet been identified in this small subgroup.

Clinical Features

In general, the same considerations apply as have been discussed earlier (see pp 931–932), but some points need emphasizing in relation to CML.

- **Splenomegaly** is nearly always present in CML (95% of cases) and the spleen is often massive. It has been suggested that the larger the size of the spleen, the worse is the prognosis, but this is by no means universally accepted. The spleen size is, however, said to correlate with the degree of increase in the white cell count.
- **Hepatomegaly** is noted in just under half the cases.
- **Sternal tenderness** is a rather characteristic sign (present in 78% of patients).
- **Fatigue** is a presenting symptom is 81% of cases.
- **Weight loss** is experienced in 61% of patients.
- **Priapism** is a rare but distressing event in some patients with CML.

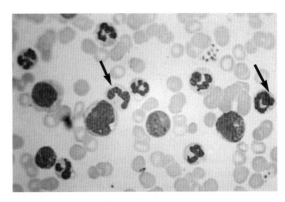

FIGURE 41.33 *Blood film in chronic myeloid leukaemia. Note the large numbers of relatively mature neutrophils and the occasional more primitive myeloid cells (arrows).*

Most patients show some degree of **anaemia** at the time of diagnosis. This is usually of the normochromic normocytic type.

The platelet count is high in about half the patients.

Laboratory Findings

The bone marrow is grossly hypercellular; neutrophils and their precursors predominate. The proportion of immature to mature neutrophils is higher in the marrow than in the blood, suggesting that there is some persistence of the normal barrier against the release of immature cells.

The cytoplasm of the immature cells appears to be maturing more rapidly than the nucleus so that there may be promyelocytes with more cytoplasmic granules than would be expected at this stage. Blast cells from these patients can also be shown to be functionally more mature, in terms of motility and phagocytosis, than expected.

The cells of the neutrophil series show decreased intracellular concentrations of alkaline phosphatase and, in just under 20% of cases, myeloperoxidase levels are also decreased. Intracellular lactoferrin levels are decreased in a majority of cases. Both the last findings probably reflect release of these compounds from the cells rather than decreased synthesis, as plasma concentrations are higher than normal.

In the **blood**, the characteristic finding is marked leucocytosis (*Fig. 41.33*). The white cell count usually exceeds $50 \times 10^9/l$ and counts as high as $500 \times 10^9/l$ have been recorded. All stages of the neutrophil series are generally present. In addition, the absolute number of circulating basophils increases fairly early in the course of the disease; this has been suggested as the explanation for these patients' increased risk of peptic ulceration (the basophils can release large amounts of histamine).

Variants of Chronic Myeloid Leukaemia

Juvenile CML

Fewer than 5% of patients with CML are children. A significant number of these have an atypical form in which the Ph chromosome is absent; this has been called **juvenile CML**. This variant is most common in children aged between 1 and 2 years. Typical clinical and laboratory features include:

- a very marked degree of splenomegaly and hepatomegaly
- lymph node enlargement
- a desquamating skin rash
- thrombocytopenia
- a white cell count tending to be lower than in those with typical CML
- a normal level of neutrophil alkaline phosphatase
- an increase in the proportion of fetal haemoglobin, which may be as high as 85% of the total

The response to treatment is usually poor.

Chronic Eosinophilic Leukaemia

In some patients, who otherwise appear to have typical CML, a striking degree of eosinophilia may be present. As with the neutrophil population, both mature and immature eosinophils may be present. The Ph chromosome may or may not be present.

Chronic Basophilic Leukaemia

Some patients with the typical picture of CML show a marked increase in the number of basophils in the blood. Not all these patients have the Ph chromosome, but in other respects the condition does not appear to behave differently from typical CML.

Chronic Neutrophilic Leukaemia

This is a very rare syndrome in which there is a marked increase in the number of circulating neutrophils without a corresponding increase in immature neutrophils. The bone marrow shows a marked degree of hyperplasia of the granulocyte series. The Ph chromosome has not been found in the small number of patients studied and the neutrophil alkaline phosphatase content is not decreased. The liver and spleen are enlarged and show foci of extramedullary haemopoiesis. Despite this rather benign blood picture, the median survival, admittedly based on a very small series, is only 2 years.

Natural History

In the chronic phase there is usually a good response to chemotherapy and 20% of patients survive as long as 10 years. The median survival time is 3–4 years.

Death may occur as a result of:
- 'blast' transformation
- infection
- haemorrhage

'Blast' Transformation

Blast crisis or transformation is one of the most important causes of death in CML. Its defining criterion is the conversion of CML into a disease with an acute leukaemic picture. The latter falls most often into the group of acute myeloblastic leukaemias, but in some 30% of patients a lymphoblastic transformation may occur. The cause of blast transformation is unknown but is associated with the appearance of new chromosomal abnormalities in cultured cell lines.

Laboratory Findings

Findings suggestive of acute transformation include:
- a degree of anaemia out of proportion to the white cell count
- thrombocytopenia
- increasing numbers of immature cells in the blood and bone marrow. There are differences of opinion at what the threshold level should be for the diagnosis of blast transformation. Some propose a proportion of 20% of blasts in the blood and 30% in the bone marrow but this is not universally accepted
- the appearance of fibrosis in the bone marrow
- the appearance, on cytogenetic studies, of new chromosomal abnormalities, such as duplication of the Ph chromosome
- an increase in the neutrophil alkaline phosphatase content

CHRONIC LYMPHOCYTIC LEUKAEMIA

CLL is characterized by proliferation and accumulation of **relatively mature lymphocytes** in the blood, bone marrow, spleen, liver, lymph nodes and other tissues. It is the commonest form of leukaemia in the Western world, accounting for about 30% of all cases, but is distinctly rare in Asia. It is a disease of later life: patients are typically older than 50 years. Men are affected more frequently than women (M : F ratio 2 : 1).

As is the case with all leukaemias, CLL represents a monoclonal proliferation. In about 95% of cases it is a disease of B cells.

Chromosomal Abnormalities

Several chromosomal abnormalities have been described, of which trisomy in respect of chromosome 12 is the commonest. This may occur as an isolated phenomenon or in association with other abnormalities such as:
- a translocation between chromosomes 11 and 14, seen most often in association with B-prolymphocytic leukaemia
- a t(14;18) translocation, which is common in follicular lymphoma but rather rare in CLL

Clinical Features

In about 25% of cases, the diagnosis is made on the basis of finding lymphocytosis on a blood count, the patients being symptom-free. Less frequently, patients may present with:
- fatigue
- lymph node enlargement
- evidence of infection

On clinical examination there may be enlargement of lymph nodes, liver and spleen. The degree of enlargement of the spleen is modest compared with that seen in CML. Tonsillar enlargement is not uncommon.

Laboratory Findings

The International Workshop on CLL has proposed the following diagnostic criteria for B-cell CLL:
- **lymphocytosis**: an absolute, sustained, peripheral blood lymphocyte count of 10×10^9/l, **most of the cells having the appearance of mature lymphocytes**
- bone marrow in which **lymphocytes account for at least 30% of the nucleated cells**
- a majority of the peripheral blood lymphocytes showing B-cell markers

The Lymphocytes in B-cell CLL

The lymphocytosis in CLL represents expansion of a single clone. This is shown by light chain restriction in respect of the surface immunoglobulin expressed by these cells: either κ or λ, but never both, is expressed.

In addition to normal B-cell markers, the B cells in CLL are unusual in that they characteristically express the CD5 molecule. This is normally associated with mature T cells and is also expressed weakly on thymocytes. Recent studies have shown that there is a subpopulation of B cells expressing CD5; these cells are normally found in the mantle zones of follicle centres. CD5-expressing lymphocytes are also found in the blood of patients with autoimmune diseases such as systemic lupus erythematosus and rheumatoid disease, and also after allogeneic bone marrow transplantation. Among the leukaemias, **the expression of CD5 is unique to B-cell CLL**; some go so far as to say that this disorder should not be diagnosed in the absence of CD5 expression. One exception that should, however, be made is with respect to the **prolymphocytic variant of CLL**, in which CD5 is not expressed.

B cells from patients with CLL show certain functional abnormalities possibly related to the increased risk of infection from which these patients suffer. Immunoglobulins may be present in the plasma in abnormally low concentrations or may even be absent. The pathogenesis of this is poorly understood.

Features of autoimmunity are fairly common in CLL. Some 15–35% of patients have an autoimmune haemolytic anaemia due to antibodies reacting specifically with antigens of the rhesus group. The development of antibodies against platelets and neutrophils has also been reported, and thus patients with CLL may present with autoimmune thrombocytopenia or neutropenia.

Staging and Prognosis in CLL

Two staging systems have been proposed in an attempt to assess the severity of the disease in an individual. The first of these, the Rai system, divides CLL into five grades (0–IV) of differing severity. Stage 0 in this system equates with survival of 12 years or more, whereas in stage IV survival times fall to 2.5 years. More recently, a simplified staging system has been introduced, the details of which are given in *Table 41.30*.

Variants of Chronic Lymphocytic Leukaemia

Prolymphocytic Leukaemia

This is characterized by florid proliferation of lymphocytes larger and less mature in appearance than those seen in typical CLL. The nuclear chromatin appears rather condensed and nucleoli are prominent. It is an aggressive disorder in which the lymphocyte count is very high (in excess of 150×10^9/l) and in which massive enlargement of the spleen is seen. Curiously, lymph node enlargement is trivial or absent. Large amounts of surface immunoglobulin are expressed but **CD5 expression, so characteristic of chronic B-cell leukaemia, does *not* occur**. A T-cell variant of prolymphocytic leukaemia can occur.

Hairy Cell Leukaemia

This is a chronic lymphoproliferative disease with a **male : female ratio of 4 : 1** and a peak age for diagnosis of 40–60 years. It is characterized by:

- **splenomegaly**
- **no evidence of lymph node enlargement**
- **differing degrees of pancytopenia**
- **proliferation of a line of lymphocytes that have a characteristic irregular or 'hairy' outline of the plasma membranes.** These are mononuclear cells with abundant pale blue-grey cytoplasm in which granules are not seen. The plasma membrane shows a variable number of elongated projections, giving the cell its name. The nuclei show a chromatin pattern that is more lightly staining than that of a normal lymphocyte, and nucleoli are prominent. **An important diagnostic feature is the presence of tartrate-resistant acid phosphatase within the hairy cells** (acid phosphatase isoenzyme 5). This is said to be present in more than 95% of cases.

It is not a very common variant, accounting for about 10% of cases of CLL. **The hairy cell is believed to be**

Table 41.30 Binet Staging System for CLL		
Stage	Features	Survival (months)
A	Haemoglobin ≥ 100 g/l Platelets $\geq 100 \times 10^9$/l **Fewer than three areas involved (number of nodes, spleen, liver)**	> 120
B	Haemoglobin ≥ 100 g/l Platelets $\geq 100 \times 10^9$/l **Three or more areas involved**	61
C	Haemoglobin < 100 g/l, or Platelets < 100×10^9/l, or **both of these**	32

a B cell, although it does show some markers normally associated with T cells and monocytes. The T-cell marker most commonly expressed is **CD25**, the receptor for **interleukin (IL) 2**, although, curiously, these cells do not proliferate in response to IL-2.

Clinical Features

The clinical picture is classically one of weakness and fatigue. On examination, **splenomegaly** is usually found. The marrow shows a striking infiltrate of abnormal lymphoid cells and a mild to moderate degree of **fibrosis**, and this last feature may be responsible for a 'dry tap' on attempted marrow aspiration. The pancytopenia causing most of the symptoms is due partly to failure of production of haemopoietic cells and partly to pooling of blood cells in the greatly enlarged spleen. Occasionally a monoclonal immunoglobulin is present in the serum.

Treatment

Splenectomy is a recognized line of treatment because it removes one important contributory factor to the pancytopenia – sequestration or pooling of blood cells in the spleen. There appears to be a definite advantage in splenectomy so far as survival is concerned. More recently there has been considerable interest in the use of **interferon** α in the treatment of hairy cell leukaemia. Some 80–90% of patients respond to this form of treatment, even though complete remission occurs in only 5–10%. It is suggested that the interferon interferes with an autocrine loop in which tumour necrosis factor α is the growth factor.

THE MYELODYSPLASTIC SYNDROMES

This is a set of disorders characterized by:
- **refractory anaemia and other cytopenias**
- **hypercellular bone marrow in which there is evidence of abnormal development of one or more of the haemopoietic cell lines**

- **evolution into acute leukaemia in some instances**

There is no universal agreement as to the fundamental nature of the myelodysplastic syndromes, although some regard them as constituting an incomplete leukaemia phenotype in which the picture is dominated by a block to normal differentiation.

Classification

As in the case of the other white cell disorders, these disorders have been classified morphologically in terms of the FAB system. **The criteria used in this classification include:**
- **the proportion of blast cells** found in the blood and bone marrow
- **the number of ring sideroblasts seen in the bone marrow.** A ring sideroblast is an erythroblast in which haemosiderin granules are arranged in a ring around the margins of the nucleus.
- **the number of monocytes** seen in the blood and of blasts in the bone marrow
- the presence of **Auer rods**

Using these criteria five subtypes have been defined, as shown in *Table 41.31*.

Aetiology and Pathogenesis

The myelodysplasias are believed to arise on the basis of an acquired abnormality in the multipotent haemopoietic stem cell; a defect at this level would explain the fact that multiple cell lineages may be affected.

The cause is unknown, although there may be a history of:
- aplastic anaemia
- paroxysmal nocturnal haemoglobinuria
- exposure to potential mutagens such as benzene and alkylating agents used in cancer chemotherapy

Myelodysplastic syndromes are disorders of the elderly (median age at diagnosis 65 years); this may be because of the increased likelihood for spontaneous mutations to occur as one gets older.

Table 41.31 Subtypes of the Myelodysplastic Syndromes

Type	Blasts in marrow (%)	Ring sideroblasts in marrow (%)	Blasts in blood (%)	No. of monocytes in blood
RA	< 5	< 15	< 1	–
RARS	< 5	≥ 15	< 1	–
RAEB	5–20	–	< 5	–
RAEB-t	> 20–30 and/or Auer rods	–	< 5	–
CMML	≥ 20	–	≤ 5	> 1 × 10⁹/l

RA, refractory anaemia; RARS, refractory anaemia with ring sideroblasts; RAEB, refractory anaemia with excess blasts; RAEB-t, refractory anaemia with excess blasts in transformation; CMML, chronic myelomonocytic leukaemia.

Cytogenetics

Chromosomal abnormalities have been found in 50% of patients with myelodysplastic syndromes; most are of the type in which chromosomal material is either lost or gained. Thus, the commonest abnormalities seen in this group of diseases are partial or total losses of chromosomes 5, 7 and Y, and trisomy 8. Loss of part of the long arm of chromosome 5 occurs in:

- 70% of cases of RA
- 30% of cases of RARS
- 30% of cases of RAEB and RAEB-t
- less than 5% of cases of CMML

The 5q Syndrome

When the only chromosomal defect is loss of part of the long arm of chromosome 5, the clinical features are remarkably constant. Most of these patients are elderly women with a refractory macrocytic anaemia. The natural history is long and tends to be uneventful, although the patients do need occasional blood transfusions. Splenomegaly occurs in nearly half the cases. The platelets are normal in number or may show some increase, and in the marrow the megakaryocyte nuclei have a smaller number of lobes than usual.

The proximal breakpoint on chromosome 5 is at or near 5q 13.3 and the distal one is at or near 5q 31.1. The genes for five important haemopoietic growth factors lie in this region:

- interleukins 3, 4 and 5
- granulocyte–macrophage colony-stimulating factor (GM-CSF)
- the proto-oncogene *c-fms*, which encodes the M-CSF receptor

Clinical Features

The clinical features of myelodysplastic syndromes are shown in Table *41.32*.

The frequency of different blood pictures is shown in *Table 41.33*.

Not only may there be a reduction in the number of neutrophils but their morphology and function may be abnormal. Single or bilobed nuclei may be seen instead of the normal multilobed neutrophil nucleus (the

Table 41.32 Clinical Features of Myelodysplastic Syndromes

Feature	Mechanism
Weakness and fatigue	Gradual onset of anaemia
Easy bruising or abnormal bleeding	Thrombocytopenia
Increased susceptibility to infection	White cell abnormalities

Table 41.33 Blood Picture

Blood picture	Frequency (%)
Anaemia	90
Pancytopenia	50
Anaemia and thrombocytopenia	20–25
Neutropenia	5–10

Pelger abnormality) and there is a decline in such functions as:

- the response to chemotactic signals
- adhesion to appropriate ligands
- phagocytosis

Myeloproliferative Disorders

The myeloproliferative disorders are a set of closely related diseases with a **common element: proliferation of one or more haemopoietic cell lines**. In many cases these proliferations are clonal and neoplastic. They represent, as do the myelodysplastic syndromes, **part** of the leukaemic phenotype, which in **this instance is growth expansion, cell differentiation being quite normal**.

The diseases included under this rubric are:

- **polycythaemia rubra vera (PRV)**
- **myelofibrosis**
- **essential thrombocythaemia**

It is a striking feature of the natural history of these diseases that:

1) **one entity may become transformed into another** (for example, 30% of patients with PRV develop myelofibrosis)

2) **there is a tendency for some patients to develop acute myeloid leukaemia** (10–20% of patients with either PRV or myelofibrosis)

POLYCYTHAEMIA RUBRA VERA

This is a disorder of unknown origin with, usually, an insidious onset. It is characterized by:

- **an increase in the number of red blood cells (RBCs), resulting in an increased red cell volume.** This increase in RBC number reflects a greater than normal rate of formation.
- **an increase in the number of white cells and platelets**, suggesting either that there has been removal of a block to excessive proliferation of multipotent stem cells, or that there has been some abnormal drive to make these cells proliferate.

Epidemiology

PRV occurs principally in later life. The mean age at the time of diagnosis is 60 years. It is rare in children. Some genetic element is likely because PRV is distinctly rare in Afro-Caribbeans. Amongst Caucasians, Jews show an increased risk, the prevalence being about twice as great as among non-Jews.

Clinical Features

The clinical picture in patients with PRV is predicated by the great increase in red cell mass and blood volume, and the resulting hyperviscosity of the blood, which produces a slowing of the circulation and an increased risk of thrombosis.

- **Headache, dizziness and tinnitus** are common symptoms and are believed to reflect the expansion in blood volume.
- **A common and striking symptom is severe itching of the skin after a hot bath.** This symptom is clearly related in some way to the RBC mass because it tends to disappear after treatment inducing a decline in the latter. When relapses occur, the itching returns.
- **Visual disturbances** are common. These are probably due to episodes of ischaemia and, indeed, vascular lesions in the brain constitute the most dangerous complication. On examination of the eye, the conjunctiva is reddened and swollen, and ophthalmoscopy shows the retinal vessels to be engorged and tortuous.
- **Dyspepsia is common** and the **risk of duodenal ulcer is about four times as great as in the non-polycythaemic population**. Varicosities not uncommonly develop in the gut; these may rupture, leading to severe haemorrhage.
- **Patients may complain of dyspnoea** but the degree of oxygen saturation is usually normal.
- **The skin is reddened** (hence the use of the word rubra), particularly at the tip of the nose, the lips, ears, cheeks and neck. The distal parts of the limbs are also severely affected and may show cyanosis.
- **The spleen** is said to be **enlarged** in 65–90% of cases. The splenomegaly is usually moderate; at post-mortem examination, the spleen is smooth and firm due to engorgement with blood, although the splenomegaly may be contributed to by extramedullary haemopoiesis. Splenic infarction is not uncommon and is accompanied by pain and, in some cases, a friction rub audible over the splenic region.
- **Hepatomegaly** occurs in over 40% of cases.

Laboratory Findings
- **The red cell count is strikingly increased**: values of $7–10 \times 10^{12}/l$ are not uncommon. The morphology of the red cells is, for the most part, normal. An occasional normoblast may be seen and this, in the presence of a normal or increased RBC count, should arouse suspicions of PRV.
- **There is an increase in the number of circulating white cells.** Counts of $25 \times 10^9/l$ are not uncommon. Myeloid cells show a relative, as well as an absolute, increase. There is a 'shift to the left' in the myeloid series, an increase in myelocytes and metamyelocytes being noted.
- **The number of circulating platelets is usually increased.** This is usually moderate, but in some instances very high platelet counts of $3000 \times 10^9/l$ or greater are recorded. The marrow megakaryocyte mass is increased in patients in whom this has been determined.
- **The total blood volume and, in particular, the total red cell volume is greatly increased.** In PRV the red cell volume can range from 38.8–93.9 ml/kg body-weight (normal average 29.9 ml/kg body-weight).
- **The blood viscosity may be five to ten times normal.**
- **Hyperuricaemia is present in from half to three-quarters of patients.**

There is an increased risk of both arterial and venous thrombosis. The complications of these are the cause of death in many instances. In addition, there appears to be an increased risk of hypertension.

The object of treatment in PRV is to reach and maintain an approximately normal red cell mass, represented by a packed cell volume of about 45%, and a normal platelet count.

Natural History

Treatment has increased median survival time to 10–15 years. About 10% of patients treated with ^{32}P develop haematological malignancy, although a much smaller percentage has been reported in patients treated with venesection alone. Thrombosis and haemorrhage remain significant causes of death.

Secondary Polycythaemia

Secondary polycythaemia affects only the red cells, the other haemopoietic cell lines being normal. It is due to an increase in the drive that erythropoietin exerts on red cell precursors. Such increases in erythropoietin activity may be deemed **appropriate** (in response to an increased demand for red cells) or **inappropriate**, where no such increased demand exists.

Appropriate increases in erythropoietin secretion occur principally when there is an increased demand for oxygen-carrying capacity, as is seen in:
- individuals living at very high altitudes
- congenital heart disease in which right to left shunts are present

- hypoxia associated with chronic airflow obstruction
- heavy smokers

Inappropriate increase in erythropoietin secretion resulting in polycythaemia is one of the paraneoplastic syndromes. It occurs in association with:

- some massive uterine leiomyomas
- some liver cell carcinomas
- some renal cell carcinomas
- cerebellar haemangioblastoma

'Stress Polycythaemia'

In addition to secondary polycythaemia, a syndrome that has been termed 'stress' or 'pseudo' polycythaemia exists. In this, the increase in red cell mass is relative rather than absolute and results from a decrease in plasma volume. No obvious cause for the contraction of plasma volume is present. The condition, which is far from uncommon, affects chiefly young and middle-aged males and may be seen in association with cigarette smoking and treatment with diuretics.

IDIOPATHIC MYELOFIBROSIS

Idiopathic myelofibrosis is another clonal neoplastic disorder involving haemopoietic stem cells; as its name implies, it is associated with marrow fibrosis. The term 'idiopathic' is used here because many other conditions, both malignant and non-malignant, may be associated with marrow fibrosis.

Stem cell proliferation with spill-over into the circulating blood and colonization of tissues leading to extramedullary haematopoiesis are integral features of the condition. Intravenous injection of radiolabelled iron is followed by localization of the isotope in areas where haemopoiesis is occurring. In normal individuals this iron localizes almost exclusively to the bone marrow. In myelofibrosis, however, there is extensive localization to the spleen and liver, indicating active haemopoiesis in these tissues. The fibrosis is believed to be due to the action on marrow fibroblasts of platelet-derived growth factor secreted by abnormal megakaryocytes in the marrow, although growth factors are also synthesized and secreted by macrophages and these too may play a part in the fibrosis.

Clinical Features

Myelofibrosis, for the most part, affects the elderly; its onset is insidious. In some individuals the course is prolonged for up to 15 years.

The most common presentation is with symptoms referable to anaemia or the characteristic, massive splenomegaly. Increased cell turnover, if present, is reflected by hyperuricaemia which may be sufficiently severe as to cause gout or renal colic due to urate stones (gout has been reported in 6% of patients and renal colic in 4%).

On examination the chief, indeed in some cases the only, abnormal finding, other than evidence of anaemia, is massive splenomegaly. The spleen may be so large that its lower border extends to the pelvic brim and its right border can be palpated on the right-hand side of the abdominal midline. In non-tropical regions, the commonest causes of such massive splenomegaly are myelofibrosis and chronic myeloid leukaemia. Hepatomegaly is present in about 50% of cases. Sternal tenderness, in contrast with chronic myeloid leukaemia, is unusual.

Laboratory Findings

Blood Picture

Anaemia is present at the time of diagnosis in most cases. This is multifactorial in origin. In part it is due to sequestration of RBCs in the spleen, in part to an increased rate of RBC destruction and in some patients to a decreased rate of erythropoiesis.

Blood films show a **leucoerythroblastic anaemia (i.e. the presence of nucleated red cells coupled with the presence of immature neutrophils)**. Many of the red cells have a characteristic 'tear drop' shape; such platelets as are seen on the blood film are larger than normal. The white cell and platelet counts are often raised (in about 50% of cases; in 25% the white cell numbers are decreased). In about two-thirds of patients the neutrophil alkaline phosphatase content is increased. The increased platelet count at the time of diagnosis is not permanent and, with the passage of time, thrombocytopenia often develops.

Bone Marrow

Attempts to aspirate marrow often fail (so-called 'dry tap') and, even in cases where aspiration is successful, the appearances may not be diagnostic. There is generally an increase in both myeloid and megakaryocyte precursors; the megakaryocytes themselves frequently appear abnormal, variations in size and increased degrees of polyploidy being seen quite commonly.

To confirm myelofibrosis, a biopsy is required. Characteristically there is variable and patchy fibrosis, shown well by the use of silver salts which bind to the reticulin fibres. There is an increase in the number of megakaryocytes and these often show morphological abnormalities. Within the small blood vessels in the marrow cavity, clear evidence of haemopoiesis can be seen.

Biochemical Changes in Serum

The principal biochemical changes in myelofibrosis reflect:

- **increased turnover of the haemopoietic cell population**
- increased concentrations of lactic dehydrogenase and β-hydroxybutyrate dehydrogenase

- **increased formation of new bone**
- increased concentration of alkaline phosphatase, which reflects the greatly increased osteoblastic activity. This finding is present in about half the patients.

Microscopic Features

A striking feature is the presence of **osteosclerosis** (increased laying down of new bone). This is sufficiently severe as to be detected radiologically in 30–70% of patients. The process affects chiefly the axial skeleton and the proximal portions of the long bones.

Bony trabeculae are abnormally thick and irregular in shape and, in some areas, the marrow cavity may be virtually obliterated.

Sections of spleen invariably show many foci of extramedullary haemopoiesis, believed to account for the splenomegaly. The liver also shows extramedullary haemopoiesis; this phenomenon can be found in virtually any organ or tissue, including such unexpected places as the breast and dura.

Natural History

Common causes of death in patients with myelofibrosis include:

- infection
- evolution into acute leukaemia
- haemorrhage
- cardiac failure
- portal hypertension, which is seen occasionally. This may be due to intrasinusoidal haemopoiesis, compression or thrombosis of the portal vein, or thrombosis occurring in the hepatic venous drainage (Budd–Chiari syndrome).

ESSENTIAL THROMBOCYTHAEMIA

This disorder is characterized by an abnormal clonal proliferation of megakaryocytes and a resulting significant increase in platelet count. It should be regarded as a neoplastic disorder in which there is growth expansion without loss of differentiation, much in the same way as PRV. Clinically, it is expressed in the form of:

- **abnormal bleeding**, especially in the form of easy bruising, gastrointestinal haemorrhage and epistaxis
- **an increase in the risk of thromboembolic events**

The pathogenesis of the haemorrhage is not clearly understood, although some have suggested that it is the expression of qualitatively abnormal platelet function. The increased risk of thrombosis is believed to be the result of the increased platelet mass and, indeed, platelet counts in excess of $1000 \times 10^9/l$ have been recorded. The locations of the thrombi tend to be unusual; frequently affected vessels include:

- the splenic vein
- small vessels of the fingers and toes
- intracranial vessels

Thus, attacks of painful ischaemia of the fingers and toes and transient cerebral ischaemic attacks are quite common.

The spleen is enlarged significantly in about 80% of cases, although in the later stages of the disease splenic atrophy may occur. Enlargement of the liver is also a fairly common finding.

Although the commonest cause of death is thromboembolism, as in the other myeloproliferative disorders thrombocythaemia may terminate in acute myeloid leukaemia. In some cases, the terminal haematological event is red cell aplasia.

Laboratory Findings

- **A greatly increased platelet count.** This is mirrored morphologically by clumps of platelets in blood films. The platelet size and shape are abnormal in many cases.
- **Some increase in the neutrophil count** associated with a 'shift to the left' is often seen.
- **Not surprisingly, in view of the grossly raised platelet counts, the bone marrow shows the presence of a marked proliferation of megakaryocytes**, sheets of megakaryocytes being seen in some areas.

Treatment

In severe cases (i.e. patients with a platelet count above $1000 \times 10^9/l$ or a history of recurrent thrombosis or haemorrhage) it is necessary to reduce the increased platelet mass. This may be done by the use of myelosuppressive agents such as busulphan but many now favour the use of hydroxurea or interferon α, which are believed to be associated with fewer long-term complications.

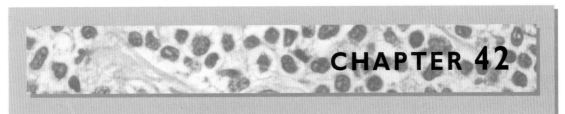

CHAPTER 42

The Lymphoreticular System

The Thymus

The thymus is pivotal to normal function of the immune system. It has a key part to play in relation to T-lymphocyte differentiation and maturation. Bone marrow-derived stem cells become immunocompetent T cells in the thymus.

NORMAL STRUCTURE AND FUNCTION

In structural terms, the thymus is partly epithelial and partly lymphoid in nature. The epithelial component is derived from the cervical sinus ectoderm and from the third and, occasionally, the fourth pharyngeal pouch endoderm, these two elements forming a tube-like structure which becomes obliterated by proliferating epithelium and which loses its connection with the pharynx by the end of the second month of embryonic life. Thymic lobes are derived from each side of the neck and fuse to form a single organ behind the sternum. At birth it weighs 20–30 g, reaching its peak at puberty with a weight of 40–50 g.

Colonization of the thymus by lymphoid cells starts at about the ninth week of gestation and part of the lymphocyte population of the thymus is derived by local cell division of these 'immigrant' lymphoid cells. From about the 13th week of gestation, export of T cells begins; these cells gain access to the bloodstream via high endothelial venules.

In its fully developed form, the thymus is a two-lobed organ, each of the lobes being subdivided by connective tissue septa into lobules. Each lobule, in turn, is divided into a cortex and a paler medulla. The tissue is highly vascular; lymphoid cells occupy the space between the small blood vessels and the basement membrane surrounding the thymic epithelium.

Thymic Epithelium

Four types of epithelial cell are recognized, each corresponding to a specific location within the thymus (see *Table 42.1*)

The cortical epithelial cells differ in their pattern of antigen expression from the other types, suggesting that there are two distinct lineages for epithelial cell development. Epithelial cells produce peptide hormones

Table 42.1 Thymic Epithelium

Type	Location and characteristics
Subcapsular	Forms a layer one or two cells thick abutting on capsular basement membrane, extending along septa to blend with perivascular epithelium
Cortical	A three-dimensional network of large cells with prominent nucleoli and cytoplasmic extensions wrapped around lymphoid precursors ('nurse cells'). In the deeper cortex, cells are smaller, are oriented more or less perpendicular to the thymic surface, and have less prominent nucleoli.
Medullary	Cells are spindle-shaped with densely staining nuclei and inconspicuous nucleoli. The cytoplasmic filaments contain contractile actin and myosin filaments and high molecular weight keratins.
Hassall's corpuscles	These are whorls of epithelial cells which, as they enlarge, become keratinized centrally, this core of keratin being surrounded by concentric layers of living epithelial cells.

which can promote the appearance of differentiation markers in T cells. These include thymulin, α_1- and β_4-thymosin, and thymopoietin, of which only thymulin and thymopoietin are exclusive to the thymus.

The Effects of Ageing

The volume of the thymus is not affected by ageing but much of its lymphoid tissue is lost and replaced by adipose tissue. Lymphoid precursors within the thymus continue to divide throughout life, although loss of thymic cortical epithelium is progressive. Half the thymic tissue has been lost by the age of 10 years and only 10% remains by the age of 35 years.

Accidental Involution

Accidental involution follows what may loosely be called 'acute stress'. It may be acute or chronic (*Fig. 42.1*). **The major mechanism leading to involution is apoptosis of cortical thymocytes**, the apoptotic bodies being phagocytosed by intrathymic macrophages. It is believed that the upregulation of apoptosis in the cortex is due to the release of large amounts of endogenous corticosteroids following 'stress'. These then bind to steroid receptors on the immature lymphocytes in the cortex. The medulla is spared because the lymphocytes here do not express the steroid receptors.

- Acute involution may occur in association with trauma, sepsis, irradiation or the acute respiratory distress syndrome (see pp 448–451).
- Chronic involution leading to a very severe degree of thymic atrophy may occur as a result of any chronic wasting disease or severe malnutrition. Very severe cortical loss occurs, not only of lymphoid cells but cortical epithelium undergoing atrophy.

IMMUNE DEFICIENCY AND THE THYMUS

Immunodeficiency may be primary or secondary, the primary forms being either genetically determined or due to fetal damage early in pregnancy. Such primary immunodeficiency may be due to defects intrinsic to

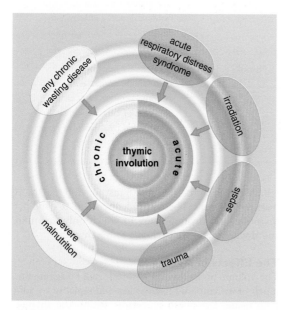

FIGURE 42.1 *Causes of acute and chronic thymic involution.*

the development of the thymus or to defects in the ontogeny of the lymphoid cells.

PRIMARY IMMUNODEFICIENCY

Di George's and Nezelof's Syndromes (see p 120)

Severe Combined Immunodeficiency Disease (SCID)

This is a set of disorders characterized by defects in both cell-mediated and humoral immunity, and usually associated with lymphopenia. SCID may be inherited in autosomal or X-linked recessive patterns.

The commonest cause is abnormal development of B and T lymphocytes from bone marrow stem cells. Thymus and peripheral lymphoid organs are largely or totally lacking in lymphocytes and affected infants show a profound lymphopenia. All immune functions are depressed and death from infection is common in the first year of life.

> ### Macroscopic Features
> The thymus is normally sited but is much smaller than normal (0.5–4 g).
>
> ### Microscopic Features
> In general terms there is:
> - loss of corticomedullary differentiation
> - absence of Hassall's corpuscles
> - marked depletion of the lymphoid cell population, lymphocytes being completely absent in some cases
>
> Several different patterns have been described, the commonest of these being termed **simple dysplasia**.

The thymic abnormalities are the expression rather than the cause of SCID. This is shown by the fact that, in most cases, immunoreactivity can be normalized by bone marrow transplantation. It is worth remembering that the morphological picture in the thymus may be complicated by the effects of intrauterine infections or by a graft versus host reaction due to maternal lymphocytes gaining access to the fetal circulation.

Autosomal Recessive SCID

Adenosine Deaminase Deficiency

About 50% of cases with the autosomal recessive form, amounting to 20% of the total, are due to deficiency in the enzyme adenosine deaminase (ADA), the gene for which is located on chromosome 2. Deletions or mutations of this gene lead to the accumulation of metabolites that are toxic to lymphocytes. These metabolites block the synthesis of DNA leading to reduced numbers of both B and T cells. Some affected individuals can be treated by transfusions of red cells containing the enzyme or with preparations of the enzyme itself, and this disease seems likely to respond to gene therapy because the cloned gene for ADA has been constitutively expressed in transfected cells.

Purine Nucleoside Phosphorylase Deficiency

More rarely, autosomal recessive SCID is caused by deficiency of the enzyme purine nucleoside phosphorylase (PNP), again leading to the accumulation of toxic metabolites in lymphocytes. T cells are more severely affected than B cells.

The 'Bare Lymphocyte' Syndrome

This disorder is characterized by failure to express normal amounts of major histocompatibility complex (MHC) class II proteins on the surfaces of lymphocytes, macrophages and dendritic cells. Thus there is a failure to present antigens to T helper cells and affected individuals are lacking both in normal cell-mediated immune responses and in antibody responses to T-dependent protein antigens.

The defect is due to a quantitative or qualitative abnormality in a DNA-binding protein which normally stimulates the transcription of MHC class II genes by binding to the 'X box' regulatory sequence 5′ of the MHC class II genes. This protein may be reduced in amount or structurally abnormal and hence inactive.

X-Linked SCID

Some cases in this group have been shown to be due to mutations in the gene coding for the γ chain of the interleukin (IL) 2 receptor, a component of high-affinity receptors for IL-2, IL-4 and IL-7. IL-7 is an important growth factor for B and T cells and thus development of a normal population of lymphocytes does not occur.

Receptor Rearrangement Failure in SCID

Many cases of SCID do not fit into any of the above categories. Their cellular and molecular bases are still unknown. It has been suggested that at least some of these cases may be due to defective rearrangement and expression of the T- and B-cell receptor genes consequent on a lack of the recombinases required for this function.

Such a situation is illustrated by an animal model, the SCID mouse, in which there is a developmental failure of both T and B cells owing to a block in maturation of bone marrow precursors. This block arises because of a defect in the DNA repair mechanisms needed for rearrangement of T-cell receptor and immunoglobulin genes. Two genes, *RAG-1* and *RAG-2* (Recombination Activating Genes) have been identified which, when transfected into mouse cells lacking in recombinase activity, restore normal activity. Proof of the existence of a homologous situation in humans has not yet been obtained. These mechanisms are summarized in *Fig. 42.2*.

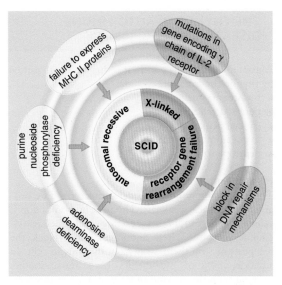

FIGURE 42.2 Mechanisms involved in the causation of severe combined immune deficiency (SCID).

Stem Cell Deficiency (Reticular Dysgenesis)

Defects in the production of stem cells in the bone marrow lead to a deficiency of B- and T-cell precursors. This situation, in its most severe form, is known as reticular dysgenesis. The development of other bone marrow cell lineages is also depressed. Affected infants have a high risk of dying from overwhelming sepsis.

SECONDARY (ACQUIRED) IMMUNODEFICIENCY

This situation is illustrated in:

- **Allogeneic bone marrow transplantation.** The associated hyperinvolution and atrophy may reflect the treatment the patient has received before the marrow transplant and the graft versus host disease, which many such patients develop.
- **Acquired immune deficiency syndrome (AIDS).** At post-mortem examination there is usually a severe degree of thymic atrophy. The thymus at this stage consists principally of strands of epithelial cells; lymphocytes and Hassall's corpuscles are absent. The thymic atrophy in AIDS precedes both atrophy of peripheral lymphoid tissue and the onset of the characteristic clinical syndromes of this disease. Loss of thymic lymphocytes is largely brought about by apoptosis. The extent and severity of thymic lymphocyte loss far exceeds the number of such cells containing the viral genome, suggesting the existence of some indirect and unrecognized mechanism to account for the upregulation of apoptosis.

THE THYMUS IN AUTOIMMUNE DISEASE

Autoimmune diseases which, it is suggested, are caused by thymic abnormalities include:
- myasthenia gravis
- pure red cell aplasia
- pancytopenia
- hypogammaglobulinaemia
- neutropenia

Myasthenia Gravis

This is an autoimmune disorder characterized by progressive muscular weakness. The muscle dysfunction is caused by autoantibodies reacting with the acetylcholine receptor. These antibodies either block the receptors or strip them away from the muscle cells. In addition, 50% of myasthenics have autoantibodies reacting with the A band of striated muscle; this antibody is present in 90% of myasthenics who have a thymic epithelial tumour (thymoma). It is unlikely to be of pathogenetic significance because the antibody may occur in normal subjects.

Some 75–85% of patients with myasthenia gravis show morphological abnormalities in the thymus. Thymectomy may reduce the plasma concentrations of autoantibody and improve the clinical picture in some cases, suggesting that the thymic changes are pathogenetically related to the disease.

Microscopic Features

Three main patterns are encountered:
- lymphoid follicular hyperplasia (thymitis)
- thymic epithelial tumour (thymoma) (see pp 946–947)
- normal or mildly atrophic thymus

Lymphoid Follicular Hyperplasia

This is associated with 50–60% of cases of myasthenia. It is commonest between 10 and 40 years; it is three times as common in females and is associated with the haplotypes A1, B8 and DR3.

The outstanding feature is germinal centres, resembling those found in peripheral lymphoid tissue (see pp 949–950). The thymus itself appears to be the main source of autoantibody in this variant of myasthenia, the antigen being found on muscle-like (myoid) cells within the thymus. Patients with this morphological picture and who have acetylcholine receptor autoantibodies in the plasma are most likely to benefit from thymectomy.

THYMIC INFECTIONS

Infections involving the thymus are very rare. Viral involvement in the course of systemic viral infections may occur as, for example, in cytomegalovirus infection in patients who have received bone marrow transplants. Examples of thymic changes in measles, varicella zoster infections and infectious mononucleosis have been recorded.

THYMIC TUMOURS AND TUMOUR-LIKE LESIONS

The origin of true neoplasms of the thymus is shown in Table 42.2.

Table 42.2 Thymic Neoplasms

Site of origin	Type
Thymic epithelium	Thymoma
	Thymic carcinoid
Lymphocytic compartment	Lymphoma
Primordial germinal rests which have not completed their journey from the urogenital ridge to the gonads during embryonic life	Germ cell tumours, benign and malignant

THYMIC EPITHELIAL NEOPLASMS

Thymoma

The commonest primary epithelial neoplasms at this site are thymomas. The term thymoma has no implications as far as the biological behaviour of these lesions is concerned.

Thymomas are also the commonest neoplasms occurring in the anterior mediastinum, accounting for 45% of primary tumours at this site. They occur chiefly in middle to later life; the mean age at diagnosis is 50 years. They are equally common in both sexes.

Thymomas give rise to clinical abnormalities either because of the presence of a mass in the mediastinum or because of their association with myasthenia gravis. The common clinical pictures are summarized in Table 42.3.

Classification

Classifying thymomas has been difficult. Rosai and Levene (1976) classified thymomas on the basis of their invasiveness and metastatic potential. Tumours that were completely encapsulated and those with a predominantly spindle cell population were regarded as benign. The remainder were divided into two categories. Category I lesions showed:
- minimal or no cytological atypia
- local invasion only

Table 42.3 Clinical Syndromes Associated with Thymoma

Clinical picture	Frequency (%)
Myasthenia with or without symptoms of a mediastinal tumour mass	Approx. 50
Symptoms of a mediastinal tumour mass	40
A non-myasthenic paraneoplastic syndrome	10

- only rare invasion of blood vessels or lymphatics

Category II lesions were:

- cytologically malignant

More recently a new histological classification based on the relationship between the predominant elements in a thymoma and their counterparts in the normal thymus has been introduced. A major advantage of this new system is a much higher degree of correlation between tumour type, degree of invasiveness and risk of associated myasthenia gravis. Some of these interrelationships are shown in *Tables 42.4, 42.5* and *42.6*, which are based on data from Muller-Hermelink *et al.*, 1994.

Macroscopic Features

Most thymomas are well-circumscribed and firm lesions; the encapsulated variants are enclosed in a fibrous capsule. The invasive examples have poorly defined edges and tend to ensheath blood vessels and neighbouring organs within the mediastinum. The tumours vary greatly in size. The average weight is 159 g but lesions weighing several kilograms have been described.

The cut surfaces show a lobular appearance produced by fibrous septa, and areas of cystic degeneration are common.

Microscopic Features

Descriptions of the variant histological forms listed are beyond the scope of a text of this length. Those interested are referred to the excellent account by Muller-Hermelink and colleagues (1994).

Table 42.4 Frequency, Sex Distribution and Risk of Myasthenia Gravis in Thymoma

Type	Frequency (%)	M : F ratio	Frequency of associated myasthenia (%)
Medullary thymoma	5.8	1 : 1.7	33
Mixed thymoma	20.0	1 : 2.1	39
Predominantly cortical thymoma	7.7	1 : 3.5	33
Cortical thymoma	41.9	1 : 1.1	66
Well-differentiated carcinoma	16.8	1 : 2.1	77
Other thymic carcinoma	7.7	3 : 1	0

Table 42.5 Types of Thymoma in Relation to their Invasiveness

Type	Stage 1 (%)	Stage 2 (%)	Stage 3 (%)	Stage 4 (%)
Medullary thymoma	66	34	0	0
Mixed thymoma	66	34	0	0
Predominantly cortical thymoma	44	44	12	0
Cortical thymoma	21	32	38	9
Well-differentiated carcinoma	0	17	57	26
Other carcinoma	0	8	59	33

Table 42.6 Relationship Between Histological Types of Thymoma and Clinicopathological Classification

Clinicopathological classification	Histogenetic classification
Non-invasive thymoma (benign)	Medullary thymoma
	Mixed thymoma
Invasive thymoma (category I)	Predominantly cortical thymoma
	Cortical thymoma
	Well-differentiated carcinoma
Thymic carcinoma (category II)	Epidermoid carcinoma
	Endocrine carcinoma
	Undifferentiated carcinoma

THYMIC LYMPHOMA

Several types of lymphoma and leukaemia may involve the thymus.

Non-Hodgkin's Lymphoma

Mediastinal involvement occurs in 18–24% of cases. Not surprisingly, most of these are T-cell lymphomas, of the lymphoblastic type. These commonly evolve into leukaemia.

Recently a large cell lymphoma arising from B cells has been described as occurring in the mediastinum of young adults. It is often associated with a marked fibrous tissue reaction, which may make the diagnosis difficult. There is a unique population of B cells in the thymic medulla and it is from this cell compartment that the B-cell lymphoma may arise.

Hodgkin's Disease

The mediastinum is a not uncommon sire for Hodgkin's disease. The majority of these cases show the nodular sclerosing form of the disease (see p 958).

GERM CELL TUMOURS

If primordial germinal crests fail to migrate from the urogenital ridges to the gonads in fetal life, rests of germinal tissue may occur; it is from these that mediastinal germ cell tumours arise.

The range of such germinal tumours mirrors that found in the gonads (see pp 727–733):

- **Seminoma.** This is the commonest germ cell tumour occurring in the anterior mediastinum. It affects males in the third decade of life.
- **Benign teratoma.** These account for about 80% of mediastinal germ cell tumours, presenting usually in the second or third decades of life.
- **Malignant teratoma.** These tumours occur almost exclusively in young males.

Lymph Nodes

NORMAL ANATOMY AND FUNCTION OF THE IMMUNE RESPONSE

This is described in Chapter 10 (see pp 98–101) and is broadly summarized in *Fig. 42.3*.

NON-NEOPLASTIC DISORDERS OF LYMPH NODES

Non-neoplastic pathology of lymph nodes can be considered in various ways:

- **reaction pattern of the node.** This may be the expression of **two sets of basic processes**:
  1) **the inflammatory response, either acute or chronic**, which is elicited by a wide range of injurious factors, many but not all of which are infections
  2) **an increase in immunological reactivity** as a result of presentation of antigen within the affected node
- **effects of known aetiological agents on the node**
- **pathological entities, the cause of which is not yet known**

ACUTE AND CHRONIC INFLAMMATORY RESPONSES IN LYMPH NODES (LYMPHADENITIS)

Acute lymphadenitis is most commonly seen in association with infections by pyogenic microorganisms such as the pharyngitis caused by β-haemolytic streptococci or skin lesions resulting from infection by *Staphylococcus pyogenes aureus*. Nodes draining the sites of infection become enlarged and tender.

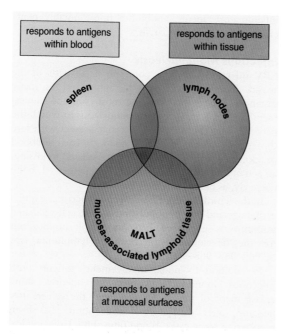

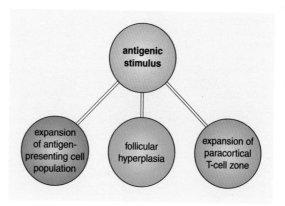

FIGURE 42.4 Morphological patterns of enhanced immunological reactivity in lymph nodes.

FIGURE 42.3 Principal compartments of the peripheral lymphoid system.

As the cause of the lymphadenopathy is usually obvious on clinical examination, lymph node biopsy under these circumstances is performed only rarely. The microscopic appearances show the expected changes of acute inflammation in any tissue: **oedema, hyperaemia and emigration of neutrophils from the microvasculature into the nodal parenchyma**. With the introduction of antibiotic treatment, suppuration within nodes leading to abscess formation has now become very rare.

Chronic lymphadenitis, like any other chronic inflammatory process, may be the sequel of acute inflammation or may be chronic *ab initio*. In the first instance, scarring of the node is a common feature and may be associated with sinus histiocytosis (an accumulation of macrophages within the sinuses).

Many infections elicit a reaction in the tissues which is dominated very early on by the features of chronic inflammation such as granuloma formation. Some of these are discussed in the section dealing with the nodal reactions encountered as a result of certain specific agents.

LYMPH NODE ENLARGEMENT DUE TO ENHANCED IMMUNOLOGICAL REACTIVITY

The appearances seen when antigenic stimulation occurs depend largely on the nature of the responsible antigen. Thus proliferation and activation can take place in any of the nodal cell compartments concerned in regulation of the immune response

or in more than one of them. The morphological correlates (*Fig. 42.4*) may therefore be:

- **follicular hyperplasia**
- **expansion of the paracortical T-cell zone**
- **expansion of the antigen-presenting cell population, with a marked increase in macrophages. This can occur either within the sinuses, which are lined by such cells, or within the lymph node pulp.**

Follicular Hyperplasia and an Increase in the Plasma Cell Population

Follicular hyperplasia is the morphological correlate of an immune response mediated predominantly by B cells. It is characteristic of the reaction elicited by many bacterial antigens and also by some non-living antigens. It may occur in nodes draining some local inflammatory reaction but also in some systemic disorders such as **rheumatoid arthritis, systemic lupus erythematosus** and in the **early phase of HIV infection**.

Microscopic Features

- an increase in both number and size of the follicles
- enlarged germinal centres which can be distinguished with ease from the smaller and more darkly staining cells of the mantle zone (*Fig. 42.5*)
- evidence of an increase in cell turnover in the germinal centre in the form of large numbers of 'tingible body macrophages' which contain nuclear debris

---

In some instances the B-cell reaction culminates in the differentiation of large numbers of the proliferated cells into plasma cells, both within the medulla and, to some extent, within the follicles. These plasma cells are polytypic and thus show no evidence of light chain restriction of their cytoplasmic immunoglobulin (i.e. both κ and λ light chains are expressed).

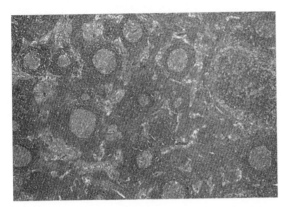

FIGURE 42.5 *Follicular hyperplasia occurring in a node from a patient with rheumatoid arthritis. The enlarged germinal centres show up as well-demarcated pale areas and vary somewhat in size.*

In some instances, the degree of follicular hyperplasia may be so great as to make the distinction between a reactive condition and follicle-centre cell lymphoma difficult. Features suggesting follicular hyperplasia rather than lymphoma are:

- Nodal architecture is preserved and there is no loss of the sinus pattern.
- The reactive follicles show marked variation in size and shape.
- The germinal centres tend to be well demarcated from the surrounding portion of the follicle.
- The reticulin fibre framework of the node is preserved.
- There is evidence of active phagocytosis of cell debris by macrophages in the germinal centres.
- There is a moderate to pronounced degree of mitotic activity in the reactive germinal centre.
- Molecular genetic studies show no evidence of the typical translocations between chromosomes characteristic of follicle-centre cell lymphoma.

Paracortical Hyperplasia: a Predominantly T-cell Immune Response

Expansion of the paracortical or T-cell zones may occur in either nodular or diffuse patterns. As this part of the node expands, some of the follicles may atrophy. T-cell zone expansion is, of course, due to cell proliferation, the increased cell population consisting chiefly of small T cells and T immunoblasts, with large nuclei and prominent centrally placed nucleoli. This T-cell response is associated with increased prominence of the high endothelium venules.

Diffuse paracortical hyperplasia occurs most frequently in certain viral infections, most notably with Epstein–Barr virus (EBV) infections leading to **infectious mononucleosis**. Paracortical expansion may also be seen as a reaction to certain drugs, such as hydantoin and its derivatives, non-steroidal anti-inflammatory agents, antibiotics (most notably penicillin) and some antimalarials.

Infectious Mononucleosis

EBV infections are very common in all parts of the world. The infection may be subclinical in many instances, and in the West the most common clinical manifestation is infectious mononucleosis in which the patients, who are usually adolescents, present with sore throat and swelling of cervical nodes. In late childhood or adolescence, infection is said to be related to kissing, an activity which at that time of life is perceived, quite correctly, as being extremely enjoyable.

In the Third World, EBV infections occur at a much earlier age and this, in populations where cell-mediated immunity is suppressed, has considerable implications for the development of Burkitt's lymphoma (see pp 962–963, 968–969).

In addition to nodal involvement, patients with infectious mononucleosis not infrequently show enlargement of the spleen and liver; the spleen may become softer than normal and rupture has been reported in some cases. Blood films show large atypical lymphocytes. These are T cells that have undergone blast transformation as a result of recognizing virally coded neoantigens on the infected and proliferating B cells. At this stage the Paul–Bunnell test, which detects heterophile antibody, becomes positive.

Although diagnosis is usually made without resort to node biopsy, the nodal changes may be very striking and can be confused with those of malignant lymphoma because of the blurring of normal node architecture and the marked proliferation of immunoblasts and immature plasma cells (*Fig. 42.6*). There may also be infiltration of the node capsule and the perinodal adipose tissue by these cells.

Features suggesting a viral reaction rather than a malignant lymphoma include:

- the predominant distribution of the immunoblasts within the nodal sinuses

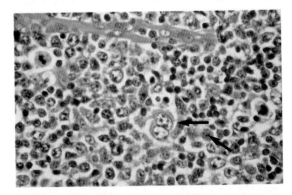

FIGURE 42.6 *Node from a patient with infectious mononucleosis showing large immunoblasts (arrowed) in the centre and some immature plasma cells with basophilic cytoplasm (arrowed).*

- the coincident presence of follicular hyperplasia with a marked degree of mitotic activity within the germinal centres
- an intact sinus pattern showing that the effacement of node architecture is more apparent than real

Expansion of the Antigen-presenting Cell Population: Increase Predominantly in Macrophages

This reaction pattern occurs in two main forms:

1) **The increase in macrophages (histiocytes) is found chiefly within the sinuses.** This pattern is known as 'sinus histiocytosis'.

2) The increase in macrophages involves chiefly the nodal tissue **between** the sinuses, although the latter may also be involved to some extent. This is known as 'pulp histiocytosis'.

Sinus Histiocytosis

This term describes a situation in which the number of macrophages within the sinuses increases with an accompanying increase in the phagocytic activity of these cells. **The sinuses are distended by these large and active macrophages.** Care must be taken to distinguish this condition from one to which it bears some morphological resemblance: a sinus B-cell reaction. Here the sinuses are also distended, not by macrophages but by B cells that have a morphological resemblance to monocytes (**monocytoid B lymphocytes**). The true nature of these cells can be determined by the fact that they express markers typical for B cells of a rather distinctive phenotype. This accumulation of monocytoid B cells within nodal sinuses is especially likely to be seen in toxoplasmosis and in acquired immune deficiency syndrome (AIDS).

Sinus Histiocytosis with Massive Lymphadenopathy (Rosai–Dorfman Disease)

This disorder, which usually occurs within the first two decades of life, is characterized clinically by:

- massive, painless, bilateral lymph node enlargement in the neck
- fever, leucocytosis, a raised erythrocyte sedimentation rate and polyclonal hypergammaglobulinaemia
- spontaneous resolution in most cases

The condition occurs more commonly in Afro-Caribbeans than in Caucasians; in addition to nodal involvement, other tissues such as the orbit, upper respiratory tract, central nervous system, salivary glands, skin, bones and other tissue may be affected in up to 25% of cases.

Microscopic Features

Affected nodes are very much enlarged and the sinuses are enormously distended, resulting in atrophy of other nodal elements. Most of the cells occupying the sinuses are macrophages with a large vesicular nucleus and abundant cytoplasm in which lipid is not infrequently seen. In addition, many of these macrophages contain intact lymphocytes, a process to which the term **emperipolesis** has been applied. The macrophages express the protein S-100 and some of them contain immunoglobulin which has, presumably, been endocytosed.

The cause is unknown and there is no specific treatment. In many cases, resolution occurs quite quickly, but in a minority the disorder drags on for years.

'Pulp' Histiocytosis

Insoluble material may produce a reaction characterized by emigration of macrophages from the sinuses into the paracortical zone. The most common example of this is the accumulation of carbon and certain other dusts within hilar and mediastinal nodes in exposed individuals. A similar picture due to the introduction of foreign material to the host may be seen in the form of silicon elastomers, used for prosthetic joints, and radio-opaque contrast media, used in lymphangiography. Similar paracortical macrophage accumulations may be seen in Whipple's disease and in certain storage diseases arising from the absence of particular lysosomal enzymes.

Dermatopathic Lymphadenopathy

This occurs in the superficial nodes of patients with certain skin diseases. These include psoriasis, chronic exfoliative dermatitis and mycosis fungoides (see pp 969–971, 990–994), and any other condition in which itching and scratching are prominent clinical features. A common feature of all these is breakdown of epidermal cells; the resulting debris is taken up by macrophages which then migrate to draining nodes. These macrophages contain large amounts of lipid (derived from cell walls) and melanin. This leads to a marked expansion of the paracortical zone as a result of infiltration by large pale cells (*Fig. 42.7*). Some are true macrophages containing the breakdown products of the epidermal cells, whereas others are **interdigitating reticulum cells**, which are not phagocytic. Plasma cell infiltration and follicular hyperplasia may accompany this paracortical expansion.

EFFECTS OF SPECIFIC AETIOLOGICAL AGENTS ON LYMPH NODES

INFECTIVE AGENTS: BACTERIAL

Mycobacterial Lymphadenitis (e.g. Tuberculosis)

Nodal involvement by tuberculosis is seen especially in cases where a **'primary complex'** develops. This consists essentially of a small parenchymal lesion in the

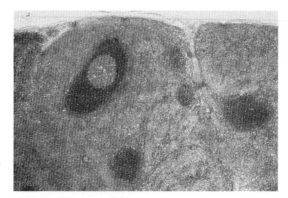

FIGURE 42.7 Dermatopathic lymphadenitis. There is marked expansion of the paracortical area by an infiltrate of pale cells (principally macrophages) against which the dark lymphocytes of the cortical follicles stand out.

affected organ or tissue which soon becomes associated with massive enlargement of the draining nodes. Because the primary portal of entry of the organisms is most commonly the lung, it is the hilar and mediastinal nodes that are most often affected in this way. In children, especially in regions where the prevalence of tuberculosis is high, it is not uncommon to see enlargement of cervical nodes due to ingested mycobacteria. The organisms presumably pass from the pharynx to the draining nodes and set up a caseating granulomatous response in these nodes. The old term for this was **scrofula**.

Macroscopic Features

The enlarged nodes are matted together due to the formation of adhesions between their capsules. On section, the typical 'cheesy' lesions of caseating tuberculosis may be seen if involvement is severe.

Microscopic Features

Numerous granulomas, composed principally of epithelioid cells (macrophages that show a secretory rather than a phagocytic phenotype), are seen. The centres of some or all of these undergo caseation necrosis with replacement of their cell population by featureless areas of eosinophilic necrosis with a high lipid content. The extent and severity of the necrosis correlates with the degree of tissue hypersensitivity to antigenic components of the mycobacterium.

Lymph nodes may be involved by infections caused by mycobacteria other than *Mycobacterium tuberculosis*.

Mycobacterium Avium Intracellulare (MAI)

MAI belongs to the large group of mycobacteria inhabiting soil and water. As a result this microorganism is frequently inhaled or swallowed. MAI may produce:

- enlarged caseating cervical lymph nodes (scrofula), clinically and pathologically indistinguishable from that caused by *M. tuberculosis*
- an infection characterized by dissemination of infected macrophages throughout the body. This is seen in patients in whom cell-mediated immunity is suppressed and, therefore, is particularly likely to be encountered in patients with AIDS. Because of defective cellular immunity, the usual T cell-mediated activation of macrophages does not take place and affected nodes merely show infiltration by large numbers of macrophages which do not form granulomata. Appropriate special stains show the infiltrating macrophages to be filled with numerous bacilli; the appearance of these cells mimics that of those seen in lepromatous leprosy.
- a pulmonary lesion similar to that seen following primary tuberculosis, in which the lesions tend to localize in the upper pole of the lung and to be associated with a high grade of hypersensitivity leading to extensive necrosis.

Yersinial Lymphadenitis

Enlargement of mesenteric nodes may occur in gut infections caused by two species of *Yersinia*: *Y. pseudotuberculosis* and *Y. enterocolitica*. These are Gram-negative coccoid or oval organisms normally carried by wood pigeons and rats. The patients, usually children, present with a clinical picture not unlike that of acute appendicitis. The ileocaecal nodes are most often affected and are enlarged.

Microscopic Features

Microscopic examination shows oedema, an increase in immunoblasts and plasma cells in both cortical and paracortical zones, follicular hyperplasia and dilatation of sinuses containing many large lymphocytes. If the responsible organism is *Y. pseudotuberculosis*, small granulomas and abscesses are present.

Cat-scratch Disease

Cat-scratch disease is characterized by a **primary skin lesion and enlargement of the draining lymph nodes**. It is believed to be caused by a coccobacillary, extracellular organism (*Bartonella henselae*), identifiable in biopsies by silver staining methods such as the Warthin–Starry stain. As its name implies, cat-scratch disease occurs in households where cats are kept as pets, although it is not necessary for a bite or a scratch to be sustained for the infection to be acquired.

Microscopic Features

The nodal lesions in cat-scratch disease are really characteristic only in the late stages when abscess formation has taken place. These abscesses have a typical pattern in which

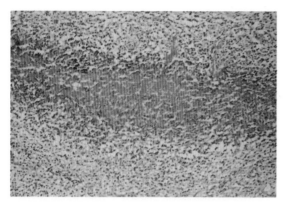

FIGURE 42.8 Cat-scratch disease. The centre of the field is occupied by an eosinophilic necrotic zone containing cellular debris and surrounded at its periphery by macrophages.

there is central necrosis often with a star-like outline. The necrotic tissue contains neutrophils and neutrophil debris, and is surrounded by macrophages arranged in a palisaded fashion (*Fig. 42.8*). Abscesses with a similar appearance may be seen in the nodes of patients suffering from lymphogranuloma venereum. The nodal sinuses in patients with cat-scratch disease are often distended with monocytoid B cells, a feature also seen in toxoplasmosis.

INFECTIVE AGENTS: VIRAL

HIV-related Lymphadenopathy

AIDS is caused by a C-type retrovirus, the **human immunodeficiency virus (HIV) types** 1 and 2. Patients with AIDS may show a wide spectrum of lymph node pathology including opportunistic infections and malignant lymphoma, nodes in the early stages of the disease show a florid form of reactive hyperplasia.

Clinically, affected individuals present with a generalized, painless lymphadenopathy which may be accompanied by fatigue and listlessness. The nodal enlargement often persists for months and this clinical stage is thus referred to as **persistent generalized lymphadenopathy**.

Microscopic Features

Biopsy material usually shows a striking degree of follicular hyperplasia, which may be associated with collections of monocytoid B cells within the sinuses.

In many cases a curious appearance is seen in which mantle zone lymphocytes appear to invade the germinal centres. This is associated with disorganization of the germinal centres themselves, giving a 'moth-eaten' appearance. These follicles may in time shrink and disappear.

Ultrastructural examination of the nodes at the early stages of follicle lysis shows a great prominence of follicular dendritic cells with alterations in the appearance of their processes. This feature has been interpreted as evidence of preferential infection of these cells by the virus.

INFECTIVE AGENTS: PROTOZOAL

Toxoplasmosis

This is caused by the common protozoon, *Toxoplasma gondii*, which parasitizes both humans and a number of other species. **In the UK the commonest reservoir is the domestic cat.** Many individuals show significant titres of *Toxoplasma* antibodies in the serum, despite the absence of a history of any clinical features suggestive of infection; **it is clear that many, perhaps the majority, of *Toxoplasma* infections are subclinical**.

In those in whom the disease surfaces above the clinical horizon, **the commonest manifestation is the appearance of a painless lymphadenopathy**, a common site being nodes in the posterior triangle of the neck. **The disease is not dangerous unless infection occurs during pregnancy, in which case the fetus can become infected and may be born with serious eye and brain defects. However, in individuals in whom cell-mediated immunity is suppressed, most notably sufferers from AIDS, severe, sometimes fatal, infections occur.** These patients may present with a number of clinical syndromes including **encephalitis, pneumonitis** and **choroidoretinitis**.

Microscopic Features

Classically, nodal pathology in toxoplasmosis is characterized by three major morphological changes:
1) follicular hyperplasia with evidence of rapid cell turnover in the form of many mitoses and abundant nuclear debris phagocytosed by macrophages
2) small epithelioid cell granulomas situated both within the hyperplastic follicles and at the periphery of the affected node
3) distension of sinuses by monocytoid B cells (*Fig. 42.9*)

These appearances in a lymph node biopsy are *not* specific and should prompt confirmation of the diagnosis of toxoplasmosis by serological methods. The Sabin–Feldmann dye test depends on the appearance in the patient's serum of antibodies that render the membranes of cultured *T. gondii* impermeable to alkaline methylene blue so that they fail to stain in the presence of serum from an infected individual. A number of other immunological tests have now been developed which makes it unnecessary for laboratory scientists to be exposed to the danger of handling live *T. gondii*.

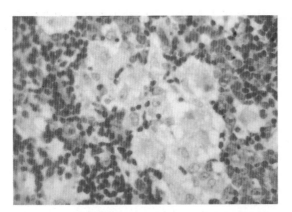

FIGURE 42.9 *Toxoplasmosis in a lymph node. The sinus shown in the centre of the field is distended by large monocytoid cells.*

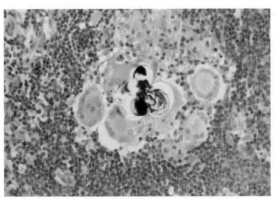

FIGURE 42.10 *A sarcoid granuloma in a lymph node. The lesion, which occupies the centre of the field, consists of several Langerhans-type multinucleate giant cells. One of these contains laminated purple-staining material (conchoidal bodies), which are frequently seen in this condition.*

PATHOLOGICAL ENTITIES OF UNKNOWN AETIOLOGY

Sarcoidosis

Sarcoidosis is a disorder of unknown, possibly infective, aetiology, characterized morphologically by numerous small, well-defined, non-caseating granulomas. These lesions can occur in virtually every tissue and the clinical manifestations depend on their localization and the extent of involvement in the affected organ or tissue.

In Europe, inhabitants of Scandinavian countries have an increased risk of developing sarcoidosis, and in the USA the disease is 10 to 15 times more frequent in Afro-Americans than in Caucasians.

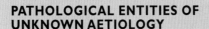

Microscopic Features

In lymph nodes, as in other tissues, small, very well-demarcated granulomas are seen. These consist of epithelioid cells with which a few Langhans-type multinucleate giant cells and helper T cells may be associated. Necrosis is absent or takes the form of central fibrinoid necrosis not difficult to distinguish from the caseation necrosis so typical of tuberculosis. The giant cells sometimes contain one of a number of different types of inclusion, such as:

- Schaumann bodies (rounded, laminated bodies containing iron and calcium) (*Fig. 42.10*)
- star-shaped ('asteroid') bodies made up of criss-crossing bundles of collagen fibres
- crystals of calcium oxalate

None of these is specific for sarcoidosis, and its diagnosis by histopathologists is really one of exclusion, as this histological picture may be encountered in a wide variety of other conditions both infective and non-infective. These include tuberculosis, brucellosis, some fungal infections, leishmaniasis, leprosy, tularaemia, atypical mycobacterial infection, zirconium granuloma, chalazion in the eyelid, Hodgkin's disease and nodes draining a carcinoma.

The cause of sarcoidosis is still not known. The macrophages in the granulomas are clearly activated, because they express two activation markers, interleukin (IL)1 and the ligand that binds the antibody Ki-67. Some workers have suggested that sarcoidosis represents a quantitative disturbance in the response to antigen, which may well be mycobacterial in nature. For further discussion of sarcoidosis see pp 168–169.

Necrotizing Lymphadenitis of Unknown Cause

Kikuchi's Disease

This disorder, which also labours under the name 'histiocytic, necrotizing lymphadenitis without granulocytic infiltration' is seen most frequently in young females in Japan but occurs also in Europe and North America.

Patients present with painless enlargement of lymph nodes in the neck sometimes associated with a mild fever. The cause is unknown but spontaneous recovery is the usual clinical outcome.

The affected nodes show well-demarcated foci of necrosis in the paracortical T-cell zone. These appear to occur in relation to areas of lymphoblastic transformation and are associated with abundant nuclear debris. The relative absence of plasma cells and neutrophils is a helpful diagnostic feature.

Kawasaki's Disease (Mucocutaneous Lymph Node Syndrome)

This is a disorder of infancy and early childhood best classified as a vasculitis (see pp 408–409). The affected lymph nodes are enlarged and contain irregular areas of necrosis. Because these areas are associated with thrombi in small intranodal vessels, it has been suggested that they are small infarcts.

Castleman's Disease (Giant Lymph Node Hyperplasia, Angiofollicular Lymph Node Hyperplasia, Lymph Nodal Hamartoma)

The existence of several synonyms for a single disorder is usually a strong indication that the condition is poorly understood. This is certainly true of Castleman's disease, in which both the basic nature of the clinico-pathological entity and its cause are unknown.

It is a peculiar and rather rare form of lymph node reaction, occurring as nodal enlargement **in a single site** (most commonly the mediastinum) or **in a multi-centric form** affecting nodes in several locations.

Microscopic Features

Castleman's disease exists in two principal morphological forms:

1) **hyaline vascular type.** This shows large follicles in which blood vessel proliferation is prominent. These vessels are surrounded by featureless hyaline material, giving an appearance mistaken by some as a Hassall's corpuscle of the thymus, which it most emphatically is not.

The mantle zone lymphocytes are arranged in concentric layers at the periphery of the follicle centres (*Fig. 42.11*). There is a prominent interfollicular stroma in which blood vessels of postcapillary venule type are again prominent. The cell population in these areas consists of an admixture of plasma cells, eosinophils and immunoblasts. In some instances, the mantle zones are widened and the follicle centres comparatively atrophic. This appearance may give rise to an erroneous diagnosis of follicle-centre cell lymphoma. Some 90% of cases presenting with a localized mass of enlarged nodes are of the hyaline vascular variety.

2) **plasma cell type.** This is characterized by diffuse plasma cell proliferation, seen predominantly in the interfollicular regions of the node. The prominent blood vessels in the follicle centres seen in the hyaline vascular type are absent, but amorphous eosinophilic material may be present in the follicle centres. It has been suggested that this is an admixture of fibrin and immune complex.

Clinical Features

The localized form presents as a single mass, often of impressive size (up to 15 cm in diameter). Although the mediastinum is the commonest site, such masses have been recorded in the lung, neck, axilla, retroperitoneal space, mesentery, broad ligaments and even in the limbs.

The generalized form presents with wide-spread lymphadenopathy.

In both forms there may be associated systemic disturbances such as fever, anaemia, joint pain, sweating, skin rashes and a polyclonal hypergammaglobulin-aemia, although this is more likely to occur in the multicentric form.

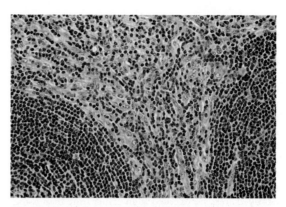

FIGURE 42.11 *Lymph node biopsy from a patient with Castleman's disease of the hyaline vascular type. Note the arrangement of the mantle-zone lymphocytes in concentric layers.*

Natural History

Surgical removal of localized nodal masses causes the constitutional symptoms of Castleman's disease to disappear, but the prognosis in the multicentric form is poor, the median survival being about 2–2.5 years. Some 20–30% of patients with multicentric Castleman's disease develop either Kaposi's sarcoma or a B-cell malignant lymphoma.

Molecular genetic analysis of affected nodes in the multicentric form has shown rearrangement of both immunoglobulin genes and genes for the T-cell receptor; this suggests that this form of the disease may be quite distinct from the localized form, and is consistent with the known tendency for some cases to evolve into a malignant lymphoma.

NEOPLASTIC DISORDERS OF LYMPH NODES

Primary neoplastic disorders are known as malignant lymphomas. They are separated into two main classes:

- **Hodgkin's disease**
- **the non-Hodgkin's lymphomas**

Hodgkin's disease is separated from all the other malignant lymphomas because its clinical and pathological features are sufficiently characteristic for it to be regarded as a distinct entity. The non-Hodgkin's lymphomas comprise a set of different neoplastic disorders of lymphoreticular tissue (nodal and extranodal) that are grouped together because of a negative defining criterion: the absence of features of Hodgkin's disease.

HODGKIN'S DISEASE

Epidemiology

A considerable degree of geographical variation exists in the prevalence of both Hodgkin's disease and non-Hodgkin's lymphoma. In general terms, malignant lymphoreticular disease occurs more commonly in less economically privileged countries and Hodgkin's disease accounts for about 50% of the cases of malignant lymphoma.

Hodgkin's disease is unusual in that the curve of age in relation to incidence is bimodal. There is an early peak in incidence in young adults in developed countries and a second peak in old age. In less developed countries, the peak in early adult life is either attenuated or absent, and there is a greater frequency in children. It has been suggested that the first peak is related to some environmental factor, possibly an infectious agent, to which the inhabitants of economically deprived areas are exposed at an earlier time than is the case in wealthier communities.

The agent most extensively canvassed as an aetiological agent for Hodgkin's disease is the Epstein–Barr virus (EBV). Evidence that lends support to this view includes the following:

- A history of glandular fever is associated with an increased risk of Hodgkin's disease.
- Patients with Hodgkin's disease more frequently have antibodies against EBV in the plasma than do age-matched controls, and the antibody titres, when present, are higher in patients with Hodgkin's disease.
- Molecular biological studies show the presence of part of the EBV genome in the tumour cells of patients with Hodgkin's disease, the Reed–Sternberg cells. In addition, latent membrane protein, one of the gene products of the EBV, has also been localized to Reed–Sternberg cells. It is thought that this protein plays a significant part in EBV-related cell transformation.

Macroscopic Features

Hodgkin's disease usually manifests in the first instance as enlargement of a **single group of lymph nodes**, the cervical nodes being most frequently affected. The individual nodes tend to remain discrete, at least in the earlier stages of the disease, and their cut surfaces may be greyish or a pale tan colour.

The consistency depends on the amount of fibrosis associated with the process and, thus, those subtypes in which such fibrosis is a prominent feature (nodular sclerosing Hodgkin's disease), tend to be associated with considerably increased firmness of affected nodes.

Microscopic Features

The Reed–Sternberg Cell

The most reliable diagnostic indicator of Hodgkin's disease is the presence of Reed–Sternberg cells in an appropriate cellular background (*Fig. 42.12*). A histological diagnosis of Hodgkin's disease should not be made in the **absence** of

these cells, although they may be seen occasionally in conditions other than Hodgkin's disease.

The Reed–Sternberg cell, believed to be the neoplastic cell in Hodgkin's disease, is a large cell with a bilobed nucleus. **The presence of large and prominent eosinophilic nucleoli** is a characteristic feature and these nucleoli are bounded by a clear zone. The nuclear membrane is well defined and there is abundant cytoplasm which either stains deep red with eosin or binds both eosin and haematoxylin, resulting in a reddish-blue colour. Mononuclear cells with otherwise similar characteristics may also be seen in Hodgkin's disease. It has been suggested that their appearance is due to their having been sectioned in a plane that shows only one lobe of the nucleus. They are known as **Hodgkin's cells**.

The origin of the Reed–Sternberg cell has been the subject of much research and controversy. The expression of immunohistochemical markers has been studied both in those instances where Reed–Sternberg cell lines have been established in culture, and at the tissue level in biopsy material.

Both B- and T-cell-associated markers have been identified. The cells express:

- **CD15**, a carbohydrate epitope known as the X-hapten
- **CD25**, the IL-2 receptor
- **CD30**, a marker of activated B and T cells and which is detected by an antibody known as Ki-1. This antigen is also expressed on EBV-transformed B cells, activated macrophages, and on the cells of a large-celled T lymphoma known as Ki-1 lymphoma.

Molecular biological studies of Reed–Sternberg cell lines have shown both B-cell immunoglobulin gene rearrangements and T-cell receptor gene rearrangements. The presence of viral DNA derived from the EBV in more than 35% of these cells has already been mentioned.

On the basis of these data, and many others not quoted here, it has been suggested that **the Reed–Sternberg cell is derived from immature lymphoid cells at vari-**

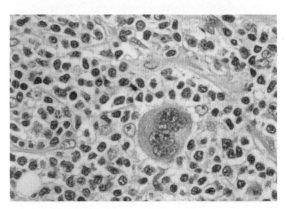

FIGURE 42.12 Hodgkin's disease. A Reed–Sternberg cell showing a lobulated nucleus and prominent nucleoli.

ous stages of differentiation which are transformed before or during B-cell immunoglobulin gene or T-cell receptor gene rearrangement. The malignant cell that results is the stimulus both for the cellular response that is part of the histological picture of Hodgkin's disease and perhaps for the systemic alterations in the immune system that contribute to the clinical picture.

Background Cellular Response in Hodgkin's Disease

Reed–Sternberg cells do not constitute proof of Hodgkin's disease because these cells can be seen in certain other conditions. **It is the combination of Reed–Sternberg cells and an appropriate cellular background that is necessary for the diagnosis to be made. This response to the neoplastic cells is always associated with distortion or, more commonly, loss of the normal architectural pattern of the node**, sometimes with the T-cell and sometimes with the B-cell zones being predominantly affected.

Several cell types make up the background to the neoplastic cells. These include lymphocytes, plasma cells, eosinophils, macrophages and granulocytes. In general, the lymphocyte population is made up of small normal-looking cells, most of which are T lymphocytes, helper cells being present in greater numbers than suppressor cells. In some cases of lymphocyte predominance subtype of Hodgkin's disease, the background lymphocytes comprise both B and T cells and may look very atypical as a result of immunological activation.

The pattern of reaction to the neoplastic Reed–Sternberg cells has important implications for the natural history in Hodgkin's disease and, indeed, is a highly significant factor in classifying Hodgkin's disease into its various subtypes. This subject is discussed in the next section. **In general terms, however, it is important to remember that prognosis worsens in cases where there are large numbers of neoplastic Reed–Sternberg cells and a weak lymphocyte response, the reverse being true in cases where lymphocytes predominate and neoplastic cells are present in relatively small numbers.**

Classification

The classification system currently used for Hodgkin's disease is based on the **Rye classification, in which four histological types are described**. This classification has now been modified with one main subtype, **lymphocyte predominance Hodgkin's disease, being further divided into three subclasses** (*Table 42.7*).

Lymphocyte Predominance Hodgkin's Disease

The defining criteria are a relatively small population of neoplastic cells and a relatively large population of reactive lymphocytes. The neoplastic cells in all the subtypes of lymphocyte predominance Hodgkin's disease differ from classical Reed–Sternberg cells. These cells, which are known as L & H or 'popcorn' cells, have multilobed nuclei in which small, usually basophilic, nucleoli are present. The cytoplasm is scanty and is usually basophilic. L & H cells express CD30, CD45 and epithelial membrane antigen but, unlike true Reed–Sternberg cells, are negative in respect of CD15. This disorder is currently grouped with the other forms of Hodgkin's disease, but an increasing body of opinion suggests that it is not, in fact, Hodgkin's disease at all but may instead be a form of B-cell lymphoma.

Nodular Form

This is the commonest form of lymphocyte predominance Hodgkin's disease. It can occur at any age but the peak incidence is in the fourth decade and it is very rare over the age of 40 years. There is a distinct predilection for males. It arises in nodes in the neck, axilla or inguinal region and, unlike certain other types of Hodgkin's disease, is rarely if ever found in the mediastinum. The nodules that give this variant its name are often very poorly delineated and in some instances may be recognized only if sections are stained with silver to show the reticulin framework of the node. The L & H cell is found in considerable numbers, often arranged in small aggregates, but classical Reed–Sternberg cells are difficult to find.

Table 42.7 Classification of Hodgkin's Disease

Rye classification	Frequency (%)	Modified Rye classification*
Lymphocyte predominance	< 10	Lymphocyte predominance: ● nodular ● diffuse ● lymphocyte predominance ('mixed')
Nodular sclerosing	50–75	Nodular sclerosing
Mixed cellularity	17	Mixed cellularity
Lymphocyte-depleted	4	Lymphocyte-depleted

*From Poppema, Lennart and Kaiserling (1979).

Apart from the neoplastic L & H cells, the nodules are made up chiefly of small lymphocytes, amongst which a number of macrophages may be seen. The macrophage population in the nodules tends to be less in the nodular than in the diffuse form of lymphocyte predominance Hodgkin's disease.

Diffuse Form

In this form, the normal lymph node structure is replaced by a diffuse infiltrate consisting predominantly of small lymphocytes. Macrophages are also present and may be distributed either randomly or in the form of small granulomas. Classical Reed–Sternberg cells are hard to find and L & H variants are scattered in a diffuse fashion through the lymphocyte infiltrate. Unlike what is found in the nodular pattern, the L & H cells do not express B-cell markers and it has been suggested that at least some of the cases diagnosed as diffuse lymphocyte predominance Hodgkin's disease are in fact T-cell lymphomas.

Nodular Sclerosing Hodgkin's Disease

This is by far the commonest histological type of Hodgkin's disease occurring in the highly developed countries of the West. It arises typically in young adults (below the age of 40 years) and shows a predilection for females. An origin in the anterior mediastinum is common but this variant can arise in other node groups as well.

Microscopic Features

In nodular sclerosing Hodgkin's disease:
- A striking fibrous tissue response is seen. The gland is divided up by bands of hyaline, collagen-rich, fibrous tissue which delineate cellular nodules.
- A variant form of neoplastic cell is found, which is known as a **lacunar cell**. This is a large cell with a multilobed nucleus, relatively small nucleoli and abundant pale-staining cytoplasm. With fixation in formaldehyde, this cytoplasm retracts from surrounding cells leaving a space or lacuna between its plasma membrane and the surrounding cellular infiltrate.
- Classical Reed–Sternberg cells may be difficult to find and, if this is the case, the presence of lacunar cells can be regarded as adequate grounds for the diagnosis.
- The reactive cellular component shows considerable variation, and areas of necrosis and granuloma formation are not infrequently seen.

In the UK, nodular sclerosing Hodgkin's disease has been subdivided into two subtypes. In type 1, tumour nodules show either lymphocyte predominance or mixed cellularity. In type 2, more than 50% of the nodules show either lymphocyte depletion or a mixed cell background associated with marked variability of the tumour cells.

Mixed Cellularity Hodgkin's Disease

This type accounts for about 17% of cases of Hodgkin's disease in the UK. The name is derived from the fact that the reactive cellular background of the neoplastic cells is, in most instances, heterogeneous. In Western countries it tends to occur chiefly in older individuals, but in Third World countries it may be seen in much younger patients.

Microscopic Features

Defining criteria are:
- a substantial number of classical Reed–Sternberg cells and Hodgkin's cells
- a cellular response including not only lymphocytes and macrophages but also significant numbers of plasma cells, neutrophils and eosinophils
- a connective tissue response which lacks the banded and hyalinized pattern seen in nodular sclerosing Hodgkin's disease and is, instead, rather disorganized.

Lymphocyte-depleted Hodgkin's Disease

This is the rarest form of Hodgkin's disease in Britain (about 4% of cases) and carries the worst prognosis. It is, however, somewhat more common in less developed countries. It is a disease of late adult life and, unlike other subtypes, quite often involves extranodal sites such as the bone marrow.

Microscopic Features

Two histological patterns exist, known as:
- **the reticular form**
- **the diffuse fibrosing form**

In the first there are sheets of rather pleomorphic Reed–Sternberg and Hodgkin's cells. The reactive cellular infiltrate shows only a poor lymphocyte response, although a considerable number of macrophages may be identified.

The diffuse fibrosing form is characterized by both pleomorphic and classical Reed–Sternberg cells set in an amorphous, collagen-poor background which is virtually depleted of reactive cells. The patients often present with systemic symptoms rather than with lymph node enlargement; bone marrow and liver involvement are common.

The frequency and natural history of the subtypes of Hodgkin's disease, as seen in the UK, are shown in *Table 42.8* and *Fig. 42.13*.

Staging

Histological subtype has an important influence on prognosis, but it is not the only factor. As with any other malignant neoplasm, the extent of spread – or 'stage' – is also significant in predicting survival.

The most widely used staging system for Hodgkin's disease is the Ann Arbor system, shown in *Table 42.9*.

Table 42.8 Natural History and Frequency of Histological Types of Hodgkin's Disease in the UK

Type	Frequency (%)	5-year survival rate (%)	15-year survival rate (%)
Lymphocyte predominance	6.2	92	64
Nodular sclerosing type 1	46.8	81	62
Nodular sclerosing type 2	26.2	66	49
Mixed cellularity	18.7	72	50
Lymphocyte-depleted	1.4	40	0

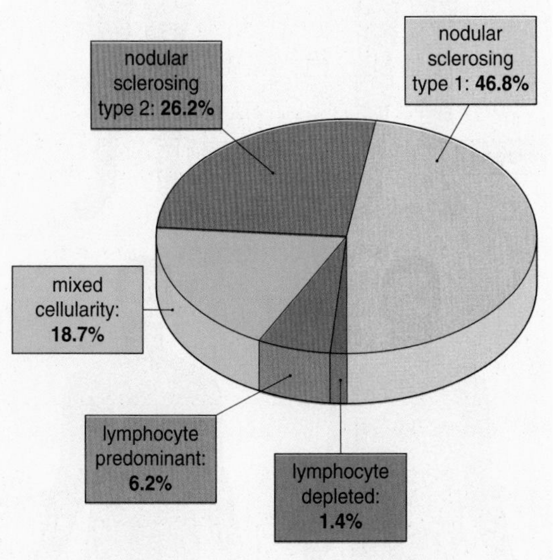

FIGURE 42.13 *Distribution of the histological types of Hodgkin's disease.*

Table 42.9 Ann Arbor System for Staging Hodgkin's Disease

Stage	Extent of spread
1	Involvement of a single lymph node region, or of a single extranodal organ or site (1E)
2	Involvement of two or more lymph node regions on the same side of the diaphragm, or of one extranodal organ plus one or more lymph node regions on same side of diaphragm (2E)
3	Involvement of lymph node regions on both sides of the diaphragm, of one extranodal site plus the lymph nodes on both sides of the diaphragm (3E), or of the spleen (3S) or both spleen (*Fig. 42.14*) and one other extranodal site (3SE)
4	Diffuse or disseminated involvement of one or more extranodal tissues with or without associated lymph node involvement (e.g. 4H = liver involvement)

Any of these stages may be followed by the suffix A or B, where:
- A is the absence of systemic clinical symptoms such as fever, etc.
- B is the presence of one or more of the following clinical features:
  1) unexplained fever above 38°C
  2) night sweats
  3) loss of 10% or more of body-weight within a 6-month period

Also important at any stage is the presence of 'bulky' disease – a nodal mass greater than 10 cm in diameter or widening of the mediastinum by more than one-third.

Staging is accomplished by means of a number of diagnostic approaches which include:
- chest radiography. This will help to detect mediastinal, lung or hilar node involvement.
- bone marrow trephine
- liver biopsy
- computed tomography (CT) or magnetic resonance

imaging. These are extremely helpful in detecting intrathoracic, intra-abdominal and pelvic masses.

Until recently, staging laparotomy, which involved splenectomy, a wedge biopsy of the liver and node sampling, was recommended for patients thought to have stage 1 or 2 disease. The increase in the power of imaging modalities such as CT, and the tendency to use not only radiotherapy but chemotherapy for patients thought to have stage 1 or 2 disease, has greatly lessened the need for staging laparotomy. Staging laparotomy is not without danger; in particular, there is a significantly increased risk of widespread sepsis as a result of splenectomy.

The Ann Arbor system of staging Hodgkin's disease is summarized in *Fig. 42.15.*

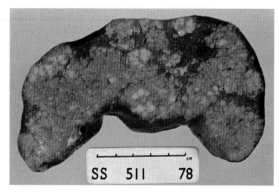

FIGURE 42.14 *Spleen showing extensive infiltration by Hodgkin's disease.*

Effect of Hodgkin's Disease on the Immune System

Irrespective of the immunosuppression resulting from treatment, it has been clear for many years that Hodgkin's disease is associated with **significant downregulation of cellular immune responses**, while, in general, humoral responses remain within normal limits. In addition, non-specific activities such as granulocyte responses to chemotactic agents are also depressed. As a result, patients with Hodgkin's disease show a significantly increased risk of infection especially with opportunistic pathogens such as fungi, viruses and mycobacteria.

Several possible mechanisms have been investigated, with rather mixed results. Currently it is suggested that depressed cellular immunity may be due to enhanced sensitivity to suppressor macrophages and suppressor T cells. In addition, there appear to be defects in IL-2 secretion by T cells. This may be purely quantitative in that synthesis and secretion are diminished, but there is also evidence that a non-functional variant of IL-2 may be produced in some cases. It is interesting that circulating, soluble IL-2 receptors are present in excess in patients with Hodgkin's disease compared with controls. These circulating receptors may interfere with IL-2-dependent stimulation of T cells and of natural killer (NK) cells.

NON-HODGKIN'S LYMPHOMA

The term non-Hodgkin's lymphoma covers a wider spectrum of lymphoreticular neoplasms than is the case with Hodgkin's disease, where the defining histological criteria are much more straightforward and much more circumscribed.

Classification

The recognition of different natural histories and different responses to treatment of neoplasms within the rubric of non-Hodgkin's lymphoma has been the dri-

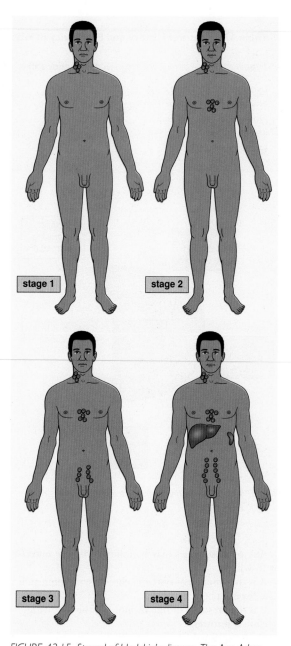

FIGURE 42.15 *Spread of Hodgkin's disease. The Ann Arbor system of staging.*

ving force to find ever better classifications of this group of neoplasms. Accurate assignment of a given lymphoma to an appropriate group may not only guide the clinician to choose the most appropriate form of treatment, but may lead to a better understanding of the biology of this fascinating set of diseases.

In earlier classification systems, the immunological functions of lymphocytes were not understood and, in particular, the existence of the two major classes of lymphocyte, the B and T cells, was not recognized. With the help of an increasingly large number of monoclonal antibodies that recognize antigens representing different stages of development and differentiation of lymphocytes, **it is now believed that the non-Hodgkin's lymphomas recapitulate to a considerable extent the ontogeny of lymphocytes, i.e. that each clonal tumour represents a stage in the development and differentiation of lymphoid cells** (*Fig. 42.16*).

Thus, in the mid-1970s, Lukes and associates in the USA and Lennert and colleagues in Germany put forward new classifications, largely based, so far as B-cell tumours are concerned, on the realization that the nodules described by others were in fact abnormal follicles

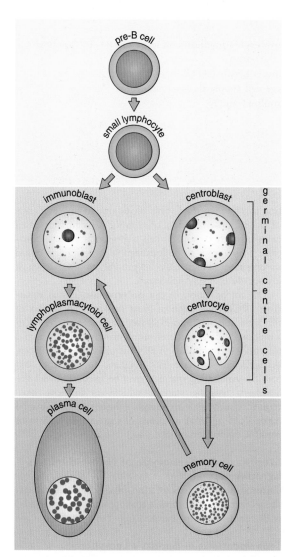

FIGURE 42.16 *Pathways of B-lymphocyte differentiation within and without the follicle centre. Clones of malignant cells may arise at any stage of differentiation.*

and that follicle centre cells played an important part in non-Hodgkin's lymphoma. In 1988, an updated version of the Kiel classification covering both B- and T-cell tumours was published (*Table 42.10*), which, on the whole, works well in relation to B-cell tumours. The proposed classification of T-cell tumours should be regarded as provisional; T-cell lymphomas are very difficult to classify because 'their microscopic appearances are inconstant, not only between cases but even in serial biopsies'(Lennert).

Working Formulation for Clinical Usage

Many other classifications of non-Hodgkin's lymphoma have been proposed. To assist oncologists who might have difficulty in comparing cases, a method for translating the results obtained with one classification to another was proposed. This is known as the **Working Formulation for Clinical Usage**. The original intentions of those who drew up the Working Formulation have been largely disregarded and it is now used simply as a pathological classification. The formulation uses criteria that are exclusively morphological, using the terms 'cleaved' and 'non-cleaved' cells instead of centrocyte and centroblast, and does not distinguish between B- and T-cell lymphomas. Nevertheless, because it is used so widely in North America, the appropriate Working Formulation (WF) term is given alongside that derived from the Kiel classification, where descriptions of individual lymphomas are given, as is that derived from the REAL classification (see below).

Revised European–American Classification of Lymphoid Neoplasms (REAL)

Recently a group of distinguished haematopathologists (International Lymphoma Study Group) put forward the view that 'the most practical approach to lymphoma categorization at this time, is simply to define the diseases that we think we can recognize with the currently available techniques'. This forms the basis of a proposed new classification, currently termed the REAL classification.

New Methods for the Study of Lymphoma

Immunophenotyping and the techniques of molecular genetics have greatly improved our ability to attribute cases of non-Hodgkin's lymphoma to various categories and have assisted our understanding of this set of disorders.

Immunophenotyping

More than 100 individual leucocyte antigens exist which can be identified by the use of monoclonal antibodies. The common nomenclature now used to identify leucocyte antigens is the **CD (cluster of differentiation)** system. The antigens expressed by an individual leucocyte provide a variety of information which includes:

Table 42.10 Updated Kiel Classification of Non-Hodgkin's Lymphoma

B-cell tumours	T-cell tumours
Low grade	**Low grade**
Lymphocytic (chronic lymphocytic and prolymphocytic leukaemia)	**Lymphocytic** (chronic lymphocytic and prolymphocytic leukaemia)
Hairy cell leukaemia	**Small cerebriform cell** (mycosis fungoides, Sézary's syndrome)
Lymphoplasmacytic/cytoid (LP immunocytoma)	**Lymphoepithelioid** (Lennert's lymphoma)
Plasmacytic	**Angioimmunoblastic**
Centroblastic/centrocytic (follicular, diffuse, follicular and diffuse)	**T-zone lymphoma**
	Pleomorphic small cell lymphoma (HTLV-positive or negative)
High grade	**High grade**
Centroblastic	**Pleomorphic medium and large cell** (HTLV-1 positive or negative)
Immunoblastic	**Immunoblastic** (HTLV-1 positive or negative)
Large cell anaplastic (Ki-1 positive)	**Large cell anaplastic** (Ki-1 positive)
Burkitt's lymphoma	**Lymphoblastic**
Lymphoblastic	
Rare types	Rare types

HTLV, human T-lymphotropic virus.

- the lineage (B cell, T cell, macrophage, red cell, platelet)
- the state of differentiation
- the state of activation (e.g. the presence of the activation marker, CD30, may indicate that aggressive behaviour is likely)
- the presence of different surface associated ligands and/or membrane-bound enzymes

Molecular Genetics

Immunophenotyping will usually reveal the **lineage of the cells in a given lymphoma**. Similarly, in many cases monoclonality of B-cell tumours can be established by immunohistological methods as **clonality is expressed by light chain restriction of the surface immunoglobulin on the neoplastic B cells (i.e. a single clone of B cells will express either κ or λ light chains but not both)**.

Establishing the clonality of T cells cannot be accomplished in this way. **Instead the receptor genes of the T cells may be studied to see whether they show rearrangement differing from that in the germ-cell line.** This is accomplished by **Southern blotting** of the T-cell DNA using probes derived from the DNA loci corresponding to the T-cell receptor genes or, in the case of B-cell tumours, immunoglobulin genes. In this way, clones which make up as little as 1–5% of the cells in a given popula-

tion can be identified. This allows one to find evidence of occult dissemination of tumour cells in individual cases of both B- and T-cell lymphomas which, clinically, may appear to be localized (e.g. peripheral blood involvement which may be present in some cases of low-grade B-cell lymphomas).

The introduction of the **polymerase chain reaction (PCR)** has been of great assistance in studies of this kind. The technique allows amplification, by up to a million-fold, of predetermined stretches of DNA, and thus only tiny amounts of DNA (from a single cell) may be sufficient to start the reaction. In addition, old paraffin-embedded material may be used. Thus all the Southern blotting studies, which up to now have required fresh tissue in adequate amounts, can now be carried out on small amounts of material derived from paraffin-embedded blocks.

Studies of the Genotype of Non-Hodgkin's Lymphomas

Chromosomal analysis of non-Hodgkin's lymphomas shows certain translocations that appear to be associated with certain specific disorders (see *Table 42.11*).

Translocations in Burkitt's Lymphoma

The first chromosomal abnormality of this kind to be discovered in malignant lymphoma was a **t(8;14)** translocation associated with a B-cell lymphoblastic

Table 42.11 Chromosomal Abnormalities in Non-Hodgkin's Lymphomas: B-cell Neoplasms

Abnormality	Lymphoma type	Oncogene	Juxtaposed gene
t(8;14)	Burkitt's lymphoma (tropical and non-tropical)	*c-myc*	Ig heavy chain
t(8;22)			Ig κ
t(2;8)			Ig λ
(8 q24 involved in all three)			
t(14;18)	Centroblastic/centrocytic	*bcl-2*	Ig heavy chain
t(11;14)	Centrocytic (intermediate cell) mainly in mantle zone	*bcl-1 (PRAD 1)*	Ig heavy chain
Trisomy 12	Small lymphocytic B-cell chronic leukaemia		
t(14;19)	B-cell chronic lymphocytic	*bcl-3*	Ig heavy chain
t(3;22)	Centroblastic/centrocytic (large celled)		Ig λ

lymphoma, Burkitt's lymphoma. This occurs preferentially, but not exclusively, in a zone that crosses equatorial Africa and appears to be related to the presence in this geographical location of endemic malaria. On culture, the neoplastic lymphoblasts contain the herpesvirus, now known as Epstein–Barr virus (EBV).

The break point in the long arm of chromosome 8 occurs at the site of the *c-myc* oncogene, which is translocated to chromosome 14 coming to lie in close proximity to the gene encoding the heavy chain of immunoglobulin. This results in loss of normal regulation of expression of the *c-myc* gene and this leads to increased proliferation of the cells of the affected clone. This translocation is present in 75% of cases of Burkitt's lymphoma whether they occur in tropical Africa or not. Other translocations that have been described in association with this tumour are **t(8;22)** and **t(2;8)**. In these variants, the *c-myc* oncogene remains in its normal position on the long arm of chromosome 8, while the genes for the κ and λ chains translocate to chromosome 8, also resulting in deregulation of the *c-myc* oncogene. Activation of the *c-myc* depends on enhancer-like elements in the immunoglobulin heavy and light chain genes which are activated by some factor(s) still unknown.

Translocations in Centroblastic/Centrocytic Lymphoma

There is a close association between centroblastic/centrocytic lymphoma and a **t(14;18)** translocation. The translocation is found in both small and large cell variants being, however, much more common in the former. Geographical location of patients with these lymphomas seems to influence the frequency with which the translocation can be identified: t(14;18) is commonest in the USA (90%), somewhat less common in Europe (70%) and least common in Japan (30%).

The translocation involves the movement of an oncogene, *bcl-2*, from the long arm of chromosome 18 to a position adjacent to the immunoglobulin heavy chain gene on the long arm of chromosome 14. The translocation is said to occur before the small lymphocyte enters its various stages of differentiation within the follicle centre.

The gene product of *bcl-2* is a 25-kDa protein, localized to the inner mitochondrial membranes and believed to prolong the cell cycle by inhibiting apoptosis. In this way, neoplastic cells with this translocation have a definite survival advantage.

A type of low-grade centrocytic lymphoma (intermediate cell lymphoma) commonly arising from lymphocytes in the mantle zone is associated with a **t(11;14)** translocation. In this, an oncogene known as *bcl-1* comes to lie in juxtaposition to the heavy chain of immunoglobulin. There is evidence suggesting that *bcl-1* is identical with a candidate oncogene known as **PRAD 1**, which is translocated to lie in proximity to the gene that codes for parathyroid hormone in a subset of parathyroid adenomas. The gene product of *bcl-1* (PRAD 1) is a protein that shows considerable similarity to the cyclins, which complex with and activate a protein kinase known as **cdc2.** This activation regulates progress through the cell cycle. The cyclin-like protein is overexpressed in lymphoproliferative disorders involving the t(11;14) translocation. These translocations are summarized in *Table 42.11*.

Chromosomal Abnormalities in T-cell Lymphomas

T-cell neoplasms have been less extensively studied in terms of non-random translocations than their B-cell counterparts. Certain translocations have, however, been identified and these seem chiefly to affect T-cell receptor gene loci. Abnormalities in the long arm of chromosome 14 have been noted in association with several different T-cell neoplasms including lymphoblastic lymphoma, T-cell acute lymphocytic leukaemia (T-ALL), adult T-cell leukaemia/lymphoma (ATLL) and T-cell chronic lymphocytic leukaemia (T-CLL). The 14q11–14 region contains the loci for the α and δ chains of the T-cell receptor.

Viral Associations with Non-Hodgkin's Lymphoma

Two viruses have been implicated in the genesis of non-Hodgkin's lymphoma:

- **EBV**
- **HTLV-1**

Epstein–Barr Virus

In African endemic Burkitt's lymphoma, EBV DNA can be found to be integrated in the neoplastic B-cell genome in 95% of cases. In contrast, only 15% of non-endemic cases show this; these findings suggest that EBV infection is not the **direct cause** of Burkitt's lymphoma. This is not to say that it is not important in the genesis of the endemic form of the disease.

Mature B cells express the antigen CD21, the receptor for EBV. In children in tropical Africa and in immunosuppressed individuals in other areas, the viral infection is usually of a latent type in which the viral number is low and cell lysis does not occur. Instead, EBV infection in these cells causes B-cell proliferation that is not ultimately halted by T cells, as in infectious mononucleosis. In those in whom cell-mediated immunity is suppressed (in tropical Africa this is probably because of endemic malaria), the virally induced B-cell proliferation proceeds unchecked. This provides favourable circumstances for c-*myc*-activating events to occur, such as one of the translocations discussed previously (*Fig. 42.17*). As a result, a neoplastic B-cell clone emerges.

Human T-cell Lymphotropic Virus

This virus is an oncogenic C-type retrovirus infecting CD4 (T helper) cells. The effect of HTLV-1 infections is probably due to the transcriptional regulators found in the long terminal repeat regions of the virus. The *tax* (transactivator) gene product enhances the expression of the genes encoding the IL-2 receptor and IL-2 itself. As a result of the increase in these two products, deregulated T-cell proliferation can occur. Initially this is polyclonal but eventually in some cases a mutational event occurs with the emergence of a neoplastic clone in the form of adult T-cell leukaemia/lymphoma. The patients usually present with enlargement of the liver and spleen. Neoplastic infiltration of the skin is common, as is hypercalcaemia and increased plasma concentrations of lactic dehydrogenase. The disease is usually rapidly fatal (see p 928).

HTLV-1 infection is endemic in certain geographical locations:

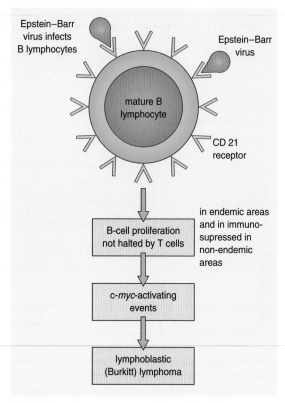

FIGURE 42.17 Pathogenetic events in Burkitt's lymphoma.

- south-western Japan, where 6–20% of the population is seropositive for HTLV-1
- the Caribbean
- New Guinea
- parts of central Africa and South America

Infection is transmitted via:

- blood transfusion
- sharing of infected needles by drug abusers
- sexual intercourse
- breast milk
- the transplacental route (rare)

Circumstances Favouring the Development of Non-Hodgkin's Lymphoma

The most important circumstance favouring the development of lymphoma is immunodeficiency. This may be congenital or 'primary', or acquired or 'secondary'.

Primary causes of immunodeficiency that have been linked with the subsequent appearance of malignant lymphoma include:

- **ataxia telangiectasia** (see p 119)
- **Wiskott–Aldrich syndrome** (see p 120)
- **common variable immunodeficiency**
- **severe combined immunodeficiency**
- **X-linked lymphoproliferative syndrome.** In this syndrome, EBV plays an important role in the

pathogenesis of lymphocyte proliferation. Infection may be followed by abnormal lymphocyte proliferation or by agammaglobulinaemia or hypogammaglobulinaemia. Some 65–70% of patients with this syndrome develop fulminating infectious mononucleosis after an EBV infection, and 25–35% develop a B-cell lymphoma. These lymphomas are usually extranodal with 75% affecting the intestine; the ileocaecal region is especially likely to be involved.

Secondary causes of immunodeficiency that have been associated with an increased risk of malignant lymphoma include:

- **organ transplants.** Organ transplantation is followed by a 30–60-fold increase in the risk of malignant lymphoma. This is due to the immunosuppressive regimens associated with allogenic grafting. Most cases are related to EBV infection occurring in an immunosuppressed individual.

- **AIDS.** The prevalence of non-Hodgkin's lymphoma in patients with AIDS is about 3–4%. Two types of lymphoma occur in AIDS sufferers:
  1) a systemic or peripheral lymphoproliferation
  2) a primary central nervous system lymphoma.
  EBV DNA sequences are found in almost all patients with this AIDS-related lymphoma in the central nervous system. In the systemic form, only 50% of the cases show integration of EBV DNA in the neoplastic B cells.

- **autoimmune diseases such as Sjögren's disease and Hashimoto's thyroiditis.** There is an increased risk of B-cell lymphomas in elderly patients with Sjögren's disease or Hashimoto's thyroiditis. **These are usually mucosa-associated lymphoid tissue (MALT) lymphomas.**

- **Hodgkin's disease.** Non-Hodgkin's lymphoma may follow Hodgkin's disease in about 1–5% of cases. Two possible sets of factors may operate in this sequence. The first is the defect in cell-mediated immunity associated with Hodgkin's disease. The second is the immunosuppressive effect of treatment. The majority of non-Hodgkin's lymphomas developing in this frame of reference are B-cell tumours.

PATHOLOGY AND NATURAL HISTORY OF B-CELL LYMPHOMAS

About 85% of non-Hodgkin's lymphomas are B-cell tumours.

Low-grade Tumours

Malignant Lymphoma, Lymphocytic (REAL – Small Lymphocytic; WF – ML Small Lymphocytic Consistent with CLL)

This is one of the commonest B-cell lymphomas and is **most frequently associated with chronic lympho-** **cytic leukaemia (CLL)**; it may be confined to nodes in a small minority of cases. It affects typically the middle-aged and elderly.

Differentiation Stage of Cells of Origin

In terms of B-lymphocyte differentiation, **the cell of origin is the small, mature B lymphocyte of the mantle zone**. Enlargement of the nodes is usually generalized and there is extensive marrow involvement, even if the malignant cells are not present in the blood. Splenic and hepatic involvement are also very common.

> ### *Microscopic Features*
>
> This is the one of the very few low-grade B-cell neoplasms that does not show a follicular or nodular pattern. **The normal node architecture is effaced completely by a diffuse infiltrate of small lymphocytes** (*Fig. 42.18*), although in some cases some remaining follicles may be seen. The sheets of small lymphocytes are usually interrupted by ill-defined focal collections of cells with larger nuclei with a more open chromatin pattern, known as **proliferation centres** (*Fig. 42.19*). In some cases, there appears to be transformation of this process into a more malignant one (known as Richter's syndrome) and in this case large bizarre lymphocytes, some multinucleated, are seen.

Immunophenotype

As the tumour arises from mature, if unstimulated, B cells, the malignant cells usually express immunoglobulin (Ig) M and IgD on their surfaces and express the B cell-associated antigens CD19, 20 and 79a. CD23 is also expressed and is useful for distinguishing this disorder from mantle cell lymphoma. The monoclonal nature of the cell proliferation can be shown by light chain restriction of surface immunoglobulin (either κ or λ light chains expressed but not both). Curiously enough, the tumour cells also express CD5, which is

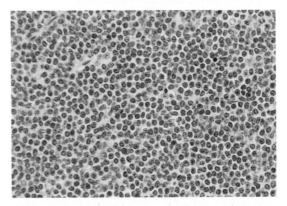

FIGURE 42.18 *Lymphocytic lymphoma (REAL – small lymphocytic lymphoma). The node is replaced by a diffuse infiltrate of small lymphocytes.*

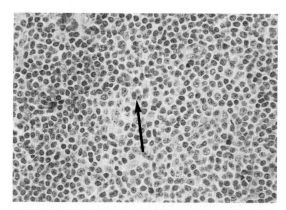

FIGURE 42.19 *Lymphocytic lymphoma. A proliferation centre consisting of somewhat larger and paler cells in the centre of the field (arrowed).*

normally associated with T cells, although a small subset of B cells may normally express this antigen.

Natural History

In general, the disease is slowly progressive and indolent, and may not necessarily cause death. Hypogamma-globulinaemia is quite commonly present, rendering patients very susceptible to bacterial infections.

Malignant Lymphoma, Lymphoplasmacytic (WF – ML Small Lymphocytic Plasmacytoid; REAL – Lymphoplasmacytoid Lymphoma)

This tumour resembles lymphocytic lymphoma but some of the cells differentiate into plasma cells (**lymphoplasmacytic**) or into cells showing some morphological features of plasma cells (**lymphoplas-macytoid**). It is much rarer than lymphocytic lymphoma and is also found chiefly in the middle-aged and elderly. Patients with this disease quite often have CLL. The majority have a monoclonal serum protein of IgM type, resulting in some in hyperviscosity of the plasma (**Waldenström's macroglobulinaemia**).

Microscopic Features

Effacement of normal nodal architecture is not complete and, in some cases, there may be proliferation of malignant lymphocytes in the interfollicular areas with some preservation of follicles. Some tumour cells will be seen to have progressed to the plasma cell stage. Their nuclei will resemble those of normal plasma cells and they have abundant basophilic cytoplasm in which periodic acid–Schiff-positive material (Russell bodies) may be present. Cells that are termed plasmacytoid show nuclei characteristic of small lymphocytes with basophilic cytoplasm similar to that of the plasma cell. Small dot-like bodies composed of immunoglobulin may be present within the nuclei of the plasmacytoid cells; these are known as Dutcher bodies.

Immunophenotype

Both the plasma cells and the plasmacytoid cells contain large amounts of intracellular IgM. IgD is not seen. Lack of CD5 and large amounts of intracytoplasmic immunoglobulin are useful in distinguishing this disorder from B-cell CLL.

Natural History

The disease is an indolent one but is generally not curable.

Malignant Lymphoma, Centroblastic/Centrocytic (WF – Follicular, Mixed Small Cleaved and Large Cell; REAL – Follicle-centre Lymphoma, Cytological Grades I–III)

This follicle-centre cell tumour is the commonest of all non-Hodgkin's lymphomas in developed countries (40% in the USA).

It is predominantly a tumour of late adult life, although occasional cases may be seen in young adults. The commonest clinical presentation is with an enlarged group of nodes or, sometimes, with generalized lymphadenopathy. Dissemination occurs early (*Fig. 42.20*); bone marrow biopsy at the time of clinical presentation frequently shows evidence of marrow involvement.

Microscopic Features

In general the lymph node shows the presence of rather closely packed follicles (*Fig. 42.21*), with obliteration of the sinuses. Mantle zones in relation to these follicles are inconspicuous or absent. This is in marked contrast to what is seen in reactive follicles. The follicles consist predominantly of centrocytes, and centroblasts may be scanty. The greater the proportion of centroblasts and the larger and more atypical the centrocytes, the worse is the prognosis. Loss of the follicular arrangement of the malignant cells with transformation to a diffuse infiltration is also an ominous sign.

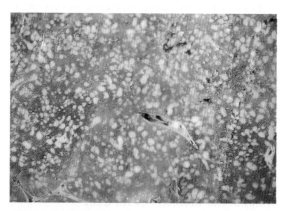

FIGURE 42.20 *Cut surface of the spleen showing numerous small deposits of follicle-centre cell lymphoma.*

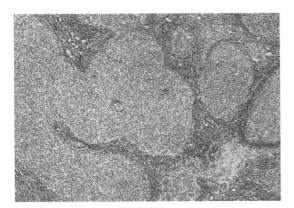

FIGURE 42.21   Centroblastic/centrocytic malignant lymphoma. Numerous closely packed follicles are present. In the left-hand side of the field the infiltration appears diffuse.

Immunophenotype

Immunohistochemical studies can be extremely useful in this disorder. Firstly they enable one, in most cases, to distinguish between reactive follicles in a node that has been antigenically stimulated and the malignant follicles of centroblastic/centrocytic lymphoma, a distinction that, on histological grounds alone, is by no means easy. Secondly they permit an appreciation of the relationship between the tumour cells and those of the normal follicle centre.

In so far as the first is concerned, the cells of the lymphoma show light chain restriction in respect of the surface immunoglobulins and Southern blotting will show the presence of the t(14;18) translocation involving the *bcl-2* oncogene, which encodes an 'antiapoptosis' protein, (see p 963) in a majority of cases (60–90%). CD5 and CD43 are absent (unlike mantle cell lymphoma) and CD10 is present (unlike marginal zone cell lymphomas).

Natural History

The clinical course is usually a long one (7–9 years) and at the time of first presentation there is usually a very satisfactory response to treatment. In most cases, however, the disease will recur, and there may be a fluctuating course with repeated episodes of recurrence and remission. Over time, the histological pattern gradually worsens, with eventual transformation to a higher grade lymphoma both in cytological terms and in terms of transformation from a follicular to a diffuse growth pattern.

Malignant Lymphoma, Centrocytic (WF – ML Diffuse, Small Cleaved Cell; REAL – Mantle Cell Lymphoma)

The cells of this variant appear to be identical with the centrocytes of the follicle centre, but it is no longer thought that centrocytic lymphoma arises from these cells. The disease may present:

- as an isolated lymphadenopathy

- as a primary lymphoma of the spleen or gastrointestinal tract
- with a leukaemic blood picture

> ### Microscopic Features
> The histological picture is distinctly variable. In many cases the normal node structure is replaced by a diffuse infiltrate of small centrocytes. In other instances the growth pattern is nodular. A further variant is seen when some normal follicles survive in the midst of the neoplastic infiltrate and mantle zone cells are replaced by the neoplastic centrocytes. The neoplastic cells are remarkably uniform in appearance, are slightly larger than small lymphocytes and have irregularly shaped nuclei.

Immunophenotype

Immunohistology supports the view that there is a difference between these cells and true centrocytes of follicle-centre origin. The tumour cells express both surface IgM and IgD, unlike true centrocytes which express only IgM. Centrocytes are CD5-positive and CD10-negative, whereas the cells of this tumour show precisely the reverse pattern, being CD5-negative and CD10-positive.

Natural History

The outlook for patients suffering from centrocytic lymphoma is somewhat worse than is the case for the B-cell tumours described in the foregoing section. Treatment usually produces remission when the patient is first seen but the disorder tends to recur and disseminate, with fatal results.

High-grade Tumours

Malignant Lymphoma, Centroblastic (WF – ML Diffuse, Large Non-cleaved Cell; REAL – Diffuse Large B-cell Lymphoma)

This neoplasm has a diffuse growth pattern; the malignant cells show a strong morphological resemblance to the centroblasts of a follicle centre stimulated by antigen. It accounts for about 30–40% of cases of non-Hodgkin's lymphoma in adults, commonly presenting with regional lymphadenopathy, although up to 40% occur extranodally. Dissemination to bone marrow and spleen has often occurred by the time the patient is first seen. The tumour may arise *de novo* in the affected nodes but may also be the result of transformation of a less aggressive follicle-centre cell lymphoma, in which case it is termed a secondary centroblastic lymphoma.

> ### Microscopic Features
> The growth pattern is a diffuse one. The cells have nuclei somewhat larger than those of a macrophage and typically show the presence of two or three small to intermediate-sized nucleoli, which may lie touching the nuclear membrane (*Fig. 42.22*).

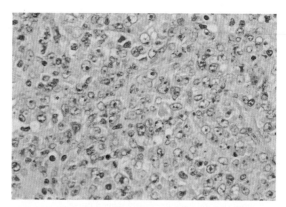

FIGURE 42.22 Malignant lymphoma, centroblastic (REAL – diffuse large B-cell lymphoma). The nuclei are large and show the presence of rather prominent intermediate-sized nucleoli.

Immunophenotype

The tumour cells are clearly B cells (CD19, CD20, CD22 and CD79a positive). They may show the presence of surface immunoglobulin and, if this is the case, light chain restriction will be present. The *bcl-2* gene is rearranged in about 30% of cases.

Natural History

Much depends on the extent of spread at the time of presentation, as modern chemotherapeutic agents are quite effective in this disorder. The Ann Arbor system, which was described in the section relating to Hodgkin's disease, is used for non-Hodgkin's lymphomas as well. In stages I and II, the chances of cure are substantial and even in more advanced disease about one-third of patients survive for 5 years.

Malignant Lymphoma, Immunoblastic (WF – ML Large Cell Immunoblastic; REAL – Large B-cell Lymphoma; Primary Mediastinal Large B-cell Lymphoma)

This is an aggressive neoplasm. The tumour cells are homologues of those that have passed through the centroblast and centrocyte phase and emigrated from the follicle centre. The tumour occurs in adult life (median age of presentation in the fourth decade) and affects females more commonly. The commonest presentation is with a locally invasive, anterior, mediastinal mass arising within the thymus and often causing compression of the airway or the superior vena cava. Relapses are likely to occur in extranodal sites such as the gut, liver, central nervous system, kidneys or ovaries. The 5-year survival rate in treated patients is of the order of 40%.

Microscopic Features

The normal node structure is infiltrated diffusely by a rather uniform large cell population. Cytologically, the constituent cell, the immunoblast, is characterized by a large nucleus with a centrally placed nucleolus and abundant cytoplasm in which a monotypic immunoglobulin can usually be detected. Surface immunoglobulin expression is weak or absent. Plasmacytoid cells may be admixed with the immunoblast population.

Malignant Lymphoma, Burkitt Type (WF – ML Small Non-cleaved Cell, Burkitt's; REAL – Burkitt's Lymphoma)

Burkitt's lymphoma is a distinctive tumour, first described in 1959 by Denis Burkitt. It chiefly affects children and occurs in an **endemic** and a **non-endemic form**.

In the endemic form, the tumour occurs in a belt stretching across equatorial Africa and in certain other locations (see pp 962–963, 964). The median age at diagnosis is 7 years. **Clinically it presents most commonly with gross enlargement and deformation of the jaw and may also involve the retroperitoneal space, the gonads and other viscera, most notably the kidneys.** Some 90% of cases show a characteristic translocation (see pp 962–963). Compelling evidence exists for the implication of EBV in the genesis of this tumour. The EBV genome can be demonstrated in most African patients and in 25–40% of non-African cases associated with AIDS.

Non-endemic Burkitt's lymphoma also affects children, although the age at presentation is somewhat greater than for the endemic tumour.

The principal target tissues appear to be the lymph nodes, gastrointestinal tract and bone marrow; jaw tumours, which are so common in the endemic form, are rare here. In the majority of cases, there is no evidence for an aetiological role for the EBV (except in relation to AIDS), although the same translocations involving the c-*myc* oncogene are present.

Microscopic Features

The affected tissues are diffusely infiltrated by a rather uniform cell population consisting of medium-sized blast cells with two to five nucleoli abutting against the nuclear membrane. There has been argument as to the nature of the tumour cell in Burkitt's lymphoma; many now regard it as arising from a B cell of unknown differentiation stage. Many mitoses show that cell proliferation is proceeding at a rapid rate. Cell death is also a prominent feature and, as a result, macrophages infiltrate the tumour and phagocytose the debris resulting from this rapid cell turnover. The presence of large pale macrophages set against a background of smaller and darker cells gives a characteristic picture, termed a **'starry sky'** pattern (Fig. 42.23).

Immunophenotype

All Burkitt's lymphomas are B-cell tumours and usually express a μ heavy chain and a single type of light

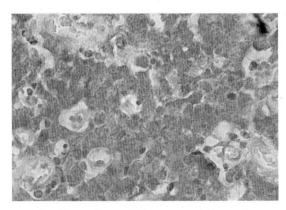

FIGURE 42.23 *Burkitt lymphoma showing the characteristic 'starry sky' appearance caused by the focal presence of macrophages set against a background of a diffuse lymphoblastic infiltrate.*

chain. Most are CD10 positive. In the endemic and AIDS-associated form, the cells show incorporation of part of the EBV genome and also express receptors for C3d.

Natural History

The outlook for patients with this tumour has been dramatically altered by chemotherapy. Before this treatment became available, the disease was uniformly and rapidly fatal, but cures can now be achieved in about 40% of cases.

Malignant Lymphoma, Lymphoblastic (B Cell) (WF – ML Lymphoblastic; REAL – Precursor B-lymphoblastic Lymphoma/Leukaemia)

Most patients who develop this tumour are children. At the time of diagnosis many will have acute lymphoblastic leukaemia, and those who are not in a leukaemic phase when first seen are very likely to develop leukaemia. The leukaemic aspect is discussed on pp 931–933. The tumour cells are CD10 positive in some instances. Those patients not expressing this antigen have a better prognosis.

PATHOLOGY AND NATURAL HISTORY OF T-CELL LYMPHOMAS

T-cell tumours are much less common than B-cell tumours in western Europe and North America, accounting for 10–15% of non-Hodgkin's lymphomas. In Asia, however, because of the relatively high prevalence of infection with the retrovirus HTLV-1, the situation is different, and in one study from Taiwan 39% of patients with non-Hodgkin's lymphoma had a T-cell tumour. EBV infection may be involved in the aetiology of some T-cell lymphomas, most notably 'lethal midline granuloma', a T-cell lymphoma occurring in the nasopharynx.

Classification

The diagnosis and classification of T-cell malignancies are difficult, although they are aided by monoclonal antibodies reacting with a number of T-cell antigens; this has greatly assisted the distinction of T-cell tumours from their B-cell counterparts. Immunochemistry in T-cell proliferations cannot prove that these are clonal. Demonstration of clonality depends on showing that clonal rearrangements of T-cell receptor genes have taken place.

Immunophenotyping of T-cell Lymphomas

T cells produced in the bone marrow undergo several stages in their maturation and differentiation, some of which occur within the thymus. Lymphomas may arise from immature T cells, which may be prethymic or thymic, and from mature (post-thymic) T cells. The various stages of maturation and differentiation are accompanied by the expression of certain antigens and an enzyme, terminal deoxynucleotidyl transferase (TdT) (*Table 42.12*). The cells of neoplasms arising from immature or mature T cells mark in the same way.

Tumours arising from immature T cells mark as either prothymocytes or thymocytes. For example, two-thirds of cases of acute T-cell lymphoblastic leukaemia mark as prothymocytes; the remainder express common thymocytic antigens. T-cell lymphoblastic lymphoma, which accounts for 80% of all lymphoblastic lymphomas, expresses the phenotype of the common thymocyte but may occasionally show either a less or more differentiated phenotype.

Many different peripheral T-cell lymphomas exist and they display several different phenotypes. These peripheral T-cell neoplasms usually lose one or more of the antigens appropriate for their stage of differentiation.

Low-grade Tumours

Malignant Lymphoma, Lymphocytic (WF – ML Small Lymphocytic; REAL – Large Granular Lymphocyte Leukaemia, T-cell and NK-cell Types)

This rare type of lymphoma is almost always associated with CLL. The lymph nodes show diffuse infiltration by small lymphocytes with irregular nuclei, which most commonly express CD2. The T-cell type also marks with antibodies against CD3 but this does not occur in NK-cell types. About one-third of cases are associated with clinical or serological evidence of rheumatoid arthritis.

Malignant Lymphoma, Small Cerebriform Cell (WF – Mycosis Fungoides, Sézary's Syndrome; REAL – Mycosis Fungoides, Sézary's Syndrome)

The term **cerebriform** is derived from the appearances of the nucleus in this form of lymphoma; the nuclear membrane is the site of a complex system of infoldings,

Table 42.12 Immunophenotyping of T-cell Lymphomas

Cell	Markers
Prothymocyte	TdT+; CD2+; CD5–; CD7+; CD1,3,4,8–
Immature thymocyte	TdT+; CD2+; CD7+; CD5,1,3,4,8–
Common thymocyte	TdT+; CD2,7,5,1,3+ (CD3 cytoplasmic); CD4,8 may be positive
Mature thymocyte	TdT+; CD2,7,5+; CD1–; CD3+ (both cytoplasm and surface membrane mark); CD4+ or CD8+ depending on differentiation
Helper/inducer T cell	TdT–; CD2+; CD7 may be positive; CD1–; CD3+ (surface membrane staining); CD4+; CD8–
Cytotoxic/suppressor T cell	TdT–; CD2+; CD7 may be positive; CD5+; CD1–; CD3+ (surface membrane stains); CD4–; CD8+

giving an appearance reminiscent of the brain to imaginative microscopists. For those addicted to eponyms, these cells are also known as Sézary–Lutzner cells.

Cerebriform cell lymphoma is expressed in two clinical forms:

- mycosis fungoides
- Sézary's syndrome

Mycosis Fungoides

The term mycosis is misleading because this disorder has absolutely nothing to do with fungal disease. It is instead a cutaneous lymphoma with, in most cases, a long clinical course which can be divided into three stages:

1) a 'patch' stage in which there are flat, scaly, reddish-brown patches on the skin
2) a 'plaque' stage in which the focal skin lesions are thickened and plaque-like in a manner not dissimilar to what is seen in psoriasis (*Fig. 42.24*)
3) a third stage characterized by the presence of ulcerated tumour nodules

Microscopic Features

In the skin, the upper dermis is the seat of a florid infiltrate of cerebriform cells admixed with macrophages and other cells including eosinophils. This cellular infiltrate breaches the dermoepidermal junction and either single cerebriform cells or aggregates of these cells are seen within the epidermis. These cerebriform cells express CD3 and CD4 antigens and are usually negative for CD8.

If clusters of the neoplastic T cells are located intraepidermally, this is termed a Pautrier microabscess, an unfortunate name because the lesion is certainly not an inflammatory one (*Fig. 42.25*). Larger, darkly staining, cells may be seen within the infiltrate and these have been called mycosis cells.

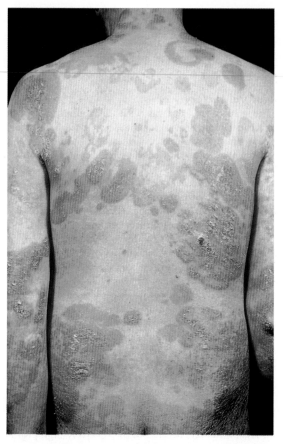

FIGURE 42.24 *Mycosis fungoides. Skin showing the 'plaque' stage of the cutaneous disease.*

Clinically evident lymph node enlargement is common in patients with mycosis fungoides. This may be due to reactive changes in the paracortical T-cell zones

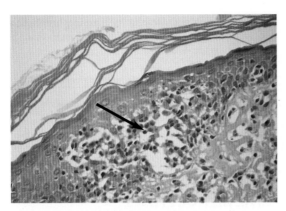

FIGURE 42.25 *Epidermis from a patient with mycosis fungoides showing the presence of infiltration by neoplastic T lymphocytes (arrowed). This feature has been termed a Pautrier microabscess.*

of draining nodes (so-called dermatopathic lymphadenopathy) or to infiltration of the node by tumour cells. Such infiltration may be inconspicuous and impossible to recognize on histological examination. The presence of infiltrating tumour cells under these circumstances can be demonstrated by use of the molecular genetic techniques described on pp 8–9 and 962, whereby clonal rearrangements of the T-cell receptor can be identified.

Sézary's Syndrome

Sézary's syndrome is characterized by red scaly skin, baldness and a leukaemic blood picture in which cerebriform T cells are present in quite large numbers in the peripheral blood.

Malignant Lymphoma, Lymphoepithelioid Type (Lennert's Lymphoma) (WF – ML Large Cell Immunoblastic, Epithelioid Cell Component)

This disorder usually presents with regional lymphadenopathy, quite often accompanied by involvement of lymphoid tissue in the tonsillar region. It is doubtful whether it should be classified as a low-grade lymphoma as it may behave in an aggressive fashion.

Microscopic Features

There is a mixed infiltrate within the affected nodes in which T cells predominate. Some of these T cells resemble Reed–Sternberg cells and mistaken diagnoses of Hodgkin's disease may be made. In addition there are many clusters of aggregated macrophages giving a somewhat granulomatous appearance, again not dissimilar to what may be seen in Hodgkin's disease.

Malignant Lymphoma, Angioimmunoblastic (WF – ML Large Cell Immunoblastic Polymorphous)

This condition was originally described under the name **angioimmunoblastic lymphadenopathy with dysproteinaemia (AILD)**, and is fairly common in Japan. Formerly it was thought to be a non-neoplastic disorder in which there might be a number of different clinical outcomes:

- spontaneous cure
- death due to immune deficiency
- the appearance of a lymphoma

It is now believed that virtually all cases of AILD are T-cell lymphomas. The patients present with a fairly abrupt onset of generalized lymphadenopathy, skin rash, and enlargement of the liver and spleen. Immunoglobulin concentrations in the plasma are often raised and the patients may present with one or more of a number of autoimmune clinical features.

Microscopic Features

There is a striking proliferation of high endothelial venules arranged in a network throughout the node. Normal nodal architecture is effaced and there is a mixed cell population between the venules in which large T immunoblasts with clear cytoplasm and prominent nucleoli are seen in fairly large numbers. The neoplastic T cells are most commonly of the helper/inducer (CD4+) type. These cells are mixed with small and intermediate lymphocytes.

Malignant Lymphoma, T-zone Type (WF – ML Large Cell Polymorphous)

In this lymphoma, there is a tendency for B-cell follicles to be preserved. Some of them may indeed be hyperplastic and mistaken diagnoses of reactive follicular hyperplasia may be made. The malignant cells are, in fact, sited within the paracortical area and the infiltrate is very similar to that seen in AILD. The disease may progress to become a high-grade lymphoma, either of diffuse T-cell type or similar to what may transpire in patients with AILD.

High-grade Tumours

Malignant Lymphoma Lymphoblastic (WF - ML Lymphoblastic Convoluted or Non-convoluted)

This tumour chiefly affects males under the age of 20 years (male : female incidence ratio 2 : 1). It accounts for only 5% of all non-Hodgkin's lymphomas, but about 40% of cases in childhood and adolescence fall into this group. It is commonly associated with acute T-cell lymphoblastic leukaemia.

Lymphadenopathy is the common presenting feature and is associated with a mediastinal mass in more than 50% of cases, owing to involvement of the thymus.

The immunophenotype is consistent with a prethymic or thymic stage of differentiation. TdT is expressed in all cases and in some patients the tumour cells mark with antibodies to CD2, CD5 and CD7, as do thymocytes. Although prothymocytes and thymocytes do not normally express differentiation antigens of either helper or cytotoxic T cells, in some cases of lymphoblastic lymphoma both of these (CD4 and CD8) are expressed together.

Microscopic Features

Normally, the pattern of infiltration of the tumour cells is a diffuse one, but occasionally in the early stages of the disease the paracortical T-cell zone appears to be particularly affected. The cells are slightly larger than small lymphocytes and their nuclei often show a convoluted appearance which, at one stage, was thought to be characteristic of T cells (hence the use of the terms convoluted and non-convoluted in the WF classification).

Natural History

The disease is an aggressive one and, if untreated, the patient pursues a rapid downhill course. Dissemination to bone marrow, blood and meninges leads to a clinical and pathological picture similar to that seen in acute lymphoblastic leukaemia.

Malignant Lymphoma, Pleomorphic (HTLV-1 Positive or Negative) (WF – ML Large Cell Immunoblastic, Polymorphous)

The characteristics of the virus and the geographical distribution of this disease are described on p 964. The disease usually pursues an aggressive course, many of the patients surviving for only a few months.

Microscopic Features

The affected nodes are diffusely infiltrated by cells that are larger, often considerably larger, than normal lymphocytes, with very pleomorphic nuclei in which prominent nucleoli can be seen. These cells are uniformly CD4 positive and CD7 negative, suggesting that they arise from post-thymic T cells of the helper/inducer phenotype.

Malignant Lymphoma, Large Cell Anaplastic (WF – ML Large Immunoblastic)

This tumour is composed of large cells with pale cytoplasm and highly atypical and pleomorphic nuclei. The tumour cells are often seen within lymph node sinuses and often show evidence of red cell phagocytosis. In immunophenotypic terms the defining criterion is the fact that the tumour cells uniformly bind the Ki-1 antibody, which reacts with the lymphocyte activation marker CD30. T-cell markers are often absent. A translocation (2;5) is often present.

Natural History

Ki-positive anaplastic lymphoma is predominantly a tumour found in the young and many cases have been reported in children. Despite its alarming histological appearances, the prognosis is slightly better than in other high-grade T-cell tumours.

EXTRANODAL LYMPHOMA

The defining criterion of extranodal lymphomas is a negative one. They do *not* arise from lymph nodes or other recognized lymphoid organs such as the thymus, spleen or tonsillar lymphoid tissue (Waldeyer's ring).

THE HISTIOCYTOSES

The histiocytoses are a set of disorders whose common feature is proliferation of cells of the mononuclear phagocyte population. Both the nomenclature and the basic understanding of this group of diseases has been very confused, as indicated by the use of the term histiocytosis X (X being the unknown quantity) as a blanket term for some of these disorders. The classification currently used is shown in *Table 42.13*.

Langerhans Cell Histiocytosis

The unifying feature of Langerhans cell histiocytosis is the presence of Langerhans cells in granulomatous lesions that may affect a wide range of tissues. The clinical features depend on the extent and anatomical location of the lesions.

Langerhans cells are normally present in skin, lymph nodes and thymus. They belong to the functional group of cells that present antigen to lymphocytes and, although, unlike macrophages, they are not phagocytes, they do appear to process antigen. They are large cells with very irregular nuclei with a fine chromatin pattern. Identification of these cells requires electron microscopy or immunocytochemistry.

On electron microscopy the defining morphological feature of the Langerhans cell is an intracytoplasmic structure known as the Birbeck

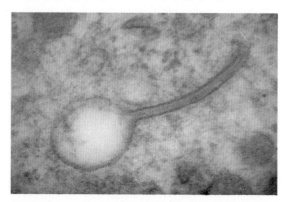

FIGURE 42.26 *Electron micrograph of a Langerhans cell showing a typical 'tennis racket'-shaped Birbeck granule.*

Table 42.13 The Histiocytoses

Group	Clinicopathological entities
Langerhans cell histiocytosis	Hand–Schüller–Christian disease
	Letterer–Siwe disease
	Eosinophilic granuloma of bone
	Self-healing cutaneous histiocytosis (Hashimoto–Pritzker syndrome)
Reactive histiocytoses	Haemophagocytic lymphohistiocytosis
	Infection-associated haemophagocytic syndrome
Neoplastic disorders	Acute monocytic leukaemia
	Malignant histiocytosis
	True histiocytic lymphoma (very rare)

Table 42.14 Langerhans Cell Histiocytoses

Syndrome	Features
Hand–Schüller–Christian disease (1921)	Enlargement of liver and spleen
	Lymphadenopathy (*Fig. 42.27*)
	Osteolytic bone lesions
	Polyuria due to diabetes insipidus in some cases with hypothalamic or pituitary involvement
Letterer–Siwe disease (1933)	Fever
	Enlargement of liver and spleen
	Lymphadenopathy
	Widespread skin rash characterized by vesicles and pustules showing marked crusting
	Osteolytic bone lesions
	Involvement of bone marrow
Eosinophilic granuloma of bone (1940)	Multiple osteolytic bone lesions **in the absence of visceral involvement**
Congenital self-healing histiocytosis (Hashimoto–Pritzker syndrome) (1973) (very rare)	Skin lesions similar to those of the acute disseminated form. Lesions present at birth or appear within 2–3 weeks. Spontaneous regression occurs usually within 3 months

granule. This is a rod-shaped organelle showing striations at right angles to the long axis. Some of these bodies terminate in an ovoid swelling, which gives the whole granule a 'tennis racket'-like appearance (*Fig. 42.26*). It is thought that Birbeck granules are an expression of invagination of the cell membranes; their significance is unknown.

A number of distinctive features can be demonstrated by immunocytochemical techniques. Langerhans cells express the marker protein S-100 and are CD1 positive, a feature that is seen in thymocytes and dendritic cells. The membranes show the presence of adenosine 5′-triphosphatase and the cells bind peanut agglutinin in a characteristic pattern.

The chief clinical expressions of Langerhans cell-containing lesions are the four syndromes listed in *Table 42.14*. They can occur at any age but are found chiefly in infants and children (the median age at diagnosis is 2–3 years). The severity ranges from an indolent localized disorder to very aggressive, widely disseminated disease.

Plasma Cell Dyscrasias

These are uncontrolled monoclonal proliferations of immunoglobulin-secreting lymphoid cells. They include:

- **multiple myeloma,** the commonest of these disorders

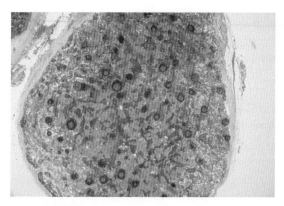

FIGURE 42.27 *Lymph node from a patient with histiocytosis X (Langerhans cell histiocytosis). The sinuses show up as large pale areas because they are stuffed with Langerhans cells.*

- **Waldenström's macroglobulinaemia**, in which the proliferated cells are lymphocytes rather than plasma cells, but secrete large amounts of immunoglobulin (Ig) M into the plasma
- **heavy chain disease**, in which the secreting cells are, once again, lymphocytes rather than plasma cells
- so-called **benign monoclonal gammopathies**

ABNORMALITIES IN PLASMA PROTEINS

Increases in the concentration of certain plasma proteins are common in this group. Because the lymphocyte or plasma cell proliferations are **monoclonal**, the excess plasma protein that occurs is **monotypic**. An increase in a monotypic immunoglobulin is diagnostically helpful; the properties of some of these proteins influence the natural history of the various diseases.

Excess proteins occur in three different forms:
- **intact immunoglobulin**
- **free light chains either alone or in combination with the intact immunoglobulin**
- **heavy chain fragments**

On serum electrophoresis, followed by densitometry, the excess protein appears as a **tall, narrow, very well-defined spike**, reflecting its monotypic nature (*Fig. 42.28*). Some M proteins have special physical and chemical properties which influence the clinical picture:
- **a high viscosity**
- **a tendency to form amyloid fibrils**
- **the ability to be precipitated at low temperatures**
- **the ability to agglutinate red blood cells in the cold**
- **the ability to form complexes with other serum proteins (including clotting factors) and with the surface membranes of platelets**

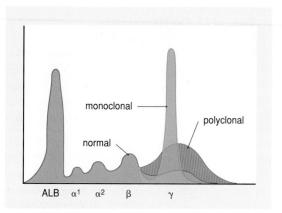

FIGURE 42.28 *γ-Globulin patterns seen on serum electrophoresis in normal subjects, in those with polyclonal increases in immunoglobulin and in myeloma. Note the tall, narrow 'spike' seen in myeloma, the appearance of which suggests the presence of a monotypic globulin.*

As a result, patients may suffer from a variety of clinical syndromes including, for example, **hyperviscosity syndrome**. This causes increased resistance to blood flow and is typically associated with:
- **visual abnormalities** due to retinal changes
- **a wide range of neurological deficits** including dizziness, stupor, fits and focal neurological abnormalities, both motor and sensory. Deafness may occur due to thrombosis in the small venules of the inner ear.
- **abnormal bleeding**

MULTIPLE MYELOMA

Multiple myeloma is a neoplasm characterized by monoclonal proliferation of mature and immature plasma cells. Its defining criteria are:
- **osteolytic lesions** due to the formation of plasma cell tumours in many bones, these sites being determined for the most part by the presence of red marrow
- **an M protein in the serum and urine**

Annual incidence in the USA is 1–2 per 100 000 in Caucasians and about double that in Afro-Americans. Multiple myeloma affects chiefly the middle-aged and elderly (mean age at diagnosis 62 years).

The cause is not known. In some cases, the tumour cells express myeloid and even erythroid markers as well as lymphoid ones, suggesting that the transforming event takes place at the stage of the haemopoietic stem cell. Chromosomal abnormalities have been found in many cases, but these have been random. Similarly there is no consistent pattern of oncogene activation, although *ras* oncogenes appear to be activated more frequently than others.

Clinical Features

The clinical picture is dominated by:

- **Bone pain and pathological fractures** due to the lytic tumours (*Fig. 42.29*). Bone destruction is almost certainly accomplished via osteoclast activation by cytokines (*Fig. 42.30*) including interleukin (IL) 1β, tumour necrosis factor α and IL-6, which is a growth factor for neoplastic plasma cells, a bone resorbing factor and a stimulus for the formation of osteoclasts.

  The resorption of bone leads to **hypercalcaemia**, which itself causes many disturbances of function (see pp 1049–1051). Occasionally, only a single plasma cell tumour is present in the skeleton. Such lesions differ from the 'punched-out' multiple lesions, often having a multiloculated 'soap bubble' appearance.

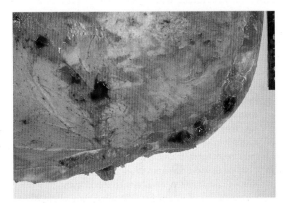

FIGURE 42.29 Multiple myeloma. Note sharply punched out lytic deposits in the cranium of this patient with myeloma.

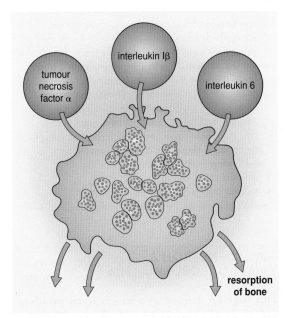

FIGURE 42.30 Bone resorption in myeloma is due to upregulation of osteoclast activity by cytokines.

- **Increased susceptibility to infection. This is one of the commonest features; infection is a major cause of death in myeloma.** Recurrent episodes of sepsis are very common; these usually are caused by virulent encapsulated microorganisms such as *Streptococcus pneumoniae* in the early phases of myeloma; later, infection with *Staphylococcus aureus* appears to predominate. Increased susceptibility to infection may have several causes of which anaemia, lack of normal immunoglobulin, and quantitative and functional abnormalities of both B and T cells are all likely candidates.

- **Involvement of the nervous system. This can occur in a number of ways:**

  1) The membranes covering the spinal cord may be invaded by tumour spreading from an adjacent vertebral body. This occurs in about 10% of patients and results in extradural compression of the cord, an extremely serious complication. Plasma cell tumours occur quite commonly in the skull and those situated at the skull base may be associated with cranial nerve palsies.

  2) In patients who develop amyloidosis as a complication of the myeloma a number of different neurological lesions can occur. These include a sensorimotor neuropathy not unlike that of diabetes mellitus. This occurs in 3–5% of patients with multiple myeloma. Carpal tunnel syndrome may occur when amyloid in the flexor retinaculum entraps the median nerve.

  3) A further 2–3% of patients with myeloma develop a polyneuropathy not associated with amyloidosis. Its mechanism is not known.

  4) **POEMS.** In a few patients with single plasma cell tumours, a curious syndrome may develop comprising:

  Polyneuropathy, which is chronic and slowly progressive

  Organomegaly, usually affecting the liver and lymph nodes

  Endocrinopathy (decreased testosterone concentrations, impotence, hypercalcaemia, hyperglycaemia and hyperprolactinaemia)

  Monoclonal protein present in the plasma

  Skin lesions (hyperpigmentation, abnormal hairiness and white nails)

  5) Multifocal leucoencephalopathy

  6) Encephalopathy due to hypercalcaemia, expressed in the form of delirium, confusion or coma

Renal Complications

Chronic renal failure is a common endpoint in myeloma. Several factors contribute. Chief among them is the filtration of large amounts of immunoglobulin light chains (Bence Jones protein) which present the renal tubules with a very large protein load for reabsorption. Some of the protein is endocytosed by renal tubular epithelial cells, in which it is seen in the form of eosinophilic inclusions, but much of the protein forms large hyaline casts which injure the lining epithelial cells. The typical microscopic findings resulting from this are eosinophilic tubular casts, showing a peripheral cuff of damaged epithelium.

Not all Bence Jones proteins are associated with this tubular reaction; the structural or charge differences between cytotoxic and non-cytotoxic varieties are not known.

Other contributors to renal failure in myeloma are hypercalcaemia and hypercalciuria resulting from bone destruction, and the high concentrations of uric acid in the glomerular filtrate. These are due to the high cell turnover within the plasma cell tumours.

These features are summarized in *Fig. 42.31*.

Complications Associated with Amyloid Deposition

These include:

- restrictive cardiomyopathy
- enlargement of the tongue
- arthropathy
- a tendency for prolonged bleeding to develop. This is due to the binding of clotting factor X by the amyloid fibrils.

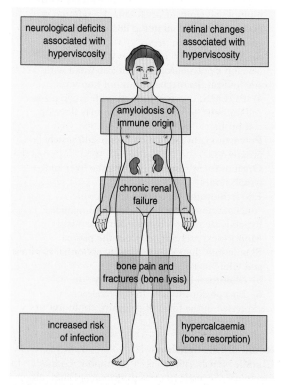

FIGURE 42.31 *Important clinical features that may occur in patients with myeloma.*

- skin changes in the form of so-called 'pinch purpura' and nodular deposits of amyloid in the upper part of the dermis

Coincident Disease in Patients with Myeloma

Patients with myeloma show an increased tendency to develop second malignancies. These may be solid epithelial tumours, most commonly breast, bowel and biliary tract cancers. An increased incidence of haematological malignancies such as acute and chronic leukaemia has also been reported.

The incidence of monoclonal gammopathies appears to be higher than expected in patients with human immunodeficiency virus (HIV) infection. The incidence in individuals with antibodies to HIV is 2–4%, whereas in those with fully established acquired immune deficiency syndrome it rises to 13%.

Laboratory Findings

The laboratory diagnosis of myeloma rests on the foundation of:

- **demonstration of a monotypic immunoglobulin peak on serum electrophoresis.** In more than 75% of patients, intact immunoglobulin is present and, of these, IgG is the commonest, the next most frequent being IgA. Normal immunoglobulin production is depressed and this, of course, may contribute to the known increased risk of infections. The urine shows light chains (either κ or λ) in about 65% of patients. In addition to the immunoglobulins, β_2-microglobulins are frequently found to be increased in patients with myeloma and other monoclonal gammopathies. This is not diagnostically helpful but gives prognostic information; survival rates are distinctly lower in patients with high β_2-microglobulin levels.
- **abnormal plasma cells ('myeloma cells') in the bone marrow** (*Fig. 42.32*). Usually the marrow contains at least 5% of such cells and concentrations of up to 30% are by no means uncommon. On immunohistological staining these atypical plasma cells show light chain restriction (either κ or λ but not both); this is strong evidence for monoclonality.

Other findings include:

- anaemia
- a raised erythrocyte sedimentation rate

WALDENSTRÖM'S MACROGLOBULINAEMIA

This may be defined as a monoclonal proliferation of B cells associated with the production of a monotypic IgM or macroglobulin. The disease is more or less confined to the elderly, the peak incidence

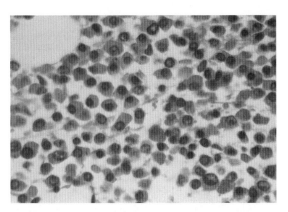

FIGURE 42.32 *Multiple myeloma. This section from a lytic bone deposit shows only plasma cells with characteristic basophilic (mauve) cytoplasm.*

being in the sixth and seventh decades. Males tend to be affected more frequently than females.

The onset of the disorder is often insidious with patients complaining of weakness and lethargy. Weight loss and a tendency to abnormal bleeding may follow. As the disease progresses, enlargement of the lymph nodes, liver and spleen become manifest and the clinical picture comes to resemble that of one of the non-Hodgkin's lymphomas. The patients may suffer from:

- **anaemia** which is multifactorial in origin. Patients may have a bleeding tendency, depressed bone marrow function, decreased survival of red blood cells, and some degree of haemodilution.
- **a bleeding tendency** due in part to binding of the macroglobulin to platelet surfaces
- **a hyperviscosity syndrome**, the principal manifestations of which have been described in an earlier section of this chapter.
- **a neuropathy**, which affects about 5% of patients
- **intestinal problems**, mainly in the form of chronic diarrhoea

Laboratory Findings
- A raised sedimentation rate and an increased tendency toward rouleaux formation may be the first expressions of the plasma protein abnormality.
- A monotypic increase in IgM concentration in the plasma can be seen on electrophoresis, where the usual tall narrow M-band is seen, and on immunoelectrophoresis which establishes the nature of the immunoglobulin.
- Liver biopsy shows a dense lymphoid infiltrate involving the periportal regions. Lymph node biopsy shows preservation of the sinuses but some degree of loss of the normal cortical follicular pattern.

The disease is usually fatal but within this bleak frame of reference there is considerable variation in the survival

time. The common causes of death are progression of the lymphoproliferative disease, infection and cardiac failure.

HEAVY CHAIN DISEASE

Heavy chain disease may be defined as a monoclonal proliferation of B cells accompanied by synthesis and secretion of monotypic protein which has the characteristics of incomplete heavy chains of immunoglobulin.

One would expect there to be a heavy chain disease to correspond with each of the immunoglobulin classes but, so far, heavy chain disease has been described only in association with α, γ, δ and μ heavy chains.

α-Heavy Chain Disease (IPSID, Immunoproliferative Small Intestinal Disease)

This is the commonest disorder within this set. Most of the patients are aged between 10 and 30 years and there is a predilection for the lesions to occur in parts of the body where IgA secretion takes place. The gut, therefore, is the principal site for the lymphoid proliferation characteristic of this disorder, although the respiratory tract may be involved in some patients.

This disease is most frequently found in individuals living in north Africa and along the Mediterranean coast and appears to be related to infestation with intestinal parasites. The importance of the latter is supported by the observation that treatment with antibiotics causes regression of the condition.

The pathological features are described in Chapter 34 (see p 530).

γ-Heavy Chain Disease

This disorder may occur over a wide age range.

The most common clinical findings are:

- lymphadenopathy, which most often involves nodes in the neck, axilla, chest, abdomen and Waldeyer's ring in the pharynx
- enlargement of the spleen
- enlargement of the liver
- fever
- symptoms referable to anaemia
- an associated autoimmune disease such as haemolytic anaemia, rheumatoid arthritis or systemic lupus erythematosus in about one-third of patients

Laboratory Findings
- **Anaemia** is present in most cases and may be severe in about 25% of patients. Thrombocytopenia is present in about 15–20%, and about 25% show the presence of abnormal plasma cells or lymphocytes circulating in the blood.

- In about 60% of patients the **bone marrow** shows an increase in plasma cells and/or large lymphoid cells or immunoblasts. These may be arranged in more or less discrete nodules or in a diffuse fashion. In some patients, the bone marrow picture is more reminiscent of myeloma or chronic lymphocytic leukaemia.
- **A monoclonal abnormal protein** can be demonstrated in about 60% of patients by means of electrophoresis and can be identified by immunoelectrophoresis. The identical protein can be seen within the cytoplasm of the abnormal lymphocytes in material stained with the appropriate immunohistological technique.

μ-Heavy Chain Disease

This is a rare disorder in which the patients present with the clinical features of a lymphoproliferative disease.

BENIGN MONOCLONAL GAMMOPATHIES (MONOCLONAL GAMMOPATHIES OF UNKNOWN SIGNIFICANCE)

These terms define a situation in which an abnormal monoclonal immunoglobulin appears in the plasma **in the absence of clinical laboratory evidence of a malignant plasma cell disorder** or **of malignant lymphoreticular disease**. The reason for the introduction of the term **monoclonal gammopathy of unknown significance** is because, in some cases, the disorder evolves into a malignant plasma cell dyscrasia such as myeloma.

Benign monoclonal gammopathy is not uncommon, showing a prevalence of 1% in individuals aged more than 25 years and of 3% in those aged more than 70 years.

A very long list of disorders of different types has been linked with the condition and, because of the diversity of these, no unifying pathogenetic concept has yet emerged.

In a patient with a monoclonal gammopathy, features that suggest a diagnosis of monoclonal gammopathy of unknown significance include:

- an M protein concentration that is usually less than 20 g/l and usually remains stationary, unlike what happens in myeloma
- absence of light chains of immunoglobulin in the urine
- normal concentrations of polyclonal immunoglobulins and, thus, normal antibody responses to infection
- absence of bone lesions
- plasma cells not exceeding 10% of the cell population in the bone marrow

Natural History

One's view of the probable course of this disorder depends very much on the length of follow-up. The proportion of patients who develop an overt plasma cell malignancy within 1 year of the original diagnosis is less than 5%. In a study in which the median follow-up was 19 years, 22% of patients developed a plasma cell dyscrasia, multiple myeloma being the commonest. The median interval between diagnosis of monoclonal gammopathy of unknown significance and diagnosis of myeloma was just under 10 years.

The Spleen

NORMAL STRUCTURE AND FUNCTION

The spleen is the largest lymphoreticular organ. It is about the size of an adult clenched fist; the median weight is 125 g in young men, and 103 g in young women. Most pathological changes are associated with enlargement. A spleen that is palpable on clinical examination implies at least a doubling of the normal weight.

Accessory spleens are common, being found in 20–30% of autopsies. They are usually small (1 cm or less in diameter). The most frequent site is the tail of pancreas or within the gastrosplenic ligament, but they can also occur in the omentum and mesentery. They may be important in cases of hypersplenism, idiopathic thrombocytopenia and hereditary spherocytosis, where splenectomy may be the treatment of choice so as to restore the blood picture to normal. If accessory spleens are present and are not removed, surgical treatment may fail.

Functions of the spleen (*Fig. 42.33*) include:
- **filtration of obsolescent red blood cells, bacteria and red cell inclusions** such as Heinz bodies and Howell–Jolly bodies
- **immunological responses** to antigens trapped in the spleen and also the formation and emigration of lymphoid cells within and from the white pulp
- **haemopoiesis.** Physiologically this occurs only during embryonic life but in severe anaemia from any cause, extramedullary haemopoiesis within the spleen is triggered.
- acting as a **storage site and reservoir for blood** elements. In normal humans the spleen contains only 30–40 ml of red cells but this can increase greatly, especially if the spleen is congested.
- **phagocytosis within the splenic cords**

This last function deserves special consideration. As the lifespan of red cells is 120 days, it must follow that 1 in 120 of the circulating red blood cells is removed from the circulation daily; this is accomplished by phagocytosis of obsolescent red cells by the mononuclear

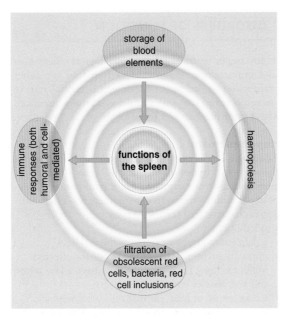

FIGURE 42.33 Functions of the spleen.

phagocyte system. About 50% of this is accounted for by splenic macrophages.

In addition, damaged or abnormal cells such as in sickle cell disease or hereditary spherocytosis, are similarly removed. Passage of red cells between the splenic cords and the sinuses depends largely on the degree of red cell deformability, because the cells must undergo a profound shape change to squeeze through the fenestrations in the sinus endothelium and basement membrane.

In the case of both damaged and intrinsically abnormal red cells, there is decreased deformability of the cell membrane and the cytoskeleton. Passage through the splenic cords in the red pulp of the spleen is significantly slowed and this increases red cell phagocytosis in this compartment.

Perhaps even more remarkable is the fact that **the macrophages in the splenic cords can remove inclusions such as Heinz bodies (portions of oxidized and denatured haemoglobin) and Howell–Jolly bodies (DNA remnants) from red cells while leaving the cells intact.** This process is known as **'pitting'**.

Splenic macrophages are also involved in the phagocytosis of bacteria, particulate material such as cell debris and certain macromolecules produced in the course of metabolism.

All the functions of the spleen are reflected in its structure. Two functional compartments are present:

1) The **white pulp**, consisting of periarterial sheaths of lymphoid cells known as **malpighian corpuscles**. Each of these measures about 2–3 mm

in diameter and can be seen with the naked eye as a whitish spot against the dark background of the red pulp.

2) The **red pulp**, consisting of an intricately branching set of sinusoids and small venules between which are splenic 'cords' where large numbers of macrophages are present

These two compartments are integrated functionally and anatomically by the vascular system of the spleen. The arterial blood supply is derived from the splenic artery entering the organ at its hilum and then dividing into smaller arteries which course along the fibrous septa derived from the capsule. These arterial branches then leave the trabeculae entering the parenchyma of the spleen as small vessels (the **central arteries**). The adventitial coat of each central artery gives way to a sheath of lymphoid cells which eventually widens to form a lymphoid follicle in which germinal centres can sometimes be seen.

The White Pulp
The lymphoid tissue is divided into three functional compartments:

1) **A T-cell area surrounding the central artery** (*Fig. 42.34*). This zone is known as the periarteriolar lymphoid sheath. About 70% of the cells in this area are T helper cells expressing the CD4 antigen; the remainder are suppressor/cytotoxic T cells (CD8). Antigen-presenting cells (dendritic cells) are also present.

2) **A B-cell area occupying the distended portion of the lymphoid sheath** (*Fig. 42.34*) and which, as already stated, may contain a germinal centre.

3) **A zone surrounding the follicle and composed of a meshwork of reticulin fibres. A moderate number of medium-sized lymphocytes expressing only immunoglobulin (Ig) M on their surfaces is present. It is in this zone that about 50% of lymphocyte traffic in the spleen occurs,** the cells passing from the blood into the white pulp. T cells return to the blood via vessels in the periarteriolar lymphoid sheath. The route taken by the B cells back to the bloodstream is not clear. T cells usually remain in the spleen for about 4 hours whereas B cells stay for about 16 hours. It is worth remembering that the spleen is not merely a visiting place for blood-derived lymphocytes but that lymphoid cells are also formed within the spleen and migrate thence to many lymphoid tissues.

The Red Pulp
The red pulp consists essentially of the sinuses and the splenic cords lying between them. The blood vessels that have initially coursed through the white pulp now form linkages with the sinusoids.

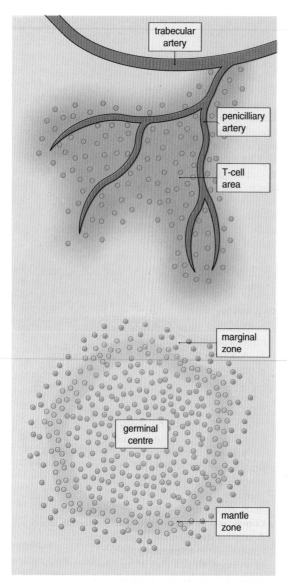

FIGURE 42.34 The white pulp of the spleen in diagrammatic form. Note the presence of both B- and T-cell areas.

The arterioles that penetrate the white pulp divide into capillaries which can either:

- enter the sinuses directly (**'closed' type of circulation**)
- open into the splenic cords (**an 'open' circulation**), the red cells from the splenic cords making their way back into the sinuses via fenestrations in the sinus endothelium. Obviously, red cell flow through this latter pathway is much slower than for the closed part of the splenic circulation and this may be relevant to the phagocytic activity of macrophages occupying the splenic cords.

DISORDERS OF FUNCTION

In any organ or tissue, clinicopathological effects may arise because one or more of its functions are either exaggerated or deficient. The spleen is no different in this respect, and there are distinct syndromes associated with **hyper**splenism and **hypo**splenism.

Hypersplenism

Pathological increase in some splenic functions is known as **hypersplenism**. It can occur in splenomegaly from any cause but is commonest in portal hypertension (congestive splenomegaly). The condition is characterized (*Fig. 42.35*) by:

- splenomegaly
- a deficiency in one or more of the cell lines normally present in the blood. Thus the affected individual may be anaemic and/or have a low white cell and platelet count.
- a marrow of, at least, normal cellularity with all three cell lines normally represented. This marrow picture indicates that there is no fault in production of blood cells, only an inappropriate degree of loss mediated by the enlarged spleen.
- reversal of the changes in the peripheral blood following splenectomy

The underlying mechanisms are still not fully understood. One suggestion is that the change in the peripheral blood picture is, in the first instance, due to the **pooling** of blood cells in the enlarged spleen. **Up to 50% of the total red cell mass can become pooled in enlarged spleens and it has been demonstrated that much the same applies in**

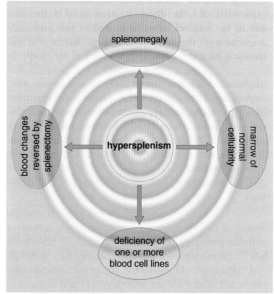

FIGURE 42.35 Basic features of hypersplenism.

respect of platelet and neutrophil pooling.
Normally about 10% of the platelet population is
pooled within the spleen; when the spleen is grossly
enlarged this proportion may rise to 90%.

In addition to pooling, **splenomegaly is associated with hypervolaemia.** Where there is a limitation on the ability of the bone marrow to respond, the
expanded blood volume comes chiefly from plasma and
the cell content of the blood is diluted.

Hyposplenism

The commonest cause of deficient splenic function is splenectomy. On rare occasions, the spleen
may be absent at birth, this being associated in most
cases with congenital cardiac defects, most commonly
those involving the atrioventricular endocardial cushions. Inadequate development of the spleen (hypoplasia) may sometimes be seen as part of the syndrome of
Fanconi's anaemia.

Acquired hyposplenism due to splenic atrophy
is a fairly common feature in **coeliac sprue, sickle
cell anaemia** and **essential thrombocythaemia**, a
condition in which there is abnormal proliferation of
megakaryocytes and consequently an overproduction
of platelets. Splenic atrophy in thrombocythaemia is
due to blocking of microvessels in the spleen by masses
of platelets.

**The haematological effects of hyposplenism
are associated with well-recognized changes in
the morphology of blood cells, especially the red
cells.** These changes include:
- nucleated red cells
- target cells
- Howell–Jolly bodies in the red cells
- iron-containing granules (Pappenheimer bodies) in
  red cells
- a high platelet count
- abnormally large platelets

Effects of Splenectomy
In addition to the haematological changes listed above,
splenectomy or atrophy of the spleen poses other dangers, described below.

Immune Functions – An Increased Risk of Infection
Splenectomy produces a fall in plasma IgM concentrations and a defect in the synthesis of antibodies directed
against carbohydrate-containing antigens such as those
in the capsules of certain bacterial species (e.g.
Streptococcus pneumoniae). This is associated with an
increased risk of infections caused by **capsulated bacteria**; in adults, the degree of such increased risk is
slight.

In children, however, splenectomy causes a significant increase in the incidence of serious, indeed life-threatening, infections. **Pneumococcal infections
are especially likely to occur** and these may be
expressed clinically in the form of meningitis or septicaemia. There is also a substantial increase in the risk of
infections caused by *Haemophilus influenzae* and *Neisseria
meningitidis*. Many advise prophylactic vaccination
against *S. pneumoniae* at least 1 month before splenectomy because of the danger of postsplenectomy infections. In tropical regions splenectomy is associated with
an increased risk of **malaria**, and in individuals who
have had previous episodes of malaria there may be
reactivation of latent infections.

Platelet Number and Function
Splenectomy may be followed by an increase in the
number of circulating platelets, presumably because
none of these can now be 'pooled' in the spleen. In
addition, the platelets may show an increased degree of
adhesiveness and the combination of these changes
increases the risk of thrombosis.

White Cell Changes
Following splenectomy there is an acute and transient
increase in the number of circulating neutrophils. This
is followed by a smaller but permanent increase in the
level of circulating lymphocytes and monocytes.

Infection in splenectomized patients produces a leucocyte response greater in degree than in those in possession of a spleen. In addition, this white cell response
is characterized by a greater proportion of less well-differentiated leucocytes.

SPLENOMEGALY

With very few exceptions, such as the atrophy associated with sickle cell disease or coeliac sprue, **pathological states in the spleen are expressed chiefly in
the form of splenomegaly**. Many groups of disorders
affect the spleen in this way (see *Table 42.15*).
Consideration of all of these is beyond the scope of this
text.

CONGESTIVE SPLENOMEGALY
The cause of congestive splenomegaly is portal hypertension (see pp 614–616) occurring in the following
forms:
- **prehepatic**, such as thrombosis in the splenic or
  portal veins, or other pathological states leading to
  obstruction of blood flow within the portal vein
- **hepatic** causes such as portal fibrosis (e.g. related to
  schistosomiasis) or cirrhosis
- **posthepatic**, such as thrombosis of the hepatic
  veins (Budd–Chiari syndrome)

The spleen may be very considerably enlarged, weighing 500–1000 g. It is characteristically very firm in consistency and the cut surface is dark red. The capsule and
fibrous tissue trabeculae derived from it are often thickened. Increased portal venous pressure is reflected in a
marked degree of dilatation of the sinuses. A further
consequence of the abnormally high pressure is sinus

Table 42.15 Splenomegaly

Mechanism	Examples
Circulatory disorders (congestive splenomegaly)	**Portal hypertension from any cause**, either presinusoidal or postsinusoidal (e.g. cirrhosis, portal fibrosis as in schistosomiasis, portal or splenic vein thrombosis, chronic congestive cardiac failure)
Viral infections	**Infectious mononucleosis**, acquired immune deficiency syndrome, cytomegalovirus infection, measles, occasionally infective hepatitis
Bacterial infections	Typhoid fever, infective endocarditis, brucellosis, tuberculosis, syphilis, septicaemia
Protozoal infections	**Malaria**, leishmaniasis (kala-azar), toxoplasmosis
Fungal infections	Histoplasmosis
Autoimmune-mediated chronic inflammatory disease	Rheumatoid disease (adult and juvenile), systemic lupus erythematosus
Storage diseases	**Gaucher's disease**, Niemann–Pick disease, some mucopolysaccharide storage diseases
Miscellaneous	Amyloidosis, tropical and idiopathic splenomegaly, cysts
Haematological and lymphoreticular disorders including malignancies	Hereditary haemolytic anaemias, **leukaemias especially chronic myeloid leukaemia**, other myeloproliferative disorders, thrombocytopenic purpura, Hodgkin's disease and non-Hodgkin's lymphomas, histiocytoses, systemic mastocytosis

rupture with intraparenchymal haemorrhage. This leads ultimately to small areas of scarring in which iron-laden macrophages are present (*Fig. 42.36*). These areas, visible as small brown nodules, are known as **Gamna–Gandy bodies** and may in due time become encrusted with calcium.

The characteristic blood picture of hypersplenism is likely to be present. In addition to pooling of blood (see pp 980–981) there may be laying down of collagen in

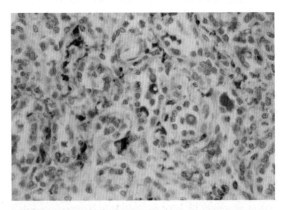

FIGURE 42.36 *Section of spleen from a patient showing the features of hypersplenism. The section has been stained by the Perl method to demonstrate the presence of haemosiderin, which shows up as blue deposits. Abundant blue-staining areas are present, indicating the presence within splenic macrophages of the iron moiety of haemoglobin derived from red cells.*

the basement membranes of the distended sinuses, making it difficult for red cells within the splenic cords to gain entry to the circulatory system; this is likely, therefore, to increase their chances of being phagocytosed within the splenic parenchyma.

SPLENOMEGALY ASSOCIATED WITH 'STORAGE DISEASES'

Massive splenomegaly may be encountered in some lysosomal storage diseases, of which at least 30 types are recognized. The defining criterion of such a disorder is abnormal intralysosomal accumulation of an intermediary metabolite.

Genetic defects lead to the absence of one or other lysosomal enzyme. Thus any metabolic block may lead to:

- **accumulation of the intermediary metabolite normally cleaved by the missing enzyme.** This may be associated with an increase in the number of 'storing' cells (i.e. fixed tissue macrophages) and can lead to enlargement of the affected organ(s).
- **absence of the normal endproduct of the metabolic pathway**
- **increased activation of some subsidiary metabolic pathway**

Most storage diseases are categorized in terms of the class of metabolite accumulating within lysosomes. Those tending to be associated with splenomegaly are shown in *Table 42.16*.

The group of storage disorders associated with massive splenomegaly is **the sphingolipidoses**. Their

Table 42.16 Some Storage Diseases

Metabolite group	Disorder	Stored metabolite	Principal organs involved
Gangliosides	GM-1 gangliosidosis	GM-1 ganglioside	CNS, liver, **spleen**, bones
Sphingolipids	Gaucher's disease (type 1)	Glucocerebroside	**Spleen**, liver, bones
	Gaucher's disease (type 2)	Glucocerebroside	CNS, **spleen,** liver, bones
	Gaucher's disease (type 3)	Glucocerebroside	CNS, **spleen**, liver, bones
	Niemann–Pick (type A)	Sphingomyelin	CNS, liver, **spleen**
	Niemann–Pick (type B)	Sphingomyelin	liver, **spleen**, lungs
	Niemann–Pick (type C)	?	CNS, liver, **spleen**
	Multiple sulphatase deficiency	Sulphate-containing glycolipids, steroids and mucopolysaccharides	CNS, liver, **spleen**, bones
Mucopolysaccharides	Hurler's syndrome	Dermatan sulphate, heparan sulphate	CNS, bones, liver, heart, **spleen**
	Hunter's syndrome	Dermatan sulphate, heparan sulphate	CNS, bones, liver, heart, **spleen**
Mucolipids	Fucosidosis	Oligosaccharides and sphingolipids	CNS, bones, liver, **spleen**

defining criterion is the accumulation of various compounds containing **ceramide** within cells and tissues.

Ceramide itself is a combination of a fatty acid and sphingosine. What makes each sphingolipid structurally and functionally distinct is the compound esterified to the first carbon atom of ceramide. Thus, for example, if this compound is glucose, the final molecule is classed as a cerebroside. Cerebroside accumulation is characteristic of the various forms of Gaucher's disease, an example of the sphingolipidoses which can be associated with massive splenomegaly.

Gaucher's Disease

This is a rare, autosomal recessive, familial disorder. Its defining characteristic is a deficiency of the enzyme β-**glucocerebrosidase** leading to intralysosomal glucocerebroside accumulation. A significant proportion of the affected individuals are Jews, especially those hailing from the Baltic seaboard, but the disorder occurs in several other groups.

There are three different forms; type 1 or 'adult' Gaucher's disease, in which the central nervous system is *not* involved, is by far the commonest. The term 'adult' is something of a misnomer because the clinical features quite often appear in childhood.

Clinical Features

Clinical features include:

- **Splenomegaly**, which is often the first manifest-

ation. The spleen may be enormously enlarged; weights of 1 kg or more are not uncommon. With splenic enlargement of this order it is not surprising that the haematological picture of hypersplenism is often present. This may be so severe, especially the striking decrease in platelet numbers, as to necessitate splenectomy.

- **Bone involvement.** The large numbers of sphingolipid-laden macrophages may destroy bone, producing striking deformities. The femur is particularly likely to be involved, showing cortical thinning and cyst formation. About 50% of patients with bony involvement complain of severe and episodic bone pain (not unlike the pain of crises of sickle cell disease). These episodes may be associated with fever, swelling and tenderness over the affected areas, leading to a misdiagnosis of acute osteitis.

- **Skin pigmentation.** Yellowish-brown skin pigmentation occurs in 45–75% of patients. This affects chiefly the skin of the face, neck and hands.

Microscopic Features

The tissue diagnosis is made by identifying glucocerebroside-laden macrophages known as **Gaucher cells**. They can be found usually in bone marrow aspirates (*Fig. 42.37*), although they are of course present in many other tissues, most notably the spleen.

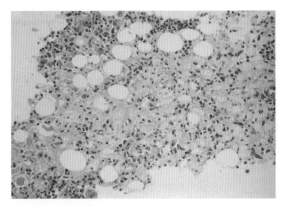

FIGURE 42.37 *Bone marrow aspirate from a patient with Gaucher's disease. Note the many, very large, pale macrophages which are distended with cerebroside.*

The cells are large (20–80 μm in diameter), staining pale blue with Romanowsky stains.

In haematoxylin and eosin-stained sections, the abundant cytoplasm of the Gaucher cell is faintly pink and appears characteristically **striated**. On electron microscopy, this appearance is seen to be due to clear, elongated, membrane-bound spaces, which are lysosomes distended by the cerebroside.

The precursor of the lipid found in the Gaucher cell is lipid derived from membranes of white cells, platelets and red cells.

'Pseudo-Gaucher Cells'

The mirror image of this situation is when abnormal amounts of lipid are taken up by macrophages because of **increased breakdown of blood cells**. The loading of macrophages with these lipids may be so great as to exceed the cells' ability to catabolize them. The end result is cells resembling Gaucher cells even though the patient's complement of lysosomal enzymes may be quite normal. This histological phenomenon occurs in such disorders as chronic myeloid leukaemia.

Niemann–Pick Disease

This sphingolipidosis reflects **a failure to catabolize sphingomyelin because of a deficiency of the enzyme sphingomyelinase**. The lipid-laden macrophages in this set of disorders (there are three types) appear foamy in histological sections rather than striated. In Giemsa-stained sections or smears, the macrophages stain blue (**'sea-blue histiocytes'**). The blue staining is due to the presence of ceroid pigment, a peroxidation product of the accumulated unsaturated lipid within the foamy macrophages. It is *not* specific for Niemann–Pick disease.

Sea-blue histiocytes may also be seen in a primary familial syndrome (sea-blue histiocytosis) characterized by:

- enlargement of the liver and spleen
- a low platelet count

They also occur as a secondary phenomenon in disorders such as idiopathic thrombocytopenic purpura, chronic myeloid leukaemia, thalassaemia, polycythaemia, sickle cell disease and various chronic granulomatous disorders including sarcoidosis.

INFLAMMATORY DISORDERS

ACUTE AND SUBACUTE INFLAMMATORY DISORDERS

In a variety of acute inflammatory systemic disorders, most particularly those associated with suppuration, the spleen may become enlarged by up to two or three times its normal weight.

At post-mortem examination, such a spleen is found to be extremely soft with a dull greyish cut surface due to a striking increase in the number of nucleated cells in the red pulp. In acute suppurative disorders, this is due largely to infiltration of the splenic cords by neutrophils, whereas in typhoid fever, for example, there is a marked increase in macrophages.

In infectious mononucleosis, often associated with splenic softening, the splenic cords are infiltrated by atypical T-cell immunoblasts, which can also infiltrate the capsule and the fibrous trabeculae.

CHRONIC INFLAMMATORY DISORDERS

Granulomatous Inflammation

Splenic enlargement is not uncommon in a wide range of granulomatous reactions. Where tuberculosis is still widely prevalent, haematogenous dissemination leading to miliary tuberculosis, is usually accompanied by large numbers of typical granulomas in the spleen. Splenic granulomas may also be found in the secondary and tertiary stages of syphilis but such cases are now rare in Western countries.

Other bacterial infections associated with a granulomatous reaction in the spleen include tularaemia, brucellosis and, very rarely, the septicaemic form of yersinial infection, which normally involves mesenteric lymph nodes.

Fungal Infections

A wide variety of fungal infections may involve the spleen. One of the most interesting is infection by *Histoplasma capsulatum*, which is fairly common in the Ohio–Mississippi valley in the USA. The end result of splenic histoplasmosis is the appearance of many foci of calcification.

Protozoal Infections

Malaria and leishmaniasis are the commonest and most important causes of splenomegaly associated with protozoal infections.

In **acute falciparum malaria** the spleen may be enlarged up to about three times its normal weight. In fatal cases, these enlarged spleens are congested and dark brown (due to a haematin-like pigment known as **haemozoin**). Non-falciparum-type malarial infections are much more benign, but are also associated with splenic enlargement.

In **chronic malaria**, the spleen may be very much enlarged, weighing 1–2 kg. While firmer in consistency than normal, it is also rather friable, and these patients have an increased risk of splenic rupture. On naked-eye examination, these grossly enlarged spleens are a slate-grey colour due to haemozoin in macrophages within the splenic cords.

'Tropical Splenomegaly Syndrome'

Chronic splenomegaly of impressive proportions (3–4 kg) may be seen in some young adults living in areas where falciparum-type malaria is endemic. The presence of high concentrations of IgM in the plasma of these patients is a characteristic finding. The level of antibodies to malarial antigens is high; treatment with antimalarial agents usually produces a significant reduction in the size of the spleen. As might be expected with a gross degree of splenic enlargement, hypersplenism is common in these individuals.

Microscopic examination of the spleen in fatal cases shows little disturbance of the normal architectural pattern. The numerous haemozoin-laden macrophages diagnostic of malarial parasitization in the spleen are not seen here.

Leishmanial Splenomegaly

Splenomegaly is a characteristic feature of visceral leishmaniasis (**kala-azar**). This is caused by *Leishmania donovani*. *Leishmania* is endemic in many parts of the world and about 12 million people are afflicted.

In visceral leishmaniasis, the disease presents insidiously with:

- fever
- anaemia
- enlargement of the spleen and liver
- increased skin pigmentation, from which the term kala-azar ('black fever' in Hindi) is derived)

The spleen may be enormously enlarged, weights of up to 4 kg being recorded in adults. The splenic cords show large numbers of macrophages, loaded with *Leishmania*, accompanied by numerous plasma cells so that the normal distinction between white and red pulp may be difficult to appreciate.

AUTOIMMUNE-MEDIATED CHRONIC INFLAMMATORY DISEASE

Rheumatoid Disease

In certain patients with chronic deforming rheumatoid arthritis (see pp 1075–1081), Felty's syndrome may occur. In addition to the joint and other extra-articular manifestations of rheumatoid disease, this includes:

- splenomegaly
- leucopenia, especially in respect of neutrophils

The splenomegaly is usually moderate (mean weight of spleen 900 g), although occasionally, huge spleens may be seen. The splenic enlargement is due mainly to expansion of the splenic cords within the red pulp by macrophages, although some hyperplasia in the white pulp has been recorded. The vessels in the white pulp may show fibrinoid necrosis and a curious laminated periarteriolar scarring, which is seen also in systemic lupus erythematosus. Splenectomy restores the white cell count to normal in nearly 90% of affected individuals, but in some the leucopenia reappears.

A small proportion (0.6%) of patients with rheumatoid arthritis may develop splenomegaly as a result of proliferation of large granular lymphocytes. This condition is distinguishable from Felty's syndrome in that lymphocyte proliferation is associated with an absolute granular lymphocytosis greater than 2000/µl and a marrow lymphocytosis. This lymphocyte population is monoclonal and shows rearrangement of the T-cell receptor gene. The distinction between this condition and Felty's syndrome is worth making because lymphocyte proliferation in rheumatoid disease is a benign and rather indolent condition.

AMYLOIDOSIS

This may be:

- focal
- diffuse

The spleen is frequently enlarged in systemic amyloidosis, although the degree of enlargement is not very great as a rule. The amyloid may be distributed chiefly within the white pulp in a focal pattern and, in this case, the cut surface of the organ shows numerous small (2–3 mm) white nodules, which has led the food school of pathologists to call this a **'sago spleen'**. Sago is a form of starch derived from the pith of certain palms and cycads; when cooked it forms glutinous granules.

Amyloid may be distributed in a different pattern in some cases. Here, the amyloid fibrils are laid down along the basement membranes of the sinuses and eventually encroach upon the splenic cords.

Splenic involvement may occur in both:

- reactive systemic amyloidosis, where the starting material for the β-pleated sheet fibrils is **serum amyloid A**
- amyloidosis of immune origin, where the amyloid is derived from the β pleating of either intact **light chains of immunoglobulin** or their aminoterminal portions

Extensive deposition within the spleen is much more common in reactive systemic amyloidosis, which may be the consequence of a variety of chronic inflammatory disorders including the infective granulomas and rheumatoid disease, certain neoplasms and the autosomal recessive disorder, familial Mediterranean fever.

The presence of large amounts of amyloid within the spleen makes the organ much more friable than normal and there is an increased risk of splenic rupture. Needle biopsy of the spleen can be hazardous in patients with splenic amyloidosis for this reason.

NON-NEOPLASTIC HAEMATOLOGICAL CONDITIONS

Haemolytic Anaemias
Splenomegaly may occur in a number of conditions characterized by excess haemolysis (see pp 889–908). This is due to the fact that red cells, either because of some intrinsic abnormality or because they are coated with antibody, tend to become sequestrated in the spleen. The splenic cords are intensely congested whereas the sinuses tend to appear empty and to be lined by cells that are larger than normal; both these factors make the affected sinuses abnormally prominent. Conditions most likely to be associated with splenomegaly are:

- **hereditary spherocytosis**
- **sickle cell disease** during the earlier phases of its natural history. If the affected individual survives for long enough, marked splenic atrophy occurs. This is because of ischaemia due to occlusion of small vessels caused by lack of deformability of the sickled cells.
- **thalassaemia** (see pp 899–903). Splenomegaly is characteristically seen in the major or intermedia type of β-thalassaemia. The splenic enlargement occurs because of excess red cell destruction within the spleen, the presence of extramedullary haemopoiesis and iron overload of the spleen.

   Other haemoglobinopathies, most notably haemoglobin C disease in West Africa and haemoglobin E disease in South-East Asia, are also associated with enlargement of the spleen.
- **autoimmune haemolytic anaemia**

Idiopathic Thrombocytopenic Purpura (ITP)
The defining criteria of this disorder are:
- immunologically mediated destruction of platelets
- absence of any specific disease that might account for this process, hence the use of the term **idiopathic**

ITP occurs mainly in the young; some two-thirds of patients are under 21 years of age at the time of diagnosis. There is a female preponderance, although there is some controversy over the order of magnitude. ITP tends to appear in autumn or winter; this is believed to be due to the prevalence of respiratory tract infections in these seasons.

Platelet survival is significantly shortened; this appears to be due to the presence of a circulating IgG antibody in the plasma. Infusion of ITP plasma into a normal control results in thrombocytopenia. In some but not all cases, the antibody binds to the IIb–IIIa glycoprotein complex which is involved in platelet aggregation.

Microscopic Features
The spleen shows hyperplastic germinal centres in the malpighian corpuscles in about half the cases, suggesting that at least some of the antibody formation is occurring within the spleen. The splenic cords show large numbers of macrophages, many of which are enlarged and vacuolated in the same way as 'sea-blue' histiocytes. The cytoplasm of these cells presumably contains lipid derived from platelet membranes.

The cardinal importance of the spleen in this disease is shown by the effectiveness of splenectomy in returning the platelet count to normal. Platelets certainly become sequestrated within the spleen in ITP and can be seen to be present both within and without macrophages on electron microscopy. When radioactive chromium-labelled platelets are injected into a patient with ITP, the radioactivity becomes concentrated within the spleen.

The Spleen in Myeloproliferative Disorders
These disorders may be associated with extramedullary haemopoiesis and this can lead to splenomegaly of impressive proportions. Disorders falling into this group (see pp 938–941) are:
- polycythaemia vera
- myelofibrosis
- essential thrombocythaemia

Splenomegaly can occur in all three but is most likely to be massive in patients with myelofibrosis. The replacement of haemopoietic cells in the bone marrow by ever-increasing amounts of fibrous tissue leads to the reinstatement of the spleen as a haemopoietic organ.

The spleen in such patients may become enormously enlarged: weights of up to 7 kg have been recorded. The organ is friable and there is an increased risk of rupture. Evidence of extramedullary haemopoiesis is conspicuous and it is obvious that all three normal haemopoietic cell lines are being produced.

NEOPLASTIC DISORDERS INVOLVING THE BLOOD OR LYMPHORETICULAR TISSUES

The spleen may be involved in lymphomas of both the Hodgkin's and non-Hodgkin's types, as well as with the histiocytoses (see pp 972–974).

Splenic involvement may be microscopic or so extensive as to lead to splenomegaly. In general, splenic infiltration by lymphoma is concentrated in the white pulp. Thus, to a considerable extent, it follows the architectural pattern of the white pulp. In some instances, however, lymphoma is expressed in the form of one or more large tumour nodules.

Splenic involvement is also common in the leukaemias, the greatest degree of splenomegaly being seen in patients with chronic myeloid leukaemia. Some 95% of patients with chronic myeloid leukaemia have splenomegaly and one of the presenting complaints may be discomfort in the left upper quadrant of the abdomen due to the splenic enlargement. In a significant proportion of patients (up to 40%), the spleen can be felt 10 cm below the costal margin. In general terms the degree of splenic enlargement is a reflection of level of the white cell count.

MASS LESIONS AND NON-HAEMATOLOGICAL NEOPLASMS OF THE SPLEEN

Splenic Cysts

Cysts in the spleen may be parasitic or non-parasitic in origin. Of the parasitic ones, the commonest is hydatid cyst resulting from infestation by the tapeworm, *Echinococcus granulosus*. The disease occurs in many parts of the world but is commonest in north Africa and the Middle-East. Splenic cysts are also seen in association with cysticercosis and, more rarely, in patients who have pentastomid larvae in their spleens.

Non-parasitic cysts are divided into two groups on the basis of whether or not they have an epithelial lining. A minority (20%) are lined by squamous epithelium; the cyst cavities may contain fatty material such as is seen in ovarian dermoid cysts. It is believed that these lesions result from metaplasia of the mesothelial cells present in the capsule of the spleen and a necessary assumption, in this case, is that some mesothelial cells have become displaced.

Cystic lesions devoid of an epithelial lining may also occur. Some are believed to be post-traumatic, whereas in others it has been suggested that they represent the end result of liquefactive changes in splenic infarcts.

Splenic Hamartomas

These are rare lesions that might be likened to intrasplenic accessory spleens in that they consist of well-defined intrasplenic nodules, ranging in size from 2 to 4 cm in diameter. These have an expansile growth pattern and thus compress the surrounding normal splenic tissue.

On histological examination, some appear to consist of tissue arranged like normal white pulp. Others show a complex array of small blood vessels set in a background of lymphocyte-infiltrated fibrous tissue.

Benign Neoplasms

Most benign neoplastic lesions in the spleen are vascular in type. Splenic haemangiomas are usually quite small (about 2 cm in diameter) and are often found incidentally. Rarely, the spleen may be involved in visceral angiomatosis in which numerous blood-filled spaces are present within the spleen, as, indeed, they are in other tissues.

Malignant Neoplasms

The commonest non-haemopoietic primary malignant tumour of the spleen is **angiosarcoma**. The lesion consists of solid areas of a frankly sarcomatous stroma interspersed with cystically dilated vascular channels. In some cases, the tumour is associated with a macrocytic anaemia, although the reason for this is not known. Other haematological abnormalities described in association with this tumour are a consumptive coagulopathy (disseminated intravascular coagulation) and a microangiopathic anaemia. Angiosarcoma is highly malignant and most sufferers are dead within 1 year of the diagnosis having been made.

Metastatic splenic deposits are found on naked-eye examination in about 4–8% of autopsies carried out on patients dying from non-haemopoietic malignant disease. The prevalence of deposits identifiable only on microscopic examination is, of course, considerably greater. The tumours most likely to give rise to splenic metastases are melanoma, lung cancer, ovarian cancer and malignant trophoblastic tumours.

RUPTURE OF THE SPLEEN

Rupture of the spleen is most commonly the result of blunt trauma to a normal spleen, such as can occur with steering wheel injuries to the upper abdomen. Large lacerations of the spleen lead to extensive intraperitoneal haemorrhage, peritoneal irritation and shock. In some instances haemorrhage into the peritoneal cavity ceases after the loss of 500–700 ml blood and a subcapsular haematoma may form, which can rupture at any time. In such cases, clinical signs of rupture may appear only some time after the injury, a phenomenon incorrectly called 'delayed rupture'.

Splenic rupture may also occur as a result of minimal trauma or, possibly without trauma, if the spleen is enlarged and abnormally soft. This is most likely to occur in patients with infectious mononucleosis but has been reported in association with measles and in pregnant women with no obvious disorder affecting the lymphoreticular system.

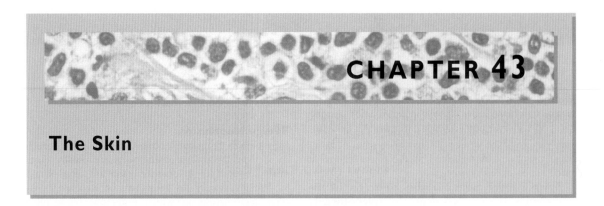
The Skin

The Skin and its Disorders

NORMAL FUNCTION

The skin is the largest organ in the body. In addition to acting as a protective covering to the tissues that lie beneath it, it has many other functions:

- formation of a physical barrier to microorganisms and certain antigens
- prevention of excessive absorption or loss of water
- prevention, as a result of the pigment within epidermal cells, of injury from ultraviolet light
- synthesis of vitamin D as a result of the interaction of ultraviolet light and 7-dehydrocholesterol within the epidermis
- regulation of temperature, by the state of tone of the dermal and subcutaneous vessels
- mediation of the sensations of light touch, pain and temperature
- mediation of immunological reactions through antigen-presenting cells known as Langerhans cells

NORMAL STRUCTURE

Skin consists essentially of three separate compartments (*Fig. 43.1*):

1) **epidermis**
2) **dermis**
3) **subcutaneous tissue**

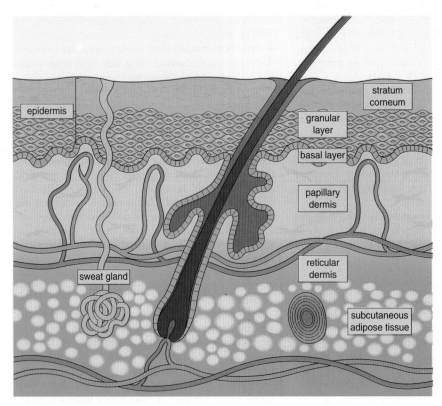

FIGURE 43.1 Normal skin showing the division into three compartments – epidermis, dermis and subcutaneous tissue – and the basic subdivisions of the first two of these.

EPIDERMIS

This is derived from the ectoderm and consists predominantly of stratified squamous epithelium (keratinocytes) (*Fig. 43.2*) in which small numbers of other cells can be identified. The latter include **melanocytes**, responsible for the synthesis of melanin, **Langerhans cells** (specialized antigen-presenting cells) (*Fig. 43.3*) and **Merkel** cells, believed to have neuroendocrine functions.

The superficial surface of the epidermis is more or less flat; the deep surface which abuts on to the dermis is undulating, as a result of the papillary folds into which the upper surface of the dermis is thrown.

The keratinocyte population is arranged in four layers. Working from the deep to superficial surfaces these are:

1) **The basal cell layer** consisting of mitotically active cells that give rise to the other keratinocytes. These are columnar to cuboidal cells with large nuclei, prominent nucleoli and basophilic cytoplasm. They are frequently pigmented because

of the transfer of melanin from adjacent melanocytes, situated normally in the basal layer.

A basement membrane separates this layer of cells from the underlying dermis, and the basal cells are attached to the membrane by special structures known as hemidesmosomes. The basal lamina region itself consists of four zones (*Fig. 43.4*):

- the plasma membrane of the epidermal cells which contains the hemidesmosomes
- an electron-lucent zone known as the **lamina lucida**, which contains the protein laminin and the bullous pemphigoid antigen (see p 997)
- an electron-dense area (**lamina densa**) consisting of type IV collagen
- a zone in which there are extensions of the lamina densa serving as attachments to the underlying dermis

2) **The squamous layer (stratum spinosum or prickle cell layer)** consists of several layers of cells which are polyhedral. The lower layers are basophilic and somewhat rounded, whereas the upper ones are more eosinophilic, flattened and oriented with their long axes parallel to the skin surface. The term 'prickle cells' has been applied to these keratinocytes because of their appearance on light microscopy. The cells look as if they are attached to each other by short processes (prickles). This appearance results from retraction of adjacent cell membranes during the process of fixation. The desmosomes, which are attachment structures, remain fixed and it is the combination of this membrane retraction and desmosome fixation that gives the 'prickle' appearance.

3) **The granular layer** is composed of one to three layers of flattened cells, the cytoplasm of

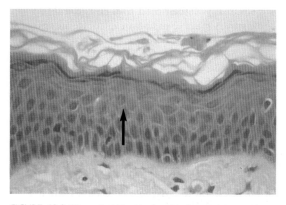

FIGURE 43.2 Normal epidermis showing the stratum corneum which is devoid of nuclei, the granular layer composed of prickle cells (arrowed) and the rather 'picket-fence'-like basal layer.

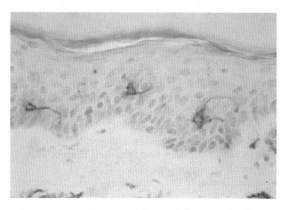

FIGURE 43.3 Epidermis immunostained to show Langerhans cells (brown) which are the 'professional' antigen-presenting cells of the skin. The characteristic Birbeck granules seen on electron microscopy of these cells are shown in Fig. 42.26.

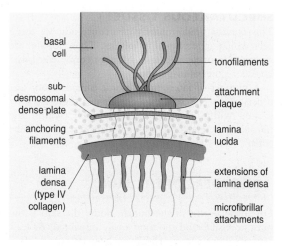

FIGURE 43.4 Zones of the dermoepidermal basement membrane and the relationships of the membrane to epidermal and dermal components.

which contains basophilic granules known as **keratohyaline**. These granules are rich in the amino acid histidine and are the precursors of a protein known as **filaggrin**, which promotes aggregation of keratin filaments.

4) The cells of the stratum corneum have lost their nuclei and cytoplasmic organelles as part of the normal maturation process. This layer is normally about three to four cells thick and has a typical 'basket-weave' appearance, as all that is left of these cells is their keratinous skeleton. The keratin is normally shed.

DERMIS

The dermis consists of a two-zoned layer of connective tissue providing a supporting matrix for the epidermis:

1) The upper zone, the papillary dermis, is configured in a series of papillae. Each papilla is separated from the one adjacent to it by a prolongation of the epidermis known as the **rete ridge**. The papillary dermis consists principally of a rather loose meshwork of collagen and some elastin fibres oriented more or less at right angles to the overlying epidermal surface. Within this matrix are loops of blood vessels and the nerve fibres that subserve the functions of light touch, pain and temperature.

2) The lower zone, the reticular dermis, is beneath an imaginary line joining the tips of the rete ridges; it consists principally of thick collagen bundles, oriented more or less parallel to the overlying skin surface. Some thick elastin fibres are also present, which often show fragmentation. Embedded within the reticular dermis are adnexal structures such as sweat glands, of both eccrine and apocrine type, sebaceous glands and hair follicles with their associated muscles, the arrectores pilorum.

SUBCUTANEOUS TISSUE

This consists predominantly of mature adipose tissue cells which are arranged in lobules. These lobules are separated from each other by bands of connective tissue known as interlobular septa.

A number of interesting chronic inflammatory disorders affect the subcutaneous tissue; these may be located within the adipose tissue itself, within the fibrous tissue septa or in both compartments of the subcutis.

DISORDERS OF THE SKIN

Of all the organs of the human body, the skin is the most accessible and the most easily inspected. At least 1000 different skin disorders have been described, often in the most arcane terms, and eponyms run wild through the field of dermatological literature.

With the possible exception of neuropathology,

dermatology causes more semantic problems to the non-expert than any other. When travelling in a foreign country, it is helpful to know something of the language; thus, the study of skin pathology can be helped by understanding some of the jargon most commonly used. It is comforting to know that, of the many skin diseases, ten account for more than two-thirds of the patients seen with skin problems (excluding skin tumours).

A short glossary of some common terms used in dermatopathology is provided in *Tables 43.1* and *43.2*.

DISORDERS CHARACTERIZED BY INCREASED EPIDERMAL CELL TURNOVER

PSORIASIS
Psoriasis is:

- **one of the commonest disorders of the skin**, affecting 0.9–2.8% of Western populations
- **genetically determined to a considerable extent.** A number of human leucocyte antigen (HLA) associations have been described, of which the strongest is **HLA-Cw6**. This antigen confers a 13-fold increased risk for the development of psoriasis. More recently another gene apparently involved in susceptibility for psoriasis has been localized to the distal region of the long arm of chromosome 17.
- **characterized clinically by well-defined pink or red plaque-like lesions covered by typical, large, silvery-white scales.** Removal of these scales sometimes shows small bleeding points. The lesions can occur anywhere on glabrous skin but are especially likely to be found on extensor surfaces, such as the elbows, and on the trunk and scalp. Lesions characteristically appear at sites where trauma has occurred (the **Koebner phenomenon**). Several clinical variants exist but the pathological features of these are essentially the same.
- **associated in about 5–10% of cases with a severe arthropathy.** The joint disease is clinically similar to rheumatoid arthritis but rheumatoid factor is never present in the serum. It belongs, therefore, to the group of conditions known as the seronegative arthropathies.
- **not confined to the skin and joints but can also affect the nail bed, the nail matrix and mucous membranes.** The nail plates characteristically show the presence of pits resulting from focal areas of parakeratosis which are shed from the nail plate. Discrete whitish-grey areas may be seen on the tongue, buccal mucosa or palate. This tends to occur in association with a variant known as pustular psoriasis.

Table 43.1 Naked-eye Morphology of Skin Lesions

Lesion	Description
Lesion	In this context, **any single, usually small, area of skin pathology**. Skin lesions are analysed in terms of their number, size, shape and colour.
Rash	**A collective noun for the totality of the lesions present.** These may extend over a wide area. The term is especially likely to be applied to lesions that are widespread, red and only slightly, if at all, raised.
Macule	**A small area of colour change.** Macules are not palpable, but, occasionally, may be slightly depressed below the surface of the surrounding skin. They are usually less than 1.5 cm in diameter.
Papule	**A small palpable lesion less than 1.5 cm in diameter.** While many papules are raised above the surrounding skin, some are not, being largely either intradermal or within the subcutaneous tissue. A subtype of papule is the wheal, in which the substance of the lesion is made up of non-loculated interstitial fluid.
Nodule	A nodule is **the lesion that results from enlargement of a papule in all three of its dimensions: length, width and height**.
Plaque	In contrast with a nodule, **a plaque is the lesion that results from enlargement of a papule in only two of its dimensions: length and width**.
Vesicle	**A small blister, less than 1.5 cm in diameter.** Some writers regard this lesion as a fluid-filled papule in which the fluid is strictly confined. As a result, if the roof of a vesicle is incised, the lesion collapses as the fluid escapes.
Pustule	**A vesicle filled with neutrophils.** As a result, this lesion is white or yellowish in colour and the fluid which it contains is turbid.
Bulla	**A blister that measures 1.5 cm or more in diameter.** In every other respect it is identical with a vesicle.
Crust	**This results from the exudation of plasma either through damaged epidermis or in an area of epidermal loss. Evaporation of plasma water leaves a deposit of dried plasma proteins at the site of the exudate.** The crust is rough to palpation and appears as an amorphous yellowish layer. If bleeding has been associated with exudation, the crust will be red, violet or black in colour, depending on its age, as a result of the presence of haem.
Scale	**A scale is formed as a result of an increase in thickness of the most superficial layer of the epidermis, the stratum corneum or keratin layer.** This may be due either to excess formation of a keratin layer or to a delay in its exfoliation. Three types of scale are recognized: • **Psoriatic** scales. These are easily visible, white, grey or silvery flakes large enough to be picked up individually. The silvery white appearance results from the fact that the scales are attached only loosely so that there are two light-refracting interfaces. • **Pityriasis**-type scales. These are too small to be distinguished individually. They cannot be seen unless the lesion is gently scraped, this yielding a fine white powder. Diseases with the word pityriasis in their names usually have this sort of scaling. • **Lichen**-type scale. This can be appreciated as a slight roughness on the surface of the affected skin. The scales are tightly adherent to the surface of the lesion and reflect light, having a shiny appearance. Lichenification of the skin is due to long-continued rubbing; the skin becomes thickened, the normal skin markings become exaggerated and lichen-type scales are present.
Erosion	The defining criterion of erosion is **loss of the epidermal surface of all or part of the lesion.** Erosions may form as a result of loss of the upper surface of a blister or as a result of external trauma, most notably scratching. The lesions are shallow, because part of the definition is that the dermis should not be involved. A special type of erosion is the **fissure**. Fissures are linear cracks seen between islands of epidermis. They are formed as a result of excessive drying which leads to shrinkage of the cells.
Ulcer	This lesion resembles an erosion in that **there is focal loss of epidermis. Dermal damage is, however, also present and this means that the lesion is obviously deeper than is the case with an erosion**.

Table 43.2 Microscopic Abnormalities in Skin Disease: the Epidermis

Abnormality	Descriptive features
Acantholysis	**Loss of cohesion between keratinocytes due to breakdown of cell–cell attachments.** This may be due to immune-mediated damage to keratinocyte plasma membranes or to desmosomes. **The result is the formation of intraepidermal clefts, vesicles or bullae, and the rounding up the damaged keratinocytes.** The level of the acantholysis within the epidermis is important in making a precise diagnosis.
Acanthosis	**An increase in the size and number of cells in the prickle cell layer (Gk. *acanthos* thorn or prickle).** Acanthosis may be due to elongation of the rete ridges, as in a **psoriasiform reaction**, or may involve the whole epidermis such as is seen in **lichenification**.
Ballooning degeneration	**Marked swelling and pallor of individual keratinocytes with loss of intercellular bridging.** This leads to the formation of blisters. It is characteristic of viral disorders affecting epithelia, such as herpesvirus infections, and may result in the formation of many large intraepidermal vesicles in which a ragged meshwork of cellular debris may be present. This appearance is known as **reticular degeneration**.
Basal cell liquefaction	This is a change that affects the basal cell layer of the epidermis. Small droplets and somewhat larger vesicles develop both within and between the basal cells, and this may be sufficiently severe as to lead to subepidermal blister formation. The melanin content of the affected cells is released and finds its way into the dermis where it is taken up by macrophages. This loss of pigment from the epidermis is known as pigment incontinence. Basal liquefaction occurs in a number of disorders including lichen planus, lupus erythematosus, lichen sclerosus and dermatomyositis.
Bullae	**A bulla is a fluid-containing cavity which may be situated within or below the epidermis.** There are several mechanisms that can lead to bulla formation within the epidermis. These include **spongiosis** (intraepidermal oedema which occurs in eczema), **reticular degeneration, acantholysis and keratinocyte destruction.** Subepidermal bulla formation may result from: • **inherited defects in the basement membrane** (e.g. epidermolysis bullosa) • **severe liquefaction degeneration of the basement membrane** (e.g. bullous lichen planus) • **inflammation involving the upper part of the papillary dermis**
Crusting	**Dried plasma protein deposits either on the epidermis or replacing lost epidermis.** Inflammatory cells and red cells are frequently seen within the crust.
Cytoid, colloid or Civatte bodies	**Homogeneous, rounded, eosinophilic bodies which result from programmed death or apoptosis of keratinocytes**, often but not exclusively in the basal layer of the epidermis. They are often seen in lichenoid processes such as lichen planus.
Dyskeratosis	**An abnormality of keratinization occurring either in association with malignant or premalignant lesions arising within the epidermis or in association with certain acantholytic disorders** such as Darier's disease (keratosis follicularis).
Microabscesses	**These are small collections of inflammatory cells found either within the epidermis or at the tips of the dermal papillae.** Varieties include: • **Munro microabscesses**: neutrophils found, as a rule, in the stratum corneum of the epidermis in chronic psoriasis • **Pautrier microabscesses**: intraepidermal aggregates of atypical lymphocytes found in cutaneous T-cell lymphomas such as mycosis fungoides

Table 43.2 Microscopic Abnormalities in Skin Disease: the Epidermis – *continued*

Abnormality	Descriptive features
Microabscesses – *contd*	• **papillary tip microabscesses**: small collections of either neutrophils or, more rarely, eosinophils within the tips of the dermal papillae. They are seen typically in dermatitis herpetiformis but may occur in other bullous eruptions.
Orthokeratosis	**Increased thickness of the stratum corneum without any retention of the keratinocyte nuclei.**
Parakeratosis	**Retention of keratinocyte nuclei within the stratum corneum.** It is normally associated with reduction of the thickness of the granular layer of the epidermis or its complete absence. It is a feature of many different types of inflammatory skin disease, especially those in which there is an increase in epidermal cell turnover, such as psoriasis and subacute eczema.
Spongiosis	**Widening of intercellular spaces in the epidermis which occurs as a result of oedema.** It is characteristically seen in acute and subacute eczematous reactions but may occur in many other skin conditions.
Saw-toothing	**The tips of the dermal papillae are widened and the rete ridges are pointed instead of being rounded.** It is typically seen in lichen planus.
Vesicle	A vesicle is a collection of fluid smaller than a bulla. The mechanisms that underlie its formation are essentially the same as those operating in bulla formation.

Microscopic Features

- Both the epidermis and the dermis are affected.
- The epidermis is thickened due to an increase in the number and size of cells of the stratum spinosum, the granular layer often being absent. As a result of this acanthosis, the rete ridges are elongated and club-shaped and, not infrequently, there is fusion of the tips of adjacent rete ridges (*Fig. 43.5*).
- The number of mitoses seen in psoriatic epidermis is about ten times that in normal epidermis.
- The epidermis between the rete ridges (i.e. the suprapapillary epidermis) is usually atrophic and shows parakeratosis, the keratin lamella often being clearly separated one from another. It is these zones of parakeratosis that constitute the typical silvery scales.
- Neutrophils may be present within the abnormal epidermis and these may collect in small foci known as **Munro microabscesses**. These neutrophils emigrate from small blood vessels within the dermal papillae and some workers envisage a regular episodic emigration of inflammatory cell from the tips of the papillae into the epidermis. This concept has led to the coining of the phrase **'squirting papillae'**.
- The dermal papillae show oedema and a mild to moderate infiltrate of inflammatory cells including macrophages arranged round small blood vessels. These blood vessels are dilated and tortuous. The dermal changes are regarded by some as the initial lesions of psoriasis, with products of the inflammatory cells 'driving' the epidermal events. In relapsing lesions, the earliest histological changes seen are swelling and separation of the endothelial cells of the small blood vessels and degranulation of mast cells.

Pathogenesis

It is still not possible to construct a model of the cause or causes of psoriasis and the pathogenetic steps involved, although some interesting evidence has accrued, which is relevant both to the microscopic features and to treatment of this distressing complaint:

- **The combination of acanthosis and an increased mitotic rate in the epidermis indicates that there is both increased cell proliferation and a reduction in the turnover time of the keratinocytes.** In respect of the latter, the normal transit time from basal layer to stratum corneum is approximately 28 days. In active psoriatic lesions this is decreased to 3–4 days. In any situation, increased cell proliferation may be the result of one or both of:

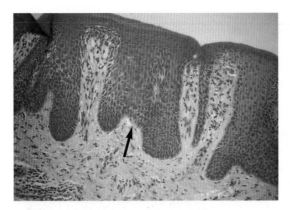

FIGURE 43.5 *Psoriasis showing hyperkeratosis (accounting for the scales) and alternating areas of epidermal atrophy and prolongation of rete pegs. Fusion of adjacent rete pegs is a prominent feature, leading to 'club-shaped' prolongation of epidermis (arrow).*

1) an increased drive
2) increased transduction of normal drive

In psoriatic skin the keratinocytes show an increase in the expression of epidermal growth factor (EGF) receptor. In addition, the EGF receptor's natural ligand, transforming growth factor (TGF) α and its messenger RNA have been identified in psoriatic lesions. Thus it seems that both the mechanisms suggested above are operating in the context of psoriasis.

- **The presence of inflammatory cells within the epidermis implies that appropriate chemoattractant signals must be generated.**
  There is an increased concentration of arachidonic acid in psoriatic skin, indicating an increase in the activity of phospholipase C which releases this fatty acid from membrane phospholipid. Arachidonic acid is the substrate for lipo-oxygenase, yielding a series of compounds including the powerful chemoattractant for neutrophils, leukotriene B_4, and also a series of hydroperoxides of eicosatetraenoic acid (HETE). Some workers have found that leukotriene B_4 is mitogenic for keratinocytes but this has not yet been confirmed. A relevant, though not predominant, role for lipo-oxygenase in psoriasis is suggested by the facts that:
  1) leukotriene B_4, when applied to normal skin, attracts neutrophils into the epidermis
  2) application of the inhibitor of 5-lipo-oxygenase, lonapalene, to psoriatic skin results in some degree of clinical improvement

  Other chemoattractants found in psoriatic skin include interleukin (IL) 8 and modified C5a.
- **A possible role for immunologically mediated mechanisms has been canvassed recently.**
  Cyclosporin A has been shown to be therapeutically effective in psoriasis, and activated T cells have been identified in the lesions. These T cells express HLA-DR molecules and also receptors for IL-2. It has also been shown that keratinocytes in psoriatic epidermis express HLA-DR antigens, although this is, of course, not the case in normal skin. Systemic administration of IL-2 to patients with psoriasis causes the lesions to worsen.

OTHER PSORIATIC ERUPTIONS

Seborrhoeic Dermatitis
Some dermatologists include seborrhoeic dermatitis as one of the psoriatic eruptions, although others maintain that it should be classified as a local eczematous reaction. It is characterized by a scaly rash in areas where seborrhoeic glands are present, most notably in relation to the scalp, eyebrows, paranasal areas, nasolabial folds, presternal area, central back and in the folds behind the ears.

The eruption may occur in a dry form with powdery scales such as are seen in its most common manifestation – dandruff – or in an oily form with greasy scales occurring on a base of reddened skin. Seborrhoeic dermatitis occurs also in infants, in whom it affects particularly the scalp, the scaly eruption on the scalp being sometimes referred to as 'cradle cap'. Spontaneous remission usually occurs within the first year of life in these affected infants and, thereafter, the disease is rare until puberty.

The histological features resemble those of psoriasis in certain respects with especial reference to the presence of parakeratotic scales in the suprapapillary regions of the epidermis. Munro microabscesses are rare and tiny.

The cause is unknown, although the view is taken by some that there is an aetiological role for the fungus *Pityrosporum ovale*; certainly, this organism is often present in the lesions. Many of the preparations that produce a clinical improvement in seborrhoeic dermatitis are antifungal agents, providing some support for a fungal aetiology.

Reiter's Disease
Reiter's disease (see also p 1083) is expressed in the skin as an eruption affecting particularly the palms and the soles. Its clinical and microscopic features closely resemble those seen in pustular psoriasis. This pattern of the disease is termed **keratoderma blennorrhagica**.

BLISTERING (BULLOUS) DISEASES OF THE SKIN CAUSED BY IMMUNE MECHANISMS

A number of diseases of the skin show blistering as their outstanding characteristic. The entities dealt with in this section are caused by autoimmune reactions, although there are some bullous disorders, for example epidermolysis bullosa, in which blistering occurs on the basis of an inherited defect.

Autoimmune bullous disorders are classified according to the position of the bullae (*Fig. 43.6*), as shown in *Table 43.3*.

As shown in *Table 43.3*, there are varieties of pemphigus **which can be divided into two groups depending on whether the intraepidermal blistering is suprabasal or more superficially situated**. In all of them, the blisters are caused by the action of **autoantibodies** either on membrane proteins or on desmosomal proteins. This results in **acantholysis**.

The archetypal lesion is a flaccid blister which may, however, rupture and crust. Microscopic diagnosis depends on identifying the level of the blistering within the epidermis and, thus, examination of lesions once they have are eroded and crusted is futile.

Pemphigus Vulgaris

Pemphigus vulgaris is the commonest of the four varieties of pemphigus. It presents with generalized blistering which is most marked within skin folds in the early stages of the disorder. Rupture of the blisters is followed by extensive crusting. In addition to the blisters, there appears to be decreased cohesion of epidermal cells in some areas of apparently normal skin; sliding pressure applied to the skin results in separation of the epidermis from the underlying tissue. This is known as **Nikolsky's sign**.

The mouth is frequently involved at an early stage (50% of cases). Because these blisters rupture easily, there is often extensive denudation of the oral mucosa associated with considerable pain. Extensive erosion of skin and mucous membranes may lead to significant protein and fluid loss and, of course, also provides a portal for secondary bacterial infection.

Aetiology and Pathogenesis

Pemphigus vulgaris has a worldwide distribution, but it tends to occur most commonly in Ashkenazi Jews. There is an increased prevalence of the HLA antigens,

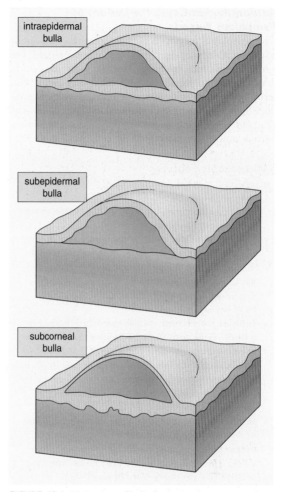

FIGURE 43.6 *Major sites of bulla formation.*

A10, A26, Bw38 and DR4, suggesting that one or more of these genes confers increased likelihood of the development of autoantibodies binding to specific epidermal antigens.

Table 43.3 Autoimmune Bullous Disorders

Epidermal or subepidermal	Location or special feature	Disease
Intraepidermal	Stratum corneum or granulosum	Pemphigus foliaceus Fogo selvagem
Intraepidermal	Suprabasal	Pemphigus vulgaris Pemphigus vegetans
Subepidermal		Bullous pemphigoid Cicatricial pemphigoid
Subepidermal	Associated with microabscesses at tips of papillae	Dermatitis herpetiformis
Subepidermal	Associated with necrosis of keratinocytes	Erythema multiforme

Autoantibodies Cause the Lesions of Pemphigus Vulgaris

The pemphigus vulgaris antigen is a normal component of the keratinocyte plasma membrane. Some regard it as a novel form of the epithelial adhesion molecule e-cadherin. Immunoglobulin (Ig)G antibodies from the serum of patients with active pemphigus vulgaris produce suprabasal clefting in cultured explants of human skin and thus appear to be responsible for the lesions and are not merely markers of the process (*Fig. 43.7*).

Microscopic Features

- The level of blister formation is just above the basal layer so that the floor of the blister shows a line of basal cells standing up like a row of tombstones above the basement membrane.
- **Within the blister cavity a moderate number of rounded, acantholytic keratinocytes are seen**; in the earlier stages of blister formation, there may be spongiosis associated with an eosinophil infiltrate in some cases. In general, inflammation is conspicuous by its absence.
- **Immunofluorescent studies show IgG bound in a linear fashion to the surface membrane of the keratinocytes; in some instances, C3 is found in an identical location.** Many regard the results of such immunofluorescence studies as being more useful diagnostically than conventional light microscopy of the lesions.
- In patients with active disease IgG antibodies, binding to the same surface membrane locations on the keratinocytes, are often but not always present in the serum. Their presence and titre may be an expression of the degree of activity of the disease.

Pemphigus Vegetans

This is a variant of pemphigus vulgaris, showing the same suprabasal bulla formation, and is the rarest of all the varieties of pemphigus.

In its early stages, pemphigus vegetans is characterized by the same flaccid blisters as are seen in pemphigus vulgaris. These blisters rupture easily but, as they heal, **warty hyperplastic masses are seen at the sites of the erosions**. It is this that has led to the term **vegetans** being applied to this disorder. These lesions are especially prone to develop in skin folds such as the groin. This naked-eye appearance reflects the presence of hyperkeratosis and epidermal hyperplasia with downgrowths of the rete ridges and a particular tendency for the epithelium of hair follicles to be involved.

Pemphigus Foliaceus

The defining criterion of pemphigus foliaceus is the level within the epidermis at which bulla formation occurs. These bullae are subcorneal and are thus smaller than the flaccid bullae so characteristic of pemphigus vulgaris. These rather

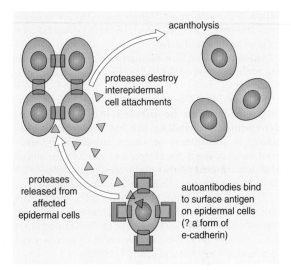

FIGURE 43.7 *A model for bulla formation in pemphigus vulgaris. Autoantibodies bind to a surface antigen on epidermal cells. This is followed by the release of proteases from the affected cells. The proteases destroy interepidermal attachments, leading to acantholysis.*

inconspicuous blisters rupture early and the disorder is expressed to a much greater extent in the form of crusted erosions than in the form of a bullous eruption. Itching is prominent and the Nikolsky sign is positive.

Pemphigus foliaceus may occur under three different sets of circumstances:

- sporadically and with no obvious association; the so-called **idiopathic variety**
- endemically in certain parts of South America, most notably in Brazil. Here the disorder is called **fogo selvagem** (wild fire). Often several members of the same family are affected and it has been suggested that this variant may be due to a viral infection, possibly transmitted via an insect bite.
- associated with the administration of certain drugs which include penicillamine (the commonest associated drug), piroxicam, the angiotensin-converting enzyme inhibitor captopril, rifampicin and phenobarbitone.

The areas of skin most likely to be affected include the face, scalp and upper part of the trunk. Indeed, the distribution is reminiscent of that seen in patients with seborrhoeic dermatitis. In patients with fogo selvagem, however, the eruption tends to be generalized.

Microscopic Features

Subcorneal acantholysis is present. IgG and C3 are found distributed in a linear pattern in relation to keratinocytes in the upper layers of the epidermis. The autoantibodies here bind to a normal component of keratinocyte desmosomes known as **desmoglein 1**.

Pemphigus Erythematosus

A variant of pemphigus foliaceus exists which is known as **pemphigus erythematosus** (Senear–Usher syndrome). These patients show, in addition to the features of pemphigus foliaceus, some of the clinical and immunological features seen in lupus erythematosus; their serum contains autoantibodies reacting in a granular discrete pattern with the lupus erythematosus antigen in the basement membrane as well as those reacting with the keratinocyte desmoglein 1.

Bullous Pemphigoid

This is a much commoner and more benign disorder than pemphigus, from which it is differentiated by the fact that the blisters occur at the **dermoepidermal junction** rather than within the epidermis.

Bullous pemphigoid affects chiefly middle-aged and elderly individuals and some degree of female preponderance is noted. Flexural areas tend to be especially affected, the inguinal regions being sites of predilection. From the groin, the blisters spread down the inside of the thighs. The blisters, which may occur on the background of normal or erythematous skin, are large and much more tense than those of pemphigus, and rupture much less easily. This is a reflection of the fact that, because the clefting occurs at the dermoepidermal junction, the roof of the blisters in pemphigoid consists of full-thickness epidermis. The Nikolsky sign is negative.

Lesions usually heal without scarring, although small so-called milium cysts may occur at the site of the blisters. In the variant known as cicatricial pemphigoid, in which the mouth, eyes and genital areas are affected, scarring is prominent.

Microscopic Features

- The bullae lie between the dermis and the epidermis. The roofs of these lesions consist of full-thickness epidermis in which there is no evidence of cellular necrosis or abnormal separation of the keratinocytes one from another.
- The cavities of the bullae contain large numbers of eosinophils.
- Direct immunofluorescent technique shows a linear deposit consisting predominantly of IgG along the lamina lucida of the basement membrane. IgM and IgA in small amounts are occasionally seen. The antigen with which the autoantibodies react appears to be a protein component of the hemidesmosomes.
- Healing may occur by the extension of new epidermal cells along the exposed dermoepidermal junction. These cells may be derived from the epidermal component of hair follicles or sweat ducts.

Dermatitis Herpetiformis

This is an intensely itchy, fortunately rare, condition characterized by groups of small vesicles on the scalp,

scapulae, extensor surfaces of the limbs, and buttocks. The vesicles contain either clear or blood-stained fluid and, because of the intense pruritus, are often excoriated due to scratching.

The disorder is not seen in black-skinned people and Asiatics, and there is an association with the HLA antigens A1, B8 and DR3. Most patients have an associated gluten-sensitive enteropathy which may, however, be asymptomatic even though the typical histological features are present in small bowel mucosal biopsies. Avoidance of foods containing gluten may bring about some improvement in the skin condition; it has been suggested that the IgA antibodies reacting with gliadin in flour also bind to connective tissue matrix proteins in the dermal papillae.

Microscopic Features (Fig. 43.8)

- small neutrophil-rich abscesses at the tips of the dermal papillae
- multilocular subepidermal bullae
- granular deposits of IgA along the dermoepidermal junction

Erythema Multiforme

This is a set of disorders in which round, fixed, erythematous lesions occur in self-limiting and/or recurrent episodes.

Microscopic Features

In microscopic terms the defining criteria of erythema multiforme are:

- epidermal cell damage consistent with cytotoxic injury
- a mononuclear inflammatory cell infiltrate suggestive of a cell-mediated immune reaction

Many factors have been suggested as possible precipitating factors, perhaps acting as antigens, for the

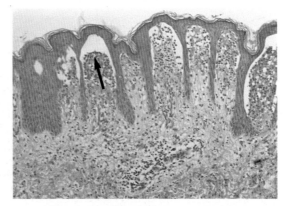

FIGURE 43.8 Dermatitis herpetiformis showing subepidermal bullae and neutrophil accumulations at the tips of the dermal papillae (arrow).

development of erythema multiforme; some of these are listed in *Table 43.4.*

Table 43.4 Precipitating Factors for Erythema Multiforme

Factor	Examples
Viral infections	Herpes simplex
	Epstein–Barr virus
	Vaccinia
Bacterial infections	Streptococci
	Yersinia
	Mycobacterium tuberculosis
	Treponema pallidum (syphilis)
Protozoal infections	*Trichomonas*
Mycoplasma infections	Primary atypical pneumonia
Fungal infections	Histoplasmosis
	Coccidioidomycosis
Immunization	Horse serum
	Various vaccines
Drugs	Sulphonamides
	Anticonvulsants
	Penicillins
	Tetracyclines
	Methotrexate
	Quinine
	Dapsone
	Cocaine
	Isoniazid
	Clindamycin
	Chlorpropamide
	Oestrogens
Contact dermatitis	Nickel
	Primula
	Terpenes
Neoplasms	Leukaemia/lymphoma
	Leiomyoma
Connective tissue diseases	Lupus erythematosus
Physical agents	Sunlight
	X-irradiation
Foods	Emulsifying agents in margarines
Inhalants	Methylparathion
Other diseases	Inflammatory bowel disease
	Sarcoidosis

Clinical Features

Three main forms of erythema multiforme are recognized, although there is a degree of overlap:

- **The iris type.** This is the commonest variant and is characterized by the presence of symmetrically distributed, round, red or purplish lesions with a central slightly raised and more erythematous area and a periphery that is less severely affected. The lesions, thus, have a target or iris-like appearance. Erythema multiforme of this type is usually self-limiting and rarely lasts more than a few weeks. The lesions tend to occur on both aspects of the hands and feet, and on the forearms and legs.
- **The vesicobullous type.** In this variant, the centre of the lesion becomes vesicular or bullous. These lesions tend to rupture, leaving painful ulcers which may involve not only the skin but also the mouth and genitalia.
- **Stevens–Johnson syndrome.** This fortunately rare variant is potentially fatal. The skin and mucous membranes are extensively involved by blistering and ulceration. A significant degree of constitutional disturbance may be present; the patient is often febrile and, because of involvement of the oral mucosa, may be unable to eat. Conjunctival involvement may be present and this can lead to corneal scarring and blindness.

Microscopic Features (*Fig. 43.9*)

- The upper dermis shows dilatation of the small blood vessels and oedema of the dermal papillae.
- The blood vessels are surrounded by inflammatory cells, the cell population consisting principally of lymphocytes and macrophages. The inflammatory infiltrate is most severe at the dermoepidermal junction.
- Some degree of necrosis of the keratinocytes is always present. This ranges from single cell necrosis to a situation in which much or all of the epidermal thickness is affected.
- Immunohistological studies show C3 distributed in a granular fashion along the dermoepidermal junction and in small blood vessels within the papillary dermis. This may be associated with the presence of IgM as well.

Pathogenesis

There is no evidence of either immune complex-related cell damage or formation of autoantibodies. Some have suggested that the pathological picture is the result of a cell-mediated immune reaction but there is still no evidence as to what has elicited such a response, and no common explanation that might account for all the circumstances associated with this condition.

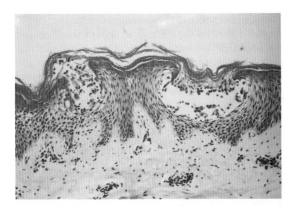

FIGURE 43.9 Erythema multiforme associated with a striking degree of necrosis of keratinocytes with the formation of large intraepidermal bullae.

NON-IMMUNE BLISTERING DISORDERS

Darier's Disease (Follicular Keratosis)

Darier's disease, an autosomal dominant disorder, is characterized clinically by the appearance of dark brown warty nodules on the skin of the hands, trunk, scalp, groins, axilla and neck. It is associated in many instances with some degree of immunodeficiency, and patients are at increased risk of developing a variety of infections.

Microscopic Features

The defining criteria of Darier's disease are histological consisting of:

- **the formation of focal suprabasal clefts due to acantholytic separation of the keratinocytes.** Some of the keratinocytes in the stratum spinosum and stratum granulosum undergo **premature keratinization** and appear as bodies known as **'corps ronds'**. These have centrally placed basophilic and somewhat shrunken nuclei surrounded by a clear halo. Later forms of the corps ronds are found in the stratum corneum in the form of small eosinophilic bodies which often show no evidence of nuclear remnants. These are known as **'grains'**.

  The acantholysis in the case of Darier's disease is believed to be due to some fault in the desmosome–tonofilament complex, the pathogenesis of which is not understood.
- **hyperkeratosis and parakeratosis involving the epidermis above the suprabasal clefts**
- **papillary downgrowths of epidermis, especially in those areas relating to sweat glands and hair follicles**
- no evidence of any antibody deposition, unlike in pemphigus.

Benign Familial Pemphigus (Hailey–Hailey Disease)

This is another autosomal dominant disorder which shares some histological features with Darier's disease. As in the case of the latter, the major defect seems to be in relation to the desmosome–tonofilament complex; as a result, there is defective adhesion between adjacent keratinocytes. Thus, in areas of friction, large flaccid blisters form, the patients generally presenting during adolescence. These blisters then become eroded and crust over, giving a clinical appearance not dissimilar to that seen in pemphigus.

Microscopic Features

- As in the case of Darier's disease, **the main pathological process is acantholysis starting suprabasally**. Unlike Darier's disease, this acantholysis affects the upper layers of the stratum spinosum as well and thus **the clefts that form are much larger than those seen in Darier's disease**.
- **Typically, the acantholysis is incomplete** and thus the degree of separation of the affected keratinocytes is, similarly, incomplete. This gives to the affected area **an appearance that has been likened to a dilapidated brick wall**.
- The hyperkeratosis and concentration on follicles, so conspicuous in Darier's disease, are not, as a rule, seen in benign familial pemphigus.
- Immunohistological studies have shown no evidence of antibody deposition in the affected areas of the epidermis.

Acantholytic Dermatosis (Grover's Disease)

Occasionally an eruption occurs in which both papules and vesicles may be seen, particularly in middle-aged men. This disorder, which is not hereditary, is known as acantholytic dermatosis. It is characterized by focal acantholysis and dyskeratosis, which is why it is grouped with Darier's disease and familial benign pemphigus, and may be precipitated by heat, exposure to sunlight and sweating.

Epidermolysis Bullosa

This is defined as a set of disorders of the skin or mucous membranes, all but one of which are inherited, in which blister formation occurs following an inappropriately small degree of trauma. The blisters all occur in the region of the dermoepidermal junction and, because knowledge of the precise level of clefting is needed for accurate diagnosis, it may be necessary to examine biopsies by transmission electron microscopy.

Classification

Epidermolysis bullosa is classified on the basis of a number of criteria:

- the pattern of inheritance
- the parts of the skin most affected
- the precise level within the skin where clefting occurs
- the age of onset

There are three principal forms of inherited epidermolysis bullosa: epidermolysis bullosa simplex, and junctional and dystrophic epidermolysis bullosa.

Epidermolysis Bullosa Simplex

This is inherited in an **autosomal dominant** fashion, and there are several variants. The commonest, known as the Weber–Cockayne syndrome, generally appears shortly after birth and affects principally the hands and feet.

The blisters are often large and are filled with clear fluid. They generally heal without scarring or hyperpigmentation. Clefting occurs either at the level of the basal cells or immediately above the basal layer.

Junctional Epidermolysis Bullosa

This disease is inherited in an **autosomal recessive** pattern and has a number of phenotypic variants. In its more severe forms there is involvement of tissues outside the skin, for example the gastrointestinal tract, as a result of which malabsorption may occur. The nails may be absent or otherwise abnormal. Pitting of the teeth is a common clinical feature.

Blister formation occurs at the level of the lamina lucida and the abnormal skin fragility is believed to be due to a defect in the hemidesmosomes.

Dystrophic Epidermolysis Bullosa

There are two major forms of dystrophic epidermolysis bullosa, one of which is inherited in an autosomal dominant pattern and the other in an autosomal recessive form. Both may cause extensive and widespread blistering. Characteristically, healing of these blisters is associated with scarring and the appearance of tiny white 'milium' cysts. In general, the autosomal recessive form is associated with more severe manifestations, and in this form significant extracutaneous involvement is much more common than in the dominant variety. Extensive involvement of mucous membranes may occur and there may be serious systemic effects such as growth retardation and severe anaemia. A rather unusual but characteristic feature of the recessive form of this disease is fusion of the skin between the digits. If this is not corrected at an early stage, the fingers and toes become encased in a keratinous wrapping. The graphic term 'mitten deformity' has been given to this malformation.

The clefting in dystrophic epidermolysis bullosa occurs at a deeper level than in the other two forms, the target area being the upper part of the papillary dermis. It is suggested that anchoring fibrils between the basement membrane and the dermis are defective. In the recessive form of the disease, an abnormal collagenase has been detected in the skin which, it is believed, has type VII collagen as its substrate. This finding has also been made in some patients with the junctional form of the disease. This finding has practical application because the anticonvulsant drug phenytoin is an inhibitor of collagenase synthesis and has produced clinical improvement in these patients.

Epidermolysis bullosa can also occur in an **acquired form**. This has been reported in patients with inflammatory bowel disease, various types of autoimmune disease and internal malignancies. The clefting occurs below the lamina densa of the basement membrane and is believed also to be associated with damage to type VII collagen.

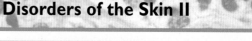

Disorders of the Skin II

ECZEMA (DERMATITIS)

Eczema, like jaundice or anaemia, is not a specific disease entity; rather, it is **a set of different disorders of the skin which have in common:**

- certain **clinical features**, which depend on the stage of the disease (see *Table 43.5*)
- certain **histological features** which include (again depending on the stage of the disease) those shown in the box

Table 43.5 Clinical Features of Eczema/Dermatitis

Stage	Clinical picture
Acute	Intensely itchy papules, vesicles and blisters from which watery fluid exudes
Subacute	Redness, scaling and crusting of the skin (*Fig. 43.10*)
Chronic	Thickened, dry, scaly and sometimes fissured skin in which the normal skin markings are exaggerated (**lichenification**). Much of this is due to rubbing and scratching. In some cases, fibrotic nodules are present (**prurigo nodularis**) and there may be areas of increased or decreased pigmentation.

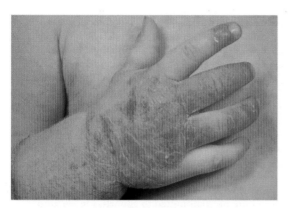

FIGURE 43.10 *Infantile eczema showing typical redness, scaling and crusting.*

Microscopic Features

- **spongiosis.** This intercellular oedema is one of the earliest changes seen in eczema. With increasing severity, intraepidermal vesicles form.
- **acanthosis**
- **hyperkeratosis** and **focal parakeratosis**
- **a predominantly lymphocytic perivascular reaction in the upper dermis**

It should be remembered that, because the eruption is always intensely itchy, the signs described above are often overshadowed by **the effects of scratching and/or infection**, and it is, in fact, rare to see a biopsy sample of an uncomplicated eczematous reaction.

Aetiology

Eczematous reactions may occur as a result of:

- **exposure of the skin to allergens or irritating substances ('contact dermatitis')**
- **some endogenous problem**

Clinical and/or pathological entities that are included under these two rubrics are shown in *Table 43.6*.

Atopic Eczema

This is a disorder that:

- shows the clinical and pathological features described in *Table 43.5*.
- has a chronic natural history punctuated by relapses and remissions but which eventually is self-limiting in most cases
- has a significant genetic component
- is associated with other features of **atopy** such as **asthma, urticaria or hay fever**

Atopy

Atopy, a form of Gell and Coombes' type I hypersensitivity, is expressed as an **inappropriate degree of immunoglobulin (Ig) E response to one or more of a number of intrinsically harmless antigens** such as pollens and grasses or animal danders.

Mast cells bind this IgE, and when the allergen is encountered on a subsequent occasion pharmacologically active compounds are released from the mast cells. These include histamine and lipid-derived inflammatory mediators such as leukotrienes. The ability to bind to mast cells is a function of the Fc portion of immunoglobulin.

A raised level of IgE in the plasma of a child suspected of having atopic eczema supports a diagnosis of atopy, but normal IgE concentrations do not exclude atopy. **IgE production is controlled by T suppressor cells, possibly via the production of glycosylation inhibiting factors, influencing the relative amounts of IgE-enhancing and IgE-suppressing**

Table 43.6 Types of Eczematous Reaction

Endogenous eczematous reactions	Eczematous reactions due to exposure to allergens or primary irritants
Atopic eczema Adult seborrhoeic eczema Discoid eczema Pompholyx eczema (confined more or less to the hands and feet) and characterized by blistering Juvenile plantar dermatosis Lichen simplex Lichen striatus Eczematous reactions due to venous stasis	**Dermatitis due to repeated contact with irritants** such as urine (napkin rash in infants) and cleansing agents such as detergents and shampoos A variant of this, known as **asteatotic eczema**, occurs in elderly people who may develop excessive drying and fissuring of the skin under conditions of cold or following frequent washing of susceptible areas of the skin. **Allergic contact dermatitis**, which is an expression of delayed hypersensitivity due to cell-mediated reactions. Once the patient is sensitized to a skin allergen, the allergen must be avoided because the potential to react abnormally is permanent.

factors released by T helper cells. Thymectomy or thymic irradiation of adult animals causes an enhancement and prolongation of IgE production, which is, however, not seen in relation to other immunoglobulin classes. Excess IgE production appears to be linked with abnormalities of loci on the long arms of chromosomes 5 and 11.

In patients with atopic eczema, **a combination of raised concentrations of IgE and decreased numbers of T suppressor cells is not infrequently seen**. In 1996 an association was described between a polymorphism affecting the gene (on chromosome 14) encoding mast cell chymase and atopic eczema. This association is lacking in respect of allergic rhinitis or atopic asthma.

The term **atopy** describes the clinical syndrome in patients with a personal or family history of such allergic manifestations. **There is a strong hereditary influence**; a child with one parent who has a history of an atopic disorder has a 60% chance of showing manifestations of atopy. If both parents are atopic, the risk rises to 80%.

The existence of an eczematous reaction implies local sensitization within the affected areas of the skin. For this to occur, proteinaceous allergens must be able to enter the skin and this suggests increased skin permeability in sufferers of atopic eczema.

Water within the stratum corneum enhances the barrier functions of the skin and, thus, an abnormal degree of drying of the skin is likely to be associated with increased permeability. On clinical examination, all patients with atopic eczema are said to show dry skin, and both normal and eczematous skin in such patients shows increased water loss across the epidermis.

Clinical Features

The disorder is common, affecting more than 1% of children in the UK. The skin lesions appear about the age of 3 months and affect principally the face, especially the eyelids, skin flexures such as elbows, knees and ankles, and the posterior gluteal folds. The eruption is usually symmetrical and, because the lesions are intensely itchy, scratch marks are common.

Complications

Children with atopic eczema are prone to develop bacterial or viral infections due, at least in part, to disruption of the normal barrier function of the skin as a result of the eczema.

The principal bacterial infection is with *Staphylococcus aureus*; the skin of patients with atopic eczema becomes colonized, with subsequent penetration of this organism through the skin barrier and resulting in the formation of numerous yellow pustules superimposed on existing skin lesions.

The principal viral infections in these patients are with:

- **herpes simplex.** This is the commonest viral infection in eczematous patients. The lesions may be local or generalized, this (usually due to herpesvirus type I) being known as **Kaposi's varicelliform eruption (eczema herpeticum)**. It is characterized by the presence of extensive vesiculation of the skin and a high fever. In rare instances, this disease may be fatal.
- **papillomavirus**
- **molluscum contagiosum.** This is caused by an, as yet, unclassified member of the poxvirus group which produces a benign epidermal tumour, only in humans. The virus can neither be grown in tissue culture nor transmitted to animals. On electron microscopy it is seen to be a brick-shaped structure somewhat resembling the vaccinia virus.

  Small, pink, wart-like lesions appear on the face, arms and buttocks. They tend to have a dimpled surface and, on incision, an amorphous yellowish-white material can be squeezed out. The histological picture, characterized by large viral inclusions, is very easy to recognize (*Fig. 43.11*).
- **Vaccinia** infections, once well recognized in atopic patients, are no longer seen, now that vaccination against smallpox is no longer practised.

Contact Dermatitis

The term contact dermatitis is defined as a set of disorders morphologically identical to atopic eczema but caused by exposure of the skin to either an exogenous allergen or an irritant substance.

Delayed (Cell-mediated) Type of Allergic Reaction following Exposure of the Skin to Exogenous Allergen

Almost any chemical species may act as an allergen in this context (*Figs 43.12* and *43.13*). Those most frequently implicated include **nickel, rubber, various preservatives, certain plants, such as**

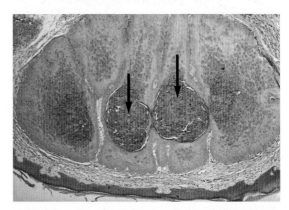

FIGURE 43.11 Section of lesion from patient with molluscum contagiosum. Note the hyperplasia of the epidermis and the numerous eosinophilic bodies (arrowed) which represent accumulations of virus.

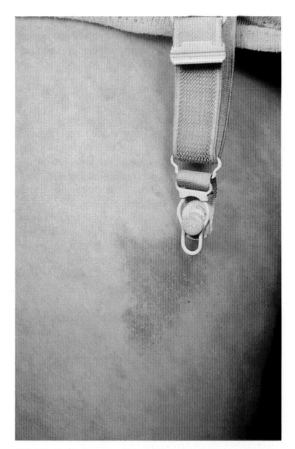

FIGURE 43.12 *Contact dermatitis. Note the red patch on this patient's thigh, caused by nickel in the suspender.*

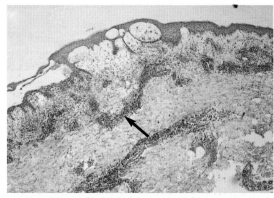

FIGURE 43.13 *Contact dermatitis. Note the subepidermal blistering and the focal, chiefly perivascular, inflammatory infiltrate (arrowed).*

poison ivy and poison oak, nail varnish, perfume and certain drugs. It is important to identify the allergen by patch testing at the earliest possible stage, because the inflammatory process may become chronic and lichenified. Removal of the allergen from the patient's environment, once lichenification has occurred, may come too late for the process to be reversed. Avoidance of the allergen, although the most rational measure, is not always easy to accomplish and may involve a considerable degree of disturbance to the affected individual's way of life, especially if the allergen is one encountered in the working environment.

The areas of skin affected may provide useful clues as to the type of eczematous reaction. If cosmetics are responsible, the head and neck are commonly involved, whereas such allergens as permanent wave lotions or shampoos produce a reaction on the scalp of the recipients and on the hands of the hairdressers.

The responsible chemical is usually of low molecular weight and, in immunological terms, acts as a hapten. These small molecules penetrate through the stratum corneum and bind to carrier proteins believed to be on the surface of the Langerhans cells. The Langerhans cells are derived from the bone marrow and express major histocompatibility complex (MHC) class II proteins and the cortical thymocyte antigen CD1. They also have receptors for the Fc portion of immunoglobulin and for complement components.

These cells migrate from the epidermis to the T-cell areas of regional lymph nodes, where presentation of the antigen occurs. Langerhans cells can reach the nodes as little as 4 hours after initial application of the sensitizing agent. Changes in the skin brought about by the migration of sensitized T helper cells into the upper dermis are fully developed within 48–72 hours.

Effect of Exposure of the Skin to Irritant Substances

The immune system is *not* involved in this form of contact dermatitis, which constitutes about 80% of the cases, although atopic individuals are more at risk. Provided the dose of the responsible agent is sufficiently large or repeated often enough, eczematous reactions can occur. **A major factor in the causation of this type of inflammatory reaction is degreasing of the skin; this leads to excessive dryness** and, ultimately, to the appearance of cracks and fissures.

CONTACT URTICARIA

Contact urticaria is another common and important set of reactions following exposure of the skin to various stimuli, not all of which are chemicals. The basic lesion is an exaggerated **wheal and flare** reaction. Urticaria affects the dermis and is the result of:

- dilatation of the vessels in the upper part of the dermis
- a change in the permeability of these blood vessels
- dermal oedema

Contact urticaria may result from immunological or non-immunological reactions.

Non-immunological Urticaria

This is usually mild and localized in most instances to the site of contact. The defining criterion is the fact that **lesions can occur without previous exposure to the offending agent**.

It seems likely that the substances responsible penetrate through the epidermis and directly affect the perivascular mast cells and/or the endothelial cells of the small blood vessels. Mast cell activation leads to release of preformed mediators such as histamine and tryptase. The latter cleaves C3 and thus activates complement via the alternate pathway. In addition, lipid-derived mediators such as prostaglandins, leukotrienes and platelet-activating factor are synthesized and released, and some types of non-immunological urticaria can be aborted by administering cyclo-oxygenase inhibitors such as aspirin or indomethacin.

'Injuries' implicated in this form of urticaria include:

- insect bites
- stinging nettles
- various marine organisms such as 'bluebottles'
- chemicals used as preserving or flavouring agents in foods or medicines. For example, 45% of individuals exposed to benzoic acid or cinnamic acid show an urticarial reaction within less than 1 hour of the skin contact.

Immunologically Mediated Urticaria

This occurs only after previous sensitization. The skin lesions may be local or generalized and there may be an associated systemic anaphylactic response characterized by laryngeal oedema, bronchial asthma or gastrointestinal symptoms. Part of this reaction is certainly due to an IgE-mediated type I hypersensitivity, although complement activation via the classical pathway has also been implicated.

There is a very long list of substances that can elicit immunologically mediated contact urticaria. Many of these are proteins contained in various foodstuffs of either plant or animal origin.

PAPULOSQUAMOUS DISORDERS

Papulosquamous disorders of the skin are characterized by the presence of a **scaly** (hence 'squamous') papular eruption.

Lichen Planus

One of the most striking disorders is **lichen planus**. This is a common disorder involving both skin and mucous membranes. Its peak incidence is between the ages of 30 and 60 years; males and females are equally affected. All races are affected, although it is said that Nigerians are, for some unknown reason, more susceptible than other groups.

Clinical Features

Lichen planus is expressed as an intensely itchy eruption characterized by polygonal flat-topped papules of a purplish ('violaceous') colour. The papule surfaces are covered by a lacy network of white lines known as **Wickham's striae**. As with psoriasis, trauma to the skin leads to the Koebner phenomenon (see p 990).

Areas of skin particularly likely to be affected include the wrists, forearms, ankles, lumbosacral region, male genitalia (where the lesions tend to be circular), the pretibial regions and the dorsa of the hands. Mucous membrane involvement is very common, the oral mucosa being affected in 50% of cases. A wide variety of clinical variants has been characterized.

The outlook for patients with acute lichen planus is good. Most cases clear within 18 months and half will do so within 9 months. Where there is erosive disease affecting mucosal surfaces, the course of the disease tends to be more prolonged.

Microscopic Features

- **Hyperkeratosis** but *no* evidence of parakeratosis
- Focal and irregular **thickening of the granular layer**
- A combination of irregular acanthosis and degeneration of the basal cells giving **a characteristic 'saw-tooth' appearance** (*Fig. 43.14*). If the basal layer damage is extensive, subepidermal clefting sufficiently severe as to present as blister formation may occur.
- The loss of basal cells probably occurs via increased apoptosis; the remaining apoptotic bodies appear as **eosinophilic globules called colloid, cytoid or Civatte bodies**.
- A **'band-like' infiltrate of inflammatory cells** is present which appears to 'hug' the dermoepidermal junction. Activated T helper cells are prominent in this infiltrate. The possibility of an immune-mediated pathogenesis is supported by the finding of increased numbers of Langerhans cells in the epidermis and dermis in affected areas of the skin.
- **Melanin is released from irreversibly damaged keratinocytes** and accumulates within dermal macrophages.
- A **linear deposit of fibrin is often present along the dermoepidermal junction**, and IgM and, less often, other immunoglobulin types and C3 may be found within the colloid bodies.

These microscopic features are highly characteristic but it should be borne in mind that rather similar changes may be seen in graft versus host disease, lupus erythematosus, drug-induced lichenoid reactions such as are caused by gold and mepacrine, and dermatomyositis.

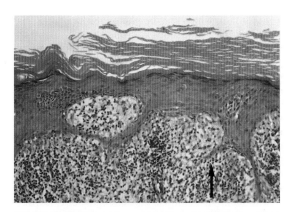

FIGURE 43.14 *Lichen planus. Note the marked hyperkeratosis, the florid band-like infiltrate which 'hugs' the basal layer of the epidermis, and the degeneration of the basal layer which leads to a typical 'saw-tooth' appearance (arrowed).*

Pathogenesis

The combination of prominence of the antigen-presenting Langerhans cells and the large local population of T helper lymphocytes suggests that immune mechanisms are involved in the production of the skin lesions. This view is strengthened by the close morphological resemblance between the lesions of lichen planus and those of graft versus host disease. A genetic component may well be involved as lichen planus is particularly associated with a haplotype that includes the class II genes DR1 or Dqw1.

Lupus Erythematosus

Lupus erythematosus is an autoimmune disease which can involve many organs including the skin. It ranges in severity from a potentially life-threatening multisystem disorder (see pp 688–690) to one that may affect only the skin. It is characterized by the formation of antibodies directed chiefly against 'self' nuclear antigens. This results in the formation of circulating immune complexes which may be deposited in a wide variety of anatomical situations where they trigger tissue-damaging inflammation.

At some time during the course of the disease, the skin is affected in 70–80% of patients, and skin disease is the presenting feature in about 25% of cases. The major types of skin disease seen are:

- **discoid lupus erythematosus**, a chronic scarring eruption usually occurring in patients with little or no systemic disease
- **acute cutaneous lupus erythematosus**, tending to occur in patients with active systemic forms of the disease
- **subacute cutaneous lupus erythematosus**, which has a more prolonged course and is associated with milder forms of systemic disease. The eruption is photosensitive and heals without scarring.

Discoid Lupus Erythematosus

This form tends to occur in early adult life and is more common in women (female : male ratio 2 : 1). The lesions are largely confined to the face, scalp and ears. It has been suggested that there are several different genotypes conferring increased susceptibility; this is supported by the fact that there are several different histocompatibility antigens associated with increased risk. These include HLA-B7, B8, Cw7, DR2, DR3 and DQW1. The combination in an individual of more than one of these antigens increases the relative risk still further.

The classical lesions are inflammatory plaques most commonly occurring in a 'butterfly' distribution across the bridge of the nose and cheeks. The lesions are characterized by:

- **redness** with, on some occasions, hyperpigmentation at the margins and central loss of pigment
- **plugging of follicles**
- **scarring associated with atrophy of the affected areas of skin.** In lesions occurring on the scalp this scarring is associated with permanent loss of hair at the sites of lesions.

Microscopic Features (*Figs 43.15* and *43.16*)

- **hyperkeratosis with follicular plugging and atrophy of the pilosebaceous apparatus**
- **focal epidermal atrophy due to damage to the basal cells** and associated with focal lymphocytic infiltrates. Focal basal cell liquefactive degeneration is present in these areas and occasional apoptotic bodies may be seen.
- **a lymphocytic infiltrate affecting any level of the dermis but usually concentrated in the middle third.** This cell infiltrate extends upwards to the epidermis in some areas and it is here that basal cell degeneration tends to occur.
- **thickening of the basement membrane**
- **degenerative changes in the dermal connective tissue** consisting of oedema, hyalinization and some fibrinoid change
- **a linear deposit of IgG and IgM at the dermal–epidermal junction** (this may be seen also in clinically normal skin in these patients, the so-called **'lupus band'**). In about 70% of cases properdin is also seen, as may be C3. C1q is seen in something over 25% of immunofluorescence-positive cases, compared with 90% in patients with systemic lupus. Its presence suggests an increased risk of systemic lupus in the future.

Subacute Cutaneous Lupus Erythematosus

About 10% of patients with lupus erythematosus have skin lesions falling into this group. The lesions may be either:

- a non-scarring papulosquamous eruption which occurs in two-thirds of these patients

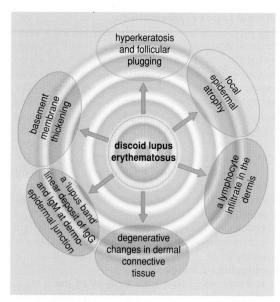

FIGURE 43.15 *The characteristic cluster of morphological features seen in discoid lupus erythematosus.*

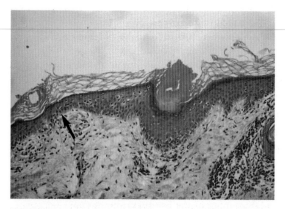

FIGURE 43.16 *Chronic discoid lupus erythematosus. Note the keratin plug within the mouth of a hair follicle, the focal atrophy of the epidermis (arrowed), and perivascular and periappendageal inflammatory infiltrate.*

- ring-shaped lesions usually above the waist,

involving especially the neck, trunk and outer arms

Follicular plugging is uncommon in this variant and the lesions heal without scarring, although their 'ghosts' may still be seen in the form of small areas of hypopigmentation. In about 50% of the patients the skin lesions appear to be sensitive to sunlight and diffuse non-scarring alopecia occurs in a similar proportion. Mouth ulceration, particularly affecting the palate, is not uncommon.

About half the patients satisfy the criteria of the American Rheumatism Association for a diagnosis of systemic lupus erythematosus. This requires four or more of the following to be present:

- arthritis
- serositis
- a skin rash, which may be photosensitive
- oral ulcers
- renal disease as manifested by proteinuria or the presence of cellular casts in the urine
- haemolytic anaemia
- the presence of non-organ-specific antibodies in the serum
- fits or a psychosis
- leucopenia and/or thrombocytopenia
- false-positive syphilis serology

Of the systemic manifestations listed above, arthritis is the one most frequently seen in subacute cutaneous lupus. Renal disease is uncommon and tends to be mild.

The skin lesions show a greater degree of epidermal atrophy than is usually seen in the discoid form of the disease, but the other morphological features described in the previous section are milder than in discoid lupus erythematosus. Deposition of immunoglobulin at the dermal–epidermal junction is moderately frequent (60%) but is seen less often than in the other variants of the disease.

Pityriasis Rosea

This is a common papulosquamous dermatosis which typically (75% of cases) affects children and young adults, although it can occur at any age.

It has a curious pattern of clinical onset in that the eruption, which predominantly affects the 'vest and underpants' area, is preceded by a single red papular or plaque-like lesion much larger than those that appear subsequently. This is commonly known as a **'herald patch'**. The herald patch starts as a small reddish papule which rapidly enlarges to reach a size of 2–10 cm in diameter. It is most commonly seen on the trunk, but it may occur in other parts of the skin. Some 3–14 days after the patch has appeared, crops of erythematous lesions erupt involving the trunk and the proximal parts of the limbs in a fairly generalized and diffuse pattern.

The lesions of pityriasis rosea are typically round or oval. A highly characteristic type of scale extends round the periphery of the lesion in a curious frilly pattern known as a 'collarette'. This is due to the fact that the scale is free on its central aspect and attached at the periphery of the papule.

Microscopic Features

The histological features are similar to those seen in eczema, with mild acanthosis and spongiosis and a cellular infiltrate in the dermis consisting of lymphocytes and macrophages. The lymphocytes are mainly T helper cells. As the disorder is easy to diagnose clinically, biopsy material is not often submitted.

Aetiology and Pathogenesis

The cause of pityriasis rosea is still unknown, although the possibility that it is due to viral infection has been widely canvassed. This is largely because of the age group predominantly affected, the acute course, the tendency for the disorder to occur in the autumn and winter, and the rarity of recurrence.

The mechanism of lesion production is believed to be immune mediated, because of the nature of the cellular infiltrate and the fact that the T cells in the infiltrate show activation markers. Further support for an immune mechanism comes from the observation that several drugs produce a reaction clinically identical with pityriasis rosea. These include gold, barbiturates, captopril, β-blockers, isoniazid, non-steroidal anti-inflammatory agents and metronidazole.

Pityriasis Rubra Pilaris

This is an uncommon dermatosis, found in between 1 in 3500 and 1 in 5000 patients referred to skin clinics, and characterized by:
- red plaques in which prominent scaling is present (hence **rubra** and **pityriasis**)
- hyperkeratosis of the palms and soles
- follicular plugging (hence **pilaris**)

It affects both sexes equally and has a bimodal age distribution, individuals in the first and fifth decades being particularly likely to be affected. Several different clinical types have been described, some of which are chronic and may require systemic treatment.

> ### Microscopic Features
> - keratin plugs in the follicles with parakeratosis in the perifollicular epidermis
> - diffuse hyperkeratosis and mild acanthosis affecting the epidermis **between** the follicles
> - a mild chronic inflammatory infiltrate surrounding the blood vessels in the upper dermis

The microscopic features are not diagnostic and biopsy is carried out chiefly to differentiate this disease from psoriasis and certain types of eczema.

Aetiology and Pathogenesis

The only relevant functional abnormality so far identified is a marked **increase in the proliferative activity of the epidermal cells in the affected areas**. This is of some interest, in view of the known effects of vitamin A and its analogues on cell proliferation and differentiation, because the condition has been found to respond favourably to oral treatment with retinoids such as isotretinoin.

ACNE VULGARIS

Other than viral warts, this condition is responsible for more dermatological consultations than any other skin disorder, because it is almost universal among adolescents. The prevalence of the disorder is equal in the two sexes, but males are usually more severely affected than females.

It is a chronic disorder of the pilosebaceous apparatus in which the outstanding features are:
- an increased secretion of sebum
- blockage of the pilosebaceous duct by a plug which consists partly of sebum and partly of keratin
- a polymorphic skin eruption in which there may be papules, pustules, dermal nodules and cystic lesions

Sebum Secretion in Relation to Acne

Acne vulgaris, not surprisingly, usually presents during adolescence, because the sebaceous glands, apart from a burst of activity in early infancy, do not secrete until puberty. The glands are largest and occur in the greatest number on the scalp, face, neck and trunk. In these sites they are associated with the hair follicles and share with them a common exit to the skin surface, the **pilosebaceous duct**.

Sebum is a holocrine secretion in which cells of the sebaceous glands are broken down and release a complex mixture of lipids. The physiological role of sebum is poorly understood. It prevents the growth of certain fungi that affect the skin and this, presumably, is why scalp ringworm is so rare after puberty, but its other functions, if any, are unknown. Sebum secretion is increased in individuals with acne but is not of itself sufficient to cause acne. In acromegaly and Parkinson's disease there is an increase in sebum secretion, but no acne, and acne vulgaris itself tends to remit in the early twenties even though there is no concomitant fall in sebum secretion at that time.

Possible Role for Bacterial Lipases in Acne

Increased amounts of free fatty acids released from sebum act as irritants and appear to promote the formation of the lesions of acne (comedones). If they are injected into areas of normal skin they produce a mixed inflammatory cell infiltrate similar to that seen in acne. The skin surface and pilosebaceous duct are colonized by the organisms *Propionibacterium acnes, Staphylococcus epidermidis* and the yeast *Pityrosporum ovale*. The microorganism population is dominated by *P. acnes* and it has been suggested that this organism secretes a **lipase** which releases large amounts of proinflammatory and comedogenic free fatty acids from the sebum. A pathogenetic role for these organisms is suggested by the fact that treatment with antibiotics that reduce their number improves the condition of the skin.

THE LESIONS OF ACNE

Non-inflammatory Lesions

This term is something of a misnomer as these lesions are usually associated with a lymphocytic infiltrate in the dermis surrounding the pilosebaceous duct. However, clinical signs of inflammation are, in general, lacking. Two types of lesion are seen:

- **open comedones (known as 'blackheads').** These result from pilosebaceous orifices widely distended by keratin plugs in which there is abundant oxidized melanin pigment. In these lesions the melanocytes forming part of the epithelial lining of the duct are highly active and produce abundant pigment. It is this that accounts for the typical appearance of a blackhead.
- **closed comedones ('whiteheads').** In these lesions there is no macroscopically visible pilosebaceous orifice and, indeed, the follicular plug appears to be trapped within the duct. The distended pilosebaceous duct is more likely to rupture in this situation than in closed comedones; if this happens, ductal contents released into the dermis elicit a florid inflammatory reaction.

Inflammatory Lesions

These may be:

- **superficial**, consisting of reddened papules and pustules
- **deep**, in which case nodules, cysts and, occasionally, deep pustules are seen

Nodulocystic Acne

This is the most severe variant of acne vulgaris, from which it may be distinguished by its **chronicity** and by **deep and painful papules and nodules**. Healing of these lesions is associated with excessive scarring, causing considerable disfigurement. Unlike the more common types of acne vulgaris, the disease does not remit in the early twenties but may persist into middle life. The use of retinoids can produce a remarkable degree of improvement.

ROSACEA

This affects both sexes equally and tends to appear at any time from the fourth decade onwards. Four sequential clinical phases may occur:

1) frequent episodes of flushing
2) persistent erythema associated with obvious dilatation of small cutaneous blood vessels
3) development of small papules and pustules in the affected areas of skin
4) hypertrophy of the sebaceous glands and surrounding connective tissue. This is associated with vascular dilatation and some lymphoedema.

All these microscopic features are expressed clinically in the form of a red lobulated thickening of the skin (*Fig. 43.17*). The lower portion of the

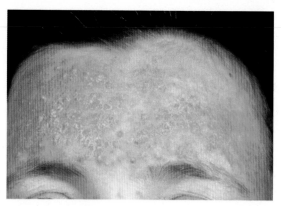

FIGURE 43.17 Rosacea affecting the forehead. Note the persistent erythema and the numerous papules that are typical of this condition.

nose is the area most commonly affected, although similar changes may occur in the cheeks, ears, chin and forehead. This striking condition is known as **rhinophyma** and is the rarest manifestation of the rosacea syndrome. It occurs almost exclusively in males.

In most instances the disorder does not progress beyond the second clinical phase. In some cases there is associated involvement of the eyes, the patient complaining of a gritty feeling in the eyes. This may be due to conjunctivitis, inflammation of the eyelids (blepharitis) or corneal inflammation (keratitis).

The cause of rosacea is unknown but there appears to be an element of vasomotor instability, changes of temperature (in either direction) being marked by facial flushing. Any vasodilator can exacerbate the condition, the classical one being alcohol. Many of the affected individuals are steady 'social' drinkers who imbibe three or four glasses of wine (or the equivalent) daily. It is not related to acne, although older texts refer to it as acne rosacea.

Microscopic Features

These vary with the clinical stage of the disease. In all stages the dermal blood vessels are dilated, the architecture of the dermal connective tissue fibres is disrupted and there is a mixed lymphocyte and macrophage infiltrate arranged round the dermal blood vessels. With the exception of rhinophyma, in which there is sebaceous gland hyperplasia, the hair follicles and sebaceous glands are not involved in rosacea.

Infections, Infestations and Non-infectious Granulomatous Disorders

INFECTIONS

It is difficult to infect the skin under normal circumstances where:

- the skin is intact
- the host is immunocompetent
- skin structures such as the sebaceous glands, which secrete antibacterial substances, are functionally normal

BACTERIAL INFECTIONS

Bacteria are normally present in the skin. These include organisms such as aerobic and anaerobic diphtheroids, *Staphylococcus epidermidis*, a small number of anaerobic staphylococci and some Gram-negative bacilli. The organisms, however, that cause clinically significant infections in the skin are *not* normally resident there and are most often acquired by person to person contact. The basic responses of the skin to bacterial infection, as in other anatomical situations, are of two types:

- **acute inflammation**
- **chronic inflammation (mostly granulomatous)**

Acute Bacterial Infections

The organisms most commonly involved are:

- *Streptococcus pyogenes* (**Lancefield group A**)
- *Staphylococcus aureus*

The clinical and pathological picture that can result from such infections depends partly on:

- the skin **level** targeted by the organisms
- the range of toxins produced by the invading bacteria

Thus a spectrum of lesions may be seen, ranging from the superficial pustular vesicles of impetigo to a destructive and life-threatening cellulitis, or, if the subcutaneous tissues are involved, necrotizing fasciitis.

Impetigo

This is an acute superficial infection of the skin caused by *S. pyogenes*, *S. aureus* or a combination of the two. It is extremely contagious and thus outbreaks may occur in nurseries and primary schools; in one striking incident, impetigo developed in many of the members of two opposing rugby teams. Impetigo chiefly affects children, especially those living in warm and humid climates.

The lesions consist, for the most part, of small, thin-walled, pus-containing vesicles which rupture with the formation of yellow-brown crusts representing dried exudate. The condition responds well to systemic antibiotics and the lesions tend to heal without scarring. In some instances, the inflammatory process tends to spread a little more deeply with shallow ulcers developing under the crusts. This variant is known as **ecthyma**. Rarely, if the impetigo has been caused by a nephritogenic strain of *S. pyogenes*, affected individuals may develop acute proliferative glomerulonephritis (see pp 661–664).

A **bullous** form of impetigo may occur in certain staphylococcal infections where a toxin is secreted that causes splitting of the epidermis just below the stratum corneum.

Staphylococcal Scalded Skin Syndrome (Lyell–Ritter's Disease)

This is a fortunately uncommon condition affecting infants and young children. It is caused by a group 2 staphylococcus (phage type 71) producing a toxin that damages the granular layer of the epidermis without eliciting an inflammatory reaction. Not all individuals so infected develop the scalded skin syndrome, suggesting that an idiosyncratic host factor may be involved.

The syndrome begins with acute diffuse tenderness of the skin followed by redness and widespread desquamation of the superficial parts of the epidermis, which come off in large sheets leaving a raw, red underlying surface resembling scalded skin.

Furuncles and Carbuncles

These terms are applied to **staphylococcal infections affecting hair follicles** and causing acute inflammation which spreads to the surrounding dermis.

- In the case of **furuncle** (or boil), a **single** hair follicle is the site of infection and an inflammatory mass develops round the affected follicle with a pustular centre through which the hair shaft passes.
- In the case of **carbuncle**, which tends to occur most commonly on the back of the neck, **several** adjacent hair follicles are affected and pus is discharged from many of these follicle orifices. Carbuncles are more common in diabetics than in the general population.

Folliculitis

Folliculitis is an acute inflammatory process affecting the opening of the hair follicle and associated with blockage of the follicle mouth and the formation of pustules confined to the hair follicles. In children, folliculitis occurs mainly on the scalp, whereas in adults it is the limbs (especially in hirsute individuals) and the beard area that are affected.

A type of folliculitis due to infections with *Pseudomonas aeruginosa* has been reported, most frequently in the USA, associated with contamination of whirlpool baths and jacuzzis. The onset is usually acute with crops of pustular lesions developing on the torso and limbs.

Erysipelas and Cellulitis

Both of these are, in most cases, the result of infections by **β-haemolytic streptococci**. They are distinguished from each other by the **level** in the skin and subcutaneous tissues affected:

- Erysipelas affects the dermis and the most superficial parts of the subcutaneous tissue.
- Cellulitis may involve the entire thickness of the subcutaneous tissue.

The pathogenetic mechanism underlying these spreading lesions is the synthesis and secretion by the streptococcus of enzymes such as hyaluronidase, facilitating the spread of the organisms through tissue planes.

These processes are associated with significant **systemic** clinical manifestations such as high fever, tachycardia, confusion and low blood pressure.

The involved areas of the skin are red, tender and oedematous and obvious lymphangitis and enlargement of regional nodes are often present. In erysipelas it is said that there is usually a sharp demarcation between involved and uninvolved skin but in practice it is not always easy to distinguish between erysipelas and cellulitis.

Necrotizing Fasciitis

In some cases, infection is associated with necrosis of subcutaneous tissues and the underlying connective tissue fascia. This is known as **necrotizing fasciitis** and, although it may be due solely to a β-haemolytic streptococcal infection, it is often the result of infection with a combination of β-haemolytic streptococci and anaerobic bacteria.

The most common site for this to occur is the extremities, the second most common being the perineum, where surgery, a perirectal abscess or infection of periurethral glands may precede the condition. Where the male genitalia are involved, the term **Fournier's gangrene** is often applied.

Necrotizing fasciitis causes severe pain in the affected areas. The patients are febrile and show evidence of systemic toxaemia. The skin over the affected areas shows the classical signs of acute inflammation, being red, hot, tender and oedematous.

The inflammatory process spreads rapidly into surrounding, previously uninvolved, areas and the skin itself may show:

- purple discoloration
- bullae
- dermal crepitus due to the formation of gas bubbles in the necrotic tissue
- superficial gangrene

It is important to distinguish necrotizing fasciitis from uncomplicated cellulitis because the former requires surgical removal of the affected soft tissues as well as antibiotic treatment, if a life-threatening situation is not to develop. Features suggesting the much more dangerous necrotizing fasciitis include:

- oedema beyond the apparent limits of the infective process
- dermal gangrene
- gas in the soft tissues
- pain, disproportionately severe in relation to the clinical signs
- pus obtained on needle aspiration of the inflamed area

Chronic Bacterial Infections

Most entities covered under this rubric are **granulomatous** lesions, of which tuberculosis and leprosy, although now rare causes of skin disorders in the Western world, are important members.

Cutaneous Tuberculosis

As in other anatomical sites, tuberculous lesions of the skin may be the expression of:

- the dose and strain of the infecting mycobacterium
- the degree of immunity as expressed in enhanced ability to clear the organism from the tissues
- the degree of local tissue hypersensitivity

Lesions of the skin associated with tuberculosis may be the result of either **exogenous** or **endogenous** infections, and may occur either in individuals previously exposed to mycobacterial antigens or in those with no previous experience of such antigens. No really satisfactory classification of skin tuberculosis exists, although a considerable number of different clinical entities have been ascribed to tuberculosis. One widely used classification, shown in *Table 43.7*, is based on a combination of the route of infection and the immune status of the host.

Tuberculous Chancre

This is now very uncommon and arises from **direct inoculation of the bacillus into the skin of an individual without immunity against *M. tuberculosis*.** Such lesions have followed ritual circumcision, ear-piercing and similar types of trauma, although the majority of infections are acquired through unnoticed minor abrasions or cuts. It is obviously most likely to occur in children and is found most often in communities with a high prevalence of mycobacterial infection.

Microscopic Features

The first reaction of tuberculous chancre is a neutrophil infiltration followed by necrosis, at which time numerous bacilli are present. Over the next 3–6 weeks a typical macrophage granuloma develops and caseation appears, this event coinciding with disappearance of the organisms from the lesion.

The lesion starts as a nondescript papule which undergoes ulceration, the latter healing very slowly over several months in the absence of appropriate treatment.

Not surprisingly, because the tuberculous chancre is a 'primary' infection, the local lesion is associated with enlargement of the draining nodes and this may be more obvious than the original skin lesion in some cases.

Warty Tuberculosis

This is a rather indolent, warty, plaque-like lesion, the expression of direct inoculation of organisms into the skin in an individual with a moderate or high degree of acquired immunity against *M. tuberculosis*.

Table 43.7 Classification of Cutaneous Tuberculosis

Type	Route of infection	Type of lesion
I	Inoculation tuberculosis (exogenous infection)	**Tuberculous chancre** (individual has no immunity against *Mycobacterium tuberculosis*) **Warty tuberculosis** (individual previously infected and has moderate to high degree of immunity) Some cases of **lupus vulgaris** (individual has moderate to high degree of immunity)
II	Endogenous infection in previously infected individuals	**Scrofuloderma** (spread from adjacent caseous lymph nodes) Some cases of **lupus vulgaris** **Miliary tuberculosis**
III	Blood spread from a primary focus	**Tuberculous 'gumma'**
IV	Eruptive tuberculosis (so-called tuberculides), representing skin reactions to an internal tuberculous focus	**Lichen scrofulosorum** **Papular or papulonecrotic tuberculides** **Erythema induratum** (Bazin's disease)

The most common origin for this lesion is accidental infection from an external source, encountered in certain specific occupations such as butchery and post-mortem examination. Occasionally, patients with active tuberculosis may infect themselves via contact between their own mycobacterium-containing sputum and the skin.

Microscopic Features

Histological examination shows an intense mixed inflammatory cell infiltrate within the dermis, well-formed tuberculous granulomas being scanty. Possibly because of the release of growth-promoting cytokines from inflammatory cells, there is a marked hyperplasia of the epidermis overlying the inflammatory infiltrate and it is this so-called 'pseudoepitheliomatous hyperplasia' that accounts for the warty appearance of the lesion.

Lupus Vulgaris

This is a form of skin tuberculosis occurring in individuals, especially women, with a moderate to high degree of immunity against the mycobacterium.

In lupus vulgaris, the bacilli may gain access to the skin via:

- inoculation from an external source
- spread from adjacent nodes showing tuberculous lymphadenopathy
- the bloodstream
- lymphatic spread from tuberculous lesions in the mucous membranes of the nose or throat

It presents most commonly as a reddish-brown, well-demarcated plaque on the face. When this lesion is pressed with a glass slide, small rather translucent nodules can be seen ('apple jelly'). This plaque-like lesion is not the only expression of lupus vulgaris and several other forms have been described which result from combinations and permutations of extensive tissue destruction and scarring, the latter leading to severe contracture of the affected tissues. Squamous carcinoma has been recorded as a late complication of such scarring.

Microscopic Features

The microscopic appearances of lupus vulgaris may be as variable as the naked-eye appearances of the lesions. In most cases it is possible to recognize well-formed macrophage granulomas but the responsible organisms are not usually seen. Indeed, when portions of the lesions of lupus vulgaris are cultured in appropriate special media, mycobacteria are found to be present in only about 6% of cases, thus confirming the presence of effective clearing of the organisms from the infected host's tissues.

The Tuberculides

The term tuberculide is applied to any one of a set of disorders characterized by the appearance of an eruption, usually symmetrical and widespread, in the presence of an internal tuberculous focus. By implication these are reactive lesions, rather than the result of direct infection, but they usually clear with antituberculous treatment.

The tuberculides may present as:

- papules, as, for example, in papulonecrotic tuberculide
- nodules, as, for example, in erythema induratum (Bazin's disease), which some regard as the only true nodular tuberculide

Papulonecrotic Tuberculide

This presents as crops of papules, most commonly situated on the extremities, distributed symmetrically for the most part. Within a short time the papule centres become necrotic and break down. Bacilli are never found on microscopic examination of the lesions or on culture; but within a few days of starting antituberculous therapy no new lesions appear and the existing lesions start to heal with central scarring. The pathogenesis is not clear but it has been suggested that the lesions may be due to haematogenous dissemination of mycobacterial antigens.

Young adults are most likely to be affected (two-thirds of patients in an African series were aged under 30 years at the time of diagnosis). The legs, knees, elbows, hands and feet are the most favoured sites but the lesions may also affect the face, buttocks and genitalia.

Microscopic Features

The most striking feature of papulonecrotic tuberculide is a central zone of coagulative necrosis surrounded by chronic inflammatory cells. The lesion is initially a dermal one but the necrosis extends upwards to involve the overlying epidermis and may spread downwards to the more superficial parts of the subcutaneous tissue. In large lesions activated macrophages may be found surrounding the necrotic centre in a palisaded fashion. Small blood vessels in the surrounding tissue show changes ranging from infiltration by lymphocytes to full-blown vasculitis with fibrinoid necrosis and secondary thrombosis.

Nodular Tuberculide

The only true example is believed to be **erythema induratum (Bazin's disease)**.

Its defining criteria are persistent or recurrent nodular lesions, most commonly localized to the backs of the lower legs, usually in females with tuberculosis elsewhere in the body. Mycobacteria are seldom recovered from the lesions and recognition of an association with tuberculosis elsewhere may depend on the skin lesions clearing as a result of antituberculous therapy. The pathogenesis is not understood but immune complex deposition is likely to play a part.

Microscopic Features

The microscopic features of nodular tuberculide are similar to those of a nodular vasculitis, with inflammatory involvement of medium and small blood vessels in the connective tissue septa within the subcutaneous adipose tissue. Extensive, rather non-specific, necrosis is usually present and the diagnosis is clinched by seeing tuberculoid granulomas admixed with the other features listed.

Fish Tank and Swimming Pool Granuloma

This results from infection with a mycobacterial species known as *Mycobacterium marinum* (synonym. *balnei*), which may contaminate water in fish tanks and swimming pools. The organism gains access to the human host via abrasions in the skin.

The infection is expressed in the form of itchy purplish-red nodules appearing initially at the site of some trivial skin injury. The lesions may be warty in appearance and, not infrequently, ulcerate. Additional lesions may develop along the line of lymphatic drainage from the primary lesion. The diagnosis is most commonly made by biopsying one of the lesions. These show the presence of non-specific chronic inflammation in the early stages, and of granulomas in which a few acid-fast bacilli may be identified in the later ones.

VIRAL INFECTIONS

Herpes Simplex

The commonest acute viral skin infections are caused by the herpes simplex virus (HSV). They are characterized by crops of small painful vesicles on an erythematous base. Individual episodes are self-limiting but recurrence is characteristic. The lesions can occur anywhere but it is commonest to find HSV-1 associated with infections of the mouth and lips and HSV-2 with infections in the genital regions.

The principal reaction pattern seen is a combination of ballooning and reticular degeneration with the production of intraepidermal vesicles which contain a meshwork of cellular debris. Intranuclear inclusions, which stain red with eosin (Cowdry type A), are commonly present, as are very large multinucleated cells. These last two features may be identified in cytological preparations of vesicle fluid (the Tzanck test) and the virus itself may be identified morphologically by transmission electron microscopy of the fluid.

Primary infections with HSV may be clinically obvious or subclinical. In the latter case patients may experience recurrent crops of lesions with no previous history of a primary infection.

Clinical Features of a Primary Infection

At the onset, which is usually sudden, a group of macules appears at the affected site. These macules rapidly become vesiculated and painful, and rupture of the vesicles with subsequent crusting is a typical event. In HSV-2 infections, usually affecting the genital region and/or buttocks, there are often systemic manifestations such as fever and enlargement of the draining nodes.

An interesting variant of primary HSV infection is **herpetic whitlow**, first described following an outbreak of what appeared to be purulent lesions on the fingers of nurses in a neurosurgical centre. Investigation of these lesions showed them to be herpetic in origin and to have been acquired from patients. Since then, many other cases have been reported, most of them in medical or dental personnel. Such infections may be avoided by wearing protective gloves in the course of certain patient procedures (e.g. cleaning endotracheal tubes).

Newborn infants have no natural immunity to herpes simplex infection and may acquire the infection in the course of their passage through the birth canal. If the mother is known to have an active infection at the time of delivery, a caesarean section may be advisable because infection in the infant may be disseminated and fatal.

Clinical Features of Recurrent Herpes Simplex

HSV can enter into a lifelong latency stage within the nuclei of neural ganglia, during which time virus cannot be recovered from these cells. The establishment of latent infections in sensory neurones appears to be due to a lack of viral immediate–early (IE) gene expression following initial infection. In cultured neuronal cell lines it has been shown that this lack of IE gene expression is due to a repressor factor specific for neuronal cells. This repressor binds to a particular sequence in the IE promoter and thus prevents its transcription.

The factors interrupting latency are identical with those described on pp 187–188. The patient experiences tingling or discomfort in the skin, followed by the appearance of a crop of painful vesicles. The attack lasts 5–10 days and the lesions heal without scarring, although some hyperpigmentation may persist at the site of the vesicles.

Herpes Zoster

Herpes zoster (commonly known as shingles) is characterized by groups of small painful vesicles on an erythematous base. The lesions are usually localized to one or two dermatomes and do not cross the midline. **They result from reactivation of latent varicella zoster virus in neural ganglia.** Reactivation appears to be associated with a decline in cell-mediated immunity and increases in frequency with increasing age of the at-risk population. Any immunosuppressed individual has an increased risk for developing zoster.

The first symptom is pain and discomfort, limited to one side of the body. This is followed by the appearance of the typical eruption described above. **Live virus is present in the crusting lesions and thus these patients constitute a source of infection for individuals who have not had chickenpox**, the other disease caused by the varicella zoster virus.

Widespread dissemination may occur, fortunately in a minority of patients who, usually, are immunosuppressed. About 15% of patients affected in this way die, usually from varicella pneumonitis.

The cranial nerves may be involved in some instances, the trigeminal nerve being affected most commonly. If the ophthalmic branch of this nerve is affected, ocular complications are likely in 30–50% of patients.

The most difficult clinical problem arising from attacks of zoster is pain, which is most severe in the older patients. Postherpetic neuralgia (defined as

pain lasting for more than 1 month) is seen in 10–15% of victims of zoster. This resolves within 2 months in 50% and within 1 year in 75%, but in a small proportion of individuals it may persist for years.

Microscopic Findings

The microscopic findings in herpes zoster infection, especially if samples are taken at the vesicular stage of the disease, are identical with those described for HSV infections. In addition, however, the sensory nerves and ganglia in the affected dermatomes show acute inflammation and some evidence of necrosis.

Varicella

This results from primary infection with the varicella zoster virus, also known as herpesvirus 3. In varicella (chickenpox), infection is spread by droplets and the route of infection is believed to be the respiratory tract mucosa. This is followed by a viraemic stage and the virus then localizes in the skin, although internal visceral involvement, most notably in the lungs, can occur.

The microscopic appearance of the skin lesions are more or less identical with those seen in HSV infections.

Exposure to the virus is followed by an incubation period of 14–21 days. The earliest symptoms are malaise and fever, followed by the appearance of crops of first papular and then vesicular lesions, distributed, for the most part, in a centripetal fashion; the trunk and the face are the first regions affected. Successive crops of fresh vesicles occur over the first 3–5 days so that lesions at different stages of their development are commonly seen.

Complications are rare, although encephalitis, which has a mortality rate of about 10%, does sometimes occur about 5–10 days after the appearance of the rash. Neonatal varicella, contracted from the mother just before or at the time of delivery, is, however, a dangerous disease with a mortality rate as high as 20%. Children who are immunosuppressed or who have inherited immune deficiency states have a high risk of developing fatal disseminated varicella infections.

Viral Warts

Warts are common skin lesions produced by direct inoculation with human papillomaviruses (HPV). They account for 10–25% of all skin outpatient attendances. They occur most commonly in children and adolescents, the peak incidence being between the ages of 12 and 16 years. About 10% of the population at risk is affected.

HPV is a DNA virus with a circular genome; at least 50 different types have been identified, some of which appear to play an oncogenic role in relation to squamous carcinomas of both male and female genital tracts. Viral replication takes place only in fully differentiated keratinocytes and thus the target cells for these infections are the superficial epidermal cells. Different types

Table 43.8 Human Papillomavirus Warts

Virus	Type of wart
HPV-2	Mosaic warts Common warts
HPV-3	Plane warts
HPV-6	Genital warts
HPV-1	Plantar warts Common warts

of HPV appear to be related to different types of wart, as shown in *Table 43.8*.

Wart virus infection in the skin results from direct inoculation; the lesions are the expression of the interaction between the dose of infecting virus and the degree of host cell-mediated immunity. The importance of cell-mediated immunity is emphasized by the observations that 40% of individuals who have received allogeneic transplants and immunosuppressive drugs have skin warts and that there is a marked increase in the frequency of warts in patients who, for whatever reason, have defective cell-mediated immunity.

Microscopic Features (*Fig. 43.18*)
- acanthosis
- papillomatosis
- hyperkeratosis
- koilocytosis
- the presence of inclusion bodies in the stratum corneum. This gives an appearance which to a certain extent mimics that of parakeratosis but the inclusion bodies are rounded rather than elongated, as are the nuclei that persist in parakeratotic epidermis.

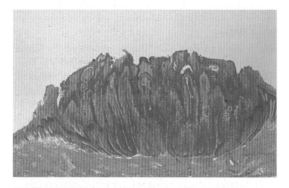

FIGURE 43.18 *Viral wart. Note the marked degree of epidermal hyperplasia with a striking prolongation of the rete pegs. The thickened rete pegs slant inwards as if towards a hypothetical centre point.*

Several clinically well-recognized variations on the theme of warts exist.

Common Warts (Verruca Vulgaris)
The hands and fingers are most frequently affected. Lesions appear as flesh-coloured papules with a rough surface due largely to hyperkeratosis.

The epidermal hyperplasia causes the surface of the lesion to be elevated in a series of cone-shaped projections, thus giving a hill and valley effect. The granular layer in the 'valleys' shows a marked degree of hyperplasia whereas the tips of the papillae tend to be covered only by a thin layer of parakeratotic epidermis. A rather striking feature is the way in which the rete ridges appear to be oriented towards the centre of the area of dermis under the lesion.

Plane Warts
A decrease in the degree of papillomatosis makes the surface of a common wart smoother and gives the lesion the configuration of a plane wart. These are either flesh coloured or a very light brown; they are seen to have a flat top on naked-eye examination and, in comparison with common warts, are only very slightly raised above the surface of the surrounding skin.

Plane warts constitute about 3% of warts. They can occur in any part of the skin but are especially common on the face, hands and fingers. Because they do not look particularly 'warty' they are often misdiagnosed and may be treated with topical steroids, which tends to promote spread. Plane warts are one of the group of quite disparate skin lesions showing the Koebner phenomenon (i.e. they tend to occur in areas where there has been some minor skin trauma).

Mosaic Warts
These are areas of roughened skin usually found on the soles, heels, palmar surfaces of the hands or in relation to the nails. In these areas a number of individual small warty lesions can be seen. They tend to be rather resistant to treatment.

Plantar Warts
These are discrete lesions which are only just raised above the surface of the surrounding skin. The commonest site for these lesions is on the sole of the foot, where they penetrate quite deeply because of the pressure of the body-weight. The infection is often contracted in swimming pools or shower rooms.

The proliferated epidermis is surrounded a collar of thick translucent keratin and when the latter is pared away the wart itself, often small, is seen.

Epidermodysplasia Verruciformis
This is a curious condition which has a variable inheritance pattern, although the majority of cases are inherited in an autosomal recessive fashion.

Affected individuals show a marked predisposition to

widespread and persistent infections with multiple types of HPV, giving rise to a complex skin picture with plane warts, reddish plaques and lesions resembling those seen in pityriasis versicolor.

This lack of resistance to HPV infection presumably indicates an impairment of cell-mediated immunity. Impairment of T helper cell function is certainly seen in some cases but is by no means always present.

Malignant transformation of some of the lesions occurs in 30% of patients with epidermodysplasia verruciformis, the most common tumour by far being squamous cell carcinoma. Sunlight appears to play a synergistic role in this phase of the disease, as tumours are confined to sun-exposed areas of the skin.

FUNGAL INFECTIONS

In many instances the outcome of fungal infection in a human host depends on the latter's degree of cell-mediated immunity. Pathogenic fungal infections in the skin may be divided into two main groups:

- **superficial** fungi which colonize the superficial layers of the skin (including hair and nails); in immunocompromised individuals, they may penetrate more deeply.
- **deep** fungi which involve the deeper parts of the dermis and the subcutaneous tissue, often with the production of granulomatous and abscess-like lesions. These are comparatively rare outside tropical areas.

Superficial Fungal Disorders

Pityriasis Versicolor

This is a common infection caused by *Pityrosporum orbiculare* (formerly *Malassezia furfur*). **This fungus, in the form of a unicellular yeast, is a normal skin commensal and becomes pathogenic only when budding occurs.** Such budding is favoured by a high environmental temperature and the disease is therefore far commoner in hot climates than in temperate ones, and in summer rather than in winter.

Lesions are distributed chiefly over the torso as small patches, showing either hyperpigmentation or hypopigmentation (hence use of the term *versicolor*). The lesions are associated with the presence of fine scales (pityriasis). As with other superficial fungal disorders of the skin, confirmation of the diagnosis is obtained by scraping the lesions and treating the scales with 30% potassium hydroxide. Microscopic examination of such preparations shows more or less spherical yeasts and elongated hyphae, giving an appearance graphically described as 'spaghetti and meatballs'.

Infections Caused by Dermatophytes

The dermatophytes are a set of related fungi with an ability to colonize keratinized tissue such as hair, nails and the stratum corneum of the skin. Three genera are involved in human disease:

1) *Microsporum*
2) *Trichophyton*
3) *Epidermophyton*

Some members of these genera reside predominantly on human skin, some in the soil and some on the skin of other animals. In the first case, infection causes little or no inflammatory response, but in the case of the other two infection elicits a florid inflammatory reaction.

When the hyphal elements of one of these fungi invade hair shafts, they are termed **endothrix** organisms, whereas those that remain on the outer surface of a hair shaft are called **ectothrix** organisms.

Clinically the dermatophyte infections are classified according to the part of the body affected and the species of fungus found. The clinical appearance of lesions and treatment are all modulated by the anatomical location.

Tinea Capitis, Tinea Corporis (Ringworm) and Tinea Pedis (Athlete's Foot)

The fungi involved, the area of skin affected and the characteristics of the lesion are shown in *Table 43.9*.

Candida Albicans Infections (Candidiasis)

Candida species, most often *C. albicans,* often infect the mouth, genitalia, skin flexures and nails. *Candida* is a normal commensal in the oropharynx, gut and vagina in about 80% of individuals, but does not usually colonize normal skin.

Candida **infections usually occur against a background of one or more predisposing causes:**

- **systemic,** such as any form of defect in cell-mediated immunity, diabetes, Cushing's syndrome, systemic administration of corticosteroids, malignancy, administration of antibiotics altering the normal flora and neutropenia. Infection is more likely at the extremes of age and during pregnancy.
- **local.** Any factor damaging the stratum corneum is associated with an increased risk of cutaneous candidiasis. This includes obesity, which increases the amount of friction at skin folds, and the presence of indwelling devices such as catheters.

It is the ability of the fungus to adhere to epithelial surfaces that changes it from a harmless commensal to a virulent organism. Adhesion is accomplished through the medium of various receptor–ligand interactions involving molecules on the surfaces of the fungus and the host cells. At least three categories of adhesion molecules are found on *C. albicans.* These are:

1) **a β_1-integrin** binding to RGD (arginine–glycine–aspartic acid) sequences such as are found in C3b, fibronectin, laminin, fibrinogen, fibrin and collagens types I and IV.
2) **lectins** which recognize sugar moieties on the host cell membranes
3) **carbohydrates** recognizing host cell membrane receptors, not as yet identified

Table 43.9 Characteristics of Tinea

Responsible fungus	Area of skin involved	Appearance of lesions
Tinea capitis		
Microsporum canis; *Trichophyton tonsurans* (now the commonest fungus involved)	Scalp hair	**Non-inflammatory lesions**: well-demarcated patches of scaling extending peripherally; the hair appears grey and lustreless and there are black dots in the lesion centre where hair shafts have broken off level with the skin surface.
		Inflammatory lesions vary from small pustules to large, boggy, suppurating lesions known as **kerions**. Tinea capitis is rare in adults and is more often found in black than in white children in the USA.
Tinea corporis		
T. rubrum; *T. mentagrophytes*	Non-hairy, smooth skin	Single or multiple, circular papulosquamous lesions with a raised red scaling edge and central clearing with scale formation. The lesions affect the trunk and limbs. In some cases they have a greater inflammatory component with formation of vesicles and pustules.
Tinea pedis		
T. rubrum; *T. mentagrophytes*; *Epidermophyton floccosum*	Interdigital spaces on feet; occurs only in those who normally wear shoes	A variety of morphological appearances may present. The commonest lesion is a boggy fissured lesion involving the toe webs, especially between the fourth and fifth toes. In some cases there are reddened scaly patches which may spread to involve much of the skin surface of the foot, whereas in others there are inflammatory lesions with vesicles and pustules that are prone to undergo secondary bacterial infection.

Other correlates of virulence, so far as the fungus itself is concerned, include the ability to secrete **a proteinase** that can destroy connective tissue proteins and the secretion of **adenosine**, which interferes with neutrophil function.

Candidiasis may be associated with a wide spectrum of clinical presentations.

Oral Candidiasis
For a fuller description of this condition (see p 485).

Candidal Intertrigo
The commonest sites for candidal infections of keratinized skin are skin folds such as the gluteal, perineal and inguinal folds, the scrotum, axillae, the skinfolds beneath the female breast, and folds that may occur in the abdominal skin in the obese. Moisture, heat and friction are likely to be present in these areas; this causes maceration of the stratum corneum, favouring colonization by *Candida*.

Affected areas are reddened and eroded, and scales are often present at the periphery of the lesions. Vesicles and pustules may be seen, often as satellites of the main lesions.

A variant is 'nappy' dermatitis in young infants in which *Candida* colonization is present in about 80% of cases. The predisposing factors here are probably the occlusive conditions created by the presence of the 'nappy' and the exposure of the skin to ammoniacal urine. Erythematous lesions begin, usually in the perianal region, and spread to involve the groin, buttocks and medial aspect of the thighs.

Candida Affecting the Nails and Nail Beds
Infections of the nail plate and nail folds are especially likely to be associated with occupations involving prolonged and frequent immersion of the hands in water (for example, dish washers, bar-tenders and laundry workers). The nail folds become swollen, reddened and painful, and serous or purulent exudates ooze from the nail fold.

Chronic Mucocutaneous Candidiasis Syndrome
The basic features of chronic mucocutaneous candidiasis are:

- candidiasis involving skin, nails, oral or genital mucosa, and which is resistant to treatment
- a defect in anti-candidal cell-mediated immunity, which may be fairly mild
- a predilection for children under 6 years (about 65% of cases). The syndrome, in one form or other, can also occur in adults.

There is a wide spectrum of clinical presentations, usually classified into five groups as shown in *Table 43.10.*

INFESTATIONS

The most common infestations giving rise to irritative skin lesions are:

- scabies
- pediculosis (infestation with lice)
- insect bites

Scabies

Scabies is the result of infestation by the eight-legged acarid mite **Sarcoptes scabiei.** The infection is usually acquired by prolonged and intimate physical contact between individuals, although rarely individuals may become infected by contact with certain inanimate objects, most notably sleeping-bags.

The mature mite secretes a keratinolytic substance and burrows into the stratum corneum. Gravid female mites lay eggs within the stratum corneum (at the rate of about two per day for 2 months) and the larvae, which take only a short time to hatch out, leave the burrow, pass through the nymph stage and then mature, at which point the whole cycle starts again.

The clinical picture results from the allergic reaction produced by the mites and patients with scabies show an increase in the plasma concentration of both immunoglobulin (Ig) G and IgM. Patients complain of intense itching, worst at night, and there is a polymorphic erythematous papular eruption.

The most helpful diagnostic sign on examination of the skin is the presence of **'burrows'**. Burrows are serpiginous, linear tracks, a few millimetres long, and which are very slightly raised above the surface of the surrounding skin. At one end of the burrow a black spot is often seen. Burrows representing the tracks made by the mite within the stratum corneum are often found at the sides of the fingers or on the wrists but can, in fact, occur anywhere. Because the clinical picture is based on an immune reaction to the presence of the mite, the only rational treatment is the eradication of the latter.

Table 43.10 Clinical Presentation of Mucocutaneous Candidiasis

Type	Characteristics
Chronic oropharyngeal candidiasis	No specific inheritance pattern Oral mucosa involved but skin and nails are spared Oesophagus may be involved
Chronic candidiasis with endocrine abnormalities	Autosomal recessive inheritance Mucous membranes and skin involved One or more endocrine defects appear after the candidal lesions. The classical triad is candidiasis, Addison's disease and hypoparathyroidism. Autoantibodies to the affected glands are present in the patient's serum
Localized mucocutaneous candidiasis	A severe form of the syndrome with hyperkeratotic, granulomatous and vegetating features No specific inheritance pattern Usually occurs during childhood Often associated with recurrent bacterial pneumonia, suggesting a severe immune defect
Chronic diffuse mucocutaneous candidiasis	Onset in childhood A variable inheritance pattern Widespread lesions No endocrine abnormality
Adult-onset chronic candidiasis	Onset usually after the third decade Diffuse resistant infections of mucosae, skin and nails High incidence of associated thymic tumours

Pediculosis

This is defined as a set of conditions characterized by infestation with lice.

Two species of louse are important in the causation of disease in humans. These are:

- *Pediculus humanus*, affecting both the scalp (pediculosis capitis) and other parts of the body (pediculosis corporis)
- *Phthirus pubis* (the crab louse), which moves relatively little and which has as its site of predilection the pubic hair, to which it clings by crab-like claws on its legs

Pediculosis Capitis

This occurs principally in schoolchildren. The lice are usually quite easily apparent on naked-eye examination and eggs (nits) cling to the hair shafts. This form of infestation may be accompanied by intense itching and, often, there is a papular rash, occurring especially behind the ears and in the occipital region. This eruption may become secondarily infected by bacteria.

Pediculosis Corporis

Although caused by a louse similar to that implicated in pediculosis capitis, this type of infestation is rare in normal civilian practice. It tends to be associated with abnormal circumstances such as war, leading to the enforced movement of populations, gross overcrowding and the breakdown of normal hygiene. The louse itself is about twice as large as the head louse and moves rather slowly. Body lice do not glue their eggs to hair shafts; instead they adhere to clothing and this can make their eradication difficult. Bites cause an itchy, red, papular rash associated with wheal formation; the lesions are most thickly clustered on the trunk and thighs.

The body louse has played an important part in history, having been the vector for infective agents capable of causing serious epidemics of **typhus** (*Rickettsia prowazeki*), **trench fever** (*R. quintana*) and **relapsing fever** (*Borrelia recurrentis*). These organisms are acquired by the louse in the course of biting infected individuals, the organisms being present in the blood. The organisms multiply in cells lining the louse gut and are then shed into the gut lumen. When the louse bites an individual, it also defaecates and the rickettsiae are deposited on the host's skin. The louse bite is irritating, the victim scratches and the infective louse faeces are rubbed into the puncture made by the louse. The importance of body louse infestation in relation to these serious disorders is underlined by the 30 million cases of typhus in Russia and eastern Europe during the years 1918–1922, causing 3 million deaths.

Pubic Lice

The pubic louse (*Phthirus pubis*) is usually sexually transmitted. The pubic hair is primarily affected, but the louse may spread to involve hair in other parts of the body such as the axillary hair, eyebrows and eyelashes. Nits may be seen clinging to pubic hairs, but this usually requires close examination of the affected parts. The bites are associated with an intensely itchy eruption.

NON-INFECTIOUS GRANULOMATOUS DISORDERS

Granuloma Annulare

This is a fairly common self-limiting disorder of unknown aetiology. **It is characterized by the appearance of ring-shaped reddish lesions with individual papules at the margins of the rings.** Granuloma annulare affects most commonly the backs of the hands, knees, ankles and elbows. It can, however, occur in any part of the body and, in a few instances, may present as a widespread papular eruption.

It is most frequently seen in children and young adults and there is an increased risk in females. There is some evidence, not universally accepted, of an association with diabetes mellitus.

Microscopic Features

The process is characterized by a granulomatous inflammatory response in the mid and upper dermis. The centres of the lesions contain degenerate collagen, tending to stain a bluish colour on haematoxylin and eosin staining instead of the normal bright pink. The zone of damaged collagen is surrounded by a mixture of macrophages, fibroblasts and lymphocytes arranged in a palisaded fashion. A small amount of mucin is often present in the central zone.

In some instances the process may extend up to involve the overlying epidermis and may communicate with the skin surface through a defect in the epidermis. This is known as the perforating form of the disease. In others there are very large lesions lying deeply within the dermis and extending to involve the subcutaneous adipose tissue.

Necrobiosis Lipoidica Diabeticorum

This is a disorder occurring in about 0.3% of all diabetics, who account for about 75% of cases of this condition. The diabetes is usually well developed at the time of the appearance of the skin lesions, but in about 14% of the diabetic cases, the skin lesions precede the overt onset of diabetes mellitus. It is three times as common in females as in males.

The lesions are reddish-brown to yellow plaques, often with a firm waxy consistency. The sites of predilection are the shins and feet.

As is the case with granuloma annulare, the pathogenesis remains unknown.

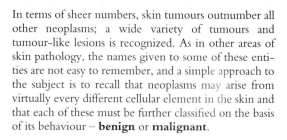

Skin Tumours

In terms of sheer numbers, skin tumours outnumber all other neoplasms; a wide variety of tumours and tumour-like lesions is recognized. As in other areas of skin pathology, the names given to some of these entities are not easy to remember, and a simple approach to the subject is to recall that neoplasms may arise from virtually every different cellular element in the skin and that each of these must be further classified on the basis of its behaviour – **benign** or **malignant**.

Aetiology

General Factors
In most cases the cause is unknown, although there are some striking associations, such as the link between acquired immune deficiency syndrome (AIDS) (especially in homosexuals) and Kaposi's sarcoma. In some common skin tumours, most notably those arising from keratinocytes, and certain types of malignant melanoma, the risk of tumour development appears to be related to the interaction of:
- **exposure to the ultraviolet rays of sunlight**
- **the degree of skin pigmentation**

In general terms, the greater the exposure and the less the pigmentation, the greater is the chance of developing skin cancer.

Thus, for example, someone living in Queensland, Australia, has a greater chance of developing skin cancer than someone living in northern Europe, and some cancers are more common in those living in a rural environment, where exposure to sunlight is likely to be greater than in city dwellers.

Similarly a red-haired, blue-eyed, fair-skinned individual whose skin tends to turn red after sun exposure rather than 'tanning', is more at risk than a dark-complexioned person. Skin cancer is much rarer in dark-skinned races than in white populations. An extreme example of the potential importance of normal skin pigmentation is the case of **albinism**. This is an inherited set of disorders characterized by absence or deficiency of tyrosinase in the melanocytes and, thus, an inability to synthesize melanin. Individuals so afflicted

have a very high incidence of sunlight-related damage to the skin (solar keratosis), basal cell carcinoma and squamous cell carcinoma.

Morphological Effect of Chronic Sun Exposure on the Skin (Actinic Keratosis) In areas of skin exposed to sunlight over a long period of time, changes may occur:
- the epidermis may show atrophy
- aberrant differentiation, atypia and hyperplasia may occur
- the papillary dermis shows degenerative changes with fragmentation and basophilia of the collagen fibres

The orderly maturation of the epidermal cells is disturbed and the superficial keratin layer becomes markedly thickened and parakeratotic. Those areas over the follicles and the intraepidermal portions of the sweat ducts are usually spared.

In some cases of actinic keratosis, the overproduction of keratin is so great as to produce a projecting mass known as a cutaneous horn (*Fig. 43.19*). (This may also be the end result of other proliferative processes affecting the epidermis and should not, *per se*, be regarded as a consequence necessarily of actinic keratosis.) The

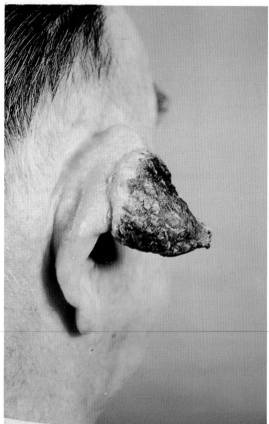

FIGURE 43.19 *Severe actinic keratosis leading to the formation of a cutaneous horn.*

keratinocytes may show a considerable degree of cytological atypia and the condition should be regarded as at least potentially malignant.

Other Aetiological Factors

Inability to Repair DNA (Xeroderma Pigmentosum) This is a rare condition inherited in an **autosomal recessive** fashion. Affected individuals are normal at birth but react abnormally to exposure to sunlight, developing large numbers of freckles on exposed areas of skin. These freckles are associated with dryness of the skin and abnormal dilatation of blood vessels. The eyes are also commonly affected and the patients show photophobia, conjunctival inflammation and ulceration.

The basic defect is the inability to excise and repair segments of DNA altered by exposure to ultraviolet light. The effect of ultraviolet light on keratinocytes is to produce abnormal linkages between adjacent base pairs (chiefly thymine). The degree of such change is, at least in part, related to the degree of ultraviolet light-absorbing melanin pigment in the skin. **In normal individuals, the altered segments of DNA in which the thymine dimers are present are excised by endonucleases and then repaired, but these enzymes are missing in the cells of patients with xeroderma pigmentosum.** As a result DNA abnormalities persist in succeeding generations of keratinocytes.

The risk of developing either squamous or basal cell carcinoma is increased by 1000-fold and there is also a greatly increased risk of malignant melanoma. In contrast to the normal age distribution of keratinocyte-derived tumours, which tend to occur in later life, patients with xeroderma develop tumours during childhood, at a median age of 8 years.

Exposure to Chemical Carcinogens The observation in 1775 by Pott, a well-known London surgeon, that there was a high prevalence of cancer of the scrotal skin in young chimney sweeps marked the beginning of the study of chemical carcinogenesis.

During the early phases of the industrial revolution in Britain, a similarly high prevalence of skin cancer was found in association with a number of occupations, all of which involved exposure to coal tar or its derivatives. Ultimately this led to the recognition that many polycyclic hydrocarbons had a carcinogenic potential, this being associated with the formation of active epoxides from these compounds catalysed by mixed-function oxidases. These epoxides can bind to DNA; the degree of binding correlates with the carcinogenic potential of the hydrocarbon.

An increased risk of skin cancer may also be conferred by some dermatological treatments, past and present. For example:

- In the early part of the century oral preparations of arsenic were used quite widely and there are still some elderly individuals alive who were treated in this way and who developed multiple skin malignancies.
- Another example of a dermatological treatment that may increase the chances of developing skin cancer is PUVA. This acronym stands for a combination of **psoralen** plus long-wavelength ultraviolet light (UVA). It has been used for severe cases of psoriasis and also in patients with the cutaneous T-cell lymphoma, mycosis fungoides. There is some evidence that recurrent low-dose treatment is associated with an increased risk of skin cancer.

Radiation-induced Tumours The increased frequency of squamous carcinoma of the skin of the hands in radiologists during the pioneering days of X-ray examination constitutes the first evidence that ionizing radiations are a risk factor for the development of skin cancer. Ionizing radiation kills cells (usually by inducing double-strand breaks in DNA) but also causes non-lethal damage, incorrect excision and repair of which leads to mutations that may be oncogenic.

Chronic Inflammatory Processes Associated with a Severe Degree of Scarring (Marjolin's Ulcer) The mean interval between sustaining an injury and developing a cancer at the same site is about 36 years, although there is enormous scatter in the duration of such intervals. The two most common precursor lesions are:
1) burns
2) chronic stasis ulcers associated with venous insufficiency in the lower limbs, which is by far the commonest site for all injury-associated skin cancers

The importance of burning is also shown by the existence of the Kangri burn cancer seen in India and the Kairo burn cancer seen among Japanese. Both of these are squamous cell carcinomas and in both there is a history of utensils containing hot coals being applied to the skin of the abdomen. It has been suggested that burning may be an **initiating** factor in relation to neoplastic transformation. This is supported by an experimental study in which skin tumours were induced in 47% of mice that had been burned and the burned areas subsequently treated with croton oil (a known tumour promoter). In burned mice not treated with croton oil, tumours developed in only 7%. The mechanisms that mediate this increased local risk are still unknown but the tumours themselves behave in an aggressive way with a higher incidence of tumour dissemination and a higher mortality rate than is usually seen in epidermal cancers.

Renal Transplantation About 7.5% of individuals with renal allografts develop neoplasms, and of these almost three-quarters affect the skin. The incidence of such tumours appears to be related to the length of time that has elapsed from transplantation and also to the degree of exposure to sunlight.

BENIGN SKIN TUMOURS AND TUMOUR-LIKE LESIONS

Epidermal Cyst

This is extremely common and is found most frequently on the face and trunk. It presents as a smooth dome-shaped, somewhat rubbery, nodule often with a central punctum. From this punctum cheesy cyst contents, consisting largely of keratin, may be expressed. The cyst wall is composed of keratinizing stratified squamous epithelium and the cyst cavity is filled with well-defined keratin lamellae. Rupture of the cyst wall due to the cyst being squeezed occurs quite often, and the release of the keratinous contents into the dermis results in a florid chronic inflammatory response in which multinucleated foreign-body giant cells are prominent.

Epidermal cysts may occur in relation to suture lines and there is an increased risk in individuals who have nodulocystic acne, although, in the majority of cases, there is no clue as to their origin.

Pilar cyst (Also Known as Trichilemmal or (Incorrectly) 'Sebaceous' Cyst)

These cysts are derived from the outer root sheath of the hair follicle and occur predominantly on the scalp, face and neck. Clinically they closely resemble epidermal cysts, a distinguishing feature being the lack of a punctum.

Microscopic Features

The cyst wall consists of a tough basement membrane (which makes rupture less likely and which allows the cysts to be shelled out fairly easily) and a stratified epithelial lining which shows the pattern of keratinization characteristic of hair sheath rather than epidermis. In this trichilemmal form, there is an abrupt transition from epidermal cells to keratin in the absence of a granular layer. Most of the epithelium consists of large pale cells which do not flatten in the same way as epidermal keratinocytes do. These bulky cells are desquamated into the cyst cavity.

Steatocystoma Multiplex

This condition, inherited in an autosomal dominant fashion, presents with multiple cystic lesion about the time of puberty. The lesions occur most commonly on the neck, sternal region, axillae and scrotum. The cysts are lined by stratified squamous epithelium and can be distinguished from other keratinizing cysts by the presence of lobules of sebaceous epithelium in their walls.

Basal Cell Papilloma (Syn. Seborrhoeic Keratosis)

This is one of the commonest skin neoplasms. It consists essentially of a mass of proliferating basal cells and mature keratinocytes (with the former predominating) and is often pigmented. The lesions may be single or multiple and occur most frequently on the trunk of middle-aged and elderly adults. The basal cell papilloma has a curious 'stuck-on' appearance and protrudes rather abruptly above the surface of the surrounding skin. The degree of pigmentation varies from a light tan colour to deep black (*Fig. 43.20*). In the latter event there may be some clinical confusion between this lesion and malignant melanoma.

Basal cell papillomas are normally without any ominous significance. However, the sudden appearance of a lesion or an increase in the size and number of basal cell papillomas may be a sign of internal malignancy **(the Leser–Trélat sign)**.

Microscopic Features

Basal cell papilloma consists predominantly of basal cells, presumably because of a maturation defect affecting the stem cell compartment of the epidermis. Keratin-filled cystic spaces are interspersed with these basal cells (*Fig. 43.21*). Some of the basal cells contain melanin pigment acquired from neighbouring melanocytes. 'Eddies' of mature squamous cells are not infrequently seen, especially when the lesions have been irritated.

POTENTIALLY MALIGNANT EPIDERMAL CHANGE

Bowen's Disease

Bowen's disease is a form of intraepidermal squamous neoplasia similar to that seen in other sites such as the uterine cervix or anus. The condition consists of indolent, scaly, red plaques occurring predominantly in those areas of the skin *not* exposed to sunlight.

Histologically the lesions show a variety of forms of keratinocyte atypia, including nuclear hyperchromatism, individual cell keratinization and an increased number of mitoses, some abnormal.

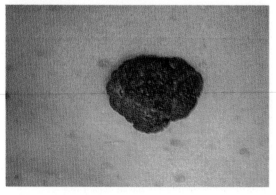

FIGURE 43.20 Seborrhoeic keratosis. Note the marked degree of pigmentation and the 'stuck-on' appearance of the lesion.

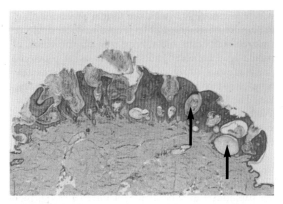

FIGURE 43.21 Seborrhoeic keratosis. Here, the superficial nature of the lesion is very apparent. The lesion consists of proliferated basal cells admixed with several keratin-filled cystic spaces (arrowed).

The change may involve virtually the entire thickness of the epidermis but a little evidence of surface maturation is usually present.

Lesions showing identical microscopic changes occur in sun-exposed areas of the skin and are most appropriately labelled as **actinic keratoses** of bowenoid type.

MALIGNANT EPIDERMAL NEOPLASMS

Squamous Cell Carcinoma (SCC)

Most of these are related to sunlight exposure. More than 80% are well differentiated with easily identifiable 'prickles' between the cells, and obvious keratin production (*Fig. 43.22*). SCC is typically seen on the backs of the hands, skin of the face (*Fig. 43.23*) and lips.

Strictly speaking, the diagnosis of squamous carcinoma should not be made in the absence of invasion of

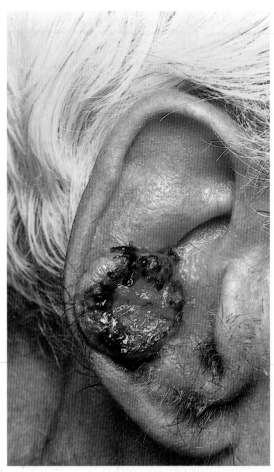

FIGURE 43.23 Ulcerated squamous carcinoma affecting a sunlight-exposed area. Note the typical everted edges of the lesion.

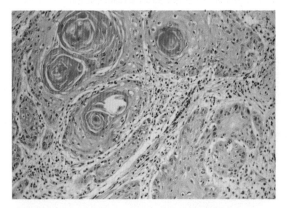

FIGURE 43.22 Invasive squamous carcinoma. This section shows the dermis infiltrated by islands of fairly well differentiated squamous epithelium in which foci of keratinization (so-called keratin pearls) are prominent.

the underlying dermis. However, an objective assessment of this is not always easy and one pathologist's 'superficially invasive squamous carcinoma' may be another's 'florid actinic keratosis with marked cellular atypia'. As local excision is the appropriate treatment in either case, this is not serious.

The existence of other microscopic variants of SCC may, on occasion, give rise to diagnostic difficulties, for example if the cells are spindle-shaped, or arranged in a pseudoglandular pattern owing to breakdown of cell cohesion caused by a defect in, or loss of, the desmosomal attachment points. In these cases the use of immunohistochemical techniques for identification of the high molecular weight keratins found in squamous epithelium may be helpful.

Basal Cell Carcinoma (BCC)

This is the most common form of skin cancer, with 500 000 cases occurring each year in the USA. It is so-called because of the similarity of the tumour cells to those of the normal basal layer of the epidermis. There is a strong relationship to sun exposure, although the lesions may develop in areas of skin normally protected from sunlight, in association with chronic venous stasis of the lower limbs, scars, irradiation and ingestion of small doses of arsenic.

The clinical appearances are extremely variable (*Fig. 43.24*). The lesions are described as:

- superficial
- nodular
- ulcerative
- erythematous
- sclerosing
- pigmented

BCC arises from stem cells in the basal layer of the epidermis and the pilosebaceous unit and differentiates, albeit incompletely, in the direction of various adnexal structures. A wide variety of microscopic patterns is seen. The tumour cells are small and darkly staining and a characteristic feature is the presence of **palisading** cells at the periphery of the islands of tumour (*Fig. 43.25*).

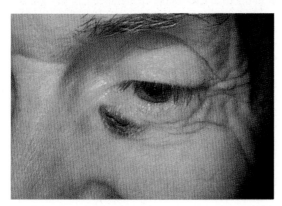

FIGURE 43.24 *Ulcerated basal cell carcinoma (so-called rodent ulcer). This lesion, like many basal cell tumours, shows a considerable degree of melanin pigmentation.*

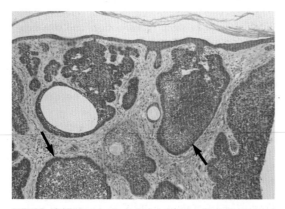

FIGURE 43.25 *Basal cell carcinoma. Islands of neoplastic basal cells are invading the dermis. Note the typical picket-fence arrangement of the cells at the periphery of the islands of tumour (arrowed).*

The presence of mitoses and of cellular atypia is without significance.

Low molecular weight cytokeratins are present within the tumour cells but the binding of antibodies against epithelial membrane antigens, carcinoembryonic antigen and involucrin, a feature of squamous carcinoma, is not seen.

Multiple BCC may occur as a part of Gorlin's basal cell naevus syndrome which is, in addition, characterized by the presence of palmar pits, dural calcification, keratinous cysts in the jaws, skeletal anomalies and occasional abnormalities in the central nervous system. In this syndrome the tumours tend to be of the superficial multicentric type, and osteoid metaplasia in the stroma is an occasional feature.

Biological Behaviour

Most BCCs show no tendency to metastasize and their growth tends to be slow. However, the tumour cells do possess the ability to invade locally and, if they are neglected, can cause extensive tissue destruction with most unpleasant cosmetic effects.

Adnexal Neoplasms

A wide variety of adnexal neoplasms exists. These involve hair follicles, sweat glands and ducts, and sebaceous glands. The only one considered here is **keratoacanthoma**. This lesion is thought to represent a neoplastic proliferation of the infundibular portion of the hair follicle and may be confused both clinically and microscopically with squamous carcinoma. Keratoacanthoma presents characteristically as a dome-shaped lesion in which there is a central crater filled with keratin. The male : female ratio is 3–4 : 1.

The most useful diagnostic feature on histological examination is the **architectural** pattern of the lesion, as seen on cross-section:

- overhanging edges
- a half-moon shape to the lesion as a whole
- a large central crater filled with keratin

Cytological criteria are essentially unhelpful in distinguishing keratoacanthoma from SCC. Most of the proliferating epithelium is well differentiated, and the cells have a rather 'glassy' cytoplasm. The growing aspect of the lesion is usually of the 'pushing' rather than of the infiltrating type, but in some instances there may be considerable infiltration into the deeper dermal tissues. In these cases the distinction between SCC and keratoacanthoma may be difficult. It has been suggested that, in such cases, the immunohistological demonstration of the histidine-rich protein, **filaggrin**, may be useful because it is usually present in the cells of a keratoacanthoma and is seen only rarely in squamous carcinoma.

Biological Behaviour

In its classical form, keratoacanthoma arises from a previously normal portion of skin, waxes rapidly over the next 4–6 weeks and then regresses over a further 4–6 weeks, leaving a depressed scar. However, a considerable degree of variation exists; some lesions grow slowly, some do not regress and others occur in areas of skin that have undergone actinic change.

TUMOURS DERIVED FROM NEUROENDOCRINE CELLS

The Merkel Cell Tumour

This comparatively rare lesion occurs for the most part on the face and extremities in middle-aged and elderly patients. It most commonly presents with a reddish or violet nodule which may ulcerate. On histological examination, the common appearance is of a uniform proliferation of small, round, dark cells, this being responsible for the not infrequent misdiagnosis of cutaneous lymphoma.

Merkel cell tumours may sometimes be seen associated with squamous carcinoma or with areas resembling basal cell tumours; this has been adduced as evidence for an origin from multipotent stem cells in the basal layer. Histochemically and immunologically, the cells react in the same way as neuroendocrine cells in other situations (*Fig. 43.26*): they are argyrophilic and bind antibodies against neurone-specific enolase. A few cases have been recorded where the tumour cells have contained peptide hormones such as vasoactive intestinal peptide, calcitonin, pancreatic polypeptide and somatostatin.

Biological Behaviour

Merkel cell tumours behave aggressively. Spread to regional lymph nodes is common and lung, liver and bones may be involved by metastases.

TUMOURS OF MELANOCYTIC ORIGIN

Malignant melanocyte-derived tumours present one of the most challenging problems in oncology. They are

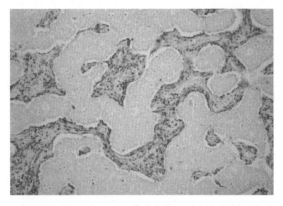

FIGURE 43.26 *Merkel cell tumour. The section has been treated with an antibody that binds to cells with neuroendocrine features.*

increasing in frequency more rapidly than any other malignant tumour. In 1935, malignant melanoma affected one person in every 1500; in the 1990s the risk is of the order of 1 in 135, and it has been projected that by the end of the century 1 in 90 inhabitants of the USA will develop melanoma.

Because malignant melanoma behaves more aggressively than most other skin tumours, early diagnosis is important. Since the 1950s there has been a considerable improvement in 5-year survival rates of patients with malignant melanoma (81% compared with 49%) but, because of the steep increase in the number of individuals afflicted, the number of deaths due to this tumour has increased by about 150%.

Benign melanocytic tumours are very common and are known as **moles** (common acquired melanocytic naevi). Their differentiation patterns mirror, to some extent, the embryonic development of the melanocytes.

Melanocytes, of which there are some two billion, lie:

- in the basal layer of the epidermis and of the skin adnexal epithelium
- in the choroid of the eye
- in some mucous membranes
- in the nervous system

Their function is to produce the insoluble ultraviolet light-absorbing pigment **melanin**, which protects the epidermal cell nuclei against the effects of the sunlight. Melanocytes can be identified immunohistologically within the basal layer using antibodies against the neurally derived proteins S-100 and neurone-specific enolase.

MELANOCYTIC NAEVI

Most people have small melanocytic naevi (moles). Often these are multiple (there may be as many as 20 to 40) and appear, as a rule, between 2 and 6 years of age. They are found most commonly on the skin of the face, neck and trunk.

Melanocytic naevi are said by some to occupy the middle ground between malformations and true neoplasms, and most of them have a rather predictable pattern of evolution.

Basically they are classified according to the **level** within the skin where the melanocytic proliferation is predominant. The commonest variants are described below.

Junctional Naevi

These are flat, or very slightly elevated, brown patches, usually less than 5 mm in diameter. The earliest stages are characterized by **an increase in the number of melanocytes in the basal layer with, at this point, no clustering of these cells**. Such a pattern of proliferation is called **lentiginous**.

As the lesions progress the proliferating cells form distinct clusters or 'nests' at the tips of the epidermal

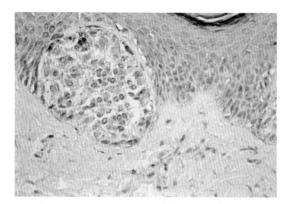

FIGURE 43.27 *Junctional naevus showing the typical nesting of proliferated melanocytes at the dermoepidermal junction.*

rete pegs, these nests being on the epidermal side of the basement membrane (*Fig. 43.27*). Most junctional naevi are benign but malignant transformation can occur in some instances.

Intradermal Naevi

In this lesion some of the proliferated melanocytes have 'dropped off' or emigrated across the basement membrane into the dermis; there is no longer any evidence of basal layer proliferation or 'junctional activity'. Small clusters of well-differentiated melanocytes (or naevus cells) are present within the dermis (*Fig. 43.28*), the degree of cellularity and pigmentation differing widely from lesion to lesion. With time, the deepest portions of the naevus tend to become less cellular and to contain a major spindle cell population arranged in a fashion that recalls the pattern of nerve sheath.

Compound Naevi

These combine the features of both junctional and intradermal naevi. As age increases, so the number of moles with an active junctional component

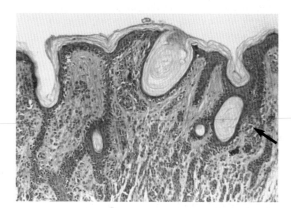

FIGURE 43.28 *Compound melanocytic naevus. Some junctional activity is still present (arrowed) but the majority of proliferated melanocytes form islands within the dermis.*

decreases. The exception to this is in the skin of the soles and palms where age does not appear to affect the capacity of naevi to show junctional activity.

Some Rarer Forms of Naevus

Blue Naevus

This is a small, darkly pigmented, lesion found most commonly on the skin of the head, neck and upper limbs. **Histologically it is characterized by an ill-defined intradermal proliferation of elongated melanocytes in which melanin is generally present in large amounts. There is a band of non-involved dermis between the lesion and the overlying epidermis, and junctional activity is never seen.**

Cellular Blue Naevus

This is a distinct subgroup of blue naevi which may give rise to suspicion of malignancy because of their large size and intense degree of pigmentation. **They are found most commonly on the buttock or in the sacrococcygeal region.**

Microscopically they are extremely cellular but show no evidence of junctional activity, cellular atypia or abnormal mitoses. Their biological behaviour is invariably benign but a few cases have been recorded in which local recurrence and regional lymph node involvement have occurred.

Spitz Naevus (Spindle Cell Naevus)

This is a lesion occurring characteristically before puberty but which can also be seen in adult life. It was at one time called juvenile melanoma but this term can give rise to confusion between this benign lesion and malignant melanoma, which is very rare in children. **The commonest clinical presentation is in the form of a raised pink or red nodule found most often on the skin of the face.**

Microscopic Features

Most Spitz naevi are **compound in pattern** with a prominent intraepidermal component; 5–10% are purely junctional and 20% are intradermal. They are composed either of **spindle cells**, many arranged more or less perpendicular to the epidermal surface as if 'raining down', or of so-called 'epithelioid'-type cells, which are large and polygonal with abundant eosinophilic cytoplasm. Multinucleate giant melanocytes may be seen and mitoses are found in up to half the cases, although atypical ones are rare.

The behaviour of Spitz naevi is almost always benign but a few cases have been documented in which aggressive behaviour with both local and distant spread has occurred.

MALIGNANT MELANOMA

Risk Factors
Several risk factors have been recognized in relation to melanoma. These include:

- **Adulthood.** Melanoma is very rare before the age of 15 years; the median age at diagnosis is 53 years and the adult risk is about 88 times as great as that in childhood.
- **The presence of pre-existing melanocytic lesions.** Included under this rubric are:
  1) **dysplastic naevi with a history of familial melanoma.** This syndrome, which is inherited in an autosomal dominant pattern, is an extremely powerful risk factor, the relative risk being 148 times as great as for an individual without this risk factor.
  2) **dysplastic naevi with *no* history of familial melanoma.** A wide range of relative risk (7–70-fold) is quoted for this syndrome. This reflects, at least in part, the different definitions of this risk factor.
  3) **the presence of a large congenital mole** (relative risk 17–21-fold)
  4) **the presence of the lesion termed lentigo maligna** (see below) (relative risk 10-fold)
  5) **the presence of a large number of benign melanocytic naevi.** Again, a wide range is quoted for the relative risk. There is still considerable controversy as to what proportion of malignant melanomas arise in previously benign moles.
- **Being white rather than black skinned** (a 12-fold relative risk)
- Other factors include immunosuppression, a previous history of melanoma in the individual concerned, a history of melanoma in a parent, sibling or child, **excessive exposure to sun and sun sensitivity. Sun-related burning of the skin appears to be most critical as a risk factor if it occurs during childhood or adolescence and if it is intermittent (such as during holiday periods).**

Dysplastic Naevus Syndrome
Studies of families with a high incidence of melanoma show that there is a distinctive type of naevus apparently associated with a high risk of familial melanoma. These naevi are known as **dysplastic naevi** and the tendency to develop these is inherited in an autosomal dominant fashion. Some regard these lesions as being the histogenetic precursors of malignant melanoma in families with a high risk of melanoma and, at a clinical level, they serve as markers of increased risk of malignant melanoma. The chance of an individual from a melanoma-prone family who has dysplastic naevi of developing malignant melanoma is almost 200-fold greater than that of an individual without such a family

history. Available data suggest that 5–10% of all malignant melanomas occur on a familial basis. The differences between dysplastic naevi and common acquired naevi are shown in *Table 43.11*.

Classification
Four main types of malignant melanoma are recognized. These are classified by the following criteria:
1) **the presence or absence of a component adjacent to the main mass, known as the radial growth phase (RGP)**
2) **the histological characteristics of the RGP**
The biological behaviour of a malignant melanoma depends to a considerable extent on whether the tumour shows a RGP only, at the time of diagnosis or whether there is evidence of a much more sinister pattern, known as the vertical growth phase (VGP).
- Where only a RGP was present at the time of diagnosis in a large series of cases followed for 7 years, **no metastases** either to local lymph nodes or to distant sites were recorded.
- The presence of a VGP correlates with competence of the tumour cells to metastasize.

The occurrence of a VGP is synonymous with acquisition by the tumour cells of the ability to metastasize. Thus the diagnosis and treatment of malignant melanoma while still in the RGP (more than 80% of lesions have such a phase) is very important.

Radial Growth Phase
Although radial growth phase (RGP) is a biological term, it has fairly precise histological correlates. It is not synonymous purely with peripheral growth.

> ### Microscopic Features
> - **Tumours may be present in the epidermis alone (an *in situ* lesion) or in the dermis as well.**
> - **The tumour cells in the dermis:**
>   1) resemble closely those involving the epidermis
>   2) are usually confined to the papillary dermis
>   3) are disposed in small clusters 10–15 cells wide
>   4) show no evidence that any individual cell cluster or nest has an apparent growth advantage over any other cluster
>   5) very uncommonly form clusters that exceed the size of the intraepidermal cell nests

Biological characteristics of such cells include the following:
1) Cell lines may be established in culture only with difficulty.
2) The cultured cells from the radial phase are not tumorigenic in nude (immunocompromised) mice.

Table 43.11 A Comparison between Common Acquired Naevi and Dysplastic Naevi

Common acquired naevi	Dysplastic naevi
Lesions absent at birth	Lesions absent at birth
First appear in early childhood	Increased number of morphologically normal naevi present between 5 and 8 years of age
Increase in number until middle adult life and decline in number thereafter	At puberty both number and appearance of naevi change significantly
Average of 10–40 lesions per person	Morphologically atypical naevi increase throughout adult life with no decline in number at older ages
Predominate in sun-exposed skin above the waist	Dysplastic naevi are typically but not inevitably larger than common acquired naevi (range 6–15 mm in diameter)
Rare in scalp or in 'bathing suit' area	
Round or oval in shape; have a smooth border and are well-demarcated from surrounding skin	Number of naevi usually of order of 25–75 per person but up to 100 is not unusual
Maximal diameter is 4–6 mm in most cases	In addition to sites mentioned for common naevi, dysplastic naevi are often found on scalp, buttocks and breast
Pigmentation of individual lesions is usually uniform	Lesions have an irregular border and a margin that is indistinct, fading into the surrounding skin. The surface is 'pebbly'
	The pattern of pigmentation is often mixed with tan, brown, dark brown and pink areas

3) The cells show non-random abnormalities in chromosome 6.

Vertical Growth Phase

The term describes the focal appearance, either within an established RGP, or *ab initio* (as in nodular melanoma), of a new population of cells growing as an **expanding spheroidal nodule** and which have a distinct growth advantage over the cells of the radial phase.

Microscopic Features

- The cells appear different from those in the radial growth phase (e.g. the VGP cells are often amelanotic whereas the cells of the RGP contain pigment).
- The cellular aggregates that characterize the VGP are larger than the clusters of intraepidermal or intradermal cells found in the RGP.
- The tumour cells extend into the lower half of the reticular dermis.
- The host's lymphocyte and macrophage response to the presence of tumour is absent at the base of the tumour cells forming the VGP.

Biological characteristics of the cells of the vertical growth phase include the following:

1) Cells cultured from the VGP very readily form permanent cell lines and often do not require supplementary growth factors.

2) Cells cultured from the VGP are tumorigenic in nude mice.
3) Non-random abnormalities are found in chromosomes 1, 6 and 7.

Classification depends, at least in part, on the presence or absence of a RGP. Thus, we have the following four main types of melanoma:

- **radial growth phase present:**
  1) **superficial spreading melanoma (67%)**
  2) **lentigo maligna melanoma (9%)**
  3) **acral lentiginous melanoma (4%)**
- **radial growth phase absent:**
  4) **nodular melanoma**

Superficial Spreading Malignant Melanoma

This is the commonest form of malignant melanoma and the one increasing most rapidly in frequency.

Macroscopic Features

In terms of colour, the appearances of superficial spreading melanoma may be variable, the commonest being bluish admixed with shades of brown (*Fig. 43.29*). The surface is usually slightly elevated above that of the surrounding skin. In some lesions, white depigmented patches may be seen. These correspond to areas of regression in which tumour cells have been destroyed by activated T lymphocytes and macrophages. In some instances complete regression of such lesions may occur. The outline of superficial spreading

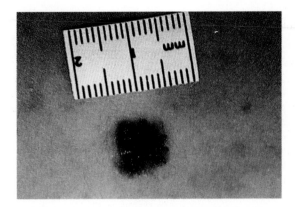

FIGURE 43.29 Superficial spreading malignant melanoma.

melanoma is irregular. Deep dermal invasion (indicative of a VGP) is generally associated with the appearance of a nodule on the surface of a previously flat lesion.

Microscopic Features

The areas at the periphery of the lesion (the component used for classification), where there is no dermal invasion, show atypical melanocytes invading the epidermis at different levels, either in clusters or in the form of single cells. This pattern of intraepidermal spread is termed **pagetoid** (*Fig. 43.30*) because of the resemblance to the intraepidermal pattern seen in Paget's disease, for example of the breast (see p 812).

If a VGP has supervened, the cells are usually epithelioid (with abundant cytoplasm) and form one or more nodules significantly larger than the small clusters of invasive cells characteristic of the RGP.

Lentigo Maligna (Hutchinson's Melanotic Freckle)

The proportion of these behaving in a malignant and invasive fashion is quite small (about 5%) and in these cases

the duration of the benign phase may range from 5 to 40 years. Lentigo maligna, which is commoner in women than in men, usually occurs in sun-exposed regions of the skin of elderly Caucasians, the malar and temple regions of the skin being the most common sites. It is a flat pigmented lesion (*Fig. 43.31*) which grows slowly and has the best prognosis of the four main types of melanoma.

Microscopic Features

The lesion of lentigo maligna is characterized by proliferation of melanocytes in a lentiginous pattern, the atypical melanocytes being confined during the preinvasive period to the basal layer of the epidermis. These melanocytes are distributed either singly or in the form of small cell clusters. If an invasive lesion develops on the basis of lentigo maligna it is generally of the spindle cell type and tends not to behave in a very aggressive fashion.

Occasionally, an aggressive melanoma does develop on the basis of lentigo maligna. Such lesions are associated with a marked degree of reactive dermal fibrosis and have been called desmoplastic melanomas.

Acral Lentiginous Melanoma

This is the rarest of the four main types of malignant melanoma (about 4% of the total). Some 90% of these lesions occur on the feet and about 16% of them are found beneath one of the nails (subungual) (*Fig. 43.32*).

Microscopic Features

Acral lentiginous melanoma has an intraepidermal component of lentiginous type which is similar in many respects to that seen in lentigo maligna. In contrast to the latter, the intraepidermal melanocytes tend to be bizarre in appearance; the epidermis is hyperplastic rather than atrophic, and the papillary dermis tends to be broadened and inflamed.

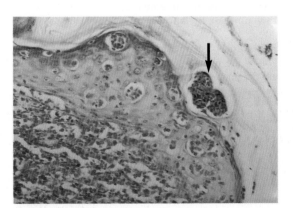

FIGURE 43.30 Malignant melanoma. This section shows upward invasion of the epidermis by malignant cells. Note the clusters of pigmented cells (arrowed) within the keratin layer.

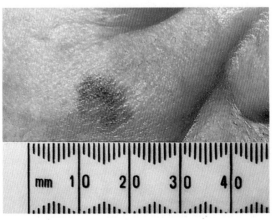

FIGURE 43.31 Typical flat lentigo maligna on the face of an elderly person.

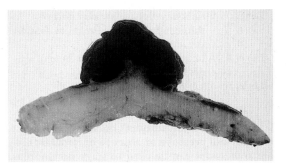

FIGURE 43.33 *Nodular malignant melanoma. Note how the lesion projects from the skin surface.*

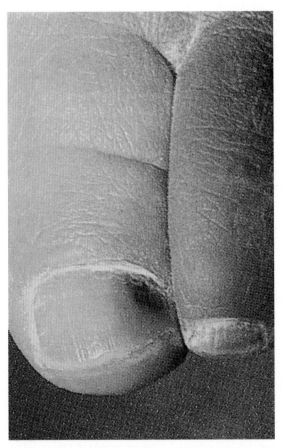

FIGURE 43.32 *Subungual malignant melanoma. This lesion is easily confused with a subungual haematoma.*

other types the significance has not yet been determined. It is a valuable criterion because it is objective. Measurement should be made vertically from the upper level of the granular epidermis to the deepest part of the tumour. The relation between tumour thickness, metastatic spread and survival is shown in *Tables 43.12* and *43.13*.

At diagnosis nodular melanomas are much thicker than the superficial spreading variety: only 25% of nodular melanomas fall into the group less than 1.69 mm in thickness in contrast with 77% of superficial spreading melanomas. The prognostic implications are obvious.

- **Level of invasion.** The prognostic implications of different levels of tumour invasion in the skin were described by Clark. Five such levels are recognized:

Level 1: tumour cells confined within the epidermis

Level 2: tumour invades the papillary dermis

Acral lentiginous melanoma is commonest in dark-skinned races. If diagnosed early, the prognosis is good (90% 5-year survival rate), but once the lesion has progressed to stage 2 (see below for staging criteria) the outlook is very poor with a 5-year survival rate of only 8%.

Nodular Melanoma

Nodular melanoma has little or no adjacent component (no more than three rete ridges involved at the periphery). It is, by definition, a lesion that is in a virtually pure vertical growth phase (VGP) *ab initio*. The lesion presents as a nodule which is red, grey or black (*Fig. 43.33*) and there is no evidence of peripheral extension of the pigmentation at the margins. A polypoid appearance may be present and ulceration is not infrequent.

Prognosis

Criteria used to assess the prognosis in individual lesions of malignant melanoma include:

- The presence or absence of a **VGP**
- **Tumour thickness.** This is the single most important prognostic indicator in patients with superficial spreading and nodular melanoma. For

Table 43.12 Melanoma Thickness and Metastasis

Thickness (mm)	Nodal metastases (%)	Distant metastases (%)
< 0.76	2–3	—
0.76–1.5	25	8
1.5–4.00	57	15
> 4.00	62	72

Table 43.13 Thickness and Survival

Tumour thickness (mm)	7-year survival rate (%)
≤ 1.69	88
1.70–3.99	61
> 4.00	32

Level 3:   tumour cells have invaded down through the papillary dermis to abut on the reticular dermis

Level 4:   tumour cells have invaded the reticular dermis

Level 5:   tumour cells have invaded right through the reticular dermis and can be seen within the subcutaneous tissues

A combination of tumour thickness, level of invasion and presence or absence of nodal or distant metastases can be used to stage melanomas (see *Table 43.14* **and** *Fig. 43.34*).

In stage I cases, the presence of **ulceration** significantly reduces the 10-year survival rate. The **growth pattern** also has prognostic significance, even in stage I. The best prognosis is associated with lentigo maligna melanoma, the next best with superficial spreading melanoma and the worst with nodular melanoma. Females with stage I tumours have a somewhat better prognosis than males. The anatomical location of the lesions also has prognostic value; those on the lower extremity do best.

Other prognostic factors include:

- **The anatomical site of the tumour.** Given an equivalent thickness of tumour, those on the scalp, hands and feet appear to have a poorer prognosis.
- **Age.** Older patients do worse than younger ones.
- **Sex.** Women have a somewhat better prognosis than men.

Table 43.14 Staging of Melanoma

Stage	Characteristics	10-year survival rate (%)
1A	Tumour invading papillary but not reticular dermis (levels II and III); not more than 1.5 mm thick	> 80
1B	Tumour invading reticular dermis or subcutaneous tissue (levels IV or V); more than 1.5 mm thick	
II	Regional lymph node spread	60
III	Juxtaregional lymph node spread	25
IV	Distant metastases	10

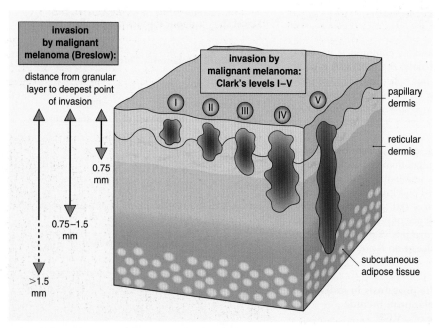

FIGURE 43.34 *Local spread in the prognosis of malignant melanoma. The extent of invasion may be assessed by measuring the thickness of the lesion, as described by Breslow (left side of diagram) or by determining the anatomical level that has been reached, as described by Clark (right-hand side of diagram).*

- **Histological features.** Those suggesting a worse prognosis include:
  a) a high mitotic rate
  b) a large tumour volume
  c) the presence of satellite nodules (i.e. discrete nodules of tumour more than 0.05 mm in diameter in either the reticular dermis or the subcutaneous adipose tissue and separated from the main tumour mass).

Chromosomal Changes in Malignant Melanoma

The short arm of chromosome 9 contains a susceptibility gene which is mutated in more than 50% of all malignant melanoma cell lines. This mutation appears to play a significant role in tumorigenesis, especially in the case of familial melanoma. Abnormalities at this locus have been described in many other tumour types.

The abnormality is usually a deletion; this suggests the existence of a tumour-suppressor gene at this site. Early in 1994 the protein product of this gene was identified and called **p16**. It exerts its effect by binding to one of the cyclin-dependent kinases driving cell cycling (**cdk4**), binding inhibiting kinase activation by cyclin D_1. This is the first suppressor gene product shown to act directly on the cell cycle. Deletions of the *p16* gene have been shown to be present in 50% of all cancers. In only two types of tumour, colorectal cancer and neuroblastoma, have *p16* deletions not been found.

CONNECTIVE TISSUE TUMOURS

Dermal connective tissue shows the same range of neoplasms as connective tissue in other sites (see pp 1092–1106). One neoplasm that has greatly increased in frequency in the past 10 years is **Kaposi's sarcoma**.

Kaposi's Sarcoma

Moritz Kaposi, born Moritz Kohn, as a career move, took a new surname from his home town of Kaposvar in Hungary. The tumour bearing his name was formerly infrequent in most Western countries, although it was found in fairly large numbers in a belt across sub-Saharan tropical Africa (**the endemic form**) and in smaller numbers among eastern Europeans and in the peoples of the Mediterranean basin (**the sporadic form**).

The incidence of Kaposi's sarcoma has now increased many 100-fold in the West; this increase has been confined, for the most part, to patients with AIDS, although the lesion may also occur in other immunosuppressed patients. In the case of human immunodeficiency virus (HIV)-associated Kaposi's sarcoma, it always seemed likely that some agent was involved other than the virus, because there is a striking difference between the prevalence

of Kaposi's sarcoma in HIV-positive homosexuals (36%) and in haemophiliacs who have seroconverted as a result of receiving HIV-infected Factor VIII (1.6%).

It has now been shown that there are sequences present in Kaposi's sarcoma suggesting infection by a novel form of herpesvirus, which has provisionally been termed herpesvirus VIII.

In the classical type of Kaposi's sarcoma, the lesion presents as multiple bluish plaques or nodules on the skin of the lower extremities. Where the tumour is endemic, in patients with HIV infection and in those who are immunosuppressed for other reasons (such as following renal transplantation), the lesions are more variably distributed and behave aggressively. In these groups the finding of regional node and visceral involvement is by no means uncommon.

> **Microscopic Features** (*Fig. 43.35*)
> The most characteristic feature is the presence of red cell-containing slits in the dermis. These are lined either by abnormal endothelial cells or by spindle-shaped cells; the spaces appear to cleave the dermal collagen. The precise differentiation of this lining cell is controversial. Some show markers suggestive of endothelium but this is not uniform or constant. Forming a background to the vasoformative element is an infiltrate of lymphocytes, iron-laden macrophages and other inflammatory cells.

Fibrous Histiocytoma (Dermatofibroma, Sclerosing Haemangioma)

This is a common lesion occurring most frequently on the lower leg. It presents clinically as a papule or, less often, as a nodule moving freely within the skin. It is often quite deeply pigmented, giving rise to suspicions of melanoma.

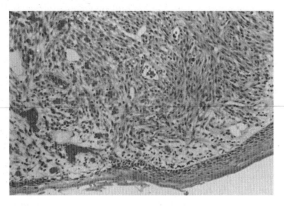

FIGURE 43.35 *Kaposi's sarcoma in a patient with AIDS. The lesion consists of bundles of spindle cells in which the presence of blood-filled clefts is very characteristic.*

Dermatofibrosarcoma Protuberans

This lesion, usually seen in the middle-aged, presents initially as a plaque-like thickening which can be mistaken for a hypertrophic scar or a keloid. The commonest site is the trunk. With the passage of time the lesion enlarges and protrudes much more obviously and with this enlargement comes bluish or red discoloration.

Microscopic examination shows the tumour to consist predominantly of spindle cells arranged in a storiform pattern. The tumour arises within the dermis but may spread downwards to involve the subcutaneous adipose tissue. Mitoses are moderately frequent. Local recurrence, if surgical removal has been inadequate, is not uncommon but the tumour rarely metastasizes.

Tumours and Tumour-like Lesions Arising from Blood Vessels (Haemangiomas)

Haemangiomas are very common. Many are hamartomas rather than true neoplasms, although the latter certainly exist in both benign and malignant forms. A large number of histological entities have been delineated under this rubric of vascular tumours. It is beyond the scope of a work of this size to refer to more than a few of the commonest variants.

Pyogenic Granuloma

The term **pyogenic granuloma** is an outstanding example of misuse of language, because this lesion is neither due to infection nor is it a granuloma. It is a highly vascular nodule developing rapidly, sometimes, but not always, at a site of injury to the skin. It is believed to represent a reaction to some angiogenic stimulus, the nature of which is not clear. The initial growth phase is rapid, but after a few weeks growth ceases. Spontaneous regression can occur but is uncommon.

Juvenile Haemangioma

Juvenile haemangioma (also known as 'strawberry naevus') is common, occurring in about 1 in 200 infants. It

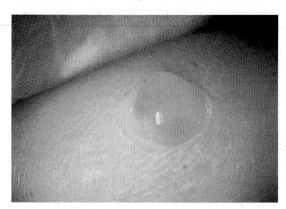

FIGURE 43.36 *Pyogenic granuloma on the finger.*

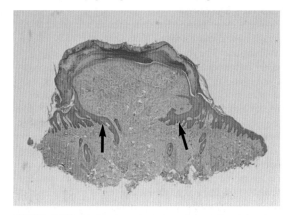

FIGURE 43.37 *Section through a pyogenic granuloma showing the exuberant nodule composed of proliferating capillaries. Note the characteristic epidermal 'collarette' at the margins (arrowed).*

presents, usually within the first few weeks of life, as a red macule which becomes elevated and usually reaches its maximal size at about the age of 6 months. Most lesions then start to regress, the presence of focal areas of a greyish white colour indicating fibrosis, and by the age of 7 years complete involution will have taken place in about 75% of cases.

In histological terms the lesion is a capillary haemangioma (*Fig. 43.38*), but in its early stages the proliferated blood vessels are inconspicuous, the predominant element being closely packed spindle cells in which mitoses may be seen in moderate numbers. The lesion is perfectly benign and, in most cases, no treatment is necessary.

Cherry Angiomas (Campbell de Morgan Spots)

This is another very common hamartoma affecting skin blood vessels. The lesions, which are multiple, make their first appearance in adult life, and are small, measuring only a few millimetres along their longest axis. They are usually very well demarcated papules with a cherry-red colour.

Histological examination shows the presence of focal aggregates of dilated thin-walled blood vessels in the upper dermis. The overlying epithelium often shows flattening.

Cavernous Haemangioma

The defining criterion of a cavernous haemangioma is the presence of aggregates of large dilated blood vessels lined by flattened endothelium. In the skin, these lesions are usually found in the deep dermis and may, in some instances, be associated with juvenile haemangioma. They occur most commonly during infancy and may grow to a very considerable size. Rarely, if the lesions are very large, sequestration of platelets may occur within the abnormal blood vessels, causing thrombocytopenia. This is known as the Kasabach–Merritt syndrome. Cutaneous cavernous haemangiomas are also found in a rare autosomal dominant condition known as the **'blue rubber bleb naevus syndrome'**. In this, cavernous haemangiomas are found in the skin, gut and other organs. The typical presentation is recurrent gastrointestinal bleeding.

Glomus Tumour

This is a comparatively rare lesion arising from the neuromyoarterial glomus, which consists of a complex system of anastomosing channels between the digital arterioles and the digital venules. Normal glomus cells surround these vascular channels and, because they contain both myosin and vimentin, they may well be related to smooth muscle cells. In most cases the lesions are single and sporadic but, rarely, multiple tumours may occur in several members of one family, the inheritance pattern suggesting that an autosomal dominant genetic factor may be operating in these cases.

The solitary tumours are pink nodules ranging in size from 1 to 20 mm. They are characteristically associated with pain, which may be spontaneous or elicited by direct pressure or changes in skin temperature. Glomus tumours are most frequently found in the extremities and the nail bed is a particularly common site. The nail bed glomus tumours are often very painful and patients thus present for treatment while the lesions are still very small.

Microscopic examination shows the lesions to be sited in the dermis. There is considerable variation in the morphological appearances but the typical lesion shows the presence of dilated vascular channels with rows of cuboidal glomus cells arranged round them.

Angiosarcoma

Somewhere between one-third and one-half of all angiosarcomas occur in the skin. The head and neck regions are especially likely to be affected and the

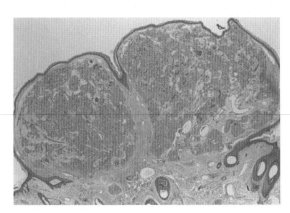

FIGURE 43.38 Benign haemangioma. This is a hamartomatous lesion consisting of a mass of proliferated capillaries, many of which appear to have no lumen.

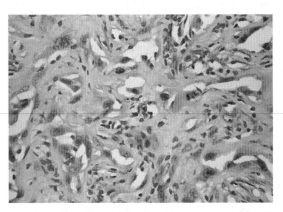

FIGURE 43.39 Angiosarcoma. Vascular spaces are obvious in this field. They are lined by large cells with rather bizarre, hyperchromatic nuclei.

tumours are much more common in elderly individuals. Angiosarcoma can occur in assocation with long-standing lymphoedema, as in patients who have undergone radical mastectomy for breast cancer. The cells of the angiosarcomas in these individuals express Factor VIII-related antigen and must be deemed to arise from blood vessel rather than lymphatic endothelium.

Most examples form easily recognizable vascular spaces which are lined by cells with large hyperchromatic nuclei (*Fig. 43.39*). The tumours are highly aggressive and the prognosis is, in general, poor.

CHAPTER 44

The Skeletal System

Bone

The skeleton has three functions. It is:

1) **a structural framework**, light enough to be mobile and support the limbs, and strong enough to protect the brain, spinal cord and thoracic viscera. These demands are met by bone's basic structure. **It is a mixture of tough type I collagen fibres, which can resist pulling forces, and of mineral particles (calcium phosphate in the form of hydroxyapatite crystals), which can resist compression.** The collagen fibres and the mineral occupy roughly equal volumes.

2) **a reservoir for almost all the body's calcium and much of its phosphorus and magnesium**

3) the chief site for **haemopoiesis**

NORMAL ANATOMY AND DEVELOPMENT

Macroscopically there are two major bone types:

- **Cortical bone** is dense and compact, forming the rigid outer shell which defines the shape of individual bones. It predominates in the shafts of the long tubular bones.
- **Cancellous bone** appears spongy, owing to its trabecular arrangement.

Microscopically, bone can also be classified on the basis of its organization into two types:

- **Woven bone** occurs normally in embryonic life and childhood. **It is characteristic of a situation where the bone formation is rapid.** In the context of bone disease, woven bone is seen in the circumstances listed in *Table 44.1*. Woven bone is characterized microscopically by a random meshwork of birefringent collagen fibres, as seen in polarized light.
- **Lamellar bone** is characteristic of adult bone, both compact and cancellous. It occurs typically where bone formation is slow. Under polarized light the collagen fibres are seen to be arranged in parallel bundles and sheets. The fibre direction of successive sheets alternates, giving rise to the layered pattern seen in polarized light.

Table 44.1 Disorders Showing Woven Bone

Age	Disorder
Childhood	Osteogenesis imperfecta
	Scurvy
	Rickets
Childhood and adult life	Fracture callus
	Bone-forming tumours
Adult life	Paget's disease of bone

Bone Development in the Fetus

In the fetus, bone is formed from undifferentiated mesenchymal tissue in two ways. These are **intramembranous** and **endochondral** ossification, and both may occur in the same bone. Mature bone can only grow by **apposition** (i.e. the deposition of new layers of bony material on preformed surfaces). However, in fetal life and postnatally up to puberty, there is a clear need for an increase in **bone length**. Such increases cannot occur as a result of appositional growth and thus there must be some other mechanism. This is **endochondral ossification**.

Intramembranous ossification is the process where the bone is formed directly from the mesenchyme; endochondral ossification involves an additional intervening step, the formation of cartilage, before bone is formed.

Intramembranous bone formation is the dominant process in the formation of the calvarium and the clavicle. At genetically determined sites, known as **ossification centres**, the mesenchymal cells proliferate and differentiate into osteoblasts. These secrete the collagen-rich bone matrix or **osteoid**, which becomes mineralized, the result being an island of **woven bone**. These islands enlarge and then fuse to form large sheets.

Most of the fetal skeleton, however, is derived from cartilage, which forms a set of minute scale models of the bones. These tiny cartilage masses grow through the interaction of growth and erosion of cartilage and deposition of bone; these processes are so exquisitely coordinated that the eventual adult bones differ little in shape from the original tiny cartilage models.

These 'models' grow initially by proliferation of cartilage cells (chondrocytes) and an increase in their matrix. In long bones, ossification starts in the midshaft. This is known as the **primary ossification centre**, and it is here in the fibrous capsule of the cartilage (the **perichondrium**) that woven bone is deposited in a sleeve-like fashion. Simultaneously, chondrocytes proliferate, enlarge and eventually die, their matrix becoming calcified. Blood vessels now grow into the centre of the cartilage, some of the mesenchymal cells differentiate into **osteoclasts** and these resorb the cartilage centre, converting it into a hollow cylinder. The deposition of bone matrix is carried out by another differentiation product of the pluripotential mesenchymal cells: the osteoblasts, which also enter the cartilage along with the ingrowing capillaries.

A similar series of events occurs at the ends of long bones (**the secondary ossification centre**). Chondrocytes grow in long columns that have a spiral arrangement. These columns are surrounded by cartilaginous matrix (rich in collagen type II). In due time, the matrix calcifies, some chondrocytes die and invasion by blood vessels and mesenchyme takes place, before deposition of woven bone on the surfaces of the matrix cores. Most of the prepubertal lengthening of bones occurs at the ends of the bones as a result of the growth in a cylinder of cartilage known as the epiphyseal growth plate. Both horizontal and longitudinal growth occur here and account both for the increase in bone length and for the fact that the ends of long bones are characteristically wider than the shafts.

The anatomical regions of a long bone are defined in terms of their relationship to the epiphyseal growth plate. Thus the **epiphysis** is the region of bone that is between the growth plate and the articular cartilage. The **metaphysis** includes that part of the growth plate furthest away from the joint and also the funnel-shaped area that joins the epiphysis to the main shaft or **diaphysis**. The metaphysis is that part of the bone in which most cell proliferation and, thus, most bone lengthening occurs.

DISORDERS OF BONE DEVELOPMENT

The chief disorders of bone growth arise from:
- disorders of the epiphyseal plate
- defects in the structure of the collagenous matrix or in the amount of such matrix secreted

DISORDERS OF THE EPIPHYSEAL PLATE

Achondroplasia

Achondroplasia is one of the commonest causes of **dwarfism**. It may be **familial** with an autosomal dominant inheritance, or **sporadic**, presumably due to a new mutation.

The growth plate is thinned and the zone in which cartilage cells normally proliferate is much shallower than normal.

Intramembranous ossification is unaffected and thus the thickness of bones is normal. The head is disproportionately large with a typical depression of the bridge of nose and a bulging forehead. There is marked shortening of the limbs but the spine is normal in length.

Morquio's Syndrome

This one of the inherited systemic disorders that result from **defective enzymic catabolism of intracellular carbohydrates** (the glycosoaminoglycans). This disorder has an autosomal recessive inheritance and is characterized by the accumulation of **keratan sulphate** within many cell types, including cartilage. The excess keratan sulphate interferes with the function of chondrocytes. Both the spine and the limb bones are affected by the growth retardation. Other clinical features include **dental defects, learning disabilities and corneal opacities**.

OSTEOGENESIS IMPERFECTA

Osteogenesis imperfecta is a set of disorders with *two* shared features:
1) **abnormal fragility of bones**
2) **the presence of a structural defect in the molecule of type I collagen or production of inadequate amounts of normal protein**

Incidence

The frequency of osteogenesis imperfecta is not easily determined because mildly affected individuals may go undetected. The reported incidence, based largely on the occurrence of fractures in the neonatal period, varies from 1 in 20 000 to 1 in 60 000 live births.

Clinical Features

> **KEY POINTS: Findings in Osteogenesis Imperfecta**
>
> The range of clinical abnormalities includes:
> 1) **fragile bones.** This is the dominant clinical expression despite the fact that osteogenesis imperfecta is a **systemic** disorder of connective tissue. The severity of osteogenesis imperfecta is directly correlated with the degree of bone fragility.
> 2) **osteoporosis**
> 3) **hyperextensible joints**
> 4) **blue sclerae.** This may be due to narrower than normal scleral fibres and poor development of Bowman's and Bruch's membranes.
> 5) **abnormalities in tooth formation due to lack of adequate amounts of normal type I collagen in the dentin.** This leads to fractures in the enamel

and exposure of dentin. In due time, the affected tooth may wear down to the gum.

6) **onset of deafness in adult life**. This is more commonly sensory rather than conductive.

These features are summarized in *Fig. 44.1*.

Genetics

Osteogenesis imperfecta is genetically heterogeneous. There may be a large number of genetic abnormalities producing only a limited number of clinical phenotypes. Within each phenotype, considerable variation of the expressivity of the abnormal gene is commonly found.

The bases of the abnormalities occurring in osteogenesis imperfecta are still not understood completely. **For this reason, the classifications used currently are based on the clinical features and, where known, on the inheritance patterns.** (*Table 44.2*). Some cases arise as a result of new mutations and it may be difficult accurately to assign an individual case to the most appropriate category.

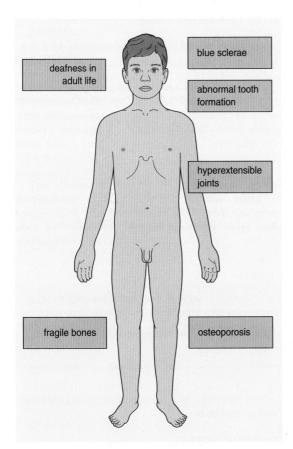

FIGURE 44.1 *Clinical manifestations of osteogenesis imperfecta.*

deafness in adult life

blue sclerae

abnormal tooth formation

hyperextensible joints

fragile bones

osteoporosis

Pathogenesis

The pathogenesis of osteogenesis imperfecta is related to abnormalities in the structure and biosynthesis of type I collagen.

It is now clear that **various mutations in the genes for type I collagen underlie the genesis of osteogenesis imperfecta**. The biosynthesis of collagen involves at least 15 stages from initial gene transcription to the final incorporation of the molecule into the typical cross-linked fibril, and thus there are many possibilities for faults to arise in the system.

There are at least 12 collagen types. In osteogenesis imperfecta, only type I collagen is qualitatively or quantitatively abnormal and thus it is only those tissues in which type I collagen is present in large amounts that are affected in osteogenesis imperfecta. **These are bones, tendons, skin, ligaments, dentin and sclerae.**

The basic unit of the **collagen fibre** is the **microfibril**, which consists of five **collagen molecules** arranged in a three-dimensional cylindrical structure. Each collagen molecule has a 'staggered' relationship to its immediate neighbour and it is this that gives the collagen fibre its periodicity when viewed with the electron microscope.

The collagen molecule itself is composed of three polypeptide chains (α chains) arranged in a tight triple helix. The molecule is a heterotrimer consisting of two identical α_1 chains and a structurally different α_2 chain. **Substitution of any other amino acid for glycine in an amino acid triplet repeated 330 times along the molecule will disrupt the highly ordered structure of collagen. Such mutations form the basis for the more severe forms of osteogenesis imperfecta.** In the case of the much commoner type I, the abnormality is a **decrease in the production of type I collagen** rather than a structural change in the protein molecule.

BONE REMODELLING

NORMAL

Like most other tissues, bone is removed and replaced in an orderly fashion, this process being known as 'bone remodelling'. Some 5–10% of the skeleton is 'turned over' in this way each year.

Bone remodelling is a series of coordinated events (*Table 44.3*) **which involves a group of cells called the basic multicellular unit (BMU).**

The normal adult skeleton contains from 10^5 to 10^6 BMUs, the cellular elements of which are osteoclasts, osteoblasts and some less well characterized mononuclear cells.

The common disorders of bone – osteoporosis, osteomalacia, Paget's disease of bone and hyperparathyroidism – are expressions of deficiencies or excess activity of these processes.

Table 44.2 Classification of Osteogenesis Imperfecta

Type	Frequency (%)	Features
I – Mild, non-deforming	60	Mildest form; fractures unusual before infants start walking and fracture risk declines after puberty Blue sclerae in all cases Some deafness in 70% Dental abnormalities in 25% Inherited as an autosomal dominant disorder
II – Neonatal, lethal	10	Most severe, lethal in most cases Multiple fractures in fetal life; neonates severely deformed with short limbs Rather 'floppy' infants, feed poorly and develop respiratory problems Extracellular matrix lacking in type I collagen and gravely impaired formation of lamellar bone Inherited as an autosomal recessive disorder
III – Severe, non-lethal	20	Fractures present at birth with deformities of long bones Marked growth retardation Severe scoliosis, which may cause respiratory problems and cor pulmonale In familial cases, inheritance shows an autosomal recessive pattern
IV – Moderate, deforming	10	Clinically, spans the gap between mild and severe types Sclerae blue in infancy and then become white Moderate growth retardation Deformities of limbs may be severe enough to require braces Most cases inherited in an autosomal dominant pattern

Table 44.3 Processes Involved in Bone Remodelling

Process	Description
Resorption	Osteoclasts attach to the bone surface and first mobilize the mineral and then digest the organic matrix, usually to a depth of 40–60 µm. Erosion is a function of metalloproteinase secretion and can be inhibited by proteinase inhibitors. Resorption in cortical bone takes the form of tunnels which originate from the haversian canals; in trabecular bone the osteoclast-mediated erosion forms depressions known as Howship's lacunae.
Reversal phase	Cells resembling macrophages modify the resorbed surface and lay down a collagen-poor basophilic layer, which is known as a 'cement line'.
Matrix formation	Osteoblasts now differentiate at the resorption sites and start to deposit organic bone matrix (osteoid), which consists of a mixture of proteins of which type I collagen is the most prominent.
Mineralization	Calcium in the form of hydroxyapatite is deposited in the new matrix and the BMU enters a resting phase.

In early life the processes of resorption and new bone formation are in equilibrium, but after the age of 30–35 years, each remodelling cycle is accompanied by a small nett loss of bone. Thus bone remodelling over a long period of time has significant decremental effects on **bone mass**.

The cells responsible for remodelling are **osteoclasts and osteoblasts**.

OSTEOCLASTS
Osteoclasts are formed by the fusion of precursor cells at the bone surface, which is the target for

resorption. They are derived from granulocyte–macrophage colony-forming units (CFUs) in the bone marrow, and the same cytokines and colony-stimulating factors involved in haematopoiesis are also involved in the development of osteoclasts.

Bone resorption will be increased:

- if more osteoclast precursors differentiate into osteoclasts
- if protease secretion by differentiated osteoclasts is increased

---

KEY POINTS: Factors Causing Upregulation of Osteoclast Differentiation and thus Increased Numbers

- interleukin (IL)-1
- IL-3
- IL-6
- IL-11
- tumour necrosis factor (TNF)
- granulocyte–macrophage colony-stimulating factor (GM-CSF)

Of these, IL-6 is particularly interesting because it synergizes with IL-3 to stimulate the development of the granulocyte–macrophage CFU in the bone marrow and, by itself, also stimulates bone resorption and osteoclast formation. IL-6 is produced by osteoblasts and marrow stromal cells, this production being stimulated by a number of factors known to promote bone resorption, including parathyroid hormone (PTH), parathyroid hormone-related peptide (PTHRP), IL-1 and TNF.

KEY POINTS: Factors Downregulating Osteoclast Activity

- calcitonin
- prostaglandins (with the exception of those of the E series)
- tissue inhibitors of metalloproteinases (TIMPs)

KEY POINTS: Factors Upregulating Osteoclast Activity

- IL-1
- TNF-α
- parathyroid hormone (via messages secreted by osteoblasts)
- interferon γ
- IL-6
- TNF-β

OSTEOBLASTS

Osteoblasts are primarily responsible for bone matrix formation. They cannot undergo mitotic division; thus any local increase in osteoblasts represents increased mitosis at a precursor cell stage. They are derived from a stem cell common to chondroblasts, fibroblasts and adipose tissue cells. Once new bone is laid down, some of the osteoblasts lose their ability to form bone and become incorporated into the new bone as osteocytes.

In addition to their role in the synthesis of new bone matrix, osteoblasts elaborate short-range chemical messages that mediate the responses of the osteoclast to bone-resorbing agents, such as PTH, and also secrete other substances that play a part in bone remodelling.

Growth Factors in Bone

There is clear evidence for the existence of chemical messengers that regulate bone growth. Most of such data have been derived from cell culture studies, and it is uncertain as to how far they should be extrapolated to the *in vivo* situation. A discussion of these factors is beyond the scope of this text.

DISORDERS OF BONE REMODELLING

The four most commonly encountered systemic bone disorders in which some disturbance of remodelling occurs are listed in *Table 44.4* (see also *Fig. 44.2*).

KEY POINTS: Morphological Criteria

Four simple morphological criteria enable one to understand and recall the pathological changes in these disorders. These are:

- **bone mass**
- **degree of mineralization of the osteoid matrix**
- **degree of osteoclast-mediated resorption of bone**
- **preservation or loss of normal lamellar architecture**

Table 44.4 Disorders of Bone Remodelling

Disorder	Processes involved
Osteoporosis	Excess osteoclastic resorption
	Deficient osteoblast matrix formation
	Both of these
Osteomalacia or rickets	Deficient mineralization
Paget's disease of bone	Excess osteoclastic resorption
	Excess new matrix formation
	Loss of normal lamellar architecture
Hyperparathyroidism	Excess osteoclastic resorption

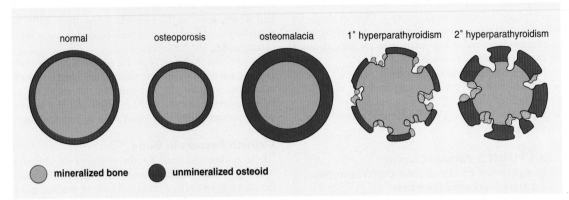

FIGURE 44.2 Important disorders of bone remodelling. These disorders can be delineated by considering the cardinal criteria of bone mass, the amount of unmineralized osteoid matrix and the degree of osteoclastic resorption.

Osteoporosis

● **Characterized by a decrease in bone mass**

Osteoporosis may be defined as a disorder in which there is an absolute decline in the bone mass sufficient to lead to fractures occurring as a result of minimal trauma.

Osteoporosis is common and dangerous. The sites of predilection for osteoporosis-related fractures are shown in *Table 44.5.*

One woman in three over the age of 65 years will have a vertebral fracture, and by extreme old age one in three women and one in six men will have had a hip fracture. Some 12–20% of such hip fractures will prove fatal and half the survivors will need long-term nursing home care. The economic consequences of osteoporosis, therefore, are staggeringly high. In the UK, 150 000 osteoporosis-related fractures occur annually at a cost, in money terms alone, of £742 million.

In young people, bone loss and bone formation are normally tightly coupled in the course of each remodelling cycle. **Bone loss implies an uncoupling of these phases of remodelling** either because of an **excessive amount of osteoclastic resorption or an impairment of osteoblast-mediated bone formation, or both of these processes** (*Fig. 44.3*).

Aetiology

The two main aetiological factors in the majority of cases of osteoporosis are **increasing age** and **the female menopause**.

Age-related Bone Loss (Type II or Senile Osteoporosis)

In osteoporosis there appears to be a **two-phase pattern of bone loss.** The first is a **slow phase which affects both sexes and which appears to correlate best with increasing age**. At about the age of 30 years a loss of trabecular bone starts, cortical bone mass not being affected until after the age of 40 years. In women, about 50% of the trabecular and 35% of the cortical bone is lost over a lifetime, whereas men lose about two-thirds as much as women. Trabecular bone is found in the largest amounts in the vertebral bodies, pelvis and other flat bones, and cortical bone occurs in the greatest amounts in the long bones.

The functional defect in the slow-phase, age-related loss of bone is an impairment of bone formation, with a failure to fill the normal-sized resorption cavities with new bone.

Menopause-related Bone Loss (Type I Osteoporosis)

The second phase is **an accelerated one which has its onset in women after the menopause and which lasts for about 8–10 years**. In respect of cortical bone, the advent of the menopause in females involves an extra loss of 2–3% per year, decreasing to the same rate as the slow phase after 8–10 years. The rate of loss of trabecular bone in the postmenopausal phase is greater initially than that of cortical bone but is of shorter duration. **The post-menopausal bone loss is associated with an increased rate of bone turnover. Osteoclasts are present in greater numbers than normal and the resorption cavities they form are similarly deeper than normal.**

Table 44.5 Sites of Osteoporosis-related Fractures

Site	Frequency (%)
Vertebrae	44.8
Hip	18.9
Colles' fracture	14.3
Other limb bones	23.6

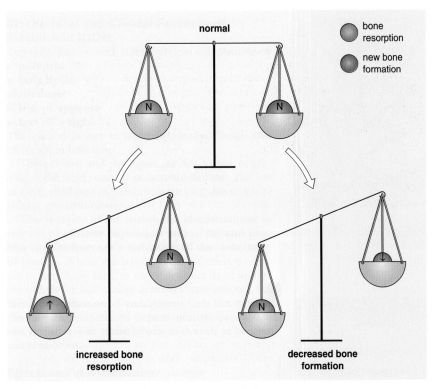

FIGURE 44.3 *The basic pathogenetic model implicated in osteoporosis is uncoupling of the normal dynamic equilibrium between bone formation and bone resorption that occurs in each remodelling cycle. Such uncoupling can be the expression of either increased bone resorption (as seen in the postmenopausal state) or decreased bone formation.*

Fractures in Osteoporosis

The anatomical and age patterns of osteoporotic fractures reflect the timing and rate of bone loss. The menopause is associated with fractures of the vertebral bodies and of the distal radius (Colles' fracture). These vertebral fractures are usually of the 'crush' variety and cause considerable pain. In old patients, vertebral fractures are more commonly of the 'wedge' variety and cause deformities such as the familiar 'dowager's hump' (kyphosis of the dorsal vertebrae). Vertebral fractures go on increasing after the age of 65 years, whereas Colles' fracture frequency appears to plateau at this age. Hip fractures, on the other hand, increase slowly in frequency until late in life, and then increase exponentially.

These epidemiological data suggest that **there are at least two distinct syndromes of osteoporosis** (not related to the presence of other disorders, drugs etc.). These are type I and type II osteoporosis.

Type I Osteoporosis In this type of osteoporosis, fractures occur characteristically 15–20 years after the onset of the female menopause. In addition to fractures involving sites where trabecular bone predominates, tooth loss may also occur. The rate of trabecular bone loss is three times normal while cortical bone loss is only slightly above normal. Osteoclastic resorption may

be so active that perforation of some trabecula takes place and this may be followed by cessation of new bone formation in the affected trabecula. Iliac crest biopsies in such patients show much widened intratrabecular spaces due to disappearance of some of these perforated trabecula (*Fig. 44.4*).

The relationship of the menopause to this type of osteoporosis is exemplified in women who have had a bilateral oöphorectomy in the premenopausal period. They have lower bone density in later life than controls; oestrogen therapy slows the rate of this bone loss. Most of our knowledge of the effect of oestrogen on bone cells is derived from studies with cultured cells and may be summed up as shown in the box.

KEY POINTS: Effects of Oestrogen Loss on Bone

- Oestrogen loss causes a **decrease in the secretion of transforming growth factor (TGF) β by osteoblast-like cells in culture**. TGF-β is a potent stimulator of proliferation of osteoblast precursor cells and also promotes the deposition of the protein matrix of bone.
- Oestrogen loss results in an increase in IL-6-mediated **osteoclast** differentiation.

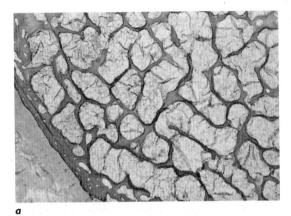
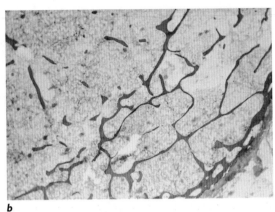

a   b

FIGURE 44.4 **a** and **b** These two sections of biopsies from the iliac crest compare the appearances seen in normal and osteoporotic bone in two age-matched individuals. In **b** (derived from osteoporotic bone) the trabecula are both scantier and smaller than those seen in normal bone (**a**).

- Oestrogen loss causes an increase in synthesis and secretion of lysosomal enzymes by cultured osteoclasts.

IL-6 production is normally restrained by oestrogen via an oestrogen receptor-mediated effect on the transcriptional activity of the IL-6 promoter.

In contrast, the osteoporosis associated with ageing in both sexes is believed to be due to an **impaired ability of the bone marrow to produce osteoblast precursors**.

Type II ('Senile') Osteoporosis This usually affects individuals who are older than 70 years. The female : male ratio is 2 : 1, in contrast with type I where it is 6 : 1. This persisting female preponderance in type II osteoporosis is probably due in part to the residual effects of the menopause occurring many years before, and in part to the fact that **women have a lower peak bone mass than men**.

The chief clinical expressions are hip and vertebral fractures, although fractures of other bones are quite common as well. Bone biopsies from the iliac crest show thinning of the individual trabecula, although the trabecular perforation occurring in type I osteoporosis is not seen.

Other Factors Affecting the Occurrence and Severity of Osteoporosis

Initial Bone Density
There is a threshold of bone mineral density below which fracture risk increases sharply. Given two individuals in whom the **rate of bone loss is equal**, it is clear that **the one in whom the initial bone mass was less is more likely to suffer from osteoporosis-related fractures in later life**. The observed influence of race, sex and heredity on osteoporosis can be explained, at least in part, on this basis. **The bone density achieved in early adult life is a major determinant of the risk of osteoporotic fracture.** Several common allelic variants exist for the gene encoding the vitamin D receptor. The presence or absence of certain variants appears to predict quite well for peak bone density in early adult life.

Osteoblast Function
From the fourth decade onwards, there is a steady uncoupling of bone remodelling in the sense that less new bone is formed than is resorbed. The osteoblasts function normally in response to local stimuli so that fracture healing does not seem to be impaired with ageing, and it has been suggested therefore that the deficiency in bone growth seen in senile osteoporosis may instead reflect deficiencies in factors that stimulate osteoblasts.

Calcium Absorption
Calcium absorption declines with ageing, and is most marked over the age of 70 years. This may reflect lowered calcitriol concentration, which declines by about 50% with ageing. The ageing kidney is less effective in 1α-hydroxylation of 25-hydroxycholecalciferol and the normal rise in 1,25-dihydroxycholecalciferol which occurs following infusion of parathyroid hormone is blunted in elderly humans. The recommended daily allowance for calcium is currently 800 mg but it is known that most middle-aged and elderly women consume only about 550 mg/day. Some trials have shown that dietary calcium supplements slow bone loss. The beneficial effect, however, is less than can be achieved by treatment with oestrogen.

Calcitonin
Calcitonin powerfully inhibits the resorptive function of osteoclasts and several groups have shown that, at all

ages, **women have lower plasma concentrations of immunoreactive calcitonin than men**.

Obesity

This appears to protect against bone loss, presumably by increasing skeletal loading stress.

Exercise and Bone Loss

Skeletal stresses occurring as a result of both weight bearing and muscle contraction stimulate osteoblastic activity and there is a direct positive correlation between muscle mass and bone mass.

Cigarette Smoking and Heavy Consumption of Alcohol

Both appear to act as risk factors for the development of osteoporosis.

Secondary Osteoporosis

Osteoporosis occurs as a secondary phenomenon in the context of certain disorders or as a result of administration of certain drugs or treatments. The most common associations are:

- early oöphorectomy
- male hypogonadism
- hyperthyroidism
- Cushing's syndrome
- subtotal gastrectomy
- chronic obstructive airflow disease
- treatment with glucocorticoids
- treatment with certain anticonvulsants
- disuse, such as occurs in hemiplegia and paraplegia

Osteomalacia

- **Characterized by defective mineralization of osteoid matrix**

Osteomalacia is the common endpoint of several metabolic abnormalities which result in the slowing down or actual stoppage of mineralization of newly formed organic bone matrix or osteoid. It is characterized, therefore, by **an increased amount of unmineralized osteoid tissue in relation to what is seen in bone samples from healthy age-matched controls**. The homologue of osteomalacia in children is rickets, in which there is also a disturbance in the endochondral ossification responsible for the growth of long bones.

The failure to fill resorption cavities with normally mineralized bone involves:

- **a reduction in the mineralization of newly formed osteoid matrix**
- **a slowing down in the actual deposition by the osteoblasts of osteoid**

Of these two processes, the first is always the dominant one.

Unmineralized Osteoid

The presence of some unmineralized osteoid in relation to trabecular bone is not abnormal.

Unmineralized osteoid is a normal component of healthy bone and as much as 15% of the trabecular surface area may be covered by osteoid. After resorption, it takes about 3 months for the lost bone to be replaced by new bone matrix, as osteoblasts deposit new osteoid lamellae at a mean rate of a little less than 1 μm per day. Mineralization lags behind osteoid formation by about 10 days. The mineralization occurs in a band at the interface between previously mineralized bone and the osteoid seam – **the mineralization front**. In normal bone the linked sequence of osteoid deposition and mineralization continues, so that the width of the unmineralized seam of osteoid remains constant as the amount of new bone laid down increases. In osteomalacia this normal coupling is lost so that osteoid volume and seam width must increase. In normal bone all osteoid is eventually mineralized; in early osteomalacia some remains unmineralized; and in severe long-standing osteomalacia little or none of the deposited osteoid becomes mineralized.

> **KEY POINTS: Biochemical Disturbances Producing Osteomalacia**
> There are three biochemical contexts in which osteomalacia or rickets occur:
>   1) hypocalcaemia
>   2) hypophosphataemia
>   3) local disturbances in bone mineralization (such as hypophosphatasia)

Hypocalcaemic Osteomalacia

Role of Vitamin D

Vitamin D is one of the main endocrine signals involved in calcium homoeostasis (in which its effect on calcium absorption from the gut plays a major part) and the control of bone growth. Together with PTH, vitamin D is also involved in the regulation of inorganic phosphorus metabolism. The causes of hypocalcaemic osteomalacia and rickets can best be understood and recalled against the background of the synthesis and metabolism of Vitamin D (*Fig. 44.5*).

Synthesis in the Skin

More than 90% of circulating vitamin D is derived from the interaction between ultraviolet light derived from the sun and a steroid molecule, **7-dehydrocholesterol**, in the epidermis. This reaction yields pre-vitamin D_3, which isomerizes to vitamin D_3 at body temperature. **The amount of ultraviolet radiation within the epidermal cells is likely to be less in people living in northern latitudes or who, like the elderly and infirm, are housebound or institutionalized; similarly, dark skin pigmentation also lessens vitamin D_3 formation in the skin. Thus, it is not surprising that people who fall**

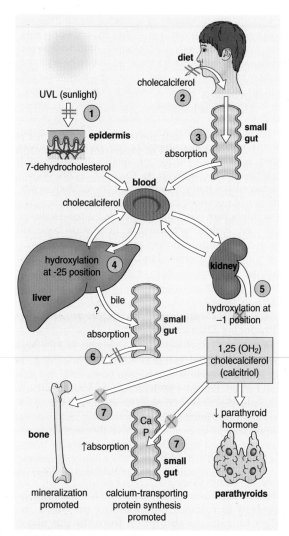

FIGURE 44.5 Steps involved in the synthesis, activation, metabolism and action of vitamin D. The causes of osteomalacia can be understood most easily against this physiological background, as defects may occur in any of the steps outlined.

into one or more of these categories form a substantial fraction of those with osteomalacia and rickets.

Dietary Vitamin D

The role of dietary intake is a secondary one, and relatively small amounts of vitamin D are derived from the normal adult diet. It must be said, however, that the introduction of dried milk and infant foods fortified with vitamin D during the Second World War virtually eradicated infantile rickets from the UK.

Rickets and osteomalacia do occur in people whose exposure to sunshine is adequate and in these the diet seems to play an important part. **A high-risk diet in**

relation to rickets and osteomalacia is one that is rich in high extraction cereals (with a high fibre content) and poor in meat, fish and dairy products. One view of this is that there is an enterohepatic circulation for vitamin D, with some of the vitamin D from the blood appearing in the bile and then being reabsorbed from the gut lumen. Fibre proteins such as lignin bind bile acids and increase their faecal excretion and, thus, the faecal loss of vitamin D.

Absorption and/or Loss of Vitamin D from the Small Gut

Any disorder associated with malabsorption and steatorrhoea, such as coeliac disease, interferes with the absorption of vitamin D (which is fat soluble) and is liable to be complicated by osteomalacia. Osteomalacia is not the only, or even the most common, metabolic bone disorder to occur in malabsorption, many such patients presenting instead with osteoporosis.

Hydroxylation of Vitamin D in the Liver

Vitamin D synthesized in the skin is transported in association with a specific vitamin D-binding protein, whereas vitamin D absorbed from the proximal part of the small gut is transported within chylomicrons. Newly synthesized vitamin D has no biological activity and further metabolic steps are needed for activation. The first of these is hydroxylation at the 25 position, carried out in the liver cells. The liver is also involved in the enterohepatic circulation of 25-hydroxycholecalciferol, mentioned in a preceding section. **Chronic liver diseases of different types, such as alcoholic liver disease and primary biliary cirrhosis, have been reported as being complicated by osteomalacia, but this is not common. Indeed, as in the case of small gut malabsorption syndromes, osteoporosis is more commonly seen in patients with chronic liver disease.**

An association has been reported between prolonged treatment with anticonvulsant drugs, such as phenytoin and phenobarbitone, and osteomalacia. Such treatment may be associated with subnormal plasma concentrations of vitamin D and with decreased serum calcium levels. This has been ascribed to induction by the drugs of enzymes that promote biliary excretion of vitamin D metabolites.

Hydroxylation at the 1α Position

25-Hydroxycholecalciferol undergoes further hydroxylation at the 1α position. **The resulting compound is calcitriol (1,25-dihydroxycholecalciferol), the most active form of vitamin D.** Normally, hydroxylation takes place almost exclusively in the mitochondria of proximal renal tubule epithelium, the hydroxylase activity being modulated in two ways:

1) **by PTH**, the release of which is controlled by plasma calcium concentrations and circulating levels of calcitriol

2) **by the plasma phosphate concentration**, a decrease in this being followed by an increase in the activity of renal 1α-hydroxylase

Hydroxylation at the 1 position can also occur extra-renally. Cells and tissues showing this activity include:

- placenta
- osteoblasts
- keratinocytes
- normal macrophages after activation with interferon γ
- activated macrophages in granulomas such as in sarcoidosis, in which hypercalcaemia, particularly after exposure to sunshine, is a well-recognized complication.

The kidney is also a major source of an alternative form of the vitamin D molecule, 24,25-dihydroxycholecalciferol. The activity of the 24-hydroxylase is controlled by the plasma concentrations of calcium and inorganic phosphorus, higher levels of these being associated with production of 24,25-vitamin D rather than the 1,25-hydroxylated molecule. 24,25-vitamin D is eight times less effective than the 1,25-hydroxylated molecule in promoting calcium absorption from the gut lumen.

In view of the importance of hydroxylation of vitamin D at the 1 position, it is not surprising that a number of chronic renal disorders in which nephron loss occurs, show progressive bone disease, the pathological picture of which tends to be dominated by the effects of secondary hyperparathyroidism, although a marked increase in unmineralized osteoid is often present as well. This condition is known as **renal osteodystrophy**. Some 54% of patients with chronic renal failure show bone changes of hyperparathyroidism alone and 34% have a combination of osteomalacia and hyperparathyroid bone disease. Osteomalacia may also occur in association with the Fanconi syndrome (a set of disorders characterized by multiple disturbances in renal tubule function). Causes of the Fanconi syndrome include several inherited disorders but it may also occur in association with **light chain nephropathy in patients with myelomatosis, and as a result of heavy metal poisoning**.

Biological Effects of Vitamin D Metabolites

Calcitriol is secreted from the kidney and is transported to its targets in association with vitamin D-binding protein. **Its principal actions are to promote the transport of calcium from the gut lumen into the blood and to promote bone growth and mineralization.** The principal cellular targets are, thus, the small intestinal mucosal epithelium and the osteoblasts. Calcitriol receptors are present in a wide variety of other cell types including parathyroid, pancreas, pituitary, ovary, thymus, brain, skin, lymphoid cells and

bone marrow. Calcitriol has a role outside calcium transport in the gut and bone mineralization, and influences growth and differentiation of both normal and tumour cells.

In the case of the small gut, calcitriol binds to a specific receptor within mucosal cells and the sterol–receptor complex acts by initiating transcription of a gene encoding a calcium-transporting protein.

In bone, the effects of calcitriol *in vivo* are to promote bone growth and mineralization. **The successful operation of this part of the chain of vitamin D metabolism depends on successful ligand–receptor binding. There is a rare form of inherited vitamin D resistance (known as vitamin D-dependent rickets type II) in which normal or even greater than normal concentrations of calcitriol are present but are ineffective because of end-organ resistance. There is no remission if physiological doses of vitamin D are given.**

Hypophosphataemic Osteomalacia

Hypophosphataemia is the second most important biochemical cause of osteomalacia or rickets, although it is much less common than vitamin D deficiency. Patients with this variant of defective mineralization show two cardinal features:

1) sustained **low concentrations of serum phosphate**

2) relative **resistance to treatment with vitamin D**

X-Linked Hypophosphataemic Rickets

This is the commonest form of osteomalacia in patients with adequate calcitriol levels. It is one of the very few forms of X-linked disease that has a dominant inheritance pattern and is related to the presence of a mutant gene located on the short arm of the X chromosome. Unlike what is seen in hypocalcaemic rickets, the disease develops in well-nourished and healthy-looking children whose growth rate is initially normal and begins to slow only when weight bearing starts.

The hypophosphataemia is due to excessive loss of phosphate by the kidney. It reflects a specific abnormality of phosphate transport by the tubular epithelium.

Hereditary Hypophosphataemic Rickets with Hypercalciuria

A small number of children present with hypophosphataemic rickets associated with a severe loss of calcium in the urine. The hypercalciuria appears to be related to increased intestinal absorption of calcium because it disappears after 15 hours of fasting. The mechanism of the renal phosphate loss is unknown.

Tumour-associated Osteomalacia

Severe hypophosphataemic osteomalacia or rickets may be caused by certain mesenchymal

neoplasms. Resection is followed by a dramatic clinical and biochemical improvement. The disorder, which occurs equally in males and females, is commonest in adults aged over 30 years. Most of the tumours originate in bone or soft tissues, and many are vascular neoplasms with an architectural pattern described as haemangiopericytomatous.

Both serum phosphate and vitamin D levels are low. These biochemical changes appear to be due to some secretion product of the tumours, which causes increased urinary loss of phosphate and also appears to inhibit hydroxylation of vitamin D at the 1 position.

Clinical Features

> **KEY POINTS: The Osteomalacia Syndrome**
> The cardinal features of osteomalacia are:
> - bone pain
> - bone tenderness
> - muscle weakness in about 40% of patients

Severe bone deformities such as limb curvature, coxa vara and contracted pelvis may occur in adults but are now rarely seen except in countries where there is an endemic vitamin D deficiency operating from childhood to adult life.

In rickets, there is a marked disturbance of endochondral ossification in addition to failure of mineralization of osteoid. The bones chiefly affected are those that grow rapidly during childhood. **In the first year of life these are the cranium, wrists and ribs**, and rickets at this time therefore leads to:
- widening of cranial sutures
- frontal bossing
- posterior flattening of the skull
- bulging of the costochondral junctions (known as a 'rickety rosary')
- enlargement of the wrists

After the first year of life, the deformities affect chiefly those bones that both grow rapidly and bear weight, and thus the legs are most severely affected. The deformities are due to pressure on weakened growth plates and the effect of weight bearing on shafts of severely affected long bones. If not treated, lasting deformities may dog the patient into adult life. Muscle weakness may be found both in osteomalacia and rickets, and in infants the resulting muscle hypotonia may cause a lax and protuberant abdomen. In some patients the muscle weakness may dominate the clinical picture and the patients may be severely disabled. As yet, its mechanism is not understood.

Radiological Findings

Radiological findings in osteomalacia are usually much less pronounced than in rickets. Generalized osteopenia (reduction in bone density) is commonly present but the most characteristic feature is the **Looser's zone** or

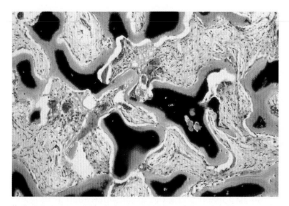

FIGURE 44.6 *Section of bone from a patient with osteomalacia. The section has been stained with a silver salt which shows mineralized bone as black; the unmineralized osteoid matrix stains pink. This pink osteoid is much thicker than normal and covers a greater area of the trabecular surfaces than normal.*

pseudofracture. The commonest sites for these are the medial edges of the shafts of long bones. They are linear areas of increased radiolucency roughly at right angles to the long axis of affected bones.

In advanced rickets, the classical finding is widening of the ends of the metaphyses; the usually straight transverse margin of the metaphysis becomes concave and cup-like.

> ### Microscopic Features
> The characteristic histological feature of osteomalacia is **an increase in the amount of osteoid** (*Fig. 44.6*), measured in terms of:
> a) **the osteoid volume**, expressed as the percentage area of the total trabecular bone
> b) **the osteoid seam width**, which can be measured in relation to all trabecula. In sections examined in polarized light, collagen lamellae of the unmineralized osteoid show up because of their birefringence. An osteoid seam with more than three or four such lamellae is regarded as being abnormal
> c) **the osteoid surface**, expressed as the fraction of the total perimeter length of all the trabecula in a section that is covered by osteoid
> Indices of mineralization are gained by examining biopsies from patients who have had time-spaced doses of tetracycline, which is deposited at the mineralization fronts. The site of deposition of the tetracycline can be seen by examining the sections in ultraviolet light as the tetracycline is fluorescent. The partial or complete absence of a tetracycline label along the interface between calcified bone and osteoid indicates a defect in mineralization.
>
> **Low serum levels of active vitamin D and calcium stimulate the production of PTH**, and this sec-

ondary hyperparathyroidism leads to increased osteoclastic resorption in order to release calcium from the storage pool in bone. Thus, depending on the duration and severity of the process in such cases of osteomalacia, the histological features of hyperparathyroidism will be added to the increase in unmineralized osteoid already described. **This is particularly evident in cases of renal osteodystrophy.** In pure hypophosphataemic states, on the other hand, because the serum calcium is usually normal there will be *no* secondary hyperparathyroidism and the histological picture will reflect only the mineralization failure.

In children with rickets, the regions of endochondral ossification are severely affected. The growth plate is widened due to disarray of normally regular columns of cartilage cells; the columns themselves are much longer than normal. The zone of provisional calcification disappears and thus the orderly progression of cartilage to primary spongiosa of bone does not occur. Instead, large irregular projections of unmineralized cartilage are seen deeply situated within the metaphysis. Such changes cannot, of course, occur after the epiphyses have fused following cessation of endochondral ossification.

Hypophosphatasia

This very rare condition, believed to be inherited in an autosomal dominant fashion, usually presents in early childhood with defective bone mineralization. Because the defect is an inability to mineralize either bone or growth cartilage at the metaphyses, the histological appearances are identical with those of rickets, although there is *no* decline in serum concentrations of calcitriol and, thus, histological features due to secondary hyperparathyroidism are not seen. Serum alkaline phosphatase levels are usually depressed and there is often a concomitant increase in urinary phosphoethanolamine levels.

Hyperparathyroidism

- **Characterized by excessive osteoclastic resorption of bone**

This set of disorders is best understood against a background of the secretion and action of PTH.

PTH is the most important regulator of calcium concentration in the blood and extracellular fluid. Its secretion is upregulated by low plasma calcium levels. It increases plasma calcium concentration via **three main targets**:

1) **The kidney, in which reabsorption of calcium in the proximal and distal tubules is increased** and phosphate reabsorption in the proximal tubule is decreased. In addition PTH upregulates 1α hydroxylation, thus increasing calcitriol concentrations.

2) **The skeleton, in which bone resorption is increased.** PTH causes recruitment of osteoclast precursors and activation of resident osteoclasts. The current view is that this effect is mediated by the PTH binding to osteoblasts, which release osteoclast-stimulating products.

3) **The small gut, in which calcium absorption is increased.** This is mediated indirectly through the PTH-stimulated increase in plasma calcitriol levels described above.

Regulators of PTH Secretion

The chief determinant of PTH secretion is the plasma calcium concentration, which seems to act predominantly on **secretion** rather than on synthesis. Small changes in the calcium concentration of the extracellular fluid are reflected rapidly within the cytosol of the parathyroid cells, and the release of PTH is inversely proportional to this cytosolic calcium concentration. High extracellular fluid calcium levels not only inhibit PTH secretion but promote cleavage of intact hormone to inactive fragments within the parathyroid glands.

Phosphate concentrations can also cause an increase in PTH secretion by lowering plasma ionized calcium concentrations, although phosphate concentrations may have some direct effect as well.

Calcitriol concentrations also affect PTH secretion, apparently by influencing the messenger RNA levels of prepro-PTH within the cells, which fall as the calcitriol levels rise.

PTH is coded for by a gene on the short arm of chromosome 11 and the amino-terminal fragment is responsible for its biological activity, some of the immunoreactive hormone in human blood being the inert carboxy-terminal.

Hyperparathyroidism is classified as being **primary, secondary (to chronic hypocalcaemia) and tertiary**.

Primary Hyperparathyroidism

Primary hyperparathyroidism may be defined as hypersecretion of PTH outside the control of normal negative feedback mechanisms. It is relatively common, particularly in elderly women. It occurs in three pathological contexts:

1) **In the presence of a benign functioning tumour (adenoma), the responsible lesion in about 80% of cases.** The vast majority are single; cases in which multiple adenomas are diagnosed are probably examples of nodular hyperplasia.

Adenomas are not always easily distinguishable from focal nodular hyperplasia, although the cells in adenomas are monoclonal and those in hyperplasia are polyclonal.

Adenomas usually weigh between 0.5 and 5.0 g (normal gland 25–50 mg) and are commonest in the inferior glands. In a small minority, the adenoma is located ectopically in the thymus, thyroid or mediastinum.

The aetiological factors involved are unknown, although there are weak associations with previous irradiation of the neck, with hyperthyroidism and with the administration of lithium for depression.

2) **In the presence of diffuse chief cell hyperplasia, which is responsible for about 15% of cases**

3) **In the presence of a malignant functioning neoplasm (carcinoma).** This is distinctly rare, accounting for 0.5–4% of cases.

Both adenoma and, more particularly, hyperplasia may occur as part of the **multiple endocrine neoplasia (MEN) syndrome**, most commonly with type I and rather uncommonly with type II.

Type I is associated with pancreatic adenomas and pituitary adenomas; type II is associated with phaeochromocytoma, medullary carcinoma of the thyroid and, sometimes, mucosal neuromas. Recently, a growth factor, apparently related to the fibroblast growth factor family, which stimulates mitosis of parathyroid cells in culture has been identified in the serum of some patients with

MEN I. Curiously enough, the target cell for this growth factor is the parathyroid endothelial cell. Fibroblast growth factor is the gene product of the proto-oncogene *int-2*, and the mutant gene in MEN I is localized to the pericentric region of chromosome 11, which is very near *int-2*.

Clinical Features

Clinical features of primary hyperparathyroidism are shown in *Table 44.6* and *Fig.44.7*.

The classical descriptions of primary hyperparathyroidism are of **a syndrome mediated by prolonged osteoclastic resorption of bone and hypercalcaemia and summed up as: 'bones, stones, abdominal groans and psychic moans'.**

Most patients with hypercalcaemia due to primary hyperparathyroidism are asymptomatic at the time of diagnosis. This is due to the use of multichannel analysers in clinical chemistry and consequent screening of serum calcium levels.

With the exception of bone disease, all the clinical features are the result of hypercalcaemia, although it is

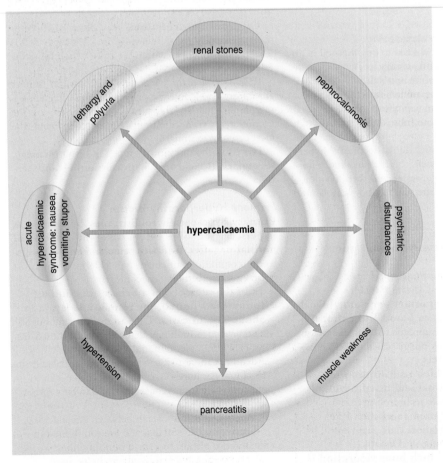

FIGURE 44.7 Clinical effects of hypercalcaemia.

Table 44.6 Clinical Features of Primary Hyperparathyroidism

Finding	Frequency (%)
No symptoms	57
Acute hypercalcaemia syndrome. Here there is a sudden steep rise in serum calcium concentration and a rapid deterioration in renal function. Nausea, vomiting, drowsiness and stupor are common.	14
Lethargy, polyuria, etc.	8
Renal (stones or nephrocalcinosis)	7
Psychiatric disturbance	5
Hypertension	5
Gastrointestinal symptoms	4
Bone disease	0

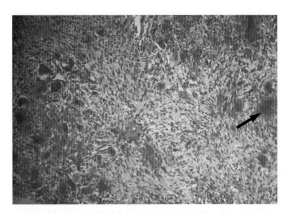

FIGURE 44.8 Section from a so-called 'brown tumour' in a patient with primary hyperparathyroidism. No bony trabecula can be seen in this field, which is composed of spindle cells and numerous multinucleated osteoclasts (arrowed).

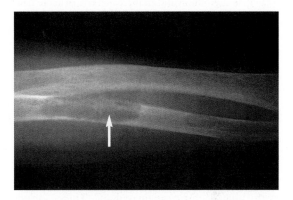

FIGURE 44.9 Radiograph of an arm, showing the lesion depicted in Fig. 44.8. Note the large area of radiolucency in the ulna (arrowed).

not always easy to understand the pathogenetic relationship between raised serum calcium levels and the clinical disturbance.

Bone Changes

As stated above, symptoms related to bone disease are rare in primary hyperfunction of the parathyroids, but, if present, take the form of bone pain and, occasionally, pathological fracture.

Microscopic Features

On histological examination of biopsy material the most prominent feature is an obvious **increase in osteoclastic resorption of bone**. The normally smooth outline of the bony trabecula shows deep jagged indentations, filled with well-vascularized connective tissue. Where diagnosis is made very late, severe bone changes, described by von Recklinghausen under the name **'osteitis fibrosa cystica'**, may occur. Rather like the Holy Roman Empire, which was neither Roman nor an empire and certainly not holy, osteitis fibrosa cystica is neither inflammatory nor cystic. The lesions, which have also been misnamed 'brown tumours', consist of areas in which trabecular bone has been completely eroded away, being replaced by vascular fibrous tissue in which many osteoclasts can be seen (*Fig. 44.8*). On radiography, such lesions are seen as rounded, well-defined areas of increased radiolucency (*Fig. 44.9*). In less severe bone disease, the classical radiological feature is subperiosteal resorption, which most typically affects the radial surfaces of the middle phalanges of the second and third fingers.

Renal Complications

The major effects of hypercalcaemia on the kidney are:
- **the formation of calcium-containing renal calculi**
- **nephrocalcinosis**
- **changes in renal tubular function**

As diagnosis is now made earlier, stone formation is a much less frequent occurrence in primary hyperparathyroidism than previously. About 5–10% of patients with recurrent calcium-containing renal calculi have primary hyperparathyroidism.

Nephrocalcinosis is rather rare and occurs in patients with long-standing disease. It is due to the precipitation of calcium and phosphate in the renal tubular epithelium.

A number of functional changes in the renal tubules may also be seen. These include:
1) **metabolic renal acidosis due to the impairment of bicarbonate reabsorption**

caused by excess PTH. This bicarbonate wasting leads to hyperchloraemic acidosis.
2) phosphaturia, aminoaciduria and glycosuria in some patients
3) a failure to concentrate urine. This is believed to be due to an impairment in the capacity of antidiuretic hormone to cause water reabsorption in the collecting tubules.

Gastrointestinal Complications

Peptic Ulcer Some studies have reported that 10–20% of patients with primary hyperparathyroidism have peptic ulcers, but this is not universally accepted. Hypercalcaemia causes an increase in gastrin secretion and thus a resulting increase in basal gastric acid secretion.

Pancreatitis A clear association exists between primary hyperparathyroidism and an increased risk of acute pancreatitis, the degree of risk is positively correlated with the serum calcium concentration. The responsible mechanism is still unknown.

Neural and Muscle Disorders

Weakness associated with atrophy of proximal muscle groups, especially in the lower limbs, may occur in hyperparathyroidism. It is associated with pathological features resembling those seen in denervated groups of muscle fibres.

Psychiatric Changes

Many psychiatric symptoms are described in patients with primary hyperparathyroidism. These include depression, memory impairment and emotional lability. They are due to hypercalcaemia and occur in patients with hypercalcaemia from other causes.

Other complications, less frequently seen, include skin necrosis associated with precipitation of both calcium and phosphorus in the dermal and subcutaneous tissues, and 'band keratopathy', the deposition of calcium and phosphorus in the cornea.

Secondary Hyperparathyroidism

- Characterized histologically by excess osteoclastic resorption of bone and defective mineralization of osteoid matrix

Secondary hyperparathyroidism is the result of chronic hypocalcaemia. Initially the feedback of low serum calcium concentration leads to an increase in PTH secretion without any morphological change, but in due time parathyroid hyperplasia supervenes.

It occurs in patients suffering from chronic renal failure, small gut diseases associated with defective calcium absorption and inborn disorders of vitamin D metabolism. Clearly **hypercalcaemia, which is a cardinal feature of primary hyperparathyroidism, is not**

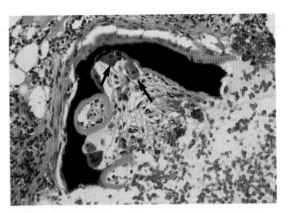

FIGURE 44.10 *Bone in secondary hyperparathyroidism. The bony trabeculum, which occupies the centre of the field, shows irregularities in its outline as a result of excess resorption by osteoclasts (arrowed). There is a definite margin of pink-staining osteoid in this trabeculum, suggesting that a degree of osteomalacia is also present. The section was derived from a patient in chronic renal failure.*

present in the secondary form, and the chief expression of PTH oversecretion is bone disease. Because of the initiating hypocalcaemia, the histological picture also shows the features of osteomalacia (*Fig. 44.10*).

Tertiary Hyperparathyroidism

In patients with long-continued secondary hyperparathyroidism due to chronic hypocalcaemia, hypercalcaemia occasionally occurs. This was originally ascribed to the development of 'autonomous' adenomas in a hyperplastic parathyroid, but this is no longer a generally held view and many doubt the existence of tertiary disease.

Hypercalcaemia

Hypercalcaemia causes considerable morbidity and may kill. In the general population, hyperparathyroidism accounts for most cases, but **in the hospital population the commonest cause of hypercalcaemia is malignancy.**

Cancers of the lung and breast account for 59% of such patients (lung 35%; breast 24%) and haematological malignancies are the next most frequent (14%).

Mechanisms causing hypercalcaemia in malignant disease include:

1) **Local lytic resorption of bone in relation to secondary tumour deposits.** This is most commonly seen in disseminated breast cancer.
2) **A generalized increase in bone resorption caused by release of circulating factors that stimulate bone resorption and may also increase tubular reabsorption of calcium by the renal tubules.** This is termed **humoral hypercalcaemia of malignancy** and occurs most frequently with squamous carcinomas of the lung, head and neck, and carcinomas of the ovary and

pancreas. Lung and head and neck tumours account for the majority of such cases.

3) **Bone resorption associated with an inability to excrete the consequently increased renal load of calcium.** This is the situation in patients with myelomatosis who develop hypercalcaemia.

4) **Bone resorption associated with increased absorption of calcium from the gut.** This is seen in some cases of malignant lymphoma and leukaemia, possibly due to the secretion of vitamin D metabolites by malignant cells.

Humoral Hypercalcaemia of Malignancy

This is due to increased bone resorption. Microscopy shows excess osteoclastic resorption, and increased amounts of hydroxyproline are lost in the urine. Drugs that inhibit osteoclastic activity, such as bisphosphonates, calcitonin and mithramycin, often decrease the raised serum calcium concentrations.

Patients show:
1) an increase in phosphate excretion
2) an increase in cyclic $5'$-adenosine monophosphate (cAMP) levels in the urine
3) increased renal calcium reabsorption

This suggests **a mechanism of action similar to that of PTH**. In contrast with hyperparathyroidism, plasma bicarbonate levels are high in humoral hypercalcaemia of malignancy, and chloride levels are low.

Tumours that produce this type of hypercalcaemia, secrete a chemical message which is not PTH but which acts through the PTH receptor. This message is known to be **parathyroid hormone-related peptide** (see *Fig. 26.2*), an 18-kDa protein encoded by a gene on the short arm of chromosome 12 (PTH itself is encoded by a gene on chromosome 11). In its pure form it is six to ten times more active than PTH, with which it shows some homology.

Transforming Growth Factor α

PTHRP may not cause all the features of humoral hypercalcaemia of malignancy and may interact with other bone-resorbing factors. These include **TGF-α**, a small polypeptide showing 40% homology with epidermal growth factor (EGF) and which acts by binding to the EGF receptor. It can stimulate osteoclastic resorption and substantial experimental evidence exists for a role in hypercalcaemia of malignancy.

Other factors suggested as playing a role in humoral hypercalcaemia of malignancy include IL-1, TNF-α and TNF-β, GM-CSF and prostaglandins. The evidence in favour of prostaglandins is not convincing, although they may well be involved in hypercalcaemia occurring in association with osteolytic metastases.

Hypercalcaemia due to Osteolytic Metastases

Many carcinomas metastasize to bone, among the most common of these being carcinomas of the breast and kidney, which give rise to lytic metastases, and carcinoma of the prostate, which is associated with sclerotic metastases. Breast cancer is second only to lung cancer as a cause of malignancy-associated hypercalcaemia but, unlike what occurs in lung cancer, most cases of breast cancer-related hypercalcaemia are due to the presence of destructive bony metastases.

Local bone destruction caused by tumour deposits could occur via several mechanisms, which include:
- release from the tumour cells of directly osteolytic molecules
- release from the tumour cells of molecules such as TGF-α, which stimulate osteoclastic resorption of bone

Hypercalcaemia Associated with Haematological Malignancy

The association between hypercalcaemia and haematological malignancy is quite common. It is most strongly expressed in **myeloma**, where 20–40% of the patients are hypercalcaemic. In these cases, there is an increased degree of bone resorption, which, however, is not believed to be sufficiently severe to account for the hypercalcaemia. **The additional element is an impairment of glomerular filtration occurring as a result of tubular obstruction by light chain casts (Bence Jones protein) or by uric acid.**

Some transformed lymphocytes secrete a factor that stimulates bone resorption. This, **osteoclast-activating factor** is known to consist of **a set of lymphokines with bone-resorbing activity**. These include IL-1, TNF-α and TNF-β.

Other haematological malignancies complicated on some occasions by hypercalcaemia include:
- acute lymphoblastic leukaemia
- Hodgkin's disease
- Burkitt's lymphoma
- adult T-cell lymphoma

The case of adult T-cell lymphoma is particularly interesting in the context of hypercalcaemia. This is a retrovirus-associated malignancy (human T-lymphotropic virus type 1), occurring in clusters in the southern part of Japan and in the West Indies, and in which hypercalcaemia is common. Raised calcitriol levels are found in some cases and serum levels of both calcium and calcitriol decline after chemotherapy. This suggests that the source of the excess 1,25-dihydroxyvitamin D_3 is the tumour cell, a suggestion supported by studies in which lymphocytes have been infected with this virus.

Paget's Disease of Bone

> #### KEY POINTS: Characteristics of Paget's Disease
> - excessive resorption of bone by osteoclasts
> - increase in bone mass in affected bones
> - loss of normal lamellar architecture

This condition, first described by Sir James Paget in 1877 as **'osteitis deformans'**, is characterized by enlargement and deformities of affected bones. In terms of process, it is the end result of repeated episodes of:

- **intense local resorption of bone by large numbers of giant osteoclasts (up to 200 μm), which contain many more nuclei than do normal osteoclasts**
- **subsequent reparative phases in which there is intense osteoblastic activity resulting in overproduction of new bone and an increase in bone mass. Much of this new bone is woven bone, of the type seen in early fracture healing, in which the normal lamellar architecture is lost. While the bone mass in affected areas is increased, its capacity for weight bearing is greatly decreased and severe deformities result.**

Epidemiology

Paget's disease is fairly common, affecting 3–4% of the population over the age of 45 years; its frequency increases with advancing age (it occurs in approximately 9% of those aged over 85 years). There are distinct geographical variations in prevalence. Paget's disease occurs most commonly in the USA, Britain, France, Germany, Australia and New Zealand, and is rare in East Asia, Scandinavia and countries bordering the Mediterranean. Even within a particular country, prevalence seems to be non-uniform, the reason for this being quite unknown. A positive family history has been reported in as many as 25% of cases of Paget's disease, although the reason for this clustering is still not clear. HLA DQW1 and its associated antigens DR1, DR2 and DRW6 are more common in patients than controls, raising the possibility of some HLA-linked disorder of immune regulation. An association between dog ownership and the risk of developing Paget's disease has also been suggested but there is little 'hard' evidence for this.

Table 44.7 Sites Affected in Paget's Disease

Site	Frequency (%)
Spine	76
Skull	65
Pelvis	43
Femur	35
Tibia	30
Clavicle	11
Sternum	7
Humerus	2

Anatomical Distribution of Lesions

Paget's disease may affect only one bone or many bones. The frequency with which various sites are affected is shown in *Table 44.7* and *Fig. 44.11*).

Bony Lesions

The pathological picture in Paget's disease of bone is dominated by a general disorganization which affects cortical as well as trabecular bone.

Macroscopic Features

The bones are enlarged and thickened. This can be seen most strikingly in the skull where the calvarium may be 2–3 cm thick and the normal distinction between the inner and outer tables and the diploë is largely lost. At the same time, the bone is softer than normal. A considerable degree of bony deformity may be present which is due partly to the mechanical strains of gravity and partly to the pull of muscles on weakened bone.

Deformities of the skull may be striking. Protuberance of the frontal bones may be prominent and softening of the skull over time may lead to a severe deformity in which the head appears to sink into the shoulders. Skull deformities are associated quite frequently with narrowing of the foramina of cranial nerves and resulting neuropathies. Deafness, which may be sensory, conductive or mixed, is a common complication, occurring in 30–50% of cases where skull lesions are present, and vestibular dysfunction may also be present. Inability to smell, facial nerve palsies and trigeminal neuralgia have also been observed.

In the long bones of the lower limbs, bowing may develop, and is most commonly anterior or lateral. Widening of the angle between the shaft and neck of femur (a **coxa vara deformity**) is not uncommon.

Microscopic Features

Microscopic examination shows the trabecula to be markedly enlarged and grossly irregular in outline (*Fig. 44.12*). Evidence of excessive bone remodelling is prominent:

1) Resorption involves over 20% of the trabecular surface, compared with about 3% in controls, and there are approximately three osteoclasts per mm^2 of bone in comparison with a mean of 0.2 per mm^2 in normal bone. In addition to this increase in the number of osteoclasts, the osteoclasts themselves are clearly abnormal being much larger than normal and containing many more nuclei (in some instances over 100 nuclei).

2) An equally florid degree of osteoblastic activity is present. Osteoid covers about 50% of the trabecular surface, compared with 16% in controls, and the osteoid volume is more than twice as great as in normal bone. The number of osteoblasts is increased, as is the size of individual cells.

apparently divide up the trabecula into irregular portions (see *Fig. 44.12*). These lines represent the remains of mineralization fronts and are another index of the intense degree of bone remodelling that dominates this disorder. This appearance is seen especially in the mixed or osteoblastic phases of Paget's disease, when the osteoclastic phase in that area of affected bone is either nearing its end or has reached a 'burned-out' stage.

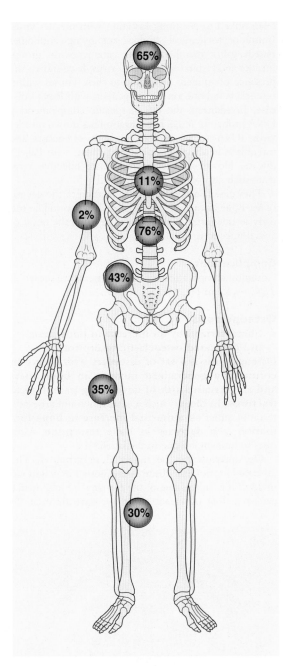

FIGURE 44.11 *Sites of predilection for bone lesions in Paget's disease of bone.*

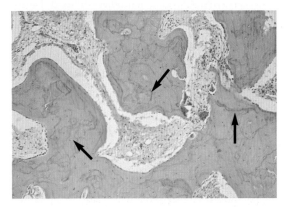

FIGURE 44.12 *Large irregular bony trabecula in Paget's disease of bone. Note also the fine blue lines which give the bone a mosaicized appearance (arrowed).*

Biochemical Changes

The high turnover of bone in Paget's disease is reflected in high plasma concentrations of bone-derived alkaline phosphatase, an expression of osteoblastic activity. The alkaline phosphatase concentration is probably the most sensitive criterion of

3) The large irregular trabecula, when examined in polarized light, can be seen to consist predominantly of lamellar bone but definite areas of woven bone are also present (*Fig. 44.13*). The trabecula have a curious mosaic-like appearance owing to the presence of numerous bluish so-called 'cement' lines which

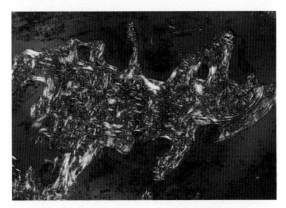

FIGURE 44.13 *Paget's disease of bone. Here, an abnormal portion of trabecular bone has been photographed in polarized light. Collagen, which is birefringent, shows up against the dark background. In Paget's disease, instead of being arranged in concentric lamellae, the collagen exists in the form of small irregular bundles. This is characteristic of woven bone.*

disease activity. Osteoclastic resorption leads to an increased plasma level of hydroxyproline and an increase in the amount of hydroxyproline lost in the urine. The positive correlation that exists between plasma alkaline phosphatase levels and the degree of hydroxyprolinuria points to a coupling between bone formation and resorption.

Aetiology

Many possibilities have been suggested, but it is fair to say that the aetiology of Paget's disease of bone remains a mystery. Morphological and other studies of Pagetic osteoclasts have raised some interesting possibilities.

Role of the Osteoclast

Pagetic Osteoclasts Contain Inclusions Resembling Paramyxovirus Nucleocapsids

It seems clear that the natural history of this disease begins with abnormal activation of the osteoclasts and a consequent gross increase in bone remodelling.

The morphological appearances of the osteoclasts in Paget's disease are abnormal. Electron microscopy shows that many osteoclasts contain inclusions, the majority of which are intranuclear. These are made up of microfilaments, some of which are arranged in a paracrystalline array resembling the nucleocapsid structure of paramyxoviruses such as measles virus (*Fig. 44.14*). Similar structures have been seen in the multinucleated cells in the brain of patients suffering from subacute sclerosing panencephalitis, a disease that has

been linked to persisting infection with measles virus. Immunocytochemical studies employing antibodies raised against members of the paramyxovirus group, measles and respiratory syncytial virus, have shown the presence of antigens belonging to these viruses within osteoclasts in bone samples of patients with Paget's disease. In addition, the use of specific complementary DNA probes for *in situ* hybridization has shown measles virus RNA to be present in both osteoclasts and osteoblasts in affected bone from patients with Paget's disease. However, attempts to isolate infective virus from such samples have, so far, failed.

The role of such infections in relation to the genesis of the bone disease remains unclear, and it is still far too early to categorize Paget's disease as being the result of a viral infection.

Complications

Common complications of Paget's disease are shown in *Table 44.8* and *Fig. 44.15*.

Osteopetrosis

- **Characterized by an increase in bone mass and decreased osteoclastic resorption**

Osteopetrosis is a set of disorders which have in common a generalized increase in bone mass and an increased risk of developing pathological fractures. In theory, such a situation could arise as a result of either **an abnormal increase in bone formation** or **a decrease in bone resorption**. Most cases in humans are due to the latter.

Osteopetrosis can be inherited or acquired. The inherited forms of the disease may present in childhood or adult life. In the case of the former, the inheritance pattern is that of an autosomal recessive disorder. In

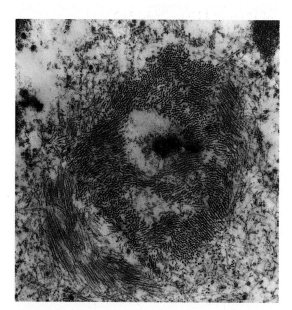

FIGURE 44.14 *Electron micrograph of an osteoclast in a biopsy of pagetic bone. The field is occupied by a paracrystalline array of structures, highly reminiscent of the appearance of a paramyxovirus (e.g. the virus causing measles or canine distemper).*

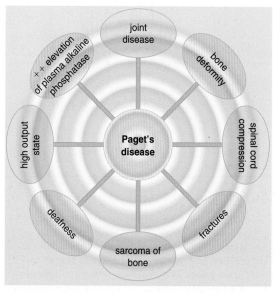

FIGURE 44.15 *Clinical features of Paget's disease of bone.*

Table 44.8 Complications of Paget's Disease

Complication	Findings
Joint disease	Up to 60% of patients develop joint problems, these being most likely to occur in weight-bearing joints such as the hip
Fractures and fissures	The bones are relatively weak and do not withstand weight-bearing and bending forces normally. This leads to fractures in 9–28% of patients, common sites being the long bones of the lower limb and the pelvis
Neurological disorders	Neurological deficits in relation to involvement of the skull have already been mentioned. If the atlas and axis invaginate through the foramen magnum, severe brainstem and cerebellar dysfunction may occur. In view of the frequency with which the spine is affected, it is not surprising that spinal cord compression, often at more than one site, is also a well-recognized complication.
Neoplastic change	The risk of developing bone sarcoma is about 30 times as great as in age-matched controls, about 1–2% of patients being affected. The anatomical distribution of these sarcomas of bone corresponds more or less with the frequency with which individual sites are affected in Paget's disease, with the exception of the humerus which appears to be at higher risk for developing malignant tumours than would be expected on this basis. Osteogenic sarcoma is the commonest tumour, followed by fibrosarcoma and chondrosarcoma. The prognosis in the context of Paget's disease for all of these is very poor.

most instances the disease is severe and likely to be fatal. In adults, inheritance may be either recessive or dominant, and the disorder tends, in general, to be less severe than the juvenile form.

All osteopetroses share five common features:
1) A radiological picture of a generalized increase in bone density together with absence or delayed appearance of marrow cavities.
2) Large bone trabecula with either normal or increased numbers of osteoblasts, or normal or decreased numbers of osteoclasts. Thus a common radiological pattern may be the expression of different histological appearances depending on the particular mutation in a single patient.
3) A reduced hypercalcaemic response to known stimulators of bone resorption such as PTH
4) Absent or delayed eruption of teeth
5) Decreased resorption of bone

Neoplasms of Bone

Neoplasms in bone may be **benign or malignant** and **primary or secondary**, the latter being far more common in adults. Neoplasms can arise from any of the stem cell populations in bone and may differentiate in different ways. **These differentiation patterns con-** stitute the basis for the classification of primary neoplasms.

PRIMARY TUMOURS AND TUMOUR-LIKE LESIONS

When haematological neoplasms arising from bone marrow are excluded:
- 21% show evidence of **cartilaginous differentiation** (*Table 44.9*)
- just over 19% of primary neoplasms are **bone forming** (show osteoid) (*Table 44.10*)

In a patient presenting with a bone tumour, two criteria give information that can be of considerable diagnostic value. These are:

Table 44.9 Tumours Showing Cartilaginous Differentiation

Benign (60%)	Malignant (40%)
Osteochondroma	Primary chondrosarcoma
Chondroma	Secondary chondrosarcoma
Chondroblastoma	Dedifferentiated chondrosarcoma
Chondromyxoid fibroma	

Table 44.10 Bone-forming tumours

Benign (13%)	Malignant (87%)
Osteoid osteoma	Osteosarcoma
Osteoblastoma	

1) **the age of the patient**
2) **the site of the lesion**

This is illustrated below in relation to **the commonest primary malignant neoplasms of bone, listed in descending order of frequency in** *Table 44.11.*

BENIGN CARTILAGE-FORMING TUMOURS

Osteochondroma (Exostosis)

Definition
These are bony lesions with a cartilage cap, projecting from the metaphyses of long bones; they are usually solitary. They are believed to be hamartomas rather than true neoplasms. Multiple osteochondromas may occur in childhood in the autosomal dominant condition **osteochondromatosis**.

Age and Sex
Solitary lesions are most common in adolescence. There is pain, local swelling or a localized deformity. Males are affected three times as commonly as females.

Site
The lesion may arise from any long tubular bone, but is most common in the femur, tibia and humerus. The pelvis, ribs and scapula are less common sites and osteochondroma is distinctly uncommon in the small bones of the hands and feet.

Macroscopic Features
Lesions may grow to about 3–5 cm along the longest axis and project from the bone in either a sessile or a pedunculated form. They consist, for the most part, of bone covered by a cap of cartilage measuring up to 1 cm in thickness.

Microscopic Features
There is a superficial zone in the cap where chondrocytes are arranged haphazardly. Deep to this, the chondrocytes show a more ordered columnar arrangement such as is seen at the growing end of a bone, and ossification occurs deep to this.

Clinical Course
Malignant change is rare, occurring in less than 1% of cases. Multiplicity increases the risks to about 10%.

Chondroma

Definition
Chondroma is a relatively common, benign neoplasm which consists of mature hyaline cartilage.

Age and Sex
Solitary chondroma occurs at any age, although children, adolescents and young adults are most commonly affected. The incidence is equal in both sexes.

Site
Solitary lesions are most frequent within the medullary cavities of the small bones of the hands and feet. This location is the reason for their often being termed **enchondromas**. Multiple lesions may occur involving either several bones or a single bone. Multiple unilateral chondromas constitute **Ollier's syndrome**. The combination of multiple enchondromas and multiple soft

Table 44.11 Age of Patients and Site of Common Primary Neoplasms of Bone

Tumour	Age	Site
Osteosarcoma	Predominantly in adolescents and young adults (peak incidence in second decade) with exception of tumours occurring in relation to Paget's disease of bone	60% occur in relation to the knee joint, where bone growth in the young is very active
Chondrosarcoma	Occurs in the middle-aged and elderly	Occurs in proximal part of skeleton (pelvis, ribs and proximal parts of long bones)
Ewing's tumour	80% occur under the age of 20 years	Most common site is diaphysis
Fibrosarcoma	Most common in middle-aged and elderly patients	

tissue haemangiomas is known as **Maffucci's syndrome**. Neither is hereditary.

Aetiology and Pathogenesis

Virtually nothing is known in this regard. A possible origin from misplaced islands of cartilage cells left behind in the course of bone growth has been suggested.

> #### Macroscopic Features
>
> The lesions are well-circumscribed lobulated masses of firm, bluish, translucent cartilage showing focal calcification. As they expand, so the overlying bone becomes thinned and, in extreme cases, eroded.
>
> #### Microscopic Features
>
> The tumours consist of lobules of mature hyaline cartilage surrounded by a well-vascularized fibrous stroma. The cartilage cells are irregularly distributed in the matrix. Generally, the cells are well differentiated but, occasionally, small dark nuclei and binuclear forms may be seen. Such cytological features in childhood do not suggest malignancy but, in adults, have a more sinister significance.

Clinical Features

The lesions may be asymptomatic or cause pain, local swelling, tenderness or pathological fracture. Malignant change is rare in lesions of the small bones of the hand and foot. Such transformation does occasionally occur in flat bone and proximal limb bone chondromas. It is more likely to occur in patients with one of the multiple chondroma syndromes; the frequency of malignancy in this setting is roughly 30–50%.

Chondroblastoma

Definition

This is a rare, benign, cartilaginous tumour (less than 1% of primary bone tumours) which is usually curable by curettage, although some recur. It is characterized by the presence of benign-appearing multinucleated giant cells and islands of cartilaginous matrix in a background of small, immature, mononuclear cartilage cells, in which mitoses are present.

Age and Sex

Most patients are aged between 10 and 20 years. The male : female ratio is 2 : 1.

Site

Chondroblastomas occur typically in the epiphyseal regions of long tubular bones; the knee joint and upper end of humerus are the most common sites.

Radiological Features

The typical picture is of a central zone of bone destruction within the epiphyseal region, which is surrounded by a narrow zone of increased bone density. Large tumours cause bulging and thinning of the cortex.

> #### Macroscopic Features
>
> The tumours are usually not very large (1–7 cm in diameter) and show a pinkish-grey cut surface with occasional areas of haemorrhage or necrosis. Despite its close apposition, significant involvement of articular cartilage is uncommon.
>
> #### Microscopic Features
>
> Despite a degree of histological variability in chondroblastoma, some features are constant. The basic proliferating cells are believed to be chondroblasts, which have round to oval, indented or grooved nuclei. Except in the areas where islands of cartilaginous matrix are present, there is little stroma between the tumour cells. The presence of mitoses in some chondroblasts does not imply malignancy. Variable numbers of multinucleated giant cells with 5 to 40 nuclei each are seen, the presence of which may lead to a misdiagnosis of giant cell tumour of bone. The giant cells of chondroblastoma are usually smaller and less numerous than those of giant cell tumour.

Clinical Features

Pain and local tenderness are common. Most chondroblastomas are benign and can be cured by adequate local removal. Some very aggressive examples occur; these show local recurrence and distant spread, usually to the lung.

Chondromyxoid Fibroma

Definition

This is another rare (less than 1% of primary tumours) neoplasm showing some differentiation towards cartilage. Its recognition is important because some of the morphological features may lead to misdiagnosis of chondrosarcoma.

Age and Sex

This tumour can occur at any age from 3 to 70 years but most cases affect individuals in the second and third decades. Males are more commonly affected than females.

Site

Chondromyxoid fibroma typically develops in the metaphyseal region of long bones, although the epiphysis may be involved in some cases. The sites most frequently affected, in descending order of frequency, are the **long bones** (tibia, femur and fibula), **flat bones** (the ilium in most cases) and the **small bones of the hands and feet**. In older patients, the long bones are less often affected, a phenomenon also seen in benign chondroblastoma.

Radiological Features

Radiological examination shows a sharply circumscribed zone of rarefaction, which is usually eccentrically situated. The long axes of the rarified areas are parallel to the long axes of the bone. The epiphyseal cartilage is usually spared.

Macroscopic Features

Most chondromyxoid fibromas are fairly small (average diameter approximately 5 cm). The cut surfaces are usually lobulated and show either cartilage or glistening white fibrous tissue. Normal bone is sharply demarcated.

Microscopic Features

Histological appearances vary from area to area. In some, the appearances are frankly cartilaginous; in others, there is a vacuolated myxoid matrix and areas of fibrous tissue. There is a lobular growth pattern with a highly characteristic concentration of nuclei at the periphery of the lobules. The cells in some areas may be large and have large, darkly staining, nuclei, but viewed against the general picture these abnormalities should not be regarded as indicating malignancy.

Clinical Features

Pain is the commonest presenting feature. Chondromyxoid fibroma is classified as benign but curettage may be followed by local recurrence, and many advocate wide excision instead.

MALIGNANT CARTILAGINOUS TUMOURS

Chondrosarcoma

Definition

Chondrosarcoma is a malignant neoplasm which differentiates for the most part into abnormal cartilage, although foci of bone and fibrous tissue may occur. It is the second commonest primary malignant neoplasm of bone. The 75% of chondrosarcomas that arise *de novo* are termed **primary**. **Others develop in osteochondromas, especially of the multiple, familial type; these are secondary chondrosarcomas.**

Age and Sex

Primary chondrosarcomas tend to occur in the middle aged and elderly but secondary ones affect a younger age group (male : female ratio 3 : 2).

Site

More than 75% occur in the trunk, especially in the ribs and pelvis (*Fig. 44.16*), and in the upper ends of the femur and humerus. Despite the large numbers of chondromas found in the small bones of the hands and feet, few sarcomas arise in these sites. Tumours may

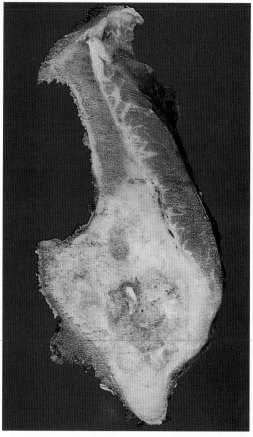

FIGURE 44.16 *Large chondrosarcoma arising from the ilium. Even at this low power it is possible to see the lobulated pattern and the greyish semitranslucent appearance of the chondroid matrix.*

occur within the medullary cavities of affected bones (**'central chondrosarcoma'**) and, rarely, within extraskeletal tissues and in teratomas.

Radiological Features

Bony destruction associated with mottled densities representing focal calcification and ossification is typically present. Central chondrosarcomas of long bones may produce a fusiform bony swelling and cortical destruction with extension of the tumour into the extraosseous soft tissues.

Aetiology and Pathogenesis

These are unknown.

Macroscopic Features

Chondrosarcomas are characteristically lobulated, the lobules varying in size from a few millimetres to several centimetres. Much of the lesions is clearly cartilaginous, although focal, central, liquefactive necrosis may occur.

Microscopic Features

Low-grade chondrosarcomas can present great difficulties in diagnosis because the features distinguishing them from benign cartilaginous tumours are subtle. It is important that the histological features are viewed in a broad context, which must include the age of the patient and the site of the lesion. Thus a cartilaginous tumour in the sternum of an adult is almost always malignant irrespective of its histology, whereas lesions in the small bones of the hands and feet may appear more malignant cytologically, but are usually benign. Features suggesting malignancy include:

- many cartilage cells with plump nuclei
- more than a few binucleated cartilage cells
- giant cartilage cells with large single or multiple nuclei

Most are well or moderately differentiated (*Fig. 44.17*) but high-grade tumours do occur. These show extreme cellularity associated with a high proportion of binucleate cells and much cellular variation.

Occasionally, histological examination shows the presence of a low-grade or well-differentiated chondrosarcoma in continuity with a highly malignant, anaplastic sarcoma. Such a lesion is termed a **'dedifferentiated chondrosarcoma'**. It accounts for 10–20% of chondrosarcomas and carries a poor prognosis (80% of patients die within 2 years). Metastases, especially to the lungs, are common; metastatic deposits always show the features of the anaplastic, spindle-cell component of the primary rather than those of the differentiated cartilaginous component.

Chondrosarcoma Variants

Mesenchymal Chondrosarcoma

This is a rare variant occurring in the young (mean age 25 years). The commonest sites are the femur, humerus, ilium and os calcis (a rare site for any bone tumour).

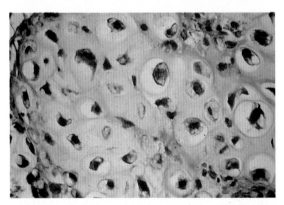

FIGURE 44.17 *Moderately differentiated chondrosarcoma. The neoplastic cartilage is hypercellular and shows the presence of pleomorphic chondrocytes in typical lacunae.*

The lesions consist of a mixture of cartilaginous tissue in various stages of differentiation and highly cellular areas in which the cell population consists of small, darkly staining, often spindle-shaped cells grouped around small blood vessels. Spread to regional and distant lymph nodes occurs commonly, this feature serving further to distinguish the tumour from common types of chondrosarcoma.

Clear Cell Chondrosarcoma

This is a tumour of rather low-grade malignancy with a male : female ratio of 2.6 : 1. It is most common at the ends of long bones, the proximal end of the femur being affected in about 60% of cases. The peak incidence is at a younger age than the usual type of chondrosarcoma: most cases occur between the ages of 20 and 40 years. Macroscopically, these lesions tend to be soft and lack the hyaline appearance of most cartilaginous tumours. Microscopically, the presence of cells with a central nucleus and apparently clear and empty cytoplasm is characteristic. The cells are arranged in small, indistinct lobules, separated by fine connective tissue strands. Most tumours contain a few benign-looking giant cells. The tumours are characteristically slow growing: 18% of patients are recorded as having had symptoms related to their lesions for more than 5 years.

Clinical Features and Natural History

Most patients with chondrosarcoma present with local swelling, pain or both. These lesions are inherently less malignant than osteosarcoma, and well-differentiated examples grow slowly and seldom metastasize, although local recurrence is by no means rare. Poorly differentiated chondrosarcomas, in contrast, grow quickly and tend to spread via the bloodstream quite early, the lung being the commonest site for metastatic deposits. Chondrosarcomas are resistant to radiation and thus surgical removal remains the mainstay of treatment.

BENIGN BONE-FORMING TUMOURS

Osteoma

Definition

The term is applied to a **set** of lesions characterized by the formation of normally arranged mature bone. These lesions constitute something of a ragbag, as some are hamartomatous, some are probably reactive, some represent osteochondromas, the cartilaginous cap of which has involuted, and a few may be true neoplasms.

They are most common in the skull and facial bones and, because they are usually very small, are asymptomatic. Some may grow into the paranasal sinuses or the orbit and cause mechanical problems. Osteomas are usually single but may occur as a component of Gardner's colonic polyposis syndrome (see p 556).

Radiological Features

These are well demarcated, markedly radio-opaque lesions, due to the prominent mature bone component.

> #### Microscopic Features
> Dense, mature, lamellar bone with well-formed haversian systems is present.

Osteoid Osteoma

Definition

This is a benign osteoblastic lesion consisting of a small rounded central area (the **nidus**) surrounded by a zone of dense sclerotic bone. This zone is a reaction to the nidus, as it tends to regress when the nidus is removed. **The classical clinical feature is pain**, which tends to be much more severe than the size of the lesion would suggest. Osteoid osteoma is relatively common (12% of all benign tumours of bone).

Age and Sex

It affects the young: 80% of patients are aged between 5 and 24 years; there is a marked male predominance.

Site

About 50% occur in the femur or tibia, affecting the ends of the shafts. The vertebrae, especially the arches, may also be affected.

Radiological Features

These are highly characteristic. The nidus appears as a small radiolucent area surrounded by a dense, markedly radio-opaque, area representing the reactive bone.

> #### Macroscopic Features
> The lesion is well defined and fleshy, usually not more than 1–1.5 cm in diameter. The nidus is redder than the surrounding bone and can often be lifted from its bed, unless extensive central sclerosis has occurred.
>
> #### Microscopic Features
> The nidus consists of interlacing, delicate bands of osteoid arranged in an apparently haphazard fashion. These osteoid seams are surrounded by plump, but otherwise normal, well-differentiated osteoblasts. The spaces between the osteoid trabeculae contain vascular fibrous tissue in which variable numbers of benign-looking giant cells may be present. Cartilaginous differentiation is never seen.

Clinical Features and Natural History

The most prominent clinical manifestation is pain, which gradually increases in severity and which may be referred to adjacent joints. Localized swelling may occur in a few cases if the affected bone is near the skin surface.

Benign Osteoblastoma (Giant Osteoid Osteoma)

Definition

This is a rare tumour, closely related morphologically to osteoid osteoma. It differs from the latter in respect of:

- **size,** usually being larger (≤ 1.5 cm)
- **site.** Unlike most primary neoplasms of bone, benign osteoblastoma shows a marked tendency to occur in the vertebral column. It may occur also in the bones of the hands and feet, sites that are rarely affected by other primary bone-forming tumours.
- **reaction of surrounding bone.** The conspicuous dense bone sclerosis surrounding the central nidus of osteoid osteoma is generally lacking in benign osteoblastoma, although it may be seen occasionally when the tumour occurs in long bones.

Age

The age distribution is similar to that of osteoid osteoma.

> #### Macroscopic Features
> The lesions are usually well demarcated from the surrounding bone and have a granular, friable, cut surface with focal haemorrhage.
>
> #### Microscopic Features
> These are similar to those of osteoid osteoma with osteoid seams surrounded by plump, but otherwise normal, osteoblasts. The intervening stroma is vascular and this accounts for the loosely woven appearance of the osteoid trabecula. Mitoses may be present but are not often atypical. In some cases large dilated vascular channels and multinucleated giant cells may be seen, these areas strongly resembling another benign bony lesion – **aneurysmal bone cyst**.
>
> Examples showing atypical osteoblasts and a poorly demarcated edge tend to recur, although metastases have not been recorded. These are called **aggressive osteoblastomas**.

MALIGNANT BONE-FORMING TUMOURS

Osteosarcoma

Definition

Osteosarcoma is the commonest primary malignant neoplasm of bone.

KEY POINTS: Osteosarcoma
The defining criteria of osteosarcoma are:
- **the presence of a frankly sarcomatous stroma**
- **evidence of the direct formation of neoplastic osteoid and bone by the malignant connective tissue cells**

Several histological variants are described:
- **osteoblastic**, in which osteoid formation predominates
- **chondroblastic**, in which formation of neoplastic cartilage is prominent
- **fibroblastic**, in which the cells resemble those seen in fibrosarcoma and produce abundant collagen

Diagnosis depends absolutely on the certain identification of bone or osteoid formation by the tumour cells. This is not always easy because other material, such as hyalinized collagen, may be difficult to distinguish from osteoid, and special staining methods may be required.

Age and Sex
Osteosarcoma is rare before the age of 10 years. The peak incidence is between 10 and 25 years, after which the frequency falls sharply. Osteosarcoma of the jaw tends to occur at a somewhat older age. Cases occurring in middle-aged and elderly people are associated with Paget's disease of bone. Males are more frequently affected than females.

Site
The site of predilection is the metaphyseal region of the long bones (about 80%), with roughly half the tumours being located in the region of the knee (*Fig. 44.18*). Any bone may be involved; the commonest sites, in descending order of frequency, are:
- the lower end of femur
- the upper end of the tibia
- the upper end of the humerus
- the ilium

Multicentric, very aggressive, osteosarcomas occur occasionally in childhood.

Most osteosarcomas arise from within the medullary cavity and spread to invade the cortical bone. A small minority arises from within the cortex and these tend to occur within the diaphysis rather than the metaphysis.

Aetiology and Pathogenesis
The vast majority of osteosarcomas arise apparently *de novo*, although some are associated with a pre-existing bone disease or previous exposure to radiation.

Deletions or Mutations of Suppressor Genes such as the Retinoblastoma Gene and p53
Children who have survived the hereditary form of

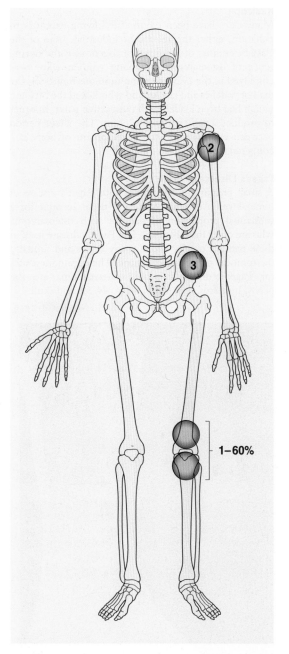

FIGURE 44.18 *Sites of predilection for osteosarcoma.*

retinoblastoma have a risk of subsequently developing osteosarcoma many times that of children without this history; the cells of the osteosarcoma show the same deletions in the q14 region of chromosome 13 as are seen in retinoblastoma.

Similarly, rearrangement of the *p53* gene, another important suppressor gene, which is either deleted or mutated in many human malignancies, has been observed in a number of cases of osteosarcoma.

Radiation

Many cases have been reported following exposure to radiation, either therapeutic or industrial. One of the classic examples of industrial oncogenesis is the occurrence of osteosarcoma in young women who were employed in the 1920s to paint luminous figures on the dials of watches and clocks, and who licked the brushes, which had been loaded with radioactive paint, in order to produce a sufficiently fine point. The latent period between exposure and the development of bone sarcoma ranged from 10 to 15 years.

Paget's Disease of Bone

A small proportion of patients with Paget's disease of bone develop osteosarcoma, and these account for a substantial proportion of patients with osteosarcoma who are older than 40 years. The Paget's disease itself in these patients usually affects many bones and similarly the tumours may be multicentric. The commonest sites for Paget's disease-associated osteosarcoma are the pelvis, humerus, femur, tibia (*Fig. 44.19*) and skull.

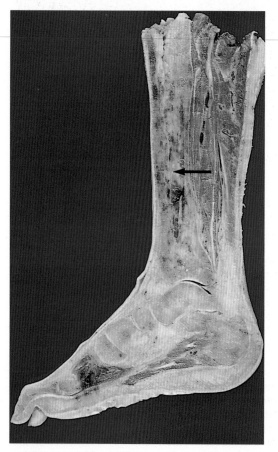

FIGURE 44.19 *Osteosarcoma of the tibia occurring in a patient with Paget's disease of bone. The tumour (arrowed) involves the shaft of the tibia and has extended into the soft tissue.*

Radiological Features

These vary depending on the relative amounts of bone destruction and new bone formation. There are several natural pathways for local spread and this, too, will influence the radiological and macroscopic appearances. The cortex is almost always penetrated by tumour. This causes **elevation of the periosteum**, the basis of a well-known radiological sign known as Codman's triangle. The two long sides of the triangle are formed by the elevated periosteum and the underlying bony cortex; the space between these is often filled with reactive new bone, the spicules of which are arranged roughly at right angles to the original cortex. This is not pathognomonic for osteosarcoma nor, indeed, for malignancy, as it can be seen in any process involving periosteal elevation.

Macroscopic Features

These depend on:

1) **The degree of bone destruction**
2) **The predominant differentiation pattern with respect to bone, cartilage and fibrous tissue formation.** Thus the tumours may be soft and friable at one extreme and range through lesions that are firm and fibrous and that may show areas of cartilage formation, to a hard form in which new bone formation predominates. The bone formation is usually most marked in the central portion of the tumour and there are usually soft areas at the margins which can be sampled for microscopic examination.
3) **The pattern of local spread.** Local spread may involve:

- extension of the malignant tissue down the medullary cavity of the bone
- penetration of the cortex with subsequent elevation of the periosteum
- extension into the epiphysis
- extension into joint spaces
- extension into adjacent soft tissue
- the appearance of separate nodules of tumour tissue (so-called 'skip metastases') within the bone in which the main tumour mass has arisen

See *Figs 44.20* and *44.21*.

Microscopic Features

Histological diagnosis depends on the recognition of a frankly malignant connective tissue stroma, the cells of which are forming new bone or osteoid. It is critically important that no mistake should be made in relation to the identification of the osteoid. Typical osteoid seams are eosinophilic, have irregular outlines and are surrounded by a rim of malignant osteoblasts (*Fig. 44.22*).

The sarcomatous stroma shows considerable variations.

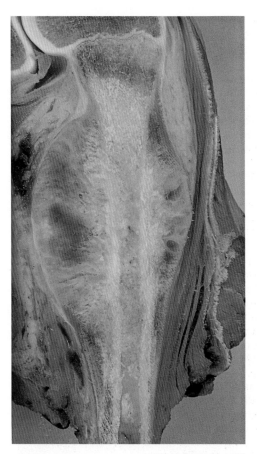

FIGURE 44.20 *Osteosarcoma of the tibia showing characteristic periosteal elevation and the 'sunburst' effect produced by new bone formation.*

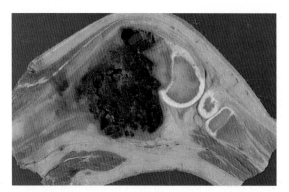

FIGURE 44.21 *So-called telangiectatic variant of osteosarcoma involving the knee joint and showing a strikingly haemorrhagic cut surface.*

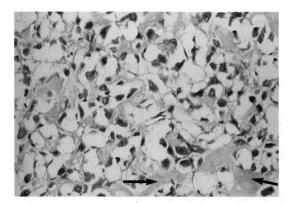

FIGURE 44.22 *Osteosarcoma showing seams of pink-staining osteoid (arrowed) and pleomorphic tumour cells.*

Osteoclast-like giant cells are present in about a quarter of the cases and in some areas may occur in large numbers. **At the histochemical level the tumour cells contain large amounts of alkaline phosphatase** and this feature may be useful in assessing completeness of excision. A large number of other conditions, some of which are non-neoplastic, may have to be excluded before a confident diagnosis of osteosarcoma is made, not the least important of which are exuberant fracture callus and areas of myositis ossificans, a reactive process that shares many features with fracture callus.

Osteosarcoma Variants

Several variants have been described. Some of these have been defined purely on the basis of their histological appearance, whereas others are distinctive in terms of their location, radiological appearance or natural history.

Parosteal (Juxtacortical) Osteosarcoma

These tumours occur in slightly older people and arise in a juxtacortical position in the metaphyseal region. They grow very slowly, sometimes over a period of many years, forming large lobulated masses tending to encircle the shaft of the affected bone. Microscopically, well-formed bone and osteoid is seen, set in a spindle cell stroma in which cytological signs of malignancy are scanty. The prognosis, with adequate resection, is very good. The chief differential diagnosis is myositis ossificans, from which it can usually be distinguished on histological examination by the orderly maturation of the new bone seen **at the periphery of the lesions** in myositis. In contrast, osteosarcomas show central bone maturation (if at all). It is important to remember that a juxtacortical location *per se* **does not automatically carry with it a good prognosis**. Some 'usual' osteosarcomas may be located in a juxtacortical position and these tumours, known as 'high-grade surface osteosarcomas' behave as aggressively as any osteosarcoma arising in the medullary cavity.

Periosteal Sarcoma

This tumour is also located superficially. Common sites are the upper shaft of the tibia or femur. Lesions show areas of radiolucency on the bone surface, associated with spicules of new bone arranged at right angles to the shaft just below the periosteum. The lesions are usually confined to the cortex. On microscopic examination, they show a frankly malignant stroma in which islands of cartilage are conspicuous. The prognosis is better than for 'usual' osteosarcoma arising in the medullary cavity.

Osteosarcoma Arising in the Jaw

These occur in somewhat older patients than the usual osteosarcoma (mean age 34 years) and areas of cartilaginous differentiation are common. Common sites are the body of the mandible and the alveolar ridge of the maxilla. The prognosis is relatively good.

Natural History

Osteosarcomas are, in general, highly malignant, tending to metastasize early via the bloodstream. Chief targets for such secondary deposits are the lung (98%), other bones (37%), pleura (33%) and heart (20%). Lymph node metastases are extremely rare.

Factors affecting the prognosis are shown in *Table 44.12*.

Overall 5-year survival rates used to be about 20%. In the past few years, presumably as a result of combined treatment with chemotherapy followed by surgery, there has been a substantial improvement and many studies have reported 5-year survival rates of 50% or more.

GIANT CELL TUMOUR OF BONE

Definition

This is so named because of the presence of numerous multinucleated or 'giant' cells. Multinucleated giant cells occur, however, in other bone disorders and the bulk of giant cell tumours are composed of mononuclear, spindle-shaped or round stromal cells. Their origin and differentiation pathway are unknown, and thus this tumour cannot be tidily assigned to any major category such as osteoblastic or chondroid tumours.

Giant cell tumours account for just under 5% of primary bone tumours and for about 21% of the benign neoplasms. More than 80% of the patients are older than 19 years, with peak incidence in the third decade. There is a slight female preponderance which is more marked in patients under the age of 20 years. Although it is generally classified as benign, giant cell tumour may be locally aggressive and a proportion undergo malignant transformation.

Site

These tumours are most common in long bone epiphyses. Common sites, in descending order of frequency, are the knee (more than 50%), the lower end of the radius and the sacrum. Tumours may spread locally from the epiphysis into the metaphysis, or break through the cortex with, in some instances, involvement of a joint space. In about 1% of cases, tumours are multiple.

Radiological Features

The lesion is bone destroying and thus the radiographic appearances are those of a lytic and radiolucent lesion that expands the affected area.

Macroscopic Features

Size varies from case to case. The cut surface is heterogeneous, showing grey and red areas, and there may be small blood-filled cysts. The overlying cortical bone is thinned, mirroring the expansile and destructive growth pattern (*Fig. 44.23*).

Table 44.12 Factors Affecting the Prognosis in Patients with Osteosarcoma

Factor	Findings
Presence of Paget's disease	Usually highly malignant; most cases have proved fatal
Location of the tumours	Osteosarcoma of the jaw (5-year survival rate 80% or less); osteosarcomas of the extremities of the limbs (below the knees and elbows) behave better than more proximal tumours. Vertebral and skull tumours (other than the jaw) carry a very poor prognosis
Multifocal tumours	Carry a very poor prognosis
Histological variants	Differentiation patterns do not affect the prognosis materially. One variant, the so-called telangiectatic osteosarcoma containing large blood-filled cysts, is more aggressive than 'usual' osteosarcoma
Parosteal or periosteal osteosarcomas	Better prognosis than conventional osteosarcoma

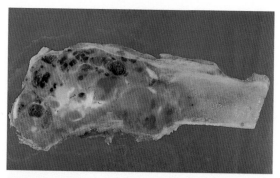

FIGURE 44.23 Giant cell tumour of bone showing expansion of the affected area with cortical thinning and numerous blood-filled cysts.

Microscopic Features

Two main elements are seen:

1) **stromal cells**, which are the basic component. These have a round to oval nucleus, surrounded by ill-defined cytoplasm. Mitoses may be present but are not, as a rule, atypical. Microscopic grading has not been found to be reliable in predicting behaviour unless the lesions are frankly sarcomatous.

2) **giant cells**, which are usually large and have, on average, 20 to 30 nuclei. The nuclei of these giant cells resemble those of the stromal cells, but mitotic figures and atypia are not seen. These cells may very well not be neoplastic at all, as both osteoclasts and giant cells in giant cell tumours express macrophage markers absent from the stromal cells.

Diagnosis

A 'knee-jerk' diagnosis of giant cell tumour should not be made simply on the basis of numerous multinucleated giant cells in a bony lesion. Any bone disease in which destruction is occurring may show an increased number of osteoclasts (as, for example, in prolonged hyperparathyroidism), and lesions such as **benign chondroblastoma, aneurysmal bone cyst and non-ossifying fibroma are also noteworthy for the presence of giant cells**.

A diagnosis of giant cell tumour of bone is likely to be wrong if:

1) the patient is a child
2) the lesion is sited in the metaphysis or diaphysis of a long bone
3) multiple lesions are present
4) the lesion is located in the vertebrae (apart from the sacrum), the jaw (except in association with Paget's disease) or the bones of the hands and feet

Natural History

If the initial surgery has been adequate, the prognosis is relatively good; recurrence is five times less likely after wide resection than after curettage. Radiotherapy is not indicated; the tumours are not radiosensitive and there is a risk of a later malignancy occurring as a result of the irradiation.

Malignant change occurs in about 10% of cases, manifesting itself in the form of uncontrollable local recurrence or metastatic spread.

EWING'S TUMOUR OF BONE

Definition

Ewing's tumour belongs to the group of **small round-cell tumours of childhood**. These include **neuroblastoma, poorly differentiated rhabdomyosarcoma, Ewing's tumour** and **malignant, small, round-celled tumour of the thoracopulmonary region in childhood (Askin tumour)**.

The link between these is the presence of some degree of neural differentiation, this being least evident in Ewing's tumour. These tumours are therefore believed to represent primitive neuro-ectodermal neoplasms.

Some 85% of Ewing's tumours characteristically show a reciprocal translocation of material between chromosomes 11 and 22. This has been found also in some extraskeletal small round-cell tumours and may serve to define a single histogenetic group. **Ewing's tumour itself accounts for 4.7% of all primary neoplasms in bone and 6.1% of primary malignant tumours of bone.**

Age and Sex

Generally, **this tumour affects younger patients than other primary bone tumours. Peak incidence is between the ages of 5 and 20 years**; it is rare over the age of 30 years and under the age of 2 years. There is a distinct **male preponderance**.

Site

Almost any bone can be affected. The long bones of the lower limbs and the pelvic girdle account for about 60% of cases and the ribs are the third most frequently affected site. In long bones, the tumour arises from the medullary cavity and grows outwards through the cortex. Invasion of the soft tissue is an ominous prognostic feature.

Radiographic Features

The tumour causes lytic destruction of the bone with widening of the medullary cavity. Often a considerable length of the shaft is involved. With cortical infiltration, gradual elevation of the periosteum occurs, associated with the laying down of periosteal new bone either roughly parallel to the cortex in an 'onion skin' fashion or at right angles to the cortex giving a 'sun-ray' appearance similar to that seen in osteosarcoma.

Macroscopic Features

Viable tumour shows a glistening, greyish white, cut surface. Focal necrosis, which may be soft and 'pus-like', and haemorrhage are quite common. The degree of bone invasion is usually greater than appears on radiological examination.

Microscopic Features

The characteristic picture is of sheets of small, uniform, round cells divided into irregular islands by fibrous tissue septa. **One of the most important diagnostic criteria is the presence of droplets of glycogen in the cytoplasm of the tumour cells.** These may be recognized either on light microscopy by the presence of periodic acid–Schiff-positive material, removable by diastase, or on electron microscopy where small electron-dense particles may be seen.

Clinical Features and Natural History

Pain and swelling are the commonest symptoms. Fever and a raised erythrocyte sedimentation rate may be present and misdiagnoses of osteitis have occurred.

In general, the tumour is very aggressive and metastatic spread to the lungs, pleura, other bones (especially the skull) and central nervous system is common.

A formerly bleak 5-year survival rate (5–8%) has been improved by high-dose irradiation followed by chemotherapy, the actuarial 5-year disease-free survival rate being put at 75%.

FIBROBLASTIC TUMOURS

Malignant Fibrous Histiocytoma

Definition

This neoplasm accounts for less than 1% of primary malignant tumours of bone and is much more commonly encountered in soft tissues. The term was originally applied to a group of soft tissue tumours characterized by a cartwheel-like or 'storiform' growth pattern. Despite the name **histiocytoma**, which suggests macrophage differentiation, the tumour cells lack most of the markers that define the monocyte–macrophage, and are most likely to be related to fibroblasts.

Age and Sex

The mean age at presentation is 40 years; just over half the patients are male. About 30% of cases are associated with the presence of foreign bodies, infarcts of bone, Paget's disease of bone or previous irradiation to the affected part.

Site

About 60% of the lesions occur in long bones but they have been reported also in the skull, jaw and sacrum.

Radiographic Features

Malignant fibrous histiocytoma destroys bone, thus the appearances are those of a lytic lesion.

Macroscopic Features

These are variable. If collagen formation has been abundant, the tumours are firm; if not, they tend to be soft. In some instances lipid is abundant and these lesions have a yellowish colour, whereas in others the tumour may be brownish-grey.

Microscopic Features

The growth pattern shows a cartwheel-like appearance and the cell population is characteristically pleomorphic. Some of the cells are plump spindle cells appearing fibroblastic; multinucleate giant cells and foamy macrophages containing lipid may be seen. Very large, atypical cells with marked nuclear atypia, the appearances of which suggest (rightly or wrongly) some differentiation towards muscle, may be prominent. Mitoses are fairly common.

Clinical Features and Natural History

Pain and swelling are the commonest presenting features. Behaviourally, malignant fibrous histiocytoma is highly aggressive. In one series, 56% of the patients died as a result of the tumour.

Fibrosarcoma

Definition

This is a malignant spindle cell neoplasm which may or may not produce collagen but does *not* produce osteoid or bone. **It constitutes about 3% of malignant primary tumours of bone.**

Age and Sex

The incidence is evenly distributed from the second to the seventh decade of life. Males and females are equally affected.

Site

More than 50% occur in long bones, the principal site being the metaphysis. Just under 30% occur in the region of the knee.

Radiographic Features

The tumour causes destruction both of medullary and cortical bone and thus appears lytic on radiological examination, having a 'soap-bubble' appearance. Low-grade tumours tend to have a well-defined margin, whereas more aggressive examples permeate cortical bone.

The appearances of fibrosarcoma depend to a considerable extent on the amount of collagen produced by the cells. If this is large, the tumours are firm and greyish-white in colour; if collagen production is scanty, the lesions are soft, friable and fleshy.

Microscopic Features

Variation from one tumour to another is common and reflects variations in the differentiation of the tumour fibroblasts. In highly differentiated examples, the cells show a 'herring-bone' pattern with abundant collagen arranged in bands and whorls. In others, there is a high degree of cellular and nuclear pleomorphism with many atypical mitoses.

Clinical Features and Natural History

Patients present with pain and localized swelling of the affected bone. Metastatic spread is common, although the overall prognosis tends to be somewhat better than that of osteosarcoma, with 5-year survival rates of about 25%. A further 25% of these survivors die from the tumour.

OTHER TUMOURS

Chordoma

Age and Sex

As their name implies, these rare neoplasms arise from the remains of the primitive skeleton or notochord. Males are affected more often than females, and cases are rare below the age of 30 years.

Site

The most frequent site is the sacrum but chordomas in the spheno-occipital region are not uncommon.

Clinical Features and Natural History

Sacral examples cause symptoms and signs because of the pressure they exert on the cauda equina or on nerve roots. Intracranial examples produce the same disturbances as any other expanding intracranial mass. They grow slowly and infiltrate extensively. They do not metastasize but the prognostic outlook is, on the whole, bleak.

Macroscopic Features

The tumours are usually lobulated and appear well encapsulated. The cut surface is gelatinous and bluish-grey and may show focal haemorrhage and cystic change.

Microscopic Features

The tumour cells are round or polyhedral and grow in clumps or cords. Typically they are vacuolated, which has given rise to the descriptive term physaliphorous (bubbly) (*Fig. 44.24*). They are set in an abundant mucin-rich stroma and may show superficial resemblances to cartilaginous tumours. The cells, however, express cytokeratins and epithelial membrane antigen.

LESIONS IN BONE THAT MAY SIMULATE PRIMARY NEOPLASMS

Fibrous Dysplasia of Bone

Fibrous dysplasia of bone is a non-neoplastic condition in which well-demarcated, localized areas of bone are replaced by fibrous tissue containing spicules of woven bone. It is relatively common and occurs in three main forms, as shown in *Table 44.13*.

Occasionally, the polyostotic form is associated with skin pigmentation and endocrine abnormalities, the most common of which is the development of precocious puberty. The skin and bone lesions are usually on the same side. Skin lesions tend to be large irregular areas with differing degrees of pigmentation. This combination is known as the McCune–Albright syndrome. Females are affected much more commonly than males.

Radiological Features

On radiography, the affected areas of bone appear cystic, but this is a false impression because the radiolucent areas are, in fact, occupied by masses of fibrous and bony tissue.

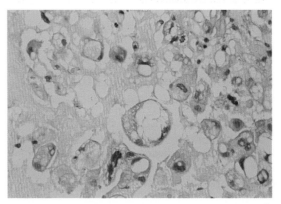

FIGURE 44.24 *Chordoma showing the typical plump, eosinophilic cells containing numerous vacuoles which give them a bubbly (physaliphorous) appearance.*

Table 44.13 Types of Fibrous Dysplasia of Bone

Type	Frequency (%)	Age	Sites
Monostotic	70	Older children and adolescents	Ribs, femur, tibia, maxilla, mandible and humerus
Polyostotic	25	Younger children	Femur, skull, tibia and humerus. In about 50%, facial involvement is present and this may cause deformities. In both forms, the male : female incidence is roughly equal
Polyostotic and endocrine abnormality (McCune–Albright syndrome) and patchy skin pigmentation	3–5		See below

Microscopic Features

Histological examination shows the presence of sheets of mature cellular fibrous tissue containing trabeculae of woven bone which have a peculiar sickle or fish-hook shape (*Fig. 44.25*). These trabeculae never mature into lamellar bone and lack the rim of osteoblasts that normally surrounds bony trabeculae.

Natural History

The natural history of these lesions is highly variable. Many of the monostotic lesions are asymptomatic and are detected in the course of radiological examination undertaken for some other reason. If the lesions are large, pathological fractures may occur, and if there is extensive involvement of the cranial and facial bones, quite severe deformities may result. Twelve cases of associated bone sarcoma have been reported, of which eight were osteosarcomas.

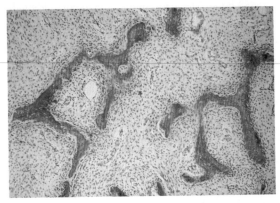

FIGURE 44.25 *Fibrous dysplasia of bone. Note the very cellular background in which curved or sickle-shaped trabecula of bone are set.*

Miscellaneous Bone Disorders

ISCHAEMIC NECROSIS OF BONE

Ischaemic necrosis of bone is common, accounting for more than 10% of the 0.5 million joint replacements performed in the USA annually.

It occurs in a number of settings:

- as a isolated event
- as a complication of local irradiation
- as a result of treatment with corticosteroids

In all these, the basis of the ischaemia is understood most easily against the background of the anatomy of the blood supply of bone.

Long bones derive their blood supply from *two* sources:
1) the nutrient artery, which enters the bone via a foramen and penetrates through the cortex to reach the medulla. Once there, the artery divides to form a plexus supplying the medulla and the inner (endosteal) half of the cortex.
2) periosteal blood vessels, which perforate the cortex more or less at right angles to the bone surface and, within its depths, anastomose with small branches of the nutrient artery. Within the cortex, blood vessels may run either parallel to the long axis of the bone (haversian canals) or at right angles to the long axis (Volkmann's canals).

Interruption of the blood supply can occur under *four* sets of circumstances:

1) **Mechanical interruption**, as in the course of a fracture or dislocation

2) **Thrombosis or embolism**, including:
- nitrogen embolism (seen in deep sea divers)
- sickle cell crises
- fat embolism

3) **Non-traumatic injury to the vessel.** This may occur in:
- vasculitis
- local irradiation
- chemically induced vasospasm (as in Gaucher's disease crises)

4) **Venous occlusion.** In closed systems, a rise in venule pressure to a level greater than that in the arterioles will result in a fall in arterial perfusion. This occurs mostly in the region of the hip joint, which is perfused largely by small vessels coursing through the subcapsular tissues. A joint effusion may be sufficient to impair venous drainage and thus may increase venular pressure to dangerous levels.

Effects of Ischaemia on Bone

Ischaemia may result in:
- infarction of **medullary** bone, which is usually silent clinically
- infarction of both **medullary** and **cortical** bone. This is most frequently seen in the femur just below the articular cartilage of the hip and knee joints and in the upper portion of the humerus. It is much more serious and usually presents with severe pain.

Ischaemia affects both marrow and bone. In fatty marrow the adipocytes die and release fatty acids, leading to the formation of soaps as the fatty acids combine with calcium in tissue fluid.

The presence of infarcted bone elicits an inflammatory response, demolition of both dead bone and exudate, and some degree of replacement by new woven bone. The late stages of these processes may be associated with stress fractures or with collapse and distortion of the infarcted area beneath the articular cartilage. This will lead ultimately to severe osteoarthritis of the affected joint.

Ischaemic necrosis of bone may occur in both adults and children. In the latter it is part of a group of disorders affecting the epiphyses of a number of different bones and given the generic name **osteochondritis juvenilis**.

There is controversy as to which members of this group are caused by ischaemic necrosis, but there does seem to be general agreement that this is the case in respect of:
- **Legg–Calvé–Perthes disease.** This disorder affects the femoral head. There is a family history in just under one-third of cases and males are more commonly affected than females. The peak incidence is between the ages of 5 and 11 years. The necrosis leads to a gradual collapse of the femoral head and affected patients often have severe osteoarthritis in later life.

- **Kienboeck's disease**, where the lunate bone in the hand is the target
- **Kohler's disease**, which affects the navicular bone in the foot
- **Frieberg's disease**, affecting the head of one of the metatarsal bones

INFLAMMATION IN BONE

The term **osteomyelitis** covers all infection-mediated inflammations of bone. It may be classified as **acute, chronic** (occurring on the basis of a pre-existing acute osteomyelitis) or **chronic granulomatous** which, like other granulomata, is destined from its start to become chronic.

Acute Osteomyelitis

This is an acute pus-forming inflammatory process in which infection may occur in two ways:

1) The organisms may penetrate bone **directly**. This can occur in:
- compound fracture
- penetrating wounds over bones without fracture
- surgical operations on bone, especially if metal plates or pins are inserted

2) Organisms may reach the bone via the **bloodstream** (haematogenous osteomyelitis). This occurs most commonly but not exclusively in association with **staphylococcal** infections, the primary foci of which may be trivial (such as a skin pustule) or in which no primary focus may be identified. Patients with sickle cell disease have an increased risk for acute osteitis. In this case, however, the organism most frequently responsible is one of the **salmonellae**.

Peak incidence is in the first two decades of life; the male : female ratio is 3 : 1. The bones affected are, in descending order of frequency, the **femur, tibia, humerus and radius**. In adults the vertebrae may be involved and this may be very serious because the intervertebral discs do not act as a barrier for the spread of the inflammatory process.

Pathology and Natural History of Acute Haematogenous Osteomyelitis

The prime target in long bones is the **metaphysis**. This is probably due to the microanatomy of the local blood supply. Arteriolar branches of the nutrient artery enter the calcified portion of the epiphyseal plate and then form sharp loops in the course of draining into rather large-calibre veins in which blood flow is sluggish. **These loops are sites of predilection for the impaction of pyogenic microorganisms**, which multiply and cause acute pyogenic inflammation.

The important determining factor of the natural history of acute osteomyelitis is the rigid nature of bone. A given volume of inflammatory oedema in bone causes a much greater rise in interstitial pressure than it would in soft tissues, and this steep pressure rise compromises the local blood supply and thus favours bone necrosis around the initial microabscess. Other factors promoting bone necrosis are the release of lysosomal enzymes from inflammatory cells and the secretion of bone-resorbing cytokines. Early diagnosis and vigorous intravenous antibiotic treatment may abort the process and avoid the need for surgery.

From this point, the natural history depends on the interactions between spread of inflammation, bone necrosis and reparative new bone formation.

Spread of Inflammation

If the process is not halted, the original microabscess expands, and both organisms and inflammatory cells may enter the endosteal vessels. This allows spread to occur both in the haversian and Volkmann's canals and the inflammation can thus extend along both the length and thickness of the bone, invading the cortex to reach the subperiosteal space. Once pus reaches this space, the periosteum, loosely attached to the underlying bone in childhood, lifts away and pus, in direct communication with the medullary cavity of the bone, accumulates beneath the periosteum. The periosteal elevation may have two effects:

1) Periosteal blood vessels supplying the cortex can shear off, leading to **ischaemic necrosis of cortical bone**.
2) A natural pathway is created for the inflammatory process to spread and this, in children, can lead to direct extension to the joint cavity, producing septic arthritis.

Further spread can now occur with perforation of the periosteum, and the pus may track through the soft tissues overlying the bone and may eventually burst through the skin forming a sinus track (**cloaca**) between the inflamed bone and the skin surface. Through this, portions of dead bone may be discharged on to the skin.

Bone Necrosis and Bone Formation

Bone necrosis in acute osteomyelitis is due to the combined effects of ischaemia and the local release of mediators that may either destroy the bone directly (such as lysosomal enzymes) or stimulate resorption, as can occur with cytokine release. Portions of dead bone often separate from adjacent viable bone; these are called sequestra. A **sequestrum** may, in time, become resorbed, may remain at the site of its formation or may be discharged on to the skin surface through cloacae.

Reparative formation of new bone starts early, intramedullary abscesses being surrounded by some new woven bone. In some instances, the acute inflammation halts at a stage when an intramedullary abscess is surrounded by a cuff of dense new bone, the radio-logical appearances showing some resemblance to an osteoid osteoma. This lesion is termed a **Brodie's abscess**.

The other source of new bone formation is the periosteum. Abundant bone formation may occur here, the sequestrum being surrounded by new bone. Such a sheath of new bone is called an **involucrum**. In preantibiotic times, when very extensive subperiosteal tracking of pus was common, much of the cortical surface might show involucrum formation with many cloacae passing through the latter.

Pyogenic Osteomyelitis Involving the Vertebrae

Vertebral osteomyelitis occurs mainly in adults. About 50% of cases are due to infection with *Staphylococcus aureus*, 20% to infection by enteric organisms, and the vertebrae are also the target in most cases of osteomyelitis caused by *Brucella* infections.

Unfortunately, the intervertebral disc does not act as a barrier for bacterial infections and thus infection in one vertebral body may spread directly to other vertebrae via this route.

Patients present with back pain and localized tenderness. A low-grade fever is usually present and diagnosis is not easy. The natural history, as in the case of long bones, depends on the extent of spread and the degree of bone destruction. Thus the complications may include:

a) extension to the dura with epidural abscess formation
b) vertebral collapse, which may be associated with paravertebral abscess formation
c) compression of the spinal cord as a result of collapse of the affected vertebral bodies

Complications

The complications of pyogenic osteomyelitis may be systemic or local.

Systemic Complications

1) **Spread of infection to the bloodstream**, where the responsible organisms may multiply, giving rise to **septicaemia**.
2) **Reactive systemic amyloidosis with deposition of the AA type of amyloid protein** in a wide variety of tissues. This occurs only if the osteomyelitis becomes chronic.

Local Complications

1) **Chronicity.** This tends to occur if diagnosis and treatment have been delayed, and is most commonly associated with the persistence of sequestra.
2) **Acute bacterial arthritis.** This occurs most commonly in children and may lead to destruction of the articular cartilage and severe osteoarthritis in the future.

3) **Pathological fractures**

4) **Malignancy.** Squamous carcinoma of the skin surface may occur after many years if sinuses have remained present; sarcoma has occasionally been recorded in scar tissue within bone.

Chronic Granulomatous Osteitis

Tuberculous Osteitis

Tuberculous inflammation in bone is almost always due to blood-borne infection and is most frequent in children and young adults. Common sites are the vertebrae and the bones of the hip, knee, ankle, elbow and wrist. In long bones, the epiphysis and synovium are quite often involved, in contrast with acute pyogenic osteomyelitis.

The lesion is typically an area of bone destruction associated with granulomatous lesions in which moderately extensive caseation may be present. The process is dominated by bone destruction and very little new bone formation is seen, again in contrast with acute pyogenic inflammation. If the process extends into the joint, the attachments of the synovium to the articular cartilage are destroyed; cartilage is deprived of perfusion from the synovial vessels and is destroyed.

Tuberculosis of the spine (syn. **Potts' disease**) usually starts in vertebral bodies and extends into disc spaces. The bone destruction leads to sharp anterior angulation of the spine (**kyphosis**), producing severe deformities.

Caseation may spread through the vertebral body to reach the periosteum, and caseous material then tracks down under the periosteum causing periosteal displacement. In some instances the caseous material gains access to the soft tissues and may track down within the sheath of one of the muscles attached to the spine, most often the psoas muscle. Once within the muscle sheath there is a cleavage pathway for the caseous material, which may eventually point as a soft subcutaneous mass beneath the inguinal ligament.

Joints

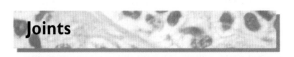

NORMAL STRUCTURE AND FUNCTION

The structure of joints is admirably adapted to their functions. Joints are connections between different bones which:

- may move freely in relation to one another (**diarthroses**)
- are fixed and rigid such as the sutures of the skull (**synarthroses**)
- have a slight degree of movement seen, for example, in intervertebral joints (**amphiarthroses**)

This chapter is concerned primarily with disorders that affect the diarthrodial or synovial joints.

SYNOVIAL JOINTS

Synovial joints have a wide range of movement. Thus adjacent bones are reasonably widely separated and there is a fairly large joint cavity. The cavity margins are defined partly by articular cartilage covering the ends of the adjacent bones, and partly by a tough fibrous capsule fused to the periosteum at or near the margins of the articular surfaces of the bones. The capsule's inner surface is lined by well-vascularized connective tissue, composed partly of fibrous and partly of adipose tissue. This is lined by a layer of covering cells composed of two functional groups:

- **type A cells**, apparently belonging to the macrophage family and which also produce hyaluronic acid, an important constituent of synovial fluid
- **type B cells**, which are basically fibroblastic but also produce non-collagen proteins

Normally, the synovial lining cells are no more than one or two layers thick. There is no basement membrane beneath these cells, facilitating the transfer of water, solute and protein between the blood and fluid within the joint cavity.

Articular Cartilage

Articular cartilage is distinctive in terms of both composition and function. It is composed of cartilage cells (chondrocytes) embedded in an abundant extracellular matrix. Chondrocytes cannot communicate directly with one another because they are not in physical contact; articular cartilage is avascular, and the cells must therefore be nourished by diffusion.

The matrix consists principally of:

- a meshwork of collagen fibres oriented differently at different levels within the cartilage
- large amounts of hydrophilic proteoglycans entrapped within the collagen meshwork
- a small amount of other proteins

Collagens of Articular Cartilage

Of the 13 different collagens so far recognized, four types are present in articular cartilage. Three of these are unique to this location:

- **Type II collagen** (approximately 90% of articular cartilage collagen) forms the fibrils that 'hold' the proteoglycans and is responsible for providing the tensile strength of the tissue.
- **Type IX collagen** (10% of the collagen content) is present on the surface of the type II fibres. It is believed to play a role in cross-linking collagen fibres to one another and to other extracellular matrix molecules.
- **Type XI collagen** (about 5% of the collagen content) is thought to play a part in determining the diameter of type II collagen fibrils.

Proteoglycans of Articular Cartilage

Proteoglycans are critical to the function of articular cartilage, giving the tissue its ability to absorb loading forces. Proteoglycans are complex macromolecules in which glycosoaminoglycan chains are covalently attached to a protein core.

The major proteoglycan of articular cartilage is **aggrecan**. This has a protein core but consists mostly of glycosoaminoglycans, of which keratan sulphate and chondroitin sulphate are the chief constituents. At the amino-terminal of the core protein are two domains, one binding to hyaluronan; the other (called the link protein) stabilizes this binding reaction and enables the aggrecan to form large aggregates.

Aggrecan is in a state of constant slow turnover, accomplished by cleaving the molecules near the amino-terminal. The responsible enzymes are derived from the chondrocytes; these cells are stimulated to increase matrix breakdown by cytokines such as interleukin (IL) 1 and tumour necrosis factor (TNF) α. These cytokines also inhibit protein synthesis by chondrocytes and thus have a double action in depleting articular cartilage of some of its important constituents. This may well be an important element in cartilage destruction in both osteoarthritis and rheumatoid disease.

JOINT DISORDERS

OSTEOARTHRITIS

Osteoarthritis (OA) is the commonest of the joint diseases, affecting 14% of the adult population. Its prevalence increases with advancing age, the slope of increase becoming much steeper after the age of 50 years; at its peak, the prevalence, as determined radiologically, may be as high as 75%.

The onset is insidious and the aetiology and pathogenesis are poorly understood. This is especially regrettable because OA not only causes much suffering but also consumes a considerable fraction of the healthcare budget.

OA is traditionally regarded as **a disorder in which the primary process is breakdown of the articular cartilage with exposure of underlying bone**; indeed, it is likely that changes in the biochemical composition and function play significant roles in impairing the load-absorbing qualities of articular cartilage. Both the genesis and severity of many disorders depend on the severity of the 'injury' and the 'resistance' of the tissue concerned. Thus OA may result from one or both of the following:

- **recurrent increased load-bearing on normal articular cartilage**
- **normal load-bearing on weakened articular cartilage**

Classification

OA is classified into *two* main groups:

- **primary**, in which there is no known associated condition that might cause the arthritis
- **secondary**, in which a known associated event or disease is causally related to the arthritis (see *Table 44.14*)

Aetiology

Individual risk factors may operate, either by increasing susceptibility to the condition or by increasing load on the articular cartilage.

Obesity

Some claim that there is a close association between obesity and OA involving the knee, whereas others claim that the obesity seen in these patients is related to lack of exercise owing to a stiff painful knee.

Genetic Factors

Data from family and twin studies suggest that there is a genetic component in the **polyarticular** form of OA. An hereditary form of OA is recognized in mice and, recently, some studies have shown abnormalities in genes coding for collagen in certain families in whom many cases of OA have occurred.

Influence of Sex

There is a marked female predominance in polyarticular OA; this has led some to suggest that OA may be hormonally determined.

Influence of Osteoporosis

Hip OA is negatively associated with osteoporotic fractures at this site; indeed, in osteopetrosis (increased bone density), there is an increased likelihood of OA.

Cigarette Smoking

Analysis of population-based data sets suggests that cigarette smoking exerts some protective action against OA. This effect appears to persist even when possible confounding variables such as body mass are taken into account.

Mechanical Factors

These include:

- trauma
- joint shape, which can vary the loading forces on articular cartilage
- occupation, which may involve repetitive trauma
- sporting injury (e.g. in footballers in whom there is an increased risk of OA of the knee)

Macroscopic and Microscopic Features

Changes are seen in the:
- articular cartilage matrix
- chondrocytes within the articular cartilage
- subchondral bone

Table 44.14 Causes of Secondary Osteoarthritis

Group	Examples
Post-traumatic	
Congenital or developmental	**Localized** Hip diseases such as Legg–Calvé–Perthes disease, congenital hip dislocation, shallow acetabulum, slipped femoral epiphysis Local mechanical factors such as unequal length of lower limbs, extreme valgus–varus deformity, scoliosis, obesity (?) **Generalized** Dysplasias such as epiphyseal dysplasia Metabolic disorders such as haemochromatosis, Gaucher's disease, haemoglobinopathies
Calcium deposition diseases	Calcium pyrophosphate deposition (pseudo-gout)
Other bone and joint diseases	Avascular necrosis of the femoral head Rheumatoid arthritis Gout Septic arthritis Paget's disease of bone Osteochondritis
Other diseases not primarily of bone	Endocrine diseases Neuropathic arthropathy (Charcot's joints) Caisson disease Kashin–Beck disease (an endemic form of the disease found in Siberia, northern China and Korea). It is believed to occur as a result of eating bread contaminated with fungi producing an unknown toxin causing epiphyseal and metaphyseal dysplasia. The disease appears as a rule in children of school age.

There is an **increase in the amount of water** in the articular cartilage and a **decrease in the proteoglycan content**.

Erosive changes occur in the cartilage, known collectively as 'fibrillation' (*Fig. 44.26*), and lead to flaking off of small portions of cartilage. With continuing movement of the joint, there may be complete loss of cartilage in certain load-bearing areas with exposure of the underlying bone (*Fig. 44.27*).

Some of the chondrocytes undergo necrosis, but more commonly focal proliferation of chondrocytes occurs, forming aggregates. Metachromatic stains show large amounts of matrix in these areas. These appearances represent an attempt by the chondrocytes to 'repair' the damaged cartilage.

Bone exposed due to focal loss of cartilage becomes polished by the continual friction. It develops a very smooth ivory-like surface ('eburnation') (*Fig. 44.28*).

Thickening of the subchondral bone plate occurs; this is seen also in the cancellous bone underlying the subchondral plate. Increased bone density tends to increase still further the load on the articular cartilage. Small fractures may occur through the subchondral plate, allowing synovial fluid, under pressure, to enter into the small defects in the bone. This results in the formation of small subchondral pseudocysts.

At the margins of the articular cartilage, bony outgrowths, known as **osteophytes**, develop, often associated with a mild to moderate synovial inflammatory reaction (*Fig. 44.29*).

Clinical Features

Symptoms

The principal, indeed the only, important symptom is **pain**, usually insidious in onset. Articular cartilage itself is devoid of pain-transmitting fibres and it has been

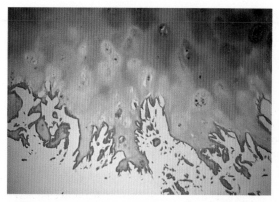

FIGURE 44.26 *Articular cartilage in osteoarthritis showing a severe degree of fibrillation with many deep indentations in the cartilage.*

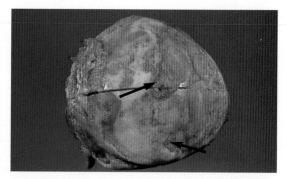

FIGURE 44.28 *Femoral head in osteoarthritis showing several areas of erosion of cartilage (arrowed).*

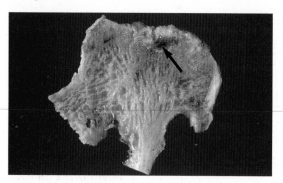

FIGURE 44.27 *Severe osteoarthritis showing virtually complete loss of articular cartilage and some small cystic areas in the underlying bone (arrowed).*

suggested that the pain may be due to several mechanisms, including:

- **stimulation of pain fibres in the joint capsules as a result of a rise in pressure within the joint space**
- **stimulation of pain fibres in the periosteum as a result of an increase in pressure within the subchondral bone**
- **subchondral microfractures**
- **bursitis occurring as a result of muscle weakness, structural changes within the joint and alterations in the way the joint is used**

Functional Impairment

Both the pain and the reduction in the range and degree of control of movement cause disability of differing degrees of severity.

Signs

The structural changes in the joint are responsible for:

- **joint deformity**
- **crepitus (a creaking sound heard on movement of the joint)**
- **limitation of movement**

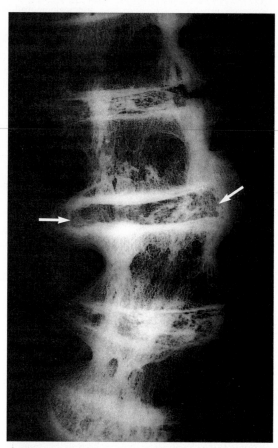

FIGURE 44.29 *Radiograph of vertebrae in severe osteoarthritis showing narrowing of the joint spaces, subchondral cystic spaces and osteophyte formation (arrowed).*

Variants of Osteoarthritis

Many workers now regard osteoarthritis as a set of disorders with certain common features rather than as a single entity. As a result, several subsets have been defined. To describe them all is beyond the scope of a general text but the commoner of these subsets are worthy of some attention.

Nodal Generalized Osteoarthritis

This is characterized by:

- female preponderance
- polyarticular involvement of the interphalangeal joints of the fingers
- peak onset in middle age
- a good functional outcome so far as the finger joints are concerned
- a predisposition for subsequent development of osteoarthritis of the knee, hip or spine
- Heberden's or Bouchard's nodes (bony swellings related to the distal interphalangeal joints (Heberden) or the proximal interphalangeal joints (Bouchard)). Initially they are red and tender but this evidence of inflammation is only transitory.

It is possible that autoimmune mechanisms are involved in this form because:

- **there is a positive association with HLA-A1 and HLA-B8**
- **immune complexes are present in the cartilage and synovium of affected joints removed at surgery**
- **immunoglobulin (Ig) G rheumatoid factor is more prevalent than in other forms of arthritis**

Neuropathic Joints

Severe disorganization follows loss of the normal nerve supply of joints. This was first described by Charcot in relation to patients with tabes dorsalis, a manifestation of tertiary syphilis. Similar changes can be seen occasionally in severe diabetic neuropathy and, in the upper limb, neuropathic arthropathy may be encountered in syringomyelia.

In tabes dorsalis, the most commonly affected joint is the knee, but the hip, ankle and shoulder may be involved in some cases. The patients complain of recurrent swellings of the joint due to effusions, and mechanical problems are common. Degenerative changes occur in the ligaments and tendons and, as a result, the joint may become abnormally mobile and subluxation may occur.

In the early stages, there may be some resemblance to osteoarthritis but as the disorder progresses there is extensive destruction of the articular cartilage and subchondral bone, and fractures may occur at the latter site.

RHEUMATOID ARTHRITIS

This is a common multisystem disease affecting 1–2% of the population. Its cause is unknown but it is currently believed that it results from an interplay between:

- genetic factors
- sex hormones (which would explain the female preponderance)
- a putative infectious agent

These act together to trigger an **autoimmune disease mechanism** resulting in inflammation of the synovium and destruction of the articular surfaces (*Fig. 44.30*).

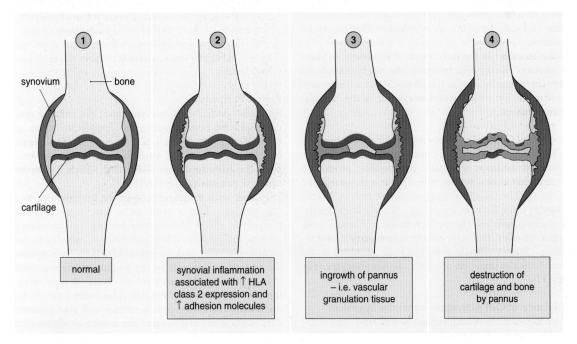

FIGURE 44.30 *Sequence of pathological changes in rheumatoid arthritis.*

Joint Abnormalities

The principal targets, so far as the arthritis is concerned, are the synovial joints. Those most commonly involved are the:

- small joints of the hands and feet
- knees
- hips

Joint involvement is frequently symmetrical.

Unlike OA, where the articular surface is primarily affected, **rheumatoid arthritis (RA) is expressed initially in the form of abnormalities of the synovium and its secretions**.

Synovial Fluid

Volume is increased and there is a striking increase in the number of cells present. The predominant cell is the neutrophil, a cell seen only rarely in the synovial membrane. In acute cases, there may be 10^6 neutrophils per ml and $1-3 \times 10^5$ macrophages per ml. The increase in inflammatory cells is accompanied by a marked increase in the protein content, and polymerized fibrin may be present within the joint cavity.

Synovial Membrane Changes

Proliferation of Synovial Cell Lining

The cellular lining of the synovium, normally no more than two cells thick, is considerably thickened. Both the A cells and the B cells are increased in number. This is accompanied by a change in the surface architecture, the synovium being thrown into folds.

Increased Vascularity

The inflamed synovium appears much more vascular than normal. It is not clear whether this represents dilatation of pre-existing vessels or whether there is an actual increase in the number of small vessels. In some instances, the vessels resemble the high endothelial venules normally seen in lymph nodes, which represent the route by which lymphocytes leave the vascular compartment.

Increased Cellularity within the Synovial Membrane

The deeper layers of the synovium are hypercellular. The cell infiltrate is initially perivascular; prominent lymphoid follicles, with germinal centres in some cases, develop. The follicles and aggregates are rich in T_H cells though some T_C cells are present, mainly between the lymphoid follicles. The markers found on these T cells, most notably CD45RO, indicate a **memory** subpopulation. Plasma cells are found in large numbers in the interfollicular areas, as are some B lymphocytes (*Fig. 44.31*).

Evidence of Cell Activation within the Synovium

Cell activation is prominent in the inflamed synovium:

- **HLA class II expression is found on nearly all the cell types present; the level of expression**

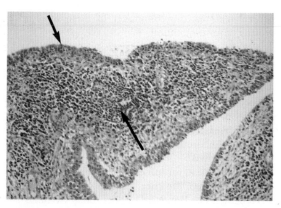

FIGURE 44.31 Synovium in rheumatoid arthritis showing hyperplasia of synovial lining cells (arrowed) and a florid inflammatory infiltrate in which lymphocyte aggregates are present (arrowed).

of these antigens is much greater than is seen in normal or osteoarthritic joints. HLA-DQ antigens are expressed in RA to a much greater extent than in other arthritides. It has been suggested that HLA-DQ T cells are part of the suppressor system of immune regulation.

- **Endothelial cells show a marked upregulation of adhesion molecules such as intercellular adhesion molecule 1 (ICAM-1) and E-selectin**, and macrophages show a similar degree of upregulation of integrin expression. Both these phenomena indicate increased inflammatory cell–endothelial cell interaction and, by implication, an increased release of the cytokines that trigger the expression of these molecules. The majority of the cells also show upregulation of the tumour necrosis factor (TNF) receptor, another reliable marker of activation.

Pannus Formation

The junction between the synovium, the articular cartilage and the bone is where the destructive aspect of the inflammatory process is first evident. **This area becomes covered by vascular tissue continuous with the inflamed synovium and which has been termed pannus** (*Fig. 44.32*).

Pannus leads to degradation of the underlying articular cartilage. This is likely to be due, in part, to the proteolytic effects of metalloproteinases and cytokines such as interleukin (IL)-1 and TNF-α, which can be identified within, and are released from the cells within the pannus, and in part to the pannus interfering with the nutrition of the cartilage, this being derived from the synovial fluid (*Fig. 44.33*). The bone adjacent to the pannus becomes demineralized and also porotic. This is not surprising because the cytokines mentioned above are known to stimulate osteoclastic resorption.

Permanent damage to the joints results from the

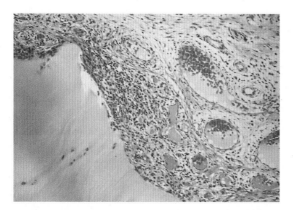

FIGURE 44.32 *Pannus consisting of inflamed, very vascular, granulation tissue.*

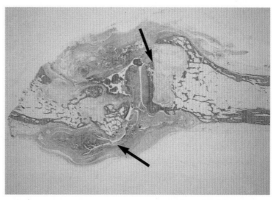

FIGURE 44.34 *Small joint in a hand severely affected by rheumatoid arthritis. The synovial lining and joint capsule are thickened and inflamed (arrow) and pannus has spread into the joint space, causing severe cartilage erosion (arrow).*

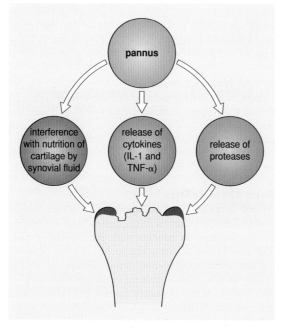

FIGURE 44.33 *Possible pathways of cartilage and bone destruction by pannus in rheumatoid arthritis.*

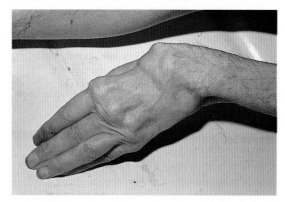

FIGURE 44.35 *Hand deformities in a patient with severe rheumatoid arthritis.*

action of the pannus (*Fig. 44.34*); the loss of articular cartilage may be followed by the formation of fibrous adhesions which severely limit joint movement. In some instances the fibrous adhesions across the joint space are replaced by metaplastic new bone (bony ankylosis). This rare complication is most likely in the small joints of the hands and feet.

Pannus also affects the joint capsule and periarticular tendons. This may lead to striking deformities, seen especially in the small joints of the hands (*Fig. 44.35*) where there may be marked ulnar deviation of the fingers; rupture of tendons can also occur. Such damage can be life threatening as, for example, in the cervical spine where atlantoaxial subluxation can occur with resulting compression of the spinal cord.

Pathological Changes Outside the Joints

Rheumatoid Nodules

Rheumatoid nodules occur in about 30% of patients, showing a predilection for pressure areas such as the extensor areas of the forearm. **Nodules consist of a central area of coagulative necrosis which is markedly eosinophilic, suggesting a fibrinoid type of necrosis. This necrotic zone is surrounded by macrophages and fibroblasts arranged in a palisaded fashion** (*Fig. 44.36*). HLA-DR expression is seen in these cells, suggesting that the central necrosis is due to the synthesis and secretion of proteases by the macrophages.

Occasionally, the skin over the nodules ulcerates. This is serious as it is likely to indicate necrotizing vasculitis. Nodules are most likely to occur in patients in whom the disease is severe and aggressive, and in whom **rheumatoid factors** are present.

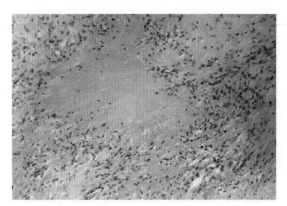

FIGURE 44.36 *Rheumatoid nodule consisting of a central eosinophilic zone of necrotic collagen. This is surrounded by a palisade of inflammatory cells.*

Rheumatoid Vasculitis

This is fortunately a relatively uncommon manifestation of rheumatoid disease. **It is associated with:**
- **high titres of IgG and IgM rheumatoid factors (so-called seropositive disease)**
- **cryoglobulinaemia**
- **hypocomplementaemia**
- **circulating immune complexes within the plasma.** It is thought that the vasculitis is due to deposition of immune complexes, formed in the zone of antigen excess, within blood vessel walls. As with other immune complex-mediated vasculitides, complex deposition is preceded by a local increase in vessel wall permeability. Immune complex deposition leads to complement activation via the classical pathway, and C5a and possibly C3a cause neutrophils to accumulate at the site of complex deposition. The release of enzymes from activated neutrophils causes damage to the blood vessel wall and this may be followed by thrombotic occlusion and ischaemic damage to the tissues downstream of the occlusion.

Microscopic examination of affected vessels shows fibrinoid necrosis associated with a neutrophil infiltrate. This affects all layers of the vessel wall. Thrombosis may or may not occur, and with time the affected segment of the vessel becomes occluded by vascular granulation tissue.

The clinical features depend on the size and site of the blood vessels affected. Thus:
- involvement of **capillaries** is associated with a 'glove and stocking' type of peripheral neuropathy
- damage to **arterioles** produces cutaneous ulceration, which may or may not be associated with rheumatoid nodules
- if **small to medium arteries** are affected, the patient may present with evidence of compromise of the function of some specific organ

- involvement of **veins** is associated with palpable purpura and with recurrent episodes of wheals in the skin

Lung Changes

Pleurisy is common but does not, as a rule, cause any symptoms. Rheumatoid nodules in the lung may occur in seropositive cases and they, too, are often asymptomatic. They may be single or multiple and may cause diagnostic problems because they show up as shadows on chest radiography. Rarely, diffuse interstitial fibrosis or fibrosing alveolitis may occur, particularly in patients with HLA-DR3 and the *PiZ* gene.

Cardiac Abnormalities

Asymptomatic pericarditis is common in patients with rheumatoid disease. Rheumatoid nodules in relation to conduction pathways may cause conduction disturbances; vasculitis, if it affects the coronary arteries may cause myocardial ischaemia and there may be aortic root dilatation leading to aortic incompetence in some cases.

Lymph Node Changes

Lymph node enlargement is common in rheumatoid disease but is rarely sufficiently marked as to render the nodes palpable. In a few cases the disease may present with widespread palpable nodes; histological examination shows a picture not greatly dissimilar from that seen in Hodgkin's disease.

Bone Abnormalities

As well as the localized osteoporosis that occurs in relation to actively inflamed joints, generalized osteoporosis may be seen in patients with rheumatoid disease. This may be due in part to the decline in physical activity that often accompanies active disease, or to the release of osteoclast-activating cytokines such as IL-1 and TNF-α. If it is necessary to treat the patients with glucocorticoids, the situation is obviously likely to be aggravated.

Eye Involvement

Rheumatoid vasculitis causes a severe inflammation of the sclera (scleritis), and rheumatoid disease is one of the common causes of scleritis. The eye is very painful and vision may become blurred. Rheumatoid nodules may be present in the affected sclera and may occasionally cause secondary glaucoma and, very rarely, perforation of the sclera.

Complications of Rheumatoid Disease

Amyloidosis

In Europe, rheumatoid disease is the commonest cause of reactive systemic amyloidosis, occurring in 2–5% of cases. Years may elapse before any clinical signs of amyloidosis appear, although this complication is more likely in chronic active disease in which an increase in the plasma concentration of **serum amyloid A protein** has been present.

Many tissues can show amyloid deposition, but kidney failure is the major hazard and overt manifestations of renal dysfunction due to amyloidosis have, until recently, carried a poor prognosis. It is now believed that active antirheumatoid treatment may improve the prognosis.

Felty's Syndrome

Felty's syndrome describes the triad of:
- **RA**
- **splenomegaly**
- **neutropenia**

It may occur in both adult and juvenile forms of rheumatoid disease and is fortunately rare (about 1% of hospital patients with RA).

The joint disease is characteristically active with much destruction of cartilage, and systemic manifestations are common. More than 50% of the patients with Felty's syndrome develop a secondary Sjögren's syndrome, and other not uncommon signs are enlargement of the liver and lymph nodes and pigmentation of the skin.

The defining criteria for diagnosis are the finding on three occasions at least of:
- **splenomegaly**
- **a white blood cell count of less than 2×10^9 per litre**

Serological Abnormalities in Felty's Syndrome
- **A high titre of IgG rheumatoid factor** is present in more than 90% of cases.
- **Granulocyte-specific, complement-fixing antinuclear antibodies** are present in many patients. Plasma from patients fails to stimulate colony formation in bone marrow cells in culture. Administration of granulocyte–macrophage colony-stimulating factor to patients with Felty's syndrome corrects the neutropenia but also causes an increase of IL-6 activity and a worsening of the arthritis.

These extra-articular events are summarized in *Fig. 44.37*.

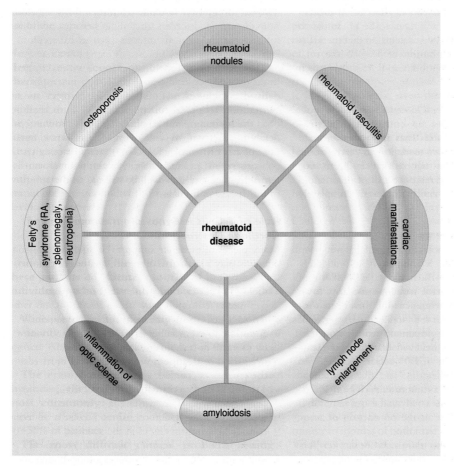

FIGURE 44.37 *Extra-articular manifestations of rheumatoid disease.*

Aetiology and Pathogenesis

The cause of rheumatoid disease is still unknown. It can be regarded as **an immunologically mediated disease involving both effector arms of the immune system (humoral and cellular). This occurs in a genetically primed host responding to a specific stimulus, which may well be an infective agent.**

Genetic Factors

The possibility of a genetic component was first suggested by a slight increase in the frequency of the disease in the first-degree relatives of patients with RA. Further support came from the observation that there is a 30% concordance of risk in monozygotic, compared with 5% in dizygotic twins.

With the advent of tissue typing, it was found that 60–70% of patients with rheumatoid disease expressed the major histocompatibility complex class II antigen HLA-DR4 (20–25% in the general population). Several subtypes of DR4 have now been defined; only some of these have a positive association with an increased risk of RA. The latter subtypes have a common feature in the form of **a substitution of glutamine and lysine at positions 70 and 71** of the HLA-DRβ1 chain. This is part of the class II protein concerned with binding of antigen to be presented to the T lymphocytes. It has been calculated that the HLA genes may make a contribution of 37% to the total genetic influence on susceptibility to RA; clearly much remains to be discovered.

Influence of Sex

RA occurs three times as commonly in premenopausal females as it does in males; women who take oral contraceptives appear to have some degree of protection. This suggests that sex hormones, presumably oestrogens, increase the risk of rheumatoid disease, although the mechanism is completely unknown.

Possible Infectious Agents

Despite much effort, no infectious agent has yet been identified beyond doubt. In human RA, one likely candidate is the **Epstein–Barr virus** (EBV). One of the EBV capsid antigens has a sequence similarity to an HLA-DR susceptibility sequence; this has been suggested as an explanation for the increased persistence of EBV in the B lymphocytes of patients with rheumatoid disease. In addition, it is believed that there is cross-reactivity between certain EBV nuclear antigens and collagen, actin and cytokeratins, and that this might lead to the induction of autoimmunity within joints. EBV is well known to be a polyclonal activator of B cells and this might influence the production of autoantibodies within the affected joints.

Other aetiological agents canvassed are the 65-kDa heat shock protein which is found in many cell types as well as in *Mycobacterium tuberculosis* and *Proteus mirabilis*.

IgG antibodies which react with *Proteus* have been reported in patients with RA but not in control subjects or in those with ankylosing spondylitis. Proof of an aetiological role is still lacking.

Goats develop an arthritis very similar to the human disease; this has been shown to be due to a retroviral infection. Some samples of human synovial tissue from patients with rheumatoid disease have been shown to contain retroviral *gag* proteins, and a transgenic mouse carrying human T-lymphotropic virus 1 has been reported as developing an arthritis similar to RA.

Production of Autoantibodies within the Joint

Synthesis of **rheumatoid factors (autoantibodies principally of IgM type reacting preferentially with determinants on the Fc portion of IgG)** is characteristic in rheumatoid disease; rheumatoid factors are found in the serum of 80% of patients with RA. These patients are termed seropositive. Seropositivity is associated with severe and aggressive disease, an increased likelihood of systemic manifestations and a poorer prognosis. Rheumatoid factor is, however, **not diagnostic** of rheumatoid disease because it may also be found in systemic lupus erythematosus, dermatomyositis, progressive systemic sclerosis and a number of non-rheumatic disorders including hepatic cirrhosis, infective granulomatous diseases such as tuberculosis, leprosy and pulmonary fibrosis, to name but a few.

The production of rheumatoid factor within affected joints may reflect local release of **IL-6**, a macrophage-derived cytokine that stimulates antibody production. In addition to the rheumatoid factors, antibodies in both the synovium and subchondral bone show a tendency to react with type II collagen, a major component of articular cartilage. IgG antibodies reacting with collagen type II produce arthritis when passively transferred to mice and may well contribute to the severity of the disease in humans.

Role of T Cells in Synovial Inflammation and Cartilage Destruction

Many pieces of evidence support the idea that T lymphocytes play a key role in the pathogenesis of rheumatoid arthritis:

- CD4 (T$_H$) cells are the principal T cell type in pannus.
- These T cells show numerous activation markers.
- A decline in the number of T cells brought about by thoracic duct drainage, total lymphoid irradiation or treatment with cyclosporin A lessens the severity of the disease.
- Treatment of patients with diphtheria toxin conjugated with IL-2, which binds with high specificity to the IL-2 receptor on T cells, produces considerable improvement in the arthritis.
- Injection of T cells reacting with collagen type II into joint cavities in rats produces a long-lasting and severe arthritis.

- Many of the T cells seen in the inflamed synovium are **memory cells** that release comparatively little IL-2 but promote monokine release from macrophages and the production of antibody from plasma cells.

> **KEY POINTS: Mechanisms of Joint Destruction in Rheumatoid Arthritis**
> - Pannus formation is promoted by activated macrophages which secrete angiogenic factors.
> - The newly formed blood vessels enhance invasion of the synovium by inflammatory cells and deliver nutrients and oxygen to these cells.
> - Immune complexes activate complement via the classical pathway and attract neutrophils. These neutrophils release large amounts of proteases and tissue-damaging oxygen free radicals.
> - Synovial lining cells and macrophages within the inflamed synovium release proteinases such as collagenase and stromelysin, and this contributes significantly to cartilage and bone erosion.
> - Clotting cascades involved in the coating of the synovium by fibrin promote further injury (e.g. fibrinopeptides attract neutrophils).
> - IL-1 causes a decrease in cartilage matrix production by the chondrocytes.
> - IL-1 and TNF-α activate osteoclasts and contribute to subchondral bone erosion and generalized osteoporosis.

JUVENILE RHEUMATOID ARTHRITIS

Juvenile rheumatoid arthritis (JRA) is not merely RA that affects juveniles, although one of its defining criteria is that the disease starts in individuals who are less than 16 years old. Some features of JRA, such as disturbances of skeletal growth, are related to the age of the patient whereas others seem to be intrinsic to this condition. The latter include:
- high spiking fever
- high white cell counts which may mimic leukaemic states
- a characteristic macular rash, the macules varying in diameter from 2 to 5 mm. The rash affects chiefly the trunk and limbs, although it may also occur on the face, palms and soles. Each macule is salmon pink in colour and is surrounded by a zone of pallor. The rash often appears in the afternoon accompanied by fever and may have vanished by the next morning.
- a predilection for the arthritis to affect the temporomandibular joints, the cervical spine and the wrists
- radial rather than ulnar deviation of the fingers
- involvement of the distal interphalangeal joints
- high prevalence of chronic iridocyclitis
- relative rarity of seropositivity

- rarity of rheumatoid nodules

Clinically, JRA shows considerable heterogeneity, leading some to suggest that it is a set of disorders rather than a single disease. Three main presentations have been described:

1) **Systemic onset JRA (Still's disease).** These patients have systemic manifestations at the time of onset of the disease. These include **enlargement of the liver, spleen and lymph nodes, and a typical 'rheumatoid rash'**. This presentation is seen in 20% of patients diagnosed as having JRA.

2) **Polyarticular onset.** These patients (40%) have numerous joints involved. This variant most closely resembles adult RA. Many of the patients are seropositive.

3) **Pauciarticular onset.** In this variant, accounting for the remaining 40% of patients, no more than four joints are involved at the time of presentation. Early-onset pauciarticular JRA affects young girls most commonly. The patients often show antinuclear antibodies in the serum and frequently suffer from chronic iridocyclitis (50% of cases). Late-onset pauciarticular disease affects boys more often than girls. Sacroiliac involvement is common and some go on to develop ankylosing spondylitis.

THE SPONDYLOARTHROPATHIES

The spondyloarthropathies are a set of disorders that may present purely as arthropathies or as arthropathies associated with disease in other systems. They share a number of striking features, shown below:

- **A strong association with class I histocompatibility antigens, most notably HLA-B27. This association varies from 50% in the arthritis associated with psoriasis and chronic inflammatory bowel disease, to more than 95% in the case of ankylosing spondylitis.** In normal healthy Caucasians, the frequency of HLA-B27 is 6–14%; in normal healthy black-skinned people it is 1–4%.
- **The arthritis tends particularly to affect the sacrum and the vertebral joints.**
- **Rheumatoid factors and any other serological markers of rheumatoid disease are not seen.** This has led to this group being called the **seronegative** arthropathies.
- The pathological changes affect especially **insertions of ligaments or tendons into bone** (entheses).
- There is a good deal of clinical overlap between the various spondyloarthropathies.
- There is a tendency for these conditions to aggregate within families.
- Evidence of involvement of other systems is found in the **eye, aortic valve and ascending aorta, skin and lung**.
- Amyloidosis of the reactive systemic variety may complicate any of this group of disorders.

The Spondyloarthropathies and their Relationship with HLA-B27

This is shown in *Table 44.15.*

HLA-B27

While the strength of the association of HLA-B27 with the spondyloarthropathies is well recognized, its role in their pathogenesis is still unknown. Possession of this haplotype is not of itself sufficient to account for the occurrence of these diseases. It is interesting, however, that transgenic mice carrying the human HLA-B27 gene develop a disorder not dissimilar from human ankylosing spondylitis, provided they are not kept in a germ-free environment.

Current hypotheses relating to HLA-B27 suggest that:

- **HLA-B27 might act as a receptor for certain microorganisms**; individuals with HLA-B27 who encounter the infectious trigger develop the disease.
- **Only HLA-B27 accepts the peptide that results from processing of a putative infectious agent within an antigen-presenting cell.**
- **'Molecular mimicry'.** The peptide antigen derived from processing of an organism within an antigen-presenting cell might have homology with part of the HLA-B27 molecule. This peptide is therefore not recognized as being foreign, no immune reaction occurs and the disease develops. Alternatively the peptide could be recognized as being foreign and an immune reaction mounted. This immune response could, however, damage cross-reacting 'self' tissue elements. There is, for example, some sharing of amino acid sequences between certain regions of the HLA-B27 molecule and certain regions of *Klebsiella pneumoniae* nitrogenase.

Ankylosing Spondylitis

The defining criteria of ankylosing spondylitis are:
- limitation of movement of the lumbar spine in three planes

- pain in the lumbar spine or dorsolumbar junction
- limitation of chest expansion to less than 2.5 cm
- radiological evidence of severe sacroiliitis

Epidemiology

The prevalence of ankylosing spondylitis appears to be about 0.25–1% of the population, with a peak of 2% found in the northern part of Norway. Most Caucasians who develop ankylosing spondylitis are HLA-B27 positive; the strength of this association is much less in black-skinned people. Some 5–20% of HLA-B27-positive individuals will develop the disease. Males are affected more often than females, the ratio being 2.5 : 1. In addition, the disease appears to pursue a more aggressive course in males. Ankylosing spondylitis makes its appearance most commonly in late teenage or early adult life.

Pathological Features

The pathological changes are characterized by ossification of the discs, the sacroiliac joints and the epiphyseal joints, this being initiated by lesions at the site of ligamentous insertions.

The target zone in which pathological changes occur is the enthesis. This is the area in which ligaments, tendons and capsules are inserted into bone and in which there is a change from the fibrous connective tissue structure characteristic of these first to fibrocartilage and then to bone. In the acute stages there is a plasma cell infiltrate and considerable amounts of the cytokines TNF-α and transforming growth factor (TGF) β are present in the affected tissues. TGF-β is a 'reparative' cytokine and may be responsible for the overgrowth of connective tissue matrix that occurs in this disease.

In the affected entheses scarring and bone formation take place and there is no destruction as such of affected joints. In the vertebral column the fibrosis and ossification affect the outer parts of the annulus fibrosus and this results in a curious 'squaring' of the vertebral bodies, destruction of the endplates of the vertebrae and

Table 44.15 Frequency of HLA-B27 in the Spondyloarthropathies

Disease	Frequency of HLA-B27 (%)
Ankylosing spondylitis	95 in Caucasians; 50 in non-Caucasians
Reactive arthropathy or Reiter's syndrome	80 in Caucasians; 50 in non-Caucasians
Enteropathic spondyloarthropathy (Crohn's disease, ulcerative colitis)	50
Psoriatic arthropathy	50–60
Uveitis	40–50

formation of bony outgrowths, which link up the adjacent vertebrae and immobilize the spine.

Some 20–40% of patients develop arthritis in peripheral joints; those most commonly affected are the hip and shoulder. This is most likely to occur in those who have developed the disease early (i.e. as teenagers).

Extra-articular Manifestations

- Many patients show **constitutional symptoms such as low-grade fever, fatigue, weight loss, a raised erythrocyte sedimentation rate and either hypochromic or normochromic anaemia**.
- **Iritis** occurs in up to 40% of patients and does not appear to be related to the activity of the joint disease.
- **Chronic infiltrative and fibrotic lesions in the upper lobes of the lungs** occur in some cases and may be associated with cough, dyspnoea and the production of large amounts of sputum. The histological appearances are non-specific, being similar to those described for other fibrosing lung diseases.
- **Cardiovascular complications** occur in a small proportion of patients who have had the disease for 15 years or more. **Aortic incompetence, cardiomegaly and persistent defects in conduction** are the most commonly encountered problems.

Reactive Arthropathies

This group of disorders is defined as **aseptic arthritides due to infections occurring outside the joints (e.g. *Shigella* species)**. As with ankylosing spondylitis, there is a strong association (in Caucasians) with HLA-B27.

Reiter's Syndrome

This archetype of reactive arthropathy has been described briefly in the section relating to psoriasis (see p 994); in this section attention is confined to the joint manifestations.

Three syndromes related to the joints may be seen:

1) **A peripheral arthritis syndrome**, in which two to four joints, chiefly the ankles and knees, are affected. Small joints of the hands and feet may also be involved; a sausage-like swelling of a digit (due to involvement of the tendon sheath) is very characteristic.

2) **An enthesopathic syndrome**, in which entheses of various bones become painful. Heel pain is particularly common.

3) **A pelviaxial syndrome**, in which dorsal, low back or buttock pain occurs. This is seen in about 50% of patients with a reactive arthropathy.

The extra-articular clinical features are many and various. They include **urethritis, cervicitis and diarrhoea**. Mucocutaneous problems such as balanitis and keratoderma blenorrhagicum, which resembles pustular psoriasis, occur. The eye is frequently affected; conjunctivitis is a common feature in the early stages of the natural history of the disease.

The first episode of oligoarticular arthropathy usually subsides within 3–6 months, although small joint disease and heel pain tend to persist for much longer. Balanitis and psoriatic lesions also tend to be stubborn. When all features are taken into consideration, 75% of the patients will be in remission by the end of 2 years. Relapses generally begin 3–4 years after the first episode.

Enteropathic Arthropathy

This may occur in association with:

- clinically overt inflammatory bowel disease such as ulcerative colitis or Crohn's disease
- mild gut symptoms or with mild histological evidence of gut inflammation not producing symptoms

In addition, arthritis may also occur in patients with Whipple's disease, jejunocolic bypass and collagenous colitis. These last three conditions do not, however, appear to be related to the spondyloarthropathies.

Psoriatic Arthropathy

This occurs in about 7% of inpatients with psoriasis, and affects males and females more or less equally. The prevalence in outpatients is said to be higher. The peak incidence is in the third and fourth decades of life.

The arthritis may affect any peripheral joint as well as the axial skeleton and the sacroiliac joints. The patients often complain of morning pain and stiffness, which gradually improve as the day goes on.

The disorder may be differentiated from RA by:

- psoriatic skin and nail lesions
- frequent involvement of the axial skeleton and sacroiliac joints
- frequent asymmetry of the distribution of affected joints
- erythema over the affected joints
- the rarity of rheumatoid factors in the serum of patients with psoriatic arthritis (about 10%)

INFECTIVE ARTHRITIS

Infective arthritis may be caused by bacteria, viruses and, rarely, by fungi. **The defining criterion is the presence of multiplying organisms within the joint**; this serves to distinguish infective arthritides from reactive joint disorders associated with infections at distant sites, such as Reiter's syndrome.

Common routes of infections are:

- by blood spread from a distant infected site
- by direct penetration through the skin to the joint cavity, as may occur in penetrating trauma
- by direct spread from a contiguous infected site such as is seen in the septic arthritis associated with adjacent osteomyelitis occurring in young children.

Blood spread is by far the most common. Micro-organisms can easily leave the bloodstream and gain access to the synovial membrane and, once there, may invade the joint cavity. Bacteraemia is an essential pre-requisite for such an arthritis to occur, but it is by no means always sufficient to trigger the inflammatory process, and several conditions are likely to increase the chances of acute arthritis. These include:

- **any pre-existing structural abnormality in the joint.** Thus a patient with any type of chronic arthropathy is at increased risk of developing septic arthritis.
- **the characteristics of the infecting organisms.** Organisms such as *Staphylococcus aureus* or *Neisseria gonorrhoeae*, which are common causes of bacterial arthritis, are either better able to adhere to synovial tissue or produce toxins that facilitate colonization.
- **the state of host immunity.** Compromised host immunity increases the likelihood of successful invasion of the tissues by microorganisms.

The acute inflammatory reaction elicited by the presence of bacteria multiplying within the synovial membrane and the joint cavity is associated with the release of large amounts of bacterial products and also of lysosomal enzymes released from dying neutrophils. These can have a profoundly damaging effect on the underlying articular cartilage. In animal models the presence of multiplying pathogenic microorganisms within the joint cavity reduces the proteoglycan content of cartilage by as much as 40% within 48 hours of the infection having become established. Such data point to the importance of early diagnosis of acute bacterial arthritis in humans.

Gonococcal and Non-gonococcal Arthritis

N. gonorrhoeae is the commonest cause of acute infective arthritis in adults. The conditions under which it occurs and its clinical features are distinct from those of non-gonococcal bacterial arthritis; the features that distinguish the two types are shown in *Table 44.16*.

Table 44.16 Features of Gonococcal and Non-gonococcal Arthritis

Non-gonococcal	Gonococcal
Seen most commonly in the very young and very old Pre-existing joint abnormality common; 10% of all cases of non-gonococcal arthritis occur in patients with RA	Peak incidence between 15 and 30 years (75% of cases) Victims are predominantly healthy and sexually active Usually no pre-existing joint disease
Predilection for males	More common in females
Hip likely to be site of infection in about 20% of cases Knee involved in 50% of cases	Hip involvement is uncommon
Usually monoarticular arthritis (80%)	Migratory involvement of several joints is common. In this variant the joint effusions may not be purulent Some patients present with single joint involvement and a purulent effusion resembling that seen in non-gonococcal disease
May be evidence of associated infection of skin, lung or urinary tract	Fever, a rash and tenosynovitis are common in the large group who present with polyarthritis
Organisms identifiable by Gram stain in synovial fluid in 50–65% of cases (75% in staphylococcal infections; 50% in infections by Gram-negative bacilli	Organisms identifiable by Gram stain in synovial fluid in 25% of cases
Positive culture of synovial fluid in 90% of cases	Positive culture of synovial fluid in 50% of cases
Marked increase in lactate concentrations in synovial fluid	No increase in lactate concentration in synovial fluid
Response to antibiotics often slow and open drainage may be required	Rapid response to antibiotics
Mortality rate of about 10%, and roughly 30% have residual joint damage after resolution of the inflammatory process	Full recovery in most cases
	Increased risk of *Neisseria* infections in individuals with terminal complement deficiencies (C5–C9)

Causes of Acute Non-gonococcal Bacterial Arthritis

A wide variety of organisms has been cultured from infected joints. The most common pathogens and the frequency with which they are found are shown in *Table 44.17*.

Tuberculosis and Joint Disease

Tuberculosis involves the joints either by:
- haematogenous dissemination of the organisms
- spread from adjacent bone in which tuberculous osteitis is present

Osteoarticular tuberculosis may be expressed in the form of a number of clinical syndromes:
- **tuberculous spondylitis** (Pott's disease of the spine)
- **peripheral arthritis**
- **tuberculous osteomyelitis**
- **dactylitis** (osteomyelitis affecting the long bones of the hands and feet)
- **tenosynovitis and bursitis**
- **Poncet's disease** (a somewhat controversial entity in which an aseptic polyarthritis develops in the presence of tuberculous lesions elsewhere in the body)

Tuberculous osteitis and spondylitis are discussed elsewhere (see p 1071), and in this section only peripheral arthritis is considered.

This is almost always associated with infection due to haematogenous dissemination. It is believed that low-grade trauma may play some part in the pathogenesis because there is a predilection for weight-bearing joints. The knee, hip, elbow and ankle are involved, in descending order of frequency.

The most common clinical presentation is the insidious development of joint pain associated with limitation of movement. Swelling is usually marked due to a combination of synovial hyperplasia and a large joint cavity effusion. Other cardinal signs of inflammation are mild or sometimes absent. The synovial fluid is hypercellular and, interestingly, in view of the usual macrophage response to the presence of *M. tuberculosis*,

the majority of the cells are neutrophils. Synovial biopsy shows the typical granulomatous lesions of tuberculosis in more than 90% of cases. Acid-fast bacilli are seldom identified in either synovial fluid or synovial tissue, but culture on Lowenstein–Jensen medium yields a positive result in about 80% of cases.

Lyme Disease

Epidemiology

Lyme disease is a disorder normally endemic in mammals, especially rodents in North America and Europe. It is caused by a spirochaete known as **Borrelia burgdorferi**, transmitted to humans via tick bites. It is the leading vector-borne disease in the United States, some 9600 cases having been reported there in 1992 alone.

Transmission

Several different species of tick transmit the disease to humans. They include the Eurasian species **Ixodes ricinus** and **persulcatus**, and the North American species **Ixodes dammini** (also known as **scapularius**) and **pacificus**. After the tick feeds on blood of an infected animal, *Borrelia* penetrates the mucosa of the mid-gut wall and is disseminated into other tissues including the salivary glands. This process takes 24–72 hours. When the infected tick bites a human, the organism is probably transmitted via saliva. Many tick bites are painless and about half the patients with Lyme disease have no memory of having been bitten.

Lyme disease affects many tissues. These include:
- the skin
- the nervous system
- the heart
- the joints

All age groups are affected and the early stages of the disorder are seen most commonly between June and October, when both activity of the nymph stage of the ixodid ticks and outdoor activities of humans are at their height. Later manifestations are present in the community throughout the year.

Clinical Features

Three clinical stages have been delineated. Not all of these necessarily appear in an orderly pattern within a single patient and they show a considerable degree of overlap. The first two stages occur early in the course of the disease, manifesting within a few weeks or months of infection. The third stage makes its appearance after 6–12 months or even some years, and clearly represents the late stage of the disorder.

Lyme disease has been compared by some to syphilis in that it is caused by a spirochaete, and can be expressed as both an acute and a chronic multisystem disorder. Like syphilis, the causative organism disseminates widely from the site of infection; cytokines and

---

Table 44.17 Frequency of Non-gonococcal Bacterial Causes of Arthritis

Organism	Frequency (%)
Staphylococcus aureus	40–50
Staphylococcus epidermidis	10–15
Streptococcus pneumoniae	2
Other streptococcal species	20
Gram-negative bacilli	15
Haemophilus influenzae	2
Various anaerobic species	5

autoimmune mechanisms may be implicated in the pathogenesis of the later stages.

The growth of the responsible *Borrelia* can be inhibited *in vitro* by a variety of antibiotics, which include doxycycline, tetracycline, amoxycillin, cefuroxime, erythromycin, ceftazidime, azithromycin and imipenem. These appear to be effective agents in infected humans.

Stage I

Typically the early localized stage of Lyme disease is marked by the development of a macular skin lesion known as **erythema migrans**. It occurs in 60–80% of patients and is usually accompanied by a low-grade fever, headache, shifting arthralgia, muscle pain and enlargement of regional lymph nodes.

This skin lesion can appear from 3 days to 16 weeks after infection, the mean time being about 10 days. It is a round to oval macule with a well-demarcated edge. It is quite large, the median size being 15 cm in diameter, although occasionally smaller lesions may occur. The initial erythematous lesion then expands and may reach a diameter of more than 30 cm, the centre appearing to clear, at least in part. After 3 or 4 weeks, erythema migrans usually resolves, although it may recur.

Stage II (Early Disseminated Form)

Dissemination of the *B. burgdorferi* from the site of the tick bite usually occurs within days to weeks of infection. As spread is via the bloodstream, the clinical manifestations may be wide ranging.

Skin Multiple ring-like lesions occur which are generally smaller than the primary lesion. Fever and its associated constitutional symptoms are still present at this stage. Some patients develop a peculiar skin lesion which is known as a borrelial lymphocytoma. This occurs most commonly in the nipples or ear lobes and is a bluish-red nodular infiltrate. This lesion occurs most commonly in stage II but can be seen in any stage.

Nervous System The commonest evidence of involvement of the nervous system during the early localized and early disseminated phase of Lyme disease is cranial neuritis. This is most frequently manifested in the form of facial palsy which may be bilateral. Peripheral neuropathies and/or lymphocytic meningitis or meningoencephalitis may also occur. In Europe, the commonest neurological abnormality is said to be Bannwarth's syndrome, a combination of severe root pain, commonly experienced at night, and an increase of lymphocytes in the cerebrospinal fluid (CSF), without, however, any overt signs of meningitis.

Heart A small proportion of patients with Lyme disease (about 8%) develop varying degrees of atrioventricular block, which in some cases is so severe as to need the insertion of a temporary pacemaker.

Stage III

Clinical features of chronic disease may occur months to years after the initial infection, and again, not surprisingly, several quite disparate clinical syndromes may develop.

Chronic Arthritis Chronic arthritis is fairly uncommon in patients with Lyme disease, being reported in 10% of North American patients who have had erythema migrans, although transient arthritis is much more frequently encountered. The arthritis usually involves only a few joints and is asymmetrical in distribution. Large joints, especially the knee, are involved, others being, in descending order of frequency, the shoulder, ankle, elbow and wrist. Patients with chronic Lyme disease-related arthritis often have the haplotype HLA-DR4, which is also said to be associated with a poor response to antimicrobial treatment.

Microscopic examination of the synovium shows a florid degree of synovitis associated with villus hypertrophy, fibrin deposits and an increase in vascularity. Plasma cells and macrophages predominate in the synovial inflammatory infiltrate and lymphoid aggregates similar to those that occur in rheumatoid arthritis may be present.

The joint fluid is typically inflammatory in that there is usually a considerable increase in cells, the majority of which are neutrophils.

Nervous System Expressions of chronic involvement of the nervous system include a subacute encephalopathy presenting clinically in the form of cognitive disturbance and disturbances of mood and sleep. Unlike chronic arthritis which usually 'burns out' after a few years, chronic neurological disease may persist for more than 10 years. In these patients, perivascular lesions may be detected by the use of magnetic resonance imaging. These lesions can be distinguished from those of multiple sclerosis by the presence of antibodies against *Borrelia* in the CSF and by a higher cell count in the CSF.

Skin The skin lesion characteristically associated with chronic Lyme disease is known as **acrodermatitis chronica atrophicans** (ACA). These lesions start as bluish-red areas with a somewhat 'doughy' consistency and become progressively atrophic, the skin in the affected areas becoming wrinkled. ACA may be accompanied by rheumatological manifestations which differ significantly from the chronic arthritis of Lyme disease described above. In patients with ACA small joint involvement is common and this may lead to subluxation of the small joints of the hands and feet. ACA is uncommon in the USA but has been reported not infrequently in northern Europe.

CRYSTAL ARTHROPATHIES

This is a set of disorders in which the deposition of various crystals in the joints and in periarticular tissues produce acute and chronic arthritis, periarthritis and tendinitis. Such crystals may be endogenous or exogenous in origin. The more common and important crystal-mediated joint disorders arise on a basis of endogenous crystal deposition. The pathogenic endogenous crystals are:

- monosodium urate
- calcium pyrophosphate dihydrate
- basic calcium phosphate (hydroxyapatite)

Monosodium Urate Deposition: Gout

Gout is a very ancient disease but its association with deposition of urate crystal from a supersaturated solution was not recognized until 1859.

Gout should be regarded not as a single disorder but rather as a set of diseases with the common features of:

- deposition of monosodium urate monohydrate crystals within the tissues
- abnormally high concentrations of uric acid in body fluids

Hyperuricaemia

Hyperuricaemia is defined as a serum urate level greater than two standard deviations from the mean. The upper limit of normal for an adult male in the UK and USA is 7 mg/dl, and that for a female is 6 mg/dl. Serum is saturated with urate at a concentration of 7 mg/dl but it is possible for much higher concentrations to remain in stable supersaturated solutions for quite long periods.

The concentration of uric acid in body fluids depends on the balance between purine ingestion and synthesis on the one hand and uric acid elimination (two-thirds of which is carried out in the kidney) on the other. Thus hyperuricaemia may be the result of:

- increased purine synthesis
- increased purine ingestion
- decreased renal elimination of uric acid
- a combination of decreased uric acid elimination plus one or more of the others

Prolonged hyperuricaemia is usually necessary before tissue deposition of urate crystals and clinical manifestations of gout occur, but hyperuricaemia alone may not be sufficient to precipitate clinical disease. There is no doubt that the higher the uric acid concentrations, in males at least, the greater is the risk of developing gout. Thus the 5-year cumulative incidence of gout in males whose uric acid level is less than 6 mg/dl is 0.5%. In those whose uric acid concentration is greater than 10 mg/dl, the incidence is 30.5%.

Serum urate concentrations are distributed within populations as a continuous variable, with mean values being higher in males than in females and a broader distribution curve in males. At puberty the serum levels rise in boys and then remain more or less constant. In girls, there is a smaller rise associated with the menarche and the serum concentrations of urate start to approach those obtaining in males only after the menopause. Population studies suggest that there is some polygenic control of urate levels, but there are some clear differences within single ethnic groups, suggesting that environmental factors play a significant part in determining the concentrations of urate. These factors probably include:

- a high dietary intake of purine and proteins
- high alcohol consumption
- high body-weight and bulk

Uric Acid Excretion

When the diet is unrestricted in terms of protein and purine intake, about 1000 mg uric acid is excreted in the urine each day. A four-component system is involved in the renal handling of uric acid:

1) Glomerular ultrafiltration is complete as urate is not bound to plasma proteins.
2) Urate is then reabsorbed in the proximal tubule via an active transport mechanism closely linked with that responsible for the tubular reabsorption of sodium.
3) Active secretion of urate into the tubule then occurs more distally.
4) Postsecretory reabsorption then occurs.

Renal clearance of urate in normal individuals is of the order of 6–9 ml/min, thus being much less than the clearance of creatinine or inulin.

Which of the Possible Mechanisms is/are involved in the Pathogenesis of Gout?

- In 75–90% of patients with so-called 'primary' gout, the hyperuricaemia is associated with a decreased fractional excretion of uric acid. Uric acid clearance is reduced to about 3.6 ml/min whereas creatinine clearance remains normal. This is likely to result from decreased urate secretion or increased urate reabsorption, or a combination of these.
- Increased uric acid production and excretion are found in 10–15% of cases of gout. In most of these the cause of the increased purine synthesis is not known but, in a minority, there is evidence of a specific inherited enzyme defect related to purine synthesis or metabolism.
- In about 10% of patients with gout there is evidence that the hyperuricaemia is due either to increased cellular turnover or to increased catabolism of purines.
- Secondary hyperuricaemia and gout have many causes. The hyperuricaemia is the expression of changes in renal blood flow, tubular reabsorption and secretion of uric acid. A wide variety of diseases may cause secondary gout, including chronic renal disease of all types. In addition several drugs are known to produce hyperuricaemia. Amongst them

are thiazide diuretics, salicylates in low doses, ethambutol and pyrazinamide.

Inborn Errors of Metabolism and Gout
Three single gene defects have been identified which lead to severe gout as a result of increased purine synthesis.

1. The Lesch–Nyhan Syndrome
This disease results from an X-linked deficiency of the purine 'salvage' enzyme **hypoxanthine guanine phosphoribosyl transferase (HPRT)**. This is involved in the recapture of free purine bases derived from the breakdown of endogenous or exogenous nucleic acid. Absence of this enzyme, and the resulting failure in the salvage of these purine bases, leads to an increased *de novo* synthesis of purine nucleotides and a very significant increase in uric acid concentrations.

The syndrome, first described in 1964, is characterized by primary purine overproduction, hyperuricaemia and gout, associated with a bizarre neurological syndrome:
- choreoathetosis
- mental deficiency of differing degrees of severity
- spasticity
- a strange behavioural disturbance characterized by self-mutilation

In a significant proportion of cases, macrocytosis and megaloblastic anaemia are present.

The clinical expression of the disease is, not surprisingly, confined to males. Affected infants appear quite normal at birth but mothers may comment on the presence of orange crystals in the napkins. By the age of 3 months a delay in motor development is obvious and over the next year extrapyramidal signs gradually appear. The compulsive behavioural disturbance may become evident any time between 2 and 16 years. Gouty arthritis and tophi are also seldom seen before puberty.

The biochemical basis for the neurological abnormalities is unknown. A number of chemical species including dopamine, homovanillic acid, tyrosine hydroxylase and dopa decarboxylase are present in decreased amounts in the putamen of affected individuals, but these findings still await interpretation.

Drugs such as allopurinol lower the uric acid levels, although total purine excretion is not affected as in other patients with gout. Such treatment prevents the development of gouty arthritis and the other manifestations of gout but, alas, has no effect on the neurological syndrome or behavioural abnormality.

Partial HPRT Deficiency A partial deficiency of HPRT has been described in which severe familial X-linked gout occurs. In 75% of these cases there are no neurological disturbances; in the remainder such disturbances are present but are mild.

2. Phosphoribosyl Pyrophosphate Synthetase
An X-linked syndrome exists in which there is severe overproduction of purines associated with a mutation resulting in increased activity of the enzyme PP-ribose-p synthetase. Affected boys develop gout or renal stones in childhood or early in adult life. Deafness may be seen both in the affected children and their heterozygous mothers but the basis for this is unknown.

3. Glucose-6-phosphatase
Glycogen storage disease type I (von Gierke's disease) is due to a severe deficiency of glucose-6-phosphatase and this is associated with severe hyperuricaemia. Gouty arthritis may become manifest before the end of the first decade and, in patients who survive to adult life, chronic tophaceous gout with kidney involvement may be a major clinical problem.

Pathogenesis
Hyperuricaemia will not lead to acute gouty arthritis unless monosodium urate crystals are deposited in the tissues from a supersaturated solution. The factors that control this deposition are poorly understood.

A long period of 'silent' hyperuricaemia always precedes the development of acute gouty arthritis and during this phase some degree of crystal deposition may occur in relatively avascular areas such as tendons. Local metabolic alterations or trauma may lead to such crystals escaping from their connective tissue sheaths, and in such patients an attack of acute gouty arthritis may occur at a time when the uric acid is not raised.

Factors triggering acute attacks of gout are believed to include **alcohol, dietary indiscretions, trauma, surgery and infection**. In the case of infection, it has been suggested that the attacks are initiated because of the release of the proinflammatory monokine IL-1 from activated macrophages.

Once microcrystals of monosodium urate have been deposited, they absorb immunoglobulin, fibrinogen, fibronectin and some complement components on to their surfaces. These proteins act as opsonins and facilitate the phagocytosis of the crystals by neutrophils and macrophages. The presence of the crystals within phagolysosomes leads to rupture of the organelle membrane with consequent spillage of the lysosomal contents. This is accompanied by complement activation and the release of a large number of acute inflammatory mediators.

The neutrophil plays a dominant role in the process of acute gouty arthritis and, indeed, **the effectiveness of colchicine in acute gout is due to its inhibitory effect on the migration of neutrophils to the site of crystal deposition** and on other neutrophil functions as well. It must be said, however, that acute gouty arthritis can occur in the absence of a significant neutrophil infiltrate. In such circumstances, it is likely that monocytes and resident macrophages are responsible for the inflammatory reaction. It is worth remembering also that **monosodium urate crystals can themselves stimulate IL-1 and TNF-α production by monocytes and macrophages**, and thus may trigger an inflammatory reaction in the absence of neutrophil phagocytosis. **It is clear, therefore, that crystal deposition is necessary for the full expression of acute gout but not necessarily sufficient for it.**

Clinical Features
There are four stages in the natural history of gout, not all of which will necessarily be present in any individual sufferer.

1. Hyperuricaemia with No Symptoms
Many years of asymptomatic increase in uric acid levels may precede the clinical presentation of gout; it is said that 19 of 20 individuals with hyperuricaemia remain free from symptoms of gout throughout their lives.

2. Acute Gouty Arthritis
This is the classical clinical manifestation of gout and is eight times as common in males as in females. As Hippocrates stated, it is rare in males before puberty and equally rare in females before the menopause. The peak incidence in males is between 30 and 60 years.

The metatarsophalangeal joint of the big toe is the commonest site (70%). Other sites include the ankle, knee, wrist, elbow and small joints of the hands and feet, in descending order of frequency.

The onset of the pain is usually sudden; the affected joint shows the classical signs of acute inflammation, becoming red, hot, swollen, painful and tender. Often the attack starts at night, the patients being woken from sleep by the pain. Both the synovium and the joint fluid usually show large numbers of infiltrating neutrophils. Clusters of urate crystals may be seen within the synovium and individual crystals may be identified within the cytoplasm of the neutrophils. Left untreated, the acute attack usually resolves spontaneously; this may take hours, days or weeks depending on the severity of the attack.

3. The Intercritical Phase
This is the asymptomatic period between episodes of acute arthritis, and may last months or even years. Some unfortunate individuals have recurrent attacks of gouty arthritis with progressive shortening of the intercritical period.

4. Chronic Tophaceous Gouty Arthritis
This follows recurrent episodes of acute gouty arthritis and is characterized by asymmetrical swelling of the affected joints. A **tophus** is a large yellowish-white mass of urate crystals easily visible with the naked eye. It elicits a mixed inflammatory reaction consisting of macrophages, foreign body-type giant cells and lymphocytes.

Tophi are found typically in the periarticular tissues, bursae, tendon sheaths and cartilage of the outer ear. Rare sites include the eye, skin, tongue, larynx and heart, where they may interfere with cardiac conduction. Tophaceous gout may be associated with progressive erosion of cartilage and bone, and joint function can become progressively and irreversibly limited.

Effect of Gout on the Kidney
Gout affects the kidney in three ways:
1) **Acute uric acid nephropathy.** Acute renal failure may occur when there is sudden precipitation of urate crystals in the renal collecting ducts and ureters. It is most likely to occur in patients with leukaemia treated with cytotoxic agents and who thus may have secondary gout. The development of acute renal failure is favoured if the patient has been allowed to become dehydrated and acidotic. It is an entirely preventable problem. The sharp rise in uric acid levels due to the cytotoxic drug-mediated cellular breakdown may be prevented by giving the patient the competitive inhibitor of xanthine oxidase, allopurinol. This syndrome can occur in patients with primary gout also especially if the latter is associated with greatly increased *de novo* synthesis of purines.
2) **Chronic renal disease.** It is now believed that chronic renal failure occurs, for the most part, in those whose gout is due to inherited abnormalities of metabolism with overproduction of purines and those with rare forms of inherited renal disease.
3) **Uric acid stones.** These are discussed in the section dealing with renal calculi in general (see p 698).

Some Other Clinical Associations of Gout
In males gout is often associated with:
- obesity
- a substantial intake of alcohol
- hypertriglyceridaemia
- impaired glucose tolerance (which in any case is associated with the type IV hyperlipidaemia)
- hypertension and ischaemic heart disease

Some of these associations are explored in *Table 44.18*.

Calcium Pyrophosphate Dihydrate Deposition: Pseudogout and Chondrocalcinosis
Calcium pyrophosphate dihydrate (CPPD) crystals may be deposited within:
- synovium, giving rise to acute inflammatory arthritis (**pseudogout**)
- articular or meniscus cartilage (**chondrocalcinosis**), in which case the affected persons may develop chronic arthritis that can resemble RA or OA.

Table 44.18 Associations with Gout in Males

Condition	Frequency and Findings
Obesity	This may be the major linking factor in this set of associations. Gouty males are, on average, 15–20% above their ideal weight, and the greater the degree of overweight, the greater is the proportion of males who are hyperuricaemic
Hypertriglyceridaemia	Some 75% of men with gout are hypertriglyceridaemic and 75% of hypertriglyceridaemic men have hyperuricaemia. Non-gouty members of the family are not affected; heavy alcohol intake and obesity appear to contribute to the hyperlipidaemia
Hypertension	This is seen in 25–50% of gouty individuals

Pathogenesis

Two questions need to be posed in any attempt to explain the joint pathology in this set of disorders:

1) **Why is the concentration of pyrophosphate raised in the joints of individuals who suffer from pseudogout or chondrocalcinosis?**

2) **Why and how does the presence of raised intra-articular pyrophosphate cause joint disturbances?**

There is no doubt that increased levels of pyrophosphate are found in the synovial fluid of patients suffering from these conditions and there is a direct relationship between the concentration of pyrophosphate and the severity of the underlying joint disease. It must be noted, however, that similar increases may be found from time to time in patients with other arthropathies.

Joint pyrophosphate is derived from the hydrolysis of nucleoside triphosphates, this being carried out in the cartilage cells rather than in those of synovium or bone. Normally the large amounts of pyrophosphate generated within mammalian cells are cleaved by pyrophosphatases. The fact that chondrocalcinosis is a disorder found principally in the elderly suggests that declining levels of these enzymes may be a cause of the raised intra-articular levels of the pyrophosphate.

The presence of CPPD crystals within meniscus or articular cartilage is not associated with acute inflammation. However, when crystals are shed from the cartilage into the joint cavity, acute attacks of pseudogout usually occur. Such crystal shedding may follow trauma or may, in some cases, be associated with a sudden decrease in the concentration of calcium or pyrophosphate in the joint cavity following parathyroidectomy.

Another circumstance leading to CPPD accumulation within the synovial cavity is the presence of an acute infective arthritis in an individual with chondrocalcinosis. The enzymes and cytokines released may 'strip out' the crystals from articular cartilage. Once the crystals have gained access to the joint cavity, the events that follow are thought to be similar to those occurring in acute gouty arthritis.

CPPD disease may occur under four circumstances:

1) sporadic disease, the cause of which is not known but which is clearly associated with ageing
2) familial disease
3) associated with one of a number of metabolic disorders
4) following trauma or surgery to the joints

Chondrocalcinosis, as diagnosed on radiography, is rare below the age of 40 years; its prevalence increases steadily after that, as shown in *Table 44.19*.

Familial CPPD Disease

Hereditary chondrocalcinosis has been reported in about 50 families. The disorder appears to be inherited in an autosomal dominant fashion. No consistent genetic marker has been identified. Clinically, these patients tend to present with severe polyarticular disease, starting as early as the third decade.

CPPD Disease Associated with Metabolic Disorders

These are described in *Table 44.20*.

Basic Calcium Phosphate (Hydroxyapatite) Deposition

Hydroxyapatite is a normal, indeed an essential, constituent of bone and teeth. Its deposition in soft tissue or

Table 44.19 Influence of Age on Prevalence of Chondrocalcinosis

Age (years)	Radiographic evidence of chondrocalcinosis (%)
65–74	15
75–84	36
> 84	44

Table 44.20 Metabolic Disorders Associated with CPPD Disease

Disorder	Findings
Hyperparathyroidism	Hyperparathyroidism is found in 10% of patients with CPPD disease, and one-third of patients with primary hyperparathyroidism have age-related chondrocalcinosis. CPPD disease does not appear to be caused by the hypercalcaemia as it does not occur in most other hypercalcaemic states.
Haemochromatosis	Radiological evidence of chondrocalcinosis is found in 25% of patients with haemochromatosis, and arthropathy, without radiological evidence of CPPD deposition in 50%. Transfusion siderosis can also be associated with chondrocalcinosis. Divalent iron inhibits pyrophosphatase activity and ferric iron salts promote the growth of CPPD crystals *in vitro*.
Hypophosphatasia	This rare disorder is associated with attacks of both pseudogout and chondrocalcinosis. Plasma and urine concentrations of inorganic pyrophosphate are raised.
Hypomagnesaemia	Familial hypomagnesaemia is regularly associated with chondrocalcinosis. CPPD disease is also occasionally seen in other conditions associated with low plasma levels of magnesium due to increased renal loss, such as Wilson's disease and Bartter's syndrome. *In vitro*, magnesium salts are known to promote the solubility of CPPD crystals.
Ochronosis (alkaptonuria)	Disc degeneration and a severe arthropathy of large joints is seen in this condition and may be associated with CPPD deposition.
Hypothyroidism	Evidence of hypothyroidism has been found in 11% of patients with CPPD disease.

within joints may be associated with acute or chronic arthropathy or with painful syndromes related to ligaments and tendons such as supraspinatus tendinitis or rotator cuff injuries. Hydroxyapatite crystal deposition may be seen also in connective tissues in a wide variety of other disorders, but this appears to be a secondary phenomenon.

TUMOURS AND TUMOUR-LIKE LESIONS OF JOINTS

True neoplasms of joints and tendon sheath are rare and the majority are benign. Synovial sarcoma can and does undoubtedly occur in these locations in some instances, but is more common in soft tissues and will be considered under the rubric of soft tissue tumours.

Pigmented Villonodular Synovitis and Giant Cell Tumour of Tendon Sheath

Despite its misleading name, pigmented villonodular synovitis is almost certainly a benign neoplasm rather than a reactive or inflammatory condition. Support for this view comes from the observation of **non-random chromosomal aberrations in this lesion, trisomies 5 and 7 being the most characteristic**.

Pigmented villonodular synovitis and giant cell tumour of tendon sheath have more or less identical morphological features and probably represent expressions of the same process. The former usually involves the synovium of the affected joint **diffusely**; the latter usually forms a discrete nodule on one of the tendon sheaths, the hands being most frequently affected.

Pigmented villonodular synovitis occurs most frequently in the knee joint (80% of cases), although the lesion may also be seen in the hip, toes, ankle, wrist, elbow and small joints of the hands. The peak incidence is between the third and fifth decades, and the sexes are equally affected. Symptoms, if present, usually take the form of mild pain, swelling and tenderness of the affected joint.

Radiological examination often shows erosion of the articular cartilage and underlying subchondral bone. Aspiration of the joint usually reveals a brown-coloured or frankly blood-stained synovial fluid. On arthroscopy the synovium is seen to be thickened and to be thrown into small villous folds. The term 'mossy' has often been applied to the macroscopic appearance of pigmented villonodular synovitis.

Microscopic Features

Examination shows numerous macrophages with finely vacuolated cytoplasm, presumably due to lipid. The synovial lining cells, macrophages and spindle-shaped stromal cells usually contain abundant haemosiderin. Lymphocytes are present in moderate numbers and the number of multinuclear giant cells differs from case to case and from area to area within individual lesions.

> **The presence of haemosiderin alone within the synovial tissues is not diagnostic of pigmented villonodular synovitis** because several other conditions, including haemochromatosis, haemophilia and rheumatoid disease, may show iron deposition. As there is a distinct tendency for pigmented villonodular synovitis to recur, it is important to make a correct diagnosis on the initial biopsy.

Giant Cell Tumour of Tendon Sheath

This is the term applied to the localized form of the process described above. Although it may occur within a joint, this lesion is most frequently found in the tendon sheaths of the hands. The lesions are well-defined, lobulated masses which have a greyish cut surface in which localized areas of yellow (indicating accumulated lipid) or brown (indicating the presence of haemosiderin) discoloration may be seen.

Microscopic Features

There is a dual cell population, consisting of spindle-like fibroblasts and macrophages. Many of these macrophages contain large amounts of lipid and therefore have a 'foamy' appearance. Multinucleate giant cells are often abundant; some degree of haemosiderin pigmentation is usually present.

Synovial Chondromatosis

Synovial chondromatosis is a set of disorders with the common feature of islands of cartilage within the synovium.

Primary synovial chondromatosis is a benign, slowly progressive, condition in which metaplastic islands of cartilage form within the synovial tissue. Some of these may become detached and are released into the joint cavity where they may give rise to mechanical problems characterized by pain, stiffness and swelling. The hip and knee are most frequently involved, although the condition may also affect other joints.

Microscopic Features

Cartilaginous islands are seen **within the synovium**. These islands have a rather disorganized appearance with clustering of chondrocytes and some degree of cellular atypia. Despite this, the lesion has a benign natural history. Occasionally the islands of cartilage undergo ossification (synovial osteochondromatosis).

Islands of cartilage may also be found within the synovium as a secondary phenomenon associated with a variety of joint diseases. In these conditions, which include osteochondritis dissecans and both inflammatory and non-inflammatory joint disease, portions of articular cartilage may become detached and embedded within the synovial tissues. In this site, some of the fragments continue to grow.

Ganglion

A ganglion is a thin-walled cyst containing mucoid fluid. It is seen most commonly on the extensor surfaces of the hands and feet, with a particular predilection for the wrist. It may arise from joint synovium or from areas of myxoid degeneration in the connective tissue of the tendon sheath.

Tumours and Tumour-like Lesions of Soft Tissue

Soft tissue neoplasms are those arising in non-skeletal mesodermal tissues such as adipose tissue, muscle, fibrous tissue, blood vessels and, despite their neuroectodermal origin, peripheral nerves. Malignant soft tissue tumours (sarcomas) account for less than 1% of all invasive neoplasms, and their often highly malignant behaviour is shown by the fact that they are the cause of at least 2% of all deaths from malignant disease.

Soft tissue neoplasms are named according to the mature tissues they most closely resemble (e.g. a malignant tumour that resembles adipose tissue is called a liposarcoma). However, in some cases the lesions are so undifferentiated as to make a morphological diagnosis very difficult. It is important also to realize that, although a given neoplasm recapitulates, in part, the structure of a certain soft tissue element, **this does not mean that it originates from that element**. Indeed, in some instances tumours may develop at sites where the tissue that they resemble is completely absent. This situation is exemplified by extraosseous osteosarcomas and chondrosarcomas, which occur at sites where neither bone nor cartilage is present.

The most commonly occurring sarcomas are listed in *Table 44.21*. No other single histological type accounts for more than 4% of all soft tissue sarcomas, and 10–15% remain unclassifiable.

Aetiology

The aetiology of the vast majority of these lesions is totally unknown, although a few interesting associations exist:
- **Genetically determined syndromes.** These include such entities as:
  1) type I neurofibromatosis (von Recklinghausen's disease) which, in addition to the presence of

Table 44.21 Commonly Occurring Sarcomas

Tumour type	Frequency as a percentage of histologically classifiable sarcomas
Liposarcoma	17
Leiomyosarcoma (smooth muscle)	14
Rhabdomyosarcoma (striated muscle)	12
Malignant fibrous histiocytoma	11
Malignant nerve sheath tumour	9.5
Synovial sarcoma	6

multiple neurofibromata, may be complicated by malignant schwannoma

2) hereditary haemorrhagic telangiectasia (Osler–Weber–Rendu syndrome)

3) Gardner's syndrome, in which the intestinal polyps are associated with fibromatosis

- **Radiation.** There is convincing evidence that some soft tissue sarcomas can arise on the basis of previous therapeutic radiation. Those most commonly reported are malignant fibrous histiocytoma and extraosseous osteosarcoma. The latent period between irradiation and the appearance of the tumours is about 10 years on average; the outlook for these patients is poor.
- **Foreign bodies.** Some cases have been reported of

soft tissue sarcomas developing in relation to long-implanted foreign material such as bullets, shrapnel and some surgically implanted material. The latent period in these cases ranges from 2 to 50 years and the tumours most frequently seen are malignant fibrous histiocytoma and angiosarcoma.

Cytogenetic Aberrations in Soft Tissue Neoplasms

The morphological diagnosis of many soft tissue neoplasms presents a considerable challenge to the pathologist. Thus any ancillary investigations that might increase the precision of diagnosis could be of great value in surgical pathology practice. Certain chromosomal rearrangements are consistently described in some soft tissue neoplasms. These are listed in *Table 44.22*.

General Morphological Correlates of Behaviour in Soft Tissue Neoplasms

These include:

- **Size.** The larger the lesion, the more likely is it to behave in an aggressive fashion.
- **Position.** Superficial lesions are likely to behave less aggressively, whereas deeply situated lesions are more likely to metastasize.
- **Growth rate.** Tumours that grow rapidly, as evidenced by large numbers of mitoses and by areas of necrosis, are likely to behave aggressively.
- **Cellularity**
- **Histological type and subtype**

General Morphological Guides in Diagnosis

There are a few morphological features that can help in the correct classification of some fairly common soft tissue neoplasms. These include:

Table 44.22 Chromosomal Abnormalities in Soft Tissue Tumours

Tumour type	Chromosome abnormality
Synovial sarcoma	Translocation (X;18)
Ewing's sarcoma and peripheral primitive neuroectodermal tumour	Translocation (11;22)
Alveolar rhabdomyosarcoma	Translocation (2;13)
Myxoid liposarcoma	Translocation (12;16). This is associated with a rearrangement of the gene encoding CHOP, a protein believed to be involved in growth arrest. Translocation leads to a fusion between CHOP and a gene provisionally named *TLS* (**translocated in liposarcoma**). The *TLS* gene product resembles *EWS*, a gene commonly translocated in Ewing's sarcoma. The role of the fusion protein CHOP–TLS is not yet understood.
Poor-prognosis neuroblastoma	Deletion of short arm of chromosome 1
Malignant pleural mesothelioma	Deletion of 1p and/or 3p and/or 22

- **the cell type**
- **the pattern in which the cells of the tumour are arranged**

Combining these criteria in the first diagnostic 'trawl' may be quite helpful in certain cases. (see *Table 44.23*)

Diagnosis should always be made in the context of the patient's clinical picture (which includes **age** and **sex**), the site of the lesion and the length of the history. Light microscopy alone may be diagnostic but there are many neoplasms in which the morphological features differ subtly or not at all. In such cases electron microscopy, immunohistochemistry and cytogenetics must be used.

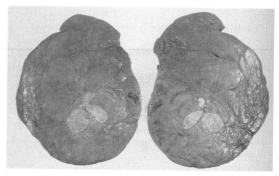

FIGURE 44.38 *Benign lipoma of neck. This is a large well-encapsulated lobulated mass of adipose tissue.*

TUMOURS WITH ADIPOSE TISSUE DIFFERENTIATION

BENIGN TUMOURS (LIPOMA)

Lipomas are the commonest soft tissue tumours in adult life. Most present as soft, slowly growing masses in the subcutaneous tissue of the trunk or limbs in the middle-aged or elderly (*Fig. 44.38*). They measure 1–20 cm in diameter and for the most part are painless; one variant, however, **angiolipoma**, is painful in about 50% of cases. Local recurrence after excision is uncommon and lipomas almost never undergo malignant transformation. A small minority (about 2%) occur within or

Table 44.23 Cell Type and Pattern in Soft Tissue Tumours

Tumour	Cell type	Pattern
Fibrous	Spindle cell: rod-shaped nucleus Long axis of cell twice as great as short axis	A palisaded or 'herring bone' pattern with the nuclei being arranged in columns
Fibrohistiocytic	Spindle cell Multinucleated tumour giant cells Large macrophage-like (histiocyte) cells with granular eosinophilic cytoplasm	A 'storiform' pattern with short fascicles of spindle cells arranged in a whorled fashion
Smooth muscle	Spindle cell Occasionally large cells with abundant cytoplasm and centrally placed nucleus (epithelioid)	Bundles of tumour cells intersecting more or less at right angles
Schwann cell	Spindle cell Epithelioid cell	A palisaded pattern with columnar arrangement of nuclei
Rhabdomyosarcoma	Small round cell Large eosinophilic cells with abundant cytoplasm and pleomorphic nuclei	One variant (alveolar type) shows small round cells arranged in nests or sheets of fibrous septa. Some of the nests show central loss of cellular cohesion giving an appearance somewhat reminiscent of lung alveoli.
Primitive neuroectodermal tumour	Small round cell	
Endothelial	Epithelioid cell	
Epithelioid sarcoma	Epithelioid cell	

between muscles. These lesions may have an infiltrating rather than a 'pushing' edge and some 15% will recur unless widely excised. **Microscopic examination of lipomas shows well-defined lobules of mature adipose tissue.**

Several interesting variants of lipoma exist.

Angiolipoma

These lesions account for up to 10% of lipomas. They occur predominantly in young or middle-aged adults and are most frequent in the upper limb, although they may occur in any anatomical location. About 50% of the lesions are painful. Other than this, their biological behaviour does not differ from that of common lipoma.

Microscopically, a complex network of thin-walled blood vessels occupying significant portions of the lesions differentiates them from common lipoma.

Angiomyolipoma

These are essentially hamartomatous rather than neoplastic lesions. They are commonest in the kidney but may be seen also in extrarenal locations.

Spindle Cell Lipoma

This lesion accounts for less than 2% of all lipomas. It is a tumour of middle and old age, occurring most commonly in males aged 50–80 years. The commonest site is the back of the neck or upper part of the back. In the vast majority of cases these lesions cause no symptoms and behave in a perfectly benign fashion.

Microscopic Features

Microscopically, they contain a mixture of:

- mature adipocytes
- short bundles of collagen
- small, rather uniform and basophilic spindle cells. These cells are believed to represent either uncommitted mesenchymal cells or very primitive fat cells. No mitoses or areas of necrosis are present.

Pleomorphic Lipoma

This lesion is clinically and, on the whole, histologically similar to spindle cell lipoma. **On microscopic examination the principal difference is the presence of bizarre multinucleate giant cells. Occasionally a few lipoblasts with multiple small intracytoplasmic vacuoles may be seen.**

Lipoblastoma

This is a rare tumour found exclusively in infants. The commonest site is the limbs, and the tumours may be either encapsulated or diffuse. They present with slowly growing, painless masses. The behaviour of this variant is perfectly benign, local recurrence being very uncommon.

Microscopic Features

Microscopic examination shows lobules of adipocytes in which there is a spectrum of differentiation ranging from the most primitive forms (prelipoblasts) to mature adipocytes. A complex network of thin-walled blood vessels is often present. Evidence of malignancy in the form of atypical mitoses, pleomorphism or areas of necrosis is not seen.

Lipomatosis

This is a rare condition characterized by overgrowth, in a diffuse pattern, of mature adipose tissue.

Hibernoma

This lesion shows differentiation into 'brown fat', normally found only in the fetus and young infants. The cells of brown fat contain many more mitochondria than do mature adipocytes and are believed to be concerned in heat production.

The tumours occur in middle-aged adults of either sex, and are most common between the shoulder blades, in the neck or in the axilla. These are sites in which brown fat is abundant in the fetus.

In morphological terms the tumour is well encapsulated and, not surprisingly, appears brown. The cells are usually multivacuolated or granular.

MALIGNANT TUMOURS (LIPOSARCOMA)

Liposarcoma is the commonest malignant connective tissue neoplasm. It is extremely rare in children but can occur at any time during adult life, the peak incidence being from 40 to 60 years. There is a slight male predominance.

The commonest sites are the lower limb (*Fig. 44.39*)

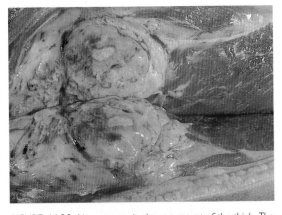

FIGURE 44.39 *Liposarcoma in the upper part of the thigh. The cut surface of the tumour shows a highly variegated appearance which is, in part, due to focal necrosis and haemorrhage within the substance of the lesion. The surface appears shiny owing to the relatively large amounts of connective tissue mucins present.*

Table 44.24 Histological Subtypes of Liposarcoma

Subtype	Prognosis	Features
Well-differentiated	The prognosis of well-differentiated liposarcomas of this type, arising within the limbs is excellent.	This group is subdivided into four types of which by far the commonest is known as 'lipoma-like'. As its name implies, it is made up of cells that resemble mature adipocytes, only a single droplet of fat being present within most of the cells. Only occasional multivacuolated lipoblasts and a few stellate or spindle cells are noted.
Myxoid	Myxoid liposarcoma has a good prognosis, metastases being rare.	This is the commonest histological subtype of liposarcoma. Microscopic examination shows the presence of small undifferentiated mesenchymal cells and variable numbers of multivacuolated lipoblasts set in a myxoid stroma. The principal component of this stroma is hyaluronic acid, which may be present in such abundance as to give the cut surface of the lesion a mucinous consistency. These tumours are well vascularized, having a complex anastomosing network of capillaries (the so-called 'chicken wire appearance').
Round cell	These tumours metastasize commonly and have a 5-year survival rate of about 20%.	This is a relatively uncommon variant. It is composed for the most part of a uniform population of small to medium, round, basophilic cells with little cytoplasm. Recognizable lipoblasts are few and far between.
Pleomorphic	Metastasis is a frequent occurrence.	As implied by their name these tumours have a mixed cell population in which there are spindle cells, numerous tumour giant cells and small numbers of multivacuolated lipoblasts which may be difficult to find. Mitoses are often present in large numbers, this being the only variant of liposarcoma in which this feature occurs.

and the retroperitoneal space. Any symptoms experienced are due to the presence of a mass in the particular anatomical location. **The site of a liposarcoma is one of the two significant factors in the natural history of the disease (the other being the histological subtype).** Thus retroperitoneal tumours have a 5-year survival rate of only 35%. This is due to the fact that they are difficult to excise completely and thus recur repeatedly, involving vital structures as they do so. In contrast, well-differentiated liposarcomas of the limbs are relatively easy to excise completely and have a good prognosis, metastases being rare.

Liposarcoma exists in a number of subtypes but **the key diagnostic feature on microscopic examination is multivacuolated lipoblasts, cells characterized by two or more lipid-filled droplets within the cytoplasm**. This feature is associated with large darkly staining nuclei showing indentations produced by the lipid droplets.

Liposarcoma is divided into *four* principal histological subtypes, these having a significant effect on prognosis (see *Table 44.24*).

SMOOTH MUSCLE TUMOURS

BENIGN TUMOURS (LEIOMYOMA)

Because smooth muscle is so widely distributed, it is not surprising that smooth muscle cell tumours should occur in many anatomical locations including:

- uterus
- gut
- dermis and subcutaneous tissue
- deep soft tissue (an uncommon site)

Smooth muscle tumours of the uterus and gut have been described in the sections on gastrointestinal and gynaecological pathology (see pp 518–519, 771–773).

In the **skin and subcutaneous tissue** leiomyoma occurs in *two* forms: **angioleiomyoma** and **pilar leiomyoma**.

Angioleiomyoma

This arises from the smooth muscle component of blood vessels. It is fairly common, usually presenting as a single nodule in one of the limbs. Its peak incidence is in middle age; females are affected more commonly than males. In about 50% of cases, pain is experienced when the lesion is compressed. Its biological behaviour is perfectly benign.

Microscopic Features

On microscopic examination angioleiomyoma is a well-circumscribed lesion. It is composed of bundles of well-differentiated smooth muscle cells oriented around thick-walled blood vessels which may show compression of their lumina.

Pilar Leiomyoma

This lesion is much less common than angioleiomyoma. The tumours are usually multiple, occurring on the limbs or trunk of young adults. In about 15% the disorder appears to be inherited, the inheritance pattern being autosomal dominant. The lesion arises from the arrector pili muscles and thus may occur in the skin, nipple, scrotum and labia. Recurrence after excision has been recorded but these lesions do not undergo malignant transformation.

Microscopic Features

Microscopically the pilar form differs from angioleiomyoma in that it has an infiltrative rather than a well-circumscribed edge. It is composed of interlacing bundles of well-differentiated smooth muscle cells which have brightly eosinophilic cytoplasm, distinct cell boundaries and blunt-ended nuclei.

MALIGNANT SMOOTH MUSCLE TUMOURS (LEIOMYOSARCOMA)

Leiomyosarcoma may occur within the muscular wall of a hollow viscus such as the uterus or stomach, or in non-visceral soft tissue. It is with this latter group that this section is concerned.

Non-visceral leiomyosarcoma may occur in the following locations:

- **Within the abdomen** (usually in the mesentery or in the retroperitoneal space). This is a relatively common site. The tumour, which has a slight predilection for females, tends to occur in late adult life. It is difficult to remove completely and the survival rate is low (20%). Death may be due to metastatic disease or recurrence with involvement of vital structures.

- **In the dermis.** These tumours, which are believed to originate from the arrector pili muscles, are usually less than 3 cm in diameter. They tend to occur in the limbs of middle-aged males; pain is a common symptom. If incompletely excised, the tumour recurs but its metastatic potential is low.
- **In subcutaneous tissues or intramuscularly.** Tumours in this situation are encountered in the same age group as dermal leiomyosarcoma. The lesions tend to be larger and up to 40% metastasize and thus have a fatal outcome.
- **In blood vessels.** Vascular leiomyosarcoma involves the walls and lumina of blood vessels as well as the soft tissues. The blood vessels involved tend to be large veins such as the saphenous and femoral veins and the inferior vena cava. Females are affected more commonly than males; the peak incidence is from 40 to 60 years. These tumours tend to metastasize early and the outlook for these patients is, in general, very bleak.

Diagnosis

Diagnostic problems relating to these tumours are twofold:

1) Identification of the tumour cells as showing smooth muscle differentiation
2) Assessment of the malignant potential of an individual lesion

Difficulties relating to the first of these may be resolved by the use of:

- **Electron microscopy** shows thin myofilaments, so-called dense bodies, which are electron-dense areas at the periphery of the cells, and a basal lamina.
- **Immunohistochemistry.** The two most useful immunohistochemical reagents are antibodies raised against the intermediate filament protein **desmin** and **smooth muscle actin**. Use of both of these gives the best chance of an accurate diagnosis.

Assessment of the Malignant Potential

Features associated with malignancy include:

- **large size.** For example, a diameter greater than 7.5 cm in a retroperitoneal smooth muscle tumour indicates malignancy.
- **a high mitotic rate.** In the skin and/or subcutaneous tissue, a mitotic rate greater than two per ten high-power fields is a definite indicator of malignancy. In the case of retroperitoneal tumours a mitotic rate of five per ten high-power fields should be regarded as malignant.
- **areas of necrosis**
- **marked cellular pleomorphism**

TUMOURS OF SKELETAL MUSCLE

This term does not mean those neoplasms that necessarily arise in voluntary muscle, but those showing striated muscle cell differentiation. This set of tumours comprises:

- rhabdomyoma
- rhabdomyosarcoma

BENIGN RHABDOMYOMA

This is an extremely rare lesion, constituting only 2% of primary muscle tumours, the remainder being sarcomas. Three principal types have been described.

1. Adult Type

This tumour is found most commonly in the head and neck of middle-aged individuals; the mean age at presentation is 50 years. Males are affected four times as commonly as females. It is probably best regarded as a hamartomatous malformation rather than as a true neoplasm, and has a benign natural history on the whole, although some may recur after excision.

The tumour presents as a solitary polypoid lesion of the larynx, pharynx, palate or mouth, or, sometimes, as an intramuscular mass within the tongue, cheeks or lateral muscles of the neck.

Microscopic Features

Microscopic examination shows the tumour to consist of a well-circumscribed mass of large round or polygonal cells with eosinophilic cytoplasm and abundant intracytoplasmic glycogen. Cross-striations are rare but other morphological features indicative of voluntary muscle differentiation are present.

2. Fetal Type

This is the rarest form of rhabdomyoma. It occurs almost exclusively in boys aged less than 3 years. The head and neck (especially the postauricular region) are the sites most frequently involved.

On microscopic examination, the lesion is seen to consist of a mixture of immature skeletal muscle and a loose, rather myxoid, stroma.

3. Genital Type

This lesion presents as a polypoid growth of the cervix, vagina or vulva in middle age. It appears to be benign and does not recur after excision.

Microscopic Features

Microscopic examination shows a mesenchymal stroma in which large rhabdomyoblasts with cross-striations and intracytoplasmic bodies are present. It is a benign lesion and must not be confused with botryoid rhabdomyosarcoma.

Cardiac Muscle: Cardiac Rhabdomyoma

This is a rare lesion occurring in infancy and, as a rule, proving fatal by the age of 5 years. An association with tuberous sclerosis is seen in about 50% of cases and other congenital abnormalities are present in 14%.

The lesions are usually multiple and involve the right

and left ventricles with equal frequency. In about 30% of cases, the atria are affected. The lesions are typically within the walls of the cardiac chambers but, occasionally, they may protrude into the ventricular or atrial cavities and cause obstruction.

Macroscopic Features

On naked-eye examination the lesions appear as well-defined, rounded nodules seldom exceeding 1 cm in diameter.

Microscopic Features

They consist of large polygonal cells which have a central mass of eosinophilic cytoplasm. From this, narrow striated processes extend to the periphery of the cell, where there is a narrow zone of striated cytoplasm. Much of the cytoplasm thus appears clear, the clear areas, in fact, being occupied by glycogen. This cell has, quite appropriately, been given the name 'spider cell' and is said to resemble the P cells of the sinoatrial node, and also normal cardiac myoblasts.

RHABDOMYOSARCOMA

This is the commonest malignant soft tissue tumour in infants and young children. Most childhood rhabdomyosarcomas occur outside muscle. Rhabdomyosarcoma is much less common in adults, the adult tumours tending to be intramuscular in location. **Correct diagnosis of this group of tumours depends on the demonstration of rhabdomyoblasts, which indicate striated muscle differentiation.** In some cases this is possible on conventional light microscopy but in others the aid of immunohistochemistry and/or electron microscopy is necessary.

The types of rhabdomyosarcoma recognized currently are shown in *Table 44.25*. Botryoid rhabdomyosarcoma is a variant of the embryonal type and not a distinct type.

Embryonal Rhabdomyosarcoma

Embryonal rhabdomyosarcoma and its variant, the botryoid tumour, account for about two-thirds of all rhabdomyosarcomas. Most cases occur before the age of 6 years. Males are affected more frequently than females. Common sites in descending order of frequency are listed below. **Of these, the two most common are the orbit and the paratesticular region.**

- **the head and neck region:**
  a) orbit
  b) nasopharynx
  c) middle ear
- **the genitourinary system:**
  a) prostate
  b) paratesticular region (upper pole of testis, spermatic cord, epididymis)
  c) urinary bladder
- **the limbs**
- **the retroperitoneal space**

Table 44.25 Rhabdomyosarcoma

Type	Features
Embryonal rhabdomyosarcoma	This is primarily a tumour of early childhood and, histologically, is said by some to resemble developing muscle.
Botryoid rhabdomyosarcoma	The term **botryoid** (grape-like) is applied to embryonal rhabdomyosarcomas with a polypoid configuration and a myxoid consistency. They occur in mucosa-lined organs.
Alveolar rhabdomyosarcoma	This tumour almost invariably arises within voluntary muscle and typically presents between the ages of 10 and 20 years. This tumour has a characteristic morphological pattern with small cells being arranged in sheets or nests separated by fibrous tissue septa.
Pleomorphic rhabdomyosarcoma	This is the rarest subtype tending to arise in the limbs of adults and children. It is usually intramuscular in position.

Microscopic Features

There is a considerable degree of heterogeneity. In some cases the tumour consists principally of small rounded or spindle-shaped cells which have basophilic cytoplasm and darkly staining nuclei. These are set in a myxoid matrix. In others there are bundles of spindle cells giving a picture somewhat reminiscent of a smooth muscle cell tumour (*Fig. 44.40*). A third variant shows the presence of stellate tumour cells arranged in a reticular pattern.

Rhabdomyoblasts, the defining diagnostic criterion, may be seen in numbers that differ from lesion to lesion and from area to area within a single tumour. These large cells may be round, elongated or oval, and have eosinophilic cytoplasm in which a fibrillated appearance may be noted. The purely descriptive but quite evocative terms 'tadpole cells, strap cells and racket cells' have variously been applied to these rhabdomyoblasts. Cross-striations of the kind seen in mature voluntary muscle are present in the rhabdomyoblasts in about 50–60% of cases of embryonal rhabdomyosarcoma.

In so far as the tumour cell population is concerned, botryoid tumours show a similar spectrum of cytological appearances. A myxoid stroma is a prominent feature, as is the presence of a concentration of tumour cells below the overlying mucosa. This cellular zone is known as the cambium layer and is separated from the surface epithelium by a narrow tumour-free zone.

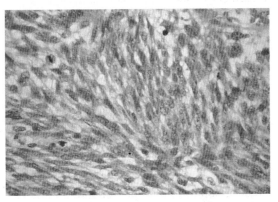

FIGURE 44.40 *Embryonal rhabdomyosarcoma showing both rounded and spindle-shaped tumour cells.*

Microscopic Features

The tumour has a characteristic pattern of honeycomb-like spaces bounded by fibrous tissue septa. The spaces are lined by small, poorly differentiated, round or oval tumour cells in which mitoses are frequent (*Fig. 44.41*). In the centre of these alveolus-like spaces, where loss of cellular cohesion has taken place, large multinucleate giant cells with peripherally arranged nuclei may be present. Both within the spaces and within the stroma, occasional strap-like rhabdomyoblasts may be present, although they tend to occur in smaller numbers than in the embryonal type of tumour.

Alveolar Rhabdomyosarcoma

About 25% of cases of rhabdomyosarcoma fall into this group. The tumour is almost always intramuscular in location, the limbs, especially the arm and the trunk, being the commonest sites. The typical age at presentation is between the ages of 10 and 20 years.

Pleomorphic Rhabdomyosarcoma

This is the rarest of the subtypes tending to occur in the limbs. Rhabdomyosarcomas in adults are most frequently of this type.

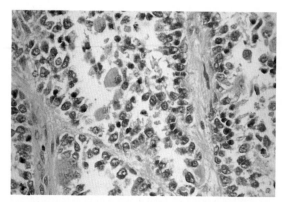

FIGURE 44.41 *Alveolar rhabdomyosarcoma showing the typical picture of a lesion divided by fibrous tissue septa, the spaces between these being lined by rounded tumour cells.*

Microscopic Features

This variant is composed principally of large cells with eosinophilic cytoplasm and either single or multiple highly atypical nuclei. Large 'tadpole' or 'strap' cells are also present but cross-striations are virtually never seen.

Natural History and Prognosis

In the mid-1960s, the 2-year survival rate of patients with rhabdomyosarcoma was less than 20%. Now, as a result of combination treatment involving surgery, radiotherapy and chemotherapy, this survival rate has risen to over 70%. Prognosis depends on:

- **the clinical stage**
- **the anatomical site of the tumour**
- **the histological subtype.** This appears to be a significant factor only in relation to alveolar rhabdomyosarcoma, which is associated with a shorter survival time than other variants. This difference is seen chiefly in patients in whom the tumour is still localized at the time of presentation.

Clinical Staging and Anatomical Location in Prognosis

A currently used system for clinical staging is shown in *Table 44.26*.

Anatomical Location

With the treatment currently available, group I and II tumours involving the orbit, head and neck, and some genitourinary tumours, have a 3-year survival rate of 70–100%. The prognosis is less favourable for patients with tumours at a more advanced stage or with lesions located in the limbs. In the case of tumours located near the meninges (e.g. those in the paranasal sinuses or middle ear) there is a substantial chance (35%) of spread into the central nervous system, and this is usually fatal within 1 year.

Table 44.26 Clinical Staging of Rhabdomyosarcoma

Stage	Characteristics
I	Localized disease completely excised
II	Localized disease; microscopic evidence of residual tumour after excision Tumour has spread to lymph nodes; no residual tumour after excision Tumour has spread to nodes; microscopic evidence of residual tumour after excision or involvement of most distal node
III	Incomplete resection with macroscopic evidence of residual tumour
IV	Distant metastases at time of presentation

TUMOURS OF UNCERTAIN ORIGIN AND DIFFERENTIATION

Synovial Sarcoma

The term synovial sarcoma is a misnomer because there is little evidence to suggest that it is either derived from or differentiates into synovial lining cells. Nevertheless it does appear to be a well-defined clinicopathological entity and for this reason the name has been retained.

There is a wide range of ages at which this tumour can present, although the peak incidence is from 15 to 35 years. Origin within a joint is rare, 90% occurring in an extra-articular location within soft tissue, often near joint capsules and tendons or their sheaths. The lower limb is the most frequently affected extremity (60–70% of cases), the knee and thigh being sites of predilection. More rarely, the tumour may occur in the head and neck area (for example, in the pharynx, larynx or oesophagus) or in the abdominal wall.

Microscopic Features

Classically, synovial sarcoma has a biphasic histological appearance. The tumour consists of:

1) **an epithelial element** consisting of either nests or gland-like spaces composed of cells that have oval, pale-staining nuclei, abundant cytoplasm and quite distinct cell borders

2) **a spindle cell component**, the cells of which are arranged, most commonly, in sheets, although they may, in some cases, be grouped round blood vessels, giving the so-called haemangiopericytomatous pattern. Mitoses are present, usually in this spindle

cell component, but their numbers differ from lesion to lesion.

In addition there is a mast-cell infiltrate, the significance of which is not known, and focal areas of calcification or ossification. This feature, which is found in about 40% of cases, may be so prominent as to show up as spotty areas of calcification on radiological examination.

Up to one-third of cases lack the classical biphasic histology and present to the pathologist as a monophasic spindle cell tumour.

While it is true that a spindle cell sarcoma occurring near a joint in a young patient is nearly always a synovial sarcoma, this is not a basis for making a definitive tissue diagnosis and ancillary methods of investigation must be used. These include: **cytogenetic techniques, immunohistochemistry and electron microscopy**.

Cytogenetic Techniques

Both biphasic and monophasic synovial sarcomas show the presence of a specific chromosome translocation between the short arms of chromosomes X and 18 (t(X;18) (p11.2;q11.2)). The chromosomal abnormality can be detected in sections of paraffin-embedded material by fluorescent *in situ* hybridization.

Immunohistochemistry

The majority of synovial sarcomas show epithelial antigens. The most useful markers are cytokeratins and epithelial membrane antigen (EMA). Cytokeratins can be identified in about 75% of synovial sarcomas (100% of biphasic tumours); the epithelial cells are strongly positive but isolated spindle cells also show these antigens. Some tumours show only one epithelial marker so it is generally thought wise to use antibodies against both epithelial membrane antigen and the cytokeratins. In relation to the origin of these lesions it is interesting that synovial lining cells never express these epithelial antigens.

Electron Microscopy

The epithelial cells lining the gland-like spaces in biphasic tumours are indistinguishable from those seen, for example, in adenocarcinoma. Microvilli that protrude into the lumen are very characteristic and may be seen occasionally in the monophasic spindle cell in relation to slit-like spaces between tumour cells.

Natural History

Synovial sarcoma, in general, does not carry a good prognosis, the overall 10-year survival rate being about 30%. Local recurrence occurs in about 50% of cases, often within 2 years of the primary excision but sometimes much later than this. In cases where metastatic disease develops, the common sites for secondary deposits are:

Table 44.27 Prognostic Criteria in Synovial Sarcoma

Criterion	Effects on prognosis
Size	Less than 4 cm along the longest axis is regarded as a favourable sign
Calcification	Tumours with extensive calcification carry a better prognosis
Vascular invasion	This carries an unfavourable prognosis
Mitotic rate	More than two mitoses per high-power field is regarded as an unfavourable sign
Age	Those who develop synovial sarcoma in childhood tend to have a better prognosis (7-year survival rate quoted as 63%)

- the lungs   94%
- regional nodes   21%
- bone   17%

Until recently, all synovial sarcomas were regarded as high-grade tumours but it now realized that criteria exist that have a bearing on the prognosis for the individual patient. These are shown in *Table 44.27*.

Alveolar Soft Part Sarcoma

This is a rare lesion accounting for less than 1% of sarcomas; its origin and differentiation pattern are mysterious. Males and females are equally affected; peak incidence is from 20 to 29 years.

The tumours are usually situated deep within soft tissues. In descending order of frequency, the commonest sites are:
- the buttock and thigh   39.5%
- the popliteal region   16.6%
- the chest wall and trunk   12.9%
- the forearm   9.7%

Other reported sites are the arm, back, neck, tongue and retroperitoneal space.

Macroscopic Features

The tumours are often quite large (more than 5 cm in diameter). They are firm in consistency and often variegated in colour owing to areas of haemorrhage and necrosis.

Microscopic Features

The microscopic features are highly characteristic. The tumour cells are large and rounded or polygonal in shape and have eosinophilic, granular cytoplasm. This cytoplasm contains periodic acid–Schiff-positive material, which is diastase resistant and is thus not glycogen. In about 20% of cases this material is arranged in the form of crystalline structures of differing shapes.

The fundamental architectural unit in which the cells are arranged is a 'ball', the centre of which often becomes necrotic, giving the so-called 'alveolar' pattern (*Fig. 44.42*). In some instances, the tumour nests appear to bulge into vascular spaces ('glomeruloid' pattern).

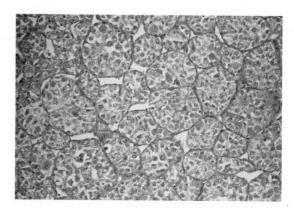

FIGURE 44.42 *Alveolar soft-part sarcoma. This section shows the characteristic appearance of a tumour composed of nests of cells separated by small blood vessels. The cells have uniform round nuclei and rather granular eosinophilic cytoplasm.*

Natural History

As the tumour is rare, it is difficult to collect adequate follow-up data. At the Sloan-Kettering Cancer Center 91 patients with a diagnosis of alveolar soft part sarcoma have been followed, a few of them for more than 20 years.

If there was no evidence of metastatic disease at the time of diagnosis, the median survival times was 11 years. If metastases were present at this time the median survival rate dropped to 3 years.

Epithelioid Sarcoma

This is a relatively rare neoplasm with a peak incidence at the age of 15–35 years. Males are affected more commonly than females.

Most present as multinodular masses in the dermis or subcutaneous tissue of the limbs, the wrist and hand being sites of predilection.

Microscopic Features

The tumours are composed of nodules, often showing central necrosis. The tumour cell population consists in part of plump, polygonal, epithelium-like cells. These usually show none of the cytological features of malignancy other than fairly frequent mitoses. At the periphery of the nodules the cell population tends to change, being composed of eosinophilic spindle-shaped cells. Because of the nodular architecture and the tendency for central necrosis to occur, this lesion has in the past been misdiagnosed as a granuloma and rhabdomyosarcoma. Metastatic carcinoma and large cell lymphoma are included in the differential diagnosis.

Immunohistochemistry shows **vimentin** (a common mesenchymal marker) and epithelial cell antigens, both epithelial membrane antigen and cytokeratin being present in many cases.

Ultrastructural studies show cells with a range of differentiation patterns; it has been suggested that epithelioid sarcoma is a primitive tumour in which multidirectional differentiation is taking place.

Natural History

Local recurrence is common, occurring in about 75% of cases. In about 40% distant metastasis, via lymphatic and blood vessel pathways, occurs, although the course of the illness may be quite prolonged.

FIBROHISTIOCYTIC TUMOURS

The term fibrohistiocytic has descriptive value but tells us little or nothing about the derivation of this large set of tumours. It was coined on the basis of an apparently mixed population of tumour cells, some of which appear fibroblastic whereas others resemble macrophages (histiocytes). Extensive ultrastructural and immunohistochemical studies have so far failed to provide any evidence that the tumour cells are of monocyte–macrophage lineage. The current view is that these lesions are derived either from fibroblasts or from a mesenchymal stem cell giving rise to a tumour cell population, some of which express phenotypic features of macrophages.

Several benign lesions are classified as fibrohistiocytic lesions; the most common, benign fibrous histiocytoma (dermatofibroma and many other synonyms) and giant cell tumour of tendon sheath, are described on pp 1031–1032, 1091–1092.

MALIGNANT FIBROUS HISTIOCYTOMA

Many regard malignant fibrous histiocytoma as the commonest sarcoma of adult life. It is still not clear, however, whether it is a specific pathological entity, a non-specific morphological pattern or, indeed, both of these. What is certain is that:
● the histological pattern called malignant fibrous histiocytoma accounts for a substantial number of all cases diagnosed as soft tissue sarcoma, especially in adults.

- several different histological subtypes are classified under this rubric and that assigning an individual tumour to one or other of these subtypes has clinical and prognostic implications.

Five histological subtypes have been recognized:

1) **pleomorphic/storiform**   60–70%
2) **myxoid**   10–20%
3) **giant cell**   5–15%
4) **inflammatory**   5–10%
5) **angiomatoid**   1–3%

Pleomorphic/Storiform Malignant Fibrous Histiocytoma

This is the commonest variant. As with all these histiocytomas, with the single exception of the rare angiomatoid variant, this is a tumour of late adult life, the peak incidence being in the seventh decade.

Site

Limb skeletal muscles, especially those of the thigh, are most frequently affected. The retroperitoneal space is the second most favoured site.

Clinically, patients present with a history of a slowly growing painless mass which may have been present for months.

> **Macroscopic Features**
>
> The lesion is usually an infiltrating, multinodular, greyish-white mass in which areas of haemorrhage and necrosis may be seen.

> **Microscopic Features**
>
> The tumours are composed of irregularly arranged, plump, eosinophilic, spindle-shaped cells with darkly staining and often bizarre nuclei (*Fig. 44.43*). Numerous mitoses, both typical and atypical, are seen. Interspersed among the tumour cells are macrophage-like cells (some containing abundant lipid) and chronic inflammatory cells.
>
> In some areas the tumour cells are arranged in the whorled pattern to which the term storiform has been applied (from the Latin *storia* – woven hemp or a mat). Invasion of blood vessels and perineural spaces is not uncommon.

Natural History

Local recurrence after excision occurs in about 45% of cases and metastasis in 42%. The 5-year survival rate is about 50%.

Myxoid Malignant Fibrous Histiocytoma

Site

Most cases occur in the limbs, often in the subcutaneous tissue.

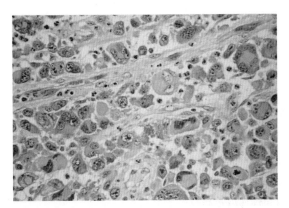

FIGURE 44.43 *Malignant fibrous histiocytoma showing numerous pleomorphic cells with bizarre angulated nuclei. Many tumour giant cells are present.*

> **Macroscopic Features**
>
> The distinguishing feature of this variant is its mucoid or myxoid cut surface.

> **Microscopic Features**
>
> The chief difference between this variant and the more common pleomorphic malignant fibrous histiocytoma is the stroma, which contains large amounts of connective tissue mucin, most of which appears to be hyaluronic acid.

Natural History

Local recurrence is common, occurring in 66% of cases. Metastasis, however, is distinctly less frequent, occurring in only 23%.

Giant Cell Malignant Fibrous Histiocytoma

Site

The commonest site is in the limb muscles, especially in the leg. However, up to one-third of cases occur in the subcutaneous tissue.

> **Macroscopic Features**
>
> The tumour is a multinodular mass in which haemorrhage tends to be more prominent than in other variants.

> **Microscopic Features**
>
> The basic histological features of this variant do not differ materially from those already described. The defining criterion, however, is osteoclast-like giant cells. In addition, in about half the cases, foci of osteoid or mature bone are present, situated at the periphery of the tumour nodules.

Natural History

Recurrence rates of 30–50% have been quoted. The site appears to influence the prognosis: metastasis is much rarer in subcutaneous tumours (20%) than in deeply situated ones (75%).

Inflammatory Malignant Fibrous Histiocytoma

Site

This tumour shows a striking predilection for the retroperitoneal space, although it may also occur in the limbs.

> #### Macroscopic Features
> Because these lesions contain large numbers of lipid-laden macrophages (xanthoma cells), their cut surfaces tend to show yellow areas.
>
> #### Microscopic Features
> The histological appearances of this variant are dominated by the xanthoma cells. Typically, the tumour is composed of sheets of xanthoma cells mixed with inflammatory cells, most of which are neutrophils. The whole cell population is set in a rather featureless hyaline matrix, and cells showing cytological evidence of malignancy may be hard to find. In some cases, there are transitions between the predominantly xanthomatous pattern and areas that resemble pleomorphic malignant fibrous histiocytoma; this can be of great help in histological diagnosis.

Natural History

Because of its tendency to occur within the retroperitoneal space, the tumour is difficult to remove completely. Recurrence is therefore common. Metastases occur in about 30% of patients and the 5-year survival rate is only about 30%.

Angiomatoid Malignant Fibrous Histiocytoma

This differs from all other variants in that the peak incidence is in the first and second decades of life.

Site

The lesion occurs most commonly in the dermis and subcutaneous tissues of the limbs, especially the upper limb.

> #### Macroscopic Features
> The tumour presents as a slowly growing mass. This is readily felt because it is not, as a rule, deeply situated. The tumour mass often appears well defined and shows cystic changes and haemorrhage.
>
> #### Microscopic Features
> The tumour is characterized by sheets of eosinophilic histiocytes intimately related to large blood-filled spaces, intense inflammation and extensive scarring. Although the blood-filled spaces resemble vascular channels, they are without any endothelial lining.

Natural History

Recurrence is by no means uncommon (approximately 60%), but metastasis is comparatively rare.

FIBROBLASTIC LESIONS: NON-NEOPLASTIC AND NEOPLASTIC

Fibroblastic processes capable of causing nodules or masses may be divided into *three* basic groups:

1) **Benign fibroblastic lesions. These are almost certainly not neoplasms but are reactive or reparative in nature.** They include such entities as **keloid, hypertrophic scar, nodular fasciitis, proliferative fasciitis and myositis, and elastofibroma**.

2) **The fibromatoses. This term is used to designate a group of lesions that are intermediate between benign and frankly malignant lesions so far as their biological behaviour is concerned.** Many, perhaps the majority, are hamartomatous in nature. Some can behave very aggressively with respect to infiltration and recurrence, but they do not metastasize. Under this rubric are included superficial lesions such as **palmar, plantar and penile fibromatosis**, and deep ones such as **abdominal wall, intra-abdominal and extra-abdominal desmoid fibromatoses**.

3) **Fibrosarcoma**

BENIGN FIBROBLASTIC LESIONS

These reactive lesions are benign but may cause problems in relation to the histological diagnosis. In some there is a clear association with preceding trauma.

Keloids and Hypertrophic Scars

Amongst the commonest reactive fibroblastic processes are keloids and hypertrophic scars. Despite the fact that they both represent an excessive connective tissue response to quite minor degrees of trauma, there are some important differences between them, as shown in *Table 44.28*.

Nodular Fasciitis

The term fasciitis is a misnomer because the process is not inflammatory but a primary fibroblastic proliferation.

It occurs most commonly in adolescents and young adults, and presents clinically as a **rapidly growing** nodule usually located within the subcutaneous adipose tissue. Few sarcomas, in fact, grow with the rapidity of nodular fasciitis, which usually reaches its maximal size of a few centimetres in diameter within 3 months. The volar surface of the forearm is the commonest site but lesions also occur not infrequently in the trunk and lower limbs.

Table 44.28 Keloids and Hypertrophic Scars

Keloid	Hypertrophic scar
Commonest in adolescents and young adults	
Show a marked predilection for Negroes	Show no predilection for Negroes
Females affected more often than males	No sex difference
Commonest in region of face, neck, sternum, forearms and lobes of ears	May occur in any site
Smooth plaques that are frequently itchy or tender	Not often symptomatic
Typically extend beyond the margins of the antecedent trauma	Do not extend beyond the boundaries of the antecedent trauma
Consist, in the early stages, of cellular fibrous tissue arranged partly in nodules and partly in interlacing bundles. Normal mitoses often present	
In late stages consist of hyalinized, brightly eosinophilic, collagen which is relatively acellular	Persist as nodules of relatively cellular fibrous tissue. Collagen does not undergo hyalinization
Tend to recur after excision	Recur only very occasionally

Macroscopic Features

Lesions appear well circumscribed, although microscopic examination often shows that they have an infiltrating margin.

Microscopic Features

In the early stages the lesions are composed of plump immature fibroblasts arranged in short bundles and whorls. The lesions are cellular and normal mitoses are fairly numerous. Unlike malignant fibrous histiocytoma, cellular pleomorphism is not present. As the lesions mature, pools of myxoid material accumulate, forming microcysts. The presence of lymphocytes, red blood cells and multinucleated giant cells makes the histological picture a very variable one. In the late stages, the lesion becomes progressively hyalinized and the stromal blood vessels, which are numerous earlier on, undergo atrophy.

Natural History

In the vast majority of cases excision is curative; only 1% of lesions recur after surgery.

A number of other forms of fasciitis exist. Description of these is beyond the scope of this text.

Elastofibroma

This is an interesting benign lesion, usually presenting just below the scapula in late adult life. There is a marked predilection for females. The clinical presentation is that of a long history of a slowly growing, ill-defined mass which may be bilateral. It has been suggested that the lesion is the result of prolonged trauma between the lower border of the scapula and the chest wall.

Microscopic Features

The characteristic appearance is of irregular fascicles of collagen within the subcutaneous adipose tissue. These are associated with many short, rather thick, elastic fibres with a beaded or sometimes a globular appearance.

FIBROMATOSES

Superficial Fibromatoses

Included under this heading are:
- **palmar fibromatosis** (Dupuytren's contracture)
- **plantar fibromatosis**
- **Peyronie's disease** (fibromatosis involving the penis see p 741).
- **fibromatosis colli** (occurring in the sternocleidomastoid muscle of neonates; some 10% go on to develop permanent torticollis (**wry neck**))

Microscopic Features

These lesions are all characterized by nodules of well-differentiated fibroblasts arranged in long sweeping bundles. Nuclear pleomorphism and mitotic activity are trivial in degree, a useful distinction from fibrosarcoma.

In the later stages of the natural history, contracture, which is the most bothersome effect, develops, leading to flexion deformities in the metacarpophalangeal joints of the hand and abnormal curvature of the penis. Curiously, fibromatosis in the subcutaneous tissue of the soles of the feet is not associated with contracture.

Palmar fibromatosis (Dupuytren's contracture) is seen most frequently in middle-aged men. While there may well be a genetic basis, this disorder is also associated with an increased frequency of alcohol abuse, diabetes mellitus and epilepsy in affected individuals. Local recurrence is common; plantar fibromatosis, for example, recurs in about one-third of cases after excision.

Deep Fibromatoses (Desmoid Fibromatoses)

The general features of this group of conditions include:

- **a typically deep intramuscular location**
- **generally, large size (up to 10–15 cm)**
- **an infiltrative growth pattern**
- **a high risk of recurrence after excision**

Desmoid Fibromatosis of the Anterior Abdominal Wall

This lesion is somewhat less common than its extra-abdominal counterpart. It usually develops in the rectus abdominis muscle of young adults, more particularly in women who have borne children. Indeed, many of these lesions are detected in the peripartum or postpartum period. Abdominal wall desmoid fibromatoses may also occur in surgical scars.

Intra-abdominal Desmoid Fibromatoses

This is a relatively rare lesion occurring most frequently in the mesentery, although the retroperitoneal space may be involved. The lesion most commonly occurs in young adults and there is a clear association with Gardner's syndrome (see p 556).

In these patients there is usually a history of previous abdominal surgery, the tumour being located within the operative field.

Extra-abdominal Desmoid Fibromatoses

This is the most aggressive of the fibromatoses. Males and females, principally in the third and fourth decades of life, are equally likely to be affected. There is no relationship with previous trauma, surgical or otherwise. The pectoral and pelvic girdles are sites of predilection

and the lesions grow slowly but relentlessly to form large masses which can be removed only by radical surgery. The recurrence rates are high, ranging between 60 and 70%.

FIBROSARCOMA

Modern aids to histological diagnosis, such as immunohistochemistry, have led to many spindle cell sarcomas, formerly diagnosed as fibrosarcomas, being classified under other rubrics, such as synovial sarcoma or malignant schwannoma.

Fibrosarcoma falls naturally into two groups distinguishable on the basis of:

- age at presentation
- biological behaviour

Adult Fibrosarcoma

These most commonly present as painless masses, deeply situated in the soft tissues of the lower limbs or trunk of middle-aged adults. There appears to be no special predilection for either sex. Occasional cases have been recorded as following therapeutic irradiation.

Local recurrence occurs in about half the cases. Five-year survival rates are of the order of 40% and after 10 years just under 30% are likely to be alive.

Infantile Fibrosarcoma

This tumour occurs typically within the first 2 years of life and may be present at birth. It is more common in males than in females and is located either in the subcutaneous tissue or within muscle. The limbs are the most common anatomical location, the distal portions being especially likely to be affected.

Infantile fibrosarcoma behaves in a much more benign fashion than its adult counterpart. Local recurrence rates are approximately 20% and metastasis occurs in only 10–15%.

Microscopic Features

The tumour consists of bundles of spindle-shaped cells arranged at angles to one another, giving a so-called 'herring bone' pattern.

Differing amounts of stromal collagen are present; the larger the amount, the better the prognosis. Mitoses are frequent and a proportion of these are abnormal. The tumour differs from malignant fibrous histiocytoma in that there is little or no nuclear pleomorphism and multinucleated giant cells are not seen.

CHAPTER 45

The Nervous System

Central Nervous System Disorders

INTRODUCTION

Most organs show uniformity in the functions of their parenchyma. Thus the **site** of injury to or loss of tissue will not necessarily affect the **pattern** of functional disturbance. Similarly, the **degree** of such disturbance is likely to reflect the **amount** of functioning tissue lost.

The situation in the central nervous system (CNS) is quite different because the brain is divided into many functionally quite separate areas. Thus, the effect of diseases in or of the CNS reflects the interplay of:

- the **site** of injury
- the **type** of injury
- the **reaction pattern** within the nervous system. In this connection it is worth remembering that the repertory of reactions within the brain is limited.

Diseases of the CNS fall basically into *two* classes:

1) basic pathological processes occurring **in any organs or tissues** such as ischaemia, haemorrhage, infection, trauma or neoplasm
2) conditions **unique to the nervous system**. In most cases the aetiology and pathogenesis of these are unknown but most are expressed in one of two forms:

- **degeneration of neurones affecting particular systems (i.e. areas of the brain with anatomical and functional connections)**
- **loss or alteration of the myelin that ensheaths the axons**

Many of the disorders unique to the CNS are very rare, but unfortunately some, such as **Alzheimer's disease** (the commonest cause of dementia), **Parkinson's disease** and **multiple sclerosis**, are not.

Many find neuropathological jargon impenetrable. The following glossary is appended in an attempt partly to overcome this difficulty.

Importance of Intracranial Pressure in CNS Disorders

The natural history of intracranial disease is strongly influenced by certain **anatomical** features unique to the brain. The most important of these is the fact that, **once the skull sutures have fused, the brain is virtually enclosed within a rigid container**. The cranium itself is divided into compartments by unyielding folds of dura mater constituting the tentorium cerebelli and falx cerebri. Thus:

- A given rise in the volume of intracranial contents

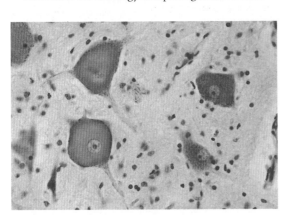

FIGURE 45.1 *Chromatolysis. This term refers to a series of changes in the neurone that result from injury to its axon. The cell body becomes rounded and the Nissl granules around the nucleus disappear. In sections stained with cresyl violet, as this one has been, the central part of the cytoplasm stains pink.*

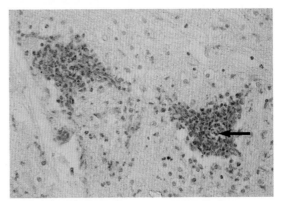

FIGURE 45.2 *Neuronophagia. This term describes the invasion of the neuronal cell body and dendrites by inflammatory cells following neuronal death. In this field, the nucleus of one of the two neurones shown can still be seen (arrowed) but the cell body is invaded by large numbers of microglial cells.*

A Glossary of Neuropathological Terms

Cell/Reaction/Syndrome/Lesion

Astrocyte	One of the three cells types derived from the neuro-ectodermal spongioblast and constituting the glial cells. The others are the oligodendroglia and the ependymal cells. Astrocytes are classified into two main types: Protoplasmic astrocytes, found mainly in the grey matter and Fibrous astrocytes found mainly in the white matter. Both have round or oval nuclei and processes which require special staining to be visible in tissue sections. They contain bundles of filaments composed of an acid protein known as glial fibrillary acid protein (GFAP). In fetal life they guide migrating neurones to their permanent position. In post-natal life they play a role in healing in repair after damage in the CNS. Glial cells also have metabolic functions in that they regulate the ionic content of the extracellular fluid and influence calcium and neurotransmitter metabolism.
Astrocytosis	Hypertrophy and hyperplasia of astrocytes as a response to a wide variety of injuries in the CNS. This occurs in both acute and chronic processes. In oedematous white matter around abscesses or tumours, the astrocytes become enlarged and rounded and have homogeneous, eosinophilic cytoplasm in which there is abundant GFAP. These cells are termed **gemistocytic** astrocytes.
Axonal bulb	Disruption of an axon is followed by swelling of both the proximal and distal severed ends. These swellings are known as axonal bulbs and consist of neurofilaments, mitochondria, microtubules etc. They result from the anterograde and retrograde axonal flow which continues for some time despite the axonal damage.
Basket brain	The presence of extensive, bilateral, developmental cysts (porencephalic) in the brain so that large frontal and occipital cystic cavities are connected by a thin rim of tissue.
Blepharoplast	Basal bodies within ependymal cells from which the ependymal cilia originate.
Boutons terminaux	Structures of the neuronal processes which form synapses on the dendrites and perikarya of other neurones.
Bunina bodies	Small eosinophilic inclusions seen in surviving neurons in patients with motor neurone disease.
Cephalohaematoma	A collection of blood seen in neonates between the surface of a calvarial bone and its pericranial membrane. Occurs in about 2.5% of all births; most likely following use of forceps or a vacuum extractor.
Carpal tunnel syndrome	A neuropathy affecting the median nerve. Not uncommonly associated with amyloid deposition in the nerve sheath.
Cerebellar cortex-microglial shrubwork	A proliferation of microglial cells occurring in the cerebellar cortex as a response to the presence of degenerating dendrites of Purkinje cells.
Cerebral cortex foliation	The development of cortical folds in the course of fetal development.
Ceroid	A pigment derived from the incomplete oxidation of lipids which accumulates within neurones, retinal cells and extraneural tissues in the hereditary neuronal storage disease – Batten's disease – one of the group of disorders associated with blindness formerly known as amaurotic family idiocy. The pigment is stained positively with PAS and Sudan Black.
Cervical spondylosis	Narrowing of the cervical disc spaces associated with disc degeneration. Associated with a reactive formation of osteophytes and thickening of the intervertebral ligaments.
Chorea	Brief, sudden, jerky involuntary movements of an irregular pattern. These occur classically in Huntington's disease and in some cases of acute rheumatic fever (Sydenham's chorea).

A Glossary of Neuropathological Terms – *continued*

Cell/Reaction/
Syndrome/Lesion

Chromatolysis	A reaction to axonal injury which causes the cell body of the neurone to become rounded, the Nissl granules to break up and disappear leaving only a thin rim of cytoplasm at the periphery of the cell. The central part of the cell becomes pale and stains pink with cresyl violet (see *Fig. 45.1*).
Constructional apraxia	A sign of parietal lobe disease in which loss of body image and spatial orientation occur in the non-dominant cerebral hemisphere. Patients are unable to carry out simple constructional tasks e.g. drawing a star.
Corpora amylacea	Rounded laminated bodies measuring 10–15 microns in diameter. They are often present in the peri-ventricular and sub-pial white matter and are believed to be the expression of end-stage degeneration of astrocytes.
Craniorrhachischisis	A combination of anencephaly with complete spina bifida.
Dacryoliths	A mass of inspissated mucus found in the lacrimal sac. It occurs usually as a reaction to the presence of a nidus of foreign material which becomes infected.
Dendrites	Branched, non-myelinated neuronal processes usually confined to the vicinity of the perikaryon (cell body) of the neurone and which receive impulses afferent to the neurone.
Diastematomyelia	A malformation of the spinal cord in which there are two hemi-cords either within a single dural sac or in two separate dural sacs.
Ependyma	The cell lining of the cerebral ventricles and the central canal of the spinal cord. Cilia project from the surfaces of these cells.
Etat criblé	The presence of many small perivascular cavities, due to irregular rarefaction and disintegration of the parenchyma around small blood vessels, in the centrum semiovale and other richly myelinated regions.
État lacunaire	The presence of many small perivascular cavities of identical pathogenesis to those described above, but located in the grey matter.
État marbre	The presence of whitish spots or streaks in the lateral parts of the corpus striatum or, more rarely, the thalamus giving a 'marbled' appearance. It is due to an abnormal distribution of myelinated fibres and is seen in neonates who have suffered from hypoxic-ischaemic damage to the brain.
Ferrugination (neuronal)	Encrusting of neurones in the vicinity of old infarcts with iron and calcium.
Finnish snowballs	Granular osmiophilic, lipid deposits seen by electron microscopy in a wide variety of cell types in Batten's disease.
Glioma-Rosenthal fibres	Bodies formed in the perikarya and processes of astrocytes. They are rather structureless, eosinophilic structures which may be rounded, oval, elongated or club shaped. They are believed to consist in part of degenerate astrocytic protein filaments and in part of a conjugate of ubiquitin and GFAP.
Gliomatosis	A neuroepithelial tumour of uncertain origin frequently occurring in the brainstem and the spinal cord. The affected area of the brain or cord is expanded and firm and the lesion is very poorly demarcated from the surrounding tissue.
Gliosis	A reaction to damage in the CNS characterized by hypertrophy and hyperplasia of astrocytes.
Haematomyelia	Haemorrhage within the spinal cord.

A Glossary of Neuropathological Terms – *continued*

Cell/Reaction/
Syndrome/Lesion

Hepatolenticular degeneration	Wilson's disease in which a defect in copper metabolism is associated with chronic liver disease leading to cirrhosis and neuronal loss and reactive astrocytosis in the basal ganglia.
Hirano body	An ovoid eosinophilic structure seen most commonly in the pyramidal cells of the hippocampus. Increasing numbers of these structures appear to be associated with increased age.
Hypermyelination	Increased thickness of the myelin sheath of peripheral nerves seen in certain hereditary neuropathies and in the neuropathy associated with paraproteinaemia.
Hyponatraemic central pontine myelinolysis	Symmetrical demyelination occurring in the central part of the pons most commonly in middle aged individuals who are alcoholics or who are malnourished or otherwise debilitated. There is a strong association with hyponatraemia especially where the latter has been corrected rapidly.
Kernohan lesion	Infarction of the contralateral cerebral peduncle due to tentorial herniation in patients with supratentorial expanding lesions.
Leukoaraiosis	Changes associated with rarefaction of the periventricular white matter seen on CT scans in both demented and intellectually normal old people. It represents partial infarction of the white matter.
Leukomalacia	The presence of ill-defined white spots in the periventricular white matter seen quite commonly in the brains of premature infants at autopsy. It represents white matter infarction due to lack of perfusion along the boundary zones between arterial territories.
Lissencephaly	A condition characterized by absence of gyri in the brain. It may be either familial or sporadic and half the cases are associated with a deletion in the short arm of chromosome 17.
Lymphorrhage	The presence of clusters of lymphocytes between muscle bundles in the extra-ocular muscles. It is strongly suggestive of endocrine exophthalmos.
Megalencephaly	Enlargement of the brain, defined in adults as a brain weighing more than 1700 g or more than 2.5 standard deviations from the mean normal for individuals of that age and gender. The primary form may occur as an isolated phenomenon or be associated with achondroplasia or endocrine disease. Secondary megalencephaly may be seen in association with storage disorders such as Tay-Sachs disease and with tuberous sclerosis.
Microcephaly	A reduction in size of the head secondary to a reduction in the size of the brain (less than 1000 g in adults and less than 2 standard deviations below the mean normal for an individual of that age and gender). There are many causes including congenital infections such as rubella, toxoplasmosis or cytomegalovirus and it may also be associated with intra-uterine growth retardation, phenylketonuria and the fetal alcohol syndrome.
Myelitis	Inflammatory process within the spinal cord.
Neuronophagia	The process in which microglial cells surround dead neurones like a capsule and invade the neurone body at a few places (see *Fig. 45.2*).
Neurone-dark cell change	Shrinkage of neurones near the surface of the brain associated with deep staining of their nuclei and a corkscrew-like twisting of their axons and dendrites. This is an artefact of fixation and may be mistaken for ischaemic neuronal damage.
Neurone-deafferentation	If the synaptic input to a neurone decreases, the neurone either atrophies and eventually dies, being replaced by gliosis or, less commonly enlarges and shows vacuolation of its cytoplasm.

A Glossary of Neuropathological Terms – *continued*

Cell/Reaction/ Syndrome/Lesion	
Neurone-dying back	A degeneration of nerve fibres, often caused by toxins, which gradually progresses upwards towards the parent cell body.
Neurone-granulovacuolar degeneration	The presence of vacuoles measuring 3–4 microns in diameter, within the cytoplasm of neurones, especially the pyramidal cells of the hippocampus. Each vacuole contains a small centrally placed inclusion. This change may be seen in the brains of intellectually normal elderly individuals but is especially common in Alzheimer's disease and may also be seen in some cases of progressive supranuclear palsy.
Neuropil	The intercellular matrix of the CNS consisting of a complex of glial and neuronal processes and myelin.
Neurulation	The formation of the axial neural tube from the primitive, two-dimensional neural plate.
Nissl substance	Basophilic granular, peri-nuclear material in neurones. It is made up of stacks of rough endoplasmic reticulum and intervening groups of polyribosomes.
Oligodendrocyte	The sub-class of glial cell which forms and maintains myelin with the CNS.
Opalski cell	Globoid cells measuring up to 35 microns in diameter which have an eccentric nucleus and somewhat foamy cytoplasm. They are believed to be derived from altered astrocytes and are seen in the brains of patients with Wilson's disease.
Pachygyria	A reduction in the normal number of gyri which, in addition are broader and shallower than normal.
Perineuronal satellite cell	An oligodendroglial cell found in grey matter and closely related to a neurone.
Polymicrogyria	A developmental abnormality in which there are large numbers of small closely packed gyri giving the surface of the brain an appearance which has been likened to that of 'cobblestones'.
Porencephaly	Cysts within the CNS which are not lined by ependymal cells.
Psammoma bodies	In the context of the CNS these are whorls of meningothelial cells which have become calcified.
Reich granules	Laminated bodies derived from lipid which are found in the cytoplasm of normal Schwann cells.
Remak fibres	This term is sometimes used to describe a Schwann cell together with its associated axons.
Subependymoma	Tumours arising deep to the ependyma most often in the lateral or fourth ventricles. They protrude as firm nodules into the affected ventricle.
Tuffstone bodies	Small amounts of cerebroside sulphate seen on electron microscopy of Schwann cells in patients with metachromatic leukodystrophy.
Ulegyria	An appearance seen in hypoxic/ischaemic damage to the infant brain in which neuronal loss and poor myelination lead to thinning of the convolutions and widening of the sulci.
Zebra bodies	An inclusion seen by electron microscopy in neurones in patients with one of the severe mucopolysaccharidoses. The Zebra body consists of irregular arrays of transverse dark and light lamellae with a periodicity of 5–7 microns, the lamellae being enclosed in a single unit membrane.

causes a much greater rise in pressure within the cranium than would be the case in another anatomical site.

- A rise in intracranial pressure causes displacement of the cerebrospinal fluid (CSF) followed by compression of the ventricles. This causes displacement of the brain, most commonly downwards and backwards towards the foramen magnum. Portions of brain **herniate** under the tentorium or falx and may become compressed against the sharp edge of the dural folds, thus sustaining damage.

Another important factor affecting intracranial pressure is the CSF. **The CSF is produced by the choroid plexus; normally the rate of formation by the choroid plexus equals the rate of absorption by arachnoid villi.** In an adult the normal CSF volume is about 140 ml; approximately 20 ml are formed and absorbed per hour. Absorption occurs via the arachnoid granulations associated with major venous sinuses and the sleeves of spinal nerve roots. The arachnoid granulations function as one-way valves which respond to pressure differences between the CSF and the dural venous sinuses.

Any disturbance in this equilibrium leads to **hydrocephalus**, expressed in the form of:
- **an increase in the volume of CSF**
- **dilatation of the cerebral ventricles** (*Fig. 45.3*).

This theoretical model of hydrocephalus being due either to overproduction of CSF or to defective absorption is correct in principle, but in fact the vast majority of cases are due to defective absorption. **The only instance of overproduction of CSF being the cause of hydrocephalus occurs in cases of the benign neoplasm, choroid plexus papilloma** (see p 1164).

Defective absorption of CSF occurs:
- **if there is obstruction to the flow pathways of the CSF** within either the ventricular system or the subarachnoid space. This accounts for most cases of hydrocephalus and is termed **obstructive hydrocephalus**.

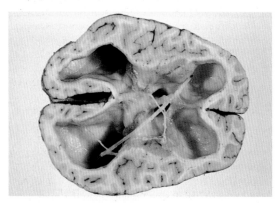

FIGURE 45.3 *Hydrocephalus showing a gross degree of dilatation of the lateral ventricles.*

- **in a small number of cases where there is either defective absorption of fluid by the arachnoid villi or in the presence of venous hypertension leading to decreased venous drainage**

Obstructive Hydrocephalus
Obstructive hydrocephalus is subdivided into **two** classes, this division being made in relation to the **site** of obstruction.

1) Where this occurs **within the ventricular system**, most commonly at points where the pathway narrows, such as the foramen of Monro, the aqueduct of Sylvius or the exit foramina from the fourth ventricle, the condition is termed **non-communicating hydrocephalus**. This term is derived from the fact that dye injected into the lateral ventricles does not appear in the lumbar CSF.

2) **When the obstruction is located within the subarachnoid space (communicating hydrocephalus)**, the dye appears in the lumbar CSF very soon after intraventricular injection. The distinction between these two types of obstruction is of practical use in relation to the location of shunts inserted to relieve the obstruction.

Obstruction may be congenital or acquired.

Congenital or Infantile Hydrocephalus
This is usually due to developmental malformations such as one of the variants of the Chiari malformation, isolated stenosis of the aqueduct of Sylvius, the Dandy–Walker malformation (see below) or obstruction of the foramina of Magendie or Luschka as a result of fibrous organization of cerebellar haemorrhage.

Effects of Infantile Hydrocephalus
In young infants in whom fusion of the skull sutures has not occurred, cranial enlargement results from hydrocephalus. Insertion of a shunt into the distended ventricles serves to drain off the excess fluid. If this is not done, irreparable brain damage may ensue, leaving the child with a severe degree of learning disability.

Very young infants (less than 2 months old) who have relatively little myelin at this stage of development tolerate ventricular distension better than slightly older children (more than 6 months old) in whom development of myelin is further advanced. Revision of the shunts is necessary from time to time as the child grows and infection is an ever-present danger.

Acquired Hydrocephalus
This may be the result of a focal lesion such as a tumour (especially lesions in the posterior fossa), an abscess or a haematoma, or of a diffuse process such as meningitis or subarachnoid haemorrhage.

Effects of Acquired Hydrocephalus
The **clinical effects** of such hydrocephalus depend largely in whether it is associated with a rise in intra-

cranial pressure or not. Symptoms and signs associated with raised intracranial pressure include mental dullness, nausea, vomiting and papilloedema.

In some instances the hydrocephalus stabilizes through small changes in the rates of production and absorption of CSF. In these patients the intracranial pressure becomes normal again but the patient may be left with a crippling syndrome consisting of:

- dementia
- a disorder of gait
- urinary incontinence

This situation is termed **'normal pressure hydrocephalus'**.

Hydrocephalus *Ex Vacuo*
This term is applied to a dilatation of ventricles seen either after loss of brain tissue as a result of ischaemia or of atrophy associated with dementia. In this situation, there is, of course, *no* rise in pressure of the CSF.

Raised Intracranial Pressure
The significance of various levels of intracranial pressure is shown in *Table 45.1*.

In addition to the absolute level of pressure, **the rate of increase is also an important factor**: the more rapid the rise, the more severe are the clinical effects. Causes of raised intracranial pressure are shown in *Table 45.2*.

Pathological Features
The main pathological effect of raised intracranial pressure is displacement of brain:

- **Supratentorial lesions cause downward and backward displacement of brain.** Vessels passing from basilar artery to brainstem may rupture leading to haemorrhage in the brainstem (Duret's haemorrhages) and foci of ischaemic necrosis. This is a common cause of death in patients with raised intracranial pressure. The uncinate gyrus of the temporal lobe may herniate through the tentorium

Table 45.2 Causes of Raised Intracranial Pressure

Type	Causes
Obstructive hydrocephalus	Developmental malformations (see p 1114) Tumour, abscess, haematoma Late results of meningitis or subarachnoid haemorrhage
Local space-occupying lesions	Neoplasm Infection Ischaemic necrosis (infarction)
Cerebral oedema	Vasogenic (breakdown of blood–brain barrier) Cytotoxic (intracellular) Associated with infection Post-traumatic Hypercapnia in chronic obstructive airflow disease

leading to stretching of third nerve with ptosis, lateral displacement of the eye (due to unopposed action of sixth nerve) and dilatation of the pupil. Compression of the pyramidal tract in the crus cerebri of the opposite side against the sharp edge of the tentorium may produce **motor paralysis on the same side as the expanding lesion**.

The **cingulate gyrus** may herniate beneath the falx. This can lead to infarction in the territory supplied by the **pericallosal arteries**, resulting in weakness or sensory loss in one or both legs.

- **Infratentorial lesions (posterior fossa) cause herniation of the cerebellar tonsils through the foramen magnum.** This can also occur in association with some supratentorial lesions. Tonsillar herniation produces **grooving on the ventral aspect of the medulla** where it has been compressed against the anterior edge of the foramen magnum. There is normally some variation in the configuration of the tonsils and this may give rise to a false impression of grooving. **Absolute confirmation of the presence of herniation depends on the presence of haemorrhagic necrosis at the tips of the cerebellar tonsils.** Tonsillar herniation adversely affects the respiratory centres, leading to apnoea and death. Performing lumbar puncture in patients with greatly raised intracranial pressure may lead to such herniation.

Table 45.1 Effects of Raised Intracranial Pressure

Pressure (kPa)	Effects
0–1.3 (0–10 mmHg)	Normal
2–3	Mild; no treatment required
4	Moderate; treatment required
> 5	Severe; associated with some cerebral ischaemia and decline of electrical activity of brain
> 8	Very severe; invariably fatal

Apart from the displacement, the brain appears swollen and, because it is compressed against the skull, the gyri are flattened and the sulci narrowed.

Clinical Features

- **Headache.** This is worst in mornings and is often described as 'bursting'. It is a result of tension in dura and distortion in cerebral vessels, both of which are pain sensitive.
- **Vomiting.** Vomiting occurs as a result of distortion or ischaemia of the lower part of brainstem.
- **Papilloedema.** This is swelling of the optic disc, as seen on ophthalmoscopy. It is due to the accumulation of axoplasm in the optic disc owing to blocking of the normal flow of axoplasm from retinal ganglion cells along the optic nerve.

CONGENITAL AND GENETIC DISORDERS

MALFORMATIONS

Neural Tube Defects

Early in life, the neural plate folds along its length to form the neural tube. The surrounding mesoderm ultimately forms the skull and vertebral column. Defects in closure of the neural tube are most common at the lower end, producing **spina bifida**, a set of disorders in which the posterior arches of the lowest lumbar vertebrae are not fused.

Patients may be mildly or severely affected depending on the type of defect:

- **Spina bifida occulta.** This is the mildest form in which only the vertebral arches are affected. Overlying skin may show a dimple, a patch of hair or a nodule of adipose tissue.
- **Meningocele.** This lesion is more severe: a CSF-filled sac of meningeal tissue protrudes through the vertebral defect.
- **Meningomyelocele.** This is still more severe: the sac contains part of the spinal cord. It is associated with major neurological defects affecting the lower limbs, and bladder and rectal function.
- **Spina bifida aperta.** This is very rare and is the most severe form. There is complete failure of fusion of caudal end of the neural plate. The unfused plate lies exposed on the skin surface. Severe neurological defects affecting lower limbs, bladder and rectum are present.

Failures of closure do occur at the cranial end of the tube but are less common. Anencephaly, which is incompatible with life, occurs as a result of complete failure of development of the cranial end of the neural tube. Meningoceles may occur in the occipital region, as may **encephaloceles** which contain brain tissue and are the homologue of meningomyelocele.

Arnold–Chiari Malformations

Four types are described:
1) **Ectopia of cerebellar tonsils**, which may herniate through the foramen magnum and be associated with arachnoiditis and thickening of the meninges. This defect may be associated with **syringomyelia**: the development of fluid-filled spaces in the spinal cord.
2) **Elongation of the medulla** with or without an S-shaped deformity, and prolongation and herniation of the vermis of the cerebellum into the foramen magnum (*Fig. 45.4*). This defect may be associated with meningomyelocele. Hydrocephalus develops, especially if the meningomyelocele is repaired.
4) **Cervical spina bifida in which the cerebellum herniates through the foramen magnum and forms part of a myelocerebellomeningocele**
4) **cerebellar hypoplasia**

Dandy–Walker Malformation

This is a rare cause of hydrocephalus in early life. Typically, three abnormalities are present:
- a malformed cerebellar vermis
- obstruction to fourth ventricle foramina with cystic dilatation of the fourth ventricle
- an elevated tentorium

INFECTIONS OF THE CNS

Infections of the nervous system are, by convention, classified as affecting:
- the **meninges and CSF (meningitis)**
- the **parenchyma of the brain** itself (**encephalitis**)

This classification is convenient but it should not be forgotten that, in some infections, both meninges and brain are involved (meningoencephalitis).

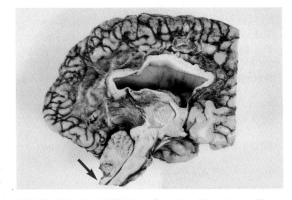

FIGURE 45.4 Arnold–Chiari malformation. Note the peg-like projection of the cerebellar tonsil (arrowed), which is protruding downwards. This is characteristic of Chiari-type malformations and, as seen here, is associated with hydrocephalus.

MENINGEAL INFECTIONS
These may be either acute or chronic.

Acute Meningitis

Acute meningitis usually involves the **leptomeninges**: the **pia mater** and the **arachnoid**. The fact that these membranes are bathed in CSF means that **dissemination of acute meningeal infections within the cranial cavity is almost inevitable**. Infections of the dura do occur (**pachymeningitis**). This may result from spread of infection from a cranial or cervical spinal osteomyelitis, or from an epidural abscess. Tertiary syphilis, now very rare, typically results in pachymeningitis.

Acute meningitis may occur as a result of either:

- **bacterial infections, in which the exudate is usually purulent**
- **viral infections, which elicit a cellular reaction that is almost entirely lymphocytic in nature**

Organisms Responsible for Acute Bacterial Meningitis

The organisms likely to be found in a given case of acute meningitis vary with the **age** of the patient and the **route** of infection:

- *Streptococcus pneumoniae* is the commonest cause of acute meningitis and especially affects the very young and the very old. The source of infection is likely to be pneumonia, endocarditis or sinusitis. Alcoholics and splenectomized patients also show an increased risk of pneumococcal meningitis.
- **Meningococcal** meningitis can occur in epidemics (caused by *Neisseria meningitidis* group A or C) or may be sporadic (group B). Group B infections have been increasing in frequency over the past 20 years. They are commonest in children under 5 years but are increasing in prevalence in the second decade of life.
- *Haemophilus influenzae* is the commonest cause of bacterial meningitis in children up to the age of 6 years but it can also occur in other age groups. It usually results from spread **from pharyngeal or middle ear infections**. There is a considerable risk of intellectual impairment in children who survive this type of meningitis.
- In the **neonatal period,** *Escherichia coli* is the organism most commonly responsible for acute bacterial meningitis. Low birth-weight, prematurity or the presence of congenital malformation seem to increase the risk of such meningitis.

The above infections account for about 40% of all cases of bacterial meningitis.

- *Listeria monocytogenes* can cause meningitis in healthy adults but is more important as a cause of disease in neonates; the infants become infected by organisms in the genital tract of the mother. A moderately high risk of *Listeria* infection exists in immunosuppressed patients.

L. monocytogenes is a Gram-positive bacterium found in plant material, soil and water. It causes a number of diseases in sheep and cattle; **the route for human infection is via food, especially unpasteurized milk and cheese**. In human adults, *Listeria* infections are often symptomless and the organisms reside in the genital and gastrointestinal tracts. Like mycobacteria, *Listeria* tends to be **intracellular** and can multiply unhindered within the cytoplasm of macrophages. This comfortable state of affairs (for the *Listeria*) is brought to an end if the macrophages become activated by lymphokines derived from specific T helper cells. Very occasionally, *Listeria* may cause a severe inflammatory process within the substance of the brain and spinal cord, associated with extensive areas of necrosis.

Possible Routes of Infection in Acute Meningitis

- **Via the bloodstream** (major route). *N. meningitidis* and *H. influenzae* colonize the nasopharynx and, if meningitis occurs, it is usually related to recent colonization in this site. *Neisseria* and *Haemophilus* attach themselves to nasal epithelium by their **pili**. New strains appear frequently and are spread by close contact such as is found in camps, hostels, etc. Organisms colonizing the nasopharynx may be ingested by macrophages and carried in these cells in the bloodstream until they reach the CNS. The mechanism by which the organisms actually gain access to the CSF is unknown but it has been suggested that it may be via the choroid plexus where the CSF is secreted.
- **Direct spread from infection in the sinuses or middle ear**
- **Direct implantation in the course of trauma or manoeuvres such as lumbar puncture or the insertion of ventricular shunts to relieve hydrocephalus**
- Certain viruses spread along nerves to reach the brain, notably rabies and herpes simplex.

Macroscopic Features

In fatal cases of acute meningitis the brain shows loss of the normal transparency of the leptomeninges. The resulting opacity is due to the presence of inflammatory exudate within the subarachnoid space (*Fig. 45.5*); the colour of the exudate may give some clues as to the aetiology. For example, pus in a pneumococcal exudate has a greenish tinge.

The location of the exudate may also vary from case to case. The exudate in pneumococcal meningitis is usually most obvious over the cerebral hemispheres, whereas that in *Haemophilus* infections is most marked at the base of the brain.

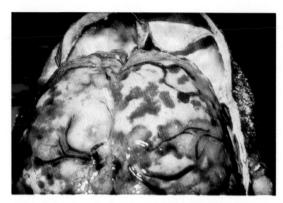

FIGURE 45.5 *Acute bacterial meningitis. The leptomeninges are obscured by a yellowish purulent exudate in which some foci of haemorrhage can be seen.*

Microscopic Features

There is vasodilatation and a large number of inflammatory cells within the subarachnoid space and extending into the sulci. The predominant cell type depends on the stage at which the brain is examined. In the early phases most of the inflammatory cells are polymorphs, but in longer-surviving patients the macrophage becomes the dominant cell type.

In some cases the inflammatory reaction extends into the underlying brain tissue, and inflammatory cells may be seen in the perivascular spaces within the parenchyma.

Complications

Complications of acute meningitis include:

- **cerebral oedema, which is usually generalized**
- **involvement of small blood vessels within the subarachnoid space by the acute inflammatory process.** This may lead to thrombosis and the production of small ischaemic lesions in the underlying brain.
- **cranial nerve palsies**, due to involvement of certain nerves (especially the sixth nerve) as they pass through the inflamed subarachnoid space
- As in any other inflammation, if the exudate is not completely removed by macrophage action, **scarring can occur and this may cause blockage of some of the foramina and the development of hydrocephalus**.
- **ependymitis.** The infection may spread to involve the ependymal lining of the ventricles. This is fortunately rare – it is usually fatal. The surface of the ventricle appears roughened and the ventricle itself may contain pus.

Diagnosis

The clinical diagnosis of meningitis is based on signs of meningeal irritation:

- headache
- neck stiffness
- photophobia
- fever
- in some cases, clouding of consciousness

Confirmation of acute bacterial meningitis depends on examination of a sample of CSF obtained at lumbar puncture.

Laboratory Findings

Macroscopically, the fluid is cloudy and microscopic examination of a smear of the fluid, or of the spun-down deposit, shows the presence of numerous acute inflammatory cells. The use of the Gram stain may show the organisms (e.g. intracellular Gram-negative diplococci in neisserial meningitis). Progress towards a rapid bacteriological diagnosis can be made by using agglutinating antisera, which are available for **Neisseria meningitidis, Streptococcus pneumoniae** and type B **Haemophilus influenzae**. Confirmation of the identity of the infecting organisms can then be obtained by culture of the CSF.

Alteration in some of the biochemical characteristics of CSF are also found in acute bacterial meningitis:

- **The protein concentration is greatly increased (to more than 5 g/l).**
- **There is a sharp fall in the concentration of glucose which, in normal CSF, is about two-thirds that in blood.** The fall in glucose concentration, presumably due to its use as a nutrient by the proliferating organisms, may bring its concentration down to less than 50% of the level in blood.

Chronic Bacterial Meningitis

Tuberculous Meningitis

Tuberculous meningitis has a much more insidious onset than the acute pyogenic meningitides. Often there is a rather non-specific prodrome lasting for 2–3 weeks in which patients, often infants or children, may show anorexia, malaise and episodes of vomiting. This is followed by the onset of symptoms and signs of meningeal irritation, but often these are less marked than in acute bacterial meningitis. A similar clinical picture may be seen in the commonest form of fungal meningitis, which is caused by *Cryptococcus neoformans*.

CSF Changes in Tuberculous Meningitis

Unlike pyogenic meningitis, the CSF in tuberculous meningitis is usually clear, although the protein content is raised and a delicate clot may be seen in the fluid. Both glucose and chloride concentrations are lowered; the reduction in glucose concentration is much less than that in the pyogenic meningitides. The cell population, which, compared with normal, is increased by a factor of approximately ten, may be a mixed one comprising both polymorphs and lymphocytes, although the former usually predominate.

Macroscopic Features

Although the entire surface of the brain may be involved, the area most severely affected is the base of the brain; the subarachnoid space may be filled with rather gelatinous, greyish-green material in which blood vessels at the base of the brain and the emerging cranial nerves are embedded.

Scarring at these sites is likely to lead to cranial nerve palsies. In some instances this exudate is associated with ischaemic lesions in the underlying brain. This results from involvement of penetrating blood vessels by the inflammatory process in the subarachnoid space leading to thrombosis or to a fibromuscular intimal response which reduces the vascular lumen.

Microscopic Features

Histologically, the diagnosis is not always straightforward as well-formed granulomas may be present in only very small numbers, and the inflammatory reaction may appear rather non-specific with many macrophages and plasma cells arranged in a somewhat haphazard fashion. If the degree of local tissue hypersensitivity is marked, there may be evidence of abundant caseation necrosis and scarring, the latter leading to hydrocephalus as a result of blockage of CSF flow.

Other chronic meningitides are caused by *Treponema pallidum* and a variety of fungi.

Syphilis and the CNS

The lesions of tertiary syphilis occurring in the CNS fall into two distinct groups:

1) Lesions involving the meninges and their small blood vessels lead to a chronic meningitis, patchy gummatous necrosis and severe narrowing of arterial lumina as a result of swelling of endothelial cells. Lesions tend to occur early in the tertiary stage and have even been recorded in the secondary stage of the disease.

2) So-called **parenchymatous neurosyphilis** occurs late in the tertiary stage and involves degeneration of the neuronal elements themselves.

Meningovascular Syphilis

Syphilis may involve either the leptomeninges or the pachymeninges, the former being more frequently affected.

Leptomeningitis occurs most often at the base of the brain; the meninges become swollen and thickened, and occasionally small patches of gummatous necrosis may be seen. Cranial nerve involvement is not uncommon and the process may also obstruct the foramina of the fourth ventricle and thus cause hydrocephalus.

Pachymeningitis may occur over the surface of the cerebral hemispheres and also in relation to parts of the spinal cord, where the blood vessel involvement can cause patchy necrosis. These conditions are now rarely seen.

Viral Meningitis

Acute Lymphocytic (Viral) Meningitis

Viral infections produce a number of different pathological effects on the cells and tissues of the CNS, one of which is **acute leptomeningitis**.

The clinical presentation is usually acute with:
- fever
- drowsiness
- headache
- neck stiffness
- nausea and vomiting

Examination of the CSF reveals a picture somewhat different from that seen in bacterial meningitis:
- There is an increase in the number of cells, the majority of these being **lymphocytes**.
- The protein concentration is slightly raised.
- The glucose concentration is usually normal.

The commonest viral infections causing acute meningitis are:
- **enteroviruses**: coxsackievirus and echoviruses
- **mumps virus** infection with or without parotitis

Somewhat less common are infections with:
- **herpes simplex type 2**
- **varicella zoster**
- the **arenavirus** causing lymphocytic choriomeningitis

In about 30% of cases of acute lymphocytic meningitis it is not possible to identify an aetiological agent.

PARENCHYMAL INFECTIONS OF THE BRAIN (ENCEPHALITIS)

These may be bacterial, viral, fungal or protozoal. The spongiform encephalopathies, which are transmissible but almost certainly not caused by a living agent, are discussed in the section on the pathology of dementia (see pp 1141–1143).

Viral Encephalitis

Viral encephalitis is an unusual complication of common viral infections; it is certainly true that the ratio of patients with systemic viral infections to those in whom obvious clinical disease of the CNS develops is high.

The viral encephalitides can be divided into **three** main groups, largely on the basis of their cause or pathogenesis:
- **acute viral encephalitis**
- **postinfectious encephalomyelitis** (see p 1134)
- **persistent viral encephalitis**
- **slow viral infections of the CNS**

A very wide range of viruses can cause encephalitis;

only a few of the commoner ones are considered here. Epidemics of acute viral encephalitis are most likely to be due to insect-borne infections; sporadic cases can be due to many different viruses, of which the most common is herpes simplex.

Routes of Infection

Viruses generally reach the CNS and gain access to it by one of two routes:

1) **The most common is via the bloodstream.** The viruses may reach the blood via lymphatic drainage from the sites of infection (e.g. the respiratory tract in the case of mumps, measles or varicella zoster infection, or the gastrointestinal tract in the case of enteroviruses such as poliovirus or the echoviruses). Obviously, infection with insect-borne viruses is mediated by the bites of the arthropod vectors concerned.

2) **Via nerves.** This is the pathway used by the rabies virus, but there is also increasing evidence that the far more common (in the UK) herpes simplex encephalitis may arise as a result of transport of the virus along nerve pathways in the olfactory tract.

The precise sequence of events between the occurrence

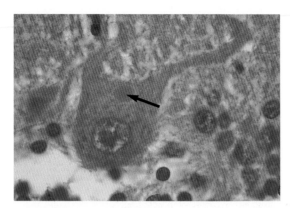

FIGURE 45.8 *Rabies showing an intracytoplasmic inclusion (Negri body, arrowed) in a Purkinje cell.*

of viraemia and the entry of the viruses to the brain parenchyma is not clear. Obviously the viruses cross the endothelial cell lining, but whether this is the result of passive pinocytotic transport or of viral proliferation within the endothelial cells is not certain. Whatever the truth may be, changes in endothelial cell morphology are present in most cases of encephalitis.

Acute Viral Encephalitis

Microscopic Features

- **Perivascular 'cuffing'**: small vessels within the brain are surrounded by a lymphocyte and plasma cell infiltrate (*Fig. 45.6*) filling the Virchow–Robin space. In severe cases the basement membrane marking the boundary between the perivascular space and the surrounding brain tissue breaks and the inflammatory cells stream out into the brain substance.
- **Neuronal changes.** Neurone loss occurs and many neurones may show the presence of shrunken, darkly staining, nuclei and eosinophilic cytoplasm.
- **Inclusion bodies** may be seen within affected cells. In herpes simplex encephalitis the inclusions are intranuclear and are referred to as **Cowdry type A** inclusions (*Fig. 45.7*). In rabies, the pathognomonic change is the presence of the **Negri body** (*Fig. 45.8*). This is a cytoplasmic inclusion measuring 1–7 μm in diameter. It stains red with eosin and is rounded or oval in shape. The largest Negri bodies occur in the pyramidal cells of the hippocampus, in Purkinje cells in the cerebellum and in anterior horn cells within the spinal cord.
- **Tissue necrosis** can be extensive in herpes simplex encephalitis (*Fig. 45.9*), typically affecting the temporal lobes most severely. Phagocytosis of necrotic neurones by microglial cells (macrophages) is seen, and is termed **neuronophagia**.

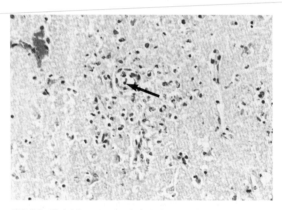

FIGURE 45.6 *Herpes encephalitis showing a perivascular inflammatory focus. The central capillary is arrowed.*

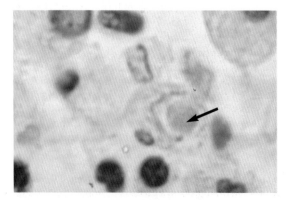

FIGURE 45.7 *Herpes encephalitis showing a typical intranuclear inclusion.*

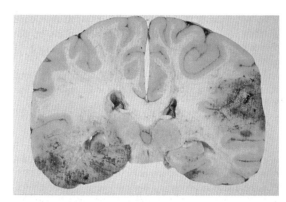

FIGURE 45.9 Herpes encephalitis showing large areas of necrosis associated with some haemorrhage. Macroscopic evidence of damage is rare in viral infections of the CNS, with the exception of herpes simplex virus.

Persistent Viral Encephalitis

Subacute Sclerosing Panencephalitis

A characteristic type of chronic infection is seen in a small number of patients as a result of infection with **measles virus**. The disease that follows the very long-continued localization of measles virus in the brain is known as **subacute sclerosing panencephalitis**. The peak incidence of this, happily rare, condition is during adolescent life. Affected patients present with increasing reduction of intellectual function, motor abnormalities and fits. An inexorable downward path is followed by death within 1 year of the appearance of symptoms. The patients' brains show degenerative features with loss of myelin and a mild increase in the supporting glial fibres. There is also evidence of an encephalitis in the form of a perivascular lymphocytic infiltrate (*Fig. 45.10*). CSF contains high titres of measles antibody

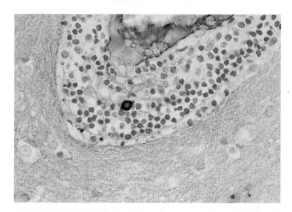

FIGURE 45.10 Subacute sclerosing panencephalitis following measles. The section has been treated with an antibody reacting with immunoglobulin A. The binding sites show up as brown area in the centre of the field. This is surrounded by a florid inflammatory reaction within the perivascular space, this indicating the presence of subacute encephalitis.

and viral antigen, and nucleocapsid material can be identified in cells within the brain as well as within lymph nodes. It has been suggested that the disorder is an expression of an aberrant T-cell response to the presence of virus in the brain, but this is still a matter of debate.

Slow Viral Infections

Progressive Multifocal Leucoencephalopathy

Slow viral infection in the human CNS is exemplified by **progressive multifocal leucoencephalopathy**, a rare disease of the brain leading to focal demyelination in many areas of the white matter. It is caused by infection with members of the **papovavirus** group and occurs only in patients who are immunosuppressed. Such immunosuppression may be seen in patients with neoplastic disease involving the lymphoid system, such as Hodgkin's disease, and also in those who are receiving cytotoxic chemotherapy in the course of treatment for malignant disease.

The papovaviruses that have been isolated from the brains of affected individuals (JC viruses) are widespread, at least in Europe and the USA, as evidenced by the fact that 70–80% of adult serum contains specific antibodies to the virus. Papovavirus infections, in the general population, are usually acquired fairly early in life.

Macroscopic Features

Many small grey foci are distributed throughout the brain. The white matter is chiefly affected but lesions also occur in the basal ganglia. Some lesions coalesce and cyst formation may occur.

Microscopic Features

Many foci of demyelination are present, associated with lipid-containing macrophages, large atypical astrocytes and abnormal oligodendroglial cells.

Electron microscopy shows virions in the abnormal oligodendrocytes. Viral antigen can be recognized by a variety of methods and JC virus can be cultured from the lesions.

NEUROPATHOLOGY OF ACQUIRED IMMUNE DEFICIENCY SYNDROME

Many of the conditions affecting the nervous system in patients with **acquired immune deficiency syndrome (AIDS)** are dealt with separately in this chapter, but there is some advantage in briefly reviewing this aspect of neuropathology in a discrete section. Some 40–50% of patients with AIDS have been reported as having neurological symptoms; in some cases these symptoms may represent the first signs of the disease. Post-mortem examination of the nervous system of patients with AIDS shows morphological abnormalities in roughly 80%.

Changes seen in the brain in AIDS fall into **three classes, being due to**:

1) the interaction of human immunodeficiency virus (HIV) type 1 with the CNS

2) opportunistic infections occurring as a result of the immune deficiency

3) an increased risk of certain neoplasms as a result of the immune deficiency

Changes Directly Due to Presence of HIV-1 in the Brain

Subacute Encephalitis (AIDS Encephalopathy)

Subacute encephalitis is recognized by the presence in the brain of one or both of **two** histological features:

1) **microglial nodules.** These are small clusters of lymphocytes and macrophage-like cells seen in the white matter, basal ganglia, pons and cerebellum, and, more rarely, in the cortex.

2) **multinucleated giant cells**, marking with antimacrophage antibodies

The frequency of subacute encephalitis, which, clinically, is associated with AIDS-related dementia, depends on the diagnostic criteria used. If numerous microglial nodules are the sole criterion, the reported frequency varies from 45 to 69%. When multinucleated giant cells are the sole criterion, the reported frequency drops to 28%.

In subacute encephalitis, the presence of the virus can be established either by seeing budding retroviral particles on electron microscopy, or by the use of immunohistochemistry or *in situ* hybridization.

Once the virus reaches the brain, macrophages become affected; some express the CD4 molecule for which the virus has selective tropism. How HIV enters the brain is still unknown.

Vacuolar Myelopathy

This condition was first described in 1985 in patients with AIDS. It is characterized by vacuolation in the spinal cord predominantly involving the lateral and posterior columns of the thoracic portion. The lesions start as swellings within the myelin sheath and this progresses to severe vacuolation with secondary degeneration of the axons.

The pathological findings are similar to those seen in subacute combined degeneration of the cord in patients with pernicious anaemia, but there is no evidence of abnormalities in the serum vitamin B_{12} or folic acid levels. Vacuolation of myelin has also been reported in toxic reactions to certain drugs.

Opportunistic Infections

Parasitic Infections

The most common of these in AIDS is the ubiquitous intracellular parasite **Toxoplasma gondii**; more than 10% of patients are affected. Most infections with *Toxoplasma* are subclinical but encysted forms of the parasite persist in tissue and may be reactivated in patients whose immune system is depressed.

The brain lesions may be widespread, involving both white and grey matter, and have been classified on the following basis:

- the **degree of acuteness** of the typical small necrotizing lesions surrounded by a cuff of macrophages
- the **frequency with which the parasite can be recognized** at the periphery of the areas of coagulative necrosis

Sometimes the lesions are atypical consisting either of a diffuse encephalitis or of encysted forms of the *Toxoplasma* with no necrosis and no inflammatory response. In such instances it may not be possible to make a diagnosis unless immunohistochemical methods or electron microscopy are used (*Fig. 45.11*).

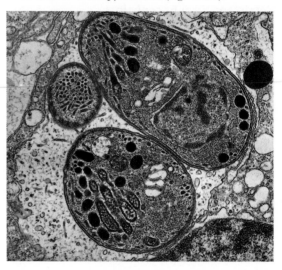

FIGURE 45.11 *Endozoites of* Toxoplasma gondii *found in the brain.*

Fungal Infections

Fungal infections are surprisingly rare in the CNS of patients with AIDS compared with their frequency in other parts of the body. The commonest are infections by **Cryptococcus neoformans**, which has been found in 2.6% of brains from patients with AIDS examined at autopsy.

C. neoformans (also known as *Torula histolytica*) is a saprophyte widely distributed in soil, fruit, milk and bird droppings. The cryptococcus usually produces a basal meningitis. The organism can be identified in CSF and in the meninges by staining its carbohydrate-rich capsule with the periodic acid–Schiff method, or by adding a few drops of Indian ink to CSF. In the latter case the capsules are seen, on microscopy, to stand out as clear halos against a dark background (*Fig. 45.12*). In the early

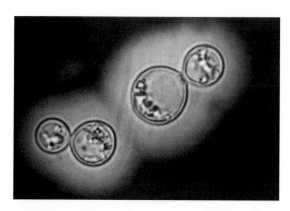

FIGURE 45.12 *CSF from a patient with meningitis due to Cryptococcus neoformans. Indian ink has been added to the sample and the organisms are identified by the presence of well-defined pale areas against the dark background, which are due to the presence of cryptococcal capsules.*

stages, the presence of the fungi may be associated with little or no inflammatory response, but as the condition progresses necrotic lesions appear which may be associated with either a mixed inflammatory cell infiltrate or a frankly granulomatous response.

Other fungal infections that have been seen more rarely include candidiasis, aspergillosis, coccidiomycosis and histoplasmosis.

Bacterial Infections
Pyogenic infections of the CNS occur only seldom in patients with AIDS, but infections with **Mycobacterium avium intracellulare** have often been reported. In such instances the brain involvement is usually part of a systemic mycobacterial infection.

Viral Infections
CNS infections by **cytomegalovirus** (CMV) are the most common, having been reported in 26% of patients with AIDS. Infection of the brain with CMV does not produce consistent clinical or pathological effects and, in some instances, may be asymptomatic.

Microscopic Features
The lesions range from isolated cells in which typical viral inclusions can be seen to areas of frank necrosis which can affect either the periventricular regions of the brain or the spinal cord and nerve roots.

The main diagnostic feature on light microscopy is intranuclear inclusions, which may be eosinophilic or basophilic, in cells of various types including vascular endothelium. It is, however, worth remembering that CMV viral antigen can be demonstrated in cells that do not show the typical inclusions and thus some infections may be missed if there is complete reliance on conventional histological methods.

The mode of entry of the virus to the CNS is not known but the presence of inclusions in vascular endothelium and in the choroid plexus suggests that the portal of entry is across small blood vessel walls.

The spread of herpes simplex virus infections (HSV-1 and HSV-2) to involve the CNS is also favoured by the depression in cell-mediated immunity which is the hallmark of AIDS. Such involvement may lead to encephalitis or, as with CMV, to inflammation in the cord or nerve roots.

CNS Neoplasms Associated with AIDS

Lymphoma
Primary cerebral lymphomas are relatively common in patients with AIDS, affecting 5–10% of patients. Most are high-grade B-cell lymphomas. Some are true Burkitt lymphomas associated with Epstein–Barr virus (EBV) infection, positive serology for this virus being extremely common in patients with AIDS. It has been suggested that EBV-infected B cells can cross the blood–brain barrier, and certainly EBV-specific antibodies can be detected in the CSF in some instances.

Kaposi's Sarcoma
This is the commonest neoplasm associated with AIDS but has been reported as occurring only rarely in the CNS and then only when the patients had disseminated tumour involving several viscera.

BACTERIAL INFECTIONS OF THE BRAIN PARENCHYMA

Cerebral Abscess
The pathogenesis of brain abscess is similar to that of meningitis. The infection may be the result of:

- **direct spread from infective inflammatory lesions in the middle ear, mastoid air cells or, more rarely, paranasal sinuses.** The microorganisms that spread from such foci tend, not surprisingly, to involve adjacent parts of the brain. Thus the cerebellum is likely to be the site of abscess when spread occurs from the mastoid air cells, the temporal lobe when the origin has been a suppurative otitis media, and the frontal lobe when the infection originated in the frontal sinus. Such locally derived abscesses are almost always single and, as such, present a less difficult neurosurgical challenge than abscesses forming as a result of blood-borne infection, which are often multiple.

- **blood spread.** This has become relatively less common in parallel with the decreased incidence of suppurative bronchiectasis, lung abscess and empyema. Acute infective endocarditis, caused by highly pathogenic organisms such as *S. aureus*, is a not uncommon source of parenchymal brain infections. As stated elsewhere (see pp 380–381), cyanotic congenital heart disease, most notably tetralogy of Fallot, is a risk factor for the development of blood-borne intracerebral infections.

- In a proportion of cases, the pathogenesis of brain abscess may remain unknown.

Pathogenesis

The formation of an abscess is preceded by a focal acute encephalitis ('cerebritis'), usually sited in the less vascular white matter. As in any other inflammatory reaction elicited by pyogenic microorganisms, neutrophils migrate from the affected capillaries and the white - matter becomes oedematous and then undergoes necrosis.

Macroscopic Features

The commonest sites are the frontal, temporal and parietal lobes, and the cerebellum is also commonly affected. Where the origin of the abscess has been local (e.g. mastoiditis), adhesions between the brain and overlying dura will be present and it may be possible to detect a track between the abscess and the local inflammatory lesion.

The abscesses themselves vary greatly in size. They are usually oval and often multilocular. In the earlier stages of development, the surrounding white matter often shows small foci of suppurative encephalitis or microabscess formation. The abscess wall is, at first, poorly defined (*Fig. 45.13*). Later it becomes thicker and firmer and can then be stripped away from the surrounding brain tissue.

Microscopic Features

A well-established abscess shows five concentric zones:
  1) a central necrotic area containing debris, pus cells and foamy macrophages
  2) granulation tissue containing new capillaries and proliferating fibroblasts
  3) granulation tissue showing a local immune reaction in the form of a lymphocyte and plasma cell infiltrate
  4) dense collagenous fibrous tissue
  5) oedematous white matter in which reactive gliosis is present

Natural History

First and foremost, brain abscesses behave as mass lesions that expand and cause raised intracranial pressure and its consequences, as discussed elsewhere in this chapter. Infection may spread through the abscess capsule resulting in a diffuse suppurative encephalitis. Rupture of the abscess may occur, either into the cerebral ventricles, producing acute purulent ventriculitis, or into the subarachnoid space, resulting in acute meningitis. Thrombosis of intracranial sinuses such as the sigmoid sinus may occur and this may be followed by embolization of the pulmonary circulation.

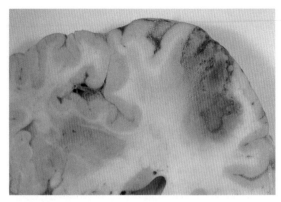

FIGURE 45.13 *Embolic abscess. The lesion shows the presence of a central yellowish-brown necrotic area surrounded by a narrow zone of congestion.*

Tuberculoma

A tuberculoma is a localized mass of caseation necrosis which is usually well encapsulated. The lesions may be single or multiple and constitute a common cause of expanding mass lesions in the brain in populations where there is a high prevalence of tuberculosis. The cerebral hemispheres are commonly affected in adults; in children the cerebellum is a site of predilection.

Parenchymatous Neurosyphilis

Two quite distinct sets of lesions and clinical syndromes can be encountered. The first of these is termed **tabes dorsalis**.

Macroscopic Features

Tabes dorsalis is characterized by degeneration of certain sensory fibres in the posterior nerve roots and in the posterior columns of the spinal cord. This leads to atrophy; the posterior columns are seen to be shrunken and greyish in colour (instead of white) at post-mortem examination. The overlying leptomeninges are thickened and the posterior nerve roots are also atrophic.

Microscopic Features

The posterior columns show fibre loss and demyelination. Similar changes may occur in more proximally situated parts of the nervous system (e.g. the optic discs and the third cranial nerve).

The degeneration leads to severe loss of function, especially in relation to deep pressure sensation, vibration sense, position sense and coordination. The patients may develop a characteristic unsteady and 'stamping' gait because they cannot feel the ground beneath their feet. Deep tendon reflexes disappear and there may be episodes of very severe shooting pains in the limbs, known as 'lightning pains'. The lack of sensation may lead ultimately to disorganization of large joints such as the knee (**Charcot's joints**).

The pathogenesis of tabes dorsalis is still unknown. It is not likely to be related to proliferation of the organisms at a time when cell-mediated immunity is deficient, because organisms are very scanty in the lesions.

The second type of parenchymatous lesion seen in neurosyphilis is known as **general paresis of the insane**. This was once one of the commonest causes of long-term admission to mental hospitals, but is now rare.

General paresis of the insane is a chronic treponemal inflammatory disorder in which, in contrast to tabes dorsalis, it is reasonably easy to identify the organisms. The brain becomes shrunken and the cerebral cortices are disorganized, the graphic term 'windswept cortex' being applied by some writers. The structural changes in the brain consist essentially of degeneration of nerve cells and their fibres, especially in the grey matter, with an associated proliferation of astrocytes and glial fibres. The small intracerebral blood vessels show the expected perivascular cuffing by lymphocytes and plasma cells, and swelling of the endothelial lining.

In the early stages the clinical picture is characterized by deterioration in personality and changes in mental function. This may express itself in the form of delusions, which may be at once bizarre and grandiose. If unchecked by treatment, the mental changes may proceed inexorably to complete dementia. Disturbances related to other functions may also be seen. These include tremors of the lips and tongue, general weakness, minor convulsive seizures and disturbances of finer movements.

FUNGAL INFECTIONS OF THE BRAIN PARENCHYMA

Fungal infections of the brain are usually secondary to fungal disease elsewhere in the body (most frequently the lung), the infections reaching the brain via the bloodstream. In some instances the 'primary' infection may be inconspicuous, the brain appearing to be the only site affected.

Infection with *C. neoformans* is discussed in the section devoted to the neuropathology of AIDS (see pp 1120–1121). Cryptococcal infections can and do occur also in individuals who are not immunocompromised.

Other fungal infections of the CNS are summarized in *Table 45.3*.

PROTOZOAL INFECTIONS

Malaria

Malaria affects many organs and tissues, but its most baneful effect is on the brain. For this reason, the aetiology and pathogenesis of malaria are dealt with here.

Epidemiology

About 60 000 000 cases of malaria occur every year, causing more than 1 million deaths. The incidence of malaria is now increasing in the tropics, largely due to the emergence of resistant strains of parasites and of resistant strains of anopheline mosquitoes.

Cases of malaria do occur in areas where the disease is *not* endemic. These most often affect individuals who have travelled through endemic areas. The disease can also be transmitted via infected blood transfusions (the commonest cause of malaria in the USA in those who have not travelled to endemic areas).

Aetiology

Malaria is caused by various *Plasmodium* species. These intracellular protozoal parasites are usually transmitted by the bite of one of the strains of *Anopheles* mosquitoes found in Africa, Asia and South America. The plasmodia implicated in human malaria are:

- *Plasmodium falciparum* (responsible for most malaria deaths)
- *Plasmodium vivax*
- *Plasmodium malariae*
- *Plasmodium ovale*

In sub-Saharan Africa, Papua New Guinea and Haiti the predominant strain is *P. falciparum*; in North Africa, Central America and part of South America, the Middle East and the Indian subcontinent, *P. vivax* is more common. These two strains occur about equally in East Asia, Oceania and parts of South America. *P. malariae* can occur in any area, but is relatively rare outside Africa, and *P. ovale* is common only in West Africa.

The plasmodia must undergo certain developmental stages in the mosquito before being transmissible to humans. This development (sporogony) cannot take place:

- in mosquitoes living at altitudes above 2000 metres
- at temperatures below 16°C
- in mosquitoes whose lifespan, after ingesting infected blood, lasts less than 7 days

The likelihood of developing malaria depends on the characters of:

- the insect vector
- the parasite
- the state of immunity of the host. Immunity to the protozoon is less well developed in infants and young children than in older children and adults. They are more susceptible to infection and tend to have a higher load of parasites. Babies seldom develop severe malaria, being partially protected by maternal antibodies and by the relatively high concentrations of haemoglobin F in their red cells. Thus children constitute both the main reservoir for infection and the main target group for infection.

The presence of parasites in the blood and malaria-related splenomegaly in children aged 2–9 years are used as indices of the degree of endemicity in a given geographical location (see *Table 45.4*).

In regions of very high endemicity the chief targets are children less than 5 years old, whereas in regions of

Table 45.3 Fungal Infections in the CNS

Fungus	Specific location	Route of infection	Clinical background	Pathology
Coccidioides	Semi-arid climates; SW United States, Mexico, South America	Usually by inhalation. Fungus spreads from granulomatous foci in lung via bloodstream		Granulomatous meningitis with occasional granulomas in brain. Lesions resemble those of tuberculosis. Fungi present in giant cells in the form of spherules
Blastomyces	USA, Canada, Mexico	Inhalation		Either granulomatous meningitis with fungus present as yeast forms in macrophages or as abscesses which may be single or multiple
Histoplasma	USA, southern Africa, South America	Inhalation of spores from contaminated bird manure		Diffuse granulomatous meningitis with occasional granulomas in brain. The fungus appears as a small ovoid body with buds
Actinomycetes (*Nocardia* rather than a true fungus)				Multilocular abscesses in which branching hyphae can be identified
Candida			Classically opportunistic infection, common in the immuno-compromised	Abscesses showing some of the features of haemorrhagic infarcts. Blood vessels are necrotic and there is a mixed acute and chronic inflammatory cell infiltrate. Fungus appears most commonly as a yeast form with pseudohyphae which almost replace necrotic vessel walls
Aspergillus			Classically opportunistic	Appearances as above; fungus appears as branching septate hyphae with no yeast forms
Nocardia asteroides			Classically opportunistic	Pathological changes as above. Organisms appear as delicate branching hyphae
Mucor			Especially seen in uncontrolled diabetics	Acute necrotizing meningitis with abscess formation in some cases. There is marked necrosis of vessel walls. Fungi appear as non-branched hyphae

Table 45.4 Endemicity of Malaria

Endemicity	Splenomegaly (%)	Parasites in blood (%)
Hypoendemic	0–10	0–10
Mesoendemic	10–50	10–50
Hyperendemic	50–75	50–75
Holoendemic	> 75	> 75

low endemicity the disease affects all age groups. Where endemicity is high, the frequency of the disease is reduced after the age of 5 years even though malarial parasites may still be present in these older individuals. This degree of **clinical immunity** is never attained in regions of low endemicity.

Genetically Determined Protection Against Malaria

Individuals heterozygous for certain red cell abnormalities show some resistance against malaria. This is strongest in the cases of the sickle cell trait (see pp 896–899) and a type of ovalocytosis found in Melanesia. Red blood cells from individuals with the sickle cell trait resist invasion by the parasites and, when they are invaded, undergo sickling. This promotes the removal of the parasitized cells by the reticuloendothelial system. Thalassaemia and glucose-6-phosphate dehydrogenase deficiency also confer some protection but this is weaker than in the case of the above-mentioned factors.

Certain human leucocyte antigens also are associated with some degree of resistance against malaria. These are HLA-Bw53 and HLA-DR B1 1302. HLA-Bw53-restricted cytotoxic T cells recognize a peptide expressed by plasmodia during their intrahepatocyte development.

Pathogenesis

There are three stages in the development of human malaria.

1. Pre-erythrocytic Schizogony

The parasite, at the stage in its development known as a **sporozoite**, is injected into the blood by an infected mosquito as it bites, and enters the liver cells where it undergoes asexual reproduction. This is known as pre- or extra-erythrocytic development. This stage lasts from 5 to 15 days depending on the plasmodium involved. It is shortest in infections with *P. falciparum* and longest in those caused by *P. malariae*.

The sporozoites either enter liver cells by binding to appropriate receptors or are cleared from the circulation within less than 1 hour. The asexual division occurring in the liver cells leads to the formation of a mass of parasites called a **schizont**. At this point the plasmodia within the schizont are called **merozoites**; many thousands of merozoites may be released into the circulation from a single infected liver cell (up to 30 000 in the case of *P. falciparum*).

In the case *P. vivax* and *P. ovale*, a proportion of the plasmodia within infected liver cells do not develop into merozoites and remain dormant for weeks or months. These dormant forms are known as **hypnozoites**. They may enter the phase of asexual reproduction at any time, and this is responsible for the relapses seen in individuals infected by *P. vivax* or *P. ovale*.

2. Erythrocytic Schizogony

The plasmodial forms released from liver cells (**merozoites**) invade red blood cells where they multiply asexually. After an interval, which varies according to the species, the plasmodia are released into the blood and invade other red blood cells. This stage is known as **erythrocytic schizogony**.

The terminology used to describe the fever patterns in the different forms of malaria are related to the length of erythrocyte schizogony. Thus *P. malariae* schizogony takes 72 hours and the bouts of fever (in untreated individuals) occur every 4 days (**quartan malaria**). The other plasmodia have a 48-hour asexual cycle in red blood cells and the fever occurs every third day (**tertian malaria**).

P. falciparum can invade red blood cells of all ages but shows a preference for young cells; *P. vivax* and *P. ovale* invade reticulocytes and *P. malariae* shows a preference for senescent cells.

How the merozoite (an ovoid motile parasite) binds to red cells in the case of all the plasmodia is still unknown. *P. vivax* attaches to the Duffy blood group antigens (Fy^a or Fy^b) and individuals lacking these antigens are resistant to infection with *P. vivax*. Such resistance is seen in the Duffy-negative inhabitants of West Africa.

As the motile parasites within the red blood cells divide, they lyse the haemoglobin in order to use the amino acids so released for their own protein synthesis. The haem is oxidized to its ferric form. The toxicity that would result is avoided by polymerization with the formation of an inert crystalline black or brown pigment, **haemozoin**.

Eventually the whole of the parasitized red cell is occupied by merozoites and the cell ruptures, releasing the merozoites into the circulation. These merozoites invade other red cells and start another cycle of asexual reproduction.

These events are illustrated in *Figs 45.14* and *45.15*.

Production of Symptoms The clinical syndromes of malaria result from:
- destruction of red blood cells in the asexual phase of reproduction within red cells
- release of material from the red cells and the parasites into the circulation with the consequent generation and release of cytokines

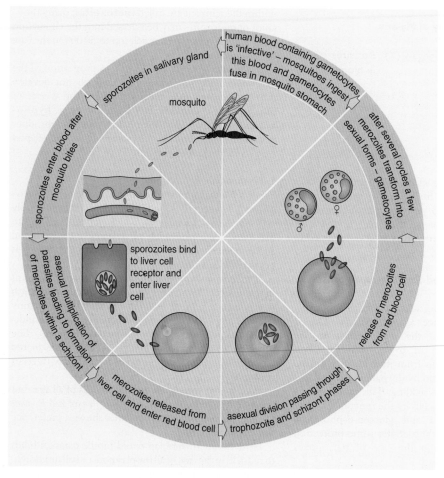

FIGURE 45.14 Malaria. Sequence of events following the bite of an infected mosquito.

- sequestration of red cells parasitized by *P. falciparum* interfering with flow through microvessels of vital organs

Cytokine Release The release of merozoites into the bloodstream has an effect similar to that of endotoxin. This is due to the presence on the surface of the released parasites of a glycolipid which causes mono-cyte-derived macrophages to release tumour necrosis factor (TNF) α and interleukin (IL)-1. This is followed by the release of IL-6 and IL-8.

The characteristic 'malarial paroxysm' of *P. vivax* malaria (shivering, headache, chills and sometimes rigors) is almost certainly the expression of raised TNF-α concentrations in the circulation.

Cytokines are probably also involved in:
- upregulation of endothelial ligands for red cells, parasitized by *P. falciparum* (see below)
- suppression of red cell formation
- inhibition of gluconeogenesis
- placental dysfunction

- activation of white cells to release toxic, oxygen free radicals and nitric oxide

Sequestration of Infected Red Blood Cells and P. Falciparum *P. falciparum* differs from the other types in its effect on parasitized red cells. Some 24 hours after invasion of the red cells, *P. falciparum* starts to express a high molecular weight specific antigen on the surface of the infected red cells. This antigen expression is accompanied by the appearance of knob-like projections from the red cell surface.

The specific antigen is known as **P. falciparum erythrocyte membrane protein 1 (PfEMP-1)** and it mediates the adhesion of red cells parasitized by *P. falciparum* to postcapillary venular endothelium in a number of organs, including **heart, lung, small gut** and, most importantly, the **white matter of the brain**. This process, in which parasitized red cells disappear from the circulating blood, is known as **sequestration**, and it is what makes *P. falciparum* infection so liable to cause death, this being most frequently due to cerebral

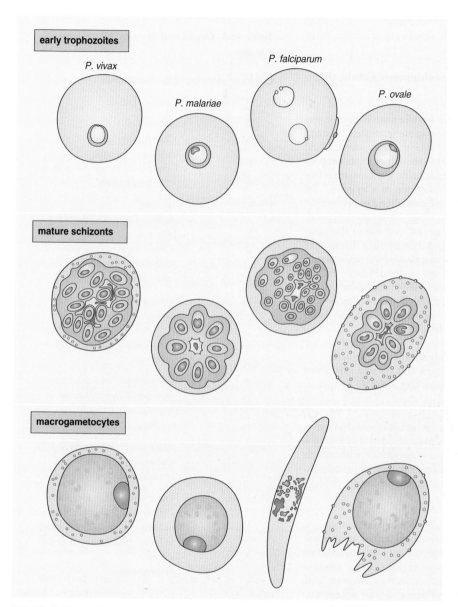

FIGURE 45.15 Morphology of malarial parasites in early trophozoite, schizont and macrogametocyte phases.

malaria in which obvious evidence of cerebral dysfunction is present.

In addition to sequestration as a result of endothelial binding, parasitized red cells may adhere to uninfected red cells, this being known as **rosetting**. Rosetting is associated with cerebral malaria and may encourage adhesion to endothelial cells by reducing blood flow through microvessels.

Ligands for PfEMP-1 Parasitized red blood cells adhere to a number of different ligands expressed on vascular endothelium. These include:

- **the leucocyte differentiation antigen CD36**

(GPIIb) located on the surface of endothelial cells, monocytes and platelets. CD36 binds specifically to the knob on the surface of red cells parasitized by *P. falciparum*.

- **intercellular adhesion molecule (ICAM) 1**, which belongs to the immunoglobulin gene superfamily of proteins
- **thrombospondin**, a multifunctional, multidomain protein which binds many different ligands

The adherence phenotype of the plasmodia varies considerably from isolate to isolate. It has been suggested that **intracerebral sequestration is due mainly to binding of PfEMP-1 to ICAM-1**. In falciparum malaria, CD36 binding does not correlate with cerebral malaria but does so with significant dysfunction in organs other than the brain.

3. Gametogeny and Development within the Mosquito (Sporogony)

Following repeated asexual cycles within red blood cells a subpopulation undergoes transformation into sexual forms (**gametocytes**). These gametocytes are ingested by female mosquitoes in the course of a blood meal, and within the gut of the mosquito the gametocytes become activated. Fusion of female and male gametocytes is followed by meiosis and the formation of a **zygote**. The zygote becomes motile (an **oökinete**) and penetrates the wall of the mosquito midgut where it becomes encysted. Within this cyst (**oöcyst**) asexual division of the parasite occurs. The oöcyst enlarges, reaching a diameter of about 500 μm and then bursts, releasing the malarial parasites (**sporozoites**) into the coelomic cavity of the mosquito. The sporozoites migrate to the salivary glands from which they may be inoculated into another human host. This phase of development in the mosquito (**sporogony**) takes 8–35 days.

Organ and System Involvement in Malaria

In severe malaria many organs and systems may show dysfunction. This is summarized in *Table 45.5*.

Cerebral Malaria

This is the most frequent and most dangerous manifestation of severe falciparum malaria. Strictly speaking it is defined as unrousable coma in association with malaria but, in practice, any malarial patient with impaired consciousness should be treated most vigorously.

Clinical Features

Affected patients are usually febrile and unrousable. There is no evidence of meningeal irritation or papilloedema but retinal haemorrhages may be seen in about one in six cases. Focal neurological deficits are uncommon. Patients may show phasic increases in tone with extensor posturing of either decorticate or decerebrate types, and opisthotonos may occur.

Macroscopic Features

The brain is slightly swollen and the cut surface shows multiple petechial haemorrhages in the white matter (an appearance not dissimilar from that seen in fat embolism).

Microscopic Features

Most microvessels are packed with red blood cells containing mature forms of *P. falciparum*. Haemozoin pigment is seen both within and outside the red cells, and accumulations of glial cells may be seen in relation to haemorrhagic foci associated with rupture of vessels blocked by parasitized red cells (*Fig. 45.16*).

Table 45.5 Organ and System Involvement in Malaria

Organ or system	Manifestations
Brain	Cerebral malaria
Blood	Anaemia
Coagulopathy and thrombocytopenia
Severe intravascular haemolysis ('Blackwater fever')
Liver	Jaundice
Reduced synthesis of clotting factors
Reduced gluconeogenesis
Reduced clearance of antimalarial drugs
Kidney	Acute renal failure due to a number of mechanisms
Nephrotic syndrome occurring in association with *P. malariae* infection
Spleen	Splenomegaly associated with evidence of hypersplenism (tropical splenomegaly syndrome; see p 985)
Lung	Acute pulmonary oedema (rather similar to adult respiratory distress syndrome)
Metabolic	Lactic acidosis due to aerobic glycolysis in tissues, production of lactate by parasites and failure of lactate clearance by liver and spleen
Hypoglycaemia

Natural History

The mortality rate in untreated cases is virtually 100%. Where appropriate treatment is given, about 15% of affected children and 20% of adult patients die. In adults the risk of dying is increased to about 50% in pregnancy. In patients who recover, about 3% of adults and 10% of children suffer from residual neurological impairment.

Blackwater Fever

This is an acute, rapidly progressive, illness in which the characteristic features are:
- fever
- severe intravascular haemolysis leading to haemoglobinuria and hyperbilirubinaemia

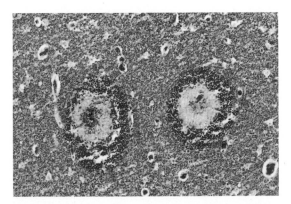

FIGURE 45.16 *Perivascular 'ring' haemorrhages in the white matter in cerebral malaria.*

- vomiting
- circulatory collapse
- acute renal failure

The disease derives its name from the brown-red colour of the urine caused by haemoglobinuria. It occurs only in association with falciparum malaria and may be precipitated in quinine-sensitive individuals by small doses of quinine.

Toxoplasmosis

The general pathology of toxoplasmosis is discussed in the chapters relating to lymph nodes (see pp 953–954) and *Toxoplasma* infections in the CNS of patients with AIDS are dealt with in a preceding section of this chapter (see p 1120). Rarely, older children infected by this protozoon develop acute encephalitis.

The CNS may also be affected in **congenital toxoplasmosis**, which occurs in 1–2 per 1000 live births. It results from *Toxoplasma* infections in pregnant women; in about one-third of cases such infections are transmitted to the fetus. Fetal infection causes a smouldering meningoencephalitis, leading to a classical set of CNS abnormalities associated with intellectual impairment:

- **hydrocephalus**
- **megaloencephaly** (enlargement of the brain to more than 2.5 standard deviations above the mean for age and sex)
- **choroidoretinitis**
- **calcification within the brain**

Amoebiasis

Amoebae cause two types of disease in the CNS:

1) meningoencephalitis
2) brain abscess

Meningoencephalitis is caused most often by *Naegleria fowleri*, the infection being acquired by swimming in warm lakes or pools contaminated by the amoeba. Spread occurs via the nasal passages and, as a result, the olfactory bulbs are often involved by the purulent meningitis that can result. The inflammation

can spread into the cerebral cortex where a necrotizing vasculitis may occur.

Amoebic brain abscess is caused by *Entamoeba histolytica*, which more commonly causes colitis. Cerebral abscess is rare and is likely to occur only if there are amoebic abscesses in the liver from which haematogenous dissemination may occur.

Trypanosomiasis

Diseases caused by trypanosomes are endemic in central Africa and South America.

- In Africa the parasites involved are *Trypanosoma gambiense* which classically causes 'sleeping sickness' and *T. rhodesiense*. They are transmitted to humans by the bite of the tsetse fly.
- In South America trypanosomiasis is caused by *T. cruzi*, which causes Chagas' disease. *T. cruzi* is transmitted to humans by house bugs.

African Trypanosomiasis

Both varieties of African trypanosomiasis may be characterized by a combination of pancarditis (more conspicuous in *T. rhodesiense* infection) and subacute encephalitis (more characteristic of *T. gambiense* infection).

> ### Microscopic Features
>
> The features are those of meningoencephalitis characterized by a striking infiltration of lymphocytes and plasma cells. These cells are arranged like a 'cuff' around small intracerebral blood vessels and extend outwards into the surrounding brain tissue.
>
> The sites principally affected are the deep white matter, the basal ganglia, the brainstem and the cerebellum. In severe cases there may be aggregates of inflammatory cells and microglial cells within brain tissue not related to blood vessels, and plasma cells distended with immunoglobulin may be seen (morular cells).
>
> Parasites are not found in brain tissue; a definitive diagnosis depends on their demonstration within the blood.

African trypanosomiasis may be complicated by the effects of the arsenical compounds used in treatment. Some patients develop an acute encephalopathy characterized by convulsions, which may be fatal. Post-mortem examination of the brain in such cases shows hypoxic brain damage or acute haemorrhagic changes within the white matter.

South American Trypanosomiasis (Chagas' Disease)

Infection usually occurs in childhood. The disease may present acutely soon after infection, but in many cases the infection remains dormant for years. In the latter case the heart and other hollow muscular viscera are principally affected.

In acute cases, encephalitis may occur. Post-mortem

samples show focal inflammation of white matter with small aggregates of lymphocytes, plasma cells and microglia.

NUTRITIONAL AND TOXIC DISORDERS

Serious disorders affecting both central and peripheral nervous systems may arise either because of:
- **deficiencies** of certain nutrients, most importantly, vitamins
- **toxic effects** of a wide range of chemical species

VITAMIN DEFICIENCIES

The important neurological effects of vitamin deficiencies are shown in *Table 45.6*.

Vitamin B₁ Deficiency

Wernicke's Encephalopathy

In Western populations deficiency of this vitamin is most commonly associated with chronic alcoholism and resulting malnourishment. Deficiency causes impairment of oxidation of pyruvate, the most frequent neuropathological effect being the development of Wernicke's encephalopathy. This condition may also be due to excessive vomiting, as sometimes occurs during pregnancy, and to malabsorption caused by small gut disease.

The characteristic clinical features in the acute stages are:
- disturbances of consciousness
- paralysis of extraocular muscles
- nystagmus

Macroscopic Features

The parts of the brain affected are the mamillary bodies, anterior nucleus of the thalamus, walls of the third ventricles, periaqueductal tissues and floor of the fourth ventricle. In the acute stages the mamillary bodies are congested and show petechial haemorrhages. In chronic cases there is atrophy of the mamillary bodies.

Microscopic Features

In the acute stages neurones and axons are preserved but small haemorrhages are prominent. In chronic cases, there is loss of mamillary body myelin and some reactive gliosis. Previous haemorrhage is marked by haemosiderin-laden macrophages.

Korsakoff's Psychosis

This syndrome is characterized by serious defects in short-term memory and with confabulation (remembering past events that have not actually occurred). It is not uncommonly associated with Wernicke's syndrome but may occur in association with other disorders affecting the diencephalon. Even when treated with adequate doses of thiamine, the memory loss may be irreversible.

Vitamin B₂ Deficiency

Pellagra

Pellagra is characterized by:
- dermatitis
- diarrhoea
- dementia

Table 45.6 Neurological Effects of Vitamin Deficiency

Deficient vitamin	Disorders
Vitamin B₁ (thiamine)	Wernicke's encephalopathy
	Korsakoff's psychosis
	Neuropathy associated with 'dry' beriberi
Vitamin B₂ (nicotinic acid)	Pellagra in which damage to neurones and degeneration of long tracts may occur and in which dementia is a characteristic feature
Vitamin B₆ (pyridoxine)	Peripheral neuropathy, most often associated with drugs that interfere with metabolism of vitamin B₆ (e.g. penicillamine, isoniazid)
Vitamin B₁₂	Subacute combined degeneration of the spinal cord as seen in pernicious anaemia (see p 882) or conditions in which intrinsic factor production is normal but there is impaired absorption of vitamin B₁₂
Vitamin E	Produces distal axonopathy (see pp 1171–1173)

It is due to a deficiency in either nicotinic acid or its precursor tryptophan. It was formerly common in populations whose diets consisted principally of maize (relatively lacking in tryptophan). However, enrichment of cereal diets with vitamin B_2 has reduced the incidence. In Western populations it is associated with:

- antibiotic-related abnormalities of normal bacterial flora
- massive resection of small gut
- some chronic diarrhoeal disorders

Cells in many parts of the CNS may be affected. These include the Betz cells, cells in many nuclei, anterior horn cells in the spinal cord, pyramidal cells in the hippocampus and Purkinje cells in the cerebellum. Long tract degeneration occurs in some cases, as does peripheral neuropathy.

Vitamin B_6 Deficiency

There are many enzyme reactions in the CNS that depend on adequate amounts of pyridoxine phosphate (the active form of vitamin B_6). Some of these are concerned in the decarboxylation of amino acids whereas others are involved in amine formation (noradrenaline, adrenaline, 5-hydroxytryptamine and dopamine) and γ-aminobutyric acid (GABA) synthesis. Thus deficiencies may affect several chemical messenger systems within the CNS and peripheral nervous system.

Deficiency of vitamin B_6 in Western populations is most often due to drugs (see *Table 45.6*). It has also been suggested that the neuropathy of acute intermittent porphyria may be due to excess amounts of pyridoxal phosphate being used by δ-aminolaevulinic acid, thus leading to a deficency of the former.

Vitamin B_{12} Deficiency

This is discussed in the section on pernicious anaemia (see pp 879–883).

Vitamin E Deficiency

Vitamin E deficiency occurs in:

- chronic malabsorption
- any condition resulting in a deficiency of bile salts in the small gut
- abetalipoproteinaemia in which there is failure of apoprotein B_{48} in the epithelium of the small gut and thus a failure of chylomicron formation (see pp 525, 1178–1179)

A 'dying back' type of neuropathy affects both central and peripheral axons of sensory ganglion cells.

TOXIC DISORDERS

Many chemical species can adversely affect the nervous system. These include commonly used substances, dangerous only in excess, such as alcohol, industrial chemicals, metals and various therapeutic agents. Some important toxic injuries to peripheral nerves are discussed on pp 1172–1173; this section is concerned only with toxins affecting the CNS, the effects of which are summarized in *Table 45.7*).

DEMYELINATING DISORDERS

Demyelinating disorders are characterized by loss of the myelin ensheathing the axons, without the axons themselves showing any evidence of damage. These changes could be caused by:

- damage to the myelin-forming oligodendrocytes
- direct injury, perhaps toxic, perhaps immunologically mediated, to the myelin sheaths themselves

Many disorders, both in the central and peripheral nervous systems, show evidence of demyelination; by convention, the term is **restricted to diseases in which the demyelination appears to be the chief pathological process involved**.

The chief members of this group are:

- **multiple sclerosis** (MS), which has a number of different variants
  a) classical (Charcot type)
  b) acute (Marburg type)
  c) diffuse cerebral sclerosis (Schilder type)
  d) concentric sclerosis (Baló type)
  e) neuromyelitis optica (Devic type)
- **acute perivenous encephalomyelitis**

Multiple Sclerosis

This is the commonest demyelinating disease. About 800 new cases are recognized annually in Britain where, at any one time, there are between 40 000 and 50 000 affected individuals.

Epidemiology

Risk rises steeply from early adolescence to a peak in the twenties or early thirties. After the age of 30 years, the risk declines steeply so that onset of MS is rare after 60 years of age.

There is a **distinct geographical distribution**, the frequency of the disease increasing with the distance from the equator; this is much more marked in the northern hemisphere. The highest prevalence rates are in the North-East of Scotland (144 per 100 000 population) and the highest incidence rates are in the Orkneys (9.3 per 100 000 per year). This compares with a prevalence of 10 per 100 000 and an incidence of 0.4 per 100 000 per year in New Orleans. MS is generally less common in the southern hemisphere and distinctly rare in Japan and the tropics. Emigration from a high-risk to a low-risk area before the age of 15 years is associated with a reduced risk. After this age the emigrant appears to carry his/her degree of risk to the new country. This has been interpreted as suggesting that the disorder starts with an infection in early life, although no organism has ever been identified as being responsible.

Genetic factors also appear to play a part; for

Table 45.7 Toxic Damage to the Central Nervous System

Toxin	Associated disorders
Ethyl alcohol	**Wernicke's encephalopathy** **Korsakoff's psychosis** These are mediated via nutritional deficiency (see p 1130) **Cerebral atrophy associated with dementia.** White rather than grey matter is lost and there is a tendency for selective atrophy of the anterior portion of the superior vermis of the cerebellum to occur. **Fetal alcohol syndrome.** One of the leading causes of birth defects associated with intellectual impairment (1 in 600 live births in USA, France and Sweden). The most common abnormality is **microcephaly**.
Methanol	Damage produced by the catabolites formaldehyde and formic acid. Blindness occurs frequently due either to degeneration of retinal ganglion cells or to swelling of axons in the optic disc. Necrosis of basal ganglia and deep white matter in both cerebrum and cerebellum is reported.
Ethylene glycol	Swelling, congestion and petechial haemorrhages seen in the brain; acute inflammation is present in meninges and around small intracerebral blood vessels. These may be associated with calcium oxalate deposition.
Phenytoin	Atrophy of cerebellum with diffuse loss of Purkinje cells
Amphetamines and cocaine	May cause intracranial haemorrhage due to hypertension, which these compounds can produce; the bleeding is usually in the region of the thalamus and basal ganglia but may also occur in the subarachnoid and subdural spaces.
Neuroleptics used in long-term treatment of psychosis	Can cause **tardive dyskinesia** (abnormal smacking of lips, grimacing, and contortion of face and neck). This is associated with neuronal loss, increased amounts of lipofuscin in basal ganglia, substantia nigra and midbrain, and satellitosis.
Clioquinol (used in amoebiasis)	**Toxic encephalopathy** **Isolated optic atrophy** **Subacute myelo-optic neuropathy (SMON syndrome).** This occurs almost exclusively in the Japanese. Lesions are found in the spinal cord, spinal nerve roots, autonomic ganglia and, to a lesser extent, peripheral nerves.
Methotrexate	**Arachnoiditis** **Disseminated necrotizing leucoencephalopathy** (multiple yellowish-grey lesions in the white matter of cerebral hemispheres, brainstem and cord). The lesions are areas of coagulative necrosis with little or no inflammatory response. In some cases fibrinoid necrosis of small blood vessels is present.
Morphine, heroin and methadone	Addiction may be associated with a characteristic pattern of ischaemic damage involving the globus pallidus, deep white matter of the cerebral hemispheres and, sometimes, the thoracic part of the spinal cord.
Carbon tetrachloride	May cause changes to small blood vessels in the white matter
Toluene	Causes a peripheral neuropathy and cerebellar ataxia
Toxic oil syndrome (related to consumption of contaminated rapeseed oil in Spain)	Causes chromatolysis of anterior horn cells in the spinal cord and of neurones in the brainstem nuclei. Also produces an inflammatory vasculitis

Table 45.7 Toxic Damage to the Central Nervous System – *continued*

Lead	**Inorganic lead** in excess causes acute encephalopathy characterized by swelling of the brain associated with congestion and petechial haemorrhages. The microscopic appearances suggest selective damage to the capillary endothelial cells, particularly in the cerebellum.
	Organic lead poisoning occurs from inhaling tetraethyl or tetramethyl lead compounds. Acute damage is characterized by cerebral swelling, congestion and petechial haemorrhages. Chronic damage shows, in addition, atrophy of the cerebellar folia.
Manganese	May cause psychiatric disturbances and parkinsonian-like extrapyramidal dysfunction. The latter is associated with loss of neurones in the lentiform and subthalamic nuclei, and also in the substantia nigra.

example, the disease is rare in Bantu, Eskimos and oriental races. In most European groups there is an association between the risk of MS and HLA-DW2 and DR2; in Japan there is an association with DR6 and BW22. This association with major histocompatibility complex class II antigens suggests that helper T cells (CD4) are involved in the pathogenesis of MS.

Clinical Features

The mode of onset and the rate and degree of progression are variable. Most patients in the early stages present with a single focal neurological deficit such as blurring of vision, double vision or blindness (30%) or limb weakness (50%). Others may suffer from tremor, vertigo or sensory symptoms. These deficits commonly remit, either completely or partially, and the remissions may be quite long lasting. Occasionally, severe cases starting in adult life run a relentlessly progressive course with no remissions.

Macroscopic Features

The major feature distinguishing MS from other CNS lesions is **sharply defined plaques of demyelination in the brain and spinal cord with, in most cases, relative preservation of the axons**. The lesions can be seen in magnetic resonance imaging scans; this mode of imaging often shows some plaques that are clinically 'silent'.

The plaques appear as **well-demarcated** grey or translucent areas ranging in size from a few millimetres to several centimetres along their longest axis; they are best seen in sections of fixed brain. This appearance is seen in the brains of cases of long standing. In the few patients dying soon after the onset of the disease, the lesions are difficult to see and appear as soft pink or yellow granular areas.

Any area of the brain can be affected but the areas bordering the ventricles, the optic nerves, chiasm and optic tracts, cerebellum, cerebral white matter, brainstem and spinal cord are all sites of predilection.

Microscopic Features

The outstanding features are:

- Sharply defined areas in which loss of myelin has occurred. This can be seen well in paraffin sections when dyes (such as Luxol-Fast blue) that stain normal myelin are used (*Figs 45.17* and *45.18*). In frozen sections the degenerate myelin is positively stained by fat-soluble dyes such as Oil red O because the breakdown in myelin is accompanied by the release of lipid, including large amounts of esterified cholesterol, which accumulates within phagocytic cells in the demyelinated area.

- 'Cuffing' of small venules by lymphocytes, plasma cells and macrophages. This is seen in acute lesions. Most of the lymphocytes are T cells with T suppressor/cytotoxic cells being present in the perivenular spaces and T helper cells being seen at the edges of the plaques. The T-cell population contains a greater number of CD4+ cells (helper/inducer cells) than suppressor/cytotoxic T cells (CD8+) and the same change in T-cell subsets is seen in the CSF.

  Interestingly, the number of CD8+ T cells in the blood also diminishes during exacerbations of the disease, suggesting that defective T-cell suppressor function may play a role in the pathogenesis of the disease. The majority of the plasma cells in the acute lesions contain immunoglobulin (Ig) G but small amounts of IgA may also be seen.

- Blood vessels in the lesions are surrounded by reactive astrocytes which are larger than normal. Their processes appear to weave between the demyelinated axons (which are preserved) and the inflammatory cells mentioned above. The astrocytes sometimes contain serum proteins derived from oedema fluid accumulating within the plaques. The presence of this oedema indicates local breakdown of the blood–brain barrier. In chronic lesions, a reduction of oligodendroglial cells (which are responsible for the synthesis of myelin) is seen.

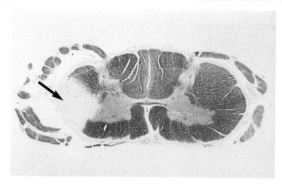

FIGURE 45.17 *Cervical spinal cord in a case of multiple sclerosis. The section has been stained by the Luxol-Fast blue method, which stains myelin blue. Note the extensive loss of myelin (arrowed) on the left side of the field.*

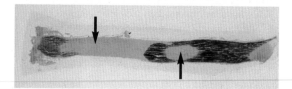

FIGURE 45.18 *Optic nerve from a patient with multiple sclerosis. The section has been stained by the Luxol-Fast blue method. The nerve shows extensive but patchy loss of myelin.*

CSF Changes in Multiple Sclerosis

The CSF shows an increase in the concentration of IgG, which is present in the form of **oligoclonal bands**. This is not specific for MS as a number of other conditions affecting the CNS, such as **subacute sclerosing panencephalitis (SSPE), syphilis and the Guillain–Barré syndrome**, may also show this feature. Unlike what occurs in SSPE, the antigen reacting in MS has not been identified and is certainly *not* myelin. The presence of this immunoglobulin is likely to represent an epiphenomenon and does not indicate a pathogenetic role for IgG.

Aetiology and Pathogenesis

A number of features suggest that the pathogenesis of MS is immunologically mediated. These features include:

- **the association with certain haplotypes.**
  Support for a genetic factor is strengthened by the finding of a 25% concordance for the presence of MS in monozygotic twins.
- **the nature of the cellular infiltrate** in acute and subacute lesions
- the fact that **demyelination can be produced in the CNS of a variety of animals by injection of an emulsion of brain tissue in Freund's adjuvant**. This is known as **experimental allergic encephalomyelitis**. The antigen responsible

appears to be myelin basic protein and the lesion is believed to be due in part to the activity of sensitized T cells and in part to an antibody-mediated reaction to a lipid hapten. The transfer of T cells sensitized to myelin basic protein from one animal to another results in the production of areas of demyelination in the recipient.

Acute Perivenular Encephalomyelitis (Acute Disseminated Postviral Encephalomyelitis)

This is a progressive illness characterized by extensive, acute, irreversible demyelination in the cerebral white matter and spinal cord. It may follow a variety of viral infections after an interval of a few days to 3 weeks. Before the introduction of vaccination against **measles** and **mumps**, these were the commonest viral antecedents with a mortality rate, in the case of encephalitis following measles, of about 40%. About 1 in 1000 patients with measles develop this complication. The reason for this immunoregulatory failure is not known. Currently **varicella** is the most frequently recognized preceding infection; the disease also occurs in a few patients after immunization against smallpox (now no longer practised), rabies and whooping cough. T lymphocytes from these patients show sensitization to myelin basic protein.

BASAL GANGLIA AND BRAINSTEM DEGENERATIONS

Parkinsonism

Parkinsonism is a clinical syndrome characterized by:

- **tremor**
- **rigidity**
- **inhibition of movement (bradykinesia)**
- **dementia (in some cases)**

Parkinsonism derives its name from the clinical account by James Parkinson in 1817 (*A Treatise on the Shaking Palsy*) and has a number of different causes all with a single functional target, **the dopaminergic system in the substantia nigra and the corpus striatum. The severity of the syndrome is proportional to the decline in dopamine concentrations in the affected areas of the brain. Up to a point, this functional deficiency can be remedied by treating the patients with levodopa, which can cross the blood–brain barrier, something that dopamine itself cannot do.**

Parkinsonism may occur in several circumstances.

Idiopathic Parkinson's Disease

This is a disorder most commonly appearing in late middle life and affecting both sexes equally. The cause is unknown; although some clustering occurs within families, there is as yet no evidence of an obvious genetic component. This is the commonest form of parkinsonism.

Free Radicals as a Pathogenetic Factor in Parkinsonism

It has been suggested that oxidative damage due to free radicals in the striatonigral region is responsible for the neuronal damage in this area. Chemical oxidation of dopamine produces potentially toxic semiquinones, and monoamine oxidase B produces hydrogen peroxide from dopamine. Certainly, post-mortem material from the affected regions of the brain shows evidence of:

- increased lipid peroxidation (a marker of oxidative damage)
- a decrease in reduced glutathione concentration, supporting the idea that oxidative stress has occurred

Some clinical data exist which show that treatment with Deprenyl, an inhibitor of monoamine oxidase type B, delays the development of disability in patients with parkinsonism, and this has been interpreted by some as indicating an actual slowing of disease progression.

Postencephalitic Parkinsonism

This occurred in considerable numbers in the 1940s as a consequence of an epidemic of encephalitis lethargica. The vast majority of these patients have now died and new cases of this kind are rare.

Drug-related Parkinsonism

The syndrome of parkinsonism can occur as a result of the administration of a number of different compounds. One that has excited much attention is the synthetic (and illicit) compound MPTP (1-methyl-4-phenyl-1,2,3,6-tetrahydropyridine), a contaminant of a synthetic form of heroin, which has caused acute parkinsonism in a number of young drug users. When this compound is administered to animals it produces the functional picture of parkinsonism and causes selective damage to the neurones in the substantia nigra. The mechanism underlying this selective targeting is not known for certain, but it may be related to oxidative stress.

Therapeutic agents associated with the appearance of parkinsonism in some cases include the phenothiazines (e.g. chlorpromazine), the butyrophenones (e.g. haloperidol), reserpine, α-methyldopa and procaine.

Miscellaneous Disorders

- **toxic damage** following exposure to carbon monoxide, cycad poisoning and chronic manganese poisoning
- **damage due to chronic cerebral injury in boxers**
- **ischaemic damage** in the basal ganglia
- **striatonigral degeneration**, which produces a syndrome clinically similar to that of Parkinson's

disease. The pathological changes (see below) are, however, different, and there is no clinical improvement with levodopa treatment.

- **the Shy–Drager syndrome**, in which there is a combination of the clinical features of parkinsonism and those of autonomic dysfunction, such as postural hypotension, inability to sweat, urinary incontinence, and impotence

Postencephalitic parkinsonism, the 'punch-drunk' syndrome in boxers and the parkinsonism–dementia complex seen in the Chamorro people of Guam, in addition to neuronal loss, show the presence of neurofibrillary tangles similar to those described in Alzheimer's disease.

Macroscopic Features

The only naked-eye abnormality seen in the brains of patients with Parkinson's disease is pallor of the substantia nigra (*Fig. 45.19*) **and of the locus ceruleus,** this, of course, being due to a loss of pigmented neurones in these areas.

Microscopic Features

The macroscopic picture is mirrored by the microscopic changes, **the chief abnormality being a decrease in the number of pigmented neurones; other neurones in the same region show shrinkage and vacuolation. The loss of neurones elicits a macrophage response; the macrophages infiltrating the area of neuronal loss contain dark pigment (neuromelanin). A marked degree of astrocytic gliosis is also present.**

Lewy Bodies

A highly characteristic feature is the presence of concentrically ringed hyaline bodies known as Lewy bodies, in some affected neurones. They are quite large, measuring 20 μm or more in diameter; usually there is only one Lewy body within a single cell. The body has a dark eosinophilic central core surrounded by rings of apparently structureless material (*Fig. 45.20*). When trichrome staining methods are used, such as Lendrum's Martius scarlet-blue, the dark central core stains red and the outer rings are light blue. The Lewy body appears to contain some neurofilament material but how it is formed and what it means in either pathogenetic or functional terms is quite unknown. It is a useful, if not absolutely specific, marker for Parkinson's disease, being present in at least 90% of cases of idiopathic parkinsonism. Interestingly, Lewy bodies are very rare in postencephalitic parkinsonism, striatonigral degeneration and the Shy–Drager syndrome.

Lewy bodies are not always confined to the substantia nigra but may also be seen in the cerebral cortex and even in peripheral ganglia. A condition known as **'diffuse Lewy body disease'** has recently been identified as a relatively common form of dementing disease. Some of the patients in whom Lewy bodies are found in the cortex, present with Parkinson's disease and become demented later, some present with dementia and later in the course of the illness develop the features of Parkinson's disease; and others are demented but show no evidence of Parkinson's disease. In Lewy body dementia there is loss of cortical neurones, and Lewy bodies are present both within the cortex and in areas usually affected in Parkinson's disease.

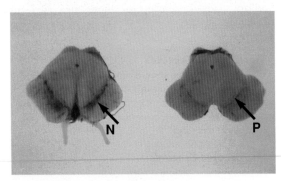

FIGURE 45.19 Parkinson's disease. The block on the left is normal (N) and shows a well-pigmented substantia nigra; that on the right (P) comes from a patient with Parkinson's disease and shows marked loss of pigmentation.

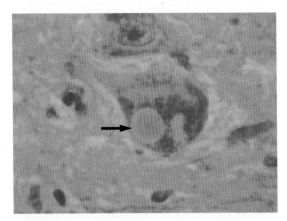

FIGURE 45.20 Lewy body in Parkinson's disease. The cytoplasm of the neurone in the centre shows a characteristic intracytoplasmic body which has an eosinophilic central core surrounded by an unstained zone.

PRIMARY 'DEGENERATIVE' DISORDERS AFFECTING CEREBELLAR FUNCTION

Several system disorders affecting the cerebellum and its connections have been described. Some are secondary, either to extracranial disorders such as small cell carci-

noma of the bronchus, or to toxic states associated, for example, with alcoholism or chronic poisoning with mercury. Others, however, are provisionally regarded as being primary.

Classifying these primary ataxic disorders is not easy because of their heterogeneity. They include:

- **congenital ataxias of unknown cause**
- **ataxias with recognized metabolic causes**, such as ataxia telangiectasia, xeroderma pigmentosum, Hartnup disease, abetalipoproteinaemia and urea cycle enzyme deficiencies
- **early-onset ataxia, which appears to be inherited in an autosomal recessive fashion. Friedreich's ataxia is a good example.** The classical clinical syndrome includes unsteadiness and dysarthria, starting in childhood, and progresses, with most patients being wheelchair-bound by their twenties. The prevalence in Europe is of the order of 1–2 per 100 000 population and the gene frequency is 1 in 110. Skeletal deformities such as kyphoscoliosis and pes cavus are not uncommon, being caused by imbalance of opposing muscle groups; cardiomyopathy is also a recognized feature. The chief targets for the disease process in Friedreich's ataxia include the cells of Clarke's column and the spinocerebellar fibres; sensory ganglion cells and their projections in the posterior columns of the spinal cord; pyramidal tracts and the dentate nuclei of the cerebellum.
  Friedreich's ataxia is associated with a mutation of a gene known as *X25*, situated on chromosome 9. The mutation consists of an abnormal number of repeats of the triplet GAA. Strangely, this abnormality appears to affect neither the coding nor regulatory sequences of the gene.
- **late-onset ataxias inherited chiefly, but by no means exclusively, on an autosomal dominant basis.** The collective term for these is olivopontocerebellar atrophy (OPCA). Cerebellar ataxia is a constant feature but, apart from this, the group exhibits a bewildering degree of clinical and thus neuropathological heterogeneity.
  At necropsy, obvious shrinkage of the pons and cerebral peduncles is seen and cerebellar cortical atrophy may be present. Atrophy of the inferior olives and of the olivocerebellar fibres is a prominent feature. Some suggest links between OPCA and defects in mitochondrial function.

DEGENERATIVE DISORDERS OF THE PYRAMIDAL SYSTEM: MOTOR NEURONE DISEASE

The term motor neurone disease encompasses a set of disorders that have a devastating effect on motor function but spare intellect, sensation and sphincter function. The aetiology and pathogenesis are unknown, although in one instance, the parkinsonism–dementia complex seen in the Chamorros of Guam, the development of the lesion has been ascribed to a toxic effect of a compound contained in the false sago palm (a cycad). It has been suggested that the compound, B-*N*-methylamino-L-alanine, acts as an excitotoxin. There is no evidence for anything similar in the environment of sufferers from motor neurone disease outside Guam.

Moter neurone disease has a worldwide distribution and occurs more commonly in males than in females (1.7 : 1) except in the familial form of amyotrophic lateral sclerosis where the sex incidence is equal. Onset is rare before the age of 35 years. The disease is progressively crippling and, eventually, fatal due to loss of either or both upper or lower motor neurone innervation of the muscles. The average duration is 2–3 years but some patients survive for 5–10 years. Classification is based on the areas that are primarily involved.

Amyotrophic Lateral Sclerosis
This is so termed because degeneration affects the corticospinal tracts, which are laterally placed in the cord. There is loss of **both upper and lower motor neurones**. The first leads to spasticity, hyperreflexia and an abnormal plantar reflex.

The lower motor neurone damage is evidenced by atrophy of muscles and fasciculation (muscle twitching). In some cases, cells of the motor cortex are lost; in others, the pyramidal tract degeneration begins below the decussation.

The disease is reasonably common; the incidence in the United States is much the same as that of MS. Familial cases make up 5–10% of the total, and linkage analysis suggests that there is an abnormal gene on the long arm of chromosome 21 which may play a causal role.

Some of the familial cases are associated with mutations of the gene encoding the cytosolic form of the enzyme copper–zinc superoxide dismutase (SOD) 1, which detoxifies superoxide anion. This led to the suggestion that damage to motor neurones in amyotrophic lateral sclerosis may be due to free radical-mediated injury.

It is not known whether such damage is related to loss of the dismutase function or whether the mutated enzyme might itself be harmful. Support for the latter view comes from studies in which transgenic strains of mice have been developed which possess extra copies of the normal SOD-1 gene or of the mutated gene found in patients with amyotrophic sclerosis. In mice that expressed the **mutated SOD-1 protein**, a disorder developed that clinically resembled amyotrophic lateral sclerosis and which was associated with severe motor neurone loss in the spinal cord.

These results suggest that the product of the mutated SOD-1 gene possesses some, as yet undefined, neurotoxic property.

Macroscopic Features
The most obvious changes are in the spinal cord, where the shrunken, greyish, atrophic anterior nerve roots contrast strikingly with normal-sized, white posterior roots.

Microscopic Features
This atrophy is due to loss of large myelinated nerve fibres originating from motor neurones in the anterior horn of the spinal cord. The lateral columns in the cord appear chalky and the use of myelin stains shows that extensive myelin loss has occurred, accompanying the axonal loss (*Fig. 45.21*). Muscles originally supplied by the affected neurones are shrunken and pale.

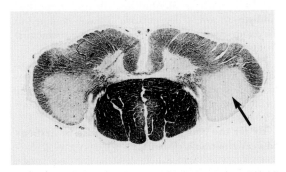

FIGURE 45.21 Spinal cord in a case of motor neurone disease (amyotrophic lateral sclerosis), showing loss of myelin on the right side (arrowed).

Progressive Muscular Atrophy
This variant occurs as a result of preferential degeneration of anterior horn motor neurones. This causes lower motor neurone (flaccid) paralysis. Muscle fasciculation is a prominent feature, caused by irregular discharge from the degenerating neurones.

A similar syndrome (**Werdnig–Hoffman disease or infantile progressive spinal muscular atrophy**) occurs as a sporadic or as an autosomally recessive or dominant disorder in infants. The infants may be 'floppy' at birth, or the muscular weakness, which is rapidly progressive, may present within the first few months of life. In familial forms of the disease, the onset tends to be earlier than in sporadic cases. The affected children usually die from respiratory infection by the age of 18 months.

Progressive Bulbar Palsy
Here, the degeneration affects the medullary motor nuclei and leads to **lower motor neurone paralysis** of the jaw, tongue and pharyngeal muscles.

DEMENTIA

Dementia is defined as **an acquired global impairment of intellect, memory and personality, but** without impairment of consciousness. It involves differing degrees of loss of higher cortical functions such as the correct performance of the tasks of daily life and the control of emotional reactions.

Dementia increases in frequency with advancing age. **Severe dementia will be seen in about 1 in 20 subjects aged more than 65 years; probably something like twice that number will show evidence of mild or moderate dementia.** More than 20% of individuals above the age of 85 years show some evidence of dementia. There are already some 880 000 people in this age group in the UK.

There are more than 50 recorded causes of dementia. These range from disorders arising primarily outside the brain, such as **alcoholism, drugs, hypothyroidism**, to severe 'degenerative' diseases, confined to the brain, associated with well-recognized structural changes.

In **histologically proven** cases of dementia in patients over the age of 65 years, the most common causes are as shown in *Table 45.8*. New techniques may reveal neuronal degenerations which have hitherto gone unrecognized.

By far the commonest single cause of dementia is Alzheimer's disease.

Alzheimer's Disease

This was first described by Alois Alzheimer in 1907 in relation to a patient with presenile dementia. For some time it was thought that senile dementia and the presenile variety were different entities. The pathological changes are, however, identical and it is clear that they represent the same disorder.

Epidemiology

Alzheimer's disease affects about 5% of people in their sixties, increasing to about 15% of subjects older than 80 years. The female : male ratio is 2 : 1 and this increases still further in the seventies. Presenile

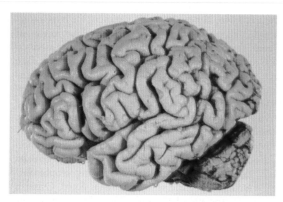

FIGURE 45.22 *Alzheimer's disease. The brain is atrophic, as evidenced by the widening of the sulci and thinning of the gyri.*

Alzheimer's disease usually starts in the fifties, but may be seen occasionally in much younger patients.

Some 5–10% of cases are **familial**. Both dementia and the histopathological features of Alzheimer's disease are seen in virtually all individuals with Down's syndrome who survive into early middle life.

Macroscopic Features

The outstanding feature is brain **atrophy**, expressed in the form of:

- a reduction in the weight of the brain, often to less than 1 kg (normal weight 1200–1300 g). The atrophy usually involves the whole of the brain, although it may be more pronounced in the frontal and temporal lobes.
- dilatation of the ventricles; in some instances the ventricular volume may be twice as great as normal.
- widening of the sulci, this being particularly marked in relation to the Sylvian fissure (*Fig. 45.22*)

However, these signs are **diagnostically unreliable** and Alzheimer's disease may be found in the presence of normal brain weight and ventricular volume, and individuals with small brains may have shown no evidence of dementia.

Microscopic Features

The 'gold standard' for a diagnosis of Alzheimer's disease is a combination of characteristic features, including **loss of neurones and disorganization of the cerebral cortex**. Areas in which neuronal loss is particularly conspicuous are within **the hippocampus, the noradrenergic locus ceruleus in the brainstem and the cholinergic basal nucleus of Meynert in the basal forebrain.**

Histological features include:

- **neurofibrillary 'tangles' within cortical neurones**
- **neuritic (senile) plaques**
- **amyloid deposition within the walls of small blood vessels, mainly in the grey matter**

Table 45.8 Frequency of Causes of Dementia

Type of dementia	Frequency (%)
Alzheimer's disease	> 50
Vascular disease (multiple small infarcts)	15
Alzheimer's disease with vascular disease	10
Pick's disease / Cerebral neoplasia	4
No definite histological diagnosis	15

- **granulovacuolar degeneration in hippocampal neurones**
- the presence within certain neurones (largely in the hippocampus) of **eosinophilic rod-shaped or pyramidal bodies which consist of cytoskeletal elements and are known as Hirano bodies**. They may be found in old people who are intellectually normal but appear to increase markedly in number in the brains of demented patients.

Neuritic (Senile) Plaques

These are rounded areas in the cortex, difficult to see in ordinary haematoxylin and eosin-stained sections but well demonstrated by staining with silver salts. They may measure up to 150 μm in diameter and consist of a **central dense core of amyloid fibrils surrounded by a cuff of abnormally distended degenerating nerve cell processes intermingled with glial processes** (*Fig. 45.23*).

As the plaque ages, the proportion of central amyloid increases. The plaques are found in the whole of the cerebral cortex, although the main motor and sensory areas tend to be spared; the hippocampus, basal nucleus of Meynert and the amygdala tend to be affected severely. Occasionally identical plaques are found in the brains of non-demented elderly subjects but the **number is much greater in those who are demented and there is a rough correlation between the number of plaques and the degree of cognitive impairment**.

Neurofibrillary Tangles

This term is applied to bundles of filaments within the cytoplasm of affected neurones. They stain positively with silver salts and contain amyloid. Electron microscopy shows the tangle to consist of masses of paired helical filaments, some elements of which are derived from the cytoskeleton of the cell. Immunological studies have shown the tangles to consist of a mixture of antigens, one of which appears to be the **tau** protein, which is concerned in microtubule assembly. Neurofibrillary tangles are *not* specific for Alzheimer's disease, being found in other disorders of the CNS including *SSPE* (see also p 1119).

The Amyloid of Alzheimer's Disease

Amyloid deposition is an integral part of the development of both the senile plaques of Alzheimer's disease and the identical cerebral lesions seen in long-surviving cases of Down's syndrome. The amyloid cores of the senile plaques and the vascular deposits of amyloid in the meninges and cerebral cortex appear to contain the same protein. This is a small molecule (about 4 kDa) known as **β protein (or A4 protein), which exists in three variants**. The gene encoding β protein has been mapped to the long arm of chromosome 21, an interesting finding in view of the development of Alzheimer-type lesions in patients with long-standing Down's syndrome, and of the fact that DNA polymorphisms affecting chromosome 21 have been shown in some cases of familial autosomally dominant Alzheimer's disease, in which the onset of the disease is often fairly early. The possible reasons for the conversion of this protein to a β-pleated (amyloid) form are discussed in the section dealing with pathogenesis.

Granulo-vacuolar Degeneration

This change is found mainly in the hippocampus in the cytoplasm of pyramidal neurones. A single cell may contain many vacuoles (measuring 3–5 μm in diameter). In the centre of each vacuole is a tiny dot which stains with silver salts and can be shown to contain abnormal phosphorylated proteins.

Aetiology and Pathogenesis

The cause of Alzheimer's disease is unknown and although a number of functional biochemical abnormalities have been identified in the brains of affected subjects, the relevance of these to both the aetiology and pathogenesis remains uncertain.

- **A cholinergic deficit is present in Alzheimer's disease. A regular finding in the brains of patients is a deficiency in acetylcholine synthesis which is associated with reduced amounts of the synthesizing enzyme choline acetyltransferase.** The cholinergic innervation of the cortex comes mainly from the basal nucleus of Meynert, which, as already stated, is one of the sites of predilection for neuronal loss to occur. In addition, recent studies point to a deficit in postsynaptic cholinergic receptors.
- **Other neurotransmitter deficits have also been recorded**, involving both the noradrenergic and serotoninergic systems. There appear to be changes in the amount of somatostatin and

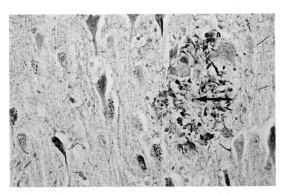

FIGURE 45.23 *Alzheimer's disease. A neuritic plaque in the hippocampus. The section is stained with a silver salt which shows up the nerve processes as black. The plaque consists of a single core of amyloid surrounded by a ring of swollen and deformed neurites.*

neuropeptide Y, and some cortical areas show the presence of reduced amounts of GABA.

These findings seem more likely to be consequences of the pathological state rather than factors bringing it about.

Is There a Role for Toxic Substances in Alzheimer's Disease?

There have been repeated suggestions that a high intracerebral concentration of aluminium might be involved in the pathogenesis of Alzheimer's disease. This is based primarily on the finding of high levels of this metal in the brains of patients, especially in areas where there are many neurofibrillary tangles. The suggestions have been made that:

- aluminium may interfere with DNA synthesis, leading to the production of abnormal proteins
- aluminium deposits may in some unspecified manner initiate the formation of neuritic plaques. High aluminium concentrations may occur in patients on chronic renal dialysis and this can be associated with dementia, although here the tissue changes of Alzheimer's disease are not seen.

Apolipoprotein E Alleles and Alzheimer's Disease

Apolipoprotein E (ApoE), an important constituent of 'remnant' particles in the exogenous cycle of lipid metabolism, exists in three different molecular forms known as E_2, E_3 and E_4. Recent studies have shown an increased frequency of the E_4 variant in patients with late-onset sporadic or familial Alzheimer's disease and it is asserted that about half the cases of late-onset disease can be attributed to the presence of E_4.

ApoE is unique amongst the apoproteins; it has a special relevance within the nervous system, in relation to **repair and growth of myelin and nerve cell membranes, both within their developmental stages and after injury**. ApoE can bind to β amyloid to form a stable adduct and can be identified in neuritic plaques. It has been suggested that the normal age-related decline in cell number and lipid content in the brain is somehow exacerbated by the presence of the E_4 allele.

Recently it has been suggested that both $ApoE_4$ and $α_1$-antichymotrypsin act as chaperones which promote the folding of the β protein amyloid precursor into a β-pleated (amyloid) form, and that it may be the presence of these chaperones rather than that of the amyloid precursor protein that determines the regional distribution of the lesions of Alzheimer's disease.

In **familial Alzheimer's disease**, a significant number of cases is associated with mutations in the **presenilin 1** gene (*PS-1*), located on chromosome 14. Many mutations have been described, the effects of which seem to be largely on messenger RNA splicing. Recently an association has been described between homozygosity of one of the alleles on the *PS-1* gene

and an increased risk of sporadic late-onset Alzheimer's disease as well.

Dementia as a Manifestation of Vascular Disease

Vascular disease is the second most common cause of dementia; the basic pathological change in the brain which is responsible for the dementia appears to be **multiple small areas of infarction**. Focal neurological signs are often present in addition to the dementia; the onset of the condition is much more abrupt than is the case with Alzheimer's disease. The underlying cause for this multi-infarct state is often hypertension.

The small infarcts can be readily identified in life by computed tomography; relatively few detailed pathological studies exist. The onset of the dementia is often sudden and the illness follows a fluctuating course, with some day to day variation in the degree of cognitive disturbance.

Binswanger's Disease

A second pathological picture may be seen in dementia associated with hypertension. Here, the **ischaemic lesions are seen in the deep white matter with the cerebral cortex being relatively well preserved**. The deep white matter is reduced in amount and cystic cavities may be seen within this region.

Huntington's Disease

This particularly cruel disease is a **hereditary form of chorea associated with severe mental deterioration. It appears for the most part in middle life and then progresses relentlessly, reducing the patient to a quivering wreck of his/her former self.** The average age of onset is in the mid-forties and the disease may last anything from 5 to 30 years, with 15 years being the average.

Molecular Genetics and Aetiology

The disorder is inherited as an **autosomal dominant with the gene having a very high penetrance (almost 100%)**; thus roughly half the children of an affected parent will develop the disease. In northern Europe, prevalence rates are between 4 and 7 per 100 000, this being much lower in Afro-Americans and in the Japanese. In early-onset cases the abnormal gene is most likely to have been inherited from the father, but when the disease develops in adult life there is no such bias in the pattern.

The genomic abnormality appears to be located **near the end of the short arm of chromosome 4**. A large gene has been identified at this site which has been named *IT15*. It spans 210 kilobases and encodes a previously unrecognized protein, **huntingtin**. The striking feature of the *IT15* reading frame is that it contains a polymorphic $(CAG)_n$ trinucleotide repeat, which in normal chromosome 4 has 11–34 copies. In chromosome 4 from patients with Huntington's disease, **there** is an increase in the number of copies of the tri-nucleotide repeat, with a range of 42–66 copies. The greater the number of copies of the trinucleotide, the earlier is the onset of disease. The function of the gene product is still unknown.

Microscopic Features

The most severe changes are seen in the **putamen and caudate nucleus, both of which show a severe degree of atrophy due to loss of neurones accompanied by gliosis**. There appears to be a selective loss of small neurones, which are normally the most numerous within the corpus striatum, with relatively good preservation of the larger cells, although some loss of these also occurs.

Biochemical examination of affected brains shows a marked decrease in GABA (an inhibitory neurotransmitter) and its synthesizing enzyme, glutamic acid decarboxylase, within the corpus striatum and the substantia nigra. Kainic acid, an analogue of glutamate, is known to be a powerful neurotoxin and produces biochemical and histological changes similar to those seen in Huntington's disease when injected into the corpus striatum of rabbits. It has been suggested, therefore, that in Huntington's disease there may be an endogenous overproduction of a kainic acid-like compound which could overstimulate the corticostriatal system and lead to loss of neurones within it.

Pick's Disease

This is a rare form of dementia, occurring for the most part in the sixth decade. Patients die 1–10 years from the onset. Women are affected slightly more often than men and some familial cases have been reported.

The clinical picture is essentially no different from that of Alzheimer's disease, but the pathological changes are.

Macroscopic Features

There is usually severe **localized** atrophy of the brain, most often involving the frontal and temporal lobes. The sulci are much widened and the gyri, particularly near their tips, show very severe atrophic change, giving an appearance that has been compared to that of a 'walnut'.

Microscopic Features

These are dominated by severe neuronal loss, mainly in the outer parts of the cortex, associated with reactive gliosis. Some of the surviving neurones show a rather characteristic appearance in which the cells swell up, becoming round or pear-shaped. The nucleus tends to be pushed to one end of the cell and the abundant cytoplasm appears uniformly eosinophilic.

Some of these cells contain intracytoplasmic inclusions staining positively with silver stains. These are known as

Pick bodies and can be shown by use of the appropriate antibodies to contain antigens characteristic of both neurofilaments and neurofibrillary tangles.

TRANSMISSIBLE SPONGIFORM ENCEPHALOPATHIES

Creutzfeldt–Jakob disease (CJD) is a rare dementing disorder which has an unremitting course and a uniformly fatal outcome. Together with **kuru**, the **Gerstmann–Sträussler–Scheinker syndrome** and **fatal familial insomnia** in humans, which may exist in either familial or sporadic forms, and **scrapie** in sheep and goats, **transmissible encephalopathy in mink** and **bovine spongiform encephalopathy**, it exhibits a triad of features:

1) **a common histological picture** characterized by:
   - loss of neurones
   - a spongy appearance of the affected parts of the brain caused by the development of small cystic cavities in the cortical substance (*Fig. 45.24*)
   - a brisk astrocytic response
   - amyloid plaques and, in some instances, amyloid deposition in blood vessels. Amyloid deposits are usually present in the Gerstmann–Sträussler syndrome and, less often, in CJD.

These features make up the pathological picture of 'spongiform encephalopathy'.

2) **transmissibility.** All these conditions are transmissible. The infective agent or agents appear to be unique in that, unlike all known microorganisms, **they have not been shown to possess any nucleic acid** and are not inactivated by circumstances that normally inactivate bacteria or viruses. The term '**prion**' (small *proteinaceous infectious* particle) has been coined for these novel transmissible agents.

3) **modification of the same host precursor protein in all species into amyloid fibrils.** This

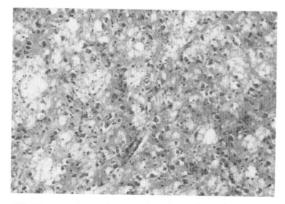

FIGURE 45.24 Spongiform encephalopathy. Sporadic Creutzfeldt–Jakob disease showing the typical spongiform appearance of the neuropil.

amyloidogenic protein or prion protein, known as PrP 27–30, is encoded for by a normal cellular gene and again, unlike any 'normal' infective agent, it elicits no inflammatory or immune response when transmitted from one animal to another. The gene coding for human PrP (*PRNP*) is located on the short arm of chromosome 20. In its native form, the prion protein is a glycoprotein anchored to the cell membrane in most cell types including neurones. Its biological function is still unknown but it has some structural resemblance to a protein modulating acetylcholine receptors.

The message that appears to be emerging is that mutations leading to an altered protein correlate with the pathological lesions of spongiform encephalopathy and that, amazingly, the mutations are associated with the protein becoming **transmissible**. At least six disease-associated mutations in the PrP gene have been described. Two of these have been insertional mutations where extra copies of a novel coding sequence appear in the gene and, in these instances, the disease pattern has been atypical. In other cases, point mutations in the gene have been associated either with the Gerstmann–Sträussler–Scheinker syndrome or with an increased risk of CJD.

When the scrapie-associated form of prion protein, derived from scrapie-infected hamster brain, is incubated with normal prion protein in a cell-free system, the normal protein assumes the configuration of the scrapie-associated protein, which has a large proportion of β-pleated sheets. This implies that the transmissibility of the scrapie-associated agent depends on a direct protein–protein interaction.

Creutzfeldt–Jakob Disease

CJD is a rare, usually sporadic, dementia. In some cases there appears to be a familial incidence, with a pattern suggesting autosomal dominant inheritance.

Clinical Features

There is a rapidly progressive global dementia, myoclonus, and severe and progressive motor dysfunction. The disease is usually fatal within 1 year.

Transmissibility

Brain tissue (even after prolonged fixation) from humans with CJD can transmit the disease to various types of monkeys, cats, guinea-pigs, Syrian hamsters and mice; the pathological changes in the brains of these animals are identical to those seen in brains from humans with CJD. Originally it was thought that intracerebral inoculation of infective material was necessary, but this is now known to be incorrect: CJD can be transmitted by a variety of routes including by mouth.

CJD has been transmitted from human to human via the use of intracerebral electrodes previously used in patients with CJD and via transplants of cornea and human dura; more alarmingly, there are now reports of a considerable number of cases of CJD developing in young humans treated with human growth hormone (prepared from pooled human pituitary tissue obtained at post-mortem examination) during childhood and adolescence (*Figs 45.25* and *45.26*). Those who have become 'infected' in this way show an **increased prevalence of methionine or valine homozygosity at codon 129 of the PrP gene**, suggesting that host factors may be of critical importance in the susceptibility of humans to transmission of spongiform encephalopathies.

Mutations in the PrP gene are found in familial CJD; a particular variant, a lysine substitution at codon 200, has been found in Libyan Jews among whom the disease occurs 30 times more frequently than in the world population.

Bovine Spongiform Encephalopathy and CJD

Bovine spongiform encephalopathy (BSE) has affected large numbers of British cattle in the past 15 years. It is believed to have arisen as a result of including scrapie-

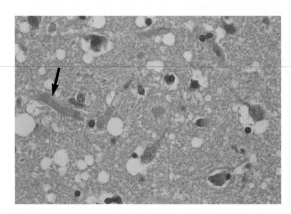

FIGURE 45.25 Creutzfeldt–Jakob disease following the administration of growth hormone. In addition to the spongiform change, some amyloid is seen in relation to one of the small blood vessels (arrowed).

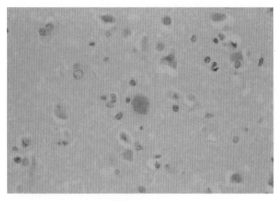

FIGURE 45.26 Section from the brain of a patient with spongiform encephalopathy stained with an antibody against prion protein. This shows up as a rounded portion of brown-staining material in the centre of the field.

infected material in cattle feed, the animal protein contributing to an increased milk yield.

It is almost certain that some cases of CJD, especially in the young, may have been due to eating products of cattle with BSE which have entered the food chain. The pathological appearances in the few cases examined so far, differ from those seen in sporadic CJD or in the inherited spongiform encephalopathies in that there are many more plaques containing PrP. In the cases suspected of being associated with BSE, **methionine homozygosity** at codon 129 of the open reading frame of the PrP gene occurs. Such homozyosity is present in about 38% of the UK population. This **'new variant' CJD** is associated with a unique and highly consistent appearance of protease-resistant PrP on Western blots; this involves a characteristic pattern of glycosylation. This pattern is identical with that seen in the brains of cats that have acquired BSE and in inbred mice to which BSE has been transmitted. These data suggest that 'new variant CJD' is very likely to be due to ingestion of abnormal prion proteins in beef or beef products.

Gerstmann–Sträussler–Scheinker Syndrome

This presents as a dementing illness associated with cerebellar ataxia. It is often familial, being transmitted vertically with an autosomal dominant pattern. Histological examination shows spongiform changes similar to those seen in CJD (*Fig. 45.27*), amyloid plaques and amyloid changes in small blood vessels, although this last feature is not present in all cases. In affected families, several different mutations have been found in the PrP gene, producing, for example, a leucine substitution at codon 102; like CJD, this disorder is transmissible.

When cloned genes producing mutant prion proteins, with a mutation homologous to that found in patients with Gerstmann–Sträussler–Scheinker syndrome, were transfected into mouse oöcytes, thus producing **'transgenic'** mice, the mice developed the pathological changes of spongiform encephalopathy, although the characteristic amyloid fibrils seen in human disease were not present. Material from these affected transgenic mice is transmissible to other animals and produces spongiform changes in their brains.

Kuru

Kuru is a disease characterized clinically by:

- cerebellar ataxia
- severe tremor
- progressive motor dysfunction associated with dysarthria which progresses to death within 1 year of the onset of symptoms

Kuru is confined to the Fore tribe in highland New Guinea (kuru = shivering or trembling in the Fore language). It was common in children and women but rare in males. During the past 25 years the disease has been gradually disappearing. As with the other diseases in this group, kuru can be transmitted to a variety of animal species via the inoculation of 'infective' material.

Both the distribution and the declining incidence have been ascribed to the unusual nature of post-funeral Fore catering, the 'funereal baked meats' consisting of the remains of the deceased. The practice of ritual cannibalism 'as a mark of mourning and respect for dead kinsmen' has now ceased. The removal of the brain was usually carried out by women (with, of course, ungloved hands) and the brain was scooped, again by hand, into bamboo cylinders. Thus, it is not difficult to see how inoculation of infected material via skin abrasions might occur.

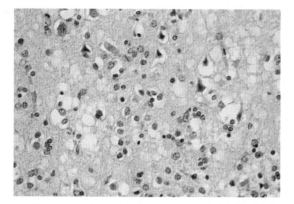

FIGURE 45.27 *Spongiform encephalopathy. Frontal cortex from a patient with Gerstmann–Sträussler–Scheinker syndrome. This is associated with a point mutation at codon 102 in the gene encoding the prion protein.*

Vascular Disorders of the Central Nervous System

STROKE

Stroke is an old-fashioned but graphic clinical term encompassing:

- **the sudden onset of focal loss of neurological function lasting longer than 24 hours**
- **a vascular origin, the brain damage being due to either ischaemia or haemorrhage**

Severe ischaemic cerebral damage can also occur as a result of **hypoxia**, but this is not stroke as hypoxia causes global rather than focal abnormalities.

Epidemiology

It is difficult to exaggerate the importance of stroke as a cause of severe disability and death in Western populations. **In the UK, stroke ranks third among causes of death, being responsible for 10% of all deaths.** Half a million new cases of stroke occur every year in the USA, and 50% of these patients die. Of the remainder, 50% are left with permanent disability and only 10% regain full function. Although the elderly are most commonly affected, about 30% of cases of strokes occur in people between the ages of 35 and 65 years.

Aetiology

Causes include infarction and haemorrhage (*Fig. 45.28*).

Infarction due to ischaemia accounts for 84% of cases of stroke. The ischaemia is due to:

- **thrombosis** in arteries supplying the brain (53%)
- **emboli** impacting in the cerebral circulation (31%). Such emboli may be derived from two main sources:

  1) the **heart**, in which thrombosis may occur under a number of circumstances including **valvular disease** (chronic rheumatic disease, infective endocarditis and 'floppy valve') associated with endocardial erosions, **abnormal flow patterns** as seen in atrial fibrillation and dilated cardiomyopathy, and the presence of **myocardial infarction**.

  2) the **neck arteries**, in which complicated atherosclerotic plaques with superficial plaque cap injury and resulting platelet-rich mural thrombi are not uncommon.

Rarer causes of cerebral ischaemia include **vasospasm** associated with hypertensive encephalopathy, **venous occlusion** due to hypercoagulability or severe dehydration, and **inflammatory diseases of supplying arteries** such as polyarteritis nodosa.

Transient ischaemic attacks (TIAs), which cause focal neurological deficits lasting only a very short time, are considered separately.

Haemorrhage is responsible for 16% of cases of stroke:

- **intracerebral haemorrhage** (10%)
- **subarachnoid haemorrhage** (6%)

The most important association by far with intracerebral haemorrhage is **hypertension**.

More rarely, haemorrhage may be associated with **vascular malformations, vascular neoplasms** or **abnormal bleeding tendencies** such as occur in clotting factor deficiencies, thrombocytopenia (from whatever cause) or somewhat overenthusiastic anticoagulant treatment.

Risk Factors for Stroke

Important factors increasing the risk of stroke are:

1) **The severity of atherosclerosis in the neck and intracranial arteries**. Thus all the inherited and environmental factors believed to have an incremental effect on atherogenesis, and thus to increase the risk of ischaemic heart disease, also increase the risk of stroke.

The existence of ischaemic heart disease is itself a powerful risk factor for stroke, increasing the risk, compared with that in control populations, by 2–5 times. Cardiac failure and atrial fibrillation also increase the risk of stroke, presumably because of the increased frequency of systemic emboli. Of the **environmental** factors positively correlated with risk of arterial disease, **cigarette smoking** appears to act most powerfully.

2) **Hypertension.** The presence of high blood pressure is associated with a sixfold increase in the risk of stroke.

3) **Diabetes mellitus** increases the risk of stroke by 2–4 times. This may be due to the twofold effect of diabetes: an increase in the extent and severity of atherosclerosis, and a greater likelihood of high blood pressure due to diabetic renal disease.

Cerebral Blood Supply

Understanding the pathology of stroke is helped greatly by some knowledge of the arterial blood supply and venous drainage of the brain.

Four large arteries provide the brain with blood:

- two internal carotid arteries
- two vertebral arteries

The carotid vessels supply the major part of the cerebral hemispheres; the vertebral arteries supply the base of the brain and the cerebellum. These two systems are connected at the base of the brain by the anterior and posterior communicating arteries to form the circle of Willis.

The anatomy of the circle of Willis in any individual plays an important part in modulating the size and location of ischaemic lesions because the circle, via its communicating arteries, helps to ensure a well-distributed blood supply to the brain. The effect of this collateral

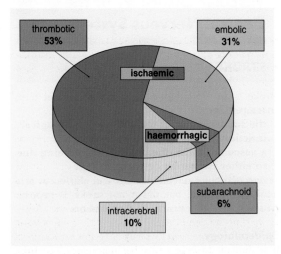

FIGURE 45.28 Relative frequency of the causes of stroke.

circulation is to make ischaemic lesions due to arterial occlusion **smaller** than the territory supplied by the occluded vessel.

Anatomical variations in the circle are common; only about 50% of the population have 'normal' circles of Willis, and the prevalence of such variations is even higher in patients with stroke who come to necropsy. From the circle of Willis are derived:

- **paramedian vessels perforating the base of the brain and supplying structures near the midline**
- **long circumferential anterior, middle and posterior cerebral arteries supplying the cortex and its underlying white matter**
- **short circumferential vessels supplying the basal ganglia**

Collateral Vessels

The main vessels supplying the cerebellum and brainstem are derived from the **vertebrobasilar system**. The vertebral arteries often show a major degree of asymmetry but anatomical variations affecting the basilar artery are rare.

The existence of a collateral circulation has clinical relevance only when there are stenosing lesions of large vessels such as the internal carotids. **If the circle of Willis is anatomically normal and is free from significant degrees of atherosclerosis**, then one internal carotid artery can be occluded without any resulting ischaemia in the territory supplied by this vessel. The vertebrobasilar system has a less well developed anastomotic circulation and, hence, **occlusion of the basilar artery always has very severe effects**.

The **small cerebral vessels** also have little or no collateral circulation and thus stenosis or occlusion of these vessels inevitably cause ischaemic lesions which, depending on their localization, may have devastating functional consequences.

PATHOLOGY OF CEREBRAL INFARCTION

Infarcts vary greatly in size from a few millimeters in diameter to massive lesions involving the whole territory of the artery that has become occluded. The infarct may be **'anaemic'** (pale) or **haemorrhagic** (classically associated with embolic occlusion of arteries or with venous thrombosis (*Fig. 45.29*)). Following embolic impaction, the embolus may become fragmented and there may also be some relaxation of arterial tone at the site of impaction. When this happens the embolus may be freed to travel further along the artery, and reperfusion takes place behind it. The reperfusing blood flows through vessels damaged by ischaemia. These are abnormally leaky and allow blood to ooze through the vascular wall into the surrounding infarcted brain tissue.

The histopathological appearances of a cerebral infarct depend on the time that has elapsed between the onset of ischaemia and examination:

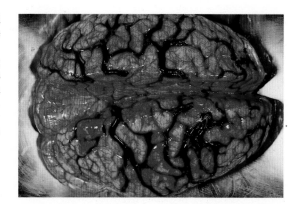

FIGURE 45.29 Extensive venous thrombosis following thrombosis of the sagittal sinus. The affected brain becomes swollen and congested, and haemorrhagic infarction supervenes.

Morphological change = Injury × Time

This relationship between time elapsed and pathological changes in the brain is shown in *Table 45.9*.

Cerebral Oedema Associated with Ischaemia

The swelling associated with infarcts is due to cerebral oedema of the cytotoxic type. A large infarct, for instance affecting most of one cerebral hemisphere (see *Fig. 45.30*), can behave as a space-occupying mass; increasing oedema causes herniation of the ipsilateral medial temporal lobe (uncal herniation) with a fatal outcome.

It should be remembered that herniation itself can cause ischaemia as a result of compression of the vessels related to the herniated portion of the brain. For example, the posterior cerebral or the superior cerebellar arteries can be affected in this way if tentorial herniation occurs.

Anatomical Patterns of Ischaemic Damage
The effects of occlusion of arteries supplying the brain are heavily dependent on the vessel occluded.

Internal Carotid Occlusion

In 80% of cases this is due to thrombosis; embolism can occur, the most common site of impaction being the upper end of the internal carotid. Blood flow through the internal carotid does not fall significantly until the lumen of the vessel is reduced by 80–90% and thus only a small proportion of radiologically demonstrable stenoses will produce overt cerebral ischaemia. When symptoms do appear in patients with mild carotid stenosis they are usually secondary to the formation of small mural thrombi and subsequent embolism from these sites.

Table 45.9 – Relationship Between Elapsed Time and Morphology in Stroke

Elapsed time	Macroscopic	Microscopic
0–6 hours	No gross change noted. At this stage the symptoms and signs are due largely to oedema which will resolve, this being associated with gradual clinical improvement (*Fig. 45.30*).	From 4 to 6 hours there is evidence of neuronal necrosis. Affected cells show intense eosinophilia of the cytoplasm, which is often vacuolated, and poor nuclear staining.
24 hours	There may be some **loss of demarcation between grey and white matter**; the affected area of brain feels softer than normal.	There is evidence of later stages of neuronal necrosis, with decreasing ability of the cells to bind dyes so that they appear rather 'ghost-like'. The neuropil looks spongy due to a combination of swelling of axons and cell processes of astrocytes. Demyelination occurs within the infarct and by 18–24 hours it is possible to see a sharp demarcation between abnormal myelin within the lesion and normal myelin at its periphery. At the edge of the infarct, large numbers of neutrophils may be seen.
4 days	The degree of **softening** seen on the cut surface of the brain is now much greater and the centre of the infarct may have begun to break down, the early **coagulative** necrosis now becoming **liquefactive**.	Macrophages are seen to have invaded the infarct in fairly large numbers and to have become foamy as a result of phagocytosis of lipid derived from broken-down myelin. In haemorrhagic stroke, iron from the red cells within the infarct is also phagocytosed.
Weeks to months	In most instances the infarcted area becomes converted to a cyst (*Fig. 45.31*) which, in haemorrhagic stroke, shows reddish yellow iron pigment in its walls.	At the edges of the lesion there is proliferation of fibre-forming astrocytes and the abundant new glial fibres wall off the cystic area from the surrounding brain. It is incorrect to compare this process of **gliosis** to scar formation in sites other than the brain. Unlike collagen fibres and other matrix proteins, which are extracellular, glial fibres, produced as part of the reaction to tissue injury, remain confined within the membranes of the astrocyte and its processes.

Five patterns of ischaemic brain damage may occur as a result of severe stenosis or occlusion of the internal carotid artery:
1) **massive infarction involving the whole territory of the middle cerebral artery**
2) **infarction of the cortex round the Sylvian fissure, with or without involvement of the internal capsule and the basal ganglia**
3) **infarction restricted to the internal capsule**
4) **small infarcts within the white matter supplied by the middle cerebral artery**
5) **infarcts occurring in the boundary zone between the territories supplied by the middle cerebral and the anterior cerebral arteries** or, less commonly, in the boundary zone between the territories of the middle and posterior cerebral arteries. Boundary zones, the areas furthest from two neighbouring arteries, are termed 'watershed areas' (*Fig. 45.32*).

Subclavian Artery Occlusion

Obstruction of the subclavian and innominate arteries may cause the **'subclavian steal syndrome'**. Occlusion of either of these vessels proximal to the origin of the vertebral artery may lead to retrograde flow of blood down the vertebral artery in order to supply the vessels of the arm. Thus blood is 'stolen' from the basilar artery and the circle of Willis. If the arm muscles

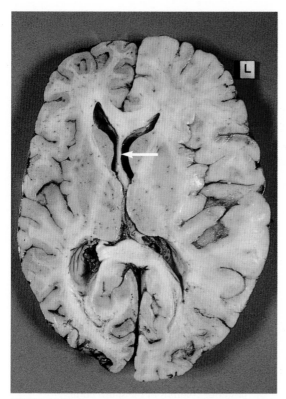

FIGURE 45.30 *Recent ischaemic infarction of the left cerebral hemisphere. Note the gross degree of associated oedema which is deforming the lateral ventricle on the affected side and which has pushed over the septum pellucidum (arrowed).*

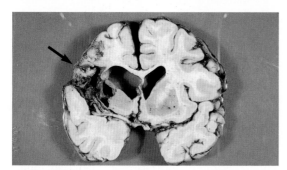

FIGURE 45.31 *Old infarction (8 years previously). There is marked loss of brain tissue on the affected side with cystic change lateral to the basal ganglia.*

are exercised, there is an up to fourfold increase in blood flow to the upper limb and this can precipitate cerebral ischaemia.

Vertebrobasilar System
The vertebral arteries have a complicated anatomical pathway through the foramina of the transverse processes of the cervical vertebrae, then curving behind

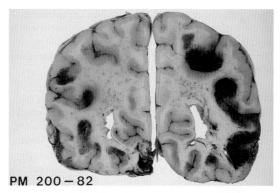

PM 200–82

FIGURE 45.32 *Multiple haemorrhagic infarcts in a 'watershed' area of the brain. Watersheds are areas of the arterial territory most remote from the parent arterial stems and are thus most vulnerable to the effects of cerebral underperfusion.*

the lateral mass of the atlas to enter the skull via the foramen magnum. Because of this, flow may be compromised as a result of a number of processes other than atheroma and thrombosis. These include **severe cervical osteoarthritis, sudden hyperextension of the neck, subluxation of the atlanto-occipital joint in rheumatoid arthritis, and damage sustained as a result of twisting and traction of the neck of infants in the course of delivery**.

In the basilar artery itself, atherothrombosis is the most common cause of occlusion. Vertigo and nystagmus are common in vertebrobasilar insufficiency; this may be associated with cranial nerve palsies and with difficulties with speech (dysarthria) and swallowing.

Basilar artery occlusion (*Fig. 45.33*) **leads to:**
- **flaccid quadriplegia**
- **coma**
- **bulbar palsy**

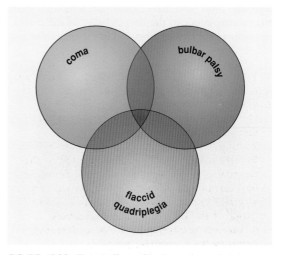

FIGURE 45.33 *Clinical effects of basilar artery occlusion.*

Some patients develop the **'locked-in' syndrome**, a dreadful state in which a conscious but mute patient is completely paralysed apart from some eye movements. The pathological basis for this is **extensive infarction of the ventral part of the pons**.

Middle Cerebral Artery Occlusion

This vessel is the commonest site of intracranial arterial occlusion. **Embolism is of major importance, accounting for up to two-thirds of cases.** Occlusion causes contralateral hemiparesis and contralateral cortical-type sensory loss. Because the speech area is in the territory of this vessel, there is expressive aphasia if the occlusion occurs on the left side; if the optic radiation is involved, the patient may have hemianopia.

Embolic Stroke

Most data suggest that embolism accounts for about 30% of strokes, although some maintain that the incidence is much higher. As with embolic syndromes in general, most emboli are derived from thrombi, the sites and origin of which have been mentioned above. As in other vascular beds, emboli may be gaseous (air or nitrogen), fat or rarer entities such as aggregates of tumour cells, parasitic larvae, clumps of meconium and keratinocytes, such as is seen in amniotic fluid embolism.

Fat Embolism

In patients dying 3–4 days after the occurrence of cerebral fat embolism, **the white matter of the brain is diffusely studded with tiny petechial haemorrhages** (*Fig. 45.34*). Staining frozen sections of the affected white matter with fat-soluble dyes shows many globules of fat within capillaries and, in some instances, the capillary walls may be necrotic. In the grey matter, the fat globules are equally numerous but haemorrhages and tissue damage do not occur because the capillaries here are short and have many anastomoses. Small infarcts may occur in the deeper layers of the cortex, especially in the frontal lobes and in the brainstem and

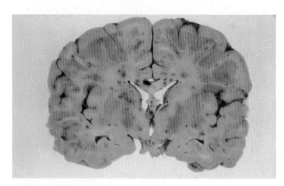

FIGURE 45.34 Fat embolism showing small haemorrhages in the white matter.

pons. In some long-term survivors of severe acute cerebral syndromes caused by fat embolism, extensive atrophy of the white matter may be seen.

Air Embolism

Cerebral air embolism may complicate cardiac, brain or pulmonary surgery and catheterization procedures.

If death occurs within a few minutes the brain shows no structural abnormalities. In patients who survive long enough for lesions to develop, areas of ischaemic damage may be found localized to the arterial boundary zones in the cerebral hemispheres.

Nitrogen Embolism

Nitrogen embolism can occur under two circumstances:

1) **hyperbaric decompression.** This takes place when **there is a reduction from an abnormally high atmospheric pressure to normal**, such as occurs after deep-sea diving or working in a caisson. If the return to normal atmospheric pressure is too rapid, nitrogen comes out of solution and forms bubbles within the circulation, which can obstruct flow, chiefly in small vessels.

In fatal cases, if death has been rapid, the brain is congested. In those who survive for longer, multiple small infarcts may be found, principally in the posterior columns of the spinal cord.

2) **hypobaric decompression.** This term describes the situation when **a reduction occurs from a normal atmospheric pressure to an abnormally low one**. Damage to the central nervous system is expressed in the form of multiple small areas of ischaemic damage, chiefly in the grey matter of the cerebral hemispheres or in the spinal cord.

Transient Ischaemic Attacks

TIAs are distinguished from full-blown stroke in that the focal neurological deficits occurring are fully reversible and usually last no more than a few minutes; occasionally the duration may be prolonged for up to 24 hours.

TIAs are important because they constitute an advance warning of future cerebral infarction. The quantification of risk of strokes occurring after TIA is not easy. Estimates of risk vary from 13% to 50%, the truth probably lying somewhere between these two extremes.

Three mechanisms may be involved in the pathogenesis of TIA:

1) **breaking off of small portions of mural thrombus** from the surface of atherosclerotic plaques or heart valves, these emboli then impacting in small cerebral vessels
2) **sudden decline in cardiac output** with resulting cerebral underperfusion
3) **hypercoagulable and high blood viscosity** states as is seen in polycythaemia

INTRACEREBRAL HAEMORRHAGE

Intracerebral bleeding may be divided into **two basic types**:

- So-called **'primary'** haemorrhage, usually found in the presence of **hypertension**. This accounts for 80% of intracerebral bleeds.
- So-called **'secondary'** haemorrhage due to either local or systemic disease. Lesions such as **aneurysms, neoplasms, vascular malformations and amyloid affecting the intracerebral vessels** fall under the rubric of local disease, while **bleeding disorders associated with inadequate numbers of platelets or deficiency in certain clotting factors** constitute the cases associated with systemic disease. In this last connection one should not forget that overenthusiastic anticoagulant or thrombolytic treatment carries a risk of intracerebral haemorrhage.

Primary Intracerebral Haemorrhage

This event occurs most commonly in late middle age. The common sites of bleeding are:

- the region of **the lentiform nucleus** (so-called 'capsular' haemorrhage). This accounts for 80% of cases.
- **the pons or white matter of the cerebellum**; these sites account for the remaining 20% (*Fig. 45.35*).

Pathogenesis

The most favoured suggestion is that these haemorrhages are due to rupture of tiny microaneurysms (Charcot–Bouchard aneurysms, miliary aneurysms) measuring 1–2 mm in diameter. These occur in small arteries (100–300 µm in diameter) in the areas of the brain most susceptible to primary haemorrhage. They are present in about 50% of hypertensive individuals, compared with 5% of non-hypertensive subjects; **90% of patients who die from hypertensive cerebral haemorrhage show microaneurysms**.

Hypertension appears to be the cause because **the number of aneurysms is related to the severity and duration of the high blood pressure**. The prevalence of microaneurysms also increases quite markedly with increasing age, being found in 70% of hypertensive patients over the age of 60 years in contrast with those aged under 50 years in whom the prevalence is only 5%.

Rupture of the aneurysms is likely to be the result of sudden rises in blood pressure occurring against an already hypertensive background. This idea gains some support from the intracerebral and subarachnoid haemorrhages occurring when patients, taking monoamine oxidase inhibitors eat foods rich in tyramine (such as cheese, yeast extracts or chocolate) or are given sympathomimetic drugs like ephedrine or amphetamines. Very sharp rises in blood pressure occur under these circumstances and may lead to haemorrhage.

Macroscopic Features

Large haematomas, whether due to rupture of microaneurysms or the other causes listed, produce deformation and some degree of destruction of the brain tissue (*Figs 45.36a* and *b*). They tend to track down within the brain along the lines of least resistance, splitting and separating, rather than destroying, white matter. Not infrequently the haematoma **bursts** either into one of the **lateral ventricles** or into the **subarachnoid space**.

Functionally, a large bleed acts as a space-occupying lesion which rapidly increases in size. This causes raised intracranial pressure with displacement downwards and backwards; the resulting herniation through the tentorium often leads to secondary bleeding in the brainstem.

If the patient survives, the haematoma gradually becomes absorbed and all that may be seen at necropsy is a cavity, the walls of which are coloured orange-brown by iron pigment derived from haemoglobin. The margins of these lesions, when examined microscopically, show many iron-laden macrophages and the area tends to be separated from the surrounding brain tissue by a zone of gliosis.

Clinical Features

One of the most striking aspects of the clinical picture associated with massive intracerebral haemorrhage is the speed of its evolution; a complex array of different neurological deficits can appear in rapid succession over minutes or hours:

- There may be severe headache, and loss of consciousness develops rapidly.
- Depending on the location of the lesion, there may be hemispheric, brainstem or cerebellar signs.

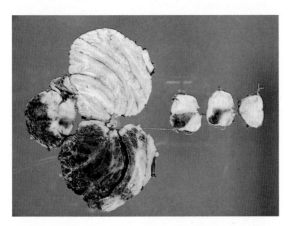

FIGURE 45.35 Haemorrhagic infarction affecting the cerebellum and pons.

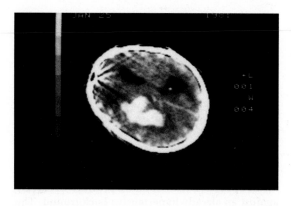

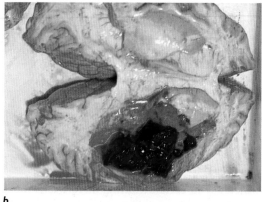

a   *b*

FIGURE 45.36 **a** *Computed tomogram of the brain in a patient with stroke. There is a large haemorrhage in one cerebral hemisphere.* **b** *Brain of the patient shown in* **a** *at post-mortem examination. The presence of a large recent haemorrhage is confirmed.*

- If the haemorrhage is large, most of the patients die, frequently within the first few days. If the haemorrhage is smaller, a clinical picture similar to that seen in cerebral infarction may be seen.

SUBARACHNOID HAEMORRHAGE

Spontaneous subarachnoid haemorrhage accounts for approximately 6% of cases of cerebrovascular disease, with a peak age of 55–60 years. Its incidence in the USA is 11–12 per 100 000 per year.

It is a serious disorder; as summarized in *Table 45.10*, many patients die within 24 hours of the bleed and the overall mortality rate for the first week is 27–30%. About one-third of the patients will have another bleed within the first month and, if this occurs, the mortality rate is 42%. The risk of recurrence is greatest between days 5 and 9. The risk of recurrence then begins to fall and, of those who have survived for 6 weeks, about 10% will have a recurrent bleed within the next year.

After the first year there is a 5% risk of recurrence for each year that passes and about half these patients will die as a result of these recurrent bleeds.

In patients who die within the first few hours, massive bleeding with rupture into the ventricular system is usually present. Other deceased patients show a mixture of:

- subarachnoid blood clot
- cerebral infarction
- intracerebral haematoma

Pathogenesis

Spontaneous subarachnoid haemorrhage arises on a basis of one of the following, as shown in *Table 45.11.*

Table 45.10 Features of Subarachnoid Haemorrhage

Proportion of total stokes	6%
Incidence	11–12 per 100 000 per annum
Mortality in first week	27–30%
Risk of recurrent bleed in first month	30%
Risk of recurrence in first year	10%
Risk of recurrence in each year thereafter	5%
Peak age	55–60 years

Table 45.11 Causes of Subarachnoid Haemorrhage

Cause	Frequency (%)
Rupture of a saccular aneurysm of one of the major cerebral arteries	65
Bleeding from an arteriovenous malformation	5
Bleeding secondary to a blood dyscrasia	2.5
Extension of an intracerebral bleed into the subarachnoid space	2.5
Rupture of 'mycotic' aneurysm	Rare
No cause found	25

Saccular Aneurysms (syn. Berry Aneurysms)

Saccular aneurysms are rounded focal defects involving only part of the circumference of a vessel wall. In the cerebral circulation the most common sites for these lesions are as shown in *Table 45.12* and *Fig. 45.37*.

Aneurysm Formation

Berry aneurysms arise on the basis of focal defects in the muscular tunica media of cerebral arteries at junction points or 'carinae'. It is incorrect to call them 'congenital' aneurysms, as is often done, because they are not present at birth, although the muscular defects are. Aneurysms are found in 1–2% of the population, being much less frequent than defects in the media at points of branching. They are commoner in females than in males.

Table 45.12 Sites for Rupture of Saccular Aneurysm

Site	Frequency (%)
Junction of the internal carotid and the posterior communicating artery	40
Junction of the anterior cerebral and the anterior communicating artery	30
Main bifurcation of the middle cerebral artery in the Sylvian fissure (*Fig. 45.38*)	20
Point where the basilar artery divides into the posterior cerebral arteries	4

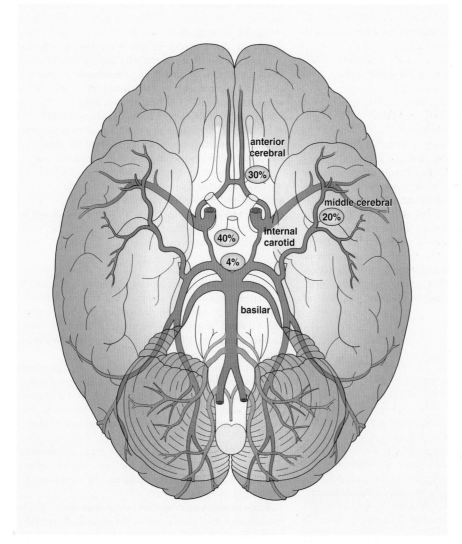

FIGURE 45.37 Common sites for aneurysm formation in intracranial arteries.

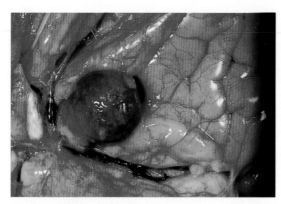

FIGURE 45.38 *Large saccular aneurysm of middle cerebral artery within the Sylvian fissure.*

Most saccular aneurysms in the cerebral circulation are sporadic but certain associations have been noted in respect of some cases. These include:

- coarctation of the aorta
- autosomal dominant form of polycystic kidney
- some forms of the connective tissue disorder (Ehlers–Danlos syndrome, most notably type IV)
- Marfan's disease
- type 1 neurofibromatosis

The mechanisms underlying rupture are not clear. Many patients are hypertensive when admitted to hospital after a subarachnoid bleed but in many instances the raised blood pressure returns to normal within a few days, and there is no clear relationship between sustained hypertension and the risk of rupture. **Transient** hypertension may be important, this being suggested by the many instances, especially in younger adults, of rupture associated with episodes of physical exertion or at times of heightened emotional tone. In this connection it is not without interest that recent heavy use of alcohol (binge drinking) is said to increase the risk of aneurysm rupture.

Microscopic Features

The aneurysm wall consists of fibrous tissue lined by a single layer of endothelial cells; no muscle or elastic tissue can be identified. As the aneurysm diameter increases, so does the risk of rupture; it is estimated that the critical diameter is about 8–10 mm, at which time the wall thickness is likely to be about 40 μm. Occasionally there are much larger aneurysms which have not ruptured; the lumina of these are usually filled with layered thrombus. These large aneurysms, although not constituting a great risk for subarachnoid bleeding, may call attention to themselves by acting as space-occupying lesions.

Pathological Consequences of Aneurysm Rupture

Early

The consequences depend on whether the haematoma is localized to the neighbourhood of the ruptured aneurysm or whether, as is more common, the blood has spread throughout the subarachnoid space. It is not always easy to identify the aneurysms because they often collapse after rupture. If the aneurysm is embedded in the underlying brain, the bleeding may be largely intracerebral with all the complications that this may bring in its train (see pp 1149–1150). Aneurysms on the anterior communicating artery may rupture into the third ventricle, thus producing massive intraventricular haemorrhage.

Late

Cerebral infarction is a common complication. The lesions may be patchily distributed and are difficult to recognize in unfixed brains. They occur most commonly in the territory of the artery on which the aneurysm occurs, but infarcts may also be seen in other areas, the genesis of these being contributed to by:

- arterial compression by the haematoma
- vasospasm, which can be demonstrated angiographically in patients with subarachnoid bleeds. Its importance as a mediator of neurological deficit in these patients is suggested by the results of a study in which the incidence of such deficits was reduced by treating patients with the powerful vasodilator, calcitonin gene-related peptide.
- the effects of raised intracranial pressure

Hydrocephalus may occur as a result of blockage by blood clot of the channels though which the cerebrospinal fluid passes.

Mycotic Aneurysms

This term describes aneurysms caused by infection of the artery wall. Most cases of intracranial mycotic aneurysm are due to impaction of infected emboli derived from 'vegetations' occurring in infective endocarditis; about 3–10% of patients with endocarditis are said to develop this complication.

Because the artery wall distal to the impacted embolus undergoes necrosis, one would expect endocarditis due to pyogenic bacteria, such as *Streptococcus pyogenes* and *Staphylococcus aureus*, to be most frequently associated with mycotic aneurysm, and this is the case.

About 65% of these aneurysms draw attention to themselves by rupture within the first 5 weeks of the endocarditis, and when this happens the mortality rate is high (up to 80%).

True fungal aneurysms are sometimes seen. These result from fungal meningitis or fungal emboli from the heart valves. *Aspergillus* is the species most commonly involved.

Fusiform Aneurysms

Fusiform aneurysms, **those in which the whole circumference of the affected segment of artery is involved**, are most commonly seen in the basilar artery and are associated with atherosclerosis in this vessel. The abnormalities of flow brought about by this dilatation predispose to thrombus formation, and TIAs affecting the territory supplied by the basilar artery may occur. Occasionally thrombotic occlusion of the segment may take place and, more rarely, these aneurysms may rupture, leading to subarachnoid bleeding.

Arteriovenous Malformations and Cavernous Haemangiomas

Arteriovenous malformations usually present some time in the second to fourth decades of life with recurrent episodes of subarachnoid or intracerebral haemorrhage. They are most common in relation to the cerebral hemispheres and may lie on the surface of the brain or penetrate some distance into its substance (*Fig. 45.39*).

On microscopic examination they appear as a meshwork of rather poorly formed vessels (both arteries and veins) surrounded by brain tissue showing gliosis and the presence of iron-laden macrophages. The latter are the markers of previous haemorrhage.

Cavernous haemangiomas are found in the white matter of the brain and tend to present clinically in the third to fifth decades. They are associated with a number of neurological syndromes which include:

- epilepsy (38%)
- intracranial bleeding (23%)
- headache (28%)
- focal neurological deficits (12%)

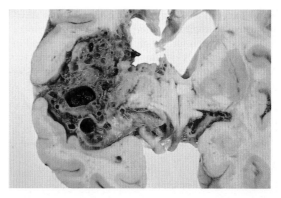

FIGURE 45.39 *Large angiomatous malformation showing a complex leash of abnormally large and interconnected blood vessels.*

HYPOXIC INJURY TO THE BRAIN

The degree of oxygenation of any tissue depends on two factors:

1) **the amount of blood flowing through that tissue**
2) **the oxygen content of the blood**

Thus, irreversible brain damage occurs when cerebral perfusion drops below a certain critical level, when there is insufficient oxygen in the blood, or when there is a combination of both these factors.

The degree of metabolic activity in the brain is more or less constant and thus the **cerebral blood flow needs to be regulated within rather narrow limits. Autoregulation within the cerebral circulation is mediated via changes in resistance of the cerebral arterioles.** Therefore, as the systemic blood pressure falls, the cerebral arterioles dilate and thus the cerebral blood flow remains constant down to a systolic pressure of 50 mmHg. Similarly there is an upper limit of autoregulation, which is about 160 mmHg. Above this pressure the cerebral arterioles cannot vasoconstrict further. Cerebral blood flow increases to undesirable levels and dysfunction develops in the blood–brain barrier, leading to the syndrome of hypertensive encephalopathy.

Cerebral arterioles also change their calibre in response to blood gas levels. Both hypoxia and hypercapnia lead to arteriolar vasodilatation and, hence, to an increase in cerebral blood flow.

These important autoregulatory functions can be disturbed in patients following anaesthesia, head injury or a stroke.

Categories of Hypoxia

- **Stagnant hypoxia.** The brain or some part of it receives an inadequate blood flow (e.g. cardiac arrest, cardiac arrhythmias)
- **Anoxic or hypoxic hypoxia.** Oxygen levels in the blood are inadequate to meet the metabolic demands of the brain.
- **Histotoxic hypoxia.** Both cerebral blood flow and oxygen content of the blood are normal but there is a failure to use the oxygen as a result of poisoning of the respiratory enzymes in the brain (e.g. cyanide poisoning).
- **Anaemic hypoxia.** Here, the oxygen content of the blood is reduced because of inadequate amounts of haemoglobin as a result of blood loss or anaemia. This situation is mimicked in carbon monoxide poisoning in which there is a decrease in the amount of haemoglobin that can combine with oxygen. Carbon monoxide poisoning is the only type of anaemic hypoxia that can produce lesions in both grey and white matter.
- **Hypoxic damage resulting from hypoglycaemia.** The deficiency of substrate leads to an inability to use oxygen.

Brain Damage Secondary to Cardiac Arrest

Irreversible damage to the brain is likely if the period of 'shut-down' (interruption of blood

flow) exceeds 5–7 minutes at normal body temperature. Recognizable morphological changes in the brain are not seen for 36–48 hours after the period of absent perfusion. It is clear that there are areas in the brain that show greater susceptibility to anoxia or hypoxia than others.

Macroscopic Features

It may be just possible to identify some patchy or laminar necrosis in the depths of the sulci and in the CA1 region of the hippocampus.

Microscopic Features

There is diffuse neuronal necrosis with certain areas more severely affected than others. In addition to the sites given above, the Purkinje cells in the cerebellum are severely and diffusely affected. Damage to the brainstem nuclei can also occur, and is more severe in infants and young children than in adults.

Severe brain damage due to cardiac arrest is usually fatal within a few days but some unfortunate patients survive for months or more with very severe neurological deficits, leading a more or less 'vegetable' existence.

At necropsy the brains from these survivors show a marked degree of atrophy as evidenced by **a decrease in brain weight and enlargement of the ventricles**. The cortex of the parietal and occipital lobes appears to be particularly severely affected.

Brain Damage due to Hypotension

Damage under these circumstances tends to be concentrated in the arterial boundary zones between the main cerebral and cerebellar artery territories. The lesions have been described in patients:

- undergoing neurosurgical procedures in the sitting position (the patient, not the neurosurgeon)
- experiencing a sudden decrease, for any reason, in arterial pressure
- after occlusion of a carotid artery
- undergoing dental anaesthesia in a semirecumbent position
- following severe 'non-missile' head injuries
- having overenthusiastic treatment for systemic hypertension

Infarcts of varying size develop, damage being most likely to occur in the parietal and occipital lobes (i.e. in the common boundary zone of the anterior, middle and posterior cerebral arteries). There is variable involvement of the basal ganglia, and the hippocampus and brainstem are usually spared.

Brain Damage due to Carbon Monoxide Poisoning

Carbon monoxide poisoning can be accidental or related to suicide. Once 30% of the haemoglobin has combined with carbon monoxide, the patient experiences severe headache, fatigue and impaired judgement. A concentration of 60–70% carboxyhaemoglobin leads to loss of consciousness, and more than 70% is rapidly fatal.

If death has occurred within a few hours of carbon monoxide exposure, the brain shows the bright red-pink colour typical of carboxyhaemoglobin, but no other changes are noted. If the patient had survived 36–48 hours after exposure, the brain shows congestion and there are often petechiae in the corpus callosum and in other parts of the white matter.

'Respirator Brain'

This term is synonymous with **'brain death'** and is used to describe the severe and extensive changes seen in the brains of patients who have been kept 'alive' by mechanical ventilation.

The electroencephalogram in such patients is isoelectric and brainstem reflexes are abolished, although spinal reflexes may persist. **The failure in brain function is caused by an arrest of cerebral circulation due to severe brain swelling.** This perfusion failure is shown by failure of contrast medium to enter the brain in the course of cerebral angiography.

Macroscopic Features

Absence of cerebral circulation causes the brain to undergo a process analogous to **autolysis**. The brain usually shows an increase in weight due to oedema (*Fig. 45.40*); it is soft and diffluent, and may pour out of the opened skull rather like porridge. Herniation of the cerebellar tonsils through the foramen magnum is commonly seen as a result of cerebral oedema and consequent rise in intracranial pressure. The combination of cerebellar herniation and the softness of the tissue may lead to portions of the cerebellum breaking off; these are then forced down the vertebral canal.

On section, the brain shows blurring of the normally distinct boundary between the grey and white matter.

Microscopic Features

There is severe and extensive neuronal necrosis, the dying cells showing marked cytoplasmic eosinophilia. The necrosis elicits no tissue reaction.

HEAD INJURY

Head injury is a major cause of death and disability, causing about 1% of all deaths in the UK. It is responsible for 25% of all deaths due to trauma and for 50% of those resulting from road traffic accidents.

In addition to the deaths caused by head injury, there are many patients who suffer from prolonged post-traumatic disabilities, and it is estimated that **1 in 300**

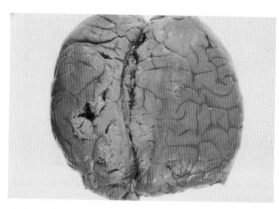

FIGURE 45.40 'Respirator brain', showing marked swelling with flattening of the gyri and obliteration of sulci. As can be seen from the tear produced in the course of removing the brain from the skull, the brain tissue, under these circumstances, is extremely friable and sometimes pours out of the skull like a stream of thick porridge.

families in Britain has a member disabled as a result of head injury.

There are two main types of head injury:
- **blunt or 'non-missile' injury** in which there is sudden acceleration or deceleration of the head
- **missile head injury**

The damage that results from these may be:
- **primary**, occurring at the moment of injury and expressed in the form of scalp injuries, skull fracture, cerebral contusion, intracranial haemorrhage and diffuse axonal injury
- **secondary**, comprising the complications of the primary injury brain damage due to raised intracranial pressure, hypoxia, brain swelling and infection

NON-MISSILE INJURY

The mechanisms underlying brain damage in non-missile injury are complex. Experimental studies in primates show that all types of brain damage occurring in humans from non-missile trauma can be reproduced in non-human primates. The results suggest that there are **two** main mechanisms responsible for the features of non-missile injury:

1) **Contact effects**, resulting from an object striking the head (or the reverse); they consist essentially of **local** effects such as scalp injury, skull fracture, extradural haematoma, intracerebral haemorrhage and some varieties of brain contusion. Lesions due to contact are usually **focal**.

2) **Acceleration effects**, produced by rapid movement of the head in the instant after the blow. Acceleration leads to shear, tensile and compressive strains, and also to changes in intracranial and intracerebral pressure. These cause two serious types of damage:
- **acute subdural haemorrhage**, resulting from tearing of subdural bridging veins

- **diffuse axon damage**, ascribed to shear strains generated within the brain as a result of angular acceleration of the head at the moment of impact. In experimental situations, it is not necessary for anything to strike the head or for the head to strike anything in order to reproduce the changes seen in human brain injury. It can all be accomplished by modulation of the acceleration–deceleration conditions. Lesions due to acceleration are most commonly **diffuse**.

Focal Injuries

Haemorrhage

Extradural Haematoma
This occurs in about 2% of cases of head injury. It is most often associated with skull fracture, especially if the fracture involves the groove in which the middle meningeal artery runs. This vessel is the commonest source of post-traumatic extradural bleeding (70–80% of cases).

In children, extradural haematoma occurs not uncommonly without skull fracture. The initial injury may seem trivial and there is often a lucid interval before the effects of the haemorrhage make themselves apparent in the form of declining levels of consciousness and, ultimately, coma.

As the blood clot enlarges, it peels away the dura from the underlying skull, forming an ovoid mass which compresses the underlying brain (*Figs 45.41b* and *45.42*).

Subdural Haematoma
Subdural haematomas are said to occur in 26–63% of cases of non-missile head injury. They most commonly result **from a fall or from a blow to the head**.

Subdural haemorrhages are also found in a proportion of battered babies. In these cases, the haematomas are usually chronic and are expressed as collections of yellow-stained fluid in the subdural space. Such children often have lesions of diffuse post-traumatic brain damage as well.

In contrast with extradural haematoma, the initial injury is often severe and the clinical syndrome may be that of an unconscious patient whose condition deteriorates.

The neurosurgical classification depends on the composition of the haematoma:
- **acute** – the haematoma is made up of dark red, semiliquid blood (*Fig. 45.41c*)
- **subacute** – there is a mixture of clotted and fluid blood
- **chronic** – the contents consist of dark, turbid fluid and some fresh blood

The **pathogenesis** of subdural haemorrhage is believed to be **tearing of the bridging veins in the subdural space as a result of rapid acceleration or deceleration**. This explains the association between the risk of

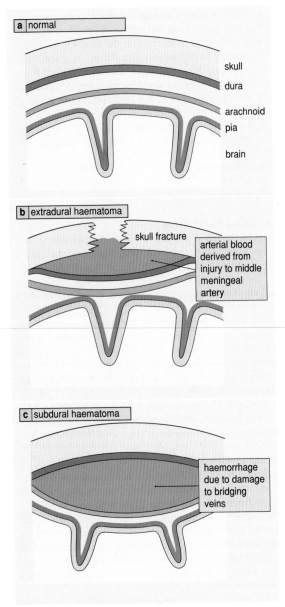

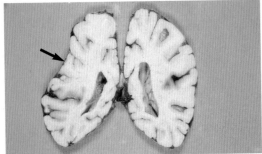

FIGURE 45.42 Deformity of the brain caused by an extradural haematoma.

lobes and the subfrontal region. The pathogenesis is uncertain but it is thought that these haemorrhages result from **rupture of small intracerebral blood vessels at the time of injury**.

Cerebral Contusion

Contusions are post-traumatic, haemorrhagic lesions in the brain substance occurring in the presence of an **intact pia–arachnoid**, this last feature distinguishing them from cerebral lacerations, where there is a direct tearing injury into the brain. They are caused by the brain surface impacting on bony protuberances in the skull.

Cerebral contusions are characteristically haemorrhagic (*Fig. 45.43*) and affect principally the crests of the gyri, although they may sometimes be seen to extend into the sulci and gyral white matter. When healed, they may be identified as golden-brown shrunken scars.

Distribution Pattern of Contusions

Chief targets for contusion injury are:

- the frontal lobe poles
- the orbital gyri
- the cortex above and below the Sylvian fissure. In

FIGURE 45.41 **a–c** Extradural and subdural haemorrhage.

subdural haematoma and falls or blows to the head, because these injuries involve very high speed angular acceleration or deceleration.

In contrast, chronic subdural haematoma may present weeks or months after fairly trivial injury to the head. There is some association with coagulation defects such as haemophilia or long-standing anticoagulant therapy, but this is by no means invariable.

Intracerebral Haemorrhage

Intracerebral haemorrhages occur in about one in six **fatal** head injuries. The principal sites are the temporal

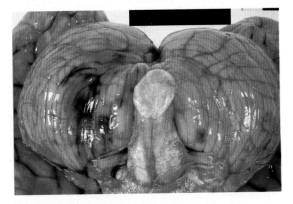

FIGURE 45.43 Cerebellar contusion. Note the focal haemorrhages at the tips of the cerebellar tonsils.

this region, the brain lies in close contact with the lesser wings of the sphenoid bone.

- the temporal lobe poles
- the lateral and inferior aspects of the temporal lobes

Contusions may be classified into four groups based on the **site of the contusion** and the **site of the injury to the head**:

1) **'coup'** contusions occurring **at the site of impact** in the absence of a fracture
2) **'contrecoup'** contusions occurring **diametrically opposite the site of impact**
3) **'herniation'** contusions occurring where the medial parts of the temporal lobe are pushed up against the edge of the tentorium, or where the cerebellar tonsils are forced down into the foramen magnum at the moment of injury
4) **'gliding'** contusions, which are focal haemorrhagic lesions in the cortex and underlying white matter along the margins of the cerebral hemispheres. In contrast to other forms of contusion, gliding contusions are not thought to be due to impaction against bone but to rotational stresses on the brain.

Diffuse Injury

Diffuse brain injury is the pathological correlate of immediate prolonged unconsciousness not associated with an intracranial mass lesion such as a haematoma.

It occurs in almost half the patients with severe head injury and is responsible for just over one-third of all deaths from head injury. It is believed to result from severe shearing strains on nerve fibres within the substance of the brain at the moment of injury and does not appear to require changes in intracranial pressure or hypoxia for its development.

There are three diagnostic pathological features of diffuse axonal injury (two are macroscopic and one microscopic).

Macroscopic Features
- **focal haemorrhagic lesions in the region of the corpus callosum.** These may extend forward and backwards for a distance of several centimetres and often involve the interventricular septum
- **focal lesions of different sizes in the dorsolateral quadrant of the rostral brainstem adjacent to the superior cerebellar peduncles**

Microscopic Features
Evidence of severe diffuse damage to axons.

The microscopic picture of diffuse axonal damage depends on the length of time the patient has survived after injury:
- If survival has been a matter of days, numerous eosinophilic swellings on nerve fibres are seen in sections stained with haematoxylin and eosin. These are somewhat more easily seen if silver stains are used, which stain the axons and axonal swellings black.
- If the patient has survived for a few weeks, the principal microscopic finding is many clusters of microglial cells scattered throughout the white matter. In addition, fat-laden macrophages (the fat presumably being derived from degenerate myelin) and reactive astrocytes may be seen.

Clinically, patients with diffuse axonal injury form a somewhat distinct group. There is a high prevalence of injury due to road traffic accidents and a low prevalence of any lucid interval.

Pathologically, there is a relative paucity of focal cerebral injuries other than gliding contusions.

The presence or absence of diffuse axonal injury is probably the most important prognostic factor in non-missile head injury.

Neoplasms of the Nervous System

In the cranium, the anatomical site of a tumour is a key factor in the clinical outcome. This is because:
- it may be impossible, because of their location, to remove certain benign neoplasms
- quite small and/or benign neoplasms may exert very severe clinical effects because of their location (e.g. tumours in the floor of the fourth ventricle which obstruct cerebrospinal fluid (CSF) circulation).
- even relatively well-differentiated examples of certain neoplasms (e.g. ependymomas, astrocytomas) may infiltrate widely, thus making complete excision impossible

Classification
The classification of primary neoplasms of the central nervous system (CNS) is based on their microscopic appearance; the assignment of a neoplasm to one or other group often gives valuable prognostic information. This prognosis based on the tumour type may, of course, be modified by factors such as the anatomical location of the lesion, age of the patient, etc.

Difficulties not infrequently arise in histological interpretation which is based, for the most part, on conventional light microscopy; here immunocytochemistry can be valuable. For example, a fibrillary astrocytoma may resemble certain varieties of meningioma. The former, however, expresses the tumour marker **glial fibrillary acidic protein (GFAP)**, whereas the latter does not.

The types of primary tumour occurring in the CNS are shown in *Tables 45.13–45.17*.

Pathophysiology

Intracranial neoplasms exert their effects (*Fig. 45.44*) via a combination of:

- Expansile growth causing **compression** of the adjacent or subjacent brain tissue. The neurological deficits caused by this may be reversed if the lesion can be removed early enough.

Table 45.13 Neuroectodermal Tumours

Basic type	Variants	Site/age
Astrocytoma	Pilocytic (well differentiated)	In the cerebrum in young adults. In children they occur mainly in the cerebellum, pons, medulla and spinal cord
	Fibrillary	As above
	Protoplasmic	As above
	Anaplastic	Mainly in the cerebrum in adults
Glioblastoma multiforme	Commonest primary neuroectodermal tumour in adults	Usually in the cerebrum in middle-aged and elderly adults
Oligodendroglioma	Well differentiated	Cerebrum, chiefly in adults
	Anaplastic	As above
Ependymoma	Well differentiated	Ventricles and spinal cord of adults and children
	Ependymoblastoma	Cerebrum and spinal cord of children and adults
	Anaplastic	As above
	Myxopapillary	Lower end of the spinal cord; thought to arise from filum terminale
Choroid plexus tumours	Well-differentiated papilloma	In ventricles, all ages
	Poorly differentiated papilloma	As above
Primitive neuroectodermal	Medulloblastoma	Cerebellum, mainly in children; occasionally in adults
	Neuroblastoma	Cerebrum in children
Tumours of neurones	Gangliocytoma	Cerebrum in both adults and children
	Ganglioglioma	As above
	Ganglioneuroblastoma	As above
	Paraganglioma–ganglioneuroma	Cauda equina
	Anaplastic gangliocytoma and ganglioglioma	Cerebrum in children and young adults

Table 45.14 Meningeal Tumours

Basic type	Variant	Site/age
Meningeal tumours	Meningioma	Cranial and spinal meninges in adults
	Malignant meningioma	Cranial meninges in adults

Table 45.15 Nerve Sheath Tumours

Basic type	Variant	Site/age
Nerve sheath	Neurilemmoma (usually benign but rare malignant variants exist)	Spinal and cranial nerve roots at all ages but mainly in adults. Occurs also in peripheral nerves
	Neurofibroma	As above

Table 45.16 Primary CNS Lymphomas

Basic type	Variant	Site/age
Lymphoma	Cerebral	Adults
	Spinal	Adults; usually extradural

Table 45.17 Blood Vessel Neoplasms and Malformations

Basic type	Variants	Site/age
	Haemangioblastoma	Cerebellar and spinal cord examples
	Cavernous haemangioma	chiefly in adults. Brain and meninges
	Capillary telangiectasia	affected in both children and adults
	Arteriovenous malformation	
	Venous malformation	

- Infiltrative growth causing **destruction** of brain tissue and hence irreversible functional effects.
- **Obstruction** to the flow of CSF if the lesion blocks the foramen of Monro or is situated in the posterior fossa; hydrocephalus may result.
- **Oedema.** A malignant intracerebral neoplasm depends for its continuing growth on the ingrowth of new blood vessels. The blood–brain barrier in these patients is frequently defective and thus quite severe oedema can develop in the lesion itself and in the brain around it.
- **Irritative** effects on neural function. These can result from a neoplasm whether its growth pattern is expansile (as in benign meningioma) or infiltrative (as in glioma). Irritative effects are expressed in the form of **focal epileptiform seizures**.

The combination of:
- the space actually occupied by the neoplasm
- cerebral oedema elicited by the lesion in many instances
- hydrocephalus, if present

often leads to **raised intracranial pressure**.

NEUROECTODERMAL TUMOURS

ASTROCYTOMAS
Well-differentiated astrocytomas of the cerebellum and brainstem account for 45% of primary neuroectodermal tumours in children and for 10% in adults. Most adult astrocytomas occur in

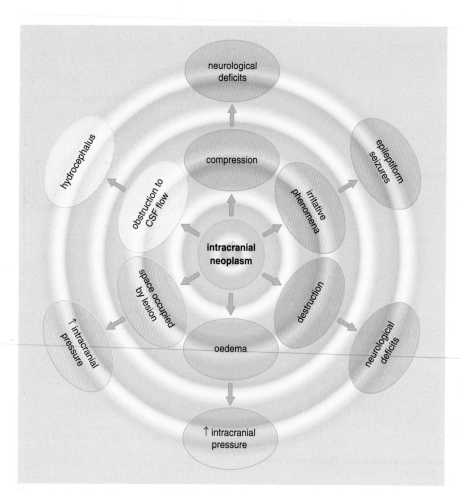

FIGURE 45.44 *Pathophysiological effects of intracranial neoplasms.*

the cerebral hemispheres of individuals under the age of 30 years.

Despite being well differentiated initially, many astrocytomas later develop anaplasia, with a much more ominous prognosis. Malignant glial tumours account for 2.5% of all deaths due to cancer and constitute the third most common cause of death from malignant disease in young people aged 15–34 years.

Clinical Features

These depend very largely on the **location**. Thus a brainstem lesion will show the insidious development of a spastic quadriparesis, whereas one in the cerebellum is likely to present with ataxia.

Site also plays an important part in prognosis. Well-differentiated cerebellar astrocytomas of the pilocytic type (see below) can be excised completely in about 70% of cases; if excision is complete, the 25-year survival rate is 90%. If anaplasia is present in the excised tumour, the survival rate falls steeply to 30–40%. In contrast with cerebellar lesions, brainstem astrocytomas cannot be removed because vital structures would be damaged in the course of surgery. They are, therefore, treated by irradiation and are associated with a 5-year survival rate of only 15–20%. Cerebral astrocytomas often infiltrate widely and thus can seldom be removed completely. However, surgical debulking of the tumour is a perfectly practical option and this can be followed by irradiation. A period of remission can be gained in this way and subsequent deterioration may be fairly slow, giving a life expectancy of 5–10 years.

Classification

Assigning an individual astrocytic tumour to an appropriate prognostic grade has been a controversial issue; several classifications have been proposed, most of which do not correlate particularly well with clinical behaviour.

A commonly used system divides astrocytic tumours into three grades of malignancy:
1) **well-differentiated Astrocytoma**
2) **anaplastic astrocytoma**
3) **glioblastoma multiforme**

Most recently, a new four-grade system has been proposed, which is based on the criteria of:

- nuclear atypia
- mitoses
- endothelial cell proliferation
- necrosis

With this system, the median survival time for patients with grade 2 lesions is about 4 years, for those with grade 3 lesions 1.6 years, and for those with grade 4 tumours 0.7 years.

Well-differentiated Astrocytomas

Macroscopic Features

Well-differentiated astrocytomas are usually white ill-defined masses; it is impossible, because of the infiltrative nature of their growth, to see the boundary zone between normal brain and tumour tissue.

Pilocytic variants are usually firm, whereas **protoplasmic** astrocytomas are soft and gelatinous. Cerebellar astrocytomas are often cystic. Sometimes there is a single large cyst with a small nubbin of solid tumour tissue on one aspect; tumours may also be polycystic.

If the tumour is large, it will displace other parts of the brain (e.g. midline structures may be shifted to one side) and in cerebral neoplasms there may be compression of the lateral ventricle on the side of the tumour to a slit-like cavity. With significant increases in intracranial pressure, parts of the brain may herniate, the pattern depending on the location of the tumour above or below the tentorium.

Microscopic Features

Protoplasmic astrocytomas consist of stellate cells with fine processes in which glial fibrils can be identified. Small cystic spaces are common and give the tumour a spongy appearance.

Fibrillary astrocytomas have rather more in the way of glial fibre content and **pilocytic** astrocytomas (**found most commonly in the cerebellum of children and adolescents**) are composed of elongated tumour cells with long thin processes containing glial fibrils. Some of the tumour cells contain long, brightly eosinophilic, club-like structures known as **Rosenthal fibres**.

Polar spongioblastoma is an uncommon astrocytic tumour occurring in the first or second decade of life. The architecture and cells are characteristic, the cells being arranged in a distinctive palisaded fashion. Their clinical behaviour is variable. Some undoubtedly behave in a malignant fashion but long survival in some individuals has also been reported (*Fig. 45.45*).

A change seen occasionally in some well-differentiated astrocytomas is so-called **gemistocytic** change, in which the tumour cells become large and plump with abundant cytoplasm.

In patients with the inherited disorder **tuberous sclerosis**, which can occur either as an autosomally dominant

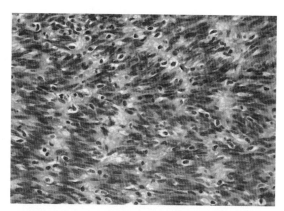

FIGURE 45.45 *Polar spongioblastoma showing the typical arrangement of the tumour cells in parallel rows with conspicuous 'palisading' of their nuclei.*

disease complex or as a new mutation, a rather characteristic type of astrocytoma is seen. This usually occurs in the region of the thalamus and is composed of large astrocytes with eccentrically situated nuclei. These are called **subependymal giant-celled astrocytomas**; they grow slowly and have a relatively good prognosis.

Anaplastic Astrocytomas

These are believed to arise from previously well-differentiated astrocytomas.

Anaplastic astrocytomas usually occur in the cerebral hemispheres of adults and are uncommon in the cerebellum and brainstem. They are associated with a worse survival rate than well-differentiated astrocytoma (approximately 50% at 2 years) but a better one than glioblastoma multiforme, where only 10% of the patients are alive at 2 years.

Microscopic Features

Two elements are usually present – a well-differentiated astrocytoma and tumour showing anaplasia in the form of:

- increased cellularity
- increased pleomorphism
- a substantial mitotic rate
- blood vessels that are more prominent than usual because of capillary endothelial cell proliferation

Glioblastoma Multiforme (also known as Grade IV Astrocytoma)

This is the commonest primary neuroectodermal tumour affecting principally middle-aged and elderly patients. About three-quarters of these lesions occur in the frontal and temporal lobes, and a further 20% in the parietal lobes. The peak incidence is in the sixth decade (7.3 per 100 000 per year). **This tumour has a poor prognosis: the majority of the patients are dead within 1 year.**

Macroscopic Features

On sectioning fixed brain, **glioblastoma multiforme** appears as a large greyish yellow mass (*Fig. 45.46*), often appearing better defined at its edges than other tumours of astrocytic lineage. Central necrosis may be a very obvious feature. The tumour may be confined to one cerebral hemisphere but may spread across the midline to form a 'butterfly'-shaped mass. Very rare examples of distant spread to lymph nodes and lungs have been reported but, characteristically, tumour cells spread via the CSF to involve diffusely, other parts of the brain and the spinal cord.

Microscopic Features

The word 'multiforme' evokes an image of great variability, and this is quite accurate. The outstanding histological features are:

- **Cellular pleomorphism** including giant cells with bizarre darkly staining nuclei (*Fig. 45.47*). Abnormal mitoses may also be seen.
- **Necrosis** which, with or without haemorrhage, is a very prominent feature. Large dilated tumour blood vessels are sometimes occluded by thrombus, leading to infarction of the central zone of the tumour.
- **Capillary endothelial proliferation**; this is seen frequently and is often striking in degree. The abnormal blood vessels have many thick-walled branches terminating in a tangle of capillaries. These have an appearance somewhat reminiscent of renal glomeruli and are called 'glomeruloid areas'.
- **Pseudopalisading.** This term describes the appearance of serpiginous areas of necrosis surrounded by tumour cells with rod-shaped nuclei, arranged roughly perpendicular to the necrotic area.
- **Small rod-shaped anaplastic cells** are very frequently seen in glioblastoma; studies of radioactive thymidine uptake suggest that these constitute the actively dividing fraction of the cell population. This fraction is quite large (12–19%). Less than 1% of the cells in the much more benign juvenile pilocytic astrocytoma are in this state.

Glioblastomas Show the Presence of Many Genomic Alterations which may be of Functional Relevance

Chromosomal abnormalities in glioblastoma most commonly affect chromosome 7, in which an increase in material is found, and chromosomes 9 and 10, where there are deletions. A deletion has also been reported in respect of chromosome 17p and it is possible that this relates to the p53 gene. Abnormalities have also been recorded in chromosomes 1, 6, 19 and 22. About 33%

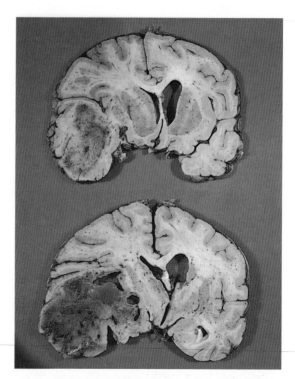

FIGURE 45.46 *Large glioma in the form of a greyish-brown mass. The tumour is occupying a large part of the hemisphere and its presence is associated with marked distortion of surrounding structures; the ipsilateral lateral ventricle shows compression.*

of glioblastomas show the presence of deletions or translocations, and 10% show double minutes suggesting gene amplification.

Oncogene Expression

Most glioblastomas express the oncogene **c-sis**, which encodes the B chain of platelet-derived growth factor;

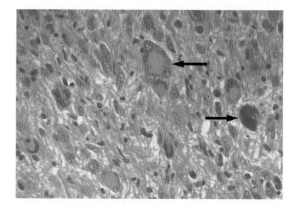

FIGURE 45.47 *Glioblastoma multiforme showing marked variation in the size and shape of tumour cells. Some so-called 'tumour giant cells' are present (arrowed).*

30% express **c-erbB** encoding the epidermal growth factor receptor, and some express **c-myc, gli** or **H-ras**.

OLIGODENDROGLIOMA

These account for about 3–6% of all glial tumours; they may occur at any age, but are far more common in adults, only 6% being found in children. Oligodendrogliomas occur most commonly in the cerebral hemispheres. Many grow slowly but there are anaplastic variants and, interestingly, astrocytomatous areas are found in about 50% of cases if adequate sampling of the lesion is undertaken. The commonest clinical presentation is with focal neurological deficit or adult-onset epilepsy; later, signs of raised intracranial pressure develop. Most oligodendrogliomas show evidence of spotty calcification and this is a useful radiological feature.

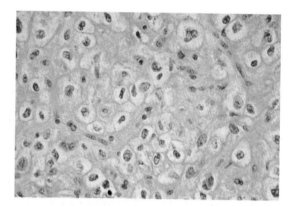

FIGURE 45.48 *Oligodendroglioma. The tumour cells show acute swelling of the perinuclear zones giving them a characteristic 'poached egg-like' appearance.*

Macroscopic Features

The tumours often have a characteristic plum-coloured appearance and appear fairly well demarcated. The tumour may extend to involve the surface of the brain, but does not spread diffusely over the surface in the manner of glioblastoma.

Microscopic Features

Most are composed of a rather uniform cell population with **small round nuclei, a well-defined plasma membrane and clear cytoplasm**, this last feature giving the nuclei a very typical **'boxed'** appearance (*Fig. 45.48*). This clearing of the cytoplasm is an artefact of histological preparation, but from the diagnostic point of view is very useful.

A fine network of capillaries divides the tumour cell population into small clusters. Small areas of focal calcification are distributed through the lesions.

Tumours in which the cellularity is low tend to have a moderately good prognosis (median survival 91 months) with a 5-year survival rate of 67%. Patients with highly cellular lesions, particularly if areas of necrosis are present, have a median survival time of only 18 months and the 5-year survival rate is 9% (*Fig. 45.49*).

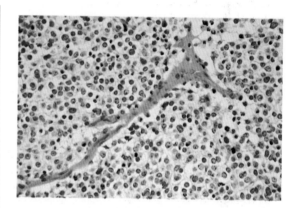

FIGURE 45.49 *Malignant oligodendroglial tumour. This lesion is markedly hypercellular but does not show the areas of necrosis often seen in malignant variants.*

EPENDYMOMA

About 4% of gliomas are ependymal in origin. These tumours arise from the ependyma lining the ventricles and also from the spinal cord and cauda equina. They have a bimodal age distribution. There is a sharp peak at about 5 years of age followed by a second broader peak in adult life. In children, ependymoma accounts for 10% of all intracranial tumours; 60% of these arise above the tentorium and the remainder below. In childhood, most ependymomas are intracranially located, whereas in adults they are divided more or less equally between the spinal cord and cranium.

The topographical distribution, irrespective of age, is shown in *Table 45.18.*

Table 45.18 Distribution of Ependymomas

Site	Frequency (%)
Floor of fourth ventricle	38
Cerebral ventricles	20
Cervicothoracic spinal cord	14
Cauda equina	28

The clinical presentation is determined by the site of the tumour:

- There may be hydrocephalus due to blockage of the fourth ventricle, leading in time to a rise in intracranial pressure.
- If the floor of the fourth ventricle is invaded, there may be focal neurological deficits related to the brainstem.
- The nerve roots of the spinal cord and, especially, of the cauda equina may be involved. These

patients will have backache and show signs of lower motor neurone-type weakness.

- Infiltration within the spinal cord may lead to long tract signs.

Most ependymomas behave in a benign fashion, but some develop anaplasia, grow rapidly and have a poor prognosis.

Macroscopic Features

Ependymomas may appear as pale pink or cream tumours within the ventricles or coating the spinal cord or cauda equina.

Microscopic Features

Ependymomas show patterns that vary not only from tumour to tumour but within individual lesions. Uncommonly, the lesions may be very well differentiated; they show well-formed rosettes lined by ependymal cells which have either retained their cilia or show small basal bodies, into which cilia are normally inserted. These are known as blepharoplasts.

Much more common is the formation of pseudorosettes, which are aggregates of ependymal cells arranged around blood vessels, with fine fibrillary processes abutting on the blood vessel wall (*Fig. 45.50*). Thus, in a section stained with haematoxylin and eosin, the tumour cell bodies and nuclei appear to be separated from the blood vessel by a pale pink halo, in which neuroglial fibrils can be seen in sections treated with antibodies against GFAP. Occasionally the tumour cells are arranged in a papillary pattern and this appearance may give rise to confusion with choroid plexus papilloma.

Myxopapillary Ependymoma

This is a distinctive variant, the occurrence of which is virtually restricted to the region of the cauda equina. It

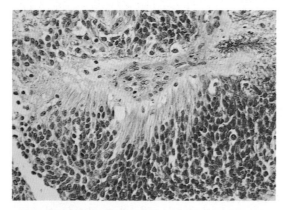

FIGURE 45.50 *Ependymoma. This section has been stained by the phosphotungstic acid–haematoxylin method, which reveals the long processes of the ependymal tumour cells attached to the periphery of blood vessels.*

originates from the conus medullaris or the filum terminale.

Myxopapillary tumours are usually found in patients aged between 20 and 40 years but they also are seen from time to time in children.

Macroscopic Features

Symptomatic examples are large sausage-shaped masses, often with a somewhat nodular surface. They compress or may even envelope the roots of the cauda equina.

Microscopic Features

The tumour is composed of well-defined cuboidal or low columnar cells surrounding central cores of acellular hyaline connective tissue in which small blood vessels can be seen. The central connective tissue core often contains some mucin. Solid masses of polygonal cells are also found away from the papillae, and more rarely there is evidence of tubule formation, the tubules being lined by tumour cells.

The tumours appear benign and behave accordingly, unless the degree of involvement of the cauda equina is so great as to make it impossible to remove the tumour completely. In this case, recurrence is likely.

CHOROID PLEXUS TUMOURS

Choroid plexus papilloma is a rare lesion (less than 1% of all intracranial tumours), usually occurring in the cerebral ventricles. Some 50% occur in patients below 20 years of age at presentation. The vast majority are benign but malignancy is found in a very small proportion of cases (choroid plexus carcinoma). The main clinical effect is hydrocephalus, resulting either from obstruction to the flow of CSF or to overproduction of CSF by the tumour cells.

Macroscopic Features

The appearances are those of a well-vascularized and, hence, pink papillary mass growing into the ventricular cavity. The stroma may be calcified and this gives these tumours a gritty feel.

Microscopic Features

Examination shows papillae composed of well-vascularized connective tissue covered by columnar or, less often, low cuboidal epithelium (*Fig. 45.51*). Immunocytochemistry shows the presence of carbonic anhydrase C (which distinguishes it from well-differentiated papillary ependymoma) and S-100 protein. Focally, these tumours also mark for epithelial cytokeratins and GFAP.

PRIMITIVE NEUROECTODERMAL TUMOURS

These are the **small blue cell tumours** of the nervous system and include:

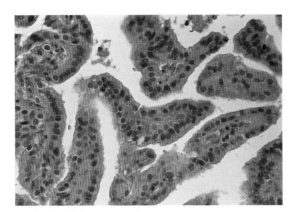

FIGURE 45.51 *Choroid plexus papilloma. Note the delicate frond-like processes of which this lesion is composed. These consist of fibrovascular cores covered by cuboidal and/or columnar cells.*

- **neuroblastomas** arising from autonomic ganglia in the abdomen
- **aesthesioneuroblastomas** of the nasal mucosa
- **retinoblastoma**
- **medulloblastoma**
- **cerebral neuroblastoma**
- **pinealoblastoma**

Microscopic Features

These tumours show a common microscopic picture:
- **Cells have a high nuclear : cytoplasmic ratio and fine fibrillary processes which can be seen in silver-stained sections.**
- **The nuclei are small, oval and darkly staining.**
- **Mitoses are common.**
- **Many show evidence of neuronal, glial or ependymal differentiation.**

Medulloblastoma

This is the commonest primary brain tumour in childhood. Some 43% of cases occur under the age of 15 years and there are two incidence peaks at 3–4 years and 8–9 years.

The name is unfortunate because medulloblasts have been neither identified nor characterized. It is believed that the stem cell of origin may be found in the external granular layer of the cerebellum.

The site of origin is characteristic. In childhood, medulloblastomas arise almost exclusively in the vermis in the midline of the cerebellum, but a more lateral site of origin – the cerebellar hemispheres – is seen in young adults.

The site of the tumour predicates the clinical presentation. Patients present either with ataxia due to cerebellar damage, or with hydrocephalus due to obstruction to the flow of CSF through the fourth ven-

tricle. If the floor of the fourth ventricle is affected, brainstem signs may be present.

Treatment by partial surgical removal followed by irradiation has greatly improved the outlook for patients with medulloblastoma. Some 40–55% of those treated in this way survive for 5 years, and 30–40% for 10 years.

Microscopic Features

The outstanding feature of the medulloblastoma is extreme **cellularity**. Every field is packed with small cells with scanty and poorly defined cytoplasm (*Fig. 45.52*). The nuclei are round or oval and stain very darkly with haematoxylin because of their high chromatin content. Mitoses are usually plentiful.

In many cases there is no architectural pattern, but sometimes the cells may be arranged in rosettes (Homer Wright rosettes) in which the cells are arranged so that their nuclei are at the periphery, with the centre of the rosette being occupied by long tapering cytoplasmic processes. Silver-staining neurofibrils can sometimes be identified in these processes.

If the tumour abuts on the meninges, a striking connective tissue response takes place which may mimic sarcoma, but this is purely a reaction to the presence of medulloblastoma cells in the meninges. This variant is called a desmoplastic medulloblastoma.

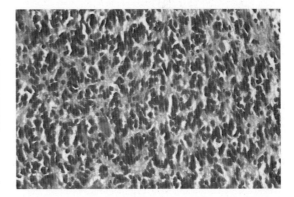

FIGURE 45.52 *Medulloblastoma from cerebellar vermis of a child. The salient feature is the extreme cellularity of the lesion. The field is packed with small dark cells in which the cytoplasm is both scanty and poorly defined. The nuclei stain darkly with haematoxylin because of their abundant coarse chromatin.*

TUMOURS OF THE MENINGES

MENINGIOMA

Meningiomas arise from cells of the arachnoid. They account for some 15% of all primary intracranial neoplasms in western Europe and North America but are more common in Africa. There is a marked difference in the prevalence between males and females with regard to both cranial (F:M ratio 2.5:1) and spinal (F:M ratio 9:1) meningiomas. Many meningiomas express receptors for oestrogens and progesterone, and there is a curious association with breast cancer. They are most common in middle age, the peak incidence in Britain being in the sixth decade.

The clinical effects depend on the rapidity of growth and site of origin. Thus tumours occurring at the base of the brain may cause focal neurological deficits by pressing on cranial nerves or structures in the cerebellopontine angle. Those over the convexity of the cerebral hemispheres and arising from the falx cerebri may grow to a very considerable size (a large orange) before drawing attention to themselves by increasing intracranial pressure.

Meningiomas arising within the vertebral column are especially common in women and cause compression of the long tracts.

Rarely, meningiomas may arise outside the cranium, the commonest sites for this being the nose, orbit, eye, skin, various viscera and extraspinal tissue.

Cytogenetic analysis has shown the occurrence of multiple deletions on chromosome 22. About 80% of patients with meningioma are heterozygous with respect to a marker on chromosome 22.

Macroscopic Features

Typically, meningioma is a firm, rounded, well-encapsulated lesion (*Fig. 45.53*) with a cream or pink cut surface. It usually adheres to the dura and can be fairly easily separated from the underlying brain. Falcine meningiomas may invade the superior sagittal sinus and this may prevent their removal, as excision of the sinus can produce venous infarction of the cerebral hemispheres. Some meningiomas, especially those in the vertebral canal, are gritty and this is due to calcified (psammoma) bodies.

Microscopic Features

Several histological variants have been described. For the most part, there is a rather uniform cell population with pale open nuclei in which one or two small nucleoli can be seen. The cytoplasm has a delicate fibrillary pattern and the tumour cells form curved bundles or whorls (*Fig. 45.54*). The most common histological variants are:

- **meningothelial.** Here sheets of tumour cells are seen and whorls may or may not be present. Cell borders may be rather indistinct giving a syncytial pattern, and there is little or no reticulin between the bundles of tumour cells.
- **fibroblastic.** There are sheets of cells which, although they have the typical nuclear appearances of arachnoid cells (see above), are elongated and show no evidence of whorl formation.
- **transitional.** Transitional tumours show features of both the meningothelial and fibroblastic type, together with typical whorls.

- **psammomatous.** Here, calcified laminated spheres (psammoma bodies) are present in large numbers (*Fig. 45.55*). The bodies probably represent dystrophic calcification occurring in bundles of collagen produced by the tumour cells. This is a common pattern in spinal meningioma.

Natural History

Meningiomas tend to be slow growing; the majority are benign so that complete excision leads to cure. Very occasionally metastases may be seen (about 1 in 1000 cases). Certain histological varieties, most notably the angioblastic and papillary types, are more likely to recur than others, and large numbers of mitoses, cellular atypia and areas of necrosis are sinister signs of a tendency to invade the underlying brain, to recur and to metastasize. The lesions are usually solitary but multiple meningiomas do sometimes occur; this is particularly likely to happen in patients with multiple neurofibromas (von Recklinghausen's disease).

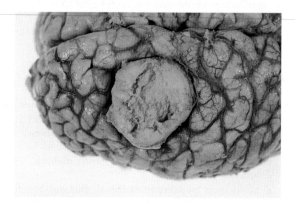

FIGURE 45.53 Meningioma. This tumour was found unexpectedly at post-mortem examination. It shows the characteristic appearance of a well-defined greyish mass rather like a bun, which is compressing the underlying brain tissue.

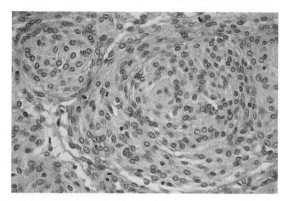

FIGURE 45.54 Meningioma showing the typical whorled appearance of the meningothelial type. The structures show some resemblance to arachnoid granulations.

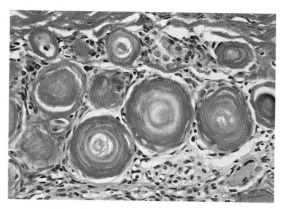

FIGURE 45.55 *Psammomatous meningioma showing numerous laminated psammoma bodies. These consist of concentrically arranged collagen fibres in which calcium and iron can be demonstrated.*

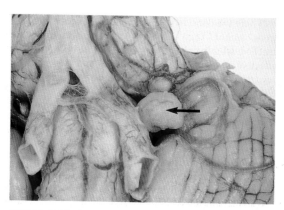

FIGURE 45.56 *Acoustic nerve schwannoma (arrowed). The lesion is well circumscribed and almost certainly encapsulated.*

NERVE SHEATH TUMOURS

The commonest neoplasms to arise from nerves are **schwannoma (syn. neurilemmoma, neuroma) and neurofibroma**.

Schwannoma

Schwannomas account for about 8% of intracranial tumours and about 25% of intraspinal lesions. They are most frequently seen in middle age.

Clinical Features

These, as always, depend on the site of the lesion. Some 80% of intracranial schwannomas arise from the vestibular portion of the eighth nerve, so the most common complaint is deafness and tinnitus on the affected side. However, if the tumour grows to a sufficient size before detection, it may cause hydrocephalus by distorting the brainstem.

Macroscopic Features

Schwannomas are smooth lobulated lesions which may be soft or rubbery in consistency. They are usually attached to a nerve or a nerve root (*Fig. 45.56*).

Microscopic Features

Two major patterns are recognized in schwannomas:

1) **Antoni type A.** This term describes compact areas in which regular interlacing bundles of uniform fusiform cells are present. Often there are foci of palisading in which there are apparently cell-free areas surrounded by palisades of banded nuclei separated by fine processes. Sometimes these palisades are arranged in a regular repetitive array, these being termed Verocay bodies.

2) **Antoni type B.** This describes much looser, more open, areas in which the cells are small with rounded nuclei and fine cytoplasmic processes. Mast cells are common in these areas, but are not seen in association with Antoni type A areas.

Typically the schwannoma is attached to one side of the nerve. This differs from the neurofibroma which infiltrates and expands the substance of the affected nerve. In tumours of long standing, some of the cells may contain large, darkly staining, atypical nuclei. This may give rise to fears of malignancy, which, unless large numbers of mitoses are seen, are quite unfounded. Secondary changes such as the accumulation of fat-laden macrophages, fibrous scarring and hyaline thickening of blood vessels are quite common.

Neurofibroma

While the schwannoma is usually solitary, neurofibromas are not infrequently multiple and may form part of the inherited syndrome of **von Recklinghausen's disease** (multiple cutaneous neurofibromas plus so-called café au lait spots on the skin, the latter usually arising in childhood). Rarely, there may be overgrowth of soft tissue around the enlarged nerve trunks so that the skin may hang in folds. This condition is known as **elephantiasis nervosa** and is what affected the patient known as 'the elephant man' described by Sir Frederick Treves. Bluish hamartomas of the iris, also known as Lisch nodules, may occur.

Von Recklinghausen's disease is not uncommon, occurring in 1 per 3000 live births. It is inherited as an autosomal dominant disorder with high penetrance but variable expressivity. In peripheral neurofibromatosis, there is a deletion localized to the **long arm of chromosome 17** near the centromere. The gene product NF1 (known as neurofibromin) normally promotes the guanosine 5′-triphosphatase activity of the *ras* protein and thus regulates the transduction of mitogenic signals within the cells.

There is a considerable spectrum of severity, ranging from minor skin lesions to gross disfigurement. Intellectual impairment may be found in up to 45% of affected subjects, 10% have epilepsy and 12–40% are reported to have kyphoscoliosis with spinal nerve root compression.

Other neoplastic complications include:
- optic nerve glioma in 15% of cases
- intracranial tumours, including glioma, in 12–20%
- sarcomatous changes in the plexiform neurofibromas arising in the peripheral nerves in 11–30% of cases.

Another variant of inherited neurofibromatosis is described below.

Central Neurofibromatosis (Bilateral Acoustic Neurofibromatosis)

This is very much rarer than peripheral neurofibromatosis, having a prevalence of 0.1 per 100 000. The patients present with multiple intracranial and intraspinous tumours, which may be schwannomas or meningiomas. Bilateral acoustic schwannomas are common in this syndrome.

Chromosome analysis of the tumour cells shows a deletion on **chromosome 22** which is associated with some abnormality of the activity of glial growth factor (NF2).

Microscopic Features

In the skin the tumours are usually poorly delimited and are composed of loosely packed bundles of spindle cells. Nerve fascicles which have been expanded by the lesion can often be seen and their axons can be demonstrated by use of appropriate silver stains. Nerve fibres within the lesions distinguish neurofibroma from schwannoma, which typically **displaces** nerve fibres rather than infiltrates them.

Malignant transformation may be detected by the presence of an increase in mitotic activity and by nuclear pleomorphism.

Disorders of Peripheral Nerves

NORMAL STRUCTURE AND FUNCTION

The functions of the peripheral nerves are to carry:
- **motor commands from the anterior horn cells to the muscles**
- **signals to the effector organs controlled by the autonomic nervous system**
- **afferent signals from sensory transducers in the skin, muscle, joint and other organs to the central nervous system (CNS)**

To carry out these tasks, nerves must be able to:
- **transmit signals very rapidly over long distances**
- **carry materials (derived from the neuronal cell body) that maintain the integrity of the nerve and are necessary for cell to cell transmission**
- **regenerate to a certain degree and thus repair minor degrees of damage (liable to occur because of the relatively exposed position of the peripheral nerves). In contrast, regeneration mechanisms have been lost in the CNS in the course of evolution.**

The nerves consist of bundles of axons (fascicles) connecting the periphery to neurones in the CNS. The functional elements of the nerves are nerve fibres consisting of axons and their associated Schwann cells.

In each fascicle, the nerve fibres are embedded in a highly specialized connective tissue known as the **endoneurium** and are surrounded by a sheath of cells, the **perineurium**. The perineurial cells are flattened cells connected by tight junctions and they are arranged in layers, each layer being separated by sheets of collagen.

Perineurium

This is the cylindrical sheath of perineurial cells, which is continuous with the pia–arachnoid of the CNS. It functions as:
- **a protective layer**
- **a diffusion barrier** (because of tight junctions between the perineurial cells and the fact that the perineurium is surrounded by basement membrane)

Endoneurium

The endoneurium is a specialized extracellular space providing an appropriate milieu for axons and their associated Schwann cells. It consists of longitudinally oriented collagen fibres embedded in a mucopolysaccharide-rich matrix. It provides a lubricant for the longitudinal movement of nerve fibres and also assists in maintaining an appropriate ionic environment for them.

In addition, the endoneurium contains capillaries providing oxygen and essential nutrients for the nerve fibres. There are tight junctions between capillary endothelial cells providing a blood–nerve barrier of the same type as the blood–brain barrier in the CNS. This barrier is, however, less effective in the region of the sensory ganglia where there are some fenestrations in the capillary endothelium. Thus certain chemical species in the blood, such as diphtheria toxin, may gain access to the extracellular space surrounding the sensory ganglion cells and affect them.

Epineurium

The epineurium is the outermost sheath surrounding peripheral nerves. It is rich in collagen fibres between which fibroblasts and occasional mast cells are present, as is a vascular bed in the form of small arteries, veins and lymphatics. Its chief function is to protect the nerve fibres from stresses related to movement of the parts of the body through which they run.

Myelinated and Unmyelinated Nerve Fibres

Nerve fibres themselves fall into two principal groups:
- **myelinated**
- **unmyelinated**

Based on size, there are two populations of myelinated fibres. There are small axons with a mean diameter of 4 μm and larger ones with a mean diameter of 11 μm. The former are about twice as numerous as the latter. Large myelinated fibres conduct nerve impulses at high speed (about 100 m/sec). They are particularly concerned with motor functions and light touch. The smaller myelinated fibres conduct impulses more slowly (12–30 m/sec) and are especially related to pain and temperature.

Unmyelinated fibres are more numerous than myelinated ones. They range in size from 0.2–3 μm. Each unmyelinated fibre is enveloped in the cytoplasm of a single Schwann cell, which separates the unmyelinated fibres from each other. Unmyelinated fibres conduct slowly (0.3–1.6 m/sec). They carry pain sensations and also constitute the postganglionic autonomic axons.

Myelination and the Schwann Cell

Myelin consists of lipid bilayers in which transmembrane proteins are embedded. The signal for myelinogenesis comes from the axon; the thicker the axon, the thicker is the myelin sheath and the greater the length of each myelinated segment. The axon segment myelinated by a single Schwann cell is the **internode**. The myelin sheath is, therefore, interrupted at regular intervals where one Schwann cell abuts on another; this point, which has a highly organized structure, is known as the **node of Ranvier**. In the fibres of largest diameter, the length of a single internode may be greater than 1 mm, whereas in the smallest fibres it may be only 100 μm. Under normal circumstances, all the internodes along a single nerve fibre are the same length. The myelin sheath is the means by which the velocity of impulse conduction is increased, and thus demyelination can have a devastating effect on conduction.

In the peripheral nervous system each Schwann cell myelinates only one segment of an axon. Myelination starts at about the 17th week of gestation. As each axon enlarges, it becomes enveloped by a chain of Schwann cells lying at intervals of about 200 μm along the axon. Each Schwann cell then spins out a spiral of plasma membrane which wraps itself round the axons. As this process goes on, the cytoplasm is extruded from the spirals; plasma membranes of the compacted Schwann cell form the myelin sheath.

REACTIONS OF PERIPHERAL NERVES TO INJURY

As there are only two functional elements in the nerve fibres, the axon and the Schwann cell, it follows that there are two main targets for injury. Thus, although there are many causes of peripheral neuropathy, two basic reaction patterns predominate:
1) damage to the neurone or axon, leading to **axonal degeneration**
2) damage to the Schwann cell, leading to **segmental demyelination**

Axonal Degeneration

Axonal degeneration results from injury:
- to the neurone (**neuronopathy**) as in poliomyelitis or motor neurone disease
- to the axon itself (**axonopathy**), as in trauma to the nerves, toxic damage or metabolic disorders such as diabetes mellitus. In generalized axonopathies there is usually distal degeneration which then extends proximally towards the neuronal cell body ('**dying back**').

The features of degeneration were first described in the context of **axonal interruption** by Augustus Waller in 1850, and are still termed wallerian degeneration.

Microscopic Features

Axonal Fragmentation

Changes are seen first in the portion of axon distal to the injury. The axon itself becomes fragmented and the myelin sheath retracts from the underlying degenerating segment(s). The axon itself tends to break at the nodes of Ranvier.

Engulfment of Debris

The axonal debris and globules of myelin start to accumulate within the Schwann cells but within a short time this role is taken over by macrophages, which not only engulf damaged axonal material and myelin but actively degrade it. The complex myelin lipid breaks down and, after 6–7 days, cholesterol esters are formed which may be identified within macrophages by using fat-soluble dyes such as Sudan III or IV.

Proximal Axonal Swelling

During the first few days after axonal interruption, axonal transport still continues in the proximal segment and thus the most distal 4 mm or so of the proximal segment, representing six to eight internodes, becomes swollen because of many mitochondria and vesicles derived from the endoplasmic reticulum. Such swellings may have a diameter of 50–100 µm.

Schwann Cell Proliferation
Within about 36 hours of nerve injury, the Schwann cells in the affected area start to multiply until they form a continuous column ensheathed by their basement membrane. These columns of Schwann cells (known as bands of Büngner) serve two functions. First, they act as a guide for newly regenerating axons and, second, they provide myelin sheaths for these axons. If no regenerating axons penetrate these cell columns, the latter undergo atrophy.

Regeneration of Axons
Axonal regeneration starts about 1 week after injury. It is preceded by a highly characteristic series of morphological events in the cell body of the neurone from which the damaged axon is derived. This is known as the **axon reaction**.

Microscopic Features
The neural cell body swells, with displacement of the nucleus away from the axon hillock. The Nissl substance (granular endoplasmic reticulum) fades away, especially in the centre of the cell, and there is an increase in the production of ribosomal RNA and protein.

Regenerating axons arise either at the site of interruption or from the preterminal nodes of Ranvier. They grow along the bands of Büngner and, if they reach a sufficiently large size, become myelinated, if this is appropriate. Their growth rate may be of the order of 2–5 mm per day. If they reach their appropriate end-organ, they may grow to a normal size, although their new internodes are shorter than normal.

The effectiveness of regeneration depends on the size of the injured nerve and the severity of the injury. Thus, in the case of a large nerve, severely damaged by trauma or ischaemia, the chances of restoration of function are quite slim.

In some cases of nerve transection, scar tissue grows between the proximal and distal ends of the affected nerve. Regenerating axons sprouting from the proximal portion may therefore be unable to make a connection with the distal end of the nerve and, instead, spread out randomly into the surrounding connective tissue forming a tangle of small fibres around the proximal stump of the transected nerve. This is what is known as a 'stump' or 'amputation' neuroma and can produce quite unpleasant sensations.

Segmental Demyelination
This is defined as loss of one or more segments of myelin from a nerve fibre in the absence of any damage to the axon. In primary Schwann cell disorders, the disintegrating myelin is first engulfed by the Schwann cells themselves. Later in the process, the damaged myelin accumulates within macrophages. When the demyelination is due to autoimmune mechanisms, such as in experimental allergic neuritis or its human homologue, the Guillain–Barré syndrome, macrophages appear to play a more active role. They insert their processes through the Schwann cell membrane and attack the myelin sheath, giving an appearance of 'stripping' the myelin away from the underlying axon.

The loss of myelin from axonal segments causes the latter to stimulate the process of remyelination. This is preceded by proliferation of Schwann cells which move along the denuded segment of axon and line up along it. New nodes of Ranvier form where these cells abut and thus new internodes are defined before the process of remyelination has really got underway. As the new myelin forms, it becomes apparent that the new internodes are shorter than the original ones and the remyelinated segments vary in length, in contrast to the normal state in which the internodes in a single fibre are equal in length.

If there are repeated episodes of demyelination and remyelination, excess Schwann cells may be produced. These arrange themselves in a whorled pattern round the axon ('onion bulbs'), an appearance that is best appreciated on transverse section. These structures are seen in several **hereditary neuropathies associated with demyelination**, such as **Charcot–Marie–Tooth disease**, and, not surprisingly, in sporadic relapsing, segmental, demyelinating neuropathies.

CLASSIFICATION OF PERIPHERAL NEUROPATHIES

Peripheral neuropathies may be classified in two main ways: **clinical** and **pathological**.

CLINICAL
This is based firstly on the **distribution of the lesions**. Thus the following may be encountered:

- a **mononeuropathy** in which a single nerve only is involved as, for example, the median nerve in carpal tunnel syndrome
- **mononeuritis multiplex** in which there is asymmetrical involvement of several isolated nerves, which may be due to vasculitis as, for example, in polyarteritis nodosa or before the acquired immune deficiency syndrome phase of human immunodeficiency virus infection
- **polyneuropathy**, which is usually a diffuse symmetrical process starting distally and then extending proximally. It may be acute, subacute or chronic. Acute inflammatory polyneuropathy (Guillain–Barré syndrome) is a classic example.

Clinical classification is modulated by **the type of fibre predominantly affected**, because this determines the functional effects. Thus the afflicted individuals may have:

- sensory neuropathy
- motor neuropathy
- mixed sensorimotor neuropathy
- autonomic neuropathy

PATHOLOGICAL

Here, the neuropathies are divided into neuronopathies and axonopathies, as shown in *Tables 45.19* and *45.20*.

MECHANICAL INJURY

The fact that mechanical trauma can give rise to peripheral nerve dysfunction has been known for more than a century. The natural history is related to the severity and type of injury affecting the nerve.

In ascending order of severity, nerve injury may be classified as:

- **neurapraxia**
- **axonotmesis**
- **neurotmesis**

Table 45.19 The Neuronopathies

Anatomical location	Disorder
Spinal cord	Loss of anterior horn cells (e.g. poliomyelitis)
	Motor neurone disease
	Spinal muscular atrophy of different types
	Spinal cord tumours
	Paraneoplastic encephalomyelitis
	Syringomyelia
	Meningomyelocele
Dorsal root ganglion cells	Virus infections
	Hereditary sensory neuropathies
	Ataxia telangiectasia
Autonomic nervous system	Diabetes mellitus
	Amyloidosis

Table 45.20 The Axonopathies

Anatomical location	Disorder
Spinal or cranial nerve roots	Prolapsed intervertebral disc
	Spinal osteoarthritis
	Spinal trauma
	Vertebral collapse
	Neoplasms
	Bacterial meningitis
	Arachnoid adhesions
Peripheral nerve trunks	Direct trauma
	Compression
	Vascular disorders, especially the vasculitides
Distal axonopathies	Toxins (e.g. organophosphorus compounds)
	Nutritional (e.g. vitamins B_1, B_6, B_{12})
	Drugs (e.g. isoniazid)
	Infections (e.g. leprosy)

Neurapraxia

This is the mildest degree of peripheral nerve dysfunction due to trauma. It is expressed in the form of a focal conduction block associated with some degree of disorganization of the paranodal structure. Demyelination and axon degeneration are not seen in the majority of cases.

Neurapraxia results, as a rule, from mild compressive injuries. These include such entities as injury to the radial nerve due to sleeping with the arm incorrectly positioned (so-called 'Saturday night palsy'), or the mild dysfunction occurring as a result of application of a tourniquet. Recovery may take several weeks but is usually complete.

The pathological correlate of this clinical disturbance is believed to be retraction of myelin in the nodal region. If the injury is more severe, there may be segmental demyelination of the affected internode. This may be repaired either by the Schwann cell producing an extension of the existing myelin to cover the defect or by insertion of a new short internode.

Axonotmesis

This is defined as an injury in which there is axonal as well as myelin damage. The basal lamina sheath of the Schwann cells remains intact. Wallerian degeneration takes place distal to the lesion, and signs of denervation such as muscle atrophy develop. Regeneration starts quite rapidly and is aided by preservation of the connective tissue framework of the nerve; functional recovery is thus a very real possibility.

Axonotmesis is likely to occur with persistent nerve compression or entrapment of the nerve within a defined anatomical compartment such as the carpal tunnel.

Microscopic Features

A zone of narrowing is seen in the nerve with expansion of the endoneurium on both sides of the compression but particularly on the proximal side. Compression leads to impairment of axonal transport and thus the axons on the proximal side show the presence of bulbous swellings. In contrast, the axons on the distal side of the compression start to undergo atrophy.

Demyelination and axon degeneration may be seen at the compression site. At a later stage, the nerve fascicle becomes scarred with proliferation of both Schwann cells and fibroblasts. Within the endoneurium, deposits of mucopolysaccharide may be seen and curious ovoid hyaline structures known as Renaut bodies appear in the endoneurium.

Carpal Tunnel Syndrome

In clinical practice, the commonest entrapment neuropathy is the carpal tunnel syndrome in which the median nerve is compressed within the anatomical compartment defined by the transverse carpal ligament.

The condition, which may be bilateral, manifests as tingling and pain in the hand (and sometimes in the lower part of the forearm). This is followed by weakness and later atrophy of the thenar muscles supplied by the median nerve. Examination shows sensory loss in the palm and in the three and a half fingers on the radial aspect of the hand.

In many patients the cause is not apparent; recognized associations, however, include:

- pregnancy
- hypothyroidism
- rheumatoid disease
- diabetes mellitus
- acromegaly
- amyloidosis. This is particularly likely to occur in patients on renal dialysis in whom β_2-microglobulin is deposited in the soft tissues.

Neurotmesis

This occurs when **nerve continuity (including that of the connective tissue sheaths) is interrupted**, either by a penetrating wound or by severe stretching injury. The absence of intact basal lamina sheaths in effect removes the tubes that guide regenerating nerve fibres and thus the chance of a full functional recovery is much reduced.

TOXIC NEUROPATHIES

Many industrial chemicals and drugs cause neuropathies. Most produce a sensorimotor neuropathy associated, pathologically, with a distal axonopathy, but many variations are present within this group. It is beyond the scope of this text to mention more than a few of these neurotoxins.

Acrylamide

This flocculating and grouting agent is widely used in a polymerized form, but it is the monomer that is neurotoxic.

Clinically, it produces a distal sensorimotor neuropathy associated with ataxia of the limbs. Tendon areflexia is noted even in mild cases and the patients complain of excessive sweating.

Nerve biopsy shows selective loss of myelinated fibres; unmyelinated fibres are affected only in very severe cases.

Hexacarbons

n-Hexane is widely used as a solvent in glues (reported as producing neuropathies in 'glue-sniffers') and n-butyl-ketone was used in the manufacture of polyvinyl chloride. It is not known exactly how these compounds produce their effects, although the toxic effect appears to be a property of their common metabolite, 2,5-hexanedione.

The clinical features are those of a distal sensorimotor neuropathy developing slowly and progressing for about 4 months after exposure to the compound has ceased.

In pathological terms, the neuropathy is characterized by focal axonal enlargement with some of the neurofilaments measuring up to 10 nm in diameter. This appearance is associated with thinning of the myelin sheath. It has been suggested that this may be due to abnormal cross-linking of the neurofilaments.

Organophosphorus Compounds

Organophosphorus compounds are used as high-temperature lubricants, as insecticides and as softeners in the manufacture of plastics. They have diverse effects on both the central and peripheral nervous systems, attributed to their ability to phosphorylate and thus inhibit esterases. The compound most commonly implicated in human disease is tri-orthocresyl phosphate. Most human cases have resulted from one single large oral dose.

The axonopathy occurring from exposure to these compounds has a curious lag phase in its development: abnormalities do not occur until 7–21 days have elapsed following a single dose.

The neuropathy presents initially with the abrupt onset of distal limb paraesthesiae followed by the development of a predominantly motor neuropathy. Not infrequently this leads to atrophy of the leg muscles and of the interosseous muscles of the hand. Signs of corticospinal tract dysfunction are common so that the clinical picture may show evidence of both upper and lower motor neurone involvement.

The microscopic picture is that of a distal axonal degeneration associated with axonal loss in the corticospinal tract and gracile fasciculi.

Drugs

Several drugs have been implicated in peripheral neuropathy. These include **isoniazid, vincristine, nitrofurantoin, chloroquine, amiodarone, metronidazole and gold**.

Most produce chronic and progressive sensorimotor polyneuropathies. A wide variety of pathological appearances and pathogenetic mechanisms is involved in this set of neuropathic disorders.

In the case of the **vinca alkaloids**, there is an accumulation of neurofilaments and of paracrystalline material in both neuronal cell bodies and axons. This is believed to be due to the fact that the alkaloids bind to tubulin and interfere with microtubule assembly. The functional defect is believed to be a failure of axonal transport.

INFECTIVE AXONOPATHY

Leprosy

The peripheral nerves constitute an important target for damage in the course of leprosy. As in other tissue, the pathology of leprous neuropathy depends on the immune reaction of the host to *Mycobacterium leprae*; the two extremes of the reaction pattern, lepromatous and tuberculoid leprosy, have their counterparts in the peripheral nerves.

In lepromatous leprosy there is a diffuse neuropathy; the distribution of lesions is predicated largely by the requirements of the bacilli for a low temperature if they are to proliferate. Thus the changes are maximal in colder areas of the body such as the distal extremities of the limbs, the nose, ears, supraorbital regions and the skin over the zygomatic arches.

Sensory loss affects temperature and pain sensation, and may lead to severe mutilation because injuries may go unheeded. The peripheral nerves become thickened and this may aggravate the clinical picture because of the superimposition of entrapment neuropathy.

Microscopic Features

Microscopic examination of the affected nerves in the early stages of the natural history shows an inflammatory reaction within the perineurium and the epineurium, and it is this that ultimately produces the nerve thickening. Numerous bacilli are present in fibroblasts within the perineurium and epineurium, within macrophages and within Schwann cells. Loss of myelinated and unmyelinated axons is present and there is evidence of demyelination as well as axon loss.

Tuberculoid leprosy tends to pursue a more benign course in respect of the peripheral neuropathy than does the lepromatous form.

Localized areas of skin anaesthesia occur, the margins of which are sharply demarcated. Anhidrosis is present in the same areas. The cutaneous nerves are often thickened and there may be lesions within the nerve that resemble so-called 'cold abscesses'.

Microscopic Features

The basic pathological lesion is an epithelioid cell granuloma. In contrast to what occurs in the lepromatous form of the disease, it is extremely difficult to identify any mycobacteria within the lesions. In the late stages of the disease, extensive and severe endoneurial scarring develops and this is associated with severe disorganization of the nerve architecture.

PERIPHERAL NEUROPATHIES CHARACTERIZED BY DEMYELINATION

These may be acquired or hereditary. Causes of the acquired form are shown below.

ACQUIRED

- **Acute inflammatory demyelinating polyneuropathy (Guillain–Barré syndrome).** May follow infection but involves an immune attack on myelin sheaths.
- **Chronic inflammatory demyelinating polyneuropathy.** Clinical features similar to those of Guillain–Barré syndrome but follows a chronic and relapsing course.
- **Diphtheria.** Nerve damage is due to the action of a bacterial exotoxin with a particular affinity for both dorsal and ventral nerve roots, possibly due to a less effective blood–nerve barrier in these locations.
- **Diabetes mellitus.** A complex set of neuropathies exists with symmetrical predominantly sensory and autonomic polyneuropathy on the one hand, and focal or multifocal neuropathies on the other.
- **Immunoglobulin (Ig) M paraproteinaemia.** This occurs in older patients, predominantly men, who have a benign monoclonal paraproteinaemia. IgM can be found on the myelin sheaths of affected nerves and it has been suggested that it acts as an autoantibody. The demyelination may be associated with loss of myelinated axons.

Acute Inflammatory Demyelinating Polyradiculoneuropathy (Guillain–Barré Syndrome)

With the virtual disappearance of poliomyelitis, the Guillain–Barré syndrome is the commonest acute neuropathy and the commonest cause of paralysis in both Europe and the USA. The peak incidence is in **men** aged 20–50 years. About two-thirds of patients give a history of some infection 1–4 weeks before the appearance of the neuropathy. This antecedent illness may vary from relatively trivial upper respiratory and gastrointestinal infections to cytomegalovirus, Epstein–Barr virus or mycoplasma infections. A fairly large outbreak in the USA was associated with a programme of immunization against influenza.

Clinical Features

The symptoms are predominantly those of a **symmetrical motor weakness associated with early loss of tendon reflexes. Distal muscle groups are affected initially but this tends to be followed by an ascending paralysis which may cause respiratory paralysis necessitating ventilation, sometimes for quite long periods.** Distal sensory loss, sometimes associated with tingling paraesthesiae, and autonomic abnormalities may also be seen. The American novelist Joseph Heller suffered from Guillain–Barré syndrome and wrote a vivid description of this experience from the point of view of the patient.

The cerebrospinal fluid (CSF) protein concentration is characteristically raised but this is not accompanied by an increase in the cell content of CSF.

Electrodiagnostic studies show a significant reduction in nerve conduction velocity and conduction block, and signs of denervation are also present. Recovery may take 3–6 months or even longer. The rather high mortality rates of earlier years have fallen considerably, but fatalities do still occur, due chiefly to respiratory paralysis and its complications.

Microscopic Features

The nerves show an inflammatory reaction, lesions being widely distributed throughout the peripheral nervous system. The inflammatory cells are initially perivascular but migrate rapidly into the endoneurium.

Macrophages dominate the cell population; these appear to be directly involved in demyelination. The macrophages insert processes into the myelin sheath and strip away the lamellae of myelin from the underlying axons. The segmental demyelination is followed by Schwann cell proliferation and remyelination, as described earlier. There may be secondary axonal loss but usually axons remain intact. Nerve function is disturbed because of the conduction block caused by demyelination.

Aetiology and Pathogenesis

The cause is not known but it is believed that an autoimmune process is involved in which both cellular and humoral mechanisms play a part. Support for this view comes from **experimental allergic neuritis**, a disorder produced in rodents within 2 weeks of injecting them with peripheral nerve myelin protein together with Freund's adjuvant. The ensuing T-cell response is accompanied by segmental macrophage-mediated demyelination, as occurs in the Guillain–Barré syndrome in humans.

T lymphocytes taken from patients with Guillain–Barré syndrome can produce demyelination in cultured myelinated nerve fibres. Antineural antibodies are also present in the plasma of these patients and appear to have a pathogenetic role, as plasma exchange appears to be of benefit in severe cases.

Chronic Inflammatory Demyelinating Polyradiculoneuropathy

The clinical features are similar to those of the Guillain–Barré syndrome but they follow a chronic relapsing or chronic progressive course. An association with the M3 allele of the α_1-antitrypsin system on chromosome 14 and a possible association with HLA-DR2 have been reported, and this suggests that genetic factors may be involved.

Microscopic Features
Widespread demyelination can be seen in the peripheral nerves and spinal roots, associated with variable degrees of inflammation. Oedema may be seen within the myelin sheaths, giving the myelin a curious 'bubbly' appearance and, in some cases, there is evidence of recurrent episodes of demyelination and remyelination in the form of 'onion bulbs'.

Diabetic Neuropathy
Diabetes is one of the commonest causes of neuropathy, which is responsible for much morbidity in diabetics. The neuropathy falls into two main groups:

1) **a symmetrical polyneuropathy involving predominantly sensory and autonomic nerves.** This form of diabetic neuropathy is believed to be metabolic in origin.

2) **an asymmetrical focal or multifocal neuropathy** believed to be vascular in origin. This may be expressed in the form of cranial nerve lesions, a thoracoabdominal neuropathy, focal lesions in the nerve supply to the limbs and the syndrome of proximal lower limb motor neuropathy, which some have termed diabetic amyotrophy.

Symmetrical Polyneuropathy
Symmetrical polyneuropathy is associated with loss of axons. This change is most prominent distally but may also affect the dorsal nerve roots. Total myelinated fibre density may be much reduced and in some instances a 'dying back' phenomenon may be noted, where initially distal changes spread proximally up axonal pathways. Loss of dorsal root ganglion cells and of anterior horn cells is also seen. In some cases there is evidence of segmental demyelination and, very occasionally, small 'onion bulbs' are noted.

Clinical Features
The earliest clinical features are:
- **loss of vibration sense**
- **loss of pain sensation (deep pain sensation is lost before superficial)**
- **loss of temperature sensation**

This picture is commonest in the feet but, at a later stage, the hands may be involved as well, giving rise to a neuropathy with a so-called 'glove and stocking' distribution. The loss of sensation is particularly baneful in the feet where absence of recognition of trauma may lead to the formation of chronic and deeply penetrating ulcers. This is made worse by atrophy of the interosseous muscles of the feet occurring as a result of motor neuropathy. This muscle loss leads to a failure to counter the activity of the long flexor muscles of the foot and this

results in a high arch and clawing of the toes. The end result of this is increased pressure on the first metatarsal head and on the tips of the toes; both of these are likely to promote the development of foot ulcers.

Some patients develop a diffuse painful neuropathy, experiencing a peculiar 'burning' or 'crawling' pain, maximal in the feet, shins and the anterior surfaces of the thighs and worst at night, being aggravated by pressure from the bedclothes.

Biopsy of nerves in such patients shows active fibre breakdown and some workers have reported a selective attack on small myelinated fibres.

Autonomic neuropathy may give rise to a variety of potentially disabling clinical abnormalities. These include:
- **cardiovascular abnormalities.** The patients may have tachycardia and there may be loss of normal sinus rhythm. In very severe cases, the heart may become effectively denervated. Postural hypotension is quite common as a result of the loss of sympathetic control of arteriolar tone.
- **urinary bladder abnormalities.** Loss of tone may occur with resulting failure to empty the bladder completely on micturition. The resulting urine stasis promotes the risk of infection.
- **gastrointestinal tract abnormalities.** Damage to the vagal supply of the gut may lead to gastroparesis which can be associated with intractable vomiting. Diarrhoea secondary to autonomic neuropathy may also occur.
- **impotence**

The features of peripheral and autonomic neuropathy are summarized in *Fig. 45.57*.

Pathogenesis of Symmetrical Diabetic Polyneuropathy
This is a difficult and controversial question. Many workers believe that the principal factor is diabetic microvascular disease affecting the endoneurial capillary network. It has been suggested also that this form of neuropathy is due to metabolic abnormalities (see p 853).

Focal Neuropathy in Diabetics
This may occur in either an acute or a chronic form. In the former, the neuropathy affects particularly nerves supplying the lower limb and cranial nerves, most notably the third nerve.

In the chronic mononeuropathies, more than 50% show involvement of either the radial or ulnar nerves.

Focal demyelinating lesions are seen in affected cranial nerves and a variable degree of fibre loss is seen in the focal and multifocal neuropathies. The endoneurial blood vessels show basement membrane thickening, presumably of the same type and pathogenesis as in diabetic microvascular disease in general.

HEREDITARY DEMYELINATING PERIPHERAL NEUROPATHIES
The causes of this group are shown below.

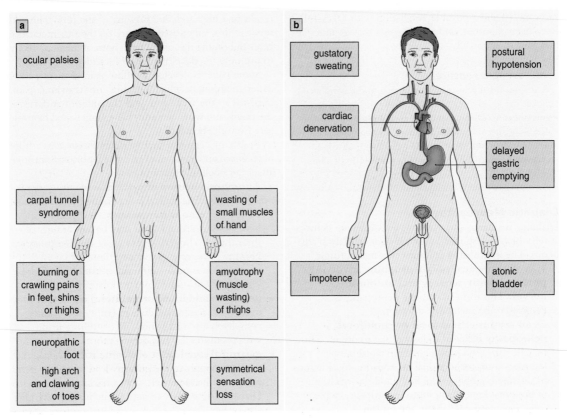

a

ocular palsies

carpal tunnel
syndrome

wasting of
small muscles
of hand

burning or
crawling pains
in feet, shins
or thighs

amyotrophy
(muscle
wasting)
of thighs

neuropathic
foot

high arch
and clawing
of toes

symmetrical
sensation
loss

b

gustatory
sweating

postural
hypotension

cardiac
denervation

delayed
gastric
emptying

impotence

atonic
bladder

FIGURE 45.57 **a** *and* **b** *Clinical features of somatic and autonomic neuropathy.*

Hereditary Sensorimotor Neuropathies

Type I: Charcot–Marie–Tooth Disease; Roussy–Lévy Syndrome

This type of neuropathy is autosomal dominant in most cases; a recessive form may be seen rarely. The disease presents in childhood with foot deformities (pes cavus) and difficulty in walking. Distal weakness, muscle wasting and sensory impairment develop, and may spread to involve the upper limbs. Ataxia and upper limb postural tremor, in addition to the above, define the Roussy–Lévy syndrome.

Nerve biopsy shows segmental demyelination, loss of myelinated fibres and, typically, the presence of 'onion bulbs' due to repeated episodes of demyelination and remyelination. The nerve trunks may be enlarged and thickened, this being so severe as to make them palpable in some instances.

This appears to be a genetically heterogeneous disorder, the commonest abnormality being a mutation on chromosome 17 of a gene coding for a myelin-specific protein, PMP-22. Another locus that may be altered exists on chromosome 1. An X-linked form of the disease also exists, the mutation here affecting the gene that codes for the gap junction protein, connexin.

Some affected families, however, show no linkage with any of these sites.

Type II: So-called Neuronal Charcot–Marie–Tooth Disease

This is a progressive axonal disorder presenting somewhat later in life and less severe than the type I disorder. Both autosomal dominant and autosomal recessive pedigrees have been reported, the latter tending to be more severely affected.

Nerve biopsies show axonal loss with relatively little demyelination. Clusters of regenerating axons may be present. Autopsy studies have shown loss of anterior horn cells and dorsal root ganglion cells.

Type III: Déjérine–Sottas Disease

This rare progressive condition is inherited in an autosomal recessive fashion. It presents in childhood with delayed motor development limb weakness, skeletal deformities and ataxia. Nerve conduction velocities are very severely reduced, suggesting a defect in myelination.

Peripheral nerves are grossly thickened and are often palpable. This is due to the extensive development of 'onion bulbs'. The central axons have either a very thin myelin sheath or no myelin at all and there is evidence of extensive axonal loss.

Hereditary Sensory and Autonomic Neuropathy

Type I
This disorder is inherited in an autosomal dominant fashion. It usually presents in the second decade or later. The principal manifestation is a sensory neuropathy expressed as loss of appreciation of pain and temperature, especially in relation to the feet. This may lead to recurrent ulcers on the soles of the feet and also to stress fractures.

These symptoms are explicable on the basis of degeneration of cells in the dorsal root ganglia. Initially this affects those in the lumbosacral region but later the ganglia supplying the upper limbs may also be involved.

Nerve biopsies show loss of small myelinated and unmyelinated axons. Large myelinated fibres are less severely affected.

Type II
This is a recessively inherited disorder differing from the type I disease in that presentation usually occurs in infancy. There is a severe and widespread sensory loss affecting all types of sensation, and the lips and tongue may become mutilated as a result of the sensory loss affecting these locations. Loss of autonomic function is restricted to anhidrosis and the occurrence of gustatory facial sweating.

There is a severe loss of myelinated fibres, with relative preservation of unmyelinated axons.

Type III (Riley–Day Syndrome)
This is a recessively inherited disorder most often affecting children of an Ashkenazi Jewish background. Affected children have difficulty in feeding during infancy, associated with frequent vomiting and an increased risk of developing lung infections. A wide range of autonomic disturbances are seen, including defective tear formation, postural hypotension, episodic hypertension and defective temperature control. Tendon areflexia and loss of pain sensation are present from birth.

The pathological basis is an aplasia of small sensory and autonomic neurones with the sympathetic nervous system being more severely affected than the parasympathetic. Biopsy of sensory nerves shows a loss of small myelinated axons, and both sensory and autonomic ganglia show a decrease in the number of neurones present.

Other Inherited Neuropathies

Friedreich's Ataxia
This is a degenerative spinocerebellar disorder. Patients in the early stages experience impaired joint position and vibration sense, and tendon areflexia.

So far as the peripheral nervous system is concerned, no abnormalities are usually seen in the somatic motor fibres and the neurones from which they originate. However, degeneration of sensory fibres, dorsal nerve roots and cells of the lower lumbosacral ganglia is a constant finding. Thick myelinated fibres suffer particularly badly and fine unmyelinated axons tend to be preserved.

Hereditary Liability to Pressure Palsies
This autosomal dominant disorder is characterized by recurrent nerve palsies. These appear to be related to mild mechanical compression which would normally not cause neuropathy. Nerve conduction studies show that there is an underlying, mild, generalized neuropathy.

Examination of affected nerves shows the presence of focal, sausage-shaped areas of hypermyelination. This is due to the presence of redundant folds and loops of myelin. Paranodal and segmental demyelination may also occur. Whether this myelin is abnormally sensitive to mechanical damage is not known.

Familial Amyloid Polyneuropathies
The familial amyloidoses affecting the peripheral nervous system are all inherited in an autosomal dominant fashion. Seven variants have been described. In five of them the amyloid is derived from an abnormal form of the transport protein **transthyretin**, a point mutation being present on the encoding gene. In two, the amyloid is not derived from transthyretin. In type III (the van Allen type), the amyloid comes from a variant apolipoprotein A_1, and in type IV (Finnish type) gelsolin appears to be the 'starter' protein. Only four types have been studied in any detail; the features are listed in *Table 45.21*.

HEREDITARY METABOLIC NEUROPATHIES

Several hereditary neuropathies exist that result from known metabolic abnormalities.

Neuropathies Related to Disturbances in Lipid Metabolism

Metachromatic Leucodystrophy
This is a set of recessively inherited disorders **associated with the accumulation of sulphatides due to a deficiency of the enzyme, aryl sulphatase A.** Demyelination occurs in both the central and peripheral nervous systems; in the latter, there is a decrease in the number of myelinated fibres.

The identifying morphological feature is metachromatic membrane-bound inclusions in the Schwann cells. These inclusions are clearly lysosomal in nature. The mechanism of the demyelination is not known.

Table 45.21 Hereditary Amyloid Neuropathies		
Type	Clinical features	Molecular basis
Type I (Portugese)	Polyneuropathy	Valine → leucine transposition at position 30 of transthyretin
Type II (Indiana)	Carpal tunnel syndrome; later a generalized polyneuropathy develops	Serine → isoleucine substitution at position 84 of transthyretin
Type III (van Allen)	Symmetrical polyneuropathy, often with duodenal ulceration and renal failure	Variant form of apolipoprotein A$_1$ with an arginine → glycine substitution at position 26
Type IV (Finnish)	Cranial neuropathy Lattice corneal dystrophy	Gelsolin is precursor molecule

Krabbe's Globoid Cell Leucodystrophy

This a recessive disorder in which the CNS is more severely affected than the peripheral nervous system. **It is due to a deficiency of the lysosomal enzyme galactocerebroside-β-galactosidase.** This causes accumulation of galactocerebroside in very large macrophage-like cells, known as globoid cells, which stain positively with the periodic acid–Schiff stain. The peripheral nerves show demyelination with endoneurial scarring, but the globoid cells, so typical in the CNS, are not present in the affected peripheral nerves. Schwann cells and also macrophages may contain characteristic inclusions, which can be seen on electron microscopic examination.

Adrenoleucodystrophy

This is an X-linked disorder affecting both the nervous system and the adrenal cortex. The biochemical basis and pathological features are described in the chapter on the adrenal (see pp 839–840).

Refsum's Disease

This is a recessive disorder expressed in the form of a chronic, distal, symmetrical sensorimotor neuropathy. It is associated with pigmentary degeneration of the retina and with ataxia. It is due to the accumulation of a long-chain fatty acid, **phytanic acid**. This is derived from phytol in the diet and is stored because it fails to undergo α-oxidation.

The affected nerves are enlarged. This is due partly to an accumulation of mucoid material within the endoneurium and partly to Schwann cell hyperplasia with the formation of 'onion bulbs'. The number of myelinated fibres is decreased.

Fabry's Disease

This is an X-linked recessive disorder in which there is a deficiency of **ceramide-trihexoside-α-galactosidase A**. The disorder is a multisystem one involving the skin, eye (cornea), heart, nervous system and kidney. Peripheral nerve involvement is expressed in the form of a mild sensory and autonomic neuropathy but superimposed on this are episodes of very severe pain in the limbs (Fabry crises). The skin involvement is expressed in the form of dark-red telangiectatic lesions (hence the alternative name **angiokeratoma corporis diffusum**).

The affected nerves show a loss of small axons, both myelinated and unmyelinated. Within endothelial and perineurial cells characteristic inclusions are present which show alternating dark and light lines. These consist of accumulated glycosphingolipid.

Tangier Disease (Hereditary Deficiency of High Density Lipoprotein)

This autosomal recessive disorder is named after an island in Chesapeake Bay rather than the North African city of that name. It is characterized by an absence of apolipoprotein A$_1$ and the affected individuals, therefore, have very low plasma concentrations of high-density lipoprotein. Although there is no increase in plasma cholesterol concentration, large amounts of cholesterol esters are deposited in the tissues, particularly in the tonsils (which are enlarged and yellow in colour), the spleen, lymph nodes, bone marrow, skin and the gastrointestinal tract submucosa.

About 50% of affected individuals have a neuropathy, which may be of several different patterns. Biopsy shows severe depletion of small myelinated and unmyelinated axons. Schwann cells show the presence of droplets of neutral lipid and cholesterol ester.

Abetalipoproteinaemia (Bassen–Kornzweig Disease)

This rare autosomal recessive disorder is due to a failure of synthesis of apolipoprotein B$_{48}$ in the intestinal lining cells. As a result, chylomicrons cannot be formed and dietary fat accumulates within the intestinal wall. The syndrome that develops is characterized by malabsorption, red blood cells with abnormal morphology (acanthocytes), pigmentary retinal degeneration and a symmetrical distal neuropathy. The neuropathy appears to be due to a secondary deficiency of vitamin E and can be prevented by prophylactic administration of vitamin E. It has been suggested that the myelin damage in this disorder, as well as in other forms of malabsorption, is mediated by free radicals which, in the absence of adequate amounts of vitamin E, are not 'scavenged'.

Demyelination and loss of axons have been reported in the affected peripheral nerves.

The Porphyrias

Peripheral nerve involvement may occur in the hepatic porphyrias:

- acute intermittent porphyria
- variegate porphyria
- hereditary coproporphyria (rare)
- porphyria cutanea tarda

The first three of these can present acutely, whereas porphyria cutanea tarda is usually non-acute. All the hepatic porphyrias, with the single exception of the very rare amino-laevulinic acid dehydratase deficiency, are inherited in an autosomal dominant fashion.

Acute Intermittent Porphyria

This presents in early adult life and females are more frequently affected than males.

Alcohol, barbiturates and oral contraceptives are well known triggers but, in fact, a large number of lipid-soluble compounds may act in this way.

Patients present with:

- abdominal pain and vomiting (90%)
- a sensorimotor peripheral neuropathy (70%)
- tachycardia and raised blood pressure (70%)
- neuropsychiatric disorders ranging from depression to frank psychosis

The pathological changes are those of a distal axonopathy of 'dying back' type.

Variegate Porphyria

This syndrome consists of a combination of features of acute intermittent porphyria with those of porphyria cutanea tarda. These patients develop a bullous skin eruption as a result of the effect of ultraviolet light on porphyrins deposited in the skin.

MISCELLANEOUS NEUROPATHIES

Neoplasm-associated Neuropathies

Neuropathies may arise in association with malignant disease as a result of direct invasion of nerve trunks as, for example, in the diaphragmatic paralysis caused by invasion of the phrenic nerve by bronchial carcinoma or the brachial plexus abnormalities that may be seen with the same tumour.

It is clear also that a variety of neuropathies arise as non-metastatic complications of malignant disease. These include:

- **a sensorimotor neuropathy** affecting principally the lower limbs. This is seen most frequently in patients with carcinoma of the lung, especially the small cell variety.
- **a subacute sensory neuropathy**, even more strongly associated with small cell carcinoma of the lung. In this variety, there is loss of fibres in both the peripheral nerves and the sensory roots. Extensive loss of ganglion cells is seen in the dorsal nerve roots and the affected ganglia show a perivascular infiltration of lymphocytes.

This last morphological feature suggests that immune mechanisms may be involved in the pathogenesis of this neuropathy. Some support for this comes from the observation that a polyclonal IgG, complement-fixing antibody, known as anti-Hu, is consistently present both in the serum and CSF of patients with subacute tumour-associated sensory neuropathy. This antibody binds with a 35–38-kDa protein expressed in the nuclei of neurones and also by the tumour cells.

Uraemic Neuropathy

Severe chronic renal failure may be associated with a symmetrical, distal, sensorimotor neuropathy. This is far from uncommon, occurring in about two-thirds of patients with chronic renal failure. The mechanism is unknown but it may be due to retention of some neurotoxic metabolite.

Autopsy studies have shown axonal degeneration, which is most severe distally. This is associated with axonal reactions in the anterior horn cells. In addition to the axonal changes, secondary demyelination is noted.

Skeletal Muscle

NORMAL MICROANATOMY AND PHYSIOLOGY

Muscle fibres are very large cells with a diameter of 50–100 µm. Their length varies from cell to cell, in some instances being more than 1000 times greater than the diameter. Each fibre develops by fusion of several fetal cells (the myoblasts); the nuclei of these original cells persist, lying just beneath the plasma membrane of the skeletal muscle cells. These multiple nuclei are easily seen on light microscopy whether the muscle cells are sectioned transversely or longitudinally.

Muscle fibres are grouped into bundles (fascicles), the number of fibres varying from case to case.

- Each individual fibre is enclosed in a delicate fibrous tissue covering known as the **endomysium**, in which capillaries are present.
- Each fascicle is bounded by a delicate fibrous tissue layer known as the **perimysium**.
- Groups of fascicles lie in fibroadipose tissue in which larger blood vessels and lymphatics run. This is known as the **epimysium.**

On light microscopy the most characteristic feature of skeletal muscle is its striated appearance. This is due to the way in which the individual myofibrils are organized. Each myofibril consists of a number of functional units known as **sarcomeres**, about 2.2 μm long. Low-power electron microscopy shows alternating dark and light bands in the sarcomere; it is these, made up of contractile filaments arranged parallel to the long axis of the sarcomere, that give muscle its typical striated appearance:

- **The dark (A) bands consist of thick filaments composed predominantly of myosin.**
- **The light (I) bands are made up of thin actin filaments attached to a Z disc, marking the end of the sarcomere.**

Sliding of Actin and Myosin Filaments Past Each Other is Responsible for the Contraction of a Myofibril

Shortening of a myofibril is caused by shortening of each individual sarcomere. This is accomplished by a mechanism in which **the individual actin and myosin filaments slide past each other without any alteration in filament length**. The morphological basis for this sliding filament action lies in the myosin II heads on the myosin filaments. These are tiny side-arms or cross-bridges extending outwards from the surface of the myosin filaments for a distance of about 13 μm. Contraction of a muscle is brought about by the cyclic action of these side-arms, which act 'like a bank of tiny oars' (Alberts *et al.*, 1994).

Contraction of myofibrils occurs only when a signal passes from the motor nerve to the muscle cell. The signal from the nerve generates an action potential in the plasma membrane of the muscle cell and this is spread into the depths of the cell. Spread occurs via invaginations of the plasma membranes known as the T tubules, extending round each myofibril. The T tubules, are separated by only a very small gap from an anastomosing system of flattened vesicles ensheathing the myofibrils, known as the sarcoplasmic `reticulum. A number of calcium-releasing channels extend from the membrane of the sarcoplasmic reticulum facing the T-tubule membrane. As the action potential spreads along the T-tubule membrane, it activates certain voltage-sensitive proteins triggering the release of calcium from the sarcoplasmic reticulum into the cytosol of the muscle cell. It is this movement of calcium ions into the cytosol that initiates the contraction of each myofibril.

Muscle Fibres within a Single Muscle Show Physiological Differences

Muscle fibres differ from one another in respect of their twitch speed and fatiguability; these differences correlate with differences in the enzyme profile, as demonstrated histochemically. When the myosin adenosine 5′-triphosphatase (ATPase) reaction is used, *three* different types of fibre can be identified:

- **Type 1:** slow twitch, fatigue resistant
- **Type 2A:** fast twitch with intermediate fatiguability
- **Type 2B:** fast twitch fibres which rapidly become fatigued

The myosin ATPase reactions shown by the different fibre types vary with the pH at which the test is carried out, as shown in *Fig. 45.58* and *Table 45.22.*

The muscle cells within a single motor unit are of the same type but fibres consist of many units, and thus a normal fibre shows a mosaic-like pattern. In some disorders there is a selective type of fibre atrophy (e.g. myotonic dystrophy) and the same selectivity can be seen to operate in muscle wasting due to infections or certain systemic disorders in which type 2B fibres appear particularly to be the target for atrophy.

MUSCLE DISORDERS

The number of pathological reaction patterns seen in skeletal muscle is limited and **it is seldom that a cor-**

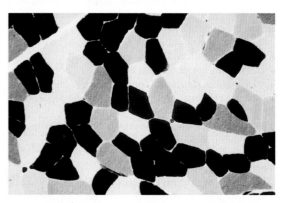

FIGURE 45.58 Normal muscle stained to demonstrate ATPase at pH 4.5. The darkly stained fibres are type 1 muscle fibres.

Table 45.22 ATPase Reactions in Different Fibre Types

Fibre type	pH 9.4	pH 4.6	pH 4.3
Type 1	Pale	Dark	Dark
Type 2A	Dark	Pale	Pale
Type 2B	Dark	Intermediate	Pale

rect diagnosis can be reached on the basis of histological examination alone. It is an area of practice in which close cooperation between clinician and pathologist is essential if the best interests of the patient are to be served. Muscle can exhibit most of the morphological changes seen in other tissues, but it can be helpful to have some idea of the spectrum of structural abnormalities occurring in muscle disease and also to have some acquaintance with the vocabulary used to describe this set of disorders (*Table 45.23*).

Table 45.23 Pathological Reactions Seen in Muscle

Condition	Features
Hypertrophy	**An increase in calibre of the fibre beyond its normal limits.** This may be due to increased muscular activity, to a hormonal stimulus or, sometimes, as a compensatory reaction to muscle weakness (e.g. Duchenne-type muscular dystrophy in its earlier stages).
Atrophy	**Atrophy: a decrease in the size of a fibre that was previously normal in size.** This is a common finding in many types of muscle disease. True atrophy follows denervation and **the presence of large groups of atrophic muscle fibres on biopsy strongly suggests a diagnosis of peripheral neuropathy or motor neurone disease** (amyotrophic lateral sclerosis). Where the atrophy is of this type, there may be sprouting of new nerve fibres from adjacent healthy subterminal fibres. Thus a denervated motor unit may become reinnervated by fibres from another motor unit. This collateral reinnervation may mask the presence of a neurogenic disorder such as motor neurone disease, which can remain clinically silent as long as the collateral reinnervation continues. **Small group atrophy and single fibre atrophy** can occur in neurogenic disorders but are not specific for this group because they may also occur in primary myopathies.
Necrosis, phagocytosis, regeneration	**Necrosis of skeletal muscle with subsequent phagocytosis of muscle debris by macrophages, followed by some regenerative activity, occurs principally in the actively progressive myopathies**; Duchenne-type muscular dystrophy and polymyositis are outstanding examples. In many cases the precise mechanism of the initial cell damage is unknown. It has been suggested that a cardinal event is sarcolemmal damage resulting in the flooding of the cell with excess calcium. The necrosis may affect a whole cell or merely a segment of that cell. In either case there is likely to be escape of water-soluble enzyme from the damaged muscle cells, reflected by an increase in the plasma concentration of creatine phosphokinase. In segmental necrosis, the affected part of the muscle cell appears either granular or eosinophilic and structureless (hyaline change). Several days later, macrophages invade the damaged cells and phagocytose the necrotic contents. Meanwhile there is some regenerative activity expressed in the form of proliferation of myoblasts lying just beneath the basal lamina. Regenerated cells are smaller than normal and appear basophilic compared with normal muscle cells. Segmental necrosis and its consequences are seen mainly to affect either single fibres or small groups of fibres.
Fibre splitting	**This term describes clefts in the individual muscle fibres.** It is a rather common and non-specific finding as it can occur in ageing muscles, in abdominal muscle as an association of pregnancy and in some slowly progressive muscular dystrophies.

Table 45.23 Pathological Reactions Seen in Muscle – *continued*

Condition	Features
Malposition of nuclei	**Normally skeletal muscle nuclei are situated peripherally and only about 3% lie internally between the myofibrils. In some congenital myopathies, the nuclei lie in a central position. Internal nuclei (i.e. those not in the normal subsarcolemmal position) may be seen in many primary muscle disorders, most notably those associated with myotonia** (the persistence of muscle contraction after the voluntary effort has ceased).
Ring fibres	**A ring fibre is a muscle cell in which peripheral myofilaments have become reoriented so that they run circumferentially.** When the affected fibres are sectioned transversely, this reorientation shows as a peripheral ring. Ring fibres occur in small numbers in several different myopathies and are seen in fairly large numbers in myotonic dystrophy. They also occur in sites of focal regeneration, especially following trauma to the muscle.
Cytoplasmic bodies	**Cytoplasmic bodies are composed of actin filaments packed together to form a central mass from which less densely packed filaments radiate.** They may be found in almost any muscle disorder.
Nemaline bodies	**Nemaline bodies are rod-shaped or thread-like bodies about 2 μm in length, occurring between the muscle fibres in a congenital myopathy** to which the bodies have given their name (**nemaline myopathy**); (see p 1187).
Cores and related abnormalities	Cores are well demarcated areas seen in type 1 fibres stained to show oxidative enzymes. The cores show up as areas of pallor in which, however, myofibrils still persist. They occur in a specific myopathy known as central core disease but are also seen in muscle derived from patients with **malignant hyperthermia**, a condition in which generalized muscle contracture may occur as a result of induction of anaesthesia with halothane. The generalized contracture is associated with hyperpyrexia and the condition, which is inherited, carries a high mortality rate. The term **'moth-eaten'** fibre is used to describe a muscle cell in which, as in core myopathy, there are areas of pallor in sections stained to show oxidative enzymes. Moth-eaten areas, however, have very irregular edges, which distinguishes them from cores. This appearance is due to a combination of an absence of staining of myofibrils and sarcoplasm and loss of mitochondria. It is a rather non-specific abnormality which can occur in denervated fibres as well as in some myopathies. **Target fibres**, variants of cores, show a central granular mass within the muscle fibres surrounded first by a clear halo and then by normal myofibrils. They are seen in cases of motor neurone disease and may also be present in some cases of slowly progressive denervation.
Vacuoles	Vacuoles are spaces within muscle cells. They vary in size and content. They were first seen in a rare dystrophy but have been identified in other conditions, including muscle ischaemia, inflammatory myopathies, systemic lupus erythematosus and certain toxic changes in muscle such as the myopathy associated with chloroquine.
Contraction bands	These are segments where the muscle fibres stain intensely with eosin. They are the result of an influx of calcium ions which activate myosin ATPase, leading to segmental hypercontraction.

CLASSIFICATION OF MUSCLE DISORDERS

The two major classes into which muscle disorders fall are:

- **myopathies**, in which muscle is the primary target
- **neurogenic muscle disorders**, in which the muscle changes are essentially secondary to **denervation** or to **failures in neuromuscular transmission**

MYOPATHIES

The list of these is long and only a few can be considered in a text of this length (see *Tables 45.24* and *45.25*).

Table 45.24 Destructive Myopathies

Group	Examples
The dystrophies (genetically determined, destructive and progressive muscular disorders which may be inherited in an X-linked or autosomal pattern)	Duchenne-type muscular dystrophy Becker-type muscular dystrophy Limb girdle dystrophy Facioscapulohumeral dystrophy Oculopharyngeal dystrophy Scapuloperoneal dystrophy
Inflammatory myopathies	Dermatomyositis associated with polymyositis. This may be idiopathic, associated with collagen disorders such as polyarteritis nodosa (*Fig. 45.59*) or with malignancy
Infections	Bacterial or viral infections (e.g. Coxsackie) or infestations Sarcoidosis
Toxic or drug-induced myopathies	Alcohol Emetine Penicillamine

Table 45.25 Non-destructive myopathies

Group	Example
Genetically determined myotonic syndromes	Myotonic dystrophy Congenital myotonia
Myopathies associated with selective type 2 fibre atrophy	Polymyalgia rheumatica Steroid myopathy Endocrine myopathies: • thyroid disease • acromegaly • osteomalacia • hyperparathyroidism
Metabolic myopathies	Glycogenosis (McArdle's disease) Periodic paralysis Malignant hyperthermia
Congenital myopathies	Centronuclear myopathy Central core disease Minicore disease Nemaline myopathy Mitochondrial myopathy

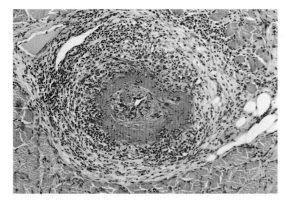

FIGURE 45.59 *Muscle biopsy in a case of polyarteritis nodosa. The vessel in the centre of the field shows obvious fibrinoid necrosis, being intensely eosinophilic and having a 'smudged' appearance. There is a brisk inflammatory infiltrate around the affected vessel.*

NEUROGENIC MUSCLE DISORDERS
1) **Spinal cord disorders**
- **syringomyelia**
- **spina bifida (neural tube defect) in its more severe forms**
- **neoplasms**
2) **Diseases of motor neurones**
- **motor neurone disease**
- **spinal muscular atrophy of various types**
- **poliomyelitis**
3) **Peripheral neuropathies of various types**
4) **Disorders of motor nerve roots**
5) **Disorders of neuromuscular transmission**
- **myasthenia gravis**
- **other myasthenic syndrome such as the Lambert–Eaton syndrome**

THE MUSCULAR DYSTROPHIES

The defining criteria of the muscular dystrophies are that they are:
- **genetically determined**
- **destructive**
- **progressive**

There is considerable variation in the natural histories of these disorders. Some, like the Duchenne type, are rapidly progressive: the patients are usually unable to walk by the time puberty is reached and most die by the age of 20 years. Others are much more slowly progressive and have little or no effect on life expectancy.

Duchenne-type Muscular Dystrophy (DMD)
This is an X-linked recessive disorder with an incidence of roughly 1 in 3500 live male births and a prevalence of about 3 per 1000 population. It is due to an abnormality in a gene located on the short arm of the X chromosome in the Xp21 region. DMD can occur occasionally in girls who have a translocation on the short arm of the X chromosome, the breakpoint being at the Xp21 region. Sporadic mutations in this region are common and account for a substantial proportion of cases of DMD; in others the mother shows the mutation in one of her X chromosomes.

Clinical Features
DMD appears in early childhood, usually by the age of 4 years. The pelvifemoral group of muscles seems to be affected earliest, giving rise to clumsiness of the gait, frequent falls and difficulty in rising. Characteristically the calf muscles are hypertrophic but this disappears as the disease progresses. **In the early stages, there is already a gross increase in the plasma concentrations of creatine phosphokinase (CPK) (10 000 iu/l; normal level 60 iu/l), indicating necrosis of muscle fibres with loss of the enzyme into the extracellular fluid.** As the muscle mass becomes severely depleted in the course of the disease, the raised CPK concentration gradually declines.

The weakness first seen in the proximal muscles of the lower limbs, then affects other muscle groups, such as those of the shoulder girdle, arms, neck and trunk. These unfortunate boys generally become wheelchair bound between the ages of 10 and 12 years. Death usually occurs before the age of 20 years. It may be due to:
- the onset of fatal cardiac arrhythmias, the hearts of most of the patients showing focal fibrosis in the presence of normal coronary arteries
- respiratory difficulties and, eventually, fatal pneumonia

Microscopic Features
The fundamental process in DMD is segmental necrosis of muscle fibres followed by invasion of the affected cells by macrophages and subsequent phagocytosis.

Small clusters of muscle cells are generally affected (*Fig. 45.60*). Regeneration follows the segmental necrosis of muscle cells but fails to compensate for fibre loss and this imbalance leads to the appearance of muscle weakness.

The endomysium and perimysium show fibrosis quite early in the course of the disease, and in the later stages there is extensive replacement of muscle by fibroadipose tissue.

In addition to the obviously necrotic fibres, there are also occasional enlarged and rounded fibres showing homogeneous, deeply eosinophilic staining of the cytoplasm. These fibres, known as 'hyaline' fibres, represent areas of hypercontraction associated with an increased intracellular calcium content.

In the early stages of the disease there is variation in fibre size. Groups of small regenerating fibres can be seen, these groups being delimited by a delicate connective tissue stroma.

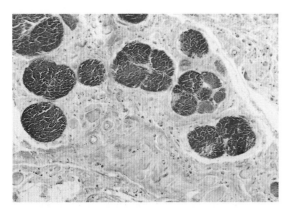

FIGURE 45.60 *Muscle biopsy from a patient with Duchenne-type muscular dystrophy. The section is stained by the PTAH method (Phosphotungstic acid-haematoxylin), which stains the fibres a purplish colour. There has been marked drop-out of muscle fibres, only a few surviving in this field.*

Pathogenesis

DMD is due to a lack of production of the protein dystrophin. Our understanding of the pathogenesis of DMD has advanced considerably in recent years. This can justly be regarded as a triumph for modern molecular genetics.

In DMD the fundamental biological fault is absence of the gene product of a large 2000-kilobase gene situated in the Xp21 region. This gene product is known as **dystrophin**, a large rod-shaped protein located on the inner surface of the sarcolemma. In the milder Becker type of dystrophy, dystrophin is synthesized but is abnormal, being either larger or smaller than normal. It has been suggested that **the difference in dystrophin production seen in these two conditions depends on the site of the mutation or deletion in the dystrophin gene**. If an open reading frame (ORF) is affected, the dystrophin is simply not synthesized, but if the ORF is preserved then protein synthesis occurs, although the protein may be too little in amount or prematurely truncated.

Dystrophin can be identified in frozen sections of muscle biopsies treated with an antidystrophin antibody:

- **Normal muscle shows the presence of dystrophin in all cells; it is localized in a subsarcolemmal position.**
- **Muscle biopsies from patients with DMD show absence of bound antibody in all muscle cells.**
- **Muscle biopsies from patients with Becker-type dystrophy show weak and patchy immunofluorescence and some of the fibres show no dystrophin.**
- **Muscle biopsies from carriers of the abnormal gene show two populations of cells, some with and some without dystrophin.** The carrier state can be diagnosed directly by identifying

restriction fragment length polymorphisms and by a new non-radioactive direct test based on competitive polymerase chain reaction amplification.

It has been suggested that **the function of dystrophin is to act as a transmembrane connector between the contractile fibrils within the muscle cells and elements of the basement membrane outside the cell**. The dystrophin molecules are believed to impart flexibility to the cell membrane and thus to protect it during contraction and relaxation of the muscle cell. If this flexibility is not present, small defects occur in the cell membrane during contraction. These may allow excess amounts of calcium to enter the affected cells and thus to trigger hypercontraction and, ultimately, coagulative necrosis.

Becker-type Muscular Dystrophy (BMD)

This is also an X-linked recessive disorder resulting from a mutation of the dystrophin gene, different to that causing DMD.

The clinical picture is qualitatively similar to that seen in DMD but is much milder. The onset of muscle weakness is delayed, in some cases to the second decade of life, and the course is much more benign; some patients reach the age of 50 years. In some, the plasma CPK concentrations are as high as those in DMD. In others, the CPK levels are only ten times as high as normal.

The relative mildness of the clinical course is paralleled by milder changes in the morphology of affected muscles. Necrosis and phagocytosis are much less prominent than in DMD, although the variation in fibre size seen in that disease also occurs in BMD. An additional feature is fibre splitting, which appears to increase in amount as the disease progresses. Extensive fibrosis and replacement of muscle by fibroadipose tissue tend to occur only in the end stages of the disease.

GENETICALLY DETERMINED MYOTONIC SYNDROMES

Myotonic Dystrophy

Myotonic dystrophy is a disorder **inherited in an autosomal dominant fashion**. It usually makes its appearance after the age of 20 years. Congenital myotonic dystrophy is seen occasionally. It occurs only in children born to mothers with the disease, even though clinical expression in the mother may be mild. The clinical hallmarks of myotonic dystrophy are:

- **myotonia (prolongation of muscle contraction after voluntary effort has ceased).** This can be demonstrated by asking the affected individual to grasp one's hand and then to relax the grip. This cannot be effected voluntarily, the grip being prolonged until **involuntary** relaxation takes place.

- **muscle weakness** in the early stages of the disease, affecting the facial muscles and anterior neck muscles as well as distal muscle groups of the limbs. Ptosis is a common early sign.

Involvement of cardiac or smooth muscle does occur in some of the myopathies, but **myotonic dystrophy is unique in that it is truly a multisystem disease involving organs and tissues that have no apparent relation to muscle**. Thus, in addition to the abnormalities of skeletal muscle function, the syndrome may include:

- frontal **baldness**
- **cataract** (present in 90% of cases)
- **diabetes mellitus** and other endocrine abnormalities
- **cardiomyopathy** leading to cardiac arrhythmias
- **mitral valve prolapse**
- **association with multiple pilomatrixomas** (a benign tumour of the skin formerly known as benign calcifying epithelioma of Malherbe)
- **gonadal atrophy**
- **dementia**
- **smooth muscle cell dysfunction** in some cases giving rise, for example, to dysphagia

The cause of the disease is a mutation of a gene known as *MyD* on the long arm of chromosome 19 (19q13.3). The mutation is an expansion of a CTG triplet in the gene encoding an adenosine 3′,5′-cyclic monophosphate-dependent protein kinase. The larger the number of repeats, the greater is the clinical severity of the disease. This is a situation not dissimilar to that in Huntington's disease and the fragile X syndrome.

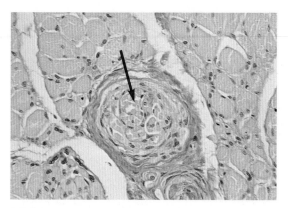

FIGURE 45.61 *Dystrophia myotonica. The muscle spindle seen in the centre of the field (arrowed) shows interesting changes with an increase in the number of intrafusal fibres, believed to be due to longitudinal fibre splitting as a consequence of the abnormal tension on the spindle produced by sustained muscular contraction.*

Muscle biopsy in these children shows a histological picture characterized by immaturity of muscle rather than the microscopic features described above.

Microscopic Features

One of the earliest muscle abnormalities in myotonic dystrophy is a **selective atrophy of type 1 fibres** (*Fig. 45.61*). This is accompanied by hypertrophy of type 2 fibres.

Central nuclei are also seen at an early stage of the disease. At this point only a few fibres are affected but with time the proportion of affected fibres increases significantly.

The myosin ATPase reaction shows **many ring fibres**.

Blebs appear on the sarcolemma. These appear to contain eosinophilic cytoplasm staining positively with periodic acid–Schiff (PAS) stain (which stains 1–2 glycol groups) but no myofibrils.

Necrosis of muscle cells is rare and the obvious wasting of muscle seen in affected areas is due to atrophy.

In the congenital form, hypotonia rather than myotonia is often seen during the neonatal period and the affected infants may also show severe respiratory difficulties. Motor development may be delayed and some degree of intellectual impairment is often present.

CONGENITAL MYOPATHY

This is a group of rare, often familial, diseases manifesting in early childhood with:

- **hypotonia**
- **a delay in motor development**
- **proximal muscle weakness**
- **facial weakness in many instances**
- **death in infancy, often due to respiratory failure**

This clinical picture is common to a number of congenital myopathies. In contrast, their histological appearances are quite distinctive.

Centronuclear Myopathies

This is a heterogeneous group. The more severe form is an X-linked recessive disorder, but a milder form exists and is inherited in an autosomal dominant pattern. In the more severe X-linked form (also known as myotubular myopathy), the infants are strikingly hypotonic and are at risk of dying from respiratory failure early in life.

Microscopic Features

The muscle fibres show centrally placed nuclei (*Fig. 45.62*) and, in sections stained to show myosin ATPase, there is a perinuclear halo which is unstained. Type 1 fibres predominate.

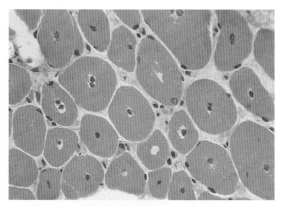

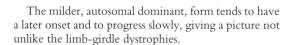

FIGURE 45.62 *Centronuclear myopathy showing, as the name of the disorder suggests, nuclei in the centre of the muscle cells rather than at the periphery.*

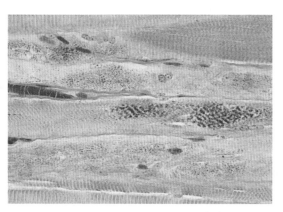

FIGURE 45.63 *Nemaline (rod body) myopathy showing numerous tiny rods and granules (composed of Z-line material) within the muscle fibres.*

The milder, autosomal dominant, form tends to have a later onset and to progress slowly, giving a picture not unlike the limb-girdle dystrophies.

Microscopic Features

Microscopic examination also shows central nuclei but the muscle cells are larger and more mature in appearance than those of the X-linked syndrome.

Nemaline Myopathy

The term nemaline is derived from the Greek *nema* meaning a worm. It is used because of a fancied resemblance of the typical inclusions seen within muscle cells to threads.

This is again almost certainly **a set of disorders** with a single histological pattern. There is evidence of both autosomal dominant and autosomal recessive transmission, and some studies show a preponderance of females. Affected infants tend to present with hypotonia and muscle weakness so severe that they may die from respiratory failure during infancy. Skeletal abnormalities such as kyphoscoliosis and a high arched palate may be seen and, in some instances, the muscles of the face may be affected particularly severely.

Microscopic Features

The histological picture is highly characteristic, consisting of a combination of a predominance of type 1 fibres and very large numbers of small rod-shaped bodies within the sarcoplasm (*Fig. 45.63*). It is necessary to employ trichrome stains on biopsies from suspected cases, because the bodies do not always show up in sections stained with haematoxylin and eosin.

On electron microscopy the rod bodies are seen to show the same periodicity and lattice structure as Z discs,

from which they are believed to be derived. Rods have been described in a number of different neuromuscular conditions but not in large numbers and not in this clinical frame of reference.

Central Core Disease

Genetic heterogeneity is a feature of this condition. It may be sporadic or inherited in either an autosomal dominant or an autosomal recessive pattern. This suggests that it is not a single disorder. This is a comparatively mild disorder in clinical terms; the onset of muscle weakness is delayed as a rule until the child has started walking and may, in some cases, be much later.

Microscopic Features

Microscopic examination shows a great preponderance of type 1 fibres. The cores which give this disorder its name are well-demarcated, centrally located zones of pallor, most easily seen when stains to demonstrate oxidative enzymes are used. The myofibrils within the cores may be disrupted or normal but there is a distinct lack of mitochondria and/or of the junctions between T tubules and the sarcoplasmic reticulum.

Mitochondrial Encephalomyopathies

A wide spectrum of encephalomyopathies due to defects in mitochondrial metabolism exists. This ranges from neonatal onset of severe and fatal disease to a mild myopathy, in which ptosis is prominent, appearing in adult life. Some clearly defined syndromes associated with mutations in the mitochondrial genome include:

- **chronic progressive external ophthalmoplegia (CPEO). This is characterized by ptosis and** ophthalmoplegia which is followed by weakness in the muscles of the shoulder girdle and upper limbs.

- *m*yopathy, *e*ncephalopathy, *l*actic *a*cidosis, *s*troke (**MELAS**)
- *m*yoclonic *e*pilepsy and *r*agged *r*ed *f*ibres (**MERRF**)

MERRF and MELAS are associated with point mutations on certain mitochondrial genes and CPEO with large deletions. The first two are inherited through the maternal line. CPEO is, however, sporadic as the large deletions are incompatible with ovum survival. It is interesting that the cells most severely and commonly affected are 'permanent' cells such as neurones, cardiac muscle and skeletal muscle. This may be a reflection of the possibility that, in cell populations where there is a regular 'turn over', cells with large numbers of abnormal mitochondria are eliminated.

Mitochondrial proteins are derived from two sources:

1) **the DNA of the cell's nucleus.** These proteins are transported across the mitochondrial membrane from the cytosol. This transport is in one direction only, there being no evidence that proteins coded for within the mitochondria are exported from it.

2) **the mitochondrial DNA, which shows a strictly maternal rather than a mendelian pattern of inheritance**, and in which the genetic code differs from that of nuclear DNA. Various antibiotics such as chloramphenicol, tetracyclines and erythromycin inhibit mitochondrial protein synthesis, as they do in chloroplasts. It is believed that the differences in protein synthesis reflect the fact that mitochondria evolved from bacteria endocytosed more than one billion years ago.

Microscopic Features

The defining morphological criterion of mitochondrial myopathies is the ragged red fibre. This is a muscle fibre containing large aggregates of peripheral and interfibrillar mitochondria, seen as granular red staining deposits in frozen sections of muscle stained with a modification of the Gomori trichrome stain. These collections of mitochondria can also be demonstrated by stains for succinate dehydrogenase, an exclusively intramitochondrial enzyme.

The abnormal fibres also show more fine droplets of neutral lipid than do normal muscle fibres and an excess of glycogen. In some ragged red fibres, **there is an absence of cytochrome *c* oxidase**; this is particularly likely to occur in patients with:

- **progressive external ophthalmoplegia**
- **a fatal infantile myopathy**, which may be associated with the Fanconi syndrome or hypertrophic cardiomyopathy

- **Leigh's syndrome**, a complex and variable combination of intellectual impairment, fits, anorexia, vomiting, cerebellar ataxia, intention tremor, nystagmus, optic atrophy, deafness, ptosis, hypotonic weakness, spasticity and peripheral neuropathy

On electron microscopic examination, a wide range of abnormalities has been described. Individual mitochondria may be grossly enlarged and show abundant cristae in which complex branching may be seen. Many intramitochondrial inclusions have been described, the most common of which have a paracrystalline structure (*Fig. 45.64*).

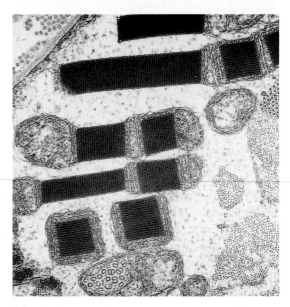

FIGURE 45.64 *Mitochondrial myopathy. Electron micrograph showing the curious intramitochondrial bars seen in this group of disorders.*

METABOLIC MYOPATHIES

This term is applied to specific enzyme defects interfering with normal energy production in muscle cells. Glycogen, glucose and free fatty acids constitute the main source for muscle energy and a number of errors in the metabolism of glycogen and lipid affects muscle. Clinically, these disorders are expressed in two main forms:

1) **progressive weakness**
2) **muscle cramps induced by exercise and which may or may not be associated with muscle necrosis and myoglobinuria**

Although the various metabolic abnormalities affecting energy pathways in muscle have been well explored, the basis of the clinical syndromes listed above is still not clear. It is clearly too simplistic to attribute them to an acute or chronic energy deficit.

- **Muscle-specific enzyme defects. If the defective or absent enzyme exists as a muscle-specific isoform, then the clinical expression of the defect will be confined to muscle.**
- **Non-muscle-specific enzyme defects. If the enzyme is not muscle specific then the metabolic defect will present as a multisystem disorder.**

In general terms the distinguishing microscopic feature of these disorders on light microscopy is the presence of vacuoles within the muscle cells. While these vacuoles appear empty in haematoxylin and eosin-stained sections, they contain either accumulated **carbohydrate** substrates (as shown by a magenta colour when sections are stained by the PAS method)

or **lipid**, which can be demonstrated by a variety of fat-soluble dyes. A considerable variation exists in the severity with which muscle cells are affected and this is reflected in a similar degree of variation in the degree of vacuolation.

It must also be borne in mind that defects in mitochondrial metabolism may cause accumulation of carbohydrate and lipid substrates in addition to the mitochondrial morphological abnormalities to which reference has been made in the preceding section.

The Glycogenoses

There are several well-recognized enzyme defects affecting glycogen metabolism or glycolysis in muscle. These are listed in *Table 45.26*.

Table 45.26 The Glycogenoses

Type	Enzyme	Eponym	Clinical and pathological features
II	Acid maltase	In infantile form – Pompe's disease	Acid maltase deficiency causes two main syndromes: • **the infantile form (Pompe's disease)** is generalized and usually fatal. Affected infants are 'floppy' and there is massive cardiomegaly and somewhat less pronounced hepatomegaly. Death due to cardiac or respiratory failure occurs before the age of 2 years. • **the childhood and adult forms present as a myopathy without cardiac involvement.** In the childhood form there may be calf hypertrophy similar to that seen in Duchenne-type dystrophy. Death may occur in the second or third decade in the childhood form, generally as a result of respiratory failure. In the infantile form vacuoles in the muscle fibres are very numerous but this is less marked in the childhood and adult forms. The accumulated glycogen is stored within lysosomes and in the cytoplasm, where it may form large pools.
III	Debrancher deficiency	Cori–Forbes disease	A benign disease of childhood characterized by hepatomegaly, failure to grow normally and fasting hypoglycaemia. A significant myopathy is uncommon but some affected individuals develop a disorder in the third or fourth decade associated with wasting of leg muscles and of intrinsic muscles of the hand. Muscle biopsy shows severe vacuolar myopathy with PAS-positive material in the vacuoles.
IV	Branching enzyme deficiency	Andersen's disease	This variant is dominated by liver disease progressing to cirrhosis. Death usually occurs by 4 years either from liver failure or from bleeding associated with portal hypertension. On electron microscopic examination of muscle, an abnormal polysaccharide with a filamentous and/or granular structure is seen and this is expressed in the form of basophilic PAS-positive deposits on light microscopy.

Table 45.26 The Glycogenoses – *continued*

Type	Enzyme	Eponym	Clinical and pathological features
V	Muscle phosphorylase	McArdle's disease	This causes exercise intolerance characterized by muscle pain, abnormally early fatigue and muscle cramps. Symptoms may be caused by intense brief exercise such as lifting weights or more sustained, less intense, exercise such as walking up a hill. Many patients typically experience a 'second wind' if they slow down at the first sign of muscle pain, but some go on to develop muscle necrosis and myoglobinuria. Permanent muscle weakness is also seen in some patients, this being more common in older patients.

Muscle biopsy shows the presence of glycogen vacuoles in both subsarcolemmal and interfibrillar locations, although the amounts of such glycogen may be small. Histochemical studies show complete absence of myophosphorylase. The disorder is inherited in an autosomal recessive pattern; the gene encoding the enzyme is located on the long arm of chromosome 11. |
| VII | Muscle phospho-fructokinase | Tarui's disease | This has a clinical picture similar to that in McArdle's disease, although myoglobinuria and hence muscle necrosis are less common. Differentiation from McArdle's disease requires biochemical studies of muscle. Some degree of clinical heterogeneity is present; some patients have late-onset proximal weakness with no cramps and in some there is a fatal infantile myopathy.

Microscopic appearance of muscle biopsies resembles McArdle's disease.

The inheritance pattern is autosomal recessive. |
IX	Phosphoglycerate kinase		This may be clinically silent or present in one of two main forms: • intellectual impairment, seizures and haemolytic anaemia in infancy or early childhood • exercise intolerance and recurrent episodes of myoglobinuria in childhood or early adult life There is no muscle-specific isoform but, despite this, muscle alone has been involved in some patients.
X	Phosphoglycerate mutase		This is extremely rare. The patients thus far described have all shown intolerance to intense exercise, associated with muscle pain, cramps and myoglobinuria.
XI	Lactic dehydrogenase		This is also extremely rare and presents with intolerance to exercise and recurrent myoglobinuria.

Disorders of Lipid Metabolism

Long-chain fatty acids constitute an important source of energy for muscle, especially under the following circumstances:

• **fasting**, when glycogen stores become depleted
• **during prolonged exercise** which cannot be sustained by carbohydrate fuels

The fatty acids are transported to the muscle in the

form of free fatty acids bound to albumin or as very low density lipoprotein. Once within the muscle cells, a number of metabolic steps occur requiring:

- carnitine
- carnitine palmitoyltransferase I
- carnitine palmitoyltransferase II

The long-chain fatty acids in the form of LC AcylCoA (long chain) and within the mitochondria are now ready to undergo **β-oxidation**.

- **The first step in this process requires short-, medium- and long-chain acylCoA dehydrogenases.**
- **The second step requires an enoylCoA hydratase.**
- **The third step requires two nicotinamide adenine dinucleotide (NAD)-dependent 3-hydroxyacylCoA dehydrogenases.**
- **The fourth and final step requires a number of ketothiolases.**

Absence of any relevant substrate or enzyme may lead to one of a number of muscle disorders.

INFLAMMATORY MYOPATHIES

The inflammatory disorders peculiar to muscle are:

- **dermatomyositis**
- **polymyositis**
- **inclusion body myositis**

The histological appearances of the first two show some resemblances and for a long time they were thought to be variants of the same disorder. The resemblances are in fact more apparent than real and it is now appreciated that the pathogenetic mechanisms involved are quite different.

Clinically, all the inflammatory myopathies present with gradual and insidious onset of muscle weakness, the precise manifestations depending on the muscle groups involved. For example, dysphagia, which is a well-recognized clinical feature, reflects involvement of the pharyngeal muscles, and difficulty in combing the hair indicates shoulder girdle involvement. In some instances, the affected muscles may be painful. Plasma concentrations of CPK are raised, the degree of increase reflecting the severity of muscle cell injury.

Dermatomyositis

Dermatomyositis affects both sexes and may occur at any age, in contrast to polymyositis which appears to be a disease of adult life only. In the older patients, about 15% show an association with malignancy: adenocarcinomas of the stomach, breast, ovary, lung and colon are the most common. In some, resection of the neoplasm has been followed by regression of the dermatomyositis.

In dermatomyositis, biopsy material shows all stages of segmental necrosis and regeneration of the fibres.

The inflammatory infiltrate is composed chiefly of B lymphocytes and is concentrated in the perimysial connective tissue where perivascular aggregates of the lymphocytes are not infrequent. T lymphocytes, mainly CD4 (helper) cells, are seen in the endomysial region.

Areas of necrosis involve small groups of fibres in a pattern suggesting ischaemic damage (*Fig. 45.65*). This view is strengthened by the relative decrease in capillaries in the affected areas. The combination of these last two morphological features with the B-cell predominance in the perimysium suggests that **the muscle necrosis is secondary to ischaemia due to an antibody-mediated attack on capillaries**. Supportive evidence derives from the fact that components of the membrane attack complex of complement can be identified on the capillary walls early in the disease.

Skin changes accompanying the muscle disorder are either those of a non-specific dermatitis or similar to those seen in lupus erythematosus.

Polymyositis

In this condition, the inflammatory infiltrate is predominantly lymphocytic (*Fig. 45.66*). There is no evidence

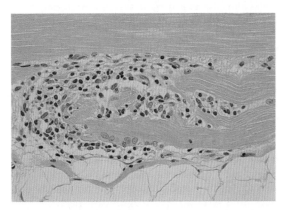

FIGURE 45.65 Inflammatory myopathy showing focal necrosis of muscle and a brisk inflammatory cell response.

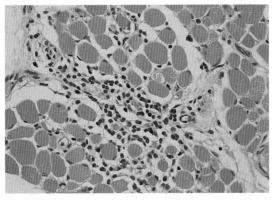

FIGURE 45.66 Focal lymphocytic infiltrate seen in polymyositis.

of damage to small blood vessels. **It is believed that the muscle cell injury is the result of an attack by cytotoxic T lymphocytes**, which, accompanied by macrophages, invade the muscle fibres. Major histocompatibility complex class I antigens are expressed on the sarcolemma of the muscle fibres, something not seen in normal skeletal muscle cells. In the early stages of the disease, before there is evidence of muscle cell necrosis, healthy muscle fibres are surrounded by CD8+ T cells and macrophages. The inflammatory infiltrate is predominantly endomysial in position and is focal.

Inclusion Body Myositis

Inclusion body myositis is a disorder affecting principally the elderly. It has an insidious onset and can be distinguished clinically from the inflammatory myopathies described above by failure to respond to steroid treatment.

In part, the histological picture resembles that seen in polymyositis in that the inflammatory process is localized chiefly to the endomysial region and cytotoxic T cells make up the most significant element in the inflammatory cell population.

The defining criteria, however, are:

- **vacuoles bordered by basophilic material within muscle fibres, and which are believed to be lysosomal in origin**
- **eosinophilic inclusions within affected muscle cells.** These may be found either within or closely related to the vacuoles described above. Electron microscopy shows these inclusions to consist of very numerous electron-dense fibrils. Similar inclusions have been found in the rare oculopharyngeal muscular dystrophy and some other equally rare distal myopathies.

It has been suggested that these histological features are consistent with self-digestion of affected muscle cells (autophagy) in which the lysosomal system plays a significant part.

RHABDOMYOLYSIS

This is a severe form of diffuse muscle necrosis. In its acute form, it is characterized by:

- sudden onset of severe muscle pain
- flaccid paralysis of the affected muscles
- myoglobinuria which may be sufficiently severe to cause acute renal failure

As might be expected with extensive necrosis of muscle fibres, the plasma concentration of CPK is greatly raised.

Acute rhabdomyolysis is sometimes associated with influenza. Many drugs and toxins have also been implicated. However, it is still unclear as to whether these compounds exert a directly toxic effect on the muscle cells or produce their effects indirectly. For instance, it

has been suggested that the rhabdomyolysis following alcohol or drug overdose may be due to muscle compression and ischaemia as a result of prolonged unconsciousness and immobility.

Muscle biopsy shows coagulative necrosis of muscle fibres which has elicited a mild interstitial inflammatory cell infiltrate in which macrophages are prominent. If a considerable time has elapsed since the insult that led to the necrosis, signs of regenerative activity may be present.

EFFECTS OF DENERVATION

In contrast to the myopathies, **the pathology of denervated muscle is the expression of a very limited range of reaction patterns**. It results from **damage to the lower motor neurone** of several different types. It is usually possible on muscle biopsy to make a diagnosis of denervation atrophy but not of the cause of the denervation.

Microscopic Features

The microscopic picture of denervation change in muscle is a combination of:

- **atrophy of muscle fibres.** A single anterior horn cell innervates many muscle cells. While they are close to one another, they are intermingled with fibres supplied by other motor units. Damage to either the anterior horn cell or the proximal axon will cause all contraction in this group of muscle fibres to cease and thus the **group** of muscle cells will become atrophic (*Fig. 45.67*). As the myofibrils and myofilaments of an individual fibre atrophy, that fibre becomes compressed by adjacent fibres and assumes an angular shape. If there is ineffective reinnervation, the fibre eventually becomes completely atrophic and the nuclei condense to form aggregates.
- **cytoplasmic changes. When sections are stained to demonstrate oxidative enzymes, the cells appear to stain more darkly than normal muscle cells.** This is because the site of the reaction is the extrafibrillar cytoplasmic constituents which become condensed in denervated fibres as a result of the loss of myofibrils.

Target fibres (see *Table 45.23*) occur in up to 20% of cases. Numerous target fibres constitute a very reliable indicator of neurogenic change in muscle. The target change occurs soon after denervation and its presence therefore acts also as an indicator of **activity of the denervating process**.

EFFECTS OF REINNERVATION

Denervated muscle fibres act as a stimulus for the sprouting of new nerve fibres from the preterminal

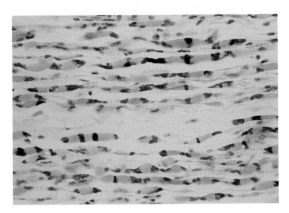

FIGURE 45.67 Total denervation atrophy. All the fibres in this field show severe and uniform atrophy; very little sarcoplasm remains.

regions of adjacent normal axons. This sprouting is associated with branching of preterminal axons so that a single axon may now supply a number of muscle fibres. The motor units are thus increased in size.

The physiological functions, and hence the enzyme pattern of individual muscle fibres, depend on the electrical stimuli received from the motor nerves. Thus reinnervation can lead to a change in the muscle fibre type; this is expressed in muscle biopsies by the formation of quite large groups of muscle fibres, uniform in terms of their enzyme pattern. This change is referred to as **type grouping**. Rapidly progressive disease is reflected by type 1 fibre predominance, whereas chronic, slowly progressive denervation is usually associated with type 2 fibre grouping.

DEFECTS IN NEUROMUSCULAR TRANSMISSION

Myasthenia Gravis and Other Myasthenic Syndromes

Myasthenia is expressed in the form of:
- **abnormal muscle fatiguability**
- **muscle weakness**

It is a set of acquired autoimmune disorders in which autoantibodies bind either to the acetylcholine receptor on the motor endplate (myasthenia gravis and neonatal myasthenia) or to the presynaptic membrane with blockage of the release of acetylcholine (Lambert–Eaton syndrome associated with malignancy).

Myasthenia gravis may affect the extraocular and/or bulbar muscles predominantly, or may be systemic. In the latter case the respiratory muscles may be severely affected and the patient may need mechanical ventilation.

Pathogenesis

In myasthenia gravis and neonatal myasthenia, immunoglobulin (Ig) G autoantibodies are present in the serum of the affected individual. These bind to various epitopes on the acetylcholine receptor. A pathogenic role for these antibodies is indicated by the fact that clinical features of the myasthenic syndrome can be induced by passive transfer of the antibodies to experimental animals. **Binding of autoantibodies to the acetylcholine receptor not only blocks the receptor so that acetylcholine cannot bind to it, but also binds complement, leading to destruction of some of the receptors.**

Electron microscopy shows changes in the postsynaptic membrane and in the junctional folds of the motor endplate.

Myasthenia Gravis Shows a Strong Association with Abnormalities in the Thymus

Up to 40% of patients with myasthenia gravis have an associated thymoma and, in many of these, the myasthenic syndrome will be relieved by thymectomy. Of the remaining cases, 75% show thymic hyperplasia and here, too, thymectomy may lead to disappearance of the clinical features of myasthenia. The presence of a thymoma is likely to be associated with an HLA-B12 haplotype and with autoantibodies binding to cardiac and skeletal muscle, as well as those that react with the acetylcholine receptor. The thymus plays an important part in the pathogenesis of myasthenia gravis, but how it does so is not at all clear. It is true that some muscle cells with acetylcholine receptors are present within the thymus and may act as the immunogen source in this disorder, but the reason for this, if it occurs, is still not known.

Neonatal Myasthenia Gravis

This occurs in a small proportion (10–15%) of the infants born to mothers with myasthenia gravis. It is further evidence of a pathogenic role for the IgG anti-acetylcholine receptor antibodies which, of course, can cross the placenta. The risks of such an infant developing transient myasthenia correlate with the concentration of the antibodies in the mother's serum.

The Lambert–Eaton Syndrome

This myasthenic syndrome is associated with wasting of the proximal limb muscles and the muscles of the trunk. It is one of the **non-metastatic manifestations of malignancy**. The neoplasm most commonly expressed in this way is **small cell carcinoma of the lung**.

The myasthenia is due to an autoantibody that binds to an antigen on the presynaptic membrane and inhibits the release of acetylcholine from the nerve terminals. It has been suggested that the binding site for this autoantibody is a calcium channel on the presynaptic membrane, but this is not yet certain.

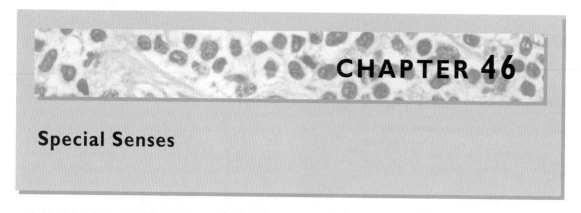

CHAPTER 46

Special Senses

The Eye

The pathological conditions affecting the eye are many and various. They are most easily approached on the basis of the anatomical locations which constitute the particular targets for eye diseases.

THE EYELIDS

Because the eyelid consists largely of skin, it can be affected by many of the disorders that affect the skin elsewhere. These are not discussed here. Disorders *peculiar* to the eyelid may arise as described below.

Developmental Abnormalities

Dermoid cysts often affect the upper lid. The lesions are rounded and usually not greater than 1 cm in diameter. They are soft and non-tender, and rest on, or are attached to, the periosteum of the orbital ridges. Microscopic examination shows them to be lined by well-differentiated epidermis; their lumina are filled with keratinous debris.

Inflammation (Acute and Chronic)

Inflammation of the lids (blepharitis) can arise on the basis of all the known causes of inflammation. Common varieties include:

- **Sty (hordeolum)** – an acute suppurative inflammation involving the hair follicles or the ducts of either sebaceous or apocrine glands. *Staphylococcus aureus* is frequently implicated in the pathogenesis of sty. The lesion is red and tender, and pus may be discharged though the site of the affected eyelash follicle.
- **Chalazion** – a chronic inflammatory lesion involving the meibomian glands which normally drain via an opening just posterior to the hair follicle of the eyelash. The basic pathological process is obstruction to the drainage of these glands. Pressure therefore rises within the duct system and rupture eventually occurs releasing the lipid-rich contents of the meibomian gland epithelium into the extraductal tissues. This elicits a florid inflammatory reaction in which lipid-laden macrophages, lymphocytes and plasma cells are present.

Cysts

Apart from the developmental dermoid cysts described above and acquired epidermal cysts (the commonest variety seen in the eyelids), cysts of Moll's glands occur. These present as thin-walled transparent blister-like lesions at the free margin of the lid. Microscopic examination shows them to be unilocular cysts lined by atrophic cuboidal epithelium or, less frequently, by flattened epithelial cells.

Tumours and Tumour-like Nodules

All the tumours of skin tissues described in another section (see pp 1019–1032) can and do affect the eyelid. The most frequent of these is basal carcinoma. One lesion worth commenting on in this context is the pigmented melanocytic naevus known as the **naevus of Ota** (congenital oculodermal melanosis). This is believed to be an extrasacral form of mongolian spot involving the skin supplied by the first and second branches of the trigeminal nerve. It occurs most commonly among Orientals and Afro-Caribbeans.

A common non-neoplastic nodule is the **xanthelasma**. This is a yellow, plaque-like lesion occurring on the medial aspect of both lids. Microscopic examination shows these lesions to consist of aggregates of lipid-filled macrophages. In the young, they tend to be associated with hyperlipidaemic states, but their appearance in the middle aged and elderly may be without significance in relation to lipid metabolism.

THE CONJUNCTIVA

The conjunctiva is affected by the following major classes of disorder:
- degenerative
- inflammatory
- neoplastic

DEGENERATIVE CONJUNCTIVAL DISORDERS

Pinguecula

This is a common process affecting the subepithelial connective tissue of the bulbar conjunctiva in the interpalpebral area. The lesion presents as a small yellowish area of thickening.

Microscopic examination shows elastosis in the subepithelial tissues similar to that seen in skin after long periods of exposure to ultraviolet light. There is hyalinization of the interfibrillar ground substance. In some cases the overlying epithelium is atrophic but in others it is so thickened as to give rise to suspicions of epithelial malignancy.

Pterygium

This lesion is in many ways similar to pinguecula but occurs at the junction between the sclera and the cornea and frequently spreads to involve the corneal conjunctiva. Microscopic examination again shows some actinic elastosis but there is also some new blood vessel formation and chronic inflammation. As the lesion spreads over the cornea it causes opacification and visual impairment.

Squamous Metaplasia

The conjunctival and corneal epithelia are normally thin and non-keratinized. They may be replaced by thick, opaque, keratinized squamous epithelium (squamous metaplasia).

Squamous metaplasia occurs under a number of different circumstances:

- the 'dry eye' syndrome where there are no tears, such as occurs in Sjögren's syndrome
- in vitamin A deficiency. Here the process often spreads to involve the cornea, the corneal areas of opacification being known as Bitot's spots
- in severe exophthalmos where the eyelids cannot close and the conjunctiva is exposed to excess amounts of irritation
- where there is paralysis of the muscle of the eyelid so that eyelid closure cannot take place
- in graft versus host disease

INFLAMMATORY CONJUNCTIVAL DISEASE

Inflammation may involve:

- the conjunctiva alone (conjunctivitis)
- the cornea alone (keratitis)
- both (keratoconjunctivitis)

The causes of conjunctival inflammation are summarized in *Table 46.1*.

NEOPLASTIC CONJUNCTIVAL DISEASE

Papilloma of the Conjunctiva

This is a relatively common lesion which tends to recur after excision. In children, the lesions tend to be multiple. Microscopic examination shows the typical appearances of a papilloma in which varying degrees of keratinization and acanthosis are encountered. The finding of koilocytosis (see p 769) in the epithelial cells suggests a viral origin. This has been confirmed: human papillomavirus types 6 and 11 has been found by *in situ* hybridization.

Intraepithelial Carcinoma (Carcinoma *In Situ*)

This is a well-recognized entity in the conjunctiva and cornea, presenting as a leukoplakic area, a papillary lesion or a complication of pterygium. The microscopic features are identical with those of carcinoma *in situ* in any mucous membrane.

Invasive Squamous Carcinoma

This is rare but more common than basal cell carcinoma of the conjunctiva. Invasive carcinomas at this site are seldom seen because the lesions tend to be treated at an earlier stage of their natural history. Many of the invasive tumours tend to show features similar to those of mucoepidermoid carcinoma of the salivary glands.

Melanocytic Naevi and Malignant Melanoma

Melanocytic naevi are not uncommon at this site. They are invariably either junctional or compound in nature (see pp 1024–1025) and often show cystic epithelial inclusions. Malignant melanoma is very rare.

THE CORNEA

NORMAL STRUCTURE

- The outer surface of the cornea is covered by flattened, non-keratinizing, squamous epithelium.
- Deep to this is an acellular region measuring 10–16 μm, known as Bowman's membrane. **If Bowman's membrane is damaged, healing of keratitis is likely to be accompanied by scarring and hence by impairment of vision.**
- the corneal stroma lying deep to Bowman's membrane is made up of regularly arranged collagen fibres embedded within a proteoglycan-rich matrix. A small cell population resembling fibrocytes is present in the stroma.
- The posterior surface of the stroma is lined by a basement membrane known as Descemet's membrane.
- Descemet's membrane is covered by a layer of endothelial cells which effectively control the fluid content of the corneal stroma.

DISORDERS OF THE CORNEA

Keratoconus

This is a congenital ectasia of the central part of the cornea which usually manifests within the first decade of life. It is often associated with atopy and tends also to occur in patients with Down's syndrome. Breaks appear in Bowman's membrane and there is thinning of the stromal component of the cornea.

Fuchs' Endothelial Dystrophy

This is an age-related disorder affecting principally the endothelium and Descemet's membrane. Loss of

Table 46.1 Inflammation of the Conjunctiva and/or Cornea

Basic group	Causes
Bacterial	Acute bacterial conjunctivitis is common, especially in childhood. Common causes include *Haemophilus aegyptius*, staphylococci and *Streptococcus pneumoniae*. Conjunctivitis due to *Neisseria gonorrhoeae* most commonly affects the newborn, maternal–fetal infection being likely to occur during delivery. Congenital syphilis affects the cornea, producing an interstitial inflammation lasting 2–3 months and followed by new blood vessel formation.
Viral	The viruses most commonly implicated are herpesviruses and adenoviruses (see pp 192–193); herpesviruses are particularly liable to damage the cornea severely and cause corneal ulceration (see below). Measles is commonly associated with a mild to moderate conjunctivitis during the prodromal period of the illness. In sub-Saharan Africa this is frequently associated with corneal ulceration which leads to scarring and blindness.
Chlamydial	**Trachoma** is the single most important cause of blindness in developing countries. It is caused by *Chlamydia trachomatis*, mainly serotypes A, B and C. Infection is spread via eye to eye contact through the agency of flies. The inflammation is characterized by the formation of lymphoid follicles which enlarge, develop germinal centres and then undergo central necrosis. Characteristic cytoplasmic inclusions can be found in the conjunctival epithelial cells. The cellular infiltrate is gradually replaced by granulation tissue which becomes converted to scar tissue and may produce severe distortion of the lids and the lacrimal ducts. **Chlamydial ophthalmitis in neonates** is caused generally by serotypes D–I. Infection is usually acquired during passage through the birth canal. This is now the commonest form of neonatal ocular inflammation.
Protozoal	*Acanthamoeba castellani* and *A. polyphaga* can cause a severe and intractable keratoconjunctivitis. These parasites have brackish or sea water as their natural habitat but can contaminate contact lens cleaning fluid. The repetitive minor trauma associated with the wearing of contact lenses may promote infection.
Helminthic	**Onchocerciasis** (loa loa) is caused by infestations with the worm *Onchocerca volvulus*. This worm is currently believed to infest more than 17 million people, most of whom live in sub-Saharan Africa. Blindness affects particularly those living in the savannas rather than the rain forests. Infection is transmitted by blackflies which inject larvae into the human host's dermis in the course of a blood meal. Eye disease is caused by microfilariae, which migrate from the skin of the face. All eye tissues can be affected. The conjunctiva and cornea show fluffy opacities in the cornea which leads to scarring.
Chemical	Any strong chemicals (alkalis, acids, fixatives, etc.)
Sunlight	Keratoconjunctivitis can occur after severe ultraviolet light exposure, as for example in 'snow blindness'
Trauma	
Immune	Allergic conjunctivitis typically occurs when contamination of the atmosphere by pollens is greatest. This so-called 'vernal conjunctivitis' is usually bilateral and is characterized by flat-topped papillae of oedematous conjunctiva containing a cellular infiltrate rich in eosinophils. Phlyctenular conjunctivitis represents a delayed hypersensitivity response to antigens of *Mycobacterium* and *Staphylococcus aureus*. It is expressed in the form of tough, roughly triangular, areas at the limbus of the cornea. These break down but the ulcers heal within 2–3 weeks.

endothelium leads to a failure of control of the fluid content of the cornea which becomes grossly oedematous. Occasionally this situation appears to be precipitated by cataract surgery and blisters appear in relation to the epithelium. In this context the corneal endothelial changes are termed aphakic bullous keratopathy.

Inherited Corneal Dystrophies

These are familial syndromes in which abnormal material is deposited within the cornea. Three principal types are recognized:

- **Lattice dystrophy** is inherited in an autosomal dominant fashion. It is characterized by the deposition of amyloid within the stroma and scarring which affects Bowman's membrane.

- **Granular dystrophy** is also an autosomal dominant disorder in which masses of protein crystals are deposited deep to Bowman's membrane in the central part of the cornea.
- **Macular dystrophy** is an autosomal recessive disease in which there is cloudiness of the cornea due to the deposition of masses of glycosoaminoglycan which is rich in keratan sulphate. These patients usually show serious impairment of vision by the age of 30 years.

Inflammatory Ulceration of the Cornea

Herpes simplex virus infections and fungal infections may cause serious damage to the cornea. Such infections may manifest as dendritic ulceration or stromal keratitis.

Dendritic Ulceration

Here the inflammation and associated damage is largely confined to the epithelial layer. The associated ulcers have a branched appearance (dendritic) which can be

recognized if fluorescein is instilled into the eye, as the fluorescein stains the exposed Bowman's membrane. As stated above, if Bowman's membrane is intact, healing takes place without scarring.

Stromal Keratitis

Both the epithelium and the stroma show oedema. Bowman's membrane frequently shows evidence of damage and there is a patchy infiltration by neutrophils and lymphocytes. Characteristic Cowdry type A intranuclear inclusions may be found in the epithelial cells in cases of herpetic keratitis. Giant cells are found characteristically in relation to Descemet's membrane. In fungal keratitis it is possible to demonstrate the fungal hyphae (*Fig. 46.1*).

Recurrent episodes lead to corneal scarring which can be treated rationally only by corneal transplantation.

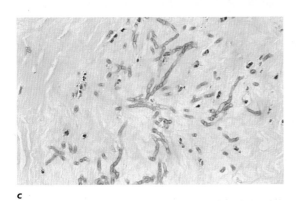

a

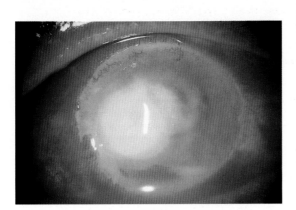

c

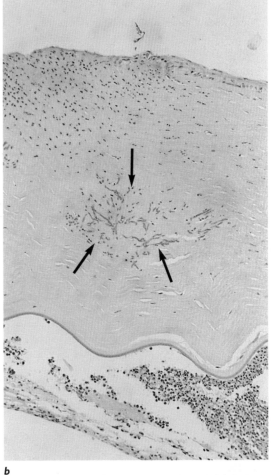

b

FIGURE 46.1 **a** *Herpes simplex keratitis. The sclera is markedly reddened; the cornea is opaque and oedematous, and the large white area seen centrally represents a corneal abscess.* **b** *A full-thickness section through the cornea in a case of fungal (Aspergillus fumigatus) keratitis. There is some subepithelial inflammation and a 'colony' of fungal hyphae in the centre of the cornea (arrows). Below Descemet's membrane, a collection of acute inflammatory cells can be seen (arrow).* **c** *A higher-power view of the section shown in* **b** *in which the fungal hyphae can be seen clearly.*

THE LENS

NORMAL STRUCTURE

The lens is a biconvex object formed by epithelial cells which contain lens protein. The whole structure is enclosed in an elastic membrane. Fine focusing is brought about by forces exerted on the equatorial portion of the lens by the ciliary muscles.

DISORDERS OF THE LENS

Cataract

This term is used to describe opacification of the lens. Such opacification can arise in many different ways (see *Table 46.2*).

Table 46.2 Causes of Cataract

Cause	Key features
Genetic	Autosomal dominant; cataract inherited alone
Genetic and systemic syndrome	Occurs in Alport's and Marfan's syndromes
Congenital	Consequence of rubella infection Associated with trisomy 13
Galactosaemia	Dulcitol accumulates in lens and creates a powerful osmotic gradient with much fluid collecting in lens
Diabetes	Poorly controlled diabetes mellitus is a powerful incremental factor in cataract formation. Operation of the polyol pathway (see p 853) leads to the accumulation of sorbitol, which produces fluid accumulation within the lens
Drugs	Long-term treatment with steroids Also induced by the uncoupling agent dinitrophenol
Long-term exposure to ultraviolet light or irradiation	
Trauma	
Age related	

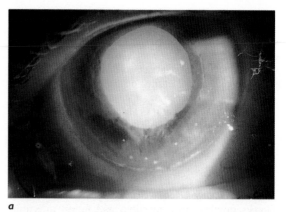

a

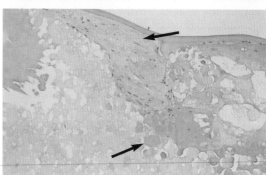

b

FIGURE 46.2 *a* A very advanced cataract. Note the white pupil. This case was complicated by glaucoma. *b* Section of a cataract showing the fibrous tissue plaque at the periphery of the lens (arrow) and the globule formation that has occurred within the lens substance (arrow).

The commonest types of cataract are those associated with ageing and/or diabetes. Because of the opacification of the lens, the pupil appears white and opaque (*Fig. 46.2a*). Four histological variants of cataract are described. The one illustrated here is an anterior subcapsular cataract in which the lens epithelial cells first proliferate, and then secrete a collagenous layer. Development of the cataract is characterized by the formation of clefts within the lens substance, which become filled with globules known as morgagnian globules (*Fig. 46.2b*)

THE UVEAL TRACT

UVEITIS

The uveal tract consists of the **iris, ciliary body and choroid. The pathological process most often affecting the uvea is inflammation** (uveitis), and the terminology used reflects the portion of the tract most affected. Thus inflammation of the iris is termed **iritis**, that of the ciliary body is **cyclitis**, and that of the choroid is **choroiditis**.

Most uveal tract inflammation produces:
- a red, painful eye
- sensitivity to bright light
- blurring of vision
- slight pupillary constriction
- in some cases, collections of pus in the anterior chamber of the eye. This is termed a hypopyon. Following iritis, adhesions may form between the iris and the lens (**posterior synechia**) or between the anterior chamber angle and the most peripheral part of the iris (**anterior synechia**).

Uveitis may occur either as an isolated phenomenon or as part of some other disease. In the former case, the cause is unknown but the proportion of affected individuals with human leucocyte antigen (HLA)-B27 is high.

Systemic associations of uveitis include Reiter's syndrome, ankylosing spondylitis, ulcerative colitis, juvenile rheumatoid arthritis and Behçet's syndrome.

Sympathetic Ophthalmitis
This term describes a fortunately rare condition in which penetrating injury of the eye involving uveal tract tissue protrusion is followed by uveal tract inflammation in the uninjured eye. The lag phase between injury and the appearance of inflammation, first in the injured eye and then in the other eye (the sympathizing eye), is usually 4–6 weeks but intervals of months or even years have been recorded.

Removal of the injured eye inhibits the development of inflammation in the second eye. However, removal is effective only if carried out before the onset of sympathetic inflammation; after this, removal of the injured eye has no effect.

The inflammation is granulomatous and affects the choroid. Sympathetic ophthalmitis is believed to be an autoimmune reaction. For a long time the responsible antigen was believed to be related to the choroid, but it has now been suggested that the S antigen of the retina is responsible for eliciting the response.

GLAUCOMA: A DISORDER OF RAISED INTRAOCULAR PRESSURE
Exchange of fluid and solutes between the blood and aqueous humour occurs in the ciliary body and iris. Ciliary epithelial cells have tight junctions which control the passage of macromolecules across the blood–aqueous humour boundary.

Pressure within the eye is regulated by:
- the rate at which secretion occurs from the ciliary body
- the rate of outflow of aqueous humour into the canal of Schlemm

Aqueous secretion is maintained at a constant level, thus **the principal factor controlling intraocular pressure is the rate of outflow of the aqueous**. If aqueous outflow is impaired, the pressure within the eye rises. Eventually it reaches a level that exceeds the

perfusion pressure in the small vessels supplying the neural tissues of the eye. Perfusion will fall and irreversible ischaemic damage may occur leading to blindness. The disorders leading to such pathological levels of intraocular pressure are classified as **glaucoma**.

Obstruction to the outflow of aqueous may occur in the following contexts:

'Open Angle Glaucoma'
This is due to increased resistance to outflow in the trabecular meshwork. This occurs in two forms:

1) **Primary.** This is a disorder of insidious onset which most commonly affects the elderly. In many instances there is evidence of familial disease but the mode of inheritance is not clear. The pathological changes leading to increased resistance to outflow are not understood.

2) **Secondary.** This occurs as a result of blockage of the trabecular meshwork. The blockage may be due to:
- red cells or cell debris following trauma
- macrophages filled with lens protein following rupture of a 'hypermature' cataract. This is termed phacolytic glaucoma.
- flakes of glycoprotein exfoliated from basement membranes

Closed-Angle Glaucoma
In this form, the trabecular meshwork is obstructed by the root of the iris. In individuals with shallow anterior chambers, the iris and the lens may be forced into contact when the iris is half dilated. Closed-angle glaucoma also occurs in primary and secondary forms; the former, which is rare, tends to have an acute onset. Secondary closed-angle glaucoma is due to adhesions between the peripheral part of the cornea and the iris (posterior synechia).

Effects of Raised Intraocular Pressure
Abnormally high levels of pressure in the eye produce damage to the **cornea, retina and optic nerve**. The endothelial layer lining the posterior surface of the cornea is susceptible to the rise in pressure, and degenerates. Thus the normal control of fluid levels within the cornea is lost and the cornea becomes oedematous. Ganglion cells are lost from both the retina and the optic nerve. In the nerve, this is associated with atrophy of some axons. An additional striking feature is outward displacement of the cribriform plate which produces a 'cupped' appearance of the optic disc.

THE RETINA

VASCULAR DISEASES
Vascular disease affecting the retina may result from:
- occlusion of the central **artery** of the retina
- occlusion of the central retinal **vein**

- systemic hypertension
- diabetes mellitus
- retrolental fibroplasia
- vasculitis, most notably giant cell arteritis (see pp 403–404)

Occlusion of the Central Artery

This is most commonly caused by the impaction of an embolus. Emboli, as in other types of occlusive disease of the intracranial arterial tree, usually arise from the left side of the heart (e.g. infective endocarditis, atrial myxoma) or from atherosclerosis involving the carotid vessels. Fat or air emboli are occasionally involved in central retinal artery occlusion. The artery is commonly obstructed at the point at which it and the optic nerve pass through the sclera. This is presumably because the retinal artery is narrowest at this point.

Because the central artery of the retina is an anatomical 'end artery', irreversible ischaemic damage leading to permanent blindness follows, if the obstruction is not relieved rapidly.

When the affected eye is examined with an ophthalmoscope, the retina appears very pale owing to the marked degree of oedema that develops, and the arterial branches appear thread-like as they are poorly filled. Pallor is particularly marked in the macular region. The well-vascularized choroid lying just deep to the macula is visible as a central red spot (a 'cherry-red spot').

A cherry-red spot also occurs in certain lysosomal storage diseases such as Tay–Sachs' disease. This is due to the extreme pallor of the retina caused by the accumulation of gangliosides within the retinal cells.

The onset of visual symptoms in central artery occlusion is usually sudden. If the ischaemia is of very short duration, as may occur in transient ischaemic attacks, the visual disturbance is fleeting (**amaurosis fugax**).

Occlusion of the Central Retinal Vein

This tends to occur in the elderly. Glaucoma, hypertension and atherosclerotic disease all increase the risk of such venous occlusion.

The impairment of venous drainage resulting from central vein occlusion leads to:
- **marked engorgement of the retinal veins draining into the central vein.** Because of the very high pressure in the local venous bed, haemorrhage is likely to occur and may be very striking in extent and degree.
- **severe retinal oedema** secondary to the high pressure within the retinal veins

In about 20% of affected individuals, there is a growth of new blood vessels which may affect the anterior surface of the iris. Associated with this is anterior synechia formation, which may narrow the drainage angle and lead to severe closed-angle glaucoma. This tends to occur 2–3 months after occlusion of the central vein.

Diabetic Retinal Vascular Disease

This is discussed in the section dealing with diabetes mellitus (see p 855).

Hypertensive Retinal Disease

The retina is a well-recognized target in untreated systemic hypertension. The basic changes affecting the retinal vessels are the same as those occurring in other systemic vessels of the same size, and are described in the section dealing with hypertension (see pp 683–688).

The changes due to hypertension that can be seen on ophthalmoscopic examination include:
- arteriolar narrowing of differing degrees of severity
- small infarcts in the superficial nerve fibre layer of the retina (so-called 'cotton wool' spots) which result from swelling within the axons of the optic nerve branches
- flame-shaped haemorrhages within the nerve fibre layer
- microaneurysms

Retrolental Fibroplasia

This disorder is virtually restricted to premature infants. It results from exposure to high concentrations of oxygen. At one time, before this was realized, retrolental fibroplasia was a common cause of blindness in infants.

The high concentration of oxygen leads to obliteration of developing blood vessels within the retina as a result of vasospasm. Normal vascularization of the peripheral part of the retina does not occur. From the ischaemic portion of the retina a vascular growth factor is liberated and there is a florid overgrowth of new blood vessels. This may lead to traction on the retina, detachment of the retina and blindness.

INHERITED RETINAL DISORDERS

Retinitis Pigmentosa

This term covers a set of disorders all characterized by:
- degeneration of the photoreceptor cells, initially in the peripheral part of the retina
- accumulation of pigment within the retina

As the disease progresses, the visual fields become ever more limited until eventually the affected individuals become blind. A noteworthy feature on fundoscopic examination is the intense pallor of the optic nerve. This appears to be associated with relative attenuation of the retinal blood vessels.

Retinitis pigmentosa may be inherited as an autosomal recessive disease or, less commonly, in an autosomal dominant or X-linked recessive pattern. Similar retinal changes may be encountered in a variety of other inherited syndromes such as Usher's syndrome in which retinitis pigmentosa is associated with nerve deafness.

Senile Macular Degeneration

Pathological changes affecting the pigmented epithelial layer in the macular region are not uncommon causes of visual impairment in the elderly. As the macular region is the principal target, affected individuals experience loss of central vision, peripheral vision being preserved for long periods.

The cause of senile macular degeneration is unknown. It is characterized by the accumulation of incompletely degraded lipid-rich material in the pigmented epithelial cells. Some of this material, which may represent a functional failure of lysosomes, is deposited on Bruch's membrane. This membrane is the limiting zone between the pigmented epithelium and the retina proper. Loss of retinal pigment epithelium and new blood vessel formation in the subretinal area are associated with degeneration of the photoreceptors. Fibrous scars are seen within the affected retina and there are basal laminar deposits in relation to Bruch's membrane (*Fig. 46.3*).

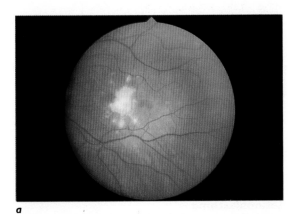

a

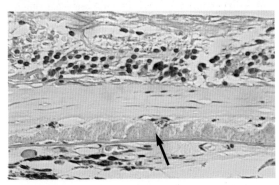

b

FIGURE 46.3 *a* A case of senile macular degeneration associated with ageing and showing a characteristic white disciform scar. *b* Section of macular in a case of age-related degeneration. The surviving retina (see top of picture) is atrophic and overlies a fibrous scar. Beneath this some eosinophilic basal laminar deposits can be seen in relation to Bruch's membrane (arrow).

Retinal Detachment

Normal retinal function depends on contact being maintained between the neural retina and the pigmented epithelial layer. The pigmented epithelium provides metabolic support for the neural retina. Loss of such contact, with either pushing forward or pulling forward of the neural retina, leads to necrosis and fragmentation of the outer layers of the neural retina. If contact between the separated layers is not restored, permanent loss of vision in the affected eye results.

Retinal detachment is classified as being:

- **rhegmatogenous (due to a combination of a break within the retina and some degree of traction from the vitreous).** The risk of this form of retinal detachment is increased as a result of:
  a) a high degree of myopia (short sightedness)
  b) a form of retinal degeneration known as **lattice degeneration** in which some of the neural cells are replaced by glial fibres
  c) trauma to the eye
  d) cataract surgery
- **tractional.** This occurs particularly when there has been vascular and fibrous tissue proliferation within the vitreous such as in diabetic retinopathy associated with neovascularization, retrolental fibroplasia or scarring within the vitreous following inflammation.
- **exudative.** This occurs when the retina is pushed forward as a result of the accumulation of blood-derived fluid behind the retina, in patients with uveitis, choroidal tumours or retinoblastoma.

On ophthalmoscopy, the detached part of the retina is grey in colour and may be seen to undulate with movements of the eye (*Fig. 46.4a*). Vitreous fluid seeps through holes or tears in the retina and accumulates in a subretinal position (*Fig. 46.4b*).

INTRAOCULAR MALIGNANT NEOPLASMS

Malignant Melanoma

In adults, the commonest intraocular malignant neoplasm is the malignant melanoma that is derived from the pigment-producing cells of the uveal tract. It is believed that many of these tumours arise on the basis of a pre-existing melanocytic naevus (see pp 1024–1025). The most frequently affected sites are the choroid (85%) and ciliary body (10%), although tumours of the iris also occur. Choroidal melanoma tends to produce retinal detachment of the exudative type. It is the visual disturbance caused by this retinal detachment that leads most frequently to the diagnosis of tumour (*Fig. 46.5a*).

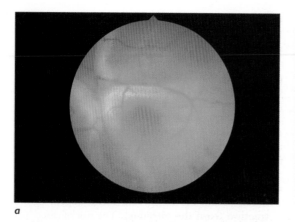

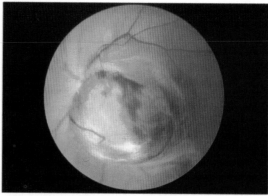

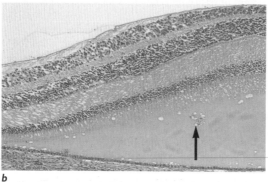

FIGURE 46.4 **a** Retinal detachment showing the folded appearance of the detached tissue. **b** Retinal detachment occurring in the macular region and showing a large subretinal accumulation of fluid (arrow).

FIGURE 46.5 **a** Melanoma of the optic disc appearing as a large pigmented mass protruding into the vitreous. **b** Spindle cell B variant of intraoptic melanoma.

Microscopic Features

It is traditional to classify intraocular melanoma into three varieties:

- **spindle cell A.** These consist of slender cells with relatively small fusiform nuclei and no nucleoli.
- **spindle cell B.** Spindle B cells are larger and more pleomorphic. They have large ovoid nuclei in which prominent nucleoli are seen. The number of mitoses is much higher than in the spindle cell A variety (*Fig. 46.5b*).
- **epithelioid.** Epithelioid cells are the largest of all and markedly irregular in appearance. They possess abundant cytoplasm and often contain multiple nuclei of bizarre appearance.

These may occur as single entities or, more commonly, in combination.

Natural History

The tumours are treated by enucleation of the affected eye. Death may be caused by metastasis and occurs in 46% of cases within 15 years of enucleation. Important prognostic factors are listed in *Table 46.3*.

Retinoblastoma

This is the commonest intraocular tumour occurring in childhood. The epidemiology and molecular genetics of this lesion are discussed in the chapter dealing with tumour suppressor genes (see pp 282–283).

The commonest presenting feature is a 'white' pupillary reflex (the pupil appears white when a light is shone into it) or, less commonly, as squint when the tumour is sited in the macular region. When enucleated eyes are examined, the tumour mass is seen to occupy a considerable part of the globe (*Fig. 46.6a*).

Microscopic Features

The tumour is composed of dense masses of small round cells with darkly staining nuclei and very little cytoplasm. In more differentiated examples, some of the tumour cells are arranged in rosettes (*Fig. 46.6b*). Patchy necrosis is common and, where this has occurred, darkly staining debris is deposited in and around the walls of small blood vessels.

Table 46.3 Prognostic Factors in Intraocular Melanoma

Feature	Prognostic significance
Cell type	Epithelioid cell melanomas in the eye carry the worst prognosis (25–33% 5-year survival rate). Spindle cell A tumours can be regarded, for all practical purposes, as benign. The 5-year survival rate for spindle cell B tumours is 66–75%.
Size of tumour	The larger the lesion, the worse the prognosis.
Site of tumour	Tumours situated in the iris have the best prognosis.
Extrascleral invasion	Extrascleral invasion doubles the 5-year mortality rate.
Necrosis	This is an indicator of poor prognosis.
Prominence of nucleoli	The greater the area occupied by nucleoli, the worse is the prognosis.

Natural History

The tumour may invade the optic nerve and from there either spread in continuity to the brain or be carried to various parts of the brain by the cerebrospinal fluid.

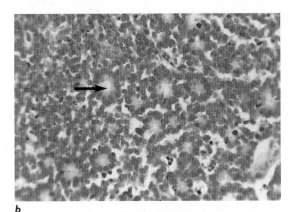

a

b

FIGURE 46.6 **a** *Retinoblastoma. The tumour appears as a cream-coloured mass protruding into the vitreous.* **b** *Section of a retinoblastoma showing the characteristic small dark tumour cells and the so-called Flexner–Wintersteiner rosettes which are characterized by a well-defined circular lumen.*

Metastases may be confined to the cranium or involve extracranial sites, most frequently the skeleton. Uveal tract invasion is also common.

If treatment is adequate, the survival rate for unilateral retinoblastoma is high (more than 90%). The survival rate for patients with bilateral tumours is a little lower. Survivors are at increased risk of developing other malignant neoplasms such as osteosarcoma. This applies only to cases in which the retinoblastoma is of the familial type in which one of the *RB-1* gene alleles is inactivated in the germ cell line (see pp 282–283).

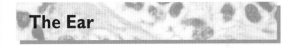

The Ear

Disorders of the ear can be related most conveniently to the anatomy of the ear, which is divided functionally into three distinct regions: the external ear, the middle ear and the inner ear.

NORMAL STRUCTURE

The External Ear

This consists of the pinna and the external auditory meatus, a canal extending from the pinna to the tympanic membrane. The pinna is a skin-covered appendage which otherwise consists largely of cartilage. Both the pinna and the meatus are lined by stratified squamous epithelium; in addition there are glands opening on to the meatal surface which secrete a waxy substance (cerumen).

The Middle Ear

This is a cavity separating the tympanic membrane from the semicircular canals and cochlea which constitute the inner ear. The middle ear communicates anteriorly via the eustachian tube with the pharynx, and posteriorly with the mastoid air cells. This anatomical arrangement renders the middle ear liable to infection spreading up the eustachian tube from the pharynx and opens up the possibility of spread from the middle ear to the mastoid air cells, a common complication in the preantibiotic era. It contains three small bones – the stapes, incus and malleolus – which transmit sound waves from the tympanic membrane to the cochlea.

The Inner Ear

This consists of the semicircular canals and cochlea. Vestibular and auditory nerves arise from the inner ear and travel to the brainstem via the internal auditory meatus.

DISORDERS OF THE EXTERNAL EAR

Pathological processes may affect the epithelial surface, the cartilage of the pinna and the ceruminous glands, and may be considered under the following headings.

DEVELOPMENTAL ANOMALIES

Preauricular Sinus

The commonest disorder under this rubric is preauricular sinus. This arises as the result of abnormal fusion of the facial folds producing a blind-ending epithelial track opening on to the skin just anterior to the external auditory meatus. If this opening becomes obstructed, a keratin-filled epidermal cyst may result. If the track becomes infected an abscess with or without a discharging sinus may occur.

Diagonal Ear Lobe Crease

Certain individuals show a crease of the ear lobe running downwards and backwards from the external auditory meatus. This minor abnormality is of interest purely because it is associated with an increased risk of death from cardiovascular disease, most notably ischaemic heart disease.

INFLAMMATORY DISORDERS

Inflammation may affect either the pinna or the external auditory meatus and may be acute or chronic and infective or non-infective. A variety of organisms – bacterial, viral or fungal – may cause inflammation in the meatus. Amongst bacterial causes, *Pseudomonas aeruginosa* is not uncommon and very severe otitis externa can occur, especially if the inflammatory process has spread from the middle ear to the external auditory canal.

The viral infections most commonly encountered include herpes simplex types 1 and 2. These produce painful blisters in the canal and meatus. Varicella zoster infections may also involve the pinna and meatus as a result of spread from nerve ganglia in which the virus has been latent. Spread from the geniculate ganglion produces a striking pattern of involvement including the pinna, external auditory canal, postauricular skin, uvula, palate and anterior portion of the tongue. Occasionally zoster in this distribution is combined with involvement of the eighth nerve ganglion, giving rise to disturbances in hearing and balance (Ramsay Hunt syndrome).

Non-infective inflammatory disease arises most commonly on the basis of foreign bodies within the tissues of the external ear. This may occur:

- following local treatment with antibiotics when the vehicle in which the antibiotic is administered may cause a foreign body reaction
- when hairs escape from their follicles in a manner analogous to what occurs in pilonidal sinus

Relapsing Polychondritis

This is a disorder in which cartilage, eye and heart are affected. In the external ear, the process presents with reddening, swelling and pain of the pinna, followed by atrophy and distortion as the cartilage is destroyed. Relapsing polychondritis is believed to be an autoimmune disorder which may be related to, and sometimes seen at the same time as, autoimmune vasculitis.

POST-TRAUMATIC DISORDERS

Cauliflower Ear

This is a thickening and distortion of the pinna caused by partial organization of repeated haematomas secondary to trauma. It is seen most commonly in boxers.

Chondrodermatitis Nodularis Chronica

This disorder presents with a small painful nodule usually on the superior portion of the helix. Often there is ulceration of the skin extending down to degenerate and eosinophilic cartilage and associated inflammation in the perichondrium. It is believed to be secondary to trauma but the evidence for this is not strong.

NEOPLASMS

For the most part neoplasms affecting the external ear are the same as those affecting any area of exposed skin, i.e. basal and squamous carcinoma and malignant melanoma (see pp 1019–1032). The exceptions arise from the ceruminous glands found in the external auditory canal. Most of such neoplasms are benign. Ceruminous gland adenoma usually presents with blockage of the external auditory canal and unilateral deafness. Rarely, malignant examples are encountered.

DISORDERS OF THE MIDDLE EAR

INFLAMMATORY DISORDERS

Otitis Media

Usually bacterial in origin, otitis media is common in children. It often follows viral infections of the upper respiratory tract. The major pathogenetic factor is impaired drainage of the middle ear as a result of blockage of the opening of the eustachian tube into the nasopharynx. Impaired drainage in many locations favours secondary bacterial infection, and the ear is no exception. Organisms frequently implicated in acute otitis media include *Streptococcus pneumoniae* and *Haemophilus influenzae*.

The affected children suffer severe earache. Examination with an otoscope reveals a reddened and tense tympanic membrane. If the infection is not treated promptly, central perforation of the tympanic membrane may occur with release of the middle ear inflammatory exudate into the external auditory canal. Such perforations usually heal by scarring within a few days.

Complications of Acute Otitis Media

Spread to the Mastoid Air Spaces

Before the introduction of antibiotics, bacterial infection of the middle ear was followed not infrequently by extension of the infection and inflammation into the mastoid air spaces within bone. This was a potentially sinister complication because further spread to involve the meninges and brain could then occur, with the formation of a brain abscess.

Chronic Otitis Media

Chronic otitis media often develops without a preceding acute phase. The organisms commonly involved include various *Proteus* species and *Pseudomonas aeruginosa*. Affected individuals may present with:

- persistent earache
- conduction deafness
- a chronic discharge from the external auditory meatus

The mastoid air cells and the tubotympanic region of the middle ear are most commonly involved. The chronic inflammation may be associated with abundant granulation tissue formation, and this may protrude through a tympanic membrane perforation as a polypoid mass (aural polyp). As in any other chronic inflammatory process, there is evidence of the triggering of repair mechanisms, both the mastoid air cells and the tympanic cavity showing evidence of scarring and new bone formation. This new bone is laid down in a woven pattern similar to that seen in healing fractures and in Paget's disease. Cholesteatoma and cholesterol granulomas are not infrequently associated with chronic otitis media.

Cholesterol Granuloma

Yellow nodules may be seen both within the tympanic cavity and in the mastoid. These consist of masses of cholesterol crystals which have elicited a chronic inflammatory cell response including foreign-body giant cells. Such granulomas are usually the consequence of previous haemorrhage, the lipid being derived from cell membranes.

Tympanosclerosis

This term is applied to a special form of scarring associated with chronic otitis media. It is characterized by the laying down of large amounts of dense hyalinized collagen within the middle ear lining. The tympanic membrane itself and the crura of the stapes are especially likely to be affected. Dystrophic, rather spotty, calcification is often seen and there may be deposits of new bone within the plaques of fibrous tissue.

Otitis Media with Effusion (OME or 'Glue Ear')

OME is a common cause of impaired hearing in children. It is characterized by an effusion in the middle ear behind a non-perforated tympanic membrane and is usually not accompanied by any clinical features of acute otitis media. The effusion is often thick and rather sticky (hence the term glue ear). Because drainage via the normal pathway (the eustachian tube) is impaired, the condition is often treated by the insertion of grommets through the tympanic membrane.

Cholesteatoma

Cholesteatoma is the term applied to **a mass of actively growing, keratinizing, stratified, squamous epithelium** within the middle ear and often extending into the mastoid air cells. It is neither a true neoplasm nor an epidermoid cyst and, at least in the acquired form, is usually associated with chronic otitis media. Cholesteatoma may exist either as a 'closed' cystic mass or in an 'open' form in which the keratin squames are discharged into the middle ear cavity.

Cholesteatomas are classified as being either:

- The **congenital** form, which is believed to arise from an epithelial cell rest in the developing middle ear. These rests always occur in the same position – where the middle ear epithelium joins that of the eustachian tube, and this is the commonest site for congenital cholesteatoma.
- **Acquired** forms, which occur usually in the upper and posterior portion of the middle ear but often expand to fill most of the cavity.

The clinical importance of these, otherwise trivial, lesions resides in their ability to expand, thus eroding adjacent bony structures such as the ossicles or the labyrinth and surrounding soft tissue including, for example, the facial nerve.

Table 46.4 Causes of Conduction Deafness

Cause	Features
Accumulations of wax occluding the external auditory canal	Commonest cause of temporary loss of hearing. Normal hearing restored after removal of wax
Acute otitis externa	Occurs if there is marked inflammatory oedema of tissues of external auditory canal
Otitis media	Both the fluid accumulations of acute middle ear disease and the granulation tissue masses and effusions of the chronic forms may cause some loss of hearing
Blast injuries	These may cause perforations in the tympanic membrane and injury to the ossicles. In the latter case, hearing loss is likely to be permanent
Otosclerosis	Hearing loss due to fixation of stapes footplate

Table 46.5 Causes of Sensorineural Deafness

Cause	Feature
Presbycusis	This, the commonest type of hearing loss, is associated with ageing. Degenerative changes in various parts of the cochlea have been described, one of the most striking being loss of the outer hair cells. At the lower end of the basal coil of the cochlea, both inner and outer layer hair cells are lost in old people.
Excessive noise exposure over long periods	Currently this may be seen in young adults who have become addicted to the use of personal stereo reproducers played at very high volume. The pathological correlate is not known.
Toxic damage from drugs	Injury to the inner ear can result from drugs of a number of different classes. These include: • aminoglycoside antibiotics such as gentamicin • loop diuretics • salicylates • quinine • cytotoxic drugs such as cisplatin Several different sites in the inner ear appear to be susceptible to damage by such compounds.
Menière's disease	Both hearing and balance are affected in this condition. Patients present with episodic deafness, tinnitus and vertigo – a disabling combination. Excess fluid accumulates in the endolymphatic spaces of the cochlea, leading to their distension. The elastic Reissner's membrane bulges into the vestibular cavity and, in some cases, perforates. The cause is unknown. The disorder is more common in males than in females and is bilateral in about 20% of cases.
Infection	Certain viruses may reach the inner ear via the bloodstream (cytomegalovirus, measles, rubella and mumps viruses). The developing ear is particularly sensitive to such infections and these viruses may cause congenital deafness. Meningitis may also cause sensorineural deafness, and is not an uncommon cause of such deafness in children.
Acoustic neuroma	Tumours arising from the Schwann cells of the eighth nerve may cause deafness. Most are unilateral but nearly 10% are bilateral. Such bilateral tumours are characteristic of neurofibromatosis type 2, and show a characteristic deletion on chromosome 22 (see p 1168).

DISORDERS OF THE OSSICLES

Otosclerosis

This is the commonest disorder affecting the bones of the middle ear and is an important cause of conduction deafness (failure of transmission of sound waves) (see *Table 46.4*). It affects principally the cochlea and the footplate of the stapes. This causes fixation of the stapes with a resulting loss of transmission of sound vibrations. To restore such transmission, the stapes must be removed and replaced with a prosthesis.

Histological examination of the stapes footplate following stapedectomy shows an appearance closely resembling that of Paget's disease of bone. There are foci of woven rather than normal lamellar bone and numerous 'cement lines' are present. As in Paget's disease, electron microscopy shows structures that resemble the nucleocapsid of measles virus, and nucleocapsid antigen has been identified in otosclerotic lesions.

NEOPLASMS OF THE MIDDLE EAR

Paraganglioma (Glomus Jugulare Tumour)

This is the commonest neoplasm in the middle ear. Most paragangliomas arise from paraganglionic tissue in the wall of the jugular bulb; a few arise from a paraganglion sited near the middle ear surface of the promontory. The former tend to invade the petrous bone; the latter remain localized to the middle ear.

The tumours are slow growing but nevertheless may invade deeply into the petrous temporal bone, reaching the intracranial cavity in some cases. Clinically they present as red masses either behind the tympanic membrane or protruding out into the external auditory canal. Metastasis occurs only rarely but recurrence is common.

Microscopic Features

Paragangliomas in all sites have a common microscopic appearance. Well-defined nests of catecholamine-containing cells are separated from each other by highly vascular fibrous tissue septa. The extreme vascularity is the reason these tumours bleed so freely during surgical removal. The paraganglionic cells are surrounded by a second cell population, the sustentacular cells. These do not contain catecholamine but react with antibodies against the neural marker S-100.

DISORDERS OF THE INNER EAR

The inner ear subserves the functions not only of hearing but of balance. Thus disorders of this part of the ear present with hearing loss, tinnitus and/or vertigo. The causes of sensorineural deafness, due to pathology either in the inner ear or in the nerves that transmit sound messages to the brain, are shown in *Table 46.5*.

FURTHER READING

Chapter 1: Introduction

Kleiner, D.E. *et al.* Necropsy as a research method in the age of molecular pathology. *Lancet* 1995; **346**: 945–948.

Mehregan, D. and Mehregan, D. Immunohisto-chemistry: a prognostic as well as a diagnostic tool? *Semin. Cutan. Med. Surg.* 1996; **15**: 317–325.

Miettinen, M. Immunohistochemistry in tumour diagnosis. *Ann. Med.* 1993; **25**: 221–233.

Naber, S.P. Molecular pathology – diagnosis of infectious disease. *N. Engl. J. Med.* 1994; **331**: 1212–1215.

Taylor, C.R. The status of immunohistochemical studies in lymphoma diagnosis. *Biotech. Histochem.* 1997; **72**: 62–77.

Chapters 2 and 3: Cell and Tissue Injury and Death

Berke, G. The Fas-based mechanism of lymphocytotoxicity. *Hum. Immunol.* 1997; **54**: 1–7.

Desbarats, L. *et al. Myc*: a single gene controls both proliferation and apoptosis in mammalian cells. *Experientia.* 1996; **52**: 1123–1129.

Finlay, B.B. and Cossart, P. Exploitation of mammalian host cell functions by bacterial pathogens. *Science* 1997; **276**: 718–725.

Finlay, B.B. and Falkow, S. Common themes in microbial pathogenicity revisited. *Microbiol. Mol. Biol. Rev.* 1997; **61**: 136–139.

Floyd, R.A. The effect of peroxides and free radicals on body tissue. *J. Am. Dent. Assoc.* 1997; **128** (Suppl): 37S–40S.

Furie, M.B. and Randolph, G.J. Chemokines and tissue injury. *Am. J. Pathol.* 1995; **146**: 1287–1301.

Galan, J. and Bliska, J.B. Cross-talk between bacterial pathogens and their host cells. *Ann. Rev. Cell Dev. Biol.* 1996; **12**: 221–255.

Goody, R.S. How G proteins turn off. *Nature* 1994; **372**: 220–221.

Halliwell, B. Free radicals, proteins and DNA; oxidative damage versus redox regulation. *Biochem. Soc. Reans.* 1996; **24**: 1023–1027.

Hancock, J.T. Superoxide, hydrogen peroxide and nitric oxide as signalling molecules: their production and role in disease. *Br. J. Biomed. Sci.* 1997; **54**: 38–46.

Hughson, F.M. Penetrating insights into pore formation. *Nat. Struct. Biol.*; 1997; **4**: 89–92.

Kerr, M.E., Bender, C.M. and Monti, E.J. An introduction to oxygen free radicals. *Heart Lung* 1996; **25**: 200–209.

Kukreja, R.C., Kontos, M.C. and Hess, M.L. Free radicals and heart shock protein in the heart. *Ann. N.Y. Acad. Sci.* 1996; **793**: 108–122.

Majno, G. and Joris, I. Apoptosis, oncosis and necrosis. An overview of cell death. *Am. J. Pathol.* 1995; **146**: 3–15.

Mathes, S.J. and Alexander, J. Radiation injury. *Surg. Oncol. Clin. North Am.* 1996; **5**: 809–824.

McConkey, D.J. and Orrenius, S. Signal transduction pathways in apoptosis. *Stem Cells.* 1996; **14**: 619–631.

McManus, M.L., Churchwell, K.B. and Strange, K. Regulation of cell volume in health and disease. *N. Engl. J. Med.* 1995; **333**: 1267–1272.

Nagata, S. Fas-mediated apoptosis. *Adv. Exp. Med. Biol.* 1996; **406**: 119–124.

Rice-Evans, C.A. and Gopinathan, V. Oxygen toxicity, free radicals and antioxidants in human disease: biochemical implications in atherosclerosis and the problems of premature neonates. *Essays Biochem.* 1995; **29**: 39–63.

Samali, A., Gorman, A.M. and Cotter, T.G. Apoptosis – the story so far . . . *Experientia.* 1996; **52**: 933–941.

Sears, C.L. and Kaper, J.B. Enteric bacterial toxins: mechanisms of action and linkage to intestinal secretion. *Microbiol. Rev.* 1996; **60**: 167–215.

Wong, B., Park, C.G. and Choi, Y. Identifying the molecular control of T-cell death; on the hunt for killer genes. *Semin. Immunol.* 1997; **9**: 7–16.

Wyllie, A.H. Death from the inside out: an overview. *Phil. Trans. R. Soc. Lon.* 1994; **345**: 237–341.

Chapters 4–9: Acute and Chronic Inflammation and Wound Healing

Ali, H. *et al.* Mechanisms of inflammation and leukocyte activation. *Med. Clin. North. Am.* 1997; **81**: 1–28.

Bazzoni, F. and Beutler, B. The tumour necrosis factor ligand and receptor families. *N. Engl. J. Med.* 1996; **334**: 1717–1725.

Bevilacqua, M.P. *et al.* Endothelial-leukocyte adhesion molecules in human disease. *Annu. Rev. Med.* 1994; **45**: 361–378.

Border, W.A. and Noble, N.A. Transforming growth factor β in tissue fibrosis. *N. Engl. J. Med.* 1994; **331**: 1286–1292.

Boros, P. and Miller, C.M. Hepatocyte growth factor: a multifunctional cytokine. *Lancet* 1995; **345**: 293–295.

Chapple I.L. Reactive oxygen species and antioxidants in inflammatory diseases. *J. Clin. Periodontol.* 1997; **24**: 287–296.

Denzlinger, C. Biology and pathophysiology of leukotrienes. *Crit. Rev. Oncol. Hematol.* 1996; **23**: 167–223.

Dinarello, C.A. and Wolff, S.M. The role of interleukin-1 in disease. *N. Engl. J. Med.* 1993; **328**: 106–113.

diPietro, L.A. Wound healing: the role of the macrophage and other immune cells. *Shock* 1995; **4**: 233–240.

Frenette, P.S. and Wagner, D.D. Adhesion molecules – Parts 1 and 2. *N. Engl. J. Med.* 1996; **334**: 1526–1529; **335**: 43–5.

Grande, J.P. Role of transforming growth factor beta in tissue injury and repair. *Proc. Soc. Exp. Biol. Med.* 1997; **214**: 27–40.

Greenhalgh, D.G. The role of growth factors in wound healing. *J. Trauma.* 1996; **41**: 159–167.

Henderson, B., Poole, S. and Wilson, M. Microbial/host interactions in health and disease: who controls the cytokine network? *Immunopharmacology* 1996; **35**: 1–21.

Koj, A. Initiation of acute phase response and synthesis of cytokines. *Biochim. Biophys. Acta.* 1996; **1317**: 84–94.

Linares, H.A. From wound to scar. *Burns* 1996; **22**: 339–352.

Nodder, S. and Martin, P. Wound healing in embryos: a review. *Anat. Embryol. (Berlin)* 1997; **195**: 215–228.

Pataroyo, M. Adhesion molecules mediating recruitment of monocytes to inflamed tissue. *Immunobiology* 1994; **191**: 474–477.

Polla, B.S. and Cossariza, A. Stress proteins in inflammation *EXS* 1996; **77**: 375–391.

Schaffer, C.J. and Nanney, L.B. Cell biology of wound healing. *Int. Rev. Cytol.* 1996; **169**: 151–181.

Slavin, J. The role of cytokines in wound healing. *J. Pathol.* 1996; **178**: 5–10.

Stossel, T.P. The machinery of cell crawling. *Sci. Am.* 1994; **271**: 40–47.

Van den Berg, W.B. and Van Lent, P.L. The role of macrophages in chronic arthritis. *Immunobiology* 1996; **195**: 614–623.

Wahl, S.M. *et al.* Role of transforming growth factor β in the pathophysiology of chronic inflammation. *J. Periodontol.* 1993; **64** (5 suppl.): 450–455.

Wong, M.E., Hollinger, J.O. and Pinero, G.J. Integrated processes responsible for soft tissue healing. *Oral. Surg. Oral Med. Oral. Radiol. Endod.* 1996; **82**: 475–492.

Chapters 10–13: The Immune System and its Disorders

Abbas, A.K., Lichtman, A.H. and Pober, J.S. (eds) Congenital and acquired immunodeficiency. In: *Cellular and Molecular Immunology*, pp. 410–430. Philadelphia: W.B. Saunders, 1994.

Armitage, J.O. Bone marrow transplantation. *N. Engl. J. Med.* 1994; **330**: 827–838.

Asghar, S.S. Membrane regulators of complement activation and their aberrant expression in disease. *Lab. Invest.* 1995; **72**: 254–271.

Attfield, D.C. Cellular immunity: the final paradigm. *Immunol. Cell Biol.* 1997; **75**: 96–101.

Baggiolini, M. and Dahunden, C. CC chemokines in allergic inflammation. *Immunol. Today* 1994; **15**: 127–133.

Beverley, P.C. Generation of T cell memory. *Curr. Opin. Immunol.* 1996; **8**: 327–330.

Brenna, F.M. and Feldmann, M. Cytokines in autoimmunity. *Curr. Opin. Immunol.* 1996; **8**: 872–877.

Brown, E and Hogg, N. Where the outside meets the inside: integrins as activators and targets of signal transduction cascades. *Immunol. Lett.* 1996; **54**: 189–193.

Dennert, G. Molecular mechanisms of target lysis by cytotoxic T cells. *Int. Rev. Immunol.* 1997; **14**: 133–152.

Drachman, D.B. Myasthenia gravis. *N. Engl. J. Med.* 1994, **330**: 1797–1810.

Fazekas-de St Groth, B. *et al.* The role of T cells in the regulation of B cell tolerance. *Int. Rev. Immunol.* 1997; **15**: 73–99.

Ferra, J.L. *et al.* The immunopathophysiology of acute graft-versus-host disease. *Stem Cells* 1996; **14**: 473–489.

Goodnow, C.C. Balancing immunity, autoimmunity and self tolerance. *Ann. N.Y. Acad. Sci.* 1997; **815**: 55–66.

Hayry, P.Y. Pathophysiology of chronic rejection. *Transplant. Proc.* 1996; **28** (6, suppl. 1): 7–10.

Knol, E.F. *et al.* The role of basophils in allergic disease. *Eur. Respir. J.* 1996; **22**: 126S–131S.

Kroemer, G. *et al.* Differential involvement of Th1 and Th2 cytokines in autoimmune diseases. *Autoimmunity* 1996; **24**: 25–33.

Liu, C.C., Young, L.H. and Young, J.D. Lymphocyte-mediated cytolysis and disease. *N. Engl. J. Med.* 1996; **335**: 1651–1659.

MacLennan, I.C.M. Germinal centers. *Ann. Rev. Immunol.* 1994, **12**: 117–139.

Mackay, I.R. and Gershwin, M.E. The nature of auto-immune disease. *Semin. Liver Dis.* 1997; **17**: 3–11.

Marboe, C.C. Pathology of lung transplantation. *Pathology Phila.* 1996; **4**: 73–101.

Marcellus, D.C. and Vogelsang, G.B. Graft versus host disease. *Curr. Opin. Oncol.* 1997; **9**: 131–138.

Nilsson, G. and Metcalfe, D.D. Contemporary issues in mast cell biology. *Allergy Asthma Proc.* 1996; **17**: 59–63.

Pathogenesis of AIDS: A special report. *Sci. Am. Sci. Med.* 1997, **4**: 410–430.

Rohn, W.M., Lee, Y.J. and Benveniste, E.N. Regulation of class II MHC expression. *Crit. Rev. Immunol.* 1996; **16**: 311–330.

Reeves, W.H. *et al.* Initiation of autoimmunity to self proteins complexed with viral antigens. *Ann. N.Y. Acad. Sci.* 1997; **815**: 139–154.

Schafer, R. and Sheil, J.M. Superantigens and their role in infectious disease. *Adv. Pediatr. Infect. Dis.* 1995; **10**: 369–390.

Shoenfeld, Y. and George, J. Induction of autoimmunity. A role for the idiotypic network. *Ann. N.Y. Acad. Sci.* 1997; **815**: 342–349.

Sneller, M.C. and Fauci, A.S. Pathogenesis of vasculitis syndromes. *Med. Clin. North. Am.* 1997; **81**: 221–242.

Sanfilippo, S. and Baldwin, W.M. Antibody and complement in graft rejection. *Transplant. Proc.* 1997; **29**: 179–180.

Thorsby, E. HLA associated diseases. *Hum. Immunol.* 1997; **53**: 1–11.

von Boehmer, H. Aspects of lymphocyte developmental biology. *Immunol. Today* 1997; **18**: 260–262.

Walport, M.J. *et al.* Complement deficiency and auto-immunity. *Ann. N.Y. Acad. Sci.* 1997; **815**: 267–281.

Weenink, S.M. and Gautam, A.M. Antigen presentation by MHC Class II molecules. *Immunol. Cell Biol.* 1997; **75**: 69–81.

Zinkernagel, R.M. and Hengartner, H. Antiviral immunity. *Immunol. Today* 1997; **18**: 258–260.

Chapters 14 and 15: Granulomatous Inflammation

Auriault, V.C. *et al.* Cellular immune response and pathology in schistosomiasis. *Parasite* 1996; **3**: 199–208.

Britton, W.J. Immunology of Leprosy. *Trans. R. Soc. Trop. Med. Hyg.* 1993; **87**: 508–514.

Bucala, R. MIF rediscovered: cytokine, pituitary hormone and glucocorticoid-induced regulator of the immune response. *FASEB J.* 1996; **10**: 1007–1014.

Chrousos, G.P. The hypothalamic–pituitary–adrenal axis and immune-mediated inflammation. *N. Engl. J. Med.* 1995; **332**: 1351–1362.

Colston, M.J. The molecular basis of mycobacterial infections. *Mol. Aspects. Med.* 1996; **17**: 383–454.

Filley, E.A. *et al.* The effect of Mycobacterium tuberculosis on the susceptibility of human cells to the stimulatory and toxic effects of tumour necrosis factor. *Immunology* 1992; **77**: 505–509.

Flesch, I.E. and Kaufmann, S.H. Role of cytokines in tuberculosis. *Immunobiology* 1993; **189**: 316–339.

Romagnani, S. The Th1–Th2 paradigm. *Immunol. Today* 1997; **18**: 263–266.

Rook, G.A. and Hernandez-Pando, R. T helper cell types and endocrines in the regulation of tissue damaging mechanisms in tuberculosis. *Immunobiology* 1994; **191**: 478–492.

Rook, G.A. and Hernandez-Pando, R. The pathogenesis of tuberculosis. *Ann. Rev. Microbiol.* 1996; **50**: 259–284.

Chapter 16: Amyloid and Amyloidosis

Falk, R.H., Comenzo, R.L. and Skinner, M. The systemic amyloidoses. *N. Engl. J. Med.* ; 1997; **337**: 898–909.

Kyle, R.A. Monoclonal proteins and renal disease. *Ann. Rev. Med.* 1994; **45**: 71–77.

Maury, C.P.J. Molecular pathogenesis of beta-amyloidosis in Alzheimer's disease and other cerebral amyloidoses. *Lab. Invest.* 1995; **72**: 4–16.

Tan, S.Y and Pepys, M.B. Amyloidosis. *Histopathology* 1994; **25**: 403–414.

Chapter 17: The General Pathology of Viral Infections

Copeland, K.F and Heeney, J.L. T helper cell activation and human retroviral pathogenesis. *Microbiol. Rev.* 1996; **60**: 722–742.

Favre, M., Ramoz, N. and Orth, G. Human papillomaviruses: general features. *Clin. Dermatol.* 1997; **15**: 181–198.

Liebowitz, D. Epstein-Barr virus – an old dog with new tricks. *N. Engl. J. Med.* 1995; **332**: 55–57.

Pattison, J.R. Human parvovirus B19. *Br. Med. J.* 1994; **308**: 149–150.

Rehermann, B. Immunopathogenesis of viral hepatitis. *Baillière's Clin. Gastroenterol.* 1996; **10**: 483–500.

Schalling, M. *et al.* A role for a new herpes virus (KSHV) in different forms of Kaposi's sarcoma. *Nat. Med.* 1995; **1**: 707–708.

Vousden, K.H. and Farrell, P.J. Viruses and human cancer. *Br. Med. Bull.* 1994; **50**: 560–581.

Weber, T. *et al.* Human retroviruses. *Baillière's Clin. Haematol.* 1992; **5**: 273–314.

Welsby, P.D. The herpes virus. In: Lawson, D.H. (ed.) *Current Medicine*, vol. 4, pp. 65–81. Edinburgh: Churchill Livingstone, 1994.

Chapter 18: Disorders of Blood Flow: A Basis

Allaart, C.F. *et al.* Increased risk of venous thrombosis in carriers of hereditary protein C deficiency. *Lancet*, 1993; **341**: 134–137.

Eby, C.S. A review of the hypercoagulable state. *Haematol. Oncol. Clin. N. Am.* 1993; **7**: 1121–1142.

Hajjar, K.A. Factor V Leiden – an unselfish gene? *N. Engl. J. Med.* 1994; **331**: 1585–1587.

Ware, J.A. and Heistadt, D.D. Platelet–endothelium interactions. *N. Engl. J. Med.* 1993; **328**: 628–635.

Weinmann, E.E. and Salzman, E.W. Deep vein thrombosis. *N. Engl. J. Med.* 1994; **331**: 1630–1641.

Chapters 22–29: Neoplasia: Disorders of Cell Proliferation and Differentiation

Arends, M.J., Wyllie, A.H. and Bird, C.C. Papillomaviruses and human cancer. *Hum. Pathol.* 1990; **21**: 686–698.

Boon, T. *et al.* Tumor antigens recognized by T lymphocytes. *Ann. Rev. Immunol.* 1994; **12**: 337–365.

Bornkamp, G.W., Polack, A. and Eick, D. *c-myc* deregulation by chromosomal translocation in Burkitt's lymphoma. In: G. Klein (ed.) *Cellular Oncogene Activation*, pp. 223–273. New York: Marcel Dekker, 1988.

Cantley, L.C. *et al.* Oncogenes and signal transduction. *Cell* 1991; **64**: 281–302.

Cirisano, F.D. and Karlan, B.Y. The role of the HER-2/neu oncogene in gynecologic cancers. *J. Soc. Gynecol. Investig.* 1996; **3**: 99–105.

Cowell, J.K. and Onadim, Z. The Li-Fraumeni cancer family syndrome. *J. Pathol.* 1990; **161**: 1–2.

Dalmau, J.O. and Posner, J.B. Paraneoplastic syndromes affecting the nervous system. *Semin. Oncol.* 1997; **24**: 318, 328.

Dreher, D. and Junod, A.F. Role of oxygen free radicals in cancer development. *Eur. J. Cancer.* 1996; **32A**: 30–38.

Evan, G. *et al.* Integrated control of cell proliferation and cell death by the *c-myc* oncogene. *Philos. Trans. R. Soc. Lond.* 1994; **345**: 269–272.

Folkman, J. Clinical applications of research on angiogenesis. *N. Engl. J. Med.* 1995; **333**: 1757–1763.

Hall, P.A. and Coates, P.J. Assessment of cell proliferation in pathology - what next? *Histopathology*, 1995; **26**: 105–112.

Hart, I.R. and Saini, A. Biology of tumour metastasis. *Lancet* 1992; **339**: 1453–1457.

Holmgren, L., O'Reilly, M.S. and Folkman, J. Dormancy of micrometastases: balanced proliferation and apoptosis in the presence of angiogenesis suppression. *Nature Med.* 1995; **1**: 149–153.

Jaspers, N.G. DNA repair genes, enzymes, patients and mouse models. *Recent Results Cancer Res.* 1997; **143**: 329–335.

Key, T.J. Hormones in human cancer. *Mutat. Res.* 1995; **333**: 59–67.

Klein, G. Rejection antigens in chemically induced tumours. *Proc. Soc. Natl. Acad. Sci. U.S.A.* 1997; **94**: 5991–5992.

Lane, D.P. p53 and human cancers. *Br. Med. Bull.* 1994; **50**: 583–599.

Levine, A.J. The tumour suppressor genes. *Annu. Rev. Biochem.* 1993; **62**: 623–651.

Liotta, L.A., Steeg, P.S. and Stetler-Stevenson, W.G. Cancer metastasis and angiogenesis: an imbalance of positive and negative regulation. *Cell* 1991; **64**: 327–336.

Maeurer, M.J. and Lotze, M.T. Tumor recognition by the cellular immune system: new aspects of tumor immunology. *Int. Rev. Immunol.* 1997; **14**: 97–132.

Marchioli, C.C. and Graziano, S.L. Paraneoplastic syndromes associated with small cell lung cancer. *Chest Surg. Clin. North Am.* 1997; **7**: 65–80.

Morgan, D.O. Principles of CDK regulation. *Nature* 1995; **374**: 131–134.

Oliner, J.D. The role of p53 in cancer development. *Sci. Am. Sci. Med.* 1994; **1**: 16–25.

Polverini, P.A. Cellular adhesion molecules. Newly identified mediators of angiogenesis. *Am. J. Pathol.* 1996; **148**: 1023–1029.

Rabbitts, T.H. Chromosomal translocations in human cancer. *Nature* 1994; **372**: 143–149.

Royds, J.A. *et al.* NM23 "anti-metastatic" gene product expression in colorectal carcinoma. *J. Pathol.*, 1994; **172**: 261–266.

Sato, H. *et al.* A matrix metalloproteinase expressed on the surface of invasive tumour cells. *Nature*, 1994; **370**: 61–65.

Smith, M.L. and Fornace, A.J. The two faces of tumor suppressor p53. *Am. J. Pathol.* 1996; **148**: 1019–1022.

Steel, C.M. Identification and characterisation of cancer genes. *Br. Med. Bull.* 1994; **50**: 536–559.

Stanley, L.A. Molecular aspects of chemical carcinogenesis: the roles of oncogenes and tumour suppressor genes. *Toxicology* 1995; **96**: 173–194.

Strauss, G.M. and Skarin, A.T. Use of tumor markers in lung cancer. *Hematol. Oncol. Clin. North Am.* 1994; **8**: 507–532.

Su, L.K., Vogelstein, B. and Kinzler, K.W. Association of the APC tumor suppressor protein with catenins. *Science* 1994; **262**: 1734–1737.

Taylor, A.M.R. and McConville, C.M. Cancer and DNA processing disorders. *Br. Med. Bull.* 1994; **50**: 708–717.

Weber, B.L. Susceptibility genes for breast cancer. *N. Engl. J. Med.* 1994; **331**: 1523–1524.

Weidener, N. Intratumor microvessel density as a prognostic factor in cancer. *Am. J. Pathol.* 1995; **147**: 9–19.

Wiseman, H. and Halliwell, B. Damage to DNA by reactive oxygen and nitrogen species: role in inflammatory disease and in progression to cancer. *Biochem. J.* 1996; **313** (Pt 1): 17–29.

Wolf, C.R. and Smith, C.A.D. Metabolic polymorphisms in carcinogen metabolizing enzymes and cancer susceptibility. *Br. Med. Bull.* 1994; **50**: 718–731.

Wood, R.D. DNA repair in eukaryotes. *Annu. Rev. Biochem.* 1996; **65**: 135–167.

Chapters 30 and 31: Genetic Disorders

Beutler, E. Gaucher disease, a paradigm for single gene defects. *Experientia* 1995; **51**: 196–197.

Chard, T. and Macintosh, M.C. Screening for Down's syndrome. *J. Perinat. Med.* 1995; **23**: 421–436.

Flint, J. *et al.* Why are some genetic diseases common? Distinguishing selection from other processes by molecular analysis of globin gene variants. *Hum. Genet.* 1993; **91**: 91–117.

Hall, J.G. Genomic imprinting: nature and clinical relevance. *Annu. Rev. Med.* 1997; **48**: 35–44.

Latchman, D. Transcription factor mutations and disease. *N. Engl. J. Med.* 1996; **334**: 34–41.

Majzoub, J.A. and Muglia, L.J. Knockout mice. *N. Engl. J. Med.* 1996; **334**: 904–907.

Onodera, K. and Patterson, D. Structure of human chromosome 21 for an understanding of genetic disease including Down's syndrome. *Biosci. Biotechnol. Biochem.* 1997; **61**: 403–409.

Patterson, D. The integrated map of chromosome 21. *Prog. Clin. Biol. Res.* 1995; **393**: 43–55.

Payne, R.M. *et al.* Towards a molecular understanding of congenital heart disease. *Circulation* 1995; **91**: 494–504.

Saenger, P. Turner's syndrome. *N. Engl. J. Med.* 1996; **335**: 1749–1754.

Shuldiner, A.R. Transgenic animals. *N. Engl. J. Med.* 1996; **334**: 653–655.

Tomlinson, I.P. and Bodmer, W.F. The HLA system and the analysis of multifactorial genetic disease. *Trends Genet.* 1995; **11**: 493–498.

Tycko, B. Genomic imprinting: mechanism and role in human pathology. *Am. J. Pathol.* 1994; **144**: 431–443.

Wells, R.D. Molecular basis for genetic instability of triplet repeats. *J. Biol. Chem.* 1996; **271**: 2875–2878.

Chapter 32: Disorders of the Cardiovascular System

Busse, R. and Fleming, I. Endothelial dysfunction in atherosclerosis. *J. Vasc. Res.* 1996; **33**: 181–194.

Califf, R.M. and Bengtson, J.R. Cardiogenic shock. *N. Engl. J. Med.* 1994; **330**: 1724–1730.

Davies, M.J. and McKenna, W.J. Dilated cardiomyopathy: an introduction to pathology and pathogenesis. *Br. Heart J.* 1994; **72**: S24.

Davies, M.J. and McKenna, W.J. Hypertrophic cardiomyopathy: pathology and pathogenesis. *Histopathology* 1995; **26**: 493–500.

Davies, M.J. and Woolf, N. Atherosclerosis: what is it and why does it occur? *Br Heart J* 1993; **69** (suppl. 1): 3–11.

Ernst, C.B. Abdominal aortic aneurysm. *N. Engl. J. Med.* 1993; **328**: 1167–1172.

Fuster, V., Badimon, L., Badimon, J.J. and Chesebro, J.H. The pathogenesis of coronary artery disease and the acute coronary syndromes, Parts 1 and 2. *N. Engl. J. Med.* 1992; **326**: 242–250, 310–318.

Glauser, M.P. The inflammatory cytokines: New developments in the pathophysiology and treatment of septic shock. *Drugs* 1996; **52** (suppl. 2): 9–17.

Gourdin, F.W. and Smith, J.G. Jr. Etiology of venous ulceration. *South. Med. J.* 1993; **86**: 1142–1146.

Kelly, D.P. and Strauss, A.N. Inherited cardio-myopathies. *N. Engl. J. Med.* 1994; **330**: 913–919.

Kushwaha, S.S., Fallon, J.T. and Fuster, V. Restrictive cardiomyopathy. *N. Engl. J. Med.* 1997; **336**: 267–276.

Maxwell, S.R. and Lip, G.Y. Reperfusion injury: a review of the pathophysiology, clinical manifestations and therapeutic options. *Int. J. Cardiol.* 1997; **58**: 95–117.

Olinde, K.D. and O'Connell, J.B. Inflammatory heart disease: pathogenesis, clinical manifestations and treatment of myocarditis. *Ann. Rev. Med.* 1994; **45**: 481–490.

Parrillo, J.E. Pathogenetic mechanisms of septic shock. *N. Engl. J. Med.* 1993; **328**: 1471–1477.

Parums, D.V. The arteritides. *Histopathology* 1994; **25**: 1–20.

Ross, R. The pathogenesis of atherosclerosis. *Nature* 1993; **362**: 801–809.

Ross, R. Atherosclerosis: a defense mechanism gone wrong. *Am. J. Pathol.* 1993; **143**: 987–1002.

Scandinavian Simvastatin Survival Study Group. Randomized trial of cholesterol lowering in 4444 patients with coronary heart disease: the

Scandinavian Simvastatin Survival Study (4S). *Lancet* 1994; **344**: 1383–1389.

Veasey, L.G. and Hill, H.R. Immunologic and clinical correlations in rheumatic fever and rheumatic heart disease. *Pediatr. Infect. Dis. J.* 1997; **16**: 400–407.

Wannamethee, G. and Shaper, A.G. The association between heart rate and blood pressure, blood lipids and other cardiovascular risk factors. *J. Cardiovasc. Risk* 1994; **1**: 223–230.

Westhuyzen, J. The oxidation hypothesis of atherosclerosis: an update. *Ann. Clin. Lab. Sci.* 1997; **27**: 1–10.

Wolf, G. Nitric oxide and nitric oxide synthase: biology, pathology and localization. *Histol. Histopathol.* 1997; **12**: 251–261.

Woolf, N. and Davies, M.J. Arterial plaque and thrombus formation. *Sci. Am. Sci. Med.* 1994; **1**: 38–47.

Chapter 33: Disorders of the Respiratory Tract

Barkley, J.E and Green, M.R. Bronchioalveolar carcinoma. *J. Clin. Oncol.* 1996; **14**: 2377–2386.

Barnes, P.J. Pathophysiology of asthma. *Br. J. Clin. Pharmacol.* 1996; **42**: 3–10.

Bartlett, J.G. and Mundy, L.M. Community-acquired pneumonia. *N. Engl. J. Med.* 1995; **333**: 1618–1624.

Buhl, R., Meyer, A. and Vogelmeier, C. Oxidant–protease interaction in the lung. Prospects for antioxidant therapy. *Chest* 1996; **110**: 267S–272S.

Cagle, P.T. Molecular pathology of lung cancer and its clinical relevance. *Monogr. Pathol.* 1993; 133–134.

Celli, B.R. Pathophysiology of chronic obstructive pulmonary disease. *Chest Surg. Clin. North Am.* 1995; **5**: 623–634.

Chapman, H.A., Riese, R.J. and Shi, G.P. Emerging roles for cysteine proteases in human biology. *Annu. Rev. Physiol.* 1997; **59**: 63–88.

Cosio, M.G. and Majo, J. Overview of the pathology of emphysema in humans. *Chest. Surg. Clin. North Am.* 1995; **5:** 603–621.

Fleming, M.V. and Travis, W.D. Interstitial lung disease. *Pathology* 1996; **4**: 1–21.

Hoidal, J.R. Pathogenesis of chronic bronchitis. *Semin. Respir. Infect.* 1994; **9**: 8–12.

Huang, L. and Stansell, J.D. AIDS and the lung. *Med. Clin. North. Am.* 1996; **80**: 775–801.

Kamp, D.W. and Weitzman, S.A. Asbestosis: clinical spectrum and pathogenic mechanisms. *Proc. Soc. Exp. Biol. Med.* 1997; **214**: 12–26.

Kane, A.B. Mechanisms of mineral fibre carcinogenesis. *IARC Sci. Publ.* 1996; **140**: 11–34.

Kollef, M.H. and Schuster, D.P. The acute respiratory distress syndrome. *N. Engl. J. Med.* 1995; **332**: 27–37.

Kumar, A. and Busse, W.W. Airway inflammation in asthma. *Sci. Am. Sci. Med.* 1995; **2**: 38–47.

Lynch, J.P. Pulmonary sarcoidosis: current concepts and controversies. *Compr. Ther.* 1997; **23**: 197–210.

McFadden, E.R. and Gilbert, I.A. Asthma. *N. Engl. J. Med.* 1992; **327**: 1928–1937.

Manning, H.L. and Schwartzstein, R.M. Pathophysiology of dyspnea. *N. Engl. J. Med.* 1995; **333**: 1547–1553.

Miller, Y.E and Franklin, W.A. Molecular events in lung carcinogenesis. *Hematol. Oncol. Clin. North. Am.* 1997; **11**: 215–234.

Poulter, L.W. Basic concepts in lung immunology. *Res. Immunol.* 1997; **148**: 8–13.

Rahman, I. and MacNee, W. Role of oxidants/antioxidants in smoking-induced lung diseases. *Free Radic. Biol. Med.* 1996; **21**: 669–681.

Rubin, L.J. Primary pulmonary hypertension. *N. Engl. J. Med.* 1997; **336**: 111–117.

Salvaggio, J.E. Extrinsic allergic alveolitis (hypersensitivity pneumonitis): past, present and future. *Clin. Exp. Allergy* 1997; **27** (suppl 1): 18–25.

Shelhamer. J.H. *et al.* NIH conference. Airway inflammation. *Ann. Intern. Med.* 1995; **123**: 288–304.

Silver, R.M. Scleroderma: clinical problems. The lungs. *Rheum. Dis. Clin. North. Am.* 1996; **22**: 825–840.

Tuomanen, E.I., Austrian, R. and Masure, H.R. Pathogenesis of pneumococcal infection. *N. Engl. J. Med.* 1995; **332**: 1280–1284.

Vuitch, F. *et al.* Neuroendocrine tumours of the lung. Pathology and molecular biology. *Chest Surg. Clin. North Am.* 1997; **7**: 21–47.

Williams, C.L. Basic science of small cell lung cancer. *Chest Surg. Clin. North Am.* 1997; **7**: 1–19.

Wright, J.L. Emphysema: concepts under change – a pathologist's perspectives. *Mod. Pathol.* 1995; **8**: 873–880.

Chapter 34: Disorders of the Gastrointestinal Tract

Brandtzaeg, P. *et al.* Immunopathology of human inflammatory bowel disease. *Springer. Semin. Immunopathol.* 1997; **18**: 555–589.

Christ, A.D. and Blumberg, R.S. The intestinal epithelial cell: immunological aspects. *Springer Semin. Immunopathol.* 1997; **18**: 449–461.

Cunningham, C. and Dunlop, M.G. Genetics of colorectal cancer. *Br. Med. Bull.* 1994; **50**: 640–655.

Fearon, E.R. and Vogelstein, B. A genetic model for colorectal tumorigenesis. *Cell* 1990; **61**: 759–767.

Fishel, R. *et al.* The human mutator gene homolog MSH2 and its association with hereditary non-polyposis colon cancer. *Cell* 1993; **75**: 1027–1038.

Hanauer, S.B. Inflammatory bowel disease. *N. Engl. J. Med.* 1996; **334**: 841–848.

Ireland, A.P., Clark, G.W and DeMeester, T.R. Barrett's oesophagus. The significance of p53 in clinical practice. *Ann. Surg.* 1997; **225**: 17–30.

Isaacson, P.G. Intestinal lymphomas and enteropathy. *J. Pathol.* 1995; **177**: 111–114.

Jen, J. *et al.* Allelic loss of chromosome 18q and prognosis in colorectal cancer. *N. Engl. J. Med.* 1994; **331**: 213–221.

Laine, L. and Peterson, W.L. Bleeding peptic ulcer. *N. Engl. J. Med.* 1994; **331**: 717–727.

Levine, D.S. Barrett's esophagus. *Sci. Am. Sci. Med.* 1994; **1**: 16–25.

Parsonnet, J. *et al. Helicobacter pylori* infection and gastric lymphoma. *N. Engl. J. Med.* 1994; **330**: 1267–1271.

Royds, J.A. *et al.* NM23 "anti-metastatic" gene product expression in colorectal carcinoma. *J. Pathol.* 1994; **172**: 261–266.

Rustgi, A.K. Hereditary gastrointestinal polyposis and non-polyposis syndromes. *N. Engl. J. Med.* 1994; **331**: 1694–1702.

Sartor, R.B. Current concepts of the etiology and pathogenesis of ulcerative colitis and Crohn's disease. *Gastroenterol. Clin. North. Am.* 1995; **24**: 475–507.

Scott, H. *et al.* Immunopathology of gluten-sensitive enteropathy. *Springer. Semin. Immunopathol.* 1997; **18**: 535–553.

Smyrk, T.C. Colon cancer connections: cancer syndrome meets molecular biology meets histopathology. *Am. J. Pathol.* 1994; **145**: 1–6.

Young, M.A., Rose, S. and Reynolds, J.C. Gastrointestinal manifestations of scleroderma. *Rheum. Dis. Clin. North. Am.* 1996; **22**: 797–823.

Williams, G.R. and Talbot, I.C. Anal carcinoma – a histological review. *Histopathology* 1994; **25**: 507–516.

Wyatt, J.I. Histopathology and gastroduodenal inflammation: the impact of *Helicobacter pylori*. *Histopathology* 1995; **26**: 1–15.

Chapter 35: Disorders of the Liver, Biliary System and Exocrine Pancreas

Anthony, P.P. *et al.* The morphology of cirrhosis: definition, nomenclature and classification. *Bull. WHO* 1977; **55**: 521–540.

Caraceni, P. and Van Thiel, D.H. Acute liver failure. *Lancet* 1994; **345**: 163–169.

Degos, F. Natural history of hepatitis C virus infection. *Nephrol. Dial. Transplant.* 1996; **11** (suppl. 4): 16–18.

DeLeve, L.D. and Kaplowitz, N. Mechanisms of drug-induced liver disease. *Gastroenterol. Clin. North Am.* 1995; **24**: 787–810.

Desmet, V. and Fevery, J. Liver biopsy. *Baillière's Clin. Gastroenterol.* 1995; **9**: 811–828.

Donaldson, P.T. Immunogenetics in liver disease. *Baillière's Clin. Gastroenterol.* 1996; **10**: 533–549.

Goldin, R. The pathogenesis of alcoholic liver disease. *Int. J. Exp. Pathol.* 1994; **75**: 71–78.

Halliday, J.W. and Searle, J. Hepatic iron deposition in human disease and animal models. *Biometals* 1996; **9**: 205–209.

Howard, T.J. Pancreatic adenocarcinoma. *Curr. Probl. Cancer* 1996; **20**: 281–328.

Jansen, P.L. Genetic diseases of bilirubin metabolism: the inherited unconjugated hyperbilirubinaemias. *J. Hepatol* 1996; **25**: 398–404.

Jalan, R. *et al.* Pathogenesis and treatment of chronic hepatic encephalopathy. *Aliment. Pharmacol. Ther.* 1996; **10**: 681–697.

Johnston, D.E and Kaplan, M.M. Pathogenesis and treatment of gallstones. *N. Engl. J. Med.* 1993; **328**: 412–421.

Kaplan, M.M. Primary biliary cirrhosis. *N. Engl. J. Med.* 1996; **335**: 1570–1580.

Knox, T.A. and Olans, L.B. Liver disease in pregnancy. *N. Engl. J. Med.* 1996; **335**: 569–576.

Krawitt, E.L. Autoimmune hepatitis. *N. Engl. J. Med.* 1996; **334**: 897–903.

Lee, W.M. Drug-induced hepatotoxicity. *N. Engl. J. Med.* 1995; **333**: 1128–1134.

Lee, Y-M. and Kaplan, M.M. Primary sclerosing cholangitis. *N. Engl. J. Med.* 1995; **332**: 924–933.

Lieber, C.S. Medical disorders of alcoholism. *N. Engl. J. Med.* 1995; **333**: 1058–1067.

Lieber, C.S. Role of oxidative stress and antioxidant therapy in alcoholic and non-alcoholic liver diseases. *Adv. Pharmacol.* 1997; **38**: 601–628.

Marcos Alvarez, A. and Jenkins, R.L. Cholangiocarcinoma. *Surg. Oncol. Clin. North Am.* 1996; **5**: 301–316.

Nagorney, D.M. and Gigot, J.F. Primary epithelial hepatic malignancies: etiology, epidemiology and outcome after subtotal and total hepatic resection. *Surg. Oncol. Clin. North. Am.* 1996; **5**: 283–300.

Perlmutter, D.H. α-1-anti-trypsin deficiency: biochemistry and clinical manifestations. *Ann. Med.* 1996; **28**: 385–394.

Renner, E.L. Liver function tests. *Baillière's Clin. Gastroenterol.* 1995; **9**: 661–677.

Robinson, W.S. Molecular events in the pathogenesis of hepaDNAvirus-associated hepatocellular carcinoma. *Ann. Rev. Med.* 1994; **45**: 297–323.

Scheuer, P.J. *et al.* Histopathological aspects of viral hepatitis. *J. Viral. Hepat.* 1996; **3**: 277–283.

Steer, M.L., Waxman, I. and Freedman, S. Chronic pancreatitis. *N. Engl. J. Med.* 1995; **332**: 1482–1490.

Stern, R.C. The diagnosis of cystic fibrosis. *N. Engl. J. Med.* 1997; **336**: 487–491.

Teli, M.R. *et al.* Determinants of progression to cirrhosis or fibrosis in pure alcoholic fatty liver. *Lancet* 1995; **346**: 987–990.

Warshaw, A.L. and Fernandez-del-Castillo, C. Pancreatic carcinoma. *N. Engl. J. Med.* 1992; **326**: 455–465.

Welsh, M.J and Smith, A.E. Cystic fibrosis. *Sci. Am.* 1996; **273**: 36–43.

Chapter 36: Disorders of the Kidney

Abt, A.B. and Cohen, A.H. Newer glomerular diseases. *Semin. Nephrol.* 1996; **16**: 501–510.

Atkins, R.C. *et al.* Modulators of crescentic glomerulonephritis. *J. Am. Soc. Nephrol.* 1996; **7**: 2271–2278.

Cavalle, T. Membranous nephropathy. Insights from Heymann nephritis. *Am. J. Pathol.* 1994; **144**: 651–658.

Coppes, M.J., Haber, D.A. and Grundy, P.E. Genetic events in the development of Wilms' tumour. *N. Engl. J. Med.* 1994; **331**: 586–590.

Couser, W.G. New insights into mechanisms of immune glomerular injury. *West. J. Med.* 1994; **160**: 440–446.

Gabow, P.A. Autosomal dominant polycystic kidney disease. *N. Engl. J. Med.* 1993; **329**: 332–342.

Korbet, S.M., Schwartz, M.M. and Lewis, E.J. The fibrillary glomerulopathies. *Am. J. Kidney Dis.* 1994; **23**: 751–765.

Mallick, N.P. Recent approaches to understanding clinical glomerular disease. *Ren. Fail.* 1996; **18**: 705–709.

Mills, J.A. Systemic lupus erythematosus. *N. Engl. J. Med.* 1994; **330**: 1871–1879.

Motzer, R.J., Bander, N.H. and Nanus, D.M. Renal cell carcinoma. *N. Engl. J. Med.* 1996; **335**: 865–875.

Ostendorf, T., Burg, M. and Floege, J. Cytokines and glomerular injury. *Kidney Blood Pressure Res.* 1996; **19**: 281–289.

Papyianni, A. Cytokines, growth factors and other inflammatory mediators in glomerulonephritis. *Ren. Fail.* 1996; **18**: 725–740.

Peten, E.P. and Striker, L.J. Progression of glomerular disease. *J. Intern. Med.* 1994; **236**: 241–249.

Remuzzi, G., Zoja, C. Bertani, T. Glomerulonephritis. *Curr. Opin. Nephrol. Hypertens.* 1993; **2**: 465–474.

Robertson, S., Isles, C. and More, I. Glomerular disease made easier, Parts 1, 2, 3, *Br. J. Hosp. Med.* 1995; **53**: 261–266, 323–326, 379–386.

Rockall, A.G. *et al.* Haematuria. *Postgrad. Med. J.* 1997; **73**: 129–136.

Rupprecht, H.D., Schocklmann, H.O. and Sterzl, R.B. Cell–matrix interactions in the glomerular mesangium. *Kidney Int.* 1996; **49**: 1575–1582.

Stockand, J.D. and Sansom, S.C. Regulation of filtration rate by glomerular mesangial cells in health and diabetic renal disease. *Am. J. Kidney Dis.* 1997; **29**: 971–981.

Thadhani, R., Pascual, M. and Bonventre, J.V. Acute renal failure. *N. Engl. J. Med.* 1996; **334**: 1448–1460.

Weight, S.C., Bell, P.R. and Nicholson, M.L. Renal ischemia-reperfusion injury. *Br. J. Surg.* 1996; **83**: 162–170.

Williamson, K.A. and Van Heyningen, V. Towards an understanding of Wilms' tumour. *Int. J. Exp. Pathol.* 1994; **75**: 147–155.

Chapter 37: Disorders of the Lower Urinary Tract

Amin, M.B. and Young, R.H. Intraepithelial lesions of the urinary bladder with a discussion of the histogenesis of urothelial neoplasia. *Semin. Diagn. Pathol.* 1997; **14**: 84–97.

Badawi, A.F. Molecular and genetic events in schistosomiasis-associated human bladder cancer: role of oncogenes and tumor suppressor genes. *Cancer Lett.* 1996; **105**: 123–136.

Boorman, G.A., Wood, M. and Fukushima, S. Tumours of the urinary bladder. *IARC Sci. Publ.* 1994; **111**: 383–406.

Cohen, S.M. Cell proliferation in the bladder and implications for cancer risk assessment. *Toxicology* 1995; **102**: 149–159.

Cohen, S.M. and Johansson, S.L. Epidemiology and etiology of bladder cancer. *Urol. Clin. North Am.* 1992; **19**: 421–428.

Eble, J.N. and Young, R.H. Carcinoma of the urinary bladder: a review of its diverse morphology. *Semin. Diagn. Pathol.* 1997; **14**: 98–108.

Grignon, D.J. and Sakr, W. Inflammatory and other conditions that can mimic carcinoma in the urinary bladder. *Pathol. Annu.* 1995; **30**(1): 95–122.

Jones, P.A. and Droller, M.J. Pathways of development and progression in bladder cancer: new correlations between clinical observations and molecular mechanisms. *Semin. Urol.* 1993; **11**: 177–192.

Kroft, S.H. and Oyasu, R. Urinary bladder cancer: mechanisms of development and progression. *Lab. Invest.* 1994; **71**: 158–174.

Maher, E.R. Genetics of urological cancers. *Br. Med. Bull.* 1994; **50**: 698–707.

Oliva, E. and Young, R.H. Nephrogenic adenoma of the urinary tract, a review of the microscopic appearances of 80 cases with emphasis on unusual features. *Mod. Pathol.* 1995; **8**: 722–730.

Rosin, M.P., Anwar, W.A. and Ward, A.J. Inflammation, chromosomal instability, and cancer: the schistosomiasis model. *Cancer. Res.* 1994; **54** (7, suppl.): 1929s–1933s.

Shirai, T. Etiology of bladder cancer. *Semin. Urol.* 1993; **11**: 113–126.

Weinstein, R.S. Genetics of tumorigenesis and multidrug resistance in urinary bladder cancer. *Monogr. Pathol.* 1992; **34**: 54–76.

Young, R.H. Pseudoneoplastic lesions of the urinary bladder and urethra: a selective review with emphasis on recent information. *Semin. Diagn. Pathol.* 1997; **14**: 133–146.

Chapter 38: Disorders of the Male Reproductive System

Angell, S.K., Pruthi, R.S. and Merguerian, P.A. Pediatric genitourinary tumors. *Curr. Opin. Oncol.* 1996; **8**: 240–246.

Bajorin, D.F. and Motzer, R.J. Germ cell tumours. *Curr. Ther. Endocrinol. Metab.* 1997; **6**: 387–392.

Bosl, G.J. and Motzer, R.J. Testicular germ cell cancer. *N. Engl. J. Med.* 1997; **337**: 242–253.

Damjanov, I. Pathogenesis of testicular germ cell tumours. *Eur. Urol.* 1993; **23**: 2–5.

Gleason, D.F. Histologic grading of prostate cancer: a perspective. *Hum. Pathol.* 1992; **23**: 273–279.

Griffin, J.E. Androgen resistance – the clinical and molecular spectrum. *N. Engl. J. Med.* 1992; **326**: 611–618.

Grigor, K.M. A new classification of germ cell tumours of the testis. *Eur. Urol.* 1993; **23**: 93–100.

Isaacs, W.B. *et al.* Molecular biology of prostate cancer. *Semin. Oncol.* 1994; **21**: 514–521.

Oliver, R.T. Testicular cancer. *Curr. Opin. Oncol.* 1996; **8**: 252–258.

Oosterhuis, J.W. and Looijenga, L.H. The biology of human germ cell tumours: retrospective speculations and new perspectives. *Eur. Urol.* 1993; **23**: 245–250.

Rukstalis, D.B. Molecular mechanisms of testicular carcinogenesis. *World J. Urol.* 1996; **14**: 347–352.

Scardino, P.T., Weaver, R. and Hudson, M.A. Early detection of prostate cancer. *Hum. Pathol.* 1992; **23**: 211–222.

Scher, H.I. and Fossa, S. Prostate cancer in the era of prostate-specific antigen. *Curr. Opin. Oncol.* 1995; **7**: 281–291.

Ware, J.L. Prostate cancer progression. Implications of histopathology. *Am. J. Pathol.* 1994; **145**: 983–993.

Chapter 39: Disorders of the Female Reproductive System and Breast

Berkowitz, R.S and Goldstein, D.P. Chorionic tumours. *N. Engl. J. Med.* 1996; **335**: 1740–1748.

Boyd, J. and Rubin, S.C. Hereditary ovarian cancer: molecular genetics and clinical implications. *Gynecol. Oncol.* 1997; **64**: 196–206.

Braunstein, G.D. Gynaecomastia. *N. Engl. J. Med.* 1993; **328**: 490–495.

Cannistra, S.A. and Niloff, J.M. Cancer of the uterine cervix. *N. Engl. J. Med.* 1996; **334**: 1030–1038.

Griep, A.E and Lambert, P.F. Role of papillomavirus oncogenes in human cervical cancer: transgenic animal studies. *Proc. Soc. Exp. Biol. Med.* 1994; **206**: 24–34.

Harris, J.R. *et al.* Breast cancer, Parts 1, 2 and 3. *N. Engl. J. Med.* 1992; **327**: 319–328, 390–398, 473–480.

Honore, L.H. Pathology of female infertility. *Curr. Opin. Obstet. Gynecol.* 1997; **9**: 37–43.

Lage, J.M., Bagg, A. and Berchem, G.J. Gestational trophoblastic disease. *Curr. Opin. Obstet. Gynecol.* 1996; **8**: 79–82.

Lawrence, W.D. Non-neoplastic epithelial disorders of the vulva (vulvar dystrophies): historical and current perspectives. *Pathol. Annu.* 1993; **28** (Pt 2): 23–51.

McCormack, W.M. Pelvic inflammatory disease. *N. Engl. J. Med.* 1994; **330**: 115–119.

Rose, P.G. Endometrial carcinoma. *N. Engl. J. Med.* 1996; **335**: 640–649.

Sharpe-Timms, K.L. Basic research in endometriosis. *Obstet. Gynecol. Clin. North. Am.* 1997; **24**: 269–290.

Snedeker, S.M. and Diagustine, R.P. Hormonal and environmental factors affecting cell proliferation and neoplasia in the mammary gland. *Prog. Clin. Biol. Res.* 1996; **394**: 211–253.

Stratton, M.R. and Wooster, R. Hereditary predisposition to breast cancer. *Curr. Opin. Genet. Dev.* 1996; **6**: 93–97.

Weber, B.L. Susceptibility genes for breast cancer. *N. Engl. J. Med.* 1994; **331**: 1523–1524.

Chapter 40: Disorders of the Endocrine System

Atkinson, M.A. and Maclaren, N.K. The pathogenesis of insulin-dependent diabetes mellitus. *N. Engl. J. Med.* 1994; **331**: 1428–1436.

Brent, G.A. The molecular basis of thyroid hormone action. *N. Engl. J. Med.* 1994; **331**: 847–853.

Dayan, C.M. and Daniels, G.H. Chronic autoimmune thyroiditis. *N. Engl. J. Med.* 1996; **335**: 99–107.

Eng, C. The RET proto-oncogene in multiple endocrine neoplasia type 2 and Hirschsprung's disease. *N. Engl. J. Med.* 1996; **335**: 943–951.

Francomano, C.A. The genetic basis of dwarfism. *N. Engl. J. Med.* 1995; **332**: 58–59.

Haller, H., Drab, M. and Luft, F.C. The role of hyperglycaemia and hyperinsulinaemia in the pathogenesis of diabetic angiopathy. *Clin. Nephrol.* 1996; **46**: 246–255.

Kaplan, M.M. (ed.) Thyroid carcinoma. *Endocrinol. Metab. Clin. N. Am.* 1990; **19**: 469–761.

Le Roith, D. Insulin-like growth factors. *N. Engl. J. Med.* 1997; **336**: 633–640.

Melmed, S. (ed.) Acromegaly. *Endocrinol. Metab. Clin. N. Am.* 1992; **21**: 483–761.

Oelkers, W. Adrenal insufficiency. *N. Engl. J. Med.* 1996; **335**: 1206–1212.

Orth, D.N. Cushing's syndrome. *N. Engl. J. Med.* 1995; **332**: 791–803.

Polonsky, K.S., Sturis, J. and Bell, G.I. Non-insulin-dependent diabetes mellitus – a genetically programmed failure of the β-cell to compensate for insulin resistance. *N. Engl. J. Med.* 1996; **334**: 777–783.

Reaven, G.M., Lithell, H. and Landsberg, L. Hypertension and associated metabolic abnormalities – the role of insulin resistance and the sympathoadrenal system. *N. Engl. J. Med.* 1996; **334**: 374–381.

Vance, M.L. Hypopituitarism. *N. Engl. J. Med.* 1994; **330**: 1651–1662.

White, P.C. Disorders of aldosterone synthesis and action. *N. Engl. J. Med.* 1994; **331**: 250–258.

Chapter 41: Disorders of the Haemopoietic System

Arya, R., Layton, D.M. and Bellingham, A.J. Hereditary red cell enzymopathies. *Blood. Rev.* 1995; **9**: 165–175.

Bertina, R.M. *et al.* Mutation in blood coagulation factor V associated with resistance to activated protein C. *Nature* 1994; **369**: 64–67.

Bunn, H.F. Pathogenesis and treatment of sickle cell disease. *N. Engl. J. Med.* 1997; **337**: 762–769.

Cline, M.J. The molecular basis of leukemia. *N. Engl. J. Med.* 1994; **330**: 328–336.

Cobbe, S.M. Thrombolysis in myocardial infarction. *Br. Med. J.* 1994; **308**: 216–217.

Cook, J.D. Iron-deficiency anaemia. *Baillière's Clin. Haematol.* 1994; **7**: 787–804.

Falcon, C.R. *et al.* High prevalence of hyperhomocystinemia in patients with juvenile venous thrombosis. *Arterioscl. Thromb.* 1994; **14**: 1080–1083.

Furie, B. and Furie, B.C. Molecular and cellular biology of blood coagulation. *N. Engl. J. Med.* 1992; **326**: 800–806.

Green, A.R. Pathogenesis of polycythaemia rubra vera. *Lancet* 1996; **347**: 844.

Harker, L.A. Platelets and vascular thrombosis. *N. Engl. J. Med.* 1994; **330**: 1006–1997.

Hassouna, H.I. Laboratory evaluation of hemostatic disorders. *Haematol. Oncol. Clin. North Am.* 1993; **7**: 1161–1250.

Howard, G.C. and Pizzo, S.V. Lipoprotein (a) and its role in atherothrombotic disease. *Lab. Invest.* 1993; **69**: 373–386.

Hoyer, L.W. Hemophilia A. *N. Engl. J. Med.* 1994; **330**: 38–47.

Huisman, T.H. The structure and function of normal and abnormal haemaglobins. *Baillière's Clin. Haematol.* 1993; **6**: 1–30.

Ketley, N.J. and Newland, A.C. Haemopoietic growth factors. *Postgrad. Med. J.* 1997; **73**: 215–221.

Krantz, S.B. Erythropoietin and the anaemia of chronic disease. *Nephrol. Dial. Transplant.* 1995; **10** (suppl. 2): 7–10.

Kyle, R.A. Monoclonal gammopathy of undetermined significance (MGUS). *Baillière's Clin. Haematol.* 1995; **8**: 761–781.

MacLennan, I.C.M., Drayson, M. and Dunn, J. Multiple myeloma. *Br. Med. J.* 1994; **308**: 1033–1036.

Masey, J.A. The myelodysplastic syndromes. *Br. J. Biomed. Sci.* 1997; **54**: 65–70.

May, A. and Fitzsimons, E. Sideroblastic anaemia. *Baillière's Clin. Haematol.* 1994; **7**: 851–879.

Oski, F.A. Iron deficiency in infancy and childhood. *N. Engl. J. Med.* 1993; **329**: 190–193.

Pui, C.H. Childhood leukaemias. *N. Engl. J. Med.* 1995; **332**: 1618–1630.

Ranney, H.M. The spectrum of sickle cell disease. *Hosp. Pract.* 1992; 133–163.

Ridker, P.M. *et al.* Mutation for the gene coding for coagulation factor V and the risk of myocardial infarction, stroke and and venous thrombosis in apparently healthy men. *N. Engl. J. Med.* 1995; **332**: 912–917.

Rozman, C. and Monserrat, E. Chronic lymphocytic leukaemia. *N. Engl. J. Med.* 1995; **333**: 1052–1057.

Schafer, A.I. Hypercoagulable states: molecular genetics to clinical practice. *Lancet* 1995; **344**: 1739–1742.

Young, N.S. Aplastic anaemia. *Lancet* 1995; **346**: 228–232.

Warrell, J.P., De-The, H. and Wang, Z.Y. Acute promyelocytic leukaemia. *N. Engl. J. Med.* 1993; **329**: 177–189.

Wickramasinghe, S.N. Morphology, biology and biochemistry of cobalamin- and folate-deficient bone marrow cells. *Baillière's Clin. Haematol.* 1995; **8**: 441–459.

Chapter 42: Disorders of the Lymphoreticular System

Adal, K.A., Cockerell, C.J. and Petri, W.A. Cat scratch disease, bacillary angiomatosis and other infections due to Rochalimaea. *N. Engl. J. Med.* 1994; **330**: 1509–1515.

Burg, G. *et al.* Pathology of cutaneous T-cell lymphoma. *Hematol. Oncol. Clin. North Am.* 1995; **9**: 961–995.

Chan, J.K.C. *et al.* A study of the association of Epstein-Barr virus with Burkitt's lymphoma occurring in a Chinese population. *Histopathology* 1995; **26**: 235–239.

De Vita, V.T and Hubbard, S.M. Hodgkin's disease. *N. Engl. J. Med.* 1993; **328**: 560–565.

Farhi, D.C. and Ashfaq, R. Splenic pathology after traumatic injury. *Am. J. Clin. Pathol.* 1996; **105**: 474–478.

Gaidano, G. and Dalla-Favera, R. Molecular pathogenesis of AIDS-related lymphomas. *Adv. Cancer Res.* 1995; **67**: 113–153.

Harris, N.L. A practical approach to the pathology of lymphoid neoplasms: a revised European-American classification from the International Lymphoma Study Group. *Important Adv. Oncol.* 1995; 111–140.

Isaacson, P.G. Malignant lymphomas with a follicular growth pattern. *Histopathology* 1996; **28**: 487–495.

Isaacson, P.G. Recent developments in our understanding of gastric lymphomas. *Am. J. Surg. Pathol.* 1996; **20** (suppl. 1): S1–S7.

Isaacson, P.G. and Spencer, J. Gastric lymphoma and Helocobacter pylori. *Important Adv. Oncol.* 1996; 111–121.

Koss, M.N. Pulmonary lymphoid disorders. *Semin. Diagn. Pathol.* 1995; **12**: 158–171.

Muller-Hermelink, H.K. *et al.* Advances in the diagnosis and classification of thymic epithelial tumours. In: Anthony, P.P. and MacSween, R.N.M. (eds). *Recent Advances in Histopathology*, vol. 16. London: Churchill Livingstone, 1994.

Ratech, H. Molecular pathology of low grade malignant lymphomas. *Med. Oncol.* 1995; **12**: 167–176.

Reed, J.C. Bcl-2: prevention of apoptosis as a mechanism of drug resistance. *Haematol. Oncol. North. Am.* 1995; **9**: 451–473.

Rice, E.O. *et al.* Gaucher disease: studies of phenotype, molecular diagnosis and treatment. *Clin. Genet.* 1996; **49**: 111–118.

Sandler, A.S. and Kaplan, L. AIDS lymphoma. *Curr. Opin. Oncol.* 1996; **8**: 377–385.

Sandlund, J.T., Downing, J.R. and Crist, W.M. Non-Hodgkin's lymphoma in childhood. *N. Engl. J. Med.* 1996; **334**: 1238–1248.

Segal, G.H., Perkins, S.L. and Kjeldsberg, C.R. Benign lymphadenopathies in children and adolescents. *Semin. Diagn. Pathol.* 1995; **12**: 288–302.

Smith, M.R. Non-Hodgkin's lymphoma. *Curr. Probl. Cancer* 1996; **20**: 6–77.

Webb, D.K. Histiocyte disorders. *Br. Med. Bull.* 1996; **52**: 818–825.

Chapter 43: Disorders of the Skin

Ahmed, I. Malignant melanoma: prognostic indicators. *Mayo Clin. Proc.* 1997; **72**: 356–361.

Berwick, M. and Halpern, A. Melanoma epidemiology. *Curr. Opin. Oncol.* 1997; **9**: 178–182.

Bielsa, I. *et al.* Histopathologic findings in cutaneous lupus erythematosus. *Arch. Dermatol.* 1994; **130**: 54–58.

Bisno, A.L. and Stevens, D.L. Streptococcal infections of the skin and soft tissue. *N. Engl. J. Med.* 1996; **334**: 240–245.

Callen, J.P., Bickers, D.R. and Moy, R.L. Actinic keratoses. *J. Am. Acad. Dermatol.* 1997; **36**: 650–653.

Cochran, A.J. and Heenan, P. The classification of melanoma: time for a further revision? *Melanoma Res.* 1997; **7**: 4–9.

Cooper, K.D. Cell-mediated immunosuppressive mechanisms induced by UV radiation. *Photochem. Photobiol.* 1996; **63**: 400–406.

Epstein, E.H. Jr. The genetics of human skin diseases. *Curr. Opin. Genet. Dev.* 1996; **6**: 295–300.

Farber, E. The step by step development of epithelial cancer: from phenotype to genotype. *Adv. Cancer Res.* 1996; **70**: 21–48.

Feliciani, C., Gupta, A.K. and Sauder, D.N. Keratinocytes and cytokine/growth factors. *Crit. Rev. Oral. Biol. Med.* 1996; **7**: 300–318.

Fry, L. Dermatitis herpetiformis. *Baillière's Clin. Gastroenterol.* 1995; **9**: 329–350.

Greene, M.H. Genetics of cutaneous melanoma and nevi. *Mayo Clin. Proc.* 1997; **72**: 467–474.

Heasley, D.D. Toda, S. and Mihm, M.C. Jr. Pathology of malignant melanoma. *Surg. Clin. North Am.* 1996; **76**: 1223–1255.

Korge, B.P. and Krieg, T. The molecular basis for inherited bullous diseases. *J. Mol. Med.* 1996; **74**: 59–70.

Korman, N.J. Bullous pemphigoid. *Dermatol. Clin.* 1993; **11**: 483–498.

Kraemer, K.H. Lessons learned from xeroderma pigmentosum. *Photochem. Photobiol.* 1996; **63**: 420–422.

Kraemer, K.H. Sunlight and skin cancer: another link revealed. *Proc. Natl. Acad. Sci. USA.* 1997; **94**: 11–14.

Meola, T, and Lim, H.W. The porphyrias. *Dermatol. Clin.* 1993; **11**: 583–596.

Nickoloff, B.J. and Foreman, K.E. Charting a new course through the chaos of KS (Kaposi's sarcoma). *Am. J. Pathol.* 1996; **148**: 1323–1329.

Nousari, H.C. and Anhalt, G.J. Bullous skin diseases. *Curr. Opin. Immunol.* 1995; **7**: 844–852.

Ortonne, J.P. Aetiology and pathogenesis of psoriasis. *Br. J. Dermatol.* 1996; **135** (suppl. 49): 1–5.

Paller, A.S. Lessons from skin blistering: molecular mechanisms and unusual pattern of inheritance. *Am. J. Pathol.* 1996; **148**: 1727–1731.

Phillips, T.J. and Dover, J.S. Recent advances in dermatology. *N. Engl. J. Med.* 1992; **326**: 167–178.

Porter, S.R. *et al.* Immunologic aspects of dermal and oral lichen planus: a review. *Oral Surg. Oral. Med. Oral Pathol. Oral Radio. Endod.* 1997; **83**: 358–366.

Preston, D.S. and Stern, R.S. Non-melanoma cancers of the skin. *N. Engl. J. Med.* 1992; **327**: 1649–1662.

Thivolet, J. Pemphigus: past, present and future. *Dermatology* 1994; **189** (suppl. 2): 26–29.

Uitto, J. and Christiano, A.M. Molecular genetics of the cutaneous basement membrane zone. Perspectives on epidermolysis bullosa and other blistering skin diseases. *J. Clin. Invest.* 1992; **90**: 687–692.

Wick, M.R. *et al.* Immunopathology of non-neoplastic skin disease: a brief review. *Am. J. Clin. Pathol.* 1996; **105**: 417–429.

Chapter 44: Disorders of the Skeleton, Joints and Soft Tissues

d'Amore, E.S and Ninfo, V. Soft tissue small round cell tumours: morphological parameters. *Semin. Diagn. Pathol.* 1996; **13**: 184–203.

Delmas, P.D. and Meunier, P.J. The management of Paget's disease of Bone. *N. Engl. J. Med.* 1997; **336**: 558–566.

DeMarco, D. and Zurier, R.B. Cytokines and rheumatic diseases. In: Kunkel, S.L. and Remick,

D.G. (eds), *Cytokines*, pp. 371–395. Marcel Dekker, New York: 1992.

De Vernejoul, M.C. Dynamics of bone remodelling: biochemical and pathophysiological basis. *Eur. J. Clin. Chem. Clin. Biochem.* 1996; **34**: 729–734.

Econs, M.J. and Drezner, M.K. Tumour-induced osteomalacia – unveiling a new hormone. *N. Engl. J. Med.* 1994; **330**: 1679–1681.

Fam, A.G. Calcium pyrophosphate crystal deposition disease and other crystal deposition diseases. *Curr. Opin. Rheumatol.* 1992; **4**: 574–582.

Goodlad, J.R and Fletcher, C.D. Recent developments in soft tissue tumors. *Histopathology* 1995; **27**: 103–120.

Grimelius, L. and Johansson, H. Pathology of parathyroid tumours. *Semin. Surg. Oncol.* 1997; **13**: 142–154.

Maini, R. The role of cytokines in rheumatoid arthritis. The Croonian lecture 1995. *J. R. Coll. Physicians Lond.* 1996; **30**: 344–351.

Mankin, H.J. Non-traumatic necrosis of bone (osteonecrosis). *N. Engl. J. Med.* 1992; **326**: 1473–1479.

Quinn, J.M.W. *et al.* Cellular and hormonal mechanisms associated with malignant bone resorption. *Lab. Invest.* 1994; **71**: 465–471.

Riggs, B.L. and Melton, L.J. The prevention and treatment of osteoporosis. *N. Engl. J. Med.* 1992; **327**: 620–627.

Teitelbaum, S.L. and Ross, F.P. Mechanisms of tumor-induced osteolysis. *Lab. Invest.* 1994; **71**: 453–455.

Sewell, K.L. and Trentham, D.E. Pathogenesis of rheumatoid arthritis. *Lancet* 1993; **341**: 283–285.

Smith, R. Osteogenesis imperfecta: from phenotype to genotype and back again. *Int. J. Exp. Pathol.* 1994; **75**: 233–241.

Sreekantaiah, C., Ladanyi, M., Rodriguez, E. and Chaganti, R.S. Chromosomal aberrations in soft tissue tumors. Relevance to diagnosis, classification and molecular mechanisms. *Am. J. Pathol.* 1994; **144**: 1121–1134.

Zvaifler, N.J. Rheumatoid arthritis: the multiple pathways to chronic synovitis. *Lab. Invest.* 1995; **73**: 307–310.

Chapter 45: Disorders of the Central and Peripheral Nervous Systems and Muscle

Benveniste, E.N. Role of macrophages/microglia in multiple sclerosis and experimental allergic encephalomyelitis. *J. Mol. Med.* 1997; **75**: 165–173.

Bronner, L.L., Kanter, D.S. and Manson, J.E. Primary prevention of stroke. *N. Engl. J. Med.* 1995; **333**: 1392–1400.

Brown, G.K. and Squier, M.V. Neuropathology and pathogenesis of mitochondrial diseases. *J. Inherit. Metab. Dis.* 1996; **19**: 553–572.

Coyle, P.K. The neuroimmunology of multiple sclerosis. *Adv. Neuroimmunol.* 1996; **6**: 143–154.

DeArmond, S.J. and Prusiner, S.B. Etiology and pathogenesis of prion diseases. *Am. J. Pathol.* 1995; **146**: 785–811.

Hardy, J. The Alzheimer family of diseases: many etiologies, one pathogenesis. *Proc. Natl. Acad. Sci. USA* 1997; **94**: 2095–2097.

Hughes, R., Sharrack, B. and Rubens, R. Carcinoma and the peripheral nervous system. *J. Neurol.* 1996; **243**: 371–376.

Jenner, P. and Olanow, C.W. Oxidative stress and the pathogenesis of Parkinson's disease. *Neurology* 1996; **47** (suppl. 3): S161–S170.

Knight, J.A. Reactive oxygen species and the neurodegenerative disorders. *Ann. Clin. Lab. Sci.* 1997; **27**: 11–25.

Larner, A.J. Physiological and pathological interrelationships of amyloid beta peptide and the amyloid precursor protein. *Bioessays* 1995; **17**: 819–824.

Lipton, S.A. and Rosenberg, P.A. Excitatory amino acids as a final common pathway for neurologic disorders. *N. Engl. J. Med.* 1994; **330**: 613–622.

Liu, D. The roles of free radicals in amyotrophic lateral sclerosis. *J. Mol. Neurosci.* 1996; **7**: 159–167.

Mark, R.J., Blanc, E.M. and Mattson, M.P. Amyloid beta peptide and oxidative cellular injury in Alzheimer's disease. *Mol. Neurobiol.* 1996; **12**: 211–224.

Murakami, T. *et al.* Charcot–Marie–Tooth disease and related inherited neuropathies. *Medicine* (Baltimore) 1996; **75**: 233–250.

Owen, F. The molecular biology of the transmissible dementias. In: Owen, F., Itzhaki, R. (eds) *Molecular and Cell Biology of Neuropsychiatric Diseases*, pp. 110–132. London: Chapman and Hall, 1994.

Pasloske, B.L. and Howard, R.J. Malaria, the red cell and the endothelium. *Ann. Rev. Med.* 1994; **45**: 283–295.

Plotz, P.H. *et al.* Myositis: immunologic contributions to understanding cause, pathogenesis and therapy. *Ann. Intern. Med.* 1995; **122**: 715–724.

Ropper, A.H. The Guillain–Barré syndrome. *N. Engl. J. Med.* 1992; **326**: 1130–1136.

Schievink, W.I. Intra-cranial aneurysms. *N. Engl. J. Med.* 1997; **336**: 28–40.

Small, D.L. and Buchan, A.M. Mechanisms of cerebral ischemia: intracellular cascades and therapeutic inteventions. *J. Cardiothorac. Vasc. Anesth.* 1996; **10**: 139–146.

Thal, L.J. Neurotrophic factors. *Prog. Brain Res.* 1996; **109**: 327–330.

The Huntington's Disease Collaborative Research Group. A novel gene containing a trinucleotide repeat that is expanded and unstable on Huntington's disease chromosomes. *Cell* 1993; **72**: 971–983.

Trapp, B.D., Haney, C. and Yin, X. Molecular pathogenesis of peripheral neuropathy. *Rev. Neurol. Paris.* 1996; **152**: 314–319.

van der Meche, F.G. and van Doorn, P.A. Guillain–Barré syndrome and chronic inflammatory demyelinating polyneuropathy: immune mechanisms and update on current therapies. *Ann. Neurol.* 1995; **37** (suppl. 1): S14–S31.

White, R.F and Proctor, S.P. Solvents and neurotoxicity. *Lancet* 1997; **349**: 1239–1243.

Wu, J.K. and Naber, S.P. Molecular biology of brain tumours. *Neurosurg. Clin. N. Am.* 1994; **5**: 127–133.

Chapter 46: Disorders of the Organs of Special Senses – Eye and Ear

D'Amico, D.J. Diseases of the retina. *N. Engl. J. Med.* 1994; **331**: 95–106.

Quigley, H.A. Open-angle glaucoma. *N. Engl. J. Med.* 1993; **328**: 1097–1106.

Michaels, L. The Ear. In: Sternberg, S.S. *et al.* (eds) *Diagnostic Surgical Pathology*, 2nd edn, pp. 917–947. New York: Raven Press, 1994.

Page numbers in **bold** refer to major discussions in the text, those in *italic* refer to figures or tables.